Hardy's Textbook of Surgery

Edited by **James D. Hardy,** M.D.

PROFESSOR AND CHAIRMAN, DEPARTMENT OF SURGERY
UNIVERSITY OF MISSISSIPPI SCHOOL OF MEDICINE;
SURGEON-IN-CHIEF
UNIVERSITY HOSPITAL
JACKSON, MISSISSIPPI

With 114 contributors

Editorial **John S. Kukora,** M.D.
Assistants ASSISTANT PROFESSOR OF SURGERY
UNIVERSITY OF MISSISSIPPI SCHOOL OF MEDICINE
JACKSON, MISSISSIPPI

Harvey I. Pass, M.D.

ASSISTANT PROFESSOR, CARDIOTHORACIC SURGERY
MEDICAL UNIVERSITY OF SOUTH CAROLINA;
CHIEF OF CARDIAC SURGERY
CHARLESTON VETERANS ADMINISTRATION HOSPITAL
CHARLESTON, SOUTH CAROLINA

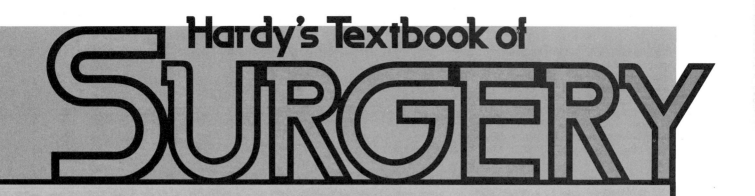

Hardy's Textbook of SURGERY

J. B. LIPPINCOTT COMPANY

Philadelphia

London / Mexico City / New York / St. Louis / São Paulo / Sydney

Acquisitions Editor: Stuart Freeman
Sponsoring Editor: Richard Winters
Manuscript Editor: Janet H. Baker
Indexer: Barbara S. Littlewood, Ph.D.
Art Director: Maria S. Karkucinski
Designer: Patrick Turner
Production Supervisor: N. Carol Kerr
Production Coordinator: Charlene Catlett Squibb
Compositor: Monotype Composition Company, Inc.
Printer/Binder: The Murray Printing Company

3 5 6 4 2

Library of Congress Cataloging in Publication Data
Main entry under title:

Hardy's textbook of surgery.

Includes bibliographies and index.
1. Surgery.   I. Hardy, James D., DATE
II. Kukora, John. III. Pass, Harvey.   [DNLM:
1. Surgery.   WO 100 T3555]
RD31.H34 1983   617'.9   82-14015
ISBN 0-397-52108-1
ISBN 0-397-50614-7 (pbk.)

The authors and publisher have exerted every effort to ensure that drug selection and dosage set forth in this text are in accord with current recommendations and practice at the time of publication. However, in view of ongoing research, changes in government regulations, and the constant flow of information relating to drug therapy and drug reactions, the reader is urged to check the package insert for each drug for any change in indications and dosage and for added warnings and precautions. This is particularly important when the recommended agent is a new or infrequently employed drug.

To All Students of Surgery

contributors

Joaquin S. Aldrete, M.D.
Professor of Surgery, University of Alabama School of Medicine, Birmingham, Alabama

James F. Arens, M.D.
Professor and Chairman, Department of Anesthesiology, University of Texas Medical Branch, Galveston, Texas

J. Bradley Aust, M.D., Ph.D.
Professor and Chairman, Department of Surgery, University of Texas Health Science Center at San Antonio; Chief of Surgery, Bexar County Hospital District Hospitals, San Antonio, Texas

Charles M. Balch, M.D.
Professor of Surgery, Associate Professor of Microbiology, University of Alabama in Birmingham School of Medicine; Chief, Section of Surgical Oncology, Associate Director for Clinical Studies, Comprehensive Cancer Center, Birmingham, Alabama

Walter F. Ballinger, M.D.
Professor of Surgery, Washington University School of Medicine, St. Louis, Missouri

Arthur E. Baue, M.D.
Donald Guthrie Professor of Surgery; Chairman, Department of Surgery, Yale University School of Medicine; Chief of Surgery, Yale–New Haven Hospital, New Haven, Connecticut

John M. Beal, M.D.
J. Roscoe Miller Distinguished Professor and Chairman Emeritus, Department of Surgery, Northwestern University McGaw Medical Center, Chicago, Illinois

Harry C. Bishop, M.D.
Professor of Pediatric Surgery, University of Pennsylvania School of Medicine, Philadelphia, Pennsylvania

George L. Blackburn, M.D., Ph.D.
Associate Professor of Surgery, Harvard Medical School, Boston, Massachusetts

Scott J. Boley, M.D.
Professor of Surgery and Chief of Pediatric Surgical Services, Albert Einstein College of Medicine–Montefiore Hospital and Medical Center, New York, New York

Lyman A. Brewer III, M.D.
Clinical Professor of Surgery, University of California School of Medicine at Irvine, Irvine, California; Clinical Professor of Surgery, University of Southern California School of Medicine; Emeritus Clinical Professor of Surgery, Los Angeles, California

Henry Buchwald, M.D., Ph.D.
Professor of Surgery and Biochemical Engineering, University of Minnesota School of Medicine, Minneapolis, Minnesota

John F. Burke, M.D.
Helen Andrus Benedict Professor of Surgery, Harvard Medical School; Chief of the Trauma Services, Massachusetts General Hospital, Boston, Massachusetts

Darrell A. Campbell, Jr., M.D.
Assistant Professor of Surgery, Co-Director of Transplantation Service, University of Michigan Medical School, Ann Arbor, Michigan

Carlos M. Chavez, M.D.
Professor of Surgery, Texas Tech University, Lubbock, Texas; active staff, Brownsville Medical Center and Valley Community, Brownsville, Texas

Laurence Y. Cheung, M.D.
Associate Professor of Surgery, Washington University School of Medicine, St. Louis, Missouri

John J. Collins, Jr., M.D.
Professor of Surgery, Harvard Medical School; Chief, Division of Thoracic and Cardiac Surgery, Brigham and Women's Hospital, Boston, Massachusetts

Fred A. Crawford, Jr., M.D.
Professor of Surgery; Professor of Pediatrics; Chief, Division of Cardiothoracic Surgery, Medical University of South Carolina, Charleston, South Carolina

Michael H. Crawford, M.D.
Professor of Medicine (Cardiology), University of Texas Health Science Center at San Antonio, San Antonio, Texas

Anatolio B. Cruz, Jr., M.D., M.S. (Surg.)
Professor of Surgery, Chief, Head and Neck Surgical Oncology Services, Department of Surgery, University of Texas Health Science Center at San Antonio, San Antonio, Texas

Jerome J. DeCosse, M.D., Ph.D.
Professor and Associate Chairman, Department of Surgery, Cornell University Medical College; Chairman, Department of Surgery, Memorial Sloan-Kettering Cancer Center, New York, New York

William C. DeVries, M.D.
Assistant Professor of Surgery; Head of Division of Cardiovascular and Thoracic Surgery, University of Utah School of Medicine, Salt Lake City, Utah

Alan R. Dimick, M.D.
Associate Professor of Surgery, University of Alabama in Birmingham, School of Medicine; Director, Burn Service, University of Alabama Hospitals, Birmingham, Alabama

Arthur J. Donovan, M.D.
Professor and Chairman, Department of Surgery, University of Southern California School of Medicine, Los Angeles, California

William R. Drucker, M.D.
Professor and Chairman, Department of Surgery, University of Rochester; Surgeon-in-Chief, Strong Memorial Hospital, Rochester, New York

L. Henry Edmunds, Jr., M.D.
W. M. Measey Professor, Department of Surgery; Chief, Division of Cardiothoracic Surgery, University of Pennsylvania School of Medicine, Philadelphia, Pennsylvania

H. Clark Ethridge, Jr., M.D.
Resident in Anesthesiology, University of Texas Medical Branch, Galveston, Texas

H. Pat Ewing, M.D.
Assistant Professor of Surgery, University of Mississippi School of Medicine, Jackson, Mississippi

Luther C. Fisher III, M.D.
Assistant Professor, Division of Orthopaedic Surgery, University of Mississippi School of Medicine; Chief of Pediatric Orthopaedic Section, University of Mississippi Medical Center, Jackson, Mississippi

Charles T. Fitts, M.D.
Professor of Surgery, Medical University of South Carolina; Director of Transplant Unit, Medical University Hospital, Charleston, South Carolina

Lewis M. Flint, Jr., M.D.
Professor of Surgery; Chief of Surgery, University Hospital/Louisville General Hospital, University of Louisville School of Medicine, Louisville, Kentucky

Thomas J. Fogarty, M.D.
Director, Cardiac Surgery, Sequoia Hospital, Redwood City, California

Irwin N. Frank, M.D.
Professor of Urology, Department of Surgery, Strong Memorial Hospital, Rochester, New York

Alan E. Freeland, M.D.
Associate Professor, Division of Orthopaedic Surgery, University of Mississippi School of Medicine, Jackson, Mississippi

Stanley R. Friesen, M.D., Ph.D.
Professor of Surgery and Lecturer in the History of Medicine, University of Kansas School of Medicine, Kansas City, Kansas

Richard E. Fry, M.D.
Assistant Instructor, Department of Surgery, Southwestern Medical School of the University of Texas Health Science Center at Dallas, Dallas, Texas

William J. Fry, M.D.
Professor and Chairman, Department of Surgery, Southwestern Medical School of the University of Texas Health Science Center at Dallas; Chief of Surgical Services, Parkland Memorial Hospital, Dallas, Texas

Joseph C. Gabel, M.D.
Professor and Chairman, Department of Anesthesiology, University of Texas Medical School at Houston, Houston, Texas

Donald S. Gann, M.D.
James Murray Beardsley Professor of Surgery and Chairman, Section of Surgery, Brown University; Surgeon-in-Chief, Rhode Island Hospital, Providence, Rhode Island

Richard D. Goodenough, M.D.
Instructor in Surgery, University of Rochester, Rochester, New York

Lazar J. Greenfield, M.D.
Stuart McGuire Professor and Chairman, Department of Surgery, Medical College of Virginia, Richmond, Virginia

Ward O. Griffen, Jr., M.D.
Professor and Chairman, Department of Surgery, and Professor of Physiology and Biophysics, University of Kentucky College of Medicine, Lexington, Kentucky

Hermes C. Grillo, M.D.
Professor of Surgery, Harvard Medical School; Chief of General Thoracic Surgery, Massachusetts General Hospital, Boston, Massachusetts

John W. Hammon, Jr., M.D.
Assistant Professor of Surgery, Department of Cardiac and Thoracic Surgery, Vanderbilt University, Nashville, Tennessee

James D. Hardy, M.D.
Professor and Chairman, Department of Surgery, University of Mississippi School of Medicine; Surgeon-in-Chief, University Hospital, Jackson, Mississippi

Jules Hardy, M.D.
Professor and Chairman, Department of Surgery, Division of Neurosurgery, Faculty of Medicine, University of Montreal, Montreal, Quebec, Canada

Karen B. Harvey-Wilkes, B.S.
Research Assistant, Nutrition/Metab-

olism Laboratory, New England Deaconess Hospital and Harvard Medical School, Boston, Massachusetts

Frederick R. Heckler, M.D.
Clinical Associate Professor of Surgery (Plastic), University of Pittsburgh School of Medicine; Head, Division of Plastic Surgery, and Director, Plastic Surgery Research Laboratory, Allegheny General Hospital, Pittsburgh, Pennsylvania

James W. Holcroft, M.D.
Associate Professor of Surgery, University of California, Davis School of Medicine; Director, Surgical ICU, and Chief, Vascular Surgical Service, University of California, Davis, and Sacramento Medical Center, Sacramento, California

John M. Howard, M.D.
Professor, Department of Surgery, Medical College of Ohio, Toledo, Ohio

James L. Hughes, M.D.
Professor and Chairman, Division of Orthopaedic Surgery, University of Mississippi School of Medicine, Jackson, Mississippi

Michael E. Jabaley, M.D.
Clinical Professor of Surgery (Plastic), University of Mississippi School of Medicine, Jackson, Mississippi

E. Thomas James, M.D.
Clinical Assistant Professor, Division of Orthopaedic Surgery, University of Mississippi School of Medicine, Jackson, Mississippi

George Johnson, Jr., M.D.
Roscoe B.G. Cowper Distinguished Professor of Surgery; Chief, Division of General Surgery; and Vice-Chairman, Department of Surgery, University of North Carolina School of Medicine, Chapel Hill, North Carolina

George L. Jordan, Jr., M.D.
Professor of Surgery, Baylor College of Medicine, Houston, Texas

Paul H. Jordan, Jr., M.D.
Professor of Surgery, Baylor College of Medicine; Chief of Surgery, Veterans Administration Hospital, Houston, Texas

M. J. Jurkiewicz, M.D., D.D.S.
Professor of Surgery and Chief, Division of Plastic and Reconstructive Surgery, Emory University School of Medicine; Chief of Plastic and Reconstructive

Surgery, Emory University Affiliated Hospitals, Atlanta, Georgia

Mark A. Kelley, M.D.
Assistant Professor of Medicine and Associate Chairman, Department of Medicine, University of Pennsylvania School of Medicine, Philadelphia, Pennsylvania

Robert L. Kistner, M.D.
Director of Surgical Education, Straub Hospital, University of Hawaii Integrated Surgical Residency Program; President/CEO, Straub Clinic & Hospital, Inc., Honolulu, Hawaii

John W. Konnak, M.D.
Associate Professor of Urology, University of Michigan Medical School, Ann Arbor, Michigan

Albert Kreutner, Jr., M.D.
Clinical Associate Professor of Pathology, Medical University of South Carolina, Charleston, South Carolina

John S. Kukora, M.D.
Assistant Professor of Surgery, University of Mississippi School of Medicine, Jackson, Mississippi

Henry L. Laws, M.D.
Associate Professor of Surgery, University of Alabama School of Medicine, Birmingham, Alabama

John R. Lurain III, M.D.
Assistant Professor of Obstetrics and Gynecology, Associate Director of Gynecologic Oncology, and Associate Director, Trophoblastic Disease Center, Northwestern University Medical School, Chicago, Illinois

James W. Maher, M.D.
Assistant Professor of Surgery, University of Mississippi School of Medicine, Jackson, Mississippi

James A. Majeski, M.D., Ph.D.
Assistant Professor of Surgery, Medical University of South Carolina, Charleston, South Carolina

Arlie R. Mansberger, Jr., M.D.
Professor of Surgery and Chairman, Department of Surgery, Medical College of Georgia; Chief of Surgery, Eugene Talmadge Memorial Hospital, Augusta, Georgia

G. Robert Mason, M.D., Ph.D.
Professor and Chairman, Department of Surgery, University of California, Irvine, Irvine, California

Kenneth L. Mattox, M.D.
Associate Professor, Department of Surgery, Baylor College of Medicine, Houston, Texas

Sue McCoy, M.D., Ph.D.
Resident in General Surgery, Hospital of the University of Pennsylvania; Assistant Instructor in Surgery, University of Pennsylvania, Philadelphia, Pennsylvania

Gérard Mohr, M.D.
Assistant Research Professor, Department of Surgery, Division of Neurosurgery, University of Montreal, Montreal, Quebec, Canada

Joseph A. Molnar, M.D.
Research Fellow, Department of Surgery, Massachusetts General Hospital; Harvard Medical School, Boston, Massachusetts

Frank G. Moody, M.D.
Professor and Chairman, Department of Surgery, University of Texas Health Science Center at Houston, Houston, Texas

Richard B. Moore, M.D.
Assistant Professor of Medicine, University of Minnesota School of Medicine, Minneapolis, Minnesota

Louis Morales, Jr., M.D.
Assistant Professor of Plastic Surgery, University of Utah Medical College; Chief of Plastic Surgery, Veterans Administration Hospital, Salt Lake City, Utah

Winsor V. Morrison, M.D.
Professor of Surgery and Chief, Division of Otolaryngology, University of Mississippi School of Medicine, Jackson, Mississippi

G. Arnold Mulder, M.D.
Assistant Clinical Professor of Surgery, University of Southern California, Los Angeles, California

George L. Nardi, M.D.
Professor of Surgery, Harvard Medical School, Boston, Massachusetts

Norman C. Nelson, M.D.
Vice-Chancellor for Health Affairs, University of Mississippi; Dean and Professor of Surgery, University of Mississippi School of Medicine, Jackson, Mississippi

Michael Newton, M.D.
Professor of Obstetrics and Gynecology and Head, Section of Graduate Education, Department of Obstetrics and Gynecology, Northwestern University Medical School; Director, Division of Gynecologic Oncology, Prentice Women's Hospital and Maternity Center of Northwestern Memorial Hospital, Chicago, Illinois

Moreye Nusbaum, M.D
Professor of Surgery, University of Pennsylvania School of Medicine, Philadelphia, Pennsylvania

C. Thomas Nuzum, M.D.
Associate Professor of Medicine, University of North Carolina School of Medicine at Chapel Hill, Chapel Hill, North Carolina

James A. O'Neill, Jr., M.D.
Professor of Pediatric Surgery, University of Pennsylvania School of Medicine; Surgeon-in-Chief, Children's Hospital of Philadelphia, Philadelphia, Pennsylvania

Harvey I. Pass, M.D.
Assistant Professor, Cardiothoracic Surgery, Medical University of South Carolina; Chief of Cardiac Surgery, Charleston Veterans Administration Hospital, Charleston, South Carolina

Richard M. Peters, M.D.
Professor of Surgery and Bioengineering and Co-Head, Division of Cardiothoracic Surgery, University of California Medical Center, San Diego, California

Hiram C. Polk, Jr., M.D.
Professor and Chairman, Department of Surgery, University of Louisville School of Medicine, Louisville, Kentucky

Herbert J. Proctor, M.D.
Professor of Surgery, University of North Carolina School of Medicine, Chapel Hill, North Carolina

John H. Raaf, M.D., D.Phil.
Associate Professor of Surgery, Cornell University Medical College; Director of Surgical Education, Cornell University Medical College Program, Memorial Hospital; Assistant Attending Surgeon, Memorial Sloan-Kettering Cancer Center, New York, New York

Seshadri Raju, M.D.
Professor of Surgery, University of Mississippi School of Medicine; Director,

Doppler Laboratory; Director, Mississippi Transplant Program, University of Mississippi Medical Center, Jackson, Mississippi

Jonathan E. Rhoads, Jr., M.D.
Associate Professor of Surgery, Medical College of Pennsylvania; Chief, MCP Division, Surgical Service, Veterans Administration Medical Center, Philadelphia, Pennsylvania

Charles G. Rob, M.D.
Professor of Surgery and Director of the Clinical Vascular Laboratory, Department of Surgery, School of Medicine, East Carolina University, Greenville, North Carolina; formerly Professor and Chairman, Department of Surgery, University of Rochester School of Medicine and Dentistry, Rochester, New York

Richard D. Rucker, Jr., M.D.
Medical Fellow, University of Minnesota School of Medicine, Minneapolis, Minnesota

Fred W. Rushton, M.D.
Assistant Professor of Surgery, University of Mississippi School of Medicine, Jackson, Mississippi

Robert F. Ryan, M.D.
Professor of Surgery and Head of Section (Plastic Surgery), Tulane University School of Medicine; Chief, Division of Plastic Surgery, Touro Infirmary, New Orleans, Louisiana

Louise Schnaufer, M.D.
Associate Professor of Pediatric Surgery, University of Pennsylvania School of Medicine, Philadelphia, Pennsylvania

Thomas W. Shields, M.D.
Professor of Surgery, Northwestern University Medical School; Chief, Surgical Service, Veterans Administration Lakeside Medical Center, Chicago, Illinois

Perry M. Shoor, M.D.
Surgical Staff, Stanford University Hospital, Palo Alto, California, and the Sequoia Hospital, Redwood City, California

Robert R. Smith, M.D.
Professor and Chairman, Department of Neurosurgery, University of Mississippi School of Medicine; Head, Neurosurgical Service, Hospital of the University of Mississippi and Veterans Administration Hospital, Jackson, Mississippi

D. E. Strandness, Jr., M.D.
Professor of Surgery, University of Washington School of Medicine, Seattle, Washington

John M. Templeton, Jr., M.D.
Assistant Professor of Pediatric Surgery, University of Pennsylvania School of Medicine, Philadelphia, Pennsylvania

Colin G. Thomas, Jr., M.D.
Professor and Chairman, Department of Surgery, University of North Carolina at Chapel Hill, Chapel Hill, North Carolina

Jesse E. Thompson, M.D.
Clinical Professor of Surgery, University of Texas Southwestern Medical School; Chief of Surgery, Baylor University Medical Center, Dallas, Texas

Hilary H. Timmis, M.D.
Clinical Associate Professor of Surgery, Wayne State University; Attending Staff Surgeon, Division of Cardiovascular Surgery, William Beaumont Hospital, Royal Oak, Michigan

J. Kent Trinkle, M.D.
Professor of Surgery and Head of Cardiothoracic Surgery, University of Texas Health Science Center at San Antonio, San Antonio, Texas

Donald D. Trunkey, M.D.
Professor of Surgery and Vice-Chairman, Department of Surgery, University of California, San Francisco; Chief of Surgery, San Francisco General Hospital, San Francisco, California

Jeremiah G. Turcotte, M.D.
F. A. Coller Professor of Surgery and Chairman, Department of Surgery, University of Michigan Medical School; Director, Surgical Transplant Program, University of Michigan Medical Center, Ann Arbor, Michigan

Richard L. Varco, M.D., Ph.D.
Formerly Professor of Surgery, and Director, Thoracic and Cardiovascular Surgery Training Program, University of Minnesota School of Medicine, Minneapolis, Minnesota

Frank J. Veith, M.D.
Professor of Surgery and Chief of Vascular Surgery, Albert Einstein College of Medicine–Montefiore Hospital and Medical Center, New York, New York

Michael P. Vercimak, M.D.
Resident in Plastic Surgery, Tulane University School of Medicine, New Orleans, Louisiana

E. Frazier Ward, M.D.
Assistant Professor, Division of Orthopaedic Surgery, University of Mississippi School of Medicine, Jackson, Mississippi

W. Lamar Weems, M.D.
Professor of Surgery (Urology) and Director, Division of Urology, University of Mississippi School of Medicine; Chief, Urology Service, Veterans Administration Hospital, Jackson, Mississippi

Raymond R. White, M.D.
Assistant Professor, Division of Orthopaedic Surgery, University of Mississippi School of Medicine, Jackson, Mississippi

Moritz M. Ziegler, M.D.
Assistant Professor of Pediatric Surgery, University of Pennsylvania School of Medicine, Philadelphia, Pennsylvania

R. E. Zierler, M.D.
Staff Surgeon (Vascular Surgery Service) and Associate Investigator, Peripheral Vascular Surgery, Veterans Administration Medical Center, Seattle, Washington

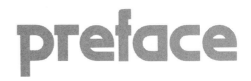

preface

This textbook represents a new departure from standard textbooks of surgery. It is a trim volume of under 1400 as compared to the usual 2000 to 2500 pages, but it is complete. The principles of core surgery, including supportive science as well as the management of specific lesions and conditions, are all covered. The thrust has been to emphasize what is clinically relevant.

The Plan. The guiding principle has been to present the material as succinctly as possible. The detailed outline of the entire book was developed as follows: First, the Editor and the Editorial Assistants and their staff—representing experience from several universities—drew up a list of topics that they considered pertinent. Next, other standard textbooks of surgery were consulted. When this consolidated outline had been completed, the segment covering each chapter was sent to the author(s) contributing the given chapter as points to be included in the chapter along with those additional items that the author deemed important. In this way serious omissions and inappropriate duplication were avoided.

The comfortable moderate length of this comprehensive book was achieved in the following way. First, again nonessential duplication was avoided. Next, the references selected were limited to the documentation of important original contributions and to ones that afforded access to further information in the field. Extensive discussion of conflicting theories or alternatives was avoided in favor of limited terse acknowledgment that such exist. Subjects such as legal medicine were omitted. The illustrations were developed in a way that each made specific points in a space appropriate for the value of the message conveyed.

The volume has been brought out rapidly and is up to date in all respects.

The key word for this volume is *accessibility.* We have endeavored to enhance access to facts by using color, by placing a detailed outline at the beginning of each chapter with factual topic discussion in sequence, by the use of shaded boxes to project "the essence," and by providing a comprehensive index.

The *authors* were selected on the basis of recognized authority and teaching experience, and they comprise a national mix to afford an overall cross-section of regional orientations. Each has adhered to the guiding philosophy and has also remained within the original space allotment.

The *audience* anticipated for this textbook represents all students of surgery: medical students, surgical residents taking in-training examinations and boards, and the more advanced surgeon who seeks a current update on surgical subjects. The book is not an atlas of surgical technique, but in most instances the basic operative steps for the management of the specific surgical entities are illustrated.

Acknowledgments. Many individuals have contributed much to this textbook. The authors have been most generous with their time and expertise, and their contributions are uniformly outstanding. Special acknowledgment must be tendered to Mrs. Virginia W. Keith and Mrs. Sandra M. Day at the University of Mississippi Medical Center and the entire participating staff at the J. B. Lippincott Company, particularly Mr. J. Stuart Freeman, Jr., Mr. Richard Winters, and Mrs. Janet H. Baker. Drs. Kukora and Pass and I extend our keen appreciation to all.

James D. Hardy, M.D.

contents

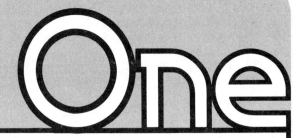

Basic and Support
Considerations

William R. Drucker/Donald S. Gann/Sue McCoy

Response to Surgery: Neuroendocrine and Metabolic Changes, Convalescence, and Rehabilitation

1

"There is a circumstance attending accidental injury which does not belong to disease—namely, that the injury done has in all cases a tendency to produce the disposition and the means of cure."

—JOHN HUNTER 1794

"Life thrives on controlled processes and properties. No living being exists without regulations. . . . Certain regulations tend to keep a designated activity or property constant whereas other regulations tend to disturb constancy. . . . No one regulation can operate in the absence of other regulations. . . . Eventually some indispensable regulation ceases to operate; the individual dies. Only rarely can the coroner decide which regulation it was that failed first" (Adolph, 1968). All organs are involved in the reaction to major accidental injury, operation, or sepsis.

A study of the metabolic response to injury provides an excellent opportunity to gain better insight into the complex regulatory processes controlling the kinetics of substrates essential for the production of energy during times of adversity. For many years, the wealth of literature germane to this subject too often provided a compendium of seemingly unrelated observations frequently misleading for the lack of physiological perspective. More recently, the role of the neuroendocrine response to injury has become recognized as the intrinsic regulatory mechanism controlling and directing the complex sequence of interrelated metabolic alterations that develop after injury. Relatively unanswered, however, is the largely philosophical question of the purpose of the observed alterations. Most students of the subject believe today that the metabolic changes are not simply by-products or signals of disoriented cellular processes but rather are part of a highly organized regulatory system designed to prolong survival. The genesis of this teleological concept is worthy of consideration because it provides an essential perspective for this subject. It also helps to point the direction for continued study.

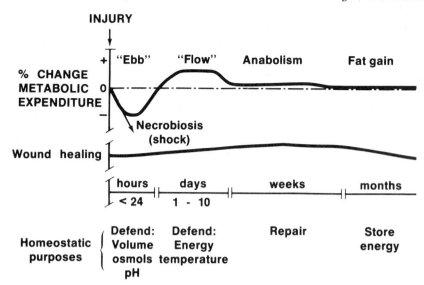

Fig. 1-1. The phases of uncomplicated convalescence. These events are paralleled by subjective sensations of emotional and physical well-being. (Adapted from Cuthbertson DP, Stoner HB, Kinney JM, in Porter R, Knight J (eds): Energy Metabolism in Trauma, p 98. London, J & A Churchill, 1970)

HISTORICAL BACKGROUND

The first organized study of metabolism in the injured human is credited to Sir David Cuthbertson; shortly after World War I, at the Glasgow Royal Infirmary, he set out to determine why fractures of the lower third of the femur are slow to heal. His findings of negative balance for calcium, phosphate, sulfur, and nitrogen in patients with fractures made it evident that it was also necessary to study the fundamental problem of changes in metabolism produced by immobilization. His results led to the hypothesis that an injured animal, as a consequence of its injury, may be faced with a diminished food supply. Therefore, Cuthbertson maintained, "the necessity is urgent and the body may require to catabolize its reserves to meet both the exigencies of repair and of maintenance." The sulfur/nitrogen and phosphorus/nitrogen ratios suggested that the material catabolized consisted mainly of muscle following the earlier and more rapid exhaustion of the carbohydrate reserves. Thus, catabolism or cannibalism of body protein was postulated to be part of a primitive survival reflex to nourish the body from endogenous resources at a time when injury precluded search for food.

Cuthbertson was not the first, however, to become interested in the metabolic alterations produced by injury. More than a half century earlier, Bernard had observed the prompt development of hyperglycemia after hemorrhage. Shortly before the turn of the century, Malcolm had found evidence of increased nitrogen metabolism in patients following surgery. Severe infections, such as typhoid fever, were found to produce wasting of body protein with large urinary losses of nitrogen proportional to losses of other intracellular compounds, such as sulfur and phosphorus. These losses were greater than those produced by starvation alone. During World War I, extensive studies of injured men were made by a group consisting of such notables as Dale and Bayliss from England and Cannon from the United States. It was Cuthbertson, however, whose systematic study of metabolism in the injured human placed the observed alterations into a temporal and physiological perspective. His concept of successive phases of metabolism following injury has proved to be exceptionally helpful in providing the background for interpretation of the complex sequence of metabolic and neuroendocrine changes elicited by injury.

The advent of quantitative clinical chemistry fostered by Peters at Yale and Van Slyke at the Rockefeller Institute in New York provided a degree of precision in the measurements required for assessing the metabolic alterations. A generation of students has been guided through complexities of fluid and electrolyte disorders by the quantitative diagnostic analyses of the biochemical alterations of extracellular fluid developed by James Gamble. The monumental clinical studies of F. D. Moore, starting in mid century, awakened further interest in the quantitative study of injured humans. While countless significant investigations have amplified Cuthbertson's original observations, the detailed biochemical studies by Stoner and the serial assessment of energy expenditure in the injured human by Kinney were primarily responsible for relating the phases of postinjury metabolic alterations to homeostatic priorities (Fig. 1-1).

The concept of homeostasis was developed by Cannon from a separate line of inquiry during the time that Cuthbertson was involved with his studies of the metabolic response to injury. The genesis of the concept of homeostasis can be traced principally to Charles Darwin in England and Claude Bernard in France.

In the opinion of many experts, general thinking about the world has been changed more by Darwin's book on evolution than by any other book, with the possible exception of Sir Isaac Newton's *Principia*, which propounded the theory of universal gravitation. At the time Darwin's book was published, it was widely believed that each species was a separate immutable entity that had maintained a constant form since creation. By the time of Darwin's death a century ago, the theory of evolution with survival of the fittest was accepted by practically all scientists. Bernard, generally regarded as the originator of the discipline of physiology, was a contemporary of Darwin. He believed that all living processes are composed of chemical reactions. His study of the chemical composition of the body fluids, which constitute the environment of cells, led to the hypothesis that the internal environment of the body is maintained in a constant state by autoregulatory mechanisms; constancy of the internal environment (*le milieu intérieur*) is the condition of free and independent life.

It remained for Walter Cannon, a generation later, to bridge the concepts of Darwin and Bernard. He originated the term *homeostasis* to describe the physiological and biochemical responses that return the internal environment to a normal steady state after an acute challenge such as injury. The degree to which these autoregulatory adjustments maintain a constant *milieu intérieur* is an index of the fitness of an organism to survive.

Homeostasis is not attained, however, without a cost. Adolph speculated that no coordinating force originated with an end in view. Rather, natural selection, by a process of optimization, developed a system in which regulatory mechanisms are compatible with one another. A system of priorities developed among the many regulatory processes. Certain regulatory activities tend to keep a designated activity or property constant, and in doing so the cost may be for other regulatory activities to give way and thereby disrupt constancy. No better example exists than that of the protection of circulatory volume at the expense of the regulation of osmolality. In the presence of hypovolemia, antidiuretic hormone (ADH) release is stimulated and water is retained, even at the expense of hyposmolality. The regulatory systems can be exhausted, however. Their constant prolonged activation leads to loss of their integration and to their ultimate death. A well-studied example is prolonged hypovolemic shock, which ultimately leads to deterioration of the mechanisms supporting circulatory volume. This is manifest when hemoconcentration replaces hemodilution, and it heralds impending death.

The regulatory neuroendocrine system with its attendant metabolic alterations does not remain constant in its response to injury. Priorities for regulation change with time and with the effectiveness of the body's response to support processes most critical for survival. With the advent of less cumbersome techniques, a wealth of laboratory information has been derived from injured patients, often without reference to the existing physiological response or to the time elapsed following injury. Cuthbertson's concept of sequential metabolic "ebb–flow" phases emphasizes that defense of homeostasis is a dynamic series of interrelated neuroendocrine, biochemical, and physiological events. These can be discovered only by an integrated study of the successive alterations of the neuroendocrine regulatory system in relation to corresponding changes in metabolism. The response of regulatory systems to trauma is not unique; rather, it is inherent in the defense against all stresses. The responses differ only in regard to the stimulus involved. Thus, a study of homeostasis provides insight into and understanding of mechanisms relevant to defense against illness as well as injury. It would be a mistake to assume that the metabolic alterations constitute the only adjustments in support of homeostasis. They occur concomitantly with numerous other physiological and biochemical adaptations designed to promote and protect the function of vital organs such as the heart, lungs, brain, and kidneys. In this chapter, attention is focused on the metabolic changes because they provide the energy that constitutes an essential prerequisite for the effective function of all other mechanisms supportive of homeostasis.

NEUROENDOCRINE RESPONSE TO INJURY

STIMULATION OF NEUROENDOCRINE CHANGES

Injury sets in motion a complex set of neural and hormonal changes. These changes are commonly regarded as the direct result of the "stress" associated with surgery or trauma.

Historically, this view developed out of the work of Selye, who spoke precisely of stress as the response to the action of one or more "stressors." Operationally, a stressor is recognized by a response of increased secretion of cortisol or its analogues from the adrenal cortex. Thus, a stressor is a stimulus that can lead to increased adrenocortical secretion. This precision of definition is important because, as will be shown, much of what is considered good surgical practice leads to diminution or reversal of the neuroendocrine response to injury. It is convenient to consider the stimuli as primary stimuli initiated by the injury itself or as secondary stimuli brought about in part by the response to injury. Furthermore, it is clear that the effectiveness of the various stimuli may be modulated by a group of factors.

PRIMARY STIMULI

Hypovolemia

Blood loss is a factor in most injury. However, even when there is no significant blood loss, there may be significant hypovolemia because of the sequestration of extracellular fluid. The pioneering work of Blalock in the 1930s established the fact that fluid accumulates in an injured area and is thus lost to the functional extracellular fluid volume, that is, that portion of extracellular and extravascular fluid that can exchange with the vascular compartment. Such fluid is generally termed the *third space*, to distinguish it from functionally exchangeable cellular and extracellular fluid. In addition, Shires and co-workers demonstrated in the early 1960s that additional extracellular fluid accumulates within the cells in various forms of shock. Although the volume of such fluid is believed to be somewhat less than originally thought, this sequestration is qualitatively important because it results in a decrease in tissue hydrostatic pressure. The resultant imbalance of the Starling forces can impair the body's own defenses that normally act to restore functional blood volume.

The circulating blood volume may be measured either as the amount of blood reaching the heart (*i.e.,* the venous return) or as the amount of blood leaving the heart (*i.e.,* the cardiac output). The former is sensed by stretch receptors located in the atria, which measure the degree and rate of atrial filling. The latter is sensed by stretch receptors located in the carotid arteries and aorta, which measure the degree and rate of stretch of those vessels. Nerves arising from both sets of these receptors course in the vagi and glossopharyngeal nerves to end in the nuclei of the solitary tract in the medulla of the brain. The brain stem is organized so that the activity of these nervous signals inhibits a variety of brain functions. As volume decreases, so does the nervous activity in the vascular afferent nerves. The inhibition is released, and the neuroendocrine response to injury is set in motion. There are two principal sets of projections from the solitary nuclei. One reaches the lateral reticular nuclei of the medulla, as well as the dorsal motor nuclei of the vagus nerves. These nuclei represent the principal origins, respectively, of the sympathetic and parasympathetic nervous systems. The other principal outflow from the solitary nuclei ascends to and through the locus ceruleus and adjacent areas of the pons and then ascends farther to the hypothalamus in three major tracts. These include the medial forebrain bundle, the dorsal longitudinal fasciculus, and the central tegmental tract. These pathways terminate in specific hypothalamic nuclei involved in the control of specific neural and hormonal functions, as indicated below. Functionally, some ascending pathways have been shown to stimulate hormonal secretion whereas others are inhibitory.

Pain

Pain accompanies most injuries. Even in the presence of unconsciousness, the nociceptive pathways that mediate afferent pain information may be activated and may contribute to the neuroendocrine response. Injury leads to the formation and release of a number of tissue factors, including histamine, kinins, and prostaglandins. It seems likely that the latter activate directly the endings of pain-afferent nerves. These synapse in the substantia gelatinosa of the spinal cord and then ascend in the spinothalamic tracts to enter the gigantocellular tegmental fields of the medulla and pons. Recent evidence suggests that they then may join some of the volume-sensitive pathways ascending from the locus ceruleus to the hypothalamus. In addition, projections to the midline raphe nuclei in the pons and midbrain may activate descending pathways that involve the endogenous opiates of the brain, the enkephalins, and that limit the flow of pain information through the primary pain-afferent endings in the substantia gelatinosa of the spinal cord.

Hypoxia

A variety of injuries leads to a decrease in the oxygen content of arterial blood. This content is sensed by chemoreceptors located primarily in the carotid and aortic bodies and in the area postrema of the medulla. These areas are also sensitive to changes in hydrogen-ion concentration of the blood and to the partial pressure of carbon dioxide. The afferent pathways terminate in the nuclei of the solitary tract, where they appear to interact with the baroreceptor and atrial afferents.

Emotional Factors

The perception of injury or of the threat of injury sets in motion a variety of emotional changes, including fear, anxiety, and, at times, anger. Such emotional changes are reflected in changes in neural activity in areas of the limbic system of the brain, including principally the septal, hippocampal, and amygdaloid nuclei. These project to the hypothalamic nuclei through the fornix or through the medial forebrain bundle and may also descend through the latter to reach lower brain-stem nuclei, including the lateral reticular nucleus and the dorsal motor nucleus of the vagus. The pathways outlined above constitute the principal neural substrates by which the primary stimuli set in motion the neuroendocrine response to injury.

SECONDARY STIMULI

The neuroendocrine response to injury interacts with the injury itself to bring about certain changes that themselves modify autonomic nervous activity and hormonal secretion. Because these signals depend upon the neuroendocrine response they may be viewed as secondary rather than as primary results of the injury itself.

Temperature

Body temperature falls in the period immediately following injury. Severe hypovolemia may lead to a decrease in hepatic blood flow with a resultant decrease in thermogenesis. This primary effect may be augmented by reflex splanchnic vasoconstriction, which is dependent both upon increased sympathetic nervous activity and upon the action of the hormones vasopressin and angiotensin II. In addition, va-

soconstriction may be inadequate in the skin during shock states, augmenting heat loss. The resultant decrease in core body temperature may be detected both peripherally and centrally, in the preoptic area of the hypothalamus, and may mediate a variety of hormonal responses.

Glucose

A large number of hormones have been implicated in the increase in plasma glucose that routinely follows injury. Changes in plasma glucose concentration in turn are detected by cells in the hypothalamus and pancreas and initiate a wide variety of hormonal changes. The hyperglycemic response to injury thus becomes an important controlling factor in determining the pattern and magnitude of the neuroendocrine response to that injury.

Blood Volume Restitution

Just as a loss of functional blood volume is a principal factor that sets in motion the neuroendocrine response, so the replacement of that volume is a major factor in attenuating or limiting that response. One of the major effects of the sympathetic response to injury is to lower capillary pressure and thus initiate plasma refill. In addition, the earliest metabolic changes that follow injury involve the release of solute, principally from the liver. As described later, this solute mediates a shift of fluid out of cells that also contributes to the restoration of plasma volume and protein. As blood volume is restored, a principal signal for the neural and hormonal changes is reduced or even eliminated. Thus, this secondary stimulus can be viewed as a sort of negative feedback aimed at terminating the signal as hypovolemia is corrected.

MODULATION

A large number of factors can modify the neuroendocrine response to the primary and secondary stimuli. The most important of these are the therapeutic maneuvers commonly used in the management of surgical patients. Thus, the administration of blood and fluids to restore and maintain blood volume, the administration of oxygen, and the use of anesthetics and analgesics can all be expected to reverse some or all of the primary stimuli. Other maneuvers commonly associated with good surgical practice fall in the same category. Thus, hemostasis, asepsis, antisepsis, and the gentle handling of tissues, while directed initially at other purposes, all serve to limit the neuroendocrine response to injury or surgery. The Trendelenburg position and the pneumatic antishock trouser may be viewed in the same regard because they shift blood volume centrally.

Several important hormonal interactions also modulate the response. The best known of these involves cortisol. Its negative feedback effect on adrenocorticotropic hormone (ACTH) is well known, although limited in injury. However, in addition, cortisol can inhibit release of vasopressin and possibly of prolactin and growth hormone. It also increases release of glucagon and renin. Angiotensin II increases release of vasopressin, ACTH, and the catecholamines. Vasopressin inhibits release of renin. These are simply examples of interhormonal interactions, since investigation in this area has just begun to scratch the surface.

Sepsis is an all too common concomitant of injury and may be associated with a variety of hormonal responses. Several mechanisms may be involved. Bacterial endotoxin, for example, can stimulate release of ACTH. Circulatory changes associated with sepsis, in part related to changes

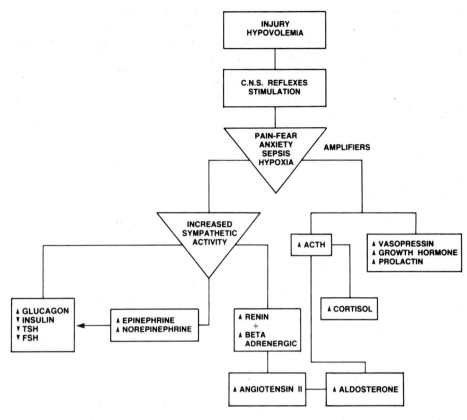

Fig. 1-2. Cascade of neurohumoral response to injury and hypovolemia induced by central nervous system (CNS) stimulation. The stimulus is amplified by factors in the triangles and modulated by the increase in sympathetic activity. (*ACTH*, adrenocorticotropic hormone)

in thromboxanes and prostacyclin, may produce hemodynamic stimuli to hormonal release. Autonomic responses to infection are well known and may stimulate hormonal secretion directly.

It has been demonstrated that the response to a second injury may differ substantially from the response to a first. This may be particularly important in the case of trauma, in which a surgical intervention frequently follows the primary injury by a matter of hours and sepsis frequently intervenes at a later time. Specifically, greatly augmented responses of catecholamines and cortisol and modest increases in ACTH have been demonstrated at times up to 1 day following an initial hemorrhage or surgical injury. Similarly, the hormonal response to a variety of stimuli may be modified by the time of day. The well-known circadian rhythms in hormonal release appear also to involve the responsiveness of hormonal control systems, so injury may produce different patterns and degrees of hormonal response when inflicted at different times. Our understanding in this area is just beginning, but it appears that there may be optimal times of day to carry out elective surgical interventions if we could determine the biologic implications of different kinds of neurohormonal responses.

THE NEUROENDOCRINE RESPONSE

One must keep in mind that nerves and hormones are not ends in themselves but are means of conveying messages between organ systems. Thus, the neuroendocrine response to injury is a means of initiating circulatory and metabolic responses to the stimuli outlined above. Although metabolic effects are not instantaneous, they tend to persist for some time after the initiating signal has disappeared, although this persistence rarely lasts as long as a matter of days. Most of the studies of neural and hormonal responses to stimuli

involved in injury have been conducted during the acute phase of injury or immediately thereafter. This time frame corresponds to the ebb phase of the metabolic response to injury. The few studies that have involved long time spans have been related to burns; in these cases, the injury itself appears to persist and the ebb phase is prolonged. Nonetheless, it is commonplace to see attempts to relate the hormonal changes involved in acute injury to the metabolic changes seen during the flow phase of the metabolic response. This is probably not legitimate, and the lack of temporal correlation between hormonal changes and metabolic changes during the flow phase represents a serious gap in our knowledge. The summary of the neuroendocrine response that follows must be viewed as describing only acute changes (Fig. 1-2).

PITUITARY HORMONES

Vasopressin

Injury leads to the secretion of both arginine vasopressin from the posterior pituitary and a battery of anterior pituitary hormones. The signals arising from injury reach the hypothalamus by the pathways outlined above, and these pathways are probably shared. Vasopressin release is dependent primarily on hypovolemia, but this release may be augmented by pain and emotional factors, as well as by the hyperosmolarity that commonly follows injury. Vasopressin is synthesized in the supraoptic and paraventricular nuclei and then transported to and stored in the posterior pituitary until its release is stimulated.

ACTH

ACTH is the classic hormone released in reaponse to injury. Its release from the anterior pituitary is stimulated by corticotropin-releasing factor (CRF), a large polypeptide recently identified in the hypothalamus. The action of CRF is potentiated by vasopressin. ACTH is synthesized from a large precursor molecule that can be processed not only into ACTH but also into β-endorphin or β-lipotropin. These substances may be cosecreted with ACTH in response to injury. β-Endorphin is one of the natural opiates produced in the body and may serve to limit the perception of pain. Recently, it has been implicated in a number of the deleterious cardiovascular changes in various forms of shock.

Growth Hormone
Growth hormone is released from the anterior pituitary under the control of both stimulatory and inhibitory factor from the hypothalamus. Growth-hormone-releasing factor has not yet been purified. The inhibitory factor is somatostatin.

Prolactin
Prolactin is released rapidly from the anterior pituitary following injury. Its release is also under dual control from the hypothalamus. The release of prolactin is inhibited by the neurotransmitter dopamine, and this is the principal mode of control. In addition, however, prolactin release is stimulated by the neurotransmitter thyrotropin-releasing hormone (TRH).

Thyroid-Stimulating Hormone (TSH)
The secretion of thyroid-stimulating hormone (TSH) from the anterior pituitary is unaffected by injury. Although cold can stimulate the release of TSH by elevating TRH release in neonates, this response is apparently lost in adult human beings. Changes in thyroid function are probably independent of changes in TSH.

Gonadotropins
Following an initial surge, the release of follicle-stimulating hormone (FSH) and luteinizing hormone (LH) is inhibited by injury. This is thought to be associated with decreases in the corresponding hypothalamic-releasing hormones. The underlying neural mechanisms relating the stimuli involved in injury to these hormonal changes have not been explored.

TARGET ENDOCRINE ORGANS

Adrenal Cortex
The secretion of cortisol by the zona fasciculata of the adrenal cortex is primarily under the control of ACTH and is a uniform concomitant of injury. Stoner has shown that there is a close correlation between the extent of injury as reflected in the injury severity score and the degree of elevation of cortisol. Recent studies have indicated that, in addition, there are one or more factors that may alter the sensitivity of the adrenal to ACTH. These factors also appear to be augmented by injury. Therefore, following injury, cortisol increases in large measure as a result of ACTH release but also in response to increased sensitivity to ACTH.

The secretion of aldosterone after injury is mediated by several interacting factors. These include angiotensin II (a hormone formed in the blood in response to the release of renin from the kidney), ACTH, and potassium released from cells in response to direct injury and as a result of acidosis that may follow hypoperfusion. Any of these factors is sufficient to produce an elevation in aldosterone during the acute period.

Thyroid
Thyroxine (T_4) and triiodothyronine (T_3) are secreted by the thyroid gland in response to the action of TSH from the pituitary. This secretion is apparently augmented by a β-adrenergic sympathetic mechanism. The secretion of the thyroid hormone is unaltered after injury. Triiodothyronine is the principal active thyroid hormone; for most sites of action, T_4 must be converted to T_3 to become active. This conversion, which occurs in most tissues, is regulated in part by the alternative conversion of T_4 into reverse T_3. There is some evidence that after injury the conversion favors the inert reverse T_3 rather than active T_3. This process then leads to a decrease in the availability of active thyroid hormone after injury.

Gonads
The secretion of the sex hormones is under the control of FSH and LH from the pituitary. Secretion of both androgens and estrogens is depressed by injury, presumably as a result of decreased secretion of these pituitary hormones.

SYMPATHETICALLY MEDIATED HORMONES
A number of hormones are secreted primarily as a result of direct neural control through the sympathetic and, to a lesser extent, parasympathetic nervous systems. Increased sympathetic activity is a fundamental component of the neuroendocrine response to injury, as has been described.

Catecholamines
The prime example of direct neural control of hormonal secretion lies in the secretion of norepinephrine and epinephrine from the adrenal medulla. The synthesis and secretion of the catecholamines are controlled directly by a cholinergic mechanism in the adrenal medulla. In addition, catecholamine secretion can be potentiated by the actions of angiotensin II and some of the prostaglandins. The relative importance of these mechanisms in the catecholamine response to injury has not been defined.

Glucagon
Glucagon is secreted by the alpha cells of the pancreatic islands in response to hypoglycemia or arginine. These responses may be augmented by α-adrenergic stimulation, which may also be sufficient to induce glucagon release, even in the face of hyperglycemia. Glucagon secretion may be inhibited by the action of somatostatin released from adjacent cells of the islands. Glucagon is secreted in a variety of forms of injury, including burns, surgical trauma, and hemorrhage. There is some evidence for hypothalamic control of glucagon secretion, through both sympathetic and parasympathetic pathways. In addition, circulating catecholamines may increase release of glucagon.

Insulin
Insulin is secreted by the beta cells of the pancreatic islands in response to hyperglycemia and parasympathetic activity. Leucine and arginine also increase insulin secretion. Insulin secretion may be inhibited by somatostatin, as well as by α-adrenergic activity. In injury, there are therefore opposing stimulatory and inhibitory influences on insulin secretion. Circulating catecholamines and adrenergic nerves act to inhibit insulin secretion, whereas hyperglycemia acts to stimulate it. Under most circumstances, the result is that insulin secretion may be elevated, but not as much as would be expected for the degree of hyperglycemia.

Renin

Renin is an enzyme of the kidneys secreted by the juxtaglomerular apparatus; it is controlled by a complex set of interacting signals. The juxtaglomerular apparatus functions as a sort of baroreceptor and may be stimulated directly by hypotension. The apparatus is also innervated by β-adrenergic nerves and may be stimulated by circulating epinephrine and by increased sympathetic activity. In addition, the macula densa of the distal nephron stimulates the release of renin in response to decreased chloride delivery to that segment of the nephron. Delivery of chloride is decreased when glomerular filtration falls, as in profound hypotension, or when proximal reabsorption of NaCl is enhanced, either by increased efferent arteriolar constriction or by decreased natriuretic factor. Increased efferent arteriolar constriction, in turn, may be stimulated through an α-adrenergic mechanism. Thus, in injury with hypovolemia, all three mechanisms may play a role in stimulating renin release. On the other hand, the release of renin is inhibited by vasopressin and increases in potassium ion. As indicated above, both of these influences are also accentuated in injury. Nonetheless, when severe hypovolemia accompanies injury, increased release of renin regularly occurs. This enzyme then leads to the splitting of an α_2-globulin, angiotensinogen, to form angiotensin I. This decapeptide is split to form the active octapeptide angiotensin II in response to the action of converting enzyme, present primarily in the endothelium of the lung and secondarily in the plasma itself. As indicated above, angiotensin II stimulates secretion of aldosterone by the zona glomerulosa of the adrenal cortex, enhances release of catecholamines, stimulates release of vasopressin, and augments release of ACTH. Its action on a variety of other hormones has not been explored fully.

NEUROHUMORAL INTEGRATION

As studies of hormonal control are extended, the basic pattern exhibited by the pancreatic islands appears to be much more generalized. That is, there are circulating, neural facilitory, and neural inhibitory factors mediating the release of virtually every hormone and there are multiple interhormonal interactions. These clearly have a modulating effect on the hormonal pattern after injury, but understanding of the full range of these modulations and of their biologic significance awaits further exploration.

METABOLIC RESPONSE TO INJURY

In his pioneering studies, Cuthbertson defined three phases of injury: an ebb and a flow of vitality, followed by an anabolic phase. For our discussion, however, convalescence is considered to begin at the time of injury and extend through complete recovery. This entails four phases (ebb, flow, anabolic, and fat gain), with frequently imprecise transitions (see Fig. 1-1). The metabolic events of convalescence are dynamic and largely operational without conscious recognition by the patient. Although numerous factors influence the inception, continuation, and ultimate completeness of convalescence, a reasonably uniform sequence of events can be identified in the process: (1) the several signals indicative of injury, that is, hypovolemia, pain, anxiety, tissue damage, infection, and immobilization, (2) are perceived, and a response is organized by the neuroendocrine system which (3) results in physiological and biochemical alterations designed to promote recovery and survival of the organism. Each phase of convalescence can be considered in terms of metabolic alterations serving homeostatic priorities of the organism to defend the stability of the internal environment, although the mechanisms by which this is accomplished frequently are not clearly understood. The constellation of these responses over the four phases of convalescence constitutes the biologic response to injury.

If our teleological hypothesis is valid, it is an oversimplification to consider the metabolic alterations of carbohydrate, fat, and protein as separate entities or to imply that a sharp difference in metabolic events separates the successive phases of convalescence. The metabolic changes are interdependent through their regulation by neuroendocrine factors to support homeostatic priorities, as illustrated in Figures 1-1 and 1-2. The metabolic changes reflect a dynamic balance between several signals of stress and feedback from the homeostatic mechanisms or therapeutic interventions.

Today, after several decades of study, a reasonable consensus exists in regard to a description of the alterations that develop in the metabolism of protein, fat, and carbohydrate after injury. Less clear, however, are the mechanisms responsible for these changes and the purpose or significance of the successive changes. It is not surprising that the greatest interest has centered on the ebb and flow phases, which follow most closely after injury, since this is the time of maximal metabolic disturbance. Drawing on these studies, it is possible to construct a conceptual framework relating the metabolic alterations observed in these phases to the homeostatic mechanisms they may serve.

EBB PHASE (DEFENSE OF CIRCULATORY VOLUME)

The immediate response to injury is organized to defend circulatory blood volume as the first priority of homeostasis. Until this need is satisfied, other priorities, such as regulation of the composition, osmolality, and pH of body fluids, as well as of body temperature and energy production, may be sacrificed or curtailed. After many injuries, the ebb phase does not occur because circulatory volume is not reduced or therapy adequately restores the lost volume. Without therapy, the initial or ebb phase of convalescence is brief after most injuries. It lasts no more than 24 to 36 hours, during which the mechanisms involving several organs and tissues unite to restore adequate circulation to peripheral tissues, while maintaining perfusion of those tissues most critical to survival. Despite the increased activity of the sympathetic nervous system elicited during this phase and its known effect on increasing the metabolic rate of most tissues of the body, both heat production and respiratory quotient are depressed. While the decreased consumption of oxygen probably simply reflects reduced tissue perfusion, this change can lead to a dangerous oxygen debt if circulatory volume is not restored. Stoner concluded from his extensive studies in rats that the decline in heat production characteristic of this phase represents a transient impairment of the thermoregulatory capacity of the hypothalamus. The extent of this impairment is determined by the severity of the injury. For the surgical patient, factors such as the ambient temperature of the operating and recovery rooms and the anesthetic agents employed determine whether or not the decline in heat production is associated with an actual fall in body temperature.

NECROBIOSIS (SHOCK)

In the event that the homeostatic responses are not equal to the severity of the illness or injury, the path toward convalescence is diverted into a preterminal period termed *necrobiosis* by Stoner. The initial ebb phase may be overlooked by the onset of necrobiosis when circulatory volume loss is extreme or when the resistance to injury is marginal. The endocrine and metabolic alterations found during the period of necrobiosis are characteristic of hypovolemic shock.

A reasonable consensus accepts the definition of *shock* as a state of persisting deficiency of peripheral perfusion. An alarming chain of events develops; reduced peripheral perfusion causes anaerobic metabolism, resulting in an increased acid load and an inefficient energy production terminating in death unless appropriate therapeutic measures are undertaken promptly.

METABOLIC ALTERATIONS DURING THE EBB PHASE OF CONVALESCENCE

Carbohydrate

While hyperglycemia is characteristic of the metabolic response to injury during both ebb and flow phases of convalescence, the mechanisms responsible for this change and the homeostatic priorities served by it differ significantly. Over a century ago, Bernard found a rapid doubling of the concentration of glucose in the blood in dogs subjected to experimental hemorrhage. This observation has been confirmed repeatedly and extended to the injured patient. In the nondiabetic, uncomplicated postoperative patient, only minimal hyperglycemia develops. By contrast, if an ebb phase occurs, there is a prompt and often marked rise in blood glucose; the magnitude of the rise generally reflects the degree of hypovolemia. If hypovolemia persists, the concentration of glucose in the blood begins to decline and may reach hypoglycemic levels shortly before death occurs. There is fair correlation between the decline in glucose concentration and the progressive loss of effective support of circulatory homeostasis. Coupled with hyperglycemia is a progressive rise in the plasma concentration of pyruvic and lactic acids, organic phosphorus, total amino acids, and, often, glycerol. The concentration of most of the hormones of the body, with the exception of insulin, increases in the plasma. In time, the *p*H falls, reflecting the steady increase in plasma of organic and inorganic acids.

The mechanisms responsible for the changes in carbohydrate metabolism have been clarified by experimental studies. Clearly the successive changes in plasma concentration of glucose must represent a balance between hepatic output of glucose from gluconeogenesis and glycogenolysis and peripheral uptake of glucose. While the relative contribution of gluconeogenesis to the hyperglycemic response to hypovolemia is uncertain, rapid glycogenolysis is a significant factor in the initial increased hepatic output of glucose. Hyperglycemia does not develop and the survival time in shock is significantly reduced in animals fasted sufficiently to deplete hepatic stores of glycogen. Findings indicate, however, that the reduced survival time more nearly reflects the dehydration that frequently accompanies fasting. The significant rise in the plasma levels of hormones known to be capable of activating gluconeogenesis and glycogenolysis, such as cortisol, epinephrine, and glucagon, indicates that these metabolic changes are in response to hormonal regulation.

Less direct evidence for increased hepatic output of glucose during shock comes from the numerous studies that indicate that peripheral tissues maintain or even increase their uptake of glucose during the early hyperglycemic period of hypovolemic shock. There is not uniform agreement, however, because Stoner found impaired uptake of glucose in his studies of tourniquet shock. Evidence for an increased uptake of glucose during hypovolemia and some insight into the mechanisms by which this may occur are derived from several studies performed during the past three decades. Randle and Stadie independently demonstrated an increased non-insulin-dependent uptake of glucose by tissues under hypoxic conditions. In elegant studies, Russell demonstrated an increased rate of removal of glucose and a more rapid rise in plasma levels of pyruvic and lactic acids in eviscerated rats, lacking circulation through pancreas and liver, when they were subjected to hemorrhage. Drucker found an increased uptake of glucose in diaphragms removed from rats subjected to hemorrhagic shock sufficient to reduce the mean arterial pressure to 50 torr. Clarissa Beatty demonstrated that an increase in the arteriovenous difference for glucose developed in the blood perfusing the hind limb of hypovolemic animals. When Shearburn extended these studies to measure the blood flow through the hind limb, he found significantly increased uptake of glucose during the initial 3 hours of hemorrhagic shock, with a return to preshock levels when the hyperglycemia began to decline. A similar, although less marked, increase in peripheral uptake of glucose was found in alloxan diabetic dogs, indicating that removal of glucose occurs during shock without a rise in plasma insulin in response to hyperglycemia and tissue hypoxia. Chaudry and Baue found that an isolated soleus muscle removed from bled animals had a normal rate of glucose uptake but that it was refractory to the influence of exogenous insulin. In the whole animal (hypovolemic dogs), however, exogenous insulin administered after the onset of deterioration of homeostasis has been found to accelerate significantly glucose disappearance from the blood.

Thus, during the ebb (hypovolemic) phase of convalescence, there is an increased hepatic output of glucose associated with a continuing or even increased peripheral removal of glucose. Since hyperglycemia develops in the well-fed animal or person subjected to shock, the hepatic output must surpass the peripheral uptake of glucose. The progressive rise of pyruvic and lactic acids is most likely indicative of a shift to glycolysis in support of energy needs in the poorly perfused peripheral tissues.

Protein

Most of the extensive literature about the alterations in protein metabolism following injury relates to the flow or catabolic phase rather than to the ebb phase. In the flow phase, findings show that both sepsis and injury are associated with a net shift of protein in the form of amino acids, predominantly alanine, from the skeletal muscle to the viscera. Unhappily, in the ebb phase of shock, the results are not as definitive. In his summary of the extensive studies of the metabolic alterations produced by shock during World War II, Engel concluded that an observed progressive rise in total α-aminonitrogen reflected an increased peripheral catabolism of protein. This belief was based on findings from an eviscerated preparation in a rat in which shock accelerated the rise of α-aminonitrogen in plasma. However, Levenson found that wounded soldiers, not all of whom were in shock, exhibited no significant rise in the free amino acids in the plasma, although there was an increase in phenylalanine, tyrosine, lysine, taurine, and, perhaps most important, alanine, with a decrease in other amino acids. McCoy confirmed Engel's observation of rising α-amino-acid concentration in blood during hypovolemia, but she found no significant increase in output (arteriovenous concentration difference times flow) from peripheral tissues. The marked reduction in peripheral flow during shock could account for these results. Elwyn concluded from studies of the interorgan transport of amino acids in hemorrhagic shock that little change occurs until the later stages of shock, when a rise in plasma concentration of amino acids reflects hepatic protein catabolism with decreased hepatic uptake and net peripheral release of amino acids.

Fat

Since both plasma levels of catecholamines and sympathetic activity are elevated and insulin does not increase in the plasma of primates directly after injury, an increase in lipolysis would be expected to occur during the ebb phase. This would lead to a greater availability of glycerol for gluconeogenesis and release of free fatty acids. Owing to the curtailed perfusion of adipose tissue during hypovolemia, however, few studies have been conducted on the metabolic flux of lipids during this phase. Kovach found a rise in arterial glycerol concentration and attributed the unchanged concentration of free fatty acids to reduced perfusion of adipose tissue. The earlier findings of Russell and colleagues, which suggested that ketones are consumed during shock, have received recent support from Barton, who found that the contribution of ketones to whole-body oxygen consumption is increased twofold after the onset of tourniquet shock. On the other hand, Beisel suggested that sepsis increases the flow of acetyl-CoA toward the synthesis of new fatty acids rather than toward ketogenesis. This mechanism also could explain a decline of ketones in sepsis or hypovolemic shock.

SIGNIFICANCE OF METABOLIC ALTERATIONS DURING THE EBB PHASE OF CONVALESCENCE

One of the important concepts resulting from the extensive studies of metabolism during World War II was the belief that tolerance for hypovolemia is directly related to the capacity of an organism to maintain its supply of energy. Direct measurement of energy stores demonstrated a progressive decline of hepatic adenosine triphosphate (ATP) and phosphocreatine (PC) as shock continues. A plausible hypothesis in keeping with the metabolic alterations noted is that glucose becomes the uniquely usable source of fuel owing to the shift to anaerobic glycolysis in support of energy needs during the ebb phase. When hypovolemia is severe or prolonged, protein and fat cannot contribute to the energy requirements of hypoxic tissues. Since glycolysis is a relatively inefficient source of energy production, the demand for glucose is increased. Nevertheless, fat continues to provide the major share of calories for nonhypoxic tissues. Gluconeogenesis is fostered by the return to the liver of the products of glycolysis, pyruvic and lactic acids, by way of the Cori cycle; by new carbon atoms derived from the catabolism of protein in peripheral tissues brought to the liver primarily as alanine; and by lipolysis, which contributes glycerol for re-formation into glucose. Liver glycogen is rapidly depleted as it contributes to the increased hepatic output of glucose. Thus, all energy substrates are diverted to meet the need for production of glucose to be used in hypoxic tissues (Fig. 1-3).

The endocrine environment is completely conducive to this goal, with the seeming exception of insulin. The low plasma concentration of insulin, however, allows the counterregulatory hormones to stimulate gluconeogenesis and glycogenolysis. At the same time, the potential inhibitory effect from the high plasma concentration of these hormones on glucose uptake, unopposed by a rise in insulin, is overcome by hypoxia, which fosters the entrance of glucose into cells. The relative deficiency of insulin output in response to hyperglycemia may actually represent, therefore, a well-tuned homeostatic device that promotes, through these mechanisms, an increased hepatic output of glucose for use by peripheral tissues during shock (Fig. 1-3).

If hypovolemia persists, the hepatic glycogen stores become depleted and gluconeogenesis is inadequate to surpass the peripheral assimilation of glucose. The resultant progressive decline in hyperglycemia is associated with deterioration of other defense mechanisms that depend on a continuing supply of energy. For instance, defense of plasma volume is compromised, as reflected by a change from hemodilution to a gradual increase in hemoconcentration. Several mechanisms have been suggested to account for the nonerythrocyte fluid lost from the circulation in this late stage of shock, including the development of cellular edema.

Based on numerous studies, Baue has postulated that a vicious cycle of events develops from an intracellular "energy crisis" initiated by ischemia. Reduced energy stores alter cellular permeability; this is reflected by a decreased transmembrane potential. The cellular responses are altered to such hormones as insulin, glucagon, corticosteroids, and catecholamines. Cellular edema develops with further depletion of substrates through a more permeable membrane and further loss of energy levels within the cell. To correct this abnormality, Baue and many others have begun to administer ATP-MgCl$_2$ as ancillary therapy for experimental shock due to such causes as hemorrhage, sepsis, burns, and peritonitis. Others, however, have not been able to confirm the beneficial effects of this therapy. Also, Shires has found that in septic and hypovolemic shock, the reduction of transmembrane potential leading to cellular edema occurred before the onset of hypotension or a discernible change in the cellular content of high-energy phosphates. These studies suggest that an impaired use of ATP could account for the maintenance of seemingly normal levels of ATP at a time when there is progressive systemic, cellular, and subcellular derangement of energy metabolism. Inhibition of the sodium–potassium pump in the cell membrane, perhaps owing to defective binding of ATP to sodium–potassium ATPase, could explain the cellular edema, with its disastrous consequences. An example of these consequences has been found by Saba, who, in extending the work of the late Sam Powers, found that resuscitated post-traumatic patients may suffer from defects in peripheral oxygen use owing in large measure to tissue edema that separates the capillaries from the mitochondria. Thus, while it is reasonably well established that cellular edema can develop in the ebb phase, if the ebb phase is sufficiently prolonged or severe, the mechanisms responsible for this alteration require further clarification.

FLOW PHASE (DEFENSE OF ENERGY NEEDS)

With uncomplicated convalescence, the ebb phase is followed within 24 to 36 hours after injury by a flow phase

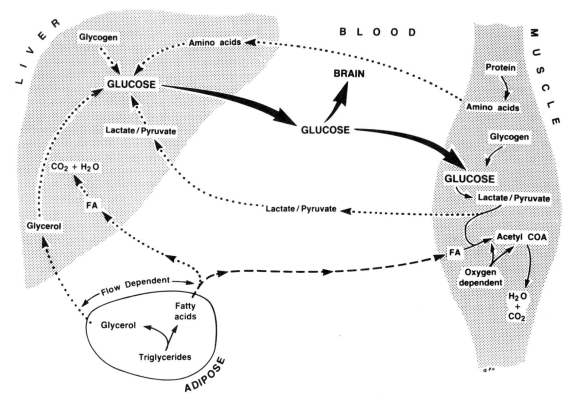

Fig. 1-3.   Major pathways for energy production during the ebb phase.

characterized by generalized catabolism and increased heat production (Fig. 1-4). The changes confined to this period commonly are known as the *acute* metabolic responses to injury. Their intensity, duration, and interrelations are determined by the prior condition of the body and the nature of injury, and they can be influenced to a great extent by medical intervention. This phase may last only a day or as long as 10 to 14 days. The observed changes are frequently considered in terms of energy metabolism, since they suggest that the priority of this phase is to provide substrate for energy and metabolic needs at a time when the body cannot acquire food owing to injury. Even in the absence of an exogenous diet, the capacity of the body to provide endogenous energy resources to maintain homeostasis is clearly evident from studies of well-nourished subjects demonstrating survival in good condition for 4 days or more without postoperative administration of food or fluid. The definitive studies of Kinney and associates, using indirect calorimetry, have made it clear that convalescence following uncomplicated operations requires an increase of no greater than 10% in resting metabolic expenditure of energy (RME), or heat production. Abbott, however, demonstrated that a marked increase in energy expenditure occurs when any febrile complication develops. A similar increase occurs following burns or fractures of long bones. Fractures commonly cause an increase of 10% to 25% in RME during the initial 2 to 3 weeks. Significant infections will increase RME by 15% to 50%. The most notable increase follows burns with sustained hypermetabolism that may be 40% to 100% above normal values until the burned surface is covered with skin. The total increase in energy expenditure, however, is not sufficient to account for the weight loss that occurs after a major injury. The extent of weight loss generally parallels the severity of the injury.

This loss, averaging 200 g to 800 g/day, is largely due to excretion of water bound to carbohydrate and protein and to combustion of fat. The loss of nitrogen is paralleled by losses of sulfur and phosphorus, suggesting breakdown of intracellular materials as well. Energy can be derived from the products of glycogenolysis, proteolysis, and lipolysis. The contribution of protein over a 3-week period after injury accounts for 10% to 14% of the weight loss, whereas fat accounts for 18% to 25% of the loss. These losses are similar to those observed after 3 weeks of starvation alone. Thus, all three nutrients, carbohydrate, protein, and fat, contribute to the provision of energy during the catabolic flow phase unless the patient obtains nutrition commensurate with the preinjury intake.

There may be, however, an intrinsic and as yet ill-defined effect of injury that causes a greater increase in metabolic expenditure than can be accounted for by a reduced nutritional intake and a slight increase in energy needs for survival and recovery. The extent to which trauma or a stress effect intensifies the catabolic responses beyond those produced by starvation is indicated by the development of fasting hyperglycemia, marked elevation of plasma free fatty acids, and increased proteolysis. These changes are in excess of needs for energy, with nitrogen losses sometimes reaching 20 g to 25 g/70 kg of body weight per day. There is also an increase in urea synthesis and in urinary excretion of creatine and creatinine. The hypermetabolic response to burns and sepsis persists as long as inflammation is present, whereas with fractures, after the initial hypermetabolic response, there may be a decline to values 10% to 20% below the preinjury level. To a great extent, however, the metabolic alterations of the flow phase reflect simply the combined influence of a reduction in dietary intake, bed rest, drugs, and ambient temperature, and they rarely exceed 10% of

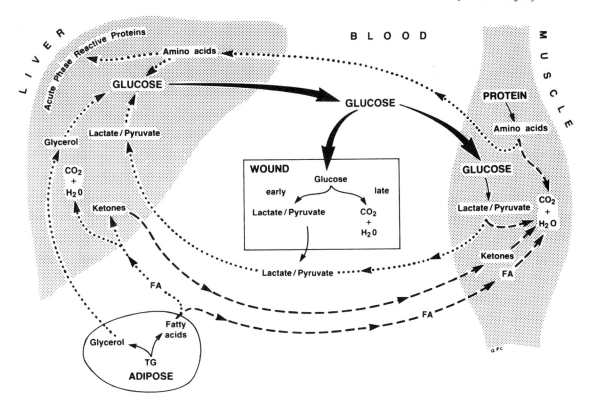

Fig. 1-4. Major pathways for energy metabolism during the flow phase.

the preinjury level. There seems little reason, therefore, to provide supplementary alimentation following soft-tissue injury with uncomplicated convalescence, whereas the value of hyperalimentation in the treatment of severe or complicated injuries and burns is widely recognized.

METABOLIC ALTERATIONS DURING THE FLOW PHASE OF CONVALESCENCE

Carbohydrate

Most injured patients, including those with a relatively minor injury such as a herniorrhaphy performed under spinal anesthesia, become transiently diabetic for 3 or 4 days. The slight hyperglycemia, delayed rate of assimilation of an infused glucose load, and glycosuria, but rarely ketosis, have been termed *diabetes of injury;* the extent of alteration is roughly proportional to the severity of injury. Similarly to diabetics, the postoperative patient has a normal tolerance for fructose at a time when glucose tolerance is markedly altered. This suggests that insulin deficiency or resistance impairs the peripheral uptake and use of glucose in the postoperative patient. In contrast to insulin-deficient diabetics, however, these patients usually have elevated plasma levels of insulin, exhibit a greater than normal rise in plasma levels of pyruvate and lactate during infusions of glucose, and rarely develop ketosis. Comparable changes are found in patients with Cushing's syndrome or steroid diabetes.

By using an isotopic tracer technique to follow the dynamic changes in carbohydrate metabolism during the flow phase after injury, Long, Kinney, and their associates found that hyperglycemia results from an increased flow of glucose, that is, an increase in synthesis or production of glucose relative to an increased turnover rate. In contrast to previous beliefs, neither injury nor sepsis was found to impair the ability of the body to oxidize glucose. Hepatic catheterization studies by Gump demonstrated an increased output of glucose in the postoperative patient despite the presence of hyperglycemia. Only recently, Elwyn found that infusions containing as much glucose as 600 g/day were required to overcome the heretofore seemingly nonsuppressible gluconeogenesis that develops during this phase of convalescence.

By studying insulin response to glucose infusions before and after injury, Giddings and co-workers demonstrated that the postoperative alteration in glucose tolerance is more likely to be due to the increase in gluconeogenesis than to any decrease in peripheral uptake and use of glucose. Support for this finding was provided by Wilmore's detailed studies of glucose kinetics in burn patients. He found that increased hepatic output accounted for the elevated glucose levels rather than any reduction in the rate of peripheral removal of glucose. Increased glucose flow from the liver in the burn patient correlated well with increased resting oxygen consumption and a return to the liver from the periphery of the 3-carbon compounds that support gluconeogenesis. It is noteworthy that despite the significant turnover of glucose, the respiratory quotient of these burn patients was uniformly low consequent to the use of fat as their primary fuel. During the early phase of sepsis, Wolfe and associates found not only an increase in gluconeogenesis, causing an increase in hepatic glucose output despite hyperglycemia, but also an increase in the rate of glucose uptake.

In marked contrast to patients in the ebb phase, when insulin secretion and action are inhibited by catecholamines and other counterregulatory hormones, a rise in plasma insulin usually occurs during the flow phase of convalescence. The persistence of gluconeogenesis in the presence of hyperinsulinemia and an increase in the insulin/glucose ratio are regarded as indications that insulin resistance is a characteristic feature of this phase of convalesence. In view of the concepts advanced by Kahn, this phase should more properly be regarded as one of reduced sensitivity to insulin rather than insulin unresponsiveness. This may be viewed as a mechanism to augment the supply of glucose as the preferential substrate for energy metabolism during the flow phase of convalescence.

Protein

A brief review of protein metabolism in the nonstressed person is essential for understanding the mechanisms involved in the breakdown of body protein that occurs during the flow phase following injury. Protein is distributed about equally between the extracellular mass and the body cell mass. The body cell mass is the metabolically active component of the body; about 60% is skeletal muscle, and the remainder is composed of viscera (20%–30%), body cells and the cellular components of adipose tissue, connective tissue, and the skeleton. The extracellular mass is not metabolically active, inasmuch as it does not perform work or consume oxygen in fulfillment of its tasks, structure, transport, and supply. It is largely fluid, but it does contain such solid components as collagen, tendon, and skeleton.

Protein metabolism is relatively inert in the extracellular mass, in contrast to the body cell mass, where protein metabolism is a dynamic process involving a constant interchange between whole proteins and amino acids. A continuous process of synthesis and degradation of protein (protein turnover) with uptake and release of amino acids in the liver, other viscera, and peripheral tissues permits rapid shifts from one protein pool to another in response to various needs.

Protein accounts for 15% to 20% of total body weight. About 300 g to 400 g of protein turnover occurs each day in the nonstressed person. Free amino acids are contributed to the pools from dietary and endogenous sources to form "labile pools of amino acids," and they are removed by synthesis to protein or degradation for excretion. Equilibrium between the several labile pools is so rapid that they can be considered a single pool of constant size which constitutes only 1% of total body amino acids. In this dynamic process, an amino acid spends only a few minutes in the pool. The fate of these amino acids for synthesis or catabolism largely determines the nitrogen balance of the organism. In the nonstressed, well-fed person, this balance remains in equilibrium.

Clearly, inability to obtain food is often a component of the total stress of injury for animals. Perhaps less obvious, but equally conducive to metabolic alterations, is the abrupt reduction in caloric intake that occurs in patients following an operation. In considerations of the metabolic response to injury, therefore, it is essential to distinguish between the alterations induced by fasting and those produced by injury. Failure to make this distinction has contributed to confusion and controversy about the sequence and significance of the changes in the metabolism of protein, fat, and carbohydrate during convalescence.

Within 24 hours after the onset of fasting, the meager glycogen stores of the body become depleted, causing endogenous protein and lipid to supply the fuel needs of the body. Cahill found that during the early days of starvation in an unstressed reference man weighing 70 kg, approximately 75 g of protein derived primarily from skeletal muscle is converted to glucose. The consequent daily excretion in urine of 12 g of nitrogen represents a loss of about 300 g/day of body cell mass. Since the muscle can recover completely without any residual evidence of damage following refeeding, it is probable that the muscle cells survive intact despite considerable loss of their protoplasm and protein. Simultaneously with the loss of protein, approximately 160 g of adipose tissue is consumed, because fat becomes the primary source of calories for the body's energy requirements during starvation—the protein being used for gluconeogenesis. With continued starvation, adaptation occurs by a decrease in the need for gluconeogenesis and an increase in the relative consumption of endogenous lipids. This spares the rapid loss of protein from the body cell mass to support gluconeogenesis, as reflected by a reduction of urinary nitrogen to the level of 3 g to 5 g/day, indicative of a breakdown of only 20 g to 30 g of protein.

In contrast to the nonstressed fasted person, injury or sepsis inhibits the adaptation to starvation, thereby allowing hypercatabolism to proceed. During this catabolic or flow phase after injury, an increase in the urinary excretion of nitrogen occurs in association with an increase in urinary sulfur, phosphorus, potassium, magnesium, and creatinine. While the source of the nitrogen and other intracellular constituents is not clear, the ratio of nitrogen/sulfur and nitrogen/potassium in the urine strongly suggests that the loss is from muscle. Further, there is little evidence that protein catabolism following injury is at the expense of the protein in such viscera as the heart, liver, kidneys, or gastrointestinal tract.

Lacking adequate nutritional intake, the postoperative patient enters a phase of negative nitrogen balance and weight loss. The amount of nitrogen lost in the urine depends on the severity and duration of injury, the prior nutritional status, and whether or not nutrition is provided after the injury.

A characteristic feature of this alteration in protein metabolism after injury is the increased rate of protein turnover. Although the kinetics of protein metabolism are very complex, studies with isotopically labeled amino acids have demonstrated an increase in both synthesis and degradation of protein. Since synthesis is usually increased less than breakdown, there is a net release of amino acids into the pools of labile amino acids and the body cell mass decreases. The increase in RME during this flow phase may be due primarily to the heat resulting from the increased deamination of protein and from use of the non-nitrogenous residues as a source of energy.

Amino acids that are catabolized in muscle are first deaminated by a transfer of the amino group to pyruvate or glutamate. The alanine formed in this way from pyruvate plus the alanine released from proteolysis is cleared from the blood by the liver, where the amino group is converted to urea or ammonia and the carbon skeleton becomes a substrate for gluconeogenesis. Thus, the alanine cycle is a pathway for converting muscle protein into new glucose, as well as functioning in concert with the Cori cycle as a pathway for conserving the partially oxidized glucose by returning pyruvic and lactic acids to the liver for gluconeogenesis.

By application of multiple isotopic dilution techniques for study of body composition, Moore concluded that the catabolic processes that produced shrinkage of the body cell mass were associated with an absolute or relative expansion of extracellular or supporting volume and its constituents.

Thus, body weight does not accurately reflect the protein loss and reduction in body cell mass after injury. Since the contribution of protein to total caloric expenditure is normally only 12% to 15% and after injury rarely more than 20%, it also is unlikely that the weight loss during this period indicates only use of endogenous protein as fuel. Rather, after an initial fluid loss, a decrease in body weight is due primarily to combustion of fat, which, following depletion of glycogen stores, contributes 70% to 90% of the total calories used postoperatively. While the two carbon fragments derived from fatty acids provide a generally usable substrate for energy needs, fat cannot contribute to a net gain of carbohydrate. Thus, protein is the only sizable reserve of carbohydrate intermediates and glucose precursors. Kinney, Long, and Duke have evidence that protein is more likely used for the production of carbohydrate essential for survival rather than to meet whole-body energy requirements. In addition, the carbon skeleton derived from protein catabolism promotes the synthesis of nonessential amino acids, which in turn support the resynthesis of protein most in demand during this period. They also foster the formation of glycerol for the synthesis of triglycerides.

It must be stressed that the protein catabolism during the flow phase is nutritionally dependent. It does not occur after injury in chronically starved or protein-depleted patients, and it is significantly less evident when a second operation closely follows the initial procedure. Under these circumstances, protein turnover is less likely to be accelerated. An acute reduction in protein intake without surgery, or simply staying in bed for more than 48 hours, induces a nitrogen loss similar to that noted after most uncomplicated injuries. In the well-nourished patient, the negative nitrogen balance can be greatly modified or prevented, however, by continuation of a high caloric and protein intake following an operation or injury. This strongly suggests that the net loss of protein is more an indication of acute undernutrition than a seemingly obligatory response to injury. Elevation of the ambient temperature to the range of 30°C also reduces the negative nitrogen balance after injury. On the other hand, an extensive injury such as a burn or a fracture of the long bones, or any febrile complication, induces a significant and sustained increase in nitrogen loss that cannot be overcome by nutritional intake. Cumulative nitrogen losses can reach 300 g or more in seriously ill or injured patients. These changes are distinctly different from those of starvation.

Fat

All of the energy substrates respond to the special requirements induced by injury. Caloric requirements are supplied almost entirely by the metabolism of fat. Even after excessive burns, with an increase in metabolic expenditure of 30% to 40%, the respiratory quotient falls within a range of 0.70 to 0.76, indicative of the shift to primary dependence on fat for energy needs.

Within 24 hours after injury, lipolysis of triglycerides causes a rapid rise and subsequent fall in the plasma level of free fatty acids to provide a source of energy for all tissues of the body except the central nervous system. The magnitude and duration of the response, which usually does not persist beyond the first week of the flow phase, reflect a balance between stimuli for lipolysis (*e.g.*, catecholamines, glucagon, and, possibly in humans, ACTH and cortisol) and inhibitors of lipolysis (*e.g.*, insulin, glucose, pyruvate, lactate, and ketone bodies). If hypovolemia is extreme, the initial rise in plasma levels of free fatty acids may not occur, owing to marked reduction of peripheral perfusion, whereas a slight injury may be insufficient to stimulate any rise in free fatty acids. During the first week of convalescence, there is ordinarily a decline in the level of cholesterol; this correlates with a fall in plasma albumin and suggests a common mechanism. However, the plasma level of triglycerides does not change.

A sustained slight increase in the plasma level of free fatty acids is not surprising during convalescence, when, in the absence of endogenous sources of nutrition, the main energy needs are met by lipolysis. The magnitude of the rise in free fatty acids can be reduced by maintaining the patient in a warm environment or providing calories in the form of an intravenous infusion of a fat emulsion, thereby possibly reducing the demand on the body for the endogenous production of energy. The capacity of the body to assimilate exogenously infused lipids is increased during the early phases of convalescence, and studies in severely injured patients indicate that fat is a well-tolerated calorie source that helps to modify the catabolic phase of convalescence. However, a syndrome of excess mobilization of free fatty acids has been described in many experimental studies, and this may have relevance to the clinical complications of fat emboli after injury.

SIGNIFICANCE OF METABOLIC ALTERATIONS

The flow phase can be regarded as a state of insulin resistance in the sense that generalized catabolism of all energy substrates develops during this period aided and abetted by the counterregulatory (catabolic) hormones, whereas insulin, the anabolic "banker hormone," which promotes the storage of these nutrients, does not increase to a comparable degree in the plasma. The mechanisms responsible for these alterations, which reach their peak within the first 4 to 8 days of convalescence, and their value for homeostasis are not clearly defined. Certain features have theoretical and practical importance. It is possible, of course, that the catabolic phase is simply a constant, nonbeneficial, nonobligatory, biologic response to injury with no value for convalescence. Or, it may be simply a prompt response to an endogenous need for fuel. Certainly, severe trauma in animals, and often in humans, is followed by a period of food deprivation accompanied by a variable increased demand by the body for metabolic fuel. The changes probably are more complex than combustion of fuel directly for energy needs. The alterations that develop in protein and carbohydrate metabolism do not appear to be essential for recovery because convalescence can proceed in their absence in the acutely starved and in many undernourished patients. For a given uncomplicated operation, the best-nourished patient is most likely to have the greatest nitrogen loss postoperatively. Fatty acids are the chief fuel in the flow phase, as reflected by the relatively low respiratory quotient in patients during this phase. The large loss of protein from body cell mass after severe injury does not seem to inhibit wound healing or repair of fistulas or the subsequent phase of anabolism.

Within the context of our convalescent model, wound healing actually begins during the ebb phase (see Fig. 1-1). Complete watertight epithelialization may be achieved in 24 hours; several days may be necessary for more complex wounds. Extensive burns are in a unique category of injury because of the severity and ongoing stress of the injury with an appreciable daily loss of protein through the open wound and the ever-attendant possibility of complicating infection. Ordinarily, wound healing continues during the catabolic phase regardless of the general metabolic condition of the patient. It is at the time of the body's general catabolism that the wound, through anabolism, develops both its tensile and its burst strengths. Only in the most protein-deficient person will a wound not heal.

In this reparative or flow phase of convalescence, the wound nevertheless may have a direct effect on metabolism. Not only do open wounds continue to leak protein, but during the early phase of the repair, the cellular elements of wounds require glucose as their specific fuel because energy is derived only through anaerobic glycolysis. Reparative tissues consume glucose with little or no oxygen and produce lactate. There seems little doubt that a burn wound creates a significant metabolic demand to replace the protein that is lost and for glucose as an energy substrate. The influence on metabolism of less extensive tissue destruction and from closed wounds, however, has not been quantitated as clearly in terms of both protein and glucose requirements. It has been suggested that a circulating protein derived from a wound signals the need for metabolic adaptation. The extensive studies by Kinney and associates indicate that the protein degradation that occurs after injury is directed less to meet whole-body requirements than to provide carbohydrate intermediates for hepatic gluconeogenesis, to supply the needs of red blood cells, wounds, and neural tissues.

In the injured patient, protein provides a source of carbon skeletons not only for the formation of new glucose but also as the source for glycerol required for synthesis of triglycerides and as a source for the synthesis of proteins that participate in convalescence. The plasma proteins that increase after injury have been termed *acute phase reactants*. Although studied extensively, the role of these proteins in convalescence is not completely defined. It is known that when the body cell mass is depleted, the synthesis of these proteins may become impaired, usually without harm to wound healing. Although the stimulus to do so is unknown, muscle protein can be considered to undergo catabolism to provide fuel or substrates for reparative processes in this phase. This is in marked contrast to the ebb phase, at which time muscle catabolism is viewed as the primary source of carbon to support the urgent need for formation of glucose to be used as a fuel through glycolysis in tissues with compromised circulation.

There is evidence, however, that under certain circumstances, protein may participate directly as a source of fuel in the flow phase. In sepsis and possibly after injury, the lack of locally available energy leads to the oxidation within muscle of the branched-chain amino acids (BCAA), leucine, isoleucine, and valine, derived from its own substance. If prolonged, this autocannibalism could cause further breakdown of muscle to provide the complement of BCAA required by the liver for its synthesis of high-priority proteins. The accumulation of a residue of nonessential amino acids following the consumption of the BCAA may be sufficient to stimulate by mass action their deamination and oxidation as energy substrates.

The purpose of glucose intolerance during the flow phase is still not altogether clear. Altered insulin sensitivity primarily affects muscle and liver. In muscle, which can use alternative energy substrates, the effect of insulin deficiency is to decrease glucose uptake, while in liver, the effect is to increase glucose output. The net effect is conservation and further production of glucose, leading to hyperglycemia.

This assures a continuing supply of glucose and a concentration gradient to promote uptake of glucose for those tissues with an absolute or preferential requirement for glucose, namely, cells in the healing wounds, neural tissue, erythrocytes, and renal medulla. It should be noted that these tissues do not normally respond to insulin and are, therefore, not directly affected by the "pseudodiabetes" after injury.

Thus, the flow phase is a period of intense metabolism to provide appropriate energy substrates for each tissue type, a state reflecting the preponderance of catabolic hormone activity (*e.g.*, steroids, catecholamines) over anabolic hormone activity (*e.g.*, insulin). This hormonal and metabolic emphasis during the flow phase can be attenuated by exogenous energy substrates (nutritional support) but cannot be entirely obliterated.

ANABOLIC PHASE (RESTORATION OF DEPLETED PROTEIN)

After the initial priorities of maintenance of circulatory volume and energy production and regulation of *p*H, osmolality, and thermoneutrality have been satisfied, the anabolic phase begins. Clearly, the first two phases of convalescence can be curtailed by exogenous provision of fluids and electrolytes to defend circulatory volume, osmolality, and *p*H, and of nutrients to support energy needs. But the recurring theme in studies of convalescence is the great inborn capacity that the body possesses to achieve these ends unassisted. Onset of the anabolic phase may be abrupt and even quite dramatic, particularly in patients who have experienced a demanding period of catabolism. The metabolic turning point from catabolism to anabolism is characterized by psychological and social phenomena reflecting the restoration of normal physiological processes. The patient often feels better and wants to be up and about. In the absence of specific disorders or surgical manipulation of the intestines, the normal processes of absorption become active early during the catabolic flow phase, usually within 1 or 2 days after surgery. The traditional custom of prescribing an oral intake that progresses from liquids to purees to soft, bland diets culminating at least in a "house diet" has little support from a physiological standpoint. Only limitations of the patient's desire or the culinary capacity of the health-care institution should curtail postoperative dietary intake except in those circumstances in which a particular illness may dictate nutritional constraints. A renewed appetite, the presence of active bowel sounds, and passage of flatus indicate transition to the anabolic phase. Weight gain during this period is frequently slow, since the reparative process must restore the muscle mass lost during catabolism. The rate of protein restoration is finite. It is estimated that nitrogen does not exceed 3 g to 5 g/70 kg of body weight/day; therefore, the total time for recovery may be significantly longer than the period of nitrogen loss directly after injury. Knowledge of the total nitrogen loss during the catabolic flow phase permits an estimation of the duration of the anabolic reparative phase; there is a weight gain of approximately 1 kg/week at maximum efficiency. Thus, a loss of 50 g of nitrogen, which may occur during a 3- or 4-day period after injury, would necessitate 10 days for anabolism to repair the losses at the maximum rate of 5 g/day.

Most patients do not require hospitalization during this phase and experience more expeditious rehabilitation if permitted to return home. The decision to resume work, however, must be delayed until the weakness resulting from this phase is overcome and when both personal and societal expectations of performance can be satisfied. An accelerated hematopoiesis during this phase compensates for any reduction in the red blood cell mass that occurs with acute injury.

While relatively little research has been directed to the neuroendocrine activity during the anabolic phase of convalescence, the marked metabolic alterations observed during the flow phase are largely terminated. The very essence of the anabolic phase, protein anabolism, indicates heightened insulin activity. Insulin, the banker hormone, is the key to reversing the manyfold metabolic alterations of the catabolic phase. Thus, insulin promotes deposition of glycogen in liver and muscle, inhibits gluconeogenesis, enhances cellular uptake of amino acids for synthesis into protein, and, by inhibiting lipolysis, sets the stage for storage of fat. In essence, the body fuels are conserved and storage of reserves is begun.

FAT PHASE (STORAGE OF ENERGY RESERVES)

After the protein lost has been restored, the final phase of convalescence is characterized largely by restoration of lost body fat, sometimes in excess of the preinjury state, and a more rapid gain in body weight. Patients who restricted their dietary intake preoperatively may experience a sometimes unhealthy accumulation of fat as they eat with abandon following surgical correction of their disorder. Others, who suffer from injuries that restrict their physical activity, such as extensive fractures or paralysis, may gain excessive weight owing to an imbalance between their customary dietary intake and a reduced energy expenditure. This phase begins when the basic priorities for homeostasis have been met. The intake of food now reflects the cultural and emotional needs and habits of the patient more than a response to physiological priorities for recovery.

REHABILITATION

The role of the health-care team is to promote convalescence by shortening its duration and minimizing its consequences. To achieve this goal, a plan for medical assistance must begin as early as possible, occasionally even in the preoperative period, and must continue through total convalescence until a maximum physical, emotional, social, and vocational capacity has been attained. In many surgical patients, this involves a cohesive, interdisciplinary team of physicians, nurses, speech pathologists, social workers, prosthetists, orthotists, vocational counselors, special educators, and physical, occupational, and recreational therapists. Appropriate rehabilitation of surgical patients, therefore, represents nothing less than comprehensive medical care in a continuous and dynamic fashion. There is a close correlation between the end results obtained and the time elapsed between the onset of injury and the implementation of suitable rehabilitative procedures. There are numerous variables that affect the convalescence–rehabilitation continuum; these include environment, prior physical status, nutrition, anesthesia and medications, and bed rest.

A fascinating observation is the effect of an increase in ambient temperature to the range of 30°C in abolishing or greatly curtailing the nitrogen loss during the flow phase. Although mechanisms responsible for this effect of temperature on protein catabolism are unknown, the therapeutic implications are obvious and have been applied in the treatment of extensive burns, fractures, and some injuries.

Of all factors influencing convalescence, perhaps none has more potential for adverse influence than the immobilization and decrease in the effects of gravity associated with complete bed rest. Although rest protects and fosters the healing of an injured organ, disuse of a normal organ leads to the progressive loss of its functional capacity. With a fracture, there is no option; muscle atrophy is accepted as a consequence of the immobilization required for healing. But total body inactivity neither facilitates wound healing nor reduces the presumed disparity between postoperative energy needs and supply. In fact, prolonged bed rest has no discernible value for patients capable of ambulation and it has many dangers.

The consequences of continued bed rest may develop within the short span of 4 days, and they become increasingly serious as bed rest is prolonged. Despite an adequate nutritional intake, deleterious metabolic responses to bed rest develop even in the absence of injury. The basal metabolic rate is reduced by 7%. There is an increased urinary loss of nitrogen and sulfur (N/S) and of potassium and phosphorus (K/P) in ratios indicating that muscle protoplasm is the source of the loss. A continuing urinary excretion of calcium may result in osteoporosis. Even if caloric intake is not reduced during this transition from daily activity to bed rest, body weight usually is not altered, owing to a change in body composition. The positive caloric balance that might be expected to cause weight gain may be masked by deposition of adipose tissue, with its high potential energy, replacing the catabolized muscle mass. Atrophy and shrinking muscle circumference reduce endurance and predispose to muscle contractures. Myasthenia develops, with a 10% to 15% loss of muscle strength per week of inactivity.

Most organ systems are not spared the serious consequences resulting from the recumbency of bed rest. Simply remaining in bed will cause a progressive increase in cardiac rate by one half beat/minute/day, a decrease in heart size and heart volume, and probably a reduction in resting cardiac output, although the blood pressure is not altered. The most notable consequence of bed rest is a marked loss of orthostatic tolerance and a reduction in work capacity. Cardiac performance under stress is significantly less efficient. The physiological mechanisms responsible for these adverse effects are not completely clear; however, there is marked individual susceptibility determined by the patient's physical fitness. The decrease in orthostatic tolerance, which is noticeable within 3 or 4 days, requires a much longer period for recovery. No definite correlation has been established between the loss of orthostatic tolerance and a decrease in blood volume.

For quite unexplained reasons, bed rest causes a reduction in plasma and blood volume, red blood cell mass, and extracellular fluid but a rise in hematocrit. Total body water, as judged by imprecise measurements, is not changed. Since the greatest loss occurs in plasma volume and there is usually no change in body weight, the rise in hematocrit suggests an intracellular shift of water. The relevance of the reduction of blood volume to the development of venous thrombosis and the danger of pulmonary embolism during prolonged inactivity is not known. There are, however, no consistent alterations in blood coagulation during bed rest.

In the urinary system, calculi might be expected to develop owing to stasis, an increased calcium concentration, and an alkaline urine. This complication rarely occurs in the absence of infection, and the use of an indwelling catheter to facilitate care of the immobilized patient inevitably risks this development.

Although no consistent changes in tests of respiratory function have been observed, a recumbent posture predisposes the patient to atelectasis and bronchial pneumonia, owing to difficulty in clearing bronchial secretions.

No complication of bed rest can be more disturbing than the development of a decubitus ulcer. Sustained pressure causes ischemia of underlying tissues and ultimately results in necrosis and development of an ulcer. This is more likely to occur in areas of anesthesia or analgesia that overlie a bony prominence. Malnourishment, which also predisposes to the development of these ulcers, becomes increasingly severe because large quantities of protein can be lost through the open wound. The occurrence of an ischemic ulcer can only be considered the result of neglect, lack of concern, and poor medical and nursing care.

Prevention of the deleterious effects of bed rest is the best therapy. Administration of steroids, having the patient use an oscillating bed or a G-suit, and having the patient exercise in bed have been tried with variable success. Simply moving a patient from bed to chair has minimal if any beneficial effects; in fact, it is potentially harmful, since the greater dependency of legs in a sitting posture may intensify the predisposition to venous stasis and thrombosis. Furthermore, all of the alterations in metabolic and organ systems observed with bed rest can be induced by immobilization in a chair.

EMOTIONAL RESPONSE DURING CONVALESCENCE

The most common emotional reactions of the patient following injury are fear, anxiety, and depression. These are highly variable in both pattern and degree and seem most related to the severity of the injury, fear of mutilation, and uncertainty regarding future functioning. The intensity of these reactions also varies according to the psychological defenses available to the patient. Most use *denial*, both a conscious and an unconscious effort to minimize the severity of injury, whereby the patient appears cheerful and relatively unconcerned about his physical status and convalescence. This defense allows for periods of good mood and low anxiety, a welcome relief to the patient. While helpful, if denial is sustained, it may prove detrimental because the patient may develop unrealistic attitudes toward his injury, hospital care, and ultimate rehabilitation.

The level of dependency the patient assumes after prolonged confinement to bed is an important consideration in total hospital management. The patient who assumes an exclusively dependent position presents problems of motivation in rehabilitation, since he anticipates that all of his needs will be met by others. The medical staff may become frustrated with the patient's inability to participate in his own treatment. The contrasting patient is hyperindependent and resents or refuses care; frequently, such a patient threatens to leave the hospital against medical advice. To manage these reactions effectively, one must understand the patient's current feelings and the experiences that have provoked and perpetuated such reactions. This understanding may require collaboration with a psychiatrist to assist the patient in resolving problems of inappropriate dependence or independence.

BIBLIOGRAPHY

Neuroendocrine Response to Injury

BYRNES GJ, PIRKLE JC JR, GANN DS: Cardiovascular stabilization after hemorrhage depends upon restitution of blood volume. J Trauma 18:623, 1978

CASLEY-SMITH JR: The functioning and interrelationships of blood capillaries and lymphatics. Experientia 32:1, 1976

FELIG P, SHERWIN RS, SOMAN V et al: Hormonal interactions in the regulation of blood glucose. Recent Prog Horm Res 35:501, 1979

FRANCHIMONT P: The regulation of follicle stimulating hormone and luteinizing hormone secretion in humans. In Martini L, Ganong WF (eds): Frontiers in Neuroendocrinology, p 331. New York, Oxford University Press, 1971

GANN DS: Endocrine control of plasma protein and volume. Surg Clin North Am 56:1135, 1976

GANN DS, CARLSON DE, BYRNES GJ et al: Impaired restitution of blood volume after large hemorrhage. J Trauma 21:598, 1981

GANN DS, DALLMAN MF, ENGELAND, WC: Reflex control and modulation of ACTH and corticosteroids. Int Rev Physiol 24:157, 1981

GANN DS, WARD DG, CARLSON DE: Neural control of ACTH: A hemostatic reflex. Recent Prog Horm Res 34:357, 1978

GERICH JE, LORENZI M: The role of the autonomic nervous system and somatostatin in the control of insulin and glucagon secretion. In Ganong WF, Martini L (eds): Frontiers in Neuroendocrinology, p 265. New York, Raven Press, 1978

HEMS DA, WHITTON PD: Control of hepatic glycogenolysis. Physiol Rev 60:1, 1980

MARTIN JB: Brain regulation of growth hormone secretion. In Martini L, Ganong WF (eds): Frontiers in Neuroendocrinology, p 129. New York, Raven Press, 1976

MENGUY R, MASTERS YF: Influence of hyperglycemia on survival after hemorrhagic shock. Adv Shock Res 1:43, 1979

SHIRES GT, CUNNINGHAM JN, BAKER CRF et al: Alterations in cellular membrane function during hemorrhagic shock in primates. Ann Surg 176:288, 1972

TAYLOR AE: Capillary fluid filtration: Starling forces and lymph flow. Circ Res 49:557, 1981

UTIGER RD: Assay and secretory physiology in man. In Werner SC, Ingbar SH (eds): The Thyroid, p 196. Hagerstown, Harper & Row, 1978

Metabolic Response to Injury, Convalescence, and Rehabilitation

ABBOTT WE, ALBERTSON K: The effect of starvation, infection and injury on the metabolic processes and body composition. Ann NY Acad Sci 110:941, 1963

ADOLPH EF: Origins of Physiological Regulations. New York, Academic Press, 1968

ALLISON SP, TOMLIN PJ, CHAMBERLAIN MJ: Some effects of anesthesia and surgery on carbohydrate and fat metabolism. Br J Anaesth 41:588, 1969

BARTON RN: Ketone body metabolism after trauma. In Porter R, Knight J (eds): Energy Metabolism in Trauma, a Ciba Foundation Symposium, p. 173. London, J & A Churchill, 1970

BEISEL WR, SAWYER WD, RYLL WD: Metabolic effects of intracellular infections in man. Ann Intern Med 67:744, 1972

BERNARD C: Leçons sur le Diabete et le Glycogenese Animale. Paris, J B Bailliere, 1877

BERNARD C: An Introduction to the Study of Experimental Medicine. Green HC (trans): New York, Macmillan, 1927

CAHILL GF: Starvation in man. N Engl J Med 282:668, 1970

CANNON WB: The Wisdom of the Body. New York, W W Norton & Co, 1939

CARLSON LA: Mobilization and utilization of lipids after trauma: Relation to caloric homeostasis. In Porter R, Knight J (eds): Energy Metabolism in Trauma, a Ciba Foundation Symposium. London, J & A Churchill, 1970

CHAUDRY IH, CLEMENS MG, BAUE AE: Alterations in cell function with ischemia and shock and their correction. Arch Surg 116:1309, 1981

CHAUDRY IH, SAYEED, MM, BAUE AE: The effect of insulin on glucose uptake in soleus muscle during hemorrhagic shock. Can J Physiol Pharmacol 53:67, 1975

CHOBANIAN AV, LILLE RD, TERCYAK A: The metabolism and hemodynamic effects of prolonged bed rest in normal subjects. Circulation 49:551, 1974

CLOWES GHA, JR, O'DONNELLY TF, BLACKBURN GL et al: Energy metabolism and proteolysis in traumatized and septic man. Surg Clin North Am 56:1169, 1976

CUTHBERTSON DP: Post-traumatic metabolism: A multidisciplinary challenge. Surg Clin North Am 58:1045, 1978

DARWIN C: On the Origin of the Species by Means of Natural Selection, or, The Preservation of Favoured Races in the Struggle for Life. London, John Murray, 1859

DEITRICK JE, WHEDON GD, SHORR E: Effects of immobilization upon various metabolic and physiologic functions of normal man. Am J Med 9:3, 1948

DRUCKER WR: Carbohydrate metabolism: Traumatized versus normal states. In Cowan GFM, Scheetz WL, (eds): Intravenous Hyperalimentation. Philadelphia, Lea & Febiger, 1972

DRUCKER WR, CHADWICK CDJ, GANN DS: Transcapillary refill in hemorrhage and shock. Arch Surg 116:1344, 1981

DRUCKER WR, DeKIEWIET JC: Glucose uptake by diaphragms from rats subjected to hemorrhagic shock. Am J Physiol 206:317, 1964

DRUCKER WR, HOWARD PL, McCOY S: The influence of diet on response to hemorrhagic shock. Ann Surg 181:698, 1975

ELWYN DH, KINNEY JM, JEEVANANDAM M et al: Influence of increasing carbohydrate intake on glucose kinetics in injured patients. Ann Surg 190:117, 1979

ENGEL FL: The significance of the metabolic changes during shock. Ann NY Acad Sci 55:383, 1956

FLEAR CTG, BHATTACHARYA SS, SINGH CM: Solute and water exchanges between cellular and extracellular fluids in health and disturbances after trauma. JPEN 4:98, 1980

FREUND H, YOSHIMURA N, LUNETTA L et al: The role of the branched-chain amino acids in decreasing muscle catabolism in vivo. Surgery 83:611, 1978

GIDDINGS AEB, MANGNALL D, ROWLANDS BJ et al: Plasma insulin and surgery: I. Early changes due to operation in the insulin response to glucose. Ann Surg 186:681, 1977

GIDDINGS AEB, ROWLANDS BJ, MANGNALL D et al: Plasma insulin and surgery: II. Later changes and the effect of intravenous carbohydrates. Ann Surg 186:687, 1977

GUMP FE, LONG, CL, KILLIAN P et al: Studies of glucose intolerance in septic injured patients. J Trauma 14:378, 1974

HOLDEN WD, KRIEGER H, LEVEY S et al: The effect of nutrition on nitrogen metabolism in the surgical patient. Ann Surg 146:563, 1957

ILLNER HP, SHIRES GT: Membrane defect and energy status of rabbit skeletal muscle cells in sepsis and septic shock. Arch Surg 116:1302, 1981

JOHNSON PC, DRISCOLL TB, CARPENTER WR: Vascular and extravascular fluid changes during six days of bed rest. Aerospace Med 42:875, 1971

JOHNSTON IDA, ROSS H, WELBORN TA et al: The effect of trauma on glucose tolerance and the serum levels of insulin and growth hormone in combined injuries and shock. In Schildt B, Thoren L (eds): Proceedings of the Symposium on Combined Injuries and Shock. East Orange, NJ, Upsala College, 1968

KAHN CR: Insulin resistance, insulin insensitivity and insulin unresponsiveness: A necessary distinction. Metabolism 27:1893, 1978

KINNEY JM, FELIG P: The metabolic response to injury and infection. Endocrinology 3:1963, 1979

KINNEY JM, GUMP FE, LONG CL: Energy and tissue fuel in injury and sepsis. Adv Exp Med Biol 33:401, 1972

KOVACH AGB: Metabolic changes in hemorrhagic shock. Adv Exp Med Biol 23:275, 1972

LONG CL, SPENCER JL, KINNEY JM et al: Carbohydrate metabolism in man: Effect of elective operation and major injury. J Appl Physiol 31:110, 1971

McCOY S, CASE SA, SWERLICK RA et al: Determinants of blood amino acid concentration after hemorrhage. Am Surg 43:787, 1977

MILLER LL, JOHN DW: Nutritional, Hormonal and Temporal Factors Regulating Net Plasma Protein Biosynthesis in the Isolated Perfused Rat Liver: Effects of Feeding or Fasting Liver Donors and of Supplementation With Amino Acids, Insulin, Cortisol and Growth Hormone: Plasma Protein Metabolism. New York, Academic Press, 1970

MILLER PB, JOHNSON RL, LAMB LE: Effects of four weeks of absolute bed rest on circulatory functions in man. Aerospace Med 35:1194, 1964

MOORE FD: The Body Cell Mass and Its Supporting Environment, 1st ed. Philadelphia, W B Saunders, 1963

MOORE FD, BALL MR: The Metabolic Response to Surgery. Springfield, IL, Charles C Thomas, 1952

PETERS JP, VAN SLYKE DD: Quantitative Clinical Chemistry. Baltimore, Williams & Wilkins, 1931

RANDLE PJ, SMITH GH: Regulation of glucose uptake by muscle: I. The effect of insulin, anaerobiosis and cell poisons on the uptake of glucose and release of potassium by isolated rat diaphragm. Biochem J 70:490, 1958

RICHARDS JR: Current concepts in the metabolic responses to injury, infection and starvation. Proc Nutr Soc 39:113, 1980

SCHLOERB PR, SIERACKI L, BOTWIN AJ et al: Intravenous adenosine triphosphate (ATP) in hemorrhagic shock in rats. Am J Physiol 9:R52, 1981

SHAH DM, NEWELL JC, SABA TM: Defects in peripheral oxygen utilization following trauma and shock. Arch Surg 116:1277, 1981

SHEARBURN EW, CRAIG WD, MAITLAND CL et al: Hemodynamic and metabolic alterations in peripheral tissues during hemorrhagic shock. Am Surg 41:696, 1975

SIEGEL JH, CERRA FB, COLEMAN B et al: Physiological and metabolic correlations in human sepsis. Surgery 86:163, 1979

SPITZER JJ, WIENER R, WOLF EH: Non-esterified fatty acid (FFA) metabolism following severe hemorrhage in the conscious dog. Adv Exp Med Biol 33:221, 1973

STADIE WC, ZAPP JA: The effect of insulin upon the synthesis of glycogen by rat diaphragm in vitro. J Biol Chem 170:55, 1947

STEIN TP, BUSBY GP: Protein metabolism in surgical patients. Surg Clin North Am 61:519, 1981

STONER HB: Carbohydrate metabolism after accidental injuries. Acta Chir Scand (Suppl) 498:48, 1980

SWERLICK RA, DRUCKER NA, McCOY S et al: Insulin effectiveness in hypovolemic dogs. J Trauma 21:1013, 1981

WILKINSON AW: Restriction of fluid intake after partial gastrectomy. Lancet 2:428, 1956

WILMORE DW, AULICK HL, GOODWIN CW: Glucose metabolism following severe injury. Acta Chir Scand (Suppl) 498:43, 1980

WILMORE DW, AULICK HL, MASON AD et al: Influence of the burn wound on local and systemic responses to injury. Ann Surg 186:444, 1977

WOLFE RR, ALLSOP JR, BURKE JF: Experimental sepsis and glucose metabolism: Time course of response. Surg Forum XXVIII:42, 1979

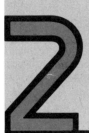

Herbert J. Proctor

Fluid and Electrolyte Management

Although Claude Bernard's concept of *le milieu intérieur* is generally listed as one of the earliest treatises dealing with fluid and electrolytes, Latta, as early as 1832, had some perception of body homeostasis when he infused salt solutions into victims of cholera with good results. From these early beginnings, the recognition of body fluid compartments, the mechanisms that govern the exchange of ions and fluid between these compartments, and the alterations imposed by disease and surgery have come to form an integral part of preoperative, intraoperative, and postoperative care.

In this chapter, all discussion focuses on the adult. Although much of the information applies also to the pediatric patient, a standard pediatric treatise should be consulted for different dosages and those specific problems arising in infants.

It is hoped the beginning student will concentrate on mechanisms and rationale for therapy rather than long lists of electrolytes committed to memory. Intelligent care of the patient is not achieved by cookbook formulas.

NORMAL BODY FLUID COMPARTMENTS

Although the term *compartment* is used as if it were a well-defined anatomical space, the so-called compartments are really phases without rigid boundaries. The differences in volume and solute concentration between phases are maintained by both active and passive forces. These compartments are measured by a variety of tracers, which are assumed to distribute themselves throughout the compartment in question. The following general formula is used to define the volume in question:

$$\text{volume} = \frac{\text{amount of tracer given} - \text{amount of tracer excreted}}{\text{concentration}}$$

TOTAL BODY WATER

Total body water, literally all the water lost from the body if the body were converted to ash, varies between 45% and 75% of the body weight. This variation results from the quantity of fat, which contains relatively less water per gram of solid than does lean muscle. Thus, fat persons tend toward a lower percentage of body weight composed of water, and thin persons tend toward a higher percentage. Although the total body water can be measured accurately for exper-

---

FLUID AND ELECTROLYTE MANAGEMENT IN SURGICAL PATIENTS

The major fluid compartments of the body are the intravascular, extracellular, and intracellular volumes, and together they comprise the total body water. Distribution of fluid, ions, and protein between the intravascular and extravascular spaces is on the basis of passive forces described by the modified Starling equation and the Gibbs-Donnan equilibrium. Distribution of fluid and ions between the intracellular and extracellular compartments is primarily on the basis of active transport, most notably the sodium pump.

Aldosterone and antidiuretic hormone (ADH) are the major hormonal influences on fluid and electrolyte metabolism and are active in compensating for variations in intake and output.

The normal adult daily fluid and electrolyte requirements are 2000 ml to 2500 ml, with 75 mEq Na, 40 MEq K, and 100 g glucose. Postoperative fluid requirements reflecting interstitial ("third space") loss generally necessitate a larger volume (4000 ml–5000 ml) and an increased requirement for Na.

Specific deficits in fluid volume and electrolyte composition may be approached by knowledge of the altered physiology leading to the deficit, calculation of the volume of the deficit by body weight and urinary output, and calculation of the quantity of electrolyte required based on knowledge of the distribution of the ion in question.

---

imental purposes, practically speaking, when confronted with the need to know the total body water for a particular patient, an educated guess is usually all the clinician can muster.

The total body water may be subdivided into a variety of component compartments.

EXTRACELLULAR FLUID VOLUME

The first major subdivision of the total body water is the extracellular fluid. Defined as all the fluid outside the cell, it comprises some 17% to 26% of the body weight and includes within it its own subdivisions: the intravascular volume (5% of the body weight), the lymphatic volume (2% of the body weight), and the interstitial volume (10%–12% of the body weight).

INTRACELLULAR VOLUME

The second major subdivision of the total body water is the intracellular volume. This volume is measured by subtracting the extracellular volume (defined by such tracers as sulfate, bromide, and inulin) from the total body water. Estimates for intracellular water vary from 30% to 40% of the total body weight.

THIRD SPACE

A final fluid compartment that plays a significant role in homeostasis in surgical patients has been called third space. During normal health, this space is comparatively small and consists of the intestinal contents, pleural fluid, pericardial fluid, joint fluid, and intravascular fluid. All are components of the total body water but are relatively unresponsive to the physiological mechanisms governing the other compartments. In the postoperative or diseased state, this com-

partment may increase enormously, consisting of such pathologic fluid collections as ascites, pleural effusion, pericardial effusion, edema, and abnormally large volumes of fluid sequestered within the gastrointestinal tract due to ileus.

FACTORS AFFECTING FLUID AND ION DISTRIBUTION

As has been mentioned, the fluid compartments should be thought of not as having rigid anatomical boundaries but rather as a given volume of fluid that is maintained in a given phase by a series of active and passive forces. Although under normal conditions the various phases are in equilibrium with one another, this does not imply that there are not large concentration gradients between adjacent phases. These concentration gradients are able to be achieved by virtue of membranes that have varying permeability to solutes and that are the location of various active transport sites.

INTRAVASCULAR–INTERSTITIAL VOLUME BOUNDARY

STARLING FORCES

The capillary basement membrane and the junctional zone between endothelial cells constitute the division between the intravascular, or plasma, volume and the interstitial volume. Starling was among the first to describe the forces causing exchange of fluid between these two spaces (Fig. 2-1). Starling's hypothesis was that at the arterial end of a capillary, the hydrostatic pressure (approximately 45 torr) forced fluid out of the capillary. This fluid supposedly exited the capillary through small pores large enough for water and ions (Na^+, K^+, Cl^-, and HCO_3^-) but too small to allow passage of proteins such as albumin. As plasma progressed to the venous end of the capillary, the protein concentration became progressively higher as fluid was lost, raising the intravascular colloid osmotic pressure. The increased colloid osmotic pressure then exceeds the hydrostatic pressure, which is lower at the venous end of the capillary (10 torr to 15 torr), thus promoting the return of fluid and ions to the capillary.

MODIFICATIONS OF THE STARLING EQUATION

Several studies subsequent to Starling's original work have caused modifications in the original Starling hypothesis. The first is that rather than extravasation and reabsorption of protein-depleted fluid occurring at different ends of the same capillary, it is more likely that while a given capillary bed is being perfused, it leaks fluid from end to end. After a minute or so, due to precapillary sphincters, capillary perfusion will cease for this network and be diverted elsewhere. During the no-flow period, which may last for several minutes, reabsorption occurs over the entire capillary.

A second area of modification stems from the characteristics of the junctional zone between endothelial cells as described by Fishman, who showed that capillaries also leak proteins through the junctional zone in quantities somewhat proportional to hydrostatic pressure.

Starling originally assumed a perfect balance between extravasation and reabsorption. It is now known that all the extravasated fluid need not be reabsorbed, because the lymph circulation is available to handle some excess.

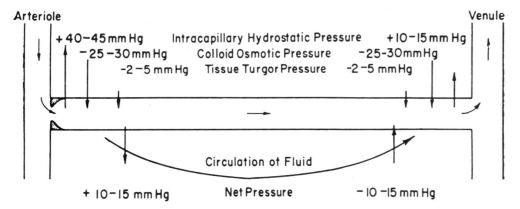

Fig. 2-1. These are the forces governing exchange of fluid between the intravascular and the extravascular fluid compartments, as described by Starling. (Pitts RF: Physiology of the Kidney and Body Fluids, 3rd ed. Chicago, Year Book Medical Publishers, 1974)

Modern versions of the Starling equation also contain an additional term, the *reflection coefficient,* a factor that describes the relative capillary permeability to proteins. A reflection coefficient of 1 would imply that the capillary was totally impermeable to protein molecules. Conversely, a reflection coefficient of 0 implies no barrier to protein. The reflection coefficient for normal capillaries is generally believed to be 0.8, but in a variety of conditions described in subsequent chapters (burns, peritonitis, the pulmonary capillaries in adult respiratory distress syndrome), the reflection coefficient is lower, thus describing a capillary with increased permeability to protein molecules.

GIBBS-DONNAN EQUILIBRIUM

Although the capillary normally allows free passage of ions, other physical forces control their distribution between the intravascular and interstitial spaces. Despite the passage of some protein outside the vascular space, most protein is retained within the intravascular space. Since these proteins have a negative charge, ions are subjected to two forces governing their distribution, a concentration gradient and an electrical gradient. Of the two, the need to achieve electrical neutrality is the more powerful, giving a predilection to retain cations within the intravascular space at the same time sacrificing equal concentration across the capillary membrane. One of the more prominent cations distributed in this fashion is H^+. As a consequence, the plasma is slightly more acid than the interstitial space. Although a real phenomenon, this distribution of ions, described first by Gibbs and Donnan, causes only a small difference in concentration and has little or no impact on clinical fluid and electrolyte therapy.

Thus, over the years, although Starling's law has not been repealed, considerable modification has occurred. It remains, nonetheless, a very useful cognitive aid.

INTERSTITIAL–INTRACELLULAR BOUNDARY

FACTORS THAT GOVERN ION EXCHANGE

Four factors govern the flow of ions through the cell membrane that separates the interstitial and intracellular spaces: (1) transmembrane concentration differences, (2) the cell membrane as a friction-retarding force, (3) transmembrane potential differences, and (4) active transport mechanisms, particularly for Na^+ and K^+.

SODIUM PUMP

Although at one time it was thought that the cell membrane was relatively impermeable to Na^+ and freely permeable to K^+, thus accounting for high intracellular K^+ and high extracellular Na^+ concentrations, it is now established that Na^+ can freely diffuse along a concentration gradient into the cell and that the low intracellular Na^+ concentration is a function of active extrusion of Na^+ by a metabolic, energy-dependent process, the so-called sodium pump. As Na^+ is transported out of the cell, K^+ is exchanged and enters the cell. Based on the work of Shires, this is not always a one-for-one exchange, and the process by which additional Na^+ is extruded into the interstitial space has been labeled the "electrogenic pump." Direct measurements of the transmembrane potential in the resting steady state are in the range of -90 mV, very closely approximating the potential equilibration of K^+; this suggests that the outward diffusion of K^+ is principally responsible for the transmembrane potential difference. The Nernst equation describes this distribution of cations and anions across the cell membrane.

DARROW-YANNET RELATIONSHIP

Suffice it to say that as a result of the four factors mentioned governing the distribution of ions intracellularly and extracellularly, Na^+ achieves a high extracellular concentration relative to within the cell and is the major ion governing the distribution of water between the intracellular and extracellular compartments, according to Darrow and Yannet. The Darrow-Yannet diagram demonstrates the calculated shift of water from the intracellular to the extracellular space after the addition of 500 mOsm NaCl to the latter and the reversed movement following the withdrawal of a comparable quantity of NaCl (Fig. 2-2). The importance of the Darrow-Yannet phenomenon will be seen in a subsequent section of this chapter dealing with the calculation of Na^+ deficits.

MAINTENANCE OF NORMAL BODY FLUID COMPARTMENTS

In the foregoing section, the body fluid compartments have been characterized and some of the forces governing the distribution of volume and composition outlined. One of the characteristics of health is the successful maintenance of these compartments in the face of wide variations in intake and output. The burden of this regulation falls upon

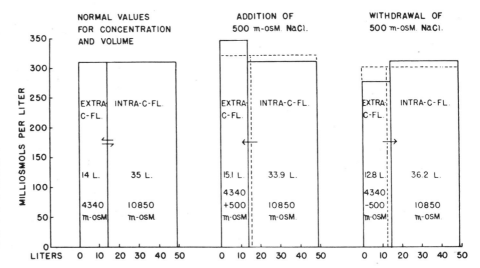

Fig. 2-2. Diagram depicts the addition and subtraction of 500 mOsm NaCl and the resulting effect on intracellular and extracellular fluid volume as described by Darrow and Yannet. (Gamble JC: Chemical Anatomy, Physiology, and Pathology of Extracellular Fluid, 6th ed. Cambridge, Harvard University Press, 1958)

the kidney, as it acts in response to arterial pressure, venous pressure, perfusion, and two major extrarenal hormones, ADH and aldosterone.

The presence or absence of a functioning gut also has an obvious impact on body fluid and electrolyte homeostasis. The role of the gastrointestinal tract is largely passive. Within limits, the kidney and gut, in conjunction with ADH and aldosterone, can maintain body homeostasis during periods of fluid and electrolyte excess or deprivation; however, these limits are frequently exceeded as a result of abnormal losses of gastrointestinal juices through vomiting, diarrhea, and fistulas, and the surgeon is called in to assist in maintaining homeostasis.

ALDOSTERONE

Aldosterone, discovered in 1952 and originally named electrocortin, is produced in the zona glomerulosa of the adrenal gland. A major role of aldosterone is the maintenance of circulating volume during times of decreased intravascular volume after dehydration or hemorrhagic shock. This is achieved by increased reabsorption of Na$^+$ by the kidney. Although aldosterone may be thought of as affecting the rate of active Na$^+$ reabsorption in the renal tubule, it should be understood that this is merely an augmentation of a process that occurs independently of the presence or absence of aldosterone. Aldosterone is released in response to Na$^+$ deprivation and as a result of adrenocorticotropic hormone (ACTH) secretion. Under ACTH influence, aldosterone is released in relative proportion to other adrenocorticoids. Release of aldosterone as a result of Na$^+$ deprivation is indirectly linked to decreases in circulating intravascular volume. Experiments in which the infrarenal inferior vena cava is ligated, for example, thus "damming" back blood in the lower part of the body, are associated with increases in aldosterone secretion. Although the total intravascular volume remains normal under these circumstances, there is a relative reduction in volume in the chambers of the heart and in the carotid distribution, and it has been hypothesized that "stretch" receptors are responsible for triggering aldosterone release. More conclusive work has demonstrated that a reduction in renal blood flow to the juxtaglomerular apparatus in the kidney cortex causes renin release. Renin, through the angiotensin axis, is a potent stimulator of aldosterone release.

Although Na$^+$ concentration *per se* does not alter aldosterone release, such is not the case with K$^+$ concentration. Experiments by Moran in which serum K$^+$ concentration was increased to 6 mEq/liter were associated with an increase in aldosterone concentration in adrenal vein effluent.

ADH

As a result of active transport mechanisms, Na$^+$ and Cl$^-$ are actively reabsorbed from the glomerular filtrate in the renal tubules and Henle's loop. The interstitial Na$^+$ concentration is increased in the region of Henle's loop to a final tissue concentration of 1400 mOsm. ADH controls the permeability of the collecting ducts to water, with increased permeability resulting from increased concentrations of ADH. With permeability increased, water is reabsorbed from the collecting duct into the interstitium by virtue of the osmotic gradient.

ADH is elaborated in the paraventricular and supraoptic nuclei of the hypothalamus and then is transported down the axons of these cells in combination with a larger molecule of "neurosecretory material" and finally released into the capillaries surrounding the neurohypophysis. A variety of stimuli will result in the release of ADH. Verney, in 1925, demonstrated that ADH was produced by pain, fear, hemorrhage, emotional stimuli, or injury of any magnitude. Verney also discovered that injection of NaCl into the carotid arteries of dogs produced antidiuresis, giving rise to the concept of osmoreceptors within the distribution of the internal carotid artery.

Infusion of volumes of isotonic fluid also promotes diuresis, indicating that, in addition to osmolality, ADH release must be governed by intravascular volume. That positive-pressure ventilation affected ADH secretion led Harry and Gainer to look for an intrathoracic "volume sensor" and culminated in the direct-measured decreases in ADH following balloon distention of the left atrium.

ACID–BASE BALANCE

A third major area of homeostasis is the maintenance of *p*H. Normal plasma *p*H is between 7.35 and 7.45. This is achieved through the interactions of a number of buffer systems within the body, the ability to raise or lower arterial P$_{CO_2}$ by altering ventilation, and the excretion or retention

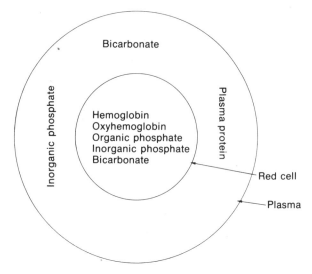

Fig. 2-3. Schematic location of eight principal buffer systems.

of acid or base by the kidney. When the ability to compensate is not adequate to keep pH normal or near normal, the surgeon may wish to intercede with a therapeutic maneuver.

Although there are eight buffer systems within the body, only the HCO_3 system and the hemoglobin (Hb) system are of major concern (Fig. 2-3). Systems such as the phosphate system and intracellular proteins other than Hb, while involved in buffering short-term acid loads, are of major importance for more long-term problems, such as renal tubular acidosis or prolonged ingestion of alkali.

HENDERSON-HASSELBALCH EQUATION

The general relation described by the Henderson-Hasselbalch equation states that pH is equal to a constant (pK) plus the log of the dissociated form of a given buffer divided by the nondissociated form. This equation for the HCO_3 system is written as follows:

$$pH = pK_{(bicarb.)} + \log \frac{HCO_3}{H_2CO_3}$$

For practical purposes, H_2CO_3 is nonexistent and is dependent upon the concentrations of dissolved CO_2. This in turn is dependent on the P_{CO_2} in the alveoli times the solubility coefficient of CO_2 in plasma. Thus, the equation may be modified to read

$$pH = pK_{(bicarb.)} + \log \frac{HCO_3}{.03 \cdot P_{CO_2}}$$

HCO_3–Hb BUFFER SYSTEMS

Hemoglobin is the other major fast-acting buffer. Just as for the HCO_3 system, an equation may be written:

$$pH = pK_{(Hb)} + \log \frac{Hb}{HbO_2}$$

Since the pH in both equations is the same (*i.e.*, the pH in the plasma in which both the red cells are suspended and the CO_2 is dissolved), a combined equation may be written:

$$pH = pK_{(bicarb.)} + \log \frac{HCO_3}{.03 \cdot P_{CO_2}}$$

$$+ pK_{(Hb)} + \log \frac{Hb}{HbO_2}$$

REGULATION OF HCO_3^- AND P_{CO_2}

The above combined equation has three constants ($pK_{(bicarb.)}$, $pK_{(Hb)}$, and .03) plus three easily measured variables (pH, P_{CO_2}, and Hb, frequently estimated as HCT/3) and allows the calculation of HCO_3 excess or deficit. This information is important for the clinician, since it is known that the ratio of HCO_3^- to dissolved CO_2 is 20:1. A report from the blood gas laboratory of a base deficit of, for example, 10 mEq/liter has the implication that taking into account the buffering contribution of Hb, restoration to a normal 20:1 ratio may be achieved by increasing the concentration of HCO_3^- by 10 mEq/liter in the volume of fluid normally occupied by the HCO_3^- ion. The HCO_3 space is the extracellular space that is normally between 17% and 26% of the body weight. Presented in a subsequent section of this chapter is how this information is used to treat patients by calculating the amount of HCO_3^- that needs to be administered.

The 20:1 ratio of HCO_3 to dissolved CO_2 is normally maintained by the lungs, regulating the H_2CO_3 (P_{CO_2}) through altering ventilation, and by the kidneys, increasing or decreasing the rate of HCO_3 excretion.

COMPENSATED ACIDOSIS AND ALKALOSIS

A respiratory acidosis or alkalosis is defined as too little or too much ventilation, thus altering the 20:1 ratio by changing the denominator. A metabolic acidosis or alkalosis is defined as decreases or increases in the 20:1 ratio caused by changes in the numerator. The most immediate response to an alteration in the 20:1 ratio (*i.e.*, a change in pH) is to alter ventilation to restore the ratio to normal. In this respect, the lungs and changes in arterial P_{CO_2} are the first-line system for restoring pH to normal. Alterations in ventilation may compensate for changes in pH due to disturbed metabolism. The result is called a compensated metabolic acidosis or alkalosis. Conversely, when pulmonary function is inadequate, even though renal excretion of HCO_3 may not occur as rapidly as changes in P_{CO_2}, the kidneys can still compensate for a respiratory acidosis or alkalosis by altering HCO_3^- excretion. It should be emphasized that it is the ratio of the dissociated to the nondissociated (in the HCO_3 systems the ratio of HCO_3^- to H_2CO_3) that establishes the pH, not the absolute quantity of either the numerator or the denominator.

COMMON CLINICAL PROBLEMS

In this section a series of commonly encountered clinical situations are presented to illustrate how an understanding of the altered physiology can be used to treat the patient.

NORMAL PERSON

As the simplest fluid and electrolyte problem, suppose a normal 70-kg person is placed at bed rest and allowed nothing by mouth for 10 days. Accepted is the fact that he will lose weight, as sufficient calories to maintain weight

TABLE 2-1	MINIMAL NORMAL DAILY BODY FLUID LOSSES AND COMMON REPLACEMENT VOLUMES*	
	OUTPUT	**ADMINISTERED**
urine	600 ml to 800 ml	1000 ml
insensible (lung)	600 ml to 800 ml	1000 ml
perspiration and feces	250 ml	250 ml
	Total	2250 ml

* The administered volume should include 75 MEq Na⁺, 40 mEq to 60 mEq K⁺, and 100 g glucose. (See text for explanation.)

will not be provided. Lack of weight loss may be achieved by intravenous hyperalimentation. The problem is to provide only sufficient fluid and electrolyte of appropriate type to maintain body homeostasis. Persons maintained in this fashion will lose about 1 pound or 0.5 kg/day as a result of inadequate caloric intake. Thus, if the patient weighs the same at the end of 10 days as he did at the outset, he has obviously been gradually overhydrated at a rate of 500 ml/day. An easy way to keep track of this situation would have been to weigh the patient at intervals, perhaps even daily, to keep track of his fluid balance.

NORMAL DAILY LOSSES

A second way of approaching the problem is to calculate fluid losses per 24 hours. By infusing an equal volume, the patient should stay in volume balance. Fluid losses for a normal 70-kg person are listed in Table 2-1. It should be noted that two volumes are included, the actual physiologic minimums and what clinicians tend to administer. For each category, the administered amount equals or exceeds the minimum. This is because given a patient with normal kidneys, it is safer to infuse slightly in excess than not enough, since the kidneys can be relied upon to save what the body needs and excrete the excess.

The minimum quantity of urine excretion per 24 hours to prevent uremia is derived from the fact that a certain number of grams of solute are filtered by the glomerulus and from the necessity to dissolve that solute in a volume of water such that the osmolality does not exceed 1400 mOsm, the renal interstitial fluid osmotic pressure and thus the maximum concentrating ability of the kidney. Since patients cannot be relied upon to have normal kidneys, plus the fact that any increased catabolism tends to increase the quantity of solids eliminated through the kidneys, 1000 ml of urine is recommended as a desirable quantity per 24 hours. The reason for exceeding the generally accepted figure of 600 ml to 800 ml for insensible loss is that many patients may be mildly febrile, which raises evaporative losses. The 250 ml listed for perspiration and feces is an average figure and may vary from day to day.

REPLACEMENT

As mentioned at the very outset of the chapter, the student should not commit to memory lists of figures because they will vary from patient to patient. Rather, at this point, he should have the feeling that somewhere between 2000 and 2500 ml of fluid are lost from a person every 24 hours and

that to maintain fluid volume balance, an equal volume of fluid should be administered.

Having arrived at what volume of fluid is to be administered, other needs must be considered. Sodium is an obvious necessity. Because of the efficiency of the aldosterone mechanism, almost all the Na⁺ can be reabsorbed from the urine such that a patient can survive on as little as 10 mEq/day. This requires normal kidneys functioning at maximal efficiency, a state patients frequently do not achieve; consequently, clinicians are more liberal in their Na⁺ administration, usually giving it in the range of 75 mEq/day. Assuming ample Na⁺ intake and no volume restriction (therefore no aldosterone-mediated K⁺ excretion), patients will excrete 15 mEq to 20 mEq/day, which must be replaced as part of intravenous therapy. In usual practice, 40 mEq to 60 mEq should be equally distributed in intravenous fluids to make it as dilute as possible, since concentrations of K⁺ in excess of 40 mEq/liter cause pain at the infusion site and are not tolerated. Rapid administration of K⁺ is also contraindicated because of the risk of cardiac arrest. Chloride is excreted in conjunction with Na⁺ and K⁺. Replacement of Na⁺ and K⁺ is usually done with NaCl and KCl, which more than replaces Cl⁻ loss.

If no source of calories is included as part of maintenance intravenous therapy, the patient will not only lose weight as he rapidly depletes his glycogen stores and then starts using fat and protein for energy but will also become ketotic. This is a consequence of fats and amino acids being converted to 2-carbon fragments (ketones). Metabolism cannot proceed further unless adequate concentrations of Krebs' cycle intermediates are present to accept the ketones and prevent a functional block in fat and protein metabolism. Gamble was among the first to recognize that unless at least 100 g glucose was provided daily to ensure adequate Krebs' cycle intermediates, ketosis would result.

In Table 2-2, adequate daily intravenous therapy in terms of volume and constituents is presented as being administered by the infusion of either D_5W (dextrose, 5% by weight in 1000 ml water) or normal saline (0.9% NaCl). Administration in this fashion is possible in the adult because the normal body homeostatic mechanisms prevent alterations in the *milieu intérieur* despite variations in input. Presentation in this fashion is also useful from an educational point of view. From examination of the volumes in Table 2-2, it is evident that the end result is not far from 25% normal saline, 75% water, with 100 g glucose and K⁺ added. A commercial product, D_5 ¼ NS (dextrose, 5% by weight in 1000 ml of 0.23% NaCl), is available and is frequently administered at a rate of 100 ml/hour, thus approximating the requisite volumes and constituents for maintenance

TABLE 2-2	AVERAGE DAILY INTRAVENOUS FLUID THERAPY
1000 ml D_5W with 20 mEq KCl	
500 ml normal saline	
1000 ml D_5W with 20 mEq KCl	

Each liter of D_5W contains 50 g glucose; the 500 ml normal saline contains 77 mEq NaCl. Approximately the same ingredients may be administered as D_5 ¼ NS with 20 mEq KCl/liter. (See text for explanation.)

TABLE 2-3   ROUTINE POSTOPERATIVE FLUID REPLACEMENT (CHOLECYSTECTOMY)

	OUTPUT	REPLACED AS
urine	1000 ml	250 ml D_5W
		750 ml NS
insensible	1000 ml	1000 ml D_5W
third space	1000 ml	1000 ml D_5S
nasogastric suction	200 ml	200 ml NS
		1250 ml D_5W
		950 ml NS
		1000 ml D_5S
		3200 ml

KCl, 40 mEq to 60 mEq, is distributed among the above intravenous fluids.

therapy. Although this is usually acceptable in normal persons, too often the administration of $D_5 \frac{1}{4}$ NS is carried out day after day without a true appreciation of the reason and in pathologic states may be contraindicated.

POSTOPERATIVE PATIENT

A cholecystectomy is now performed on the patient. Assume that all blood lost during surgery and all evaporative loss from the open abdomen are replaced by the anesthesiologist. A nasogastric tube is inserted, the patient is in the recovery room, and fluid orders are being written to cover the ensuing 24 hours.

The fluid and electrolyte requirements are summarized in Table 2-3. If it is desirable for a normal person to excrete 1000 ml of urine, then certainly with the increased catabolism in the postoperative patient, 1000 ml of urine is desirable.

ABNORMAL LOSSES AND REPLACEMENT

An important difference has occurred, however, as a result of surgical trauma. Urine volume is composed of the volume to clear free water plus the volume to clear a solute load. The patient was anxious about the pending surgery, received a preoperative sedative and then a general anesthetic, had his bowel retracted for exposure, has postoperative pain, and is probably receiving a narcotic. All of these factors are potent stimuli of ADH. Thus, the postoperative patient will not have the capability of excreting much free water. The length of the ADH response may vary from one day to several days, depending upon the magnitude of the stress. Therefore, if 1000 ml of urine per 24 hours is desired, it must be achieved by infusing some solute such as saline. Measurements of urine Na^+ in postoperative patients have demonstrated a uniformly high Na^+ concentration, often as high as 125 mEq/liter, nearly the composition of normal saline.

The postoperative patient will also have an insensitive loss of a magnitude at least equal to a normal person (*i.e.*, 1000 ml). Since there is no electrolyte in this loss, it may be replaced as D_5W.

THIRD SPACE

A major additional fluid compartment in the postoperative patient is the so-called third space, consisting of wound edema and secretions sequestered in the gastrointestinal tract as a result of ileus. In the clinical setting, this volume can only be estimated. Patients having operations involving extensive retroperitoneal dissection, such as abdominal aneurysm repair or pancreaticoduodenectomy, will have much greater third space loss than will the patient undergoing cholecystectomy. For this patient, it would not be unreasonable to estimate a third space loss of 500 ml to 1000 ml during the first 24 postoperative hours. Since this will have an Na^+ concentration approximating that of plasma (140 mEq/liter), appropriate replacement is with either normal saline or a balanced salt solution such as Ringer's solution, which has a composition approximating interstitial fluid (Table 2-4).

During the first 24 hours, gastric secretion may be reduced below normal. The composition of normal gastric secretion is listed in Table 2-5. Measured losses may be restored every 4 hours, or replacement of an anticipated 100 ml to 200 ml may be incorporated into the postoperative orders. Due to the kidney's ability to save what is needed and excrete the excess, the replacement fluid need not be an attempt to replicate gastric juice. Some Na^+-containing fluid such as saline is adequate. Sufficient K^+ should be added to the intravenous fluids to compensate for the normal obligatory loss plus the additional amount lost through nasogastric suction and sequestered within the intestines.

COMMON ERRORS

Once again, the aim is not to have the student commit the above postoperative fluid requirements to memory. Rather, two facts deserve emphasis: First, the volume of intravenous fluid required by the postoperative patient, particularly those undergoing abdominal surgery, is greater than that required for normal maintenance by virtue of the third space requirements and second, more Na^+-containing fluids need to be used because of the need for adequate urinary output as well as replacement of the third space loss.

TABLE 2-4   COMPOSITION OF 1 LITER OF RINGER'S LACTATE

Sodium	130 mEq
Potassium	4 mEq
Calcium	3 mEq
Chloride	109 mEq
Lactate*	28 mEq

* Or equivalent organic molecule

TABLE 2-5   COMPOSITION OF SECRETIONS FROM SURFACE EPITHELIAL CELLS OF THE HUMAN STOMACH

COMPOSITION	ESTIMATED LEVEL
Sodium	150 mEq to 160 mEq/liter
Potassium	10 mEq to 20 mEq/liter
Calcium	3 mEq to 4 mEq/liter
Chloride	125 mEq/liter
Bicarbonate	45 mEq/liter
pH	7.67

FLUID AND ELECTROLYTE MANAGEMENT

I. Normal

	Water (ml)	Na⁺ (mEq)	K⁺ (mEq)
A. Daily Gains			
Liquid intake	1700		
Hydrated foods	550–650	50–90	34–40
Water of metabolism	150–250		
Total	2500	50–90	34–40
B. Daily Losses			
Urine	1500	10–40	40
Feces	200	0–20	2–3
Insensible			
Lungs	400		
Skin	400	10–60	1–2
Total	2500	50–90	40–45

C. Intravenous fluid therapy for patients without abnormal losses:
Daily infusion
  1. Water: 2500 ml/day
  2. Na⁺: 50 mEq to 90 mEq/day as 2 liters D_5W and 500 ml normal saline (NS) or 2500 ml ¼ NS (39 mEq/liter)
  3. K⁺: 40 mEq to 50 mEq/day; add 20 mEq to each liter of fluid.

II. Fluid and Electrolyte Disequilibrium

	Water (ml)	Na⁺ (mEq)	K⁺ (mEq)
A. Daily Gains			
(Excesses usually due to overly aggressive intravenous therapy)			
B. Daily Losses			
Gastric (nasogastric tube)	100–3000	60–300	10–40
Biliary (T tube)	500–2000	145–300	10–15
Pancreatic (fistula)	1000–1500	140–210	10–15
Intestinal secretion	up to 3000	300–350	20–60
Proximal bowel fistula	up to 10,000	650–1000	50–130
(− Intestinal conservation)	(− 8000 ml)		
Distal bowel fistula (or ileostomy)	2000–2500	110–150	20–30
Third space loss (pancreatitis, bowel obstruction, edema, ascites)	up to 20,000	up to 800	up to 30
Abnormal skin (burn)	up to 10,000	up to 800	up to 30
High-output renal failure	up to 10,000	> 40 mEq/liter	< 40 mEq/liter

C. Intravenous fluid therapy for patients with abnormal losses:
  1. Water: Determine approximate deficit; replace half of it over 8 hours and the remainder over the next 16 hours.
  2. Na⁺: Determine approximate deficit; choose appropriate Na⁺ concentration for water replacement fluid (NS, ½ NS, and so forth)
  3. K⁺: Determine approximate deficit; replace by adding to intravenous regimen after determining that renal function is intact. Do not add more than 40 mEq/liter of fluid or more than 15 mEq to 1 hour's infusion.

The consequences of an attempt to maintain a postoperative patient on D_5 ¼ NS at 100 ml/hour are also pertinent. Inadequate volume would be administered, and three quarters of what was given would be water. This leads to inadequate urinary output as a result of the patient's inability to excrete free water and dilutes what Na⁺ the patient already has at a time when he needs more Na⁺ to make up for deficits created by third space losses. As a result, the serum Na⁺ concentration would be decreased on postoperative day 1. When inadequate Na⁺ is administered, the diminished urinary output is frequently interpreted as hypovolemia, and this mistaken assumption leads to challenging the patient with a rapid infusion of intravenous fluid. Normal saline or Ringer's solution is usually selected as the test fluid, and urinary output increases not because hypovolemia is rectified, as the unwary might suspect, but because sufficient solute has now been administered. This therapeutic maneuver may be repeated several times until an adequate volume of Na⁺-containing fluid has been administered, albeit for the wrong reason.

PROLONGED VOMITING

In the above two fluid and electrolyte problems, the surgeon is starting with a normal balanced situation and, based on his knowledge of physiology, is projecting future fluid and electrolyte requirements for the ensuing 24 hours. A different problem is encountered when the patient arrives in the emergency department with a deficit created either by failure of replacement of normal losses or by an unusual site or volume of fluid loss. The surgeon is then faced with replacing the deficit in addition to providing maintenance fluids.

Pyloric obstruction with prolonged vomiting, a common problem, produces dehydration, sodium-chloride–potassium depletion, and a state of metabolic alkalosis. *Small bowel obstruction* with vomiting produces a more balanced electrolyte loss.

DEHYDRATION (INCLUDING "WATER INTOXICATION")

Prolonged vomiting over several days will frequently produce dehydration, since the patient is unable to ingest sufficient fluids to compensate for the losses of gastrointestinal fluid, as well as to meet normal daily fluid requirements. Dehydration may be categorized as hypertonic, isotonic, or hypotonic. Hypertonic dehydration occurs when electrolyte is replaced but an inadequate volume of water is ingested; an example is the football player who takes salt pills but is not allowed to drink adequate quantities of water. A patient such as this will present with decreased body fluid, both in the intravascular and in the extravascular compartment, increased concentrations of electrolyte in the serum, and an increased serum osmolality. Isotonic dehydration occurs when the patient's losses are isotonic with respect to body compensation and, despite the right concentration of electrolytes, volume replacement is inadequate. Such a patient will have normal serum electrolyte concentrations but will still have a volume deficit. This illustrates why measuring serum electrolyte concentration does not necessarily indicate the status of hydration, since the values reflect concentration (milliequivalents per liter) and what is at question is the number of liters. Hypotonic dehydration is the most common type, especially in conjunction with abnormal gastrointestinal losses. Typically, after diarrhea or vomiting, with the inability to retain oral fluids, the patient feels thirsty. The fluids selected to quench the thirst usually do not contain adequate concentrations of electrolyte to replace that which was lost, nor can the patient retain enough oral fluid to replace the volume deficit. Any volume that is retained, since it is low in electrolyte, tends to dilute existing body electrolytes. Hypotonic dehydration is characterized by both a low serum electrolyte concentration and a volume deficit. The stomach tends to add electrolytes and water to ingested material to render it more or less isotonic. By ingesting fluid low in electrolyte and then vomiting, the patient is lavaging his stomach and causing even further electrolyte loss. Severe hypotonicity can lead to water-intoxication coma, best treated by withholding nonelectrolyte fluids and administering NaCl solutions.

ESTIMATING THE VOLUME DEFICIT

The following patient illustrates a management problem associated with fluid and electrolyte loss. A 48-year-old woman with known duodenal ulcer disease began to vomit 5 days prior to admission. She attempted to drink ginger ale but was able to retain only a little. Hypotonic dehydration was anticipated on the basis of the history. The initial problem becomes one of estimating first the extent of the volume deficit. There are several methods. The first is physical examination. The mucous membranes are usually dry, and the skin classically has poor turgor. In the face of poor oral hygiene and an elderly patient, neither of these two signs is particularly reliable. Orthostatic hypotension, another method, is not seen until nearly 20% to 30% of the circulating blood volume is lost; thus, it is not a very sensitive indicator. Although one can estimate that 500 ml of intravascular volume is lost for every three-point rise in hematocrit, another method, this presupposes some knowledge of the patient's starting hematocrit and, like orthostatic hypotension, does not assess deficits in fluid compartments other than the intravascular compartment.

The two most reliable measures of volume deficit are

	ASSESSMENT OF PATIENT'S FLUID BALANCE	
	DEHYDRATION	**OVERHYDRATION**
History	Vomiting, diarrhea, blood loss, thirst, oliguria, lethargy	Orthopnea, edema, dyspnea, normal urine output or oliguria
Physical	Dry mouth, poor skin turgor, peritonitis or other site of fluid sequestration, tachycardia, hypotension, collapsed veins, cold extremities, weak pulses	Distended veins, rales and wheezes, edema, tachycardia, S_3 gallop, brisk pulses
Laboratory	Urine specific gravity > 1.015; hematocrit (HCT), blood urea nitrogen (BUN) elevated	HCT, BUN normal or low
Therapy	How much? Of what solution? How fast? Specific ion deficits? Intravenous crystalloid solution, monitor urine output, ↑ pulmonary artery wedge or central venous pressure	Fluid restriction, diuretics, ↓ pulmonary artery wedge or central venous pressure

body weight and urinary output. If, for example, the patient's normal weight is 70 kg, and she weighs only 65 kg in the emergency department, one might reasonably assume that one is dealing with a volume deficit in the range of 5000 ml. Regardless of what arithmetical value is derived, an intravenous infusion will be started and some fluid administered. If, after administration of a liter or so of intravenous fluid, the urinary output exceeds 50 ml/hour, it does not matter what the calculated deficit is, the patient is telling you that at that moment she has all the intravascular volume she needs; persisting in administering more runs the risk of creating congestive heart failure. The patient may really have a 5000-ml deficit, but what is happening is that the fluid is being administered faster than it can equilibrate with the extravascular compartments. After all, it took the patient 5 days to lose the fluid; it does not have to be replaced in 2 hours.

REPLACEMENT THERAPY

Now comes the problem of calculating what quantity of electrolytes to administer. Serum electrolytes should be obtained. A representative set of values might include Na$^+$, 129 mEq/liter; K$^+$, 2.8 mEq/liter; Cl$^-$, 88 mEq/liter; and total CO$_2$, 31 mEq/liter. It should be reemphasized that the values represent concentrations (mEq/liter), and to calculate the number of milliequivalents to be administered, the volume of body fluid into which they will be distributed needs to be known.

SODIUM DEFICIT

There are several methods to estimate Na$^+$ deficits, and the one presented merely represents my preference. Historically, it was thought that Na$^+$ was distributed in the total body water. On this basis, the Na$^+$ deficit was calculated as follows:

$$
\begin{array}{ll}
70 \text{ kg} & = \text{body weight} \\
\times\ .60 & = \text{fraction of body weight representing water} \\
\hline
42.00 & = \text{liters of total body water} \\
\times\ 11 & = (140 - 129 = 11) \text{ mEq/liter Na}^+ \text{ deficit} \\
\hline
42 & \\
42 & \\
\hline
462 & = \text{mEq of Na}^+ \text{ to be administered}
\end{array}
$$

For years, this was found to be a reliable method. In fairness, it was recognized that part of the ability to achieve a normal serum Na$^+$ concentration using this technique resulted from the ability of the kidneys to excrete any excess inadvertently given. It subsequently became apparent that Na$^+$ did not distribute equally through the total body water but in fact was mainly extracellular. Calculation of the Na$^+$ deficit on this basis then would proceed as follows:

$$
\begin{array}{ll}
70 \text{ kg} & = \text{body weight} \\
\times\ .20 & = \text{fraction of body weight representing} \\
 & \quad \text{extracellular water} \\
\hline
14.00 & = \text{liters of extracellular water} \\
\times\ 11 & = (140 - 129 = 11) \text{ mEq/liter Na}^+ \text{ deficit} \\
\hline
14 & \\
14 & \\
\hline
154 & = \text{mEq of Na}^+ \text{ to be administered}
\end{array}
$$

SODIUM DISTRIBUTION

Practical experience has demonstrated that the administration of such a small quantity of Na$^+$ will not correct the majority of Na$^+$ deficits. How then to resolve the difference between practical experience and scientific fact? The answer is theoretical but probably represents a true state of affairs. Referring back to the Darrow-Yannet diagram, it can be seen that as Na$^+$ is lost from the extracellular compartment, for example, in vomiting, the intracellular compartment is left relatively hypertonic. To maintain osmotic equilibrium across the cell membrane, water moves from the extracellular to the intracellular compartment. The longer and more pronounced the extracellular Na$^+$ deficit, the more water will move intracellularly. Conversely, as Na$^+$ returns to the extracellular space, for example, as the result of intravenous administration, water returns to the extracellular compartment, continually diluting the administered Na$^+$; in the end, the quantity of Na$^+$ required to achieve a normal extracellular concentration approaches a quantity such as if the Na$^+$ were going into the total body water. An appropriate way to think about this problem is first to recognize that at the bedside there is no way to know what quantity of water has gone intracellularly and therefore no way to determine precisely how much Na$^+$ is required. The 462-mEq value represents the absolute maximum amount of Na$^+$ required, the 154-mEq value represents the absolute minimum quantity of Na$^+$ required, and the true amount required lies somewhere between the two extremes. Generally speaking, the more chronic the Na$^+$ deficit, the closer to the 462-mEq end of the spectrum will be the true value.

POTASSIUM DEFICIT

There is no way to estimate the quantity of K$^+$ to be administered. This is because nearly all the K$^+$ is within the cell and the concentration sampled in the serum represents only a small fraction. After it has been established that the patient has the ability to excrete urine, K$^+$ should be administered at a concentration of 40 mEq/liter of fluid; the serum K$^+$ concentration should be checked intermittently until such time as the concentration returns to the normal 3.5-mEq to 4.5-mEq/liter range. Experience has shown that the amount of K$^+$ necessary under these circumstances may be in excess of 150 mEq to 200 mEq.

Little attention is paid to calculating the requirements of Cl$^-$ because the Na$^+$ and K$^+$ are administered in the form of Cl$^-$ and at least equivalent concentrations of Cl$^-$ are necessary to correct the deficit. We will see that vomiting causes a large loss of Cl$^-$. Once again, the kidney may be relied upon to excrete any administered excess.

RENAL AND GASTRIC CONTRIBUTION TO HYPOKALEMIC METABOLIC ALKALOSIS

Inspection of the total CO$_2$ reveals this value to be increased, consistent with a metabolic alkalosis, which was clinically suspected in view of the history. A rather simplistic way to view the total CO$_2$ is to remember that it represents all the *C's* and *O's* and that any physiological abnormality increasing them, such as respiratory acidosis (increased Pco$_2$) or metabolic alkalosis (increased HCO$_3^-$), will elevate the total CO$_2$; conversely, respiratory alkalosis (decreased Pco$_2$) or metabolic acidosis (decreased HCO$_3^-$) will lower the total CO$_2$.

Since the patient has a metabolic alkalosis, why not treat with intravenous acid? To answer this, it is necessary to understand the mechanism by which these electrolyte abnormalities occurred. Simple loss through vomitus is not an adequate explanation, since it is evident from Table 2-5 that there is surprisingly little K$^+$ in gastric secretion. Dilution by ingestion of fluid low in Na$^+$ and K$^+$, although contributing to the decreased serum Na$^+$ and K$^+$, also does not totally explain the abnormal serum concentrations. Intracellular migration of K$^+$ due to alkalosis is also only a partial explanation.

A useful approach to the problem is to reenact the sequence of events that led to the present altered serum concentrations. Vomiting is associated with fluid loss which, once the swallowed contents of the stomach are evacuated, represents fluid that had its origin from the intravascular compartment. Both Na$^+$ and H$^+$ ions, in variable quantities, are lost as part of the vomitus. In general, there is an inverse relationship between the concentration of Na$^+$ and H$^+$ ions. Thus, vomiting can lead predominantly to a loss of salts (NaCl, KCl) plus water or the loss of hydrochloric acid in addition to the loss of salt. With the excretion of H$^+$ ions into the lumen of the stomach, there is a corresponding shift of HCO$_3^-$ ions into the plasma. To preserve electrical neutrality, these changes are balanced by the movement of Cl$^-$ ions from the blood across the gastric wall and into the stomach lumen. With vomiting and the loss of Cl$^-$, HCO$_3$ accumulates in the blood. This accumulation tends to occur regardless of the amount of hydrochloric acid lost, since in gastric juice, depending upon the concentration of H$^+$, the concentration of Cl$^-$ is either equal to or in excess of the

TABLE 2-6   NORMAL VOLUMES AND ELECTROLYTE COMPOSITIONS OF ALIMENTARY TRACT FLUIDS

	VOLUME (ml/24 hr)	SODIUM (mEq/liter)	POTASSIUM (mEq/liter)	CHLORIDE (mEq/liter)	BICARBONATE (mEq/liter)
Salivary	1500	10	26	10	30
	(500–2000)	(2–10)	(20–30)	(8–18)	
Stomach	1500	60	10	130	
	(100–4000)	(9–116)	(0–32)	(8–154)	
Duodenal		140	5	80	
	(100–2000)				
Ileal	3000	140	5	104	30
	(100–9000)	(80–150)	(2–8)	(43–137)	
Colonic		60	30	40	
Pancreatic		140	5	75	115
	(100–800)	(113–185)	(3–7)	(54–95)	
Bile		145	5	100	35
	(50–800)	(131–164)	(3–12)	(89–180)	

Na^+ concentration, whereas in the blood, Cl^- is normally less (140 mEq Na^+, 100 mEq Cl^-).

The initial stages of vomiting thus result in hypovolemia, hyponatremia, loss of H^+ ion, and accumulation of HCO_3, both the latter acting synergistically to produce a metabolic alkalosis. The hypovolemia is a potent stimulus for aldosterone secretion. Under the influence of aldosterone, Na^+ reabsorption in the kidney increases. Since H^+ ions, which normally compete with K^+ for exchange with Na^+, are depleted by loss of vomitus, K^+ becomes the predominant cation exchanged in the renal tubule for Na^+. Adrenocortical stimulation promotes the loss of K^+ in the urine at the same time causing reabsorption of HCO_3, thus worsening the alkalosis once K^+ depletion has occurred. At this stage, the urine will be alkalotic. As extracellular K^+ is depleted, H^+ ions become the predominant cation exchanged for Na^+, further exacerbating the alkalosis. Although the blood is alkalotic, the renal loss of H^+ ions now causes an acid urine, a situation called paradoxical aciduria. The depletion of K^+ that results from prolonged vomiting has led to a special name for this type of metabolic alkalosis, hypokalemic metabolic alkalosis. It is evident why administration of only acid or Cl^- will not correct the situation, since H^+ ions will continue to be lost in the urine until adequate K^+ has been provided to exchange for $Na.^+$

MAGNESIUM DEFICIT

The deficit from vomiting, in summary, is volume, Na^+, K^+, and Cl^-. Therapy, therefore, is the administration of volume, Na^+, K^+, and Cl^-. Rarely, an Mg^{2+} deficit may occur in the presence of massive fluid losses such as are seen with a high small-bowel fistula. The symptoms and signs are the same as for Ca^{2+} deficiency. Therapy consists of the administration of $MgSO_4$.

FISTULAS

External gastrointestinal fistulas may also contribute to severe electrolyte and fluid deficits. Knowledge of normal concentrations of electrolytes and volumes of secretion of the various fluids found in the intestinal tract contributes very little to the care of the patient with an external fistula (Table 2-6). This is because (1) the volume lost from the body may vary enormously, depending on whether the fistula represents complete or partial diversion of intestinal contents to the exterior, (2) the concentrations of electrolytes comprise a varied mixture of gastrointestinal organs (stomach, bile, pancreatic, duodenal, and jejunal in the case of, for example, an ileal fistula), and (3) the volume and concentration of electrolytes lost are a reflection in part of the modification imposed by intestinal absorption and secretion proximal to the fistula. A few general facts are useful, however. Once water reaches the small intestine, it is rapidly absorbed; most of the salt and water are absorbed by the time the ileum is reached. Although the contributions of bile and pancreatic juice to the duodenum are alkaline, upper jejunal contents tend to be acid and have a high Na^+ content. (Large concentrations of Na^+ exist in pancreatic juice.) As the fluid progresses through the small intestine, there is a gradual exchange of Na^+ for K^+ and of luminal Cl^- for HCO_3 from the blood. Thus, upon arrival in the ileum, volume is decreased and the fluid is alkaline and high in K^+. This exchange of Na^+ for K^+ and Cl^- for HCO_3 continues, albeit at a slower pace, in the colon. In general, high intestinal fistulas will cause hyponatremia and metabolic alkalosis and low intestinal fistulas will cause hypokalemia and metabolic acidosis. *Pure biliary or pancreatic fistulas* will cause hyponatremia and acidosis.

Awareness of these facts will perhaps assist the physician in understanding the metabolic problems of the patient, but when the physician is confronted with a fistula of sufficient magnitude to necessitate the administration of supplemental volume and electrolyte, the wisest course is to send a sample to the laboratory for analysis.

In addition to ascertaining the electrolyte content, careful attention needs to be devoted to the volume of the fistula by collecting and measuring the lost volume. Daily weights provide a useful check on the adequacy of volume replacement, and periodic serum electrolytes check on the appropriateness of replacement.

SHOCK

Shock is generally defined as inadequate perfusion to maintain normal cell metabolism. In shock of nearly all etiologies (hemorrhagic, neurogenic, septic, and some cardiogenic), a disturbance can be demonstrated between the quantity of fluid in the intravascular compartment and the size of the anatomical boundary of the compartment. For example, in hemorrhagic shock, despite compensatory vasoconstriction, the loss of blood leads to inadequate volume to fill the vascular space. In neurogenic and early septic shock, there is no loss of fluid but vasodilatation has increased the size of the vascular compartment and again there is inadequate volume to fill the space. It is not the intent of this section to cover the treatment of shock but only to use shock as a method of introducing the fluid and electrolyte abnormalities associated with a period of hypoperfusion and of developing a rational plan of therapy.

It would seem appropriate that if the problem is too little volume in the intravascular compartment, the solution should be to infuse the fluid most apt to remain within the vascular space, that is, a colloid. However, in the mid 1960s, from the work of Shires and others, it was demonstrated that there was also an interstitial fluid compartment deficit. Some of this fluid had obviously gone from the interstitial to the intravascular compartment in response to the lowered hydrostatic pressure in the intravascular space, according to the Starling hypothesis mentioned earlier. It is generally accepted, however, that there is an additional loss from the interstitial space and that this fluid goes into the intracellular space. The hypothesis to account for this intracellular movement is that with hypoperfusion and inadequate delivery of O_2 and substrate, active transport of Na^+ from within to without the cell stops, leaving an unopposed leak of Na^+ down the concentration gradient from the interstitial to the intracellular compartment. An osmotic imbalance occurs that is satisfied by isotonically obligated water moving intracellularly.

CRYSTALLOID REPLACEMENT

The presence of the interstitial fluid deficit has led some to recommend that volume restoration in shock should be accomplished using crystalloid solution such as normal saline or lactated Ringer's solution. Lactated Ringer's has an advantage over saline in that its electrolyte composition more closely approximates the composition of plasma and interstitial fluid and the organic molecule, lactate, may be metabolized by the liver to produce HCO_3, thus reducing the metabolic acidosis resulting from anaerobic metabolism and lactic acid buildup secondary to inadequate O_2 delivery to the cell. The assumption is that with restoration of perfusion, there is adequate O_2 to metabolize the lactate.

DISTRIBUTION OF CRYSTALLOID

As a result of the physical forces described previously, the normal distribution of any crystalloid between the intravascular and extravascular spaces is 1:4 (*i.e.*, for every 5 liters administered, 1 liter remains intravascularly and 4 will be extravascular). The initial distribution in the treatment of shock, however, tends to favor retention of more of the fluid within the vascular compartment than occurs normally. This is because when the patient is in shock at the time the initial infusion of a crystalloid solution starts, the hydrostatic pressure is low, colloid oncotic pressure is normal, and much of the capillary bed is not being perfused; thus, there is not much filtration surface area available through which the salt solution may leak. As resuscitation with a crystalloid solution continues, conditions gradually favor more extravasation as hydrostatic pressure increases, colloid oncotic pressure decreases as protein is diluted, and more capillary beds open up and are perfused.

METABOLIC ACIDOSIS

During the period of hypotension and poor perfusion of tissue, inadequate O_2 was provided to the cell to achieve aerobic metabolism. More precisely, increasing quantities of lactate developed, since, in the absence of O_2, the reaction

$$NADH \xrightarrow[\text{pyruvate} \rightleftharpoons \text{lactate}]{O_2 \downarrow} NAD \text{ (nicotinimide = adenine dinucleotide)}$$

could not proceed at a normal rate. The resulting lactic acidosis causes an imbalance in the acid–base status of the patient. The final common clinical problem to be discussed is the correction of acid–base abnormalities.

CALCULATION OF BASE DEFICITS

An arterial blood sample is analyzed for blood gases, an imprecise term, since, in addition to a Po_2 and a Pco_2, there is also a determination made of arterial pH. Many laboratories will also calculate the base (HCO_3) excess or deficit. This is usually done from a nomogram, which allows the solution of the simultaneous pH equation mentioned previously, taking into account both the HCO_3 and the Hb buffer systems (Fig. 2-4). A representative set of values for the patient in hemorrhagic shock might be as follows (line A, Fig. 2-4):

$Po_2 = 60$ torr

pH = 7.28

$Pco_2 = 31$ torr

$HCO_3 = $ deficit, -11 mEq/liter

Fig. 2-4. Modified Siegaard-Andersen nomogram for computing acid–base status.

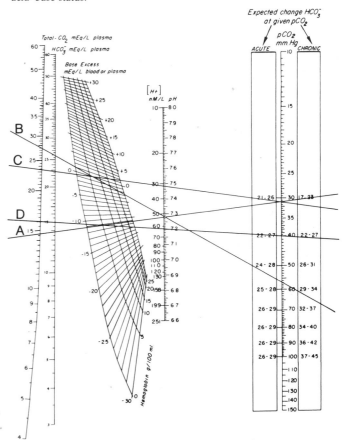

The P_{O_2} does not have any direct effect on the corrections of the acid–base abnormality and may be disregarded at this point. The first value that should be examined is the *p*H. Is the patient acidotic or alkalotic? It can be seen that the value of 7.28 is lower than the normal range of values, 7.35 to 7.45. Having established that the patient is acidotic, the next step is to decide whether the acidosis is on a respiratory or metabolic basis. If it were on a respiratory basis, we would expect a greater than normal quantity of dissolved CO_2 reflected in a high P_{CO_2}. The treatment would be to ventilate the patient to lower the P_{CO_2}. In fact, to cause a *p*H of 7.28 on a purely respiratory basis, the P_{CO_2} would have to be 57 (line B, Fig. 2-4). Not only is the P_{CO_2} not elevated in the example, it is less than the normal P_{CO_2} (40 torr). Also, there must be some element of metabolic acidosis present, since a P_{CO_2} of 31 torr with no associated metabolic acidosis should be associated with a *p*H of 7.48 (line C, Fig. 2-4). The only way a *p*H of 7.28 could occur in the presence of a P_{CO_2} of 31 torr is if a base deficit of 11 mEq/liter HCO_3^- were present, assuming the presence of 5 g to 10 g of Hgb per 100 ml of blood (line A, Fig. 2-4). Why is the P_{CO_2} low? As was mentioned above, the lungs and kidneys work together to attempt to maintain the plasma *p*H in the normal range. As the *p*H progressively fell in response to the developing metabolic acidosis, the increasing concentrations of H^+ stimulated the respiratory center, causing hyperventilation, lowering the P_{CO_2}. Thus, the patient in the example is said to have a partially compensated metabolic acidosis, because (line D, Fig. 2-4) if there really were an 11-mEq/liter base deficit and the P_{CO_2} were normal (*i.e.*, no respiratory compensation had occurred), the *p*H would be 7.20. By working with the nomogram it is possible to solve hypothetical acid–base problems, since an identical series of steps is used to work out other problems, such as metabolic alkalosis after prolonged vomiting.

Since the patient has a metabolic acidosis (*i.e.*, a relative loss of HCO_3^- in the numerator of the Henderson-Hasselbalch equation), the therapy is logically the administration of HCO_3^-. If the cause of the metabolic acidosis is shock, with reperfusion of the tissue and restoration of O_2 delivery, the excess lactate will be converted to pyruvate and enter the tricarboxylic acid cycle with correction of the acidosis by production of HCO_3. In fact, one form of therapy for acidosis is·to administer a balanced salt solution with an organic molecule such as acetate or the more familiar lactate in Ringer's lactate, the purpose of the organic molecule being that as it is metabolized, HCO_3^- ions are produced.

A faster, more predictable method is the direct administration of HCO_3^-. The base deficit is 11 mEq/liter. The next piece of information needed is the number of liters or, more correctly, the size of the pool in which administered HCO_3^- will be distributed. In simplest terms, HCO_3 may be conveniently thought of as being distributed in the extracellular fluid space (*i.e.*, about 20% of the body weight):

$$
\begin{array}{rl}
70 \text{ kg} & = \text{body weight} \\
\underline{\times\ .20} & = \text{ECF compartment} \\
14.00 \text{ liters} & = \text{volume} \\
\underline{\times\ \ \ 11} & = \text{mEq/liter deficit of ECF} \\
14 & \\
\underline{14\ \ \ \ } & \\
154 \text{ mEq } HCO_3 \text{ necessary} &
\end{array}
$$

The body, unfortunately, cannot be viewed in the simplest terms. Estimates of the volumes of the extracellular compartment vary from 17% to 26% of the body weight. On this basis, the calculated quantity of HCO_3 to be administered might vary between 131 and 200 mEq.

Furthermore, depending on the length of time the acidosis has been present, other intracellular buffer systems may be involved and more or less of the calculated HCO_3 dose is appropriate. An additional caveat is that it is preferable to avoid overcorrecting and inadvertently making the patient alkalotic, because this is most difficult to correct to normality. In view of these unknowns, having calculated 154 mEq as the appropriate quantity of HCO_3, it is advisable to administer one half to two thirds of the calculated dose, wait 30 minutes, and recheck the acid–base status with additional blood gases.

BIBLIOGRAPHY

BERNARD C: Leçons sur les propriétés physiologies et les altérations pathologiques des liquides de l'organisme. Paris, 1859

DARIS JO: Mechanisms regulating the secretion and metabolism of aldosterone in experimental hyperaldosteronism. Recent Prog Horm Res 17:293, 1961

DARROW DC, YANNET H: The changes in the distribution of body water accompanying increase and decrease in extracellular electrolyte. J Clin Invest 14:266, 1935

DAVENPORT HW: The ABC of Acid-Base Chemistry, 6th ed. Chicago, University of Chicago Press, 1974

DAVENPORT HW: Physiology of the Digestive Tract. Chicago, Year Book Medical Publishers, 1977

GAMBLE JC: Chemical Anatomy, Physiology, and Pathology of Extracellular Fluid, 6th ed. Cambridge, Harvard University Press, 1958

GOTTSCHALK CW: Osmotic concentration and dilution of the urine. Am J Med 36:670, 1964

PITTS RF: Physiology of the Kidney and Body Fluids, 3rd ed. Chicago, Year Book Medical Publishers, 1974

SHIRES GT, CARRICO CJ, COHN D: The role of the extracellular fluid in shock. In Shock, International Anesthesiology Clinics No. 2. Boston, Little, Brown Co, 1964

SHIRES GT, WILLIAMS JA, BROWN F: Simultaneous determination of plasma volume, extracellular fluid volume, and red cell mass in man utilizing I^{131}, $S^{35}O_4$, and Cr^{51}. J Lab Clin Med 55:776, 1960

STARLING EH: On the absorption of fluids from the connective tissue spaces. J Physiol 19:312, 1896

USSING HH: The use of tracers in the study of active ion transport across animal membranes. Cold Spring Harbor Symp Quant Biol 23;193, 1948

WRIGHT HD, GANN DS: Correction of defect in free water excretion in post-operative patients by extracellular fluid volume expansion. Am Surg 158:70, 1963

Arthur E. Baue

Shock and Cardiac Arrest

3

SHOCK

DEFINITIONS

Shock is a multifactorial clinical state that occurs when cardiac output is inadequate to permit arterial perfusion of blood under sufficient pressure to provide organs and tissues with adequate blood flow. Clinically, shock must be recognized and treated rapidly since in many instances patient survival depends upon the restoration of adequate tissue perfusion within minutes. Four types of shock are recognized and described by their etiologic cause (Table 3-1).

Hypovolemic shock is characterized by loss of blood or plasma volume from the circulation. It is treated by identifying the source of the loss, by attempting to mechanically control hemorrhagic areas, and by restoring the circulating volume with Ringer's lactate solution initially and with blood if significant hemorrhage is present. Urine output, central venous pressure (CVP), and left atrial pressure are the best monitors of adequacy of volume replacement. The primary source of blood or fluid loss must be identified and corrected.

Septic shock occurs when invasive infections produce a decrease in peripheral vascular resistance and a hyperdynamic circulatory state. Treatment consists of fluid replacement until left ventricular filling pressure is adequate, evaluation of the patient for septic foci, culture and sensitivity analysis of potential septic sources, appropriate antibiotic, and surgical drainage as needed. Inotropic agents, nutritional–metabolic support, and observation for signs of progressive multiple organ failure are necessary.

Cardiogenic shock is usually due to muscular inadequacy of the heart as a pump, most commonly because of atherosclerotic coronary artery disease and myocardial infarction, myocardial failure, or pulmonary embolism. Treatment consists of assurance of adequate circulating volume, electrocardiogram (ECG) monitoring, and provision of cardiotonic agents (*e.g.,* dopamine, epinephrine, isuprel, digitalis). Oxygen administration is frequently required, and specific treatment of the underlying cause by such measures as pulmonary embolectomy should be considered.

Neurogenic shock results from impairment of central nervous system mediated vasoconstrictor activity owing to injury or medications. Treatment consists of eliminating other causes of shock and increasing circulatory volume and use of vasoconstrictor drugs.

Cardiac arrest may occur from any number of causes, but most commonly from hypoxemia, acute myocardial infarction, arrhythmia, or hemorrhagic shock. Treatment consists of establishing an airway, instituting effective ventilation, and closed- or open-chest cardiac massage. Simultaneous treatment of the underlying cause such as aspiration of pericardial tamponade or restoration of volume in a patient with hypovolemic shock is required. Successful treatment of cardiopulmonary arrest depends upon the underlying cause and the rapidity of resuscitative efforts.

CLINICAL AND HEMODYNAMIC PICTURE

The manifestations of shock will vary to some extent with the cause of the problem, its severity, and its stage (Figs. 3-1, 3-2, and 3-3). The patient may exhibit evidence of decreased blood flow to all tissues and organs and sympathoadrenal stimulation. Appearance and mental status will

TABLE 3-1   CLASSIFICATION OF SHOCK

HYPOVOLEMIC SHOCK

Type of Fluid Lost
  Blood
  Plasma
  Extracellular-extravascular fluid (salt and water loss or deficiency)
  Water

Location of Loss
  External loss—blood, water by sweating, vomitus, stool, fistulas
  Internal loss
    Traumatic—hematoma, sequestration in wounds, body cavities or bowel
    Obstructive—intestine, etc.
    Inflammatory—exudative

Etiology
  Bleeding
  Traumatic or wound shock—blood and fluid loss
  Burns
  Intestinal obstructions
  Perforated ulcer—early
  Crush injury
  Dehydration from high temperature and/or sweating
  Fistulas, diarrhea

CARDIOGENIC SHOCK

Intrinsic
  Myocardial infarction—aneurysm
  Myocardial failure, ischemia or depression from sepsis, pulmonary failure or late hypovolemia
  Myocardial contusion
  Arrhythmias
  Drugs, including anesthetic agents

Extrinsic
  Pulmonary embolism
  Cardiac tamponade
  Respiratory failure and pulmonary hypertension
  High levels of PEEP

SEPTIC SHOCK—INFECTION FROM ANY GRAM-NEGATIVE OR GRAM-POSITIVE ORGANISM AND FUNGI WITH BACTEREMIA AND SEPTICEMIA
  Peritonitis
  Late abscesses
  Genitourinary instrumentation
  Septic abortion
  Intravenous catheters
  Pulmonary or other infections

VASOGENIC OR NEUROGENIC SHOCK
  Spinal anesthesia
  Spinal cord injury
  Anaphylactic shock

be that of fatigue, anxiety, fear, or restlessness progressing to apathy and diminished responsiveness. Vertigo and faintness may occur if the patient is not recumbent. Beecher and co-workers defined three grades of shock in severely wounded soldiers. In slight shock, the blood pressure may be slightly increased and the pulse normal, but the skin is cool and pale with prolonged blanching of the skin or fingernails with pressure and a distressed mental state. With moderate shock, blood pressure is reduced 20% to 40%, pulse is

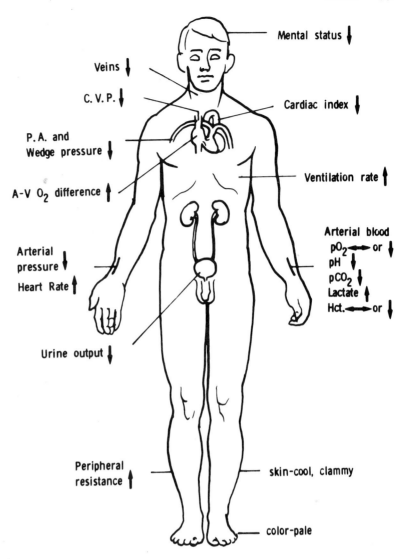

Fig. 3-1. Hypovolemic shock.

decreased in volume (thready), the skin is cool and pale with prolonged blanching, and the patient exhibits thirst and apathy. With severe shock, blood pressure is decreased 40% or more or is not recordable, the pulse is weak to imperceptible, the skin is cold and ashen to cyanotic with sluggish capillary filling, severe thirst is present, the patient exhibits an apathetic to comatose or stuporous mental status. Symptoms of fear, of feeling cold, and of weakness may be present along with thirst and nausea and vomiting. Sweating may be present, contributing to the clammy feel of the skin, along with hyperventilation and tachycardia. Neck and extremity veins will be collapsed. Body temperature may be somewhat decreased, and muscular weakness may be evident. Although much of this response after an injury in otherwise normal young individuals may be due to inadequate circulation, some may be caused by the sympathoadrenal, hypothalamic, and hypophyseal responses to injury. Some of the apathy and systemic effects may be produced by endorphin secretion from the hypothalamus.

The above picture accurately describes the patient after an injury or the patient with blood or volume loss and hypovolemic shock. The clinical appearance of a patient with cardiogenic or septic shock will be similar in the late phases. Early in cardiogenic shock, however, the major difference in clinical appearance will be fullness of neck and extremity veins and perhaps less of the anxiety produced by injury. On the other hand, the septic patient with early circulatory failure will often have had a chill with temperature elevation and will be warm and dry with the bounding pulses of a hyperdynamic circulation and high cardiac output. MacLean described the prodrome of mental aberrations, hyperventilation, and respiratory alkalosis seen in patients with sepsis as the circulation is failing. Early septic shock will produce a hyperdynamic circulation unless the patient cannot respond because of an inadequate blood volume or myocardial problems. In such circumstances, even septic shock may show the characteristic hypodynamic (low cardiac output) constricted state of hypovolemic or cardiogenic shock. All forms of shock in the terminal phases will be similar—with "cold hypotension."

INITIAL ASSESSMENT AND MONITORING

Any patient after injury, during or after a major operation, or with an illness in which the circulation may be in jeopardy, requires rapid assessment of the status of the circulation, insertion of venous and arterial conduits for therapy, and monitoring and institution of other methods of support as required. The "ABCs" of resuscitation require first the establishment of an *Airway,* if the patient's airway

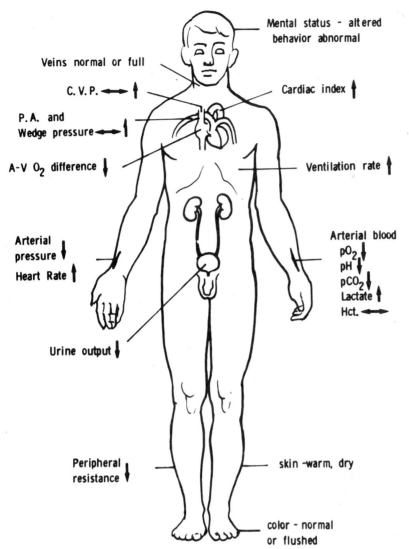

Mental status - altered
behavior abnormal

Veins normal or full

C.V.P.

P.A. and
Wedge pressure

A-V O$_2$ difference

Cardiac index

Ventilation rate

Arterial
pressure
Heart Rate

Arterial blood
pO$_2$
pH
pCO$_2$
Lactate
Hct.

Urine output

Peripheral
resistance

skin -warm, dry

color - normal
or flushed

Fig. 3-2.   Hyperdynamic septic shock.

is not adequate due to bleeding, vomiting, aspiration, coma, or cervical spine injury. Secondly, *Breathing* must be supported if spontaneous ventilation is not adequate or is in question. This may require insertion of an orotracheal or nasotracheal tube. Seldom is an emergency tracheostomy necessary unless an endotracheal tube cannot be inserted. Thirdly, the *Circulation* must be supported by intravenous conduits and fluid infusion. Detailed assessment and resuscitation of injured patients are described in Chapter 10.

Access to the circulation is provided by percutaneous insertion of catheters in major veins. Veins of the upper extremities should be used first, if possible, although they may be collapsed and difficult to cannulate. Insertion of catheters in the subclavian veins or in the internal jugular veins may be necessary (Fig. 3-4). If there is evidence for or the possibility of subclavian or jugular vein injury, veins of the lower extremity such as the femoral veins may be used. The possibility of iliac vein or inferior vena cava injury must also be considered, particularly with gunshot or stab wounds. Cutdowns for cannulation of the antecubital, external jugular, or saphenous veins at the ankle may be necessary. If shock is severe and due to hypovolemia, several large-bore #15 or larger catheters should be inserted for initial fluid, and later blood, transfusions. Initial blood samples are obtained for typing and crossmatching, and for

the laboratory for baseline blood studies, including hemoglobin, hematocrit, electrolytes, BUN, creatinine, and blood sugar. Fluids are then given unless the venous pressure is clearly elevated.

The insertion of a catheter into the right atrium percutaneously through the subclavian vein is useful in defining the problem by measurement of CVP. Since this measurement can be affected by intrathoracic and intrapericardial pressures and venomotor tone, serial measurements are required. It is more important to determine the response of CVP to fluids than to rely only on the initial measurement. A low CVP represents a low venous return volume, but a high CVP may be produced by a number of factors (see section on neurogenic shock).

Unless the patient responds rapidly to initial treatment and becomes stable, an arterial catheter should be inserted for monitoring blood pressure and obtaining blood samples for measurements of blood gas tensions and *p*H. Patency of the ulnar artery should be checked before the radial artery is cannulated. Periodic measurement of arterial blood gas tensions is necessary to be certain that ventilatory assistance is not required. Arterial *p*H and PaCO$_2$ will indicate whether the metabolic acidosis of decreased perfusion has been corrected. Persistent metabolic acidosis in a nondiabetic patient indicates the need for increased circulatory support,

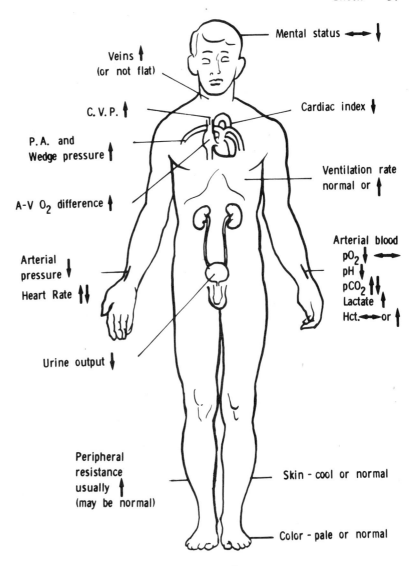

Veins ↑
(or not flat)

C. V. P. ↑

P. A. and
Wedge pressure ↑

A-V O$_2$ difference ↑

Arterial
pressure ↓
Heart Rate ↑↓

Urine output ↓

Peripheral
resistance
usually ↑
(may be normal)

Mental status ↔ ↓

Cardiac index ↓

Ventilation rate
normal or ↑

Arterial blood
pO$_2$ ↓ ↔
pH ↓
pCO$_2$ ↑↓
Lactate ↑
Hct. ↔ or ↑

Skin - cool or normal

Color - pale or normal

Fig. 3-3. Cardiogenic shock.

no matter what the blood pressure. A Foley catheter is inserted into the urinary bladder to measure urine output unless a pelvic injury or blood at the urethral meatus suggests the possibility of a urethral injury. In such a situation, it is best to obtain a cystourethrogram prior to insertion of a catheter.

Initial observation and monitoring of the major components of the circulation—arterial pressure, venous return, heart rate and rhythm, and peripheral perfusion (kidney, skin)—are necessary. If with initial therapy the patient does not respond rapidly and become stable, then insertion of a Swan-Ganz catheter should be carried out. This also allows measurement of pulmonary artery pressures and the pulmonary artery wedge pressure (PAWP) by wedging the catheter in a small pulmonary artery and inflating the balloon. The wedge pressure is a reflection of left atrial mean pressure, which is indicative of left ventricular filling pressure. A catheter that also allows measurement of cardiac output by the thermodilution technique should be used; this permits repeated measurements of cardiac output during and after various treatment programs. The initial cardiac output is not as important as is documentation of an increase in cardiac output with therapy until adequate blood flow and organ perfusion are obtained. However, there are circumstances in which the CVP does not accurately reflect

the left atrial pressure or ventricular filling pressure. These include infection, ventilatory failure, and pulmonary embolism—where pulmonary artery and right-sided pressures may be high—and cardiac disease, myocardial infarction, and long-standing shock in which left-sided pressure may be higher than suspected. The PAWP often more accurately reflects the effects of volume infusion.

The fully monitored patient and measurements to be made are shown in Figure 3-5. These are separated into critical measurements by a plus sign (+), that should be carried out in any patient with an actual or even potential circulatory problem. Measurements and calculations indicated by an asterisk (*) should be made in all patients who do not respond rapidly to treatment. Such information can be developed by automated data processing using a minicomputer, as developed by Del Guercio in the Automated Physiologic Profile, or by using a calculator, as developed by Barash in the Hemodynamic Tracking Profile. Arterial lactate is measured in some centers and has prognostic value as an indicator of the metabolic severity of shock. Measurement of blood volume by dye or isotopic dilution has limited value because the blood volume gives no indication of the size of the vascular bed which that volume must fill. Insertion of a nasogastric tube should be done to

(Text continues on p. 40)

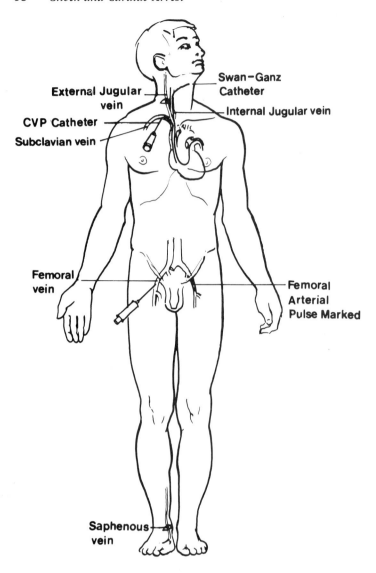

External Jugular vein

Swan–Ganz Catheter

Internal Jugular vein

CVP Catheter

Subclavian vein

Femoral vein

Femoral Arterial Pulse Marked

Saphenous vein

Fig. 3-4. Sites of access to the venous circulation.

Fig. 3-5. Monitoring and measurements in shock patients.

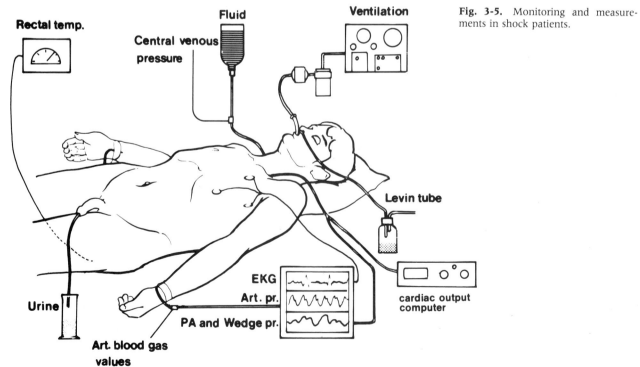

Rectal temp.

Fluid

Ventilation

Central venous pressure

Levin tube

EKG

Art. pr.

PA and Wedge pr.

cardiac output computer

Urine

Art. blood gas values

*Arterial blood pressure (BP)	95–140/70–90 torr	Pulse pressure: 40 torr Mean arterial pressure: 80–105 torr
†Positional change in BP	0	
*Heart rate and ECG	70–80/min; normal sinus rhythm and normal tracing	
*Central venous pressure (CVP)	5 ± 2 cm saline	
†Pulmonary artery pressure	20–30/7–12 torr	Mean pulmonary artery pressure: 10–16 torr
†Pulmonary artery wedge pressure (PAWP)	5 ± 2 cm saline	
†Cardiac output (CO)	4.0–6.5 L/min	Body surface area (BSA) from height, weight, and chart: M^2 Cardiac index (CI): 2.8–3.6 L/min/M^2 Stroke index: 30–65 ml/M^2 Systemic vascular resistance (SVR): 770–1500 dynes/sec/cm^{-5} Left ventricular stroke work index (LVSWI): 30–110 gm meters/M^2 Mean: 56 ± 6 gm meters/M^2 Pulmonary vascular resistance (PVR): 100–300 dynes/sec/cm^{-5} Right ventricular stroke work index (RVSWI): 6 ± .9 gm meters/M^2
§Blood volume	3 L/M^2 (8.5–9.0 % body weight)	
*Arterial blood Po_2 Pco_2 pH O_2 content ‡Lactate	 85–100 torr 39–41 torr 7.39–7.41 17–20 ml/100 ml 5–18 mg/100 ml	
†Mixed venous blood O_2 content	14 ± 1.0 ml/100 ml	Arteriovenous O_2 content difference: 4–6 ml/100 ml Oxygen consumption: 140 ± 25 ml/min/M^2
*Venous blood Hematocrit Hemoglobin †Creatinine †Osmolality	 38–42 14 ± 1 gm/100 ml 0.7–1.5 mg/100 ml 285–295 mOsm/Kg water	
*Urine Output Specific gravity †Sodium †Creatinine †Osmolality	 50 ml/hour 1.005–1.030 <20 mEq/L (with injury or operation) 75 mg/100 ml 900–1330 mOsm/Kg water	 Urine/plasma creatinine ratio > 20 Urine/plasma creatinine ratio > 3–4.7
*Observation of the patient	Appearance and sense of well-being	

* Critical measurements in patients with circulatory problems
† Important measurements in patients who do not respond rapidly to treatment
‡ Measured routinely in some centers
§ Limited value

empty the stomach, to prevent pulmonary aspiration, and to begin a program to prevent stress ulceration and bleeding unless the patient responds rapidly and can take fluids by mouth. Of greatest importance with all of these systems is that the surgeon not lose sight of the patient. Observation and communication with the patient to determine comfort, sense of well-being, mental status, and peripheral circulation can only be done by the concerned surgeon.

HYPOVOLEMIC SHOCK

The diagnosis and treatment of hypovolemia is the cornerstone of care of patients who have been injured, have acute surgical problems, or are undergoing elective operations. A decreased circulating blood volume is one of the most common results of many different disease processes. When such a decrease exceeds the ability of the individual to compensate for the loss, either because of rapidity of blood loss or continued slow loss, the circulation begins to fail, and hypovolemic shock is present. Blood volume is defined as the sum of the volume of cells and of plasma inside the circulatory system. However, all components of blood— even the formed elements—are present to some degree outside blood vessels in the lymph and interstitial or extracellular fluid. In addition, intravascular fluid is in equilibrium with the extracellular fluid, and a dynamic equilibrium is present with intracellular fluid. Thus, disorders of total body hydration seriously affect vascular volume.

BLOOD VOLUME—REGULATION AND REPLENISHMENT

Measurement of Blood Volume and Blood Loss
Blood volume was first measured by Welcker in 1854 by exsanguination and flushing out the system—the wash-out method. Now the dilution principle is used; an indicator that will mix with the plasma is injected into the bloodstream. The two indicators most commonly used are the blue dye T-1824 and albumin tagged with radioactive iodine, ^{131}I. Determination of the time concentration curve of the test substance allows the calculation of plasma volume. Total blood volume can also be determined by measuring the red-cell volume with a test substance such as red cells tagged with radioactive chromium. Measurement of the hematocrit and either the red cell volume or plasma volume alone allows the calculation of total blood volume but requires correction, both for the plasma trapped in the packed cells in measuring the hematocrit and for the somewhat higher hematocrit in venous blood drawn for the determination as compared with the entire circulation. The range of normal plasma volume is 40 ml/kg to 49 ml/kg of body weight, and the range for cell volume, 24 ml/kg to 31 ml/kg; total blood volume is 64 ml/kg to 80 ml/kg, or 4480 ml to 5600 ml for a 70-kg person. Blood volume is most closely related to lean body mass and activity and, on a weight basis, the ratio is proportionately lower in obese individuals. It decreases with bed rest and short, vigorous exercise and increases with prolonged athletic training, warm weather, higher altitudes, and pregnancy. Three fourths of the circulating blood is in the venous side of the circulation, whereas only one fifth is in the arterial system, and only about 5% is in the capillaries.

Blood loss in the operating room can be measured fairly accurately by weighing sponges and measuring the volume removed by suctioning. However, blood loss with injury or postoperatively and fluid loss, particularly into areas of a wound, soft tissues, the peritoneal cavity, and bowel, can only be estimated. Large hidden loss after injury, particularly with fractures of the femur or pelvis and with retroperitoneal hematomas, often escapes attention. Blood loss with a simple closed fracture of the femur may be as much as 1 to 2 liters. *The best estimates of the amount needed to replace lost blood volume are based on the concept of functional blood volume.* Thus, the amount of blood or fluids needed to replace a loss is that needed to restore a normal circulation. Rough estimates of some decrease in blood volume are provided by the signs of attempted compensation by the circulation, such as tachycardia, narrowed pulse pressure, cool skin and extremities, and low CVP, or by evidence of a marginal circulation, such as postural hypotension and hypotension with a Valsalva maneuver. The Swan–Ganz catheter can be used to determine left atrial filling pressures.

Adequate or Optimal Functional Blood Volume
Measurements of blood volume, although providing worthwhile information when studying groups of patients and disease processes, are not as helpful in treating the individual injured or operated patient. They do not take into account the volume of the vascular system in which that blood volume must function and the dynamics of the circulation. If the vascular bed is dilated, a measured blood volume of 6 liters may be inadequate to maintain venous return and peripheral blood flow. If the vascular bed is constricted, such a volume may be quite satisfactory. Thus, from a functional standpoint, a "normal" blood volume is not necessarily in all patients and at all times the optimal blood volume.

The essential role of the blood volume is to keep the system filled in order to maintain satisfactory venous return and volume flow of blood. Thus, optimal blood volume is that needed to provide an adequate filling pressure for both ventricles. A low right atrial pressure indicates a less than adequate circulating volume. Even if such a patient's arterial circulation is normal, he would have no reserve if circulatory demands increased. Normal atrial pressures with an adequate arterial circulation indicate an adequate blood volume. However, circulating blood volume may be low and the arterial circulation diminished, but atrial pressure may be normal because of compensating mechanisms. A high right atrial pressure indicates a higher blood volume than the heart can accept and pump, regardless of the actual blood volume or adequacy of the arterial circulation. This is true unless there is valvular heart disease, when a high filling pressure may be necessary. A few years ago, machines for measurement of blood volume were present in most intensive care units. These instruments are no longer present because the measurements were not useful in treating patients. The dynamic measurements of atrial pressures, cardiac output, and peripheral perfusion are much more helpful.

Regulation of Blood Volume
Maintenance of blood volume requires the maintenance of total body water and extracellular fluid volume by the mechanisms of antidiuretic hormone and aldosterone secretion, volume of urine production, saliva production, and thirst, sweating, red cell production and the production and mobilization of plasma proteins, particularly from the liver (Chapter 1). Maintenance of an adequate volume within the circulatory system is dependent primarily upon the

following four mechanisms: (*1*) The ability of the vascular system to decrease its volume by constriction of capacitance vessels, particularly in the splanchnic bed; (*2*) the ability to decrease blood flow to body areas and organs not so critical for immediate survival and to shift available blood flow to vital organs; (*3*) the ability of extracellular fluid to provide volume to the circulation in the capillary bed according to the Starling equilibrium concept (capillary refilling); (*4*) the replenishment of plasma proteins, which may occur with a contribution of fluid from cell water as well. The shift in the balance in the capillary circulation between filtration and reabsorption is much more sensitive to changes in venous pressure than it is to changes in arterial pressure. The interrelationship between circulatory function and body fluid volumes is a powerful regulatory system for defense of the circulation.

PATHOPHYSIOLOGY OF HYPOVOLEMIC SHOCK

The abnormalities of hypovolemia are produced by the attempts to compensate for decreased blood flow, on the one hand, and the effects of decreased blood flow on organs and tissues, on the other.

Compensation for Blood and Fluid Loss

Cardiovascular Responses. As blood volume is lost, venous return is decreased and cardiac output decreases. Small changes in arterial pressure are recognized by the carotid and aortic arch baroreceptors, and through the medullary vasomotor center they lead to decreased vagal tone and increased sympathetic nervous system activity. This results in arterial and venous constriction and an increase in heart rate and force of ventricular contractions. Vasoconstriction of capacitance vessels, particularly of veins, decreases the volume of the circulatory bed in order to provide more blood in the central circulation and to maintain venous pressure and return. In humans, the decrease in volume of the vascular bed occurs first in the splanchnic bed where 500 ml to 1000 ml of blood may be available for this purpose; it functions as a small reserve tank. Vasoconstriction in the arterial system maintains pressure in the central circulation and blood flow to certain vital organs, particularly the heart and brain, while decreasing flow to the skin, muscle, splanchnic bed, and kidneys. If the amount of blood lost is small, these compensating mechanisms may maintain a normal blood pressure, cardiac output, and even venous pressure with little or no evidence of the loss. A slow loss of 500 ml of blood may produce no overt hemodynamic changes, particularly if the patient is recumbent. Postural hypotension, syncope, or a feeling of light-headedness with sitting up rapidly may be the only evidence of loss. Loss of 1000 ml over many minutes to hours may also be compensated for, but definite evidence of postural hypotension would be evident in all patients. An abrupt loss of 1000 ml to 1500 ml of blood will produce moderate hypotension, reduced renal blood flow, oliguria, and cool skin owing to vasoconstriction. If the person is otherwise normal, is kept recumbent, and is not otherwise stressed, a loss of this magnitude could be tolerated and generally replaced by capillary refilling. Abrupt loss of 2000 ml or more is incompatible with survival if not treated.

Transcapillary Refilling of the Circulation and Protein Replenishment. The process of transcapillary refilling in hemorrhage and shock is a powerful mechanism for maintenance of blood volume. Restoration of blood volume occurs in two phases mediated primarily by Starling forces

(Fig. 3-6). In the first phase, a fall in capillary hydrostatic pressure owing to decreased blood volume, venous pressure, and arteriolar vasoconstriction produces a rapid shift of protein-free fluid from the interstitium into the capillaries. The second phase, which temporally overlaps the first, involves the return of protein to the circulation to support plasma oncotic pressure. Interstitial albumin probably accounts for most of this restoration. The protein returns by way of lymphatics and the hepatic and mesenteric capillaries. Synthesis of proteins is also increased and there is a decreased rate of breakdown. The driving force for return of protein depends on interstitial volume and pressure, which in turn depends on movement of fluid from cells to the interstitium. This phenomenon, which has been described by Gann and his colleagues, is believed to be brought about by an increase in solute (especially glucose and perhaps other osmotically active solutes) bathing the cells and drawing water out of the cells into the interstitial space. This process seems dependent on a number of factors including solute from the splanchnic bed, glucose, cortisol, perhaps epinephrine, adequate nutrition, and prior hydration. If these factors, particularly nutrition and hydration, were abnormal prior to injury, the second phase (replenishment of protein) either may be incomplete or may not occur. Then a third phase with severe or late hypovolemic shock and decompensation may develop. It consists of impaired vasomotor activity, altered interstitial macromolecules and collagen, which may allow takeup or binding of fluid, and cell swelling. With severe or late shock, the effects of norepinephrine and angiotensin production may be deleterious because they prevent capillary refilling and increase capillary fluid loss by increasing venous pressure.

Moore and Skillman and co-workers found that the loss of 500 ml to 1000 ml of blood by slow venous hemorrhage, which does not produce shock in a normal human, is followed by a net movement of water, salt, and protein into the plasma. This plasma volume refill from the capillary bed is rapid at first—as high as 2.0 ml per minute—and decreases with time, with plasma volume restored to normal in 20 hr to 40 hr. It is accompanied by increased secretion of renin, aldosterone, antidiuretic hormone, and erythropoietin, and by renal conservation of sodium and water. Cortisol secretion does not seem to increase initially. Interstitial fluid is decreased and is restored only by ingestion or injection. Albumin enters the circulation rapidly, initially at rates of up to 4.0 g per hour. A rapid arterial bleed produces even higher initial rates of capillary refilling so long as shock is not produced. If shock is produced, then adrenal release of epinephrine and adrenal and sympathetic nervous system release of norepinephrine are increased, as is cortisol secretion.

Fig. 3-6. Starling concept.

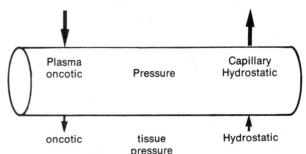

Endocrine Responses. The neuroendocrine responses to hemorrhage and blood volume loss are quite similar to those occurring in patients under the stress of injury. The stress associated with tissue injury, the need for an increased circulation, and fluid volume losses and shifts are all closely related. The neuroendocrine response to injury or stress is minimal with starvation, bed rest, and an anesthetic alone. It is not activated by a small operation, such as an inguinal hernia repair, and there are only modest changes with an injury, such as an elective cholecystectomy. It is only when there are significant tissue injury, fluid changes, and infection that the maximum response occurs (Chapter 1). The neuroendocrine response to decreased blood flow is shown in Table 3-2.

Effects of Decreased Blood Flow and Compensatory Mechanisms

If blood volume decreases more rapidly or more extensively than can be compensated for, the circulation begins to fail. There is no demonstrated stage or descriptive set of hemodynamic variables at which shock is said to be present. Suffice it to say that it is an inadequate circulation with decreased blood pressure, cardiac output, and blood flow to organs. There is decreased capillary blood flow, with all of its attendant effects. A number of vasoactive mediators are produced that have profound effects on organ and tissue blood flow (Table 3-2). The action of these mediators and the decreased blood flow affects the various organ systems and their functions, changes metabolism, alters the microcirculation, and causes changes in cell function.

Alterations in Organ Function. Changes in the various organ systems occur as organ and capillary blood flow decrease. In the kidney there is decreased renal blood flow and an alteration in the intrarenal distribution of flow from the cortex that favors the medulla. Accompanying this are decreased glomerular filtration rate and oliguria. Medullary

sodium is decreased with loss of the medullary hyperosmolar zone and of the countercurrent concentrating system. If the insult persists, tubular necrosis and acute renal failure may eventually occur. The problem of tubular ischemia is accentuated by pigments that have been filtered into the tubules, such as myoglobin, hemoglobin, and other proteins that circulate after injury. Total renal shutdown, anuria, and the rapid development of azotemia, hyperkalemia, and acidosis may follow. Renal damage due to ischemia and protein may not be severe enough to produce oliguric or anuric renal failure, but may result in high-output renal failure. This is a less severe problem, but may be difficult to recognize because the urine output may be normal or high in spite of the inability to get rid of waste products (Chapter 4).

A decrease in coronary blood flow may contribute to a further decrease in cardiac output. This is a particular hazard in patients with coronary artery disease. The coronary circulation has the capability of autoregulation, and it dilates as cardiac output decreases. However, myocardial oxygen extraction is high under normal circumstances, so that increased oxygen extraction is of limited value if increased flow is not possible. Electrocardiographic changes and myocardial ischemia may be seen, particularly if there is preexisting coronary artery disease. The ischemic heart produces lactate rather than using it in its metabolism, with altered utilization of free fatty acids. If shock persists and is severe, no matter what the initial cause, there may ultimately be depression of the myocardium. This would be expressed clinically by a low cardiac output and a high and rising venous pressure.

In the liver, the ability to metabolize lactate and to detoxify other substances decreases. The liver's synthetic activities, particularly production of albumin, are decreased. Often the effects of ischemia on the liver are not evident until later, when bilirubin is found to be elevated, albumin decreased, and globulin increased. Elevated enzyme levels,

TABLE 3-2   VASOACTIVE AND NEUROENDOCRINE MEDIATORS IN SHOCK

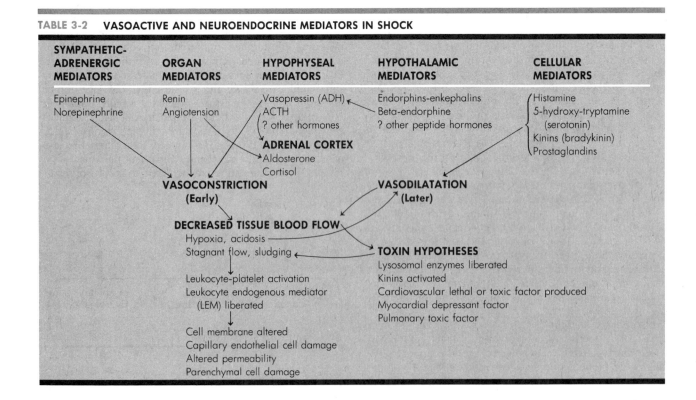

increased bromsulphalein (BSP) retention, and an abnormal cephalin flocculation test may be present. Decreased function of the gallbladder has been demonstrated in patients after ischemic injury. In the brain, the *sensorium* and electroencephalographic activity may be depressed if circulatory failure and hypotension are severe.

Gastric and salivary secretion are decreased with decreased production of hydrochloric acid, but ischemia of the gastric mucosa contributes to the development of stress ulceration and bleeding.

Much has been written about the effects of shock on the lung, leading to the creation of terms such as *shock lung.* Certainly after injury failure of ventilation and the need for ventilatory support are frequent problems. However, the lung is fairly resistant to ischemia, and it is unlikely that hypovolemic or hemorrhagic shock *per se* produces significant damage to the lung. The lung is exposed to oxygen in the air breathed, and whatever cardiac output there is passes through the pulmonary circulation, albeit with shunting. In men studied in the Vietnam conflict, hemorrhagic shock was not associated with a high incidence of pulmonary complications. However, shock with severe tissue injury of the extremities, thorax, and abdomen, and particularly with sepsis, was associated with a high incidence of pulmonary dysfunction and failure. This led to use of the term, *post-traumatic pulmonary insufficiency,* which is preferred because it indicates the setting and suggests the multifactorial nature of this problem. Shock may well make the lung more vulnerable to fluid overload and increase the likelihood of later pulmonary capillary permeability changes.

Hyperventilation occurs initially with shock due to decreased blood flow to the central nervous system and a rise in P_{CO_2} in the respiratory center. This may initially produce *respiratory alkalosis* and a further decrease in cerebral blood flow due to the fall in $PaCO_2$. Later hyperventilation occurs owing to *metabolic acidosis* from increased lactate production. Decreased blood flow in the lung and shunting may contribute to hypoxia and carbon dioxide retention.

The host defense system becomes depressed; the capacity for phagocytosis of white blood cells and macrophages of the reticuloendothelial system decreases. With injury there are circulating immunosuppressive factors that may be related to suppressor T-cell activation. Therefore, during or after shock, the patient has increased susceptibility to infection. The coagulation system may be altered; some have ascribed many of the effects of shock to intravascular coagulation. However, this does not seem to be an important factor with hypovolemic shock in humans. With tissue injury, multiple operations, and multiple transfusions, abnormalities of coagulation are frequent.

Metabolic Changes. The combination of cardiovascular responses, endocrine secretion, and decreased tissue blood flow produces metabolic changes characteristic of shock. Some of these are adaptive mechanisms to provide energy during stress; others are the result of hypoxia and ischemia. Mobilization of carbohydrate reserves, increased breakdown of protein, and lack of use of fat stores seem to be characteristic. The need for large amounts of glucose is characteristic of shock and trauma; there is hyperglycemia early in shock, but peripheral glucose utilization also increases. Hepatic glycogenolysis due to epinephrine is a major early factor in this, whereas muscle glycogen breakdown produces lactate. During and after injury and shock, patients have a diabetic glucose tolerance curve owing partly to increased glycolysis, reduced insulin secretion, and perhaps some

tissue insulin resistance as well. Late in shock, particularly shock due to sepsis, hypoglycemia may be present. This is probably due to failure of glucose production by the liver.

Both lactate and pyruvate levels rise in early shock. Later the rise in lactate accelerates, leading to metabolic acidosis. The increased lactate has been thought to be due to a shift from aerobic Krebs cycle–electron transport metabolism to anaerobic glycolytic metabolism as cellular hypoxia occurs. Certainly this is in part true with decreased oxygen consumption during shock, increased oxygen extraction, an increased A-V O_2 difference, and an oxygen debt. Much of the increase in lactate in the dog in shock is the result of epinephrine induced muscle glycogenolysis, as shown by Liddell and co-workers. Some lactate may also be due to hyperventilation unrelated to hypoxia. In an experimental shock study, the elevation of lactate did not correlate with lack of oxygen or decreased production of CO_2. MacLean and co-workers found, however, that a high lactate level on admission in patients in shock correlated closely with mortality. Thus, the increased lactate may indicate not only tissue and cellular hypoxia, but also decreased ability of the liver to clear organic acids, and altered substrate metabolism due to catecholamines. Protein synthesis is decreased, amino acid levels in the blood increase—particularly alanine—and amino acids are broken down, as indicated by increased rates of urea production. The deamination of amino acids in muscle may occur through pyruvate, available from glycolysis, accepting the amino groups. This produces alanine, which then goes to the liver for gluconeogenesis.

With modest blood loss, free fatty acids increase in man, but with shock, fat mobilization seems to be turned off. This may be related to hypoperfusion of fat deposits. With glycogenolysis there is a tendency toward hyperkalemia and decreased serum sodium. Liddell and co-workers concluded from studies of dogs in shock that high serum catecholamines cause increased blood lactate, initial hyperglycemia, and poor free fatty-acid oxidation. Cortisol and glucagon along with epinephrine were necessary to mimic the massive protein breakdown or catabolism of shock. Hypoperfusion was necessary to diminish fatty acid mobilization from fat stores. Evidence of adrenal activation is present with eosinopenia, lymphocytopenia, and reduced platelets. Other changes represent impaired organ function due to decreased blood flow to the kidneys, liver, and muscle.

Microcirculatory Changes. The microvasculature is thought of as all vessels of 100 μ or less in size, and consists of precapillary arterioles, capillaries, and venules. It is the business end of the circulation for cell nutrition, and improvement of flow in this segment of the vascular bed is the primary aim in the treatment of shock. Blood is a viscid fluid and in the microcirculation, where flow may normally be slow or stop transiently, viscosity becomes important. At low flow rates or low rates of shear, blood has the property of developing a fluid structure that is more resistant to deformation. Thus at low flow rates, blood in capillaries becomes much more viscid, up to 40 times more than in the aorta, for example. This is called the non-Newtonian behavior of blood and is due to the presence of red cells and proteins, especially fibrinogen and globulin. During shock, when blood flow in a capillary bed is decreased, rouleaux of red cells form, and some capillaries become plugged with red cell aggregates. This has been called *sludging of blood* and has been thought by some to be a pathologic event in itself, producing microcirculatory damage rather than a simple transient phenomenon of low blood flow.

The dextrans, and particularly low molecular weight dextran (average 40,000), were proposed as antisludging agents to improve microcirculatory blood flow in various situations. This effect, however, does not seem to be specific. Anything that decreases hematocrit and fibrinogen concentration will decrease viscosity and improve blood flow. Thus, saline and Ringer's lactate solution seem to be as effective as dextran in decreasing cell aggregation and improving capillary flow. Although the microcirculation is important, it has not been possible to demonstrate specific and important means of affecting it other than the general approach of giving fluids and improving flow.

Late in shock there may be a reversal of capillary fluid exchange with loss from the capillaries rather than capillary refilling. This is probably not due to a generalized change in capillary membrane permeability. Possible explanations for this reversal include persistence of increased postcapillary resistance, an alteration of interstitial collagen and other macromolecules that forms a gel to trap water and sodium, a movement of water and sodium into cells (as indicated by the work of Shires and colleagues and by our work), and a failure of capillary refilling with major hemorrhage.
Cell Abnormalities. Progressive cell injury occurs with shock and ischemia. This occurs initially in those organs where blood flow is most reduced by hypovolemia such as the kidney, liver, and skeletal muscle. Although the evidence for this and the studies pertaining to it have been primarily in experimental animals, there is now sufficient clinical correlation and evidence to indicate the importance of these phenomena. The reasons for altered hepatic function in patients after injury clearly are due to ischemic damage to hepatocytes. The changes in muscle membrane potential and decreased functional extracellular fluid in patients with severe shock have been shown by Shires and colleagues. The tissue, organ, and cell swelling that occur after injury or with ischemia are easily recognized. The use of cold, chemical cardioplegia during cardiac surgery to preserve the myocardium is an example of the use of this experimental information for practical clinical purposes. The same is true in the preservation of organs for transplantation.

The sequence of events leading to progressive cell injury is shown in Figure 3-7. Alterations occur initially at the cell membrane; membrane transport and function are altered. Hydrogen ions accumulate within the cell along with lactate. Later, membrane potential decreases; sodium enters and potassium leaves cells. The Na–K adenosine triphosphatase enzyme system is activated. Adenosine triphosphate is used, mitochondria are stimulated, but energy and cyclic adenosine monophosphate levels decrease. Calcium regulation is altered, and nuclear and protein synthesis are depressed. The cell swells, and as further deterioration occurs, lysosomes eventually leak, mitochondria are disrupted, and cell is destroyed.

Clinical examples of altered cell and organ function

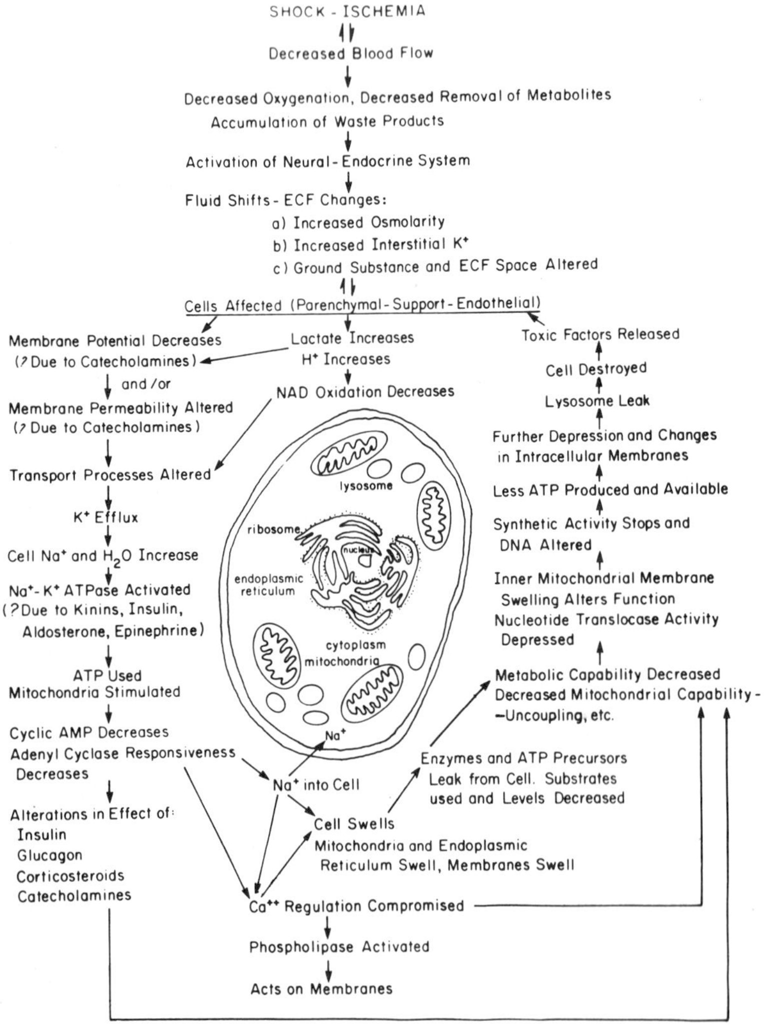

Fig. 3-7. Alterations in cell function with shock and ischemia.

owing to ischemia and shock are numerous and play a critical role in the development of multiple system failure after injury. Treatment requires rapid restoration of adequate blood flow. Whether or not additional benefit may be achieved by biochemical support of these cell abnormalities will be discussed later.

TREATMENT

Replacement Fluids

The mainstay of treatment of hypovolemic shock is volume replacement to increase the circulating blood volume (Table 3-3). As a general rule, the replacement solution should be that which the patient has lost. Thus, if oligemic shock is produced by intestinal obstruction with prolonged vomiting and sequestration of fluid in the bowel and peritoneal cavity, the replacement solution should be saline or lactated Ringer's solution. If blood has been lost in large quantities, whole blood transfusion is necessary. When blood loss has occurred, immediate resuscitation and initial support of the circulation by giving a solution such as lactated Ringer's can be quite adequate during the time that blood is being prepared in the blood bank by appropriate typing of the patient and crossmatching of donor blood. If blood loss has been 1000 ml or less, resuscitation with Ringer's lactate solution alone may be adequate, as long as the blood loss stops spontaneously or is stopped by operative intervention. A common approach used in an emergency facility for the treatment of an injured hypotensive patient is to begin a rapid infusion of Ringer's lactate solution, giving 1000 to 2000 ml over the first half hour to 45 minutes. This will serve as a therapeutic trial of the amount of blood loss and of continuing bleeding. If the patient stabilizes on this

regimen, blood loss has not been massive. This will also allow time to properly prepare crossmatched blood, should it be needed, and to carry out a full evaluation of the extent of injury. Such an approach will also reduce the amount of blood required, will help to increase the extracellular fluid volume and improve microcirculatory exchange, and will also provide a modest degree of hemodilution which reduces blood viscosity and improves flow. The potential hazard of giving lactate to a patient in shock with lactic acidosis is not a problem. Ringer's lactate is closer to arterial pH than is normal saline, and the lactate will be rapidly metabolized as the circulation is improved. Since Ringer's lactate solution fills the extracellular fluid space as well as the vascular volume, more solution must be given than the blood that is lost. Moyer and Butcher determined that a normal blood volume is maintained when after a slow loss of less than 20% of blood volume (900 ml to 1300 ml),

> volume of Ringer's lactate given = volume of hemorrhage + volume of hemorrhage × (0.035 × hematocrit of the shed blood)

This is roughly 2.5 times the volume of shed blood.

The limit in the volume of electrolyte solution to be used for blood loss before blood transfusions are used is the extent of anemia that the patient will tolerate. When the hematocrit decreases below 30, there is a progressive limitation in the amount of oxygen that arterial blood can carry. Although there are advantages to modest hemodilution, such as lowered viscosity of blood and increased capillary blood flow, these can be outweighed by decreased oxygen-carrying capacity. When the hematocrit reaches 25, even a normal person is in jeopardy, in part because the myocardium has little reserve in increasing oxygen extraction from blood.

TABLE 3-3   STEPS IN TREATMENT OF HYPOVOLEMIC SHOCK

1. Briefly assess cause of volume loss, possibility of decreasing loss from external wounds by pressure, and ventilatory and circulatory status.
2. Simultaneously withdraw venous blood sample for hematocrit, hemoglobin, electrolytes, and blood type and crossmatch, and insert large-bore intravenous cannula.
3. Begin rapid volume replacement with Ringer's lactate solution.
4. Insert Foley catheter; begin monitoring cardiovascular function.
5. Decide on need for immediate or early operative control of blood loss and proceed or plan this intervention.
6. Insert additional intravenous cannulae if needed.
7. Give supplemental O_2 by face mask.
8. Obtain an ECG and portable x-ray films as needed, *i.e.*, chest, abdomen, emergency IVP, cystogram.
9. Give furosemide, 40 mg IV, unless urine output is good.
10. Measure arterial blood gases.
11. Give $NaHCO_3$ if arterial pH is below 7.3.
12. Insert CVP catheter.
13. If patient stabilizes, decrease rate of volume replacement, continue monitoring and assess continuing loss and need for operation. If loss is continuing, consider need for angiographic diagnosis for site of bleeding.
14. If patient does not stabilize and losses continue, increase rate of volume replacement, give blood when prepared, or type-specific uncrossmatched blood, and proceed with operative control of loss.
15. If patient does not stabilize, blood or fluid loss is not continuing and central venous pressure increases to high normal or above, begin isoproterenol (or dopamine or epinephrine) 2 mg in 500 ml dextrose and water at 20 microdrops per min. Also begin digitalis as digoxin, 0.5 mg IV.
16. Reassess renal function, pulmonary function, cardiac function, electrolytes, coagulation; use appropriate agents as needed.
17. Insert Swan-Ganz catheter and measure left atrial pressure.
18. Measure cardiac output.
19. Adjust drugs and volume therapy appropriately.
20. Obtain other diagnostic studies to elucidate cause of continuing circulatory failure. Consider possibility of sepsis as a factor, or other injuries.

Blood Transfusions

For blood loss beyond 1000 ml, blood must be prepared and given as soon as it is ready after initial resuscitation with an electrolyte solution. If blood loss is massive and immediately life-threatening, such as a loss beyond 1500 ml to 2000 ml, and is continuing, maintenance of the circulation with an electrolyte solution may be impossible, and whole blood transfusions may be needed before appropriate cross-matching of donor blood can be carried out. In the past, "universal donor," type O, Rh negative, low antibody titer blood was kept on hand for this purpose. Today it seems better to use type-specific uncross-matched blood when necessary in an emergency situation. As part of the resuscitation in such a circumstance, immediate action must be taken to stop the hemorrhage as well.

The problems of blood transfusion are discussed in Chapter 5. It is important here to recognize, however, that blood from the bank, whether whole blood or packed red cells, is cold, acidotic, has a high potassium level, and contains citrate. When blood is given rapidly and in large quantities, it should be warmed before infusion. Giving cold blood rapidly can decrease myocardial temperature sufficiently to depress cardiac function and produce ventricular fibrillation. Also, when blood is given rapidly, buffering with sodium bicarbonate may be needed. Some recommend one ampule of $NaHCO_3$ (44.6 mEq) with every second unit of blood. Monitoring the arterial pH is best. In most patients, the citrate in bank blood will be metabolized rapidly by the liver. However, in certain patients with a depressed circulation or with liver disease, citrate may produce hypocalcemia. Routine administration of calcium is not recommended; rather, measurement of ionized calcium and an awareness of potential problems are preferred. The increased potassium in bank blood should not be a problem if the patient has reasonable renal function. In the past the occurrence of a shift in the oxyhemoglobin dissociation curve of hemoglobin produced by a decrease of 2, 3-diphosphoglycerate content in bank blood red cells was described. The clinical significance of this problem, however, was never documented. Now, with blood preserved in citrate–phosphate–dextrose solution (CPD) rather than in acid–citrate–dextrose solution, this should no longer be a problem.

Blood stored in a blood bank does accumulate particles made up of red cell ghosts, platelet aggregates, and other debris. This led to development of microfilters (the Swank and Pall filters) to get rid of particles down to 20 μ to 40 μ in size and to prevent microembolization in the lungs during transfusion. These microfilters have been important during extracorporeal circulation in which blood is pumped from a machine directly into the arterial circulation. Microemboli to the brain in such a circumstance are disastrous. With transfusion into the venous system, however, there is no good clinical evidence that these filters make a difference. First of all, a lot of particles still get through. Secondly, no difference in pulmonary function has been measured in transfused patients when such filters have been used. Whether or not there would be a difference in patients requiring 30 or more units of blood with massive trauma is uncertain. At present the use of microfilters should not interfere with the need to give blood as rapidly as needed.

Plasma Expanders

Through the years, studies and trials of various plasma substitutes have been carried out that now are primarily of historic interest only. At one time, plasma was used extensively for initial resuscitation and support of the circulation. However, the realization that shelf storage for a prolonged period, such as 6 mo, decreased but did not totally eliminate the threat of serum hepatitis has gradually decreased the use of plasma for this purpose. Clinical dextran has been used extensively as an initial resuscitative fluid, in part because it provides oncotic pressure, its average molecular weight of about 70,000 being comparable to that of albumin. Although it is safe to use clinical dextran in small volumes, there is no particular advantage in its use. When it is given in volumes beyond 1500 ml to 2000 ml, bleeding problems may result owing in part to dilution of clotting factors and in part to an increase in capillary blood flow. Preparations of plasma proteins, concentrated albumin, and hydroxyethyl starch have been used but also have no particular advantages. In addition to the use of Ringer's lactate solution for initial resuscitation and blood when needed, albumin has been given by some to provide colloid osmotic pressure. This approach is costly and there is little if any evidence that the albumin is needed. Moss and co-workers demonstrated that human serum albumin was not necessary for safe, effective resuscitation of patients after trauma. The organ that would seem to be most in jeopardy with a decrease in colloid osmotic pressure is the lung. However, Peters has pointed out that hemodilution-induced reduction of the intravascular protein concentrations in patients with intact capillaries does not lead to pulmonary edema. The protective factors are a drop in the extravascular concentration of protein, a rise in interstitial fluid pressure, and an increase in lymph flow. If the capillaries are damaged, then the protein leaks out and causes other problems. Immediately after certain injuries or problems in which plasma has been lost, as with a perforated ulcer, there may be a place for the use of albumin or protein as a resuscitative solution. Low molecular weight dextran with an average molecular weight of 40,000 is not a satisfactory solution for volume replacement because it is lost rapidly from the circulation and kidneys. Hemoglobin solutions for resuscitation are being studied but are not recommended for use in humans at present.

Autotransfusion has been used by suctioning blood from the operative field, adding an anticoagulant and returning the blood to the patient. This can be life-saving in an emergency and helpful in elective procedures where sudden massive blood loss is anticipated. Caution is required so that intravascular coagulation is not produced by activation of clotting factors in the extracorporeal reservoir. Unfortunately, autotransfusion cannot be used in abdominal injuries when there is a risk of alimentary tract perforation with bacterial contamination.

Rate of Fluid Administration

Blood volume must be replaced as rapidly as it is lost, or as needed and tolerated to produce a normal circulation. The sooner the circulatory deficit is corrected, the more rapidly the circulation will return to normal and correct the various metabolic and functional abnormalities produced by the low-flow state. The urgency of fluid administration or volume replacement in the hypovolemic patient must be stressed. The longer shock persists, the more devastating its effect and the more difficult treatment becomes. Five minutes of profound hypotension in the patient with coronary artery disease may be fatal. The only limitation to the rapidity of volume replacement is the ability of the heart to accept the volume load given. This may require documentation of the response of CVP and left atrial pressure to the replacement.

While shock is being treated, the wounds and sites of hemorrhage must be treated as well. If blood loss is continuing, it may not be possible to achieve normal cardiovascular function. In that circumstance, circulatory support may be sufficient only to maintain coronary, cerebral, and renal blood flow and function while the patient is transported to the operating room to remove a ruptured spleen or to suture a bleeding ulcer. With a ruptured abdominal aortic aneurysm, a normal circulation can be achieved only after definitive treatment of the aneurysm. Persistence in resuscitation and volume replacement in such circumstances will not only increase the loss but will also result in irreversible damage to organs such as the kidneys.

A common problem in patients with oligemic shock is inadequate volume replacement due to underestimating what is needed or has been lost. A patient may require replacement of a larger volume than predicted from the injury or from estimated loss. Continuous monitoring is the best guide not only to the volume of blood and fluids needed for treatment, but also to the rate of administration. Achievement of a reasonable arterial blood pressure, good urine output, and good peripheral perfusion as judged by palpable peripheral pulses, and warm, dry skin without excessive elevation of atrial pressures indicate an effective circulating blood volume.

During initial resuscitation and continuing support, various adjunctive measures may be helpful (Table 3-4).

Position

The position of the patient should be supine and horizontal. Elevation of the legs is the equivalent of a single unit blood transfusion, but lowering the head interferes with ventilation, and may be misinterpreted by the baroreceptors. The Trendelenburg position was introduced to expose the pelvic organs during an abdominal operation, not to treat shock.

Oxygen

Since one of the problems with hypovolemic shock is decreased oxygen delivery to tissues, it may be thought that supplemental oxygen would be helpful. If the lungs are normal and the patient is breathing adequately, arterial oxygenation in a patient with oligemic shock may be fairly normal, and supplemental oxygen will not add much to the oxygen content of arterial blood. However, because there may be some small advantage in increasing the oxygen dissolved in arterial blood even though partial pressures are not increased, all patients with hypovolemic shock should receive supplemental oxygen by face mask in concentrations of 40% to 50% of the inspired gas. If alveolar ventilation is inadequate or if there is arterial hypoxemia, assisted ventilation is needed.

Diuretics

Although renal function during hypovolemic shock must be restored by increasing both blood volume and renal blood flow, there may be some initial advantage in helping to protect the kidneys against the insult by giving a diuretic as well. A small dose of mannitol, an osmotic diuretic, or small doses of furosemide, a loop diuretic, may be given. The oligemic patient, however, may not respond to the diuretic until volume is restored. Whether or not hypovolemic shock by itself produces acute tubular necrosis in humans is not established. In cases of injury, in which

TABLE 3-4 VOLUME REPLACEMENT

RED BLOOD CELLS	Fresh blood Packed red cells Whole bank blood Reconstituted frozen red cells

COLLOID SOLUTIONS	Plasma
	Plasma protein preparations
	Dextrans
	   a. Clinical (70,000 mol wt)
	   b. Low molecular weight (40,000)
	Albumin

CRYSTALLOID SOLUTIONS	Lactated Ringer's solution (balanced salt solution) Normal saline (with or without glucose) 5% dextrose and saline with 2 ampules (90 mEq) sodium bicarbonate added Hartmann's solution Hypertonic saline or sodium lactate
OTHER SOLUTIONS	Stroma-free hemoglobin solution
COLLOID SOLUTIONS OF HISTORICAL INTEREST	Gelatin Gum acacia Hydroxyethyl starch

myoglobin, hemoglobin, and other proteins, in combination with decreased renal blood blow, may damage the tubules, the adjunctive use of a diuretic to help flush out the tubules initially is appropriate.

Buffers

Correction of metabolic acidosis with a buffering agent can be a helpful measure. The use of sodium bicarbonate should be monitored by measurement of arterial blood pH. Most importantly, the metabolic acidosis of hypovolemic shock must be corrected primarily by improving the circulation with volume replacement; otherwise, the acidosis, even though corrected partially or initially by sodium bicarbonate, will recur. Sodium bicarbonate is not needed if volume replacement is rapid and adequate. With severe metabolic acidosis in animals there was no difference in the hemodynamic response to saline or sodium bicarbonate, suggesting that circulatory depression by acidosis in intact animals is not a major problem.

Vasoactive Drugs

Hypovolemic shock should not be treated by the use of vasoactive drugs, particularly drugs that increase blood pressure, until volume has been restored. Vasoconstrictor drugs are contraindicated. The only circumstance in which a vasoactive drug, such as phenylephrine, that increases blood pressure may be helpful is when there is such severe hypotension that rapid elevation of the blood pressure from immediate life-threatening levels of 40 to 50 torr would be useful while volume replacement is also being provided. In most patients with hypovolemic shock, 1000 ml of Ringer's lactate solution administered rapidly (in a few minutes) will often elevate blood pressure to a less threatening level; volume replacement can then continue without the use of vasoactive drugs. If, however, volume replacement for what has seemed to be hypovolemic shock produces a high CVP, and the arterial circulation and tissue perfusion are not yet adequate, a vasoactive agent may be needed. In this circumstance a drug having an inotropic effect on the heart to increase contractility, such as dopamine, isoproterenol, epinephrine, or digitalis, would be necessary. Drugs that produce marked vasoconstriction, such as norepinephrine, may actually reduce cardiac output and blood flow to various organs and should be avoided if at all possible. The various vasoactive agents are classified in Table 3-5 and described in the section on cardiogenic shock.

There was a time when experimental animal and clinical studies suggested the use of vasodilator drugs for severe shock. The concept was that prolonged vasoconstriction was deleterious, and reversal of it would be helpful. Conceptually this may be true. However, the vasoconstriction must be reversed by improving blood flow, and not simply by blocking vasoconstriction with a drug such as phenoxybenzamine. The clinical use of these agents did not provide sufficient improvement, and decreased arterial oxygenation and increased mortality occurred in some patients. The use of a vasodilator as a general approach has now been abandoned in favor of more precise circulatory therapy with inotropic and unloading agents.

Antibiotics

Although host resistance is probably depressed by shock, the use of antibiotics with hypovolemic shock alone, such as with gastrointestinal hemorrhage, does not seem justified. Most of the time, however, there is tissue injury that produces shock. In such circumstances, antibiotics have clearly been beneficial in decreasing later wound infections and abscesses. A broad spectrum antibiotic should be given

as soon as possible after wounding, continued for 2 days, and then stopped. Antibiotics given 4 to 6 hr after tissue contamination have not been shown to influence the rate of infection.

Organ Preservation by Cooling

With severe injury, shock, and ischemia, cold saline or Ringer's lactate to protect the kidneys and liver during operative repair of these organs and other injuries has been used. This approach may have benefit, particularly if major vessel or organ injury requires temporary occlusion of the aorta or organ vascular pedicles.

Hypertonic Solutions

The swelling that occurs with burns, the cell swelling that occurs with ischemia and injury, and the concept that the major determinant of circulatory volume is the sodium ion have led to interest in hyperosmotic or hypertonic solutions. Some years ago we documented the pronounced circulatory effects of hypertonic sodium chloride and bicarbonate solutions in experimental shock in dogs; we found that a large amount of fluid could be mobilized, presumably from cells. Monafo used hypertonic saline solutions in the treatment of burn shock and found that not only were they effective in maintaining the circulation with a much smaller volume than an isotonic solution, but burn swelling was also greatly reduced. These observations have been confirmed by others. Hypertonic solutions such as mannitol have been used by Leaf and others to improve reflow to the kidney and heart after a period of ischemia, and Ames has done this with the brain. Their hypothesis that this approach reduces the endothelial cell swelling of ischemia is attractive but perhaps oversimplistic. In the kidney, mannitol affects renal hormonal regulation of blood flow and may act in this way. The late Sam Powers and his group used hypertonic mannitol to improve glomerular filtration rate in injured patients and also improved ventilation–perfusion coordination in patients

---

TABLE 3-5   AHLQUIST CLASSIFICATION OF SYMPATHETIC NERVOUS SYSTEM RECEPTORS (VASOACTIVE DRUGS)

PURE ALPHA-STIMULATING DRUGS	PURE BETA-STIMULATING DRUGS
Methoxamine hydrochloride (Vasoxyl)	Isoproterenol hydrochloride (Isuprel)*
Angiotensin II (Hypertensin)	
STRONG ALPHA DRUGS	**MIXED ALPHA AND BETA DRUGS**
(with some beta effect on the heart)	Epinephrine (Adrenalin)—5 mg/250 ml (0.003-0.1 μg/Kg/min)
Phenylephrine (Neo-synephrine)—slight cardiac effect	Dopamine (Intropin) 400 mg/250 ml (2-20 μg/Kg/min)
Metaraminol (Aramine)—some beta cardiac effect	Dobutamine (Dobutrex) 500 mg/250 ml (2.5-10 μg/Kg/min)
Mephentermine (Wyamine)—some beta cardiac effect	Norepinephrine (Levarterenol, Levophed)—some beta cardiac effect—16 mg/250 ml (0.03–1.0 μg/Kg/min)
ALPHA BLOCKING AGENTS	**BETA BLOCKING AGENTS**
Phenoxybenzamine hydrochloride (Dibenzyline)	Propranolol (Inderal)
Phentolamine (Regitine)	
(These agents are not recommended for shock treatment.)	
Thymoxamine—a competitive blocker	

* Catecholamines. Other drugs are sympathomimetic drugs. There are other drugs in each classification but they are not appropriate for use in the circulation. All infusions of these drugs should be started with a dilute solution and a microdrip infusion set, to titrate their effects.
Alpha-Receptors—Stimulatory—*Vasoconstriction*
Beta-Receptors—Inhibitory—*Vasodilatation*
Cardiac Receptors—All beta receptors, but all stimulatory—increased contractility (inotropy) and increased heart rate (chronotropy)

with respiratory distress syndrome. Peters and his group are presently carrying out a study of hypertonic sodium lactate solution for fluid replacement in patients undergoing aortic surgery. Hypertonic solutions may well be beneficial to shock patients, particularly in late shock, by utilizing the increased cell water for resuscitation and thus reducing cell swelling.

Substrates for Cell Metabolism

It is recognized that an individual or an organ will tolerate a period of shock or ischemia better if it is well nourished before the insult. Increasing the substrates available for cell function prior to an insult has demonstrated value. There is considerable evidence in animal experiments that substrates for cell metabolism given after the insult or after a period of shock are also helpful. Adenosine $3':5'$–cyclic phosphate (cyclic AMP), nicotinamide, Krebs cycle intermediates, inosine, adenosine, creatine phosphate, and allopurinol have all been used with some beneficial effects. We have evaluated the use of the high-energy phosphate compound adenosine triphosphate (ATP) complexed with $MgCl_2$ to try to provide energy directly in various experimental shock and ischemic situations. The effects in animals have been very impressive providing early improvement in function of ischemic cells. Whether or not these approaches will be valuable in humans remains to be established.

Continuing Management

After initial volume replacement has elevated arterial blood pressure to a reasonable level and urine output has begun to increase, the rate of volume replacement should be decreased until resuscitation is complete. Excessive volume replacement may result if monitoring of the patient is not done carefully. Overenthusiastic resuscitation in hypovolemic shock to support circulation and kidneys may jeopardize the lungs and contribute to posttraumatic pulmonary insufficiency. During resuscitation, pulmonary function must be monitored by arterial blood gases, by listening for rales, and by monitoring atrial pressures. However, interstitial edema of the lungs may occur with little initial change in these parameters. The measurement of CVP has greatly improved care and resuscitation of the patient in shock. A single measurement is not helpful since dynamic changes occur during volume replacement. Resuscitation should not be continued to a predetermined level of CVP if the arterial circulation seems to be returning toward normal. Large excesses of volume replacement may be given before the CVP goes above a high normal measurement. There are situations in which the measurement of both right atrial and left atrial pressures is required. As with any biological measurement, clinical judgment is needed as well.

The most frequent causes of lack of responsiveness to treatment are unrecognized volume deficits or continuing losses of blood volume and inadequate replacement of losses. There may also be myocardial failure, sepsis, peripheral pooling of blood, inadequate ventilation with hypoxia or carbon dioxide retention or both, persistent metabolic acidosis, hyponatremia, hyperkalemia, hypocalcemia, and renal failure. Other injuries producing pneumothorax, hemothorax, cardiac tamponade, gastrointestinal perforation, or increased intracranial pressure may complicate or perpetuate the problem. In the past, the term *irreversible shock* has been used for such difficult problems. This is a term brought from the experimental laboratory to describe late hemorrhagic shock in dogs. Even though some patients

may not survive an injury or shock, this term should not be used to describe humans because there is no such entity, and energetic treatment may be successful. Many of these factors are interrelated and occur more often in combination rather than as sole causes of unresponsiveness. The recognition and correction of such abnormalities will improve the rate of survival of patients in shock.

SEPTIC SHOCK

Shock due to infection is a frequent problem that is more complex and less well understood than hypovolemic and cardiogenic shock. Septic shock usually occurs in the presence of a major underlying disease that may be the critical factor in survival. Also, the response of an individual to an infection is varied, and some of the abnormalities produced by infection are still obscure. A frequent result of severe infection in a surgical patient is the development of multiple organ failure.

Circulatory failure occurring with infection was described by Laennec in 1831; in 1897, Boise published a manuscript on the differential diagnosis of shock, hemorrhage, and infection. Bloodstream invasion by gram-negative organisms, particularly after urinary-tract instrumentation, was recognized early in this century, but it did not occur frequently. There were few references to hypotension and a shocklike appearance with sepsis until Waisbren described two clinical pictures with gram-negative bacteremia; in one, the patient appeared toxic, and in the other the patient appeared to be in a shocklike state. Of 29 cases he reported, 15 patients had hypotension, cold, clammy skin, and lethargy (a low cardiac output syndrome), whereas the other 14 had the more usual manifestations of an infection with fever, bounding pulse, wide pulse pressure, and warm, flushed skin. In the same year, Borden and co-workers described fulminating circulatory failure after transfusion of blood contaminated with gram-negative bacilli. Extensive study of gram-negative infection was then carried out with the emphasis in recent years on septicemia and shock from these organisms. Shock, however, may be produced by an organism, gram-positive or gram-negative, and by fungi and yeast. It is apparent, also, that the original descriptions of a hypodynamic circulation with cold skin, vasoconstriction, and hypotension represent a late stage in septic shock. In the early stages of septic shock, no matter what the organism, the patient has a hyperdynamic circulation, unless he is not able to respond to the infection.

ETIOLOGY

Septic shock frequently occurs in a hospitalized patient; often there is an underlying disease process or injury that renders him susceptible to bloodstream invasion and septicemia. Predisposing factors include advancing age, diabetes mellitus, cirrhosis, leukemia, lymphoma, disseminated carcinoma, chemotherapy, transplantation with its associated immunosuppression, and a variety of surgical procedures and injuries that may lead to peritoneal contamination and areas of infection or abscess. The urinary tract is a frequent site of infection, and many cases in the past were preceded by instrumentation, such as catheterization of the bladder, cystoscopy, passage of a sound, or by operation. Recognition of this source of gram-negative septicemia and careful techniques for these procedures have decreased the frequency of this problem. The respiratory tract is a frequent source of such infections, particularly in the patient with a tracheostomy. The gastrointestinal tract may be a source of infection, with fecal contamination of the peritoneal cavity, the biliary tract with cholangitis, as well as the skin with burns. A number of cases result from prolonged use of intravenous infusion sites. Septic abortions and post partum infections account for a small number of such problems. Recognition of these sites as a source for invasive infection has decreased the frequency of septic shock from such problems.

The most frequent single organism has been *Escherichia coli,* followed by *Aerobacter aerogenes, Pseudomonas aeruginosa,* and *Klebsiella pneumoniae.* Proteus organisms and bacteroides have also been implicated. Gram-positive organisms such as *Staphylococcus aureus* can also produce septicemia with shock, as can *Candida albicans.* Pneumococcal and streptococcal infections can also be lethal with septicemia and shock. The capacity to treat infection by gram-positive organisms has been better in recent years and, therefore, severe shock and mortality from gram-positive infections have been less. Thus, there has been an emphasis on gram-negative organisms and their associated problems.

CLINICAL PICTURE

Gram-negative septicemia often begins with chills and an elevated temperature above 38.3° C, often to 39° C to 40° C, followed by shock, that may develop suddenly or slowly. With hypotension there may be initial changes in mental status with inappropriate behavior, followed by decreased urine output and systolic blood pressure below 70 to 80 torr. Most patients initially will have warm, dry skin despite hypotension. Vasodilatation or arteriovenous shunting in the presence of warm, dry extremities is typical of early septic shock, whereas the classic picture of shock with vasoconstriction is seen only later in the course. Heart rate may be slow, rather than fast. Vomiting and diarrhea may occur initially, with blood in the stool later, depending on the infection. It is apparent, now, that the clinical picture is determined in part by the response of the individual to infection and in part by the state or condition of the patient at the time that the septic process occurs. Thus, the response to infection with an elevation in temperature is vasodilatation and the need for an increased cardiac output and increased peripheral blood flow, perhaps to all tissues and the skin but certainly to the area of infection. If the patient cannot respond, either because of a low blood volume, low extracellular fluid volume, or limited cardiac reserve, then the initial picture of a warm, hyperdynamic, dilated patient will not be seen. If, however, the blood volume is reasonable and cardiac function is adequate initially, then a hyperdynamic circulation is characteristic of the septic process in all patients. The two varieties—the cold, clammy, hypodynamic, and hypotensive, and the hyperdynamic, warm, and dilated—are not different responses to infection but rather are determined by the condition of the patient at the time that the septicemia occurs or the stage of the insult.

Hyperventilation and respiratory alkalosis are helpful early signs in the diagnosis of serious gram-negative bacteremia. This may be a primary response to bacteremia, but it could also be due to altered cerebral or brain stem blood flow. The triad of altered sensorium, a source of gram-negative infection, and hyperventilation with respiratory alkalosis may allow the diagnosis to be made before shock and overt circulatory failure develop. MacLean and co-workers found that treatment begun during this early stage,

prior to the development of metabolic acidosis, was much more successful. In shock with gram-positive septicemia, warm, dry extremities and normovolemia have been thought to be characteristic. Again, this is an early stage of vasodilatation followed later by vasoconstriction as circulatory failure progresses. The white blood cell count is usually 15,000 to 20,000/mm³ or higher, but leukopenia may occur, particularly early in shock. There are no other characteristic laboratory findings other than progressive development of circulatory failure and its attendant features.

PATHOPHYSIOLOGICAL RESPONSE TO INFECTION

In simple terms, an infection requires an increased circulation that must be provided locally at the site of the infectious process and generally to the entire organism. If the circulation of the individual can keep up with the demands of the septic process, then a hyperdynamic but adequate circulation results. If, however, the individual's circulation cannot keep up with the demands, either because of lack of volume, excess vasodilatation, effects on the heart, or other toxic factors, then circulatory failure and septic shock will ensue. The mediators of the increased need for circulation and the various toxic factors may be complex but certainly are not mysterious.

The relatively simple phenomenon of the local response to infection helps in this understanding. The throbbing pain, heat, redness, and swelling described originally by Galen are the result of local release of substances producing vasodilatation and increased blood flow to the area with altered capillary permeability, exudation, and swelling. Heat is produced by increased blood supply, and pain from the edema and perhaps release of vasodilating polypeptides. These local effects may be due to the effects of the bacterial organism itself, from endotoxin (a high molecular weight phospholipid–polysaccharide–protein complex in the wall of gram-negative organisms) or exotoxins produced by gram-positive organisms. These interact with white blood cells, polymorphonuclear leukocytes, and macrophages that then liberate several materials, including a pyrogenic factor and leukocyte endogenous mediator. These alter the temperature control center in the midbrain and produce other effects on the individual. With the increase in temperature, the initial hemodynamic event seems to be a fall in peripheral vascular resistance. This may be brought about by release of vasodilating substances or by the increased temperature and altered neurogenic control. Accompanying this is an increase in cardiac output and the beginning of the hypermetabolic state. Chills and fever increase heat production by the body by altering skin blood-flow and attempting to regulate heat production and heat loss. Catecholamine output and protein catabolism begin. There is increased oxygen consumption. However, measurements of oxygen consumption in patients with sepsis and in animal models have shown that for every one degree centigrade rise in temperature, oxygen consumption increases only 12%. Thus, the increase in cardiac output with infection is far in excess of the increase in oxygen consumption. Therefore, the increased cardiac output is only partially related to the increase in metabolism and oxygen demand. The initial decrease in total peripheral resistance could be mediated by such endogenous substances as histamine, beta-endorphin from the hypothalamus, changes in components of the complement system (particularly C3 and C3 proactivator), or in alterations in the kallikrein system.

Characteristic of severe infection with septic shock in

humans is an increase in mixed venous oxygen content returning to the heart. This is in contrast to all other forms of shock, for which there is increased extraction of oxygen from the blood perfusing all the organ systems with decreased blood flow. This increase in venous oxygen content suggests three possible mechanisms: (*1*) an overall increase in peripheral blood flow in most areas of the body; (*2*) the opening of arteriovenous shunts; and (*3*) a direct cytotoxic effect on cells of the various organs, decreasing their capability to utilize oxygen. Although there has been some evidence that cells are unable to function and to utilize oxygen with severe infection, the major mechanism for this increase in venous oxygen content seems to be increased blood flow from vasodilatation rather than the other mechanisms. This problem, however, is still not totally solved. This hemodynamic situation does behave somewhat like an arteriovenous (AV) shunt and establishes a new steady-state equilibrium with a very high blood flow and low resistance system. If at this point of adaptation the circulation can meet the needs of the patient and of the septic process, then stability will be maintained with a hyperdynamic state. If, however, the disease process continues and septicemia or other changes ensue, then the hyperdynamic phase will slowly or rapidly progress to a hypodynamic situation. Initially cardiac output and blood pressure will fall, and as this happens, peripheral vascular resistance will increase to compensate, leading to a hypodynamic cold hypotensive state of late shock similar to other types of shock. An increase in venous capacitance could be one of the factors of infection that initiates this deteriorating state of affairs. As the hyperdynamic process continues, cardiac fatigue, with resultant toxic effects on the myocardium, produces an element of cardiogenic shock as well. Thus, septic shock may have a number of components: (*1*) loss of vascular and extracellular fluid volume into the area of infection, such as in peritonitis or in a large abscess; (*2*) peripheral vasodilatation due to a high temperature and increased blood flow from the septic process; (*3*) circulatory and cellular effects produced by the endotoxins or exotoxins of bacterial organisms, leukocyte mediators, prostaglandins, kallikreins and kinins, and other toxic factors. Furthermore, the heart, adrenals, lungs, and other organs are eventually affected and become significant factors in perpetuating or intensifying the original process.

EFFECTS OF INFECTION ON OTHER ORGANS— MULTIPLE ORGAN FAILURE

Recently the profound effects of systemic infection on the entire individual and on other organs remote from the site of the infection have been recognized. The development of multiple or sequential organ or systems failure has as its most common feature a septic process. Thus, the development of pulmonary failure, renal failure, hepatic problems with elevated bilirubin, eventual failure of the heart, alterations in coagulation, and severe demands upon metabolism all may result from a septic process in which the circulation is supported so that shock *per se* is not evident, but the effects on the other organs develop.

An infectious process such as peritonitis is frequently associated with respiratory failure. In fact, the development of respiratory failure and need for ventilatory assistance has been pointed out as an initial sign of occult infection. The reason why a septic process such as peritonitis may produce ventilatory failure is not totally clear. There is considerable experimental evidence that various factors, such as toxin

from the septic process, a polypeptide, immune complexes, aggregated white blood cells with superoxide production, complement activation, platelet and fibrin debris, kallikrein and kinin activation, and prostaglandin effects through arachidonic acid and lipoxygenases, may damage the capillary endothelium of the pulmonary microcirculation producing an increase in permeability, interstitial edema, loss of protein and eventual development of the full syndrome of the adult respiratory distress syndrome.

The kidney may be damaged directly by circulating factors from an infection and will be altered by changes in renal blood flow. With the hyperdynamic septic state in humans, renal blood flow is increased and there is increased urine production. Polyuria may occur due to damage to the juxtaglomerular apparatus, and the production of large volumes of urine is inappropriate for the level of renal blood flow and filtration. The kidney would then be very susceptible to a decrease in blood flow; such an added insult may produce acute renal failure—either high-output renal failure or anuric or oliguric renal failure—as a direct result of a septic process.

The liver is also altered; whether this is due to a direct toxic effect, decreased blood flow, or to an abnormal intrahepatic distribution of flow is not well understood. As a septic process continues, even though the circulation seems to be well supported, there is often a rise in bilirubin to fairly high levels, with clinical evidence of jaundice, a decrease in liver synthetic and detoxifying activities, and sometimes even the full picture of hepatic failure. Failure of the myocardium has previously been commented upon. Again, this may be due to the production of some toxic factor that damages the myocardium *per se* or from "fatigue" of the myocardium owing to prolonged hyperdynamic circulation.

Abnormalities of coagulation are frequent, particularly abnormalities of various levels of circulating clotting factors. Overt abnormalities in coagulation, however, are less frequent. On occasion, there is clear-cut evidence of disseminated intravascular coagulation. This occurs particularly with septic abortions and other such overwhelming problems. Changes in prothrombin time, fibrinogen levels, platelet count, and detection of fibrin split products may be found in a number of patients; but they become severe in only a few. Whether or not microscopic intravascular coagulation plays a role in the development of multiple organ failure is not well understood. There is some experimental evidence for the deposition of fibrin within the microcirculation. Whether or not this is a primary or secondary effect, however, is not well established.

The demands of an infectious process over a period of days to weeks upon overall body metabolism are overwhelming. A terminal event in such patients may well be exhaustion of the metabolic processes of skeletal muscle and the liver, which are called upon to provide the protein for glucose production and for continuation of defense against the septic process. Detailed studies of the metabolic effects of sepsis with multiple systems organ failure in patients have been described in a series of papers by Border, Cerra, and their group. They have defined a peripheral metabolic defect that reduces oxidative metabolism of conventional energetic fuels—glucose, fatty acids, and triglycerides—and enhances the catabolism of essential branch-chain amino acids. Along with this, there is reduced hepatic protein synthesis and increased albumin catabolism. This produces an autocannibalism of skeletal muscle. They ascribe the ultimate death of such a patient to metabolic exhaustion. Such studies indicate that better support might be provided by giving branch-chain amino acids along with short-chain fatty acids.

TREATMENT

The cornerstone of control of septic shock is prevention—recognizing predisposing factors, limiting prophylactic antibiotics, awareness of sites of origin of common gram-negative infections, prompt recognition of signs of gram-negative septicemia, and early treatment of all infections. Treatment has been much more successful before shock develops than afterward. Furthermore, septic shock has responded better to therapy when recognized early. With these approaches, in recent years there has been a great reduction in the incidence and frequency of overt septic shock. The problems of severe overwhelming infection and mortality from infection in surgical patients still continue. The emphasis, however, has shifted now since the prevention of septic shock has been more frequent. Now our problems concern the development of organ failure rather than of septic shock *per se*. The reason for the development of organ failure may well be decreased blood flow, in spite of what seems to be a generalized hyperdynamic circulation. Blood flow to organs such as the liver and the kidney, to the coronary circulation, and to other areas may not be adequate, and the intraorgan distribution of flow may be altered along with various toxic effects of the septic process and its metabolic breakdown products. At the present time, the measurement of organ flow in patients is difficult, and intraorgan distribution of flow impossible. Thus, maintenance of the hyperdynamic circulation with infection is imperative. Documentation of the ability to respond to skin antigens, maintenance of nutrition and acute phase protein production, and minimizing the burden of organisms and necrotic or contaminated tissues help to prevent infection.

The patient with sepsis and a failing circulation should be observed by careful and continuous arterial and central venous monitoring, urine output measurement, and electrocardiographic monitoring as previously described (Table 3-6). Temperature, arterial blood gas tensions and pH, and physical signs must also be observed. Blood and other septic sites should be cultured and appropriate antibiotics administered in massive doses systemically. If antibiotics were given previously, a new more appropriate regimen is insti-

tuted. Blood volume replacement and expansion is carried out rapidly and judiciously. If these measures do not rapidly improve the circulation, drugs will be necessary. Isoproterenol, rapidly acting digitalis preparations, and other vasoactive agents such as dopamine often help by improving cardiac efficiency when atrial filling pressures are high or rising and arterial pressure and blood flow are low. Vasopressors are avoided if at all possible. A schema for the treatment of septic shock is shown in Table 3-6. The various vasoactive drugs and their use are described in detail in the section on cardiogenic shock.

Antibiotics

It has been well established by Altemeier and his group, and by others, that selection of the most appropriate antibiotic for a patient with sepsis is the most important determinant of final morbidity and mortality. Antibiotics must be given intravenously and a broad spectrum antibiotic or combination of antibiotics in large dosages is critical. Whether or not the agent is bactericidal or bacteriostatic does not seem to be as important as is selection of an antibiotic for the organism which seems most likely, whether it be urinary tract, biliary tract, peritoneal cavity, or elsewhere. The local record of experience in the hospital and susceptibility of organisms to antibiotics should be used. In general, treatment is best started usually with an aminoglycoside such as gentamicin or kanamycin. If the infection is a gram-positive one and the organisms are known to be cocci, then a large dose of intravenous penicillin should be used as well. With peritonitis, abdominal-wall infections, fasciitis, and other infections in which anaerobes may be active, or for mixed infection including aerobes and anaerobes, a combination of gentamicin, 3 mg/Kg–5 mg/Kg, clindamycin, 600 mg/day–1200 mg/day, and 20 million units of penicillin is recommended. For potential clostridial infection, a large dose of intravenous penicillin should be given.

With enteric infections and nosocomial infections, penicillinase resistant agents should be used (*e.g.*, oxacillin) or a cephalosporin, such as cefoxitin, cefamandole or cefazolin. This should be combined with an aminoglycoside such as gentamicin or tobramycin. Clindamycin instead of a cephalosporin has been used for anaerobic infections along with an aminoglycoside. In patients who are neutropenic or when a pseudomonas infection is suspected,

---

TABLE 3-6　TREATMENT OF SEPTIC SHOCK

1. Instrumentation and monitoring as for hypovolemic shock.
2. Draw blood for cultures and other specimens for culture, as needed and available—sputum, urine, wound, abscess.
3. a. Begin fluids to increase vascular volume and raise filling pressures until they are high normal. b. At the same time begin systemic broad spectrum antibiotics based on the most likely organisms.
4. Continue intravenous fluids until the arterial circulation becomes adequate or filling pressures of the ventricles are high.
5. Evaluate need for drainage of abscesses or accumulations or abdominal exploration—ultrasound and CT scan.
6. Adjunctive measures—supplementary oxygen or ventilatory assistance, correction of acidosis, diuretics if urine output not adequate.
7. If fluids and antibiotics do not initially produce adequate blood flow, then an inotropic agent is necessary. See Table 3-8.
8. Obtain culture reports with sensitivities to determine need for different antibiotics.
9. Observe closely remote organ function for evidence of ischemia (particularly of the kidney; a low urine sodium with normal urine output indicates need for more fluid), the liver, ventilation, the heart, and metabolism with the need for nutritional support.
10. If at this point the patient is still in shock, some would use pharmacologic doses of steroids such as methylprednisolone. Some would have given steroids earlier. Others would not give steroids. It is necessary to be sure that adrenal insufficiency does not develop.

carbenicillin or ticarcillin should be used along with an aminoglycoside.

Steroids

There has been considerable disagreement about the use of steroids with severe infection and particularly with septic shock. The use of massive or pharmacologic doses of steroids has become a common practice, not because of adrenal insufficiency but because of the pharmacologic effects of these agents. This was suggested by Altemeier and Cole in 1958 after hydrocortisone seemed helpful in three patients with septic shock. No clinical or laboratory evidence of adrenal insufficiency or improvement with physiologic doses of corticosteroids has been found. In experimental animals in which steroids have been given before the insult, such as before the injection of gram-negative organisms or of endotoxin, there has been a protective effect. This has been thought to be due to membrane and lysosomal stabilization, improvement in cell function, and a decrease in the vaso-active, vasoconstrictive, and deleterious effects of materials such as endotoxin. Part of the difficulty in this area is that early in septic shock, the time at which some have recommended giving steroids, these agents are probably not necessary. Late in septic shock, the situation is complex. In reported series, it is extremely difficult to separate the effects of steroids from other treatment programs that are being carried out simultaneously. Considerable effort has been devoted to this, and many investigators have tried to document the effects of steroids. The cornerstone of treatment of sepsis and septic shock must be prevention and, next, appropriate antibiotic therapy followed by drainage of the septic process and circulatory support by volume and by other agents during this period. If a patient does not respond quickly to this regimen, then a trial of pharmacologic doses of steroids may be in order for the following several reasons: (1) Adrenal exhaustion may occur late in sepsis and such a patient may have adrenal insufficiency. It is best to try to document this, but also not withhold treatment until too late. (2) If in such a circumstance the patient has not responded to other treatment, the addition of pharmacologic doses of steroids might be helpful and should not be denied the patient simply because final results and overall effects are unclear or not agreed upon. There are few problems associated with the injection of 250 mg to 1 g of methyl prednisolone sodium succinate as a bolus injection, to be repeated in 6 hr to 12 hr and then stopped.*

Drainage

Of greatest importance in treating surgical patients is the old adage that *the sun should not set on undrained pus.* The clinician must continue to evaluate the patient to determine the presence of a localized infection that must be drained. A subphrenic abscess, an hepatic abscess, an intraloop abscess within the peritoneal cavity and empyema, a pelvic abscess, necrotizing fasciitis, or other infections should be treated early and adequately. The documentation that remote organ failure may be produced by an intraperitoneal septic process requiring surgical intervention has provided emphasis for this concept. It should now be possible to treat septic shock adequately by support of the circulation, maintenance of blood flow, and initial treatment of the

---

* Recently, the use of steroid therapy has been found to impair immunologic defenses, and continued use may be deleterious.—Ed.

septic process. The final outcome should now be dependent upon the ability of the surgeon and the patient to control the septic process by maintenance of host resistance, surgical drainage, and appropriate antibiotics. If this cannot be done, progressive, sequential, or multiple organ failure is likely to result which may then produce death.

CARDIOGENIC SHOCK

Failure of the heart to provide adequate circulation may be due to specific cardiac problems such as an acute myocardial infarct or to ventricular tachycardia. Frequently, however, in surgical patients, the problem is a nonspecific one in which the ventricles cannot meet the needs of the circulation. Whether this is due to depression of the myocardium by various diseases, by circulating factors, or by the nonspecific stress of prolonged shock, sepsis, or illness is not known. What is known is that after a severe injury, an infection, or a disease such as pancreatitis, the heart may become the limiting factor in the circulation. Thus the definition of cardiogenic shock is an inadequate circulation with inability of the ventricles to pump the blood returning to them. There may be a specific intrinsic abnormality or a nonspecific ventricular depression (Table 3-1). The failure may be due initially to the left ventricle or may be a primary right ventricular problem. Right ventricular failure may, by ventricular distention and shift of the septum, decrease the filling capacity of the left ventricle and produce what seems to be left ventricular failure as well.

The definition of shock following myocardial infarction was developed by Fishberg and associates in 1934. Harrison in 1935 and Blalock in 1940 included the term *cardiogenic shock* in the classifications of circulatory failure. Cardiac output was found to be reduced after myocardial infarction in humans by Grishman and Master in 1941, but it was not until 1952 that Freis and associates described the hemodynamic abnormalities of cardiogenic shock after a myocardial infarction. Infarction of more than 40% of the left ventricle has now been recognized as a fatal lesion. Since then, Wiggers, Guyton and Crowell, Siegel and DelGuercio, and others have emphasized the importance and potential problems of the heart in all forms of shock.

PATHOPHYSIOLOGY

There are four physiological determinants of cardiac output (Table 3-7). First is the preload or filling pressures of the ventricles during diastole. If this is inadequate, then by definition the problem is one of hypovolemia, to be corrected by volume expansion. Excess volume, on the other hand, unless it is given extremely rapidly produces more chronic heart failure or pulmonary edema and not shock, except in the terminal phase. The Frank–Starling relationship or principle states that as ventricular filling pressure increases, the length of myocardial fibers increase at the end of diastole. As this happens, the force of contraction increases, which increases cardiac output. If the optimal length of stretch of the myocardial fibers is greatly exceeded, then contractions cannot increase and myocardial failure results. Decreased ventricular filling by pericardial tamponade compressing the ventricles and not allowing them to fill or positive end-expiratory pressure (PEEP), which decreases blood return to the thorax, will produce a form of extrinsic cardiogenic shock that is truly a preload problem. The measurements needed to determine preload are the atrial pressures, which are an indication of ventricular filling pressures. Ventricular

TABLE 3-7   DETERMINANTS OF CARDIAC OUTPUT

DETERMINANT	DEFINITION	EFFECT ON CARDIAC OUTPUT	MEASUREMENT	TREATMENT
Preload	Length of myocardial fibers at end-diastole which is the result of ventricular filling pressure	Direct, up to physiologic limit	End-diastolic volume and pressure of the ventricles Pulmonary diastolic pressure Pulmonary capillary wedge pressure Direct left atrial pressure measurements CVP (right atrial)	Volume expansion Pericardiocentesis Reduction of PEEP
Contractility	The inotropic state of the myocardium; Length/tension/velocity relationship of myocardium independent of initial length and afterload	Direct	Ventricular function curves Ejection fraction Vmax Vcf PEP/LVET $\dfrac{dP/dt}{iP}$	Dopamine Norepinephrine Epinephrine Isoproterenol Dobutamine Digitalis Glucagon GKI
Afterload	Systolic ventricular-wall stress which is produced by the force against which the myocardial fibers must contract	Inverse, as long as coronary flow is maintained	Aortic pressure for left ventricle Pulmonary artery pressure for right ventricle	Diuretics Phentolamine Sodium nitroprusside Nitroglycerine Intra-aortic balloon pumping External counterpulsation

Pulse Rate	The number of cardiac systoles per min	Direct, above 60 and below 180 per min	ECG
			Count pulse
				Bradycardia:
				  Isoproterenol
				  Pacemaker
				Tachycardia:
				  Digitalis
				  Lidocaine
				  Electroversion

end diastolic pressure is the important measurement, but it is impractical to measure except during cardiac catheterization. If ventricular function is depressed by injury, operation, sepsis, or other factors, a higher preload or atrial pressure may be necessary to obtain optimal ventricular muscle stretch and force of contraction. Thus, a trial of increase in preload is always necessary even with an acute myocardial infarction. Pulmonary edema should not occur until a wedge pressure of 24 cm H_2O is reached unless colloid osmotic pressure is reduced.

Contractility is the state of health and vigor of the myocardium and can be affected by many primary and secondary disease processes. It is defined as the rate of myocardial fiber shortening independent of the initial length or afterload. Alterations in contractility are the most common problem producing cardiogenic shock. This can occur because of myocardial necrosis, ischemia, anoxia, or depression of function by drugs or diseases as well as with such problems as sepsis, peritonitis, or severe injury even in a young individual with a previously normal heart. Various aspects of ventricular function can be measured during cardiac catheterization, but during routine monitoring the measurements that can be made are more limited.

The most commonly used measurement is the ventricular function curve. Sarnoff and his group developed a family of ventricular function curves plotting changes in stroke work of the left ventricle over a range of end-diastolic volumes and pressures. Thus, the relationship of ventricular stroke work to a certain end-diastolic volume is a measure of contractility. In order to have an exact measurement of contractility, the other variables—preload, afterload, and heart rate—would have to remain constant. Obviously, in the clinical situation, this cannot be done. Therefore, an approximation of contractility is obtained by plotting the left ventricular stroke work against the filling pressure—pulmonary capillary wedge pressure (PCWP) or left atrial pressure. This point can then be compared with the curves obtained from normal ventricles. This allows an estimation as to whether contractility is in a normal or low range. If it is low, then an inotropic agent can be given and the measurement repeated to determine if there is improvement. A ventricular function diagram can also be calculated using the shape of an indicator dilution curve and relating this to ventricular work. Ventricular work is simply the product of stroke volume and arterial pressure. Ventricular contractility can also be expressed in terms of the ejection fraction, velocity of maximal shortening of cardiac muscle (V max), velocity of circumferential muscle shortening (Vcf), pre-ejection period/left ventricular ejection time (PEP/LVET), and the first derivative of the maximal rate of pressure rise in the left ventricle divided by the intraventricular pressure at that point (dP/dt/iP). Ejection fraction is the ratio of stroke volume to end-diastolic volume of the ventricle or the fraction of ventricular volume that is ejected with each beat. It can be measured with contrast angiography, echocardiography, and gated blood-pool imaging with a scintillation camera. None of these methods is easily applied in the intensive care unit. The V max is the velocity of maximal shortening of the contractile elements of cardiac muscle, but it is not independent of preload and afterload. Vcf can be obtained from analysis of the echocardiogram.

Systolic time indices such as the PEP/LVET ratio can be recorded using transducers for heart sounds, carotid pulse contours, and the ECG. The dP/dt is a good measure of contractility, but it requires a catheter-tip pressure transducer in the left ventricle, which is not satisfactory for intensive care monitoring. Function curves can also be developed for the right ventricle. The Frank–Starling mechanism is important, but the original concept and ventricular function curves related stroke work to diastolic volume. Since this cannot be measured in the intensive care unit with ease, we have had to substitute the wedge or filling pressure. This can distort our interpretation of ventricular contractility because it does not consider ventricular compliance or the effect of the state of one ventricle on the other. This is particularly true with respiratory failure, pulmonary hypertension, and reduced coronary blood flow to the right ventricle.

Alterations in contractility by myocardial infarction, ventricular aneurysms, and various forms of myocardiopathy are fairly well understood. The nonspecific depression of myocardial function that may occur with pancreatitis and other visceral diseases, sepsis such as peritonitis, or gram-negative septicemia such as with a septic abortion or after severe multisystem injury or prolonged illness, is not well understood. There have been many hypotheses and considerable evidence in experimental animals about etiologic factors involved in producing such changes. These involve the production of agents that circulate and damage the myocardium (Table 3-2). Depression of the myocardium has been found in late experimental hemorrhagic shock. Lefer and others have identified a myocardial depressant factor with experimental pancreatitis and other problems. A myocardial depressant material has also been found with experimental burns. Lysosomal enzymes from ischemic cells or leukocytes may act as primary toxins or may act upon plasma kinins (*e.g.*, bradykinin) and upon endotoxin. A cardiovascular toxic factor has also been implicated in producing myocardial depression in various situations. There is considerable difference of opinion as to the nature and significance of such substances. It has not been possible to identify them in humans, and there is little that can be done about such factors at the moment if they are present. Suffice it to say that myocardial depression may occur or develop in many seriously ill patients and must be treated appropriately by support of ventricular function.

Problems of afterload may occur in several circumstances. Decreased or low afterload or resistance is characteristic of neurogenic shock and septic shock. In certain patients with acute myocardial infarction, peripheral vascular resistance may not adjust to the decrease in cardiac output, resulting in hypotension. An acute increase in afterload can occur with aortic dissection or with cross-clamping the aorta during the treatment of an abdominal aortic aneurysm. This may result in ventricular dilatation and failure. In a damaged or depressed ventricle, even normal resistance may not be tolerated, and a reduction in afterload may be necessary for optimal ventricular performance. The corollary of this is that normal preload may also be inadequate for the abnormal ventricle. A bad ventricle may require a higher preload and a lower afterload to maintain an adequate cardiac output. Excessive afterload is a major problem for the right ventricle in pulmonary embolism.

Problems with heart rate occur at the extremes of bradycardia or tachycardia. Cardiac output will decrease at a heart rate below 60 except in trained athletes with a large stroke volume. At heart rates above 160/min, and certainly at 180/min, there is inadequate time for diastolic filling, and stroke volume and cardiac output will fall.

Once the circulation becomes inadequate, the chain of events in attempted compensation for decreased blood flow and pressure and the effects on organ function, metabolism and cellular events are similar to those with hypovolemic shock.

CLINICAL AND HEMODYNAMIC PICTURE

The clinical features of cardiogenic shock are similar to those of hypovolemia *with the exception of increased venous pressure.* This major differential point is critical in treatment. Although there may be evidence clinically of distended veins, it can escape notice unless looked for. Measurement of right atrial pressure and pulmonary wedge (left atrial) pressures is necessary. Blood pressure will be low (80 to 90 torr or less), cardiac output low (1.5 to 2.0 L/M²/min), and venous pressures, RA 8 to 10 cm H_2O and PCWP 15 to 18 cm H_2O. Initially venous pressures may not be high, but they will go up rapidly if fluid is given. Peripheral vascular resistance may be normal or increased. A cardiogenic problem may also be associated with or produce pulmonary problems leading to congestive heart failure, or pulmonary edema with dyspnea, rales, and radiographic findings of pulmonary congestion. Often the presenting symptoms of the patient with a cardiogenic problem, such as precordial chest pain, back pain, and other complaints, will suggest the cause of the problem.

TREATMENT

Proper therapy requires identification of the heart or pump as the problem, usually by the finding of a high or rising venous pressure in the face of inadequate arterial circulation or perfusion. Initial monitoring and measurement of cardiovascular function should provide this definition. It is critical to be certain that there is no volume deficit. Of even greater importance is to determine whether the patient and the circulation will improve if more fluid is given. Thus, a cautious trial of intravenous Ringer's lactate or saline solution even with an acute myocardial infarction may be helpful. If such a patient has been receiving diuretics previously with salt restriction, blood and extracellular fluid (ECF) volume may be low. Next, it is critical to determine that there is not a mechanical problem such as pericardial tamponade, which would require pericardiocentesis, or pulmonary embolism in the postoperative patient. If the problem is due to myocardial failure, then infusion of an inotropic agent is indicated. The branching logic of treatment is shown in Table 3-8. The vasoactive agents are listed in

TABLE 3-8   TREATMENT OF CARDIOGENIC SHOCK

1. Instrumentation and monitoring as with hypovolemic shock
2. Measure of right and left ventricular filling pressures (CVP–PAWP) to be certain there is no volume deficit.
3. Twelve-lead ECG for ischemia, infarction, etc.; chest x-ray, ventilation-perfusion lung scan, pulmonary arteriogram or other diagnostic studies.
4.

a. Begin intravenous infusion of an inotropic agent—dopamine, epinephrine, isoproterenol, etc.	b. Correct bradycardia by isoproterenol or pacemaker, and tachyarrhythmias by digitalis, lidocaine, cardioversion.	c. Reduce the afterload on the left ventricle by nitroglycerine paste, sodium nitroprusside or intra-aortic balloon pumping.	d. Reduce the afterload on the right ventricle by pulmonary embolectomy (after No. 6), supplementary oxygen, or ventilatory assistance	e. Ultrasound of the heart and/or diagnostic-therapeutic pericardiocentesis

5. Give a diuretic—furosemide, ethacrynic acid—if urine output is not adequate.
6. Adjunctive measures—supplementary oxygen or ventilatory assistance, correction of acidosis.
7. If there is a response to inotropic agents, give a rapid-acting digitalis preparation.
8. Consider coronary arteriography and/or cardiac catheterization and emergency value of coronary bypass procedure.

Tables 3-2 and 3-9. For rapid improvement in ventricular contractility, agents such as isoproterenol, dopamine, dobutamine, or epinephrine are preferred. Rapid acting digitalis preparations may be given, but 20 min is required for an initial effect, and several hours may be required for maximal effect.

Inotropic Agents

Digitalis compounds are important drugs when there is need for a prolonged increase in contractility. In acute situations with shock, however, it is better to use an agent that acts more rapidly and can easily be titrated intravenously. Following this, digitalis can be given and the intravenous agent discontinued. It takes some time for even the rapid-acting digitalis drugs to have an effect, and they also have a narrow therapeutic/toxic ratio. If the degree of circulatory depression is not so acute, then digoxin is the most appropriate drug.

Isoproterenol is rapid acting and has a potent inotropic effect on the heart. It increases heart rate as well. Peripheral resistance is decreased. Since myocardial oxygen consumption is determined by the heart rate, preload, contractility and afterload, and since isoproterenol increases two of these factors, there has been concern by some with its use when there is myocardial ischemia or infarction. If heart rate is increased above 130/min by this drug, it may be less effective. It is, however, a very useful agent when a primary inotropic effect with some decrease in resistance is desired. It is particularly helpful when the heart rate is not rapid.

Epinephrine can be quite helpful to provide an inotropic effect and also some increase in peripheral resistance. It has been used primarily by cardiac surgeons because of its potent effect on the ventricles. It does increase ventricular irritability and should be used with caution if there are frequent premature ventricular contractions.

Dopamine has been the most popular drug when an inotropic effect is needed but no increase in peripheral vascular resistance is desired. It has a specific effect on vascular (dopamine) receptors in the kidneys, and perhaps elsewhere as well, with a decrease in resistance. For this reason, it has been preferred in situations where decreased renal blood flow and renal failure could be a problem. It has been an extremely useful agent with few harmful side effects.

Dobutamine is similar to dopamine but with less chronotropic effect. It may be helpful in circumstances in which dopamine is not effective.

Glucagon has an inotropic effect, but it is weak and has many side effects. It may be useful with a beta-blockade from propranolol overdose.

Vasoconstrictor–Alpha Drugs

There is little place for these agents in the treatment of any form of shock, and particularly cardiogenic shock. They may be necessary with neurogenic shock when resistance must be increased and during resuscitation from cardiac arrest. The other situation in which they might be used for a brief period of time is to increase blood pressure above dangerous levels in an emergency while resuscitation and diagnosis can be carried out. If a mild increase in resistance with minimal side effects is desired, the drug of choice is neosynephrine. In contrast to norepinephrine, neosynephrine can be infused for a number of days in humans with little organ or tissue ischemia. In the past, low doses of norepinephrine were used for shock with myocardial infarction; now, dopamine is preferred.

Alpha Blocking Agents

There was a time when persistent vasoconstriction and catecholamine effects were thought to be part of the progressive pathophysiology of shock. Although this may indeed be a problem, it is reduced blood flow rather than increased resistance that is the problem. For this reason, there is little to be gained by the use of an alpha blocking agent other than for certain specific purposes. Phenoxybenzamine should not be used because it produces prolonged (24 hr) and irreversible blockade. A newer agent, Thymoxamine, however, is a competitive alpha blocker that can be given intravenously and its effects titrated. It has been shown to be quite effective in reducing afterload and increasing cardiac output after cardiac surgery.

Beta Blocking Agents

The major compound in this category, propranolol, is quite helpful for certain arrhythmias and for angina pectoris. There is no particular place for its use with cardiogenic shock.

Afterload Reduction

The major place for this treatment is in a patient with a high filling pressure (PAWP 18 cm saline), a low cardiac

TABLE 3-9   OTHER CIRCULATORY AND VASOACTIVE AGENTS

AGENT	DOSAGE
Digitalislike Compounds	
Digoxin (Lanoxin)	0.5–0.7 mg IV initially; 0.5 mg. in ½ hr–4 hr followed by 0.3–0.5 mg in 2 hr–4 hr (total 1.5 mg). Initial effect in 5 min–30 min, maximum effect in 1.5 hr–3 hr
Digitoxin	Initial effect in 30 min–120 min, maximum effect in 4 hr–8 hr
Ouabain	Same as digoxin
Deslanoside (Cedilanid-D)	Same as digoxin
Amrinone	Investigational drug, not recommended as yet
Afterload-Reduction	
Ganglionic blocking agents	Trimethaphan camsylate (Arfonad)—500 mg in 500 ml IV drip
Nitroglycerine	2% ointment on 2.5 cm–5 cm of skin
Sodium nitroprusside (Nipride)	50 mg in 500 ml—give 0.1–3 μg/kg/min
Antiarrhythmic Agents	
Digitalis	See above
Class I—interferes with depolarization of the muscle	
Lidocaine	1–2 mg/kg as a bolus IV followed by 20–50 μg/Kg/min infusion
Procainamide	100 mg IV in 1 min; repeat every 5 min as needed
Diphenylhydantoin (Phenytoin)	As with procainamide
Quinidine	Best given orally
Class II—antisympathetic activity, block or interference	
Propranolol (Inderal)	0.5 mg–0.1 mg IV every 3 min–5 min as needed
Bretylium	5 mg/kg IM or 5–10 mg/kg IV over 10 min–20 min
Class III—prolongs the action potential	
Amiodarone	
Class IV—calcium channel blockers	
Verapamil	10 mg IV bolus

output, and an arterial pressure that is fairly well maintained or not very low. This type of situation is still considered shock because blood flow is low and organ function may be affected due to ischemia of the kidneys, gastrointestinal tract, and liver. The best agent in such a situation is sodium nitroprusside, which has a balanced effect on both the arterial and venous systems. In contrast, nitroglycerin dilates primarily the venous capacitance vessels and the ganglionic blockers dilate primarily the arterioles. Intravenous nitroprusside is rapid-acting. Its side effects include hypotension due to excessive reduction in afterload, decreased cardiac output due to excessive reduction in preload, increase in pulmonary shunt, platelet malfunction, and cyanide and thiocyanate toxicity. These can be avoided by administering low doses and by careful titration. When afterload reduction with nitroprusside is used appropriately, there should be an increase in cardiac output, a reduction in venous pressure, and little change or improvement in arterial pressure.

Afterload reduction and diastolic augmentation can be achieved by the use of the *intra-aortic balloon and pump.* This approach should be considered when myocardial ischemia is a factor. The balloon pump will augment myocardial perfusion by increasing aortic diastolic pressure, and by facilitating left ventricular emptying it will decrease left ventricular diastolic pressure. This reduces myocardial oxygen requirements. This instrument has been very effective in patients before and after cardiac operations and in other patients with abdominal problems or sepsis when myocardial function has been a limitation.

Antiarrhythmic Agents

The most useful agent for most arrhythmias, particularly for the ventricular tachyarrhythmias, is lidocaine. It is given by an initial intravenous bolus injection followed by a continuous infusion. For atrial fibrillation, digoxin is the drug of choice with cardioversion used as needed. The other agents may be helpful in particular circumstances.

Combination of Drugs

To obtain the inotropic effects of norepinephrine but decrease or eliminate its strong alpha-vasoconstrictive action, this drug has been used with the alpha blocking agent phentolamine. Dopamine and sodium nitroprusside have also been used together. However, the same effects may be achieved by isoproterenol alone.

All of the catecholamines produce ventricular irritability through an excitatory effect of increasing automaticity and must be used with caution. If isoproterenol produces ventricular premature beats or incipient ventricular tachycardia, the addition of 20 mEq to 40 mEq of potassium to the infusion should eliminate this problem.

Other aspects of treatment are provided in Table 3-8. The pain of myocardial infarction must be treated by appropriate narcotics. Heparin may be helpful in reducing the problem of later pulmonary embolism. Drug therapy must be adjusted for the particular patient, and careful hemodynamic observation of responses to the drugs is essential. There is no single best drug for all circumstances, and trials of response must be carried out.

PREVENTION OF CARDIOGENIC SHOCK

In surgical patients with urgent problems requiring an operation and in elective operations, study of the patient's circulation and cardiovascular reserve is necessary. Control of hypertension, by reduction in afterload, improvement in ventricular performance if marginal by elective digitalization, reduction in high preload or congestive failure, control of or maintenance of normal rate and rhythm, and careful maintenance of oxygenation during the operation may make the difference in survival of a patient with a limited cardiovascular system or a previous myocardial infarction. Prospective consideration of these factors can be lifesaving.

NEUROGENIC SHOCK

A decrease in peripheral vascular resistance can be sudden and brief, as in fainting (syncope), or can persist due to the effects of an anesthetic agent or a central nervous system injury. With a spinal anesthetic, there is decreased vascular tone from the level of the anesthetic downward. This may not cause overt changes in the patient's hemodynamic status due to adjustments in the circulation elsewhere. A modest decrease in blood pressure may be well tolerated. If the decrease is excessive, then a drug such as Vasoxyl is used. Most anesthetic agents are associated with some decrease in blood pressure. An alteration in cardiac output is probably due to a cardiac depressant effect.

Central nervous system injury, and particularly a spinal cord injury, will reduce vascular tone from loss of sympathetic innervation. The individual may be able to compensate for this or a vasoconstrictive agent may be necessary. These forms of shock are usually not a serious problem and perhaps should not be classified as shock because they do not produce long-term depression of the circulation and other effects on organ function unless they are not corrected. The clinical picture of neurogenic shock is also quite different. Usually the pulse rate is slow, and the patient appears warm and dry. With the milder forms of neurogenic collapse, simply placing the patient supine and elevating the legs for a short time may be sufficient. If neurogenic shock, such as occurs with spinal cord injury, occurs with severe generalized trauma, then careful monitoring, resuscitation, and treatment are required, recognizing that there will be blood and fluid loss along with decreased vascular resistance and tone. Generally in such circumstances, increasing vascular volume and even overexpansion is more physiologic than use of vasoconstrictor agents. Problems such as acute gastric dilatation can also produce a form of neurogenic shock.

CARDIAC ARREST

HISTORICAL BACKGROUND

Cardiac arrest is the final common pathway for death from any cause, but the emphasis here is on cessation of cardiac contractions in a person who does not have an otherwise fatal illness or injury. This distinction, however, may be difficult to make in an emergency situation when cessation of cardiopulmonary function can be on one hand simply the definition of death, or on the other, is a potentially reversible event. The term *cardiac arrest* implies that the heart has stopped with no mechanical or electrical activity; ventricular fibrillation without contractions is considered a form of cardiac arrest. A third category is that of ineffective ventricular contractions with no evident cardiac output. Arrest of the circulation may follow ventilatory failure or if occurring initially will rapidly produce respiratory arrest. Thus, the term *cardiopulmonary arrest* is more accurate. For this reason, the team and programs for resuscitation use the term: *cardiopulmonary resuscitation* (CPR).

Elisha made the first attempt at resuscitation to improve or stimulate ventilation in a newborn Shunemite child in the eighth century B.C. As early as 1543, Vesalius resuscitated the quiescent hearts of pigs and dogs by blowing into the trachea and moving the lungs. Artificial respiration by the prone-pressure method was introduced by Schafer in 1904. This method, known as the Sharpey–Schafer method, was in vogue for over 40 years. Comroe and Dripps in 1946 questioned its effectiveness and began a return to mouth-to-mouth resuscitation. The superiority of this method was firmly established by the report of Gordon and co-workers in 1958.

Cardiac arrest was not recognized until the introduction of chloroform as a general anesthetic. The first recorded occurrence was in 1848 in a girl receiving chloroform anesthesia for removal of a toenail. A report of successful resuscitation using the closed chest technique was first provided by Konig in 1883.

Frequent problems with chloroform led to studies by Mickwitz, and reported by Boehm, in 1878 on external cardiac compression of cats asphyxiated by chloroform. Schiff carried out experiments using the open chest method and wrote in 1893, "If the thorax is opened and at the same time air is insufflated into the lungs, by rhythmical compression of the heart with the hands it is possible to reestablish the heartbeat even up to a period of eleven and one-half minutes after the stoppage of that organ." Direct massage after thoracotomy was first used successfully in humans by Igelsrud in 1901, and Lane was able to resuscitate a patient successfully by massage of the heart through the diaphragm. Hovard used compression of the thorax for resuscitation but abandoned it because of breaking several ribs. His assistant Maas, however, used the method successfully in two patients in 1891 with chloroform arrest.

The problem of ventricular fibrillation was more difficult. The demonstration by Prevost and Batelli in 1889 of defibrillation by countershock in an animal was not used successfully in humans until Beck used an internal-type alternating current defibrillator in 1946. The internal defibrillator had been developed by Hooker, Kouvenhoven, and Langworthy some years earlier. The external defibrillator was first used successfully by Zoll in 1956. The combination of external cardiac massage and external defibrillation was then established by Kouvenhoven, Jude, and Knickerbocker in 1960.

PATHOGENESIS

ETIOLOGY

A wide variety of factors, singly or together, may produce circulatory arrest. Etiologic agents, some proven and some hypothesized, are listed below. They are divided into three categories: those that are most likely to produce asystole, those that produce ventricular fibrillation, and those that lead to such a profound reduction in cardiac output that it cannot be distinguished from circulatory standstill. In most instances of cardiac arrest, the circumstances do not allow exact documentation of the cause of the arrest; thus, some of the information is speculative and many of the initiating mechanisms can produce either asystole or fibrillation.

Causes of Asystole

Hypoxemia. Most cardiac arrests are probably triggered by insidious hypoxemia. Blood gas determinations in postoperative patients have shown that critically low levels of arterial blood oxygen tension (PaO_2 less than 40 torr) can occur without clinical evidence of cyanosis or other abnormalities. Progressive bradycardia usually precedes total arrest, especially in infants and children. The degree of hypoxia tolerated without apparent effect on cardiac function varies considerably from one person to another. This suggests that other factors may play a role in the action of hypoxemia on the heart.

Acidosis. Metabolic acidosis is an early consequence of shock or cardiac arrest; there is considerable doubt about its being a primary causative factor. Severe acidosis with a *p*H below 7.1 has been demonstrated to impair myocardial contractility only slightly. Acidosis is a factor in producing hyperkalemia, however, which does induce cardiac arrest.

Hyperkalemia. A high concentration of extracellular potassium causes cardiac arrest in diastole at levels of 7 mEq/liter to 10 mEq/liter. Deliberate cardioplegia for cardiac surgery is frequently induced with this mechanism. With hyperkalemia, the action potential is shortened, conduction is slowed, and the QRS complex is prolonged. Potassium toxicity is commonly encountered in cases of renal insufficiency, severe burns, shock, diabetic acidosis, adrenal insufficiency, and an excessive rate of potassium infusion. Hyperkalemia can be induced by succinylcholine, particularly in patients with major injuries or burns.

Vagal Stimulation. The possibility that a "vasovagal reflex" may produce a cardiac arrest is somewhat controversial. Vagal stimuli can suppress sinus node rhythmicity and atrioventricular nodal conduction. This reflex can be satisfactorily blocked with atropine. Cardiac arrests have occurred in association with endotracheal intubation, extubation, bronchoscopy, endotracheal suctioning, rectal examination, prostate massage, testicular trauma, operations on the eye, and fright. The infrequency of cardiac arrest with these common stimuli casts some doubt on their significance as the sole causative mechanism. A second factor, such as myocardial ischemia or hypoxemia, may be necessary before ventricular fibrillation or prolonged asystole occurs. Many of the above procedures (*e.g.,* endotracheal suctioning) are now known to be associated on occasion with severe hypoxemia.

Stokes–Adams Attacks. The sudden onset of third-degree heart block results in asystole followed by ventricular fibrillation or by a slow idioventricular rhythm. Asystole is classically a transient happening and is followed by a return of consciousness. However, either ventricular fibrillation or prolonged asystole may cause fatal brain or myocardial injury. Autopsy studies of such patients have shown some fibrosis in and around the conduction system, but this is not a reliable basis on which to make a diagnosis of third-degree heart block as a cause of death. The conduction and rhythm abnormalities occurring in patients monitored in hospitals indicate that such problems are not infrequent.

Jaundice and Biliary Tract Surgery. These operations are thought to be associated with a higher incidence of cardiac arrest through increased vagal tone. However, this complication is not common, and documentation of its frequency is not available.

Coronary Insufficiency. A decrease in myocardial perfusion or an increase in myocardial oxygen requirement that cannot be met because of coronary artery disease may produce arrest after coronary thrombosis, embolization, hypotension, or pericardial tamponade on one hand or acute hypertension and tachycardia on the other. Ischemia due to coronary artery disease is not uniform throughout the myocardium. Thus, ventricular fibrillation is more likely to occur with ischemia than is asystole. However, asystole can result from a major infarction with heart block or ischemic depression of the sinus node.

Causes of Ventricular Fibrillation

Idiopathic Ventricular Arrhythmias. This is probably the most common cause of sudden death and may account for the majority of deaths due to coronary occlusive disease. Autopsies of patients who die suddenly without premonitory symptoms during normal activity or rest usually show varying degrees of coronary atherosclerosis. Although this provides some explanation for the death, there are often no acute changes, thrombotic occlusions, or infarctions. Thus an ischemic etiology can only be inferred.

Anesthetic Agents. Although some anesthetic agents are associated with cardiac arrhythmias, this is an infrequent occurrence. Cardiac arrests occur more frequently during the induction of an anesthetic when other factors such as hypoxemia and circulatory changes may occur. Arrhythmias are less frequent during the course of an operation unless there are complications of the procedure.

Hypothermia. Exposure to cold and immersion are associated with depression of vital functions. Respiratory arrest may occur before cardiac arrest. When massive blood transfusions are needed, core temperature may be reduced significantly if the blood is not warmed and can result in ventricular fibrillation or bradycardia and asystole. External total body hypothermia was used in the past and was on occasion associated with ventricular fibrillation at body temperatures below 27° C. Hypothermia produced by cardiopulmonary bypass more often produces bradycardia and asystole at temperatures of 26° C down to 20° C.

Catecholamines. These drugs, due to their beta-stimulating effect on the heart, stimulate the sinus node and increase conduction and ventricular automaticity. There is a wide range of dose responses in different patients and in different conditions of cardiac hypoxia and strain. Although toxicity may lead to fibrillation, these drugs may also be necessary in resuscitation.

Digitalis. Digitalis intoxication probably accounts for a number of deaths due to arrhythmias, usually from ventricular fibrillation. Although digitalis toxicity may occur with an excess dose, it is most often due to a change in the patient which alters his susceptibility. Toxic effects are increased by myocardial hypoxia or ischemia, by hypokalemia, hypomagnesemia and hypercalcemia and by reduction in renal loss of the drug such as when creatinine clearance is reduced. Measurement of blood levels does not indicate sensitivity. Electrical defibrillation during digitalis toxicity is difficult and will require correction of electrolyte imbalance and suppression of myocardial irritability with drugs.

Electric Shock. This may occur with fibrillation from electrocution in normal individuals or can occur in hospitals and operating rooms if great caution is not used in grounding, preventing current leaks, and with other electrical hazards.

Trauma. Penetrating and blunt trauma can lead to cardiac arrest or fibrillation. A severe myocardial contusion can produce arrhythmias.

Profound Shock

A massive myocardial infarction, pulmonary embolism, or hemorrhage from a major artery or ventricular wound, pericardial tamponade, and other overwhelming insults may result in no perceptible cardiac output or inadequate ventricular function that cannot open the aortic valve even though there is continued electrocardiographic activity. This must be treated in the same way as cardiac arrest, along with correction of the underlying problem.

PATHOPHYSIOLOGY AFTER CARDIAC ARREST

The effects of circulatory arrest on organs and cells are both time and temperature dependent. These events are similar to those described previously with shock except that they occur rapidly. Tissue anoxia leads to anaerobic metabolism, acidosis, changes in membrane function, and then to cell death. The metabolic needs of organs and the characteristics of their circulation determine their sensitivity to ischemia and anoxia. The cells of the cerebral cortex seem to be most sensitive with irreversible damage occurring in perhaps 4 to 10 min. One of the problems after cardiac arrest, however, is that when the circulation is restored, the blood flow to an organ such as the brain may not be normal immediately. Cell swelling in the microcirculation and other changes may produce a period of continuing ischemia. There is some evidence that this is true with the brain and the kidney. If blood flow could be returned immediately to normal, the brain could perhaps tolerate no circulation for a longer time. After the brain, the most sensitive tissues are the renal tubules, the gastrointestinal mucosa, liver cells, and the myocardium. Skeletal muscle, fat, skin and bone can tolerate ischemia for some hours. Anything that can be done to decrease the metabolic requirements of an organ, such as hypothermia, will increase the tolerance to anoxia and ischemia. Because of wide variations in susceptibility—related to cell type, metabolic activity, residual blood flow, and priority of restored blood flow—it is not possible to define or predict prospectively the potential reversibility of the anoxic period. If resuscitation of the heart and ventilation are successful and a good circulation and spontaneous ventilation are restored, frequently there will not have been irreversible damage to other systems or to the brain. Occasionally a patient who is successfully resuscitated remains unresponsive with a severe neurologic deficit. Frequently these patients will have other problems and will not survive for more than a few days. Thus, the thought of a potential decerebrate survivor should not curtail resuscitative efforts.

RESUSCITATION

Recognition and correction of the cause of the arrest are critical for successful resuscitation. Frequently, however, this mechanism is not known, and it is hoped that the resuscitative measures will correct the cause (such as hypoxemia, ventricular irritability, acidosis and hyperkalemia, and conduction defects). When myocardial or respiratory insufficiency is obviously progressive and cannot be reversed by intensive therapy, then cardiac arrest is inevitable and resuscitation at best would be only temporary. To apply the full battery of resuscitative efforts in such circumstances is inhumane and wasteful.

The standard procedures for resuscitation of a patient, other than in an intensive care area, are now well known and widely used even by laymen. Therefore, surgeons must be thoroughly familiar with these techniques, knowledgeable about the timing and priority of their application, and able to teach them to others. Briefly, these principles include the following:

1. Positioning the Patient
   Place the patient in a supine position with solid support beneath his chest and with additional support under his shoulders to allow hyperextension of the neck. It may be necessary to place a board under the patient or move him to the floor.
2. Establishing an Airway
   Establish an airway into the trachea and begin ventilation. Endotracheal intubation is the most effective measure to achieve this objective; when unavailable, the next best is an oropharyngeal tube and anterior displacement of the mandible to keep the tongue from occluding the pharynx. Mouth-to-mouth breathing while holding the patient's nose is employed if mechanical methods are unavailable (Fig. 3-8). Other airways may be used if available. An esophageal obturator airway has been helpful for use by individuals who are not trained in endotracheal intubation (Fig. 3-9). This tube has a blunt tip and can be inserted easily. A balloon prevents aspiration from the stomach and ventilation is possible.
3. Cardiac Compression
   Cardiac compression is necessary to restore circulation and cardiac function. A sharp blow to the chest after a brief period of asystole can be effective. As this is done, access to the circulation must be obtained as was described in the previous section on shock.

EXTERNAL CARDIOPULMONARY RESUSCITATION (EXTERNAL COMPRESSION OR MASSAGE)

The technique of applying arm and shoulder pressure through the "heel" of the left hand (covered by the right hand) to the lower sternum (Fig. 3-10) is usually effective, providing a modest cardiac output. However, experience with patients whose intra-arterial pressure is monitored reveals that subtle variations in location and velocity of the compression impulse can result in considerable change in the pressure generated. The most effective motion is a rapid compression of the anterior chest wall toward the spine and a quick release. It should be possible to do this without breaking ribs. After every three or four chest or cardiac compressions (at the rate of 60 to 80/min), the lungs should be quickly inflated and then massage resumed. With an endotracheal tube in place, both can be done simultaneously. Cardiac outputs have been measured in the range of 1 to 2 liters/min which is only marginal at best. The femoral artery pulse should be monitored by palpation during cardiac compression until an indwelling arterial cannula has been introduced. Because of the absence of valves between the femoral vein and tricuspid valve, large venous pulses from external compression may give a false impression of an effective arterial pulse. External compression has been facilitated by a variety of mechanical devices supplanting the human hand. These include a hand driven lever and a

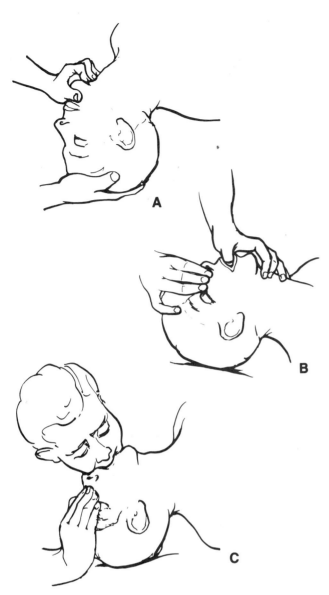

Fig. 3-8. For mouth-to-mouth ventilation, the head is tilted back (*A*), the nose is occluded with one hand, the mouth opened, and the tongue and mandible held forward with the thumb and other hand (*B*). The mouth and finger are covered with the mouth of the resuscitator, who provides forceful ventilation (*C*).

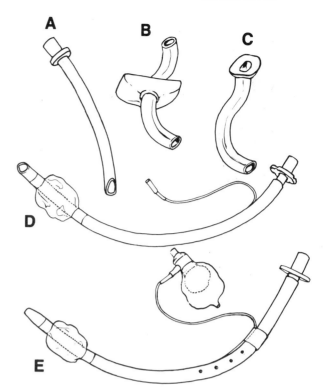

Fig. 3-9. Tubes helpful for providing an airway and ventilation include (*A*) nasopharyngeal tube, (*B*) Safar oropharyngeal tube for mouth-to-mouth ventilation, (*C*) oropharyngeal tube, (*D*) endotracheal tube, (*E*) esophageal airway with balloon to prevent gastric aspiration.

pneumatically driven compressor, each supported in a frame over the patient's chest. These have not been helpful enough to merit continued use.

In some patients with asystolic arrest, cardiovascular function may be restored by these measures alone. Therefore, drugs should not be given immediately. When circulatory arrest occurs suddenly and is recognized instantly, it is reasonable and not infrequently effective to carry out immediate defibrillation (or cardiac stimulation) even before electrocardiographic identification of the arrhythmia. A brisk blow to the precordium with the ulnar side of the hand followed by external "blind defibrillation" is worthwhile before expending valuable time on ventilation, cardiac massage, or drug treatment. The effects of hypoxia accumulate rapidly, however, and after several minutes oxygenation must be provided and acidosis corrected before electrical depolarization can be achieved.

OPEN-CHEST CARDIAC MASSAGE (INTERNAL COMPRESSION)

Effective cardiopulmonary resuscitation by external massage, defibrillation, and ventilation has been a major advance in the care of patients and has brought these techniques to the home, highway, and emergency vehicle. It has also eliminated attempts to carry out a thoracotomy in surroundings without capability for such an effort. There are still circumstances, however, when a direct approach to the heart is needed and when closed chest resuscitation is likely to be ineffective and should be abandoned in favor of opening the chest. These include

1. Failure to respond to closed-chest resuscitation if the patient is potentially viable and the support is available to open the chest
2. Pericardial tamponade
3. A flail chest
4. Chest-wall deformity so that effective massage is not possible
5. An open pericardium after cardiac surgery
6. A cardiac injury
7. Severe valvular disease—mitral or aortic stenosis
8. Refractory ventricular fibrillation.

The advantages of open-chest resuscitation are that a better cardiac output can be achieved, direct visualization of myocardial performance is possible, coronary perfusion can be augmented by temporary narrowing of the ascending or descending aorta, drugs can be injected directly into the heart, defibrillation is more effective, and ventilation can be continued more effectively along with cardiac massage.

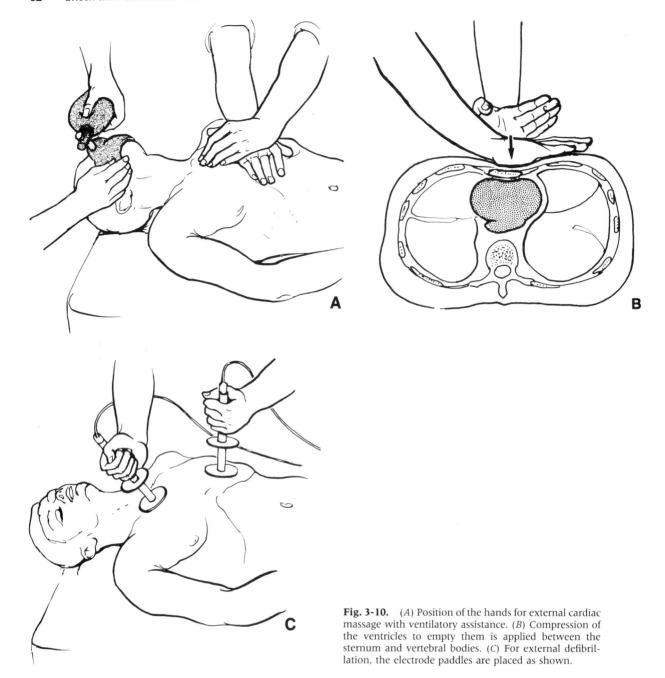

Fig. 3-10. (*A*) Position of the hands for external cardiac massage with ventilatory assistance. (*B*) Compression of the ventricles to empty them is applied between the sternum and vertebral bodies. (*C*) For external defibrillation, the electrode paddles are placed as shown.

If there has been a previous thoracic incision, it is reopened. Otherwise, an incision is made in the anterior chest just below the breast, and the chest is then opened through the fourth interspace. The fifth interspace is a bit low. The incision must be long enough to allow insertion of the hand easily and without compression of the wrist. As soon as the chest is opened, a few compressions of the ventricles through the intact pericardium should be attempted along with one attempt at internal defibrillation. If this is not immediately successful, the pericardium is opened anteriorly avoiding injury to the phrenic nerve. For optimal manual compression, the fingers are placed around the left ventricle and compression is carried out by the fingers squeezing the heart against the length of the thumb and thenar eminence. The tip of the thumb should not dig into the heart or it will perforate the ventricle or atrium. A rapid compression will give the best output. The compression

should be similar to squeezing a rubber bulb held in the palm of the hand with an attempt to squirt fluid from the bulb as high and forcefully as possible. A chest retractor will be helpful.

DEFIBRILLATION

The multifocal activity of ventricular fibrillation or ventricular tachycardia requires complete electrical depolarization to allow a conducted atrial impulse (or an idioventricular impulse) to initiate a normal coordinated contraction. The safest and most effective current to achieve that objective is a very brief high-voltage direct-current impulse applied either directly to the epicardial surface through concave disc electrodes 5 cm to 6 cm in diameter (2 cm to 3 cm in diameter for infants) or through the chest wall with larger (7 cm) flat electrodes. Most defibrillators deliver a discharge current from a condenser that can be battery-primed and, therefore, are potentially portable. Discharge currents required to defibrillate range from 10 to 200 watt-seconds for direct epicardial application or 100 to 500 watt-seconds for external application, depending on the size of the heart, the degree of damage, and the state of relative ischemia. Unsuccessful defibrillatory attempts may be due to a current that is too weak to complete the depolarization of a large ventricle. Defibrillators that deliver a maximum of 60-watt-seconds to internal electrodes are inadequate for a large heart.

Some degree of irreversible myocardial damage (largely from generated heat) may occur with each electric shock; thus, repeated attempts to defibrillate should be spaced with adequate time for heat dispersion and should be accompanied by other measures to reduce myocardial irritability. Restoration of relatively normal myocardial temperature and perfusion should precede attempts at electrical defibrillation for an optimal response. In the presence of irreversible myocardial ischemia or damage, intractable ventricular fibrillation may be encountered, but persistent efforts are justified. Successful defibrillation and ultimate survival has been achieved after 100 to 300 shocks for recurrent fibrillation over periods of several hours or days. A patient who develops ventricular fibrillation secondary to the ischemia and depressed cardiac ouput of severe bradycardia may require a pacemaker rather than chronotropic drugs.

DRUG THERAPY

Drug therapy is frequently necessary to improve the circulation if cardiac action is restored, to increase cardiac excitability if asystole persists, to improve ventricular function, to correct arrhythmias, and to counteract the metabolic effects of the arrest. Thus, a number of agents may be necessary including alkali, catecholamines, cardiotonic agents, and antiarrhythmic agents. Severe metabolic acidosis causes decreased myocardial contractility, depressed response to catecholamines, and increased difficulty in defibrillating the heart. Acidosis should be neutralized with alkali in the form of sodium bicarbonate. Sodium bicarbonate should be administered at the rate of 0.5 mEq/kg to 1.0 mEq/kg every 10 min of circulatory arrest, until an arterial sample can be obtained to measure the *p*H.

Lidocaine is the drug of choice for decreasing ventricular irritability resulting either from increased automaticity or from reentry mechanisms. Bolus doses of 1 mg per kg, repeated 3 to 4 times at 5 to 10 min intervals, will decrease the tendency to recurrent fibrillation and may enhance electrical defibrillation. This agent will not significantly increase the degree of atrioventricular block, but may suppress the ventricular escape mechanism. Lidocaine has minimal depressant effect on circulatory dynamics and its only side effect is neuromuscular seizures, which may interfere with effective ventilation of the patient. Parenteral quinidine and procaine amide produce hypotension and should be avoided if possible. Parenteral propranolol may cause marked depression of myocardial contractility. If ventricular irritability is due to digitalis toxicity, lidocaine therapy should be accompanied by administration of potassium. Potassium must be administered slowly, since potassium in high concentrations in the coronary circulation may itself produce asystole. Furthermore, acidosis secondary to ischemia may shift potassium from cells into the circulation. Thus, even with depletion of total body potassium,

which is commonly found in patients on chronic digitalis and diuretic treatment, a potassium shift across the cell membrane can rapidly alter the extracellular potassium concentration. Laboratory measurements are essential.

Ventricular asystole or marked bradycardia will respond to pacemaker stimulation but transvenous electrode placement is time consuming. Transthoracic electrodes are useful, or, if a high-voltage pacemaker is available, skin electrodes may be adequate. Pacing methods are most effective when asystole is the primary event causing the arrest and are least effective when asystole is secondary to progressive deterioration of cardiac automaticity following prolonged ischemia. In the latter case, epinephrine or isoproterenol, combined with cardiac massage and ventilation, have a greater chance of restoring rhythm and contraction. These drugs may be administered into a cardiac chamber, preferably the left ventricle, using a long needle directed cranially from the fifth left intercostal space at the sternal edge. If some circulation appears to be present, catecholamines may be given in a central vein at a rate of one or more micrograms per minute. Norepinephrine or dopamine may be useful in supporting myocardial contractility when heart rate increase is undesirable. With restoration of a heartbeat, there is often a very low blood pressure initially due to massive vasodilatation after the arrest. Vasoconstriction by a drug such as norepinephrine may be critical to increasing coronary perfusion pressure and restoring an adequate circulation.

Calcium is a potent inotropic agent without a tendency to increase heart rate. Doses of 1 mg/kg may be given at 5 to 10 min intervals. It is particularly useful after massive transfusion with citrated blood, in which hypocalcemia may play a role in the arrest. Also, in potassium intoxication (renal failure, therapeutic error), calcium is the agent of choice for reversing the cardiac effects. Calcium given to a digitalized patient may enhance the glycoside toxicity.

COMPLICATIONS

Resuscitation following cardiac arrest in a well-equipped intensive care unit of a hospital is likely to be rapid, effective, and relatively free of complications. However, outside the hospital and even on ordinary hospital wards, the resuscitative process may be associated with some degree of haste, confusion, and inexpertise. A variety of complications have been encountered that may be prevented by training and experience.

Fracture or dislocation of costal cartilages, ribs or sternum may result from vigorous external compression. A brittle chest wall in an elderly person increases the risk. Operative fixation may be required if a flail chest, respiratory impairment, pain, or bone fragments jeopardize subsequent management. Laceration of the liver may occur, and pericardial tamponade can result from a lacerated or punctured coronary artery from a needle puncture. Myocardial contusion or laceration can result either from open manual compression or even from external compression. Aspiration and pneumonitis from vomitus or other oral contents, lacerations of the oropharynx and loss of teeth during intubation, infection from unsterile procedures, phrenic nerve injury, and burns from defibrillator electrodes can all occur.

RESULTS

Survival after cardiac arrest is dependent upon a number of factors including the location where the arrest occurs and the underlying problem of the patient. In hospitals, resuscitation teams were organized in the early 1960s. It is estimated that about 30% of deaths in hospital have cardiac resuscitation attempted and three fourths of all successful efforts occur in the emergency room or intensive care units. The overall rate of successful resuscitation in hospitals varies from 12% to 20%. The major problems in trying to increase this percentage are identifying two groups of patients, those at high risk of arrhythmias who require monitoring and those with terminal illness who should not be resuscitated. The survival rate from arrests occurring outside a hospital varies from 6% to 23%, depending on the area, patient selection and emergency service capability. The critical factors in survival are

1. Was the arrest witnessed? If so, resuscitation begins sooner.
2. The cardiac rhythm—ventricular fibrillation being much more favorable than asystole
3. CPR begun by a bystander
4. Speed—paramedic response time of less than 4 min

Those individuals with a favorable score according to these four criteria have a survival as high as 70%, as compared with 1% with unfavorable findings. Advanced life-support systems are also helpful. Providing this capability is expensive and the cost-benefit effectiveness of such programs is difficult to assess.

The status of the central nervous system is of critical importance in survival. Patients who have no pupil light or corneal reflex from 6 hr after CPR do not survive. In survivors, all reflexes have returned to normal within 48 hr.

BIBLIOGRAPHY

ALBRECHT M, CLOWES GHA: The increase of circulatory requirements in the presence of inflammation. Surgery 56:158, 1964

BARASH PG, KITAHATA LM, CHEN Y et al: The hemodynamic tracking system: An aid to data management and cardiovascular decision-making. Anesth Analg (Cleve) 59:169, 1980

BAUE AE: Multiple, progressive, or sequential systems failure. A syndrome of the 1970s. Arch Surg 110:779, 1975

BAUE AE: Metabolic abnormalities of shock. Surg Clin North Am 56:1059, 1976

BAUE AE, CHAUDRY IH: Prevention of multiple systems failure. Surg Clin North Am 60:1167, 1980

BAUE AE, TRAGUS ET, WOLFSON SK JR et al: Hemodynamic and metabolic effects of Ringer's lactate solution in hemorrhagic shock. Ann Surg 166:29, 1967

BECK CS, PRITCHARD WH, FEIL HS: Ventricular fibrillation of long duration abolished by electric shock. JAMA 135:985, 1947

BEECHER HK, SIMEONE FA, BURNETT CH et al: The internal state of the severely wounded man on entry to the most forward hospital. Surgery 22:672, 1947

BERGER RL, SAINI VK, LONG W et al: The use of diastolic augmentation with the intra-aortic balloon in human septic shock with associated coronary artery disease. Surgery 74:601, 1973

BLALOCK A: Experimental shock: Cause of low blood pressure produced by muscle injury. Arch Surg 22:959, 1930

BLALOCK A: Acute circulatory failure as exemplified by shock and hemorrhage. Surg Gynecol Obstet 58:551, 1934

BOISE E: The differential diagnosis of shock, hemorrhage and sepsis. Transactions of the American Association of Obstetrics 9:433, 1897

BORDEN CW, HALL WH: Fatal transfusion reactions from massive bacterial contamination of blood. N Engl J Med 245:760, 1951

BRAUNWALD E: On the difference between the heart's output and its contractile state. Circulation 43:1971, 1971

BURKE JF, PONTOPPIDAN H, WELCH CE: High output respiratory failure: An important cause of death ascribed to peritonitis or ileus. Ann Surg 158:581, 1963

CANNON WB: Traumatic Shock. New York, D Appleton Co, 1923

CHAUDRY IH, CLEMENS MG, BAUE AE: Alterations in cell function with ischemia and shock and their correction. Arch Surg 116:1309, 1981

CLOWES G, VUCINIC N, WEIDNER N: Circulatory and metabolic alterations associated with survival or death in peritonitis. Ann Surg 163:866, 1966

CLOWES GHA JR, ZUSCHNEID W, TURNER M et al: Observations on the pathogenesis of the pneumonitis associated with severe infections in other parts of the body. Ann Surg 167:630, 1968

COMROE JG, DRIPPS RD: Artificial respiration. JAMA 130:381, 1946

COOPER A: A Dictionary of Practical Surgery, 7th ed. London, Longmans Green & Co, 1938

COURNAND A, RILEY RL, BRADLEY SE et al: Studies of circulation in clinical shock. Surgery 13:964, 1943

CRILE GW: An Experimental Research Into Surgical Shock. Philadelphia, J B Lippincott, 1899

CROWELL JW, GUYTON AC: Evidence favoring a cardiac mechanism in irreversible hemorrhagic shock. Am J Physiol 201:893, 1961

CUNNINGHAM JN JR, SHIRES GT, WAGNER Y: Cellular transport defects in hemorrhagic shock. Surgery 70:215, 1971

DANIEL AM, WOOD CD, SHIZGAL HM et al: The metabolic utilization of protein and muscle glycogen in experimental shock. J Surg Res 26:663, 1979

DELGUERCIO LRM, COOMARASWAMY RP, STATE D: Cardiac output and other hemodynamic variables during external cardiac massage in man. N Engl J Med 269:1398, 1963

DRUCKER WR, CHADWICK CDJ, GANN, DS: Transcapillary refill in hemorrhage and shock. Arch Surg 116:1344, 1981

EISEMAN B, BEART R, NORTON L: Multiple organ failure. Surg Gynecol Obstet 144:323, 1977

EISENBERG M, HALLSTROM A, BERGNER L: The ACLS Score: Predicting survival from out-of-hospital cardiac arrest. JAMA 246:50, 1981

FREIS ED, SCHNAPER HW, JOHNSON RL et al: Hemodynamic alterations in acute myocardial infarction. I. Cardiac output, mean arterial pressure, total peripheral resistance, "central" and total blood volumes, venous pressure and average circulation time. J Clin Invest 31:131, 1952

GORDON AS, FRYE CW, GITTELSON L et al: Mouth-to-mouth versus manual artificial respiration for children and adults. JAMA 167:320, 1958

HARKINS HN, LONG CNH: Metabolic changes in shock after burns. Am J Physiol 144:661, 1945

HESS ML, HASTILLO A, GREENFIELD LJ: Spectrum of cardiovascular function during gram-negative sepsis. Prog Cardiovasc Dis 23:279, 1981

HIPPOCRATES: Epidemics. In Medical Works, vol. 1. Cambridge, Harvard University Press, 1978

KOUWENHOVEN WB, JUDE JR, KNICKERBOCKER GG: Closed chest cardiac massage. JAMA 173:1064, 1960

KOUWENHOVEN WB, KAY JH: A simple electrical apparatus for the clinical treatment of ventricular fibrillation. Surgery 30:781, 1951

LAENNEC RTH: Traité de l'auscultation mediaté et des maladies des poumons et du coeur, p 138. Paris, J S Chaude, 1831

LEDRAN, HF: Traité ou reflexions tirées de la pratique sur les plaies d'armes à feu. London, 1737. Clarke J (trans).

LIDDELL MJ, DANIEL AM, MACLEAN LD et al: The role of stress hormones in the catabolic metabolism of shock. Surg Gynecol Obstet 149:822, 1979

LILLEHEI RC, LONGERBEAM JK, BLOCH JH et al: The modern treatment of shock based on physiologic principles. Clin Pharmacol Therap 5:63, 1964

MACLEAN LD, MULLIGAN WG, MCLEAN APH et al: Patterns of septic shock in man—A detailed study of 56 patients. Ann Surg 166:543, 1967

MONAFO WW, CHUNTRASAKUL C, AYVAZIAN VH: Hypertonic sodium solutions in the treatment of burn shock. Am J Surg 126:778, 1973

MOORE FD: The effects of hemorrhage on body composition. N Engl J Med 273:567, 1965

MOSS GS, LOWE RJ, JILEK J et al: Colloid or crystalloid in the resuscitation of hemorrhagic shock: A controlled clinical trial. Surgery 89:434, 1981

MOYER CA, BUTCHER HR: Burns, Shock, and Plasma Volume Regulation. St Louis, C V Mosby, 1967

OLLODART RM, HAWTHORNE I, ATTAR S: Studies in experimental endotoxemia in man. Am J Surg 113:599, 1967

POLK HC JR, SHIELDS CL: Remote organ failure: A valid sign of occult intra-abdominal infection. Surgery 81:310, 1977

PONTOPPIDAN H, GEFFIN B, LAVER MB: Respiratory failure in septic shock. In Hershey SG, DelGuercio LRM, McConn R (eds): Septic Shock in Man, p 37. Boston, Little, Brown & Co, 1971

RUSH BF JR, ROSENBERG JE, SPENCER FC: Changes in oxygen consumption in shock: Correlation with other known parameters. J Surg Res 5:252, 1965

SARNOFF SJ, MITCHELL JH, GILMORE JP et al: Homeometric autoregulation in the heart. Circ Res 8:1077, 1960

SCHAFER EA: The relative efficiency of certain methods of performing artificial respiration in man. Proc R Soc Edinburgh 25:39, 1904

SHIRES GT, CUNNINGHAM JN, BAKER CRF et al: Alterations in cellular membrane function during hemorrhagic shock in primates. Ann Surg 176:288, 1972

SKILLMAN JJ, AWWAD HK, MOORE FD: Plasma protein kinetics of the early transcapillary refill after hemorrhage in man. Surg Gynecol Obstet 125:893, 1967

VINCENT J, WEIL MH, PURI V et al: Circulatory shock associated with purulent peritonitis. Am J Surg 142:262, 1981

WAISBREN BA: Bacteremia due to gram-negative bacilli other than the Salmonella: A clinical and therapeutic study. Arch Intern Med 88:467, 1951

WIGGERS CJ: Physiology of Shock. Cambridge, Harvard University Press, 1950

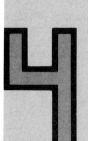

Arlie R. Mansberger, Jr.

Acute Renal Failure

PREDISPOSING FACTORS

Factors that predispose patients to acute renal failure include advancing age, volume depletion, diabetes, recent exposure to aminoglycosides or other nephrotoxic drugs, and pre-existing renal disease. Pre-existing renal disease may be due to a variety of factors including congenital renal problems (polycystic disease), longstanding obstruction with hydronephrosis from any cause, urinary tract infection, metabolic derangements and endocrinopathies (*e.g.,* nephrocalcinosis of primary hyperparathyroidism), and diseases of the glomeruli and small vessels as well as major blood vessel disease.

Certainly diseases of the glomeruli and the small and large vessels can cause acute renal failure without additional insult. However, their presence in any significant degree sets the stage for rapid deterioration of renal function leading to renal failure when ischemic disorders from any cause, especially trauma and shock or additional nephrotoxic insult, are superimposed.

In addition to major blood vessel pathology (*e.g.,* atherosclerosis and renal artery stenosis or fibrous dysplasia), the list of glomerular and small blood vessel diseases setting the stage for and leading to acute renal failure is substantial.

Renal function deteriorates with age. Consequently, acute renal failure occurs more frequently in the older age groups and the mortality rate is higher in these groups.

Drugs that impair prostaglandin synthesis that are used widely for the treatment of arthritis in the aged (*e.g.,* aspirin, indomethacin) may predispose the kidney to a more severe degree of ischemia in the presence of a hemodynamic insult.

Patients with diabetes are especially prone to the onset of acute renal failure following the use of radiologic contrast materials. This is particularly true when the diabetic patient is in the older age group (> 55 years); when there is pre-existing renal damage; when the diabetes is of 10 or more years' duration and is associated with neuropathy, retinopathy, or significant vascular disease; when proteinemia exists; and when nephrotoxic drugs have been recently administered.

PRECIPITATING CAUSES

The major disorders associated with acute renal failure (ARF) in surgical patients are well known and include dehydration, profound low perfusion states (shock), hypoxia, extensive trauma, rhabdomyolysis due to crush injuries, burns, and compartment syndromes, intravascular hemolysis owing to transfusion reactions, and sepsis from a variety of causes.

Other less well known but increasingly appreciated causes of renal failure involve a wide variety of nephrotoxic compounds. The aminoglycosides, gentamicin, kanamycin, tobramycin, amikacin, and sisomycin are all capable of impairing renal function. The increased therapeutic use of this group of compounds in the treatment of gram-negative infections has made them one of the most frequent causes of ARF. Aminoglycosides damage the proximal tubules and decrease glomerular permeability for filtration. Their neph-

FACTORS IMPLICATED IN ACUTE RENAL FAILURE
Shock
Sepsis
Hemolysis
Crush injury (rhabdomyolysis)
Nephrotoxic drugs (aminoglycosides and others)
Anesthetic agents
Radiologic contrast agents
Increasing age
Vascular disease
Diabetes mellitus

rotoxicity probably is related to their binding to renal cortical tissue; as a consequence, the renal tissue levels of aminoglycosides last much longer than blood levels. In the experimental animal, the half-life of gentamicin in renal tissue is 218 times longer than the half-life in serum.

The nephrotoxicity of the anesthetic agent methoxyflurane has been thoroughly documented and is dose-related. The nephrotoxic potential of halothane is associated with hepatic damage and the consequent release of tissue thromboplastin, intravascular coagulation, and renal cortical necrosis. The spectrum of nephrotoxins is enlarging as new therapeutic agents are introduced. Low molecular-weight dextran, once heralded as a therapeutic agent for ARF associated with intravascular hemolysis, has been implicated in its cause.

ARF induced by radiologic contrast material is well documented and has been reported following a variety of arteriographic procedures as well as following intravenous urography, cholangiography, and oral cholecystography. The popular use of radiologic contrast media in scanning techniques used with computerized axial tomography will undoubtedly have an impact on the incidence of ARF.

Other pharmacologic agents, although not directly nephrotoxic, can and do have significant effects on renal blood flow. For example, a single 100-mg dose of meperidine or thiopental anesthesia can reduce renal plasma flow by as much as 30%.

Less well known causes of ARF in the surgical patient include drug interactions. For example, cephalothin, an antibiotic rarely incriminated alone as an etiologic agent in renal failure, appears to have a much greater nephrotoxic potential when combined with furosemide or gentamicin. Similarly, the nephrotoxic potential of methoxyflurane, even in low doses, can be considerably heightened when it is combined with other nephrotoxic substances such as the aminoglycosides.

Heavy metals (*e.g.,* lead) and organic solvents (ethylene glycol) as well as certain pesticidal and fungicidal agents are nephrotoxic. Chemotherapeutic agents (cis platinum) utilized in the management of patients with malignant disease can also be nephrotoxic.

DIFFERENTIAL DIAGNOSIS

Azotemia in the surgical patient is properly classified by the anatomic site in which the initiating disturbance occurs—that is, as prerenal, postrenal, or renal (Fig. 4-1). The classes and broad causal relationships are as follows:

Prerenal azotemia results from events leading to a decrease in renal perfusion pressure, increased vascular resistance, or both; glomerular filtration is diminished to such a degree that endogenous nitrogenous waste cannot be eliminated.

Postrenal azotemia is due to obstruction in the lower or, more rarely, the upper urinary tract.

Renal azotemia results from intrarenal causes of renal failure, oliguric or nonoliguric, secondary to a wide variety of precipitating causes.

PRERENAL AZOTEMIA

The prerenal azotemic state can be corrected immediately if the extrarenal circumstance causing the decrease in renal perfusion pressure is reversed. To this end, therapy may involve increasing the extracellular fluid volume, enhancing

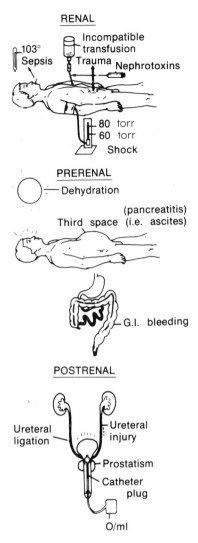

Fig. 4-1. Etiology of oliguria.

cardiac output, or correcting the cause of systemic vasodilation (*e.g.,* sepsis or excessive use of vasodilating drugs).

A careful search for the causes of prerenal azotemia utilizing the patient's history and a physical examination must constitute the initial effort in the evaluation of patients with a potential diagnosis of ARF.

The surgeon especially must recognize that dehydration from any cause with attendant reduction in renal blood flow and glomerular filtration rate, coupled with enhanced resorption of sodium and water under the influence of aldosterone and antidiuretic hormone, is a frequent and often unrecognized form of oliguria.

Third-space accumulations such as occur with pancreatitis, peritonitis, intestinal infarctions, and wide anatomic dissections (*e.g.,* pelvic exenterations) can result in oliguria by way of similar mechanisms.

Bleeding into the gastrointestinal tract is a frequent cause of prerenal azotemia. Blood in the gastrointestinal tract is acted on by urease from fecal bacteria, forming ammonia. Ammonia in turn is absorbed into the tributaries of the portal vein and converted to urea by way of the urea cycle in a single passage through the liver.

In patients with prerenal azotemia the concomitant rise in serum creatinine is usually not of the same magnitude

ACUTE RENAL FAILURE

Predisposing Factors. Advanced age, volume depletion, diabetes, small and large vessel disease, nephrotoxic agents, congenital renal problems, long-standing obstructive uropathy, metabolic derangements.

Precipitating Causes. Dehydration, shock, hypoxia, trauma, rhabdomyolysis, intravascular hemolysis, transfusion reactions, sepsis, nephrotoxic agents.

Diagnosis. Careful attention to history for screening of predisposing factors and precipitating causes. Systematic elimination of prerenal and postrenal oliguria and azotemia. Qualitative urinalysis that demonstrates a urine osmolality < 400, urine Na > 40 mEq/L, U/P creatinine ratio > 20, BUN/creatinine < 10:1, renal failure index > 2, and FENa > 2. Careful clinical trials with volume replacement and potent loop diuretics.

Treatment. *Oliguric:* Restriction of fluid intake, monitoring for and treatment of hyperkalemia, judicious use of TPN utilizing hypertonic glucose and L-essential amino acids, surgical implantation of AV shunt or peritoneal catheter using meticulous aseptic technique. Hemodialysis or peritoneal dialysis.

as the rise in blood urea nitrogen (BUN). The urinary osmolality is greater than 500 mOsm, the urine sodium value is less than 20 mEq/liter, the urine-plasma (U/P) creatinine ratio is greater than 40, and the examination of the urinary sediment shows nothing remarkable.

In some patients, the differentiation of prerenal azotemia from renal azotemia based on the above normal laboratory results may be difficult because of an overlap in laboratory values. In these instances, calculation of the "renal failure index" (U_{Na} divided by U/P creatinine ratio) and of the fractional excretion of sodium (FENa); this is arrived at by dividing the U/P_{Na} by the U/P creatinine ratio and multiplying by 100. A value of less than 1 for these two entities is characteristic of prerenal azotemia, whereas values of 2 or greater are associated with renal azotemia (ARF).

POSTRENAL AZOTEMIA

Obstruction of the bladder outlet, especially in older men, is probably the most common cause of acute oliguria or complete anuria when urinary output has been adequate previously. A history of frequency, nocturia, or gradually increasing difficulty in initiating and terminating the act of voiding should alert the clinician to the possibility of lower urinary tract obstruction in the preoperative period. When such obstruction is suspected, especially in the patient scheduled for elective surgery, its presence or absence should be carefully determined by proper diagnostic techniques (cystoscopy and catheterization for residual urine).

In these patients a urinary catheter, inserted preoperatively, will allow proper and accurate monitoring of urinary output in the postoperative period.

When a catheter is in place and urinary output ceases abruptly, catheter obstruction must be considered. An obstructed catheter should, of course, be irrigated or replaced.

Upper urinary tract obstruction is a much less frequent cause of postrenal oliguria. Although simultaneous bilateral

ureteral obstruction is rare, it must be considered in cases of unexplained oliguria. Similarly, unilateral ureteral obstruction from ligation or injury in the patient with a solitary kidney is always a potential cause of postoperative oliguria. Upper urinary tract obstruction must always be considered a possibility in patients in whom operative procedures proximal to the ureters have been carried out.

Examination of clinical parameters is less helpful in differentiating postrenal azotemia from ARF. The urine in patients with acute obstruction of the urinary tract may show a composition similar to that of prerenal azotemia for a short time. By contrast, chronic urinary tract obstruction causes tubular dysfunction, and when acute obstruction is superimposed, the urinary composition is similar to that in ARF.

RENAL AZOTEMIA

OLIGURIC

The diagnosis of ARF is based on rapid and sequential elimination of prerenal and postrenal azotemia through a history, physical examination, and laboratory tests, including a qualitative examination of the urine. Pertinent tests, as outlined in Figure 4-2, include a urine osmolality that is less than 400 mOsm, a urine sodium value that is usually greater than 40 mEq/liter, a U/P creatinine ratio greater than 20, a renal failure index greater than 2, a fractional excretion of filtered sodium (FENa) greater than 2, and a microscopic examination that is abnormal and includes brown granular casts, tubular cells, red cells, and/or protein casts.

In addition, BUN to serum creatinine ratios in renal failure do not usually exceed 10:1. In prerenal azotemia, on the other hand, the BUN-serum creatinine ratio is considerably more than 10:1. The explanation for this phenomenon is that urea clearances are flow-dependent, and therefore, the combination of decreased urine flow and intact tubular function (as in prerenal azotemia or acute urinary tract obstruction) is associated with reduced urea clearances. Creatinine clearances, on the other hand, are not flow-dependent, and the rise in urea nitrogen in prerenal and acute postrenal azotemia is therefore more rapid than the increase in serum creatinine concentration.

When ARF is suspected and postrenal etiologies have been eliminated as the cause of oliguria, a cautious fluid challenge should be administered. A simultaneous challenge with a patent loop diuretic such as furosemide that is not followed by brisk diuresis is evidence of ARF.

NONOLIGURIC

Nonoliguric ARF as a clinical entity has been recognized since 1943. Its early recognition depends on a high index of suspicion. It occurs more frequently than has previously been recognized and may be initiated by a variety of renal insults, including volume depletion, trauma (including the controlled trauma of operation), nontraumatic rhabdomyolysis, sepsis, impaired cardiac output, and the administration of a large group of nephrotoxic substances (especially antibiotics and water-soluble contrast agents) in addition to several miscellaneous factors (such as transfusion reactions, hyperuricemia, and hypercalcemia). The clinical course of nonoliguric ARF is qualitatively similar but not identical to that of the oliguric variety. Anderson et al, in a prospective study of 92 patients, compared the clinical course and urinary diagnostic indices of nonoliguric and oliguric renal

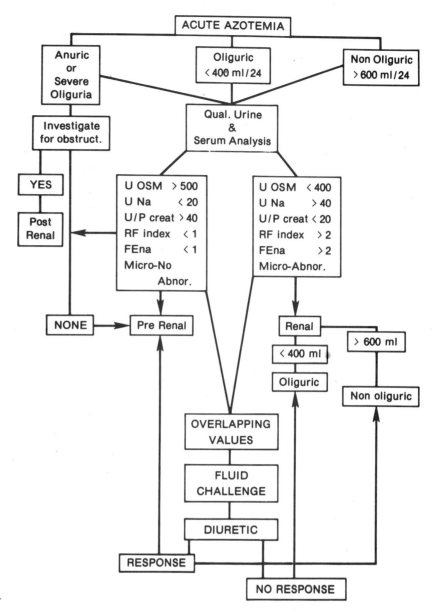

Fig. 4-2. Algorithm for differential diagnosis.

failure patients. They found that although the causes of nonoliguric renal failure varied, nephrotoxic etiologies due to antibiotics and contrast media occurred more frequently in nonoliguric than in oliguric patients ($p < 0.01$). Renal failure patients without oliguria had lower urinary sodium concentrations ($p < 0.05$) than did patients with oliguric renal failure. They also had shorter hospital stays ($p < 0.01$) and fewer episodes of sepsis, neurologic changes, gastrointestinal bleeding, and acidemia; they required dialysis less frequently ($p < 0.001$) and had significantly lower mortality rates (26% vs 50%).

TREATMENT

FLUID AND ELECTROLYTE MANAGEMENT

When prerenal and postrenal azotemia have been eliminated as causes of oliguria and the diagnosis of renal azotemia has been established, the intake of substances requiring renal excretion must be limited.

Fluid intake must be restricted and is best adjusted by obtaining the daily weight of the patient on an accurate scale. In the absence of fistulas or other causes of significant extrarenal fluid loss, daily fluid intake should rarely exceed 500 ml to 700 ml per 24 hr; in some instances as little as 300 ml to 400 ml per day is required for maintenance. Amounts must be added to the daily requirement to compensate for extrarenal losses through tubes and fistulas. The body weight should be allowed to decrease by 0.2 kg to 0.3 kg per 24 hr. Normal electrolyte patterns are desirable. When there is clear evidence that hyponatremia and hypochloremia are not dilutional, small amounts of hypertonic (3%) sodium chloride may be used for replacement on the basis of calculated deficiencies. Similarly, small amounts of sodium bicarbonate, added to the infusate as necessary in allowable doses, are beneficial in combating acidosis and hence hyperkalemia. (Care must be taken to ensure that the serum lactate level is not excessive when bicarbonate is used). Daily monitoring of electrolytes, urea, and creatinine levels is essential as a guide to judicious replacement therapy.

A significant and immediately life-threatening problem

associated with renal azotemia is hyperkalemia. Hyperkalemia occurs with both oliguric and nonoliguric renal failure, although the incidence of clinically significant hyperkalemia is less in the latter entity.

In less severe conditions, the body tolerates moderate elevations of potassium by compensation through potassium fluxes across cellular membranes. Rapidly developing increases in serum potassium content are not accompanied by the same degree of intracellular potassium flux and may alter the membrane potential severely, leading to neuromuscular dysfunction and arrhythmias.

Acute increases in serum potassium in the vicinity of 5.5 mEq/liter are generally not associated with symptoms. Peaking of T waves is commonly noted on electrocardiographic tracings. As the level of potassium rises the patient may experience fatigue, lassitude, and paresthesia. Decreased tendon reflex responses occur. When serum levels of potassium approach 7.5 to 8 mEq/liter complete neuromuscular paralysis, vascular collapse, ventricular fibrillation, and cardiac arrest are imminent.

Although there is no distinct or absolutely accurate correlation between serum potassium levels and electrocardiographic changes, definite trends may be noted. The QRS complex widens when the serum potassium level reaches 6.5 mEq/liter. As the serum potassium level rises, P-wave amplitudes decrease and the PR interval is prolonged. As the levels of serum potassium approach 7.5 mEq/liter, the P wave may disappear and the QRS complex may resemble a sine wave. A distinct bradycardia may be noted; if uncorrected, it will be followed by ventricular fibrillation or ventricular standstill.

The treatment of acute hyperkalemia should be considered in two parts as follows: (1) the treatment of hyperkalemic cardiac toxicity and (2) the immediate and long-term therapy of acute elevations of serum potassium levels.

The cardiac toxicity of acute elevations in potassium levels is best managed by the intravenous administration of a 10% calcium solution (one ampule of calcium lactate or calcium chloride) given over a 5-min to 10-min period. The infusion of calcium causes rapid reversion of the QRS complex to normal. Since the result is directly dependent on the calcium ion, the cardiac effects of calcium infusion last only as long as the Ca^{2+} levels are effectively maintained. Continuous electrocardiographic monitoring is necessary, and calcium infusions are repeated as indicated.

Hyperkalemia is treated by causing potassium flux from the extracellular to the intracellular space and by effectively lowering the total body potassium. The former is accomplished by raising the arterial *p*H and by causing the formation of glycogen. One ampule (44 millimoles [mM]) of sodium bicarbonate should be given directly intravenously over a 5-min to 10-min time span. An additional two or three ampules should be added to 500 ml of 10% glucose. Ten to 15 units of regular insulin should be given subcutaneously at the start of the infusion or added to the infusate, which should be given over a 2-hr to 4-hr period. Neither of these mechanisms reduce total body potassium. Rather, they result in a shift of potassium from the extracellular to the intracellular space. Generally speaking, the serum potassium level will be reduced by 1 mEq/liter for every 0.1 unit rise in arterial *p*H.

Total body potassium can be lowered by the administration of the cation exchange resin polystyrene sodium sulfonate (Kayexalate), which effectively exchanges sodium for potassium. Thirty grams mixed with 200 ml to 300 ml of solution are given as a high retention enema. Approximately 1 mEq of potassium is removed for every gram of polystyrene used. The process can be repeated two or three times in 24 hr. If mixed with sorbitol, the cation exchange resin can be given effectively by mouth if the patient can tolerate the oral intake. Sodium levels must be monitored as a safeguard against hypernatremia when large quantities of cation exchange resins are used to lower the total body potassium content.

Oral and parenteral administration of the potassium ion is contraindicated. Blood transfusions are omitted unless absolutely necessary. It is equally important to restrict the administration of any drugs that are eliminated by way of the urinary tract. These include digitalis, certain antibiotics, and sedative compounds.

NUTRITION

A dietary regimen of nonprotein calories in the form of carbohydrates should be used to take advantage of its protein sparing effect, thus decreasing the rate and degree of endogenous catabolism and negative nitrogen balance.

However, in surgical patients, especially postoperative or post-trauma patients, total protein restriction may compound wound healing problems and affect those protein moieties concerned with bacterial defense, thus enhancing the possibility of invasive infection and sepsis. The use of a solution of hypertonic glucose and L-essential amino acids administered via central venous lines enhances the recycling and utilization of endogenous urea nitrogen for purposes of nitrogen balance. Utilization of this technique in prospective double-blind studies has shown that those patients receiving this "renal failure fluid" have a more rapid recovery with a significant reduction in morbidity and mortality compared with patients whose caloric needs were managed in a traditional way.

DIALYSIS

Artificial methods of eliminating the end products of protein catabolism and of regulating the volume and composition of body fluids are provided through the mechanisms of hemodialysis and peritoneal dialysis.

HEMODIALYSIS

In hemodialysis, blood is passed through tubing composed of a series of semipermeable membranes that allow small-molecular-weight toxic materials to be passed from the blood to the dialysate and dialyzable material from the dialysate into the bloodstream. Thus these small-molecular-weight toxins can be removed, and acid-base balance and electrolyte homeostasis can be achieved. Volume is increased by one of three mechanisms (or various combinations of the three) as follows:

1. Addition of glucose concentrations to the dialysate to increase the osmolality (for each 100-mg% increase in glucose concentration, 5.5 milliosmoles are added).
2. Constriction of blood outflow from the dialyzer, thus increasing the peripheral resistance within the dialyzer.
3. The running of dialysate at negative pressures, thus effectively raising the filtration pressure.

To perform hemodialysis three requirements must be met: there must be (1) access to blood flow, (2) an effective dialysate, and (3) a tubing composed of semipermeable membranes.

In patients with ARF access to blood flow is achieved by the use of a surgically implanted prosthetic arteriovenous shunt. Until recently a standard Quinton-Scribner Silastic Teflon cannula was the device most widely used for this purpose. Currently, use of the Buselmeier shunt allows decreased resistance to blood flow owing to decreased tubing length and immediate access to the system without needle cannulation.

The shunts can be placed in several locations—radial artery, cephalic vein, posterior tibial artery, saphenous vein or an arterialized saphenous vein segment (superficial femoral artery), or greater saphenous vein. The upper extremity approach is the one ordinarily utilized when hemodialysis is urgent. Ideally, the dialyzer should be safe and simple, and rupture of the dialysis membrane should be rare. Dialysis must be efficient and should be accomplished with the available blood flow. Urea clearance should exceed 80 ml per min. The volume of the dialyzer should be such that ''blood priming'' of the coil is unnecessary. To avoid blood transfusion, return of blood from the dialyzer to the patient must be virtually complete.

The composition of the dialysate varies. Most dialysate solutions contain physiologic concentrations of sodium and chloride. Potassium, calcium, and magnesium concentrations can be varied as indicated. Acetate can be added for its buffering effect and glucose for its effect on osmolality of the dialysate solution.

PERITONEAL DIALYSIS

Peritoneal dialysis is a relatively safe and effective form of therapy in ARF. It is approximately 25% as effective as hemodialysis per unit time. Conditions such as dense adhesions to the anterior abdominal wall with the attendant risks of gastrointestinal injury and fistula formation negate the use of peritoneal dialysis. However, recent abdominal operations are no longer considered contraindications to peritoneal dialysis.

Among the advantages of peritoneal dialysis are the following: (1) it can be carried out in the patient's room because the mechanics are uncomplicated and commercially available materials are employed; (2) hemodynamic and biochemical changes are moderate per unit time; (3) anticoagulation and blood transfusion are unnecessary; and (4) it is less costly than hemodialysis.

The recommended frequency of dialysis varies. However, in the postoperative patient or in the post-trauma period, frequent or at times daily dialysis is indicated because of the increased catabolic rate associated with trauma and operation.

The choice of peritoneal dialysis versus hemodialysis should depend on the capacity of the method to prevent uremic symptoms of the disorder. In general, those disorders associated with severe catabolic states requiring optimal clearances will need hemodialysis, because even continuous peritoneal dialysis will be inadequate to prevent uremic symptoms. The use of continuous peritoneal dialysis should be discouraged in these patients because there is a definite relationship between the length of peritoneal dialysis and the incidence of attendant complications.

COMPLICATIONS

The hypocalcemia and hyperphosphatemia of ARF are not generally associated with symptoms. On the other hand, severe hyponatremia can accentuate renal failure and should be corrected. Hyperkalemia leads to severe cardiac problems, as outlined previously in this chapter, and must be corrected. Symptomatic hypermagnesemia occurs most commonly in patients who are receiving antacids containing magnesium as part of their therapy. The hyperuricemia of ARF rarely causes gouty arthritis, but in patients with rhabdomyolysis and ARF, treatment with a xanthine-oxidase inhibitor may be necessary.

Hypertension and cardiac failure in ARF are usually caused iatrogenically from volume overload and usually respond to appropriate dialysis. When they do not, the use of antihypertensive medication is indicated. Digoxin may be necessary, but because it is excreted by the kidneys and because of the rapid changes in plasma potassium concentration in ARF, this drug should be used very cautiously and should be reserved for those who do not respond to other forms of therapy. Gastrointestinal (nausea and vomiting), neurologic (asterixis, somnolence, coma, and neuromuscular irritability), and hemorrhagic complications should be treated or, better yet, prevented by the use of dialysis.

The anemia of ARF, hastened by bone marrow suppression and hemodialysis, does not generally require blood transfusion unless simultaneous bleeding occurs.

Immunosuppression in ARF invites infection, the major cause of death in this disease, and is not prevented by dialysis. Obviously, meticulous asepsis with respect to intravenous catheter care, wound toilet, and so on is mandatory.

The main complication of peritoneal dialysis is peritonitis. Continuous peritoneal dialysis beyond 36 hr to 48 hr is associated with a rather striking increase in the incidence of this entity. Further, peritonitis is the main complication of intermittent peritoneal dialysis. Elevation of the diaphragm and the required immobilization associated with the continuous form of dialysis predispose the patient to significant respiratory complications.

Both peritoneal dialysis and hemodialysis can impair cardiac output, but hemodynamic and cardiovascular consequences are more common with the latter method.

The requirement for heparin in hemodialysis may result in bleeding or enhancement of a bleeding tendency, especially in the post-trauma or postoperative periods.

MORTALITY

The overall mortality rate for oliguric renal failure is 50%, a figure that has not changed appreciably in the last two decades.

Nonoliguric renal failure, which comprises an increasing percentage of recognized ARF (20% to 30%), is associated with a mortality rate that is roughly half that of the oliguric variety.

ARF occurs more frequently in the geriatric population, and the mortality rate is higher in this group than in other age groups.

Patients with ARF secondary to major trauma and operation have a high mortality rate, as do those in general in whom there is a significantly accelerated catabolic state. Patients with ARF who acquire such complications as pneumonia, generalized sepsis, and gastrointestinal hemorrhage have higher mortality rates.

However, there is evidence to suggest that the extensive use of L-essential amino acids and hypertonic glucose in nutritional support of patients with ARF, particularly those with severe catabolic states and the significant complications cited above, will result in a substantial reduction of mortality in the next decade.

BIBLIOGRAPHY

ANDERSON RJ, LINAS SL, BERNS AS et al: Non-oliguric acute renal failure. New Engl J Med 296:1134, 1977

CONGER JD, SCHRIDER RW: Renal hemodynamics in acute renal failure. Ann Rev Physiol 42:603, 1980

HARRINGTON JT, COHEN JJ: Acute oliguria. New Engl J Med 229:89, 1975

HUMPHRIES AL JR, NESBIT RR JR, CARVANA RJ et al: Thirty-six recommendations for vascular access operations: Lessons learned from our first thousand operations. Am Surg 47:145, 1981

MILLER TR, ANDERSON RJ, LINAS SL et al: Urinary diagnostic indices in acute renal failure. A prospective study. Ann Intern Med 89:47, 1978

NEWMARK SR, DLUHY RG: Hyperkalemia and hypokalemia. JAMA 231:631, 1975

SCHRIDER RW: Acute renal failure. Kidney International 15:205, 1979

Kenneth L. Mattox

Disorders of Surgical Bleeding and Blood Transfusion Problems

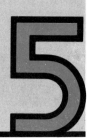

ASSESSMENT OF PERIOPERATIVE HEMOSTATIC FAILURE	
PROBLEM	**TREATMENT**
Uncontrolled vascular disruption	Explore and suture-ligate bleeding vessel
Hypothermia	Rewarm patient
Acidosis	Administer sodium bicarbonate
Factor deficiency	Check PT, PTT, platelet count; administer platelets, fresh frozen plasma

DISORDERS OF SURGICAL BLEEDING

The flow of blood and its containment within the body have always fascinated mankind. Since early Egyptian times, removing blood from a sick body was considered therapeutic. Shamans, medicine men, barbers, and later, surgeons sought techniques to stanch the flow of shed blood. These techniques included the use of ligatures, tourniquets, hot cautery, and caustics, as well as application of materials such as spider webs and portions of recently slain animals. Indirect means of stopping hemorrhage have included incantations, sand paintings, and even exorcisms. By 1906, an understanding of the mechanisms of blood coagulation emerged, with descriptions of thromboplastin, prothrombin, thrombin, fibrinogen, and fibrin. MacFarlane, in 1964, described an easily understandable model of the cascade mechanism of coagulation.

CAUSES OF SURGICAL BLEEDING

GENERAL

Intraoperative and postoperative uncontrolled hemorrhage presents frustrating dilemmas for the surgeon and progressive complications for the patient. Such bleeding may be the result of (1) lack of surgical hemostasis; (2) acquired coagulopathies from alterations in temperature, acid–base balance, serum electrolytes, platelets and clotting factors; or (3) the presence of congenital defects in clotting. The first and second of these causes are directly influenced by the surgeon, and a knowledge of congenital defects can allow for specific preoperative preparation or intraoperative therapy directed at replenishing the specific genetic defect. *The most common cause of surgical bleeding is lack of hemostasis.* Many factors—including too small an incision or lack of exposure, poor lighting, improper preparation or inadequate understanding of anatomy, too hurried an operation, poor choice of or inadequately tied sutures, poorly applied hemostatic clips, and improper reliance on electrocautery—may contribute to iatrogenic surgical bleeding. The final task prior to surgical closure is examination of the wound for retained foreign bodies or instruments and ascertaining hemostasis.

MECHANISMS OF HEMOSTASIS AND THE COAGULATION SYSTEM

Normal hemostasis relies on four interrelated components: (1) integrity of the blood vessel wall, (2) platelet function, (3) the coagulation system, and (4) the necessity for the clot to remain unlysed. The mechanisms work together and are governed both positively and negatively by scores of interrelated systems. Familiarity with the presently known major contributors to the coagulation system helps to prevent blind empirical or "shotgun" therapy.

When a blood vessel wall (be it a capillary or a major vein or artery) is disrupted, local and systemic factors interact to contract that vessel. Serotonin and catecholamines are two humoral factors that contribute to this contraction. A completely severed vessel will contract more than a partially severed vessel. The injured vessel is also affected by the mechanical trapping and clumping of platelets and the development of a fibrin clot.

Platelets are necessary for firm clot formation, the initial step being adherence of platelets to the exposed collagen. Platelet clumps form a plug in capillaries and small vessels. This reaction involves ADP and ATP in concert with thrombin, phospholipids, serotonin, and other factors. Although patients with platelet counts as low as 5000/mm^3 may survive for long periods of time without serious bleeding difficulties, platelet counts in excess of 25,000/mm^3 should be present or achieved by platelet transfusions in the patient with surgical bleeding. Platelet function is impaired by many drugs, including aspirin, Persantine, dextrans, and others. Platelets may also be reduced because of congenital or acquired diseases, including neoplasia and reticuloendothelial diseases. Platelet numbers may be depressed because of massive blood transfusions, especially transfusions of "packed" red blood cells that are depleted in platelets, either because of a prolonged shelf life or because platelets were removed during processing.

At least 13 clotting factors have been described, each with specific names and synonyms (Table 5-1). Both acquired and congenital deficits in these factors result in inability of the blood to form a clot. The coagulation factors cascade is complex, with multifactorial activation and regulatory points. The surgeon encountering a congenital or acquired deficit is well advised to seek assistance from a hematologist or pathologist with an interest in coagulation disorders. Anticoagulants (*e.g.,* coumarin), which antagonize vitamin K, depress Factors II, VII, IX, and X. A patient receiving multiple blood transfusions is deficient in Factors V, VIII, and platelets. Once a soft fibrin clot has formed, Factor XIII acts to produce a firmer clot; other factors, such as thrombin and calcium, are necessary in the development of this firm clot. Various abnormal globulins, dextrans, and other large molecules may impede the formation of this firm clot. Fibrinolysins may dissolve the mature fibrin clot, an action that is seen in patients with hemopericardium and hemothorax. Damaged endothelium itself may activate fibrinolysis, as may tissue hypoxemia. Clinically, clot lysis has occurred with streptokinase, urokinase, and even heparin. Such mechanisms are clinically useful in patients with multiple pulmonary emboli but are deleterious in troublesome surgical bleeding. Fibrinolytic syndromes are also seen in patients with abruptio placentae and occasionally following prostatic surgery. If a fibrinolytic syndrome is suspected, blood should be drawn for observation of clotting and measurement of euglobulin lysis time. Specific deficits should be sought before using drugs such as ε-aminocaproic acid.

CONGENITAL DEFECTS IN CLOTTING

Congenital disorders of blood coagulation, although less common than acquired deficits, may result in unexpected prolonged intraoperative and postoperative bleeding. At least ten congenital clotting disorders are known (Table 5-2). These factors may be replaced by administering banked blood, fresh frozen plasma, or cryoprecipitate. Factors II, VII, VIII, IX, and X are commercially available in concentrated form. Krieger et al. reviewed 42 patients undergoing 94 operations who had blood coagulation disorders; no deaths occurred, and a complication rate of only 8.4% was reported. A previously undiagnosed clotting deficit may be encountered during emergency surgery; however, most such defects may be diagnosed by carefully obtaining a complete patient history prior to surgery. When the emergency surgery patient exhibits abnormalities in partial thromboplastin time (PTT) and prothrombin time (PT) in spite of adequate replacement therapy with fresh frozen plasma, hematologic consultation should be obtained to seek specific congenital deficits in clotting factors. Adequate replacement material should be on hand for a patient with a known deficit requiring elective surgery. Furthermore, as pointed out by Krieger and colleagues, the patient's plasma level should be elevated to 100% of the known deficit just prior to surgery, and should be maintained at more than 60% for 4 days and at more than 40% until all the sutures are out.

COAGULOPATHIES

A variety of acquired coagulopathies have been described, each with complex interrelations or activation, acceleration, and inhibition by medications, sepsis, acidosis, and hypoxemia.

Disseminated intravascular coagulation (DIC) and consumption coagulopathy (CC) have been extensively reviewed, as in articles by Silver and Colman et al. Multiple factors may trigger DIC and CC, including infection, incompatible blood, cardiopulmonary bypass, many neoplasms, decreased cardiac output syndromes, endothelial damage from multiple causes, and others. Accelerated intravascular

TABLE 5-1   CLOTTING FACTORS

ROMAN NUMERAL	NAME	SYNONYM(S)	TEST FOR FUNCTION	REPLACEMENT SOURCES
I	Fibrinogen		Fibrinogen	BB, FFP, C
II	Prothrombin			BB, FFP, CA
III	Thromboplastin			
IV	Calcium		Serum Ca^{2+}	CA
V	Proaccelerin	Labile factor accelerator globulin (Ac-G)	PTT	FFP, FB
VI	Same as V (obsolete)			
VII	Proconvertin	Stable factor, serum prothrombin conversion accelerator (SPCA)	PT	BB, FFP, CA
VIII	Antihemophilic Globulin (AHG)	Antihemophilic factor A	PTT	FFP, C, CA, FB
—	Factor VIII regulator		↑ Bleeding time ↓ Factor VIII ↓ Platelet adhesiveness	FFP, C
IX	Plasmathromboplastin component	Christmas factor antihemophilic factor B	PTT	BB, FFP, CA
X	Stuart-Prower factor	Thrombokinase autoprothrombin C	PTT	BB, FFP, CA
XI	Plasma thromboplastin antecedent (PTA)	Antihemophilic factor C	PTT	BB, FFP
XII	Hageman factor	Contact factor/glass factor		BB, FFP
XIII	Fibrin stabilizing factor	Laki-Lorand factor fibrinase		BB, FFP

BB, banked blood; FFP, fresh frozen plasma; C, cryoprecipitate; CA, commercially available; FB, fresh blood

utilization of clotting factors and platelets and secondary activation of fibrinolysis occur. The microcirculation may even become obstructed by thrombi with resultant cellular and tissue death. When the etiologic stimulus is removed, the syndrome is self-limited. In DIC, many of the clotting factors are consumed and unavailable for clot formation. Although heparin has been recommended as a means of stopping or impeding the consumption process in DIC, many surgeons are reluctant to administer heparin to a patient already bleeding from every exposed capillary and every puncture site. Should a patient appear to have a DIC syndrome, consultation with an internist, hematologist, or pathologist is recommended.

Dilutional and transfusion coagulopathy is more frequently encountered than is DIC. A patient receiving more than 8 to 10 units of banked blood rapidly becomes depleted in Factors V, VIII, and platelets because the banked blood is deficient in these factors. Immediate replacement must be accomplished through transfusion of fresh frozen plasma and platelets.

OTHER ACQUIRED CAUSES

In some patients, anticoagulants are used therapeutically, either orally or intravenously. Both vitamin K antagonists and heparin act at various levels in the clotting cascade to interfere with clot formation. The citrate (ACD and CPD) used for the anticoagulation of banked blood is not used in medications. Since the body has unlimited stores of calcium, citrate intoxication syndromes produce cardiac arrhythmias rather than producing *in vivo* bleeding syndromes. A patient receiving anticoagulants should be given vitamin K or protamine to reverse the anticoagulant activity. Tests for abnormalities in bleeding secondary to these anticoagulants include PTT, PT, Lee White clotting time, and activated clotting time. Medications such as salicylates, oral antibiotics, Butazolidin, and quinidine may potentiate bleeding problems in a previously stable patient.

Biologic chemical and enzymatic reactions are best under normothermic conditions. A patient undergoing prolonged surgery whose celomic cavities are exposed to operating room temperatures of 22.2° C or who is receiving multiple units of cold banked blood rapidly becomes hypothermic. Attempts to rewarm the patient by using thermal blankets, indirect warming lights, and peritoneal, pleural, and wound lavage with warm saline help impede acquired hypothermia.

Thrombocytopenia may be secondary to a primary condition such as thrombocytopenia purpura or reduction of megakaryocytes. Secondary thrombocytopenia may result from infections, hypersplenism, DIC, or multiple medications. Thrombocythemia (increased platelet count) may be

TABLE 5-2   CONGENITAL COAGULATION DISORDERS

ROMAN NUMERAL	CONGENITAL DEFECT	GENETICS	INCIDENCE	SEVERITY FOR SURGEONS
I	Fibrinogen deficiency		Rare	
II	Prothrombin deficiency		Rare	
V	Parahemophilia (Owren's disease)	Autosomal recessive		
VII	Pseudohemophilia	Autosomal recessive	1 in 500,000 births	Mild to severe
VIII	Hemophilia A (classic hemophilia)	Sex-linked recessive	1 in 25,000 births	Serious
—	Von Willebrand's disease (vascular hemophilia)	Autosomal dominant		Mild
IX	Hemophilia B (Christmas disease)	Sex-linked recessive	1 in 100,000 births	Moderate
X	Congenital deficiency factor X	♂ = ♀		Mild
XI	Hemophilia C (Rosenthal syndrome)	Simple dominant		Mild
XII	Hageman trait			No effect *in vivo*

temporary, such as occurs following splenectomy, or sustained, as in patients with myeloproliferative disorders. Thrombocythemia occasionally leads to consumption coagulopathy. Treatment of thrombocythemia is directed toward removing the primary causes with perhaps the addition of dextrans and heparin to reduce platelet clumping.

EVALUATION OF THE SURGICAL PATIENT AS A HEMOSTATIC RISK

Except in dire emergencies, the patient with a pre-existing congenital bleeding diathesis can be detected prior to surgery and prepared so that surgical risks are reduced. The single most important factor in determining a pre-existing congenital bleeding diathesis is a complete patient and family history. Factors such as prolonged bleeding following minor lacerations or dental extractions or prolonged or excessive bleeding during menstruation or in association with previous surgery should be specifically sought. The patient may minimize or omit a family history of a known bleeding diathesis unless he is specifically questioned for such information. A patient should also be questioned about all medications being taken (prescription and nonprescription). The possibility of liver or splenic disease, neoplasia, or myeloproliferative disorders should be discussed with the patient. On physical examination, look for bruising, capillary fragility, hypersplenism, enlarged liver, presence of palpable tumors, evidence of intravascular thrombosis, splinter hemorrhages, infections, and other conditions that might predispose to DIC.

Laboratory tests routinely available in most laboratories include whole blood clotting time, activated clotting time, PTT, PT, and platelet count. The whole blood clotting time (Lee White) is somewhat insensitive and is quite variable when performed by different individuals. The activated clotting time (ACT) is more reliable than the Lee White clotting time. Easily performed at the bedside, ACT is an excellent means of assaying heparin administration. Instruments for evaluating ACT are commercially available for the operating room in cases of open heart and vascular surgery and for the intensive care unit and clinical units where heparin is administered routinely. Factors VIII, IX, XI, and XII are measured solely by PTT. PT evaluates the "extrinsic clotting system," specifically Factors I and VII. When both PTT and PT are abnormal, there are usually deficiencies in Factors II, V, and X.

Many laboratories are able to perform whole blood clot lysis time, euglobulin lysis time, bleeding time, tourniquet tests, and fibrinogen determinations, although these tests may be performed infrequently. The whole blood clot lysis time measures fibrinolysis and is relatively insensitive. The euglobulin lysis time measures plasminogen concentration by lysis of the patient's own fibrin in the absence of plasma inhibitors. Bleeding time and tourniquet tests assay vascular function and are helpful only when positive. They are quite gross in performance and interpretation and are presently performed infrequently. Fibrinogen (Factor I) may be measured directly and is the most easily determined of the coagulation factors. In the presence of fibrinolysis, low levels of fibrinogen may be artifactual. Other tests that are less frequently performed include plasminogen, fibrin plate lysis assay, and assays of Factors V, VII, XII, and XIII.

SPECIFIC PROBLEM AREAS

THE DIFFICULT CROSS-MATCH

If administered blood is incompatible with the patient's own blood, life-threatening reactions may result. Blood banks test for major incompatibilities of the ABO and Rh systems. A variety of test sera allow screening for minor incompatibilities. The presence of large molecules such as dextrans and hydroxyethyl starch in the patient's blood or the presence of disease processes, such as macroglobulinemia, cryoglobulinemia, sepsis, lupus erythematosus, and others, may make testing for incompatibility difficult if not impossible. In such instances, *in vivo* testing for incompatibilities is possible by close cooperation between the physicians in charge of the blood bank, the hematology department, and the surgeon.

RELIGIOUS OBJECTIONS TO BLOOD TRANSFUSIONS

Some individuals may have religious objections to receiving blood and blood products. Numerous reports concerning elective surgery in such individuals have appeared in the literature. Preoperative preparation with oral and intramuscular iron to elevate the hematocrit is indicated. Plasma expanders increase the intravascular volume, and meticulous hemostasis should be achieved. Autotransfusion is frequently acceptable to such individuals, as long as the autotransfusion apparatus is kept in a complete circuit, as in cardiopulmonary bypass. Individual permission should be obtained from the patient and/or the family in each case. In instances of emergency surgery, autotransfusion should be used, and rapid hemostasis may result in salvage of a patient with massive hemorrhage. In a patient with religious objections to receiving blood or blood products who also has a major congenital absence of clotting factors, both elective and emergency surgery present extremely difficult management and philosophical problems, since virtually all of the available exogenous clotting factors are products of banked blood.

THE MASSIVE BLEEDER

The surgical patient who requires more than six units of banked blood during a 2-hr to 3-hr operation or four to six units of blood postoperatively, or who requires blood replacement (during and after surgery) that exceeds the blood bank availability may be defined as a massive bleeder. Every operating room and surgeon should have a plan for managing the massive bleeder. In some instances, when type-specific compatible blood stores are depleted, a compatible alternate blood type may be chosen. Occasionally, when type O blood is given to a massively bleeding patient, it may be preferable to continue transfusion of type O blood even when the patient is found to have a different blood type. Should this occur, the blood bank should be consulted. In all cases of massive bleeding, the surgeon should consider autotransfusion as well as other treatment algorithms that are discussed later in this chapter. When massive transfusions are given, all hazards of transfusion are markedly increased. Hypothermia is very common with massive transfusion, as is the transmittal of numerous diseases. Following the administration of four to six units of banked blood, the risks of hepatitis are significant, especially non-A non-B hepatitis. Other problems associated with the massive bleeder and massive transfusions will be discussed in the sections on Blood Transfusions and Treatment Modalities.

THE UNCOOPERATIVE LABORATORY

Many intraoperative and postoperative bleeding problems occur when the laboratory is unable to provide rapid "coagulogram" results. Even when platelet counts, PTT, and PT are performed, frequently 1 hr to 4 hr elapse before the test results are available to the clinician. Although it is highly desirable to know coagulation defects, problems that arise intraoperatively and postoperatively are frequently not due to pre-existing genetic defects. Therefore, when specific laboratory tests may be delayed, arbitrary empiric therapy

includes the administration of multiple units of fresh frozen plasma, platelet packs, and in some instances, cryoprecipitate. The surgeon may draw an aliquot of blood into a tube containing no anticoagulant and then time blood clot formation and possible clot dissolution as a gross test of fibrinolysis. When they are available in the operating room or the intensive care unit, activated clotting times may be helpful in assessing excessive heparin activity.

TREATMENT

GENERAL CONSIDERATIONS

Prevention is the best approach to uncontrolled hemorrhage and bleeding problems. Expeditious surgery, normothermia maintained during a long operation, preoperative discontinuance of drugs that interfere with platelet function, prevention or rapid treatment of acidosis, and strict adherence to proper surgical techniques will in most cases prevent uncontrolled hemorrhage.

Local hemostasis is the most important single factor in the control of surgical bleeding. Adequate hemostasis through clamping and tying bleeding points prevents the necessity for blood transfusions, dilutional coagulopathies, and associated hypothermia. Electrocautery is useful in small bleeding points but should not be used on any named artery or vein. The surgical pack is a time-honored method of hemostasis and has been used in all body cavities as well as for wounds of the extremities, but such hemostasis by compressions should be used only when all other methods of hemostasis have failed. G-suits, constricting bands, lower extremity and abdominal compression trousers, and intra-abdominal packs for injuries to the liver, retroperitoneum, pelvis, and extremities have been used. These devices are not without complications, including subphrenic abscesses, rebleeding, and even loss of an extremity.

Chemical and topical agents such as thrombin, Surgicel, Surgifoam, Avitene, and others serve as a matrix upon which a clot can form more easily in a patient with oozing from the spleen, kidney, liver, and other raw surfaces. Newer waferlike starch sponges have also been used as topical hemostatic agents.

Once a patient has had six to eight units of packed red cells, the use of whole blood and even fresh whole blood should be considered. The reconstitution of whole blood in such a massive bleeder by the administration of platelet packs, packed red blood cells, and fresh frozen plasma and perhaps cryoprecipitate results in a much more costly product than if whole blood had been used originally.

Thermal control may be accomplished by a variety of techniques. Expeditious surgery, thermal blankets on the operating table underneath the patient, and external radiant heating lamps may not only prevent downward temperature drift during surgery but may also be used in rewarming the patient. Rewarming banked blood may be achieved by commercially available water baths and externally applied contact heating coils. Use of microwave ovens for reheating whole units of banked blood has resulted in occasional coagulation of the blood and, at times, massive hemolysis. In general, such microwave techniques are presently not widely applied. The use of cardiopulmonary bypass pump attached through a femoral vein to the femoral artery route in combination with a heating coil has been successful in victims of massive hypothermia and theoretically may be used in patients with hypothermia coagulopathies.

AUTOTRANSFUSION

Autotransfusion may be accomplished through a variety of techniques. Preoperatively a patient may donate a unit of his blood to be stored either conventionally or frozen. As many as six or eight units of blood can be stored in preparation for anticipated surgery. Another form of autotransfusion is performed after the induction of anesthesia when 20% of the patient's blood volume is removed and replaced with one and a half times its volume of Ringer's lactate. The operation then proceeds as usual, and during surgery the patient loses blood that has a lower hematocrit. Toward the end of the operation the units of blood that were removed prior to hemodilution are reinfused. A variety of commercially available devices may be used intraoperatively to recover shed blood. With such devices (*e.g.*, the Bentley, Sorenson, and Haemonetics Cell Saver), anticoagulation is achieved by using either citrate or heparin in the extracorporeal circuit. The blood may be processed by centrifugation and concentration or, in some cases, may be given back directly. A variation of these devices is used to recover and recycle blood shed postoperatively. Blood may be collected with mediastinal tubes or, in the patient with DIC, with tubes left in the abdomen, chest, or extremity. Survival of patients receiving more than 50 to 75 units of recycled blood during this period of coagulopathy has been reported.

TREATMENT ALGORITHM FOR INTRAOPERATIVE UNCONTROLLED BLEEDING

If a patient begins to bleed diffusely or has uncontrolled bleeding intraoperatively, a dire, life-threatening emergency is present, and the surgeon encountering this condition should immediately summon extra help and other surgeons to assist. Control of bleeding from major arteries and veins must be accomplished, and an operative plan aimed toward completion and termination of the procedure should be devised. Local laparotomy packs should be used to impede bleeding mechanically in one area while a methodical, sequential procedure is followed to achieve topical hemostasis. Acidosis and hypothermia should be corrected. The patient should immediately be given four units of fresh frozen plasma and four to six platelet packs if available. Blood should be drawn for a PT, PTT, and platelet count. Attempts to rewarm the patient should begin immediately. Intraoperative and postoperative autotransfusion should be used if possible. If hemorrhage is still present, consider resorting to placement of laparotomy packs. Then, if cessation of hemorrhage results, the abdomen is closed, and a second operation for removal of the packs is planned anywhere from 12 hr to 5 days later. In the patient who is hypotensive and requires application of multiple topical hemostatic agents, a second operation 24 hr later may be indicated.

FUTURE ADJUNCTS

A number of technical advances provide hope for the surgeon who has encountered uncontrolled bleeding. Improved rewarming devices using external radiant heat and extracorporeal rewarming devices may receive more widespread application. It is anticipated that local topical hemostatic agents at a reasonable cost will be more widely available. Dialysis may be used to increase the volume of fresh frozen plasma that may be given. Removal of fluid by dialysis prevents the development of pulmonary edema from large volumes of fresh frozen plasma containing coagulation factors. The use of hyperbaric oxygen to increase the oxygen supply and the use of hypothermia to decrease oxygen demands are presently theoretical considerations in the patient with a hemorrhagic problem.

BLOOD TRANSFUSIONS

HISTORICAL BACKGROUND

For many centuries, surgical barbers, working under the premise that "bad blood and humors" were being removed, performed bloodletting using lancets and leeches and making febrile and ill patients hypovolemic and anemic. It was not until the latter half of the 17th century that successful transfusions from animal to animal and, on at least one occasion, from animal to man were performed. In London in 1818, James Blundell performed the first man-to-man blood transfusion, and this procedure became popular in the second half of the 19th century. William Halsted transfused his own blood into his sister after she suffered a postpartum hemorrhage. Landsteiner, working from 1900 to 1940, discovered the ABO blood groups and later the Rh factor. Antiserum was later developed to test blood groups as methods of collecting and storage of blood became available.

BLOOD BANKING

In 1937 the first blood bank was established at Cook County Hospital in Chicago. Presently, blood banks are available in most cities and in most major hospitals. Many regional blood centers perform many other functions in addition to banking blood. Under the direction of a physician who is usually a pathologist or a hematologist, the blood bank is able to provide the following services: (1) consultation for patients with abnormal clotting studies or coagulopathies; (2) procurement, typing, testing, labeling, storage, crossmatching, and distribution of blood; (3) preparation of blood products such as platelets, fresh frozen plasma, and cryoprecipitate; (4) performance of plasmapheresis and plateletpheresis; (5) supervision or coordination (in some circumstances) of autotransfusion activities; and (6) performance of or cooperation with the clinical pathology laboratory in general and specific coagulation testing.

AVAILABLE PRODUCTS

According to the American Association of Blood Banks, the available products from a blood bank include red blood cells, whole blood, fresh frozen plasma, single donor plasma, cryoprecipitated antihemophilic factor (AHF), platelet concentrates, and leukocyte concentrates. Red blood cells may be distributed as leukocyte-poor, frozen, or deglycerolized. Whole blood may be modified with platelets removed, modified with cryoprecipitated AHF removed, or leukocyte-poor. Traditional blood products that may be provided are fresh whole blood, heparinized blood, albumin, and fibrinogen. Albumin preparations of plasma protein fraction (PPF), 5% albumin, 25% albumin, antihemophilic factor concentrate, and concentrates of factors, II, VII, VIII, IX, and X are available in commercially produced, off-the-shelf packages.

Red Blood Cells (Human)

Red blood cells are those that remain after the plasma has been separated from whole blood and are anticoagulated with CPD (citrate-phosphate-dextrose). One pack usually contains 200 ml of red blood cells with a hematocrit of 70% to 80%; it should raise the recipient's hematocrit approximately 3%. Red blood cells should be administered through a filter and may be warmed to a temperature not exceeding 37°C. Each unit of red cells should be administered in less than 4 hr.

Red blood cells may also be modified by the addition of glycerol as an endocellular cryoprotective agent, and cells so prepared may be frozen for storage up to 3 years. When thawed and washed to remove the glycerol, these red blood cells function and survive like nonfrozen, stored red blood cells. Once these freeze-thaw-wash red blood cells are prepared, they must be used within the period indicated and may not be refrozen.

Whole blood is similar to red blood cells except that the plasma remains. Whole blood intended to replace labile coagulation factors (Factors V, VII, and platelets) should be less than 24 hr old. Modified whole blood may have platelets or cryoprecipitated AHF removed. Heparinized whole blood is only occasionally prepared, for example, when an exchange transfusion in an adult is indicated or when blood is required to prime a blood oxygenator. Like red blood cells, whole blood should be administered through a filter.

Plasma

Single-donor fresh frozen plasma (human) is the anticoagulated plasma separated from an individual donor's blood and frozen within 6 hr of the time of collection. Plasma is a source of clotting Factors V, VIII, and fibrinogen and also provides plasma proteins for volume expansion. It should not be used to correct coagulopathy, which can be corrected by vitamin K or cryoprecipitated or antihemophilic (Factor VIII) concentrates. Although compatibility testing is not usually necessary, certain antibodies in the plasma can react with the recipient's red blood cells, causing a positive direct antiglobulin test and possible hemolysis. The usual unit for an adult contains approximately 250 ml of anticoagulated plasma with approximately 400 mg of fibrinogen, 200 units of Factor VIII, and 200 units of Factor IX. Immediately prior to administration, the fresh frozen plasma is thawed by the blood bank and then administered through a filter.

Cryoprecipitated antihemophilic factor (human) contains Factor VIII obtained from a single unit of human blood; it should not be used unless this specific coagulation defect exists. The risk of hepatitis is higher when multiple units of cryoprecipitate are administered compared with other blood products. The following formula may be helpful for calculating Factor VIII requirements: desired Factor VIII level in % × patient's plasma volume in ml divided by the average units of Factor VIII/cryo (80) × 100 = number of cryoprecipitate bags required.

Platelet concentrate (human) consists of platelets separated from a unit of whole blood collected from a single donor and suspended in a specific volume of the original plasma. This preparation is used for the correction of thrombocytopenia. The side-effects from administered platelets are similar to those from whole blood. One unit of platelet concentrate contains no less than 5.5×10^{10} platelets and will usually increase the platelet count of a 70-kg adult by 5000 microliters (μl). If the patient has sepsis or DIC, transfused platelets may be destroyed almost as fast as they are infused. In the patient with a platelet count below 25,000 μl, six to eight units are usually transfused. Platelet concentrates should be administered through a specific platelet filter. Microaggregate filters designed to remove debris and other microparticles from red blood cells also remove platelets and should not be used for platelet transfusions.

LIMITATIONS OF BANKED BLOOD

In addition to the complications and risks of blood transfusions, other limitations of banked blood exist. Routinely stored ACD and CPD blood may be used up to 21 days after it has been collected. Some blood banks are extending the functional use of red cells up to 36 days by using 0.25 mM adenine in addition to CPD. Banked blood that has been stored for more than 24 hr loses the labile coagulation factors (V, VIII, and platelets). The cost for a unit of blood ranges from $30 to $75, with similar costs for single units of platelets and fresh frozen plasma. Type-specific blood of certain ABO blood groups may be in short supply due to a shortage of available donors or predominate use, thereby causing depletion of the supply of certain blood types. Busy cardiovascular and trauma units frequently find that their stores of O-positive blood become depleted very rapidly because it is used so commonly.

CRITERIA FOR BLOOD TRANSFUSIONS

A patient with continued acute blood loss in excess of 2000 ml unquestionably requires replacement of red blood cells while the acute condition is being surgically corrected. However, patients with chronic anemia seem to tolerate operation with hematocrits of as low as 18% to 20% with very little difficulty. The optimal hematocrit required prior to surgery is under some debate. A patient whose cardiac reserve is capable of doubling cardiac output can tolerate removal of up to 20% of blood volume without any demonstrable hemodynamic or tissue deficits. Experimentally, animals have been bled to hematocrits of 5% with simultaneous expansion of blood volume with crystalloid solutions and maintenance on 100% oxygen without any demonstrable deficit in hemodynamic parameters or tissue oxygenation. Patients with fixed cardiac output who have a deficit in the oxygen delivery system and coronary artery disease or increased oxygen demands should have a hematocrit in excess of 30% prior to surgery. No arbitrary level of hematocrit concentration is required for elective surgery. In emergency surgery, as in a patient with a gunshot wound to the aorta, hemoglobin and hematocrit changes are delayed, and the initial hematocrit may be normal. In such a patient, replacement should be commensurate with blood loss, and crystalloid solution should be provided while the initial type and cross-match is being performed. Component therapy is indicated when specific factor deficits are demonstrated or when the patient sustains massive blood loss. A workable rule of thumb in the patient with massive blood loss is administration of two units of fresh frozen plasma and two units of platelet packs for every four to six units of blood or packed red blood cells given.

HOW AND WHAT TO ORDER FOR SPECIFIC PLANNED AND EMERGENCY OPERATIONS

Friedman has provided an analysis of surgical blood use for 63 commonly performed surgical procedures in the United

States that can be applied to the maximal surgical blood order schedule. This study reflects the fact that many more units of blood are ordered than are transfused in most elective surgical procedures. Individual operating room and surgeon profiles have been developed by hospital blood banks, and specific recommendations are made through utilization review and blood transfusion committees of local hospitals. For emergency operations, four to six units of blood should be cross-matched in patients with injuries due to penetrating and blunt trauma, and 10 to 15 units of blood should be cross-matched in acute cardiovascular catastrophes. These amounts allow for initiation of operation, assessment of blood loss, and timely reordering of blood if necessary.

COMPLICATIONS AND RISKS OF BLOOD TRANSFUSIONS

Assuming that the proper care has been taken in maintaining sterility, performing venipuncture, monitoring the infusion rate, and handling blood and blood products, complications that can occur include hemolytic and nonhemolytic transfusion reactions, transmitted disease, microemboli, citrate intoxication, air embolism, hypothermia, and acid-base imbalances and other metabolic derangements. Complications involving the immunization of the recipient and febrile reactions are usually self-limiting.

HEMOLYTIC TRANSFUSION REACTIONS

Hemolytic transfusion reactions are secondary to incompatibility between the donor red blood cell and the recipient plasma and occur approximately once in every 15,000 to 20,000 transfusions. The most common cause is mistaken identification or clerical error, and the potential hazards of this complication demand careful surveillance. This reaction is manifest by hemoglobinemia, hemoglobinuria, fever, chills, dyspnea, occasional renal shutdown, and even anaphylactic shock. Treatment includes immediate cessation of transfusion and judicious administration of fluids, diuretics, possibly steroids, and sodium bicarbonate intravenously to alkalinize the urine and diminish cast formation. *In vivo* (nontransfusion) hemolysis may occur secondary to the administration of hypotonic fluids, bacterial infection in donor blood, acute hemolytic anemia from any cause, and improper handling of the blood (*e.g.*, overheating and freezing). A hemolytic transfusion reaction may occur when as little as 25 ml of blood have been transfused or may not be manifest until after 500 ml have been transfused.

NONHEMOLYTIC TRANSFUSION REACTIONS

Hyperpyrexia may occur with or without chills in approximately 0.5% to 1% of all transfusions. Treatment is accomplished by antipyretic drugs. Nonhemolytic allergic reactions occur in 2% to 3% of transfused patients and are manifest by the appearance of urticaria and diffuse rash. Antihistamines and steroids are used to treat severe allergic reactions.

TRANSMITTAL OF DISEASE

Some diseases present in the donor may be transmitted to the recipient, specifically viral and bacterial diseases. By careful screening, such donors are usually eliminated. Blood banks routinely test for hepatitis B and syphilis. Despite this testing, viral hepatitis may be transmitted in 0.2% to 2% of transfusions. Non-A non-B hepatitis viruses, for which no test exists, are probably transmitted more often than is appreciated. Recent research involving liver biopsies among patients receiving more than eight transfusions revealed that the incidence of non-A non-B hepatitis exceeded 40%. Malaria, syphilis in the sero-negative phase, Epstein-Barr virus infection, cytomegalic virus infection, brucellosis, trypanosomiasis, and Colorado tick fever are other diseases potentially transmitted by homologous blood transfusion.

MICROEMBOLI

Microaggregates ranging in size from 6 μ to 160 μ have been demonstrated to occur in transfused blood that has been filtered through the routine 180 μ blood filter. The majority of microemboli that produce pulmonary problems are thought to be in the 40 μ to 80 μ range. These microaggregates consist of fibrin, white blood cells, platelets, ghosts of red blood cells, and other proteinaceous debris. Post-transfusion respiratory insufficiency is multifactorial, and the exact role of removal of microaggregates has been debated. The use of micropore filters is generally recommended in patients who are expected to require more than four to six units of banked blood. A variety of micropore filters ranging from 20 μ to 40 μ in size are available commercially and may be obtained in both grid filter and depth filter types.

OTHER COMPLICATIONS

Citrate toxicity is rare but may occur in patients with severe liver disease. Citrate toxicity may occur with autotransfusion if excessive ACD or CPD is used as an anticoagulant and there is an inadequate collected volume of shed blood to dilute and accommodate the citrate level. Intravenous calcium gluconate (0.5 ml to 1 ml of 10% solution for every 100 ml of transfused blood) may prevent citrate intoxication, although it must not be added directly to the blood pack. Air embolism has been reported when glass blood containers have been used. However, when plastic bags are used for collection and air is prevented from entering into a closed system, air embolism has been virtually eliminated. Acidosis may occur with massive transfusion, especially if the patient is hypothermic and in shock. In patients without liver disease, metabolic acidosis rarely requires treatment. In rare cases, buffers such as bicarbonate may be indicated. Another metabolic complication is hyperkalemia, especially in multiple transfusions of older banked blood. In patients with hepatic disease the use of old blood may result in hepatic coma, and therefore in these patients the freshest blood possible should be used.

SPECIAL PROBLEMS

Single unit transfusions are generally not indicated. Because of the inherent risks and complications from banked blood, patients who would benefit from a single unit and who have a normal erythropoietic mechanism should be given iron therapy rather than exogenous blood.

There are clinical situations that make it imprudent to wait for completion of optimal compatibility testing prior to administration of blood. Various blood forms are available for emergency transfusions. Group O Rh-negative (preferably low titer) blood may be issued and available immediately. Group- and Rh-specific blood is available within 5 min, a saline cross-match is available within 10 min, and a stat cross-match is available within 30 min. A complete cross-match is usually available within 1 hr. The disadvantages of group O Rh-negative blood are that it may be detrimental in approximately 55% of all patients (*i.e.*, patients in the blood groups A, B, or AB), and it does not permit detection of unexpected recipient antibodies that could be responsible for hemolytic transfusion reactions. Group- and Rh-specific blood has the advantage that incompatible alloagglutinins are not transfused into the patient, and it generally requires only approximately 5 min to obtain blood. The disadvantage of using group- and Rh-specific blood is that unexpected antibodies in the recipient as well as errors in ABO blood grouping of donor or recipient cannot be detected. The saline cross-match will detect ABO incompatibilities and can be completed in a relatively short period of time but does not detect many antibodies, especially the IgG type. Stat cross-match is relatively safe and will detect almost all unexpected antibodies, but a complete cross-match has the disadvantage of requiring more time. Most blood banks, when providing an initial and less complete cross-match, will carry the cross-match to completion. If a subsequent incompatibility is detected, the physician accepting the release of incompletely cross-matched blood will be notified immediately.

Plasmapheresis involves withdrawal of blood from a donor to obtain platelets, plasma, plasma components, or other non-red cell elements, with reinfusion of the red cells back into the donor. It is important to monitor a donor's plasma levels, because donating plasma or platelets by pheresis too frequently may result in protein depletion. Plasmapheresis principles are also being used for patients with immunologic disorders. These procedures are usually carried out in the blood bank.

Albumin is available as a plasma expander in both 5% and 25% solutions. Although the risk of hepatitis is low, albumin has the disadvantage of rapid excretion and is expensive. The value of albumin in hypovolemic shock recently has come under attack; it may not have any advantage over crystalloid solutions. Lucas and Ledgerwood have suggested that albumin actually may increase the incidence of respiratory insufficiency in patients with hypovolemic shock.

Exciting future advances in the development of oxygen-carrying artificial blood in both stroma-free hemoglobin and fluorocarbon solutions may reduce the need for banked blood.

BIBLIOGRAPHY

Becker GA, Aster RH: Platelet transfusion therapy. Med Clin North Am 56:81, 1972

Collins JA: Problems associated with the massive transfusion of stored blood. Surgery 75:274, 1974

Colman RW, Robboy SJ, Minna JD: Disseminated intravascular coagulation (DIC): An approach. Am J Med 52:679, 1972

Connell RS, Webb MC: Filtration characteristics of three new in-line blood transfusion filters. Ann Surg 181:273, 1975

Friedman BA: An analysis of surgical blood use in United States hospitals with application to the maximum surgical blood order schedule. Transfusion 19:268, 1979

Greenburg AG, Hayashi R, Siefert I et al: Intravascular persistence and oxygen delivery of pyridoxalated, stroma-free hemoglobin during gradations of hypotension. Surgery 86:13, 1979

Hewson W: An Experimental Inquiry Into the Properties of the Blood, 2nd ed. London, T Cadell, 1772

Hutchin P: History of blood transfusion: A tercentennial lode. Surgery 64:685, 1968

Krieger JN, Hilgartner MW, Redo SF: Surgery in patients with congenital disorders of blood coagulation. Ann Surg 185:290, 1977

Lucas CE, Ledgerwood AM, Higgins RF: Impaired salt and water excretion after albumin resuscitation for hypovolemic shock. Surgery 86:544, 1979

MacFarlane RG: A clotting scheme for 1964. Thromb Diath Haemorrh 17 (Suppl):45, 1965

McKittrick JE: Banked autologous blood in elective surgery. Am J Surg 128:137, 1974

Mattox KL: Comparison of techniques of autotransfusion. Surgery 84:700, 1978

Mattox KL: Blood: What's new and over the horizon. Med Instrum 15:259, 1981

Morawitz P: Über einige postmortale Blutveranderungen. Beitr Chem Physio Pathol 8:1, 1906

Nemerson Y: Diagnosis of hemorrhagic disorders. Med Clin North Am 57:531, 1974

Reul GJ, Solis RT, Greenberg SD et al: Experience with autotransfusion in the surgical management of trauma. Surgery 76:546, 1974

Schechter DC: Problems relevant to major surgical operations in Jehovah's Witnesses. Am J Surg 116:73, 1968

Scoville WA, Annest SJ, Saba TM et al: Cardiovascular hemodynamics after opsonic alpha-2-surface binding glycoprotein therapy in injured patients. Surgery 86:284, 1979

Silver D: Coagulopathies and surgeons. J Surg Res 16:429, 1974

Silvergleid AJ: Autologous transfusions: Experience in a community blood center. JAMA 241:2724, 1979

Technical Manual of the American Association of Blood Banks, 7th ed. Washington, D.C., American Association of Blood Banks, 1977

Valeri CR, Valeri DA, Dennis RC et al: Biomedical modifications and freeze-preservation of red blood cells—a new method. Crit Care Med 7:439, 1979

Youdin SS: Transfusion of stored cadaver blood. Lancet 2:361, 1937

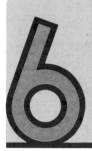

Richard M. Peters

Routine Respiratory Care and Support

An operation or accidental trauma creates stress that leads to an increase in the metabolic rate and some compromise of the efficiency of the metabolic process. As a result, there are increased demands for gas exchange. Such exchange is not only dependent on lung function but also requires an adequate cardiac output and properly functioning transport vehicles: red cells, intact lungs, and an effective ventilatory pump—the chest bellows. It is the responsibility of the surgeon to ascertain during primary evaluation whether the patient has adequate cardiorespiratory reserve to tolerate the proposed surgical procedure.

CLINICAL EVALUATION

HISTORY

A careful history is a major source of information in determining whether a patient has adequate pulmonary reserve for a given surgical operation. The pertinent questions center on the amount of activity required to produce dyspnea. If the patient is sedentary, a history of absence of dyspnea provides little information, while a vigorous jogger is unlikely to have significant dysfunction of the heart,

lungs, or chest cage. However, even for a person who performs vigorous exercise, a history must be sought of any change in level of exercise at which dyspnea occurs. Since smoking is one of the major agents that injure the lungs, ascertaining the number of pack years of smoking as well as recent smoking habits is important.

Significant disease states—asthma, pneumonia, pneumothorax—significant cough, or sputum all predict possible postoperative problems. A patient with a history of significant morning cough and sputum should be awakened early on the day of operation to cough and expectorate sputum accumulated during sleep. A history of pneumothorax signifies that positive pressure breathing during anesthesia may cause pneumothorax, and extra care is indicated to monitor tidal volume and airway pressure. The rise in pressure for a given tidal volume is increased by intrapleural air. The asthmatic patient may need bronchodilators, and some drugs may be contraindicated. The patient with recent pulmonary infection must have chest roentgenogram and careful laboratory studies to ascertain that recovery is complete.

PHYSICAL EXAMINATION

The physical examination must assess the effectiveness of the ventilatory muscles of both the chest cage and the abdomen. Inspect the chest for symmetry of motion with quiet and deep breathing. Look for any evidence of retraction in the supraclavicular area or in the intercostal spaces. Retraction is evidence of inspiratory obstruction. In the supine position inspect the degree of outward motion of the abdomen during deep breathing to assess the motion of the diaphragm. The relative anterior–posterior diameter of the chest also gives some evidence of whether emphysema is present. Wheezing on auscultation indicates the presence of bronchial obstruction, and the loudness of the breath sounds indicates the amount of air moved; coarse rales are evidence of the presence of secretions, while fine basilar rales indicate edema.

CHEST ROENTGENOGRAM

The modern surgeon must recognize that a chest x-ray film should be part of the preoperative work-up of patients with any respiratory symptoms. It is also indicated in patients over the age of 45 years and in those with a history of more than 10 pack years of smoking. The chest x-ray film should be evaluated for the degree of lung expansion, position of the mediastinum, evidence of any infiltrates, regional loss of lung volume, and the presence of fluid or air fluid levels. An air fluid level in a patient who has not had a thoracentesis is clear evidence of bronchopleural fistula. The patient is at risk of flooding the normal lung during anesthesia when cough is suppressed.

PULMONARY FUNCTION EVALUATION

It is common practice to perform many routine laboratory tests preoperatively—complete blood count, urine examination, chemistry panel, and so on. Rarely is there any routine objective measure of lung function. Patients with respiratory symptoms, 10 pack years of smoking, or evidence of abnormality on physical examination or chest radiography should have spirometric testing.

SPIROMETRY

Spirometry, a simple office form of testing, has now been made more effective by readily available automated spirometer systems. Unfortunately, the charges for these tests in many hospitals have been set far above their true cost, which discourages their use. Figure 6-1 shows a typical spirometer tracing from a patient who has performed a slow maximal inhalation followed by a maximal expiration. From the tracing, subdivisions of the lung volume can be determined. The simple tracing permits the recognition of restrictive disease. Lung disease or chest cage dysfunction characterized by an inability to take in a large volume of air is called restrictive disease and is depicted by the dotted trace. Vital capacity below 1200 cc represents severe restrictive disease (see Table 6-1). Restrictive disease can result from a number of causes, and the differential diagnosis depends on interpretation of the physical examination and the chest x-ray film. The most common cause of restrictive disease in a surgical service is restriction of motion of the chest cage due to pain. This pain produces a severe decrease in lung volume, as seen in Figure 6-2, for patients who have had a median sternotomy. Another cause is obesity. The weight of the fat must be lifted to move the chest cage, and this added effort limits ventilatory volume while increasing the work of ventilation.

Pleural effusion or pneumothorax, hemothorax, atelectasis or fibrosis, or other factors that limit lung expansion

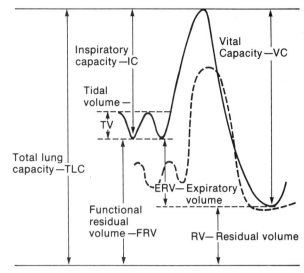

Fig. 6-1. Spirogram tracing showing the subdivisions of the lung volume. The patient first breathes quietly at the normal tidal volume (TV), then on command takes in a maximum inspiration at the end of a normal expiration, using the full inspiratory capacity (IC). The patient then breathes out slowly the total vital capacity (VC) to residual volume (RV). ERV is the expiratory reserve volume, FRV the functional reserve volume, the sum of ERV and RV. Since RV is the air left in the lungs at the end of maximum expiratory effort, it can only be measured indirectly with gas dilution or body box techniques. Total lung capacity (TLC) is the sum of RV and VC. The dotted line is an example of a tracing from a patient with restrictive lung disease. (Peters RM: The lungs. In Peters RM, Benfield JR, Peacock EE (eds): Scientific Management of Surgical Patients. Boston, Little, Brown & Co, in press)

all reduce lung volume. The differential diagnosis of the cause of the restriction depends on the interpretation of the x-ray film and the spirometric test.

To assess whether obstructive disease is present, the patient is asked to take in a deep breath and exhale as fast as he can (Fig. 6-3). The portion of air expelled in the first second is indicative of the presence of expiratory obstruction. A normal subject can expel 80% of inspired volume in the first second. First second vital capacity (FEV_1) is reduced in an asthmatic attack, in smokers, and in patients with emphysema. To be able to perform minimal activities for a comfortable life, a person must have a minimum FEV_1 of 800. Table 6-2 provides an interpretation of spirometry in assessing severity of dysfunction in patients requiring pulmonary resection. Patients with spirometric tests that place them in the moderate or severe category should have

TABLE 6-1   LUNG VOLUME

	NORMAL	ADEQUATE	MARGINAL	EMERGENCY ONLY* (POSTOP PREDICTED)
Vital Capacity (% Predicted)	≥80%	>70%	<2500 cc	<2000 cc
FEV_1	>80%	>60%	<2000 cc	<800
FEF 25–75	2 L/sec	1 L/sec	<0.8 L/sec	<0.3 L/sec
$PaCO_2$	40	<42	>45 <48	>50

* For patients in the emergency column, pulmonary resection is absolutely contraindicated.

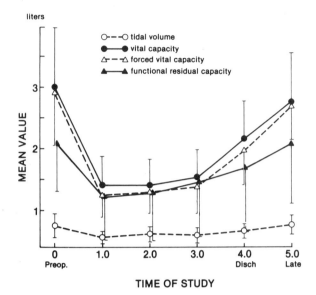

Fig. 6-2. This figure shows the result of measurement of lung volumes in postcardiopulmonary bypass patients. The periods are preoperative, postoperative days 1, 2, and 3, at time of discharge, and 6 weeks to 3 months after discharge. Vital capacity, forced vital capacity, and functional residual volume drop to approximately one third of preoperative level and return to preoperative value only at the late study. Tidal volume is about one half the preoperative value. These changes are largely the result of chest wall disruption. Similar changes would be found after posterior lateral thoracotomy. (Peters RM: The lungs. In Peters RM, Benfield JR, Peacock EE (eds): Scientific Management of Surgical Patients. Boston, Little, Brown & Co, in press)

measurement of arterial blood gases, preferably at rest and after exercise.

BLOOD GAS INTERPRETATION

The role of blood gas determination in the evaluation of pulmonary function depends on an orderly analysis of the information provided. If blood gases are abnormal, the proper interpretation can tell us whether the patient has respiratory insufficiency of some form or other. What are the indications for measuring arterial blood gas concentrations in the preoperative and postoperative periods? Figure 6-4 shows a scheme for such a decision. Blood gas determination is indicated when there is evidence from spirometry of abnormal ventilatory function. An additional indication is a roentgenogram that shows a region of unaerated lung.

Blood gas determinations provide information about

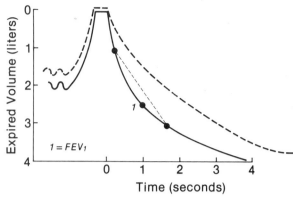

Fig. 6-3. This is the tracing for a forced vital capacity maneuver. The sequence is the same as for vital capacity measurements except that the patient is asked to expire as forcefully and as fast as he can. The percent expired in the first second, FEV_1, is noted by #1. The dotted line is the slope of volume change between 25% and 75% of VC. From this forced expired flow, the FEF^{25-75} can be derived. The heavier dotted line represents a tracing of a patient with obstructive airways disease. The slope is less and expiration is prolonged. (Peters RM: The lungs. In Peters RM, Benfield JR, Peacock EE (eds): Scientific Management of Surgical Patients. Boston, Little, Brown & Co, in press)

oxygen acquisition, carbon dioxide excretion, and acid–base status. The interpretation of blood gases depends on an understanding of acid–base chemistry and the effects of incoordination of ventilation and perfusion. The level of P_{CO_2} is an indicator of the adequacy of alveolar ventilation. This fact defines the first step in the interpretation of blood gases.

This first step is consideration of the *p*H. Is it above or below the range of 7.41–7.38? If below, the primary defect is acidosis; if above, alkalosis. The next step is evaluation of the P_{CO_2} (Fig. 6-5). Is it coordinated with the *p*H, above 40 torr with low *p*H, or below 40 torr with a high *p*H? If it is coordinated, the defect is, in part at least, respiratory. If the change is incoordinate, the primary defect is nonrespiratory, and one must decide whether the change in P_{CO_2} to compensate for a change in *p*H is appropriate in degree. Metabolic acidosis resulting from hypovolemia and a low cardiac output is a frequent problem in surgical patients. A patient with a *p*H of 7.30 and a P_{CO_2} of 38 torr has not responded appropriately. Despite the fact that the P_{CO_2} is in the normal range, the patient has a significant defect in ventilatory reserve because he or she has not increased ventilation to compensate for the low *p*H caused by metabolic acidosis. If such patients cannot hyperventilate to

TABLE 6-2   RISK FOR PULMONARY RESECTION

	HIGH RISK	MODERATE RISK	LOW RISK
Vital Capacity (VC)	<1.85 L	1.85–3.0 L	>4.0 L
First-Second Forced Expired Volume (FEV₁)	<1.2 L	1.2–3.0 L	>3.2 L
Maximum Voluntary Ventilation (MVV)	<28 L/min	>30 <80 L/min	>80 L/min
Maximum Midexpiratory Flow (FEF²⁵⁻⁷⁵)	<1.0 L/sec	>1.0 <2.0 L/sec	>2.0 L/sec

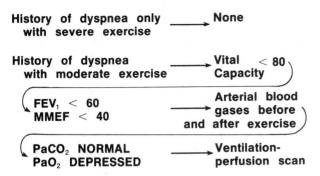

History of dyspnea only ——→ None
with severe exercise

History of dyspnea ——→ Vital < 80
with moderate exercise   Capacity

FEV₁ < 60 ——→ Arterial blood
MMEF < 40   gases before
                 and after exercise

PaCO₂ NORMAL ——→ Ventilation-
PaO₂ DEPRESSED   perfusion scan

Fig. 6-4. This figure outlines stepwise decisions for carrying out pulmonary function tests.

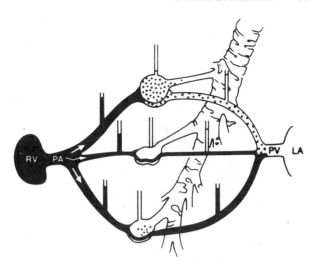

Fig. 6-6. The three types of alveoli are depicted; unsaturated blood from the right heart goes to each. *Top,* The well-ventilated alveoli fully oxygenate the blood and remove carbon dioxide. *Middle,* Collapsed alveoli provide no gas exchange but increase vascular resistance and decrease blood flow. *Bottom,* The alveolus is poorly ventilated, only partially aerating the blood perfusing it. Left heart blood is a mixture of all three. In the acute respiratory distress syndrome, the defect is perfusion of unaerated alveoli, not underventilation of perfused alveoli. LA, left atrium; PA, pulmonary artery; PV, pulmonary vein; RV, right ventricle. (Peters RM: Lifesaving measures in acute respiratory distress syndrome. Am J Surg 138:368, 1979)

partially compensate for the metabolic acidosis, they present evidence of no reserve capacity, and thus severe respiratory compromise and ventilatory support is indicated.

If P_{CO_2} is elevated above 40 torr, it signifies inadequate alveolar ventilation. In such patients a reason must be sought for this deficiency. In the preoperative patient, the most common cause is chronic obstructive lung disease. Patients with moderate elevation of P_{CO_2} (to 50 torr) will have spirometric evidence of severe obstructive disease. They may tolerate nonthoracic operative procedures if pre- and postoperative care is optimal, but pulmonary resection is absolutely contraindicated.

The interpretation of the P_{O_2} value is more complex because it can be altered by a change in F_IO_2, a decrease in alveolar ventilation, or incoordination of ventilation and perfusion. The normal range of P_{O_2} breathing air is 90 torr to 100 torr. If P_{O_2} is above 100 torr, the patient must be breathing a gas mixture enriched with added oxygen. The interpretation of P_{O_2}, therefore, requires a knowledge of P_{CO_2} and F_IO_2. If P_{CO_2} is normal, alveolar ventilation is adequate and abnormality of P_{O_2} is not caused by a decrease in alveolar ventilation. Interpretation of P_{O_2} requires a knowledge of the difference between inspired P_{O_2} ($F_IO_2 \times$ barometric pressure − P_{CO_2} − P_{H_2O}) and arterial P_{O_2}. When breathing room air, this difference should be less than 10 torr.

The most common cause of low P_{O_2} is ventilation-perfusion incoordination. Figure 6-6 shows three kinds of ratios of ventilation to perfusion—well-ventilated, well-perfused alveoli (*top*); unventilated but perfused alveoli (*middle*); and poorly ventilated perfused alveoli (*bottom*). Unventilated perfused alveoli result in venous blood reaching the arterial circulation, and poorly ventilated alveoli allow blood with incompletely removed carbon dioxide and acquired oxygen to reach the arterial circulation. In both instances, P_{O_2} will be depressed and the gradient of alveolar arterial oxygen increased. The carbon dioxide dissociation curve is a straight line, and hyperventilation of ventilated

alveoli lowers the carbon dioxide content of blood leaving them. With an intrapulmonary shunt, P_{CO_2} may be low or normal. However, P_{O_2} is depressed despite hyperventilation of well-ventilated alveoli. Because of the shape of the oxyhemoglobin curve, above 95 torr all the hemoglobin is fully saturated with oxygen and more cannot be added. Hyperventilation of aerated alveoli can remove carbon dioxide not removed by unventilated or poorly ventilated alveoli. Hyperventilation cannot compensate for oxygen not acquired (Fig. 6-7).

If an intrapulmonary shunt is present, the degree of depression of P_{O_2} is controlled by both the portion of shunted blood and the oxygen saturation of the venous blood. If cardiac output falls, resulting in increased oxygen extraction from the blood, venous oxygen saturation will fall, resulting in a fall in arterial P_{O_2}. The clinician must be aware that in the presence of a shunt, a fall in P_{O_2} can be caused by a drop in cardiac output as well as an increase in the portion of shunted blood (Fig. 6-8).

PREOPERATIVE PREPARATION

If a preoperative patient has abnormal spirometric tests or abnormal blood gases, a regimen to improve function is

Fig. 6-5. This diagram shows coordinate and incoordinate changes for respiratory and metabolic acid-base disturbances. In the coordinate column, the changes are confirmatory of the primary diagnosis. In the incoordinate column, the changes are not confirmatory of the primary diagnosis. (Peters RM: Acid-base and hemoglobin. In Peters RM, Benfield JR, Peacock EE (eds): Scientific Management of Surgical Patients. Boston, Little, Brown & Co, in press)

	Respiratory				Metabolic			
	pH,	PCO₂	HCO₃⁻	PO₂	pH,	PCO₂	HCO₃⁻	PO₂
Coordinate **Acidosis**	↓	↑	(↑)	↓	↓	(↓)	↓	—
Alkalosis	↑	↓	(↓)	—	↑	(↑)	↑	—
Incoordinate **Acidosis**	↓	=↓	↓	—	↓	↑	=↑	↓
Alkalosis	↑	=↑	↓	—	↓	↓	=↓	—

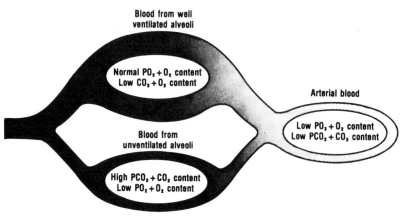

Fig. 6-7. This figure depicts the effect on the arterial blood gas oxygen partial pressure and contents of mixing blood from unventilated and well-ventilated alveoli. The ventilated alveoli are hyperventilated because of a central stimulus from the depressed arterial Po_2. The hyperventilation lowers the Pco_2 and carbon dioxide content of the blood leaving these alveoli. Because of the shape of the oxygen dissociation curve, this blood has only a normal oxygen content. Blood perfusing the unventilated alveoli has a low oxygen and high carbon dioxide partial pressure and content. In this illustration, 25% blood is perfusing the unventilated alveoli. Arterial blood, a mixture of blood from ventilated and unventilated alveoli, has low Po_2—a mixture of normal oxygen content and low oxygen content—and low Pco_2—a mixture of more low carbon dioxide content than high. This is the mechanism that results in the combination of hypoxemia and hypocapnia. (Peters RM: The lungs. In Peters RM, Benfield JR, Peacock EE (eds): Scientific Management of Surgical Patients. Boston, Little, Brown & Co, in press)

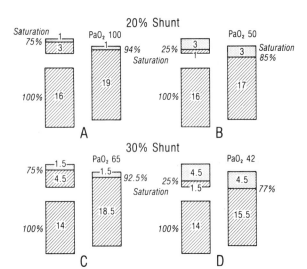

Fig. 6-8. The effect of change in venous oxygen content on arterial Po_2 and oxygen saturation. At a 20% shunt with normal venous oxygen (*left upper corner*), arterial blood is 20% blood with 75% saturation. When these are mixed (*second bar*), the result is normal or near normal Po_2 and oxygen saturation. At top right, if venous saturation falls to 25% owing to a decrease in cardiac output or increased oxygen utilization, the low venous oxygen making up 20% of the arterial blood drops the PaO_2 to 50 and the saturation to 85% (*right upper bars*). If the shunt is raised to 30%, the effects of the fall in venous oxygen are exaggerated (*lower two sets of bars*). (Peters RM: The lungs. In Peters, RM, Benfield JR, Peacock EE (eds): Scientific Management of Surgical Patients. Boston, Little, Brown & Co, in press)

indicated. The first requirement is cessation of smoking. Measuring the level of carbon monoxide in the blood can be used to monitor adherence to a no-smoking regimen. A program of graded exercise for the sedentary patient is probably the most valuable second step. A useful regimen is that of taking a walk three or four times per day, increasing the distance according to toleration of dyspnea. If a good respiratory physiotherapist is available, breathing training, particularly instruction in coughing and deep breathing, is helpful. This form of prescription without a skilled therapist

(a rare blessing in the United States but commonly available in England) is an expensive waste.

Patients with obstructive airway disease may be improved with bronchodilators and a regimen of pulmonary toilet. If there is evidence of chronic bronchitis, antibiotics are indicated. Steroids are useful in asthmatics who cannot be otherwise controlled but should be avoided if possible in surgical patients.

Since maintenance of cardiac output is critical in patients with lung disease, digitalis is indicated if there is evidence of cardiac dysfunction.

The most important factor in preparation of the patient is recognition of significant obstructive or restrictive disease so that consultation can be obtained from a competent pulmonary internist and the anesthesiologist is informed of the potential problems.

POSTOPERATIVE CARE

In discussing postoperative care it is useful to view the steps in moving the patient from complete ventilatory control by the anesthesiologist to his or her release from close supervision.

EXTUBATION

The first step is to ascertain that the effects of anesthetic agents in depressing the central respiratory drive or muscle myoneural blockade are removed. Myoneural blockade can be subjectively evaluated by the patient's ability to move. More difficult is assessment of central depression. The gold standard for this evaluation is a Pco_2 appropriate to pH, signifying that alveolar ventilation is adequate. If blood gas measurements are not available, tidal volume and rate are useful. The rate should be in the range of 15 to 25, and tidal volume should be at least 5 to 7 cc per kg of body weight. If tidal volume is low, rate should be higher.

Where does the level of PaO_2 enter in this decision? Postoperative patients can have significant incoordination of ventilation and perfusion, probably the result of poor ventilation of the basilar and posterior portions of the lung. As discussed earlier, the result can be depression of PaO_2.

Underventilation due to central depression can usually be corrected by an increase in F_IO_2 to 0.5 but low PCO_2 cannot, so the first step is to ascertain whether PCO_2 is appropriate. The high F_IO_2 may depress respiratory drive and thus alveolar ventilation in patients with obstructive disease. Therefore, F_IO_2 should be kept at the lowest level consistent with PO_2 of 100 torr. There is no advantage in keeping PO_2 above 100 torr because all hemoglobin will be fully saturated with oxygen at this PO_2.

Assessing the level of PaO_2 is not enough since the important factor to protect is the amount of oxygen delivered to the tissues, not the oxygen level in arterial blood. The amount of oxygen delivered is the amount of oxygen in the blood (the oxygen content, CaO_2) times the amount of blood flow (cardiac output, CO). This is expressed by the formula Oxygen delivery = $CaO_2 \times CO$.

If oxygen content is depressed, cardiac output should be elevated. If cardiac output is depressed, even with normal CaO_2 oxygen delivery will be depressed. If oxygen delivery is depressed, oxygen needs must be minimized. If the patient has a low cardiac output from any cause, it is advisable to continue respiratory support until the cause of the depressed cardiac output is corrected. A ventilator can perform the work of breathing for the patient and the oxygen needs of the muscles of respiration are decreased.

VENTILATORY SUPPORT

If a patient needs ventilatory support, what are the choices available? At this time there is a consensus that volume-regulated ventilators should be used. It is my firm conviction that the intermittent mandatory ventilator system (IMV) is the best postoperative method of ventilation. The IMV rate can be set to supplement the patient's own efforts to the extent needed. As the patient's strength recovers, the IMV rate can be lowered in increments until the support is no longer needed. Recent evidence clearly indicates that the strength of respiratory muscles decreases with inactivity, indicating the importance of requiring patients to provide as much ventilation on their own as they can.

The indicator of adequate alveolar ventilation is PCO_2. It should be appropriate to *pH*—*i.e.,* if metabolic acidosis is present, PCO_2 should be in the low 30s. The IMV should be adjusted to give an appropriate PCO_2. If the PO_2 is low, continuous positive airway pressure (CPAP) should be used to increase functional residual volume and expand collapsed alveoli. If shunt fraction is above 0.25, the patient needs a Swan–Ganz catheter to monitor cardiac output (CO) as CPAP is raised. CPAP can depress CO by increasing pulmonary capillary resistance and decreasing venous return to the left and right cardiac compartments.

In summary, the IMV rate, CPAP, and F_IO_2 should be adjusted to keep F_IO_2 below 0.5, PO_2 above 65 torr, and PCO_2 at 38 to 40 torr.

The usual method of weaning patients from the IMV is to lower the IMV and test the patient's response 30 min to 60 min later. Has the respiratory rate increased or the spontaneous tidal volume increased or decreased? Has PCO_2 remained appropriate? If the rate is below 25, the tidal volume above 250 cc to 300 cc, and the PCO_2 appropriate (35 to 45 torr), then the reduced rate is tolerated and in a few hours it can be lowered further. PaO_2 and calculated shunt fraction are used to adjust CPAP and F_IO_2. The first step is to keep the PaO_2 above 65 while lowering F_IO_2 to 0.30. Then CPAP can be lowered, preserving the same PaO_2

of 65. Sixty-five is chosen because that is the shoulder of the oxygen dissociation curve. Below a PaO_2 of 65, small decrements in PaO_2 result in large decrements in arterial oxygen content.

It may not be possible to wean patients who have required prolonged ventilatory support by gradually decreasing the IMV rate. Such patients allow PCO_2 to rise as the IMV rate is lowered because they will not increase their voluntary ventilation. They must be taken off the ventilator or placed on a low IMV rate for periods of increasing length during the day to provide stress for them and to increase their muscle strength. In the early stages of weaning, it is best to provide ventilator support at night to rest the patient.

Patients requiring prolonged ventilation often have been placed on hyperalimentation with very high caloric intakes. Excessive calories increase the metabolic rate and the carbon dioxide produced. The amount of hyperventilation required to excrete this carbon dioxide may exceed the patient's respiratory reserve. Lowering caloric intake can often lead to successful weaning.

REINTUBATION

Under what circumstances must a patient be reintubated for reinstitution of ventilatory support? There are two sets of requirements. The first is clinical evidence of respiratory distress that cannot be relieved—*i.e.,* tachypnea above 25 to 30 breaths per min with a low tidal volume of less than 250 cc to 300 cc per breath. Laboratory indications are acute elevation of PCO_2 above 45 torr or 50 torr, depression of PO_2 below 65 torr on F_IO_2 of 0.5, or evidence of low cardiac output.

Another question is, how long can an endotracheal airway be used for ventilatory support? There is no evidence that an endotracheal tube in place for weeks is any more hazardous than a tracheostomy tube. Our criterion for change is to perform tracheostomy only to improve patient comfort when we anticipate more than 2 weeks of ventilatory support. If a tracheostomy is required, it should be done as a carefully planned, precise operative procedure, preferably in the operating room. No tracheal wall should be excised, and the opening should not be below the third ring. Many regimens have been described for removing tracheostomy tubes using fenestrated tubes. These interval regimens are unnecessary before complete removal. In most instances, as soon as the patient can be removed from ventilation, the cuff should be deflated; if the patient can remain off the ventilator for 24 hr, the tube can be removed.

ROUTINE RESPIRATORY CARE

Fortunately, most patients do not require postoperative ventilatory support if skilled respiratory care is provided. Figure 6-2 shows the usual effects on lung volumes of surgery performed in the chest or abdomen. These restrictions are the result of postoperative pain. They result in decreased ventilation, particularly to the lower lobes. Cough is also inhibited and ineffective. These deficiencies set the stage for postoperative atelectasis. The reduction in functional residual volume due to pain results in closing of the bronchi in the basilar portions of the lungs. Basilar bronchi close at higher lung volumes in elderly patients and in those who smoke. In obese patients, functional residual capacity (FRC) is decreased preoperatively and further decreased postoperatively. A patient with bronchitis or increased secretions has an added problem. The number of these abnormalities determines the likelihood of atelectasis, usually basilar.

Postoperative care is critical in controlling these factors. Inadequate postoperative fluid replacement results in dry airways and thick sputum that is difficult to cough up. Inadequate pain control inhibits cough and increases splinting, which decreases FRC. High F_IO_2 removes the stabilizing gas N_2 from the alveoli, and brief obstruction can cause acute collapse of alveoli. Adequate analgesia is the most critical need. In elderly patients or in those with chronic obstructive lung disease (COLD), narcotics may suppress ventilatory drive and result in inadequate alveolar ventilation. The use of epidural blocks or other methods of local analgesia in patients with COLD may avoid the need for ventilatory support by removing pain and permitting effective respiratory muscle function. Patients with COLD are particularly vulnerable to drying of secretions. It is important to assure adequate hydration to patients with COLD, but it must not be neglected in others. In all postoperative patients, but particularly in those with COLD, hyperventilation is necessary to compensate for the inefficiency of the lungs postoperatively so that extra work is required and more water is evaporated from the lungs.

Patients with lung disease preoperatively are the most difficult postoperative patients, but even those with normal lungs preoperatively develop pulmonary complications if respiratory care is neglected. The greater the injury by trauma or the nearer the injury or operative incision is to the diaphragm, the greater the effect on ventilatory function.

In patients without lung disease, narcotics should be provided to control pain. A pro re necessitas order for narcotics does not necessarily assure adequate analgesia. Did the nurse inquire of the patient if he had pain? Does the staff speak the patient's language? Do they appreciate cultural differences? The physician must monitor whether his patient has received the prescribed narcotics. Narcotics should be given prior to respiratory therapy, bed making, and ambulation, not afterwards when pain is extreme.

Fever or tachycardia may indicate atelectasis. If cough and deep breathing fail to correct the symptoms, a roentgenogram should be obtained. If atelectasis is present, fiberoptic bronchoscopy is indicated, as is a regimen to correct other deficiencies that lead to atelectasis. Hydration should be checked, and the adequacy of analgesia, the amount of mobility by the patient, and the possible presence of sepsis should be reviewed.

The sophisticated devices and techniques of respiratory therapy that have been developed in the last three decades are gadgets that too often are used improperly and are substituted for effective postoperative respiratory care. Used in this way, they are harmful, not helpful. The most important factor in preventing respiratory postoperative problems is mobilization of the patient. Get him out of bed and ambulating. This increases deep breathing and cough, and changes areas of the lung that are dependent. Appropriate use of analgesics and good nursing care in helping the patient to move are the essentials of good postoperative respiratory care; they will not be replaced by any device.

ADULT RESPIRATORY DISTRESS SYNDROME— FEATURES AND MANAGEMENT

Risk Factors	Multiple organ trauma, shock, sepsis, multiple organ failure, multiple transfusions, aspiration, smoke inhalation
Pathogenesis	Incompletely understood; increased pulmonary capillary membrane permeability by uncertain mechanism(s) cause interstitial and alveolar edema, which lead to ventilation-perfusion incoordination, increased intrapulmonary shunt, and hypoxemia
Diagnosis	Tachypnea; dyspnea; increased total body weight; blood gases— ↓ Po_2; ↓ Pco_2; ↓ O_2 saturation; chest x-ray shows interstitial edema; ↓ pulmonary AV shunt; ↓ pulmonary compliance; normal to low left atrial filling pressure Increased pulmonary artery pressure.
Treatment	Treat associated problems—e.g., shock, sepsis; use mechanical ventilation—intermittent mandatory ventilation; PEEP, CPAP; place Swan-Ganz catheter to monitor PA wedge and cardiac output; monitor arterial and mixed venous blood gases. Optimize cardiac output while raising CPAP or PEEP to raise FRC and open closed capillaries. Use diuretics and inotropic agents if wedge pressure is high and cardiac output inadequate.

RESPIRATORY INSUFFICIENCY

Respiratory insufficiency is one of the most common complications of complex surgery or multiple injuries. It is also a leading cause of death in surgical patients, particularly when combined with multiple organ failure. Respiratory insufficiency has two forms: (1) that resulting from the stress of surgery aggravating pre-existing pulmonary disease and (2) acute respiratory insufficiency caused by the trauma inflicted on the patient. This latter form of respiratory insufficiency has many names—shock lung, post-traumatic respiratory insufficiency, wet lung, and adult respiratory distress syndrome (ARDS).

PRE-EXISTING LUNG DISEASE

Respiratory insufficiency is most likely to occur in patients with marginal preoperative lung function in whom the effects of operation cause a low respiratory reserve below levels that can provide adequate gas exchange. These patients develop progressive elevation of $PaCO_2$ and hypoxemia as a result of hypoventilation. The insufficiency may be worsened by pulmonary complications such as atelectasis, pneumonia, or pneumothorax. Treatment consists of endotracheal intubation and ventilatory support with a volume ventilator to assure adequate alveolar ventilation, as well as therapy of the associated problems, such as antibiotics for pneumonia or a chest tube for pneumothorax.

ADULT RESPIRATORY DISTRESS SYNDROME (ARDS)

CLINICAL PICTURE

ARDS tends to occur in patients who have had extensive operative procedures or multiple injuries. Very often there is major blood loss requiring large intravascular volume replacement. After correction of hypovolemic shock, these patients have a period of stable vital signs and apparently adequate pulmonary function. During the couse of the next 24 hr to 48 hr they develop progressive dyspnea associated with marked hyperventilation. Arterial blood gases show a low $PaCO_2$, in the mid or lower 30s, and a progressive decline in PaO_2 that is little affected by increasing F_1O_2. Cardiac output is often two to three times the normal resting level.

Pulmonary function studies show high minute ventilation, falling lung compliance, decrease in functional residual capacity, and increase in respiratory work. Serial chest x-ray films show progressive diffuse pulmonary mottling that may become confluent. Increased shunting and progressive hypoxemia are noted until the patient succumbs from hypoxemia and hyperventilatory exhaustion unless ventilatory support is provided.

PATHOPHYSIOLOGY

A number of factors have been implicated in the pathophysiology of ARDS, including fat embolus, leukocyte or platelet aggregates, circulating toxins, complement and other vasoactive substances, and excessive fluid administration. Smoke inhalation and aspiration injury, shock, multiple trauma, burns, head injuries, sepsis, cardiopulmonary bypass, and acute abdominal processes are frequently associated with the syndrome clinically.

Damage to pulmonary capillary endothelial cells alters the permeability of the capillaries. Fluid and proteins leak into the lung interstitium and move to the perivascular space, where they are removed by lymphatics. If the leak exceeds lymphatic pump capacity, the fluid accumulates in the perivascular lymphatic space. When this space is full, the fluid floods the alveoli, leading to their collapse and an increasing intrapulmonary shunt. Increase in pulmonary shunt results in a low arterial Po_2, the hallmark of ARDS.

Generally, ARDS is not due to increased hydrostatic forces causing fluid leakage from pulmonary capillaries, as may be seen, for example, with acute left ventricular failure. Lowering of plasma oncotic pressure, such as may occur with hemodilution during cardiopulmonary bypass or in cirrhotic patients with decreased albumin production, does not seem to be implicated in the etiology of ARDS. Changing circulating volume by means of diuretics alone or altering plasma oncotic pressure by administration of albumin does not seem to affect the course of the syndrome substantially.

TREATMENT OF ARDS

The most effective therapy for ARDS is the use of mechanical ventilation and positive end expiratory pressure (PEEP) or spontaneous ventilation with continuous positive airway pressure (CPAP) delivered through an endotracheal tube. These methods employ a mechanical system that prevents the airway pressure at end expiration from dropping to the ambient atmospheric pressure. This increased pressure results in an increase of functional residual capacity that prevents further alveolar collapse and opens the already collapsed alveoli. The shunt is thus diminished and oxygenation is increased. Patients with ARDS should be treated in an intensive care unit and monitored with an electrocardiogram, Foley catheter, frequent blood gas determinations such as those that can be obtained through an arterial line and a Swan–Ganz catheter for monitoring left atrial filling pressures, and, in some cases, cardiac output. The F_1O_2 should be limited to 50% or lower to prevent pulmonary oxygen toxicity. PEEP levels should be adjusted to as low a value as possible (between 5 and 30 cm H_2O) to maintain an acceptable arterial oxygen concentration (PaO_2 greater than or equal to 60 torr).

Pulmonary capillary wedge pressure should be monitored and kept as low as feasible while maintaining a level of cardiac output that assures adequate oxygen delivery despite the low arterial oxygen content. Diuretics may be useful if the patient is significantly overhydrated, though they frequently are of no use if the capillary is still leaking. Diuretics can be dangerous if they lower circulatory volume, causing a fall in cardiac filling pressures and cardiac output.

PEEP increases intrathoracic pressure and tends to decrease cardiac filling. Similarly, diuresis and secondary decreases in circulating volume impair cardiac return. Both of these factors may result in inadequate cardiac output. To increase cardiac output, the use of inotropic agents, such as dopamine, or afterload reducing agents, such as nitroprusside, may be necessary, but only if the physician is certain that filling pressures are adequate.

Treatment of underlying conditions such as sepsis is likely to shorten the duration of the ARDS syndrome. Prevention of secondary bacterial infection of the lungs by careful nursing care is similarly important.

Pneumothorax or tension pneumothorax can occur from the high ventilatory pressures associated with PEEP, which may cause alveolar rupture. Awareness of the possibility of acute tension pneumothorax should allow prompt needle or tube thoracostomy if necessary.

Changes in the radiographic appearance of interstitial edema do not closely parallel the changes of oxygen exchange dynamics in the ARDS lung. Gradual improvements of the blood gases over several days are noted as recovery from the syndrome occurs. Decreasing PEEP levels and subsequent weaning from the ventilator can be accomplished as the lung regains its normal function.

BIBLIOGRAPHY

HODGKIN JE: Preoperative evaluation of pulmonary function. Am J Surg 138:355, 1979
MACKLEM PT: Respiratory muscles. The vital pump. Chest 78:753, 1980
PETERS RM: Management of surgically treated patient with limited pulmonary reserve. Am J Surg 138:379, 1978
WEST JB: Regional differences in the lung. Chest 74:426, 1978

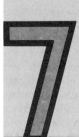

George L. Blackburn/Karen B. Harvey-Wilkes

Nutrition in Surgical Patients

METABOLIC RESPONSE TO INJURY

STRESS CATABOLISM

Surgical injury, trauma, or critical illness results in a hormone-mediated mobilization of endogenous substrates (Fig. 7-1). The catecholamines (epinephrine), corticosteroids, and glucagon stimulate a mobilization of stored protein and energy reserves in support of key pathways necessary for stabilization, host defense, and recovery. Free fatty acids, ketones, and glucose meet energy needs; amino acids are utilized for the synthesis of acute phase proteins, gluconeogenesis, and thermogenesis essential in the homeostasis of injury metabolism.

These metabolic changes are best understood as a redistribution of macronutrients from labile reserves (skeletal muscle and adipose tissue) to more active tissues (liver, bone marrow) for host defense, visceral protein synthesis, and heat production (Fig. 7-2).

Micronutrients are also redistributed. There is an increased uptake of zinc by the liver; zinc is a cofactor in several enzymatic functions required during injury. Greater amounts of iron are taken up by iron-binding proteins such as transferrin, thus reducing the amount available for iron-dependent pathogenic microorganisms.

The duration of this acute phase of the stress response depends upon the severity of injury and the presence of sepsis and associated malnutrition. The increased levels of glucocorticoids associated with severe stress such as sepsis antagonize the peripheral action of insulin (insulin resistance). In order to maintain normal blood glucose levels or to distribute a glucose load increased amounts of insulin are needed. Higher insulin levels interfere with fat mobilization and ketogenesis. Because endogenous fat makes such a major contribution to energy production, even a small reduction in fat mobilization creates a gap in the substrate supply that must be covered by increased oxidation of glucose and certain amino acids. Since glycogen stores are limited, endogenous protein is increasingly catabolized. With prolonged stress and catabolism, substrate levels (particularly amino acids) fall, resulting in decreased synthesis of plasma proteins, especially those concerned with host defense. For clinical purposes a "five-day rule" is important, at which time supplemental nutrition support should begin in order to sustain the metabolic response to injury without development of malnutrition and risk of impaired host defense and wound healing.

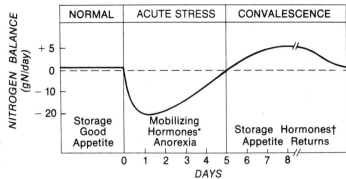

Fig. 7-1. Biphasic hormonal response to injury in the normal postoperative patient. *, Catecholamines, corticosteroids, glucagon, growth hormone, "injury" hormones, leukocytic mediators; †, Insulin.

Once the acute phase of injury has subsided, the patient enters an "adaptive" or convalescent phase; feeding should begin at this time. Catecholamine and glucocorticoid concentrations decrease, enabling insulin to promote the uptake of glucose and amino acids for storage (*e.g.*, glycogen), incorporation of amino acids into proteins, or conversion of glucose to triglycerides. If the patient is fasting, fatty acids continue to be the primary fuel. The percentage of use of free fatty acids as an energy source is reflected in the respiratory quotient (R.Q.), ketonemia, and ketonuria, which can be monitored easily using an acetone test. Although fluids, electrolytes, amino acids, vitamins, and minerals are essential components of all surgical feedings, caloric requirements vary. If after 5 days of fasting, no ketonuria exists, exogenous glucose and fat should be provided in modest amounts (*e.g.*, 25 kcal/kg/day).

The overall response to injury should not be viewed as pathogenic but rather as a finely tuned integrated series of reactions that provide adequate quantities of fuel and amino acids for visceral protein synthesis during short-term (5 days) fasting in young, well-nourished patients. Metabolically active tissues such as liver and bone marrow undergo anabolism at the expense of increased net catabolism of muscle, connective tissue, and gut mucosa. Nutritional support during this period should be directed toward supplementing the redistribution of amino acids, not blocking the process. Amino acids, fluids, and electrolytes are the quintessential nutrients for this therapy.

ENERGY EXPENDITURE

The average nonstressed individual lying quietly in bed requires 23 kcal/kg/day to maintain body weight. Limited physical activity increases this requirement to 28 kcal/kg/day. Ordinary elective surgery does not cause a significant increase in energy requirements. In the severely injured or septic patient, however, there is an increased caloric requirement secondary to the catabolic response. Needs are increased approximately 25% in skeletal trauma, 50% in sepsis, and 75% to 100% in severe burns (Fig. 7-3). Associated with an increased energy expenditure in hypermetabolic patients is an increased drain on protein stores, as previously mentioned. The following nitrogen losses are commonly seen in fasting patients:

Elective postsurgical patients	7–9 g N/day
Skeletal trauma or septic patients	11–14 g N/day
Severe burns	12–18 g N/day

The addition of exogenous corticosteroids to the high circulating levels characteristic of stress can increase nitrogen losses even further.

ETIOLOGY OF MALNUTRITION

Many patients who will develop clinically significant protein-calorie malnutrition enter the hospital with a history of weight loss resulting from the anorexia and increased

Fig. 7-2. Functional redistribution of body cell mass after injury or surgery provides nitrogen for protein synthesis. Arrows reflect the net release (−) in grams from connective tissue, gut mucosa, and muscle, as well as uptake (+) of amino acids into tissues whose net anabolism is associated with survival. The conversion of protein into glucose and urea is a minor source of energy but is an important part of the role of the liver to produce the heat necessary to maintain core temperature.

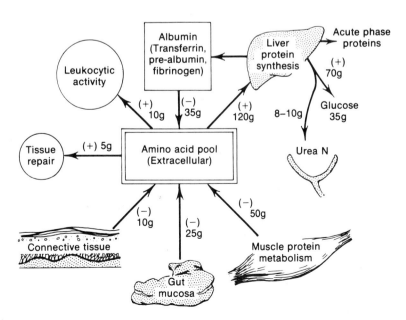

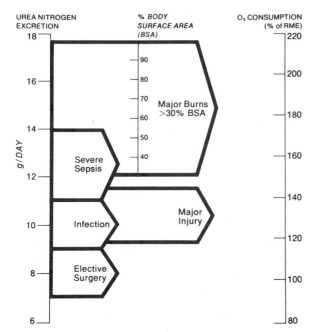

Fig. 7-3. Rates of hypermetabolism estimated from urinary urea nitrogen excretion. (Blackburn GL, Bistrian BR, Maini BS: Nutritional and metabolic support of the hospitalized patient. Journal of Parenteral and Enteral Nutrition 1:11, 1977)

catabolism associated with their underlying disease. Other patients become malnourished after admission as a consequence of the catabolic stress of surgery or sepsis and the semistarvation regimens commonly used with the very ill (*e.g.*, D₅W).

PROBLEMS WITH D₅W

D₅W solutions, providing about 100 g of glucose (400 kcal) per day, have been traditionally given with the thought that they would spare body proteins by reducing the need for gluconeogenesis. However, the 100 g of glucose is a sufficient quantity to stimulate insulin release, thereby inhibiting free fatty acid (FFA) mobilization. This reduces the contribution of FFA and ketone bodies to meet the energy deficit, causing more, not less, protein to be broken down for gluconeogenesis to meet energy needs. This process can be detected by a respiratory quotient (R.Q. > 0.76).

POSTOPERATIVE STARVATION vs. FASTING

In prolonged fasting, the ability of the body to use free fatty acids and ketone bodies as an energy source results in a high degree of glucose and protein conservation. Insulin levels are low and allow for the redistribution of fat and protein from body reserves to maintain homeostasis. Free fatty acids or ketone bodies are metabolized as an energy source by most tissues of the body (exceptions include the renal medulla, erythrocytes, bone marrow, and peripheral nerves); amino acids are used primarily for protein synthesis. Gluconeogenesis from amino acids is a homeostatic mechanism to maintain the blood glucose level once glycogen stores are depleted. Although fasting can be tolerated for several weeks, surgery inhibits adaptation (increased catecholamine levels), and the well-nourished postoperative patient can tolerate starvation for only 5 to 10 days with no clinically significant depletion of visceral protein, skeletal

NUTRITION IN SURGICAL PATIENTS

Incidence A substantial proportion of hospitalized patients are at risk nutritionally for major morbidity and mortality. The prevalence of clinically significant protein-calorie malnutrition exceeds 15% in many acute care hospitals.

Etiology Patients may enter the hospital with weight loss due to the anorexia and increased catabolism associated with their primary disease. Other patients become malnourished after admission as a result of the catabolic stress of surgery or sepsis and the semistarvation regimens commonly used in critically ill patients (*e.g.*, D₅W).

Diagnosis A complete nutritional assessment includes evaluation of visceral proteins concerned with immune competence (delayed hypersensitivity response, total lymphocyte count), substrate transport and oncotic pressure (albumin and transferrin), creatinine height index, anthropometric parameters (arm muscle circumference, triceps skinfold), and catabolic rate (urine urea nitrogen and urine creatinine). These parameters, in particular, albumin and delayed hypersensitivity response, have prognostic value in evaluating hospitalized patients, thus implicating protein-calorie malnutrition as a factor in the course of many illnesses.

Treatment Parenteral and enteral nutrition using new feeding devices, formulas, and feeding modules provide adequate amounts of protein, carbohydrate, and fat.

muscle mass, or adipose tissue. In contrast, the patient who on admission is nutritionally at risk (prolonged stress, low visceral protein levels, weight loss) cannot tolerate the further depletion that would occur with a starvation state and must receive exogenous substrates—amino acids, glucose, fat.

NUTRITIONAL ASSESSMENT

Detection of patients at nutritional risk is the first step in nutritional support. The clinically significant correlate of a depleted nutritional state is impaired host defense, which predisposes the patient to medical and surgical complications, especially those of a septic nature. A battery of nutritional assessment parameters allows one to develop a profile of the individual patient. A specific therapeutic regimen may be tailored to meet the patient's specific needs.

A complete nutritional assessment includes evaluation of visceral proteins concerned with host defense, substrate transport and oncotic pressure, and anthropometric measurements.

VISCERAL PROTEINS

HOST DEFENSE

Considerable evidence indicates that infections occur more frequently and with greater severity in malnourished individuals.

The immune system encompasses a wide variety of host defense activities—phagocytosis, antibody synthesis, lymphokine production, complement-mediated bacteriolysis, cell-mediated cytolysis, and interferon production. These functions require the interaction of three types of leukocytes: thymus-derived (T) lymphocytes, antibody-synthesizing (B) lymphocytes, and accessory cells (*e.g.,* macrophages and neutrophils). Many of these cooperative interactions and activities are dependent on protein synthesis. Nutritional depletion, resulting from anorexia, increased metabolic rate, malabsorption, or increased losses (fistulas, diarrhea), may therefore result in decreased immunocompetence (see also Chapters 9 and 10).

Immunologic assays are valuable in assessing the functional and clinically significant severity of malnutrition. Simple measurements include an enumeration of total leukocytes (*i.e.,* total lymphocyte count and total neutrophil count). Decreased lymphocyte counts (<1000/mm³) have been reported in hypoalbuminemic postsurgical patients and children with kwashiorkor but not in marasmic persons. It is suggested that rapid protein depletion due to increased protein catabolism may have a different effect on immune response than the more gradual depletion resulting from anorexia and inadequate protein and carbohydrate intake. There are other explanations for decreased counts, however, such as blood loss, migration to traumatized tissues, and sequestration in lymphoid tissues.

The nonspecific immune defense system—in particular, complement and immunoglobulins—is the primary mechanism for containing bacterial contamination and preventing colonization, infection, and sepsis. Owing to the high priority of complement and immunoglobulin synthesis with respect to amino acid availability, they are not useful in the early detection of mild or moderate nutritional deficiency in hospitalized patients. However, in cases of severe protein-calorie malnutrition, such as in burn patients, decreased complement and immunoglobulin levels may be seen.

The most widely utilized assay for the analysis of immune function before elective surgery, or before and during nutritional support, is delayed hypersensitivity (DH) skin testing, which evaluates cell-mediated immunity. A positive skin test requires functioning accessory cells, T and B lymphocytes, macrophage activation, lymphokine production, and monocyte chemotaxis (Fig. 7-4). A wide variety of metabolic systems can interfere with this complex process. Anergy has been reported not only in immune deficient

states but also in advanced age, uremia, bacterial infections, viral infections, and liver disease. Transient anergy often follows surgery or acute injury and is due to the appearance of a serum inhibitor or T-lymphocyte reactions. One should therefore wait until the seventh or eighth postoperative day before evaluating the delayed hypersensitivity reaction. Radiation and chemotherapy, as well as cancer itself, may also act to depress the DH response to recall skin antigens. Thus, protein-calorie malnutrition is not the only cause of acquired anergy in the hospitalized patient; but regardless of the etiology, depression of cell-mediated immunity as reflected by delayed hypersensitivity skin antigen testing has been associated with increased sepsis and related mortality, even though those organisms against which cell-mediated immunity is not the primary host defense are frequently the cause of the sepsis. In most patients, the infectious agents are gram-negative rods or gram-positive cocci, ubiquitous organisms generally from the patient's own flora, which are normally of low virulence in healthy, well-nourished individuals, instead of viruses, fungi, and intracellular parasites from the environment. One possible mechanism for the increased frequency of sepsis associated with anergy is that the critical number of bacteria that one would expect to be handled by the inflammatory response may be altered. DH testing does not identify the deficit; it is simply a marker that the immune system is not functioning adequately.

Because of their high metabolic priority, immune functions of lymphocytes or accessory cells may be the first metabolic system to respond to nutritional support, and thus serial measurements of immune function may be of use in determining the appropriateness and effectiveness of nutritional therapy. Serial measurements have been found to be valuable in predicting outcome (*i.e.,* mortality) of hospital therapy.

To measure the intactness of the delayed hypersensitivity response, three recall skin antigens—*Candida albicans,* mumps, and streptokinase–streptodornase—are commonly used. One-tenth milliliter of each solution is placed intradermally in the forearm area, and the reaction is examined at 24 hr and

Fig. 7-4. Mechanism of delayed hypersensitivity response to recall antigens. Nonspecific host defense functions required to produce induration in response to antigenic stimulation.

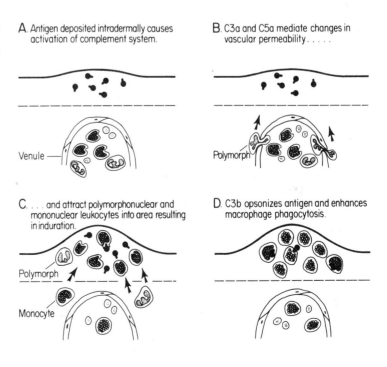

A. Antigen deposited intradermally causes activation of complement system.

B. C3a and C5a mediate changes in vascular permeability . . . . .

C. . . . and attract polymorphonuclear and mononuclear leukocytes into area resulting in induration.

D. C3b opsonizes antigen and enhances macrophage phagocytosis.

48 hr; a 5-mm induration or greater is considered positive. Immune competence is defined as a positive response to one or more of the antigens. Ninety-five percent accuracy of the test can be anticipated if the test is meticulously performed. While a negative response to recall skin antigen (particularly mumps and *Candida*) may be due to a variety of causes, a positive response followed serially can provide important knowledge about the integrity of the host defense system and the effectiveness of nutrition support therapy— parenteral or enteral or a combination of the two methods.

SERUM ALBUMIN

Serum albumin serves as the prime indicator of protein-calorie malnutrition in both medical and surgical patients. Albumin functions as the major protein in the body by maintaining colloid osmotic pressure and by transporting metals, ions, hormones, drugs, and other metabolites. Synthesized only in the liver, albumin equilibrates between intravascular and extravascular compartments so that 31% to 42% of the exchangeable albumin pool is in the plasma. The half-life of albumin is 14 to 18 days.

During prolonged fasting, albumin synthesis is depressed. The catabolic rate does not decrease immediately after protein deprivation but only after the concentration of plasma albumin has declined somewhat. Refeeding leads to rapid stimulation of synthesis, which is very sensitive to dietary amino acid supply, particularly that of tryptophan and possibly the branched chain amino acids. Under suitable hormonal control, these amino acids appear to influence hepatic free and endoplasmic reticulum-bound polyribosomal aggregation, which enhances intracellular and secretory protein synthesis.

In the patient who is stressed, either from surgical or other trauma or infection, serum albumin concentrations decrease. One probable explanation is a redistribution throughout the intravascular and extravascular spaces. The proportion of albumin in the extravascular compartment increases owing to wound edema, reduced lymphatic return, or sodium retention, all of which lead to an expansion of the extravascular compartment. This must be taken into account when interpreting serum albumin concentrations. If a preoperative or peritrauma serum albumin level is not available for evaluation, one should wait 10 days following surgery or other trauma to allow the extravascular volume to return to normal as a marker of protein-calorie malnutrition.

Low albumin levels are also seen in nephrotic syndromes, protein-losing enteropathies, and liver disease. However, it is difficult to consider a patient with hypoalbuminemia without nutritional risk, whatever the etiology.

OTHER PLASMA PROTEINS

Other plasma proteins have been used as markers of nutritional status. Transferrin ($t_{\frac{1}{2}}$ = 7 to 8 days), prealbumin ($t_{\frac{1}{2}}$ = 2 days), and retinol-binding protein ($t_{\frac{1}{2}}$ = 12 hr) have been proposed as more sensitive indicators of nutritional repletion due to their shorter half-lives than serum albumin ($t_{\frac{1}{2}}$ = 14 to 19 days). Like albumin, however, none are specific indicators of malnutrition. Depressed concentrations have been noted following surgery and other forms of stress.

Transferrin, primarily synthesized in the liver, is the major iron-binding protein. One factor that precludes its wide use as a marker of nutritional depletion is that increased concentrations are found in iron-deficient persons. *The strength of using transferrin as a parameter of protein status is in serial measurements in which the patient serves as his own control* (Table 7-1). Transferrin levels are valuable markers of plasma protein status in the patient receiving albumin infusions.

Prealbumin and retinol-binding proteins are integral parts of the vitamin A transport system. Decreased circulating levels of these two plasma proteins result in impaired transport of vitamin A from the liver and thus may precipitate vitamin A deficiency symptoms. In addition, 15% of circulating thyroxine is normally bound to prealbumin. The major restriction to clinical use of these proteins is their rapid variation in serial measurements due to very short half-lives.

Owing to the wide availability of SMA-12 screening, albumin levels are measured on most patients on admission to the hospital. In light of the unfavorable prognostic implications of a low serum albumin, there is a tendency to treat hypoalbuminemia by giving albumin; such treatment does not allow for the more general loss of function hypoalbuminemia represents. Restoration of a normal serum albumin requires adequate nutritional support in addition to reduction of the stress response. Exogenous albumin is usually not necessary until the serum albumin falls below 2.2 g/dl, and then its function is to maintain oncotic pressure.

Serum albumin concentrations are routinely measured in most clinical laboratories by a standard "salting out" technique, autoanalyzer (colorimetric), or radial immunodiffusion. Serum transferrin is measured by radial immunodiffusion. To use these parameters serially, one must obtain from the clinical laboratory the standard deviation and coefficient of variance for the assay. From these values, one can determine if a change in serum concentration is significant or within the variation of the assay.

Local standards vary, but a serum albumin value of less than 3.0 g/dl represents significant protein-calorie malnutrition, since other changes characteristic of protein-calorie

---

TABLE 7-1   SERIAL SERUM PROTEINS*

OUTCOME	ALBUMIN		TRANSFERRIN	
	Initial	Final	Initial	Final
Discharged (n = 50)	3.4 ± 0.1	$\rightarrow 3.1 \pm 0.1\dagger$	154 ± 9	$\rightarrow 177 \pm 9\dagger$
Died (n = 18)	3.2 ± 0.1	$\rightarrow 2.8 \pm 0.1\dagger$	116 ± 15	$\rightarrow 125 \pm 11$

* A group of 68 cancer patients who received nutritional support during a course of oncological therapy. A decrease in serum albumin was seen in both groups (those who were discharged and those who died during the hospitalization) despite adequate nutritional intake. In contrast, a significant increase in serum transferrin was seen in those patients who were discharged, and serum transferrin levels were maintained in those who died.
† $p < 0.05$

malnutrition occur near this level (anergy, edema), as do increased morbidity and mortality rates (Table 7-2). Serum transferrin levels of less than 150 mg/dl may similarly be considered indicative of severe depletion.

LEAN BODY MASS AND FAT STORES

CREATININE HEIGHT INDEX

Creatinine excretion and calculation of creatinine height index are useful indicators of lean body mass in the hospitalized patient. In normal, well-nourished adults creatinine excretion (a breakdown product of creatine found in muscle) correlates with muscle mass, weight, and height.

Creatinine height index (CHI) is defined as the 24-hr urinary creatinine excretion of a particular subject divided by the expected 24-hr urinary creatinine excretion of a "normal" male or female of the same height. The "normal" urinary creatinine excretion is calculated as the product of the mean creatinine on a creatine and creatinine-free diet (males: 23 mg/kg body weight; females: 18 mg/kg body weight) and the ideal weight for each height. Since height remains essentially unaltered by malnutrition and creatinine excretion continues to correlate with body cell mass, CHI can be used to estimate the degree of protein loss from the body cell mass and thus, the status of the metabolically active tissues.

ANTHROPOMETRY

The degree of depletion of fat and protein stores can be assessed from weight for height, arm muscle circumference (AMC), and triceps skinfold (TSF).

The standards used in nutritional assessment and cut-off points indicative of protein-calorie malnutrition are under debate. Historically, percentage of standard (median) values for AMC and TSF has been used, with <80% of standard taken to indicate moderate depletion. Recent surveys have suggested that, especially with respect to TSF, we may be overdiagnosing protein-calorie malnutrition (marasmus). Use of the 5th percentile from the Ten State Nutrition Survey has been proposed and appears to support this observation. The prevalence of protein-calorie malnutrition (PCM), as defined by <85% standard AMC, differs very little from that determined by the 5th percentile, but use of <85% standard for TSF overstates the prevalence of PCM as determined by the 5th percentile (Table 7-3). This supports the clinician's intuitive unwillingness to use TSF alone to diagnose protein-calorie malnutrition, since fat is a dispensable tissue, the loss of which does not correlate with a loss of function. An important function of TSF is to calculate AMC, which does correlate with serum albumin, percentage weight loss, plasma prealbumin, and hemoglobin. The AMC value characterizes the loss of functionally important body protein mass. Measurement of AMC is particularly useful in patients with fluid retention from cardiac, renal, or hepatic disease when weight for height underestimates the degree of depletion.

SURVEILLANCE

The above parameters (DH skin testing, albumin, transferrin, CHI, AMC, TSF) are used to characterize the nutritional status of the hospitalized patient. No single clinical or laboratory parameter alone will suffice. Use of such a profile of tests provides assessment of the various components of the body, that is, viscera, skeletal muscle, adipose tissue (Fig. 7-5).

On admission to the hospital all patients should be screened by the dietary department or floor nurses to identify those with possible malnutrition.

Screening identifies patients with

1. Recent involuntary weight loss exceeding 5% over 1 month or 10% over 6 months
2. History of recent physiologic stress within the last 3 months, such as major surgery or illness lasting more than 3 weeks
3. Total lymphocyte count less than 1500 cells/mm³
4. Serum albumin less than 3.5 g/dl.

Patients with positive replies to any of the above criteria may have malnutrition and should receive further assessment—skin tests, transferrin, calorie counts.

From such a nutritional assessment plan one can predict

TABLE 7-2   PROBABILITY ESTIMATES USING SERUM ALBUMIN*

	<10%	<25%	50%	>75%	>90%
Anergy	5.2	4.2	3.2	2.2	1.2
Sepsis	4.3	3.7	3.1	2.5	1.9
Death	4.9	4.0	3.2	2.3	1.5

* The probability of anergy, sepsis, and death given the serum albumin concentration. For example, an albumin of 2.1 g% is associated with a greater than 75% estimated probability of being anergic, being septic, and dying during the hospitalization.

TABLE 7-3   STANDARDS FOR ARM MUSCLE CIRCUMFERENCE AND TRICEPS SKINFOLD

	STANDARD	LOWER 5TH PERCENTILE	PERCENT OF STANDARD REPRESENTED BY 5TH PERCENTILE
Upper arm muscle circumference (mm)			
Male	270	220	81
Female	213	177	83
Triceps skinfold (mm)			
Male	11	4	36
Female	19	9	47

NUTRITIONAL ASSESSMENT FOR PROTEIN-CALORIE MALNUTRITION

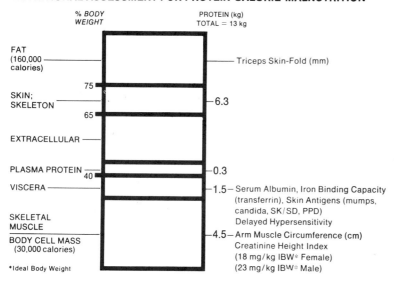

Fig. 7-5. Major parameters for the assessment of nutritional status with corresponding components of body composition. Approximate protein content and caloric reserve for a reference 70-kg man are given. (Blackburn GL, Bistrian BR, Maini BS: Nutritional and metabolic support of the hospitalized patient. Journal of Parenteral and Enteral Nutrition 1:11, 1977)

outcome (morbidity and mortality—Table 7-4) and plan appropriate nutritional therapy.

PROGNOSTIC FACTORS

Historically, hypoalbuminemia has been associated with morbidity and mortality. In 1955, Rhoads and Alexander observed an increased incidence and severity of infections and surgical complications in hypoalbuminemic patients, and Cannon et al, in 1944, commented on the necessity of adequate intake and utilization of protein in combating infections.

Recent studies have found that anergy and a low serum transferrin (<170 mg/dl) are also valuable parameters in identifying patients at risk for postoperative complications (*i.e.*, infections, respiratory failure, wound dehiscence, fistulas) and mortality. The importance of an intact host defense system in the recovery of surgical patients is reflected in the predictive value of serial delayed hypersensitivity skin antigen testing. An improvement in the response to three recall antigens has been reported by several investigators to correlate strongly with an improved outcome.

Preoperative attention to nutritional status is of particular importance in the patient who undergoes nonemergency elective surgery. If nutritional deficiencies are found, surgery can often be delayed for several weeks to allow enteral or

TABLE 7-4   PROGNOSTIC USE OF NUTRITIONAL ASSESSMENT PARAMETERS

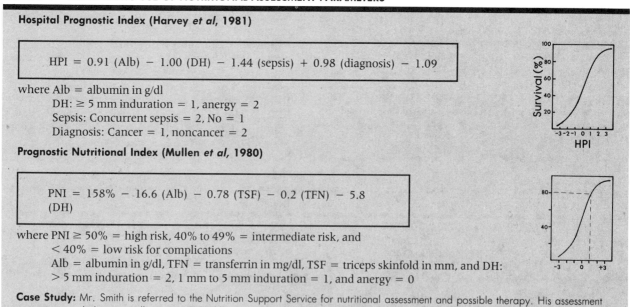

Hospital Prognostic Index (Harvey *et al*, 1981)

$$HPI = 0.91 \,(\text{Alb}) - 1.00 \,(\text{DH}) - 1.44 \,(\text{sepsis}) + 0.98 \,(\text{diagnosis}) - 1.09$$

where Alb = albumin in g/dl
  DH: $\geq$ 5 mm induration = 1, anergy = 2
  Sepsis: Concurrent sepsis = 2, No = 1
  Diagnosis: Cancer = 1, noncancer = 2

Prognostic Nutritional Index (Mullen *et al*, 1980)

$$PNI = 158\% - 16.6 \,(\text{Alb}) - 0.78 \,(\text{TSF}) - 0.2 \,(\text{TFN}) - 5.8 \,(\text{DH})$$

where PNI $\geq$ 50% = high risk, 40% to 49% = intermediate risk, and
  $< 40\%$ = low risk for complications
  Alb = albumin in g/dl, TFN = transferrin in mg/dl, TSF = triceps skinfold in mm, and DH:
  > 5 mm induration = 2, 1 mm to 5 mm induration = 1, and anergy = 0

Case Study: Mr. Smith is referred to the Nutrition Support Service for nutritional assessment and possible therapy. His assessment parameters include serum albumin = 3.0 g/dl, serum transferrin = 240 mg/dl, triceps skinfold = 20 mm, DH skin test response: < 5 mm induration to two of three antigens. He is not septic at this time and does not have cancer.
  His HPI is 1.16, which corresponds to an estimated probability of survival of approximately 80%.
  His PNI gives his estimated risk of subsequent complications as 33%.

parenteral repletion. Preliminary results with such a prophylactic approach have shown a marked improvement in morbidity and mortality.

MICRONUTRIENTS

If facilities are available, evaluation of vitamin and trace mineral stores should be included in the nutritional assessment.

VITAMINS

Several recent surveys of hospitalized patients have reported serum deficiencies of vitamins A, C, B$_6$, and folate. In most cases these deficiencies were found across a wide spectrum of underlying diseases, but of interest was the finding by Bollet and Owens that of the patients on a medical service with peptic ulcer disease, 42% had serum vitamin C levels below the lower limit of normal. This may be important since wound healing is a critical feature of response to therapy in this disease.

The availability of both multivitamin and single-vitamin preparations that may be given parenterally with nutrient solutions or orally permits restoration of normal vitamin levels—additional amounts can be given as needed.

Low serum levels may not always be due to reduced vitamin A stores. Studies in children with kwashiorkor have suggested that low serum vitamin A levels reflect a functional impairment in the hepatic release of vitamin A rather than an actual vitamin A deficiency. Hepatic release is dependent on adequate synthesis of plasma transport proteins (retinol-binding protein and prealbumin), which is in turn dependent on adequate substrate for protein synthesis. Repletion with calories and protein but not vitamin A resulted in normal vitamin A plasma concentrations in the children studied.

Thus vitamin deficiencies may be a reflection of other nutrient deficiencies. In addition to measuring trace elements and vitamin levels, attention must be paid to the larger area of protein synthesis.

TRACE MINERALS

Currently, evidence exists for a nutritional and metabolic role for 14 trace minerals in humans. Of these, iron, zinc, copper, manganese, selenium, iodine, chromium, cobalt, and molybdenum are considered to be essential; fluorine, vanadium, nickel, silicon, and tin are likely to have an important nutritional role.

Iron and zinc are the two trace minerals most frequently found deficient in malnourished patients. Iron is required for hematopoiesis. Individuals with antecedent or ongoing hemorrhage require iron replacement and maintenance. It should be kept in mind that deficiencies of other nutrients (vitamin B$_{12}$, folic acid, copper) may also impair the hematopoietic utilization of iron.

Care must be taken in the administration of iron to the malnourished patient with low plasma protein levels. Increased levels of free iron associated with low serum transferrin concentrations have been reported to cause patients to be more susceptible to bacterial and fungal pathogens. Free iron is necessary for the bacteria to synthesize substances such as endotoxin.

Zinc forms part of numerous metalloenzymes in the body. Its physiologic roles include growth, cell division, protein synthesis, vitamin A transport, retinol function, membrane stabilization, wound healing, and taste acuity.

A number of disease conditions predispose a patient to zinc depletion; catabolic stress and excessive fluid losses (fistulas, diarrhea) increase zinc requirements.

With the advent of total parenteral nutrition (TPN), in particular long-term home TPN, deficiencies of copper, selenium, molybdenum, and manganese have been inadvertently induced iatrogenically. Addition of trace minerals to the administered solutions can easily correct this problem. An expert committee of the Department of Foods of the AMA has recently published "Guidelines for Essential Trace Element Preparation for Parenteral Use."

TREATMENT

GOAL

The goal of nutritional support is to provide protein, calories, electrolytes, and vitamins in a form that can be utilized by the patient to restore and maintain the body cell mass, in particular the visceral compartment. Care must be taken to administer all nutrients in adequate amounts and proper proportions, since it is known that efficient utilization of one nutrient requires the presence of others. Knowledge of the phase of response to illness or injury, degree of nutritional depletion, and degree of hypercatabolism will influence the attainable goals and timing of therapy (Fig. 7-6).

Major consideration must be given to whether the goal of treatment is the "fed" state or the "nonfed" (starved) state and to the route of administration, enteral or parenteral. Enteral and parenteral feedings are frequently used together to obtain the appropriate protein-calorie ratios for the "fed" state.

Figure 7-7 provides a general scheme of nutritional products and feeding situations.

Fig. 7-6. Criteria for designing nutritional therapy. The timing and nature of nutritional therapy are determined by both nutritional assessment and evaluation of the degree of catabolism.

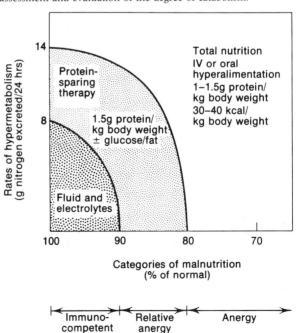

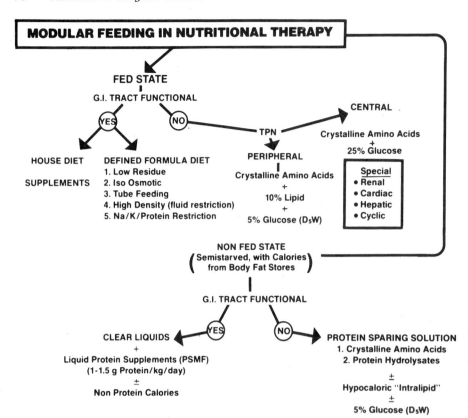

Fig. 7-7. Logic tree, depicting the use of various feeding systems in nutritional support. (Blackburn GL et al: Curative nutrition: Protein-calorie management. In Schneider HA (ed): Nutritional Support of Medical Practice. Hagerstown, Harper & Row, 1977)

INDICATIONS

ENTERAL FEEDING

The decision-making process for the application of enteral feeding requires an understanding of the functional capacity of the patient's gastrointestinal tract, the methods available to provide adequate nutrient support, and a working understanding of the various products and equipment available to make use of enteral feeding techniques. Many factors interfere with adequate voluntary feeding in the hospitalized patient. Internal factors include anorexia due to pain and depression; external factors include drugs with anorectic side-effects and restrictive unpalatable diets. If any of these factors is thought to be operative, the patient's spontaneous intake should be monitored with protein and calorie counts. Depending on the patient's degree of stress, physical strength, primary diagnosis, degree of nutritional depletion, and therapeutic plans, an appropriate level of nutritional intervention should be initiated.

In feeding the malnourished patient there are physiologic and technologic advantages of enteral over intravenous feeding. The enteral route should be used whenever possible, even if only to provide a fraction of the patient's total needs.

Enteral feeding results in higher rates of visceral protein synthesis than are seen with parenteral alimentation. This results from the delivery of all water-soluble substrates absorbed by the intestine—glucose, amino acids and small peptides, fatty acids, and monoglycerides from medium-chain triglycerides—to the liver via the portal vein. Nutrients pass into the hepatocytes where they may be stored (*e.g.,* glucose as glycogen), utilized for energy, or converted to other needed substances such as serum proteins, ketones, and creatinine.

Enteral feeding causes greater release of the gut hormones gastrin and CCK, which have trophic effects on the gastrointestinal tract. Insulin and glucagon release are also greater than that seen with an equivalent intravenous infusion. In addition, animal studies have shown that luminal nutrition is necessary to maintain the structural and functional integrity of the small intestinal mucosa. These changes are thought to be mediated by gastrin.

There are three basic criteria for the initiation of tube feeding. First, the spontaneous nutrient intake should be shown to be inadequate. Attempts should first be made to optimize spontaneous intake—changes in meal frequency and size, use of favorite foods prepared in the patient's home, careful consideration of the schedule for diagnostic and therapeutic maneuvers, supplementation of ingested foods and liquids with food modules, *e.g.,* powdered protein. If such interventions fail to increase oral intake to an adequate level, more effective means of enteral feeding must be employed.

The second criterion for the initiation of tube feeding is the determination that use of the gastrointestinal tract is, in fact, desirable in the individual patient. The patient's presenting illness may be best treated by putting the bowel to rest. Examples include gastrointestinal fistulas and inflammatory bowel disease. It may be that the intestine itself is functional but the patient's disease is best treated by avoiding stimulation of the accessory components, that is, minimizing pancreatic or biliary secretion by avoiding all enteral feedings.

The final essential criterion for initiation of tube feeding is that the gastrointestinal tract be functional. Usually this implies that the stomach is capable of accepting the delivery of tube feeding, that the feeding can empty into the small intestine, and that digestion and absorption can occur normally. Within this framework, there can be minor variations that do not entirely preclude the use of the gastrointestinal tract as the route of feeding. For example, if there is a problem with gastric emptying due to a metabolic gastropathy or to some surgical manipulation, tube feeding can be delivered into the proximal small intestine, thereby entirely avoiding the problem associated with gastric dysfunction. Another minor problem that is easy to overcome is relative lactose intolerance. The availability of lactose-free feedings circumvents problems due to congenital or transient lactose deficiency.

PARENTERAL FEEDING

Parenteral nutrition may be partial or total. In many instances the patient is able to sustain himself only partially by the oral route and needs some support or assistance. In other cases he may be totally unable to take in food via the gastrointestinal tract, and total parenteral nutrition (TPN) is necessary.

There are no hard and fast indications for parenteral nutrition—only some guidelines. In general, indications for the use of parenteral nutrition may be categorized into two groups: parenteral nutrition as supportive therapy and as primary therapy.

Patients who need parenteral nutrition as supportive therapy include malnourished or elderly surgical patients. For example, the patient with a stenosing carcinoma of the gastrointestinal tract may not have eaten an adequate diet for a prolonged period of time. A 5- to 10-day period of preoperative nutritional repletion will repair nutrient deficiencies, promote protein synthesis and host defense function, and result in fewer postoperative complications such as poor wound healing and sepsis.

Patients who have a nonfunctional gastrointestinal tract or prolonged stress response postoperatively benefit from total parenteral nutrition. Several specific categories of patients include those with ileus, stomal dysfunction, short-gut syndrome, acute pancreatitis, and severe burns.

There are several categories of nonsurgical patients who may also derive benefit from supportive parenteral nutritional therapy. Patients who receive chemotherapy or radiation therapy often suffer anorexia, mucosal inflammation, nausea, and vomiting that preclude adequate oral intake. Nutritional support may be necessary to allow continuation of therapy. In addition, radiation to the abdomen may result in radiation enteritis; treatment consists of bowel rest and TPN.

In some instances parenteral nutrition may be considered a primary therapeutic modality. In such cases all nutrients are administered by way of the intravenous route, thus allowing the gastrointestinal tract to rest while restorative and healing processes are enhanced by the provided nutrients. Several diseases frequently treated in this manner include enterocutaneous fistula, inflammatory bowel disease, chronic relapsing pancreatitis, and acute renal failure, the latter usually in conjunction with hemodialysis.

Thus, in the patient who is unable to eat by mouth and in whom tube feeding is contraindicated or has failed, parenteral nutrition is a means of restoring or maintaining visceral protein status, in particular, host defense.

COMBINATION OR TRANSITIONAL FEEDING

Frequently both enteral and parenteral techniques represent the optimal nutritional support therapy. For example, amino acid solutions may be given peripherally to increase the protein intake of a patient on tube-feeding or eating spontaneously. Also, burn patients have very high calorie requirements that often cannot be met by feeding tube alone. A combination of techniques is necessary to deliver the needed nutrients.

The inability of the gastrointestinal tract to tolerate full feedings does not preclude the use of some enteral alimentation. When practical, the clinician should take advantage of any degree of gastrointestinal function. If, for example, the patient were able to tolerate a portion of his protein and calorie requirement as tube feeding, it would reduce the amount of nutrient required by the intravenous route. The nutrients delivered enterally would be more efficiently utilized and would help promote and maintain the functioning of the gastrointestinal tract. This combined enteral and parenteral feeding is part of the orderly transition of most patients from complete intravenous nutrition to complete oral feedings. It avoids a period of inadequate nutrient intake, which frequently occurs when intravenous feeding is abruptly stopped and the patient is immediately expected to consume adequate amounts orally.

PROTEIN-SPARING

In some patients the goal of nutritional therapy need not be to provide all nutrients but rather to optimize the body's adaptation to starvation and minimize losses from the body cell mass. In the starved state substantial amounts of protein can be spared by the infusion of amino acids or oral intake of protein in amounts of 1.5 g protein/kg body weight with appropriate cofactors of vitamins, minerals, fluid, and electrolytes.

The administration of 3.5% crystalline amino acid solutions limits the antilipolytic and antiketogenic effects of increased insulin secretion that follows glucose infusions (D_5W). When infused amino acids are the only exogenous source of nutrition, endogenous fat contributes most of the body's nonprotein energy requirements, as it does during starvation. Even though total urea nitrogen excretion increases when amino acids are administered, the infused amino acids can effectively replenish the pool of amino acids available for protein synthesis, particularly the synthesis of essential visceral proteins.

Solutions of 3.5% amino acids that contain maintenance electrolytes, vitamins, and minerals are well tolerated. In fact, the mild ketosis that results causes patients to be more comfortable in the postanorectic stage of their illness by reducing hunger. One limiting factor in the administration of amino acids alone is the availability of adequate body fat. The availability of parenteral fat, however, enables one to provide calories as needed to compensate for decreased fat stores without stimulating as great an insulin response as would be seen with glucose.

Protein-sparing has been found to be useful in postoperative insulin-requiring diabetic patients. Dextrose-free solutions minimize nitrogen loss and allow for easier control of blood glucose levels (see later section, Specialized Feedings: Diabetes Mellitus).

During major injury or sepsis, the failure to adapt to a protein-sparing regimen may indicate the presence of hypermetabolism and insulin resistance secondary to sepsis. Withholding of carbohydrate allows the development of ketosis, reflecting fat mobilization. Failure to spill ketones in the urine may be used as a sensitive marker for the development of significant sepsis and signals the need for supplemental feedings of 1000 to 1500 kcal (IV fat and

10% glucose can be added to the peripheral system) to support the hypermetabolism.

OPTIMAL PARENTERAL FEEDING

Use of a formula containing 20% to 40% fat and 15% to 20% protein in amounts not to exceed the energy expenditure by more than 200 kcal/day will lessen the insulin response and lower the respiratory quotient to 0.9. The substrate and hormone profiles in the blood following infusion of such a mixture are similar to those seen in the postprandial state and are optimal for visceral protein synthesis.

This therapy is expensive and should be reserved for severely malnourished, septic, or stressed patients. Patients needing surgery, and thus accelerated wound healing and intact host defense, and patients in intensive care units benefit most from this therapy.

TECHNIQUES

ENTERAL FEEDING

The oral route is the route of choice for nutritional support whenever possible. However, failure to present nutritious food in an attractive and palatable manner is a common problem that becomes serious in the presence of anorexia associated with illness. For the patient who is unable to maintain his oral intake voluntarily, due either to anorexia or to gastrointestinal dysfunction, tube feeding is the next step.

Enteral feeding is safer than intravenous alimentation in that it does not require sterile techniques. Recent technological advances have made enteral alimentation better tolerated and more easily implemented than in the past.

Equipment

The newly available fine-bore Silastic (7–9 fr) and polyurethane tubes with mercury-weighted tips are considerably better tolerated and produce fewer complications than the more rigid Levine tubes.

The greater use of infusion pumps facilitates the utilization of continuous feeding, which is better tolerated, is associated with smaller residual volumes, reduces the possibility of pulmonary aspiration, and requires less supervision.

In a patient with ileus or delayed gastric emptying or with an increased risk of aspiration (*e.g.*, elderly, obtunded, or restrained), nutrients may be delivered directly into the jejunum using a Dobhoff (Biosearch Medical Products) or long Keofeed tube (Hedeco). When administering feedings directly into the small bowel, it is generally better to use a continuous infusion of calorically dilute solutions. Bolus feeding of hypertonic solutions is often not well tolerated, producing cramping and diarrhea.

A modification of the Hickman-Broviac silicone rubber catheter has been developed for long-term feeding (including home enteral feedings). This jejunostomy tube should be considered in all patients receiving a laparotomy, or, if short-term therapy is anticipated, a Page/Ryan needle jejunostomy using a polyvinyl #19, 9 in to 15 in IV catheter may be used.

Formulas

A series of solutions appropriate for a wide variety of disease states has developed. These solutions differ in osmolality, digestibility, caloric density, lactose content, viscosity, fat content, taste, and expense. These solutions are of three main types.

1. Elemental or monomeric formulas are residue-free, containing essential and nonessential amino acids as the protein source, oligosaccharides or monosaccharides as the carbohydrate source, electrolytes, trace minerals and vitamins, and little or no triglycerides or starch. Due to their elemental composition and high carbohydrate–low lipid content, they are rapidly absorbed over short levels of intestine without the need for intestinal or pancreatic enzymes. They contain 1 kcal/ml. Two examples of low residue, defined formula diet products are Vivonex and Flexical. Vivonex contains 90% carbohydrate as glucose and 1% fat. Flexical provides 30% of the calories as fat; 20% of this fat is medium-chain triglycerides (MCT). Other products such as Travasorb MCT are uniquely valuable, since MCT is absorbed without pancreatic lipase or bile salts and reaches the liver by way of the portal circulation. Unlike long-chain triglycerides, MCT can only be oxidized and not stored. This is important in many critically ill patients.

   Defined formula diets are of particular benefit in patients with fistulas of the large or small intestine in whom successful treatment requires control of secretions or in patients with severely compromised bowel function (extreme short bowel or extensive radiation enteritis).

   A major disadvantage of elemental diets is their high osmolarity, which requires them to be administered slowly over a prolonged period of time.

2. Nonelemental or polymeric diets contain protein, fat, and carbohydrate in high molecular-weight form and thus are lower in osmolarity. They contain 1 kcal/ml and are less expensive than the elemental diets. They require normal digestive proteolytic and lipolytic capacity. Examples include Precision LR/HN, Isocal, Ensure/Ensure Plus (1.5 kcal/ml), and Magnacal (2 kcal/ml). All of these are lactose-free and Precision is also low-fat. The atrophic small intestine of protein-calorie malnourished patients is often deficient in lactase.

3. The third type of formula available is the carbohydrate, fat, or protein modules. "Modular feeding" consists of mixing the commercially available modules with standard enteral formulas to give a solution of desired composition. As more is learned about different disease states and their respective nutritional needs, modular feeding is becoming more widely used. Examples of commonly used modules include carbohydrate—Polycose, Controlyte, and Hy-Cal; fat—Lipomul, MCT oil, corn oil, and safflower oil; protein—Casec and Pro-Mix.

Complications (Tube-Related or Metabolic)

Complications of tube feeding may be tube-related or metabolic. Tube-related problems include injury to the gastrointestinal mucosa, oropharyngeal ulceration, displacement of the tube, and aspiration. Use of the newer, soft, inert silicone rubber and polyurethane feeding tubes reduces the oropharyngeal and esophageal irritation associated with nasoenteral feedings. The weighted mercury tip allows the tube to pass through the pylorus into the duodenum with a resultant decrease in the chance of aspiration. Radiographic confirmation of the tube location will avoid inadvertent feeding into the trachea. Small-bore feeding tubes can become occluded when viscous feedings or medications are allowed to settle within the tube. Irrigating the tube with water each time feedings are stopped will help keep the tube clear.

Metabolic and physiological complications include diarrhea, dehydration, nausea, and glucosuria. Diarrhea is the most common complication associated with tube feeding. The diarrhea may be due to the formula used (rapid administration, high osmolality, lactose-intolerance) or may be unrelated to the formula, for example, concurrent medications. If the diarrhea is thought to be due to the formula, decreasing the rate or strength of the tube feeding may help. Alternatively, an opium derivative (*e.g.*, Lomotil) may be added to the feeding.

Dehydration can be a problem in elderly patients with impaired renal concentration ability or increased extrarenal fluid losses. Close monitoring of fluid balance is necessary, especially in the patient who is unconscious or confused and thus unable to express thirst.

The high carbohydrate concentrations administered in many tube feedings may precipitate glucosuria in a patient with no previous history of diabetes mellitus.

PARENTERAL FEEDING

Equipment

Most of the solutions used for total parenteral nutrition are extremely hyperosmolar (>1100 mOsm). In order to prevent or minimize damage to the vein, a central line is used for the infusion. The usual procedure is to place percutaneously a polyvinyl or Silastic catheter into the subclavian or external jugular vein and direct it into the superior vena cava. Before the catheter is used for hyperosmolar solutions one must first check that good blood return is present to prevent infusing into the mediastinum, and then its position must be verified radiographically. Alternatively, in occasional patients, a long Silastic catheter may be threaded into the superior vena cava by way of the brachial vein. In either case, placement of the central venous catheter must be done in accordance with strict aseptic techniques, in particular, mechanical cleansing to disinfect and defat the skin. Povidone-iodine ointment applied to the skin surrounding the catheter site is the least significant component of the procedure. A completely occlusive sterile dressing is desirable, and dressings are changed at least every 2 to 3 days.

Protein-sparing solutions are commonly given through a peripheral vein catheter. The maximum osmolarity that a peripheral vein can tolerate without the development of phlebitis is 600 mOsm. Procedures that will extend vein tolerance are described later under Parenteral: Complications.

Requirements and Solutions

Major changes have occurred in total parenteral nutrition. Energy requirements are considerably less than those initially used. Measured energy expenditures in hospitalized patients are rarely more than 30% above basal energy expenditure. Standard feedings should therefore provide caloric intakes no greater than 130% of the calculated basal energy expenditure. Two thousand to 2400 kcal/day meet the needs of most postsurgical, critical care, or moderately injured patients. The metabolic response to injury produces a "hypercaloremic" state, and therefore 1000 to 1500 calories often will suffice in the first few postoperative days. These modest feeding rates avoid most of the metabolic problems associated with "hyperalimentation."

Nonprotein calories may be supplied by glucose or by fat. Lipid emulsions (10% and 20%) may be "piggybacked" onto the hyperalimentation solution (amino acids and glucose) and administered by way of the central line. In addition, because the caloric value of fat is twice that of dextrose, and because emulsified fat does not exert an osmotic pressure, it is possible to administer 1500 to 2500 kcal in 2 to 3 liters (L) through peripheral veins and thus feed many types of malnourished patients.

Following infusion, the fat particles are rapidly cleared from the circulation in a way similar to chylomicron clearing. The fat emulsion is metabolized and utilized for energy; an increase in oxygen consumption and heat production and a decrease in respiratory quotient are seen.

Insulin is not required for the metabolism of fat; thus, infusions can be discontinued abruptly without the danger of hypoglycemia. This is of particular benefit in the critically ill patient who may require frequent changes in infusion composition or rate of administration.

While many adult patients can tolerate 2.5 g fat/kg/day, slow (over 8 hr) infusions of 1 to 2 g fat/kg/day will provide all the fat calories needed (usually fewer than 1000 kcal/day).

Extreme caution should be used in administering 20% fat emulsions in severely ill patients with organ failure until more experience is achieved with this new solution. New generations of fat emulsions can be expected to alter approaches to intravenous fat in the coming years.

The provision of an adequate supply of amino acids for protein synthesis is a major objective of parenteral nutrition. The Recommended Daily Allowance (RDA), calculated from balance studies in healthy adult males, is 0.8 g protein/kg body weight/day. When calculating protein needs for the hospitalized patient, additional factors must be taken into consideration. Sepsis, severe trauma, and burns dramatically increase nitrogen losses, requiring greater amino acid intake. For example, abnormal losses, such as protein-rich exudates in burns or upper gastrointestinal tract contents rich in pancreatic secretions, increase requirements to between 1.5 and 2.0 g/kg/day.

Increased amounts of amino acids are needed if caloric requirements are not met by carbohydrates and fats and if amino acids are metabolized to glucogenic precursors.

In addition, consideration must be given to the pattern of amino acids infused, since unbalanced mixtures (*e.g.*, high glycine) will not optimally support protein synthesis.

The protein intake that will permit anabolism in the nonstressed patient with no abnormal losses has been set at 1.2 to 1.5 g/kg body weight/day. Calculation of nitrogen balance allows one to fine-tune this requirement for the individual patient.

Nitrogen balance (Nbal) is equal to nitrogen intake minus nitrogen excretion and indicates whether the nutritional support has been sufficient to prevent net catabolism (Nbal = 0) or promote anabolism (Nbal > 0). Dividing the protein intake by 6.25 yields the nitrogen intake. Nitrogen excretion is the sum of the urine urea nitrogen (measured in a 24-hr urine specimen); a factor of 4 that accounts for nitrogen losses from feces, skin, and the respiratory tract; and any abnormal nitrogen losses. Abnormal losses would include exudates from burns, losses in dialysate fluids, fistulae drainage, upper gastrointestinal tract losses, and diarrhea.

Nitrogen balance

$$= \frac{\text{Protein intake (g)}}{6.25} - (\text{UUN} + 4 + \text{abnormal losses})$$

Protein needs are delivered parenterally by crystalline L-amino acid solutions containing a broad mix of essential and nonessential amino acids.

Solutions that contain only the eight essential amino acids and solutions that are rich in the branched-chain amino acids are also available for patients with renal or hepatic insufficiency respectively.

Failure to achieve nitrogen balance with a standard formula suggests stress (*e.g.,* sepsis, organ failure)-induced catabolism. This can be estimated by the catabolic index:

$$\text{Catabolic index} = \text{UUN} - [(0.5 \times N_{in})] + 3$$

The above index partitions the urea excretion into that resulting from an increase in endogenous protein catabolism and that due to dietary protein intake and obligatory urea excretion. An index of less than 0 represents no significant stress; an index between 0 and 5, moderate stress; and an index greater than 5, severe stress.

Complications (Catheter-Related, Septic, or Metabolic)

Complications associated with parenteral feedings fall into three categories: catheter-related, septic, and metabolic.

1. *Catheter-related.* Pneumothorax and thrombosis are the two most frequent catheter-related complications. Pneumothorax occurs in approximately 1% to 2% of all catheter insertions, secondary to laceration of the pleura. It often resolves spontaneously but may require needle aspiration at the second intercostal space or placement of a chest tube at the same location.

    Thrombosis of the central vein has been reported in 5% to 10% of catheters, generally in patients with a tendency to hypercoagulopathy (*e.g.,* sepsis, inflammatory bowel disease, pancreatitis, cancer). A shortened partial thromboplastin time or antithrombin factor III can be used to identify patients at increased risk.

    Central vein thrombosis can be effectively treated prophylactically. Heparin is given daily (3000 units/L hyperalimentation solution or 6000 units/day) to all patients receiving total parenteral nutrition, and coagulation factors are monitored by measuring prothrombin time, partial thromboplastin time, and antithrombin factor III. If a thrombus is suspected, a distal venogram is performed. If positive for a thrombus, the catheter is removed, peripheral vein feeding is begun, and total intravenous heparinization is accomplished. A repeat venogram is performed in 1 to 2 weeks. With such an approach the incidence of central venous thrombosis has been reduced from 5% to 10% to less than 2%.

2. *Septic.* Fungal infections have long been associated with malnourished, debilitated patients, presumably due to depressed cell-mediated immunity. In recent years, however, the reported incidence of fungal infections has fallen. Currently the predominant agents are skin contaminants and other gram-positive organisms. Impaired neutrophil function, leukocytic endogenous mediators, and nonspecific immune function are usually present. The implication is that these infections should be well-controlled by earlier detection and correction of nutritional deficiencies and by close monitoring and fastidious care of the insertion site.

The ability to change a central vein catheter by using a guidewire under sterile conditions rather than removing the catheter has changed the management of the patient with an unexplained fever. On occurrence of an unexplained fever, three steps are taken: (1) a blood culture is drawn from the central line, (2) a peripheral blood culture is drawn at the same time, (3) the catheter is changed over a guidewire, and the catheter tip is sent to the microbiology laboratory for culture.

Being able to change the line over a wire allows one to eliminate the catheter suspected of being the source of infection while maintaining central venous access during the wait for the culture results. Within 24 hr to 48 hr, preliminary results from the microbiology department will dictate the next course of action (Table 7-5). If the peripheral blood culture plus either the catheter tip or the culture drawn through the line are positive, the central line is removed and reinserted 24 hr later if the patient's fever has defervesced. A peripheral feeding regimen is used in the interim. If the peripheral blood culture is negative, but *either* the catheter tip or the blood culture drawn through the line is positive, the catheter is changed over a guidewire a second time, and the second catheter tip is cultured to see if it was contaminated during the initial line change. If it is "clean," the third catheter remains. If only the peripheral blood culture is positive, the source of infection is assumed to be systemic without colonization of the catheter. If the fever continues for several days, the central line is changed again to check for colonization.

Use of such a protocol will enable one to detect catheter sepsis early in its course and treat it before systemic complications (*e.g.,* septicemia) occur.

A reduction in catheter sepsis from 2% to 10% to 1% to 2% and central vein thrombosis from 5% to 10% to less than 2% has resulted from earlier and more frequent catheter changes using a guidewire. Time, effort, and complications from location and cannulation of central veins have also been reduced. Knowledge about the factors operative in the department of catheter sepsis and thrombi and how to control such factors makes one more likely to use central venous infusions in patients who would benefit from the nutritional support but may be at increased risk for sepsis and thrombosis.

3. *Metabolic.* This is the overfeeding syndrome. The provision of hypertonic glucose solution far in excess of energy

---

TABLE 7-5 WORKUP OF FEVER IN TOTAL PARENTERAL NUTRITION

BC-C	BC-P	CC-T	DIAGNOSIS	TREATMENT
+	+	+	Catheter sepsis	RC
+	+	−	Sepsis, ? catheter	RC
−	+	+	Catheter sepsis	RC
+	−	+	Catheter tip infection	CC
+	−	−	? Catheter tip infection	CC
−	−	+	? Catheter tip infection	CC
−	+	−	Systemic sepsis	Nothing/CC
−	−	−	No infection	Nothing

BC-C: Blood culture—catheter; BC-P: Blood culture—peripheral; CC-T: Catheter culture—tip; RC: Remove catheter; CC: Change catheter over guidewire.

requirements (*e.g.*, 700 to 900 g/day) results in respiratory quotients of greater than 1. This increase in carbon dioxide production may be significant in debilitated patients with compromised ventilatory function.

Liver dysfunction also occurs as excess carbohydrate and fat are stored in the liver. The resulting hepatomegaly leads to a marked elevation and fixation of the diaphragm, causing a reduction in tidal volume and adding to the respiratory problems due to increased carbon dioxide production.

Table 7-6 lists other metabolic complications and their treatment.

4. Peripheral vein catheter. The principal complication encountered in the use of peripheral veins for the administration of nutritional solutions is the occurrence of phlebitis. Phlebitis is most common when the solutions have an osmolarity above 600 mOsm/L and a high potassium concentration (>40 mEq/L) and when antibiotics are given through the catheter.

Efforts must be made to keep osmolarity below 550 mOsm/L and potassium less than 30 mEq/L. The addition of heparin (1000 units/L), hydrocortisone (5 mg), and ''piggybacking'' of fat emulsions all protect the vein. The use of stainless steel pediatric scalp vein needles (21-

TABLE 7-6   METABOLIC COMPLICATIONS OF INTRAVENOUS HYPERALIMENTATION

COMPLICATION	ETIOLOGY	TREATMENT
Hyperglycemia, which can progress to hyperosmolar nonketotic coma	Excessive rate of glucose administration; inadequate endogenous insulin; increased insulin needs 2° to glucocorticoids or infection	Stat subcutaneous insulin based on capillary blood sugars every 6 hr; add insulin to hyperalimentation solution after needs are established
Metabolic acidosis	Excessive chloride content of amino acid solutions or added sodium chloride; excessive base or bicarbonate loss unrelated to solution (*e.g.*, pancreatic fistula)	Decrease sodium chloride in solution, use sodium and potassium as acetate
Hypophosphatemia	Inadequate administration	Add phosphate as potassium or sodium salt
Hyperphosphatemia	Excess phosphorus administration or inability to excrete phosphorus, as in renal failure	Reduce or eliminate phosphorus in solutions
Hyperkalemia	Excess administration or inability to excrete potassium, as in renal failure	Reduce or eliminate potassium
Hypokalemia	Inadequate administration or increased losses due to excretion (stool or urine) or anabolism	Add potassium
Hypercalcemia	Excessive calcium or vitamin D administration	Reduce vitamin D or calcium
Hypocalcemia	Inadequate calcium administration or excessive phosphorus administration, particularly in osteomalacia	Increase calcium administration
Hypermagnesemia	Excess magnesium administration, especially with renal impairment	Reduce or eliminate magnesium
Hypomagnesemia	Inadequate provision of magnesium, particularly in anabolic situations	Appropriate supplementation
Essential fatty acid deficiency	Continuous feeding of hypertonic dextrose or true deficiency from prolonged severe malnutrition (rare)	IV fat emulsion or cyclic hyperalimentation for the first, IV fat emulsion for the second
Azotemia	Excessive amino acid administration or reduced renal function	Reduce amino acid load
Elevation in liver enzymes	Continuous infusion of glucose (? essential fatty acid deficiency)	Cyclic hyperalimentation Intralipid or Liposyn daily
Anemia	Excessive diagnostic blood tests; inadequate iron, copper, B_{12}, folate, protein replacement	Limit phlebotomies; appropriate supplements
Rare deficiencies (copper, zinc, chromium)	Inadequate administration	Appropriate replacement

gauge) securely immobilized with frequent (every 24 hr to 48 hr) rotation also extends the use of peripheral vein feedings.

CYCLIC FEEDINGS

The continuous administration of carbohydrate and amino acids requires that high levels of insulin be constantly maintained. If a formula (enteral or parenteral) with a high percentage of carbohydrate is used in volumes exceeding caloric needs, an appreciable conversion of exogenous carbohydrate to fat occurs in the liver. It has been estimated that in high carbohydrate diets up to one-third of the ingested carbohydrate is converted to glycogen and fat. With a normal cyclic diet (*i.e.,* three meals a day), fed and fasting phases alternate. During the postabsorptive (fasting) phases (when insulin levels fall), the fat and glycogen are mobilized as free fatty acids and glucose respectively and oxidized as an energy source. With continuous feedings, however, insulin levels remain high and prevent the release of glycogen and fatty acids. The excess fat and carbohydrate that result from overfeeding are stored in the liver as triglycerides and glycogen and result in hepatomegaly, cholestasis, and impaired structural and secretory function. If, in addition, the formula lacks or contains minimal linoleic acid, the ability to mobilize fat stores can result in essential fatty acid deficiency.

High insulin levels facilitate the preferential uptake of amino acids into skeletal muscle. Thus, secretory protein synthesis in the liver, which is primarily dependent on amino acid redistribution from muscle during the postabsorptive (low insulin) phase, is left deficient by the high insulin signal from continuous high-carbohydrate feedings.

The net result of constant high insulin levels is prompt repletion of skeletal muscle and fat stores and less effective visceral protein (albumin, transferrin, host defense) synthesis.

It therefore would appear desirable to use a therapy that approximates the normal diurnal feeding pattern. Since the state of hyperinsulinism, resulting from the continuous administration of glucose, is responsible for the unfavorable metabolic phenomena ("fatty" liver, decreased visceral protein synthesis), stopping the feeding for a period of time each day would allow insulin levels and thus the "anabolic" drive to diminish. Fat mobilization from the liver and adipose tissue would prevent the development of "fatty" liver and essential fatty acid deficiency, and endogenous amino acid mobilization would allow for increased visceral protein synthesis.

Studies comparing continuous intravenous hyperalimentation and cyclic hyperalimentation have shown that an 8-hr to 12-hr dextrose-free period leads to a significant fall in blood glucose levels and a fall in the circulation level of insulin. As a consequence of the reduced insulin level, adipose tissue triglycerides undergo lipolysis to free fatty acids, and ketogenesis occurs in the liver. A rise in the glucagon level is seen, causing the release of glycogen from liver and skeletal muscle and amino acids from skeletal muscle. During the postabsorptive phase, free fatty acids, ketone bodies, and glycogen are used to support energy requirements, and endogenous amino acids stimulate secretory protein synthesis.

Coincident with the mobilization of fat and glycogen from the liver, hepatomegaly is reduced and liver function improves.

Cyclic alimentation not only is more physiologic but also

enables the patient to be free of his feeding tube or intravenous infusion system for a portion of each day and thus aids in the patient's return to the activities of daily life. Also, cyclic feedings, particularly enteral, can be easily adapted for outpatient use.

SPECIALIZED FEEDINGS

The modular nature of parenteral and enteral formulas allows the feeding to be fitted to the individual patient's needs. Organ dysfunction is the most prevalent reason for modifying nutritional therapy.

PULMONARY DYSFUNCTION

In patients with pulmonary dysfunction it is advantageous to keep the respiratory quotient below 1.0. Most commercial enteral products contain a high carbohydrate:fat ratio, resulting in high carbon dioxide production. A fat module can be added to a standard formula when one desires to increase the calories given to a patient with pulmonary insufficiency. Likewise, in the patient receiving total parenteral nutrition, some of the dextrose calories may be replaced with IV fat.

HEPATIC INSUFFICIENCY

Alterations in amino acid profiles have been seen in patients with hepatic insufficiency. Decreased insulin degradation by the liver results in higher plasma insulin concentrations and greater deposition and utilization of branched-chain amino acids (BCAA) by muscle tissue. Lowered BCAA levels are found in the plasma. Other amino acids are only partially metabolized by the failing liver. High concentrations of the aromatic amino acids (phenylalanine, tyrosine, and tryptophan) accumulate in the plasma.

The ratio of plasma aromatic amino acids (AAA) to BCAA influences the amount of tryptophan that enters the brain. Tryptophan is the precursor of serotonin, an inhibitory neurotransmitter. In hepatic insufficiency, increased tryptophan enters the brain, resulting in increased synthesis of serotonin.

In addition, certain amines, such as tyramine, that are normally degraded by the liver, accumulate in the plasma and are transformed in the brain to octopamine. This amine acts as a false neurotransmitter by displacing dopamine, an excitatory neurotransmitter.

The accumulation of serotonin and octopamine is thought to contribute to the encephalopathy seen with hepatic failure or following a portacaval shunt.

The use of a formula high in BCAA in patients with hepatic dysfunction has resulted in less hepatic encephalopathy but has not been shown to increase survival. The patient with chronic hepatic insufficiency (*e.g.,* cirrhosis) or a portacaval shunt can be maintained on a diet with a low protein content (40 g to 60 g with a high BCAA concentration) to reduce symptoms of encephalopathy. For the patient receiving enteral feedings, carbohydrate and fat modules (70:30 ratio) can be added to a small volume of standard formula to provide adequate calories, appropriate sodium restriction, and potassium replacement. Special "liver" diets containing high BCAA content can be used to increase the percentage of BCAA.

CARDIAC DISEASE

Volume and sodium restrictions are commonly encountered in cardiac disease. By adding carbohydrate, protein, and fat modules to a small amount of standard formula one can maintain caloric (2 kcal/ml) and protein intake without excess electrolytes and volume.

In the patient receiving TPN, central vein access allows administration of a highly concentrated solution at a low infusion rate. Diuretics aid the excretion of free water and thus permit the administration of more calories.

Due to the unpalatable nature of many cardiac diets (restricted sodium and fluid, and high potassium to cover losses due to diuretic use), voluntary caloric intake is low. Tube feeding or intravenous therapy is often necessary to ensure adequate intake, especially when the goal is pre-operative repletion.

Since many critically ill patients with cardiac disease, particularly those with ischemic heart disease, have border-line myocardial perfusion and oxygenation, anaerobic glycolysis plays a significant role in the total energy expenditure of the myocardium. High doses of glucose (*e.g.*, 100 ml of 3% AA, 49% dextrose) may result in improved hemodynamic parameters and oxygen transport.

RENAL FAILURE

Total parenteral nutrition not only supplies needed nutrients in a patient with severe dietary restrictions, but recent evidence suggests that modifications in diet *per se* may serve a direct therapeutic function as well.

IV fluids that contain the eight essential L-amino acids and high carbohydrate concentrations have been used in patients with acute renal failure. The lowering of BUN level and the need for supplementation of certain electrolytes in most patients receiving this therapy suggest that this diet brings about a recycling of endogenous nitrogenous wastes into tissue protein. Adequate calories are necessary for the retention and utilization of exogenous amino acids to form protein. The uremic patient requires additional calories for the conversion of urea nitrogen to useful protein. A ratio of 1 g N:800 kcal has been demonstrated to be effective in lowering BUN levels in patients with acute renal failure.

The presence of oliguria or anuria restricts fluid intake. It is necessary to highly concentrate IV solutions, thus requiring direct superior vena cava infusion.

Enteral nutrition in the patient with renal failure is accomplished with a solution that is low in protein (25 g to 40 g with high biologic value, for example, a solution with a high BCAA/AAA ratio. BCAA are not metabolized to urea in the liver but pass through the liver and are metabolized by muscle tissues).

Formulas composed of high essential to nonessential amino acid ratios, carbohydrate, and fat in a concentrated form (*e.g.*, 2 kcal/ml), with limited magnesium, potassium, phosphate, and vitamins, allow one to nourish the patient with renal failure without excessive build-up of toxic metabolites and electrolytes.

DIABETES MELLITUS

Patients with diabetes can be difficult to manage on hyperalimentation because of the continuous delivery of glucose. For the patient receiving parenteral feedings, the provision of intravenous insulin (added to the hyperalimentation bottles) in amounts similar to prehospital needs corrected for caloric intake, appears to work well, since the average amount necessary is approximately twice that needed before hospitalization. This is a conservative approach and leads to fairly consistent underestimation of insulin requirements. Sliding scale and subcutaneous insulin are used to fine-tune the amount of insulin according to measured blood glucoses. Hyperglycemia is more apt to occur than hypo-glycemia with this protocol, but this is acceptable given that hyperglycemia is better tolerated.

Alternatively, since insulin is not required for the utilization of fat, by replacing carbohydrate calories with fat one can administer adequate calories with reduced insulin requirements. If the patient is well-nourished or obese, amino acids alone will prevent excessive protein catabolism and reduce the need for exogenous insulin. This technique is particularly helpful in the immediate postoperative period when it is especially difficult to control blood sugars due to the insulin resistance associated with the metabolic response to injury.

Further modifications in formulas are often needed given the complications of diabetes mellitus, that is, atherosclerotic vascular disease and renal failure.

BURNS

The hypermetabolism associated with severe burns results in a weight loss that is closely correlated with the extent and depth of the burn and the degree of sepsis. In large full-thickness burns, the weight loss during the recovery period is often 30% to 40% of the preburn weight. Calculation of nitrogen balance may be used to estimate the severity of the catabolic response and its duration. One gram of nitrogen lost represents 30 g of lean tissue. In the burn patient sources of nitrogen loss include exudation from the burned surfaces in addition to losses in urine and feces.

Large amounts of the energy lost by severely burned patients are secondary to the evaporative water loss from the burned surfaces. The average daily loss of water through normal skin is 960 g/m^2 with a caloric cost of 600 kcal/m^2/day, or about 21% of the daily heat loss. If the patient has a large burn, the daily evaporative loss can increase to 3000 g or more/m^2 and the associated expenditure to 6200 kcal/day. It is essential that the feeding program allow the patient to maintain his body temperature at the new "injury" set point of 28° to 32° C, and that a high humidity environment be provided to control heat and water losses.

Compounding these increased requirements are anorexia secondary to decreased mobility of the patient's arms, hands, and jaw, anxiety, sedative medications, and the large number of operative procedures (grafts, dressing changes) resulting in missed meals.

Nutrient requirements are thus much higher in the burn patient than in other surgical patients. Published guidelines suggest a caloric intake of 25 × body weight (in kg) × percent of body surface burned. Protein requirements have been set at 2 g to 4 g/kg body weight/day. Vitamin and trace mineral requirements may be met by providing 2 to 4 multivitamins/day and 1 g to 2 g vitamin C/day.

Combined enteral and parenteral regimens are frequently used in the burn patient to maintain fluid balance and meet nutritional needs.

OBESITY

The administration of amino acids alone (in the form of lean meat) represents a successful weight-reducing regimen. The resulting low insulin levels allow for the mobilization of free fatty acids from the adipose tissue and the synthesis of ketone bodies (acetoacetate and β-hydroxybutyrate) to meet energy needs. The elevated levels of ketone bodies also have a hunger-suppressing effect.

The ingestion of 1 g to 1.5 g protein/kg ideal body weight

TABLE 7-7   MONITORING OF HYPERALIMENTATION*

PARAMETER	INITIAL 72 HR	FIRST MONTH	MAINTENANCE
Serum Values			
Glucose	Every 8 hr	3 × weekly	2 × weekly
CBC	2×	2 × weekly	1 × weekly
Electrolytes	2×	3 × weekly	2 × weekly
SMA-12	2×	1 × weekly	2 × month
Folic acid, vitamin B$_{12}$	1×		
Magnesium	1×	1 × weekly	1 × month
Zinc	1×		
Iron	1×	2 × month	1 × month
Transferrin	1×	1 × weekly	1 × month
PT/PTT	1×	1 × weekly	1 × month
Nutritional Assessment			
Weight	every day	3 × weekly	2 × weekly
Creatinine height index	1×	2 × month	1 × month
Nitrogen balance		2 × weekly	1 × month
Delayed hypersensitivity skin test response	1×	2 × month	1 × month

* Special requirements and tests in patients with organ failure (*e.g.*, NH$_3$), infection or sepsis (*e.g.*, catheter culture), and hypercoagulation states (*e.g.*, antithrombin factor III).

compensates for the degradation of amino acids for gluconeogenesis, and the nitrogen balance will be close to zero. Losses of lean body mass can thus be efficiently minimized over periods of many weeks on intakes of a few hundred calories per day with adequate mineral supplements. The decrease in body weight is almost exclusively due to a temporary loss of water and to a decrease in adipose tissue mass, the latter amounting to some 200 g to 250 g/day. At the end of a period of weight reduction, the patient will not have lost his physical strength and need not attempt to restore lean body mass. A period of marked positive nitrogen balance, which brings about a rapid regain of body weight, does not occur when the patient returns to a more balanced diet.

Many of the metabolic benefits of fasting (*e.g.*, decreased carbon dioxide production, salt diuresis) result when using this diet program pre- and postoperatively in the obese patient.

MONITORING OF HYPERALIMENTATION

The success of long-term therapy is reflected in an improved prognostic index, that is, improvement in serum protein (albumin and transferrin) levels, conversion of skin antigen tests from negative to positive, return of total lymphocyte counts to ≥1500 cells/mm^3, resolution of sepsis, recovery from illness, renewed muscle strength (*e.g.*, hand grip strength), and restored lean body mass. On a day-to-day basis, calculation of nitrogen balance from urinary urea nitrogen measurements represents the only clinical tool available to evaluate the adequacy of nutritional therapy.

Table 7-7 provides a protocol for monitoring hyperalimentation. Careful monitoring, especially at the onset of therapy, will help prevent many of the complications (especially metabolic) associated with nutritional support in the hospitalized patient.

THE TEAM APPROACH

Concern about the poor nutritional status of hospitalized patients and the general lack of nutritional knowledge in both diagnosis and treatment of malnutrition has led to the development of nutrition support services in large university or tertiary care hospitals as well as in small community-based hospitals. The goal of such a service is to monitor the nutritional status of all hospitalized patients, to consult with and supervise appropriate therapeutic support in selected patients, and to provide a multidisciplinary approach to the nutritional problems that arise in the hospital. Particularly with total parenteral nutrition, a team approach and standard guidelines are needed if dangerous complications (*e.g.*, sepsis, pneumothorax, hyperosmolarity) are to be minimized.

A multidisciplinary nutrition support service, which combines the services of nursing, dietetics, pharmacy, and physical therapy with the major clinical disciplines, is also able to provide efficient outpatient nutritional support for patients receiving cancer therapy or for those with long-term nutritional problems secondary to their primary disease, *e.g.*, "short-gut" syndrome, inflammatory bowel disease, pancreatic insufficiency, renal disease, or obesity.

Clinical investigation, in-service education, and formal continuing education courses can also be effectively carried out by a multidisciplinary team.

Supported in part by grants GM-22691, GM-24401, and GM-24206 awarded by the National Institute of General Medical Sciences, DHHS, and the Center for Nutritional Research Charitable Trust.

BIBLIOGRAPHY

BISTRIAN BR: Nutritional assessment and therapy of protein-calorie malnutrition in the hospital. J Am Dietet Assoc 71:393, 1977

BISTRIAN BR: A simple technique to estimate severity of stress. Surg Gynecol Obstet 148:675, 1979

BISTRIAN BR: Anthropometric norms used in assessment of hospitalized patients. Am J Clin Nutr 33:2211, 1980

BLACKBURN GL, BOTHE A JR, LAHEY MA: Organization and administration of a nutrition support service. Surg Clin N Am 61:709, 1981

BLACKBURN GL, FLATT JP, CLOWES GHA et al: Peripheral intravenous feeding with isotonic amino acid solutions. Am J Surg 125:447, 1973

BLACKBURN GL, MAINI BS, PIERCE J: Nutrition in the critically ill patient. Anesthesiology 47:181, 1977

BOLLET AJ, OWENS S: Evaluation of nutritional status of selected hospitalized patients. Am J Clin Nutr 26:931, 1973

CAHILL GF: Starvation in man. N Engl J Med 282:668, 1970

CANNON PR, WISSLER RW, WOOLRIDGE RL et al: The relationship of protein deficiency to surgical infection. Ann Surg 120:514, 1944

CUTHBERTSON DP, TILSTONE WJ: Metabolism during the post-injury period. Adv Clin Chem 12:1, 1969

FLATT JP, BLACKBURN GL: The metabolic fuel regulatory system: Implications for protein-sparing therapies during caloric deprivation and disease. Am J Clin Nutr 27:175, 1974

HARVEY KB, MOLDAWER LL, BISTRIAN BR et al: Biological measures for the formulation of a hospital prognostic index. Am J Clin Nutr 34:2013, 1981

HEYMSFIELD SB, BETHEL RA, ANSLEY JD et al: Enteral hyperalimentation: An alternative to central venous hyperalimentation. Ann Int Med 90:63, 1979

LONG CL, BLAKEMORE WS: Energy and protein requirements in the hospitalized patient. J Parent Ent Nutr 3:69, 1979

LOWRY SF, GOODGAME JT, MAHER MM et al: Parenteral vitamin requirements during intravenous feeding. Am J Clin Nutr 31:2149, 1978

MEAKINS JL, PIETSCH JB, BUBENICK Q et al: Delayed hypersensitivity: Indicator of acquired failure of host defenses in sepsis and trauma. Ann Surg 186:241, 1977

MILLER CL: Immunological assays as measurements of nutritional status: A review. J Parent Ent Nutr 2:554, 1978

MULLEN JL, BUZBY GP, MATTHEWS DC et al: Reduction of operative morbidity and mortality by combined preoperative and postoperative support. Ann Surg 192:604, 1980

Nutrition Advisory Group, AMA Department of Foods and Nutrition: Guidelines for essential trace element preparations for parenteral use. JAMA 241:2051, 1979

OTA DM, IMBEMBO AL, ZUIDEMA GD: Total parenteral nutrition. Surgery 83:503, 1978

RHOADS JE, ALEXANDER CE: Nutritional problems of surgical patients. Ann NY Acad Sci 63:268, 1955

SCHNEIDER HA, ANDERSON CE, COURSIN DB: Nutritional Support of Medical Practice. Hagerstown, MD, Harper & Row, 1977

YOUNG GA, CHEM C, HILL GL: Assessment of protein-calorie malnutrition in surgical patients from plasma proteins and anthropometric measurements. Am J Clin Nutr 31:429, 1978

M. J. Jurkiewicz/Louis Morales, Jr.

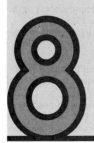

Wound Healing, Operative Incisions, and Skin Grafts

WOUND HEALING

A complex, integrated sequence of events initiated by the stimulus of injury to tissues, wound healing has evolved as an effective mechanism in preserving the physical integrity of our organ systems. Humans cannot regenerate whole organs, excepting bone and, in part, the liver. Healing, therefore, can take place only by the process of scarring. The function of a scar may be looked upon as binding injured tissues together to restore integrity—although as often as not at some cost of function.

Posthepatic cirrhosis, esophageal stricture, pulmonary fibrosis, aortic and mitral stenosis, intestinal obstruction, and burn contractures are but a few examples of the disabling consequences of scarring. Ordinarily, in wounds by clean incision, healing proceeds without consequence and normal function is restored. Contraction—which may be disabling—occurs when there is loss of substance accompanied by the inward movement of the existing tissue, with subsequent epithelialization. Knowledge of the inflammatory response, fibroplasia, contraction, epithelialization, and scar maturation is basic to the surgeon. To manage wounds is the study of surgery; to manage them correctly is the essence.

CLASSIFICATION

The healing of a wound is classified into one of three general categories: first, second, and third intention. These are dependent on the nature of the wound, on whether soft tissue has been lost, or if infection is present or likely to be present. Healing by *first intention* occurs in a surgically clean wound made by an incision and closed by suturing in the period immediately after wounding. Very little if any granulation tissue is present, and the amount of scarring is minimal. If wounding results in soft tissue loss or if a contaminated wound is left open to granulate, healing can occur by *second intention*. In the process considerable granulation is formed; there is resultant contraction and epithelialization that ultimately accounts for a closed wound. After sufficient granulation has occurred, another option is to close the wound secondarily by split-thickness skin graft. For example, an avulsion injury to the thigh with significant contamination is allowed to granulate after appropriate debridement. When clean, a skin graft may be used to close the wound. When a wound is secondarily closed 4 to 5 days after injury, it is said to have healed by *third intention*. Initially such a wound is left open because of gross contamination. After cleansing, it is kept covered with a sterile occlusive dressing. If the wound is clean in 4 to 5 days, it is closed by suture or by approximation with sterile tape. A classic example is the management of the patient with a ruptured appendix. After the pus is evacuated, the appendix removed, and the stump ligated, only peritoneum and fascia are closed to prevent evisceration. The remainder of the wound is packed loosely with sterile gauze and covered with sterile dressings. At 4 to 5 days the dressings are removed under sterile conditions; if the wound is clean with granulation tissue present, it is closed. If there is purulence present, it is left open and allowed to heal by second intention (Fig. 8-1).

GENERAL PROCESS OF WOUND HEALING

Although a complex continuum, wound healing has been divided into the following phases: (*1*) inflammatory reaction, (*2*) fibroplasia, (*3*) contraction, and (*4*) scar remodeling. These phases overlap but do serve to facilitate understanding.

Inflammation is the initial response to any type of wounding. The intensity and duration of inflammation is determined by local and systemic factors, that is, a clean or contaminated wound, a simple laceration, or an untidy avulsion. Both a vascular and a cellular phase occur in the inflammatory response to wounding. The vascular response occurs immediately after injury with transient vasoconstriction lasting 5 to 10 min. This controls bleeding to some extent, and actual vessel thrombosis may be evident. Subsequently vasodilatation of the small venules (20 μ in diameter) occurs with actual separation between the endothelial cells. This permits egress of plasma proteins, red blood cells, and leukocytes into the wound. Because vessel walls become "sticky," leukocytes adhere to the endothelium. These leukocytes migrate through the vessel wall by diapedesis and are the predominant cell in the injured area for 72 hr. The vascular changes are mediated by several substances, histamine being the most ubiquitous. Leukotaxine, kinins, and prostaglandins are all implicated in the vascular response, but their roles are less well defined.

Once the leukocytes have entered the wound, active phagocytosis occurs. Both polymorphonuclear leukocytes and monocytes are engaged in the active process of destruction and ingestion of wound debris. The short-lived polymorphonuclear leukocytes die within days, leaving the monocytes to carry on the task. Usually the inflammatory period is shortlived in a clean surgical incision. When the inflammation becomes chronic because of persistent infection or foreign body, the monocyte becomes the predominant cell. The monocyte may transform into a macrophage or become a multinucleated giant cell.

There are concurrent changes in the epithelium. Within 24 hr to 48 hr the marginal basal cells are no longer fixed to the underlying dermis. Mitosis of basal cells is remarkably increased, and the resultant daughter cells enlarge, flatten, and spread across the exposed dermis to cover the incision. Within days the wound may be epithelialized with several layers.

The fibroblast migrates into the wound at 48 hr to 72 hr to initiate the phase of fibroplasia. Local undifferentiated mesenchymal cells residing in extravascular tissues transform into fibroblasts attendant upon the stimulation of wounding. These newly-formed fibroblasts are recruited locally and migrate along fibrin strands that are thought to serve as a matrix. If there is an excessive amount of fibrin, the migration of the fibroblast is hindered and wound healing is impaired. Capillaries formed by endothelial budding follow the proliferating fibroblast. Fibrinolysin breaks down fibrin and thus assists the fibroblast in its role at the site of injury. This phase of repair usually lasts 2 to 4 wk depending on the amount of necrotic debris, hematoma, or infection.

The wound is now a highly cellular structure with fibroblasts being the dominant cell. Protein–polysaccharides and glycoproteins are present in the ground substance. By

Fig. 8-1. Classification of wound healing. *First intention*—A clean incision is made with primary closure; there is minimal scarring. *Second intention* (contraction and epithelialization)—The wound is left open to granulate in with resultant large scab and abnormal dermal–epidermal junction. *Third intention* (delayed closure)—The wound is left open and closed secondarily when there is no evidence of infection.

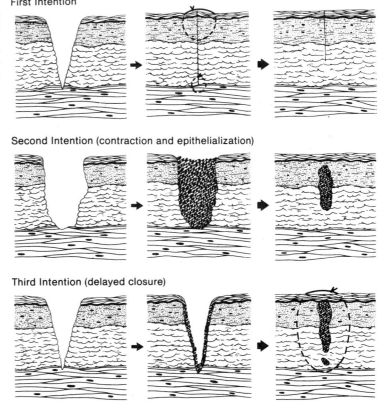

First Intention

Second Intention (contraction and epithelialization)

Third Intention (delayed closure)

the fifth to seventh day active collagen synthesis begins, and the wound gains tensile strength. This takes place at a very rapid rate, but the cellular population remains stable for several weeks. It is felt that the mucopolysaccharide that is dominant in the ground substance determines to a degree the type of collagen formed. The rate of gain of tensile strength is similar for all tissues, but overall tensile strength differs with each tissue. For example, in 3 wk skin obtains 30% of tensile strength, fascia about 20%, intestine 65%, and urinary bladder 95%. After 5 to 6 wk the fibroblasts decrease in number, the capillary network becomes organized into well-defined capillary systems, and the rate of total collagen synthesis decreases.

SCAR CHEMISTRY

The basic components of a scar include collagen and the ground substance in which the fibers are oriented. The ground substance consists of mucopolysaccharides, protein–polysaccharides, glycoproteins, electrolytes, and bound water. Although ground substance does not contribute directly to the strength of a scar, it probably does markedly influence collagen fibril aggregation and orientation, hence affecting the solidity as well as the final appearance of a scar.

There are seven substances classified as mucopolysaccharides, and each occurs in various concentrations depending on where they are found (Table 8-1). The mucopolysaccharides can be divided into sulfated and nonsulfated compounds. The nonsulfated substances comprise the gel fraction, whereas the sulfated ones are interrelated with the connective-tissue fibers. Overall, the mucopolysaccharides are quite close chemically and it has been difficult to assess their presence in different stages of wound healing as well as concentrations in different tissues. These large macromolecules are present within wounds by the fourth day and their number continues to increase until 2 to 3 wk after wounding. Depending on the site, their concentration varies; for example, dermatan sulfate is the predominant mucopolysaccharide in skin, whereas chondroitin-4-sulfate occurs predominantly in bone.

COLLAGEN AND ITS METABOLISM

Collagen, the principal component of all connective tissue, makes up approximately 20% to 30% of total body protein.

In scar tissue, it contributes most of the protein makeup and tensile strength. It is a sturdy structural protein that is found throughout the body in stress-related tissues (*e.g.,* bone, tendon, fascia). It follows, therefore, that collagen should also be the predominant component in a healing wound.

Collagen is an extracellular protein that is manufactured intracellularly by the newly transformed fibroblast. The procollagen molecule or tropocollagen is synthesized within the fibroblast and passes from the endoplasmic reticulum to the Golgi apparatus thence to the extracellular space. Here it undergoes an enzymatic cleavage of the nonhelical portion, releasing the collagen molecule. This then aggregates, forming specific fibers with aldehyde cross-bonding giving rise to a specific collagen architecture.

Tropocollagen is composed of three α-polypeptide chains in a helical structure with a molecular weight of 270,000 and a width of 15 A. There are two α_1 and one α_2 chains intertwined to form the helix. An intramolecular hydrogen bond between the α_1 and α_2 chains maintains the helical structure.

Fundamentally collagen has the following three identifying features: (*1*) three α-peptide chains in a right-handed helix; (*2*) the presence of glycine in every third position along the peptide chain; and (*3*) the presence of two unique amino acids—hydroxylysine and hydroxyproline.

Tropocollagen formed within the fibroblast is secreted as a collagen filament outside the cell. These filaments aggregate to form collagen fibers—usually 100,000 A to 200,000 A in diameter (in comparison to the 15 A-wide tropocollagen) (Fig. 8-2) Tropocollagen is soluble in water, and not until a mature collagen fiber is formed does it become insoluble.

The cross-linking of the collagen molecule is susceptible to various environmental factors. Temperature, *p*H, the presence of inorganic substances, and electrical charge all affect the bonding of these peptide chains. The most common cross-link is that formed from an aldehyde group of lysine or hydroxylysine. The resultant compound is a Schiff base. It is this cross-link that is the factor responsible for tensile strength. Aging of a collagen molecule appears to increase the number of cross-links present. The variations in cross-linking are also responsible for the appearance of a scar, its elasticity, and texture.

TABLE 8-1   MUCOPOLYSACCHARIDES OF CONNECTIVE TISSUE

	SYNONYMS	DISACCHARIDE REPEATING UNIT
Chondroitin	—	Glucuronic acid + galactosamine
Chondroitin 4-sulfate	Chondroitin sulfate A	Glucuronic acid + 4-sulfogalactosamine
Chondroitin 6-sulfate	Chondroitin sulfate C	Glucuronic acid + 6-sulfogalactosamine
Dermatan sulfate	Chondroitin sulfate B Heparin	Iduronic acid + 4-sulfogalactosamine
Heparin sulfate	Heparitin sulfate Heparin monosulfate	Glucuronic acid + glucosamine (Contains N and O sulfate groups)*
Hyaluronic acid	—	Glucuronic acid + glucosamine
Keratan sulfate	Kerato sulfate	Galactose + 6-sulfoglucosamine

* The structure of this compound is not completely clear.
(Madden JW: Wound healing: The biological aspects. In Hardy JD [ed]: Rhoads Textbook of Surgery, 5th ed. Philadelphia, J B Lippincott, 1977)

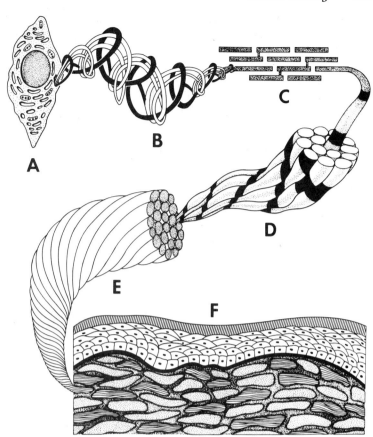

Fig. 8-2. Schema of events in the production of collagen. (*A*) Fibroblast active in protein synthesis. (*B*) Tropocollagen production with triple helix. Molecular weight is 270,000A. (*C*) Collagen filament with intermolecular bonding. (*D*) Aggregation of collagen filaments into collagen fibril. (*E*) Collagen fiber. (*F*) Mature collagen fibers arranged in connective tissue.

Several types of collagen have been discovered. At present there are four distinct types with differences in the amino acid and the carbohydrate content.

1. Type I—Conventional type with two α_1 and one α_2 chains, found in skin, tendon, cartilage, and cornea
2. Type II—Found only in cartilage and has no α_2 chain
3. Type III—Found in the aorta, lung, and embryonic dermis. There is also no α_2 chain. This is primarily an embryonic tissue collagen.
4. Type IV—Found in the basement membrane and anterior lens capsule and is composed of three identical chains

SCAR REMODELING

The overall form and bulk of a scar changes once maturation has started. Organization of the collagen fibers from their initial inchoate state occurs, providing for the continued changes in the appearance of a scar and the increase in its tensile strength. This process continues for years, resulting in a continued turnover of collagen and remodeling of the scar. The amount of remodeling is dependent upon external physical forces (*i.e.*, musculoskeletal pull) and on the age of the patient. Unanswered remains the question for the reason behind the differences between lysis and production of collagen in different scars (*i.e.*, mature soft scar versus keloid). Collagen fibers, as they become organized, are closely aligned to each other, allowing for an increase in intermolecular bonding and hence an increase in tensile strength. The strength of a scar is felt to be more dependent on these cross-links than on the amount of collagen present.

Tensile strength, measured in kilogram per square centimeter, continues to increase despite the similarities, microscopically and quantitatively, of scar that is six weeks old versus a six year old scar. It is this remodeling phase that provides for the final characteristics of a scar.

The tensile strength of scar and presumably its appearance can be altered in a profound way pharmacologically. For example, β-aminopropionitrile, found in the seeds of the sweet pea (*Lathyrus odoratus*), will increase the solubility of the collagen without altering the quantity produced. There is both an intermolecular and intramolecular interference with cross-linking. Penicillamine also appears to act in a similar fashion to prevent cross-linking. Although the side effects of these agents vitiate their routine clinical use, the possibilities of potential control of scar formation have been opened.

OPEN WOUNDS

Wounds by trauma may not be closed primarily in every instance. The open wound, whether the result of significant soft-tissue loss or of an incision that was left open to drain in a severely contaminated case, presents a significant biologic challenge to the patient and a management problem to the surgeon. These wounds can either be closed by third intention or, if necessary, by second intention. Large skin and soft-tissue losses mandate either a skin graft or a flap for closure. When spontaneous healing is permissible, the process of contraction and concomitant epithelization comes into play.

The process of contraction has been described for centuries. Prior to the advent of skin grafts and local flaps, open wounds were allowed to heal by contraction. Examples include the healed stump following guillotine amputation of an extremity shattered and contaminated in warfare, scalping injuries, or burns.

Contraction is defined as the centripetal movement of adjacent skin to either diminish the size or to close an open wound. *Contraction* is often confused with *contracture,* which is the resultant deformity that limits mobility of the part from fibrosis. Wounds should not be allowed to contract to closure over certain areas of the body because the resultant deformity is crippling. Examples include the open wound of an eyelid allowed to progress to cicatricial ectropion or a useless hand frozen by burn cicatrix.

The process of contraction begins in a fashion not dissimilar to the healing of a closed wound. However, once a wound is left open, fibrin is deposited to actually seal the wound from the environment. The fibrin cover quickly loses its water content and becomes a scab. If it is left covered with moist dressings, then a scab will not form and granulation tissue is the rule. Whether a scab is formed or not, contraction will start in 3 to 4 days after wounding. Inflammation is the initial step, with polymorphonuclears predominant, followed by lymphocytes and macrophages. Endothelial buds then appear along with the fibroblasts. Both ground substance (mucopolysaccharides) and collagen fibers are produced. It was once theorized that collagen itself was responsible for the active contraction process. It is now known that collagen contains no contractile elements and does not shorten as a living substance. Contraction has now been attributed to a very unique type of cell, the myofibroblast. Electron microscopy has revealed that this contractile fibroblast has the characteristics both of a fibroblast and of a smooth muscle cell. First identified by Gabbiani in 1971, these cells tend to be joined to one another by hemidesmosomes and by gap junctions, in contrast to the normal fibroblast. These agents that directly stimulate smooth muscle will also stimulate portions of granulation tissue excised from an open wound. Myofibroblasts reside throughout the substance of granulation tissue and are not concentrated at the periphery of the wound. Therefore, the active pull of the wound is distributed throughout its substance.

Methods of controlling contraction involve pharmacologic control of myofibroblasts, mechanical manipulation of the wound, and biochemical control of collagen. Splinting and range of motion exercises both modulate stress factors to rearrange collagen fibers while counteracting the active pull of the myofibroblast. These techniques are especially applicable in the management of injuries of the neck, hand, and extremities.

A smooth muscle inhibitor, triphenamil hydrochloride (Trocinate) has been used experimentally to inhibit wound contraction. As long as it is applied the treatment is effective; once discontinued, however, contraction immediately resumes. Colchicine and vinblastine have also been used. Each of these agents is tissue-toxic and, therefore, of little practical use in wound management.

Steroids, β-aminopropionitrile, and penicillamine all affect collagen metabolism, its maturation, and thus indirectly inhibit contraction. This may be due to the necessary organization of collagen fibers to provide for myofibroblasts to lock into them.

The best overall method to inhibit contraction in an open wound is to close the wound with a split-thickness skin graft or with a flap as soon as possible. All wounds contract to some extent—to the greatest degree when left open, less with a skin graft, and much less when skin and subcutaneous tissue are used to close the wound. Splinting of the part must be used as an adjunctive measure when indicated to prevent further contraction and hence contracture.

FACTORS AFFECTING WOUND HEALING

NUTRITIONAL FACTORS

Malnourishment, from whatever reason, alters the body's metabolic steady state with biochemical changes that may hinder the normal wound-healing process. It has been demonstrated that in the severely malnourished, both visceral and cutaneous wound healing are adversely affected. There is no doubt that in this setting hyperalimentation is essential to restore the patient's nitrogen balance to a positive state. Hyperalimentation also replenishes the indispensable essential amino acids and the unsaturated fatty acids. In those instances in which malnutrition is mild or moderate, wound healing appears to be normal. A short course of hyperalimentation prior to surgery has not been shown to favorably influence the overall healing of wounds. Although there appears to be an increase in the overall production of collagen, wound tensile strength is not increased. A decrease in serum protein levels is not well correlated with the quality of wound healing until levels of less than 2 g% protein are reached.

VITAMIN DEFICIENCIES

Ascorbic acid deficiency (scurvy) and its relationship to wound healing are well known. Ascorbic acid is a necessary cofactor that provides for the hydroxylation of proline and lysine. A deficiency state inhibits the overall production of collagen because without ascorbate, collagen synthesis proceeds to the point of proline and lysine hydroxylation and not beyond. The rapid synthesis and turnover of collagen is profoundly affected. New wounds will not heal in early scurvy. Later, old healed scars will become fragile and will finally open in the severely scorbutic state because lysis of collagen continues while all production ceases.

Established scurvy takes months to become clinically evident. Whether transient periods of undernourishment or starvation (*e.g.,* the perioperative period) result in subclinical deficiency that in turn will affect wound healing has never been established. Nonetheless, pharmacologic doses of vitamin C continue to be infused into patients convalescing from operations.

TRACE-ELEMENT DEFICIENCIES

Zinc deficiency, although uncommon except in children in the Middle East, will retard wound healing by preventing cell proliferation. Zinc is necessary in several deoxyribonucleic acid (DNA) and ribonucleic acid (RNA) polymerases and transferases; hence, a deficiency state will inhibit mitosis.

CONDITIONS THAT MAY ADVERSELY AFFECT WOUND HEALING

Ischemia	Cirrhosis
Infection	Hypercortisolism
Foreign body	Radiation injury
Malnutrition	Cytotoxic agents
Vitamin and mineral deficiency	Mechanical tension
	Renal failure
Diabetes mellitus	Malignancy

Fibroplasia is therefore retarded. Severely stressed patients, such as those with massive burns or undergoing major operations, may become deficient, and zinc supplementation may be of value. In patients with normal zinc levels, the administration of zinc will be of no advantage. In fact, excessive zinc levels may hinder macrophage migration and phagocytosis, and therefore impair wound healing.

ANEMIA AND HEMORRHAGE

Wound healing will proceed to completion in severe anemic states for both open and closed wounds if hypovolemia is not a factor. Rats that were made anemic up to 2 g% by an iron-deficiency state, hemolysis, or repeated bleeding were able to heal burns of 20% of body surface by contraction at the same rate as controls. Moreover skin grafts in such animals took just as well as in normal litter mates.

Sickle cell anemia is associated with chronic leg ulcers. Pathogenesis of the ulcer is thrombosis of nutrient vessels to skin; perpetuation relates to anoxemia.

Hemorrhage with its consequent hypovolemic state will result in a shutdown of the microcirculation. It is this microcirculation with its provision of oxygen and nutrition to the local tissues that influences wound healing. It is therefore imperative that blood volume be maintained if normal wound healing is to be achieved.

OXYGEN TENSION

Oxygen is fundamental for normal cell function and proliferation. Fibroplasia and hence collagen synthesis are dependent on available oxygen for the hydroxylation of proline and lysine. Temporary anoxia may lead to unstable collagen with resultant poor tensile strength. Injury to tissues can impair the local circulation and hinder delivery of nutrients and oxygen to the wound. Perfusion more often than not is the problem. For example, a wound of the face that is quite vascular heals rapidly, whereas a wound in a foot of a diabetic, where perfusion and hence the delivery of oxygen are impaired, heals poorly.

Wound oxygen tension below 20 torr will significantly impair collagen metabolism. Normally in wounds closed primarily the oxygen tension will exceed this critical level. Clearly, therefore, if the patient is at risk of wound hypoxia, then oxygen should be administered to increase the delivery to the tissues.

The factors that are responsible for the hypoxemia obviously should be corrected if the patient is to survive and the wound is to heal.

STEROIDS

Cortisol administered in pharmacologic doses inhibits fibroplasia and neovascularity and moderates the normal inflammatory response. This effect can be seen whether cortisone is used topically on a wound bed or given systemically for long periods. Epithelialization and contraction both are impaired. The wound may eventually heal but the time period is prolonged depending on the dosage and chronicity of steroid administration. Vitamin A given systemically or topically will reverse the effect.

Scars subject to tension over a joint or to the stimulus of thermal injury will hypertrophy. In some patients the scar will proliferate beyond the limits of the original incision or injury and become a keloid. Whether this is a failure of the normal lysis of collagen or the result of an excess production of collagen is not completely settled, but the weight of evidence indicates an excess production.

Triamcinalone, in doses of 10 mg/mm³, injected into hypertropic scar or into keloid will definitely ameliorate the condition.

ANTI-INFLAMMATORY DRUGS

Anti-inflammatory medications do not interfere with wound healing when administered at the usual daily dosages. Aspirin and indomethacin both inhibit prostaglandin synthesis. Prostaglandins are the terminal mediators of the acute inflammatory response, and if inhibited, will result in a reduction of inflammation. Nonetheless, with usual doses, wound healing will continue unimpaired, provided bleeding and hematoma are not complications.

RADIATION

The effects of radiation on tissue are classified as acute, intermediate, and chronic. Not only rapidly proliferating tumor cells but also normal cells with a high turnover rate are affected in the acute phase. These acute changes result in mucositis, desquamation of epithelium, erythema, epilation, and bone-marrow depression; thus, normal homeostasis and repair are affected. For example, Grillo found that small doses of radiation to experimental wounds resulted in better than 80% reduction in fibroblast and endothelial cell proliferation measured 5 days after wounding.

Intermediate effects of irradiation produce injury to a more slowly proliferative cell renewal system, principally endothelium and connective tissue.

The late effects, directly related to total dose, typically are manifested in connective tissues not only of skin but also of the walls of blood vessels. Wolbach described early histologic changes in the skin as swelling of the collagen. Later collagen hyalinizes, elastic fibrils rupture, become frayed, or curled, and there are bizarre dysplastic fibroblasts scattered throughout the irradiated area. Blood vessels similarly become hyalinized, sclerotic, and stenosed. Neither fibroplasia nor endothelial proliferation can proceed. Because of avascular scarring and obliterative vasculitis, repair is profoundly affected. In response to trauma, ulceration is very likely to be followed by colonization by opportunistic bacteria. The patient cannot mount an effective inflammation response. Progressive necrosis may result involving not only skin but underlying bone, hollow viscus, or lung. Sepsis, fistulas, or rupture of major vessels may occur. Such complications may occur as early as a few months to years after irradiation.

A surgeon operating in an irradiated field should allow the acute effects to subside before proceeding (*i.e.*, 3 to 4 wk) and before the intermediate effects ensue (*i.e.*, 3 to 6 mo). If an operation is to be carried out where late effects of irradiation are manifest or for radiation necrosis itself, then all damaged tissue should be removed, and tissue with intact, normal blood supply brought in to provide not only oxygen but the necessary cells for inflammation and repair. If, for example, bowel is involved by obstruction or fistula, all involved bowel must be resected if possible. Anastomosis made through normal-appearing intestine should have a proximal decompression enterostomy. The part must be covered with well-vascularized skin or skin–muscle flaps.

CYTOTOXIC AGENTS

The effects of the various cytotoxic drugs on fibroblasts, collagen deposition, and maturation are incompletely understood. There is, however, information that is useful to guide management.

The tensile strength of a healing wound is depressed by 30% when a dose of 0.3 mg/kg/d of methotrexate, a folic acid antagonist, is given, and 50% if 0.5 mg/kg/d is administered.

If leucovorin is given within 4 hr, the tensile strength of the wound approaches that of normal. This also is dose-related, with greater return of strength with higher doses of leucovorin. If methotrexate is given after wounding rather than before, the impairment of wound healing is greater.

Alkylating agents will depress rate of gain in tensile strength and will hinder formation of granulation tissue, and therefore contraction. The effect is dose-related. For example, cyclophosphamide (Cytoxan) does not impair healing, although revascularization is slightly prolonged. Cytoxan at a dose of 2 mg/kg has no effect on wound healing. At midrange, 50 mg/kg, there is significant decrease in wound tensile strength.

Doxorubicin (Adriamycin) given at a dose of 6 mg/kg will significantly impair wound healing. The wound breaking strength of Adriamycin-treated animals is about 50% of control at 21 days, and wound content of hydroxyproline is similarly reduced. There is an underproduction of collagen and also an inability of collagen fibril aggregation to reach maturation.

Clinically, skin grafts that are incompletely healed will slough completely if the patient is receiving therapeutic doses of either actinomycin D or doxorubicin. The epithelialization of skin-graft donor sites will cease and can be converted to full-thickness loss. It follows therefore that adjuvant chemotherapy, especially doxorubicin, should be given after wound repair is complete, if possible.

DIABETES

Diabetics heal poorly. Why? There are a number of reasons. The risk in diabetics of infection in clean wounds approaches five-fold the risk in nondiabetics. Impaired circulation secondary to large and small vessel occlusive disease and a decrease in the inflammatory response caused by hyperglycemia and by abnormal intermediary metabolism are major factors. Impaired sensation consequent to diabetic neuropathy renders the lower extremity blind to everyday hazards. Trauma, which is omnipresent, causes a break in the integrity of the skin; ulcers develop that are often painless and go untreated. The diabetic out of control with dorsal swelling of the foot and a trophic ulcer over the head of the second metatarsal as the signs of a plantar space abscess is classic. Control of blood sugar is essential in the patient with diabetes who is to undergo an operation. Exquisite attention to the details of handling of tissue, wound management, and control of infection are requisite for wound repair in the diabetic. Even so, failure is common enough and amputation a reality.

JAUNDICE

Jaundiced patients have been shown to have a higher incidence of abdominal wound dehiscence and wound infections. Whether this is directly related to the jaundice is uncertain. There are other hepatic disturbances and derangements of metabolism, especially hypoproteinemia, that may in effect be the primary cause of poor wound healing. Malnourishment, especially in obstructive jaundice secondary to malignancy, confuses the direct relationship. Animal studies have demonstrated that jaundice in itself is probably not the cause of poor wound healing. Clearly other derangements contribute to the failure of the healing process.

OPERATIVE INCISIONS

SKIN INCISION

Essential in preoperative planning are the type of incision, its length, and its location. Not only is exposure of paramount concern; equally important is regard for a favorable outcome of wound healing.

DIRECTION

The incision should be made in a direction that allows for adequate exposure during the operation and ready extension in an appropriate direction, if so required. For example, exploration of an injury to the axillary artery may require extension of the incision from the bracium around to the subclavicular area to obtain proximal control.

LENGTH

Many incisions made may be shorter than is optimal for safe, rapid conduct of an operation. All students of surgery, undergraduate and graduate, have heard—many times, perhaps—that "incisions heal from side to side and not from top to bottom." The thinking that a smaller incision will heal faster and appear less obtrusive is erroneous. The amount of local tissue trauma applied to a wound by an assistant tugging on a retractor or by pulling up the skin edges with forceps to provide exposure adds to local tissue ischemia and cellular destruction, factors that are known to retard repair. Furthermore, the amount of postoperative pain secondary to the stretching of muscle fibers and nerves may result in compromise to other organ systems (*e.g.*, pulmonary atelectasis secondary to an abdominal operation).

LOCATION ("WRINKLE LINES")

In 1951, C. J. Kraissl advised that elective incisions be made in the normal "wrinkle lines" if possible. Areas of least tension fall into the normal skin creases or "wrinkle lines." Incisions so placed where the tension is minimal will heal kindly. Even today students of medicine are taught that the lines of Langer are the appropriate lines to follow when making an incision. K. Langer in 1861, in the Proceedings of the Society for Natural History of Vienna, described these skin tension lines on observations made on cadavers after puncturing the body with an awl. These lines are at variance with the "wrinkle lines" of Kraissl, which are the summation of dynamic forces acting on human skin. Wrinkle lines or normal skin creases generally run perpendicular to the underlying muscle and are formed by the repetitious contraction of these muscles from daily activities. (See Figs. 8-3, 8-4, and 8-5.)

It should be emphasized that incisions should be made in wrinkle lines if a choice is possible, but there are pragmatic reasons for making exceptions to this general rule. When speed is of the essence in an emergency, or when access to a lesion is critical, then the most direct incision is applicable.

Incisions should be made with a thorough understanding of the region, the underlying muscles, nerves, and vessels; for example, incisions of the chest should parallel the ribs and should hug the superior border of the rib so as not to injure the neurovascular bundle of the rib above (Fig. 8-6).

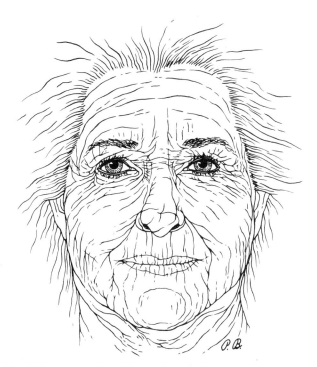

Fig. 8-3. Exaggeration of normal "wrinkle" lines, showing the variety of wrinkles present upon facial expression.

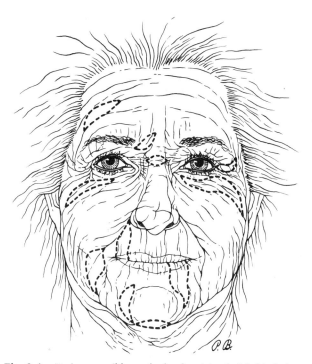

Fig. 8-4. Various possible methods of excising facial skin lesions following the normal "wrinkle" lines.

Fig. 8-5. Muscles of facial expression with the overlying "wrinkle" lines. These lines lie perpendicular to the underlying muscle fibers.

Fig. 8-6. The pattern of skin lines over the anterior thorax, abdomen, and arms. Dotted lines represent the various types of incisions in use today.

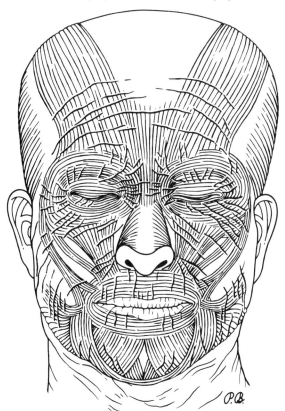

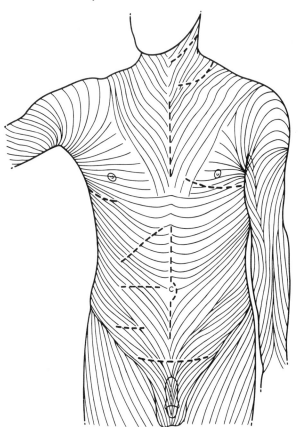

The incision is made by a single deliberate motion with a sure knowledge of the anatomy of the region and the purpose of the operation. The venturesome but intellectually impoverished operator is dangerous; the hesitant, insecure operator is a morbid factor in his patient's convalescence. Important structures should not be unnecessarily or unknowingly sacrificed.

The incision should be precise and perpendicular to the skin, allowing for easy approximation afterwards. Only those large vessels encountered should be either ligated or cauterized in a pinpoint fashion. Small oozing vessels should not be cauterized since these will usually stop by direct pressure. Haphazard clamping of vessels or generalized cauterization will lead to tissue necrosis and, hence, an increase in the infection rate. Dessication or excessive trauma are to be avoided. Blood clots, loose pieces of fat, and debris should be removed by irrigation before wound closure.

ABDOMINAL INCISIONS

Depending on the area of the body, incisions have been devised to accommodate the necessary ease in peformance, in closure, and for exposure. Abdominal incisions in general use are midline, paramedian, transverse and oblique, up or down (Fig. 8-6). The midline abdominal incision is easy to perform and is the incision of choice when speed is essential to successful outcome. It is quite versatile and if necessary can be lengthened from xiphoid to pubis for exposure. Moreover, it can be extended through an intercostal space if the chest need be entered. Incisional hernia, dehiscence, and evisceration are associated most often with midline abdominal incisions in every age group.

The transverse incision was described in 1823 by Baudelocque for cesarean sections and popularized by Pfannenstiel in 1900 for pelvic operations. It was Maylard in 1899 who first used this anatomic incision in the upper part of the abdomen, and Boeckmann later utilized the transverse incision in all types of abdominal operations in 1906.

The transverse incision in most instances is the best abdominal incision. Not only is it anatomic but is stronger and associated with few complications. The incidence of dehiscence, evisceration, and late hernia is remarkably less when compared to the midline incision. The forces of tension across the vertical incision as measured by Sloan were found to be 30 lb for a 3-in incision and 80 lb for a 5-in vertical incision. This is some 30 times greater than across a transverse incision. The sutures coapting a transverse incision will lie across the aponeurotic fibers rather than parallel to them and, hence, will tear out less easily.

The ninth intercostal nerve passes transversely across the abdomen at a point one third the distance between the umbilicus and the xiphoid. Nerves above this tend to run obliquely upward while those below run obliquely downward. The lateral transverse incision, therefore, is least likely to injure these nerves. Incisions in the upper part of the abdomen may be made obliquely downward without causing appreciable injury to nerves. Incisions in the lower abdomen should be made obliquely upward.

There are variations in the transverse incision ranging from the muscle-retracting variant to the more common incision of all layers. The left infraumbilical transverse incision gives excellent exposure for a sigmoid resection, whereas that made on the right is more than adequate for a right colectomy. If there is a narrow costal arch, then access to the upper abdomen can be facilitated by an oblique

incision. Rees and Coller state that a Kocher type of incision that lies near and parallel to the costal arch will section too many nerves and should therefore not be the incision of choice. The only problem in a transverse incision is the correct placement across the abdomen in a traumatic or acute abdominal case. If the injury or pathology is suspected to be upper abdominal but is found to be in the lower abdomen, the exposure may be less than optimum.

If a previous incision has been made, it should be reused if possible. Parallel incisions on the abdomen have been made by many surgeons in situations of necessity. It is not altogether uncommon for the strip of skin between the two incisions to die even if the time period between incisions is years. This is especially true if a paramedian incision is made hard upon a midline scar. The blood supply to the skin of the abdominal wall in general comes from perforating branches of arteries to muscle—specifically, the superior and inferior epigastric arteries. Damage to the epigastric arterial system and undermining of skin essentially will result in necrosis of this bridge of skin.

WOUND CLOSURE

Hemostasis and gentle handling of tissue proceed *pari passu* with the proper conduct of an operation. Nonetheless, prior to wound closure, hemostasis is once again checked and all loose tissue particles are irrigated from the wound.

Wound closure is best accomplished by approximating in an accurate anatomic fashion all layers that provide strength to the wound; for example, closure of a transverse abdominal incision requires suture of the posterior rectus fascia, anterior rectus fascia, and the three musculofascial layers laterally, but not the rectus muscle nor the subcutaneous layer. Careful approximation of the fascial layers with attention to preservation of their circulation is essential to lend strength to the wound.

Halsted of Hopkins at the turn of the century stated, ''To drain or obliterate with the greatest of care all of the dead spaces of a wound is still an almost universally accepted precept of surgery; and surgeons have a wholesome fear of presence of blood in wounds.'' Surgeons from that time all recommended the obliteration of dead spaces with buried sutures. Probably the first good study of the problem of closure of the subcutaneous space was that of deHoll and Rodeheaver in 1974. They demonstrated that not only did dead space increase the infection rate but that closure of the dead space with sutures was even more detrimental. The subcutaneous layer does not provide support nor does it hold sutures very well. Buried sutures often simply provide a nidus for infection. Skin and subcutaneous tissue, if undermined, are poorly vascularized by definition. Therefore, the susceptibility to infection increases. If dead space with accumulation of serum is of concern, then a closed suction apparatus is the preferred method of management.

The approximation of the skin edges of an incision is the final surgical step in an operation. The apposition of two raw surfaces by a particular suture technique with an appropriate suture should be performed without undue tension. When too tight, sutures will cut through the skin—inflamed secondary incisions invite wound complication as well as unnecessarily obtrusive scarring. As Gillies once stated, ''How tight to tie is a matter of experience and lies between that adequate to bring the edges closely apposed and that which cuts through by causing tissue necrosis. Err on the loose side. Stitch marks are indisputable evidence of a suture that has caused local pressure necrosis and its accompanying infection." Obligatory edema of the wound seen up to 48 hr postoperatively should be taken into account. Sutures should be used sparingly and spaced far enough apart to accomplish a satisfactorily sealed wound.

Skin eversion, meticulous local care of the skin edges, and approximation without tension are the hallmarks of an adequately closed wound. If possible, suture removal should be within the first week. Beyond this time suture marks are inevitable. Depending upon the region (*e.g.*, lower extremity incisions) and the dynamic forces involved, sutures may need to be left in for longer periods.

SKIN GRAFTS AND FLAPS

The simplest method to close an open wound is the skin graft. Bunger, Reverdin, Lawson, Wolfe, Ollier, Thiersch, and Krause each described successful grafting techniques of split- and full-thickness skin from 1823 through 1893. It was not until Blair and Brown in 1929 described an accurate method for cutting split-thickness skin at a consistent level of mid-dermis that large sheets of skin could be grafted. In 1939 Pagett introduced a mechanical dermatome to cut calibrated skin grafts. Since that time there have been new advances in instrumentation as well as meshing techniques—all of remarkable help in the treatment of skin wounds, particularly large, full-thickness burns.

Isologous skin grafts are free grafts that are transplanted from one part of the body to another. These free grafts can either be full-thickness or split-thickness depending on whether all of the dermis or portions of it are removed with the epidermis. The relative thickness of skin varies with location on the body. Postauricular and eyelid skin is the thinnest and the skin of the sole and palm the thickest. A child will reach adult thickness of skin at about age seven.

Fresh wounds or clean granulating wounds can be closed successfully with skin grafts. Grafts will not take on bare cortical bone but will take on cortical bone covered with periosteum. Similarly, grafts will take on paratenon but not on bare tendon; on perichondrium, but not on bare cartilage. The amount of subsequent contraction must be anticipated if function is to be restored or preserved. Once the decision to use a skin graft is made, then thickness of the graft is determined. This is dependent on the amount of anticipated contraction and the nature of the recipient bed. Little or no contraction occurs with full-thickness or thick split-thickness grafts. If, however, the recipient bed is less than optimal, then a thin split-thickness graft will be more likely to "take."

A skin graft adheres to the wound surface initially because of fibrin deposition. Serum penetrates the graft and the latter becomes edematous—the "phase of serum inhibition." Within 3 to 4 days the graft becomes vascularized by a process of capillary budding and the establishment of anastomotic connections to vascular channels within the graft, a process called *inosculation*. At approximately 24 hr to 36 hr early circulation occurs invariably within preexisting graft vessels. Initially it is a to-and-fro sluggish movement, but a steady undirected flow occurs within 6 hr to 24 hr. Once this circulation is established, neovascularity ensues followed by an alteration of the vascular architecture. Vascular proliferation reaches a peak about 10 days after grafting. If there is a limited avascular area in the recipient site, a graft may still succeed by the "bridging" phenomenon.

Nutriments may be supplied by collateral vessels of the graft to supply the avascular area. Up to 3 mm to 5 mm can be so bridged.

Skin grafts fail for the following reasons: (*1*) hematoma beneath the graft, (*2*) mobility of graft over the recipient site, and (*3*) infection as defined by bacterial counts greater than 1×10^5 per gram tissue in the host site and relative recipient site avascularity (*i.e.*, bare cortical bone, diabetic leg ulcer, irradiated chest wall). Hemostasis is essential. If small-vessel bleeding is a problem, as in tangential excision of burns, then grafting should be delayed 24 hr to 48 hr. During this time the skin may be stored on the donor site itself or wrapped in moist sterile gauze in a sterile container placed in the operating room refrigerator at 4°C. The movement of a skin graft should not be a problem if proper fixation technique and dressing and splinting procedures are carried out. If the recipient site has a bacterial count greater than 10^5, then additional débridement, continued wet-to-dry dressing changes, and appropriate topical antibiotics are indicated.

A stent dressing should be used in areas in which it is difficult to maintain a graft, for example, on the face or the axilla. In this technique, sterile petrolatum gauze is placed over the wound. A bolus of sterile resilient material such as Dacron fiber is then placed on the gauze, and sutures previously placed at the perimeter of the graft are tied over the bolus. On an extremity, an occlusive dressing appropriately splinted is most satisfactory. Skin grafts can also be left open with minimal dressing in areas too difficult to dress. Care of these grafts requires periodic inspection to roll out the accumulated serum beneath the graft. The Tanner mesher has greatly assisted the easy egress of serum through the interstices while increasing the usable width of the graft.

Pigmentation of skin grafts (especially thin grafts) is a curious and obdurate biologic problem. Grafts in patients with pigmented skin will darken while those in the fair-skinned will become yellow. Skin grafts in general will pigment in response to ultraviolet radiation and in the first year or two will hold that pigment. Thus sun screen cremes are advised for at least a year. Skin from a like donor site will match best in texture and color (*i.e.*, for the face, preauricular or postauricular full-thickness skin grafts; for the fingertip, skin harvested from the hypothenar eminence).

Skin grafts are either full-thickness or split-thickness. The full-thickness skin graft includes the entire thickness of the skin. The underlying subcutaneous fat must be trimmed for vascularization to succeed. Such a graft, because it is thick, requires an optimum bed, preferably a freshly excised wound, and effective immobilization if it is to survive transplantation. The advantages of full-thickness graft include

1. A texture more akin to normal skin
2. Normal growth of the graft in a child
3. Less tendency to pigment
4. Limited contraction.

The disadvantages include

1. Limited donor area
2. Limited size
3. Ideal recipient site and size requirements.

Full-thickness grafts are ideal to reconstruct the eyelids and face.

The split-thickness graft is harvested either by a modified razor or a mechanical dermatome at variable levels within the dermis. In so doing the donor site managed properly will reepithelialize. Thus, large sheets can be taken to close large full-thickness losses of skin. The survival of burned patients depends on the surgeon's ability to close the burn wound with sheets of split-thickness skin. The advantages of split-thickness skin grafts include

1. Any skin site is a potential donor site, including scalp, palms, soles
2. Large sheets of skin can be harvested
3. Repeated cropping is possible
4. Optimum recipient site is not required
5. Irregular contours can be closed successfully.

The disadvantages include

1. The wound so closed may continue to contract up to 60% of surface area
2. Growth potential is less than normal
3. Pigmentation is a problem
4. The graft has a glabrous surface unlike normal skin.

A composite graft refers to a graft of full-thickness skin and some other tissue. The first composite graft consisted of full-thickness skin of the ear and a portion of cartilaginous skeleton. Such a graft, limited in size, is used to reconstruct defects of the ala of the nose. It is revascularized by host vessels at the periphery of the graft.

Flaps by definition have a vascular pedicle and are composite tissues. A flap may consist of skin and subcutaneous fat, of muscle, or of muscle and overlying subcutaneous fat and skin. Omentum has served as a transposition flap to cover chest wall defects. Complex flaps may include bone, muscle, and skin and can be innervated. Survival of such flaps is provided by the vascular pedicle. The latter may remain attached, and the flap may be transposed to an adjacent wound or transferred to a heterotopic distant site. Nowadays such a transfer is best carried out by a microsurgical anastomosis of the flap vessels to vessels in the recipient site. Reconstruction of the cervical esophagus by a free flap of jejunum is a good example of such a heterotopic flap.

The blood supply to a flap is critical for its survival. Because most flaps have to do with skin and skin losses this discussion will focus on the blood supply to skin. The vascular supply to skin fundamentally is provided by (*1*) direct cutaneous vessels, (*2*) perforating branches from vessels to muscle, and (*3*) segmental vessels arising from the aorta. The forehead is supplied by the superficial temporal artery; the dorsum of the foot by the dorsalis pedis; the groin by the superficial circumflex iliac artery. These are examples of skin supplied directly by named relatively large vessels. Most of the skin is supplied by perforating branches of arteries to muscle. In general each muscle has a dominant vascular pedicle, usually proximal and usually accompanied by a motor nerve. That vessel supplies not only the muscle but also the overlying subcutaneous fat and skin. The vascular territory generally is close to twice the width of the muscle but does vary. An island of skin with the underlying muscle providing its vascular supply is called a musculocutaneous (myocutaneous) flap and can be transposed directly to adjacent wounds with great confidence. For example, the latissimus dorsi musculocutaneous flap serves admirably to supply the missing skin and muscle attendant upon a radical mastectomy and thus serves a key part in breast reconstruction. Finally, flaps supplied by segmental vessels coming directly off the aorta include intercostal flaps as well as transverse back flaps based on the direct precostal or lumbar vessels.

SKIN PREPARATION FOR OPERATION

Two discoveries made within two decades of one another irrevocably changed the scope and practice of surgery. Nitrous oxide rendered human beings insensible to their environment and to the pain of an operation (1841, Horace Wells and William Morton) and dilute phenol sprayed in operating rooms in the Glasgow Infirmary decreased the incidence of surgical wound sepsis to a remarkable degree (1865, Joseph Lister). General anesthesia and surgical antisepsis permitted the remarkable flowering of surgery as a separate discipline.

Thorough cleansing of the skin of the patient at the operative site, the hands of the surgeon, and of the operating team is requisite as the initial step of an operation. Agents currently in use include hexachlorophene, povidone-iodine, chlorhexidine, benzalkonium chloride, and pluronic F-68.

Hexachlorophene (pHisoHex) is effective against gram-positive bacteria but much less so against gram-negative bacteria and spores. While immediate reduction in bacterial count is less than with other agents it has a longer effective period. Toxic effects appear to be related to the concentration, length of exposure, and age of patient. It is not advisable to use hexachlorophene to cleanse open wounds. Encephalopathy can result from prolonged use in burned patients; similar toxic effects have been reported in premature infants. Povidone-iodine (Betadine), an iodophor, has a broad spectrum of antibacterial activity. It is active against both gram-positive and gram-negative bacteria. The immediate effect in reducing bacterial numbers is quite good but the effect is rapidly lost after 2 hr. Toxicity of povidone-iodine is dependent on the amount of iodine absorbed. For example, severe metabolic acidosis has been reported in burn patients. Despite an expected increased protein-bound iodine there are no consistent changes in thyroid function attendant upon its use. Surprisingly free from overt toxic effects to the cellular constituents of repair are wounds irrigated vigorously with dilute povidone-iodine solution.

Chlorhexidine gluconate (Hibiclens) is an excellent antiseptic against gram-positive and gram-negative bacteria and fungi. When compared to povidone-iodine and hexachlorophene its immediate effect is greater while its duration of effect is comparable to hexachlorophene. Reported toxic effects are minimal if confined to dermal use. Oral ingestion of high doses can cause liver damage. It may be ototoxic if instilled in the middle ear. Contamination of chlorhexidine solutions by pseudomonas species has been reported, but not in the usual 4% solution routinely used for antisepsis.

No antiseptic agent is ideal. Most studies disclose that by 2 to 3 hr, bacterial counts on gloved hands have increased significantly no matter what agent is used. Surgeons would do well to continue to follow the example of Mikulicz and change gloves every 2 hr in the course of a long operation.

While the method of scrubbing basically is unchanged (starting at the fingertips and going to the elbows) the duration of scrubbing has changed. Dineen evaluated the necessary time to scrub and found that 5 min was as good as 10 min regardless of the agent used. Bacterial counts obtained from individual fingertips did not disclose any significant differences up to 2 hr after scrubbing.

CARE OF TRAUMATIC WOUNDS

The nature of the injury, the degree of contamination, the amount of necrotic material and foreign body present, injury to vital structures, concomitant metabolic abnormalities, and the interval of time between wounding and treatment are factors to be taken into account in the formulation of a treatment plan for an injured patient.

Fundamental to wound care is the adequate debridement of necrotic tissues and the removal of all foreign material. A contaminated wound so treated can be converted into a relatively clean wound that can be closed either primarily or secondarily. Mechanical debridement involves the manual removal of debris imbedded in a wound, such as dirt, road debris, paint, glass, clothing, and so forth. In addition, all devitalized tissue, particularly muscle, must be removed.

Hydrodynamic debridement can complement mechanical measures in cleansing a wound. Bulb irrigations with sterile normal saline will wash away most superficial debris but will not suffice to remove fragments of devitalized tissue or deeply imbedded debris or bacteria. A forceful hydraulic lavage using a pressure of 8 to 10 pounds per square inch has been demonstrated to be much more effective in removing wound contaminants. This can easily be accomplished by using a large syringe with a 21-gauge needle. Hydraulic jet lavage systems involve a very high pressure system that can remove small particulate matter but at the expense of injury to local tissues. Wound healing can be affected adversely if sustained high pressures are used.

Use of antiseptic solutions to assist in irrigation can decrease the overall bacterial counts in contaminated wounds. Surgical scrub solutions (hexachlorophene, povidone-iodine) have deleterious effects on wounds because of the detergent. The antiseptic agent povidone-iodine is not harmful in usual concentrations in a wound and does definitely reduce bacterial numbers. A recent cleansing agent, pluronic F-68, shows promise. This surfactant agent has a very favorable reported therapeutic index.

As a rule of thumb the time period between wounding and treatment has been said to be 6 hr or less if a wound is to be closed primarily. Obviously adherence to a strict time period is totally empiric and cannot be relied upon. Certain other factors must be taken into account—the wounding agent, the energy adsorbed by the wound, the degree of tissue injury, the type and estimated size of the bacterial inoculum, injury and replacement of major vessels by alloplastic graft, age of the patient, vascularity of the part. For example, a wound with extensive tissue loss that is heavily contaminated is best treated by adequate intravascular and extravascular volume replacement, systemic antibiotics, and sterile dressings. Such a patient should be returned to the operating room within 12 hr to 24 hr for further debridement, or sooner if gas-forming infection becomes evident. Decisions of this type require a basic understanding of wound healing and surgical sepsis, and experience.

A wound inoculated by human mouth organisms should not be closed primarily. On the other hand wounds infected by dog bite can be closed if properly cleansed. Wounds in general may be closed if quantitative culture discloses less than 1×10^5 organisms per gram of tissue. In acute wounds a rapid slide technique for estimating bacterial numbers has been reported by Robson, Krizek, and others. A 500 mg sample is excised from the wound, homogenized, and suspended in 1 ml of saline. A 0.01 ml aliquot is placed on a glass slide, gram-stained, and a bacterial count is made over 10 fields under oil immersion. The following is the mathematical computation:

$$\frac{\text{No. bacteria}}{1 \text{ cm}^2} \times \frac{\text{homogenate vol (ml)}}{0.01 \text{ ml}}$$
$$\times \frac{1}{\text{sample wt (g)}} = \frac{\text{bacteria}}{\text{g tissue}}$$

This technique can rapidly (within 30 min) provide the surgeon with important data, whereas routine cultures might not be available until 24 hr to 36 hr later.

Useful in the operative assessment of blood flow to tissue are appearance, color, capillary return, bleeding, and contractility of muscle. Perfusion of tissue can be estimated by administration of fluorescein systemically. Ten minutes after administration perfusion of the part is assessed by ultraviolet light—an ordinary Woods lamp usually found in every department of dermatology is quite adequate. Highly fluorescent tissue is very well perfused and will survive; spotty fluorescence means marginal perfusion but probable survival; no fluorescence means no perfusion and thus inevitable death of the tissue.

Simple lacerations may be closed directly by appropriate suture techniques. All infected wounds must be packed open and closed secondarily. Noninfected, large exposed wounds adequately debrided should be closed by the simplest method consistent with the best functional and aesthetic result attainable. If a skin graft can be used to achieve this goal, then this is the method of choice. Rotation of local flaps, muscle flaps, and free flaps should be reserved for situations that require soft-tissue coverage overlying important structures such as tendon, nerve, bone, or major blood vessels. Indications for grafts and flaps will be covered in the section on plastic surgery.

WOUND CLOSURE

Skin edges of an open wound may be coapted by a variety of materials and techniques. Some understanding of suture material is useful to the student of surgery. Sutures are of two types, (*1*) absorbable and (*2*) nonabsorbable. Further characteristics such as breaking strength of the suture, whether it is monofilament or braided, the facility of knot-tying, and tissue reaction all enter in the choice. Nowadays most sutures are provided with a needle swaged on the suture. These needles may be cutting, tapered, easy "pop-offs," curved, or straight and of various sizes.

ABSORBABLE SUTURES

Absorbable sutures include plain or chromatized catgut, collagen, and polyglycolic acid. Catgut is obtained from the collagen of the submucosal layer of the small intestine of sheep or from the serosal layer of cattle intestine. These strips are chemically treated with dilute formaldehyde to provide resistance to enzymatic breakdown. Further resistance to dissolution is provided by chromatization. The material is sterilized by irradiation. Proteolytic enzymes in the body will digest catgut sutures, but the length of time for complete digestion is highly variable. One to two weeks is average for plain catgut. Chromatized gut will be lysed in approximately 4 wk. Sutures placed within the oral cavity or intestine will be lysed faster in comparison to those placed in subcutaneous tissues. Plain catgut provokes the most inflammatory reaction of all suture material, but less so with chromic catgut.

Collagen sutures are extruded from the tendons of cattle and chemically treated with formaldehyde and chromic salts. Collagen is used for the most part as a fine (6-0 and 7-0) suture material for the eye.

Polyglycolic acid (Dexon) and polyglactin-910 (Vicryl) are produced by polymerization of glycolic acid, extruded, stretched, and braided into various sizes. Less reaction is associated with this suture than with catgut. It is absorbed by hydrolysis over a period of 2 mo to 6 mo. It provides more strength than a comparable catgut suture. Disadvantages include a high friction coefficient, handling difficulty, and the persistence of the suture for long periods. The handling characteristics have been improved by silicone coating.

NONABSORBABLE SUTURES

The nonabsorbable sutures include silk, cotton, nylon, Prolene, Dacron, and stainless steel—either monofilament or braided. Termed *permanent,* these sutures evoke less tissue reaction and provide more tensile strength than absorbable sutures. Prolene, stainless steel, and nylon are the least reactive of the sutures. Silk and cotton provoke a greater inflammatory reaction. Postlethwait in 1969 examined the long-term characteristics of nonabsorbable sutures. Silk is slowly absorbed over years with a decrease in tensile strength after 4 wk to 60%, and after 3 mo to 20%. Cotton is truly permanent and evokes a slightly greater tissue reaction. Dacron sutures (Tevdek and Polydek) cause little reaction unless the Teflon coating is dislodged from the suture. Dacron also maintains significant tensile strength for at least 2 years. Nylon and Prolene cause the least inflammatory reaction and have excellent tensile strength. Silk and cotton have the best handling characteristics. Nylon and Prolene tend to be slippery and many knots are required to maintain a secure suture.

Although gain in tensile strength from tissue to tissue varies, as a general rule the tensile strength at 20 days is 20% of normal; at 40 days, 40%; at 90 days, 60%; and at 1 year, 70%. A wound rarely if ever attains the same tensile strength of noninjured tissue. Sutures therefore have to provide tensile strength appropriate for the part until healing has occurred and dehiscence is no longer a problem. Ideally it should then disappear quickly. Because gain in tensile strength is relatively slow in tendon, fascia, or aponeuroses, a permanent nonabsorbable suture is necessary. Polypropylene, Dacron, Tevdek, and stainless steel will maintain their tensile strength for over 2 years. Absorbable sutures lose strength rapidly and provide little support after 1 mo, although the suture material may persist within the wound long after losing its supporting strength.

In general, nonabsorbable suture is used for the reapproximation of fascia of abdominal wounds. Because there can be substantial increase in intra-abdominal pressure during the postoperative period due to ileus, coughing, and ambulation, the use of permanent sutures with high-quality tensile strength would seem obvious. Polypropylene, nylon, Tevdek, stainless steel wire, silk, and cotton are the choices. Silk and cotton have given way to synthetic monofilament suture as the material of choice.

To secure prosthetic material within the body (*e.g.,* mitral and aortic valves, aortofemoral Dacron grafts, polypropylene mesh, etc.) the surgeon must use nonabsorbable suture that can maintain its tensile strength for the duration of the patient's life. Any loss of strength or absorption could be catastrophic for the patient. Polypropylene and Teflon-coated polyester are most frequently used. One should bear in mind that the polyester suture is multifilament and the risk of infection is higher.

Repair of uterus, fallopian tubes, bladder, and bile ducts is best achieved with absorbable sutures for the mucosal layer. The knot should be tied outside the lumen to obviate the suture acting as a nidus for bacteria or for calcareous stone formation. Studies comparing various sutures in the urinary tract suggest that stone formation may be more dependent on the multifilament character of the suture than on the type of suture. Polypropylene can probably be used without adverse effects in the urinary or biliary tract.

Classically a gastrointestinal anastomosis is carried out with a running everting suture of chromic catgut for the mucosa and submucosa. The suture is locked or another started at the halfway point. The anastomosis is then completed by interrupted silk in the serosa placed so as to invert. Monofilament nylon can be substituted for silk. Many anastomoses are now being performed by stainless steel staples. These techniques have the advantage of speed and ease.

The bronchus should be closed with a permanent suture with high tensile strength. Polypropylene and stainless steel are probably the best choices. As in abdominal surgery, the stapler plays a major role, and most bronchial stumps are closed in this manner.

Peripheral nerve repair requires little strength. Critical is an accurate approximation of the epineurium or the perineurium without inciting inflammation and hence dense scar. Polypropylene and nylon again are the choices as they are the least reactive of the suture materials. Polypropylene and nylon are the suture materials of choice in peripheral vascular repairs.

ABDOMINAL DEHISCENCE AND EVISCERATION

Wound disruption is a major complication following operations on the abdomen and chest. The incidence of burst abdomen ranges from 0.3% to 5.8% and has not improved since the turn of the century. The incidence at Johns Hopkins Hospital from 1889 to 1923 was 0.18%, from 1923 to 1936, 0.86%, and in 1954, as high as 5.8%. Reports in the surgical literature give varying rates; examples include 1.1% at the University of Missouri, 1.5% at Middlesex Hospital, London, 2.5% at St. Luke's Hospital, Cleveland, and 9.36% at the University of Tennessee. Mortality rates range from 6% to 38%.

No one factor causes "burst" abdomen. The following appear to be risk factors. Mean age is usually greater than 50 years. Regardless of age, the incidence is significantly higher in midline vertical incisions (nonanatomical) than in transverse incisions (ratio of 7:1). Wound infection increases the rate two-fold. Patients with malnutrition or hypoproteinemia appear to be at higher risk. Exteriorization

---

SOME CAUSES OF ABDOMINAL WOUND SEPARATION

1. Increased intra-abdominal pressure (distention, ascites, coughing, straining)
2. Hematoma or infection
3. Imperfect operative technique
4. Metabolic causes (steroids, diabetes, uremia, cancer chemotherapy, etc.)

of a viscus through the incision increases the occurrence. Wolff reported a 5.8% incidence of disruption in such a group of patients. The triad of distension, vomiting, and coughing significantly increases the intra-abdominal pressure, which in turn will increase tension on the closure. The presence of a tracheostomy is clearly a risk factor. Other factors cited include obesity, diabetes, anemia, uremia, jaundice, malignancy, steroid therapy, reoperation through the same incision, type of closure (running versus interrupted), and type of suture. Clearly burst abdomen is higher in patients whose abdominal wounds are closed with running catgut. Technical factors also play a role. Sutures placed too close to the wound edge or at precisely the same interval in the fascia or tied too tightly predispose to wound disruption. A combination of wound ischemia or actual strangulation with acute, repeated increases in intra-abdominal pressure due either to vomiting or to coughing will lead to burst abdomen or a disrupted chest wound.

Wound dehiscence occurs within the first 2 wk with the mean being 8 days. It has been borne out over and over again that the transverse or oblique incision is more anatomic and better preserves the integrity of the fascial fibers of the abdominal wall. Singleton and Blocker reported only one dehiscence in 3,147 anatomic incisions. Sloan has demonstrated that the force (tension) produced by the abdominal musculature is 30 times greater in a vertical incision than in a transverse one. A midline incision is preferred by most surgeons when exposure is paramount and speed critical to success; for example, a ruptured abdominal aneurysm. In such patients, attention to details in wound closure, nutritional support, and postoperative care is absolutely essential for a successful outcome. In such patients, or in those for whom a colostomy is necessary, retention sutures are of help.

Retention sutures of stainless steel or heavy monofilament nylon should be placed 3 cm to 4 cm from the wound edge encompassing all layers. The wound should then be closed in the usual fashion for 10 cm to 12 cm followed by tightening of the retention suture. If the retention suture goes through the peritoneum, then care must be exercised to prevent inclusion of viscera. Rubber guards or buttons may be used for skin support. The sutures should be tied with enough tension to remove the total burden of support from the fascial stitches. An excellent method is to place retention sutures just above the level of the peritoneum. This permits good support and at the same time places a barrier between the viscera and sutures. This prevents the occasional complication of small intestine being eroded or actually caught up by a retention suture.

ABDOMINAL WALL DEHISCENCE

The cardinal sign of abdominal wall dehiscence is the issue of a large amount of serosanguineous fluid from the incision at or about 8 days after operation. Although such a wound may appear to be intact, careful inspection and gentle palpation will disclose a fascial defect. In such a situation, or if frank evisceration has occurred, the wound should be covered with a sterile towel and the patient supported by an abdominal binder. If the skin is intact, such a wound should never be explored with a hemostat on the ward. The patient should be taken directly to the operating room for inspection, irrigation, and reclosure.

ABDOMINAL HERNIA

Partial abdominal wound dehiscence or fascial weakness will result in an abdominal hernia. The incidence of abdominal hernias postoperatively ranges from 2% to 12%. At the Mayo Clinic 10.8% of all herniorrhaphies are performed to repair abdominal incisional hernias.

Most incisional hernias occur in midline incisions. Attenuation of fibers from the constant increased intra-abdominal pressure (*e.g.*, chronic obstructive pulmonary disease or benign prostatic hypertrophy) may allow protrusion of intra-abdominal content. Poor placement of sutures, poor choice of suture material with inappropriate tensile strength, infection, hematoma, and closure under tension can all contribute directly or indirectly to an abdominal hernia. Obesity clearly is a risk factor.

The actual defect of an abdominal wall hernia is usually greater than the palpable defect. In repairing such a defect the scar tissue present may be confused with the fascia. It is useful to open the hernia sac completely to adequately palpate and visualize the defect. Principles of repair are two—excision of the sac and layer closure. At times imbrication of the sac may suffice.

Suture materials and techniques for hernia repair are no different than those for closing a primary abdominal incision. If sutures tend to tear through the fascia because of undue tension, then another method of reconstruction must be resorted to lest one be confronted with a postoperative dehiscence or evisceration. Use of Prolene or Marlex mesh has contributed greatly to abdominal wall reconstruction. This synthetic mesh graft can be sutured to the fascia present and is strong enough to maintain abdominal wall integrity. Sheets large enough to cover the entire abdominal wall have been used in gastroschisis of the newborn, gunshot wound, and necrotizing fasciitis. Once the mesh has been sutured into place, the overlying skin and subcutaneous tissue can be approximated above this. If omentum is available, it should be placed between mesh and viscera.

When both fascia and skin are necessary for abdominal wall reconstruction, transposition of a musculocutaneous flap has provided excellent wound closure, stability, and contour. Such flaps are particularly applicable to repair of the abdominal wall following excision of tumors (*e.g.*, fibromas and desmoid tumors) or after stabilization of a large defect with mesh and skin graft (*e.g.*, post-gunshot wound, or post-necrotizing fasciitis). The tensor fascia lata and its iliotibial tract fit the requirements precisely. First described by Wangensteen in 1936 for repair of recurrent groin hernias, it can be rotated with its overlying skin to close defects of the lower abdomen from the umbilicus to pubis with extension across the midline. Its strong fascia can be sutured to the existent fascia of the abdominal wall. Prolene mesh may or may not be used depending upon whether further reinforcement is necessary.

The rectus abdominis muscle based superiorly or inferiorly on the epigastric arterial system can be rotated with its overlying skin to smaller defects of the abdominal wall. The external oblique muscle can also be used for small defects. Details of muscle flaps are provided in Chapter 43.

BIBLIOGRAPHY

ADAMSON RJ, ENQUIST IF: The relative importance of sutures to the strength of healing wounds under normal and abnormal conditions. Surg Gynecol Obstet, 117:396, 1963

ALLEN HE, EDGERTON MT, RODEHEAVER GT et al: Skin dressings in the treatment of contaminated wounds. Am J Surg, 126::45, 1973

BORGES AF: Elective Incisions and Scar Revision. Boston, Little, Brown & Co, 1973

BROWN RG, JURKIEWICZ MJ: Reconstructive surgery in the cancer patients. Curr Probl Cancer 2:7, 1977

BRYANT WM: Wound Healing. CIBA Found Symp 29(3):1977

DOBSON T, SHULLS WA: A study of various surgical scrubs by glove counts. Surg Gynecol Obstet 124:57, 1967

EDLICH RF, CUSTER J, MADDEN J et al: Studies in management of the contaminated wound. III. Assessment of the effectiveness of irrigation with antiseptic agents. Am J Surg 118:21, 1969

ELIAS EG: Chemotherapy and wound healing. Clin Plast Surg 6:27, 1979

GABBIANI G, RYAN GB, MAJWO G: Presence of modified fibroblasts in granulation tissue and their possible role in wound contraction. Experientia, 27:549, 1971

GOODSON WH, HUNT TK: Wound healing and the diabetic patient. Surg Gynecol Obstet 149:600, 1979

GREANEY MG, NOORT RV, SMYTHE A et al: Does obstructive jaundice adversely affect wound healing? Br J Surg 66:478, 1979

HAURY B, RODEHEAVER G, VENSKO J et al: Debridement: An essential component of traumatic wound care. Am J Surg 135:238, 1978

HUNT TK: Disorders of wound healing. World J Surg 4:271, 1980

HUNT TK: Wound Healing and Wound Infection: Theory and Surgical Practice. New York, Appleton-Century-Crofts, 1980

IRVIN TT: Effects of malnutrition and hyperalimentation on wound healing. Surg Gynecol Obstet 146:33, 1978

JOERGENSON EJ, SMITH ET: Postoperative abdominal wound separation and evisceration. Am J Surg 79:282, 1950

KAUL AF, JEWETT JF: Agents and techniques for disinfection of the skin. Surg Gynecol Obstet 152:677, 1981

KRAISSL CJ: The selection of appropriate lines for elective surgical incisions. Plast Reconstr Surg 8:1, 1951

LEE PW, GREEN MA, LONG WB III et al: Zinc and wound healing. Surg Gynecol Obstet 143:549, 1976

LEHMAN JA, GROSS FS, PARTINGTON PF: Prevention of abdominal wound disruption. Surg Gynecol Obstet 126:1235, 1968

MAGEE C, HAURY B, RODEHEAVER G et al: A rapid technic for quantitating wound bacterial count. Am J Surg 133:760, 1977

NAHAI F, BROWN RG, VASCONEZ LO: Blood supply to the abdominal wall as related to planning abdominal incisions. Am Surg 42:691, 1976

NIINIKOSKI J: Oxygen and wound healing. Clin Plast Surg 4:361, 1977

OXLUND H, FOGDESTAM I, VIIDIK A: The influence of cortisol on wound healing of the skin and distant connective tissue response. Surg Gynecol Obstet 148:876, 1979

PEACOCK EE JR, VANWINKLE W JR: Wound Repair, 2nd ed. Philadelphia, W B Saunders, 1976

REES VL, COLLER FA: Anatomic and clinical study of the transverse abdominal incision. Arch Surg 47:136, 1943

RUDOLPH R, KLEIN L: Healing processes in skin grafts. Surg Gynecol Obstet 136:641, 1973

VARMA S, FERGUSON HL, BREEN HJ et al: Comparison of seven suture materials in infected wounds—An experimental study. J Surg Res 17:165, 1974

Richard D. Goodenough/Joseph A. Molnar/John F. Burke

Surgical Infections

9

Surgical infection has been defined as an infection most effectively treated by surgery or an infection in the surgical wound or operative site. This rather restricted definition is no longer useful, for the infections now pertinent to surgical practice are not only those related directly to surgery but also those related to the surgical patient's overall state of health and ability to resist bacterial invasion (Table 9-1). Pulmonary, urinary tract, and bloodstream infections are now as important to surgical practice as are drainage of abscesses and postoperative wound infections. Extensive improvements in surgical and anesthetic management of patients during the operative period now permit the safe performance of urgent operation in patients with complicating systemic disease, including infection, but these complicating infections must be managed effectively through the operative and postoperative periods.

It should be noted that the other infectious agents, namely the viruses and fungi, continue to increase in importance in medical practice. This is occurring due to the recognition of new disease entities (*e.g.,* cytomegalovirus infections in renal transplant patients) and the increasing operative management of patients whose host resistance is compromised and who have a high susceptibility to infection by what were previously considered to be nonpathogenic microbes.

Surgical infection may therefore be broadly defined as an infection related to or complicating surgical therapy, and surgical management must take into account and deal with infectious processes that in the past would have caused patients to be considered unsuitable candidates for surgical therapy. In the context of this widened definition, surgical infections can be categorized as follows: (*1*) infections that cause disease and are effectively treated by operation (*e.g.,* abscess, trauma, cholecystitis); (*2*) infections complicating surgical treatment in the preoperative period (*e.g.,* septicemia 2° to gangrenous cholecystitis); and (*3*) infections complicating the postoperative period (*e.g.,* wound infection, subphrenic abscess).

TABLE 9-1 MEDICAL CONDITIONS THAT IMPAIR HOST RESISTANCE

ACQUIRED DEFECTS

Age extremes
Diabetes mellitus
Malignancy (especially leukemias)
Obesity
Severe trauma
Sepsis
Malnutrition of any cause
Cardiac failure
Hepatic failure
Renal failure
Active tuberculosis
Radiation sickness
Coagulopathies
Cushing's syndrome (endogenous or exogenous)
Addison's disease
Aplastic anemia
Pharmacologic immunosuppression
Hyposplenism and hypersplenism

CONGENITAL DEFECTS

White cell disorders
Agammaglobulinemia
Chronic granulomatous diseases

LOCAL DEFECTS

Regional ischemia
Rheumatic heart disease
Congenital heart and great-vessel disease
Chronic pulmonary diseases
Radiation tissue damage
Neuropathies

The clinical manifestations of bacterial infection may fundamentally be divided into *cellulitis* and *abscess formation*. *Cellulitis* represents an active spread of bacteria through the tissue spaces themselves, with a resultant intense inflammatory reaction, but without extensive tissue necrosis or suppuration. Cellulitis presents as pain, local tenderness, swelling, redness, and local heat. The basic treatment of cellulitis is limited to rest, heat, elevation, and the judicious use of antibiotics. Surgical drainage is not indicated.

Abscess formation is the local collection of necrotic tissue, bacteria, and white cells, commonly denoted as pus. Superficial abscesses may be detected by their localized erythema, their tendency to develop point tenderness, and fluctuation on palpation. However, abscesses may occur deeper within the body and can be more difficult to diagnose. For practical purposes, all abscesses should be drained or excised, for they present a considerable hazard of further bacterial spread to the patient. Therapeutic antibiotics are indicated only when systemic signs of infection are present.

Blood-borne bacterial spread is called *bacteremia* and lymphangitic spread is called *lymphangitis*. These represent specialized methods of bacterial spread that are life-threatening because of wide and rapid dissemination of bacteria to all parts of the body by way of these routes. *Bacteremia* presents as the systemic signs of infection, whereas *lymphangitis* may present as erythematous streaking of the skin with or without systemic signs. Because of the dangers of metastatic bacterial spread inherent in bacteremia or lymphangitis, vigorous treatment is always indicated, including appropriate antibiotic therapy, as well as local treatment directed at the initial lesion, and surgical drainage if abscess formation is present. *Septicemia* denotes the continuous growth of bacteria in the bloodstream and is a further progression of bacteremia. *Sepsis* is used to denote the clinical manifestation of an infectious process.

Host defense defines those factors the host organism possesses that attempt to limit microbial entry and that limit microbial growth if entry has occurred. Microbial *virulence* describes the invasiveness and toxicity of a given agent. Host defense may be divided into *specific* and *nonspecific factors*. Specific factors refer to those facets of host resistance aimed at one specific microbe and that require previous exposure to that microbe; specific immunoglobulins are examples. Nonspecific factors are those that attempt to eliminate all organisms, regardless of type. An example of a nonspecific factor is phagocytosis by macrophages.

ETIOLOGY OF BACTERIAL INFECTIONS

The opposing factors that affect the development of any infection are the number and virulence of bacteria gaining access to the host's tissues and the ability of the host to prevent their growth and eliminate them. The balance between these two sets of opposing forces leads to maintenance of normal health or to the development of an infectious disease. This host–pathogen interaction constantly occurs in normal humans as some bacteria continually gain entrance to the host from the outside environment. However, the normal and effective function of host defense can be influenced to a major extent by alterations of the normal physiologic state of the host or by the circumvention of normal defense mechanisms such as occurs during anesthesia and surgery. Care of the surgical patient, then, requires special attention to those factors that will maintain or supplement host defense because the balance of these opposing factors may frequently be tipped in favor of the development of infection by the patient's disease, the introduction of massive bacterial contamination (as in trauma), or the introduction of highly virulent and antibiotic resistant bacteria (as may occur in the hospital).

MECHANISMS OF BACTERIAL INJURY

Bacteria produce damage by elaborating toxins that act both locally and systemically. Examples include substances that impair local defenses, such as streptococcal M protein, exotoxins such as streptokinase, and the systemically active lipopolysaccharide endotoxins from the gram-negative rods. In addition, bacteria produce substances such as hyaluronidase that enhance their ability to spread through tissue. We should also note that bacteria may share adaptive properties in mixed infections, which may be synergistic in overcoming host defense. Bacteria may also adapt to environmental pressures through the development of antibiotic resistance by biochemical means and the development of L forms. Bacterial virulence, then, is a combination of a bacterium's ability to produce tissue damage from toxins, to propagate, and to spread through tissue. Bacterial virulence, therefore, presents a multifaceted threat to the surgical patient. In brief, the ability of a bacterial strain to survive in tissue may be thought of as a combination of numbers of organisms present and their virulence.

HOST DEFENSE MECHANISMS

Host defenses have evolved on two levels, those aimed at excluding microbial entry and those that attempt to control and eliminate microbes once entry is gained. The barriers to microorganism access consist of the skin and mucous membranes. When they are breached, as they are with a surgical incision, for example, the host normally responds with specific and nonspecific immune mechanisms. Specific mechanisms are learned and stored in "memory" lymphocytes. When a microorganism appears that has been previously encountered, a specific response is evoked through humoral antibodies or cell-mediated immunity. Specific immunity, however, occurs in the context of the acute inflammatory reaction, which is mostly constructed of those factors that are nonspecific.

Nonspecific factors are those that are activated in the presence of any invading microorganism without previous exposure to that organism. They are of extreme importance in the prevention of postoperative infection. Examples of these innate antimicrobial factors are phagocytosis and the complement system. It should be clear, though, that specific and nonspecific factors are absolutely intertwined. For this reason, we will consider them as they occur together in the inflammatory response.

BARRIER MECHANISMS

Host resistance has evolved into a series of "back-up" systems. The first level of resistance consists of the chemical and mechanical barriers that prevent the nonsterile outside environment from contaminating the normally sterile internal one. Keratinized skin provides an impermeable barrier and also produces lipids with antimicrobial activity. In addition, sweat glands and hair follicles have bacterial flora of low virulence that compete with pathogenic bacteria for their ecological niche. Mucous membranes have also developed antimicrobial properties. Among these are gut production of IgA, pH changes in the stomach and vagina, and the "mucociliary elevator" of the respiratory tract. Despite these barrier mechanisms, bacterial penetration does occur, and a second line of defense must then respond.

HUMORAL FACTORS

When bacteria have gained an initial foothold, they trigger local defense mechanisms by damaging tissue. The kallikrein-kinin system of the injured host cells causes marked increases in local vascular permeability, attracting the inflow of plasma immunoglobulins, complement, and clotting factors. In addition, granulocytes undergo vascular margination and diapedesis and thus invade the damaged tissue (Fig. 9-1). Clotting mechanisms are activated in an effort to wall off the process by fibrin deposition and platelet aggregation.

Once in contact with the invading bacteria, the immunoglobulins, especially IgG and IgM, react to antigenic structures on the bacterial surface. This reaction activates the complement system, which leads to direct injury to the bacterium, neutrophil chemotaxis, opsonization of the bacterial surface, and further host response by positive feedback and the further release of vasoactive substances.

CELLULAR FACTORS

The above humoral reactants affect the behavior of the phagocytic cells. When induced, these cells exhibit meaningful patterns of movement, phagocytosis of the opsonized bacteria, and increased metabolic activity as they degranulate their bacterial enzymes into the phagosomes and go about the process of intracellular bacterial digestion. The predominant phagocytic cell of the acute inflammatory reaction is the polymorphonuclear leukocyte.

Another cellular defense mechanism is embodied in the reticuloendothelial system (RES). The RES may be divided into fixed and wandering components. The fixed component consists of phagocytic cells that remove foreign elements from the bloodstream. They are located especially in the hepatosplenic circulation and lymphatics, and are important in clearing the blood when bacteremia occurs. However, when the RES is impaired or outnumbered, bacteremic symptoms supervene.

The wandering elements of the RES are comprised of the T-lymphocytes and B-lymphocytes. The B-lymphocyte is the memory cell of the immunologic humoral system. B cells produce the immunoglobulins that are instrumental to

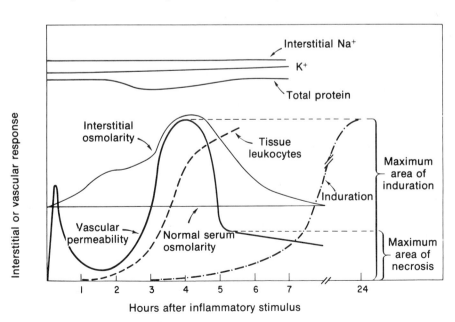

Fig. 9-1. A comparison of the time of occurrence of events of early inflammation. Changes in interstitial composition (osmolarity, electrolyte and protein concentration) are compared with changes in vascular permeability and development of induration and tissue leukocytosis. (Leak LV, Burke JF: Early events of tissue injury and the role of the lymphatic system in early inflammation. In Zweifach BW, Granl, McCluskey RT [eds]: The Inflammatory Process. New York, Academic Press, 1974)

GENESIS, PREVENTION, AND TREATMENT OF SURGICAL INFECTION

The origin of surgical infection is in the balance between host defense mechanisms and the number and virulence of the invading microbes. Host defenses have evolved as backup systems. These defenses consist of barrier, humoral, and cellular mechanisms. Compromised host resistance plays a major role in the genesis of clinical infection.

Infection is prevented by the maintenance of normal physiology, which sustains host resistance. Infection is also prevented by meticulous attention to sterile technique and by the augmentation of host resistance by the timely use of preventive antibiotics.

The clinical types of infection are cellulitis, abscess, and those that are either lymphatic or blood-borne. These frequently occur in combination. The systemic response to sepsis is most frequently manifested as fever, although cardiovascular, pulmonary, renal, and metabolic effects may become prominent as the severity of sepsis increases.

The most frequent postoperative infections are in the wound, abdomen, urinary tract, chest, and at catheter sites. Careful observation and clinical suspicion are imperative to make the correct diagnosis. Therapy for each differs, but common aspects are the selection of culture-dictated therapeutic antibiotics, restitution of normal host physiology (and defenses), the drainage of abscesses, the débridement of necrotic tissues, and the correction of the originating process.

killing bacteria and to the acute inflammatory reaction, as noted above. T cells are active in certain bacterial and viral infections, and their mechanism of immunity is cell mediated, rather than by way of humoral antibodies. They induce mononuclear macrophages to ingest and destroy those microbes to which they have been sensitized. It should be noted that in the majority of surgical infections, however, the major involvement is through the humoral immunity mechanisms.

COMPROMISED HOST RESISTANCE

Host defense mechanisms may be impaired by any of the conditions noted above (see Table 9-1). Identification of the patient at risk, due to the presence of one or more of these factors, allows clinical attention to be paid directly to those factors that are deficient. The three final common pathways of host resistance that are commonly impaired, through either congenital or acquired mechanisms, are the mediation of the acute inflammatory response, phagocytic mechanisms, and opsonization.

Common acquired conditions that impair host resistance are diabetes mellitus, atherosclerotic vascular disease, corticosteroid therapy, trauma (especially thermal trauma), alcohol abuse, protein–calorie malnutrition, uremia, radiation changes, cancer, and the use of immunosuppressive agents. In addition, patients with specific genetic defects that impair host resistance (*e.g.,* hypogammaglobulinemia) will occasionally be encountered.

PREVENTION OF POSTOPERATIVE INFECTION

Infection of any tissue can be prevented by limiting the number of bacteria to which it is exposed to a level below the number that the existing host defense mechanisms can eliminate and by increasing the host defense mechanisms. Either of these strategies will prevent infection when carried to their extremes. However, our inability to reasonably create these extreme conditions leads us to the optimization of both variables simultaneously. That is, reduction of the number of contaminating organisms by rigid aseptic technique and vigorous support of the patient's physiology, to provide as normal a state of host resistance as possible, are necessary. Furthermore, it has been clearly demonstrated that antibacterial activity, in addition to support of host defense, is effective in reducing the probability of infection. Therefore, the selective use of preventive antibiotics allows the augmentation of normal host defenses by supplementing the patient's antibacterial host defense mechanisms.

MAINTENANCE OF NORMAL PHYSIOLOGY AND HOST RESISTANCE

Normal resistance to infection is a function of normal host physiology. Significant physiological impairment, therefore, signifies a deficit in resistance. This is true on both local and whole-body levels.

While it is obvious that an adequate central blood pressure is required for normal renal, cardiac, and central nervous system function, it is not always remembered that local tissue defenses are dependent on local perfusion and that a normal central pressure does not assure a normal peripheral blood flow. The maintenance of normal local perfusion is necessary to prevent tissue hypoxia, acidosis, and electrolyte disturbances. Normal perfusion also assures a supply of the mediators of the inflammatory response. Adequate blood flow to the site of microbial inoculation is, therefore, necessary for normal host resistance at the local level.

We should also note that adequate ventilatory physiology and nutritional status are important, since decreases in oxygen delivery, acid-base disturbances, and chronic nutritional deficit impair host resistance. Nutrition and respiration, as well as cardiovascular function, must therefore be carefully monitored and corrected in order to maintain normal host resistance.

STERILIZATION AND ASEPTIC TECHNIQUES

Surgical aseptic practices, originated by Semmelweis and Lister, have allowed the development of surgery as it is practiced today by dramatically reducing the numbers of bacteria gaining access to the surgical wound. However, even with optimal aseptic technique a low level of bacterial contamination is present in the cleanest operative procedures. When host resistance is adequate, this low level of contamination usually does not exceed the threshold for the development of a clinical infection. Strict aseptic technique is essential to minimize the level of bacterial contamination during surgery in order to maintain the lowest possible surgical infection rate. It is important to keep in mind that the bacterial contamination of surgical wounds and previously clean tissues leading to wound infection usually occurs in the operating room when the wound is open during surgery.

Aseptic technique consists of preparing the patient's and scrub team's skin, the use of mechanical barriers to preserve "sterility" (masks, gloves, and drapes), the reduction of bacteria in the operating environment (air filtration, operating room cleaning, and decontamination), and sterilization of operative equipment. All facets are essential. Although it is impossible to sterilize the skin of the patient's operative site or the hands and forearms of the scrub team, proper preparation of these sites will effectively lower the bacterial population to a level where the possibility of spread of bacteria into the wound is greatly reduced. There are a number of accepted "scrub techniques." All utilize the removal of gross surface dirt and oil by a soap or detergent scrub, plus the application of a topical bactericidal agent for a period long enough to reduce the bacterial population made vulnerable by the removal of dirt and oil. These procedures must be carefully executed to achieve optimal results.

Skin bacteria can be divided into resident and transient flora. Resident flora, residing deep in the skin glands and hair follicles, cannot be eradicated using the above methods, but they are generally organisms of low pathogenicity. The transient flora consists of bacteria acquired from the environment and therefore are often highly pathogenic, hospital strains. Fortunately, they can be effectively removed or killed by mechanical scrubbing and bactericidal treatment. The surgical scrub and preparation of the patient's operative site, therefore, make up an important part of aseptic technique.

There is a further problem in the preparation of the patient's operative site. Often it is covered by a thick growth of hair which makes degerming and operation difficult. Removal of this hair is usually accomplished by shaving. Shaving inevitably causes trauma to the skin which allows bacterial growth in a matter of hours. Shaving, if it is to be carried out, is best done immediately before the skin preparation at operation.

Mechanical barriers separating nonsterile areas from the "sterile" operative field consist of head covers, masks, scrub uniforms, shoe covers, sterile gowns, gloves, and drapes. They are uniformly used. Here again, care must be exercised in their use in order to prevent penetration of bacteria and contamination of the wound.

Many innovations in operating room design attempt to reduce the bacterial content of the operative environment. Hard, smooth, easily cleanable wall and floor surfaces, reduced traffic into and out of the operating room and meticulous housekeeping following each case maintain an operating environment with a low level of bacteria. Airflow filters are necessary to prevent airborne bacteria from entering the room, and a constant room air-change removes those bacteria shed by the patient and the operating room staff. Special methods, such as the killing of airborne bacteria by ultraviolet irradiation or the use of laminar air flow, have found success in some quarters but have not been widely accepted. It is important to recognize that bacteria are much more efficiently spread by contact rather than by the airborne route. Airborne bacterial spread becomes important only after contact spread is eliminated. In the well-run operating room where contact spread of bacteria has been largely eliminated, airborne spread is of decided importance in bacterial spread.

Most sterilization of operative equipment is performed in steam autoclaves. Correct operation of these units is essential to assure sterility. Therefore, training in the theory and use of these devices is necessary for the personnel using them. In addition, heat destructible items must be sterilized by less reliable means. These include ethylene oxide and irradiation methods.

SURGICAL TECHNIQUE

Expert surgical technique is required to prevent excessive tissue damage during surgery because tissue damage results in local destruction of host resistance. Blood perfusion is absent from devitalized or frankly necrotic tissue and can markedly limit the local defenses, increasing the probability of infection. Therefore, gentle tissue-handling, the removal of foreign bodies, and the débridement of grossly contaminated tissue are of paramount importance in the prevention of infection. In addition, the careful use of electrocautery and the judicious use of ligatures will limit the amount of necrosis and number of foreign bodies. Also, close attention to hemostasis must be paid, as hematoma formation creates an excellent bacterial culture medium. The need for gentle and precise surgical technique cannot be overestimated as a requirement of infection prevention.

PREVENTIVE ANTIBIOTIC MANAGEMENT

As we have noted, normalization of the patient's physiologic state is of primary concern to the maintenance of host resistance to infection. Reduction of bacterial contamination of wounds through aseptic techniques and accurate surgical techniques are of equal importance. In addition, there is a further route of infection prevention that must be considered. Augmentation of host resistance by the use of preventive antibiotic management is indicated when the patient will not be able to handle the inherent level of bacterial contamination through normal defense mechanisms, especially when defense impairment exists.

This augmentation of host defense is carried out only during the period in which the patient is at increased risk, during surgery and anesthesia, for long-term antibiotic delivery is not an effective supplement to infection prevention. When the decision to employ preventive antibiotics is made, they are administered so that peak tissue levels are available at the time of probable bacterial contamination during the surgical procedure. This requires intramuscular injections about 2 hr prior to surgery and intravenous administration just prior to the onset of surgery. The same dose should be repeated every 3 to 4 hr until the probability of wound contamination ends (usually at the close of the surgical procedure) and host physiology has returned to normal (usually several hours postoperatively).

The choice of antibiotic used should be predicated upon the likely contaminating bacterial species. Even when properly chosen, it should be understood that these agents will help to prevent infection only during the initial period of bacterial contamination. Once the biochemical lesion due to bacterial proliferation reaches a certain threshold, preventive antibiotics will no longer obviate the development of frank infection (Fig. 9-2).

The decision to employ preventive antibiotics is made for the following groups of patients (Table 9-2):

1. Patients in whom there is likelihood of massive bacterial contamination of previously uncontaminated tissue. These patients are generally to undergo surgical treatment of existing infectious processes.
2. Patients with isolated or general defects in host resistance to infection. This category includes both congenital and acquired defects. Subcategories include patients with profound metabolic abnormalities, congenital or acquired defects in immunocompetence, diseases leaving specific organ systems vulnerable, and severely traumatized patients (see Table 9-1).

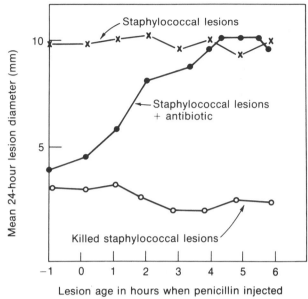

Fig. 9-2   Decreasing effect of penicillin on lesion diameter as lesion age increases. (Burke JF: The effective period of preventive antibiotic action in experimental incisions and dermal lesions. Surgery 50:161, 1961)

3. Patients who will undergo significant physiological depression due to the extent of surgery. An example of this type of indication would be cardiac surgery requiring heart-lung bypass.
4. Finally, they are indicated in patients for whom the morbidity or mortality of a postoperative infection would be very high, despite a relatively low probability of infection. Neurosurgery and the orthopedic or vascular use of prosthetics are examples of this category.

It is important to recognize that there is a cost to using preventive antibiotics indiscriminately or for extended periods of time, for they may be toxic or produce allergic reactions, even in short-term delivery. However, by rigid adherence to the concepts that (*1*) patients who require supplemental host resistance are selected, (*2*) antibiotics are given in the immediate preoperative period to ensure adequate tissue levels at the time of bacterial contamination, and (*3*) delivery is halted after the period of wound contamination and upon return of normal physiology, the toxic effects of antibiotics can be minimized and the wound infection rate will be maximally reduced. In addition, there will be patients in whom the addition of preventive antibiotics will not prevent postoperative infection. This may be due to the extent of impaired resistance or amount of contamination. However, for the patient with an indication

TABLE 9-2   **OPERATIVE WOUND CLASSIFICATION ACCORDING TO CONTAMINATION-INFECTION RISK**

CLASSIFICATION	INFECTION RATE
Clean Nontraumatic No inflammation encountered No break in technique Respiratory, alimentary, genitourinary tract not entered	**Reported infection rates are usually 1%–4%.** In general, no antibiotics are needed unless the host defenses are suppressed or unless the consequences of infection are catastrophic—heart valve replacement, etc. Drains are not used unless blood or fluid must be evacuated, and should be left in no longer than the period of accumulation (usually 24 hr).
Clean–Contaminated Gastrointestinal or respiratory tracts entered without significant spillage Appendectomy—not perforated—no cloudy peritoneal exudate Prepared oropharynx entered Prepared vagina entered Genitourinary or biliary tract entered in absence of infected urine or bile Minor break in technique	**Reported infection rates are 5%–15%.** Here the surgeon must use his judgment about using preventive antibiotics. It will probably not be necessary to use antibiotics in most cases of biliary or small intestinal surgery, unless the operation is to be carried out in the face of invasive bacterial infection or *unless* host defenses are suppressed. Cases in which the consequences of infection are trivial (*e.g.*, minor mouth procedures) do not require antibiotics. Delayed primary closure may be considered in cases with preexisting sepsis.
Contaminated Major break in technique Gross spillage from gastrointestinal tract Traumatic wound, fresh Entrance of genitourinary or biliary tracts in presence of infected urine or bile	**Reported infection rates are about 16%–25%, although many centers are reporting lesser rates.** In this category, most patients will need supplementation unless the operation is minor, as in oral surgery. Delayed primary or secondary closure techniques should be used frequently.
Dirty and Infected Acute bacterial inflammation encountered, without pus Transection of "clean" tissue for the purpose of surgical access to a collection of pus Perforated viscus encountered Traumatic wound with retained devitalized tissue, foreign bodies, fecal contamination, and/or delayed treatment, or from dirty source	**Infection rates mean little here, but are often over 25%.** Here, either preventive antibiotics or delayed closure or both should be used. Antibiotics are *not* usually necessary for drainage of a small abscess.

(Burke JF: Fundamentals of Wound Management in Surgery: Infection. New York, Appleton-Century-Crofts, 1977)

for use, preventive antibiotics usually will elevate resistance to infection high enough to prevent postsurgical sepsis.

We should also note that there is extensive research being carried out in the general concept of augmentation of host resistance to infection. Direct repair or replacement of host resistance is surely the solution. Certainly, the specific and nonspecific immunopotentiators are examples in a field promising significant contribution to this type of therapy in the future. At present, however, these factors require more testing prior to widespread clinical use.

CLINICAL CHARACTERISTICS OF INFECTION AND THEIR TREATMENT

The problems of dealing with an already established infection are completely different from those of prevention. Here the general principles of drainage, elevation, heat, and rest are cornerstones. In addition to these classic methods of dealing with bacterial infection, antibiotic therapy has added an additional specific element to control. The importance of antibiotics in the therapy of bacterial infection is impressive but can be overstated. It is wise to recognize that antibiotics in therapy, as in prevention, are adjuncts to host resistance—they do not replace it. Furthermore, in order to be an effective supplement, the antibiotic used must be selected so that it is effective against the infecting bacteria (Table 9-3). It must be used in a concentration that is bacteriocidal or bacteriostatic and given over a period of days rather than hours, as is the case in prevention. Therefore, in the treatment of any infection it is more important to restore normal physiology than merely to prescribe an antibiotic. In addition, antibiotics must be selected and dose established to avoid allergic and toxic reactions, which occasionally occur following administration of all antibiotics. Therefore, a bacterial diagnosis and sensitivity pattern of the isolated bacteria are essential for efficient treatment. Although the press of clinical disease may require the initiation of antibiotic treatment before an exact diagnosis can be established, bacterial smear may provide vital information and initial careful bacteriologic cultures should be carried out in order to allow adjustments for maximum antibiotic effectiveness to be made when definitive bacteriologic information is available.

Antibiotic treatment has been so prominent in adding to the effectiveness of the treatment of infection that it has obscured the essential nature of host resistance in the control of infection and elimination of bacteria in tissue, as noted above, and has clouded the contribution of surgical drainage and the restoration of normal anatomy in the treatment of bacterial disease. Thus, it is common to find patients with localized abscesses being treated with prolonged courses of antibiotics where simple surgical drainage would solve the problem with less morbidity and in far less time. Furthermore, patients with demonstrated anatomical abnormalities of the genitourinary tract, for example, may be treated repeatedly with antibiotic therapy when restoration of normal anatomical function is far more likely to produce a permanent cure. As noted above, the place of antibiotics in the treatment of bacterial disease must always be considered as an adjunct to host resistance, and also often as an adjunct to a surgical procedure which either eliminates the bacterial disease by excision (as in a brain abscess or acute appendicitis) or provides drainage of a closed space, allowing effective function of host resistance and healing of the wound. Surgery, therefore, has a fundamental role in the treatment of certain bacterial infections, as will be discussed below.

CELLULITIS

Although all bacterial infections that begin in tissues rather than in the bloodstream itself begin as cellulitis, only certain bacterial species usually spread through tissue as extending cellulitis (β-strep) while others usually remain localized to form abscesses (staph) if not controlled. Rest, heat, and elevation are most important in the treatment of cellulitis, for they reduce the possibility of lymphatic or blood-borne spread and allow host resistance to function optimally with an increased blood supply and without the impediment of dependent edema. The local manifestations of cellulitis are pain and local tenderness, swelling, redness, and local heat. Because there are no localized areas of pus formation, drainage is indicated only to relieve pressure that may cause ischemia. However, localized abscesses may contain surrounding cellulitis, and drainage of the localized abscess and treatment with antibiotics are essential parts of therapy (see Table 9-3).

ABSCESS

Abscess formation is the local collection of necrotic tissue, bacteria, and white cells, commonly denoted as pus. Superficial abscesses may be detected by their localized nature, their tendency to develop point tenderness, and fluctuation on palpation. For practical purposes, all abscesses should be drained or excised, for they present a considerable hazard of further bacterial spread to the patient. Because of the enzymatic processes that go on in the abscess cavity and the isolation of this degenerating material from normal tissue, there is increased osmotic pressure within the walled-off abscess cavity itself owing to the splitting of large molecules into a number of small fragments. As water migrates into the area under the generated osmotic force, considerable pressure is produced, causing the risk of bacterial spread along tissue planes or by way of blood or lymphatic vessels. Open drainage to eliminate the increased pressure in the closed space is an essential element of treatment. Furthermore, the open space must be maintained until it is obliterated by the natural healing processes, for if the space is allowed to seal, a closed space and increased pressure are again produced. Incision and prolonged drainage, with a drain tract kept free of coagulation by a saline dressing changed frequently, is a most effective method when added to rest, heat, and elevation.

BLOOD AND LYMPHATIC INFECTIONS

Bacterial infections of the lymph or the bloodstream usually result from extension of localized areas of cellulitis or abscess formation. Because of dangers of metastatic bacterial spread inherent in bacteremia or lymphangitis, vigorous treatment is always indicated, including appropriate antibiotic therapy as well as local treatment directed at the initial lesion, and surgical drainage if abscess formation is present (see Table 9-3).

INFECTIONS ASSOCIATED WITH TRAUMA

A major cause of serious bacterial infection is the contamination of devitalized or injured tissue as a result of trauma.

(*Text continues on p. 135*)

TABLE 9-3

INFECTING ORGANISM	DRUGS OF CHOICE	PARENTERAL Total Daily Dosage Range	PARENTERAL Divided Daily Dose Given at Intervals of	ORAL Total Daily Dosage Range	ORAL Divided Daily Dose Given at Intervals of	ALTERNATIVE DRUGS
Gram-negative Cocci						
Meningococcus	Penicillin G (Cryst.) PCNG	1.2–24 million units	q 4–12 h			Chloramphenicol, Sulfonamide
Gonococcus	Penicillin G (Cryst.) PCNG	1.2–24 million units	q 4–12 h			Ampicillin, Tetracycline, Amoxicillin, Cefoxitin
Gram-positive Cocci						
Staphylococcus aureus (nonpenicillinase-producing)	Penicillin G (Cryst.) PCNG	1.2–24 million units	q 4–12 h			Cephalosporin, Vancomycin, Clindamycin
	(Phenoxymethyl PCN) Penicillin V			1.6–3.2 million units	q 6 h	
Staphylococcus aureus (penicillinase-producing)	Penicillinase-resistant penicillins					
	Methicillin	4–6 g	q 4–6 h			
	Nafcillin	2–12 g	q 4–6 h	2–4 g	q 6 h	Cephalosporin, Vancomycin, Clindamycin
	Oxacillin	2–12 g	q 4–6 h	2–4 g	q 6 h	
	Cloxacillin			1–2 g	q 6 h	
	Dicloxacillin			1–2 g	q 6 h	
Streptococcus viridans	Penicillin G (Cryst.) PCNG	1.2–24 million units	q 4–12 h	1.6–3.2 million units	q 6 h	Vancomycin, Cephalosporin
		1–2 g	q 12 h			
Streptococcus pyogenes (Groups A,B,C,G)	Penicillin G (Cryst.) PCNG, Penicillin V	1.2–24 million units	q 4–12 h	1.6–3.2 million units	q 6 h	Erythromycin, Cephalosporin
Streptococcus enterococcus	Ampicillin or penicillin G (Cryst.) PCNG with gentamicin	2–12 g, 1.2–24 million units, 3–5 mg/kg	q 6 h, q 4–12 h, q 8 h			Vancomycin c̄ gentamicin

Organism	Drug	Dosage	Interval	Dosage	Interval	Alternatives
Pneumococcus	Penicillin G (Cryst.) PCNG / Penicillin V	1.2–24 million units	q 4–12 h	1.6–3.2 million units	q 6 h	Cephalosporin, Chloramphenicol, Vancomycin, Erythromycin
Streptococcus anaerobic	Penicillin G (Cryst.) PCNG	1.2–24 million units	q 4–12 h			Clindamycin, Tetracycline, Chloramphenicol, Vancomycin
Gram-negative Bacilli						
Shigella	Trimethoprim/sulfamethoxazole			0.32 g/1.6 g	q 12 h	Ampicillin, Tetracycline, Chloramphenicol
Salmonella	Chloramphenicol	30–100 mg/kg	q 6 h	30–50 mg/kg	q 6 h	Ampicillin
Escherichia coli	Gentamicin or tobramycin	3–5 mg/kg	q 8 h			Ampicillin, Ticarcillin, Carbenicillin, Amikacin, Cephalosporin
Enterobacter	Gentamicin or tobramycin	3–5 mg/kg	q 8 h			Carbenicillin, Ticarcillin, Amikacin, Cefamandole, Chloramphenicol
Klebsiella pneumoniae	Gentamicin or tobramycin	3–5 mg/kg	q 8 h			Cephalosporin, Kanamycin, Amikacin, Tetracycline
Serratia	Gentamicin	3–5 mg/kg	q 8 h			Amikacin, Carbenicillin
Proteus mirabilis	Ampicillin	2–12 g	q 6 h	2–4 g	q 6 h	Cephalosporin, Gentamicin, Tobramycin
Other proteus	Gentamicin or tobramycin	3–5 mg/kg	q 8 h			Carbenicillin, Amikacin, Tetracycline
Providencia	Amikacin	15 mg/kg	q 8–12 h			Carbenicillin
Pseudomonas aeruginosa	Gentamicin c̄ carbenicillin	3–5 mg/kg / 30–40 g	q 8 h / q 6 h			Tobramycin, Amikacin, Ticarcillin

* These are suggested dosages and depend upon bacterial sensitivities and patient physiology. Antibiotics should be tailored to each patient. (Burke JF: Fundamentals of Wound Management in Surgery: Infection. New York, Appleton-Century-Crofts, 1977)

TABLE 9-3　TREATMENT OF INFECTION CAUSED BY SPECIFIC BACTERIA: SPECIFIC BACTERIAL INFECTIONS—ANTIMICROBIAL DRUGS OF CHOICE AND DOSAGE SCHEDULE* *(Continued)*

| | | ROUTE OF ADMINISTRATION AND DOSAGE | | | | |
| | | PARENTERAL | | ORAL | | |
INFECTING ORGANISM	DRUGS OF CHOICE	Total Daily Dosage Range	Divided Daily Dose Given at Intervals of	Total Daily Dosage Range	Divided Daily Dose Given at Intervals of	ALTERNATIVE DRUGS
Yersinia pestis (bubonic plague)	Streptomycin	1–2 g	q 12 h			Tetracycline Chloramphenicol Cephalosporin
Hemophilus influenzae	Ampicillin	2–12 g	q 6 h	2–4 g	q 6 h	Amoxicillin Tetracycline
(epiglottitis or meningitis)	Chloramphenicol	30–100 mg/kg	q 6 h			Ampicillin Tetracycline
Hemophilus ducreyi (chancroid)	Trisulfapyrimidines					Tetracycline
Bacteroides	Clindamycin	1.2–2.4 g	q 6–12 h			Metronidazole Chloramphenicol Cefoxitin Penicillin G
(see also mouth and pharyngeal infections)						
Acinetobacter (Mima, Herellea)	Gentamicin	3–5 mg/kg	q 8 h			Tobramycin Amikacin
Calymmatobacterium granulomatis (granuloma inguinale)	Tetracycline	0.75–1.0 g IV	q 6–12 h	1–2 g	q 6 h	Streptomycin
Choleta vibrio (vibrio comma) (cholera)	Tetracycline	0.75–1.0 g IV	q 6–12 h	1–2 g	q 6 h	Trimethoprim Sulfamethoxasole
Legionella pneumophila	Erythromycin c̄ or s̄ rifampin	1–4 g IV	q 6 h			Tetracycline
Gram-positive Bacilli *Clostridium tetani*	Penicillin G (Cryst.) PCNG	1.2–24 million units	q 4–12 h			Tetracycline Cephalosporin
Clostridium welchii (gas gangrene)	Penicillin G (Cryst.) PCNG	1.2–24 million units	q 4–12 h			Chloramphenicol Clindamycin Cephalosporin

Organism	Drug of choice	Dose	Interval	Dose	Interval	Alternative drugs
Bacillus anthracis (anthrax)	Penicillin G (Cryst.) PCNG	1.2–24 million units	q 4–12 h			Erythromycin Tetracycline
Listeria monocytogenes	Penicillin or	1.2–24 million units	q 4–12 h			Tetracycline
	ampicillin c̄ or s̄ gentamicin	2–12 g / 3–5 mg/kg	q 6 h / q 8 h	2–4 g	q 6 h	Chloramphenicol
Acid-fast Bacilli *Mycobacterium tuberculosis*	Isoniazid c̄ ethambutol c̄ or s̄ rifampin	5–10 mg/kg	single or divided doses	5–10 mg/kg / 15 mg/kg	single or divided doses	Streptomycin Pyrazinamide Para-aminosalicylic acid
Pneumocystis *Pneumocystis carinii*	Trimethoprim Sulfamethoxazole			20 mg/kg / 100 mg/kg	q 6 h	Pentamidine
Spirochaeta *Borrelia recurrentis* (relapsing fever)	Tetracycline	0.75–1.0 g IV	q 6–12 h	1–2 g	q 6 h	Penicillin
Leptospira	Penicillin G (Cryst.) PCNG	1.2–24 million units	q 4–12 h			Tetracycline
Treponema pertenue (yaws)	Penicillin G (Cryst.) PCNG	1.2–24 million units	q 4–12 h			Tetracycline
Treponema pallidum (syphilis)	Penicillin G (Cryst.) PCNG	1.2–24 million units	4–12 h			Erythromycin Tetracycline
Rickettsia (Rocky Mountain spotted fever; endemic typhus; Q fever)	Tetracycline	0.75–1.0 g IV	q 6–12 h	1–2 g	q 6 h	Chloramphenicol
Mycoplasma *Mycoplasma pneumoniae* (atypical pneumonia)	Erythromycin	1–4 g IV	q 6 h	1–2 g	q 6 h	Tetracycline
Chlamydia (lymphogranuloma venereum)	Tetracycline	0.75–1.0 g IV	q 6–12 h	1–2 g	q 6 h	Sulfonamide Erythromycin
(psittacosis)	Tetracycline	0.75–1.0 g IV	q 6–12 h	1–2 g	q 6 h	Chloramphenicol
Chlamydia trachomatis (urethritis)	Tetracycline		1–2 g			Erythromycin

* These are suggested dosages and depend upon bacterial sensitivities and patient physiology. Antibiotics should be tailored to each patient. (Burke JF: Fundamentals of Wound Management in Surgery: Infection. New York, Appleton-Century-Crofts, 1977)

TABLE 9-3 TREATMENT OF INFECTION CAUSED BY SPECIFIC BACTERIA: SPECIFIC BACTERIAL INFECTIONS—ANTIMICROBIAL DRUGS OF CHOICE AND DOSAGE SCHEDULE* *(Continued)*

INFECTING ORGANISM	DRUGS OF CHOICE	ROUTE OF ADMINISTRATION AND DOSAGE				ALTERNATIVE DRUGS
		PARENTERAL		ORAL		
		Total Daily Dosage Range	Divided Daily Dose Given at Intervals of	Total Daily Dosage Range	Divided Daily Dose Given at Intervals of	
Actinomyces						
Actinomyces israelii	Penicillin G (Cryst.) PCNG	1.2–24 million units	q 4–12 h			Tetracycline
Fungi						
Candida albicans	Amphotericin B	0.25–1.0 mg/kg	By slow IV infusion daily			Nystatin Flucytosine
Histoplasma capsulatum	Amphotericin B	0.25–1.0 mg/kg	By slow IV infusion daily			
Aspergillus	Amphotericin B	0.25–1.0 mg/kg	By slow IV infusion daily			
Cryptococcus neoformans	Amphotericin B	0.25–1.0 mg/kg	By slow IV infusion daily			
Blastomyces	Amphotericin B	0.25–1.0 mg/kg	By slow IV infusion daily			Hydroxystilbamidine
Virus						
Herpes simplex keratitis	Vidarabine ophthalmic 3%		q 3 h			Idoxuridine
Mouth or Pharyngeal Infections						
Bacteroides	Penicillin G (Cryst.) PCNG	1.2–24 million units	q 4–12 h			
Leptotrichia buccalis	Penicillin G (Cryst.) PCNG	1.2–24 million units	q 4–12 h			Tetracycline Erythromycin
(Vincent's infection)	Penicillin V			1.6–3.2 million units	q 6 h	

* These are suggested dosages and depend upon bacterial sensitivities and patient physiology. Antibiotics should be tailored to each patient. (Burke JF: Fundamentals of Wound Management in Surgery: Infection. New York, Appleton-Century-Crofts, 1977)

In this situation, normal defenses against bacterial invasion are seriously hindered by devitalized tissue that not only interrupts blood supply but provides a medium for bacterial growth. In addition, following serious trauma, systemic abnormalities of the cardiorespiratory system are frequent and further complicate the ability of the patient to defend himself against bacterial invasion. Although the problems of trauma are dealt with extensively in other chapters, the overall problems and methods of management of sepsis following trauma are briefly outlined here.

The local treatment of the traumatic wound is of crucial importance in the successful management of sepsis associated with trauma. Here, as elsewhere in surgery, the keystone is prevention of the development of invasive infection. Wounds must be thoroughly débrided of all nonviable tissue, and the removal of foreign bodies, such as pieces of clothing, wood, metal, and dirt, is of primary importance. The complete removal of tissue that has been devitalized or injured to an extent that it cannot survive, although alive at the time of initial débridement, presents a difficult problem in clinical surgical judgment. This is particularly true in areas of trauma where loss of tissue involves the serious loss of function or the production of cosmetic abnormalities.

DELAYED CLOSURE

In traumatic and other contaminated wounds, the methods of *delayed primary or secondary closure* allow some leeway in the débridement of traumatic wounds (Fig. 9-3; see also Chapter 8). In patients in whom serious loss of function will result from wide excision of questionable tissue at the time of initial débridement, loss of function can often be avoided without the risk of invasive sepsis by allowing the questionable tissue to remain in place. It is then observed over the immediate postdébridement period and débrided again if infection intervenes. Delayed primary closure is defined as being within 3 days of the initial treatment, whereas secondary closure occurs any time after that, usually in 3 to 7 days. This technique provides reliable drainage of

Fig. 9-3. Steps in technique of delayed primary closure using allograft or fine gauze wound cover. (*A*) Allograft or gauze is placed as the usual split thickness skin graft. (*B*) Relation of debrided area to allografted surface and stay suture tract. (*C*) and (*D*) Stent holding allograft in place on debrided surface. (*E*) Allograft or gauze is removed at time of definitive closure. (*F*) Appearance of wound following definitive closure. (Burke JF: Fundamentals of Wound Management in Surgery: Infection. New York, Appleton-Century-Crofts, 1977)

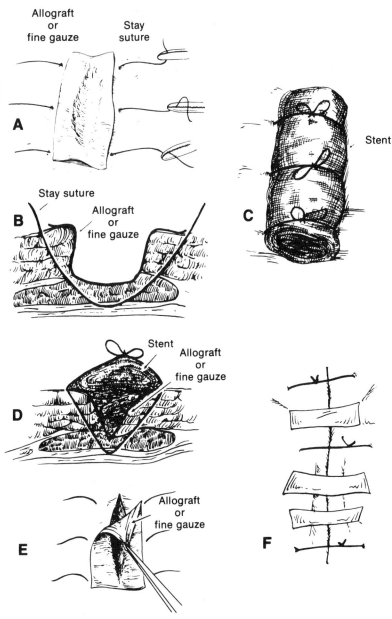

the entire wound, as well as the opportunity for easy and repeated inspection and further débridement as necessary.

In an acceptable method of delayed primary or secondary closure, the edges of the débrided wound are separated by a thin layer of fine mesh gauze or skin allograft which allows effective drainage without danger of pocketing. The wound is then covered by an occlusive dressing to prevent further bacterial contamination. If exudate, local pain, cellulitis, or a systemic reaction takes place in the following period, the wound can be examined without difficulty and further débridement carried out as necessary. If in 3 days there is no sign of suppuration or further devitalized tissue, the wound can be definitively closed with direct apposition of all layers of the tissue, including the skin.

PRIMARY CLOSURE

In the treatment of traumatic wounds, primary closure is carried out in those wounds that can be accurately and completely débrided within 6 hr to 8 hr after injury. In civilian practice, successful primary closure can often be accomplished, but careful continuous observation of the closed wound must be carried out in the immediate postoperative period.

SYSTEMIC EFFECTS OF SEPSIS

Sepsis is a continuum from the locally controlled abscess to agonal septic shock. As a patient moves toward increasing severity of sepsis, increased systemic effects become evident. Systemic injury from bacteria or bacterial products (*e.g.*, endotoxin) occurs due to their effects in the bloodstream and in distant tissues. Endotoxins and exotoxins may directly impair cellular metabolic processes and eventually, if unchecked, produce organ failure. In addition, the products of local necrosis at the site of infection may also adversely affect organ function through the activation of complement and the coagulation system. Abnormalities in capillary permeability, peripheral resistance, and disseminated intravascular coagulation are examples. Anaphylotoxins, other vasoactive peptides, bacteria, and bacterial products all cause abnormalities at the biochemical, cellular, and systemic level, affecting especially the cardiovascular, pulmonary, and renal systems. These, coupled with the production of fever and alterations in normal metabolism as described below, explain the widely varied clinical picture seen in sepsis.(Jaundice may suggest hepatic impairment.—ED)

FEVER AND ITS DIFFERENTIAL DIAGNOSIS

Fever is frequently seen in postoperative patients and is often, but by no means always, due to infection. For this reason, a febrile postoperative patient always requires an accurate diagnostic evaluation of the fever, beginning with infection as a probable cause. While any infectious agent can produce fever, the magnitude of the response depends on patient physiology and microbial pathogenicity. It is well recognized, for example, that children sometimes respond to minor infections with very high fevers whereas elderly, or immunocompromised patients, may be euthermic or even hypothermic in the presence of a wide range of infectious disease. In beginning an evaluation of the febrile postoperative patient, the type and the time of onset of the fever should be carefully noted. A spiking fever, especially associated with chills or rigor, is more suggestive of an active, invasive infection with bacteremia than is a low-grade fever, which implies a more slowly developing inflammatory process, perhaps unrelated to bacterial cause. The fever of infection itself is caused by certain agents of the bacterial wall (*e.g.*, lipopolysaccharides) that produce pyrogens when incubated with leukocytes *in vivo*. These circulating pyrogens reset the hypothalamic thermostat that regulates body temperature, and fever results when the core temperature rises in response to this change in set point. Postoperative fever, therefore, is an early and important sign of physiological abnormality and demands immediate and careful evaluation.

The differential diagnosis of postoperative fever is an important activity in postoperative care because there is a wide range of abnormalities capable of creating a postoperative febrile response that demand greatly differing treatment regimes for their correction. For example, in addition to infection, fever can be produced by atelectasis, can accompany malignancy, or be produced by drug therapy, blood transfusion reaction, dehydration, heat exposure, malignant hyperthermia, or hyperthyroidism. In addition, postoperative complications such as pneumothorax, thrombophlebitis, pancreatitis, or pulmonary emboli may cause fever. As noted above, the character of the fever and particularly the time of onset in the postoperative period are important in arriving at a correct diagnosis. Atelectasis, usually produced by anesthesia-induced bronchial mucus obstruction or by alveolar collapse, is the most common cause of fever in the immediate postsurgical period. On the other hand, fever beginning on the third postoperative day is more likely to be due to a urinary-tract infection, especially if the patient has been catheterized or is on continuous bladder drainage. A complete schematic approach to the diagnosis of postoperative fever, as suggested by Roe, is presented in Table 9-4.

CARDIOVASCULAR RESPONSE

The initial cardiovascular response to sepsis is increased cardiac output. The major portion of this increase is due to a fall in total peripheral resistance, probably secondary to the effects of vasoactive substances, autonomic nervous system activity, and the direct action of bacterial toxins. The minor portion stems from the sepsis-induced increase in metabolic rate. In extensive sepsis, the beginning of decompensation is signalled by a decrease in tissue extraction of oxygen and nutrients, possibly secondary to shunting, or direct injury to cellular metabolism. The resulting tissue hypoxia necessitates anaerobic energy-production leading to systemic lactic acidemia from anaerobic glycolysis, which may be complicated by multiple organ failure or eventual death if not promptly corrected. In frank septic shock, as noted above, lowered peripheral resistance exceeds the increased cardiac output, resulting in falling arterial pressure and all of the pathologic consequences of insufficient arterial perfusion of vital organs. In addition, direct myocardial depression can be present, along with increased pulmonary resistance, resulting in acute right heart failure as well as left heart decompensation.

Therapy of established septic shock requires the use of antibiotics, plasma-volume expansion, vasopressors, respiratory support, and, perhaps most important of all, surgical removal of the septic focus. The identification and elimination of the site of sepsis is of the utmost importance in addition to supportive measures, because appropriate, timely drainage or débridement of the origin of sepsis has been

TABLE 9-4   WORKUP FOR POSTOPERATIVE FEVER

CHART

—Is the patient receiving drugs to which he may be or is known to be allergic?

—Is the patient receiving drugs that commonly cause fevers?

—When did the fever start? Fever within the first 48 hours suggests pulmonary origin. Fever starting 6 to 8 days after surgery suggests wound infection.

—Has the patient had a blood transfusion within the last 12 hours? Look at the fluid intake and output; could the fever be associated with dehydration?

PHYSICAL EXAMINATION

Head and Neck

—Does the patient complain of earache or sore throat? Nasogastric tubes can cause inflammation and blockage of the eustachian tube and cause otitis media.

—Look in the ears; are the drums healthy?

—Check the mouth; is there evidence of monilia or other local infection? Parotitis causes pain and fever.

Upper Limbs

—Check both arms; is the site of present or recent intravenous infusions tender or inflamed?

—Is there phlebitis in the arm? Intravenous hyperalimentation catheters are commonly associated with infections and fever.

—Has there been any break in sterility, such as administration of drugs through a hyperalimentation catheter? Have the dressings been changed regularly with proper aseptic precautions? Is the fluid running freely or is there some obstruction which could be due to an infected clot?

—Fevers due to infected hyperalimentation catheters can exist even when all the above appear to be normal.

Chest

—Is expansion good?

—Are breath sounds normal?

—Are there any signs suggesting atelectasis or pneumonitis? Remember: pneumothorax by itself may cause fever.

—Is the patient dyspneic or cyanotic? Obtain blood gases and think of pulmonary embolism.

Abdomen

—Are there signs of peritonitis?

—Does the patient have bowel sounds? Absent bowel sounds are of little diagnostic value, but their presence helps to rule out peritonitis.

—Could fever be due to an anastomotic leak? (Usually 3 to 4 days after operation)

—Remember that blood in the peritoneal or pleural cavities can produce fever and pain.

—Both pancreatitis and cholecystitis can occur as postoperative complications.

—Check the serum amylase when fever is accompanied by abdominal and back pain.

—Is there CVA tenderness? Think of pyelonephritis and perinephric abscess.

—Does the patient have burning or pain on micturition?

—Is the urine cloudy?

—Has a urinary catheter been in place for more than 48 hours?

—Has the patient had a pelvic procedure which might lead to pelvic thrombophlebitis?

Lower Limbs

—Does the patient have leg pain, swelling or calf tenderness?

—Have I.V.s been placed in the lower limbs?

—Is there tenderness or redness along the course of superficial veins?

Wound

—Are the edges puffy or red?

—Is the wound area tender? Check it for crepitus, which may indicate infection with gas gangrene organisms.

—Is there a swelling under the incision?

—Are the sutures infected?

LAB AND OTHER CHECKS

The following procedures may be of value:

—Complete blood count and differential. Leukocytosis with a shift to the left is seen in most infections. This may be unreliable in elderly patients or in patients with overwhelming infections at which time a leukopenia may be found. The erythrocyte sedimentation rate is nearly always elevated in such cases.

—Get a chest x-ray film.

—Fluoroscope for diaphragmatic movement if a subphrenic abscess is suspected. Ultrasonography? CT scan?

—Send a clean-catch or catheter specimen of urine for urinalysis and culture.

—With a high fever, do repeated blood cultures (usually 3) when the temperature is as close to the peak as possible.

—Where the source of infection may be respiratory, do a sputum culture. Make sure that it is sputum and not saliva that is cultured.

—An infected wound should be cultured. Often the wound has healed over the wound abscess. It should be opened in the line of the wound with a pair of scissors and a Kelly clamp, and no local anesthesia is necessary.

—When indicated, I.V. catheters should be removed and cultured.

—It should be remembered that ventilators and other respiratory equipment can be reservoirs of infection.

(Roe CF: Fever in surgical patients. In Hardy JD (ed): Textbook of Surgery. Philadelphia, J B Lippincott, 1977)

demonstrated to be a key to survival. In the treatment of sepsis in general, postsurgical sepsis included, in addition to repair of physiological defects causing or associated with infection, the use of intravenous antibiotics is important. Until culture and sensitivity results dictate more specific choices, wide-spectrum antibiotic coverage based on the probable organisms to be encountered in the specific clinical situation should be provided. When available, therapy is modified according to direct bacterial sensitivities (Table 9-3). Accurate central arterial pressures and cardiac index should be obtained at times, necessitating the use of a pulmonary artery catheter. On the basis of these data, plasma volume expansion using lactated Ringer's solution and fresh frozen plasma or colloid solution is employed to maintain an adequate circulatory volume and perfusion pressure. The use of dopamine hydrochloride and other cardiotonic agents is frequently necessary to maintain organ perfusion and mean arterial pressure during the period of peripheral and myocardial abnormalities. In addition, there are limited data indicating that massive doses of corticosteroids stabilize capillaries and aid in diminishing the generalized shock response. Therefore, steroids are sometimes given at times when the state of sepsis is unresponsive to other measures.

PULMONARY RESPONSE

The initial pulmonary response to sepsis is a compensatory increase in ventilation to accompany the increased need for oxygen delivery and CO_2 production which are produced by an increased metabolic rate. The pulmonary response to sepsis as decompensation begins is frequently present as interstitial pneumonitis. This pneumonitis is the result of increased pulmonary arterial pressure and loss of capillary integrity, and may result from the action of bacterial toxins and circulating vasoactive substances. Right to left shunting is produced, leading to a widened alveolar arterial oxygen gradient and hyperventilation in an attempt to maintain normal arterial oxygen concentration. Also, lung compliance decreases as the parenchyma becomes more rigid as a result of increasing extravascular lung water and perhaps less surfactant. This constellation of hypoxemia, respiratory alkalosis and increased work of breathing in the face of systemic sepsis has been clinically called the *adult respiratory distress syndrome* (ARDS). In addition, direct pulmonary sepsis is often seen in the development of bronchopneumonia, further comprising pulmonary vascular physiology and pulmonary compliance. Bacteremic seeding from distant sites of infection or failure to adequately clear airway secretions due to septic inhibition of mucociliary action and a generalized compromised host defense system provide access for bacterial spread to the lungs.

The therapy for the pulmonary component of sepsis consists of (*1*) control of distant septic foci, as noted above, (*2*) maintaining PaO$_2$, PaCO$_2$, and *p*H at acceptable levels by the use of intubation, oxygen, mechanical ventilation, and positive end expiratory pressure (PEEP), as required, (*3*) close attention to fluid balance and the prevention of circulatory overloading and pulmonary edema, (*4*) maintenance of careful pulmonary toilet and prevention of aspiration, and (*5*) the diagnosis and treatment of pulmonary sepsis through the use of sputum and blood cultures, radiograms, and culture-dictated antibiotics.

RENAL AND BODY FLUID RESPONSES

Severe sepsis induces hemoconcentration and a decrease in plasma volume. The intravascular fluid lost appears as edema fluid in the extravascular space and leads to shock, loss of adequate renal perfusion, and acute tubular necrosis (ATN). At the same time, there is loss of intracellular water and potassium which also appear in the extravascular space. Hyponatremia and hyperkalemia can occur, especially if renal function is impaired. Careful fluid management is necessary to provide adequate organ perfusion, yet avoid pulmonary and peripheral edema. Furthermore, the margins of adequate renal perfusion are narrowed in sepsis. There-

fore, hypovolemia due to sepsis-induced fluid shifts may quickly produce oliguria and renal failure. In severe sepsis, glomerular filtration seems more affected than renal plasma flow, suggesting renal maldistribution of available perfusion.

Prompt fluid resuscitation, sufficient to maintain adequate cardiovascular perfusion pressures, using crystalloid and colloid solutions is imperative in the prevention of disastrous renal failure. Low-dose dopamine hydrochloride (3μg/kg/min) may augment renal bed perfusion, and diuretics, commonly furosemide, have a limited role in sustaining urine output. When acute renal failure becomes well established, however, peritoneal or hemodialysis is necessary to handle the fluid, acid, potassium, and nitrogenous loads. In the septic patient, renal failure is more effectively prevented than treated, and prevention depends on adequate renal perfusion.

ENERGY METABOLISM

Sepsis increases the metabolic rate. This is partially produced by the septic response to stress and partially produced by fever (approximately a 13% increase for each °C of increased body temperature). Therefore, in order to prevent extensive nitrogen loss secondary to stress and starvation, food intake must be maintained to avoid serious metabolic consequences. To complicate matters, oral intake of substrates for energy and protein synthesis may be markedly impaired due to paralytic ileus or intra-abdominal sepsis, or general malaise necessitating the use of parenteral hyperalimentation.

The general metabolic response to infection leads to an increase in hepatic glucose production and an elevated plasma glucose concentration. Initially, stored glycogen provides this increased endogenous glucose production if food is not taken by the patient. However, gluconeogenic sources, mainly amino acid from muscle, soon become solely responsible. Further, glucose production is not diminished by glucose infusion to the same degree as in a healthy person. This lack of hepatic gluconeogenic suppressibility, in conjunction with decreased plasma glucose clearance, provides the basis for the hyperglycemia and "glucose intolerance" seen in septic patients. Protein becomes the major gluconeogenic precursor, in part increasing protein catabolism that, if unchecked over a matter of a week or so, may cause protein wasting with its effect on wound healing and host defense mechanisms. In profound sepsis associated with shock, as noted above, hypometabolism occurs with diminished cellular extraction of oxygen and nutrients. In this situation energy production may be forced towards anaerobic glycolysis, with less energy produced per mole of glucose degraded and the production of lactic acid leading to acidosis.

The hormonal response in sepsis is a marked elevation in plasma concentrations of epinephrine, norepinephrine, glucagon, and cortisol. Plasma insulin concentrations are less predictable but are often elevated. In addition, there is a blunted response to circulating insulin, which has been called *insulin resistance* but which is not clearly understood. Despite this descriptive pattern of hormonal changes, little is known about their causal relationships to the observed metabolic changes of sepsis.

Although nutritional therapy of surgical patients is discussed at length elsewhere in this text, some guidelines on nutrition in sepsis are appropriate. Total calories provided should approximate those expended. In addition, they should be provided in the most appropriate form for energy production and protein synthesis. Recognizing the increased metabolic needs of the septic patient who is not carrying out extensive, voluntary muscular exercise, we would currently estimate his daily calorie need at twice the predicted basal metabolic requirement based on his ideal weight. Protein is given at a rate of 2.5 g/kg/day, carbohydrate at 5 mg/kg/min, and the remainder of calories would be supplied as fat.

SPECIFIC SURGICAL INFECTIONS AND THEIR TREATMENT

POSTOPERATIVE INFECTIONS

WOUND INFECTIONS

The identification of infection as an abnormal feature of wound healing is quite recent. Until the concepts of aseptic technique were fully disseminated and implemented, a suppurative wound was the expected norm. The attempt to eliminate wound infection has continued in recent years with the improvement of host defense maintenance and the use of preventive antibiotics. Further advances in the prevention of postoperative infection are currently being sought.

When considering the incidence of wound infections, it is helpful to categorize a wound by the relative amount of contamination present. Table 9-2 shows examples of clean, clean-contaminated, contaminated, and dirty wounds. Clean wounds are those in which only preoperatively sterile tissues are handled, after the skin is incised. Clean-contaminated wounds are those in which only incision into normal skin and sterile tissues, and entry into normal gastrointestinal, genitourinary, or respiratory tracts occur, without gross contamination. Contaminated wounds are those in which gross contamination has occurred, during recent trauma or operation for diseases producing a source of bacteria. Dirty wounds include heavy wound contamination from established bacterial infections, from heavily contaminated trauma, or from previous operation that has resulted in sepsis.

The incidence of clean wound infection is 1% to 5% depending upon the hospital population, the type of operations included, and the completeness of record keeping. The infection rate in dirty wounds is markedly increased and may approach 30% to 50%. These figures are the product of many variables and are necessarily different in each hospital setting. It is important to document these rates in one's own hospital so that continuing focus is kept on elimination of wound infection.

The onset of wound infection is dependent upon the virulence of the infecting organism. Classically, symptoms will appear 3 to 7 days after wounding. Local signs of erythema, edema, pain, and warmth signal an inflammatory response. Because some initial level of acute inflammation occurs as all wounds heal, the key to early diagnosis and therapy of wound infections is in repeated wound observation in the patient, carefully following the signs of normal wound healing. Changes or alterations in the course of normal wound healing are early and reliable signs of developing wound infection.

While abscess with surrounding cellulitis is the most frequent presentation of wound infection, there are other presentations. Cellulitis may be predominant as it is in some streptococcal infections. Also, bacteria may spread through deeper tissues. Such is the case in necrotizing fasciitis, acute hemolytic streptococcal gangrene, anaerobic cellulitis, and clostridial myositis. These fall into the category of severe soft-tissue infections and are discussed in a following section.

When local control of wound infection is lost, regional and systemic effects appear. Lymphangitis, lymphadenopathy, septic thrombophlebitis, and direct deeper extension of the infectious process may occur. In addition, direct access to the bloodstream may produce metastatic abscesses and the symptoms due to bacteremia and toxemia.

As we have noted, diagnosis of wound infection is directly related to clinical observation. A postoperative or traumatic wound should be observed regularly and must be suspect when fever, rigor, inflammation, or tenderness appear. Dressings are removed from primarily closed wounds within 48 hr of surgery and serial observations are made. Diagnosis of infection is confirmed by the appearance of frank cellulitis, a fluctuant tender mass, purulent drainage, or upon the needle aspiration of purulent material. Gram stain and both aerobic and anaerobic cultures must be carefully performed upon any wound drainage.

Therapy of wound abscess consists of incision and drainage. Drainage must continue until the entire cavity is closed, thus preventing the development of another closed-space infection. Therefore, after incision and drainage, wounds should not be primarily closed. Secondary closure, as was discussed in the management of traumatic wounds, is well suited to this purpose. The use of systemic antibiotics is usually limited to the appearance of invasive sepsis, such as significant cellulitis, fever, or other systemic signs of infection, especially in a patient with impaired host defense. Many well-localized infections, therefore, require only incision and drainage.

ABDOMINAL INFECTIONS

Abdominal infections are best categorized on an anatomical basis. These infections may occur as intraperitoneal, retroperitoneal, and visceral abscesses, or as generalized peritonitis. Intraperitoneal and retroperitoneal abscesses are seen most frequently and generally have a surrounding cellulitis (peritonitis), as is seen with other abscesses. Generalized bacterial peritonitis presents a different set of clinical problems and is considered separately. In general, all abdominal infections markedly prolong the hospital course and increase the chance of a fatal outcome in a patient's illness.

Types of Abscess

Intraperitoneal abscesses occur most commonly in the right lower quadrant, followed equally by left lower quadrant, pelvis, and subphrenic areas. They occur when a significant bacterial inoculum is introduced into the normally sterile environment of the peritoneal cavity. Abscesses tend to occur adjacent to the initiating organ of pathology and at the most dependent site. Frequent sources of intraperitoneal abscesses are acute appendicitis, genitourinary tract infections, pancreatic disease, biliary disease, colonic perforation, and enteroanastomotic leakage.

Visceral abscesses are confined within a given abdominal organ. They may be single or multiple and may give rise to significant organ dysfunction. They are caused by primary organ pathology (*e.g.,* hematoma, pancreatitis) or from vascular bacterial seeding from a distant site of sepsis. Visceral abscesses occur most commonly in the liver, but are also encountered in the pancreas, gallbladder, kidney, spleen, and female adnexa.

Retroperitoneal abscesses develop posterior to the abdominal cavity. *True retroperitoneal abscesses* lie between the peritoneum and transversalis fascia, and *retrofascial* abscesses are posterior to the transversalis fascia. However, these sites are often clinically indistinct and will be referred to only as *retroperitoneal*. Infection in the retroperitoneal space is seen frequently and can be secondary to renal, pancreatic, colonic, or appendiceal pathology. This group of abdominal abscesses is most severe, with high morbidity and mortality even when treated optimally.

Bacteriology

The bacteriology of abdominal infections is usually polymicrobic. *Escherichia coli,* bacteroides, the enteric streptococci, and klebsiella are frequently seen. Anaerobic species are present in two thirds of cases. For this reason, careful culture techniques are important to identify the species present and to dictate the appropriate choice of antibiotics (Table 9-3).

Diagnosis

The diagnosis of abdominal infections can be difficult because of the extreme variability in onset of symptoms. Some abscesses may produce modest, nonspecific symptoms for many months prior to proper diagnosis and therapy. Classically, fever, rigor, abdominal tenderness, ileus, jaundice, leukocytosis, and other organ dysfunction are present to varying degrees. When these signs are equivocal in an ill patient, repeated examinations are necessary, as developing abdominal sepsis must be suspected. However, abdominal infections may also present catastrophically, as is frequently seen in generalized peritonitis. In these cases, all of the signs and symptoms of severe abdominal infection may be present, in conjunction with the systemic manifestations of septic shock.

Routine abdominal films and radiological organ imaging have proven inadequate in the diagnosis of intra-abdominal abscess because surgical pathologic findings may be undetected or nonspecific in these studies. Subtraction ^{67}Ga–^{99m}Tc scans, ultrasonography, and computed tomography have been recently applied in an effort to improve our diagnostic means. While all three methods improve diagnosis over conventional methods, and all three areas have continual technical improvements with increased resolution, all three tests continue to have false negative and positive results, taken separately or in combination. Of these three, ultrasonography and computed tomography are most frequently used together, in conjunction with a high degree of clinical suspicion. As such, the diagnosis of abdominal abscess can still be an imprecise science. In the appropriate setting, suspicion is the most important diagnostic factor.

Therapy

The therapy of intra-abdominal abscess consists of surgical drainage, the administration of antibiotics, and general support of the patient. In addition, the initiating pathology needs definition and prompt attention (*e.g.,* transverse diverting colostomy in perforated sigmoid diverticulitis). A technical question to be answered is that of the method of approach to drainage. In general, extraperitoneal drainage is advantageous since it avoids potential peritoneal spread. When transperitoneal drainage is necessary, as in hepatic abscess, it is used with complete abscess evacuation, a therapeutic course of antibiotics, and the placement of drains. General peritoneal lavage should not be performed.

A notable recent advance in the therapy of abdominal abscess is drainage by percutaneous catheter insertion, guided by abscess localization with computerized tomography. While limited studies have been performed to date, this approach offers a remarkable advance in the therapy of abdominal abscesses in certain patients.

Because of the polymicrobic nature of abdominal abscess, therapeutic antibiotic choice usually requires coverage of bacteroides species, gram-negative rods, and the enteric gram-positive cocci. In a seriously ill patient, we currently would use clindamycin, gentamicin, and ampicillin delivered intravenously, until such time as definitive culture and sensitivity results are available from intraoperative abscess sampling. The antibiotic choices are then refined (Table 9-3). A full course of antibiotic therapy is always indicated in the treatment of abdominal infection. Further antibiotic therapy, or change in therapy, will be indicated by the specific patient response.

Generalized Peritonitis

Generalized peritonitis is a special case in which any intra-abdominal pathology may present as a global peritoneal infection. The wide peritoneal spread of any locally occurring process is dependent on several factors. Among these are the number and virulence of the contaminating bacteria, in addition to all facets of host resistance and the absence of a successful "walling off" process.

As we have noted, generalized peritonitis often exhibits as severe abdominal pain and rigidity, in addition to systemic hypovolemia and septic shock. The peritoneum represents a large surface area that reacts quickly to mesothelial injury with increases in vascular permeability and the resultant exudation of fluid, leukocytes, and plasma proteins. The formation of fibrin is prominent in this response and important in "walling off" bacterial infection.

In the treatment of generalized peritonitis the following four points are most important: (*1*) resuscitation to restore normal physiology; (*2*) repair of the originating process; (*3*) removal of necrotic debris; and (*4*) therapeutic systemic antibiotics. Fluid, plasma protein, and electrolyte balance must be aggressively corrected and maintained. Because the microbiology of peritonitis is identical to that of abdominal abscess, initial antibiotic choices and refinement of these choices are made in the same manner (Table 9-3).

The purpose of operative intervention in generalized peritonitis is to repair the initiating process, to débride necrotic tissue, and to reduce the bacterial load. The repair, however, is essential to the survival of the patient, as continued soilage of the abdominal cavity portends a septic death. An example of repair is a diverting sigmoid colostomy and mucous fistula in the operative treatment of perforated sigmoid diverticulitis.

As opposed to the case with abscesses, operative peritoneal lavage with saline can dilute the bacterial load in peritonitis. Fluids and electrolytes require special attention when lavage is performed, however. Also, there have been favorable reports of continuous peritoneal lavage after surgery for generalized peritonitis through catheters left in each abdominal quadrant. Continuous lavage will require further trial before it becomes widely accepted. A second controversial method, that of radical intraperitoneal débridement, has also been proposed. In this method, all fibrinous exudate and compromised tissues are excised in order to reduce the bacterial load and the available culture media. To date, this extensive operative procedure has gained little support.

URINARY TRACT INFECTIONS

Urinary tract infections are frequently seen in the care of the surgical patient. In one series of hospitalized patients with gram-negative sepsis, these infections accounted for 50% of the total. While these infections do occur in the noncatheterized patient, catheter-related infections are most common.

Catheter-related infections are a function of the number, the duration, and the management of indwelling urinary catheters. Bacteria may achieve access to the bladder by ascending outside the catheter, or through the catheter lumen as a result of being introduced by nonsterile technique or reflux of contaminated urine from the collection bag.

In order to minimize infection, catheters should be used only when strictly indicated. They are not a tool of convenience. The technique of catheterization is performed observing sterile procedure. Obvious breaks of technique during insertion require the replacement of any nonsterile equipment with that known to be sterile. The patient's skin may need to be reprepared, as well. As with other invasive devices, catheters should be removed when no longer indicated.

Catheter management requires the use of closed urinary drainage. Disconnections of this apparatus should occur only for very good reasons, and then in sterile fashion. Irrigation of the catheter must be done sterilely, and only when obstructed. Meatal and perineal care should consist of careful hygiene and the application of an antimicrobial ointment.

Surveillance for infection must be performed on a regular basis through the use of urinalysis and culture data. Samples can be drawn sterilely, through the catheter wall, with use of needle and syringe. In addition, the use of other urinary devices, such as the condom or suprapubic catheter, may be more appropriate and at less risk in certain patients.

Therapy of urinary tract infection, once it occurs, requires adequate culture and antibiotic sensitivity data. Appropriate antibiotic therapy is chosen and continued for 7 to 14 days depending on the severity of infection and response. If a catheter is present and can be removed, it is removed. If the catheter is still necessary, then it should be replaced. In addition, if the infection is difficult to clear, other predisposing patient factors, such as obstruction, congenital abnormality, or lithiasis must be considered.

RESPIRATORY INFECTION

Pneumonia intervenes in the surgical patient's course on a regular basis. The factors predisposing to bacterial pneumonia are the toxic effects of anesthesia, aspiration of oropharyngeal or gastric contents, atelectasis, and underlying disease. In addition, manipulation of the tracheobronchial tree may bypass or thwart normal defense mechanisms.

Anesthetic gases have direct toxic effects on the cells that clear mucus and particulate matter. Preanesthetic medications increase secretion viscosity, thereby increasing the difficulty of clearance. Mechanical ventilation and postoperative convalescence produce atelectasis, which predisposes to pneumonia. In addition, aspiration of gastric contents causes a chemical pneumonitis. The resultant chemical pulmonary damage markedly increases the likelihood of secondary bacterial infection. Therefore, the prevention of aspiration is important. Assuring gastric emptying prior to anesthesia and elevating the patient's head when obtunded are imperative.

Acute viral infection and chronic obstructive pulmonary disease (COPD) also predispose to bacterial pneumonia since they impair clearance and other defense mechanisms. For this reason, general anesthesia should be postponed, if possible, in the face of severe viral infection or the case of exacerbation in COPD. In both of these cases, mucus viscosity increases and transport decreases.

Careful management of the tracheostomized or intubated patient is important. Stomal hygiene must be meticulous and suctioning techniques performed in sterile fashion. The use of ventilators and nebulizing equipment carries the risk of patient cross-contamination, so that careful cleaning techniques are mandatory.

Diagnosis of pulmonary infection is as in other patients. The information obtained from chest radiogram, sputum culture and gram stain, bronchoscopy, and blood culture are all important. Therapy of pneumonia is the administration of an adequate course of culture-dictated antibiotics, careful pulmonary toilet, and physiotherapy. In addition, the identification of those factors that may have predisposed to the development of infection should be addressed and appropriate changes made.

INTRAVENOUS AND ARTERIAL LINE SEPSIS

The use of intravenous and arterial catheters produces the risk of catheter-induced infection. These infections are due to contaminated catheters, infected catheter sites, and infusion of contaminated fluids. Line sepsis is related to the success of sterile placement, catheter maintenance techniques, the length of catheterization, other sources of bacteria such as the burn wound or abdominal abscess, and the level of patient resistance.

Both central and peripheral venous catheters carry the risk of infection. The use of hyperalimentation, however, increases the risk of catheter-related infection to between 3% and 10%. Total parenteral nutrition (TPN) solutions are excellent culture media. For this reason, all handling of TPN solutions and manipulation of infusion systems must be done sterilely. Insertion of TPN catheters includes sterile procedure and dressings, and TPN solutions themselves should be mixed in laminar flow hoods. Solutions and infusion equipment are used for limited lengths of time and in-line filters are employed. Additionally, TPN catheters need to be replaced on a regular basis and should be used only for hyperalimentation. When in proximity to bacterially colonized wounds, as in burn patients, these catheters are replaced every 3 days, as the risk of associated infection increases dramatically.

Peripheral arterial catheters are less susceptible to infection than peripheral venous catheters. Steel needles harbor fewer bacteria than plastic cannulae, but both need regular replacement and inspection. Again, the careful attention to sterility of infusion apparatus and medication administration is important.

The diagnosis of catheter related infection can be difficult. The diagnosis is made when systemic signs of bacterial or fungal infection occur without anatomical source and resolve with catheter removal. Suspect catheters should be cultured and blood cultures drawn at a remote site. In addition, septic thrombophlebitis presents as an inflamed, suppurative venous infusion site.

Therapy of catheter-related bacteremia requires catheter removal. A full course of an appropriate systemic antibiotic is used when signs of sepsis do not immediately resolve or when general or regional host defenses are impaired (*e.g.,* immunosuppression in a cancer patient, rheumatic heart disease). Peripheral septic thrombophlebitis requires antibiotic therapy and the excision of the involved vein.

We also note that the use of blood products carries the finite risk of contamination and infection. The commonly encountered transmissible diseases are hepatitis, malaria, and cytomegalovirus infection.

INFECTIONS CAUSED BY SPECIFIC ORGANISMS OR AT SPECIAL SITES

STAPHYLOCOCCAL INFECTIONS

Staphylococcal infections are usually localized infections and are often characterized by cellulitis surrounding an area of central necrosis, containing thick, creamy, yellow or reddish-yellow pus that is usually odorless. Staphylococci are frequently the cause of bacterial illness, producing folliculitis, furuncles,and carbuncles, as well as more serious invasive infections. The treatment of an established staphylococcal infection usually includes surgical drainage, as well as rest, heat, and elevation. If the infection is well localized and there is no surrounding cellulitis or systemic response, antibiotic therapy adds little to effective drainage of the abscess itself. Appropriate antibiotic therapy, however, adds to the effectiveness of treatment if invasive infection is present in addition to the localized collection of purulent material (Table 9-3).

BETA HEMOLYTIC STREPTOCOCCAL INFECTIONS

Beta hemolytic streptococci produce a rapidly invasive spreading infection, tending to cause extensive cellulitis with a marked systemic response, rather than localized areas of abscess formation, as is the case with staphylococci. Erysipelas is an example of beta hemolytic streptococcal cellulitis, and the infection may be heralded by chills, high fever, rapid pulse, and severe toxemia. Purulent material, if present, is thin and watery, and invasion of the blood and lymphatic streams is frequently seen. Beta hemolytic streptococcal cellulitis is a serious infection that may develop into a life-threatening systemic infection in hours and must be treated vigorously for proper control. Antibiotic therapy, plus rest, heat, and elevation of the infected area are essential for early control of the invasive process, and in infection without a localized collection of purulent or necrotic material drainage has little to add (Table 9-3).

Acute hemolytic streptococcal gangrene is a necrotizing cellulitis that frequently follows minor, nonoperative trauma. The intense cellulitis noted above appears first, followed by cyanotic skin, the formation of blebs containing dark fluid, and eventual dermal gangrene due to thrombosis.

The differential diagnosis of acute hemolytic streptococcal gangrene includes anaerobic cellulitis and necrotizing fasciitis. Emergency longitudinal incision through superficial fascia, beyond the extent of involvement, is performed to limit ischemia by decompression. The blebs are drained, systemic penicillin is used, and the affected part is dressed, elevated and rested.

NECROTIZING FASCIITIS

Necrotizing fasciitis is an infectious process that produces rapid necrosis of tissue, spreading along fascial planes. It is most often caused by the synergism of gram-positive cocci and gram-negative rods. It presents as a sudden toxemia with fever, tachycardia, and acute hemolysis. Necrotizing fasciitis usually occurs in a postoperative wound, often after the gastrointestinal tract has been opened.

Clinical signs include easy fascial dissection when probed, little local pain, and lymphedema. Cutaneous gangrene and bleb formation may occur in more advanced cases, but are absent early. Hypocalcemia and fluid losses may be a problem.

The treatment of necrotizing fasciitis is radical incision and drainage. The overlying tissue is incised in all directions until viable fascia is found. The overlying tissues are necessarily undermined. The wound is packed open and continuously irrigated through operatively placed catheters. Repeated incision or excision may be necessary. Broad-spectrum antibiotics are employed to cover the synergistic organisms until sensitivity reports are available.

When the infection is controlled, allograft may be used to tentatively close the wound. As wound sterility is regained, the skin flaps may be approximated, as in delayed primary closure, and any defects are then autografted.

ANAEROBIC CELLULITIS

Anaerobic cellulitis is a mixed, sometimes crepitant infection often seen following wounds of the perineum, abdominal wall, buttocks, hip, thorax, or neck. Usually these wounds have been contaminated by material from the gastrointestinal, genitourinary, or respiratory tracts. No single bacterial etiology has been identified, but the mixed infection usually contains strains of the coliforms, bacteroides, anaerobic streptococci, and occasionally clostridium. The infection spreads along several tissue layers, causing progressive gangrenous changes in the skin as a result of vascular thrombosis. The purulent material is thin with a putrid odor.

Wide surgical drainage with excision of necrotic tissue is imperative for the control of this type of infection. Broad spectrum antibiotic therapy is again necessary until culture sensitivities are available. Serious depletion of circulatory volume and shock may follow these infections. Systemic support with adequate fluid replacement is therefore essential for effective treatment.

CLOSTRIDIAL MYOSITIS (GAS GANGRENE)

Clostridial organisms may produce a life-threatening gangrenous infection of muscle that is rapidly progressive and causes extensive, life-threatening systemic as well as local abnormalities. The infection usually follows injuries of the extremities, buttocks, or trunk that are associated with devitalized muscle. Delayed or inadequate surgical care provides important predisposing factors.

Pain is an early symptom of clostridial myositis, appearing usually within the first 24 hr after injury. At this time crepitus may be present in the tissue, but extensive edema may occur in clostridial myositis without gas formation. The patient develops rapidly progressing systemic and local signs; pain is prominent and a striking pallor of the face is common, with weakness, apathy, profuse sweating, prostration, and shortness of breath. The pulse is rapid and feeble, but fever is seldom over 38.5°C. The discharge is thin, watery brown, and foul smelling, usually containing many bacteria and red blood cells but few white cells.

Soluble toxins diffusing into the circulation from the involved tissue produce a severe hemolytic anemia and renal, cardiac, and hepatic damage, as well as septic shock, which may lead to death if treatment does not intervene. Laboratory data include a severe anemia and a relatively low white count, seldom exceeding 15,000 cells per mm.

The early diagnosis of gas gangrene is essential if treatment is to be successful. Early diagnosis at times may be difficult because the infection often follows treatment of a severe injury that may obscure early signs of clostridial infection. However, continued pain at the site of the injury and a rapid and faint pulse with minimal fever, combined with a rapidly spreading toxemia, are signs demanding immediate surgical exploration of the wound. Other signs of importance include a thin, watery brown, foul-smelling exudate, dusky or bronze appearance of the skin overlying the wound, with vesicles filled with dark red fluid, crepitus, and herniation of dark red discolored muscle.

Treatment includes the immediate surgical exploration of any wound in which the presence of clostridial myositis is suspected. Wide incision and débridement of involved muscle are essentials of effective treatment. Intensive antibiotic therapy should be employed, usually using penicillin intravenously. Supportive therapy is crucial for maintaining fluid and electrolyte balance, as well as to correct a severe anemia and decreased circulatory volume produced by the infection. Several authors have advised the use of hyperbaric oxygen in the treatment of gas gangrene.

TETANUS

Tetanus is caused by a toxin produced by the anaerobic bacterium *Clostridium tetani*. As the bacteria grow in the tissue, a soluble toxin is produced that diffuses, acting locally on neuromuscular end organs and causing local tonic contraction, and systemically on susceptible cells in the central nervous system, resulting in trismus, rigidity, and generalized clonic convulsions, often precipitated by external stimulation of the patient.

The successful treatment of tetanus depends on early diagnosis, neutralization of circulating toxin, elimination of the bacterial infection caused by the tetanus bacilli, and the control of systemic manifestations, such as convulsions, using sedation or curarelike drugs if necessary. Complete local excision of the tetanus infection should be carried out whenever possible. Nasotracheal intubation or tracheostomy may be considered if convulsions seriously interfere with respiration. Antibiotic therapy, although not effective in controlling the effects of tetanus toxin, should be vigorously pursued in the attempt to extirpate the bacterial lesion (Table 9-3). Human antitetanus globulin (250 units) should be used to neutralize circulating toxin, and the patient should be actively immunized with 0.5 ml of tetanus toxoid. A dose of 500 units of globulin is recommended in severe cases.

Here again, prevention of clinical tetanus is far more effective than treatment of the clinical disease. Prevention depends on adequate immunization of the population, plus expert surgical management of all traumatic wounds, no matter how minor. Patients with wounds that are grossly contaminated, in the setting of an unclear or inadequate immunization history, should also receive antitoxin therapy. The IM doses are 250 units for patients older than 10 years, 125 units for ages 5 to 10 years, and 75 units for those younger than 5 years. Active immunization with tetanus toxoid is also instituted.

GRAM-NEGATIVE BACTERIAL INFECTIONS

Gram-negative infections have steadily become more prominent over the past 10 years and now make up over half of the infections following trauma or infections complicating surgery. *E. coli, Pseudomonas aeruginosa,* strains of proteus species, and klebsiella are frequently the causative orga-

nisms. In debilitated patients, or in patients in whom debridement of dead tissue has been incomplete, invasive lesions caused by these bacteria frequently occur. These organisms often cause serious infections and they have become a frequent cause of death following trauma. The treatment of infections produced by gram-negative bacteria includes surgical incision and drainage of any abscesses, excision of necrotic tissue, and appropriate antibiotic therapy, as well as extensive systemic and nutritional support of the infected patient. Gram-negative bacteria are usually of relatively low virulence, and invasive infection with one of these organisms may indicate serious systemic or nutritional abnormalities that must be corrected before the infection can be brought under control. Systemic and nutritional support, therefore, are particularly important in patients in whom invasive gram-negative infection is present.

BACTEROIDES

A bacteroides infection may occur as a monobacterial infection or as an anaerobic component of a mixed infection. Here, careful anaerobic as well as aerobic bacteriology is important in establishing a diagnosis that will allow effective antibiotic therapy to be carried out. Again, drainage of abscesses and excision of foreign or necrotic material are essential components of therapy, for antibiotic therapy alone seldom produces a permanent cure.

INFECTIONS FOLLOWING HUMAN BITES

Human bite infections are produced by mouth organisms that cause serious invasive infection. A mixture of organisms is almost always found, consisting of aerobic nonhemolytic streptococci, staphylococci, anaerobic streptococci, or spirochetes. In human bite infections, particularly those of the dorsum of the hand, extensive débridement with wide opening of tissue planes and débridement of necrotic tissue, as well as immobilization and antibiotic therapy (usually consisting of penicillin) are essential. When the infection develops, extensive decompression of the infected area with débridement of necrotic tissue, as well as intensive antibiotic therapy, must be carried out. Immobilization, heat, and elevation add to the protection against further spread of the bacterial process.

FUNGAL INFECTIONS

In recent years, fungal infections have become more frequent in the case of seriously ill patients. This trend is due to the identification of previously unrecognized disease and as a result of the care of more debilitated patients, who previously would have died of their primary diseases.

Candida

Candida albicans sepsis is an important infectious entity. It occurs most frequently in the setting of immunocompromised, major burn injury, diabetes mellitus, central venous hyperalimentation, and long-term antibiotic therapy. Yeast colonization and invasion occur most often at catheter sites or are due to gastrointestinal overgrowth. Direct wound invasion is apparently uncommon. Candidemic seeding of secondary sites, however, creates important infections, requiring eradication. These secondary infections include candida myocarditis, osteomyelitis, endophthalmitis, and meningitis.

The diagnosis of candidemia should be suspected in susceptible population groups when the systemic signs of sepsis are uncontrolled by adequate antibacterial therapy.

Urinary budding yeast cells are almost always seen, as are positive arterial candida cultures, in clinically significant candidemia. Venous fungal cultures are inadequate due to the efficient filtering effect of capillary beds.

Therapy of confirmed candida sepsis, as outlined by Stone, includes (*1*) control of the entry, (*2*) the elimination of predisposing factors, and (*3*) consideration of the administration of a parenteral antifungal drug. Venous catheters must be removed and cultured and the gastrointestinal tract should be treated with oral nystatin. Long-term antibiotic or immunosuppressive therapy should be interrupted to allow the recovery of bacterial flora and host defense, respectively.

Amphotericin B is a valuable, though toxic, antibiotic in the therapy of severe fungal infections. The indications for the use of amphotericin B can be problematic, however. Simply removing a contaminated hyperalimentation line may be sufficient to eliminate infection in a stable patient. However, a severely compromised clinical status or a secondary candida focus, certainly require the use of parenteral therapy. An initial test dose of 1 gm of amphotericin B in dextrose solution is usually given, followed by 5 mg increments in dosages up to the daily maintenance dose. Maintenance dose will depend on patient size and tolerance. Total cumulative dose in deep-seated infections in adults approaches 2 g.

Actinomyces

Actinomyces israelii produces a mycotic infection usually characterized by the development of nodular, granulomatous areas, with eventual suppuration and discharge of purulent material through sinus tracts. The purulent discharge contains characteristic ''sulfur granules,'' which are masses of lightly entwined mycelial filaments visible to the eye. If infection runs a chronic course, it produces a burrowing process into adjacent tissues but usually does not spread along regional lymphatics. Actinomyces infections are common in the cervicofacial, thoracic, and abdominal areas, and are usually secondary to local injury or a preceding bacterial infection.

The treatment of an actinomyces infection consists of surgical incision and drainage or, if possible, excision of the entire abscess process, together with a prolonged course of antibiotic (usually penicillin).

Partially supported by USPH GM 07035 and GM 021700.

BIBLIOGRAPHY

ALEXANDER JW: Host defense mechanisms against infection. Surg Clin North Am 52:1367, 1972

ALTEMEIER WA, BURKE JF, PRUITT BA, et al: Manual on Control of Infection in Surgical Patients. Philadelphia, J B Lippincott, 1976

ALTEMEIER WA, CULBERTSON WR, FULLEN WD et al: Intra-abdominal abscesses. Am J Surg 125:70, 1973

American College of Surgeons Committee on Trauma: A Guide to Prophylaxis Against Tetanus in Wound Management. Chicago, American College of Surgeons, 1979

ANDERSON CB; MARR JJ, BALLINGER EF: Anaerobic infections in surgery: Clinical review. Surgery 79:313, 1976

BAXTER CR: Surgical management of soft tissue infections. Surg Clin North Am 52:1483, 1972

BECK WC: Aseptic barriers in surgery. Arch Surg 116:240, 1981

BERNARD HR, COLE WR: The prophylaxis of surgical infection: The effect of prophylactic antimicrobial drugs on the incidence of infection following potentially contaminated operations. Surgery 56:141, 1964

BURKE JF: The effective period of preventive antibiotic action in experimental incisions and dermal lesions. Surgery 50:161, 1961

BURKE JF: Preventive antibiotic management in surgery. Ann Rev Med 24:289, 1973

BURKE JF: Fundamentals of Wound Management in Surgery: Infection. New York, Appleton-Century-Crofts, 1977

BURKE JF: Prevention of sepsis following surgical operation: An overview. In Karran S (ed): Controversies in Surgical Sepsis. New York, Praeger Publishers, 1980

CHODAK GW, PLANT ME: Use of systemic antibiotics for prophylaxis in surgery. Arch Surg 112:326, 1977

The choice of antimicrobial drugs. The Medical Letter 22:5, 1980

CLOWES GHA JR: The metabolic effects of peritonitis and other major infections. In Hardy JD (ed): Textbook of Surgery, 5th ed. Philadelphia. J B Lippincott, 1977

CRUSE PJE, FOORD R: A five-year prospective study of 23,649 surgical wounds. Arch Surg 107:206, 1973

CURRIE DJ: Continuous peritoneal lavage. Surg Gynecol Obstet 135:951, 1972

EDLICH RF, ROGERS W, KASPER G et al: Studies in the management of the contaminated wound. Am J Surg 117:323, 1969

EDWARDS LD: The epidemiology of 2056 remote site infections and 1966 surgical wound infections occurring in 1865 patients. Ann Surg 184:758, 1976

GERZOF SG, ROBBINS AH, JOHNSON WC et al: Percutaneous catheter drainage of abdominal abscesses: A five-year experience. N Engl J Med 305:653, 1981

HAU T, AHRENHOLZ DH, SIMMONS RL: Secondary bacterial peritonitis: The biologic basis of treatment. Curr Probl Surg 16: 1979

HIRSCH EF, CLARKE JR, GOMEZ-ENGLER HE et al: The lung: Responses to trauma, surgery and sepsis. Surg Clin North Am 56:909, 1976

HUDSPETH AS: Radical surgical debridement and the treatment of advanced generalized bacterial peritonitis. Arch Surg 110:1233, 1975

KUNIN CM: Detection, Prevention and Management of Urinary Tract Infections, 3rd ed. Philadelphia. Lea & Febiger, 1979

LEAK IV, BURKE JF: Early events of tissue injury and the role of the lymphatic system in early inflammation. In Zweifach BW, Grant L, McCluskey RT (eds): The Inflammatory Process, vol 3, 2nd ed. New York, Academic Press, 1974

MOLNAR JA, BURKE JF: Nutritional aspects of surgical physiology. In Burke JD (ed): Surgical Physiology. Philadelphia, W B Saunders, 1982

NORTON L, EULE J, BURDICK D: Accuracy of techniques to detect intraperitoneal abscess. Surgery 84:370, 1978

O'LOUGHLIN JM: Infections in the immunosuppressed patient. Med Clin North Am 59:495, 1975

ROE CF: Fever in surgical patients. In Hardy JD (ed): Textbook of Surgery, 5th ed. Philadelphia. J B Lippincott, 1977

RYAN JA, ABEL RM, ABBOTT WM et al: Catheter complications in total parenteral nutrition. N Engl J Med 290:757, 1974

SHEAGREN JH: Septic shock and corticosteroids. N Engl J Med 305:456, 1981

SHUBIN H, WEIL MH: Bacterial shock. JAMA 235:421, 1976

STEPHEN M, LOWENTHAL J: Continuing peritoneal lavage in high-risk peritonitis. Surgery 85:603, 1979

STONE HH, KOLB LD, CURRIE CA et al: Candida sepsis: Pathogenesis and principles and treatment. Ann Surg 179:697, 1974

WEINSTEIN L: Tetanus. N Engl J Med 289:1923, 1973

WEINSTEIN L, BORZA MA: Gas gangrene. N Engl J Med 289:1129, 1973

WINSLOW EJ, LOEB HS, RAHIMTOOLA S et al: Hemodynamic studies and results of therapy in 50 patients with bacteremic shock. Am J Med 54:421, 1973

Donald D. Trunkey/James W. Holcroft

Trauma: General Survey and Synopsis of Management of Specific Injuries

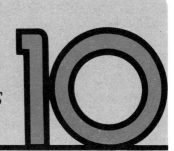

OVERVIEW

Trauma is a major health and social problem. It is the number-one cause of death for people up to the age of 38 and accounted for 164,000 deaths in 1980. The death rate due to trauma between the ages of 15 and 24 increased from 106 per 100,000 to 120 per 100,000 between 1960 to 1978, an increase of 13%. During the same period, the death rate for ages 25 to 64 declined 16%. Murders increased from 8464 annually in 1960 to 24,800 in 1980. The overall death rate for American teens and young adults is 50% higher than for their counterparts in Britain, Sweden, and Japan. Trauma affects young productive citizens, and the estimated cost for death, disability, and loss of productivity exceeds $225 million a day. The most tragic statistic is that at least half the deaths are needless and could be prevented if better programs of treatment, education, and research were linked in an operational system. Optimal trauma treatment programs include preplanned operation of an emergency medical service (EMS) system, which includes carefully defined injury levels of patients related to hospital and prehospital response capabilities.

In 1976, the American College of Surgeons' Committee on Trauma presented optimal guidelines for the care of trauma patients. These have subsequently been updated and additional guidelines presented. The intent of the guidelines is to fulfill the "three Rs": Get the *right* patient to the *right* hospital at the *right* time. The right hospital implies a facility staffed and equipped to deal with all the problems of the injured patient.

Guidelines for categorization of patients by field personnel have been developed (Table 10-1). This is a further attempt to triage patients to an appropriate facility, recognizing that most trauma victims (category 3) do not require treatment in a major trauma center.

Optimal care of the trauma patient implies rapid, prompt transportation with adequately trained field personnel to care for victims. Until recently, the United States had not had organized rotary-wing transportation as part of an organized EMS system. Fixed-wing aircraft have been available for some time on a sporadic basis. Rotary-wing aircraft have repeatedly proved their value in the transport of the seriously injured patient, both in Vietnam and in civilian situations.

There are many controversial areas in the provision of trauma care that have yet to be resolved. The first of these is whether or not it is better for ambulances to bypass certain hospitals and take the critically injured patient directly to a designated major trauma facility. This question addresses the issues involved in setting up a regionalized trauma system. The relation of mortality to the interval between injury and treatment is listed in Table 10-2, which demonstrates that mortality has dropped dramatically since

TABLE 10-2   RELATION OF MORTALITY TO INTERVAL BETWEEN INJURY AND TREATMENT

Conflict	Interval (hr)	Mortality Rate (%)
WW I	12–18	8.5
WW II	6–12	5.8
Korea	2–4	2.4
Vietnam	1–4	1.7

TABLE 10-1   FIELD CATEGORIZATION OF TRAUMA PATIENTS

System	Category 1	Category 2	Category 3
Soft tissue	Avulsion type injuries, severe uncontrolled bleeding	Soft-tissue injuries with stabilized bleeding	Soft-tissue injuries of moderate degree
Fractures	Open fractures, pelvic fractures, severe maxillofacial injuries	Single open or closed fractures	Uncomplicated fractures
Abdomen	Blunt or penetrating abdominal injuries especially when associated with hypotension	Blunt abdominal or penetrating trauma not producing hypotension	No abdominal injuries
Chest	Unstable chest injuries, respiratory rate > 30 or < 10	Multiple rib fractures without flailed segments, respiratory rate > 20 or < 10	No respiratory distress, respiratory rate 10-20
Head & neck, upper respiratory	Severe maxillofacial injuries; open penetrating and blunt trauma to face, neck, and cervical spine; multiple facial fractures; injuries affecting vision	Facial trauma with single facial fractures (without airway or major cervical vascular or cervical spine involvement)	Simple contusions of the head and neck, nasal fractures
Neurologic	Prolonged loss of consciousness, posturing, lateralizing signs, open cranial injuries, paralysis	Transient loss of consciousness, oriented to time, place, and person	No neurologic injuries
Vital signs	BP < 90 systolic P > 100 or < 60 Skin—cool, ashen, pale	BP > 90 systolic P—60-100 Skin—warm to slightly cool	BP > 100 systolic P—60-100 Skin—dry, warm

(Reprinted with permission from the February Bulletin of the American College of Surgeons, 1980)

World War I. It could be argued that this reduced mortality is in large part due to improved anesthesia, antibiotics, and other medical advances. These advances probably do contribute, but they would probably be offset by introduction of more devastating weapons and their resultant injuries. One cannot ignore that the average delivery time from injury to *definitive* care was approximately 81 minutes in the Vietnam conflict. Therefore, the military concept of bypassing the battalion aid station and the division surgical hospital and taking the victim directly to the corps surgical hospital is a valid one. The analogy is obvious: If we have rapid ground or air transportation with highly trained paramedics to initiate resuscitation and treatment, it is logical to bypass some hospitals and emergency rooms to get the victim to a definitive-care facility.

Another controversy deals with the type of personnel who care for the trauma patient. Historically and traditionally, the trauma patient has always been cared for by the surgeon. After 5 to 6 years of surgical residency, the surgeon is well suited to care for the patient who has sustained massive injury and shock. More recently, the emergency physician has assumed a more visible and important role in the initial care of the trauma patient. Probably the most important asset of the emergency physician is availability. The controversy occurs only when definitive care is delayed. Trauma is a disease that should be cared for as soon as possible by the surgeon. In large urban and suburban areas, it does not make sense that a category 1 or 2 trauma patient should stop at a hospital emergency room to be resuscitated, stabilized, and transferred. The civilian experience in various trauma centers in the United States lends credibility and support to the military concept of bypassing certain hospitals. In rural areas, the case is not as strong, and it may be more reasonable to stop at a less qualified hospital for resuscitation and stabilization and transfer to a major trauma center.

The composition of the trauma team will vary region to region and hospital to hospital. The American College of Surgeons has suggested that the trauma team include a general surgeon, anesthesiologist, neurosurgeon, orthopaedic surgeon, urologist, plastic surgeon, pediatric surgeon, thoracic surgeon, and all the consultative services normally present in a large community hospital. For major trauma facilities, it is recommended that the general surgeon and anesthesiologist be in-house 24 hours a day, with prompt response time by the other surgical specialties.

The trauma team must have a predetermined leader. This person must act as "captain of the ship" and direct the care of the patients admitted during his "tour of duty." He must also assume follow-up care and responsibility until the patient is ready for discharge or is transferred to a rehabilitation center. In most instances, this leader would be the general surgeon, and although the general surgeon may never operate on the patient, he must direct the various surgical specialities and other physicians involved in the care of the patient. Ideally, only one physician should write the orders on a patient, and the person writing the orders should be the trauma team leader. This serves to minimize errors and to personalize the care of the injured patient.

INITIAL MANAGEMENT IN THE EMERGENCY ROOM

As a result of rapid patient transport, we are now receiving seriously injured patients who in the past might have died prior to their arrival in an emergency room.

Field personnel should notify the hospital that is to receive the seriously injured patient so that a trauma team can be mobilized before the patient arrives in the emergency room. If the patient is undergoing cardiopulmonary resuscitation, the trauma team should proceed with that resuscitation. If the patient has vital signs, he should be stripped of clothing and, provided there are no contraindications, rolled from side to side to assess the back for injuries. The physician should note the pattern of breathing and the movement of the chest with breathing. He should look for injuries to the mouth and anterior neck and palpate for the carotid pulse and for the position of the trachea. He should inspect the neck veins; their character is the key in determining whether shock is based on hypovolemic or cardiogenic mechanisms. The skin of the toes and foot of one extremity should be examined; if cool, pale, and clammy, shock should be presumed.

This entire initial examination should take no longer

QUICK ASSESSMENT OF PATIENT IN PROFOUND SHOCK

Feel extremity

↓

Cool, pale
Capillary refill > 2 seconds

↓

Clinical shock

↙   ↘

Neck veins flat   Neck veins full

↓   ↓

Hypovolemic shock   Tension pneumothorax
until proven   Pericardial tamponade
otherwise   Myocardial contusion
                                       Myocardial infarct
                                       Air embolism

PRIORITIES IN EVALUATION AND RESUSCITATION OF THE TRAUMA VICTIM

First Priorities
1. Airway
2. Bleeding—control of rapid external hemorrhage
3. Cardiovascular
   a. pump
   b. volume—vascular access, fluid resuscitation

Second Priorities
4. The second examination
   a. Neurologic
   b. Orthopaedic
5. Occult hemorrhage
6. Radiologic procedures
7. Definitive diagnosis and care

than a few seconds. Attention should then be turned to the priorities of evaluation and resuscitation, with the goal being to deliver oxygen and nutrients to the heart and brain as soon as possible. Accordingly, attention should be directed first to the airway and ventilation, second to control of massive external bleeding, and third to the cardiovascular system: the ABCs of resuscitation.

AIRWAY AND VENTILATION

The first priority in resuscitating the trauma patient is to recognize and treat inadequacy of airway or ventilation or both (Fig. 10-1). The signs of airway obstruction and ventilatory insufficiency are similar: stridor, cyanosis, anxiety, intercostal retractions, use of the accessory muscles of ventilation, and tachypnea with a ventilatory rate of more than 25/minute. Sometimes the signs are subtle; as the patient weakens, he may struggle less. Unconscious patients should be intubated.

The oropharynx should be gently cleared with a tonsil sucker or the examiner's fingers. The back of the tongue should be brought forward, away from the oropharynx, by displacing the angles of the jaw anteriorly. Insertion of an oral or nasal airway sometimes helps to keep the tongue forward. In patients with massive maxillofacial injuries, the tongue itself can be pulled forward. To secure pressure on the tongue, the examiner can wrap a gauze around the tongue; the midline of the tongue may also be pierced with a towel clamp or a suture, which is then used to pull the tongue forward. The patient should be given several breaths of 100% oxygen with an ambu bag and a face mask and then intubated, through either the mouth or the nose. If attempted oral or nasal intubation fails to secure an airway within 60 seconds, and if the patient cannot be ventilated with a mask, access to the trachea should be gained through the cricothyroid membrane.

Surgeons and physicians familiar with surgical techniques should cut down on the membrane, insert the handle of

Fig. 10-1. This patient, with a gunshot wound to the face, represents a severe airway problem. The great majority of patients can be managed with orotracheal or nasotracheal intubation, as shown here.

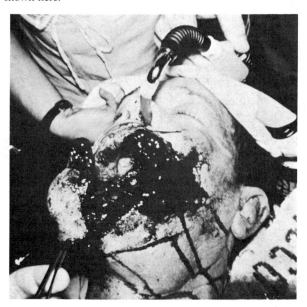

the scalpel into the trachea, twist the handle so as to enlarge the tracheal opening, and insert a tracheostomy tube or cuffed pediatric endotracheal tube. Physicians unfamiliar with surgical techniques can percutaneously insert two sharp-ended 14-gauge needles through the cricothyroid membrane into the trachea. In theory, cricothyroidostomies can lead to tracheal stenoses; in practice, short-term cricothyroidostomies rarely do, except perhaps in children. The only contraindication to a cricothyroidostomy is a complete laryngeal separation.

Cricothyroidostomies offer several advantages over the puncture technique. A tracheostomy or endotracheal tube allows suctioning of the tracheobronchial tree; needles do not. Tubes offer less resistance to airflow and ventilation than do needles. Adapters that attach mechanical ventilators to tracheostomy tubes are available in most emergency rooms; adapters for needles are often hard to find.

The same sequence of steps for securing the airway should be used in the conscious patient, but it is usually not necessary to go as far as emergency intubation. If there is no sign of head or neck injury, the patient's head can be turned to the side and the oropharynx cleared with the sucker. If the airway is still obstructed, the tongue should be brought forward by displacing the angles of the jaw forward or by inserting a pharyngeal airway. These maneuvers are usually sufficient; if not, the patient should be intubated.

Conscious patients frequently assume the position that gives them the best airway. Patients with fractures of the mandible may sit up and hang their head forward so as to let the mandible and its attached tongue fall away from the back of the throat. They should not be forced into a recumbent position.

Conscious patients frequently struggle as attempts are made to establish an airway. The physician must show fine judgment in this situation. On the one hand, many struggling patients are more than strong enough and awake enough to maintain their airway and oxygenate and ventilate themselves; too-vigorous attempts to establish an airway, with suctioning and attempted passage of endotracheal tubes, may lead to vomiting and aspiration. On the other hand, some conscious patients begin to struggle when they become hypoxemic; in this situation, the physician must be aggressive in securing the airway. To distinguish these two situations, the physician should note the struggling specifically associated with ventilatory insufficiency: stridor, intercostal retractions, use of the accessory muscles, and tachypnea. If these findings are present, he must proceed aggressively. If, on the other hand, the patient is struggling in a nonspecific manner, treatment can be more deliberate.

On a rare occasion, the physician will be forced to use a paralyzing agent in the struggling patient with an obstructed airway. If such an agent is used, the physician must be prepared to secure the airway for the patient within 60 seconds because the patient will lose his protective reflexes with the paralysis and will depend entirely upon the physician. The physician must be ready to perform a cricothyroidostomy if necessary; otherwise, he should not give the paralyzing agent in the first place.

Once the airway is established, ventilation must be ensured. Open pneumothoraces should be closed with occlusive dressings. Flail segments of the chest wall should be stabilized by placing sandbags next to the flail or by turning the patient so that the flail segment is against the mattress. Chest tubes should be inserted to evacuate pneumothoraces and massive hemothoraces. If the patient requires intubation, positive-pressure ventilation should be provided mechanically.

BLEEDING

Control of external bleeding has usually been achieved by paramedics prior to the patient's arrival in the emergency department. If not, external bleeding should be controlled simultaneously with establishment of airway and ventilation. Simple pressure directly to the bleeding site will almost always control bleeding until definitive treatment can be given. Tourniquets are rarely indicated except in the case of traumatic amputation. Wounds should not be probed, and blind clamping is contraindicated, because it jeopardizes the chance for primary vascular repair and can result in permanent nerve injury.

CARDIOVASCULAR RESUSCITATION

CARDIAC OUTPUT

The *C* of the ABCs, cardiovascular resuscitation, includes resuscitation of both the heart and the systemic circulation. Five conditions (tension pneumothorax, pericardial tamponade, coronary air embolism, myocardial contusion, and myocardial infarction) can acutely shut off cardiac output and must be dealt with promptly.

Tension Pneumothorax

A tension pneumothorax impedes venous return by increasing thoracic pressures and by shifting the mediastinum and kinking the great veins as they enter the chest. Ventilatory function is compromised because one lung is collapsed and the other is compressed. Delivery of oxygen to the tissues, the product of cardiac output and actual oxygen content, can plummet. Patients with a full-blown tension pneumothorax will be in shock and may have distended neck veins, respiratory distress, a trachea deviated away from the involved hemithorax, hyperresonance and diminished breath sounds on the involved side, and a chest radiograph demonstrating a collapsed lung with a shifted mediastinum. Patients with tension pneumothoraces may not have these signs, however. Neck veins may be flat if the patient is hypovolemic or has a fat neck that obscures the physical findings; the patient may not be lying in a perfectly symmetrical manner, so evaluation of a deviated trachea becomes difficult; noise in the examining area may make percussion and auscultation difficult; and most patients with a tension pneumothorax will be unstable, and chest radiographs cannot be obtained quickly enough. Thus, because a tension pneumothroax can kill quickly and because the diagnosis can be difficult to make, physicians treat for a presumptive tension pneumothorax even when they are unsure of the diagnosis. The tension pneumothorax can be treated on a temporary basis by inserting a 16-gauge needle in the second intercostal space in the midclavicular line of the involved side. Tube thoracostomy is the definitive therapy.

Pericardial Tamponade

Pericardial tamponade is often a life-threatening emergency. The key to making the diagnosis is a high index of suspicion when the patient is in shock with distended neck veins but no evidence of tension pneumothorax. If pericardial tamponade is diagnosed early, pericardiocentesis may be helpful in temporarily treating the patient. This is accomplished by inserting an 18-gauge spinal needle in the subxyphoid area at a 45° angle and advancing it slowly while aiming at the left shoulder. Electrocardiographic (ECG) V-lead monitoring is helpful in localizing the tip of the needle. When the needle touches the epicardium, the observed QRS complex inverts. Removal of as little as 10 ml of blood sometimes dramatically reverses hypotension.

If pericardiocentesis is unsuccessful in removing clotted blood (as is usually the case with penetrating injuries to the heart) or if the patient arrests from tamponade, immediate emergency thoracotomy is indicated. If tamponade results from penetrating trauma, the thoracotomy should be on the side of the injury; otherwise, the thoracotomy should be on the left. The incision should be started in the interstitial space just below the nipple and carried medially to the sternum, where, to facilitate exposure, the costochondral cartilages can be incised above and below the incision. The incision should then be carried laterally as far as possible. The pericardium should be opened along its anterior surface in a caudal-to-cephalad direction, avoiding the phrenic nerve, which runs along the posterior lateral aspect of the pericardium, also in a caudal-to-cephalad direction.

Clots should be quickly evacuated and any holes in the heart occluded with the physician's finger. If there is no spontaneous cardiac activity, open heart massage should be begun, using the palmar surface of the fingers and the palm. Arterial *p*H should be corrected, and epinephrine (5 ml–10 ml of a 1:10,000 solution) should be administered in an attempt to establish coarse fibrillation. Electrical defibrillation should then be attempted with internal paddles set at 20 watt-seconds to 40 watt-seconds or with external paddles set at 400 watt-seconds. If resuscitation is successful, repair of the heart can be accomplished in the emergency room or operating room.

Coronary Air Embolization

Coronary air embolization is an unusual consequence of injury to the lung parenchyma from either blunt or penetrating trauma. This condition is usually seen in patients with major lung lacerations, the lacerations being caused either by rib fractures or by a stab or gunshot wound. Institution of pressure ventilation in such patients can force air from the tracheobronchial tree into the pulmonary venous circulation, thus allowing air to gain access to the systemic circulation. Embolization of air to most organs causes few recognizable acute changes; however, embolization of air to the brain can cause hemiparesis or other severe neurologic deficits and embolization to the coronary arteries can cause cardiogenic shock. Treatment of this condition, if recognized in the emergency room, is emergency thoracotomy on the involved side; if at thoracotomy the diagnosis is confirmed, the lung hilum is occluded. Definitive therapy, lobectomy or pneumonectomy, can then be performed in the operating room.

Myocardial Contusion

Myocardial contusion is usually the result of blunt chest trauma and can cause serious arrhythmias, usually within the first hour. This injury should be suspected in any patient struck in the anterior chest and particularly in those patients with sternal fractures. In children, the physician must have a high index of suspicion for this injury because often there are no fractures, owing to the high compliance of the child's bony thorax. The ECG may show an injury pattern, and

---

PRIORITIES IN VOLUME RESUSCITATION

Access to Circulation
Cutdown—saphenous, antecubital
Percutaneous—femoral, internal jugular

Obtain Blood (approximately 40 ml)
Type and cross-match
Hematocrit
Toxicology
Consider electrolytes, blood urea nitrogen (BUN), creatinine, glucose, amylase if indicated

Start Fluid Resuscitation
Balanced salt solution
Blood

Monitor Resuscitation
Atrial filling pressure between 3 and 8 torr
Urine output > 0.5 ml/kg/hr
Reverse clinical signs of shock

---

these patients should have continuous ECG monitoring for arrhythmias. If needed, lidocaine or other antiarrhythmics should be given and inotropic support provided.

Myocardial Infarction

Myocardial infarction must be considered in the trauma patient in cardiogenic shock. The infarction may have preceded the injuries or may result from blood loss, hypoxemia, or stimulation from circulating catecholamines. Therapy is the same as for myocardial contusion.

SYSTEMIC CIRCULATION

For practical purposes, resuscitation of the systemic circulation in trauma patients consists in gaining access to the circulation and giving fluids. Inflation of a pneumatic antishock garment has also been recommended as a means of resuscitating the systemic circulation at the scene of an accident.

Vascular Access

In patients in mild shock, a 16-gauge catheter or larger should be placed percutaneously in an upper-extremity vein; in patients in moderate or severe shock, access to the vascular space should be gained by one or more cutdowns, the number depending on the clinical severity of the shock. The safest and quickest cutdown is on the long saphenous vein over the medial malleolus. An additional cutdown on the basilic vein in the antecubital space, with central passage of the catheter, allows monitoring of the central venous pressure. The inserted catheters should be as large as possible to maximize flow rates of administered fluid. Catheters inserted by cutdown in the average adult should be 14-gauge or larger. Short catheters should be used for the saphenous vein at the ankle, the shortness recommended for the purpose of maximizing flow. Long catheters are necessary for the antecubital cutdown if one is to derive the benefit of central venous monitoring. A cutoff 5 F or 8 F pediatric feeding tube serves this purpose well. Catheters should not be inserted in injured extremities. As fluid resuscitation proceeds, percutaneously placed catheters may be placed in upper-extremity veins that begin to distend.

In circumstances such as single-physician resuscitation,

percutaneous femoral vein punctures may allow rapid access to the circulation without major complications. Such punctures may also be best if the physician is uncomfortable with the surgical technique of a cutdown.

We discourage the use of central percutaneous subclavian or internal jugular punctures in hypovolemic patients. Although such punctures may be easy and safe in the quiet normovolemic or hypervolemic patient, they can be difficult and dangerous in the restless, or even combative, hypovolemic patient. The severely hypovolemic patient has empty central veins. Empty veins are difficult to cannulate by using percutaneous techniques, and several life-threatening conditions may arise if an attempted percutaneous central puncture goes awry. First, the patient will not receive the required fluids. Second, the physician cannot be sure that the catheter is properly placed until a confirmatory chest radiograph is obtained. Failure of the patient to respond to fluid administration may mean continued and concealed hemorrhage into body cavities such as the abdomen or misplacement of the catheter. The physician will not know, and diagnostic confusion results. Third, a complication of an attempted percutaneous central puncture, such as a hemothorax or a tension pneumothorax, that might be tolerated in the normovolemic patient might be fatal in the hypovolemic patient, who already has severe impairment of venous return. Finally, the catheters used for percutaneous central venous punctures are long and small. Flow rates through such catheters are limited.

Types of Fluid

Many types of solutions are available for resuscitation of patients in hypovolemic shock; the two main categories are crystalloids and colloids. In mild or moderate shock, many types of fluid may be used to restore blood volume with good results. Ringer's lactate or acetate, normal saline, plasma, or other blood products are all equally effective. Cost and availability may be factors in determining which solution to use.

WHERE IS THE BLOOD VOLUME LOSS?

External Bleeding (scalp, face, extremity)—A history can be obtained from the patient, a paramedic, or the family.

Chest—Chest x-ray is the one test mandatory for all trauma patients.

Abdomen (including pelvis)—Notorious harbinger of hidden blood loss

Serial hematocrits
Serial white blood cell counts
Serial physical examinations
Peritoneal lavage

Thigh—Usually obvious but an unsplinted femur fracture may sequester 6 units to 8 units of blood.

Intracranial blood loss and other extremity fractures are not major sources of blood loss.
If the chest and thigh can be ruled out as sources of major blood loss and the patient manifests hypovolemic shock, the source of blood loss can be assumed to be in the abdomen and exploratory laparotomy is indicated.

FLUID RESUSCITATION OF SHOCK

Crystalloids
Isotonic NaCl
Hypertonic NaCl
Balanced salt solution
Ringer's lactate
Ringer's acetate
Normosol, Plasma-Lyte

Colloids
Blood
Low-titer O-negative blood
Type-specific
Typed and crossed
Washed red cells
Fresh warm blood
Plasma
Plasma—fresh frozen
Albumin
Plasmanate
Plasma substitutes
Clinical dextran (molecular weight 70,000)
Low-molecular-weight dextran (molecular weight 40,000)
Miscellaneous
Stroma-free hemoglobin
Hemacel
Starch
Fluorocarbons

In severe shock the type of resuscitative fluid becomes important. Albumin administration should be limited because albumin leaks out of capillaries. At best, this leakage means waste of an expensive blood product; at worst, the leakage means an accumulation of protein-rich interstitial fluid that has to be removed by the lymphatics.

We initiate resuscitation from severe shock with a balanced salt solution; we favor such a solution for four reasons. First, severe shock is accompanied by a metabolic acidosis; partial correction of this acidosis can be achieved with administration of a balanced salt solution, additional correction being achieved with administration, if needed, of 1 or 2 ampules of sodium bicarbonate to bring the blood pH to 7.30. Second, a balanced salt solution, like any crystalloid, decreases blood viscosity and enhances perfusion of the microvasculature. Third, a balanced salt solution replenishes extracellular stores of sodium, chloride, and water, stores that may have been depleted because of external losses (as in hemorrhage) or because of losses into the cell (as a result of cellular membrane deterioration). Finally, the crystalloid is expendable if the patient continues to bleed; premature infusion of blood into the patient who is actively bleeding can result in the loss of limited blood-bank resources.

If the patient responds to the initial infusion of 3 liters of balanced salt solution with an improved mental status, improved skin perfusion, increased urine output, and restoration of normal vital signs, we proceed with a deliberate diagnostic workup. If the patient remains in shock, we make plans to control bleeding as needed, in the operating room, and start type-specific whole blood.

Type-specific whole blood offers several advantages in the emergency situation. Whole blood, as opposed to packed red blood cells, can be administered with rapid flow rates through intravenous lines; packed red cells tend to sludge. Type-specific blood is preferable to cross-matched blood because cross-matched blood takes too long to obtain and because type-specific blood is tolerated well by most patients. The risk of a transfusion reaction with type-specific blood is very small (see discussion of transfusion, Chapter 5).

Low-titer O-negative blood may be used in emergency situations, especially if type-specific blood is not available. Administration of such blood occasionally causes difficulty with typing and cross-matching for subsequent transfusions.

Autotransfusion also provides compatible blood with minimal delay. The most favorable situation for autotransfusion uses blood drained from hemothoraces into containers with a citrate anticoagulant. Blood can also be used from the abdominal cavity, but care must be taken to ensure that the blood is free of contamination from bowel contents, an assurance that is rare at the beginning of the operation, when the blood is needed most. Only small amounts of autologous blood can be transfused; large amounts cause coagulopathies.

Although we do not use dextrans in resuscitating patients from shock, others—particularly in Europe—do. The dextrans are relatively inexpensive and are effective blood-volume expanders. They also decrease blood viscosity. On the negative side, they may impair reticuloendothelial function. High-molecular-weight dextran coats red cells and may make crossmatching difficult; low-molecular-weight dextran coats platelets and may contribute to bleeding.

Complications of Fluid Resuscitation

Several complications are specifically associated with initial volume replacement. These complications include the inducement of metabolic abnormalities, coagulopathies, and hypothermia.

When using banked blood, multiple metabolic changes occur. Stored blood is acidic because of the citrate-phosphate-dextrose anticoagulant storage medium. The pH of a unit of blood is about 7.1. Usually, in a single pass through the liver, much of the citrate is converted to bicarbonate, resulting in post-transfusion alkalosis. Banked blood is also high in potassium. Since there is usually sodium retention after injury, and because of the metabolic alkalosis following massive transfusion, large quantities of potassium are excreted by the kidneys, often resulting in moderate hypokalemia. The anticoagulant also binds calcium and can cause hypocalcemia and arrhythmias. Ideally, one should monitor for hypocalcemia with an ECG and treat as changes develop. Overadministration of calcium is potentially lethal. If continuous ECG monitoring is not available, 1 ampule of calcium chloride is given for each 4 units to 5 units of blood transfused within 30 minutes.

Coagulopathies associated with massive transfusion are most often due to platelet abnormalities. Most blood banks remove platelets from blood for component therapy. Even if they are not removed, platelet function in cold stored blood deteriorates with time, and platelets in blood stored for more than 72 hours should be considered nonfunctional. In massive transfusions, the quantity and function of platelets are roughly proportional to the number of units of blood administered. In general, it is advisable to administer platelet packs whenever 10 units of blood have been administered in less than 1 hour (see also Chapter 5).

The importance of the labile clotting factors in blood (factors V and VIII) in post-transfusion coagulopathy is not well understood and is probably overemphasized. Factor VIII levels are elevated by hepatic production following resuscitation. Factor V is the only clotting factor reduced in the serum after massive transfusion. Fresh frozen plasma is used to provide clotting components, but its effectiveness in preventing post-transfusion bleeding is not firmly established.

Hypothermia is a frequent side-effect of receiving blood stored at 4°C. Core temperature of massively transfused patients can easily fall to 30° to 35°C. Cold patients are less able to metabolize acid and potassium, and hypothermia shifts the oxyhemoglobin curve to the left, thereby making less oxygen available to the tissues. Blood should be given through warmers, if possible. With massive transfusions, it is usually not possible to return the temperature of the blood to normal with commercial warmers. A simple, effective method to warm the blood is to pass the blood through an extension tube immersed in a bucket of water at about 44°C.

Pneumatic Antishock Garments

In modern EMS systems, the unstable trauma patient is often transported with the antishock garment in place. This device may save lives in the prehospital system. The antishock garment in theory has both a good and a bad effect on cardiac output. It can tamponade bleeding in the extremities and perhaps in the abdomen. It can also compress the veins and augment venous return. When applied at high pressures, however, its beneficial effects may be outweighed by the increase in total peripheral resistance generated by the external pressure. This increased total peripheral resistance increases the afterload to the heart and depresses cardiac function. Application of an antishock garment to the abdomen can have an added detrimental effect of compressing the inferior vena cava, increasing venous resistance and decreasing venous return. The garment may also impair motion of the chest cage and limit ventilation.

If the patient arrives with the antishock garment inflated, access to the vascular system should be obtained with upper-extremity cutdowns or with percutaneous subclavian and internal jugular punctures. At least two large-bore lines should be placed. Blood should be obtained for typing and cross-matching and resuscitation started before deflating the antishock garment. In some institutions, deflation is reserved for the operating room, where the specific injuries can be definitively treated. In general, the abdominal portion should be removed first. Acidosis and volume should be corrected and then consideration made for immediate exploratory laparotomy and vascular control before the two leg compartments are deflated. The clinician must be aware that deflation of abdominal and leg compartments at one time will result in "declamping aortic shock," with blood flow to the legs increasing to as much as 30% of the cardiac output, as compared to the normal resting leg flow of 3%. The insult of this declamping shock is thus added to the insult of the original injury.

If the patient arrives with the antishock garment in place and only minimal to modest pressures have been used (20 torr to 40 torr), the resuscitation should proceed as normal and the trousers should be deflated as the injuries are assessed and treatment is planned.

ASSESSMENT OF INITIAL RESUSCITATION

Once the airway and ventilation are established, bleeding is controlled, and resuscitation of the cardiovascular system is begun, the initial resuscitation should be assessed. This

---

INDICES OF SUCCESSFUL RESUSCITATION

1. ATRIAL FILLING PRESSURES—keep at or near normal
2. URINE OUTPUT 0.5 ml/kg/hr
3. REVERSE CLINICAL SIGNS OF SHOCK

---

assessment should include examination of neurologic status, placement of a Foley catheter in the urinary bladder, assessment of the peripheral perfusion, and evaluation of the patient's vital signs.

NEUROLOGIC EXAMINATION

The initial neurologic examination should take no more than 20 seconds. The patient's state of consciousness should be categorized as alert, responsive to vocal stimuli, responsive only to pain, or unresponsive. The pupils should be assessed for size and reactivity. The extremities should be assessed for spontaneous movement or for movement in response to command or pain. No further neurologic examination need nor should be done at this time, even if a severe neurologic deficit should be found. The purpose of the initial neurologic examination is to establish a baseline to which later neurologic examinations can be compared; it is not the purpose of the initial examination to make a definitive neurologic diagnosis.

Trauma to the brain can cause any of a number of alterations in mental status, including coma, obtundation, confusion, agitation, combativeness, delusions of paranoia, or even euphoria. All of these altered states of consciousness can also be produced by hypoxemia, hypovolemic shock, or inebriation.

The physician's first duty in treating the trauma patient with an altered state of consciousness is to recognize and treat hypoxemia and shock, should these conditions be present. His second duty is to recognize and treat brain damage. The physician should never ascribe an altered state of consciousness to brain damage or inebriation until hypoxemia and shock have been ruled out. He should never ascribe an altered state of consciousness to inebriation until brain damage has been ruled out.

BLADDER CATHETERIZATION

Urine flow should be measured in all severely traumatized patients early in the course of their resuscitation. Measurement of such flow requires passage of a Foley catheter. The catheter should be passed gently, particularly in men with pelvic fractures. Such patients may have a partial laceration of the urethra, and forced insertion of the catheter may convert the partial laceration into a complete one (Fig. 10-2). Most patients with a urethral laceration will have at least one of several physical signs. These signs include blood at the urethral meatus, blood in the scrotal sac, and a free-floating prostate, which rides high in the rectum.

An adequate urine flow is one of the best indices of an adequate resuscitation of the cardiovascular system. Resuscitation is probably adequate if an adult patient produces glucose-free urine at a flow of 50ml/hour or more. Infants up to the age of 1 year should produce 2 ml/kg/hour and children older than 1 year, 1 ml/kg/hour.

Although good urine flows usually indicate adequate resuscitation, such flows are unreliable in inebriated patients. High blood alcohol levels inhibit release of antidiuretic hormone, and inebriated patients may diurese even in the

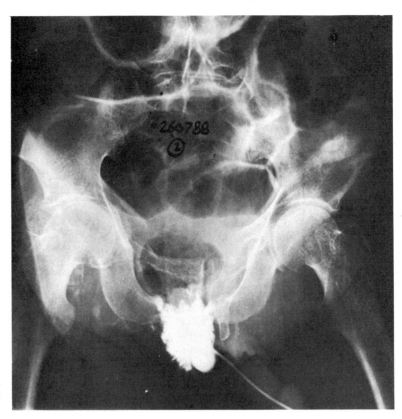

Fig. 10-2. X-ray film demonstrates extravasation of urine from the membranous urethra following rupture secondary to blunt trauma.

face of hypovolemia. Urine flows are also unreliable in diabetics or patients who have been given osmotic diuretics (*e.g.*, mannitol or radiopaque contrast agents).

SKIN PERFUSION

Skin perfusion is the most sensitive physical sign in assessing adequacy of shock resuscitation, poor perfusion indicating persistent shock. Release of catecholamines from the adrenal medulla and discharge of the sympathetic nervous system are the earliest compensations the patient makes in response to shock. The skin becomes pale, cool, and clammy. The veins collapse.

Warm, well-perfused skin indicates adequate cardiovascular resuscitation except in patients who are inebriated, who have lost neurologic control of their systemic circulation, or who have carbon monoxide poisoning. Inebriation can produce a flushed, warm skin, even in the face of hypovolemia. The patient usually is hypotensive, however, and the physician will be able to detect the hypovolemia. Patients with spinal cord trauma or who have ingested sympatholytic agents can have warm, well-perfused skin even while hypovolemic. Hypotension also helps make the diagnosis. Carbon monoxide poisoning prevents release of oxygen from the hemoglobin molecule, thus maintaining pink blood and skin even in the presence of shock and low flow. History and direct measurement of blood carboxyhemoglobin levels make the diagnosis.

Poorly perfused skin does not necessarily indicate shock. Patients who are frightened or who have suffered cold exposure may have pale, cool skin and still be normovolemic. Nonetheless, a diagnosis of fear-induced sympathetic discharge or cold-induced peripheral vasoconstriction should be made only after hypovolemia has been ruled out.

BLOOD PRESSURE AND PULSE RATE

Blood pressure and pulse rate should be measured at this time during the resuscitation. A low blood pressure or a rapid pulse indicates moderate or severe shock and will alert the physician to take further active resuscitative measures. The low pressure or rapid pulse can be especially helpful in patients who are inebriated and in patients with spinal cord trauma, because in these patients skin perfusion becomes unreliable as a physical sign.

A low blood pressure or a rapid pulse in an obtunded patient with head trauma should be presumed to be due to hypovolemia. Although severe head injuries eventually result in shock, the shock is a terminal sign and indicates irreversible brain damage. Severe shock in and of itself can cause obtundation. Sometimes obtunded patients with a low blood pressure and rapid pulse wake up when their cardiovascular status is resuscitated.

SECONDARY MANAGEMENT IN THE EMERGENCY ROOM

At times, in the seriously injured patient, the need for a rapid assessment and resuscitation conflicts with the need for a thorough assessment. The resolution of this conflict depends on the patient's condition. If the unstable trauma patient does not respond to initial resuscitation and remains in shock, diagnostic studies must be bypassed. A short history should be obtained, a rapid physical examination should be performed, a chest radiograph should be taken, and the patient should be taken directly to the operating room. On the other hand, if the patient does respond to the initial resuscitation, the work-up can proceed more deliberately. This more deliberate work-up should include a more thorough history, a more thorough physical examination, radiographs, and laboratory tests.

HISTORY

Histories should be kept to a minimum during the early phases of evaluation, but some information needs to be obtained. The past medical history should include allergies, medications, major illnesses, and major operations. The present illness should include the circumstances of the accident, the magnitude of the forces involved in the accident, the patient's condition when first seen by medical personnel, and the patient's condition while being transported to the hospital.

In all injuries, the history can be helpful, in some cases, it can be essential. With knowledge that the patient has been exposed to an electrical shock, the physician will seek out internal injuries, even though the external burn appears minor. A collapsed steering column in an accident in which the driver patient was not wearing a seat belt alerts the physician to observe the patient for a rupture of the atrium or a transected aorta, as well as other thoracic injuries that can occur with less severe thoracic trauma. A fall from a height with the patient landing upright on his heels can result in a constellation of injuries, including fractures of the calcanei, compression fractures of the lumbar spine, and fractures of the cervical spine. Head trauma that does not render the patient comatose immediately is unlikely to be associated with severe damage to the brain itself; subsequent neurologic deterioration is probably due to an expanding intracranial hematoma or cerebral edema, both treatable lesions.

Although the history in these and other cases can be helpful, only those aspects of the history that are readily available should be obtained. The physician should stay with the patient during the early stages of evaluation and resuscitation; he should not leave the patient at this time to make phone calls to the family or private physician to obtain a more complete history. Further physical examination is more likely to yield information that will benefit the patient.

PHYSICAL EXAMINATION

As the physician is taking the abbreviated history, he should be reexamining the patient.

HEAD, EARS, EYES, NOSE, AND THROAT

Brisk bleeding from the scalp or face, resulting in a blood loss of more than 100 ml/minute, should be controlled by closing the bleeding lacerations with a monofilament suture. The sutures should be placed rapidly with no attempt made to obtain a good cosmetic result; the wounds can be reclosed later with more attention to plastic technique. Brisk bleeding from the nasopharynx can be slowed by inserting a 20 F Foley catheter with a 30-ml balloon through one of the nostrils into the nasopharynx. The balloon can then be inflated and traction applied to the catheter to lodge the inflated balloon in the nasopharynx, thus tamponading the bleeding.

Once this brisk bleeding is controlled, the face and scalp should be inspected and palpated for hematomas, nonbleeding lacerations, and bony deformities. Inspection and palpation of the scalp will reveal lacerations if an effort is made to expose the skin in all areas, particularly under matted, bloody hair. Inspection and palpation of the skull can be

misleading in detecting depressed skull fractures. A subgaleal hematoma with a tear in the galea can feel like a depressed skull fracture, and the irregularity of a depressed skull fracture can be missed if there is a smooth overlying scalp hematoma. Palpation of the facial bony prominences will detect most major facial fractures. The physician should palpate the orbital rims, the zygomatic arches, the mandible, and the nose. He should also examine the maxilla for unstable fractures by grasping the upper incisors and attempting to rock the maxilla back and forth. Inspection of the face and skull in the patient with injuries more than 24 hours old may reveal Battle's sign or "raccoon eyes," presumptive evidence for a basilar skull fracture.

The ears should be examined for blood in the external canal, again presumptive evidence for a basilar skull fracture; they should also be examined for blood behind the tympanic membrane, pathognomonic evidence for a basilar skull fracture. Hearing activity can be evaluated by talking to the patient.

The eyes should be checked for extraocular movements. Limitation of upward gaze suggests a blow-out fracture of the orbit; dysconjugate gaze suggests neurologic damage. Binocular vision can be checked by asking the patient to enumerate the number of fingers displayed to him. Visual acuity can be assessed by asking the patient to read the label on a bottle of intravenous fluids. Pupils should be checked for size and reactivity, both ipsilateral and conjugal. Funduscopic examination should detect trauma to the lens. It will also reveal retinal bleeding and establish the presence or absence of retinal venous pulsations; the development of increased intracranial pressure is presumed if such pulsations are present initially and disappear during the observation period. The disks should also be checked for papilledema, a finding with increased intracranial pressure of several hours' duration.

The nose and throat should be examined for adequacy of airway. Blood issuing from the nose or a retropharyngeal hematoma warns the physician of a possible airway obstruction. Drainage of clear fluid from the nose, if proved to be cerebrospinal fluid, is another pathognomonic sign of a basilar skull fracture. The fluid can be proven to be cerebrospinal fluid, as opposed to a catarrhal exudate, if its glucose concentration approximates blood glucose levels or if, when dried on a handkerchief, it forms a thin, flaky crust.

NECK

Inspection of the neck may reveal distended neck veins, suggesting a cardiac cause of shock; flat neck veins suggest hypovolemia. Swelling of the neck indicates bleeding into one of the fascial planes of the neck. Such bleeding can obstruct the airway, and intubation can be difficult because the hematoma can displace the larynx; it is best to intubate these patients early, before laryngeal anatomy becomes excessively distorted.

Palpation may reveal a shifted trachea, suggesting a tension pneumothorax. Subcutaneous emphysema indicates a rupture somewhere in the tracheobronchial tree or, less likely, somewhere in the esophagus. Tenderness or instability of the cervical spine suggests a fracture, especially if the patient has associated major maxillofacial trauma.

CHEST

Inspection of the chest may reveal poor movement on one side, indicating either a collapsed lung or splinting associated with the pain of chest wall trauma. A flail chest may or may not show paradoxical motion when the patient presents. Inspection may also reveal chest wall abrasions or ecchymosis, alerting the physician to search for damage to underlying organs in the chest or abdomen.

Palpation of the chest wall will reveal rib fractures, even when radiographs are negative. A damped apical heart beat suggests a pericardial tamponade.

Percussion of both sides of the chest helps to make a diagnosis of a pneumothorax or hemothorax. The physician should not attempt to learn anything more from percussion: A displaced heart may indicate a shifted mediastinum and a tension pneumothorax, but a shifted trachea is a better sign; similarly, although percussion may reveal a high hemidiaphragm, there is no hurry to make such a diagnosis, and a chest radiograph obtained later will demonstrate the elevation in time.

Auscultation of the chest helps to diagnose pneumothoraces. Muffled heart tones suggest pericardial tamponade.

ABDOMEN AND LOWER CHEST

The abdomen and lower chest should be considered as a single unit in the trauma patient. Some of the most commonly injured organs in blunt trauma, for example, the spleen, liver, and kidneys, lie at least in part under the lower ribs. Penetrating injuries of the lower chest can also damage many intra-abdominal organs, perhaps the easiest injury to miss being that of retroperitoneal penetration of the left colon.

Inspection is the most important part of the physical examination. Ecchymosis and abrasions may indicate underlying organ damage. The location of penetrating injuries should be noted and an attempt made to characterize the nature of the injury, remembering that any characterization may be in error. Knife wounds that are large enough to admit the tip of a gloved finger should be gently explored with the finger, but the physician must remember while exploring such wounds that the patient's musculature may have been in a different position when the patient was stabbed; the muscles of the patient while he is being examined may cover up a penetrating tract, and the physician may underestimate the depth of the wound. Gunshot entrance wounds are usually smaller than exit wounds, and powder burns are more common around entrance wounds. These are only generalizations, however, and exceptions do occur. Trajectories of gunshot wounds should be estimated, remembering that bullets, once they enter the body, do not necessarily travel in straight lines and sometimes take remarkably erratic courses.

Inspection of the abdomen and lower chest should end with observation both of the contour of the abdomen and of movement of the abdominal musculature in response to voluntary coughing or spontaneous ventilation. Abdominal distention indicates intra-abdominal gas or intra-abdominal bleeding. Muscular splinting indicates pain from muscular trauma or from irritation of the parietal peritoneum.

Percussion of the abdomen is mainly useful in detecting gastric distention, a condition which should be promptly treated by passage of a nasogastric tube. Percussion also confirms irritation of the parietal peritoneum if the patient's muscles tighten with a light tap. A dull percussion note suggests intra-abdominal fluid, usually blood, but occasionally urine.

Palpation of the abdomen can detect hematomas in the abdominal wall. Involuntary guarding indicates irritation of the parietal peritoneum.

Auscultation of the abdomen offers little in the trauma patient. A silent abdomen may only represent a temporary ileus after extra-abdominal trauma. Conversely, there may be bowel sounds even in the presence of a ruptured or perforated viscus.

PELVIC AND RECTAL

The perineum, genitalia, and rectum will have been examined quickly during the initial resuscitation if the patient was in deep shock and required passage of a Foley catheter. If these structures were not examined initially, they should be examined at this time. The perineum should be inspected for lacerations and hematomas. The urethral meatus should be inspected for blood. The scrotum should be inspected for hematomas, an indication of a retroperitoneal hematoma. Inspection of the vagina by using a speculum is impractical in most trauma patients; the vagina can be palpated, however, for deep lacerations, and blood in the vagina will be detected on the glove of the examining hand. Blood in the rectal vault will similarly be detected during the rectal examination. The rectal examination also allows assessment of both sphincter tone and position of the prostate.

VASCULAR

The neck, supraclavicular spaces, groin, and all four extremities should be inspected for hematomas. Large expanding hematomas, in conjunction with either a nearby penetrating injury or a broken bone, frequently indicate disruption of a major artery. All four extremities should be inspected for adequacy of skin perfusion and temperature. Poor perfusion of all extremities suggests shock; poor perfusion of one with good perfusion of the others suggests an arterial injury.

The carotid, subclavian, brachial, radial, femoral, popliteal, dorsalis pedis, and posterior tibial pulses should be palpated. Blood pressures should be obtained in both arms to assess the subclavian arteries. The area around any penetrating injury should be auscultated for the continuous to-and-fro bruit of an arteriovenous fistula.

MUSCULOSKELETAL

The musculoskeletal system should be inspected for gross deformities and hematomas; the overlying skin should be inspected for ecchymosis, abrasions, and lacerations. Grossly deformed limbs should be gently straightened, especially if the limb is ischemic.

The large bones should be palpated; particular attention should be paid to bones underlying or near any abnormality detected by inspection. The head, cervical spine, and ribs will already have been palpated. The pelvis should be palpated by pressing down on the pubis and also by compressing the iliac wings toward one another. The clavicles and bones of the extremities should be palpated next.

The purpose of this initial examination is to elicit tenderness or instability. Abnormalities will prompt the physician to obtain appropriate radiographs and also to initiate treatment in some instances. Continued movement of unstable fractures of large bones can cause pain, major tissue damage, major blood loss, and, occasionally, damage to adjacent neurovascular structures; unstable fractures of large bones should be immobilized to minimize these sequelae. Open fractures should be cultured and temporarily covered with sterile dressings. Dislocations and fractures that have compromised the neurovascular supply to an extremity should be manipulated into better alignment in an attempt to reestablish flow.

NEUROLOGIC

The secondary neurologic examination should expand upon the first. The character and the adequacy of the patient's ventilation should be noted. The patient's mental status can be described using the categories of the Glasgow Coma Scale (Table 10-3).

The necessary cranial nerve examination will have been completed with the head, ears, eyes, nose, and throat examination. Particular note should be made of the presence or absence of vision, the pupil size and activity, and extraocular movements.

Neurologic examination of the extremities should assess the patient for spontaneous purposeful motor function, purposeful function to voice command, purposeful response to pain, withdrawal from pain, nonpurposeful flexion to pain, nonpurposeful extension to pain, and no response (Table 10-3). Deep tendon reflexes and a sensory examination are not necessary at this time; they should be evaluated at this point only if the preceding examination indicates an injury to the spinal cord.

As is the case with the initial neurologic examination, the major purpose of the second examination in the trauma patient is to establish a baseline for later evaluation: Deterioration in neurologic status should prompt a more thorough evaluation, including computed tomography (CT) scanning of the head. A secondary purpose of this neurologic examination is to recognize symptoms and signs of increased intracranial pressure and begin treatment. The intubated

TABLE 10-3   GLASGOW COMA SCALE

Eye Opening	
Spontaneous	4
To voice	3
To pain	2
None	1

Verbal Response	
Oriented	5
Confused	4
Inappropriate words	3
Incomprehensible words	2
None	1

Motor Response	
Obeys command	6
Purposeful movement (pain)	5
Withdraw (pain)	4
Flexion (pain)	3
Extension (pain)	2
None	1

Total GCS Points	Score
14–15	5
11–13	4
8–10	3
5–7	2
3–4	1

patient should be hyperventilated to an arterial P_{CO_2} of approximately 30 mm Hg. Mannitol may also be given after consultation with a neurosurgeon.

RADIOGRAPHY

CHEST FILM

Every trauma patient should have a chest film early in the course of his resuscitation. With only one exception, no trauma patient should go to surgery, no matter how urgent the case, without a chest film; the only exception is the patient who has had an emergency room thoracotomy.

A portable film is more than adequate. The x-ray technician should be available when the critically injured patient is brought in, and a film cassette can be laid under the patient when he is initially rolled over to examine his back or when he is transferred from the ambulance stretcher to the hospital gurney. The process of obtaining the film should take no more than 15 seconds. If the patient has to be taken immediately to the operating room, the film can be developed while the patient is being transported; the interpretation of the film can be called in to the surgeon in the operating room while he is preparing the patient for surgery.

The information obtained from the film can be lifesaving. The patient in hypovolemic or cardiogenic shock, without an obvious source of extracavitary blood loss, must be bleeding into the left side of his chest, right side of his chest, or abdomen or must have cardiogenic shock due to myocardial failure, pericardial tamponade, a tension pneumothorax, or a ruptured hemidiaphragm with displacement of abdominal viscera into the chest. The chest film can help make many of these diagnoses and will direct the surgeon to the appropriate body cavity.

The chest film may demonstrate any of a number of abnormalities, many of which can be hard to detect on physical examination. A hemothorax or a simple pneumothorax can be missed in the rushed atmosphere of a noisy emergency room. They will be obvious on the chest film. A chest film of the patient with a ruptured left hemidiaphragm may demonstrate abdominal viscera in the left side of the chest or an abnormal position of a nasogastric tube. Aortic or intrathoracic great-vessel ruptures are almost always associated with some abnormality of the mediastinum or of the aortic knob; they may also be associated with fractures of the posterior portion of the first or second ribs, apical capping, displacement of the main stem bronchi, or deviation of the nasogastric tube. With a pulmonary contusion, a lung infiltrate is typically demonstrated within 1 hour of the injury. Ruptures of the tracheobronchial tree often demonstrate mediastinal air. An enlarged heart shadow may be demonstrated in acute pericardial tamponade, but usually no abnormality is seen on the chest x-ray film. Rib fractures may be demonstrated on the chest film or they may not, even with rib details.

CERVICAL SPINE FILM

All hemodynamically stable patients with major craniofacial trauma or with physical signs of a cervical spine injury should have x-ray films of the cervical spine. The most important film to obtain is the lateral film. The seventh cervical vertebra must be visualized, because many cervical fractures involve that vertebra. It is often necessary for two medical attendants to be in the radiology suite when the x-ray film is being obtained, one to maintain the patient's head in an axial orientation and the other to pull down on the patient's upper extremities so as to expose the seventh vertebra. *All cervical vertebrae must be visualized.*

The lateral film will demonstrate misalignment in most patients with an unstable cervical spine. The anterior or posterior borders of the spinal canal may be out of line, the atlas and odontoid may be displaced, or the vertebral bodies may be compressed or fractured. The lateral film may also indicate the need for more views, such as odontoid, anteroposterior, oblique, or flexion-extension films.

ABDOMINAL FILM

In contrast to the chest film the abdominal film usually does not contribute much to the therapeutic management of trauma patients. However, if time permits, in the multiply injured patient, an abdominal film should be obtained when other x-ray films are being obtained in the radiology suite. The film may show fractures of the lumbar vertebrae or fractures of their transverse processes, both types of fractures indicating that large forces were applied to the abdomen and back. A scoliosis indicates retroperitoneal trauma and bleeding, causing spasm of the paraspinous muscles. The same injury may obliterate the psoas margins or the kidney shadows. Air around the duodenum indicates a retroperitoneal rupture of the duodenum. The radiographic signs of bleeding into the peritoneal cavity, such as fluid in the paracolic cutters or obliteration of the properitoneal fat line, become positive only with very extensive blood loss.

GENITOURINARY FILM

The excretory urogram, cystogram, and urethrogram are the mainstays for preliminary evaluation of injuries to the genitourinary tract. An intravenous pyelogram should be obtained in any stable patient with hematuria defined as more than 100 red blood cells per high-powered field in an unspun specimen. An intravenous pyelogram should also be obtained, even when there is no hematuria, in stable patients with severe blunt trauma or with penetrating injuries near a kidney or ureter.

A cystogram should be obtained in any patient with hematuria or severe lower abdominal or pelvic trauma, particularly the inebriated patient with lower abdominal blunt trauma. A urethrogram should be obtained in any patient with a suspected urethral tear, as described in the section on initial management, or in any male who presents with severe pelvic trauma.

In the adult patient, the intravenous pyelogram can be obtained by intravenously administering 100 ml of contrast material early during the course of resuscitation. The first plain film of the abdomen usually gives most of the information that will be needed. The cystogram can be obtained by infusing 150 ml of contrast material through the Foley catheter into the bladder; the infusion should be by gravity. An anteroposterior view and either an oblique or a lateral view of the bladder should be obtained. The urethrogram can be obtained by gently injecting 30 ml of contrast material into the urethral meatus. If a Foley catheter is already in place, some detail of the urethra can be obtained by injecting contrast material into the urethra, around the catheter (see Fig. 10-2).

Contrast studies of the genitourinary tract can delineate many abnormalities. The excretory urogram will show the number of functioning kidneys; a nonvisualizing kidney indicates absence of the organ or interruption of its blood supply. The degree of extravasation of contrast material will give an index of parenchymal damage.

The ureters usually are not seen in their entirety with the single-film urogram. In blunt trauma, this nonvisualization is usually not important because ureteral ruptures are rare. In contrast, in penetrating trauma near a ureter, an effort should be made to see the entire structure. Lacerations of the ureter can be small and easily missed. Bladder ruptures are frequently posterior, hence the need for oblique or lateral views.

CRANIAL COMPUTED TOMOGRAPHY

CT scans of the head should be obtained in any hemodynamically stable patient with a suspected depressed skull fracture, in any stable patient with a severe neurologic deficit, and in any stable (or even moderately unstable) patient with a worsening neurologic status. Not every obtunded inebriated patient needs CT scanning, as long as he has no neurologic deficit other than the obtundation. If the obtundation persists for more than several hours, however, CT scans should be obtained since drunkenness should lighten with time, not stay the same, or worsen.

CT scans of the head are definitive for diagnosis of depressed fractures, epidural hematomas, subdural hematomas, intracerebral hematomas, and cerebral edema (Figs. 10-3 and 10-4). It has made cerebral arteriography for trauma obsolete. Plain films of the skull have also become less important with the advent of CT scanning. If the patient has a neurologic deficit, he should have tomography, and there is no need for plain films. If the patient has no neurologic deficit, he does not need tomography and usually does not need plain films either.

Fig. 10-3. CT shows laceration of the brain (*arrow*) and a subdural hematoma (*S*).

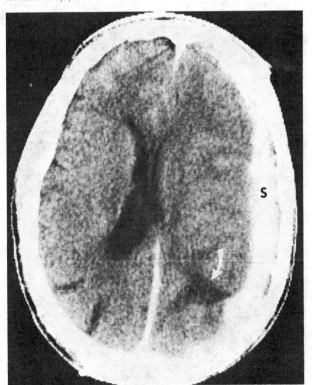

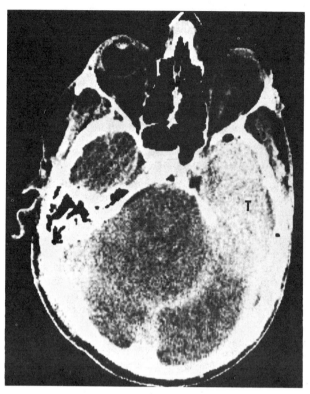

Fig. 10-4. CT scan shows intracerebral bleeding within the temporal lobe (*T*) following blunt trauma.

ABDOMINAL COMPUTED TOMOGRAPHY

CT scans of the abdomen can help evaluate hemodynamically stable patients who have been subjected to blunt trauma to the lower chest or abdomen, especially patients with equivocal indications for celiotomy or patients who are difficult to evaluate because of obtundation or spinal cord damage. Tomography can not only detect intraperitoneal and retroperitoneal bleeding but also identify the damaged organ. Tomography is most accurate in assessing those organs—the liver, spleen, kidneys, and pancreas—most likely to be damaged with blunt trauma (Fig. 10-5). Tomography is accurate in detecting retroduodenal air or edema associated with duodenal disruptions. It is also accurate in detecting free intraperitoneal air associated with rupture of the small or large intestine.

ARTERIOGRAMS

A thoracic aortogram should be obtained in any hemodynamically stable patient with a suspected disruption of the thoracic aorta or of the great vessels. The physician's suspicion should be aroused by a decreased blood pressure in the left arm or by demonstration of a wide mediastinum or obliteration of the aortic knob on chest x-ray film. Weaker indications are listed in the section on radiography of the chest.

In the stable patient, selective arteriograms may be used to evaluate suspected arterial injuries in the neck and extremities (Table 10-4). These are suggested in any patient with a penetrating injury near an artery; in any patient with a hematoma, a bruit, decreased distal pulses, diminished peripheral perfusion, or compromised neurologic function associated with a penetrating injury; and in any patient with severe blunt trauma to the region of the knee (Fig.

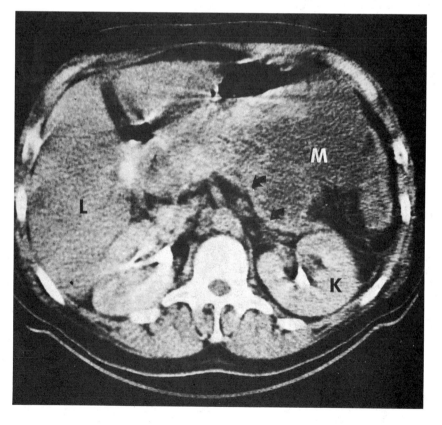

Fig. 10-5. CT scan shows contusion and bleeding within the pancreas following blunt trauma. (*K*, kidney; *L*, liver; *M*, bleeding into the mesocolon)

TABLE 10-4 INDICATIONS FOR ARTERIOGRAPHY FOLLOWING TRAUMA

Neck injuries, zones I and III
Chest injuries
    Mediastinal widening
    First rib fracture
    Deviation of trachea to the right
Abdominal injuries
    Nonvisualization of a kidney by pyelogram
    Selected pelvic fractures
All penetrating wounds of extremities in proximity to major
    vessels
Dislocation of the knee
All fractures associated with abnormal pulses

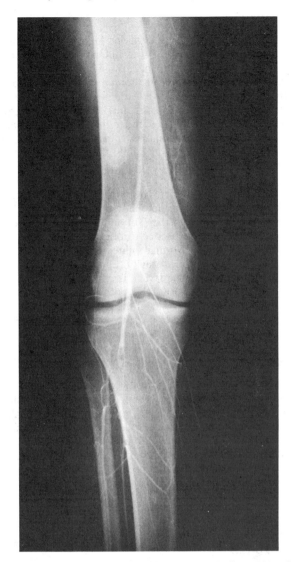

Fig. 10-6. Arteriogram shows disruption and clot within the popliteal artery in a young man following a motorcycle accident. Clinical examination had shown an unstable knee with posterior dislocation.

10-6). If arteriograms are not obtained in patients with suspected injuries to large arteries, namely, the carotids, brachials, and femoropopliteals, the vessels should be explored.

In stable patients with penetrating injuries to the base of the neck or the upper third of the neck, arteriography is preferable to exploration (Fig. 10-7). These vessels can be difficult to expose, and arteriography can help plan an operation. In penetrating injuries to the middle third of the neck and in injuries to the extremities, either arteriography or exploration can be used. Exploration of these wounds is preferred if the patient is unstable, if a hematoma is expanding, or if the extremity distal to the injury is ischemic. Exposure of the vessels in the middle third of the neck or in the extremities is usually straightforward, and no time should be lost with arteriography.

RADIONUCLIDE SCANS AND SONOGRAPHY

Echocardiography is occasionally useful in ruling out a pericardial tamponade in the stable patient. Otherwise, because they lack anatomical resolution, radionuclide scans and sonography have little to offer in assessing the trauma patient.

Fig. 10-7. Zones of the neck.

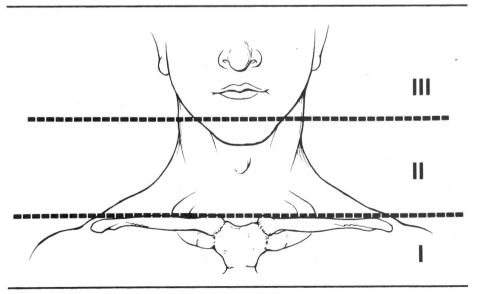

PERITONEAL LAVAGE

In the stable patient, the indications for peritoneal lavage are the same as those for CT scanning of the abdomen: equivocal findings on abdominal examination or neurologic abnormalities that preclude abdominal examination. However, tomography has two advantages; it is sensitive in detecting retroperitoneal injuries, and it localizes the injury, whether it is in the abdomen or the retroperitoneum. Lavage can miss retroperitoneal injuries, and it does not localize injuries. At best, lavage only tells the surgeon that an abdominal organ is injured.

To perform a lavage, the bladder should first be emptied by passing a Foley catheter. The skin below the umbilicus should be infiltrated with a local anesthetic, and an incision should be made through the skin and down to the fascia. The catheter should be inserted through the fascia and into the peritoneal cavity. Normal saline, 1000 ml, should be infused into the peritoneal cavity, allowed to equilibrate, and then drained off. The lavage is considered technically adequate if more than 500 ml is recovered. Injury to the abdominal viscera is suggested if the red blood cell count is greater than 50,000/mm³ or if the white blood cell count is greater than 500/mm³.

ENDOSCOPY

Pharnygoscopy and esophagoscopy can help assess injuries to the neck. Gastroscopy and duodenoscopy have no place in assessing the trauma patient: Penetrating injuries of the abdomen should be explored. Proctosigmoidoscopy should be performed in any patient with a suspected rectal injury; the study can be done in the operating room before celiotomy is performed. Appropriate endoscopy should also be performed in any patient with a suspected injury to the larynx or tracheobronchial tree.

BLOOD AND URINE TESTS

HEMATOCRIT

All patients subjected to major trauma should have hematocrit determinations of their peripheral blood, although urgent surgery should not be delayed if the result is not immediately available. The hematocrit can be determined by centrifuging a specimen of blood in a capillary tube and dividing the volume of red cells by the total volume. The hematocrit can also be determined by using the Coulter counter.

The hematocrit remains unchanged for several hours after acute hemorrhage in the patient who is given no intravenous replacement. In the patient who is given fluid replacement, the hematocrit falls rapidly and in proportion to the amount of blood lost, approximately three points for every unit of blood lost. The hematocrit eventually will fall the same amount in patients who are chronically bleeding. In patients who are not replenished, equilibration by transcapillary refill will be complete within 72 hours.

The value of the hematocrit in the trauma patient, then, is that it quantitates the amount of blood lost. It is particularly useful in following patients for occult hemorrhage into the abdomen or retroperitoneum.

URINALYSIS

All patients subjected to major trauma should have a urinalysis, but, again, surgery should not be delayed if the results are not immediately available. Microscopic examination of the urine reveals the presence or absence of red blood cells. Immersing a reagent strip (a plastic strip impregnated with specific compounds that give color reactions with specific substances) into the urine measures urine pH and detects protein, glucose, ketone bodies, bilirubin, and occult blood.

The reagent strips can also detect myoglobinuria in patients with either severe crushing injuries or burns involving muscle. The reagent for hemoglobin on the strips cross-reacts with myoglobin. This cross-reactivity, along with the insolubility of hemoglobin with ammonium sulfate, allows the physician to test for myoglobinuria. Eighty percent ammonium sulfate is added to an aliquot of urine to precipitate out any hemoglobin in the specimen. The aliquot is then centrifuged and the supernatant tested with the hemoglobin reagent part of a reagent strip. A positive reaction suggests myoglobinuria. Both positive and negative reactions should be confirmed by electrophoretic and immunochemical methods.

The urine can also be checked for drugs and other toxic substances. The surgeon should be wary in interpreting toxicology screens, however. A positive screen for drugs in an irrational, belligerent patient may suggest that the irrationality and belligerency are due to drug ingestion. Alternatively, the patient's behavior may be due to a subdural hematoma. The physician's task is to sort out those patients with correctable lesions.

GLUCOSE

Blood glucose concentrations should be measured in every patient subjected to trauma, again with the understanding that surgery should proceed even if the results are not available. Hyperglycemia of severe degree is usually picked up as glucosuria. Hypoglycemia can be missed, however, and tragedy can result if, for example, an insulin reaction is missed.

WHITE BLOOD CELL COUNT

Peripheral blood contains approximately 4,000 white cells to 10,000 white cells per microliter. More important than the total white cell count is the differential white cell count, which gives the proportions of different cell types that comprise the total number of white cells. Of primary importance in the patient who has sustained trauma is the "shift to the left," which reflects an absolute increase in the number of neutrophils, in particular, of the more immature forms. Conditions causing neutrophilia (more than 8000 polymorphonuclear/μl) are shown in Table 10-5. Serial

---

TABLE 10-5   CAUSES OF NEUTROPHILIA

Infections
    Pyogenic bacteria
    Abscess
    Septicemia
Acute inflammation or necrosis
    Infarction
    Collagen disease
    Acute hemolysis
Neoplasms
Intoxication
    Drugs
    Chemicals
Acute hemorrhage

white cell count determinations are of more value in the trauma patient than single determinations. The development of neutrophilia or the appearance of a shift to the left may give the clinician early clues that there is an inflammatory response, usually in the peritoneal cavity, that is causing early mobilization of neutrophils.

AMYLASE

Amylase is an enzyme secreted by both the pancreas and the salivary glands. It splits starch into its component sugars. Damage to either the glandular cells or the ductal systems may cause amylase to enter the bloodstream.

Elevated serum amylase concentrations, especially persistent elevations at levels of more than 300 Somogyi units/dl, suggest pancreatic injury. However, the pancreas can be seriously damaged and serum amylase concentrations remain normal. In addition, the serum amylase can be quite high transiently in patients with a nondamaged pancreas. Thus, for the most part, we do not rely on serum amylase concentrations in assessing the trauma patient.

OTHER BLOOD TESTS

Other laboratory blood tests that should be considered but that need not be performed routinely on trauma patients include serum electrolytes (sodium, potassium, bicarbonate, and chloride), BUN, creatinine, and liver function tests. After the first intravenous line has been inserted, approximately 40 ml of whole blood should be obtained rapidly; 10 ml should be sent immediately for type and cross-match and the remainder kept for further tests to be performed when indicated by history or subsequent events. Ten milliliters of blood should be kept aside for toxicology and blood alcohol determinations, which are done when the history warrants it.

ARTERIAL BLOOD GASES

Arterial blood gases, obtained anaerobically from the femoral or radial artery, include the partial pressure of oxygen (Po_2), the partial pressure of carbon dioxide (Pco_2), and blood *p*H. The arterial Po_2 is indicative of the amount of oxygen passing from inspired air into the blood. It is influenced by ventilatory capacity, pulmonary perfusing surfaces, distribution of pulmonary blood flow, and the adequacy of pulmonary and systemic circulation. The Pco_2 is a more accurate measure of ventilation, since carbon dioxide diffuses more readily across alveolar surfaces than does oxygen. Blood *p*H values accurately reflect the body's acid–base balance but do not as a single value tell the clinician whether an abnormality is due to metabolic or respiratory causes. In the severely traumatized patient, the *p*H is most commonly

below 7.4 and reflects a metabolic acidosis secondary to the accumulation of hydrogen ions. The metabolic acidosis may be altered, both by compensatory respiratory alkalosis, if the patient is spontaneously ventilating, and by the resuscitation procedure itself, which is often done with balanced salt solution containing variable amounts of base. Isolated measurements may give the clinician some index as to ventilatory status or perfusion, but serial measurements give more information.

EVALUATION AND MANAGEMENT OF SPECIFIC INJURIES

PATHOPHYSIOLOGY OF PENETRATING AND BLUNT TRAUMA

PENETRATING TRAUMA

Stab wounds are relatively benign injuries unless a major blood vessel has been lacerated or a vital structure has been injured. Rarely do these result in much morbidity. Gunshot wounds, on the other hand, may cause devastating abdominal injury, particularly if they are from high-velocity weapons or close-range shotguns. Common handguns and weapons are listed in Table 10-6 with their respective muzzle velocities.

Terminal ballistics, the amount of energy imparted to tissues by the missile, largely determines the injury and killing power. Although not all authorities agree, the most widely accepted terminal ballistic theory is the kinetic energy theory. The kinetic energy theory states that kinetic energy released to tissues equals mass times velocity squared, divided by two times the gravity. This is thought to provide the best estimate of wounding capacity, and it follows that modest increases in velocity will result in tremendous increases in the kinetic energy of the missile and the resultant killing and wounding power. Simple calculations using this formula demonstrate that a .22 Magnum is capable of eight times the energy release of a .38 revolver. Generally, those weapons capable of generating a missile velocity in excess of 2000 ft/second are said to be high velocity.

The amount of energy imparted to the tissue is estimated to be kinetic energy upon impact minus kinetic energy upon exit. Thus, bullet design becomes important; to inflict the greatest possible tissue damage, a bullet should dissipate all of its energy to the tissue with no residual exit energy. This has led to the development of missiles that disintegrate upon impact, such as soft-point and hollow-nose bullets. Increased muzzle velocity and disintegrating missiles can cause extensive tissue damage. Some missiles, for example, can create a temporary cavity 30 times the size of the entering bullet, the size of this cavity being dependent on ballistics, the type of bullet, and the tissue that is transgressed. The damage produced can be worsened by secondary missiles or fragments of disintegrating bone and other tissue.

Close-range shotgun blasts undoubtedly cause the most devastating injuries of any weapon to which civilians are normally exposed. Sherman and Parrish have classified shotgun wounds into three categories: type I shotgun injuries, sustained at long range (greater than 7 yards); type II shotgun injuries, sustained at close range (3 yards–7 yards); and type III shotgun injuries, sustained at very close range (less than 3 yards). Type I injuries usually present as scatter types and may not even penetrate visceral cavities

TABLE 10-6   EXAMPLES OF MUZZLE VELOCITY

WEAPON	VELOCITY (FT/SEC)
.22 Long Rifle	1335
.22 Magnum	2000
.220 Swift	2800
.270 Winchester	3580
.357 Magnum	1550
.38 Colt	730
.44 Magnum	1850
.45 Army Colt	850

from distances greater than 40 yards; at 20 yards, penetration is increased and yet expectant management may sometimes be warranted. Type II injuries usually involve damage to deep structures and require more aggressive management. Type III wounds produce massive tissue injury, and the mortality rate is very high (85%–90%).

BLUNT TRAUMA

Blunt injury can be caused by direct impact, deceleration, rotary forces, and shear forces. Direct impact may cause significant injury, and the severity can be estimated by knowing the force and duration of impact, as well as the mass of the patient contact area. Ejection, steering assembly impact, windshield impact, instrument panel impact, and rear collision account for the majority of the most common sites of injury from motor vehicle accidents.

Deceleration injuries are most often associated with high-speed motor vehicle accidents and falls from heights. As the body decelerates, the organs continue to move forward at terminal velocity, tearing vessels and tissues from points of attachment. Rotary forces also tend to cause tearing injuries from a tumbling type of action.

Shear forces have a tendency to produce degloving injuries such as are apt to occur when the patient is run over by a large vehicle. As the vehicle passes over the body, the skin and subcutaneous tissues are pushed ahead, tearing nutrient blood supply from its muscular sources below. Subsequent extensive soft-tissue loss is common following such injury.

Blunt trauma, under certain conditions, can result in a compartment syndrome, a syndrome of swollen necrotic muscle confined within a fascial compartment. The compartment syndrome can be caused by direct impact on the muscle or by continuous pressure. The continuous pressure can be generated by obtunded patients lying on their extremities in an awkward position; the pressure can also be generated with severe muscular exertion, metabolic disturbances, and toxicity syndromes.

The pathophysiology of compartment syndromes begins with local muscle compression, decreased capillary flow, damage to capillaries, and eventual ischemic necrosis of the compressed muscle. This in turn leads to increased permeability of capillaries. Fluid leaks into the interstitium, compartment pressure builds up, and a compartment tamponade occurs.

The symptoms and signs of an early compartment syndrome include pain and tense swelling in the affected extremity. Skin edema is frequently minimal. The patient develops a third-space loss of plasma, resulting in an increasing hematocrit, progressive hypovolemia, and oliguria.

The sequelae of the compartment syndrome are muscle necrosis, nerve damage, and paralysis. Myoglobin and hemoglobin can be released into the plasma and can precipitate in the renal tubules and cause tubular necrosis.

Treatment includes early fasciotomy, excision of necrotic tissue, and volume resuscitation. An alkalotic urine should be maintained with bicarbonate, and a diuresis should be promoted with mannitol.

GENERAL APPROACH TO THE INJURED PATIENT

PROPHYLAXIS AGAINST INFECTION

Preoperative antibiotics are useful adjuncts in the management of compound fractures, dirty soft-tissue wounds, and suspected small-bowel or colon injuries. The use of antibiotics in other trauma injuries has not been demonstrated to be efficacious. Suggested antibiotics are shown in Table 10-7. In the case in which antibiotics have been started for a suspected intestinal injury but no injury is found at surgery, the antibiotics should be stopped in the immediate postoperative period. Otherwise, the antibiotics should be given for a total of 48 to 72 hours.

Prophylaxis against tetanus should be considered for all open wounds. Guidelines have been developed by the American College of Surgeons and are listed in Table 10-8 (see also Chapter 9).

ASSIGNMENT OF PRIORITIES

A team approach is often appropriate in the patient with multiple injuries and may include simultaneous decompression of a space-occupying intracranial lesion by neurosurgeons while general surgeons explore the abdomen. In the patient with massive abdominal injuries and an associated widened mediastinum, exploration of the abdomen with repair of injuries is indicated first. Following laparotomy, an aortogram can be obtained and thoracic aortic rupture, if present, treated. If the patient has associated major vascular injuries to the extremities, control of these must be obtained prior to abdominal exploration. If the patient remains unstable, exploratory laparotomy should be done before definitive treatment of the peripheral vascular injuries.

SURGICAL PREPARATION AND EXPOSURE

The trauma patient must be prepared and draped widely so that the surgeon can gain access to any body cavity expeditiously and can properly place drains and chest tubes, if needed. The entire anterior portion and both lateral portions of the torso should be prepared with iodine paint and draped off so that the surgeon can work in a sterile field from the neck and clavicles cephalad to the groins caudad and from table top to table top laterally. Prepping should not involve

---

TABLE 10-7   ANTIMICROBIAL PROPHYLAXIS—72 HOURS OR LESS

Suspected small-bowel or large-bowel injury

  Chloramphenicol, 60 mg/kg/day, intravenously in 4 divided doses*
  or
  Cefoxitin, 150 mg/kg/day, intravenously in 4 to 6 divided doses*
  or
  Clindamycin† 40 mg/kg/day, intravenously in 3 to 4 divided doses plus tobramycin or gentamicin, 5 mg/kg/day, intravenously or intramuscularly in 3 divided doses*

Traumatic wound (compound fractures, extensive soft-tissue injury)

  Methicillin, nafcillin, or oxacillin, 1 g intravenously three to four times a day
  or
  Cefazolin, cephalothin, or cephapirin, 1 g intramuscularly or intravenously three to four times a day

* Penicillin, 200,000 units/kg/day, in 6 divided doses may be added.
† Metronidazole may be substituted for clindamycin. Give 15 mg/kg over 1 hour (loading dose), then 7.5 mg/kg every 6 hours.

TABLE 10-8 TETANUS PROPHYLAXIS

I. Persons previously immunized

A. When the attending physician has determined that the patient has been previously fully immunized and the last dose of toxoid was given within 10 years:

1. For non-tetanus-prone wounds, no booster dose of toxoid is indicated.

2. For tetanus-prone wounds and if more than 5 years have elapsed since the last dose, give 0.5 ml absorbed toxoid. If excessive prior toxoid injections have been given, this booster may be omitted.

B. When the patient has had two or more prior injections of toxoid and received the last dose more than 10 years previously, give 0.5 ml absorbed toxoid for both tetanus-prone and non-tetanus-prone wounds. Passive immunization is not considered necessary.

II. Persons not adequately immunized

A. When the patient has had no prior injection of toxoid or has received only one prior injection of toxoid, or when the immunization history is unknown:

1. For non-tetanus-prone wounds, give 0.5 ml absorbed toxoids.

2. For tetanus-prone wounds,

a. Give 0.5 ml absorbed toxoid.
b. Give 250 units (or more) of human T.A.T.
c. Consider providing antibiotics, although the effectiveness of antibiotics for prophylaxis of tetanus remains unproved.

more than a few minutes; preferably, it is carried out prior to induction of anesthesia so that should deterioration occur, immediate laparotomy or thoracotomy can be performed.

For rapid access and wide exposure of the abdomen, the midline incision is the incision of choice. Only rarely will transverse or oblique incisions be appropriate for trauma. Surgeons should be prepared to extend the midline incision up to the sternum as a sternal splitting incision or into the right or left side of the chest, if necessary. The chest should, therefore, be prepped along with the abdomen.

An abdomen filled with bright red blood indicates an arterial injury. The patient should be eviscerated, each corner of the abdomen rapidly inspected, and packs placed temporarily to control any bleeding encountered. All quadrants of the abdomen and the mesentery should be inspected on the first pass. This can be done within a minute or two so that the most major source of hemorrhage can be located and dealt with first. The application of packs will control bleeding from many arterial injuries, and if the injury can be controlled by pack or direct pressure, this should be done while volume is restored. Initially, the injury should not be exposed directly because the vascular system may suddenly decompress; massive loss of blood volume in a previously hypovolemic patient frequently leads to cardiac arrest.

If the injury appears to be arterial and in the upper abdomen, the possibility of injury to the visceral portion of the aorta or one of its major upper abdominal branches should be considered and proximal control must be ensured. If a hematoma extends into the level of the diaphragm, the left side of the chest should be opened and the aorta encircled. If the aortic hiatus is free of hematoma, the gastrohepatic ligament should be divided and the aorta encircled as it emerges through the crura of the diaphragm.

Minor injuries and minor sources of hemorrhage should not distract the surgeon from dealing with major ongoing hemorrhage, particularly venous hemorrhage. Venous bleeding may not be obvious unless looked for, since it is low pressure and may not be as dramatic or as evident as the arterial hemorrhage. Almost all venous bleeding can be controlled by the judicious application of packs, permitting time for restoration of volume.

In general, the supine position is preferred for all trauma patients. One exception is the patient with demonstrated injury to the left subclavian artery between its takeoff and the vertebral artery. In this injury, a right lateral decubitus position and left posterolateral thoracotomy is preferred.

After neurosurgical, thoracic, and abdominal injuries have been treated, maxillofacial and orthopaedic injuries are treated, in that order, often making use of the initial anesthetic. Exceptions to this general priorization occur.

HEAD INJURIES

INITIAL EVALUATION AND MANAGEMENT

Head injuries continue to be the most frequent cause of death following traumatic injury. They account for approximately half of the fatalities from trauma, and the nonfatal injuries account for over 5 million days of hospitalization and over 30 million days lost from work annually in the United States.

Evaluation and treatment of head injury become the number four priority after control of airway, control of hemorrhage, and support of the cardiovascular system. The mechanical brain damage that occurs at the moment of injury cannot be reversed by therapeutic intervention. Effective management of head injury depends on the prevention of secondary insults to the traumatized brain. Therefore, the surgeon resuscitating the trauma patient must concentrate on diagnosing and treating hypoxia and hypovolemia; as is the case in any injured patient, effective oxygen transport and blood flow must assume first priority.

The severity of brain injury can be determined in less than 1 minute by evaluating level of consciousness, high brain-stem activity, pupillary function, lateralized weakness of the extremities, and spinal cord function (Table 10-9).

Level of consciousness can be assessed either by the Glascow Coma Scale (see Table 10-3) or by a more simple method of testing appropriateness of responses to verbal and painful stimuli. The advantage of the Glascow Coma Scale is that a numerical score can be obtained, which then facilitates triage and determination of deterioration that requires surgery or further diagnostic work-up. A difference of 2 signals a change in neurologic status. A decrease of 3 usually indicates an enlarging hematoma and demands prompt treatment.

High brain-stem function is best determined by whether the patient has posturing signs such as decorticate or decerebrate posturing. The prognosis with such findings in adults is poor, since this is usually associated with parenchymal bleeding.

TABLE 10-9   CORRELATION BETWEEN CLINICAL SIGNS AND LEVELS OF BRAIN FUNCTION

ANATOMICAL REGION	NEUROLOGIC SIGN
Cerebral hemispheres	Verbal responses Purposeful movements
Brain stem	Reflex motor movements Decortication Decerebration
Reticular activating system	Eye opening
Midbrain, cranial nerve III	Reactive pupils
Pons, cranial nerves V + VII	Corneal reflex
Pons, cranial nerves VIII, VI, III, + MLF	Doll's eyes and ice-water responses
Medulla	Breathing Blood pressure
Spinal cord	Deep tendon reflexes Rectal examination Sphincter tone Bulbocavernosus reflex

Pupillary function is assessed by size, equality, and response to bright light. Although ocular injury may cause asymmetry, any observed pupillary inequality must be attributed to intracranial injury until proved otherwise.

Lateralized extremity weakness is detected in patients able to cooperate by testing motor power and in uncooperative patients by observing symmetry of movement in response to painful stimulus. As the severity of injury worsens, lateralized weakness is more difficult to appreciate, but small differences may be important.

In the unconscious patient, spinal cord function should be assessed by determining rectal sphincter tone and by eliciting the bulbocavernosus reflex. No neurologic examination is complete until the rectal examination is done.

Basilar skull fractures are diagnosed on the basis of physical findings. Unilateral or bilateral periorbital ecchymosis (raccoon eyes) is due to intraorbital bleeding from orbital roof fractures. Bleeding from the ear represents a basilar fracture through the lateral portion of the temporal bone unless there has been injury to the ear or tympanic membrane. Ecchymosis behind the pinna (Battle's sign) represents blood dissecting to the skin from a mastoid fracture. This sign is usually not present until 12 to 24 hours after injury. Cerebrospinal fluid may be detected in the nose or ears and invariably indicates meningeal disruption from a basilar fracture.

Fractures of the temporal bone may produce damage to the seventh or eight cranial nerve. Facial palsy of immediate onset represents direct facial nerve injury at the site of temporal bone fracture and requires early diagnostic evaluation and possible surgical repair. Facial palsies of delayed onset almost always resolve spontaneously.

A chest film is mandatory in all patients with head injury to rule out hemothorax, pneumothorax, or other pulmonary lesions that might lead to hypoxia or hypercarbia. Similarly, film of the lateral cervical spine is mandatory in unconscious patients with head injury or in those who manifest crepitance or pain on physical examination.

The indications for skull films remain controversial. They are not a substitute for a carefully done neurologic examination that is documented in the medical record. They may be helpful in penetrating injuries or if a fracture is suspected on physical examination. If the patient is neurologically intact following head injury without headache, nausea or vomiting, lethargy, or focal deficit, skull films are not warranted.

CT scanning of the head has proved to be an invaluable diagnostic aid. Epidural, subdural, and intracerebral hematomas, cortical contusions, cerebral edema, skull fractures of various sorts, and intracranial foreign bodies are all visualized with precision. CT scanning has become so important in the management of head injury that institutions without these devices should have transfer agreements to centers where the technique is available. CT scans should be obtained in any patient with a depressed level of consciousness or focal neurologic deficit such as hemiparesis or aphasia. Digital subtraction angiography is now being used in conjunction with CT scanning and may be a useful adjunct, since it can show displacement of cerebral vessels. Air ventriculography and radioisotope scanning have largely been replaced by CT scanning.

DEFINITIVE MANAGEMENT

After assuring adequate oxygen transport and blood flow to the patient with a head injury, attention should be directed toward treating intracranial hypertension. This can be managed best in the early phases of injury by decreasing the intravascular cerebral blood volume or by decreasing brain water. Intravascular cerebral blood flow should be decreased by controlled hyperventilation because the arterial carbon dioxide concentration is the most potent known regulator of cerebral vessel size. For severe head injury, hyperventilation to Pco_2 values in the low 20s may be necessary. Decreasing brain water may be accomplished with diuretics or hyperosmotic agents, the latter being more prompt in action. If the Glasgow Coma Scale is less than 6 or drops by 3 or more points, mannitol should be used, given as a loading bolus of at least 1 g/kg. Although some centers still advocate the use of steroids, their use is controversial and has not been proved effective in reducing brain edema following acute head injury.

The role of surgery in head trauma is to remove mass lesions and to prevent the delayed development of infection by treating open head injuries. Ideally, radiographic studies will have been obtained prior to surgery to direct the surgeon to the lesion. If the patient has arrived in an unstable state or deteriorates rapidly before diagnostic tests can be obtained, bilateral diagnostic burr holes should be placed in the temporal, frontal, and parietal regions. If the clinical examination shows evidence of transtentorial herniation, the first burr hole is placed in the temporal region on the side of the dilated pupil and quickly expanded to a small craniectomy. If no extradural hematoma is found, the dura is opened in search of a subdural hematoma. Any hematoma that is found is rapidly decompressed by suction through the burr hole. This lateral temporal decompression is designed to quickly relieve brain-stem compression. If no hematoma is discovered at the first burr hole, a temporal burr hole is placed on the contralateral side. These two burr holes are rapidly followed with bilateral frontal and parietal burr holes to exclude an extracerebral hematoma in these locations.

If a subdural or epidural hematoma is found, a frontotemporoparietal craniotomy must be performed rapidly. Acute extracerebral hematomas cannot be adequately evacuated through burr holes. Epidural hematomas usually arise from temporal skull fractures that have caused laceration of the posterior branch of the middle meningeal artery, which must be exposed and coagulated. Subdural bleeding typically arises from veins bridging from the cerebral cortex to the superior sinus, most often in the frontal region. These may also be controlled by electrocoagulation. If cortical lacerations are found, the surgeon must débride necrotic brain and secure hemostasis in the pial and intraparenchymal vessels.

Compound, depressed skull fractures require immediate operation to prevent development of late intracranial infection. These fractures are débrided and the bone fragments are washed in an antibiotic solution and reserved for immediate replacement. Dural and brain lacerations are débrided, and the dura is prepared either primarily or by the use of pericranial and fascia lata grafts. Large dural lacerations overlying basilar fractures may be repaired by onlay grafts of temporal fascia or pericranium.

Intracranial hypertension must be controlled in the postoperative period as well as in the preoperative period. A catheter can be left in the lateral ventricle or subdural space for postoperative monitoring of intracranial pressure. Alternatively, a threaded bolt can be placed through a small drill hole in the skull under which the dura has been opened. An attempt is made to keep intracerebral pressure below 20 torr. This can be achieved in some cases by moderate hyperventilation, hyperosmolar therapy, drainage of ventricular cerebrospinal fluid, head elevation, control of body temperature, and, occasionally, diuretic therapy.

Barbiturate coma has been tried both experimentally and in clinical situations. Its efficacy is not well established, and the complications may outweigh its usefulness. Dimethyl sulfoxide (DMSO) has also been tried in some clinical situations. Results are encouraging, but further clinical evaluation is required.

Other postoperative management problems include fluid and electrolyte regulation, anticonvulsive therapy, and management of late sequelae of head injury, including communicating hydrocephalus, cerebrospinal fluid leaks, and postconcussion syndrome (see Chapter 46).

SPINAL CORD INJURIES

INITIAL EVALUATION AND MANAGEMENT

Spinal cord injuries are devastating to the patient and to society. One of the most important concepts in caring for the trauma patient is to prevent further cord damage after the patient arrives in an emergency facility. It is equally important to diagnose spinal cord injury when the patient is first seen. In one series, one third of the patients were not diagnosed when first seen in the emergency room. Causes for this lack of diagnosis include patients with head injury, patients with multiple injuries (including fractures elsewhere), impaired consciousness, and intoxication with drugs or alcohol.

Cervical spine fractures and dislocations are most common after motor vehicle accidents, falls, athletic injuries, and missile wounds. In most instances, patients are conscious and give a history of pain in the back or neck, weakness, numbness, or loss of control of extremities or sphincters. If any of these symptoms exist, the patient should have immediate protection of the neck to prevent further damage until films are obtained to rule out spinal injury. Stabilization can be obtained with light halter traction and continuous supervision. Sandbags may provide additional stability. Collars provide no significant neck protection.

Of the patients who are unconscious and have a head injury, 3% will have an associated cervical spine injury. For this reason, all patients who arrive unconscious must be assumed to have cervical spine injury until ruled out by a lateral cervical spine film that includes all seven vertebrae.

Lower spine injuries are best assessed by palpation of the spinous processes to locate tenderness and swelling. Rotational deformity and gaps between the processes are indicative of posterior instability. A complete neurologic examination, including sensory and motor evaluation and anal sphincter contraction, must be given each patient. It is also important to differentiate between nerve root injuries and damage to the cord. Incomplete cord injuries show mixed motor and sensory sparing rather than a classic pattern of partial injury.

X-ray films are extremely important in evaluating the patient with spinal injury. They are of primary use in assessing damage to the vertebral column and whether the fracture is stable or unstable. They may demonstrate fractures and dislocations and potential for further cord damage. CT scanning has been extremely useful in assessing vertebral injuries. CT scan plus routine x-ray film may or may not establish whether the fracture is stable or unstable. If an unstable spinal injury is diagnosed, skeletal traction is indicated for cervical spine injuries and most thoracolumbar spine injuries as well.

DEFINITIVE MANAGEMENT

The patient who presents with quadriplegia is often hypotensive secondary to absence of sympathetic tone. This may confuse the clinical picture, causing occult blood loss to go undetected. The hypotension should be correlated with peripheral perfusion and fluid overload should be avoided to achieve "normotensive" pressures.

Respiratory failure is a common sequela following quadriplegia. This may be secondary to inability to clear secretions, atelectasis, or lack of diaphragm function. Mechanical ventilation may be necessary.

No treatment has been shown to restore cord function in complete injuries; if a cord is incompletely injured and contused, mechanical stabilization is the treatment of choice. All dislocations and angular deformities should be corrected by proper traction and positioning of the patient. Skeletal traction is best achieved with Gardner-Wells tongs or with the cranial halo. The amount of weight required varies with the level, type, and severity of injury. (For a more extensive review of spinal cord injuries, see Chapter 46.)

MAXILLOFACIAL AND NECK INJURIES

INITIAL EVALUATION AND MANAGEMENT

The first problem in patients with extensive maxillofacial and neck injuries is control of the airway. The swelling and hemorrhage associated with fractures, contusions, and lacerations of the face and neck can make such control difficult. In addition, airway control—difficult as it may be when the patient first presents—usually becomes more difficult as resuscitation and swelling progress.

The physician must recognize the signs of possible airway obstruction (stridor, cyanosis, and air hunger) and act quickly. It is far easier to secure an airway under semielective conditions, when swelling, bleeding, and anatomical distortion are minimal, than to secure it under emergency conditions.

Securing of the airway in patients with severe maxillofacial or neck trauma usually requires insertion of a tube into the trachea. In some patients, the tube can be passed through the mouth or nose; in others, it is necessary to perform a cricothyroidostomy or tracheostomy.

The second problem in patients with severe maxillofacial and neck injuries is control of bleeding. The bleeding can be formidable because of the rich vascularity of the region. Lacerations of the face can be quickly sutured. Bleeding into the posterior pharynx can be controlled with Foley balloon tamponade or formal packing.

The third problem in severe maxillofacial and neck injuries is that these patients may well have cervical spine injuries. The head and neck should be maintained in an axial orientation until such an injury is ruled out with film of the cervical spine.

DEFINITIVE MANAGEMENT

Patients with complete tracheolaryngeal separation have only a few minutes to live. They present with the signs of upper airway obstruction and, in addition, crepitance over the anterior neck. Treatment is emergency tracheostomy in the second or third tracheal ring. Coniotomy or endotracheal intubation in patients with complete separation is contraindicated because the tube will end up in the retrolaryngeal space. Patients with incomplete separation must be treated with oral or nasal endotracheal intubation or with tracheostomy. Oral or nasal endotracheal intubation should be attempted only in the presence of a physician who can perform a tracheostomy, if need be. The tracheolaryngeal separation should then be repaired in the operating room.

Facial fractures are best treated electively in the first 2 weeks after the initial swelling has subsided. Anatomical reduction and stable K-wire fixation of displaced parts to uninjured portions of the craniofacial skeleton may be accomplished through incisions that give excellent exposure with minimal resultant deformity. The stabilization of mobile portions to adjacent uninjured segments is the guiding principle for repair of these injuries.

The craniofacial skeleton is divided into thirds: cranium, maxilla, and mandible. The most common and most severe fractures of the cranium and maxilla are the Le Fort I, II, and III fractures, representing transverse alveolar, paramedian, and craniofacial separations, respectively. The fractures occur along specific tension lines of the maxilla. They should be treated with internal stabilization.

Mandibular fractures can result in significant disability, particularly with regard to occlusion. They may be treated either open or closed, depending on the nature of the injury and the favorability of mastoid muscle pull on the mandibular segments. The primary goal is to establish normal occlusion with the application of arch bars.

Fractures of the frontonaso-orbital region may involve telescoping injuries, with comminution of fragments and disruption of the medial collateral ligaments resulting in traumatic telecanthus. Assessment and treatment of the lacrimal system is required to avoid subsequent epiphora. The incidence of associated ophthalmic and neurologic injury is high, and appropriate consultations must be obtained early. Coronal and lid incisions may be used to give excellent exposure of these injuries with minimal cosmetic deformity.

CHEST INJURIES

Chest injuries account for one fourth of all civilian trauma deaths; the lethal injuries range from rupture of the thoracic aorta to severe pulmonary contusion. Successful initial resuscitation of these injuries requires particular attention to ensuring adequate ventilation and appropriate use of chest tubes and emergency thoracotomies.

INITIAL EVALUATION AND MANAGEMENT

Ventilation

In the patient with a chest injury, as in any acutely injured patient, attention should first be directed to maintaining the airway and ventilation, controlling external bleeding, and resuscitating the cardiovascular system. Patients with direct trauma to the chest are particularly at risk to develop ventilatory insufficiency. The physician must recognize that insufficiency when it occurs. Specific signs of ventilatory insufficiency include air hunger, cyanosis, use of the accessory muscles of ventilation, and a ventilatory rate faster than 25/minute. Less specific manifestations include those of a generalized sympathetic discharge: anxiety, fear, agitation, tachycardia, and cold, clammy skin.

The physician will sometimes have time to confirm ventilatory insufficiency with arterial blood gases. A Pco_2 greater than 40 mm Hg in an acutely injured patient who does not have a *documented* chronic hypercarbia must be taken as absolute evidence of ventilatory insufficiency.

Hypercarbia in patients with slow ventilatory rates is ominous because it implies depression of normal ventilatory drive; hypercarbia in patients with rapid ventilatory rates is ominous because it implies that the patient is unable to eliminate his carbon dioxide even though he is working hard to do so.

In many acutely injured patients, the physician will not have time to wait for the results of a blood gas determination. Lack of a confirmatory gas should not delay intubation and mechanical ventilation if the patient appears to have ventilatory insufficiency. Mechanical ventilation can be discontinued and the patient extubated later if he proves to have good ventilatory function.

Tube Thoracostomy

Eighty to 90% of all chest injuries, whether due to blunt or penetrating trauma, are adequately treated by insertion of one or more chest tubes and do not require open thoracotomy. Whether the injury results in hemothorax or pneumothorax, a chest tube is required to allow drainage of the intrapleural blood, monitoring of the rate of further bleeding, and evacuation of any air present. A large-bore siliconized tube (32 F–40 F) is recommended for this because blood may clot in smaller tubes, precluding their effective function. Only straight chest tubes should be used; right-angled ones are hard to place and position properly unless the chest is open.

If the patient is stable after chest trauma, one should expeditiously obtain a chest film, upright if possible, to define the intrathoracic pathology. However, if the patient is in distress and the clinical examination points to the possibility of hemothorax or pneumothorax as the cause, a chest tube should be inserted in one or both pleural spaces, as clinically indicated, without waiting to see the film.

In the trauma patient, we insert the chest tube in the midaxillary line at the level of the nipple line or higher. Insertion in the midaxillary line avoids the pectoralis and latissimus dorsi muscles; insertion at the nipple line or higher avoids the diaphragm and accidental puncture of intra-abdominal organs.

An incision is made sharply about 3 cm long and carried down through the deep fascia. A large blunt clamp is then inserted through the musculature into the pleural space and opened to bluntly create a hole large enough for insertion of the chest tube. A gloved finger is then inserted in the pleural space and swept around to ensure that the space is free and the chest tube can be inserted without entering lung parenchyma. The chest tube is then grasped at the tip with the clamp and inserted through the hole and directed posteriorly and superiorly. The tube is inserted until the most proximal hole is well inside the chest; it is then tied in place. The chest tube is sterilely connected to a three-bottle suction, and 20 cm to 25 cm water suction is applied.

Posterior tubes effectively drain both fluid and air and are therefore universally effective, whereas anterior tubes are ineffective for fluid removal. Use of the second interspace anteriorly for chest-tube placement should be condemned: It is technically more difficult, yet less effective in evacuation of fluid.

Emergency Thoracotomy

Emergency room thoracotomy offers the only chance for salvage in injured patients who have sustained, or who are about to sustain, a cardiac arrest. Closed-chest cardiopulmonary resuscitation in trauma patients is doomed to failure because of inadequate venous return and limited thoracic blood volume. Open cardiac massage is also limited by inadequate venous return, but it does effectively empty the heart of what blood it does contain.

Occasionally, thoracotomy is the best way to make a quick diagnosis of a life-threatening intrathoracic abnormality. A left thoracotomy will make the diagnosis of, and treat, a left tension pneumothorax. A right tension pneumothorax will be recognized because it pushes the heart and mediastinum into the left hemithorax. Pericardial tamponade can sometimes be recognized on opening the left side of the chest and, in any case, can always be ruled out by opening the pericardial sac.

Emergency thoracotomies succeed most often in patients with penetrating chest injuries. The patient may have a pericardial tamponade that is easy to relieve, intrathoracic bleeding that can be controlled with pressure, a continuing air embolism that can be aborted, or a massive air leak that can be controlled.

Occasionally, emergency thoracotomies succeed in patients with blunt thoracic trauma. The patient may have a controllable rupture of the thoracic aorta or of the atrium or a ruptured mainstem bronchus that will be controlled with cross-clamping of the pulmonary hilum.

Emergency thoracotomies rarely succeed in patients with penetrating extrathoracic trauma. Open cardiac massage may keep a young patient alive while he is being taken to the operating room for definitive control of an uncomplicated injury.

Emergency thoracotomies almost never succeed in patients who have exsanguinated and arrested from severe blunt extrathoracic trauma. The time involved in taking the patient to the operating room and then obtaining control of what is usually a complicated injury is almost always too long to allow salvage.

In penetrating injuries to the left side of the chest, blunt thoracic injuries, and penetrating extrathoracic injuries, a left thoracotomy should be performed. The chest should be opened in the fourth or fifth intercostal space, just beneath the nipple. The incision should be made from the sternum medially to the table top laterally; the severed internal mammary vessels should be ligated later. One or two of the costochondral cartilages at the sternum, above and below the incision, should be cut to facilitate exposure. The pericardium should be opened in a caudal-to-cephalad manner, taking care to avoid the phrenic nerve. The physician should insert his right hand behind the heart and periodically compress it against the sternum. At the same time, he should explore the hemithorax for correctable lesions.

In penetrating injuries to the right side of the chest, the physician should open that side. Although cardiac massage will be impossible, the physician may find a correctable abnormality such as a partially severed intercostal artery or an air leak. The incision can then be carried across the sternum into the left side of the chest, if need be, to initiate cardiac massage.

DEFINITIVE MANAGEMENT OF IMMEDIATELY LIFE-THREATENING INJURIES

Injuries to the chest wall and parenchyma may be subdivided into two categories, immediately life-threatening and potentially life-threatening. There are seven immediately life-threatening injuries: airway obstruction, open pneumothorax, flail chest, tension pneumothorax, massive hemothorax, pericardial tamponade, and air embolism. The six potentially life-threatening injuries are rupture of the tracheobronchial tree, pulmonary contusion, diaphragmatic rupture, esophageal perforation, myocardial contusion, and great-vessel injuries.

Airway Obstruction

The airway can be obstructed by a foreign body, secretions, severe maxillofacial trauma, or a fractured larynx. Treatment of the obstruction includes removing the foreign body, suctioning of secretions, pulling the tongue away from the posterior pharynx, and, if necessary, inserting an oral or nasal endotracheal tube. If these maneuvers fail, a cricothyroidotomy should be performed, except in the patient with a complete laryngeal fracture. Tracheostomy is rarely indicated and should only be performed by someone skilled in the method.

Open Pneumothorax

Either penetrating or blunt trauma can produce an open pneumothorax. The inability to generate negative intrathoracic pressure collapses the lung and leads immediately to ventilatory insufficiency. Treatment is that of immediate covering of the hole in the chest wall with petroleum jelly gauze or any other clean airtight dressing. A chest tube should be inserted through a separate counterincision as soon as feasible. The most important aspect of immediate treatment is closure of the chest wall opening. Reexpansion of the affected lung is of secondary importance.

Flail Chest

Flail chest results from the paradoxical movement of a portion of the chest wall when there are multiple rib fractures and usually when ribs are broken at multiple sites. The problem is analogous in many ways to open pneumothorax, in that the lungs themselves are often not severely damaged, although there may be an element of pulmonary contusion in the lung beneath the fractured segment. Respiratory difficulty occurs because the chest wall is unstable, moving inward with inspiration and outward with expiration. The development of negative intrathoracic pressure is prevented; thus, the patient cannot move air in and out of the trachea normally. Knowledge of this fact also dictates the treatment; one need only stabilize the chest wall. It does not have to be stabilized in an outward position but can be stabilized in an inward position. In an emergency, simply preventing movement of the chest wall will relieve the severe respiratory distress that these patients experience. This is most easily accomplished by turning the patient onto the affected side. If ventilatory distress continues, immediate intubation and positive-pressure ventilation are in order to achieve internal stabilization of the fractures and to ventilate the lungs adequately.

Massive Hemothorax

Massive hemothorax usually results from injuries to the aortic arch, pulmonary hilum, or systemic vessels such as the internal mammary or intercostal arteries. Rupture of large vessels is usually incompatible with survival. On the other hand, many patients present who have continuing rates of blood loss on the order of 500 ml to 1000 ml/hour. Most of the bleeding that occurs with thoracic injuries is not from the lung itself, because the lung is a low-pressure system and the average pulmonary artery pressure is only about 15 torr, not much above venous pressure. As a result, the patient who continues to bleed is usually doing so from the systemic arteries in the chest, that is, the intercostal or internal mammary arteries.

Early placement of chest tubes in any patient who has evidence of intrathoracic blood loss is essential. Monitoring of blood loss indicates how much blood volume replacement is needed and provides continuous assessment of the patient's hemodynamic status. Blood loss of more than 1000 ml to 1500 ml total or more than 300 ml/hour for 2 to 3 hours usually indicates the need for surgery. In addition, autotransfusion should be considered if the patient bleeds massively.

Tension Pneumothorax

Lacerations in the pulmonary parenchyma sometimes act like flap valves and create a tension pneumothorax. Air enters the pleural space but cannot escape. Pleural pressure rises, the lung collapses, the mediastinum shifts into the opposite hemithorax, the opposite lung becomes compressed, and the cava kinks, thus interfering with venous return. The combination of these two factors may lead rapidly to death. Treatment is immediate tube thoracostomy.

Pericardial Tamponade

Patients with pericardial tamponade typically present with shock and tightly distended neck veins. The only other conditions that present similarly in the injured patient are tension pneumothorax and myocardial failure secondary to a myocardial contusion or coronary air embolism. Of these, the cardiac tamponade and tension pneumothorax are usually easy to treat, and the physician must be sure not to miss these diagnoses. One should not miss injuries that are easy to treat.

Treatment of penetrating cardiac injuries have gradually changed from initial management by pericardiocentesis to prompt thoracotomy and pericardial decompression. Pericardiocentesis is reserved for selected patients when the diagnosis is uncertain or during preparation for thoracotomy.

The underlying cardiac injury with cardiac tamponade is usually easily repaired and does not require cardiac bypass. When suturing the wound, care must be taken not to compromise the coronary arteries with the repair sutures (see Chapter 40).

Air Embolism

Air embolism occasionally occurs after penetrating thoracic trauma and rarely after blunt. The systemic air arises from a fistula between a bronchus and a pulmonary vein. Diagnosis is difficult, at best, but should be strongly suspected in any patient who presents with penetrating chest trauma and focal neurologic findings without obvious head injury, any patient who, after endotracheal intubation and the first few breaths of positive-pressure ventilation, develops cardiovascular collapse, and any patient in whom air is found as froth in the initial set of arterial blood gases. This last condition is universally fatal in our experience.

Treatment of air embolism consists of cross-clamping the hilum of the damaged lung. Open cardiac massage sometimes breaks up air bubbles in the coronary arteries. Insertion of a needle into the apex of the left ventricle may recover air. Systemic administration of vasoconstrictors may increase the blood pressure enough to drive some of the air out of the arterioles and capillaries and into the veins.

DEFINITIVE MANAGEMENT OF POTENTIALLY LIFE-THREATENING INJURIES

Rupture of the Tracheobronchial Tree

Rupture of the tracheobronchial tree is characterized by ventilatory distress, subcutaneous emphysema, and hemoptysis. Some patients will have obstruction of their airway, depending upon the nature of the disruption. All patients will have mediastinal air on chest film, many will have a pneumothorax, and some will have a tension pneumothorax.

Treatment consists in trying to establish an airway, if possible, by passing an endotracheal tube beyond the region of the tear so that the patient can be effectively ventilated and will not aspirate blood. A chest tube is inserted to evacuate the pneumothorax when indicated. Thoracotomy is usually required to control the tear.

Pulmonary Contusion

Pulmonary contusion is usually associated with rib fractures and represents a bruise of the lung. Treatment regimens that are controversial include use of diuretics, salt-poor albumin, or steroids, or some combination of these. We recommend that none of these agents be used, as all are ineffective in improving pulmonary function and may be harmful in other ways. Our management consists in pulmonary toilet and ventilatory support.

Rupture of the Diaphragm

Rupture of the diaphragm may be quite a subtle diagnosis, and the clinician must maintain a high index of suspicion. It occurs most often on the left side when secondary to blunt trauma; it can occur in either hemidiaphragm when penetrating trauma is the cause. Although diaphragmatic rupture can be repaired easily from above or below the diaphragm, we prefer the abdominal approach in the majority of cases.

Myocardial Contusion

Myocardial contusion is analogous to pulmonary contusion and represents a bruise or intramural hematoma of the myocardial wall. It is probably underdiagnosed, and only recently, with the advent of myocardial nuclear scanning, has its incidence been appreciated. It commonly presents as arrhythmias in the period immediately surrounding the injury. These may be life-threatening, and procainamide (Pronestyl) given intravenously is usually therapeutic. Frank cardiac failure is rare, but when present it is treated with afterload reduction and inotropic support.

Great-Vessel Injuries

Patients who suffer severe deceleration injuries or penetrating injuries in the vicinity of the great vessels are at risk for injuries to those vessels. The great majority of patients with ruptures or penetrations of the great vessels die at the scene of the accident unless the hole in the artery is small or is tamponaded by the surrounding tissues.

If the patient with blunt trauma and a possible great-vessel injury arrives alive in the emergency room and is hemodynamically stable, work-up should proceed with chest films and, if indicated, a rapidly obtained arch aortogram (Fig. 10-8). Most patients with a rupture of the thoracic aorta secondary to blunt trauma have either a wide mediastinum or obliteration of the aortic knob on chest film. Other chest film findings include blood in the pleural cavities, left apical capping, and displacement of the trachea, left mainstem bronchus, or esophagus, as seen by the position of the nasogastric tube. All of these signs arise because of thoracic bleeding, either intrapleural or extrapleural. Occasionally, the patient will have a well-contained periarterial hematoma and have none of these signs at presentation. The warning to the clinician in these cases will be evidence of severe thoracic trauma, with fractures of the posterior portions of the upper ribs, multiple rib fractures, or fractures of the scapula. Arch aortograms should be obtained in these patients as well.

Patients with blunt trauma, shock, and continuing bleeding from the left side of the chest should be explored through a left posterolateral incision. Such patients usually have a transected aorta. The transection admittedly could be at the origin of the aorta or in the arch, in which cases a posterolateral incision will fail to give adequate exposure and the patient will exsanguinate. In any case, these injuries are difficult to control no matter what incision is used; such a patient who presents with active hemorrhage will probably die no matter what the surgeon does. A left posterolateral incision will provide the best exposure for disruption of the aorta just distal to the takeoff of the left subclavian. Not only is this the most likely injury with blunt trauma, but it is also the injury that the surgeon has the best chance of controlling.

Patients with blunt trauma, shock, and massive bleeding from the right side of the chest should be explored through either a median sternotomy or a right anterolateral thoracotomy. The median sternotomy should not be used if it will delay exposure; the right thoracotomy will usually be adequate.

Patients with penetrating injuries of the great vessels that do not communicate with the pleural cavity frequently survive to reach the hospital; these penetrating injuries are usually at the base of the neck. In the hemodynamically stable patient, arteriography should be obtained to guide the surgeon in exposing the injured vessel. A left postero-lateral thoracotomy should be used to expose injuries of the origin of the left subclavian artery; a median sternotomy with extensions into the neck should be used, if necessary, for the innominate artery or for the origins of the right subclavian and carotid arteries.

Patients with penetrating injuries of the great vessels that communicate with the pleural cavity almost always exsanguinate into the pleural cavity and rarely reach the emergency room alive. If such a patient does reach the emergency room alive, the surgeon will be alerted by a massive hemothorax and continuing bleeding. If the wound is in the left supraclavicular area or in the left side of the chest, an emergency left thoracotomy should be carried out, preferably a posterolateral thoracotomy with the patient in the lateral decubitus position. The posterolateral incision will offer by far the best exposure for the origin of the left subclavian artery and the descending thoracic aorta. If the wound is in the right supraclavicular area or the parasternal regions, a median sternotomy gives the best exposure for the anterior surface of the heart, the ascending aorta, the innominate artery, and the origins of the right subclavian and common carotid arteries. A right anterolateral thoracotomy may be used, if necessary, and carried upward through the sternum or across the sternum if need be. (See also Arterial Injuries in Chapter 36.)

ABDOMINAL INJURIES

INITIAL EVALUATION AND MANAGEMENT

Deaths from abdominal trauma result from either sepsis or hemorrhage, the sepsis or hemorrhage typically arising from different causes, depending upon whether the trauma is penetrating or blunt.

Penetrating Injuries

Penetrating injuries cause sepsis if they perforate a hollow viscus (Table 10-10). A full bowel, when injured, readily evacuates into the peritoneal cavity, and signs of injury are obvious. When an empty bowel is injured or when the site of penetration of the bowel involves its retroperitoneal portion, egress of bowel contents may be negligible initially and therefore give minimal findings. Increasing abdominal tenderness demands exploration. An elevated white cell count or fever appearing several hours following the injury are keys to early diagnosis.

Penetrating injuries of a major vessel or the liver cause severe and early shock; penetrating injuries of the spleen, pancreas, and kidneys usually do not bleed massively unless a major vessel to the organ (*e.g.*, the renal artery) is damaged. Control of the bleeding vessel must be obtained promptly. If the patient with a penetrating injury of the abdomen and shock does not respond to the first 3 liters of fluid resuscitation, he should be operated on immediately, delaying only for a chest film (Fig. 10-9).

The treatment of hemodynamically stable patients with penetrating injuries to the lower chest or abdomen varies from hospital to hospital. All would agree that patients who show signs of peritonitis or hypovolemia should be explored. Surgeons disagree about patients who show no signs of sepsis and who are hemodynamically stable.

We believe that most, but not necessarily all, stab wounds of the lower chest or abdomen should be explored promptly. When a hollow viscus has been injured, delay in treatment can result in progression of intraperitoneal or retroperitoneal contamination to the point of invasive infection and a high

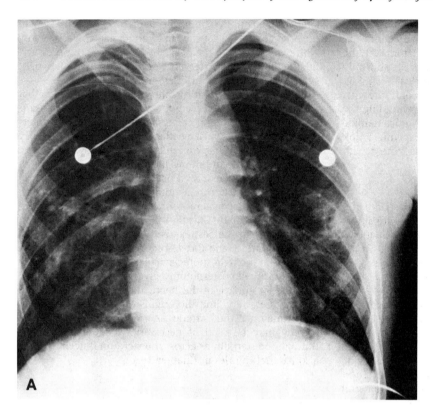

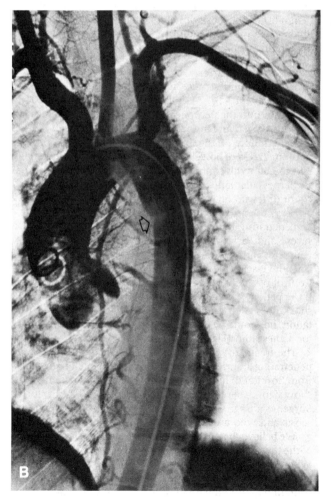

Fig. 10-8.   Patient with a deceleration injury from a motor vehicle accident. In the chest x-ray film (*A*) the mediastinum is minimally widened. Auscultation of the chest revealed an aortic click and mediastinal crepitance. (*B*) An aortogram was obtained, and the arrow marks a bulge and indentation of the descending thoracic aorta.

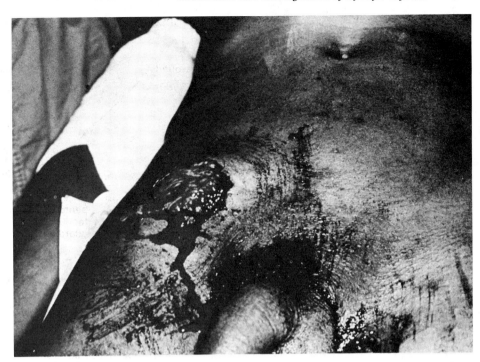

Fig. 10-9. This patient presented with a .357-magnum wound to the right lower quadrant. Injuries were extensive, including right iliac artery, right iliac vein, and extensive soft-tissue and bone injuries in the posterior pelvis.

TABLE 10-10	PENETRATING TRAUMA IN COLLECTED SERIES: THE RELATIVE INCIDENCE OF ORGAN INJURY

ORGAN	PERCENTAGE
Small bowel	30
Mesentery and omentum	18
Liver	16
Colon	9
Diaphragm	8
Stomach	7
Spleen	6
Kidney	5
Major vessels	4
Pancreas	3
Duodenum	2
Bladder	1
Ureter	1
Biliary system	1

incidence of septic complications. A guideline for management of abdominal stab wounds is presented in Figure 10-10. We believe that all gunshot wounds of the lower chest and abdomen should be explored; the incidence of injury to major intra-abdominal structures exceeds 90% with these wounds.

Blunt Trauma

Blunt abdominal trauma usually injures the solid abdominal organs: the spleen, liver, pancreas, and kidneys. Occasionally, hollow organs are injured; the retroperitoneal portion of the duodenum and the bladder are particularly susceptible (Table 10-11).

The three main indications for exploration of the abdomen in patients with blunt abdominal trauma are peritonitis, hypovolemia, and the presence of periabdominal injuries, which are known to be frequently associated with intra-abdominal injuries. Peritonitis after blunt abdominal trauma is rare but, when present, mandates exploration. The peritonitis can arise from rupture of hollow organs, such as the duodenum, bladder, intestine, or gallbladder; from pancreatic injuries; or from free retroperitoneal blood, which, in an occasional patient, can irritate the parietal peritoneum.

Hypovolemia in patients with normal findings on chest film also mandates abdominal exploration unless intra-abdominal bleeding is ruled out by peritoneal lavage or CT scanning of the abdomen or unless the physician can document enough extra-abdominal blood loss to account for the hypovolemia. The physician must put intra-abdominal bleeding as his first diagnosis in any patient with blunt trauma and hypovolemia, even patients who have no overt evidence of abdominal trauma as such. The hypovolemic patient with a large scalp laceration may be hypovolemic on the basis of bleeding from that laceration; he may also be hypovolemic because he has a ruptured spleen. Hemoperitoneum may have no associated physical signs whatsoever except for the signs of hypovolemia. The abdomen may not be distended; it may not be tender. Patients with controlled extra-abdominal bleeding should respond to the initial fluid resuscitation with a good urine output and stabilization of vital signs. If, after initial stabilization, the patient becomes hypovolemic again, there must be bleeding into his abdomen. The surgeon must consider, and reconsider, intra-abdominal bleeding in any hypovolemic patient.

Certain periabdominal injuries are frequently associated with abdominal injuries. These associated injuries include rib fractures, pelvic fractures, abdominal wall injuries, and fractures of the thoracolumbar spine. Sometimes the association between these injuries is striking. For example, 20% of patients with fractures of the left lower ribs have a ruptured spleen. If the patient has any of these periabdominal injuries, he must be observed particularly closely for abdominal injuries that may require exploration.

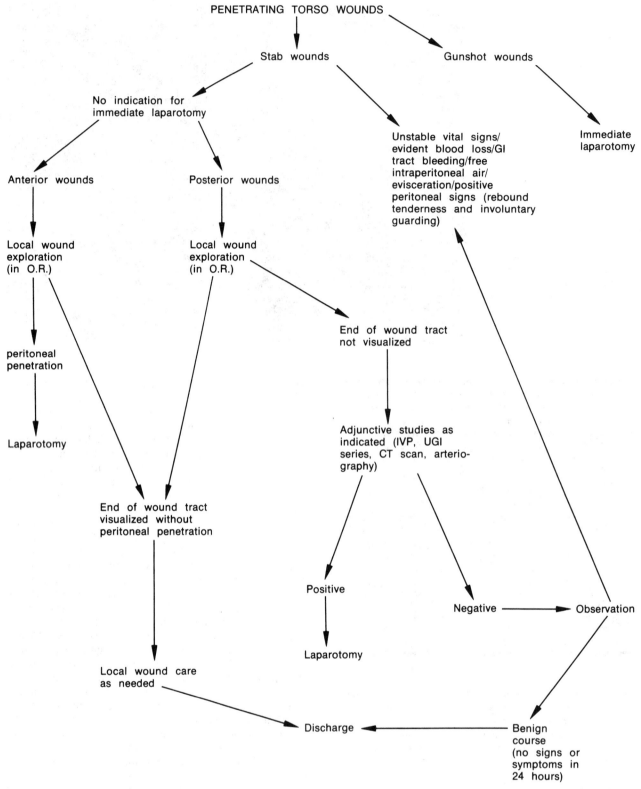

Fig. 10-10. Summary of management protocol for penetrating torso wounds.

DEFINITIVE MANAGEMENT

Abdominal Wall

Abdominal wall injuries from blunt trauma are most often due to shear forces, such as being run over by the wheels of a tractor or bus. The shearing often causes devitalizing injury to the subcutaneous tissue and skin. If these devitalized tissues are not debrided soon after the injury, the stage will be set for necrotizing infections and ultimate mortality. Penetrating abdominal wall injuries are usually straightforward. Debridement and irrigation are the hallmarks of good surgical treatment. Every effort must be made to

TABLE 10-11 **BLUNT TRAUMA IN COLLECTED SERIES: THE RELATIVE INCIDENCE OF ORGAN INJURY**

ORGAN	PERCENTAGE
Spleen	25
Liver	15
Retroperitoneum	13
Kidney	12
Small bowel	9
Bladder	6
Mesentery	5
Large bowel	4
Pancreas	3
Urethra	2
Diaphragm	2
Vessels	2
Stomach	1
Duodenum	1

remove foreign material, particles of clothing, necrotic muscle, and soft tissue. Abdominal wall defects may require prosthetic replacement or myocutaneous flaps.

Biliary Tract

Injury to the gallbladder usually requires cholecystectomy. Cholecystectomy should also be performed whenever there has been a diversion procedure on the common duct and the ampulla is no longer intact. Simple laceration of the gallbladder in conjunction with other major abdominal trauma may be treated with simple closure with an absorbable suture such as polyglycolate.

Most injuries to the common bile duct can be treated with closure and decompressive T-tube choledochostomy. Avulsive injuries of the common duct from duodenal or ampullary trauma may require choledochojejunostomy in conjunction with total or partial pancreatectomy, duodenectomy, or other diversion procedures. Segmental loss of the common bile duct can be treated with mobilization and end-to-end anastomosis with decompression diversion. Occasionally, this may require choledochojejunostomy.

Pancreas

Pancreatic injuries may be hard to detect on physical examination because the organ is retroperitoneal and damage to it may not irritate the anterior parietal peritoneum. The surgeon must suspect a pancreatic injury whenever the upper abdomen is injured, especially when the serum amylase remains persistently elevated. (See also Chapter 28.)

Gastrointestinal Tract

Most injuries of the stomach can be repaired with simple closure in a two-layer technique. Large injuries, such as from shotgun blasts, may require subtotal or total resection.

Most duodenal injuries can be treated with lateral repair, but some may require resection with end-to-end anastomosis, depending on the shared blood supply with the pancreas. Occasionally, total duodenectomy and pancreatectomy are required to manage severe injuries. Duodenostomy is useful in decompressing the duodenum and can be used to control the fistula if a suture-line leak develops. Jejunal or omental patches may also aid in preventing suture-line leak.

The great majority of small-bowel injuries can be treated with two-layer closure, although devascularizing injuries to the mesentery or small bowel require resection. The underlying principle is to maintain as much small bowel as possible.

In massive abdominal injury, the most conservative approach to large-bowel and rectal injuries is to divert the fecal stream or exteriorize the injury (Table 10-12). Primary repair and anastomosis of large bowel in the face of massive trauma or fecal contamination is contraindicated. Treatment of rectal injuries should include proximal diversion and repair with presacral drains. Irrigation of the distal stump should be considered but not done if it will further contaminate the pelvic space.

GENITOURINARY INJURIES

The work-up of genitourinary injuries consists primarily in radiologic examinations and is discussed in the preceding section on radiographic evaluation of the injured patient. The most commonly injured organs of the genitourinary tract are the male genitalia, the uterus, the urethra, the bladder, and the kidneys. Injuries to the female reproductive organs are infrequent except in combination with genitourinary or rectal trauma. Minor injuries to the uterine fundus can usually be repaired with chromic catgut sutures; drainage is not necessary. In more extensive injuries, hysterectomy may be preferable. The vaginal cuff may be left open for drainage, particularly if there is an associated urinary or rectal injury. Injuries involving the pregnant uterus usually result in death of the fetus. Bleeding may be massive in such patients, particularly in women near parturition. Cesarean section and hysterectomy may be the only alternative (see also Chapter 45).

EXTREMITY INJURIES

INITIAL EVALUATION AND MANAGEMENT

Inspection

Because the extremities are paired structures, evaluation commences by comparing the appearance, circumference. length, range of motions, and temperature of the two limbs. Characteristic positions are assumed that suggest deviation from normal. The position of function of the upper extremity favors reaching the face and perineum. It provides a comfortable and unfatiguing grip, with the elbow held at 90° and the forearm neutral between pronation and supination with the wrist extended 30° to 40° and the fingers curled into a pronate position. The position of function is the ideal to be achieved by immobilization with a splint. The position of pain of the upper extremity is one in which the wrist is flexed and grasping is awkward and fatiguing. In the position of pain, the forearm is pronated, the elbow extended; it is

TABLE 10-12 **MORTALITY FROM COLON INJURIES**

CONFLICT	MORTALITY RATE (%)
Civil War	90
Boer War	80
WW I	55
WW II	45
Korea	15
Vietnam	17

the position that the arm passively assumes after injury and paralysis.

In the position of function of the lower extremity, the thigh is slightly adducted, the knee flexed; the ankle is in a neutral position between dorsiflexion and plantar flexion. The position of pain of the lower extremity is flaccid, flexed, and dependent. It is a position assumed after paralysis, below-knee amputation, or rest pain associated with vascular insufficiency (see also Chapter 44).

Peripheral Neurologic Function

Pain in an injured extremity frequently hampers precise motor and sensory evaluation; however, with patience and gentleness, the physician can usually elicit the necessary information. Patients with injuries to the brachial plexus usually present with a mixed weakness and a mixed sensory loss in the arm, forearm, and hand. Injury of the median nerve (C5–T1) above the elbow results in inability to oppose the thumb to the other digits and paralysis of the muscles of the thenar eminence. It is associated with sensory loss over the palmar aspect of the thumb, index finger, middle finger, and radial half of the fourth finger. Injury of the radial nerve (C5–C8) results in wristdrop and inability to extend the fingers and thumb at the metacarpophalangeal joint. Radial nerve injury in the arm is associated with inability to extend the elbow. It characteristically is associated with anesthesia of the dorsum of the thumb and index, middle, long, and part of the fourth fingers. The ulnar nerve (C7–T1), when injured, results in inability to spread or close the fingers or flex the metacarpophalangeal joint, producing a claw hand. It is associated with anesthesia over the dorsal and palmar aspects of the little finger and the ulnar half of the fourth finger.

In the lower extremity, loss of the sciatic nerve results in paralysis of all the muscles below the knee. The leg is anesthetic from midcalf distally, except for a small area on the medial side of the leg. Loss of the peroneal nerve results in paralysis of the muscles in the anterior compartment. The patient is unable to dorsiflex his foot or his toes. He is anesthetic on the anterior portion of his distal leg and on the dorsum of his foot. Loss of the tibial nerve results in paralysis of the muscles in the posterior compartment of the leg. The patient cannot plantar flex his foot fully and cannot flex his toes. He is anesthetic on the plantar surface of his foot.

DEFINITIVE MANAGEMENT

Soft-Tissue Injuries

Soft-tissue injuries of the extremity without a break in the skin are common. Contusions are treated with cold compresses as initial treatment. Sprains and other stretch injuries of ligaments may require initial immobilization by cast or splint and operative repair if total tendinous disruption has occurred. Ace bandages and elevation aid in recovery and minimize discomfort.

Crush Injuries

Crush injuries of the extremities may result in death of muscle tissue from direct injury or from ischemia secondary to venous and arterial obstruction by a tight fascial compartment. The compartment pressure can be measured by several available methods, the simplest of which is to use an 18-gauge needle connected to a strain gauge. If the compartment pressure exceeds 40 torr or rises to within 30

mm of the diastolic blood pressure, fasciotomy is indicated. Although measurement of fascial compartment pressure is somewhat useful in anticipating the potential of ischemia prior to irreparable nerve and muscle injury, electromyography is probably a superior method for evaluating impending functional loss.

Crush injury of the extremity and fascial compartment syndromes are associated with myonecrosis and may cause acute renal failure by precipitation of myoglobin in the proximal renal tubules. In patients at risk for renal failure from crush injury, frequent monitoring of the urine for myoglobin is mandatory. Prophylaxis against myoglobin-induced renal failure after crush injury can be provided by an intravenous infusion of 1000 ml 5% dextrose and water, to which has been added 1 ampule of sodium bicarbonate and 1 ampule of sodium mannitol. The resultant "cocktail" is hyperosmolar and alkaline. It will promote diuresis and alkalinize the urine, preventing myoglobin precipitation. The initial liter of solution is administered at 200 ml/hour until a brisk diuresis is induced, then the rate is reduced to 100 ml/hour. While diuresis is occurring, the urine is frequently checked for myoglobin.

COMPLICATIONS OF INJURY

PHYSIOLOGICAL DEFECTS

CELL MEMBRANES

Transcellular skeletal muscle membrane potentials deteriorate in hemorrhagic and traumatic shock. Sodium, chloride, and water shift into the cell in association with the membrane deterioration; potassium may shift out. The inward flux of fluid compounds the already present intravascular hypovolemia and worsens the shock; it also contributes to the edema seen in patients who have been resuscitated from shock.

ENDOTHELIAL INTEGRITY

Patients who have been subjected to severe trauma behave as if their endothelium is damaged. Protein extravasates into the interstitium more readily than it normally does. Intravascular volume decreases and edema increases.

IMMUNE DEFECTS

Shock and trauma impair immune defenses. The reticuloendothelial system can become congested with debris that washes out of the traumatized tissue. Deposition of clot depletes plasma fibrinogen concentrations and impairs opsonization. Plasma levels of fibronectin (α surface-binding protein) decrease, thus impairing opsonization. T-suppressor-cell function is augmented and B-cell and neutrophil function are impaired, at least in some patients. The effect of all of these abnormalities is to make the patient susceptible to infection.

DISSEMINATED INTRAVASCULAR COAGULATION

Severe shock and trauma frequently lead to at least some intravascular coagulation; the process is characterized by deposition of platelet and fibrin microthrombi throughout the microvasculature. The deposition of clot can compound the inadequate tissue perfusion associated with the shock and can contribute to organ failure. Clinical manifestations of intravascular coagulation include a decreasing platelet count, a decreasing fibrinogen concentration, an increasing prothrombin time, an increasing partial thromboplastin time, an increasing activated clotting time, and an increasing bleeding time. Fibrin monomers and fibrin degradation products may be produced. The patient may develop generalized oozing.

HEMATOPOIESIS

The hematocrit of patients after severe trauma frequently equilibrates at approximately 30%.Transfusion of blood will raise the hematocrit transiently, only to have it fall back toward 30% over the next several days. Erythropoietin levels in patients who have been seriously injured appear to be low for a given hematocrit, and it appears that the hematocrit of 30% is due to the inadequate erythropoietin.

ORGAN DYSFUNCTION

LUNGS

Protein and water extravasate into the interstitium of the lungs of patients resuscitated from traumatic shock to form interstitial and alveolar edema. Although little edema is formed in patients resuscitated from pure hemorrhagic shock, large amounts of edema can form in patients resuscitated from severe traumatic shock. To further worsen pulmonary function, the edema that forms seems to be rich in protein and difficult to clear.

The cause of the increased extravasation of protein into the pulmonary interstitium in patients resuscitated from traumatic shock is unknown. It is not due to fluid overload, in most cases, and it is not due to low plasma oncotic pressures. Thus, resuscitation of patients from traumatic shock should proceed with crystalloid as needed to establish good perfusion and good urine output, even if ventilatory insufficiency develops. Ventilatory insufficiency can be treated with intubation and mechanical ventilation; treatment of renal failure is difficult.

KIDNEYS

Administration of adequate amounts of fluid early during resuscitation is almost all that is needed to prevent renal failure in the trauma patient. Renal failure should be rare.

In the early phases of resuscitation, fluid should be given until urine output responds. The physician should never use diuretics in the acute phases of resuscitation of the trauma patient. Inadequate urine output almost always means inadequate fluid replacement or inadequate control of bleeding.

In the oliguric patient with a pulmonary arterial catheter in place, diuretics may be given cautiously. Cardiac indices and filling pressures should be measured before and after administration of the diuretic.

The diagnosis of acute tubular necrosis in the oliguric patient can be established by finding tubular casts in the urine sediment and by documenting a fractional excretion of sodium that is greater than 1%. Interpretation of urinary electrolytes and fractional excretions of sodium is unreliable if the patient has been given a diuretic.

LIVER

Serum bilirubin concentrations frequently increase several days after resuscitation in severely traumatized patients. The alkaline phosphatase may also rise. The other liver function test results remain close to normal.

This cholestaticlike picture seems to be due to obstruction of the biliary canaliculi by swollen hepatocytes or by fatty infiltration of the liver. The swollen hepatocytes are probably another reflection of the generalized shock state; the fatty infiltration is sometimes due to the administration of inappropriately large amounts of carbohydrate in total parenteral nutrition. Prevention and treatment consist in rapid resuscitation and judicious use of nutritional support.

GASTROINTESTINAL TRACT

The gastrointestinal tract responds to trauma with an ileus; the stomach responds with hyperacidity and stress ulceration. The ileus should be treated with nasogastric suction; the hyperacidity should be treated with antacid neutralization.

HEART

The heart performs well in most patients resuscitated from shock. In an occasional patient with underlying disease, and in patients whose hearts were damaged by the injury, cardiac function will be marginal. Pulmonary arterial catheters should be placed in any patient in whom the question of adequacy of cardiac function arises. Measurement of filling pressures and of cardiac index will guide treatment toward more or less fluid or toward the administration of inotropes or afterload-reducing agents.

BRAIN

The brain responds to shock and tramua with the development of mental states that vary from excitation to obtundation. The physician's first duty is to be sure that the abnormal mental status is not due to inadequately treated shock.

SKELETAL MUSCLE

Patients resuscitated from severe shock and trauma frequently are weak. The weakness impairs ventilatory efforts and ability to ambulate. This weakness is presumably related to the deteriorated membrane potentials. Prevention and treatment of all the postinjury complications start with aggressive resuscitation, prompt control of hemorrhage, early immobilization of fractures, early restoration of flow to ischemic tissues, and definitive debridement of necrotic tissues.

BIBLIOGRAPHY

BAKER CC, MILLER CL, TRUNKEY DD: Predicting fatal sepsis in burn patients. J Trauma 19:641, 1979

BAKER CC, OPPENHEIMER L, STEPHENS B: Epidemiology of trauma deaths. Am J Surg 140:144, 1980

BAKER CC, THOMAS AN, TRUNKEY DD: The role of emergency room thoracotomy in trauma. J Trauma 20:848, 1980

BAKER SP, O'NEILL B: The injury severity score: An update. J Trauma 16:882, 1976

BECKER DP, MILLER DJ, WARD JD: The outcome from severe head injury with early diagnosis and intensive management. J Neurosurg 47:491, 1977

BLAISDELL FW, TRUNKEY DD: Abdominal Trauma. New York, Thieme/Stratton, 1982

CARLTON CE, JR, SCOTT R, JR, CUTHRIE AJ: The initial management of ureteral injuries: Report of 78 cases. J Urol 105:335, 1971

CLIFTON GL, GROSSMAN RG, MALEKA ME: Neurological course and correlated computerized tomography findings after severe head injury. J Neurosurg 52:611, 1980

DAUGHTRY DC (ed): Thoracic Trauma. Boston, Little, Brown & Co, 1980

DEMLING RH, MANDHAR M, WILL JA: Response of the pulmonary microcirculation to fluid loading after hemorrhagic shock and resuscitation. Surgery 87:552, 1980

DINGMAN RO, CONVERSE JM: The clinical management of facial injuries and fractures of the facial bones. In Converse JM (ed): Reconstructive Plastic Surgery, pp 646–708, Philadelphia, W B Saunders, 1977

DUCKER TB et al: Experimental spinal cord trauma: III. Therapeutic effect of immobilization and pharmacologic agents. Surg Neurol 10:71, 1978

FEUER H: Management of acute spine and spinal cord injuries: Old and new concepts. Arch Surg 111:638, 1976

FRY DE, PEARSTEIN L, FULTON RL et al: Multiple system organ failure: The role of uncontrolled infection. Arch Surg 115:136, 1980

GALBRAITH TA, ORESKOVICH MR, HEIMBACH DM et al: The role of peritoneal lavage in the management of stab wounds to the abdomen. Am J Surg 140:60, 1980

GRAHAM JM, FELICIANO DV, MATTOX KL et al: Management of subclavian vascular injuries. J Trauma 20:537, 1980

GREEN BA, CALLAHAN RA, KLOSE KJ et al: Acute spinal cord injury: Current concepts. Clin Orthop 154:125, 1981

GRIFFITH GL, TODD EP, MCMILLIN RD et al: Acute traumatic hemothorax. Ann Thorac Surg 26:204, 1978

JENNETT F, TEASDALE G: Management of Head Injuries. Philadelphia, F A Davis, 1981

KERSTER TE, MCQUARRIE DG: Surgical management of shotgun injuries of the face. Surg Gynecol Obstet 140:517, 1975

KINNEY JM, BENDIXEN HH, POWERS SR JR (eds): Manual of Surgical Intensive Care. Philadelphia, W B Saunders, 1977

LUCAS CE: The renal response to acute injury and sepsis. Surg Clin North Am 56:953, 1976

MENDEZ R: Renal trauma. J Urol 118:698, 1977

OMMAYA AK, GENNARELLI TA: Cerebral concussion and traumatic unconsciousness: Correlation of experimental and clinical observations on blunt head injuries. Brain 97:633, 1974

OPARAH SS, MANDAL AK: Operative management of penetrating wounds of the chest in civilian practice. J Thorac Cardiovasc Surg 77:162, 1979

PETERSEN SR, SHELDON GF: Morbidity of a negative finding at laparotomy in abdominal trauma. Surg Gynecol Obstet 148:23, 1979

PETERSEN SR, SHELDON GF, LIM RC, JR: Management of portal vein injuries. J Trauma 19:616, 1979

POPOVSKY J, LEE YC, BERK JL: Gunshot wounds of the esophagus. J Thorac Cardiovasc Surg 72:609, 1976

PRIEBE HJ, SKILLMAN JJ, BUSHNELL LS et al: Antacid versus cimetidine in preventing acute gastrointestinal bleeding: A randomized trial in 75 critically ill patients. N Engl J Med 302:426, 1980

RADWIN HM, FITCH WP, ROBISON JR: A unified concept of renal trauma. J Urol 116:20, 1976

REUL CJ, JR, MATTOX KL, BEALL AC et al: Recent advances in the operative management of massive chest trauma. Ann Thorac Surg 16:52, 1973

SCHULTZ RC: The nature of facial injury emergencies. Surg Clin North Am 52:1, 1972

SHEELY CH, MATTOX KL, REUL CJ JR et al: Current concepts in the management of penetrating neck trauma. J Trauma 15:895, 1975

SHER MH: Principles in the management of arterial injuries associated with fracture/dislocations. Ann Surg 182:630, 1975

SHERMAN RT, PARRISH RA: Management of shotgun injuries: A review of 152 cases. J Trauma 3:76, 1963

SHIRES GT: Care of the Trauma Patient, 2nd ed. New York, McGraw-Hill, 1979

SNYDER WH III, WATKINS WL, WHIDDON LL et al: Civilian popliteal artery trauma: An eleven-year experience with 83 injuries. Surgery 85:101, 1979

SNYDER WH III, WEIGELT JA, WATKINS WL et al: The surgical management of duodenal trauma: Precepts based on a review of 247 cases. Arch Surg 115:422, 1980

STAUFFER ES, WOOD RW, KELLY EG: Gunshot wounds of the spine: The effects of laminectomy. J Bone Joint Surg 61A:389, 1979

THAL ER, MAY RA, BEESINGER D: Peritoneal lavage, its unreliability in gunshot wounds of the lower chest and abdomen. Arch Surg 115:422, 1980

THOMAS AN, BLAISDELL FW, LEWIS FR et al: Operative stabilization for flail chest after blunt trauma. J Thorac Cardiovasc Surg 75:793, 1978

THOMAS AN, STEPHENS BG: Air embolism: A cause of morbidity and death after penetrating chest trauma. J Trauma 14:633, 1974

WALDSCHMIDT ML, LAWS HL: Injuries of the diaphragm. J Trauma 20:587, 1980

WILMORE DW, GOODWIN CW, AULICK LH et al: Effect of injury and infection on visceral metabolism and circulation. Ann Surg 192:491, 1980

ZIMMERMAN RA, BILANIUK LT, GENNARELLI T et al: Cranial computed tomography in diagnosis and management of acute head trauma. Am J Roentgenol 131:27, 1978

ZUIDEMA GD, RUTHERFORD RB, BALLINGER WF II (eds): The Management of Trauma, 3rd ed. Philadelphia, W B Saunders, 1979

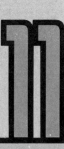

Burns and Cold Injury, and Bites and Stings

Alan R. Dimick

Burns and Cold Injury

BURNS

THERMAL BURNS

The dimensions of the thermal burn problem are readily apparent when it is realized that from 1 million to 2 million such injuries are sustained in the United States each year. This figure is much higher than perceived, since many small burns undoubtedly go unreported. Fortunately, most of these burns are relatively minor and require little attention. Even so, significant burn wounds result in a major expense and hospital time each year, far out of proportion to the actual number of such patients admitted; a 50% surface area flame burn is one of the most metabolically devastating wounds that the surgeon must treat, and the mortality rate remains substantial.

The American Burn Association has suggested the following classification: Minor burns involve less than the moderate burns and may usually be treated on an outpatient basis; erythema is prominent. Moderate burns include second-degree burns (blisters) of 15% to 25% of the total body surface area (TBSA) in adults and 10% to 20% in children; third-degree burns (full thickness—needs grafting) of less than 10% of TBSA; and burns not involving the eyes, ears, face, hands, feet, or perineum. Major burns include second-degree burns involving more than 25% of TBSA in adults and 20% in children; more than 10% of TBSA third-degree burns; all burns involving eyes, ears, face, hands, feet, or perineum; all burns with inhalation injury; all high-voltage electrical burns; burn injuries associated with fractures or other major trauma; and all poor-risk patients.

Patients with major burn injury are best treated in a burn

	THE MAJOR THERMAL BURN: A Massive Metabolic Assault
Etiology	Flame burns ignite clothing and are likely to cause full-thickness injury (third-degree) that requires skin grafting. Flash burns from explosive gas injury or hot water often cause only blisters (second-degree), and grafting is usually not required.
Dx	Immediately estimate percent body surface area burned to assess fluid requirements. How much first-degree (erythema), probable second-degree (blisters), or third-degree (full-thickness skin destruction and even deeper)? Assess prognosis based on age, extent and depth of burns, and associated injuries and health problems. Respiratory tract involved?
Rx	*Early*—fluid therapy to prevent shock; sedation? antibiotics? *Intermediate*—control infection; cover burn wounds. *Late*—further skin grafting? *Very late*—correct late burn scars and contractures.

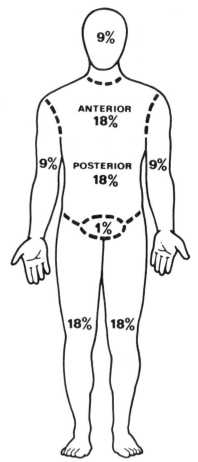

Fig. 11-1. Rule of Nines.

center, next best in a hospital with a well-staffed separate burn unit, and least effectively in a general hospital without special interest or facilities for burn management. The prognosis in the patient with a severe burn injury is influenced not only by the magnitude of the injury but also by the expertise and dedication of the personnel in attendance.

Thermal destruction causes alterations in the anatomy of the skin with a subsequent change in local and systemic physiological events unparalleled in either magnitude or duration in other types of trauma. In addition to the local wound, there are severe systemic responses and physiological alterations in almost all organ systems throughout the course of burn illness, which must be thoroughly understood to treat the patient. All members of the burn team must understand the mechanism of thermal trauma in producing such local and systemic reactions.

IMPORTANCE OF THE EXTENT OF INJURY

The magnitude of pathophysiological changes resulting from thermal burns is often directly related to the extent of the body surface area burned and, to a lesser extent, to the depth of the burn. Also, the magnitude of care appears to be directly related to the extent of body surface area burned. Therefore, accurate determination of burn size is important in evaluating the requirements for care (both physiological and technical), in anticipating life-threatening complications, and in projecting the prognosis for survival.

Extent of burn is expressed as a percentage of the TBSA involved in the burn. A good, rapid method for initial estimation of the extent of burn is the Rule of Nines (Fig. 11-1). According to this rule, the body surface is divided into regions, each of which represents 9% or a multiple of 9% of the body surface area. Accuracy is enhanced by making one estimation of the body surface involved in the burn and another of the normal unburned skin. A more nearly accurate method of determining the extent of burn, and one that makes allowances for the varying surface area

of different anatomical areas in children, is to use the Lund and Browder chart (Fig. 11-2). Another method is the use of the patient's open hand as 1% of his body surface. This can be useful when the burns are scattered over the body. The prognosis following a major burn is directly related to the percent area burned, the age of the patient, and other associated injuries or health problems (Fig. 11-3). The very young and especially the very old have a relatively high mortality rate following a burn involving a given amount of surface area.

FIRST AID, TRIAGE, AND TRANSFER OF BURN PATIENTS

Emergency first aid includes measures to minimize the magnitude of the burn by removing the patient from further contact with heat or electricity. Chemical agents should be lavaged away. Since other types of major trauma may have been sustained by the burn patient, as well as respiratory tract burn injury, the usual precautionary measures are employed as needed to prevent cardiorespiratory arrest. Most of the time the patient arrives at the hospital without intravenous fluid replacements having been started; however, if prolonged transport is anticipated, an intravenous line should be placed and Ringer's lactate solution begun for the trip.

Local Measures

The application of ice or cold water is effective in decreasing pain but should not be used unless the burns involve less than 10% of TBSA. If ice or cold water is used, the patient

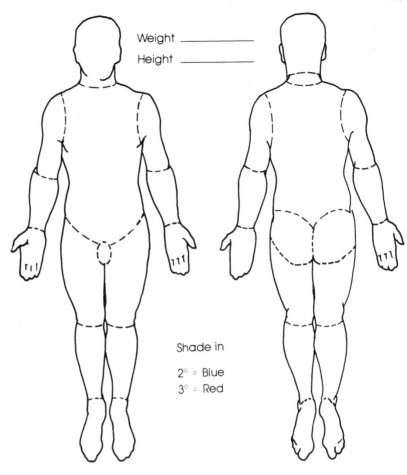

Weight _____

Height _____

Shade in

2° = Blue

3° = Red

Area	Age — Years					% 2°	% 3°	% Total
	0-1	1-4	5-9	10-15	Adults			
Head	19	17	13	10	7			
Neck	2	2	2	2	2			
Ant. Trunk	13	17	13	13	13			
Post. Trunk	13	13	13	13	13			
R. Buttock	2½	2½	2½	2½	2½			
L. Buttock	2½	2½	2½	2½	2½			
Genitallia	1	1	1	1	1			
R. U. Arm	4	4	4	4	4			
L. U. Arm	4	4	4	4	4			
R. L. Arm	3	3	3	3	3			
L. L. Arm	3	3	3	3	3			
R. Hand	2½	2½	2½	2½	2½			
L. Hand	2½	2½	2½	2½	2½			
R. Thigh	5½	6½	8½	8½	9½			
L. Thigh	5½	6½	8½	8½	9½			
R. Leg	5	5	5½	6	7			
L. Leg	5	5	5½	6	7			
R. Foot	3½	3½	3½	3½	3½			
L. Foot	3½	3½	3½	3½	3½			
					Total			

Fig. 11-2. Lund and Browder chart for determining extent of burn.

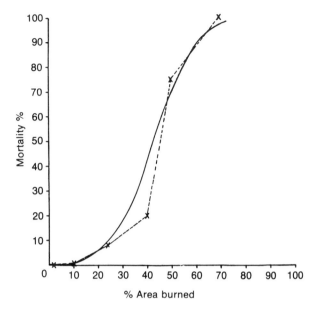

Fig. 11-3. There is a direct correlation between the percent of body surface area burned and the mortality rate. The precise survival rates have improved in recent years, but the general correlation is still quite valid. (Bull JP, Squire JR: A study of mortality in a burns unit. Ann Surg 130:160, 1949)

must be checked carefully for systemic hypothermia. With the loss of skin due to the burn, the patient is unable to maintain his core body temperature and frequently loses tremendous amounts of heat through the area of the burn. Ice or cold water potentiates this loss of heat, resulting in hypothermia and subsequent cardiac arrest. Also, prolonged application of ice or cold water to the burn area may result in frostbite in addition to the burn. Therefore, the duration of such application must be short. Because of the inherent dangers in the application of ice or cold water to burns involving more than 10% of TBSA, it is best not to use such applications on these larger burns. Also, the application of wet dressings to the burns potentiates the movement of bacteria into the burn wound, since most burn accidents occur in dirty environments. Therefore, it is best to apply only a dry, sterile dressing to the burn area and cover this with some type of insulation, such as a blanket, to maintain and conserve the patient's body heat. It is best not to apply

ointments or other medications to the burn wounds before they are covered with sterile sheets or dressings; these will have to be removed by the attending physician at the hospital after the patient arrives, so the burns can be evaluated. Dry, sterile sheets are the best dressings for these patients.

Respiratory Measures

Carbon monoxide poisoning causes hypoxemia and usually occurs in patients burned in an enclosed space. The first responder should begin the administration of 100% oxygen to accelerate the dissociation of carboxyhemoglobin in any patient suspected of having inhaled significant amounts of carbon monoxide. With severe inhalation injury or rapidly progressing edema of the upper airway, an endotracheal tube should be inserted to maintain the airway. If possible, this should be a nasotracheal tube, since it is the preferred method for long-term airway maintenance.

Fluid Administration

If the patient is more than 30 minutes' travel time from a treatment facility, the first responder, in conjunction with the medical-control physician, should decide on the institution of intravenous fluids. Ideally, this should be by a large-caliber cannula, and the infusion should be begun with a balanced salt solution, Ringer's lactate. A history should be obtained of the exact circumstances of the injury, the presence of preexisting disease, and medications taken prior to injury. This information should be provided to the physicians treating the patient at the hospital. The amount of fluid required for effective replacement of fluid sequestration of the burn wounds and other functional losses almost invariably causes the patient to gain weight during the first several days of treatment (Fig. 11-4). Later, the patient who becomes infected usually loses both body fat and lean body mass and is likely to lose some weight despite vigorous oral or intravenous alimentation.

EMERGENCY DEPARTMENT CARE OF BURN PATIENTS

Initial Evaluation

A rapid evaluation of the burn patient should be accomplished upon his arrival in the emergency department; specific emphasis should be placed on the depth of burn and the extent of burn, which can be estimated using the Rule of Nines or any of several burn diagrams available

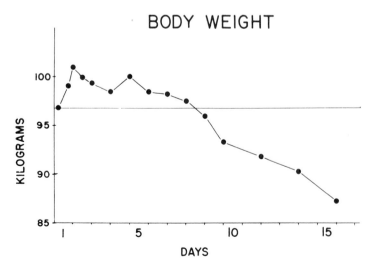

Fig. 11-4. Variations in body weight following 40% flame burn (see text). (Hardy JD (ed): Pathophysiology in Surgery. Baltimore, Williams & Wilkins, 1958)

(Fig. 11-5). Fluid needs are then estimated based on TBSA of burn and body weight, and the fluid administration is adjusted accordingly, with accurate recording of the volume and type of all administered fluids. Some have advocated that fluid replacement be achieved by mouth, but many burn patients have reported marked intestinal ileus and tolerate oral intake poorly. The pulmonary status should be carefully assessed in terms of the need for endotracheal intubation, oxygen administration, and ventilatory assistance. A urethral catheter should be placed in all patients requiring intravenous fluid therapy, and the hourly urine output should be measured and recorded. Patients with high-voltage electrical injury should have ECG monitoring for at least 48 hours after injury because of the possibility of cardiac irregularity in this interval.

After the physician is satisfied that the patient's pulmonary and cardiovascular status are stable, attention is then turned to the burn wound. The burned areas should be cleansed gently with a surgical soap or detergent and the loose, nonviable skin removed. Bullae are removed, because they easily become infected.

In patients requiring hospital care, transfer to the most appropriate treatment center as determined by the extent and complexity of the burns should be accomplished once the patient is stable.

Fig. 11-5. Patient with extensive flash burns of the arms and torso from a propane gas explosion. The burns proved to be almost entirely deep second-degree burns; the outer skin was shed, and almost no skin grafting was required.

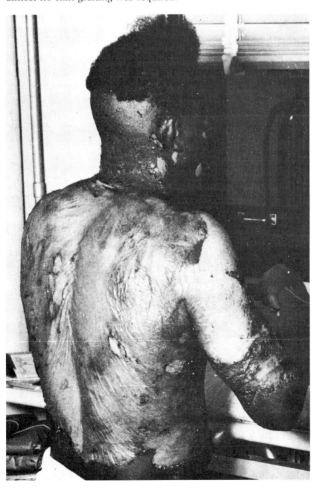

Outpatient Management

Burns of limited extent (small areas, less than 5%–10% of the body surface) are not at a significant risk of infection, and topical antimicrobial agents may or may not be used. Such small burns can be dressed with fine mesh gauze, with or without medication, and covered with a dry, bulky dressing held in place with an elastic gauze dressing. The patient is followed up as appropriate to the degree of injury and the circumstances in general, but the wounds should be inspected at least every 3 to 5 days. If healing is proceeding uneventfully and there is no infection, a dressing is reapplied as many times as necessary until healing has occurred. However, if infection is present, the patient is admitted to the hospital and topical antimicrobial therapy initiated.

Airway and Fluid Therapy

For extensive burns requiring hospital care, priority is given to the maintenance of airway and resuscitation of burn shock. Intravenous lines are established with a catheter in a peripheral or central vein. In the initial care of extensively burned patients, it is preferable to place intravenous lines through burned skin to save the veins in unburned areas for future use. A urethral catheter is required for hourly measurement of urinary output, and a nasogastric tube is inserted to relieve gastric dilatation. Burn patients are very apprehensive and usually swallow a great deal of air, which needs to be removed through the nasogastric tube. Once these measures are accomplished, a quick evaluation of the magnitude of injury is accomplished to calculate the fluid requirements and the rate of administration. Continuing evaluation of the upper and lower airway and a search for associated injuries are done. Pain associated with extensive burns can best be alleviated with small intravenous doses of morphine or meperidine. Tetanus prophylaxis is accomplished with tetanus toxoid, or, if the patient has not been immunized previously, 250 units of human tetanus toxoid. Penicillin is usually administered during the initial days of burn care for control of gram-positive infections, especially in children.

In the first 24 hours post burn, Ringer's lactate is used exclusively for resuscitation. The total amount of Ringer's lactate needed to correct the extracellular fluid volume deficit in burn patients may be calculated as follows: 4 ml per percent TBSA burns per kilogram body weight. The rate of administration is calculated from the time of the injury and not from the time of initiation of therapy, since there is always some inherent delay between the time of injury and the time of initiating fluid therapy.

One of the recommendations of the National Institutes of Health (NIH) Burn Consensus Conference in 1978 was that Ringer's lactate be used initially in the treatment of burn shock. The lactic acidosis of untreated burn shock disappears rapidly despite the large quantities of exogenous lactate from Ringer's lactate. No free water is given in the first 24 hours, since the sodium concentration of lactated Ringer's solution is 130 mEq/liter and therefore furnishes 75 ml to 100 ml of free water per liter administered. In the first 8 hours post burn, half of the calculated volume of lactated Ringer's solution is given (Fig. 11-6). In the second 8 hours, one fourth of the calculated volume is given, and in the third 8 hours, the final fourth of the calculated volume is given. Signs of successful resuscitation are clear sensorium, urinary output of 20 ml to 50 ml/hour in children and 30 ml to 70 ml/hour in adults, central venous pressure below 2, and lack of ileus or nausea.

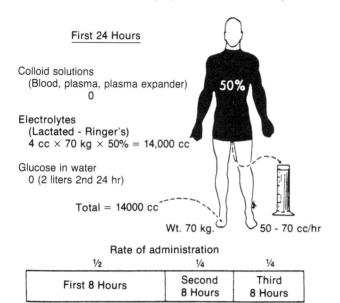

First 24 Hours

Colloid solutions
(Blood, plasma, plasma expander)
        0

Electrolytes
(Lactated - Ringer's)
4 cc × 70 kg × 50% = 14,000 cc

Glucose in water
0 (2 liters 2nd 24 hr)

        Total = 14000 cc

        Wt. 70 kg.   50 - 70 cc/hr

Rate of administration

½	¼	¼
First 8 Hours	Second 8 Hours	Third 8 Hours

Fig. 11-6. Guide to initial fluid requirements of major burns (above 20% TBSA). (Baxter CR: Pathophysiology and treatment of burns and cold injury. In Hardy JD [ed]: Rhoads Textbook of Surgery, 5th ed. Philadelphia, J B Lippincott, 1977)

In the fourth 8 hours following burn (24–36 hours), plasma expansion can and should be accomplished. Prior to 24 hours, colloids such as plasma do not effectively change the plasma deficits, because of the continuing capillary leak. At approximately 24 hours, the leak of the capillaries has sealed and whatever fluids are given remain in circulation. A guide to the quantity of plasma needed in relation to the area of burn is shown in Table 11-1. The completeness of restoration of blood volume can be judged roughly by the return of the hematocrit to normal. As might be expected, there is some biologic variation in the time capillary integrity is regained, which may result in further plasma loss. Therefore, in a few patients, the response to the administration of plasma may be delayed more than 30 hours post burn. Obviously, one must titrate these patients by measuring their vital signs and urinary output to determine what is best for each patient.

Usually after the administration of colloid (plasma), no further volume expansion is needed after 30 hours. While this guide to resuscitation is usually successful, one must remember that all fluid formulas are simply guidelines and must be adjusted to the needs of individual patients.

Insensible water losses in burn patients are severalfold

TABLE 11-1   RANGE OF PLASMA REQUIREMENTS AS RELATED TO PERCENTAGE OF TOTAL BODY SURFACE AREA (TBSA) INVOLVED IN BURNS

% TBSA BURNED	PLASMA REQUIREMENTS 70-kg man (ml)
20–40	0– 500
40–60	500–1700
60–80	1000–3000
>80	1500–3500

(Baxter CR: Pathophysiology and treatment of burns and cold injury. In Hardy JD [ed]: Rhoads Textbook of Surgery, 5th ed. Philadelphia, J B Lippincott, 1977)

higher than those through normal skin, so a basic daily water requirement of 2.5 liters must be exceeded. Free water in the form of 5% dextrose in water should be administered to maintain serum sodium levels at or near 140 mEq/liter. Potassium supplementation may be required on the second and third postburn days, but usually no other electrolyte therapy is required. The continued destruction of erythrocytes usually requires transfusions of packed red blood cells from the third day on.

Failure of this regimen of fluid resuscitation is uncommon. Unsatisfactory resuscitation occurs usually from a miscalculation of burn size, the presence of associated injuries requiring additional fluid therapy, respiratory tract injury, and burns extending deep into muscle.

PATHOPHYSIOLOGY

The burn injury produces coagulation necrosis of the skin and underlying subcutaneous tissue. The extent of the injury is dependent upon both the temperature to which the tissue was exposed and the duration of the exposure. In addition, the severe metabolic assault of burn injury produces demonstrable pathophysiologic alterations in most other organs. Mortality is related to the magnitude of burn injury, further influenced by the age of the patient, the previous state of health, the quality of care, and still other factors.

Cardiopulmonary Effects

The changes in the cardiovascular pulmonary systems are predominant at the outset and demand priority. The maintenance of the airway and the ability of oxygen to diffuse from the alveolus to the pulmonary capillary, as well as the treatment of blood-volume deficits, are of primary importance to prevent the development of burn shock. The local and general effects of burn injury result in an increased capillary permeability, which permits the loss of fluid and protein from the intravascular compartment into the extravascular compartment. These volume shifts occur in direct proportion to the extent of burn and are clinically apparent as edema, which develops in areas of thermal injury and may also occur in unburned tissues as resuscitation proceeds in patients with extensive burns (*i.e.*, those involving over 25% of TBSA). In the early postburn period, cardiac output falls as a result of the decreased blood volume, increased viscosity of the blood caused by the increased hematocrit, and aggregation of red blood cells, platelets, and white blood cells. A myocardial depressant factor in extensive burns has been implicated by some investigators, but recent findings have shown the most obvious cause of diminished cardiac output is hypovolemia causing impaired venous return. In these patients, there was no evidence of a myocardial depressant factor: All indices of myocardial function were normal or elevated. The diminished blood volume and cardiac output cause decreased blood flow and oliguria, which if not treated result in acute renal failure. Hypovolemia results in diminished flow to other organs, and restlessness is a frequent early sign of inadequate perfusion of the brain.

In addition to the loss of plasma from the circulation in the early postburn period, there is also red blood cell destruction in direct proportion to the extent of burn, particularly in the case of third-degree burn. There is also continuing red blood cell loss during the first postburn week due to a multiplicity of factors. Damaged tissue cells imbibe larger quantities of isotonic solutions through damaged cell walls. Within 24 hours of injury, platelets and leukocytes exhibit abnormal aggregation, sticking firmly to vessel walls and producing thrombosis. This progressive vascular impairment may produce an area of ischemia greater in depth than the initial cellular damage initiated by the heat. Transfer of oxygen and nutrients to damaged cells is thus impaired, enhancing the likelihood of additional cell damage. The thrombotic tendency in the burn wound is present for a minimum of 5 days. Systemic factors decreasing the arterial systolic pressure or aggravating the hypercoagulable state may further contribute to the depth of injury.

Burn Depth and Tissue Destruction

For these reasons, the depth of burn may not be clinically apparent for 3 to 5 days following the thermal insult. The final depth of tissue destruction should be strictly defined. First-degree burns are characterized by simple erythema of the skin, with destruction of only superficial areas of the epidermis. This is typical of a severe sunburn. Healing occurs in 5 to 7 days, and there is the characteristic peeling of the dead epithelium.

Second-degree burns have deeper tissue destruction, usually the entire epidermis and also the superficial areas of the dermis. Blisters are one hallmark, but blisters may obscure even third-degree burns on occasion. Although the depth of injury may vary, if epithelial elements such as hair follicles and sweat glands remain, from which regeneration can occur, the burn by definition is second-degree. Since restoration and regeneration can occur from remaining epithelial elements, second-degree burns are described as partial-thickness burns. Blister formation is the hallmark of second-degree burns. The sweat glands and hair follicles are extremely important in second-degree partial-thickness burns. These specialized skin appendages course normally through the epithelial layer into the dermis and are lined with epithelial cells. Again, in second-degree burns the existing epidermis is totally destroyed, along with the superficial portions of the dermis. It is primarily from the epithelial cells lining the hair follicles and sweat glands that the epithelial cells proliferate, resurfacing the second-degree burn.

Third-degree burns have total destruction of the epidermal and dermal elements, with all layers of the skin coagulated and destroyed. Thus, in full-thickness third-degree burns, spontaneous regeneration of epithelium is not possible. This means that the burn wound can only heal by second-intention healing or by the application of skin grafts.

Skin thickness varies in various portions of the body and also with the age of the patient. In elderly patients, in whom dermal papillae and skin appendages are atrophic, and in the very young, in whom they have yet to develop fully, deeper burns result from heat of the same intensity that produces only a second-degree burn in the average adult. Skin is thickest on the back, palm of the hand, and sole of the foot; it is thinnest on the inner arm. Epidermal appendages such as hair follicles penetrate to varying depths in different areas, such as in the scalp or the male beard, which are notably deep. Skin from the thickest areas and from areas with more epidermal appendages regenerates faster.

The pain seen with burn injury is also related to the depth of burn. In first- and second-degree burns, the nerve endings are irritated and therefore hypersensitive, with whatever stimulus they perceive being interpreted as severe excruciating pain—"nerve pain." In full-thickness third-degree burns, everything is coagulated and destroyed, including the nerve endings. Therefore, in third-degree burns, initially there is no pain, because there are no viable nerve endings to perceive pain. After several weeks, the nerve endings in full-thickness third-degree burns begin to regenerate and then become hypersensitive. After several weeks, the first- and second-degree burn injuries are healed and no longer painful.

Local Results

With burn injury, there is a loss of the functional integrity of the body's largest organ, the skin. Some of the important protective functions lost include the regulation of water evaporation from the body, defense against infection, and the loss of body fluids through an open wound.

Evaporative water loss through the intact skin in the normal man averages 10 ml/kg/day. Normal skin prevents the passage of water vapor from the saturated tissues in the body to the relatively dry external environment. In thermal injury, the protective layers of skin are lost and water may evaporate through the area of injury at the same rate as from an open pan of water. In second-degree burns, which have only a partial loss of epithelium, evaporation of water still proceeds at an accelerated rate. Accurate calculation of evaporative water losses for individual patients is extremely difficult, since the amount varies with the area exposed, the type of topical treatment, and the environmental temperature and humidity. Daily determination of serum sodium concentration and daily weights are helpful guidelines, as is the urinary sodium concentration. Large volumes of water may be required for replacement, and some patients require as much as 10 liters/day.

Excessive loss of water by evaporation has many very important consequences. If it is not recognized and restored, severe water deficiency results. Also, the evaporation of water results in a heat loss of 0.58 kcal/liter evaporated, which can result in a tremendous strain on the body to produce such heat. This caloric loss was once thought to be responsible for the hypermetabolism of the burn state. Although this question is not entirely settled, many investigators have determined that the hypermetabolism is not driven primarily by this caloric requirement. Furnishing external heat increases the comfort of the patient but has little effect on core temperature. Thus, it is necessary to supply additional calories to replace the calories used for evaporation of this water.

The first line of defense against the continual assault of microorganisms in the environment is the skin. Loss of this skin barrier results in various degrees of bacterial invasion. The coagulation of skin furnishes an almost ideal culture medium at body temperature for bacterial proliferation. The lack of an effective blood supply in the local area precludes any active humoral host resistance. The third-degree burn is characterized by extensive vascular thrombosis and no cellular inflammatory reaction. In contrast, the second-degree burn has open vasculature and an accompanying active cellular inflammatory response. However, if the second-degree burn becomes infected, there is progressive perivascular inflammation, with subsequent thrombosis. This results in infectious conversion of a second-degree burn to a third-degree burn. Therefore, it is extremely important to prevent the proliferation of bacteria in second-degree partial-thickness burns to prevent conversion to full-thickness third-degree burns.

After thermal injury, the normal bacterial flora of the skin persist deep in the hair follicles and sweat glands. As these bacteria colonize the superficial areas of burn, their concentration may reach 10^4 to 10^8 per gram of tissue. Colonization of the entire thickness of the burn, from 10^4

to 10^8, may occur by the fifth postburn day. The type of organisms first colonizing the wound is dependent upon the initial treatment and the environment of the patient. For example, burns that do not receive topical therapy usually develop streptococcal or staphylococcal colonization, whereas hospitalized patients usually become colonized with gram-negative organisms from the hospital environment.

Burn-wound sepsis has been defined as the active proliferation of bacteria in the quantity of 10^5 or more per gram of tissue. Once colonization of the burn wound has been established, rapid growth of the bacteria with invasion into adjacent tissues ensues, culminating in systemic sepsis.

Blood cultures are seldom positive in burn patients. The gram-negative bacilli invading primarily by way of the lymphatics are cultured from blood only late in the disease, and death often occurs from burn-wound sepsis without bloodstream invasion. The presence of a positive blood culture actually suggests strongly that a secondary source is producing the signs of sepsis in the burn patient. This may be due to pneumonia, urinary tract infection, or septic thrombophlebitis.

With the loss of normal skin, large amounts of fluid, proteins, and other essential materials are lost from the body. Roughly half of the protein and nitrogen losses by the body during the first few weeks is through the burn wound. Trace metals such as zinc, copper, cobalt, and magnesium, together with vitamins and electrolytes, are lost in varying amounts through the open burn wound. Obviously, this must be recognized and appropriate treatment instituted.

SYSTEMIC EFFECTS

Burn Shock
A cascade of pathophysiological changes affecting the function of almost every organ of the body is initiated by a major burn wound. The most immediate life-threatening pathologic response to burn injury is the composite syndrome of burn shock. It is well recognized that the most important component of burn shock is the loss of large volumes of both plasma and extravascular, extracellular fluid.

The classic description of burn shock has been the loss of body fluids into the burn wound. Heat damage to tissue produces a change in the molecular configuration of collagen that then chemically binds both sodium and water. Damaged cells imbibe salt and water, and the capillary leak permits plasma to flow into the area of injury. The acute hypovolemia causes decreased tissue perfusion. There is direct heat damage to the red blood cells, which decreases their half-life and results in accelerated hemolysis, contributing to the early anemia of the immediate postburn period.

The classic concept of the pathophysiology of burn shock has been challenged by recent experimental evidence that the sequence of fluid losses in burns, the changes in the formed elements of the blood, and the cardiovascular response are not as simply explained as once thought. The very rapid loss of fluid in the first few postburn hours (1–4 hours) is, for the most part, a shift of sodium and water from the extravascular, extracellular space into skeletal muscle cells throughout the body. Approximately one third of the extracellular fluid surrounding the muscle cell is shifted from the extracellular space to an intracellular location. At the same time, both extracellular fluid and

plasma are being lost into the burn wound. These findings explain the necessity of administering approximately half of the calculated fluid requirements in the first postburn hours.

Available evidence indicates that the capillary leak seals at about 24 hours postburn, limiting the rate of plasma loss. The damaged collagen and cells have sequestered fluid as obligated by their reaction to injury. Yet edema continues to accumulate in, beneath, and adjacent to the area of the burn wound, becoming increasingly severe up to 48 to 72 hours after injury. The magnitude of this edema in a burn wound exceeds that in any other type of injury except total venous occlusion of an extremity.

A possible explanation for this severity of edema in a burn wound has been found in a study of fibrinogen metabolism. An increasing concentration of fibrinogen polymers is demonstrated in the edema fluid. It is probable that these polymers produce mechanical obstruction of the lymphatics and venules draining the burn area. The rate of complete breakdown of the fibrinogen is indicated in the appearance of fibrin split products in the circulation. In the first 24 hours, little or no fibrin split products are detectable in the plasma; then an acute rise begins and a sustained level of five to ten times the normal blood concentration is reached. This level gradually diminishes over 10 to 14 days.

These experimental results suggest that the formation of burn-wound edema is biphasic: (1) The initial response is not only a loss of isotonic extracellular fluid and plasma into the area of tissue damage but also a dramatic shift of sodium and water into skeletal muscle cells throughout the body. (2) As the fluid demand in the wound increases because of obstruction of the lymphatics and venules by long-chain fibrinogen polymers, the fluid imbibed by normal cells returns to the extracellular fluid and is shifted by way of the circulation from noninjured locations into the burn wound.

Clinical Response
In addition to the fluid volume changes of the initial response to burn injury, there are significant changes in the cardiovascular system, both in myocardial performance and in formed elements of the blood. Cardiac output falls immediately following the burn to between 30% and 50% of normal in burns involving more than 30% of TBSA. With prompt, adequate fluid volume replacement, the cardiac output is restored to normal within 12 hours. In all major injuries of more than 40% of TBSA, evidence of a decrease in myocardial contractility can be demonstrated. Some investigators have identified a myocardial depressant factor of burn shock. Its exact mechanism of action is not known, but it is clinically manifest by failure of the cardiac output to respond to fluid therapy. This appears to occur in massive burns, in lesser burns in patients with preexisting heart disease, and often in elderly patients with limited myocardial reserve.

The mechanism of damage to the formed elements of the blood is only partially related to direct heat damage. Hemolysis of 3% to 15% of the red blood cell mass may occur acutely. However, the persistent shortened half-life of red blood cells is not due only to heat damage or to sequestration in the burn wound. Crossover studies of ^{51}Cr-tagged erythrocytes in burn patients and normal patients showed that the red cells from burn patients had a decreased half-life. This microangiopathic anemia persists for at least 2 weeks following burn, with a daily loss of from 3% to 9% of the red blood cell mass, requiring frequent packed-cell transfusion. Increased platelet adhesiveness and progressive platelet depletion are present for 3 to 5 days. Platelet half-life is greatly shortened. Leukocyte counts drop to mild leukopenia levels. The pathogenesis of these changes has not been fully clarified, but formed elements have been observed to stick or sludge in small vessels.

The renal response to the thermal injury is difficult to interpret, but it is quite clear that acute renal failure is rare if prompt, adequate resuscitation is accomplished. Although renal function studies in the non–steady state are difficult to interpret, there is an increase in glomerular permeability, as evidenced by protein in the urine. Although the glomerular filtration rate may fall in the first few hours following burn injury, it rapidly returns to a normal level with adequate resuscitation. Tubular integrity is usually not affected, with creatinine and urea clearances remaining essentially normal. Thus, with adequate resuscitation therapy, renal function, although temporarily deranged in some respects, usually remains adequate and returns rapidly to normal.

The lungs play a major role in the clinical response to major thermal injury, but there appears to be little effect of the peripheral burn on pulmonary function. The high incidence of pulmonary dysfunction observed in some burn series is related to direct damage produced by the inhalation of noxious gases and chemicals in smoke, including damage to the respiratory tract mucosa, atelectasis, and pneumonitis. Later in the course of hospitalization, the lungs participate significantly in the systemic response to invasive sepsis, and the incidence of pneumonia is high.

Gastrointestinal changes following thermal injury are common and are manifest by early coffee-ground gastric material in most major burns. The pathogenesis of the lesion is not clear, nor are many of the functional alterations well delineated. Acute gastric dilatation is a common accompaniment of severe stress of any nature, and total gastrointestinal ileus commonly occurs during the first 3 days following burn. These initial changes do not appear to be related directly to the later appearance of Curling's ulcer, which may be manifest by significant bleeding or perforation occurring most often in the duodenum and less frequently in the stomach.

Immunologic competence is even less well defined. The initial leukopenia was described above. Complement disappears rapidly but is reconstituted rapidly also. The bactericidal capacity of leukocytes is periodically impaired normally, but in burn patients an abrupt decrease occurs concomitant with the appearance of sepsis. Humoral immunity appears to be intact shortly after the thermal injury, but cellular immunity remains depressed, one manifestation of which is the lengthened survival of allogeneic (homograft or heterograft) skin grafts. Depression of immunoglobulins, both IgG and IgM, occurs and persists for 2 to 3 weeks following injury.

Inhalation Injury

The most immediate threats to life in burn patients are upper-airway obstruction, carbon monoxide poisoning, and inhalation damage to the lower airway. Initial examination should assure patency of the upper airway with removal of foreign bodies and secretions. The presence of singed nasal hairs, inflamed, dried pharyngeal mucosa and edema of the glottis, or hoarseness suggests potential upper-airway obstruction from direct thermal damage. Increasing hoarseness, inability to swallow secretions, or increased respiratory rate

is indication for immediate endotracheal intubation to prevent total upper-airway obstruction. Upper-airway obstruction is not usually an immediate problem; it occurs most often between 6 and 30 hours following burn. However, one must be constantly cautious to avoid it and should never feel apologetic about placement of an endotracheal tube to prevent the possibility of such obstruction. Endotracheal tubes are much easier to place and remove than tracheostomies, and if they prevent upper-airway obstruction, they may be lifesaving.

Carbon monoxide intoxication is frequently difficult to detect, since the typical cherry-red skin color may be absent in burn patients. Unconsciousness or irrational behavior, together with a history of prolonged smoke inhalation, strongly suggests carbon monoxide intoxication. Treatment with 100% oxygen by mask is indicated for carbon monoxide intoxication.

Initial damage to the lower airway is usually not obvious until 12 to 24 hours following burn; it then becomes manifest by rales, wheezing, and tachypnea. This is followed rapidly by hypoxemia, progressing to total ventilatory insufficiency. Inhalation injury may be obvious initially as florid pulmonary edema, requiring immediate endotracheal intubation and positive-pressure ventilation. Narcotics should not be given for pain or respiratory distress until therapy for shock and resuscitation has been initiated. A controversial mode of therapy has been that of administration of steroids to the patient with inhalation injury. At the NIH Burn Consensus Conference in 1978, the final recommendation was not to use steroids for pulmonary inhalation injury because of the higher propensity for generalized infection in patients receiving steroids and the lack of significant benefit for the patient.

Frequent reevaluation of the airway is necessary in patients with evidence of inhalation injury and in patients with severe burns of the face and neck. Should airway maintenance be necessary, endotracheal tubes rather than tracheostomies should be routinely employed. Tracheostomy should be employed only when endotracheal tubes cannot be placed for maintenance of the airway. If there is a continued need for ventilatory assistance after several weeks, a tracheostomy may be needed. With the newer plastic materials in endotracheal tubes, physicians can now postpone tracheostomies even longer.

INITIAL HOSPITAL MANAGEMENT

Initially, all burn wounds should be cleansed and débrided, with removal of all foreign bodies and dead skin, as gently as possible. Although many detergents and antiseptic solutions may be used, simple soap and water usually suffice. Coarse gauze sponges may be soaked in the water and gently rubbed over the surface of the wounds, producing adequate cleansing without excessive pain. Loose remnants of blisters may be removed with forceps. Initial débridement may be done after giving the patient intravenous morphine or meperidine. General anesthesia is contraindicated.

The patient should be positioned to minimize edema formation. Burns of the hands or feet should be elevated. Once the patient is no longer in shock, the head of the bed can be elevated to minimize as much as possible edema of the face.

Circumferential constricting burns of the extremities may cause circulatory embarrassment. The eschar is firm and tough, and when swelling occurs underneath it, the low-pressure venous system is rapidly occluded, resulting in diminished venous return from the involved extremity. Since the arterial inflow is at a higher hydrostatic pressure, arterial inflow continues into the extremity, resulting in further swelling until the tissue pressure equals the arterial hydrostatic pressure. If not recognized and treated, this results in ischemia, necrosis, and, eventually, gangrene. Peripheral pulses and temperature of the skin are poor indicators of blood flow in this situation. Reliable manifestations of decreased arterial perfusion include slow capillary refilling, and motor and sensory deficits in the distal extremity, and persistent deep pain. Should there be any doubt, it is best to perform incisions in the eschar (escharotomies) to alleviate this pressure. Usually, no local anesthesia is required, since the third-degree burn eschar has no viable nerves to perceive pain.

Since edema formation is the inevitable result of burn injury, in conditions in which the burn in an extremity is constricting and circumferential or has that potential, escharotomies should be accomplished to avoid gangrene of the hand or foot. Such escharotomies may be done on the medial or lateral aspect of the upper or lower extremity and should be carried from the hand or foot to the most proximal portion of the constriction. If the initial escharotomy does not provide adequate relaxation of the tissues, a second incision may be necessary on the opposite side of the extremity. Fasciotomies are usually not necessary except when muscle damage occurs. Occasionally, it is necessary to perform escharotomies over the thorax if there is constriction of the chest severe enough to prevent normal respiratory excursions. This is especially important in children whose bony rib cage is not yet ossified. Such constricting circumferential burns of the chest, especially in small children, may result in a vital capacity approaching zero. Obviously, this will cause death in minutes; therefore, rapid performance of escharotomies should be accomplished in such situations. This is usually done by incisions in the anterior axillary line bilaterally, as well as a transverse incision across the chest connecting them. This allows adequate expansion of the chest wall. Incisions in burns of the neck are usually not required to alleviate upper respiratory tract obstruction; rather, upper-airway obstruction should be treated by the placement of an endotracheal tube.

CARE OF MAJOR BURNS AFTER THE INITIAL ACUTE PERIOD OF SHOCK AND RESUSCITATION

The thrust of care after the critical period of burn shock and resuscitation is directed at closure of the burn wound as soon as possible. The method most commonly used is aggressive, daily débridement of the burn wound, employing topical and antibacterial agents for prevention and control of burn-wound sepsis while waiting for the development of granulation tissue sufficient to accept a skin graft or for the healing of partial-thickness burns. Early excision of the burn wound followed by immediate skin coverage with either an autograft or a homograft may be used in selected patients. This may be an excision of the eschar to the deep fascia or tangential excision. Enzymes may also be used in combination with topical antimicrobials to prepare the wound for early grafting. Regardless of the method chosen, the prevention and control of sepsis, the maintenance of nutrition, and meticulous attention to many details, both physiological and anatomical, are necessary for successful results. Complications are frequent and usually are related to the burn injury itself, as well as to the various methods of therapy used.

Control of Sepsis

The most important problems in burn patients who survive the initial resuscitation period are sepsis and complications related to sepsis. Successful resuscitation with sterile handling and cleansing of the burn wound minimizes sepsis. Necrotic tissue and decreased vascularity ensure colonization of bacteria in the burn wound, as previously described. Therefore, topical antibacterial agents must be used to provide direct control of colonization of bacteria in the burn wound to prevent or minimize such infection. Topical agents have reduced the mortality of burn-wound sepsis considerably. However, their effectiveness is limited by their spectrum of activity and because of certain disadvantages they possess. Since the introduction of 0.5% silver nitrate and mafenide acetate (Sulfamylon) in 1961, a variety of topical antibacterials have been used. The agents that have been most effective and that have withstood the test of time are 10% mafenide acetate and 1% silver sulfadiazine. Both of these agents may be employed by either the open or the closed method, the latter consisting of a relatively light cotton mesh dressing changed at least once daily. Both drugs may be used two or three times a day, and hydrotherapy is usually used for removal of the previously applied drug or dressing prior to reapplication. The characteristics of both drugs are shown in Table 11-2. The bacterial spectrum of each drug is limited, and resistance may develop with prolonged use. Therefore, some physicians rotate the use of these topical agents, depending upon the colonization of the burn wound.

The bacterial flora of the burn wound may be monitored by quantitative burn-wound biopsy cultures every 48 to 72 hours during the phase of eschar separation or crust healing. This method of monitoring the flora of the burn wound determines the effectiveness of the topical or systemic antibacterial therapy employed. Separation of the burn eschar is hastened by daily cleansing of the burn wound during hydrotherapy, which softens and loosens the burn tissue.

Increasing bacterial colonization of the burn wound is indicative of failure of topical chemotherapy. This may be treated by changing the topical chemotherapeutic agent but also may be treated by the use of appropriate antibiotics administered by clysis into the burn wound. Such subeschar clysis is an effective means of altering the bacterial flora. The choice of antibiotics is based on the type and sensitivity of organisms colonizing the wound. The total daily dosage of antibiotic is administered in divided doses by clysis, using 22-gauge needles at 8-cm intervals in the burn wound and delivering 25 ml of 0.5N saline containing the antibiotic into each site. This technique is effective in established burn-wound sepsis and is even more effective in preventing burn-wound sepsis when colonization is occurring rapidly.

Classic signs of sepsis usually occur late in the course of burn-wound sepsis and usually herald a lethal outcome. Disorientation, ileus, dark urine, tachycardia, and extremes of temperature (hyperthermia and hypothermia) and tachycardia followed by hypotension, oliguria, and obvious deterioration of the burn wound are late signs of invasive burn-wound sepsis. The use of systemic antibiotics, with the exception of penicillin, is reserved for patients exhibiting these signs of sepsis. Early diagnosis of burn-wound sepsis may be based on burn-wound biopsy, which provides for selection of appropriate systemic bacterial therapy. In the patient with suspected sepsis, after appropriate cultures have

TABLE 11-2   CHARACTERISTICS OF MAFENIDE ACETATE AND SILVER SULFADIAZINE*

	10% MAFENIDE ACETATE	SILVER SULFADIAZINE (SILVADENE)
Antibacterial activity	Bacteriostatic Broad spectrum	Bacteriostatic and bacteriocidal Broad spectrum
Local and systemic effects	Penetrates rapidly Rapidly oxidized (*p*-carboxy salt), absorbed, excreted as acid salt in urine Strong carbonic anhydrase inhibition Moist wound	Penetrates slowly Slowly broken down; 10% absorption of sulfadiazine Moist wound
Method of use	10% cream, applied daily 2 × Daily washing of wound Debridement	1% cream, applied daily 3 × or every 48 hr (in dressing) Wash off without débridement
Advantages	Not inactivated by pus or body fluids Nontoxic Softens wound, permitting better mobility	Same Nontoxic Softening Nonpainful
Disadvantages	Painful Sulfa sensitivities Severe acidosis with renal or pulmonary impairment	Sulfa sensitivities
Effectiveness	Partial	Partial

* All topical agents, at best, either delay colonization or suppress growth rates of organisms colonizing the burn wound. Selection of resistant organisms within burn units reduces effectiveness of each drug with length of time and intensity of use in individual units.

been taken, systemic antibiotic therapy should be initiated as soon as possible because the total course of gram-negative sepsis may be 6 to 12 hours.

In the past, antibiotics were given as recommended by the drug manufacturer. However, when actual blood levels of antibiotics, especially aminoglycosides, were measured, they were found to be very low in burn patients. With this knowledge, antibiotics are now prescribed using the knowledge of pharmacokinetics to maintain peak and trough blood levels in the therapeutic range. This technique has resulted in decreased mortality in burn patients with documented infection.

Nutritional and Metabolic Support
Burn patients have a hypercatabolic state characterized by increased oxygen consumption, marked increase in nitrogen excretion, and weight loss. This occurs with sustained increased catecholamine excretion, hyperglucagonemia, and normal or low insulin levels. The pathogenesis of the extreme hypercatabolism of burn injury remains an enigma. The increase in metabolic rate is proportional to the size of burn, reaching 2 to 2½ times the normal metabolic rate. The preferential use of the lean body mass for gluconeogenesis characterizes this hypermetabolic state. Weight losses exceeding 35% of preburn weight are generally lethal. Nutritional support should be begun at the earliest possible time post burn, since caloric and nitrogen deficits for as little as 3 days produce specific metabolic deficits. By 1 week, visceral protein is severely depleted and immunologic defects are detectable.

Nutritional support is begun by the third day. A simple formula for supplying sufficient calories to prevent weight loss is as follows: In adults, 40 calories per %TBSA burned + 25 calories/kg; in children, 65 calories/kg + 25 calories per %TBSA burned.

One gram of nitrogen per 150 calories is supplied. A balanced vitamin intake at a level 3 times the normal daily requirement for each vitamin approximates the known vitamin needs, with the exception of vitamin C, which is supplied in adults in excess of 2 g/day. Magnesium and zinc requirements are doubled, and other trace elements should also be supplied.

The gastrointestinal tract is the preferred route of administration for this tremendous caloric intake. Elemental diets administered by feeding tube can provide the necessary calories and protein in burns involving up to 40% to 50% of the body surface area. Intravenous hyperalimentation is frequently necessary in larger burns and when the gastrointestinal tract is not available. Central venous catheterization for intravenous alimentation in burn patients has a very high infection rate. The most efficient method of central venous alimentation requires changing of the catheters every 72 hours regardless of the site of placement. Bacteremia occurs frequently, causing seeding of the catheters and necessitating their frequent changing.

The increased oxygen requirements of the hypermetabolic state demand maintenance of a normal red blood cell mass. This is usually accomplished by frequent transfusions of whole blood or packed (preferably washed) red blood cells. Closing of the burn wound significantly decreases the hypermetabolic state. Therefore, every effort should be made to cover the wound as soon as possible.

AUTOGRAFTS, HOMOGRAFTS (ALLOGRAFTS), AND HETEROGRAFTS (XENOGRAFTS) IN TREATMENT AND REPAIR

Once the burn wound is cleared of necrotic tissue, it should be closed. To this date, no synthetic skin covering has been satisfactory; there is still no substitute for skin, although some newer materials appear promising. However, frequently it is not necessary to use the patient's own skin initially, particularly when the risk of graft loss is great. Under these circumstances, homografts obtained from cadaver donors may be placed over the areas from which necrotic tissue has been removed. With daily débridement, more and more of the eschar is removed and replaced by homograft. The homograft is usually changed every 2 to 3 days, or sooner if purulent collections occur beneath it.

Homografts may be placed on a freshly débrided wound in the absence of any significant granulation tissue. However, even small amounts of eschar remaining in the wound may result in the rapid collection of purulent material beneath the homograft, necessitating its removal. Once the raw area is clean, ideally the area has an autograft placed on it. If the autograft donor area is limited, a portion of the homograft may be allowed to remain and progress to homograft rejection, at which time the area can be covered with the autograft.

Porcine heterografts can be used in a manner similar to the homograft. Porcine heterografts are commercially available and currently in widespread use for the same indications as the homograft.

Homografts and heterografts can be used not only to provide temporary cover for areas of skin loss but also to test the acceptability of a recipient site for autograft. This usually occurs when there is limited donor area; therefore, failure of the initial autograft would be a disaster. Under such circumstances, temporary grafts can be placed over the recipient area, and if a good granulation-tissue bed occurs, autografts may be placed with the assurance of an excellent take. Also, reepithelialization of deep dermal burns can be hastened by the application of homografts or heterografts.

The greatest value of the homograft is its ability to temporarily close the burn wound prior to the availability of the autograft. The homograft is as effective as the autograft in preventing evaporative water loss, reducing caloric demand, diminishing pain, and preventing invasive infection of the burn wound.

Autogenous skin can be obtained by various surgical methods. How the skin is obtained is of little consequence if suitable skin coverage is provided, and the donor site heals as a second-degree burn in 10 to 14 days.

The choice of donor site is dictated by the distribution of the initial thermal injury. Certain characteristics of skin must be remembered. The skin of the back is the thickest skin in the body, while skin from the lateral aspect of the thigh and arm is somewhat less thick. The skin of patients at the extremes of age must be taken as a relatively thin sheet, since the dermal papillae and appendages are atrophic in the older age-group and less well developed in the younger.

Concerning the application of an autograft to a recipient site, it is not necessary that granulation tissue be present or that the wound be sterile. However, necrotic tissue must be absent and a good blood supply must exist. The bacteria of greatest significance in regard to skin-graft survival is the β-hemolytic streptococcus. This pathogen can cause extensive graft loss, which can be prevented by the administration of penicillin for 24 hours before and after grafting.

Donor sites classically are treated by the application of one layer of fine mesh gauze, which may then be left open. Porcine heterografts may also be used effectively as primary treatment, resulting in reduced pain and accelerated healing of the donor areas.

Fixation of the skin grafts may be with sutures, tape, or staples. The use of staples significantly shortens the operative time. The grafts may be dressed in the same fashion as were the burns prior to grafting. There is a wide variance among burn surgeons as to the types of dressings applied to skin grafts, as well as to the time these dressings should be changed postoperatively. The initial postoperative dressing change may be done any time from the first to the fifth postoperative day. The most common causes of graft failure are hematomas or seromas under the graft, lack of immobilization of the grafted area, and infection of the graft.

Depending on the preference of the surgeon and the area to be grafted, solid sheets of split-thickness skin or mesh grafts may be applied. Usually solid sheets of skin are applied to areas of cosmetic importance, such as the face. Mesh grafts may be applied to all other areas. The solid sheets of skin can be meshed with expansion ratios of 1:1.5, 1:3, 1:6, and 1:9. In patients with limited donor sites, the more expanded mesh grafts are used and required for skin coverage. Long-term results with these mesh grafts have been very satisfactory, especially when they have been used with pressure garments in the rehabilitation phase of burn care.

Excisional therapy for burns to fascia has been attempted during the past 3 decades with varying results. This usually has been done as staged procedures with excision of portions of the burn covering the cosmetic and functional areas of the body, to provide earlier skin coverage for these areas. As surgical techniques and the supporting services for surgical patients have improved, there have been better results for extensively burned patients.

LATE BURN-SCAR FORMATION AND CONTRACTURES

Unfortunately, many burn patients, for one reason or another, eventually exhibit varying degrees of scar formation and joint-skin contractures (Fig. 11-7). These deformities may require extensive plastic surgery for functional and cosmetic rehabilitation.

CHEMICAL BURNS

The incidence of chemical injuries is relatively low and the experience of individual physicians is limited. Therefore, Jelenko's review of chemicals that burn is invaluable as a reference. Since many chemical agents continue to act until neutralized or removed, emergency therapy should be rapid and specific for the offending agent when possible.

Copious lavage with water dilutes or neutralizes a wide range of chemicals effectively. The relatively more common chemical injuries that require specific therapy are summarized in Table 11-3. Except for emergency therapy to minimize the severity of chemical injury, the treatment of chemical burns is the same as that of thermal burns. All clothing saturated with the chemical should be quickly removed and copious lavage with water instituted to dilute the chemical.

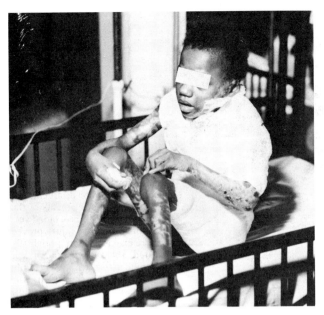

Fig. 11-7. Young girl with late contractures of the left elbow and left side of the neck preventing free movement of the head and left elbow. Movement was much improved by appropriate corrective plastic surgery.

ELECTRICAL BURNS

Electrical current produces tremendous tissue destruction, and necrosis of the deeper tissues is the predominant lesion in high-voltage injuries (Fig. 11-8). High-voltage electrical burns are characterized by wounds of entry and exit. Both are hard, leathery, charred, and cavitary, appearing to be the result of an explosion. Multiple entry or exit points may be present. There may be associated arc and flame burns. Tissue destruction is most severe at the points of entry and exit because these are the points at which the electrical current is most concentrated. There is also extensive deep-tissue injury, which is usually not obvious at the time of initial injury. The treatment of electrical injury is entirely different from that of thermal burns except for the cutaneous burns produced by the arc of the current igniting the clothing or other materials.

EMERGENCY CARE

At the scene of the injury, the primary concerns are cardiorespiratory resuscitation, protection against neurologic damage caused by fractures of the spine, and the initiation of fluid resuscitation.

Rescue personnel should ensure a safe area for the patient. Respiratory and cardiac function are initially evaluated and appropriate measures initiated. High-voltage currents usually result in cardiac standstill, whereas low voltage (below 440 volts) usually produces ventricular fibrillation. As prophylaxis for any spinal fracture that may have occurred because of severe muscle contraction or associated falls, the unconscious victim should be carefully placed on a long backboard to stabilize the spine. If the patient is conscious, details of the accident should be obtained to ascertain whether electricity actually went through the body.

IMMEDIATE HOSPITAL CARE

Unlike the case with thermal burns, the fluid-volume resuscitation cannot be calculated from the skin burns. Damage to deeper tissues is variable for each patient. Lactated Ringer's solution is given in sufficient volume to restore blood pressure and pulse to normal and establish a urine flow of 50 ml/hour. If myoglobinuria or hemoglobinuria is present, mannitol, 25 g/hour, is given beginning as soon as adequate fluid-volume resuscitation has restored vital signs. Mannitol is continued until the urine clears. In massive injuries, the tissue destruction results in release of intracellular acids and metabolites that produce a progressively severe metabolic acidosis as the circulation is restored.

TABLE 11-3 TREATMENT OF CHEMICAL "BURNS"

AGENT	INITIAL THERAPY	SPECIAL CONSIDERATIONS
Muriatic acid (HCl) Sulfuric acid (H_2SO_4) Nitric acid (HNO_3)	Soap	Then cover with Mg (OH_2) or Mg trisilicate
Oxalic acid [$2H_2O (COOH)_2$] Hydrofluoric acid (HF)	$NaHCO_3$ wash, then 0.2% hyamine in ice-alcohol	Inject Ca gluconate into area for residual pain
Chromic acid (H_2CrO_4)	Dilute Na hyposulfite wash	
Sodium hypochlorite (NaClO) (Clorox, other disinfectants, bleaches, deodorizers with chlorine)	Water wash, then 1% Na thiosulfate	
Phenol (C_6H_5OH) and cresols (sanitizers, disinfectants)	10% Ethanol	Then cover with olive, castor, or vegetable oils
Lyes (metal hydroxides), Na metal, lithium hydroxide	Dilute vinegar	Alternate with lemon juice, then cover with oil
Dichromate salts	2% Hyposulfite	
Alkyl mercury salts	Débride blisters and remove fluid	Then apply balm
White phosphorus	1:5000 $KMnO_4$	Then cover with oil
Tar	Clean with surgical antiseptic Cover with Neo-Polycin ointment	Wash off dissolved tar at 24 and 48 hours

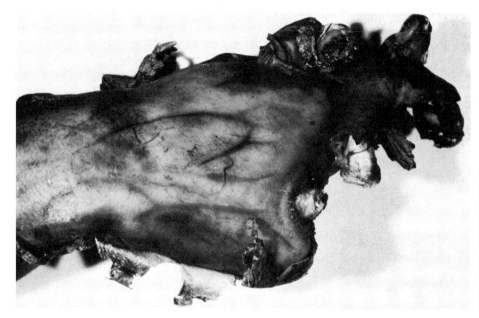

Fig. 11-8. Destroyed hand of a patient who grasped a high-tension electrical wire. Note destruction of bone and all other elements of the fingers and thrombosis of blood vessels of the hand. The injury proved far more extensive than it originally appeared to be, and amputation near the shoulder was required. (Hardy JD (ed): Pathophysiology in Surgery. Baltimore, Williams & Wilkins, 1958)

Arterial blood gases and *p*H should be obtained frequently (2-hour intervals during the first 8 hours), and sodium bicarbonate should be given to correct the base deficit.

This approach to resuscitation has resulted in virtual elimination of acute renal insufficienty as a complication of thermal injury. A severe hemolytic anemia may also be present, making it necessary to transfuse blood.

The immediate concern in wound care is preservation of adequate blood flow in the injured area. Massive edema frequently is present. Signs of adequate blood flow are evaluated on the basis of pulse volume, capillary refill, and the absence of deep, aching pain. Nerves are damaged by the electricity, with complete loss of sensation.

Fasciotomies are required throughout the extent of the wound to release tense, swollen muscles. Escharotomies do not suffice in electrical injury, because of damage to the skeletal muscle. Fasciotomies are also of diagnostic value in determining the extent of muscle necrosis in or adjacent to the obvious burn.

Electrical burn wounds are cleansed and débrided in the same manner as thermal burns. Sulfamylon is the topical chemotherapeutic agent of choice, because of its ability to penetrate deeply into the tissues. Sulfamylon is a carbonic anhydrase inhibitor, which results in a bicarbonate diuresis that causes a metabolic acidosis. This may further aggravate the acidosis caused by the original injury.

Demarcation between necrotic and viable tissue may require 7 to 10 days. Therefore, in wounds of limited extent, excisional therapy is usually accomplished between the seventh and tenth day. When massive muscle necrosis requires débridement of one or more large muscle masses or amputation, this should be done within the first 48 hours after injury. Removal of all dead tissue as soon as possible decreases the mortality and morbidity of the injury. Penicillin in significant doses is given as prophylaxis for gas gangrene. Wounds in special locations such as the hands should have early decompression with fasciotomies. The loss of skin coverage subsequent to excision and débridement results in desiccation of the tissues if not covered immediately with skin (autograft, homograft, or heterograft).

COLD INJURY

LOCAL COLD INJURY

Cold injury may have several causes. It may be due to a severe freezing environment or to prolonged immersion in cold water (trench foot, immersion foot). The most common cause is local injury to body parts exposed to low environmental temperatures. The escape of highly volatile liquids stored at low temperatures may produce a rapid freezing of tissues. Severe total-body hypothermia may result from prolonged exposure to environmental cold.

When tissues are exposed to intense cold for varying periods, frostbite occurs. The severity varies with the intensity of cold and the duration of exposure, producing four clinical types: first-degree injury, edema and redness of the affected part without necrosis; second-degree injury, formation of blisters; third-degree injury, necrosis of the skin; and fourth-degree injury, gangrene of the extremity.

The severity of injury usually cannot be made on initial examination until after rewarming. The rewarmed tissues become reddened, hot, and edematous, and the signs of the depth of the injury become apparent. Edema increases to a maximum in 24 to 48 hours and then gradually recedes. The areas of gangrene become apparent over the next few days to weeks. Fortunately, the degree of gangrene is often much less than initially feared, because the skin may be gangrenous while the underlying tissues are viable. Therefore, unless infection supervenes, amputation should be delayed until the extent of gangrene is definitely known.

Following recovery of the extremity, there is frequently a permanent increase in sympathetic tone, resulting in hyperhidrosis and an abnormal sensitivity to cold. Pain and paresthesias are common.

Rapid rewarming of the injured tissue is the most important aspect of treatment. The affected part should be placed in warm water, the temperature ranging between 40° C and 44° C. Complete rewarming usually takes about 20 minutes. Higher temperatures only cause further damage.

Blankets and other forms of rewarming are inadequate. After rewarming, the injured extremity should be elevated to minimize edema and then protected from environmental contamination by a sterile dressing, preferably using topical chemotherapeutic agents (*e.g.,* mafenide acetate or silver sulfadiazine). Blisters and necrotic skin are débrided as they separate. Hydrotherapy and physiotherapy are employed to maintain mobility of the affected parts.

There has been controversy concerning the use of heparin and sympathectomy as routine therapy for cold injuries. However, these are not currently recommended.

Rapid-freeze injuries may occur from the sudden escape of gases stored under very high pressure in liquid form. Contact produces instant freezing of varying depth. The skin is intensely blue to purple. Massive edema occurs rapidly, and pulses are frequently absent. Deep-tissue necrosis usually occurs because of ice-crystal formation. On initial examination, muscle appears viable, but within 10 days it becomes obviously necrotic. Excision of necrotic areas or amputation is best withheld until demarcation is complete, unless infection supervenes.

TOTAL-BODY HYPOTHERMIA

Severe total-body hypothermia (below 31° C) results from prolonged exposure to low environmental temperature. The patient exhibits signs of severe vasoconstriction, gray cyanosis, low respiratory and blood flow rates, hypotension, and oliguria and is comatose. Rapid rewarming by immersion in water 38° C to 40° C should be accomplished without delay. Ventilatory assistance should be provided and vital signs monitored carefully during rewarming. Large plasma losses begin during rewarming from leaks through the blood vessel walls similar to those seen in burns and should be treated in the same manner, with careful monitoring.

Fibrinogen precipitates during the hypothermia and often produces a hemorrhagic diathesis near the end of rewarming. Fresh plasma used for volume replacement usually prevents this problem. However, if there is a low fibrinogen level, several grams administered intravenously may be necessary to control hemorrhage.

Prognosis for survival in total-body hypothermia is poor. The postrewarming course is characterized by continued coma, failure of various organ systems, and bleeding tendencies.

BIBLIOGRAPHY

ALEXANDER JW, MacMILLAN BG, LAW E, et al: Treatment of severe burns with widely meshed skin autograft and meshed skin allograft overlay. J Trauma 21:433, 1981
ALEXANDER JW, OGLE CK, STINNETT JD et al: A sequential prospective analysis of immunologic abnormalities and infection following severe thermal injury. Ann Surg 188:809, 1978
ARTZ CP, MONCRIEF JA, PRUITT BA JR (eds): Burns: A Team Approach. Philadelphia, W B Saunders, 1979
BAXTER CR: Present concepts in the management of major electrical injury. Surg Clin North Am 50:1401, 1970
BURKE JF, QUINBY WC, BONDOC CC et al: Immunosuppression and temporary skin transplantation in the treatment of massive third degree burns. Ann Surg 182:183, 1975
BURKE JF, YANNAS IV, QUINBY WC et al: Successful use of a physiologically acceptable artificial skin in treatment of extensive burn injury. Ann Surg 194:413, 1981
CZAJA AJ, McALHANY JC, PRUITT BA JR: Acute gastroduodenal disease after thermal injury: An endoscopic evaluation of incidence and natural history. N Engl J Med 291:925, 1974
DAY SB, MacMILLAN BG, ALTERMEIER WA: Curling's Ulcer: An Experiment of Nature. Springfield, IL, Charles C Thomas, 1972
DIMICK AR, ROUSE RG: The treatment of electrical injury compared to burn injury: A review of pathophysiology and comparison of patient management protocols. J Trauma 18:43, 1978
GOODWIN CW JR, PRUITT BA JR: Burns. In Cagan BM (ed): Antimicrobial Therapy, 3rd ed, pp 397–408. Philadelphia, W B Saunders, 1980
GRALINO BJ, PORTER JM, ROSCH J: Angiography in the diagnosis and therapy of frostbite. Radiology 119:301, 1976
HICKS LM, HUNT JL, BAXTER CR: Liquid propane cold injury: A clinicopathologic and experimental study. J Trauma 19:701, 1979
HUNT JL, MASON AD, JR, MASTERSON TS et al: The pathophysiology of acute electric injuries. J Trauma 16:335, 1976
JELENKO C III: Chemicals that burn. J Trauma 14:65, 1974
LEVINE BA, PETROFF PA, SLADE CL et al: Prospective trials of dexamethasone and aerosolized gentamicin in the treatment of inhalation injury in the burned patient. J Trauma 18:188, 1978
LEVINE BA, SIRINEK KR, PRUITT BA, JR: Wound excision to fascia in burn patients. Arch Surg 113:403, 1978
LOEBL EC, BAXTER CR, CURRERI PW: The mechanisms of erythrocyte destruction in the early postburn period. Ann Surg 178:681, 1973
McALHANY JC, JR, CZAJA AJ, PRUITT BA, JR: Antacid control of complications from acute gastroduodenal disease after burns. J Trauma 16:645, 1976
McMANUS WF, MASON AD, PRUITT BA, JR: Subeschar antibiotic infusion in the treatment of burn wound infection. J Trauma 20:1021, 1980
MERYMAN HT: Tissue freezing and local cold injury. Physiol Rev 37:233, 1957
MOYLAN JA, CHAN CK: Inhalation injury—an increasing problem. Ann Surg 188:34, 1978
NINNEMANN JL: The Immune Consequences of Thermal Injury. Baltimore, Williams & Wilkins, 1981
O'KEEFFE KM: Accidental hypothermia: A review of 62 cases. Journal of the American College of Emergency Physicians 6:491, 1977
PRUITT BA JR: Multidisciplinary care and research for burn injury. J Trauma 17:263, 1977
PRUITT BA JR: Advances in fluid therapy in the early care of the burn patient. World J Surg 2:139, 1978
PRUITT BA JR: The burn patient: I. Initial care. Curr Probl Surg 16:4, 1979
PRUITT BA JR: The burn patient: II. Later care and complications of thermal injuries. Curr Probl Surg 16:5, 1979
PRUITT BA JR, DIVENCENTI FC, MASON AD JR et al: The occurrence and significance of pneumonia and other pulmonary complications in burned patients: Comparison of conventional and topical treatments. J Trauma 10:519, 1970
PRUITT BA JR, ERICKSON DR, MORRIS A: Progressive pulmonary insufficiency and other pulmonary complications of thermal injury. J Trauma 15:369, 1975
PRUITT BA JR, McMANUS WF, KIM SH et al: Diagnosis and treatment of cannula-related intravenous sepsis in burn patients. Ann Surg 191:546, 1980
RAYFIELD D, VAUGHT M, CURRERI PW et al: Extravascular fibrinogen degradation in experimental burn wounds: A source of circulating fibrin split products. Surgery 77:86, 1975
RICHMOND D, MARVIN JA, CURRERI PW et al: Dietary requirements of patients with major burns. J Am Diet Assoc 65:415, 1974
SCHUMAKER HB, WHITE BH, WRENN EL et al: Studies in experimental frostbite: The effect of heparin in preventing gangrene. Surgery 22:900, 1947
SEVITT S: Reactions to Injury and Burns and Their Clinical Importance. Philadelphia, J B Lippincott, 1974
SEVITT S: A review of the complications of burns, their origin and importance for illness and death. J Trauma 19:358, 1979
SHIRES GT, BLACK EA (eds): Proceedings of consensus development conference in supportive therapy in burn care. J Trauma 19:855, 1979
SHIRES GT, BLACK EA (eds): Proceedings of second conference on supportive therapy in burn care. J Trauma 21:665, 1981

SHUCK JM, PRUITT BA JR, MONCRIEF JA: Homograft skin for wound coverage: A study in versatility. Arch Surg 98:472, 1969

SORENSON B: Closure of the burn wound. World J Surg 2:167, 1978

SPEBAR MJ, PRUITT BA JR: Candidiasis in the burned patient. J Trauma 21:237, 1981

STEWART C, MUNGALL D, DIMICK AR: Ecthyma gangrenosum. Drug Intell Clin Pharm 13:692, 1979

WILLMORE DW, AULICK LH, PRUITT BA JR: Metabolism during the hypermetabolic phase of thermal injury. Adv Surg 12:193, 1978

WILTERDINK ME, CURRERI PW, BAXTER CR: Characterization of elevated fibrin split products following thermal injury. Ann Surg 181:157, 1975

ZASKE DE, CIPOLLE RJ, STRATE RJ: Gentamicin dosage requirements: Wide interpatient variations in 242 surgery patients with normal renal function. Surgery 87:164, 1980

H. Clark Ethridge, Jr.

Bites and Stings

INJURIES INFLICTED BY MAMMALS
Dog Bites
Rabies
Incidence
Rationale for Initiating Prophylaxis
Type of Exposure
Treatment
Human Bites
SNAKEBITE
Brief General Survey
Type of Snake and Bite Characteristics
Grading the Severity of the Bite
First Aid
Hospital Management
Use of Antivenin
Coral Snakes
HYMENOPTERA STINGS
Brief General Survey
Reactions
Treatment
Immunotherapy
ARACHNID INJURIES
Black Widow Spider
Brown Recluse Spider
Scorpions
INJURIES FROM MARINE LIFE

INJURIES INFLICTED BY MAMMALS

More than 1 million persons are bitten each year in the United States; bites by dogs account for about 85% to 90% of those seeking medical care. Most bites are minor, but a significant number require suturing, administration of antibiotics, and follow-up patient visits. Hospitalization is not uncommon, but fatalities are rare.

DOG BITES

Large dogs can generate tremendous pressure with their jaws, creating a crush injury with significant soft-tissue damage. Because a dog's mouth contains many bacteria, including *Staphylococcus aureus* and *Pasteurella multocida*, the potential for infection is great.

Treatment of dog bites is not much different from basic surgical principles for dirty lacerations, with a few excep-

tions. Copious, high-pressure irrigation with normal saline or dilute povidone–iodine solution is the most important aspect, along with débridement of devitalized tissue or excision of the wound. Whether closure should be primary or delayed primary is controversial. All hand wounds should be left open, packed with povidone–iodine- or iodoform-soaked gauze, and rechecked daily; delayed primary closure is accomplished when the risk of infection is over. Treatment of other wounds is at the discretion of the physician, and if any question exists, delayed closure is the preferred means of closure.

Antibiotic coverage is recommended and should cover *Staphylococcus aureus* and *Streptococcus viridans*. *Pasteurella* infections usually develop less than 24 hours after the bite and can be prevented with high-dose (8 million–12 million units/day) penicillin.

RABIES

INCIDENCE

Many thousands of persons receive postexposure rabies prophylaxis in the United States each year, although only 100 to 200 persons are bitten by animals proved to be rabid. Since the 1950s, the number of cases of rabies in domestic animals has decreased dramatically, while it has increased in wildlife to 70% of reported cases, especially in skunks, raccoons, foxes, bobcats, and bats.

The decision to administer postexposure rabies prophylaxis is difficult for the physician. The Center for Disease Control has recommended specific treatment of rabies and the rationale for initiating that treatment.

RATIONALE FOR INITIATING PROPHYLAXIS

Any bites by carnivorous wild animals, especially skunks, raccoons, foxes, bobcats, coyotes, or bats, should be treated unless the animal is killed and proved not to be rabid. Domestic animals should be confined for 10 days, and if symptoms of rabies develop, the animal should be sacrificed and the brain analyzed for rabies. If rabies is proved, treatment should be initiated. If the animal cannot be captured, treatment is based on the physician's judgment, realizing that unprovoked bites carry a higher risk than those provoked by the victim. Rodents have never been implicated in transmitting rabies to humans, and their bites should not be treated as such.

TYPE OF EXPOSURE

A bite is present when there is penetration of the skin by the teeth. Nonbite exposure involves contamination of an open cut or scratch with saliva of the rabid animal. Petting a rabid animal is not considered exposure to rabies. Human-to-human transmission of rabies virus has been documented in two cases of corneal transplants but has not been reported in any human bites.

TREATMENT

Primary treatment involves local treatment of the wound and tetanus prophylaxis. Immediate cleansing of the wound with soap and water is the most effective means of removing the rabies virus.

Immunotherapy should always consist of active (vaccine) and passive (globulin) prophylaxis and should be given as soon as possible after exposure. Human diploid cell vaccine (HDCV) is the vaccine of choice and is given with rabies immune globulin, human (RIG). If HDCV is not available, the old duck embryo vaccine (DEV) should be used. Antirabies serum, equine, (ARS) can be used if RIG is not available. Serum samples for antibody assay should be sent after completion of either of the vaccination regimens. The doses are as follows:

HDCV/RIG—RIG (20 IU/kg) is given in one dose, half around the bite and half intramuscularly. HDCV is given in six intramuscular doses of 1 ml each.

DEV/ARS—ARS (40 IU/kg) is given as one intramuscular dose. DEV requires 21 subcutaneous doses.

HUMAN BITES

The oral cavity of the human harbors a multitude of organisms that are potentially pathogenic when introduced into a wound. These include staphylococci, streptococci, clostridia, gonorrhea, spirochetes, fusiforms, and several viruses. Therefore, the potential for seriously disabling, even life-threatening, infection exists in human bite wounds.

Most wounds occur during an altercation in which the victim is usually intoxicated and does not recognize the need for medical care until infection is evident. Hand injuries, cuts associated with a striking blow, and injuries more than 24 hours old have a higher incidence of infection and complications. Copious irrigation with isotonic saline or dilute povidone solution and loose suturing of minor bites are acceptable if the patient is seen early, placed on broad-spectrum antibiotics, and seen in follow-up in 2 to 3 days.

Deep penetrating wounds, hand injuries, and more extensive wounds require excision or débridement, drainage, and closure by delayed or second intention after the threat of infection has subsided. The need for hospitalization depends on the severity of the bite, the condition of the patient (other associated injuries, inebriation), and the risk of noncompliance with outpatient care.

SNAKEBITE

BRIEF GENERAL SURVEY

There are from 6000 to 9000 venomous snakebites in the United States each year. Although only 9 to 12 deaths occur each year from these bites, the morbidity associated with severe bites is significant. One must realize that the treatment of envenomated snakebites is an extremely controversial issue from both medical and medicolegal standpoints, with morbidity occurring from delayed surgical intervention in serious bites as well as from overzealous débridement and disfigurement in minimally envenomated bites.

TYPE OF SNAKE AND BITE CHARACTERISTICS

In the United States, there are basically two groups of native venomous snakes, the pit vipers (copperhead, cottonmouth moccasin, and rattlesnakes) and the coral snake. The differentiation between poisonous and nonpoisonous snakes is depicted in Figure 11-9. The major distinguishing features are the heat-sensing facial pit, the elliptical pupils, and the venom glands on the pit viper. If the head is not presented, as in most cases, the caudal scales may be used for identification, as shown in Figure 11-9.

Fig. 11-9. Comparison of venomous and nonvenomous snakes. (Courtesy of Terry L. Vandeventer)

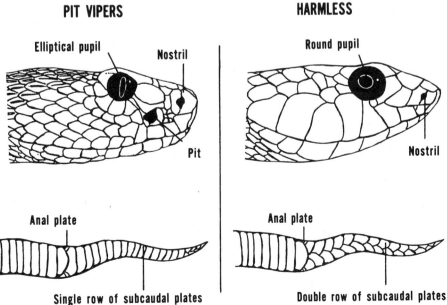

Ninety percent of snakebites occur on the extremities, two thirds on the lower extremities. Fang marks and immediate swelling and pain must be present to justify treatment as a poisonous snakebite. Nonpoisonous snakebites, as a rule, leave only superficial scratches, with minimal pain and no swelling. More than 50% of poisonous snakebites are "dry bites" (no venom is injected), and only 20% to 30% of the bites result in severe envenomation.

Early signs and symptoms of envenomation include pain similar to a bee sting, erythema, and edema. With time, the edema spreads proximally (often distally also), faint bruising and erythema spread around the bite, and often frank ecchymosis develops around the fang marks. The pain becomes deep and throbbing and can become very severe. With rattlesnake bites, localized fasciculations and paresthesias often occur and may involve other extremities and the perioral area.

With moderate to severe envenomations, systemic spread may occur and the patient may develop protracted nausea and vomiting, hypotension, coagulopathies, confusion, diplopia, tinnitus, or incontinence. Direct cardiac depression and renal failure have been reported but are less common complications.

Pit viper venoms are complex mixtures of enzymes and peptides that attack the local tissues, endothelium, and red blood cell membranes. The necrotizing potential varies among the species, with the large rattlesnakes having the most and the copperhead the least.

Taking into account the tremendous variability in snakes, victims, and quantity and quality of venom, a very generalized grouping of envenomations can be made. Copperheads, pigmy rattlesnakes, and juvenile cottonmouths usually produce only minor envenomations, while adult cottonmouths, juvenile diamondback rattlesnakes, and average-sized timber rattlesnakes produce moderate envenomations. Bites by full-sized rattlesnakes and extremely large cottonmouths often result in severe envenomations and systemic symptoms.

GRADING THE SEVERITY OF THE BITE

A more complex method of grading snakebites is prevalent in the literature but is felt by most authorities to be inadequate. I have used the following simplified system with confidence.

Grade 0—No envenomation; fang marks present, with erythema or swelling less than 1 inch from the bite

Grade I—Soft edema to, but not including, the first major joint proximal (or distal) to the bite

Grade II—Soft edema including and beyond the first major joint (minor to severe, depending on the extent of edema beyond the first joint); possible frank ecchymosis or blebs

Grade III—Systemic symptoms present, regardless of degree of local involvement

Grade IV—Cardiovascular collapse, respiratory distress, or coma

This system is used on presentation of the patient and altered if the symptoms progress during observation and treatment.

FIRST AID

The currently recommended first aid measures are less aggressive than those used in the past because most snakebite victims are now seen by the physician within 1 hour of the

---

BITES AND STINGS

Bites and stings from insects, mammals, and snakes are common injuries and in most circumstances pose little threat to the patient. Inoculation of bite wounds with bacterial organisms can produce severe local infection, and prophylactic antibiotic coverage is recommended for all animal and human bites. Infection with rabies virus from animal bites should always be considered, and the current recommendations for treatment and prophylaxis of rabies by the Communicable Disease Center should be observed.

Snakebite from a venomous snake, although rarely fatal, can cause significant morbidity and should be treated with specific antivenin whenever systemic envenomation has occurred.

Wasp and bee stings are significant because of occasional severe allergic reactions to Hymenoptera venom. Antihistamines and systemic epinephrine are required promptly to treat severe reactions. Black widow spiders, brown recluse spiders, and scorpions can produce envenomated bites that, although rarely fatal, can cause severe local and systemic complications.

---

bite. The basic measures are to calm the victim, immobilize the extremity, identify or obtain the snake, and transport the patient to a medical facility. Only in extreme envenomations with rapidly progressing symptoms or when a long time delay is expected should a constricting band or cooling of the area be used. Incisions in the field have no place in the first aid of the vast majority of snakebites.

HOSPITAL MANAGEMENT

In the emergency department, a good history and physical examination (including allergies, asthma, prior snakebites) are a must, as are routine blood work plus a coagulogram, type and match for blood, and tetanus prophylaxis.

It is imperative to base one's management on the degree of envenomation and the type of snake involved rather than to use a standard procedure for all snakebites. It is in this area that physician judgment plays a large part in decisionmaking, and the physician with little experience in snakebites risks increased morbidity to the patient from either too little or too aggressive treatment.

A summary of my grading system and basic guidelines of management is given in Table 11-4. The patient should be placed on broad-spectrum antibiotics to cover grampositive and gram-negative organisms. The bitten extremity should be kept in a neutral position, unless surgical débridement was performed, in which case elevation is recommended. The patient should be hospitalized at least until the edema is progressively subsiding.

Laboratory work for routine snakebite includes the following:

1. On admission—complete blood count (CBC), chemistry profile, urinalysis (U/A), and coagulogram, to include prothrombin time (PT), partial thromboplastin time (PTT), fibrinogen, fibrin split products (FSP), type and screen. Also electrocardiogram should be performed, if indicated by age, history, or symptoms.
2. Follow-up—CBC, U/A, PT, and PTT every 4 to 6 hours for 24 to 36 hours. Repeat fibrinogen and FSP if any of the above change.

Varying degrees of coagulopathy can be found in most pit viper envenomations, usually involving a depletion of fibrinogen with production of FSP due to a thrombin-like

TABLE 11-4 SNAKEBITE TREATMENT SUMMARY

	GRADE 0	I	II	III	IV

Symptoms	Little pain
	No edema
	Minimal erythema
		Minor pain
		Edema to 1st joint
		May have
		  Local cyanosis
		  Ecchymosis
		    at fang marks
			Moderate pain
			Edema beyond 1st
			  joint
			Cyanosis of area
			May have
			  Paresthesias
			  Blebs
			  Ecchymosis
				Severe pain
				Systemic symptoms
					Cardiovascular (CV)
					  collapse
					Possible coma
					± severe local
					  symptoms

Tetanus prophylaxis	+	+	+	+	+
Antibiotics	Oral	Oral, IV	IV	IV	IV
Hospitalization	Observe × 4 hours	Overnight	+	ICU	ICU
Antivenin	No	No	No	+	+
Débridement	No	No	±	+	+
Steroids	No	No	No	No	Possibly for CV support

peptide in the venom. Rarely does this cause significant clinical problems, and usually a rebound in the serum fibrinogen level is seen in 2 to 3 days. In severe envenomations, especially with rattlesnake venoms, hematuria, prolonged clotting times, low fibrinogen levels, elevated FSP levels, a fall in hematocrit, and sometimes a disseminated intravascular coagulation–like syndrome may occur. Treatment with large amounts of blood components rich in clotting factors is required until the venom can be neutralized with intravenous antivenin.

Débridement of grossly envenomated tissue is the major point of controversy in snakebite management. I feel that all bites of Grades III and IV should have local débridement to remove any residual venom. Grades 0 and I and certainly any nonvenomous snakebites should not be débrided. If frank ecchymosis or blebs are present, indicating severe local reaction, débridement is probably indicated.

Débridement consists of subcutaneous dissection of grossly envenomated tissue (usually limited to 2 cm–4 cm from the bite after 1–2 hours). It is often difficult to assess the viability of adjacent muscle tissue, which is usually very hemorrhagic in response to the venom. Unless there is no question that the muscle is necrotic, a second-look procedure in a few days is much more acceptable than the removal of tissue that might recover all or part of its function.

Any fasciotomy necessitated by a severe intramuscular envenomation (usually seen with large rattlesnakes) should be performed with fascial incisions that are removed from the skin incisions, thereby reducing the need for subsequent skin grafting and resultant deformities.

USE OF ANTIVENIN

The use of antivenin (Crotalidae) polyvalent is also extremely controversial in snakebite treatment. It is of definite benefit in treatment of coagulopathies and other symptoms due to systemic spread, but the controversy exists over its use in relatively minor envenomations because it has not been shown to prevent or reduce local tissue necrosis. Because allergic reactions, either immediate or delayed, are common, the risk/benefit ratio is such that it is usually reserved for patients in whom systemic symptoms are present.

A skin test for horse-serum sensitivity should always be performed, according to the instructions in the package insert. If the skin test is negative, 3 to 5 vials of antivenin are diluted in 500 ml saline or D₅W and given intravenously over the first hour. Whenever antivenin is being given, an epinephrine drip (1 mg in 250 ml) and intravenous diphenhydramine hydrochloride (Benadryl) should always be at hand to treat any allergic reactions. If the systemic symptoms abate, no further antivenin is necessary. If they progress, 2 to 3 more vials should be given over the next few hours.

The dose of antivenin should be increased 1½ to two times for infants and children, because they have a smaller blood volume for dilution of venom. In severe cases, more antivenin should be used initially and up to a total of 20 to 30 vials may be necessary.

Minor allergic reactions (flushing, wheals, pruritus) can usually be managed by slowing the infusion rate or administering intravenous Benadryl. Anaphylaxis, although rare, has occurred and should be treated with Benadryl, epinephrine, fluids, and supportive measures.

The patient with a positive skin test should be given antivenin only if limb or life is in danger. This should be done under close observation in an intensive-care setting.

CORAL SNAKES

Although bites by the small, seclusive coral snakes are rare and envenomation is even less likely, all patients suspected of being bitten by a coral snake should be observed for at least 6 to 8 hours. If any symptoms of localized or central paresthesia or paralysis develop, 3 to 5 vials of antivenin (micrurus fulvius) should be given intravenously, with more given as needed thereafter. When a definite coral snake bite has occurred and some local pain is involved, the antivenin should be given immediately and the patient placed in an intensive-care setting, with precautions for management of respiratory failure at hand.

HYMENOPTERA STINGS

BRIEF GENERAL SURVEY

Stings by members of Hymenoptera, which include bees, hornets, wasps, yellow jackets, and fire ants, are responsible for more than 40 deaths in the United States each year. It is estimated that 1 million to 2 million persons in the United States have significant allergic reactions to the venom of the insects.

REACTIONS

There are two basic types of reactions to these venoms, a local reaction and a systemic or generalized reaction. Local reactions in nonsensitive persons are characterized by pain, swelling, and redness in an area about the size of a quarter or half-dollar, which is followed by itching and resolution in 2 to 3 days. More severe local reactions include rash, massive swelling, and pain and are thought not to predispose to systemic reactions. Systemic reactions range from hives to peribronchial edema with wheezing, periorbital edema, laryngeal edema, and respiratory distress. Anaphylaxis usually appears within minutes after the sting if it is going to occur.

TREATMENT

Soothing of the local area can be achieved with ice or a paste of meat tenderizer, while antihistamines can relieve the swelling and itching that also occur. Antiseptics may be applied to prevent secondary infection.

Systemic reactions should be treated as soon as recognized with aqueous epinephrine (1:1000) administered in 0.3-ml to 0.5-ml doses subcutaneously, along with antihistamines and support for cardiovascular and respiratory complications. Steroids have no place in the immediate treatment of local or generalized reactions but may be helpful in prevention of delayed serum sickness–type reactions.

IMMUNOTHERAPY

Whole-body extract has been used for years to immunize sensitive persons but has recently been shown to be ineffective in generating sufficient levels of protective venom-specific IgG antibodies. More recently, venom immunotherapy has proved to be more effective and is the recommended method of immunizing persons who have a history of a systemic-type reaction to a Hymenoptera sting. These persons should also practice measures to avoid being stung and should have one of the prescribed kits with antihistamine and a preloaded syringe of epinephrine with them at all times.

ARACHNID INJURIES

BLACK WIDOW SPIDER

The black widow has a shiny black body with an orange to red hourglass figure on the underside. The venom is of a neurotoxic class and produces minimal local reaction. Rapid onset of localized muscle cramps and sweating is followed by severe abdominal pain suggestive of a surgical abdomen.

A specific antivenin is available for early relief of symptoms and should be given intravenously to all children and to adults with severe envenomations. Atropine sulfate may be used if antivenin is not available. Muscle cramps may be relieved with methocarbamol (Robaxin), given slowly as 60 mg/kg/day in four divided intravenous doses.

BROWN RECLUSE SPIDER

The brown recluse is about the same size as the black widow spider but lacks the shiny body and is brown. It has a darker violin- or fiddle-shaped marking on its back, hence the name fiddler spider. It is a very seclusive spider, preferring dark, moist areas, and is commonly found in closets, under houses, and in abandoned dwellings. The bite of the brown recluse is rarely noticed until hours later, when local pain, vesicle formation, and erythema appear, often accompanied by nausea, vomiting, and malaise. The classic reaction consists of a central vesicle surrounded by blanching, then erythema, resembling a bull's-eye. Necrosis of the tissues with undermining of the skin edges occurs over the next few days, hence the name necrotic arachnidism. Severe systemic symptoms are usually found in cases with minimal local changes, in children, and have an onset within 24 hours of the bite. Rapid hemolysis, thrombocytopenia, hemoglobinuria, and disseminated intravascular coagulation may occur.

There are several controversial areas in the treatment of brown recluse bites. In many bites, small necrotic areas heal with no further treatment, but many feel that excision of areas greater than 1 cm to 2 cm should be performed with primary or delayed closure. Local injection of steroids to lessen the severity of the lesion is popular, although the value of this is unproved. Frequent coagulation studies should be performed to detect any hemolysis or decrease in platelet counts. Supportive care, early massive doses of steroids (especially in children), and, rarely, exchange transfusions are the mainstay of treatment of systemic manifestations. A specific antivenin has yet to be developed in the United States for use in brown recluse envenomations.

SCORPIONS

Although scorpions are a feared species in the Southwest, less than one death per year is related to scorpion stings in the United States. Young children appear to be more susceptible to their venom; most of the deaths from scorpions in Mexico are in children.

The scorpion is not aggressive, and it usually stings only when cornered. Early local symptoms are burning and edema; ecchymosis and necrosis occur in some instances. Systemic reactions to this neurotoxin may occur, especially in children, and include sweating, nausea, salivation, headache, paresthesias, and cramping of abdominal muscles. In severe envenomations, this may progress to shock or convulsions.

Treatment of localized stings is symptomatic, with application of ice and elevation. For systemic spread, intravenous steroids, atropine, and barbiturates should be used. A specific antivenin is available from Arizona State University at Tempe. Narcotics are to be avoided because they may obscure the neurologic symptoms.

INJURIES FROM MARINE LIFE

Sharks, barracuda, killer whales, and several of the large fish can inflict mutilating injuries on humans. On-the-scene emergency care may well be a lifesaving factor, because shock may be present or pending. After initial control of hemorrhage and adequate fluid resuscitation, the mainstay of treatment is surgical irrigation and débridement of the wounds, with primary or secondary reconstruction; broad-spectrum antibiotics are given to prevent secondary infection.

The jellyfish and Portuguese man-of-war probably account for the majority of marine stings each year in the United States. Treatment is immediate rinsing of the area with the closest available fluid. Most regular beachgoers use papain (Adolph's meat tenderizer) on the wounds for relief of symptoms. Baking soda and flour are thought to assist in the removal of the tentacles.

Some forms of marine life rely on sharp spines as defense mechanisms. The list includes the starfish, sea urchins, and sea cucumbers, as well as the well-known stingray or "demon of the sea." Although pain is intense following injury from these spines, fatalities are rare and often related to arrhythmias or respiratory distress. Treatment should begin immediately with thorough washing of the area and removal of any sheath material, while papain, if available, will neutralize the venom. A constriction band should be applied proximal to the injury and the area submerged in hot water for 30 to 90 minutes to inactivate the venom. Surgical débridement, irrigation, and closure are recommended, as are tetanus and antibiotic prophylaxis.

BIBLIOGRAPHY

ANDREWS CE, DEES JE, EDWARDS RO et al: Venomous snakebite in Florida. J Fla Med Assoc 55:308, 1968

CALLAHAM M: Dog bite wounds. JAMA 244:2327, 1980

CHIPPS BE, VALENTINE MD, KAGEY-SOBOTKA A et al: Diagnosis and treatment of anaphylactic reactions to Hymenoptera stings in children. J Pediatr 97:177, 1980

GLASS TG JR: Early debridement in pit viper bites. JAMA 235:2513, 1979

HUANG TT, LYNCH JB, LARSON DL et al: The use of excisional therapy in the management of snakebite. Ann Surg 179:598, 1973

MALINOWSKY RW, STRATE RG, PERRY JF JR et al: The management of human bite injuries of the hand. J Trauma 19:655, 1979

PEEPLES E. BOSWICK JA JR, SCOTT FA: Wounds of the hand contaminated by human or animal saliva. J Trauma 20:383, 1980

Public Health Service Advisory Committee on Immunization Practices: Rabies: Risk, management, prophylaxis, and immunization. Ann Intern Med 86:452, 1977

REISMAN RE: Allergic reactions to insect stings. South Med J 71:208, 1978

RUSSELL FE: Marine Toxins and Venomous and Poisonous Marine Animals. Neptune City, NJ, TFH Publications, 1971

RUSSELL FE: Snake Venom Poisoning. Philadelphia, J B Lippincott, 1980

RUSSELL FE: Snake venom poisoning in the United States. Ann Rev Med 31:247, 1980

STOCHSKY B: Necrotic arachnidism. West J Med 131:143, 1979

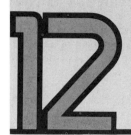

Jeremiah G. Turcotte/Darrell A. Campbell, Jr./John W. Konnak

Immunobiology and Transplantation of the Kidney

The successful transplantation of an organ allograft is one of the most satisfying experiences in clinical medicine. Success or failure depends primarily on events taking place at a cellular level. The ability to influence these events favorably is one of the most fervently sought goals in modern biology.

RENAL IMMUNOBIOLOGY

At present two general approaches are employed to improve results in organ transplantation. The first of these strategies involves the selection of donor tissue on the basis of antigenic similarity to recipient tissue. The degree to which this can be done has a most important bearing on the ultimate clinical result. Appropriate donor–recipient matching requires a detailed knowledge of transplantation antigens and an understanding of the histocompatibility relationships between cells.

The second approach to organ transplantation involves the development of drugs capable of blunting the naturally occurring immune response to an allograft. This approach has been successful in making organ transplantation a clinical reality. Unfortunately, because only a nonspecific depression of immunity is possible with presently available drugs, infectious complications associated with the immunosuppressed state still occur. Future successes in the field of organ transplantation will undoubtedly involve methods for depressing immune reactivity more specifically. Whether this will be done with drugs or immunologic manipulations, or both, remains to be seen.

TRANSPLANTATION ANTIGENS

The development of an immune response to a transplanted organ depends upon the recognition by recipient lymphocytes that the organ allograft is in fact "foreign" or "nonself." The ability of lymphoctyes to make this distinction depends upon the presence of distinctive celll-surface antigens that are called *histocompatibility antigens*. The synthesis of such antigens is governed by a specific area of chromosomal information; this area is called the *major histocompatibility complex* (MHC). Because most information about human transplantation antigens has come from the study of the mouse MHC and its antigenic products, a brief discussion of mouse transplantation antigens follows.

DEFINITIONS

Adoptive transfer. Transfer of immunocompetent cells from one animal to a histocompatible but immunoincompetent recipient.
Alleles. Any one of a series of two or more different genes that may occupy the same position or locus on a specific chromosome.

IMMUNOBIOLOGY IN RENAL TRANSPLANTATION

Results in organ transplantation depend upon interactions between donor cells expressing foreign histocompatibility antigens and recipient cells capable of recognizing these antigens. Class I transplantation antigens are expressed on all cells and serve as targets for the immune response. Class II antigens have a limited tissue distribution (B cells, some macrophages, sperm, epidermal cells) and serve as distinctive recognition structures. The immune response to cells expressing foreign transplantation antigens is dependent upon the degree of antigenic disparity appreciated. Histocompatibility testing, utilizing serologic techniques and the mixed lymphocyte culture (MLC), is used routinely to select an organ from a donor bearing antigens that are most similar to recipient antigens. When rejection of an organ transplant does occur, it may be of three types: hyperacute, acute, or chronic. Hyperacute rejection is antibody mediated and occurs within hours of transplantation. Acute rejection is primarily a cell-mediated phenomenon and typically occurs 7 to 10 days following transplantation. Chronic rejection involves both humoral and cell-mediated immunity, is far more subtle than acute rejection, and is less responsive to antirejection therapy. A well-functioning organ transplant is absolutely dependent upon administration of immunosuppressive drugs. The most important immunosuppressive protocol used includes corticosteroids (prednisone) and azathioprine (Imuran). In many instances a preparation of heterologous antiserum is also used temporarily to depress recipient immune responsiveness. Cyclosporin-A, a new drug, appears to be a very potent immunosuppressive agent of clinical importance.

Renal transplantation is a proven effective modality for the treatment of chronic renal failure, and the kidney has been the most successfully transplanted vital organ. Newer immunosuppressive techniques are constantly improving transplantation results.

Allogeneic. Pertaining to the relationship between genetically different individuals within the same species.

B cells. Lymphocytes that are precursors of immunoglobulin-secreting plasma cells. These cells can be distinguished from T cells in that, unlike T cells, they bear cell-surface immunoglobulin.

Haplotype. The complement of transplantation antigens inherited from a single parent.

Major histocompatibility complex. Area of genetic information of a chromosome that codes for the production of histocompatibility antigens.

Opsonization. The process by which bacteria or other substances are altered so that they are more readily and more efficiently engulfed by phagocytes.

T cells. Lymphocytes that are derived initially from bone marrow but undergo a process of maturation in the thymus gland. These cells are responsible for such diverse functions as allograft rejection, cell-mediated cytotoxicity, delayed hypersensitivity reactions, and graft-versus-host disease.

ANTIGENS CODED BY H-2

The mouse MHC is referred to as *H-2* and is located on the 17th chromosome. The *H-2* locus can be subdivided into a number of distinctive regions. Regions *H-2K* and *H-2D,* which are the boundaries of the *H-2* complex, code for the production of histocompatibility antigens that serve as targets for specific immune responses. Thus, immunization between mice differing at *H-2K* and *H-2D* results in the development of an antibody response to these antigens and also in the development of lymphocytes specifically cytotoxic for cells bearing these determinants. In contrast, the *H-2I* region, which is located between *H-2K* and *H-2D,* codes for antigens that are responsible for the induction of an immune response. Thus, the immune response to alloantigeneic tissue is the result of both recognition of allogeneic *H-2I* region products as "non-self" and the development of specific effector mechanisms (antibody response or development of cytotoxic "killer" cells) directed against allogeneic *H-2K*- and *H-2D*-encoded targets.

H-2K and *H-2D* region antigens differ from *H-2I* region antigens with regard to structure. *H-2K* and *H-2D* antigens (class I antigens) are composed of a 43,000 Mol wt glycoprotein and a smaller protein, a 12,000 Mol wt β_2 microglobulin. *H-2I* region antigens (class II antigens), on the other hand, are composed of two glycoprotein chains of Mol wt 33,000 and 28,000, respectively, but no β_2 microglobulin.

The tissue distribution of class I and class II antigens is also different. Class I antigens are distributed on the surface of all nucleated cells, whereas class II antigens have a much more limited tissue distribution and are found only on B cells, some macrophages, spermatozoa, and epidermal cells. Class II antigens are in general not found on resting T cells but may be expressed on T cells following specific antigenic activation and subsequent clonal expansion.

ANTIGENS CODED BY THE HLA LOCUS

The major histocompatibility complex in man is located on the short arm of chromosome 6 and is called *HLA* (human leukocyte-associated antigen). HLA is in many ways analogous to the *H-2* locus in the mouse. The HLA locus can be subdivided into four regions. The *HLA-A, HLA-B,* and *HLA-C* regions code for class I antigens. As in the mouse, these antigens serve as targets for antibody response and as targets for cytotoxic lymphocytes. The *HLA-D* region is analogous to the mouse *H-2I* region and codes for class II antigens responsible for induction of the immune response. Specific subregions within *HLA-D* have not been defined.

Characterization of *HLA-A, HLA-B,* and *HLA-C* locus products is easily accomplished using serologic techniques. For this reason these antigens are also referred to as serologically defined (SD) antigens. Until recently it has been difficult to characterize *HLA-D* locus products serologically. As will be described later, other tests, including mixed lymphocyte culture (MLC), have been used instead. *HLA-D* locus products are also referred to as lymphocyte-defined (LD) antigens.

Human histocompatibility antigens are similar in structure to their murine counterparts. Class I antigens have a Mol wt of 44,000 with a 12,000 Mol wt β_2 microglobulin subunit. Class II antigens are composed of two noncovalently linked glycoprotein chains of 34,000 and 28,000 Mol wt, respectively. The 34,000 Mol wt chain is called the alpha, or heavy, chain, and the 28,000 Mol wt chain is referred to as the beta, or light, chain. Allospecificities (alleles of the *HLA-D* locus) are thought to be present on the light chain, whereas the heavy chain is identical from individual to individual.

Each nucleated cell in humans expresses two types of antigens coded for by *HLA-A,* two types of antigens coded for by *HLA-B,* and two types of antigens coded for by

HLA-C. In addition, those cells expressing *HLA-D* locus products express two types of *HLA-D* antigens. At each locus a variety of different antigenic specificities may be expressed. There are 20 different alleles that may be inherited at *HLA-A* and 42 that may be inherited at *HLA-B.* The *HLA-D* locus is somewhat less polymorphic; only 12 possible alleles are described at present.

HISTOCOMPATIBILITY

The intensity of the allograft rejection process is directly related to the degree of antigenic disparity between donor and recipient tissue. Thus no rejection process develops at all in transplantation between identical twins, whereas marked rejection usually occurs in transplantation between unrelated individuals. It follows that attempts to minimize the antigenic disparity between donor and recipient tissue also minimize the severity of the rejection process following transplantation.

Currently, donor-recipient matching is done by comparing HLA antigenic specificities found on donor lymphocytes to the HLA specificities found on recipient lymphocytes. Although HLA codes for the most obvious transplantation antigens, it should be noted that there are other loci outside HLA which code for less obvious transplantation antigens. Such loci, called minor histocompatibility loci, have been clearly described in mouse systems but have been more difficult to characterize in humans. The presence of minor histocompatibility loci can be inferred, however, from the fact that rejection often occurs even when transplantation is done between HLA identical siblings.

PRELIMINARY TESTING

Two simple but very important tests must be carried out before an organ transplant may be done between two individuals. First, it must be established that donor and recipient are compatible for ABO blood groups. The reason is that ABO antigens are expressed on the parenchymal tissue of the organ allograft. Because humans have *isoantibodies* (naturally occurring antibodies) to blood group antigens, a transplanted organ of incompatible blood type will be the target of antibody-mediated cell killing. The clinical result is the very rapid (within hours) loss of organ function and signs of marked systemic toxicity. This syndrome is referred to as "hyperacute rejection."

In clinical practice the same rules of ABO compatibility that apply to blood transfusions also apply to renal transplants—that is, type O individuals are "universal donors" of blood and kidney transplants, while AB recipients are "universal recipients" and may receive blood or a kidney transplant from individuals of any blood type.

The second important preliminary test is the survey of the potential recipient's blood for the presence of preformed cytotoxic antibodies directed against HLA antigens of the donor. Individuals may develop anti-HLA antibodies as the result of exposure to a prior kidney transplant, exposure to HLA antigens on lymphocytes present in previous blood transfusions, or, in females, exposure to paternally derived antigens of a fetus. Hyperacute rejection results if anti-HLA antibodies specific for donor kidney cells are present at the time of transplantation. A careful test is done to ensure that a kidney is not transplanted into an individual possessing such anti-HLA antibody. This test is called a *cross match.* Lymphocytes of donor origin are incubated for 4 hr in the presence of rabbit complement. If more than 20% of donor

cells are killed at the end of 4 hr, the results are referred to as a positive cross match. Because the levels of anti-HLA antibodies may vary over time, it is standard practice to collect and freeze multiple serum samples from any potential transplant recipient. All serum samples collected from this individual must show a negative cross match with donor lymphocytes before a transplant may be considered.

DONOR-RECIPIENT MATCHING IN RELATED RENAL TRANSPLANTS

Clinical renal transplantation involves two types of transplants. Those transplants in which a relative donates a kidney to a recipient are referred to as *related donor transplants,* while transplants in which a kidney from an unrelated "brain-dead" cadaver is used are referred to as *cadaver donor transplants.* Within any family it is possible that two siblings may not share any HLA antigens. In this case related transplantation offers no clear advantage over a cadaver donor transplant. Conversely, it is possible that two siblings may be entirely HLA identical. In this case the results of related renal transplantation are excellent. It is common practice to test the immediate family of a renal failure patient serologically to make these distinctions.

The inheritance of HLA antigens follows straightforward rules of mendelian genetics. Humans, being diploid organisms, have cells that contain 46 chromosomes. When gametes are produced, these cells are haploid, that is, they contain only 23 chromosomes. The gametes produced by one individual are of two different varieties, one set representing the paternal genome and one set representing the maternal genome. The set of 23 chromosomes is often referred to as a *haplotype* (maternal or paternal). At the time of fertilization a diploid zygote results. Following the rules of independent segregation, the genome of the zygote may then be one of four different varieties, each of which will occur with equal (25%) probability. If one considers that a father (AB) makes gametes of the A or B haplotype and that a mother (CD) makes eggs of the C or D haplotype, then at fertilization a zygote of AC, AD, BC, or BD genome may result. An offspring of this union (AC, for example) has a 25% chance that two haplotypes will be shared with a sibling (HLA identical), a 25% chance that no haplotype will be shared (HLA nonidentical), and a 50% chance that one haplotype (HLA semi-identical) will be shared. Obviously, an offspring must always share one haplotype with a parent. These relationships are important because results in related renal transplantation correlate directly with the number of haplotypes shared between recipient and donor.

The haplotype status of individuals can be easily characterized using standard serologic techniques. In these types of assays antiserum having specificity for a known antigen (*typing antiserum*) is incubated with lymphocytes under study. Rabbit complement is added. If more than 20% of cells are killed after 4 hr of incubation at room temperature, it is considered evidence that the cells in question express antigen to which the typing antiserum is directed. The HLA antigens that are typed are expressed on the surface of cells in a *codominant* pattern. This means that the HLA antigens of the paternal and maternal haplotype are both equally expressed on the surface of lymphocytes. This is true for each of the four HLA regions, so that a total of eight types of HLA antigens may be expressed on a cell surface. In clinical practice information about the six *HLA-A, HLA-B,* and *HLA-C* specificities is usually obtained. Using the information about antigen specificities expressed by cells from each member of a family, it is possible to define the haplotype relationship between family members.

It has been difficult to define *HLA-D* specificities using the same serologic techniques that are used to define *HLA-A, HLA-B,* and *HLA-C* specificities. This is primarily due to the paucity of *HLA-D* antigen expression on peripheral blood lymphocytes, most of which are T cells. However, if a related donor and recipient share *HLA-A, HLA-B,* and *HLA-C* serologically defined products, one can usually infer that *HLA-D* antigens are also shared since the four regions are all located in close proximity to each other (linked) on the same chromosome. An exception to this rule may occur when there has been a crossover involving *HLA-D*.

MIXED LYMPHOCYTE CULTURE

The mixed lymphocyte culture (MLC) is an assay that is used to gain more information about *HLA-D* antigenic differences between donor and recipient. This assay takes advantage of the observation that lymphocytes will begin to proliferate markedly if they are co-cultivated *in vitro* in the presence of allogeneic lymphocytes. More precisely, recognition of *HLA-D* antigenic disparity triggers cellular proliferation. The rate of proliferation is measured and is taken as an index of antigenic differences at *HLA-D*. MLC is frequently used in clinical renal transplantation to make decisions about the appropriateness of a related donor for a given recipient. One drawback of the MLC as currently performed is that the *in vitro* incubation takes place over 5 to 6 days. Thus, MLC cannot be used in the selection of cadaver donors because the cadaver kidney may be reliably preserved for only 2 days. One example of the way in which MLC is used in the decision-making process is shown in Figure 12-1.

DR TYPING

It has become possible to define 12 different *HLA-D* specificities. Because *HLA-D* antigens are found primarily on B cells, these antigens are also generally referred to as *B-cell antigens*. Recently, it has become possible to define similar or perhaps identical B-cell specificities using serologic techniques rather than MLC. Antigens detected in this way are referred to as *HLA-DR antigens* (D-related). Whether or not these antigens are coded for by *HLA-D* or a closely linked *HLA-"DR"* locus is not known. The ability to define B-cell antigens serologically is an important advance, because the shortened time requirements of the serologic techniques versus MLC permit matching for D-locus products in cadaver recipients as well as related recipients. There is increasing evidence that careful matching of donor–recipient pairs for DR antigens improves results in renal transplantation.

DONOR–RECIPIENT MATCHING IN CADAVERIC RENAL TRANSPLANTS

Serologic definition of *HLA-A, HLA-B,* and *HLA-C* locus specificities generated with it the hope that matching donor and recipient tissues for these antigens would dramatically improve the results of cadaveric renal transplantation. In general, a substantial improvement in results using such techniques has not been realized, particularly in the United States. When the percentage of cadaver kidney transplants functioning for 1 year is used as an endpoint, the difference between very well matched donor–recipient pairs (two identical *HLA-A* and two identical *HLA-B* antigens) and entirely unmatched donor–recipient pairs (no shared *HLA-A* or *HLA-B* antigens) is only 12%. Matching for

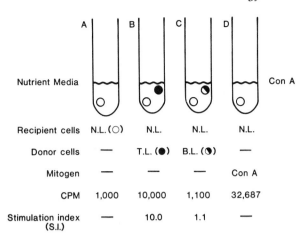

Fig. 12-1. Mixed lymphocyte culture. In the example depicted, renal failure patient N.L. has two siblings (B.L. and T.L.) who are available to donate a kidney. Serologic testing indicates that both donors share one haplotype with the recipient. The MLC is used to obtain further information about recipient compatibility with donor cells.

In a typical test N.L. cells are incubated in nutrient media under various circumstances. Panel A shows N.L. cells incubated alone, a negative control. Panel B shows N.L. cells incubated with one sibling's cells, and panel C shows N.L. cells incubated with the other sibling's cells. Panel D shows N.L. cells incubated in the presence of Con A, a nonspecific stimulator of lymphocyte proliferation. This serves as a positive control. After 6 days the rate of cellular proliferation induced in N.L. cells can be measured (in counts per minute [cpm] of tritiated thymidine incorporation). In this example donor B.L. cells would be considered less of an antigenic stimulus to N.L. than donor T.L. cells and would thus be the more appropriate donor. A stimulation index, used to quantitate these relationships, is calculated by dividing cpm generated in panel B or C by cpm generated in the negative control (panel A).

HLA may correlate better with success rates at 5 years and 10 years. Considering that the probability that two unrelated individuals will share four *HLA-A* and *HLA-B* antigens is only 0.03%, it becomes clear why attempts to match for serologically defined *HLA-A* and *HLA-B* antigens have not been more productive. An important contrast between the HLA typing of related and cadaver transplant candidates is that in the case of related donor–recipient combinations, identity for two *HLA-A* and two *HLA-B* locus antigens implies that the rest of HLA is also identical, since HLA is inherited as a single unit. In contrast, matching *HLA-A* and *HLA-B* locus antigens in cadaver donor transplant situations implies little about other areas of HLA, particularly *HLA-D*. There is optimism that selection of cadaveric donor–recipient combinations on the basis of shared DR specificities will be more successful than matching for products of *HLA-A* and *HLA-B*.

ALLOGRAFT REJECTION

The immunologic events that make up the process of allograft rejection are complex and difficult to examine *in vivo*. For this reason the process of allograft rejection has been described mostly in clinical terms.

HYPERACUTE REJECTION

Despite the careful screening of potential transplant recipients, occasionally a renal allograft is implanted into a patient possessing cytotoxic antibodies directed against donor HLA antigens. When this occurs, the resulting clinical events are dramatic. Within hours or sometimes minutes, the kidney becomes soft and blue, and urine output, if it had begun, ceases abruptly. This sequence of events, called hyperacute rejection, is the direct result of the deposition of preformed cytotoxic antibody on renal parenchymal cells expressing HLA antigens. Under these circumstances, complement is fixed and cell death rapidly ensues. Vascular endothelial cells are known to express HLA antigens and appear to be the primary targets of such a reaction. Pathologic examination of a kidney undergoing this process is characterized by a marked accumulation of granulocytes in glomerular capillaries and extensive thrombosis of small vessels. Electron microscopy often reveals marked capillary endothelial damage and exposed basement membranes. Hyperacute rejection is almost never reversible and requires prompt removal of the transplanted organ.

ACUTE REJECTION

Assuming that a transplant recipient does not have preformed cytotoxic antidonor HLA antibodies, the typical clinical course of a renal transplant is as follows. The graft is implanted without difficulty, and normal renal function ensues rather promptly. Approximately 7 to 10 days following transplantation, the patient begins to feel ill and develops fever and myalgia, and renal function begins to deteriorate. The renal transplant usually becomes noticeably larger and more tender to palpation. This clinical syndrome is called acute rejection. In contrast to hyperacute rejection, which is not treatable, acute rejection episodes are usually reversed using potent immunosuppressive drugs.

The cellular events involved in acute rejection are best considered using the rejection of skin grafts as a model. Syngeneic engrafted skin undergoes a process of revascularization 3 to 7 days following grafting. The revascularization process is followed by a week-long period of healing. If allogeneic skin is engrafted instead of syngeneic skin, revascularization occurs normally, but thereafter a prominent perivascular infiltration of mononuclear cells is seen. Thrombosis of involved vessels occurs rapidly, and sloughing

of the skin graft results 9 to 10 days following the grafting procedure. Interestingly, if allogeneic skin from the same donor is used for a second grafting procedure, the rejection process occurs more rapidly. Although such skin appears viable for 1 to 2 days, early thrombosis of vessels occurs, revascularization never takes place, and the skin graft undergoes ischemic necrosis 5 to 6 days following grafting. Because of the early thrombosis of vessels, the cellular infiltration seen in primary acute rejection does not occur. Such a phenomenon is called a "second set" rejection.

The mononuclear cell infiltrate seen in the acute rejection episode is characterized by focal deposition of cells around small blood vessels and marked interstitial edema. An example of this type of process in a rejecting renal allograft is shown in Figure 12-2. When the infiltrating cells are further characterized, most (45%) are found to be T cells, and a significant percentage (25%) are found to be macrophages. Host B cells and plasma cells are also found throughout the graft. Granulocytes are known to comprise only a small (3%) percentage of host cells infiltrating the rejected organ.

In the past the immunologic mechanism responsible for the acute rejection episode has been thought to be primarily cell-mediated. Evidence for this conclusion comes from observations that (1) immunosuppressive therapy affecting cell-mediated responses but not humoral responses is effective in reversing rejection episodes, (2) second set acute rejection responses can be transferred to unimmunized animals with cells but not with serum, and (3) allografts survive for long periods of time in animals lacking T-cell function.

T cells can be recovered in large numbers from a rejected allograft. When these cells are tested *in vitro* against various different types of allogeneic cells, antigen-specific cytotoxicity is observed; cells from the allograft donor are killed while unrelated cells are not. Such specific cytotoxicity is mediated by a specialized subset of T cells referred to as cytotoxic T cells. Other cell-mediated mechanisms involved in the rejection process are more nonspecific in nature.

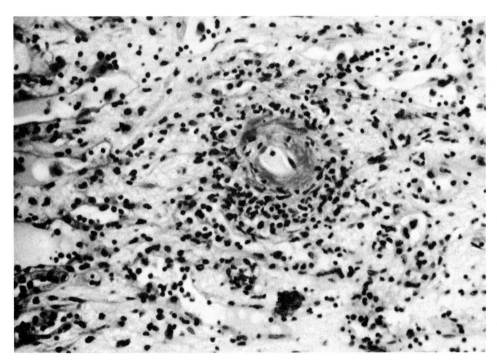

Fig. 12-2. Photomicrograph of a renal allograft undergoing acute rejection. A perivascular infiltrate of mononuclear cells associated with a vessel exhibiting fibrinoid necrosis is seen. Marked interstitial edema is also apparent. (Hematoxylin and eosin stain, original magnification × 40)

Macrophages, for example, may be recruited to perform cytotoxic functions by soluble factors (lymphokines) secreted from other cells.

Recently, interest has been directed to the role of circulating antibody in the acute rejection phenomenon. Although anti-HLA antibodies are not present at the time of transplantation (this is assured by careful cross-match testing), it is possible that these antibodies could develop subsequent to implantation of the allograft. As in the case of hyperacute rejection, these antibodies may destroy a graft through the process of antibody deposition within the kidney and complement fixation. Other types of antibody molecules function not by fixing complement but by rendering allogeneic cells more susceptible to lysis by nonsensitized cells. A role for host antidonor antibody in the acute rejection of an allograft is supported by the finding that such antibody molecules can be consistently eluted from a rejected transplant.

CHRONIC REJECTION

The process of chronic rejection of an allograft is much more subtle than the process of acute rejection. Frequently, patients experiencing chronic rejection feel entirely well and are surprised to learn that renal function is deteriorating. The microscopic appearance of a chronically rejecting allograft, however, is good evidence that important, if subclinical, immunologic events are taking place (Fig. 12-3). A characteristic finding is that of vascular sclerosis. In addition, tubular atrophy and interstitial fibrosis are seen. The mechanisms by which these changes take place are at present unknown. Unfortunately, the process of chronic rejection is difficult to reverse using conventional immunosuppressive therapy, and a slow but inexorable decline in renal function is often the clinical result.

METHODS OF CIRCUMVENTING THE REJECTION PROCESS

CORTICOSTEROID DRUGS

Clinical organ transplantation depends heavily on the immunosuppressive effects of corticosteroid drugs. Withdrawal of steroid therapy from a stable renal transplant patient, for instance, results in rejection of the transplanted organ. Likewise, tapering steroids too rapidly from large doses to small doses may precipitate a rejection episode. Against this critical requirement for steroids must be balanced an appreciation of the substantial complications associated with long-term steroid use.

The mechanism by which steroid drugs suppress the immune response is not well understood. It is known that large doses of intravenous steroids effectively lower circulating T-cell levels. Furthermore, there is some evidence that the subset of circulating T cells responsible for cell-mediated cytotoxicity is relatively sensitive to the effects of steroid administration. Stabilization of lysosomal membranes by steroid drugs may be important in limiting the cytotoxic effects of activated macrophages.

AZATHIOPRINE

Azathioprine is almost universally used (in combination with corticosteroids) as an immunosuppressive agent. An imidazole derivative of 6-mercaptopurine, azathioprine (Imuran) is an inhibitor of DNA and RNA synthesis. The immunosuppressive effects of the drug include inhibition of delayed hypersensitivity reactions, inhibition of the rejection of skin allografts, and inhibition of mixed lymphocyte reactivity.

Azathioprine and corticosteroids have a synergistic immunosuppressive effect when used in combination, but neither is sufficiently immunosuppressive when used alone to prevent rejection in most patients. The development of leukopenia, a side-effect of azathioprine, often requires a reduction in the drug dosage. Azathioprine is sometimes hepatotoxic, and cyclophosphamide may be substituted when azathioprine hepatitis occurs.

CYCLOSPORIN-A

Cyclosporin-A is a newly described fungal metabolite with potent immunosuppressive effects. One of the most important immunosuppressive effects appears to be the inhibition

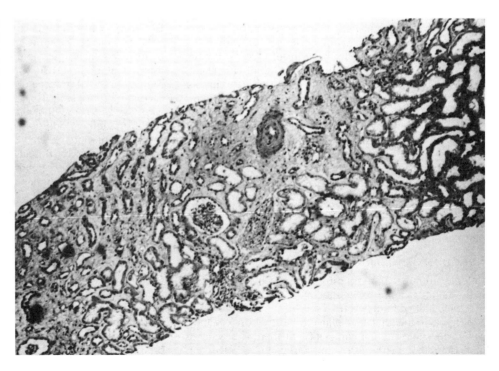

Fig. 12-3. Photomicrograph of a renal allograft undergoing chronic rejection. Tubular atrophy and marked vascular sclerosis are seen. There is no significant cellular infiltrate. (Hematoxylin and eosin stain, original magnification × 10)

of allograft rejection, although the mechanism by which this occurs is not well understood. An attractive aspect of this drug is that, in contrast to azathioprine, cyclosporin-A appears to have no significant bone marrow toxicity. Furthermore, in early trials it has been possible to maintain some renal transplant recipients on cyclosporin-A alone without steroid administration. This "steroid-sparing" effect of the drug is potentially important in clinical transplantation. Unfortunately, cyclosporin-A is nephrotoxic in high doses, so in the context of renal transplantation at least, the distinction between allograft rejection and drug-induced nephrotoxicity may be difficult. Lymphomas have occurred following cyclosporin-A administration, and the incidence of this complication is currently under study.

ANTILYMPHOCYTE SERUM

Heterologous antiserum directed against human lymphocytes is a highly effective immunosuppressive agent. Most sera are produced by injecting rabbits, horses, or goats with human lymphocyte preparations. Antilymphocyte serum (ALS) is usually administered to the transplant recipient during the first several weeks following transplantation. Although ALS has been used clinically for several years, there is still considerable debate about its usefulness in prolonging allograft survival. The disparate results probably stem from the variability inherent in the production of the agent. The type of cells used for immunization, the rate of administration of antigen, the species of animal immunized, and individual animal variations all may influence the efficacy of the ALS produced. Recent techniques that allow production of monoclonal antibodies to T-cell antigens promise to eliminate this variation. In the opinion of most observers, the use of monoclonal anti–T-cell antibodies will enhance treatment of organ transplant recipients, particularly since it is now possible to develop monoclonal antibodies that identify T-cell subsets. It seems logical to suppose, for instance, that a monoclonal antibody reagent directed against the subset of cytotoxic T cells would be particularly useful, and safer than a broadly reactive anti–T-cell sera.

THORACIC DUCT DRAINAGE

Another type of immunosuppressive technique is chronic drainage of thoracic duct lymphocytes. Because thoracic duct cells are almost entirely made up of T cells, chronic thoracic duct drainage results in a lowering of circulating T-cell levels. Although it has been shown by many investigators to prolong allograft survival, this method of immunosuppression has not gained wide acceptance, primarily because it is technically difficult to keep a thoracic duct cannula patent for several weeks.

RADIATION

X-rays delivered to the area of the rejecting allograft are sometimes used to inhibit cell-mediated mechanisms responsible for graft destruction. A typical therapeutic course would involve 150 rads given daily to the area of the transplant for 4 to 6 days.

INDUCTION OF TOLERANCE

Although immunosuppressive drugs are effective in blocking the immune response to an allograft, a far more desirable method is induction of a state of specific unresponsiveness, or *tolerance*, to the implanted allogeneic tissue. Understanding of this subject is not complete, but there is a general impression that many successful transplants involve not only potent immunosuppressive therapy but also the unwitting induction of tolerance to the transplanted graft. For this reason much attention has been devoted to the study of tolerance in animal models. Some of these insights have been applied to clinical renal transplantation.

Induction of immune nonresponsiveness on an experimental level depends upon a number of factors including the nature of the antigen used, the manner in which antigen is administered, and the genetic make-up of the animal studied. Depending on the conditions under which tolerance is induced, the phenomenon may be the result of any one of several distinct mechanisms.

Clonal Deletion

Dizygotic twins in cattle are genetically distinct but share a common intrauterine circulation. As a result the animals become hematologic chimeras; they possess circulating cells of their own as well as cells of the genetically different twin. Such animals make no immune response to shared allogeneic tissue. This observation prompted Burnett to propose the "clonal deletion" theory of tolerance, which postulates that exposure to antigen at some stage in neonatal life results in a selective deletion of the clone of cells that could ordinarily respond to that antigen. This theory has been used to explain the fact that individuals do not make immune responses directed against their own ("self") tissues; clones of cells capable of reacting with self tissues are destroyed early in fetal life. The development of autoimmune disease, according to this theory, is the result of the re-emergence of a "forbidden" clone of cells at some point in adult life.

In an experimental setting the injection of an antigen into a neonatal animal frequently results in long-lasting unresponsiveness to that antigen. Such *neonatal tolerance* may be due in some cases to a clonal deletion–type mechanism, since adoptive transfer of normal antigen-responsive cells restores responsivity. However, there are many described instances in which adoptive transfer of normal lymphoid cells does not reverse neonatal tolerance, indicating that the phenomenon may be the result of other mechanisms as well.

Blocking (Enhancing) Antibody

Rats reject allogeneic kidney transplants in the usual fashion. If, however, the recipient animal is treated with rat antiserum directed at donor MHC products and then immediately receives a renal transplant, the result is a long-lasting successful transplant. This phenomenon is referred to as *passive enhancement.* Enhancement also may result from the administration of donor-strain antigen to the recipient prior to transplantation so that the recipient produces his own anti-MHC antibody; this is called *active enhancement.* Hyperacute rejection does not ordinarily occur in the rat model, as opposed to the human situation, because of unique differences in handling of complement. Thus the rat model is ideal for the study of this phenomenon.

The mechanisms involved in the enhancement phenomenon are complex. Originally it was postulated that anti-donor MHC antibody simply masked relevant MHC antigens on the donor kidney, making them unrecognizable as targets for an immune response. Recent explanations propose a more central effect, in which antigen–antibody complexes fixed to an effector cell surface result in opsonization and removal of the effector cell by the reticuloendothelial system. Alternatively, enhancing antibodies may act through the production of suppressor T cells or the production of anti-idiotypic antibody, as will be discussed in the following sections.

Suppressor Cells

Immune unresponsiveness may be the result of active suppression of normal responsiveness. In one of the first demonstrations of this phenomenon, it was seen that adoptive transfer of spleen cells from sheep red blood cell (RBC)-tolerant mice interfered with the ability of nontolerant mice to make anti-sheep RBC antibody. This phenomenon, sometimes called *infectious tolerance,* has since been described in many different contexts. Usually antigen-specific suppression is mediated by subpopulations of T cells. Nonspecific suppression may also be mediated by T cells as well as by other cell populations, particularly macrophages. The T cells involved in suppression of responsiveness can often be identified by characteristic cell-surface markers. The mechanisms of action of suppressor cells are not well understood but involve the production of antigen-specific and nonspecific suppressor factors. Entirely cell-mediated mechanisms may be involved as well. In a recently described example, suppressor T cells accomplished suppression by the specific killing of other autologous cells participating in the immune response. Clinically, suppressor cells have been identified in renal transplant recipients who appear "tolerant" of their allografts. Such cells inhibit the *in vitro* cytotoxic T-cell response directed at donor cells but do not inhibit cytotoxic responses directed at nondonor cells.

Anti-Idiotypic Antibody

A recently described mechanism for producing tolerance involves anti-idiotypic antibody. Antibody molecules produced in response to a given antigen have combining sites specific for the antigen in question. This combining site is called the *idiotype.* Because the antigen has unique characteristics, the idiotype must also have a unique configuration that corresponds to the antigen. The host animal, which has not previously been exposed to antigen, regards it as foreign and makes an appropriate antibody response.

The host animal may also regard the unique idiotypic configuration of its own antibody as foreign and make an antibody response to it as well. Such an antibody is called an *anti-idiotypic antibody,* or *antireceptor antibody.* A primary antibody response may be limited, or "turned off," by the development of anti-idiotypic antibody because antibody blocking of an antigen receptor site would eliminate an effective antibody response to that antigen. T cells and B cells also have these cell-surface receptors for antigen. It is thus possible to inhibit cell-mediated immunity as well as humoral responses by way of the anti-idiotypic antibody mechanism. In some mouse systems it is possible to inhibit the rejection of an allogeneic skin graft by the passive administration of anti-idiotypic antibody. Whether or not such mechanisms will have practical clinical application remains to be seen.

Attempts to Induce Tolerance on a Clinical Level

Based on the previous observations in animal models, several attempts have been made to induce tolerance in human renal transplant recipients.

Enhancement. Attempts have been made to enhance actively the success of human renal allografts. In some instances human buffy coat membrane extracts of donor cells, or solubilized HLA antigens, have been given to patients prior to transplantation. Although the results have sometimes been encouraging, too few patients have been tested to draw firm conclusions. Passive enhancement has also been attempted. In human trials, passive administration of intact antidonor antibody would result in antibody deposition on the transplanted kidney, complement fixation, and the clinical syndrome of hyperacute rejection. Such a problem has been avoided by administering papain-treated antibody instead of intact antibody. Papain treatment generates antibody (F[ab']2) fragments that possess antigen combining sites but no receptor for complement. The problem of hyperacute rejection is then avoided. In six recently reported related renal transplants, the passive prior administration of antidonor MHC F(ab')2 fragments had no obvious beneficial effect. However, it is known from the study of animal models that F(ab')2 fragments are much less effective than intact antibody in mediating enhancement.

Donor-Specific Transfusions. In one of the most encouraging recent clinical trials potential related renal transplant recipients were given "donor-specific" blood transfusions, that is, blood transfusions from the related donor of the transplant, on several occasions prior to transplantation. Recipient antibody responses to donor HLA antigens were measured frequently thereafter. If antibody to donor HLA antigens developed, as it did in 30% of cases, the transplant procedure could not be performed because hyperacute rejection would have resulted. In 70% of cases antidonor antibody did not develop over a period of 8 weeks. Transplantation in these cases was extremely successful. There is a strong suspicion but no direct evidence that a form of tolerance was induced by this protocol. Simple selection process might also explain the results in that transplants were only performed when the recipient did not make a measurable antibody response when challenged with donor cells. These patients would presumably mount a less intense immune response on subsequent transplantation.

Total Lymphoid Irradiation and Allogeneic Bone Marrow Grafting. Another innovative protocol involves an attempt to induce a stable chimerism in transplant recipients. Potential recipients are treated with total lymphoid irradiation, such as that given to a patient with Hodgkin's disease. This treatment dramatically lowers T-cell levels. Thereafter, donor bone marrow is administered intravenously. The theoretic objective of such a protocol is to induce a stable chimerism in which donor bone marrow cells become "engrafted" in the recipient owing to the inability of the irradiated recipient to reject them. The patient is not immunosuppressed to the degree that graft-versus-host disease results. In several large animal models it has been possible to induce long-term stable chimerism by this method, and subsequent transplants in these cases have not been rejected. In human trials some transplants have been successful, but it has not yet been possible to demonstrate true cellular chimerism.

RENAL TRANSPLANTATION

HISTORY AND OVERVIEW

Prolongation of life through kidney transplantion represents the clinical application of knowledge obtained from several disciplines. In the early 1900s Carrel and Guthrie implanted canine renal allografts with sufficient technical skill to maintain function for several days. Abel and coworkers in 1913 established the concept of hemodialysis by removing

RENAL TRANSPLANTATION

Modern renal transplantation began with the first successful cadaveric graft implanted by David Hume in 1953. Most transplant recipients are placed on dialysis prior to transplantation. The complications associated with chronic uremia and dialysis are identified during evaluation and corrected prior to transplantation. Matching for HLA antigens correlates well with the results of related transplants. The risk to volunteers of donating a kidney is very low. A cadaveric transplant is performed when a suitably matched blood relative is not available to donate. The ability to preserve cadaveric kidneys for 48 hr to 72 hr and the acceptance of the concept of brain death have improved results and increased the number of cadaveric kidneys retrieved. Azathioprine and prednisone have been the basic drugs used for immunosuppression since the early 1960s. Transplant recipients experience the usual complications following major operations plus those directly related to transplantation and immunosuppression, such as rejection, opportunistic infection, and the side-effects of chronic steroid administration. Patient survival has markedly improved, and today 1-year survival rates of 90% to 95% for related transplants and 85% to 90% for cadaveric transplants are reported regularly. The graft survival rate at 1 year for HLA identical related grafts is 90% to 95%, for a one-haplotype related match 70% to 80%, and for cadaveric grafts 45% to 60%. More widespread use of pretransplant blood transfusions and mixed lymphocyte culture to select related donors should enhance graft survival. DR typing for matching, and cyclosporin-A, monoclonal antibody, and total lymphoid irradiation for treatment of immunosuppression are promising techniques and are under intensive investigation.

salicylate from blood perfused through semipermeable collodion tubes. Despite the hardship imposed by the German occupation of his homeland, Kolff in 1943 treated uremic patients in Holland with a crude hemodialyzer constructed of cellophane tubes. In May 1949, Merrill, a nephrologist, and Walter, a surgeon and engineer, used more modern materials to treat a uremic patient near death at the Peter Bent Brigham Hospital in Boston. Medawar, Brent, Gorer, and many other workers, basing their studies primarily on the rejection of skin grafts in inbred mice, demonstrated by the mid 1940s that rejection was an immunologic response to genetically incompatible tissue.

Thus, by the 1950s the scene was set and the support systems and basic knowledge were available for a serious trial of clinical transplantation. The principal sites for these trials were the Peter Bent Brigham Hospital in Boston and several hospitals in France, all institutions with a long-standing multidisciplinary interest in kidney failure. Some earlier surgical attempts at renal transplantation were unsuccessful: Voronoy, a Russian, transplanted an allograft for mercury poisoning in 1936; Lawler, a surgeon in Chicago, transplanted a cadaver kidney to the renal vessels and bladder of a recipient in 1950 with evidence of short-term function; in 1951, Servelle, Dubost, and Kuss of France reported separate experiences with human allografts anastomosed to the iliac vessels. It remained for David Hume, a surgeon at the Peter Bent Brigham Hospital with boundless energy, enthusiasm, and intellectual curiosity, to demonstrate that long-term function was possible. The first successful cadaver transplant was performed on February 11, 1953. This transplant, the ninth in Hume's series, was implanted into the thigh and functioned for $5\frac{1}{2}$ months

without immunosuppression. Murray, a plastic surgeon from the same hospital, performed the first successful identical twin transplant in 1954, using the iliac vessel technique described earlier by the French.

Subsequent progress focused largely on improvements in immunosuppression. Total body irradiation was used successfully by Hamburger in Paris and by Murray in Boston in 1959 with nonidentical twin transplants. During the same year Schwartz and Dameschek reported the induction of specific tolerance with the antimetabolite 6-mercaptopurine. In 1961 Calne, in an extensive series of dog experiments, demonstrated that azathioprine, an analog of 6-mercaptopurine, was effective and less toxic. Zukoski, not discouraged by the consensus that steroids held little promise, reported the use of large doses of corticosteroids to extend survival of canine renal allografts in 1963. In 1964 Marchioro, following up on Goodwin's success in reversing rejection in one patient, confirmed the efficacy of prednisone in suppressing rejection. Waksman and Woodruff experimented with a potent biologic immunosuppressant, antilymphocyte serum, and in 1967 Starzl reported its first clinical application. In 1972 Turcotte and Feduska, stimulated by the work of Kountz with direct intrarenal artery infusion, introduced "pulse" therapy, that is, the intermittent intravenous administration of pharmacologic doses of steroids as a potentially less toxic and more convenient method of reversing rejection.

During the 1960s many other clinical and basic scientists made important contributions to improvements in renal transplantation. Quinton and Scribner made vascular access for dialysis more practical with a Silastic-Teflon external arteriovenous shunt in 1960, and Brescia extended this concept with his development of an internal radiocephalic arteriovenous fistula in 1966. Terasaki's report of his microcytotoxicity method in 1964 permitted clinical application of significant advances in understanding of the HLA histocompatibility system. Bogardus, Schloerb, and Humphries investigated the efficacy of pulse perfusion, hypothermia, and oxygenation to preserve kidneys, and in 1968 Belzer reported successful 72-hr preservation of dog kidneys using cryoprecipitated plasma to perfuse the kidney and a machine that incorporated the concepts described by these early investigators.

Progress in the 1970s was largely confined to refinement of previously described techniques and improved management of patients. A more appropriate selection of recipients, better management of complications, and a more conservative approach toward the use of steroids and other immunosuppressive agents resulted in a marked diminution of patient mortality and morbidity associated with transplantation. The concept of brain death was accepted throughout the United States and led to a greater availability of well-preserved cadaveric kidneys for transplantation. In 1978 Cerilli demonstrated that the one-way mixed lymphocyte culture histocompatibility test, initially introduced by Hirschhorn and Bach in 1963, could be used to select the best related donor among volunteer family members. Najarian and his colleagues at the University of Minnesota reported good results with kidney transplantation in patients with end-stage diabetic nephropathy. By analyzing the extensive information in their transplant data bank, Terasaki and Opelz were able to determine that graft success was substantially increased in recipients who had received preoperative blood transfusion. The work of early investigators has firmly established renal transplantation as a clinical therapy and science. New histocompatibility tests and immunosuppressants are being investigated, and continued progress can be expected with great confidence.

SELECTION AND EVALUATION OF TRANSPLANT RECIPIENTS

Most patients with end-stage renal disease are potential candidates for renal transplantation. One study estimated the need at 40 renal transplants per million population per year, and since that time the indications for transplantation have broadened. Many patients are candidates for either dialysis or transplantation but often remain on dialysis because of a reluctance to undergo an operation with its attendant risk. Modern renal transplantation, however, is more cost-beneficial, has a higher rate of patient rehabilitation, and, with recent advances, is associated with no more or even less mortality and morbidity than chronic hemodialysis.

DISEASES CAUSING END-STAGE RENAL FAILURE

Glomerulonephritis is the primary renal disease in more than half of renal transplant recipients, pyelonephritis in 13%, polycystic disease in 5%, and nephrosclerosis in 5%. Some other relatively common renal diseases leading to transplantation are diabetes, congenital abnormalities of the kidney and lower urinary tract, familial and drug nephropathy, Goodpasture's disease, cystinosis, lupus nephritis, hemolytic-uremic syndrome, Alport's disease, and medullary cystic disease of the kidney.

INDICATIONS AND CONTRAINDICATIONS

Most transplant candidates are initially treated with hemodialysis. Patients are placed on dialysis when their symptoms become severe or when hyperkalemia and fluid and electrolyte balance cannot be controlled by dietary and medical management. This usually occurs when the serum creatinine level is 8 to 10 mg/dl and the blood urea nitrogen is 100 mg/dl or greater. Transplantation is also recommended to avoid the long-term complications of chronic uremia or dialysis, such as renal osteodystrophy, secondary hyperparathyroidism, peripheral neuropathy, malnutrition, dialysis dementia, and cessation of growth in children.

Most transplant candidates are 10 to 55 years of age. The ethical concern about whether it is justified to prolong life in younger children has limited the application of transplantation in this age group. It is technically feasible, however, to implant kidneys in newborn infants. Many young children have had such transplants, especially when a well-matched related kidney is available. Transplantation in older patients is associated with a higher mortality, but the physiological status of the patient is more important than his chronological age in determining suitability for transplantation.

Contraindications to transplantation include chronic infections that cannot be eliminated, cancer, the presence of another life-limiting disease that will not be corrected by transplantation, and a deteriorated physiological status that inordinately increases the risk of operation and immunosuppression. Oxalosis is an absolute contraindication. Oxalate crystals will reaccumulate in the graft and progressively impair renal function. Because immunosuppression may enhance the growth of neoplasms, transplantation is precluded in most cancer patients.

A comprehensive medical evaluation is a prerequisite for renal transplantation. The goals of the evaluation are to diagnose the primary renal disease when possible and to identify and treat any associated diseases or complications that may preclude or increase the risk of transplantation. Routine studies obtained to evaluate potential renal transplant recipients include the following:

Creatinine, BUN
Sodium, potassium, chloride, HCO_3
Calcium, phosphorus
Liver enzymes, bilirubin
Alkaline phosphatase
Total protein, albumin/globulin
Hematocrit, white blood cells, and differential
Parathyroid hormone
Uric acid
Cholesterol
24-hr urine protein
Urinalysis, urine culture
FBS and 2-hr postprandial glucose
HLA and DR typing
Cytotoxic antibody screen
Direct cross match and MLC (for related transplants)
* Lupus erythematosus preparation
* Antinuclear antibody
Hepatitis antigen and antibody
* Anti-GBM antibody
CMV antibody
Tuberculosis and histoplasmosis skin tests
TORCH screen
Electrocardiogram, electromyelogram
Chest x-ray
* Upper gastrointestinal x-ray, sinus x-rays
Oral cholecystogram
* Aortoiliac arteriogram
Oral surgery consultation
Gynecology consultation
Social service consultation
ABO red blood cell typing

Asterisks identify studies that are obtained only when clinically indicated. Other studies may be needed to evaluate specific problems (*e.g.,* echocardiograms when pericarditis is suspected; cystoscopy and cystometrics when a neurogenic or contracted bladder is present).

Several forms of glomerulonephritis are known to recur in transplanted kidneys, that is, focal glomerulosclerosis, membranous glomerulonephritis, membranoproliferative glomerulonephritis, and rapidly progressive glomerulonephritis. Even with these diseases, renal transplantation is usually indicated, since the incidence and severity of recurrence are unpredictable and low. When antiglomerular basement membrane antibody is present, transplantation is deferred until this antibody has disappeared from the serum.

COMPLICATIONS ENCOUNTERED IN UREMIC PATIENTS

Complications that occur commonly in chronically uremic patients and that should be specifically ruled out during evaluation are pneumonia and pleural effusion; bacterial infections of vascular access sites, the urinary tract, the oral cavity, and the female genital tract; viral infections; hepatitis; arteriosclerotic heart disease; uremic pericarditis; bone marrow depression with leukopenia or thrombocytopenia; peptic ulcer disease; hypersplenism; ascites; hypertension, and severe secondary hyperparathyroidism. A complete urologic evaluation is essential to confirm that the lower urinary tract is functioning adequately and to allow surgical correction prior to the transplant procedure when necessary. Most transplant candidates have significant psychological symptoms, but experience has demonstrated that a successful transplant usually relieves the symptoms and that the post-transplant psychological response cannot be predicted accurately.

OPERATIONS TO PREPARE RECIPIENTS FOR TRANSPLANTATION

A variety of operations may be indicated to prepare a patient for transplantation. Bilateral recipient nephrectomy is indicated when the patient's own diseased kidneys are thought to be the cause of hypertension or when they are the source of persistent urinary tract infections. This operation is also indicated in some cases of polycystic kidney disease when the size of the kidneys causes symptoms or when the kidneys occupy the area of the pelvis needed for the renal transplant. Recipient nephrectomy is not performed routinely, because host kidneys may be the source of erythropoietin needed for red blood cell synthesis or may excrete a significant volume of dilute urine. The presence of such host kidneys simplifies the management of patients during hemodialysis should the transplant fail. If the patient has a compromised bladder or urethra, construction of an ileal loop as a substitute bladder may be required prior to transplantation. A urethral resection, vesiconeckplasty, or other urologic procedure may also be necessary to ensure that urine from the newly transplanted kidney has adequate egress. Splenectomy is performed to treat a significant degree of hypersplenism with leukopenia or thrombocytopenia. Some transplant centers routinely remove the spleen on the basis of experimental data suggesting that immunosuppression may be more effective in the absence of the spleen. Subtotal parathyroidectomy, that is, removal of all but approximately 200 mg of parathyroid tissue, is occasionally performed in patients with severe secondary hyperparathyroidism. This complication is usually reversed with a successful transplant, and most transplant centers recommend parathyroidectomy only in very selected instances. Pretransplant vagotomy and antrectomy is performed for intractable or bleeding peptic ulcers, pericardiectomy is indicated for severe uremic pericarditis, and arthroplasty or joint replacement may be required for advanced renal osteodystrophy.

RELATED DONOR SELECTION AND NEPHRECTOMY

Counseling of the patient and family members about the benefits and risks of tranplantation is an important obligation of the transplant surgeon. The recipient and his family should be advised of the differences and prognosis between two-haplotype identical and one-haplotype identical related transplants and cadaveric transplants. The transplant team must be sensitive to pressures within the family, and it is preferable to allow family members to volunteer to donate spontaneously after initial counseling and before differences in histocompatibility matches are identified.

There is risk in donating a kidney, but it is remarkably low. Minor postoperative complications are common, but serious ones are rare. Among the thousands of related transplants that have been performed only a few deaths have been reported. The 5-year life expectancy for a 35-year-old male undergoing unilateral donor nephrectomy has been estimated at 99.1% as opposed to 99.3% for the normal age-matched control. There have been no deaths in the 370 related renal transplants performed at the University of Michigan.

Related donors must have normal renal function, no disease that may later impair renal function such as diabetes, hypertension, or a family history of polycystic disease, and no associated illnesses that significantly increase the risk of operation. Related donors are usually at the age of consent, that is, between 18 and 55 years of age. Identical twins are often allowed to donate at a younger age. In addition to a complete preoperative evaluation, a creatinine clearance study, 24-hr urine protein test, urine culture, glucose tolerance test, hepatitis antigen and antibody tests, serologic tests for syphilis, an intravenous pyelogram, and a renal arteriogram to delineate the anatomy of the renal vasculature are obtained.

Related donor nephrectomy is performed either transabdominally or through a retroperitoneal flank incision. The kidney is carefully dissected from the renal fossa with a minimum of handling and traction. The ureter is identified and freed to below the pelvic brim. The renal vessels are isolated and divided at their junction with the aorta and vena cava. Multiple or accessory renal arteries are present on at least one side in 40% of patients, and care is taken not to injure or inadvertently divide accessory vessels. Very small polar arteries may be ligated. There is free intercommunication of renal veins within the kidney, and accessory renal veins may be divided. Donors are given heparin just prior to removal of the kidney, and this is promptly reversed with protamine sulfate. The donor kidney is flushed with cold electrolyte or modified electrolyte solutions both to cool it and to remove all retained blood. The kidney is immersed in a container filled with 4° C balanced electrolyte solution and carried to the adjacent recipient operating room for transplantation.

CADAVERIC DONOR SELECTION, CADAVERIC NEPHRECTOMY, AND SHARING OF KIDNEYS

EVALUATION

Kidneys for cadaveric transplantation are retrieved from patients who have died between the age of 1 or 2 and 50. Implantation of a kidney from a young child is technically feasible, and such a kidney will provide adequate renal function for an adult. With hypertrophy renal mass will be sufficient to normalize creatinine clearance. Kidneys from aged persons are usually arteriosclerotic and do not tolerate ischemia or preservation as well.

Potential donors of cadaveric kidneys are excluded from further consideration when an underlying renal disease or a disease process that could be transmitted to the transplant recipient is identified. Common examples of these contraindications to donation are chronic renal disease, long-standing hypertension, diabetes, hepatitis, systemic or abdominal infections, and cancer. There is a tendency to be overly conservative in accepting cadaveric donors, and minor complications in terminally ill patients such as bacteriuria secondary to urinary catheters, localized pulmonary infiltrates, reversible prerenal azotemia, or a minor degree of reversible acute tubular necrosis are not contraindications. Primary brain tumors and localized skin cancers are not contraindications to donation because these tumors do not metastasize systemically.

In the United States many potentially usable cadaveric kidneys are not made available for transplantation despite a national shortage of such kidneys. As a result of public education programs, patients' families, rather than physicians or nurses, very often initiate the donation offer and frequently find solace in the knowledge that some good has been derived from what is otherwise a tragic or unexpected loss of a loved family member. The majority of cadaveric kidney donors are patients expiring from head injuries, brain tumors, hypoxic brain damage, and strokes.

BRAIN DEATH

The advent of renal transplantation was the primary motivation for developing formal criteria for brain death in this country. The same criteria are now frequently utilized in the decision to stop life-support systems in other critically ill patients. Many states have passed laws that recognize the declaration of brain death, and recently a national Uniform Determination of Death Act has been proposed: "An individual who has sustained either (1) irreversible cessation of circulatory and respiratory functions or (2) irreversible cessation of all functions of the entire brain, including the brain stem, is dead. A determination of death must be made in accordance with accepted medical standards." Usually the absence of response to all stimuli, the absence of reflexes, a flat electroencephalogram, and in some cases an angiogram demonstrating cessation of blood flow to the brain are required by hospital brain death committees as adjuncts to arriving at the clinical determination that brain death has occurred.

CADAVERIC NEPHRECTOMY

Removal of kidneys from recently deceased donors is a major operation. The procedure is performed in an operating room with all the anesthesia and other support needed for operations on living individuals. In most areas of the United States only donors who have suffered irreversible brain damage and whose cardiorespiratory functions can be maintained with the assistance of a respirator and cardiotonic drugs are selected. The procedure is accomplished through a generous vertical or cruciate abdominal incision. Usually both kidneys and ureters, the aorta, and the vena cava are removed *en bloc,* as illustrated in Figure 12-4. An alternative is to remove each kidney separately using a technique similar to that described for volunteer nephrectomy. The kidneys are flushed with cold heparinized electrolyte solution just after removal or, in some instances, just before removal from the donor and then placed on an organ preservation machine or preserved by simple hypothermia. After the kidneys have been removed the respirator support of the cadaveric donor is discontinued.

KIDNEY SHARING

Most states or regions in the United States are organized to facilitate the sharing of cadaveric kidneys. The Southeastern Organ Procurement Foundation is the largest such organization in the United States. This organization incorporates 38 transplant programs in 16 states. The Transplantation Society of Michigan is an example of a statewide organization. Between 1973 and 1980, 1307 cadaveric kidneys were retrieved, 91 were accepted from outside the state, and 1057 cadaveric transplants were performed. These organizations have several important functions including provision of a 24-hr communication network, tissue typing and cross-matching of potential donors, preservation of cadaveric kidneys, transportation of kidneys, simplifying billing procedures for hospitals and physicians, and public and professional education.

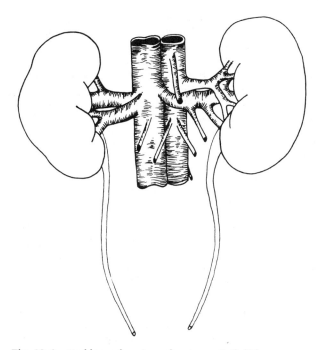

Fig. 12-4. En bloc cadaveric nephrectomy. Both kidneys, a segment of aorta and vena cava, and a long length of both ureters are removed intact. One end of the aorta is occluded and the other end is cannulated for initial flushing and then attachment to an organ preservation machine.

KIDNEY PRESERVATION

The ability to preserve kidneys has greatly expanded cadaveric transplantation. Normal kidneys will withstand 30 min of warm ischemia well, but increasing degrees of acute tubular necrosis will occur with warm ischemia of longer duration, and kidneys are not viable after 2 hr of warm ischemia. Kidneys can be preserved for up to 24 hr by flushing them with heparinized balanced electrolyte or special solutions and cooling them to 4° C. A more prolonged and, some believe, more reliable preservation can be obtained with the use of an organ preservation machine. Several models of these machines are available. All models provide hypothermia and oxygenation of the perfusate, and most incorporate pulsatile rather than nonpulsatile perfusion. Cryoprecipitated plasma or electrolyte solutions supplemented with albumin or purified protein fraction are the usual perfusates employed. Kidneys can be preserved reliably for 48 hr to 72 hr with these machines.

THE RENAL TRANSPLANT OPERATION

Although some of the first renal transplants were placed subcutaneously in the leg, it soon became obvious that a preferable location was the retroperitoneal iliac fossa. This location has the advantage of easy accessibility to the iliac vessels and close proximity to the urinary bladder. The renal transplant is protected by iliac bone and abdominal musculature. Transplants are not placed in the normal renal fossa, since this requires removal of the recipient kidney and a longer length of viable ureter than is usually available.

Transplant recipients have already undergone evaluation and treatment of associated complications as described previously. A complete history and physical examination are again performed, routine preoperative blood studies are obtained, and a chest x-ray is repeated to rule out any intercurrent infection that may have appeared since the patient was last examined. The direct donor–recipient cross-match is repeated to rule out the presence of any recently appearing antidonor antibodies. A judgment is made about the recipient's fluid and electrolyte status. Dehydration secondary to vigorous chronic hemodialysis is corrected to help avoid acute tubular necrosis in the transplanted kidney. Conversely, when cadaveric transplantation is contemplated, emergency dialysis may be necessary to remove fluid and correct electrolyte imbalances such as hyperkalemia. Most uremic patients have adapted to chronic anemia, and a hematocrit of 20 or greater is acceptable for operation.

When a choice is available, the left kidney is used because of its longer renal vein. The transplant is placed in the contralateral iliac fossa to position the renal artery anteriorly, thus facilitating the arterial anastomosis. Most transplant surgeons will use kidneys even when two or three renal arteries are present, either anastomosing the arteries to each other or constructing separate arterial anastomoses. Many variations of the classic procedure have been described to adapt to the anatomy available. The essence of the procedure is to place the kidney and the vascular and ureteral anastomosis in a comfortable position within the fossa. Drugs that require excretion by a functioning kidney should be avoided, and dosages of antibiotics and other medications should be adjusted appropriately until it is certain that renal function has been restored. A typical renal transplant operation is depicted in Figure 12-5.

Fig. 12-5. Renal transplant operation. The procedure is performed through a curvilinear incision into the retroperitoneal space extending from the iliac spine to above the pubis. When feasible, the end of the renal vein is anastomosed to the side of the external iliac vein and the spatulated end of the renal artery to the end of the divided internal iliac artery. The ureter is tunneled beneath the mucosa of the bladder to help prevent reflux by means of either an external ureteroneocystostomy on the anterior surface of the bladder (*insert*) or insertion into the posterior surface of the bladder near the trigone through a transvesical incision (Leadbetter-Politano procedure).

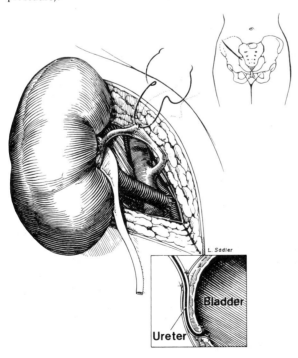

POSTOPERATIVE CARE AND COMPLICATIONS

IMMEDIATE POST-TRANSPLANT CARE

During the immediate post-transplant period special attention is directed at maintaining fluid and electrolyte balance. Varying degrees of renal function are present early, and an obligatory diuresis usually occurs in the first 24 hr to 48 hr following transplantation. This diuresis may be as great as 1000 to 1500 ml/hr. Urine volume is replaced hourly with half-strength saline solution, and a clinical estimate of needed additional fluids is made by monitoring vital signs, central venous pressure, and serum electrolytes. The urethral catheter must be kept patent, and frequent irrigation to remove blood clots originating from the ureteral or bladder anastomoses may be necessary.

Most transplant surgeons use prophylactic antibiotics but discontinue them within 3 days to avoid overgrowth by fungi and other opportunistic infections. Prophylactic oral mycostatin helps prevent monilial infections. Hypertension occurs frequently in the early post-transplant period and is controlled with appropriate drugs. Insulin is administered when steroid hyperglycemia or frank diabetes is present. Patients may be ambulatory within hours of the procedure and are usually returned to oral alimentation within 1 to 3 days. Patients are placed on a diet restricted in sodium, potassium, and protein (*e.g.*, 40 mEq of sodium, 40 mEq of potassium, and 40 g of protein for an adult) until good renal function returns.

Approximately 90% of related renal transplants and two thirds of cadaveric transplants function within hours of the transplant procedure. Renal transplants with good function will lower the serum creatinine level to below 2 mg/dl within 48 hr regardless of the preoperative level of serum creatinine. When necessary, dialysis is reinstituted promptly should the kidney not function immediately or severe rejection occur. Usually dialysis is not mandatory for at least 3 days following the transplant even when severe oliguria is present.

REJECTION

Acute tubular necrosis, rejection, ureteral obstruction, or vascular stenosis or thrombosis may occur in the early post-transplant period. The differential diagnosis between these entities can be difficult at times. Serial renal technetium-hippuran scans and ultrasound scans are useful in distinguishing ureteral obstruction from parenchymal damage and also help to determine whether the kidney is recovering or deteriorating over time. A distinction between severe acute tubular necrosis and rejection in the early post-transplant period is often judgmental and depends more upon a detailed knowledge of the circumstances surrounding the transplant rather than the interpretation of scans or other studies. Scans may suggest a compromise of the renal anastomoses or vessels, but the definitive diagnosis is made by renal arteriography. Arteriography is also useful to diagnose rejection when less invasive studies are not definitive (Fig. 12-6). Because acute rejection usually occurs in a very patchy pattern and because the histologic picture of accompanying acute tubular necrosis does not necessarily correlate with the severity of the process, most transplant groups reserve percutaneous renal biopsy for selected circumstances.

IMMUNOSUPPRESSION

The pathogenesis and signs and symptoms of hyperacute and acute rejection have been discussed in a previous section.

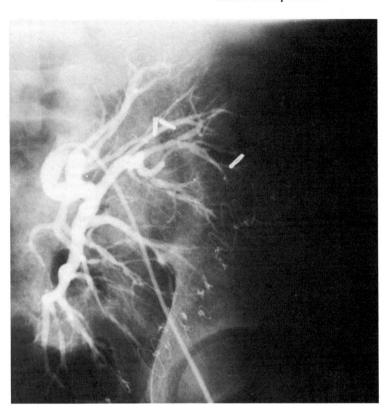

Fig. 12-6. Renal arteriogram during acute rejection. Rejection has damaged the intralobular arteries in a patchy fashion, resulting in decreased cortical flow and early "pruning" of the vascular tree.

Acute rejection is analogous to an inflammatory process initiated by the immune system. The kidney swells, becomes tender to palpation, and loses function. The patient may develop systemic symptoms such as fever, leukocytosis, hypertension, and a feeling of malaise and may gain weight from retention of sodium and water. All of these symptoms except the loss of renal function may be modified or suppressed by immunosuppressive therapy. Acute rejection is treated by administering three to five large intravenous pulses of steroid, that is, 1 to 2 g of methylprednisolone every 12 hr to 48 hr, or by temporarily increasing the dose of oral prednisone to 100 to 200 mg/day. Hyperacute or accelerated rejection occurs when, despite a negative cross-match, the recipient has been previously sensitized to donor antigens. Hyperacute or accelerated rejection is not amenable to any known treatment but does reverse spontaneously on rare occasions.

Each transplant group, on the basis of personal experience, has its own variation of a prophylactic immunosuppressive regimen to prevent acute rejection. The two drugs azathioprine and prednisone remain the mainstay of immunosuppressive protocols. All groups use these drugs at high dosages initially and subsequently taper them to the lowest levels that can be maintained and still prevent rejection or loss of renal function. Typically, 2.5 to 3 mg/kg/day of azathioprine is administered initially and is then tapered to 0.5 to 1 mg/kg/day in the late post-transplant period. Azathioprine must be stopped temporarily when leukopenia is induced. One to three mg/kg/day of prednisone is usually administered initially. The dosage is tapered beginning a few days to 3 weeks after transplantation. Patients remain on immunosuppressive therapy as long as the transplant is functioning. Most groups will not reduce azathioprine to below 25 mg/day or prednisone to below 7.5 to 10 mg/day because the risk of an unpredictable and irreversible rejection episode outweighs the minimal side-effects accompanying these low dosages. If azathioprine hepatitis occurs, cyclophosphamide may be substituted. Many groups augment their basic azathioprine and steroid program with antilymphocyte globulin for the first 1 to 3 weeks. Recently the use of cyclosporin A as a replacement for azathioprine and antilymphocyte globulin as a means of reversing acute rejection have been under investigation with encouraging preliminary results. Figure 12-7 depicts a typical postoperative course.

COMPLICATIONS

All of the complications seen after any major operation plus some unique ones associated with transplantation and immunosuppression may occur. Technical complications include leaks or stenosis of the vascular anastomoses; pseudoaneurysms secondary to infection of the arterial anastomosis; ureteral stenoses, and fistulas; and infarction of the kidney or a pole of the kidney sometimes accompanied by a pelvic or calyceal urinary fistula. A lymphocele may develop, presumably from division of the lymphatics coursing along the iliac vessels. Lymphoceles present with swelling of the leg, displacement of the bladder, and a decrease in renal function owing to obstruction of the bladder or ureter. Serial ultrasound studies have demonstrated that many lymphoceles resolve spontaneously, but sometimes aspiration, external drainage, or surgical construction of a window between the peritoneal cavity and the lymphocele is necessary. If chronic administration of high doses of steroids is required, recipients develop a Cushingoid appearance, protein depletion, osteoporosis, and other complications caused by excessive administration of corticosteroids.

Infection remains the most common and most feared complication. With the occurrence of any symptom sugges-

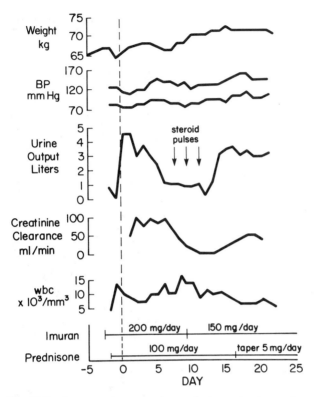

Fig. 12-7. Postoperative course in a patient experiencing a rejection episode. The transplant functioned promptly, but rejection intervened about day 6. The patient retained fluid, became moderately hypertensive, and developed a moderate leukocytosis with a diminishing creatinine clearance and urine volume. Rejection was reversed with three intravenous pulses of 30 mg/kg of methyl prednisolone administered at 48-hr intervals.

tive of infection patients should be completely evaluated and treated appropriately. Some of the more common infections encountered are staphylococcal and gram-negative pneumonias, peritransplant abscesses, wound infections, cytomegalic and herpetic viral infections, chronic viral hepatitis, and *Candida* infections. Virtually every type of bacterial, viral, or fungal infection can occur, including some very uncommon infections such as *Pneumocystis carinii* pneumonia, cryptococcal meningitis, and Legionnaires' disease. Patients with positive tuberculin tests or a history of exposure to tuberculosis are routinely placed on prophylactic medication.

TRANSPLANT NEPHRECTOMY AND SEQUENTIAL TRANSPLANTS

When the renal transplant is unsuccessful or when severe rejection later intervenes, transplant nephrectomy is often indicated. Some patients, especially after progressive chronic rejection, remain asymptomatic even when immunosuppression has been discontinued, and in these circumstances the transplant may be left in place. Another transplant may be placed either in the contralateral iliac fossa or even on the same side as the previous transplant after removal of the rejected kidney. Second and third transplants are almost as successful as primary grafts. Lower success rates are reported when the first graft has been acutely rejected in the first few months following transplantation. Especially good results with second transplants are obtained when the first graft has functioned for a long time but has failed from slow chronic rejection. As many as five renal grafts have been transplanted sequentially into a single recipient.

RESULTS

The End-Stage Renal Disease Division of the Federal Health Care Financing Administration reported that in 1979 1205 related and 3066 cadaveric transplants were performed by 148 transplant facilities in the United States. The success of renal transplantation is generally stated in terms of patient survival and graft function. Patient survival is obviously of paramount importance and has steadily improved. One-year patient survival rates of over 90% are reported regularly for related renal transplantation; a recent survey of six major renal transplant centers demonstrated a 1-year survival rate following related renal transplantation of 97%, an improvement of 10% over results obtained in these centers in 1968. Patient survival rates of over 85% at 1 year have also become the norm following cadaveric renal transplantation. The same group of six major transplant centers reported a 90% 1-year patient survival following cadaveric transplantation, representing a dramatic improvement over the 65% patient survival rate noted by these centers in 1968. These improvements have resulted from better selection and management of patients and a change in philosophy toward more rapid discontinuation of immunosuppression when severe or progressive rejection occurs.

Kidney graft function rates are reported in three major categories depending upon whether (1) the donor and recipient are HLA identical, (2) there is a one-haplotype

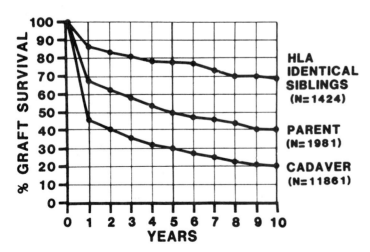

Fig. 12-8. First kidney transplant survival rates. No failures were excluded on the basis of technical error. The grafts were performed between 1969 and 1979, and the 10-year graft survival was computed by actuarial methods. (Terasaki PI, Opelz G, Mickey MR: Clinical kidney transplants. Cell Immunol 62:277, 1981)

match as in 50% of siblings and in parent–child transplants, or (3) a cadaveric graft has been used. Two-haplotype mismatched related or volunteer unrelated grafts are rarely used because the results approximate those obtained with cadaveric grafts. Paul Terasaki at the University of California in Los Angeles has collected results from many transplant centers throughout the world. Figure 12-8 illustrates the life table survival of grafts from the data in his computer registry. More recent reports indicate that 1-year graft survival is 5% to 10% better than those illustrated in Figure 12-8. Another useful actuarial statistic is the estimate of half-life of grafts. If a graft is functioning 2 years after transplantation, then the half-life from this time has been estimated to be 35 years with HLA identical grafts, 11 years with a one-haplotype match, and 7.5 years with a cadaveric graft. The preliminary results with newer methods of immunosuppression and histocompatibility typing indicate that further improvements can be expected in the future.

BIBLIOGRAPHY

Guttman RD: Renal transplantation. N Engl J Med 301:975, 1038, 1979

Hamburger J (ed): Renal Transplantation: Theory and Practice, 2nd ed. Baltimore, Williams & Wilkins, 1981

Morris PJ (ed): Kidney Transplantation: Principles and Practice. London, Academic Press, 1979

Opelz G, Terasaki PI: Dominant effect of transfusions on kidney graft survival. Transplantation 29:153, 1980

Sell S (ed): Immunology, Immunopathology and Immunity, New York, Harper & Row, 1980

Terasaki PI, Opelz G, Mickey MR: Clinical kidney transplants. Cell Immunol 62:277, 1981

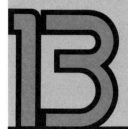

James D. Hardy

Transplantation of Organs Other Than Kidney

Clinical tissue transplantation has made enormous strides over the past 20 years and has contributed knowledge and technique to virtually every branch of medical practice. While laboratory investigation of the immunological and technical aspects of allotransplantation had been going on for decades, it was only in the 1950s that successful kidney isogeneic transplantation and allotransplantation received full attention, to be followed by the transplantation of other organs. Whereas two decades ago the role of transplantation in a department of surgery was a minor one with only minimal space and personnel devoted to this effort, clinical transplantation now has been accepted as a legitimate and formal service, division, or department in most university medical centers and, indeed, the large nonuniversity medical centers.

Transplantation of the kidney has appropriately been used as the prototype for all whole-organ transplants. For it was the basic experience with clinical transplantation of the kidney that paved the way to the clinical exploration of liver, pancreas, lung, and heart transplantation. The kidney gained this central position (a) because the clinical need for transplantation in a given patient with terminal renal failure was obvious to everyone, (b) because the kidney could be readily transplanted to the iliac fossa by many surgeons trained in vascular suturing techniques, and (c) because, if the transplant failed, the kidney could usually be removed and the patient saved by placing him back on chronic dialysis. Moreover, renal allotransplantation allowed the development of immunosuppressive techniques to prevent rejection.

In contrast to the paired kidney, which could be secured from a living donor and which in the event of failure had the backup of dialysis, transplantation of the liver, lung, or heart was very likely to result in death of the patient if the allotransplant failed, since there was no backup of chronic mechanical support for liver, lung, or cardiac function. Exploration of the clinical transplantation of these other organs was therefore approached very cautiously, despite a great deal of experience in the animal laboratory. Nevertheless, substantial progress has been achieved with clinical heart transplantation and definite but certainly considerably less success with liver, lung, and pancreatic transplantation. The basic immunopathology of the allograft rejection reaction is similar for most organs, though some are somewhat more resistant to rejection than are others. However, the clinical evidence of impending rejection is fairly specific for the given organ: decreasing renal function with the kidney, jaundice with the liver, and declining cardiac output and changes in the electrocardiogram with the heart.

The current state of the art in the transplantation of whole organs has been achieved by research performed in centers all over the world. Space does not permit acknowledgment of all contributions, but sources appear at the end of the chapter.

TRANSPLANTATION OF THE LIVER

Transplantation of the liver is a far more formidable operation than is kidney transplantation, especially in humans. Whereas auxiliary transplants were explored initially, because of the relative ease of their insertion without the need for removal of the recipient's own liver (Welch, 1955), these extra-anatomic or heterotopic transplants were less successful than the gradually developed but more difficult orthotopic transplants, placed after removal of the recipient's own liver. At present only the orthotopic method is used in the few clinical centers that have mastered the stern test of successful orthotopic liver transplantation. Contributions by many transplant teams have been and continue to be important, but the work of Starzl in the United States, Calne in Great Britain, and Pichlmayr in Germany has been outstanding.

The liver may be transplanted for a variety of pathologic conditions, including malignant tumors, terminal liver failure caused by such conditions as postnecrotic or alcoholic cirrhosis, acute liver failure from toxins, and Wilson's hepatolenticular degeneration. Since liver transplantation must still be considered an experimental procedure, it is often difficult to determine when or whether a given patient with liver disease is a justifiable candidate.

OPERATIVE TECHNIQUE

Orthotopic transplantation of the liver is carried out as shown in Figure 13-1. The liver is harvested from a brain-death heart-beating donor and immediately perfused with cold electrolyte (Collins') solution to flush out the blood and to cool the organ. Thereafter it is stored in ice-cold solution until it is inserted. Meanwhile, other members of the transplant team will perform laparotomy on the recipient and prepare the appropriate structures—hepatic artery, common bile duct, portal vein, and inferior vena cava above and below the liver—for excision of the recipient's own liver at the appropriate time, when the donor liver is sutured (orthotopically) into the same anatomical position from which the recipient's liver was excised. Naturally, the less time the cooled liver has to be stored the better, preferably not longer than six hours and certainly not more than ten.

POSTOPERATIVE COMPLICATIONS

The postoperative complications of clinical orthotopic transplantation of the liver include excessive bleeding not only because of the extensive operative dissection required for insertion of the organ, often in the presence of portal hypertension with the markedly increased venous vascularity, but also because the liver is fragile and especially susceptible to hypoxia during storage, with resulting diminished capacity to form blood-clotting elements in a patient already cold and perhaps acidotic and thrombocytopenic from sometimes massive blood transfusion during operation. Additional problems include varying degrees of liver necrosis with later abscess formation, occlusion of vascular suture lines, and still other complications. However, the most experienced liver transplant teams, transplanting a well preserved liver into a reasonably good-risk patient, have perhaps most often experienced as the major complication biliary tract anastomotic breakdown, bile leakage, and attendant infection. Finally, rejection of the allograft will almost inevitably occur eventually, and that of course must prove fatal unless another liver transplantation can be performed. However, early rejection of the liver has not usually been a major problem in the first weeks and months following transplantation.

RESULTS

Several hundred clinical liver transplantations have now been performed. The results have been encouraging, a few patients surviving several years. As would be expected, the prognosis in any given patient will be influenced by the disease for which transplantation was performed. The recurrence of malignancy in the earlier transplant recipients has tended to diminish enthusiasm for transplantation in

Fig. 13-1. Technique of liver transplantation.

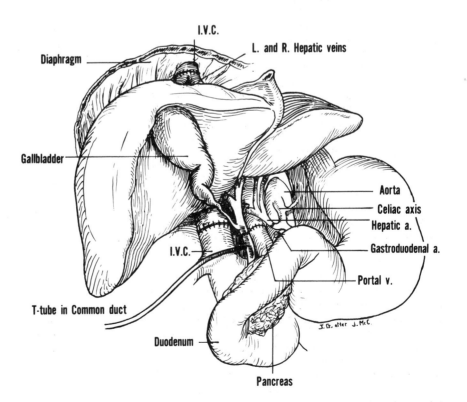

the treatment of hepatic malignancy, whereas transplantation for cirrhosis has increased.

The gradual accumulation of further knowledge by deeply experienced teams, plus the advent of the drug cyclosporin-A for immunosuppression, promises to afford still more successful clinical liver transplantation in the future.

TRANSPLANTATION OF THE PANCREAS AND OF THE PANCREATIC ISLETS

Successful transplantation of the pancreas has been difficult to achieve. While it is not essential to restore the exocrine functions of the pancreas, since these needs can be supplied by appropriate oral medication and dietary management, it still remains an earnestly sought-after objective to transplant the islets of Langerhans. For whereas theoretically diabetes and its severe attendant long-term complications should be amenable to control with the usual insulin injections and dietary management, the fact remains that it has not thus far been possible to achieve perfect control of carbohydrate metabolism. Thus, patients with juvenile or adult-onset diabetes are prone to develop such severe complications as blindness, kidney disease, and peripheral vascular disease and, to a lesser extent, heart disease. It has been estimated that in the Western world diabetes is the fifth leading cause of death from disease. It is a leading cause of new cases of blindness in adults. The use of buried subcutaneous servo-insulin infusion pumps, whose release of insulin is governed by the blood sugar level to achieve more continuous appropriate control, may prove to be a substantial improvement in preventing the complications of diabetes. However, transplantation of the pancreas appears at present to be perhaps the most feasible method for the management of diabetes if such transplantation can become more successful.

Transplantation of the pancreas is in concept a relatively simple technical operation, but long-term success, with transplantation either of the whole pancreas or of islet cells extracted from the pancreas, has been limited to date.

The first clinical allogeneic pancreas transplant was apparently that of Kelly, Lillehei, and Merkel. The operative technique has varied, but one method is to anastomose the splenic artery and the splenic vein to the iliac vessels. The pancreatic duct itself may be ligated, to produce atrophy of the acinar exocrine functions of the organ. Unfortunately, extremely few patients who received such transplants became insulin independent. The next cycle of experiments consisted of the injection of islet cells themselves, appropriately extracted from the pancreas, into the spleen or into the portal vein. Clearly, the hoped-for success would be dependent upon the number of islet cells actually transplanted in this manner, and relatively few patients became insulin independent. Ultimately, almost all failed.

At the present, the treatment of diabetes with islet cell injections has proved sufficiently unsuccessful that attention is being turned once again to transplantation of the whole or a part of the pancreas.

As a corollary to the above studies, the islet cells were extracted from the removed pancreas in total pancreatectomy for chronic relapsing pancreatitis, and these autotransplants were then infused into the portal vein. Since there was no immunological barrier to successful survival and multiplication of these infused autologous islet cells in the liver, one might expect that important evidence would be achieved regarding whether or not such injected islets would in fact survive. Here again, relatively few patients became insulin independent, but some did.

Thus, pancreatic transplantation has in general not yet proved especially successful, and at the present time such transplantation in a clinical setting must be considered still experimental. However, the fairly extensive clinical experience of Najarian and colleagues at the University of Minnesota is showing definite promise. Of approximately 50 patients who have received pancreatic transplants over the past two decades, about one fourth have been able to discontinue insulin therapy for a period of one year (personal communication).

TRANSPLANTATION OF THE SMALL INTESTINE

Transplantation of the small intestine would be a very desirable achievement. Small-bowel insufficiency is produced in a large number of patients throughout the United States and the world each year by massive resection of the gut for gangrene or for some other reason. These patients are then left with minimal digestive absorptive capacity, and only long-term or permanent intravenous alimentation lies ahead of them. Since such treatment is expensive and beyond reach of many of these individuals, many or most are doomed. There is every justification for pursuing the investigation of intestinal transplantation.

Unfortunately, as with pancreatic allotransplantation, the success of clinical allotransplantation of the small bowel has thus far been meager. Actually, it is not a difficult matter to transplant an appropriate segment of gut from one human being to another (Fig. 13-2). The blood vessels to be sutured are large enough to permit ready anastomosis, and the insertion of the transplant is achieved with relative ease.

Fig. 13-2. General concept and procedure for small bowel allotransplantation in man. (*A*) A segment of gut several feet long is removed from a living related donor, with a wedge of mesentery. Actually, it is not necessary to skeletonize the vessels to this exaggerated extent. (*B*) The donor vein and artery are anastomosed to the iliac vessels of recipient. (*C*) Both ends of the donor segment are brought out on abdominal wall for several days to establish viability. (*D*) A second operation is performed to insert the donor bowel into the alimentary tract of the recipient. (From Hardy JD: The transplantation of organs. Surgery, 56:685, 1964)

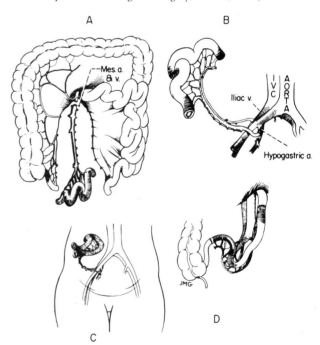

However, the long-term survival and function of small bowel allotransplants has been very limited, and this must be viewed at present as a technically feasible but otherwise experimental procedure.

TRANSPLANTATION OF THE LUNG

The widespread incidence of respiratory insufficiency owing to chronic pulmonary emphysema and other causes has been the stimulus for investigation of lung transplantation in man. As with other organs, the laboratory reimplantation and allotransplantation of the lung in various animals has provided much technical and physiological information, useful not only in explaining certain parameters of respiratory function but also in identifying optimal techniques for transplantation of the lung in humans (Fig. 13-3). Lung transplantation has now been investigated for almost 40 years. The first laboratory transplantation of lung to its usual site was apparently that performed by Demikhov in Moscow in 1947. Outstanding subsequent investigation was carried out, particularly by Blumenstock, by Alican, and by Veith, among many others. The parameters explored were the causes for the temporarily diminished function of the lung following its reimplantation orthotopically into the same

Fig. 13-3. Technique of lung transplantation. Anastomosed are the bronchus, pulmonary artery, and a left atrial cuff into which the pulmonary veins flow. (From Hardy JD, Alican F: Transplantation of the lung. In Hardy JD (ed): Human Organ Support and Replacement. Springfield, Charles C Thomas, 1971)

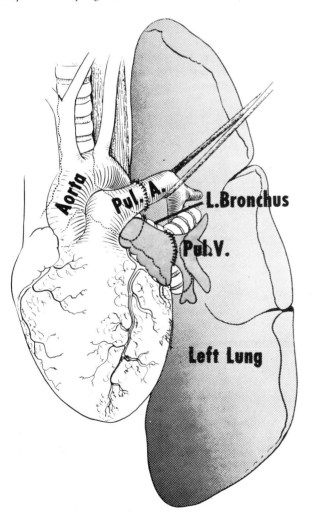

animal, the relation of pulmonary innervation to respiration, the regeneration of the pulmonary lymphatics, the several regimens available for the prevention of rejection of lung allografts, and still other studies. However, it has proved difficult to gain indefinite survival of lung allografts in the new hosts, though an average survival rate of about 35 to 50 days, and even 1 year for some dogs with bilateral lung allografts, is possible.

The first lung transplant in humans was performed by Hardy and associates in 1963, after several hundred lung transplants in the laboratory. The transplanted human lung functioned immediately as an efficient organ of respiration, and at the time of death from various causes, about 3 weeks later, there was little histological evidence of rejection of the lung allograft. Subsequently, perhaps as many as 50 human lung transplants have been performed in various medical centers around the world. The longest survival was that reported by Derom, who performed the transplant for advanced silicosis in a young man who had no evidence of chronic infection in the opposite lung. This patient lived 10 months, with the transplant representing virtually the only functioning lung tissue.

The reasons for the disappointing results with clinical transplantation of the lung are multiple. While the technical procedure is readily achieved, the patient for whom one might ethically consider a transplant will almost always have been ill for a long period of time with chronic emphysema, pneumonitis, and often cardiac difficulties and thus harbors chronic infection to some degree at the outset. Infection constitutes a major threat. In fact, it has often not been possible to determine from cytological examination at autopsy to what extent the changes in the allotransplanted lung were caused by various elements of immunological rejection and which were caused by infection.

There is some evidence still, though disputed, that the insertion of one normal lung allotransplant results in overall ventilation-perfusion disturbances between the transplanted lung and the patient's own remaining lung, in the patient with chronic pulmonary emphysema and overdistention of the remaining lung. For these various reasons the long-term results of clinical lung transplantation have been poor.

Recently, however, the clinical approach to transplantation of both lungs and the heart as a single *en bloc* anatomical and functional unit has been approached again by Shumway and his associates, largely for the management of intractable pulmonary vascular hypertension, and they have been successful in so transplanting these organs in a number of instances. In these patients, the transplanted lungs were not rejected and afforded adequate function. There is some evidence that this remarkable achievement is due to current availability of the new drug cyclosporin-A. These results are most encouraging for the long-term promise of lung transplantation itself.

TRANSPLANTATION OF THE HEART

Transplantation of the heart has offered challenge for a great many years. Carrel and Guthrie transplanted the heart heterotopically to the necks of dogs in 1905. Following these studies, other types of transplants in animals were performed and reported. Yet it was not until two major contributions occurred—the development of the pump oxygenator in the 1950s and the description by Lower, Stofer and Shumway of a new atrial suture method for orthotopic heart transplantation—that active investigation of orthotopic heart transplantation was undertaken in many laboratories.

The most outstanding studies were and remain those of Shumway and his group, but Wilman, Hanlon, and Cooper, among others, also did outstanding early work. These various studies disclosed that the heart could in fact be reimplanted and support the animal satisfactorily postoperatively; it was later shown that the heart allograft could, with appropriate immunosuppression therapy, provide long-term animal survival.

The first human heart transplant patient was that of Hardy and associates in 1964, who employed a xenograft when the prospective patient was in apparently terminal cardiogenic shock and no human heart allograft was available. (The prospective human donor remained alive on a ventilator, and neither stopping the respirator nor the diagnosis of brain death was accepted at that time to permit the harvesting of a still-beating heart.) The use of the xenograft followed the surprising early successes with lower primate kidney transplants in man. The use of the xenograft assured that a vigorous organ would be transplanted. The heart of a large chimpanzee supported the patient for about an hour and a half, after discontinuation of pump oxygenator support, but it ultimately failed, in considerable measure owing to the fact that the recipient had been in prolonged shock at the time he was placed on cardiopulmonary bypass. Nonetheless, the heart was readily inserted by the usual techniques which had been employed extensively in the animal laboratory (Fig. 13-4). It did beat immediately and supported the circulation for a period of time. But perhaps the transplant's most far-reaching contribution was to make both professionals and laymen aware that successful heart transplantation was a real and imminent possibility. The heart held at that time a special status in human concepts and emotions, far more than being just a pump, and public discussion was widespread.

The first successful heart transplantation in man was that of Barnard in 1967. Following this a considerable number of human heart transplants were performed with varying success in different centers throughout the world. The basic

operative technique described by Shumway and his associates became the standard against which other potential innovations were measured and generally discarded. During this stage of immunosuppressive therapy, few human recipients exhibited long-term survival. At the present time, however, Shumway's group at Stanford University has achieved a 1-year survival rate that compares favorably with the 1-year survival rate of cadaver kidney transplants; after performing over 200 orthotopic human heart transplants, the current survival rate is 60% for 1 year and 40% for 5 years. In addition, a number of patients have been successfully retransplanted. It is pertinent now to review some of the considerations to which this group attributes its steadily improving results.

RECIPIENT SELECTION

The guidelines employed to evaluate the suitability for transplantation of a patient with end-stage heart disease begin with the standard history and physical examination, cardiac catheterization, left ventriculography, and coronary angiography. Psychiatric evaluation must establish that the potential recipient is a sufficiently stable candidate, and careful evaluation must indicate that nontransplant modes of therapy hold out little hope for survival past the next several months. The contraindications to accepting a given potential candidate for transplantation include a severely elevated pulmonary vascular resistance unresponsive to vasodilator therapy, the presence of an active infectious process, insulin-requiring chronic diabetes mellitus, an age over 50 years, a recent unresolved pulmonary embolus or infarction, and a separate systemic disease that may be susceptible to exacerbation with immunosuppressive therapy. It is possible that the Stanford group will now be able to accept some patients with severely increased pulmonary vascular resistance in that they have currently successfully transplanted both heart and lungs *en bloc* in a number of patients.

ADDITIONAL FACTORS

One of the most important advances in obtaining a healthy cadaver heart for transplantation has been the acceptance of brain death on a firm legal basis. This allows a still-beating heart to be removed, quickly cooled, and thus preserved prior to insertion into the new host. Next, the continued experience with various immunosuppressive agents has afforded safer use of these agents, basically azathioprine (Imuran) and prednisone. Cyclosporin-A, which has recently become available, is looked upon as a still more favorable agent, in that it appears capable of suppressing the allograft rejection reaction without many of the unfavorable side-effects of both azathioprine and prednisone, in particular the impairment of host defenses against bacterial and other infective agents.

The diagnosis and treatment of rejection are managed by the Stanford group in the following manner: daily physical examination, electrocardiograms, and T-cell measurements are routinely performed. The data thus derived are then used to direct the need for and the timing of transvenous endocardial catheter biopsies. These data, in turn, while nonspecific in many instances, collectively allow the adjustment of the immunosuppressive drugs. This is important, because excessive dosages of the immunosuppressive agents azathioprine and prednisone predispose to

Fig. 13-4.   The basic Lower-Stofer-Shumway excision and suture technique. (From Hardy JD, Chavez CM: The first heart transplant in man: Historical reexamination of the 1964 case in the light of current clinical experience. Transplant Proc 1:717, 1969)

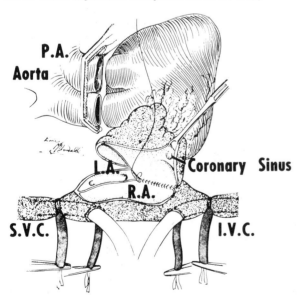

the very considerable risk of serious bacterial, fungal, and viral infections in these patients. Infections must be treated promptly and aggressively. Long-term follow-up and close observation are essential to the achievement of superior results.

COMBINED CLINICAL CARDIOPULMONARY TRANSPLANTATION

Combined cardiopulmonary transplantation has interested surgeons for many years, for there are certain pathologic conditions in which patient cardiopulmonary disorders cannot be managed successfully by transplantation of lung or heart alone. Webb and Howard in 1957 at Mississippi achieved living dogs for limited periods following orthotopic cardiopulmonary transplantation, and Castaneda and associates achieved long-term survival in baboons after cardiopulmonary replantation. Cooley and associates and Lillehei performed the operation in several patients, but with only brief survival times.

As was noted in the discussion of lung transplantation, Shumway and his group have reported very promising early clinical success with this operation in five patients using the new immunosuppressive agent cyclosporin-A. Basically, the operation is indicated for combined cardiac and pulmonary disease from a variety of causes, an outstanding one being a congenital cardiac disease with intractable severe pulmonary arterial hypertension.

MISCELLANEOUS OTHER CLINICAL TISSUE GRAFTS

Many other types of tissue are utilized clinically, with varying degrees of frequency and success. In fact, some such grafts are used so commonly that they have for many years been accepted as routine surgical therapy.

SKIN

Skin autografts have been used for centuries, and they of course survive permanently if appropriately harvested and placed on a granulating bed that is not infected. The skin itself is a remarkable organ which, among other functions, preserves heat and body fluids and affords protection against bacterial invasion. If a large skin defect is not successfully grafted or cannot finally heal in by scar tissue, it remains open and a ready avenue for bacterial invasion. To be sure, some patients live with relatively large venous ulcers of the lower leg, for example, for many years without serious bacterial invasion. Nonetheless, invasion is always possible, especially in diabetics. Skin autografts containing hair are used to restore hair to the scalp or to replace eyebrows. Free skin grafts from the vulva are used at times by plastic surgeons to replace the nipple when an amputated breast has been replaced by a mound of tissue produced by muscle transfer or by artificial prosthesis. The principal use of skin allografts, usually taken from a cadaver, has been in grafting for extensively burned patients who cannot afford enough split thickness grafts from the remaining unburned surfaces to cover the burned areas temporarily. However, such allografts are eventually rejected, so vigorous investigation has been carried on over the years to find suitable replacements.

TENDON, NERVE, AND FASCIA

Nerve and tendon autotransplants are regularly used to graft tendon and nerve losses following various types of injuries. The tendon transplants serve remarkably well, and the nerve transplants serve with reasonable success in some instances. Fascial autografts from the fascia lata of the thigh have long been used as living suture material for the repair of inguinal hernias. Such fascia may also be employed for bridging defects elsewhere.

CORNEA TRANSPLANTS

One of the most gratifying developments of transplantation has been that of transplantation of the cornea to preserve sight where the cornea of the recipient is opaque for one reason or another. The cornea is harvested from the cadaver within an hour or so after death and can be stored and then transplanted to the recipient with a high rate of success. Corneal transplants are employed far more commonly than is generally realized.

BLOOD VESSEL TRANSPLANTS

Autografts of vein and occasionally artery are used routinely in virtually every medical center in the world. The most commonly used vascular structure is the saphenous vein, which is employed variously for coronary artery bypass and for bypassing arterial occlusive disease in arteries of the neck, arm, kidney, small bowel, or legs. Autografts of the hypogastric artery have been used occasionally, but rarely today because reasonably satisfactory artificial fabric replacements are available.

Allografts of blood vessels have fallen generally into disuse. These grafts were found to deteriorate gradually, and it was difficult to harvest them from cadavers and to treat enough of them satisfactorily to supply the heavy demand. The autologous saphenous vein is now generally used for bypassing lesions at the sites where a vessel of this size is needed; otherwise, a fabric graft of one type or another is employed as a replacement for the aorta where formerly surgeons used freeze-dried allografts.

Xenografts of blood vessels and of pig aortic and mitral valves are still used to a considerable extent. Bovine arterial vessel grafts are utilized to some extent, and there is widespread use of the pig aortic and mitral valves. The porcine valve is treated with a denaturizing and preservative solution which appears largely to abolish the antigenic properties of these valves. Certainly, long-term success over a period of years has been achieved with such valves, though many centers are finding that in time they have to replace many of them because of deterioration. Nonetheless, the most striking feature of the use of porcine valves has been their progressively increased success, which may have resulted from a continuous modification of the type of preparation and subsequent storage.

BONE AND CARTILAGE

Autologous grafts of bone and cartilage have long been used with much success. Allogenic bone grafts are also stored in banks and used frequently, though they do not serve as well as do autologous bone grafts. In contrast, cartilage has a very low antigenicity, and thus cartilaginous allografts are associated with much more success.

AUTOTRANSPLANTS OF ENDOCRINE TISSUE

The transplantation of pancreatic islets was discussed previously. In addition, a considerable experience has been developed regarding the implantation of parathyroid tissue in the forearm following total parathyroidectomy for various types of hyperparathyroidism. It has been shown that these parathyroid autotransplants do survive and provide considerable parathyroid function. Parathyroid allografts excited considerable interest some years ago but were finally rejected, so such allografts were abandoned when it was not possible to demonstrate long-term success.

Adrenal autotransplantation has also been employed following total intra-abdominal adrenalectomy, with concurrent transplantation of slices of the excised hyperplastic adrenals to the muscle at some readily accessible site, occasionally to a pectoralis muscle but more often to the sartorius muscle in the thigh. These implants, which are of course autografts, almost routinely survive in varying degrees, and years later they may very occasionally have increased in their function sufficiently to produce recurrent Cushing's syndrome. The reason for preserving adrenocortical function in this way has been to preserve adequate adrenal function without the necessity for the patient's taking replacement therapy for the rest of her life (the majority of these patients are female and relatively young), to prevent the excessive pigmentation which may be observed in some white patients following total adrenalectomy and maintenance on cortical steroid replacement therapy, and, it is hoped, to prevent the development of the usually chromophobe pituitary tumor (Nelson's syndrome), which may encroach on the optic chiasm years later and cause impairment of vision. In a substantial number of patients receiving such adrenal tissue implants, it has later been possible to withdraw steroid replacement therapy completely.

BONE MARROW, THYMUS, AND SPLEEN

There has been considerable experience with the allogenic transplantation of bone marrow as replacement therapy for aplastic anemia or other blood dyscrasias. Varying degrees of success have been achieved, but intense interest continues in the investigation and improvement of this therapy.

Some children are born without adequate thymic activity and fail to develop their immune capacity through the T-cell (thymic) system. Thus they are prone to infections which commonly threaten their life. Some degree of success has been realized in allogenic thymic transplants, but this work remains under investigation.

Similarly, there has been interest in the transplantation of the intact spleen or spleen cells. Such studies are in their infancy. Splenic allografts in the animal laboratory have not been successful. There is, however, an important interest in spleen replacement, especially for children who have lost the spleen and thus have a much enhanced susceptibility to certain types of severe infections.

BIBLIOGRAPHY

Gut

ALICAN F, HARDY JD, CAYIRLI M et al: Laboratory experience with intestinal transplantation and a clinical case. Am J Surg 121:150, 1971

FORTNER JG, SHIRE MH, KUNLIN A et al: Orthotopic intestinal allografting after massive intestinal resection. Bull Soc Int Chir 31:264, 1972

OLIVIER G, RETTORI R, OLIVIER C: Homotransplantation orthotopique de l'intestin grêle et du colon droit il transverse chez l'homme. J Chir 98:323, 1969

Heart

BARNARD C: The operation. A human cardiac transplantation: An interim report of the successful operation performed at Groote Schuur Hospital, Cape Town. S Afr Med J 41:1271, 1967

BAUMGARTNER VA, BEITZ BA, OYER PE et al: Cardiac homotransplantation. Curr Probl Surg 16:1, 1979

CASTANEDA AR, ZANORA R, SCHMIDT-HABERLMANN P et al: Cardiopulmonary autotransplantation in primates (baboons): Late functional results. Surgery 72:1064, 1972

COOLEY DA, BLOODWELL RD, HALLMAN GL et al: Organ transplantation for advanced cardiopulmonary disease. Ann Thorac Surg 8:30, 1969

HARDY JD, CHAVEZ CM, KURRUS FD et al: Heart transplantation in man. Developmental studies and report of a case. JAMA 188:1132, 1964

HUNT SA, STINSON EB: Cardiac transplantation. Annu Rev Med 32:213, 1981

LOWER RR, STOFER RC, SHUMWAY NE: Homovital transplantation of the heart. J Thorac Cardiovasc Surg 41:196, 1961

OYER PE, STINSON EB, REITZ BA et al: Cardiac transplantation: 1980. Transplant Proc 13:199, 1980

REITZ BA, WALLWORK JR, HUNT SA et al: Heart-lung transplantation: Successful therapy for patients with pulmonary vascular disease. N Engl J Med 306:557, 1982

WEBB WR, HOWARD HS: Cardiopulmonary transplantation. Surg Forum 8:313, 1959

WILLMAN VL, COOPER T, CIAN LG et al: Autotransplantation of the heart. Surg Gynecol Obstet 115:299, 1962

Liver

CALNE RY, WILLIAMS R: Liver transplantation. Curr Probl Surg 16:1, 1979

MOORE FD, SMITH LL, BURNAP TK et al: One-stage homotransplantation of the liver following total hepatectomy in dogs. Transplant Bull 6:103, 1959

STARZL TE, IWATSUKI S, KLINTMALM G et al: Liver transplantation, 1980, with particular reference to cyclosporin-A. Transplant Proc 13:281, 1981

STARZL TE, KLINTMALM GBG, PORTER KA et al: Liver transplantation with use of cyclosporin-A and prednisone. N Engl J Med 305:266, 1981

STARZL TE, PORTER KA, PUTNAM CW et al: Orthotopic liver transplantation in 93 patients. Surg Gynecol Obstet 142:487, 1976

WELCH CS: A note on transplantation of the whole liver in dogs. Transplant Bull 2:54, 1955

Lung

ALICAN F, ISIN E, COCKRELL JV et al: One-stage allotransplantation of both lungs in the dog. Am Surg 177:193, 1973

DEMIKHOV VP: Experimental Transplantation of Vital Organs. New York: Consultants Bureau, 1962

DEROM F, BARBIER F, RINGOIR S et al: Ten month survival after lung homotransplantation in man. J Thorac Cardiovasc Surg 61:835, 1971

HARDY JD, WEBB WR, DALTON ML et al: Lung homotransplantation in man: Report of initial case. JAMA 186:1065, 1963

VEITH FJ: Lung transplantation. Surg Clin North Am 58:357, 1978

WILDEVUUR CRH, BENFIELD JR: A review of 23 human lung transplantations by 20 surgeons. Ann Thorac Surg 9:489, 1970

Pancreas

KELLY WD, LILLEHEI RL, MERKEL FK et al: Surgery 61:827, 1967

LARGIADER F, KOLB E, BINSWANGER U: A long-term functioning human pancreatic islet allotransplant. Transplantation 29:76, 1980

SUTHERLAND DER, GOETZ FC, NAJARIAN JS: Review of world's experience with pancreas and islet transplantation and results of intraperitoneal segmental pancreas transplantation from related and cadaver donors at Minnesota. Transplant Proc 13:l, 1981

John H. Raaf/Jerome J. DeCosse

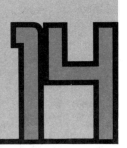

Cancer Biology and General Approaches to Management

The field of oncology is undergoing dynamic change. The precise events responsible for chromosome replication, cell division, cell dedifferentiation, and the implantation and growth of metastases are still unknown. However, recent advances in molecular biology and immunology suggest that important discoveries that will dramatically increase our understanding of neoplasia are not far away and will lead eventually to the control of cancer at a biochemical level.

Progress in the clinical care of patients with cancer is also being made in all areas, including prevention, early detection, diagnosis, and treatment. Examples include new radiologic techniques such as computed tomography (CT), better methods of nutritional support, implantation (brachytherapy) techniques for radiation therapy, and more effective, less toxic combinations of chemotherapeutic agents. The surgeon who operates on patients with neoplastic disease must incorporate these new developments into his practice to offer optimum care.

OVERVIEW OF CANCER

Cancer is a diverse group of diseases characterized by the uncontrolled growth and spread of malignant cells. *Oncology* (Gr. *onkos*—tumor; *logos*—study) is the study of these diseases. Neoplastic cells behave independently; they do not have fixed relationships to other cells and do not form organs. Tumors consisting of neoplastic cells are called benign or malignant. *Benign* implies noninvasive growth without metastases, while *malignant* means invasive growth with metastases. Actually, these two terms describe the ends of a spectrum of behavior, and it is not always possible on histologic grounds to determine if a tumor is definitely benign or malignant. For example, a gastric leiomyoma with few mitoses may eventually metastasize and then will be reclassified as a malignant leiomyosarcoma. A desmoid fibrosarcoma can be locally invasive and will occasionally metastasize, so most pathologists call these low-grade malignancies. However, a desmoid sarcoma is almost always curable by wide, soft-part resection, and therefore it could be argued that it is a benign tumor. Malignant tumors that arise from epithelium are called carcinomas, whereas those arising from connective tissue are called sarcomas (Fig. 14-1). If there is a glandular element within a carcinoma, the tumor is termed an adenocarcinoma.

BIOLOGY OF NEOPLASIA

Malignant cells tend to dedifferentiate, and in tissue culture they "pile up" because of loss of the normal mechanisms for contact inhibition, cell turnover, and cell death. A single neoplastic cell has the potential to become a clone of malignant cells, which can develop into a clinical cancer. This does not mean that all cells in a tumor are the same. On the contrary, the population of cells in a clinically detectable tumor is usually quite heterogeneous, owing to their inherent genetic instability. Only some of the cells are capable of metastasizing, and not all are sensitive to a given cytotoxic drug.

One can consider that the cells in both normal and

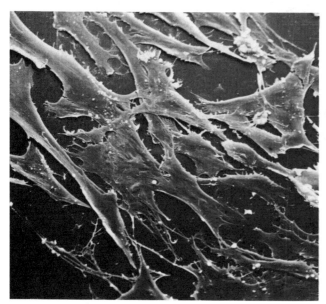 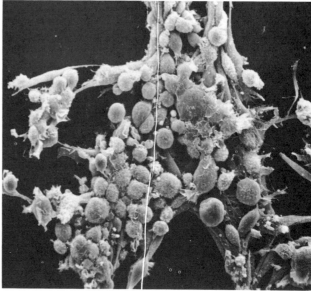

Fig. 14-1. Scanning electron micrograph of cultured fibroblasts before and after transformation by Rous sarcoma virus. Normal fibroblasts (*A*) are flat and adhere to the surface of the culture dish, while transformed cells (*B*) are round and cluster together. (Micrographs provided by J. Michael Bishop, G. Steven Martin, and Jerry Guyden)

neoplastic tissue consist of three populations: rapidly proliferating cells, which are going around the cell cycle; G_0 cells, which are quiescent but can reenter the cycle, and nondividing cells, which eventually will die. Tissue growth depends on only a few parameters: the cell-cycle time, the growth fraction, and the rate of cell loss. One might suppose that the cell-cycle time for tumor cells would be abnormally short, but this is not true. Actually, cancer cells do not proliferate faster than normal cells such as bone-marrow leukocytes or intestinal epithelium. Therefore, tumor growth depends on a high growth fraction (fraction of cycling cells in the population) and on a rate of cell loss (noted in some tumors to be substantial) that is less than the rate of cell production. The result is net growth.

The interval between malignant transformation of a single cell and when it is detected as a clinical tumor is termed the latent period. A transformed cell may lie quiescent for months or years prior to becoming clinically evident. In animal systems, very active chemical carcinogens cause a latent period of only a few months, but a mouse infected with mammary-tumor virus at birth rarely develops breast cancer before 1 year. The life span of the mouse is only about 2 years, so the equivalent latent period in the human would be 35 years. Thirty-five years is also the interval between the average age when smoking begins and the age at peak incidence of lung cancer. With such long latent periods, it is not surprising how difficult it is to implicate specific carcinogens as the cause of given tumors. Factors that influence the duration of latency are largely unknown, although hormone stimulation and immune response by the host are both suspected of playing roles.

It is convenient to express the rate of tumor growth by its doubling time (the time it takes to double in volume). The doubling time of a pulmonary metastasis, for example, can be estimated by measuring the mass on sequential chest x-ray films. If a malignant cell begins to divide and the mass of the tumor doubles with each replication, it is estimated that the latent period will constitute approximately 30 divisions. At the end of that time, the tumor will be a 1-cm nodule and will contain 1 billion cells (Fig. 14-2). Occasionally, a tumor will exhibit spontaneous regression.

The reasons for this are not known, although an immunologic response to antigens on the surface of the tumor may be responsible. In the case of regression of neuroblastoma in children, a spontaneous maturation of the tumor probably occurs.

About 4% of autopsied patients will have a small microscopic focus of papillary thyroid cancer, and about 15% of autopsied men will have a microscopic focus of prostatic cancer. These findings have been labeled "pathologist's cancer" because they have had no biologic activity of consequence to the patient. They illustrate the frequency and the extraordinarily long latent period that may be present with precancer or early cancer.

Multicentricity is a feature of cancer originating at many anatomical locations. Cancer of the oral cavity may occur in multiple sites within the mouth, and this phenomenon has been called a field effect. The patient with cancer in the oral cavity is more likely to develop cancer of the lung or esophagus. All of these epithelia are squamous, and multicentricity may be a product of a common susceptibility to a particular carcinogen, for example, a component of tobacco. About 5% to 8% of all patients with a cancer of the large bowel will develop another cancer of the large bowel either at the time of their initial presentation (called synchronous) or later in life (called metachronous). Women who develop cancer in both breasts are more likely to have multicentric carcinoma than are those with unilateral disease, which suggests that multicentricity and bilaterality are manifestations of a common process involving malignant transformation at multiple sites in the mammary glandular epithelium.

ONCOGENES AND MOLECULAR BIOLOGY

Abnormal mitotic figures have been observed in tumor cells for almost a century. As early as 1914, the German biologist Boveri suggested that mitotic errors were the cause of neoplasia. It is now known that cancer cells often have numerical abnormalities (aneuploidy) as well as structural abnormalities in their chromosomes. In fact, most human tumors exhibit chromosomal abnormalities, which usually

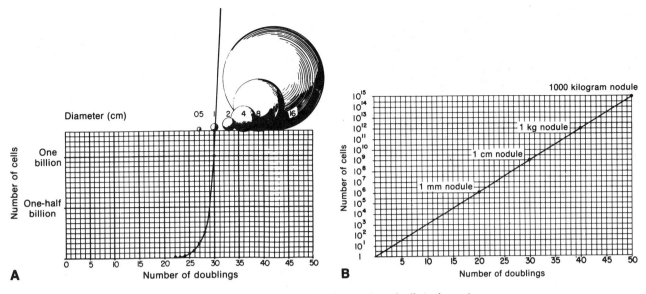

Fig. 14-2. Diagrammatic illustration of exponential tumor growth. The number of cells is shown in relationship to the number of doublings and tumor weight and diameter. (Collins VP Loeffler RK, Tivey H: Observations of growth rates of human tumors. Am J Roentgenol 76:988, 1956)

are nonrandom and occasionally are quite specific. In 1960, Nowell and Hungerford reported that the cells of chronic myelogenous leukemia (CML) were characterized by a very small chromosome, named the Philadelphia (Ph[1]) chromosome (Fig. 14-3), which is now regarded as diagnostic of CML. The Ph[1] chromosome originates by the exchange (translocation) of a terminal segment from chromosome 22 to the end of chromosome 9, giving a shortened No. 22 and a slightly elongated No. 9. The appearance of chromosomal changes in addition to the Ph[1] in the lymphocytes of a CML patient signals the onset of the blast phase, in some cases months before it becomes clinically evident.

Specific chromosomal abnormalities are also being discovered in human solid tumors. Most B cell–derived lymphomas contain a chromosome 14 that is longer than its partner. This is called the 14q+ marker, and it represents a translocation from chromosome 8. Two other specific abnormalities have recently been found: loss of chromosome 22 in benign meningiomas and a translocation involving chromosomes 6 and 14 in ovarian papillary serous cystadenocarcinoma.

The study of tumor viruses in experimental animals has been an important method for examining the molecular basis of malignant transformation. Research on deletion mutants of the Rous sarcoma virus (RSV), a ribonucleic acid (RNA) virus that causes sarcoma in chickens, has shown that 15% of its genome contains an oncogene (named src) that codes for approximately 450 amino acids. Mutant viruses that have lost the oncogene are unable to transform chicken fibroblasts in tissue culture. An enzyme, reverse transcriptase, can be used to make deoxyribonucleic acid (DNA) probes with which one can learn whether oncogenelike DNA sequences also exist in the chromosomes of normal animal cells. It appears that oncogenes are present in all cells, normal and transformed, but in normal cells these DNA sequences are not transcribed. The RSV oncogene may be a host control gene that switches on a large set of genes during embryonic development, a gene that becomes inactive when the cell undergoes maturation and differentiation.

EPIDEMIOLOGY

In the United States, cancer is the second most frequent cause of death (20.4% of all deaths), following heart disease (37.8%); it is followed at some distance by stroke (9.6%) and trauma (5.4%). The chance of developing cancer increases with advancing age, yet it is the most frequent cause of death in children between ages 3 and 14. One of four persons living in the United States will eventually develop cancer, and two of three families will be affected. Excluding nonmelanoma skin cancer and carcinoma in situ, 805,000 Americans were diagnosed as having cancer in 1981. Approximately one third of these people will be alive 5 years after treatment. If one excludes patients dying of other causes (*e.g.*, heart disease, old age), then 41% of cancer patients will live at least 5 years.

Cancer incidence according to site and sex as estimated for 1981 is shown in Figure 14-4. Female and male death rates for the most common cancers (1930–1977) are presented in Figure 14-5. Lung cancer is the most common cause of cancer death in men, and breast cancer is the most common cause in women. For both men and women, cancer of the large bowel (the second most frequent for each) is the most common cause of cancer death. It can be seen that for most types of cancer, the death rates are leveling off or declining. The single exception is cancer of the lung, for which there has been a major increase among both men and women. In 1982, more than 25% of cancer deaths in the United States were from lung cancer.

Epidemiologic studies of cancer are carried out with the hope that clues may be discovered regarding the etiology of cancers with a high incidence within a given population. These studies have identified a high incidence of liver cancer in certain parts of Africa and a high incidence of gastric cancer in Japan. This type of study often attempts to examine the diet of a population that seems prone to a certain type of tumor, but it has been difficult to establish particular dietary factors as being responsible. Such studies have provided circumstantial evidence that a high intake of fat and protein in the diet may contribute to cancer of the large

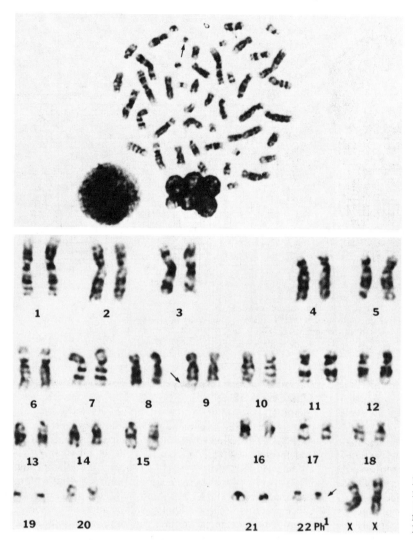

Fig. 14-3. Karyotype of patient with chronic myelocytic leukemia showing the Philadelphia (Ph[1]) chromosome, the result of a transposition from one chromosome No. 22 to a chromosome No. 9. (Courtesy of Dr. R.S.K. Chaganti)

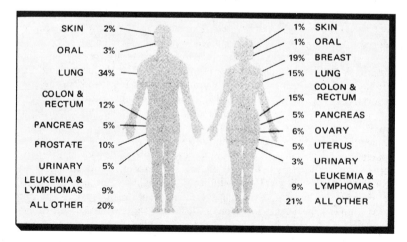

Fig. 14-4. Cancer incidence in 1981 for both sexes, shown for each primary tumor type as a percentage of all cancers.

bowel in the United States, but this has not been proved. The most convincing evidence by far is the correlation between cigarette smoking and lung cancer; cigarette smokers are ten times as likely to develop lung cancer as are nonsmokers. Epidemiologic studies have also shown that cessation of smoking results in reduced mortality from lung cancer.

CARCINOGENESIS

The exact biochemical steps leading to neoplastic transformation are not known. However, in the past 3 decades, enormous progress has been made that has increased our understanding of nucleic acids and the regulation of protein synthesis in the cell. It appears that the precise biochemical

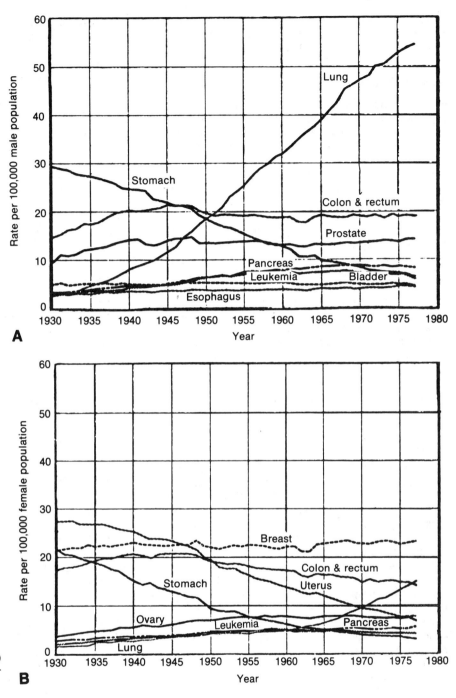

Fig. 14-5. Male (*A*) and female (*B*) cancer death rate shown for each primary tumor site.

steps involved in the initiation of chromosome replication will soon be known, as well as, perhaps, the mechanism through which many etiologic factors act to induce tumors.

Malignant transformation appears to develop as a multistep process in which there are two major stages. During initiation, there is a specific DNA mutation, usually induced by an environmental carcinogen (a virus, a chemical, or radiation). This results in escape of the target cell from its normal restriction of proliferation, which is imposed by differentiation. The cell is now "premalignant" and can progress to full malignancy through promotion, a still mysterious event that involves further mutation by environmental factors that are not necessarily carcinogens themselves. Croton oil is a classic promoter, which produces papillary tumors in "initiated" mouse skin. Colonic polyps in patients with familial polyposis behave as though they are already initiated, ready to be converted to malignancy by an as yet unidentified promoting agent.

CHEMICAL CARCINOGENS

Pott, the English surgeon, was the first to implicate a cause-and-effect relationship between a chemical substance and human cancer. In 1775, he suggested that exposure to soot was responsible for cancer of the scrotum in chimney sweeps. Yamagiwa and Ichikawa, in 1915, painted the ears of rabbits with coal tar and thereby produced tumors. It is now known that 1,2-dibenzanthracene is an important carcinogenic agent in coal tar. The nitrosamines may be important human carcinogens, since they can be formed from nitrites found in bacon, pastrami, and frankfurters.

PHYSICAL CARCINOGENS

Following the discovery of radium, it was realized that ionizing radiation can produce cancer. The high incidence of bone cancer in radium-dial painters who licked brushes containing radioactive material was recognized, as was a high incidence of lung cancer in uranium-mine workers. Japanese exposed to the atomic bomb have had a greatly increased incidence of leukemia. Also, cancer of the skin of the hands was seen with high frequency in the early physicians who used fluoroscopy without adequate protection, and, more recently, thyroid cancer is being found in adults who received irradiation to the neck during childhood for various reasons, including acne and an enlarged thymus.

The development of skin cancer, including squamous carcinoma and malignant melanoma, is more frequent in persons who spend considerable time outdoors in the sunlight. The ultraviolet component has been incriminated.

Sites of chronic irritation appear to be at a high risk for the development of carcinoma. Examples include a draining pilonidal sinus, fistula in ano, chronic osteomyelitis, chronic ulcerative colitis, and a chronically scarred esophagus following ingestion of a corrosive agent. Carcinoma also appears in old burn scars (Marjolin's ulcer) and in the schistosome-infested liver and bladder.

VIRUSES

Viruses have been shown to cause malignant transformation in cells grown in tissue culture and in several experimental animal models. In 1911, Rous found a filterable agent that produced sarcoma in chickens. In 1936, Bittner found a virus in the milk of mice that predisposes the progeny to development of carcinoma of the breast. In 1951, Gross transmitted leukemia in mice with cell-free filtrates.

No human cancer has been unequivocally identified as viral in origin. It is suspected that some human hepatic cancers result from infection with hepatitis virus. A lymphoma of the jaw in African children has been studied by Burkitt, who suggested that it may be caused by a virus carried by mosquitoes at certain geographic altitudes. It is now believed that the Epstein-Barr (EB) virus bears an etiologic relationship to Burkitt's lymphoma and nasopharyngeal carcinoma.

A new syndrome, characterized by the appearance of the lesions of Kaposi's sarcoma in the skin, lymph nodes, and gastrointestinal tract of young, sexually active homosexual men, has recently appeared. These patients, most of whom have had previous venereal infections or hepatitis, are also susceptible to opportunistic pathogens such as *Pneumocystis carinii* and cytomegalovirus. The cancer appears to be "infectious," since the responsible agent is likely passed by sexual contact. These patients are usually compromised immunologically, and it has recently been suggested that amyl nitrite may be immunosuppressive in the setting of repeated viral antigenic stimulation. Male homosexuals who are regular amyl nitrite users have abnormally low helper (OKT4)/suppressor (OKT8) T-lymphocyte ratios.

B-type virions have been found by electron microscopy in cultured human breast carcinoma cells. However, a viral etiology for human cancer is extremely difficult to prove,

since absolute proof would require isolation and identification of the organism, reproduction of the disease in a healthy person, and recovery of the same organism from the newly diseased person. This type of experimentation is obviously not possible in humans.

HORMONES

Work with animals has shown that development of tumors can be made more likely by hormonal manipulation, for example, by the long-term administration of estrogen to rats. In humans, postmenopausal use of estrogens may contribute to development of endometrial cancer, while the administration of diethylstilbestrol (DES) to pregnant women has been associated with the development, in the offspring from that pregnancy, of clear cell carcinoma of the vagina during young-adult life.

HEREDITARY FACTORS

Genetic factors are of considerable importance in carcinogenesis. Some common cancers (*e.g.*, carcinoma of the breast) occur with increased frequency in children of parents who have this type of cancer. Some families generally appear to be prone to a variety of cancers, while others are susceptible to certain less common types of tumors, for example, those of endocrine organs in the multiple endocrine neoplasia syndromes. Patients with familial polyposis of the colon are susceptible to carcinoma of the colon later in life. About 15% of all patients with cancer of the large bowel have a family history of large-bowel cancer.

ENVIRONMENTAL AND GEOGRAPHIC FACTORS

Some tumors occur with high frequency in certain populations and in certain geographic locations. Examples include the high incidence of liver cancer in Africa, stomach carcinoma in Japan, and bladder cancer in Egypt (associated with schistosomiasis). These geographic distributions of tumors are likely related to a combination of inherited traits within the population and environmental carcinogens, some of which are in the diet.

PRECANCEROUS CONDITIONS

Several benign though precancerous conditions exist that may progress to malignancy. Leukoplakia in the mucous membrane of the mouth or the skin of the vulva can develop into frank carcinoma. It is strongly suspected that large-bowel adenoma can develop into large-bowel carcinoma, and it is clear that carcinoma of the colon can develop in areas of long-standing chronic ulcerative colitis. Another example is the progression of cervical dysplasia to carcinoma of the cervix.

PREVENTION

The prevention of cancer depends upon the avoidance of carcinogens and the careful screening of high-risk patients for premalignant or early localized malignant lesions. In the latter situation, if a precancerous lesion such as leukoplakia or severe cervical dysplasia is found, adequate local destruction or excision can usually result in cure.

Exposure to industrial carcinogens is receiving closer scrutiny. As relationships become clearer, such as between mesothelioma and asbestos inhalation and between angiosarcoma of the liver and polyvinylchloride exposure, more emphasis is being placed on avoidance of these and similar materials.

A greater impact on the cancer problem could be achieved by reducing exposure to tobacco and alcohol. Of 160,000 cancer deaths in the United States in 1980, approximately 50,000 (31%) likely could have been prevented by avoidance of cigarette smoking. Other smoking-associated cancer sites include pancreas, bladder, oral cavity, kidney, esophagus, and larynx. These sites and the lung make up about 50% of cancer deaths in men and 25% in women. Lung cancer has been consistently the most common cancer in men, and it is projected that it will soon exceed breast cancer as the most common cause of cancer death in women. Several European countries are doing more than the United States to discourage smoking. Legislative action by Congress could increase the price of cigarettes, ban advertising, stop sales through vending machines, and prohibit smoking in theaters and on public transportation.

Alcohol is associated with cancer of the oral cavity, larynx, and esophagus, as well as many other health problems, and it appears that alcohol and tobacco have additive effects. The highest priority in preventing cancer, then, should be given to educating healthy people about the risk of cigarette smoking and heavy use of alcohol. Total elimination of cigarettes would not, of course, abolish all lung cancer, since it does occasionally appear in nonsmokers. Other factors, such as genetic predisposition, must also be involved.

METASTASIS

The development of a metastasis from a solid tumor is an unfavorable event that decreases the chance of curability. The mechanism by which metastases occur are still obscure. Several steps are involved, including invasion and shedding of tumor cells into blood vessels or lymphatics, invasion of these circulating cells into normal tissue at a distant site, and the securing of a new blood supply (angiogenesis) by the metastatic cells. For some tumors, the shedding of cells into the bloodstream is not a rare event, and tumor cells may easily be found by examination of the peripheral blood. However, this alone is not sufficient for the development of metastases. The number of tumor cells in the blood does not correlate with the likelihood of metastases, since many other factors influence the number and distribution of metastases. Some of these may be immunologic, and some may relate to coagulation mechanisms.

Malignant tumors can spread by direct extension, lymphatic spread, vascular spread, seeding of shed cells onto the surfaces of the pleura or peritoneum, or implantation at surgical operation (Fig. 14-6). The routes of spread of an individual tumor are determined largely by its own unique characteristics. For example, most epithelial tumors are likely to metastasize to regional lymph nodes, while sarcomas and renal carcinoma are more likely to spread hematogenously to the lungs. Tumors arising in the gastrointestinal tract and drained by the portal circulation often metastasize to the liver.

Whether tumor cell emboli within lymphatics can be trapped in lymph nodes (Fig. 14-7) is the subject of controversy. Halsted, in devising the radical mastectomy for breast cancer, advocated regional lymph node dissection based on the idea that a cancer might still be curable provided that trapped tumor cells in regional nodes were removed in addition to the primary tumor. This concept seems at least partially valid, since long-term (30-year) follow-up data, such as that published by Adair and colleagues for breast cancer, document the cure of some patients who had regional disease. However, other patients are not cured by regional node dissection, and therefore the concept of Fisher that breast cancer has already spread systemically at the time the patient appears with her primary tumor also seems valid at times. The truth may be a combination of these two views, which are not mutually exclusive.

Patients with a large primary tumor or with metastatic disease may develop systemic symptoms owing to products secreted by the tumor. These products, many of which are not yet defined biochemically, can cause abnormalities, including hyponatremia, hypercalcemia, hypoglycemia, anemia, myopathy, leukocytosis, and cachexia. Nonspecific but cancer-related lesions have also been described in the skin (acanthosis nigricans), neuromuscular system (polyneuropathy), blood vessels (thrombophlebitis and endocarditis), and skeleton (osteomalacia). These systemic effects are grouped under the heading paraneoplastic syndromes. Small-cell lung cancer is a particularly frequent cause of such disorders.

DIAGNOSIS

CLINICAL EVALUATION

The symptoms of cancer are numerous and nonspecific. Similarly, the physical signs associated with tumors can mimic many benign conditions. In an attempt to increase the awareness of the public, the American Cancer Society has publicized seven warning signals that may be the first symptoms or signs of cancer:

Change in bowel or bladder habits
A sore that does not heal
Unusual bleeding or discharge
Thickening or lump in breast or elsewhere
Indigestion or difficulty in swallowing
Obvious change in wart or mole
Nagging cough or hoarseness

In the patient suspected of having cancer, the work-up should include a thorough history and physical examination. Other methods used to evaluate cancer patients are listed in Table 14-1. The surgeon should be particularly sensitive to symptoms such as dysphagia, epigastric discomfort and indigestion, changes in bowel habits, gastrointestinal bleeding, anorexia, weight loss, hematuria, vaginal bleeding, chronic cough, and hemoptysis. Any mole that has changed size, color, or configuration or that has bled should raise the suspicion of malignant melanoma.

During the physical examination, the surgeon should routinely palpate the cervical, supraclavicular, axillary, and inguinal lymph nodes if a tumor is suspected. The liver should be palpated for masses consistent with metastatic disease. In all adult patients, a rectal examination should be performed; it may disclose carcinoma of the rectum or prostate. In women, a pelvic examination is essential. The overall "performance status" of the patient can be recorded in a quantitative manner by use of the Karnofsky scale (Table 14-2).

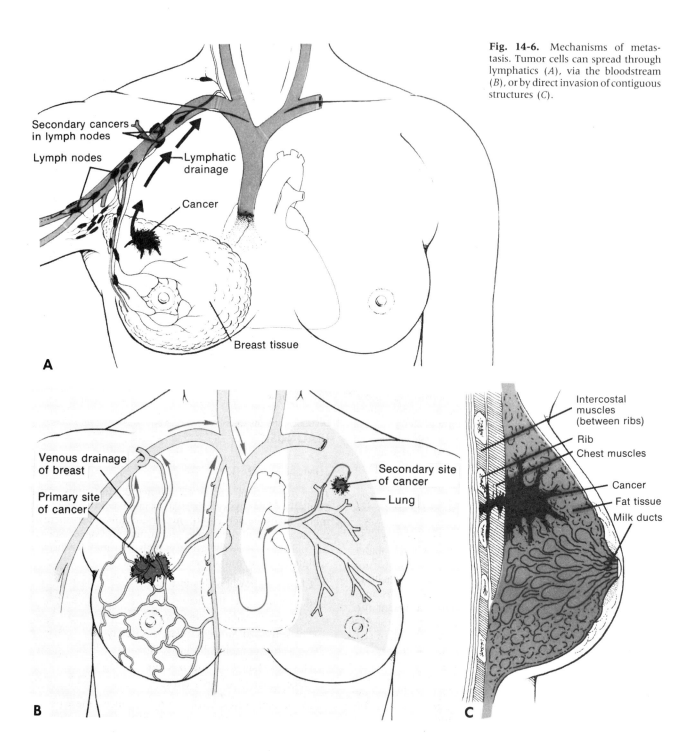

Fig. 14-6. Mechanisms of metastasis. Tumor cells can spread through lymphatics (*A*), via the bloodstream (*B*), or by direct invasion of contiguous structures (*C*).

A

- Secondary cancers in lymph nodes
- Lymph nodes
- Lymphatic drainage
- Cancer
- Breast tissue

B

- Venous drainage of breast
- Primary site of cancer
- Secondary site of cancer
- Lung

C

- Intercostal muscles (between ribs)
- Rib
- Chest muscles
- Cancer
- Fat tissue
- Milk ducts

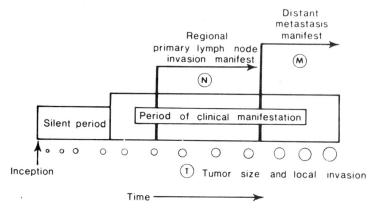

Distant metastasis manifest

Regional primary lymph node invasion manifest

(M)

(N)

Silent period

Period of clinical manifestation

Inception

(T) Tumor size and local invasion

Time ⟶

Fig. 14-7. Illustration of the classic concept of cancer metastasis by orderly spread to regional nodes and then to distant sites. (Manual for Staging of Cancer 1978, American Joint Committee for Cancer Staging and End-Results Reporting)

TABLE 14-1 ROUTINE METHODS TO EVALUATE CANCER PATIENTS AND DETERMINE THE EXTENT OF DISEASE

History
Physical examination
Chest x-ray film
Electrocardiogram
Blood tests
　Complete blood count
　Liver function tests
　Electrolytes, blood urea nitrogen, creatinine, glucose
　Tumor markers (carcinoembryonic antigen, α-fetoprotein)
Urinalysis
Cytology (Pap smear) of cervix, ascites, pleural fluid, urine (cytofluorimetry)
Nuclear scans (liver, bone, brain)
Ultrasound
Radiographic contrast studies (IVP, upper gastrointestinal series, barium enema, angiogram)
CT scan
Endoscopy (bronchoscopy, esophagogastroscopy, endoscopic retrograde cholangiographic panendoscopy, colonoscopy)
Bone-marrow aspirate
Biopsy of mass (needle, incisional, excisional)

TABLE 14-2 PERFORMANCE STATUS (KARNOFSKY SCALE)

CRITERIA OF PERFORMANCE STATUS		
Able to carry on normal activity; no special care needed	100	Normal, no complaints; no evidence of disease
	90	Able to carry on normal activity; minor signs or symptoms of disease
	80	Normal activity with effort; some signs or symptoms of disease
Unable to work; able to live at home and care for most personal needs; varying amount of assistance needed	70	Cares for self; unable to carry on normal activity or to do active work
	60	Requires occasional assistance but is able to care for most needs
	50	Requires considerable assistance and frequent medical care
Unable to care for self; requires equivalent of institutional or hospital care; disease may be progressing rapidly	40	Disabled; requires special care and assistance
	30	Severely disabled; hospitalization indicated although death not imminent
	20	Very sick; hospitalization necessary; active supportive treatment necessary
	10	Moribund; fatal processes progressing rapidly
	0	Dead

Routine evaluation of hematologic parameters and blood chemistries is performed and can disclose anemia or leukocytosis. Malignancy may be suggested by hypoproteinemia or elevation of liver function enzymes. Radiologic studies have increased the precision of diagnosis. Contrast studies, such as intravenous pyelogram (IVP), upper gastrointestinal x-ray series, barium enema with air contrast, and arteriogram, can be of value. Ultrasonography has the advantage of not exposing the patient to radiation. Nuclide scans of the liver, bone, and brain are useful, and the CT scan (Fig. 14-8) is an extremely powerful and precise tool.

BIOPSY

To be certain of a definitive diagnosis of malignant disease, a tissue diagnosis is required. The various methods of tissue biopsy are shown in Figure 14-9. Aspiration of a breast cyst is simply the insertion of a needle and withdrawal of fluid in a syringe. This fluid can be submitted for cytologic examination, although the yield of positive cytologies from such fluid is low. In these patients, a mammogram should be considered. Solid tumors such as breast carcinoma can be sampled by aspiration biopsy, simply by injection of a fraction of a milliliter of saline and vigorous withdrawal of

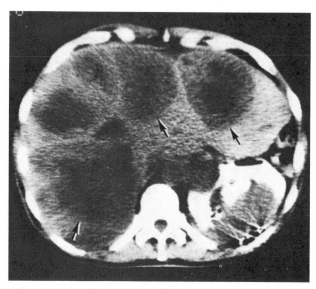

Fig. 14-8. Computed tomogram in a patient with cancer. Recurrent gastric leiomyosarcoma (*arrows*) presented as an epigastric mass, but it was shown in this study to involve much of the liver and to be unresectable.

the syringe barrel. This usually results in sufficient numbers of cells for cytologic examination.

Needle biopsy can be performed to obtain tissue from subcutaneous masses and some internal organs such as the liver. With this method, a Vim-Silverman or Tru-cut needle is used to take a core of tissue, but since the sample is small, the tumor itself (especially metastatic disease in the liver) may be missed. If the diagnosis is still in question, an open biopsy should be done. Transduodenal needle biopsy of the pancreas can be performed at laparotomy to diagnose carcinoma of the head of the pancreas without spreading tumor cells into the peritoneal cavity.

Excisional biopsy denotes the complete removal by an open technique of the lesion being biopsied, while incisional biopsy signifies that only a sample of the tumor is removed. Excisional biopsy is used for small skin lesions or small masses in the breast, and it allows the pathologist to examine the entire lesion.

An endoscopic biopsy is performed through an endoscope, usually with an alligator-type side-biting forceps.

Pathologic examination can be done using either frozen or permanent (paraffin) sections. A tentative diagnosis can be made in a few minutes for some types of tumors, using frozen section while the patient is under general anesthesia. The surgeon can then decide in consultation with the pathologist whether to proceed with a definitive resection or to close the biopsy site and wait 1 or 2 days for processing of the permanent sections.

STAGING AND GRADING

Grading of a tumor is a measurement of the degree of malignancy based on histologic appearance. Tumors are graded from 1 (least malignant) to 4 (most malignant). The finding of many mitoses suggests a high-grade cancer, as does anaplasia (Fig. 14-10).

Staging refers to the extent of local tumor and the presence or absence of metastatic cancer in regional lymph nodes or more distant sites. In general, Stage I refers to a tumor that

has not metastasized. Stage II is a tumor that has metastasized to the regional lymph nodes, while stages III and IV indicate distant metastases. The TNM system is a more sophisticated method of staging, where T represents the size of the primary tumor, N refers to the presence or absence of tumor in lymph nodes, and M indicates the presence or absence of distant metastases. The scheme for assigning TNM values to breast cancer is shown in Table 14-3.

SCREENING PROGRAMS

Cancer screening is the use of diagnostic tests in asymptomatic populations to identify patients with neoplasia. To be feasible in large groups, a relatively inexpensive and acceptable test must be initially employed. Examples are the routine chest radiograph, sputum cytology, breast mammogram, Pap smear of the cervix, and guaiac examination of the stool (Table 14-4). In the subset of persons with a positive test, more sophisticated and expensive examinations are used. Efforts are being made to define high-risk populations on the basis of known environmental carcinogens or genetic backgrounds, and screening is particularly useful in these populations.

TREATMENT

SURGERY

Operative treatment of cancer is most applicable to patients who have localized tumors without metastases. This guideline is not absolute, since surgical palliation is also possible and, occasionally, a curative attempt can be made by resection of a primary tumor plus a single metastasis in the liver or lung. However, curative surgery is more likely to be successful if the tumor is confined to the primary lesion or if spread is only to regional lymph nodes.

A major concept in the operative treatment of the cancer patient is *en bloc* resection, that is, removal of the primary tumor, the regional lymph nodes, and the intervening lymphatic channels as one specimen. This concept implies that the surgical incision and dissection be performed through normal tissue at an adequate distance from the tumor. The exact distance depends on the anatomy of the region being operated on and may need to be modified to preserve major nerves or blood vessels. The traditional method of resecting the site of a primary melanoma is to remove 5 cm of normal skin in all directions, plus the underlying fascia. However, there is little evidence that removing the fascia results in better control, and some authorities believe that the margin can be less than 5 cm for Clark's level I or II melanomas. If the surgeon is uncertain whether the margins are clear of tumor, he should remove an additional rim of normal tissue (which the pathologist can examine by frozen section), and he may wish to consider postoperative interstitial or external radiation therapy to assure local control.

The surgeon should be gentle in handling the tumor and should be careful not to spread tumor cells during the operation. When it is technically feasible, early ligation of the venous drainage from the tumor is a logical step. In operating on patients with carcinoma of the large bowel, many surgeons ligate the colon proximally and distally before manipulation of the tumor, to avoid intraluminal dissemination of tumor cells. One should avoid cutting into

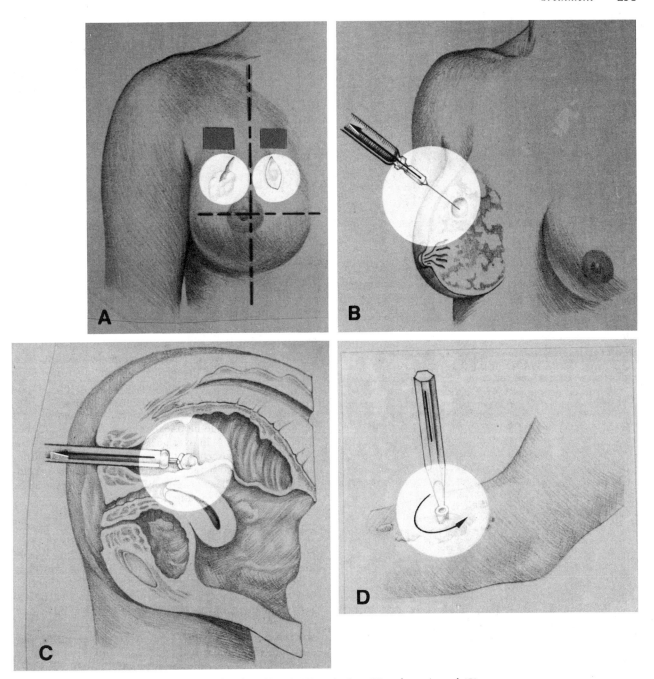

Fig. 14-9. Methods of biopsy. (*A*) incisional and excisional, (*B*) aspiration, (*C*) endoscopic, and (*D*) skin punch.

the tumor or rupturing it in such a way that tumor cells are spilled. If spillage does occur, copious irrigation of the area with hypotonic solution may destroy cells that could become implanted.

In some patients, cytoreductive surgery without total excision is performed for palliation, with the potential benefit that postoperative chemotherapy or radiation therapy will have a better chance of being effective. Such palliative surgery is justified if useful life can be prolonged, for example, for intraperitoneal ovarian carcinoma or locally recurrent soft-tissue sarcoma. However, it is the responsibility of the oncologic surgeon to advise against heroic attempts to reduce the tumor mass if this is not likely to benefit the patient for any meaningful length of time. In some circumstances, chemotherapy or radiation therapy

may produce sufficient tumor shrinkage to make surgery feasible. Surgical palliation also includes placement, in selected patients, of a chest tube to drain a malignant pleural effusion, creation of a pericardial window to relieve cardiac tamponade, or insertion of a peritoneovenous shunt for symptomatic, medically unresponsive malignant ascites.

Operative intervention can be important in the treatment of metastatic cancer. With the advent of effective chemotherapy, resection of lung metastases from cancer originating in the testis or bone is increasingly performed. Selected patients with liver metastases (solitary, or multiple in only one lobe) from cancer of the large bowel are amenable to cure by hepatic resection.

Surgery may play a crucial role in the staging of patients, for example, in those who are newly diagnosed as having

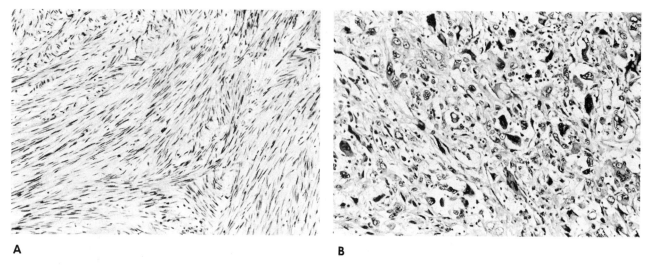

A   **B**

Fig. 14-10.   Different tumor grades. Grade 1 gastric leiomyosarcoma (*A*) is well differentiated and has mild cellular atypia and few mitoses. Grade 4 leiomyosarcoma (*B*) has severe (pleomorphic) atypia and numerous mitoses. (Lindsay PC, Ordonez N, Raaf JH: Gastric leiomyosarcoma: Clinical and pathological review of fifty patients. J Surg Oncol 18:399, 1981)

TABLE 14-3   TNM SYSTEM FOR BREAST CARCINOMA

SYMBOL	DESCRIPTION
T_1	Less than 2 cm
	No skin fixation
T_2	2 cm to 5 cm
	Skin dimpled
	No pectoral fixation
T_3	5 cm to 10 cm
	Skin infiltrated or ulcerated
	Pectoral fixation
T_4	More than 10 cm
	Skin involvement not beyond breast
	Chest-wall fixation
N_0	No nodes
N_1	Axillary nodes movable
	Not significant
	Significant
N_2	Axillary nodes fixed
N_3	Supraclavicular nodes
	Edema of arm
M_0	No metastases
M_1	Metastases including skin involvement beyond breast and contralateral nodes

FOUR CLINICAL STAGES DESIGNATED BY TNM SYMBOLS

Stage I	$T_1\ N_0\ M_0$
	$T_2\ N_0\ M_0$
Stage II	$T_1\ N_1\ M_0$
	$T_2\ N_1\ M_0$
Stage III	$T_1\ N_2$ or $N_3\ M_0$
	$T_2\ N_2$ or $N_3\ M_0$
	$T_3\ N_0\ N_1\ N_2$ or $N_3\ M_0$
	$T_4\ N_0\ N_1\ N_2$ or $N_3\ M_0$
Stage IV	Any combination of T and N symbols including M_1

(Copeland MD: American Joint Committee on Cancer Staging and End Results Reporting: Objectives and Progress. Cancer 18:1637, 1965)

Hodgkin's lymphoma. It is important to know whether the spleen, liver, or abdominal lymph nodes are involved, because if they are, the patient should be treated with chemotherapy and not radiation therapy alone. Several authors report that staging laparotomy for Hodgkin's lymphoma (which includes splenectomy, liver biopsy, and multiple lymph node biopsies) changes the stage assigned prior to laparotomy in over 30% of the patients.

Operative treatment of the cancer patient is often combined with chemotherapy or radiation therapy in a multidisciplinary approach. The nonsurgical modalities may be used before, during, or after the operation.

RADIATION THERAPY

For some tumors highly sensitive to radiation, this type of therapy should be the primary treatment (*e.g.*, in early stages of Hodgkin's lymphoma). Certain other tumors, such as carcinoma of the larynx, may be equally well treated with radiation therapy as with surgery, and radiation therapy will have the advantage of better preservation of structure and function. To avoid heavy irradiation of normal tissues, a radiotherapist often will use a cross-firing technique, in which the tumor is given a cancericidal dose from two or more beams coming from different directions.

Intracavitary radiation, a form of internal radiation therapy, is frequently used to treat cancer of the cervix. A radioactive material such as ^{137}Cs is placed, using specially designed applicators, into the uterus and vagina and left in place for a carefully calculated interval of up to several days.

The new field of brachytherapy (Gr. *brachy*—short) has to do with the delivery of radiation therapy by implanted (interstitial) sources of radiation. This is presently accomplished by implantation of seeds containing ^{125}I or by afterloading using catheters containing ^{192}Ir (Fig. 14-11). Both drawings in Figure 14-11 show a primary lung cancer with right hilar lymph node metastases. In the drawing on the left, external radiation is given using ^{60}Co and rotation; 6000 rads can be delivered to the tumor-bearing area, but the entire right lung receives at least 3000 rads, causing pulmonary fibrosis. The drawing on the right illustrates interstitial implantation, which delivers 15,000 rads to the

**TABLE 14-4 AMERICAN CANCER SOCIETY GUIDELINES
FOR THE EARLY DETECTION OF CANCER IN PEOPLE WITHOUT SYMPTOMS**

AGE 20–40	AGE 40 & OVER
Cancer-Related Checkup Every 3 Years Should include the procedures listed below plus health counseling (such as tips on quitting cigarettes) and examinations for cancers of the thyroid, testes, prostate, mouth, ovaries, skin, and lymph nodes. Some people are at higher risk for certain cancers and may need to have tests more frequently.	**Cancer-Related Checkup Every Year** Should include the procedures listed below plus health counseling (such as tips on quitting cigarettes) and examinations for cancers of the thyroid, testes, prostate, mouth, ovaries, skin, and lymph nodes. Some people are at higher risk for certain cancers and may need to have tests more frequently.
Breast Exam by doctor every 3 years Self-exam every month One baseline breast film between ages 35 and 40 Higher risk for breast cancer: personal or family history of breast cancer, never had children, first child after 30	**Breast** Exam by doctor every year Self-exam every month Breast film every year after age 50 (between ages 40-50, ask your doctor) Higher risk for breast cancer: personal or family history of breast cancer, never had children, first child after 30
Uterus Pelvic exam every 3 years Cervix Pap test—after 2 initial negative tests 1 year apart—*at least* every 3 years, includes women under 20 if sexually active Higher risk for cervical cancer: early age at first intercourse, multiple sex partners	**Uterus** Pelvic exam every year Cervix Pap test—after 2 initial negative tests 1 year apart—*at least* every 3 years Higher risk for cervical cancer: early age at first intercourse, multiple sex partners Endometrium Endometrial tissue sample at menopause if at risk Higher risk for endometrial cancer: infertility, obesity, failure of ovulation, abnormal uterine bleeding, estrogen therapy
	Colon & Rectum Digital rectal exam every year Guaiac slide test every year after age 50 Procto exam—after 2 initial negative tests 1 year apart—every 3 to 5 years after age 50 Higher risk for colorectal cancer: personal or family history of colon or rectal cancer, personal or family history of polyps in the colon or rectum, ulcerative colitis

tumor and minimal radiation to the normal lung tissue. Another advantage of brachytherapy is that even using afterloading catheters, treatment is completed in less than 1 week. External radiation therapy usually takes 3 to 6 weeks.

CHEMOTHERAPY

Chemotherapeutic agents have become part of the oncologist's armamentarium since World War II, when it was noted that nitrogen mustard, a product of chemical warfare research, could cause pancytopenia. Current classes of these agents include alkylating agents, antimetabolites, antibiotics, steroids, and miscellaneous drugs (Table 14-5, Fig. 14-12). Chemotherapy is administered either to achieve a therapeutic effect or as an adjuvant to prevent recurrent disease following definitive surgical extirpation. Chemotherapeutic agents are usually delivered orally or intravenously, although regional (intra-arterial) infusion is being explored on an experimental basis, often in combination with hyperthermia. It has been found that administering several chemotherapeutic agents, each of which is active against a particular tumor, is often more effective and less toxic than the use of a single agent alone. For example, the combination of 5-fluorouracil (5-FU), Adriamycin, and mitomycin-C (FAM) gives a response rate of 42% (*i.e.,* produces 50% or more tumor regression in 42% of the patients) for advanced gastric carcinoma, which is superior to any single drug administered alone (Table 14-6).

Much clinical research is presently being carried out to improve results of chemotherapeutic treatment. These studies are called phase I, II, or III trials. A new drug that has shown antitumor activity in an animal tumor system will then undergo a phase I trial, in which it is given in increasing doses to patients with a variety of tumor types in whom conventional types of therapy have failed. It is hoped that a tumor response will occur, but the main purpose of the phase I trial is to establish the maximum tolerated dose in humans so that major toxicity can be avoided in later trials.

The next step is for the drug to be given to patients with a single type of cancer (which is measurable) in whom treatment with other drugs has failed or for whom there is no known effective treatment. In this phase II trial, responses to the drug being tested are recorded as complete (CR), partial (PR, greater than 50% reduction of tumor mass),

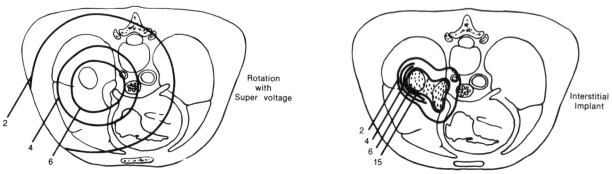

Fig. 14-11. Conventional external beam radiation therapy (*left*) compared to brachytherapy using interstitial implantation with ^{125}I seeds (*right*).

TABLE 14-5 CHEMOTHERAPEUTIC DRUGS

	ABBREVIATION	TRADE NAME		ABBREVIATION	TRADE NAME
Alkylating Agents			**Steroids and Antisteroids (cont.)**		
Nitrogen mustard (mechlorethamine)	HN$_2$	Mustargen	6-Methylhydroxypro-gesterone		Provera
Chlorambucil	CLB	Leukeran	Megestrol acetate		Megace
L-phenylalanine mustard (melphalan)	L-PAM	Alkeran	Prednisone		Meticorten
Cyclophosphamide	CTX	Cytoxan	Dexamethasone		Decadron
Triethylenethiophos-phoramide	TEPA	Thio-TEPA	Tamoxifen		Nolvadex
Busulfan	Bus	Myleran	**Plant Alkaloids**		
			Vincristine	VCR	Oncovin
Antimetabolites			Vinblastine	VLB	Velban
Methotrexate	MTX	Methotrexate			
6-Mercaptopurine	6-MP	Purinethol	**Miscellaneous**		
6-Thioguanine	6-TG	Thioguanine	L-Asparaginase	L-Asp	Elspar
5-Fluorouracil	5-FU	Fluorouracil	Carmustine	BCNU	BiCNU
Floxuridine		FUDR	Lomustine	CCNU	CeeNU
Cytosine arabinoside	Ara-C	Cytosar	Semustine (methyl-CCNU)	MeCCNU	
			Mitotane (o,p'-dichloro-diphenyl dichloro-ethane)	o'p'-DDD	Lysodren
Antibiotics					
Doxorubicin	Adria	Adriamycin	Dacarbazine (dimethyl imidazole triazeno carboxamide)	DTIC	DTIC
Bleomycin	Bleo	Blenoxane			
Dactinomycin (actinomycin D)	Dact, Act D	Cosmegen	Hydroxyurea	HU	Hydrea
Daunorubicin (daunomycin)	Daun	Cerubidine	Cisplatin (cis-platinum diamine dichloride)	Cis-DDP	Platinol
Mithramycin	Mith	Mithracin	Procarbazine	Procarb	Matulane
Mitomycin-C	Mito	Mutamycin	Hexamethylmelamine	HMM	
			Streptozotocin		Zanosar
Steroids and Antisteroids			Tegafur		Ftorafor
Testosterone propionate		Oreton	Teniposide		VM-26
Fluoxymesterone		Halotestin	Vindesine		Eldesine
Diethylstilbestrol	DES		Aminoglutethimide		
Ethinyl estradiol		Estinyl	AMSA (Amsacrine)		
Hydroxyprogesterone caproate		Delalutin	5-Azacytidine		
			Etoposide		VP16-213

minor (MR, less than 50% reduction of tumor mass), stabilization (no growth during the interval of treatment), or progression. Survival time is also measured in phase II trials, but this cannot be used to evaluate the treatment because survival is often more strongly influenced by prognostic factors than by the treatment itself. For example, patients with a good performance status who receive ineffective treatment may live longer than patients with a poor performance status who get effective therapy.

If a drug shows acceptable toxicity in a phase I trial and has antitumor activity in a phase II trial, it is ready for phase III study. In phase III trials, different forms of treatment

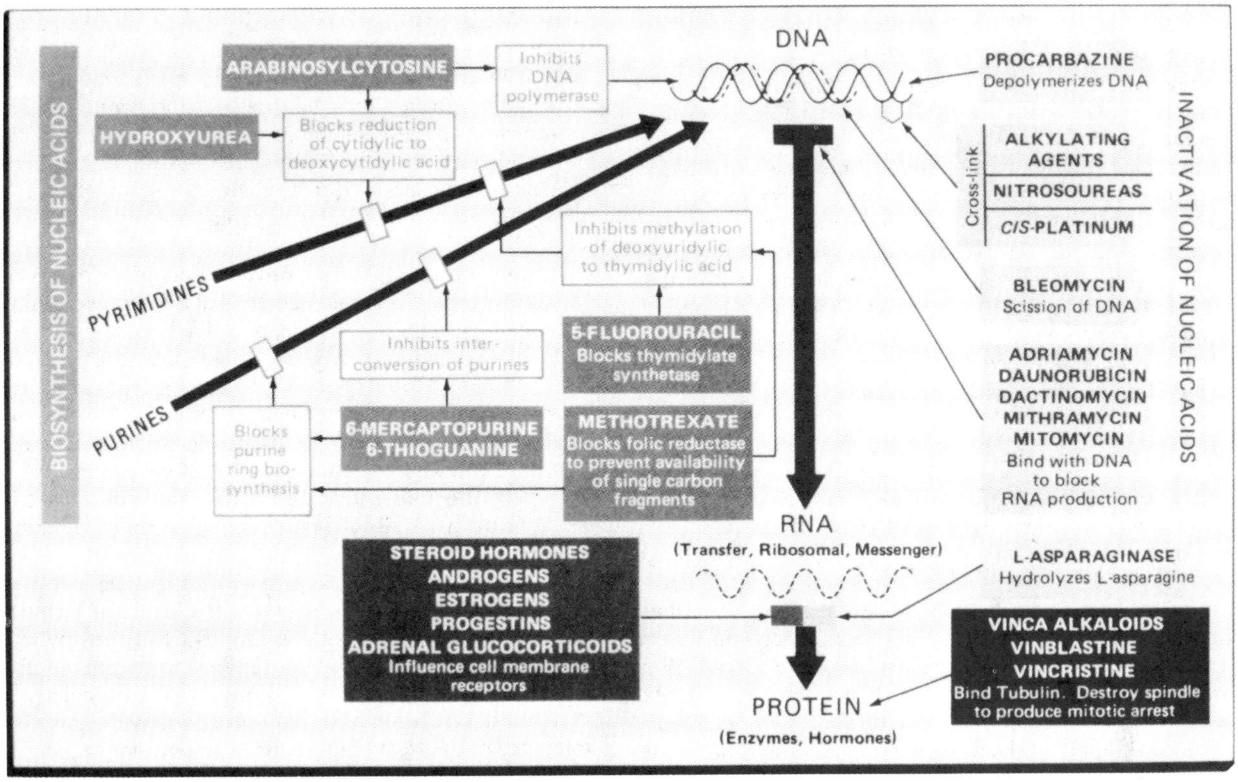

Fig. 14-12. Mechanisms of action of chemotherapeutic agents. (Krakoff IH: Cancer chemotherapeutic agents. Cancer 31:130, 1981)

are compared in two equivalent groups of patients; the patients are randomly assigned. If prognostic factors are well defined, patients can be "stratified," assuring that these factors are evenly balanced between the two groups. For example, stratification might assure equal distribution of poor-risk patients with very large or high-grade tumors. A phase III trial may compare the new drug to the best previous treatment or evaluate the addition of the new drug to a previously established treatment.

Chemotherapy given intravenously is often sclerotic to the peripheral surface veins through which it is administered. Thus, vascular access for chemotherapy can be a challenging problem; in difficult patients, this can be solved by the insertion of long-term Silastic central venous catheters (Hickman or Broviac) or by implantation of a polytetrafluoroethylene (PTFE) arteriovenous shunt.

Prior to any type of major surgery, patients who have received chemotherapy should be evaluated with particular care by the anesthesiologist, to avoid chemotherapy-related anesthetic complications. For example, doxorubicin can cause cardiomyopathy and may predispose to congestive failure; bleomycin increases the risk of pulmonary oxygen toxicity, so high levels of inspired oxygen must be strictly avoided; and cisplatin can cause renal toxicity, although renal failure can be prevented by prehydration and the use of mannitol. Halothane is avoided so there will be no confusion between possible halothane-induced hepatic toxicity and other forms of hepatic failure seen in cancer patients. Of course, patients with severe leukopenia or thrombocytopenia (perhaps resulting in nadir sepsis) due to marrow depression by cytotoxic drugs should not be operated on except in emergencies. Bone-marrow recovery

usually takes only 1 to 2 weeks, not too long an interval to postpone elective surgery.

The development of tensile strength in healing wounds can be delayed by administration of chemotherapy before wounding. However, this effect is usually not of clinical significance if sound surgical technique for wound closure is used. Nonabsorbable sutures can be left in place for several weeks if healing appears slow or the patient has been treated with steroids. One should attempt to avoid making incisions in heavily irradiated areas, even though such wounds will eventually heal.

TABLE 14-6   SINGLE AND COMBINATION CYTOTOXIC DRUG THERAPY FOR GASTRIC CARCINOMA

Drug	Response Rate (%)
5-Fluorouracil (5-FU)	21
Nitrosoureas	
1-BCNU (BiCNU)	18
1-methyl-CCNU (CeeNU)	15
Mitomycin-C (Mutamycin)	25
Doxorubicin (Adriamycin)	30
Cisplatin (Platinol)	20
5-FU plus BiCNU	41
5-FU plus Adriamycin plus Mutamycin	42
5-FU plus Adriamycin plus BiCNU	approx. 40

(Woolley PV: Gastric cancer: What chemotherapy can accomplish. Your Patient and Cancer 1:46, July 1981)

HORMONAL MANIPULATION

Patients with hormone-dependent tumors such as cancer of the breast or prostate can benefit from hormonal manipulation. Response of cancer of the breast to this form of treatment depends on the presence of steroid receptors on the tumor cells. Bilateral oophorectomy is worthwhile in premenopausal women with estrogen receptor–positive (ER+) tumors, since 50% to 60% will respond, whereas the response will be less than 10% in estrogen receptor–negative (ER−) patients. In patients who respond, further palliation can be achieved by bilateral total adrenalectomy or hypophysectomy. At present, efforts are being made to achieve comparable benefit pharmacologically with aminoglutethimide, an adrenal suppressant.

HYPERTHERMIA

Tumor cells growing in tissue culture appear to be more sensitive to heat than are normal cells. This difference in sensitivity is most marked at temperatures in the range 41° C to 44° C, a range that is lower than the threshold of thermal pain in humans (45° C). Also, since the blood flow through many tumors is reduced as compared with normal tissues, tumors may retain heat and act as heat reservoirs. These observations suggest that hyperthermia could be useful as cancer therapy, and clinical trials are under way. Methods of applying heat include regional limb perfusion (for unresectable tumors of the extremity), total-body hyperthermia (by an arteriovenous shunt connected to an extracorporeal heat exchanger, application of hot-water blankets, or immersion in molten wax), and local hyperthermia. Local heat can be produced by ultrasound, microwaves, or radio-frequency waves, while deep-seated tumors can by heated by a magnetic-loop induction coil. Heat may be combined with conventional external-beam radiation or chemotherapy. All of these hyperthermia methods are promising but still experimental.

NUTRITIONAL SUPPORT

Protein-calorie malnutrition is found in up to 30% of hospitalized patients and is especially common among patients with cancer. The cachexia associated with advanced malignancy may be due to decreased intake (secondary to anorexia, difficulty in swallowing, or gastrointestinal obstruction) or increased loss (related to malabsorption or intestinal fistula). Malnutrition contributes to anemia, hypoproteinemia, impaired healing, reduced immunocompetence, and decreased resistance to infection. A malnourished patient with cancer may tolerate poorly a major operation or a course of radiation therapy or combination chemotherapy.

Some types of cancer are especially likely to be associated with malnutrition. Tumors of the mouth, pharynx, larynx, and esophagus make it difficult for patients to eat solid food. Patients with cancer of the head and neck are often heavy users of alcohol and tobacco and frequently have a poor diet. Head and neck surgery itself may at least temporarily lead to decreased oral intake, while radiotherapy to this region can cause stomatitis, mucositis, and decreased salivary secretion. Monilial infections of the pharynx and esophagus are common during periods of leukopenia and nadir sepsis following chemotherapy. Anorexia is common in many patients with cancer and seems to be associated at an early stage with certain tumor types such as carcinoma of the lung. An alteration of taste may be contributory.

Nutritional support can be given by either the enteral route (through the intestinal tract) or the parenteral route (intravenous hyperalimentation—IVH). If the patient is not extremely sick and is well motivated, his calorie intake can usually be increased by dietary counseling and use of one of the many commercially prepared oral nutrient supplements.

In the anorexic, poorly motivated patient, or one whose disease impairs oral intake, enteral tube feedings should be tried. Soft silastic No. 8 nasogastric feeding tubes are now available, which are more comfortable than the previously used large-bore tubes. The silastic feeding tubes are carried into the duodenum or upper jejunum by means of a mercury-filled capsule attached to the tip, reducing the potential for vomiting and aspiration. Long-term enteral support is usually by gastrostomy, although a fine-bore tube placed at laparotomy as a needle-catheter jejunostomy is gaining popularity.

Parenteral nutrition is given to cancer patients with nonfunctioning intestinal tracts by the standard technique of IVH. Patients faced with strenuous treatment involving induction chemotherapy, bone-marrow transplantation, or radical abdominal or thoracic surgery are candidates for IVH. Nutritional support during this period will allow better tolerance of the treatment, reduce complications, and maximize the chance of a response.

It is obvious that nutritional support is an important therapeutic modality in treating cancer and that the method of support must be individualized for each patient.

MANAGEMENT OF PAIN

Not all cancers cause pain, but a significant number of cancer patients suffer from pain in the terminal stages of their disease. The most effective way to relieve cancer-related pain is to eradicate the tumor or reduce its size. Radiation therapy, for example, can be quite effective in palliating pain in patients with osseous metastases. However, if the patient has progressive disease that no longer responds to treatment, the pain should still be controllable by adequate amounts of analgesics. Inadequate use of these drugs by physicians is surprisingly common, reflecting misconceptions and unjustified fear of addiction, as well as lack of knowledge of analgesic pharmacology. It is important to recognize that the patient with pain due to cancer is quite different from an otherwise well drug addict. The addict is psychologically dependent on the drug, whereas the cancer patient is not. When cancer patients are sent home on large doses of oral narcotics, they rarely abuse their medication, do not attempt suicide, and can be weaned from the narcotics if necessary without significant problems. Patients must be individualized, and many will benefit if their pain medication is given regularly, around the clock, rather than on demand.

PSYCHOLOGICAL SUPPORT

The cancer patient and his family deserve to be told the truth about the diagnosis. However, this can and should be presented in as positive a manner as possible, emphasizing possibilities for successful treatment. At least initially, an attitude of uncertainty should be adopted regarding prognosis. The patient will do better if he is assured of his physician's interest and support in the future and if his hope for returning to his home and family can be maintained.

UNPROVED METHODS

The diagnosis of cancer may provoke great anxiety in the patient and the family. This, together with the misconception that cancer treatment will be intolerable in itself, makes the patient uniquely susceptible to purveyors of unproved therapy. For example, it is estimated that 70,000 American cancer patients have used the drug Laetrile (amygdalin), and Laetrile proponents have convinced 22 state legislatures to legalize its use. When an unconventional treatment achieves such widespread popularity, it is appropriate to test it in a well-controlled trial despite the lack of preliminary evidence of effectiveness. A National Cancer Institute–supported multicenter study, in which 178 patients were given Laetrile (plus "metabolic" treatment), recently demonstrated Laetrile's lack of antitumor activity in humans. Recognizing the patient's right of choice, the physician must establish a supportive relationship so he can guide the patient away from such useless and often exploitative therapy.

TUMOR IMMUNOLOGY AND IMMUNOTHERAPY

The theory of immune surveillance was proposed by Thomas and Burnett, who suggested that the purpose of the immune system might be not only to combat invading pathogens but also to attack and kill the host's own cells that had undergone malignant transformation by somatic mutation. Such cells would be recognized by the appearance of new surface tumor antigens and would be eliminated mainly by a cellular immune mechanism. Failure of immune surveillance might be due to attachment of "blocking antibodies" to tumor antigens, thereby preventing recognition of tumor cells by sensitized lymphocytes.

The idea of immune surveillance as a natural defense against cancer is attractive for several reasons. First, it can explain the occasionally observed spontaneous regression of tumors. Second, assays of immune competence, for instance delayed hypersensitivity skin testing with a *de novo* antigen, such as dinitrochlorobenzene (DNCB), or with recall antigens (*e.g.*, tuberculin, *Candida*, mumps, and streptokinase–streptodornase), show that many cancer patients have impaired cellular immunity. Anergy (lack of immune reactivity) is often found in patients with head and neck malignancy, even at an early stage of their disease. Finally, immune surveillance can explain why patients who receive long-term immunosuppressive drugs have a higher-than-normal incidence of tumors. The theory is not consistent with the observation that athymic nude mice, which lack thymus-derived lymphocytes (T cells), do not develop spontaneous or chemically induced tumors more frequently than normal mice. Nude mice do have natural killer (NK) lymphocytes, which may be capable of eliminating cancer cells.

The presence of tumor-specific transplantation antigens (TSTAs) on the cell surface of chemically induced tumors of mice can be demonstrated by rejection of these tumors after transplantation into syngeneic animals. Prehn and Main, using methylcholanthrene-induced sarcomas, showed that rejection was specific for the immunizing tumor. Unfortunately, further studies on these antigens (and also on

TSTAs in humans) have been thwarted by difficulties in producing antibodies specific for individual TSTAs. Syngeneic antiserums to mouse tumors have shown extensive cross-reactions to other tumor-associated antigens, including embryonic antigens, fetal bovine serum components in the case of cultured tumors, and murine leukemia virus–associated antigens, which are widely expressed on mouse tumors and normal tissues. It is hoped that antibodies produced by hybridoma technology will have a more highly restricted specificity for unique TSTAs on both human and animal tumors.

Many attempts have been made to stimulate patients' immunity to their cancer, mainly by administration of nonspecific immunotherapeutic adjuvants, including bacillus Calmette-Guérin (BCG), *Corynebacterium parvum*, levamisole, mixed bacterial vaccine (MBV, modeled after Coley's toxin), and polynucleotides such as poly AU. The direct intralesional injection of BCG or DNCB into a small melanoma skin metastasis is effective in creating local inflammation and bringing about the disappearance of the injected lesion. Despite extensive clinical trials, however, the overall role and value of immune adjuvants in treating or preventing human malignancy are still uncertain.

Future investigation with immunotherapy will involve treatment of patients with killed tumor cells (active immunization) and with lymphocytes previously sensitized against tumor antigens (passive immunization). Trials are in progress using another biologic-response modifier, interferon, which is not a single substance but a family of proteins produced by cells in response to viral infection or other stimuli. Interferons are now classified as alpha (formerly leukocyte interferon), beta (formerly fibroblast), and gamma (formerly immune interferon). Recombinant DNA techniques will permit the manufacture of very pure preparations of these agents. The most promising use of interferon is perhaps in those tumors strongly suspected to be associated with viruses, such as juvenile laryngeal papilloma, venereal wart (condyloma acuminatum), and Kaposi's sarcoma in homosexual males. Excellent responses have also been seen in patients with nodular, poorly differentiated lymphocytic lymphoma.

TUMOR MARKERS

Tumor markers are biochemical substances produced by a cancer and found circulating in the blood. At present, only a few are specific to a particular neoplasm, but it is likely that hybridoma techniques will lead to other more specific immunochemical assays. Tumor markers can be divided into four categories: fetal-placental markers, hormonal markers, nonspecific biochemical markers, and immunoglobulins.

Fetal-placental markers include carcinoembryonic antigen (CEA), α-fetoprotein, and human chorionic gonadotropin. CEA is a useful test to assess the presence of recurrent cancer of the large bowel. CEA is also elevated in breast cancer, and it can be moderately elevated in smokers and persons with benign liver disease. α-Fetoprotein is a marker for the presence of hepatocellular carcinoma and may also be elevated in germ cell tumors of the testis. High-risk populations for liver cancer in China are now screened with the α-fetoprotein assay, and small, curable liver tumors are being found. The β-subunit of human chorionic gonadotropin is usually positive in patients with choriocarcinoma and is commonly elevated in germ cell tumors of the testis.

Useful hormonal markers are calcitonin (medullary carcinoma of the thyroid), catecholamines (neuroblastoma and pheochromocytoma), serotonin (carcinoid), and steroid hormones (adrenal tumors). Insulin and glucagon are markers for rare pancreatic endocrine tumors.

Nonspecific biochemical markers include lactate dehydrogenase (elevated in patients with malignant lymphoma) and acid phosphatase (elevated in patients with prostatic carcinoma). Immunoglobulins are markers for multiple myeloma and Waldenström's macroglobulinemia.

PROGNOSIS

After the cancer patient is treated for cure, he and his family usually seek information about prognosis. Ordinarily, estimates are provided based on survival figures determined for cancer at that site and adjusted to grade, histology, location, and stage. These data may be useful, but they can be misleading, since there are many variables, such as the biologic characteristics of the tumor, that are presently not fully understood. Some rough quantitation is possible: Most recurrences from lung or oropharyngeal cancer will occur within 2 years, but a substantial proportion of patients with breast or large-bowel cancer will have a recurrence after 5 years.

Factors that worsen the prognosis include high-grade tumor (low degree of differentiation), presence of tumor in regional nodes or distant sites, presence of primary or metastatic tumor in vital organs (*e.g.*, brain or liver), and, perhaps most important, the biology of the histologic tumor type. For example, if the tumor is papillary carcinoma of the thyroid, it may have an indolent course for several decades, but an anaplastic carcinoma of the thyroid of the same size is much more likely to be lethal within 6 months. The primary location of the tumor is also important. Small lesions on the skin or lip are likely to be brought to the attention of the physician at an early stage, but tumors of the stomach or lung, for example, are generally not recognized until they are large; therefore, they are among the hardest to cure.

It is never possible to predict exactly how long the patient will live, and the patient who survives for 5 years without evidence of recurrence or metastasis is traditionally told that most likely he is cured. However, he should continue to receive careful follow-up care. Periodic assessment after operation depends most importantly on history of any symptoms and also on physical examination, blood tests, and radiographs. The purpose is to assure good health, identify early recurrence when it is possibly curable, and search for second primary tumors.

SURGICAL ONCOLOGY AND CLINICAL RESEARCH

The care of patients with cancer forms part of the professional activity of most general surgeons and of many surgeons who practice the surgical specialties. However, some physicians, because of particular interest or by virtue of special fellowship training, choose to limit their practice almost entirely to the treatment of cancer patients and regard themselves as surgical oncologists; often, they belong to national societies for oncologists.

The function of the surgical oncologist is not to perform all the cancer surgery in his institution but rather to be a leader in cancer-related education and research. He should keep up to date in areas of multidisciplinary treatment controversy, such as the management of carcinoma of the breast. He should interpret for his colleagues the published results of clinical trials and therefore must be familiar with biostatistical methods such as Kaplan-Meier and life-table analyses. When feasible, he should encourage suitable patients from his own institution to enter clinical studies so that further progress can be made in our understanding and management of cancer.

BIBLIOGRAPHY

ADAIR F, BERG J, JOUBERT L et al: Long-term follow-up of breast cancer patient: The 30 year report. Cancer 33:1145, 1974

American Cancer Society: 1981 Cancer Facts and Figures, 1982

BALCH CM, MURAD TM, SOONG SJ et al: Tumor thickness as a guide to surgical management of clinical stage I melanoma patients. Cancer 43:883, 1979

BASERGA R: The cell cycle. N Engl J Med 304:453, 1981

BEATTIE EJ, MARTINI N, ROSEN G: The management of pulmonary metastasis in children with osteogenic sarcoma with surgical resection combined with chemotherapy. Cancer 35:618, 1975

BECKER FF: Recent concepts of initiation and promotion in carcinogenesis. Am J Pathol 105:3 1981

BITTNER JJ: Some possible effects of nursing on the mammary gland tumor incidence in mice. Science 84:162, 1936

BURCHENAL JH, OETTGEN HF (eds): Cancer: Achievements, Challenges, and Prospects for the 1980s, 2 vols. New York, Grune & Stratton, 1981

BURKITT D: A sarcoma involving the jaw in African children. Br J Surg 46:218, 1958

BURNETT FM: Immunological Surveillance. Elmsford, NY, Pergamon Press, 1970

CLAYSON DB: Nutrition and experimental carcinogenesis: A review. Cancer Res 35:3292, 1975

COLE WH, McDONALD GO, ROBERTS SS et al: Dissemination of Cancer. New York, Appleton-Century-Crofts, 1961

COPELAND EM, DUDRICK SJ: Nutritional aspects of cancer. Curr Probl Cancer 1:1, 1976

DEVITA VT: The evolution of therapeutic research in cancer. N Engl J Med 298:907, 1978

DEVITA VT, HELLMAN S, ROSENBERG SA (eds): Cancer: Principles and Practice of Oncology. Philadelphia, J B Lippincott, 1981

DOLL R, PETO R: Mortality in relation to smoking: 20 Years' observations on male British doctors. Br Med J 2:1525, 1976

DOLL R, PETO R: The causes of cancer: Quantitative estimates of avoidable risks of cancer in the United States today. J Natl Cancer Inst 66:1191, 1981

DUNPHY JE: On caring for the patient with cancer. N Engl J Med 295:313, 1976

FARBER E: Chemical carcinogenesis. N Engl J Med 305:1379, 1981

FOLEY KM: The management of pain of malignant origin. In Tyler HR, Dawson DM (eds): Current Neurology, vol 2. Boston, Houghton Mifflin, 1979

FOLKMAN J, MERLER E, ABERNATHY C et al: Isolation of a tumor factor responsible for angiogenesis. J Exp Med 133:275, 1971

GOEDERT JJ, NEULAND CY, WALLEN WC et al: Amyl nitrite may alter T lymphocytes in homosexual men. Lancet I:412, 1982

GOLD P, WILSON J, ROMERO R et al: Immunology and colonic carcinoma: Further evaluation of the radioimmunoassay for carcinoembryonic antigen of the human digestive system as an adjunct in cancer diagnosis. Dis Colon Rectum 16:358, 1973

GRAVES G, CUNNINGHAM P, RAAF JH: Effect of chemotherapy on the healing of surgical wounds. Clin Bull 10, No. 4:144, 1980

GREEN I, COHEN S, McCLUSKEY RT (eds): Mechanisms of Tumor Immunity. New York, John Wiley & Sons, 1977

HALSTED WS: The results of operations for the cure of cancer of the breast performed at the Johns Hopkins Hospital from June 1889 to January 1894. Ann Surg 20:297, 1894

MACEK C: Oncogenes: New evidence on link to cancer. JAMA 247:1098, 1982

MARKS PA: Distinguished address: Genetic predisposition to cancer. Surgery 90:132, 1981

MILES W: Abdominoperineal operation. Cancer 2:1812, 1980

MORTON DL: Immunological aspects of neoplasia: A rational basis for immunotherapy. Ann Intern Med 74:587, 1971

OLD LJ, BOYSE EA, CLARKE DA et al: Antigenic properties of chemically induced tumors, Ann NY Acad Sci 101:80, 1962

PENN I, HALGRIMSON CG, STARZL TE: De novo malignant tumor in organ transplant recipients. Transplant Proc 3:773, 1973

POTT P: Chirurgical Observations Relative to the Cataract, The Polypus of the Nose, the Cancer of the Scrotum, the Different Kinds of Ruptures, and the Mortification of the Toes and Feet. London, Hawes, Clarke, and Collins, 1775

RAAF JH: Vascular access prostheses in the management of cancer patients. Clin Bull 10, No. 3:91, 1980

Radiologic and Other Biophysical Methods in Tumor Diagnosis. Chicago, Year Book Medical Publishers, 1975

REIF AE: The causes of cancer. Am Sci 69:437, 1981

ROUS P, KIDD JG: The carcinogenic effect of a papilloma virus on the tarred skin of rabbits: I. Description of the phenomenon. J Exp Med 67:399, 1938

RUDDON RW: Biological Markers of Neoplasia: Basic and Applied Aspects. New York, Elsevier, 1978

RUDDON RW: Cancer Biology. New York, Oxford University Press, 1981

SUGARBAKER EV: Cancer metastasis: A product of tumor-host interactions. Curr Probl Cancer III, No. 7:1, 1979

WALDENSTROM JG: Paraneoplasia: Biological Signals in the Diagnosis of Cancer. New York, John Wiley & Sons, 1978

WANGENSTEEN OH: Should patients be told they have cancer? Surgery 27:944, 1950

WHIPPLE AO, PARSON WB, MULLINS CR: Treatment of carcinoma of the ampulla of Vater. Ann Surg 102:763, 1935

WILLIAMS RR, HORM JW: Association of cancer sites with tobacco and alcohol consumption and socioeconomic status of patients: Interview study from the Third National Cancer Survey. J Natl Cancer Inst 58:525, 1977

WYNDER EL: Conference on the primary prevention of cancer: Assessment of risk factors and future directions. Prev Med 9:163, 1980

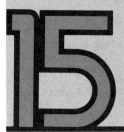

Jonathan E. Rhoads, Jr.

Preoperative Preparation of the Patient

The operation itself is the central act of surgical care, but the outcome of surgical treatment is tremendously enhanced by accurate preoperative assessment and careful preoperative preparation. (Postoperative care is of equal importance, but it is not the subject of this chapter.)

Optimal preparation of the patient depends upon a conscious assessment and integration of factors relating to the patient's illness, physical condition, related medical conditions, and current surgical diagnosis with the intention of decreasing surgical and anesthetic risks. Precise diagnosis, carefully considered therapeutic plans and goals, knowledge, skill, judgment, and experience with thoughtful doctor–patient interaction are all factors that ultimately contribute

PRESURGICAL ASSESSMENT
Respiratory status and function
Blood volume and state of hydration
Cardiac status and function
Renal status and function
Presence of endocrine problems
Nutritional status
Medications
Electrolyte and acid–base status
Coagulation status
Hepatic status and function
Other medical problems affecting surgery

to the best outcome. A well-informed, compliant, physiologically prepared patient in the hands of a knowledgeable surgeon who has a precise diagnosis and is mindful of complications and their prevention and management will make the best recovery from surgical disease.

PREOPERATIVE ASSESSMENT OF THE PATIENT

Surgical care begins with gathering information about the patient's symptoms, previous illness and treatments, and physical condition, analyzing the results of a variety of tests, x-ray films, and studies, and then arriving at a diagnosis. The extent of the disease process, its prognosis, the severity of the symptoms, and the urgency of the problem will figure prominently in arriving at a decision of whether or not to offer operative treatment, when to offer such treatment, and which operation among several available choices should be proposed.

When a surgeon is confronted with a patient whose clinical problem may require surgical intervention, his thoughts will be continuously comparing the information he receives with the immediacy of the situation, the priority of the patient's various problems, and the availability of resources and support services needed for the optimum delivery of care. A very urgent situation such as exsanguination (or the threat of exsanguination) from an injury or a ruptured aneurysm forces a surgeon to make major compromises with the usual careful preoperative evaluation and preparation for an elective operation. The overwhelming feature of the case may be the need to operate and stop the bleeding. Conversely, a patient with a recent myocardial infarction is not a candidate for any but the most urgent operative procedure because of the risk of death from recurrent infarction or other cardiac complications. The timing and extent of surgical activity will depend strongly on the clinical situation.

Although the practice of surgery reflected by the chapters in this text is the optimal state of the art available to cooperative patients in modern medical centers under ideal situations, any of a wide variety of adverse factors may force the surgeon to change the plan of care to cope with the unavailability of needed services. Some examples in the author's experience include the following: The intensive care unit is full and cannot accept your patient; the blood bank is out of blood or platelets; the operating room is not available at a time you consider optimal; the nurses or other hospital employees are on strike; a consultant cannot be located or persuaded to come to provide a needed opinion or service at short notice. The list of potential impediments to care is endless, and the probability of an impediment increases with distance from a major medical center. The availability of resources must be considered in planning the evaluation and treatment of a patient.

HISTORY

A careful history will allow the physician to make the diagnosis in many cases. In this era of highly sophisticated diagnostic measures such as sonograms, angiograms, and CT scans, a careful and complete history and physical examination remain the backbone of patient evaluation. It is this basic knowledge that leads to the appropriate evaluation and therapy. The major symptoms need to be defined as completely as possible. For example, the symptom of pain can be delineated according to its location, its direction of radiation, its quality (burning, aching, sharp, dull), its severity, its duration, its behavior in time (steady, intermittent, fluctuating, increasing, decreasing, and change in location or character, its relation to position and activity, inciting factors (eating, urinating, emotional stress), factors that relieve it, remedies that have been tried and their results, previous episodes, and its relation to other symptoms such as belching or vomiting.

Of particular interest to surgeons is precise knowledge of the pathology reports of previously removed tissues and biopsies and complete reports of previous operations, especially those in the area of the current problem. Detailed information on the amount and extent of radiotherapy is equally important. A sure knowledge of exact tissue diagnosis is so important in the management of neoplastic diseases that microscopic sections from other centers should be reviewed by one's own pathologist. A surgeon wants to know how the normal anatomy and physiology has been altered by previous surgery or radiotherapy, how much of an organ has been removed, how much function of that organ remains, and where he will encounter scarring or distortion that may exert important limitations on what surgical activity is technically feasible.

Careful elicitation and documentation of a history of allergy is extremely important. A surgeon may want to administer drugs while the patient is under anesthesia or in the postoperative period when the patient may give a poor history because he is receiving narcotics and is uncomfortable. A fatal anaphylactic reaction may occur if a drug to which the patient is allergic is administered.

PHYSICAL EXAMINATION

Physical examination is best carried out with the patient unclothed, in good light, and in a quiet, peaceful, private place. A discussion of all the details of physical examination as well as much of the art of history-taking is beyond the scope of this chapter, and the reader is referred to standard texts on physical diagnosis. Lumps and masses are of interest to all surgeons. A lump or mass should be described in terms of its location, its size, its color, its relationship to adjacent structures, and its consistency (firm, soft, fluctuant); whether it is mobile or fixed to superficial structures or deep structures; whether it is tender or not; whether it causes deformity of adjacent structures; and whether it pulsates, and if so, whether the pulsation is inherent or transmitted. Knowledge of all these factors is necessary in arriving at a diagnosis of the mass and in planning its biopsy, removal, or other treatment. Frequently a picture or diagram in the chart is useful in documenting the findings (Fig. 15-1).

LABORATORY, ROENTGENOLOGIC, AND ELECTROCARDIOGRAPHIC EXAMINATIONS

Routine evaluation of a patient includes a urinalysis, complete blood count (CBC), blood sugar, blood urea nitrogen, serum electrolytes, prothrombin time, and partial thromboplastin generation time prior to surgery. Additional tests of liver function, serum protein, serum calcium and phosphates, and uric acid are done in many patients because the currently available automatic biochemical testing equipment makes these determinations readily available. Virtually all patients admitted with upper abdominal pain should have a serum amylase determination to help evaluate the possibility of pancreatitis. A wide variety of less commonly performed measurements are also available. Analysis of gastric juice and other secretions is frequently helpful. Arterial blood gas determinations are widely performed when indications are appropriate.

It is routine to obtain a chest film for virtually all patients admitted to the hospital (possible exceptions being healthy children and young adults admitted for a routine surgical procedure such as repair of a hernia or a tonsillectomy). Additional radiologic views or techniques, films of other parts of the body, fluoroscopic examinations, and studies with radiopaque contrast materials are carried out when indicated. They give clues to the nature of the disease process, its anatomic location, and its extent. Ultrasonograms, radioisotopic scans, and CT scans give additional very useful information. Any organ that is to undergo major surgery should be adequately evaluated roentgenologically before the operation. However, multiple modalities generating the same information are costly and time-consuming and should be obtained only after careful consideration.

Electrocardiograms are performed routinely on middle-aged and elderly patients admitted to the hospital.

ENDOSCOPIC EXAMINATION

Fiberoptic endoscopes have made an increasing number of the body's epithelial surfaces available to easy, direct visualization by physicians. Many areas of the body such as the stomach, the colon, the bronchi, the bladder, and certain joints are now studied regularly prior to operation upon them.

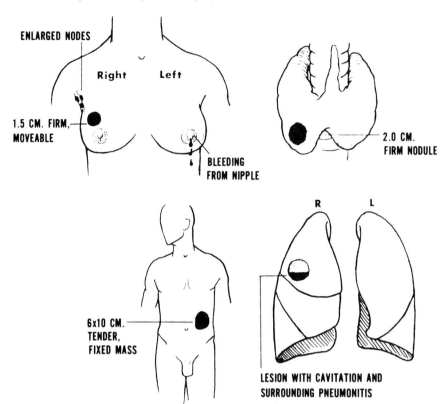

ENLARGED NODES

Right   Left

1.5 CM. FIRM, MOVEABLE

BLEEDING FROM NIPPLE

2.0 CM. FIRM NODULE

6x10 CM. TENDER, FIXED MASS

R   L

LESION WITH CAVITATION AND SURROUNDING PNEUMONITIS

Fig. 15-1. Examples of documentation of physical examination.

All of the foregoing tests are subject to errors of interpretation, and the surgeon should be aware of them.

When all data have been obtained and assembled, the surgeon has enough information to establish a diagnosis and to know something about the extent of the disease process and how it affects the patient physiologically, psychologically, and socially. The surgeon knows about the patient's concomitant diseases and is in a position to treat or modify them prior to subjecting the patient to anesthesia and operation. Finally, he is able to weigh risks and to plan the operation that is likely to benefit the patient most with the least risk.

PSYCHOLOGICAL PREPARATION OF THE PATIENT

Patients approach an operation with considerable anxiety and fear, which are reasonable. They know they will be in an environment to which they are unaccustomed, and they know they can expect a variety of painful experiences ranging from drawing blood and intramuscular injections to postoperative incisional pain. Some fear they will not have good anesthesia during the operation. Some have fears of dying and of mutilation, and some have fears of the unknown. In addition, there may be much apprehension based on fantasy, rumor, or hearsay.

The surgeon is first and foremost a physician. A physician–patient relationship begins as soon as the patient meets the surgeon. At the time of the first meeting the surgeon begins preparing the patient psychologically for his operative treatment. The surgeon has the opportunity to inspire confidence and allay fears. He should take time to answer questions sympathetically and in understandable terms. Drawings and diagrams may help the patient understand

the operation. The surgeon should be firm in matters about which he is sure and be willing to admit ignorance when the answers are not known.

Advising the patient about what he will experience at different stages of his preoperative care allays suspicion and fear and inspires confidence. It is helpful to the patient to know what routine to expect when he is admitted and that he may be examined by house officers and medical students. He needs to know what preoperative preparations will be made and what tests will be performed.

The patient needs to be told preoperatively what can be expected postoperatively: where he will be; whether he will have a nasogastric tube in place; whether there will be an endotracheal tube in his mouth to help him breathe and he will be unable to talk until it is removed; whether, if there is to be a tracheostomy or a colostomy, it will be temporary or permanent; whether an extremity will be immobilized or amputated.

The patient should know what will be expected of him in the postoperative period—for instance, he will be asked to take deep breaths and cough to minimize pulmonary complications even though these moves are painful. Some patients will have to be taught how to cough and take deep breaths, or taught the difference between clearing the throat and a vigorous cough that will remove secretions from the tracheobronchial tree. The patient may need to be taught how to use respiratory support equipment such as an incentive spirometer so that when he needs it postoperatively he knows how to use it and does not have to learn it when he is medicated, uncomfortable, and confused.

The patient should be told to expect postoperative pain and that appropriate analgesic medication is available but he may have to ask for it. Patients counselled in this way preoperatively require less postoperative analgesia.

THE OPERATIVE CONSENT

In the age of consumerism, the patient has the right to know the diagnosis of his illness, the prognosis, the nature of a proposed operation, what it is intended to accomplish, the possibility of failure, the benefits, the risks of the operation in terms of mortality and complications, and the alternative means of treatment available. The unpleasant aspects of the situation can be presented in a matter-of-fact manner and not dwelt on unnecessarily. The seriousness of the indications for surgery can be emphasized. In any case, the patient should be allowed to decide for himself on the basis of fairly presented information whether he wants to undergo the operation. There is much room for persuasion; part of the art of medicine is persuading patients to undergo treatment.

The best practice of medicine and surgery (and the best defense against a lawsuit) lies in developing a good relationship with the patient and his family and in open discussion about the possible consequences of the surgery, which must be weighed against the expected benefits. Clearly, it is possible to frighten any patient away from surgery by too much emphasis on the risks, yet the patient should not be allowed to come to the operating room blissfully ignorant of the hazards to which he will be exposed.

PHYSIOLOGICAL PREPARATION OF THE PATIENT

After the surgeon has apprised himself of the many data in the patient's initial evaluation, he must decide if the patient's condition permits operation or if any of a wide variety of abnormalities require treatment before definitive surgery can be undertaken. Sometimes such preliminary treatment requires a minor procedure such as a tube thoracotomy or a tracheostomy. In many cases there will be abnormalities that must be considered in deciding which anesthetic to use, and in other cases there will be diseases such as congestive heart failure, diabetes mellitus, or adrenal insufficiency that must be managed during the operation. To achieve consistently good results, the surgeon must make sure the patient is in optimal condition to withstand the anesthesia, the surgical procedure, and the postoperative period. The anesthesia may be a more serious physiological challenge than the surgery. A variety of measures that are important in achieving an optimal preoperative condition are discussed here. In urgent cases it may be necessary to abbreviate or forego some of the following preparatory measures. In elective cases the patients should be in optimal condition.

EMPTY STOMACH

Under anesthesia, gastric contents are likely to reflux into the esophagus and be aspirated. The use of muscle relaxants contributes to the reflux. Frequently muscle relaxants are administered to facilitate tracheal intubation. Sometimes a patient will vomit while anesthesia is being induced and his glottic reflexes are depressed, thus permitting aspiration. During abdominal surgery, the stomach may be compressed or retracted, pushing its contents into the esophagus. Aspiration is a serious complication; if the patient does not asphyxiate immediately, he may develop a serious postoperative pneumonitis to which he may ultimately succumb

or that may require prolonged postoperative respiratory support with a tracheostomy and a ventilator, leaving him with permanent respiratory impairment.

Therefore, in elective surgery cases it is routine to have the patient eat or drink nothing from midnight the night before until the operation in the morning. For operations scheduled for afternoon, a liquid breakfast may be permitted. For infants who need to eat every 4 hr, a 4 hr period without food is sufficient, and one should probably not make a baby go longer than 6 hr without food before an operation.

If the patient has inadvertently eaten, it may be wiser to postpone the procedure 6 hr or 8 hr, or until the next day, rather than risk aspiration. Some emergency cases, such as abscesses requiring drainage, may be postponed safely. Others who have just eaten, such as trauma patients, whose surgery cannot be postponed, pose a difficult problem. Sometimes one cannot wait for the stomach to empty. (Frequently after a serious injury the stomach will not empty in a normal period of time.) In such cases, one may be able to empty the stomach with a nasogastric tube. If food particles block the nasogastric tube, an Ewalt tube may be inserted to empty the stomach. If these measures are not successful, the anesthesiologist may have to intubate the patient awake.

SKIN PREPARATION

The final preoperative preparation prior to incision is to cleanse the skin with appropriate agents that will remove dirt and desquamated epithelium and kill bacteria. (See Chap. 9 for a thorough discussion.) Customarily, hair is shaved prior to cleaning the skin. This is best done immediately before the operation. If it is done the night before, skin nicks from the razor may afford bacteria an opportunity to grow near the incision, where it is difficult to eradicate them by cleansing the skin. For optimal skin preparation the patient washes with pHisoHex, Hibiclens, or Betadine (I prefer Betadine) the night before surgery, or even once or twice a day for several days preoperatively to reduce the numbers of bacteria on the skin at the time of operation.

Infected hair follicles, inflamed scratches, and pimples in the region of the incision cannot be sterilized with the skin preparation. To proceed with an operation in their presence increases the risk of infection. It is better to let them heal and reschedule the operation when the skin of the operative field is in good condition. If surgery is urgent, the incision may be placed away from the point of inflammation, or, if that is not possible, one can excise the local inflamed lesion and discard the instruments that were used for it before making the full incision. The adjunctive use of antibiotics might be considered in such a case, but antibiotics cannot be expected to eliminate the risk of infection.

CONCOMITANT INFECTIONS

In general, the presence of an infection somewhere on the body increases the risk of a postoperative wound infection. If the infection is remote, such as the contralateral leg when one is operating on the arm, the increased risk is not great.

If the operation must be carried out in an area involving the lymphatic drainage from the infection, the likelihood of wound infection is considerably greater. The greatest danger occurs when the site of infection is in the immediate vicinity of the incision. Internal infection such as urinary tract infections may be the source of a postoperative wound infection. Whenever possible, infection should be treated and eliminated prior to operation. If one must operate on a patient who harbors an infection, its bacteriology and drug sensitivities should be as well defined as possible preoperatively, and appropriate antibiotics should be administered.

PREOPERATIVE ANTIBIOTICS

Most elective surgical patients do not need antibiotic therapy. In fact, the use of antibiotics is contraindicated because of the possibilities of inducing an allergy to the drug in the patient or of provoking the emergence of organisms resistant to the drug. There are specific situations when antibiotics are indicated, such as the presence of an infection that cannot be eradicated preoperatively; operations for contaminated wounds such as compound fractures or penetrating injuries; operations that cut into or across the gastrointestinal tract, the genitourinary tract, or the respiratory tract; and implantation of a foreign body. In such cases, specific antibiotics to which the infecting organisms are known to be sensitive should be selected. If the organisms are not known, as in trauma cases or colon cases, broad-spectrum agents should be employed as well as agents effective against anaerobes. When antibiotics are to be used, they should be started preoperatively so that there will be adequate blood and tissue levels of the agents by the time contamination occurs. In patients with compound fractures and penetrating injuries, antibiotics should be started as soon as the patient is first seen because contamination has already occurred.

TEMPERATURE

A patient's temperature should be approximately normal when he comes to the operating room. When the temperature is elevated, metabolic processes are more active, more oxygen is required, the events of shock are less well tolerated, the myocardium may be more irritable, and arrhythmias are more likely. A febrile patient may be rendered euthermic by the use of aspirin or Tylenol suppositories, hydration, removal of excess clothing or covers, the use of a cooling blanket, placement of ice packs on the groin and axillae, or placement of towels soaked in iced alcohol on the patient. Shivering, which raises the temperature and may be incited by vigorous attempts at reducing temperature, may be reduced or eliminated by the use of small amounts of chlorpromazine.

HYPOTHERMIA

Although patients with fever are at excess risk for anesthesia and surgery, patients with an abnormally low temperature (*e.g.*, below 34.4° C) may also be at risk. At lower temperatures chemical reactions, including enzymatically mediated ones, proceed more slowly. Blood takes longer to clot. Patients whose body temperature is reduced, for example, by exposure to cold, are prone to develop refractory ventricular fibrillation in the presence of shock. If time permits, such patients may be warmed with a hyperthermic blanket or by immersion in a bath of 40.6° C water (never more than 42.2° C to avoid burning the patient).

CURRENT MEDICATIONS

Certain drugs may have profound physiological effects while the patient is under anesthesia. The surgeon and the anesthesiologist need to be aware of each such agent taken by the patient. Some drugs, such as monamine oxidase inhibitors, must be stopped entirely 2 weeks prior to surgery because their interactions with other drugs are so unpredictable.

CORTICOSTEROIDS

Patients who have been receiving steroids for prolonged periods of time may have atrophied adrenal cortices and be incapable of an appropriate response to stress. Anesthesia and surgery are major stresses. Such patients may develop hypotension under anesthesia unless they are given large amounts of steroid. Patients who have been treated with steroids in the past but have not been taking them for 6 months or even longer may be incapable of a brisk response to stress and should be treated much the same way as patients taking the agents at the time. As a rule of thumb, patients who have been taking steroids longer than a week should be presumed to require additional preoperative steroid support.

SHOCK

In most instances, shock is attended by poor cardiac output, poor perfusion of vital organs, and decreased oxygen utilization by tissues. In shock a wide variety of aberrations of the internal milieu are developing, and cellular and organ functions are deteriorating. Most forms of shock are exacerbated by anesthesia, surgical manipulation, and blood loss.

It is of utmost importance that shock be reversed prior to anesthesia and surgery. Failure to do so is to invite disaster in the form of a fatal outcome. The exception to getting the patient out of shock prior to surgery is the surgical problem whose nature makes this impossible. A patient who is exsanguinating internally may need to have the bleeding stopped as part of the therapy of his shock. Certain cases of septic shock will respond much better once the septic focus is drained. Special forms of shock such as cardiac tamponade and tension pneumothorax require specific treatment (described in other chapters of this book). These possibilities must be ruled out in certain patients in shock.

HYPERTENSION

A patient with elevated blood pressure will bleed more profusely during operation. His heart must work harder and is more at risk for arrhythmia, heart failure, and infarction under stress. The patient's blood pressure should be brought under control (diastolic less then 100, preferably less than 90) prior to operation.

HYDRATION

Hydration may be difficult to assess. In general, if a patient's urine output is good (40 ml/hr), if his tongue and mucous membranes are moist, and if skin turgor is good, hydration is adequate. There are exceptions to the foregoing, of course.

On the other hand, dependent or peripheral edema is a sign of overhydration. The findings may depend on how fast the patient lost water.

Patients tolerate surgery best when they are properly hydrated. A dehydrated patient is likely to develop hypotension from anesthesia and further dehydration by third space losses in dissected tissues. Mild forms of dehydration, as in the patient who has fasted overnight, are easily corrected by the anesthesiologist when he starts an intravenous infusion. More severe forms may require several hours to days to achieve hydration prior to operation. The replacement of fluid is carried out in conjunction with the restoration of electrolytes and acid–base balance. A full discussion of fluid and electrolyte management will be found in Chapter 2.

If a patient is overhydrated, fluid may be removed by diuretics, by fluid restriction and insensible loss, or by dialysis. Edematous tissues are more difficult to dissect because of their weight and stiffness, anatomic structures are harder to identify, and they heal less well. Indeed, they sometimes will not hold stitches.

Different clinical situations have different levels of optimal hydration; patients undergoing abdominal surgery require more salubrious hydration than those undergoing brain surgery. In fact, some neurosurgeons prefer to dehydrate their patients immediately preoperatively to shrink the brain. This can be accomplished by administering a large dose of intravenous urea, which promotes a profound osmotic diuresis.

ELECTROLYTES

Determination of the serum concentration of sodium, potassium, chloride, and calcium and the serum carbon dioxide combining power are readily obtained in most hospitals. Aberrations in serum sodium are closely associated with aberrations in body fluids. Hypernatremia may be corrected by administering a solution such as 5% dextrose. Hyponatremia may be corrected by fluid restriction or hypertonic saline, depending on circumstances. In patients with a diseased heart, liver, or kidney, it may be very difficult to raise the serum sodium level without risk of subsequent fluid overload.

Abnormal serum potassium levels have profound effects on the cardiovascular system. Hyperkalemia is evident on the electrocardiogram by peaked T waves and S-T segment depression. With higher levels of potassium, the T wave disappears, heart block appears, and finally, diastolic arrest occurs. Measures that will reduce the serum potassium level include withholding exogenous potassium, intravenous infusion of insulin and glucose, and the use of kayexalate by mouth or by rectum to exchange sodium for potassium. Hyperkalemia usually reflects severe renal disease, and surgery should be contemplated in such patients with caution. Most patients undergo a catabolic phase in the postoperative period that normally produces negative balances of nitrogen and potassium. If the kidneys do not function adequately, the BUN and serum potassium levels will rise, exacerbating previous derangements in these parameters.

Hypokalemia is a more common problem and is more easily managed. It may result from excessive renal excretion, movement of potassium intracellularly, prolonged parenteral administration of potassium-free fluids, gastrointestinal losses, or prolonged use of diuretics. Metabolic alkalosis contributes to it because of the renal tubular exchange of potassium for hydrogen. Hypokalemia causes failure of normal contraction of skeletal, smooth, and cardiac muscles and the signs and symptoms related to such failure. It predisposes patients to digitalis toxicity and ventricular arrhythmias. Hypokalemia should be prevented by anticipation and preoperative administration of potassium.

ACID–BASE BALANCE

In general, the *p*H should be corrected to roughly 7.4 and HCO_3 to 25 mEq/liter. The common acid–base abnormality is acidosis. Initially, a metabolic acidosis will be compensated for by hyperventilation (respiratory alkalosis); as acidosis progresses, this mechanism may fail or become inadequate, and the blood *p*H falls. The first concern is the correction of *p*H to normal, usually by administration of $NaHCO_3$ or sometimes by tris buffer. Respiratory alkalosis may occur as a result of hyperventilation secondary to hypoxia. Metabolic alkalosis may occur in patients who vomit gastric juice, for example, in cases of pyloric obstruction. Such patients have lost hydrochloride in the gastric juice and will exchange K^+ for H^+ in the kidney, becoming hypokalemic. Preoperative correction includes replacing the lost gastric secretions with normal saline solution and large amounts of potassium. In very severe cases, ammonium chloride, arginine hydrochloride, or dilute hydrochloric acid may be helpful.

NUTRITION

Patients with good nutrition can be expected to withstand a surgical procedure better than the malnourished. A desirable degree of nutrition is indicated by a previously active patient who has been able to eat and who reports eating a good, well-balanced diet. Such a patient should have good muscle mass and a reasonable but not excessive amount of subcutaneous tissue. Signs of vitamin deficiency such as fissures of the lips, petechiae, bruises, and bleeding gums should be sought. Normal levels of serum albumin and hemoglobin are usually present in well-nourished persons. Patients with major trauma, sepsis, or recent weight loss may be poorly nourished at the time of surgery. Such patients should be treated preoperatively with parenteral vitamins including vitamins B, C, and K, varying amounts of plasma or albumin, and, where indicated, whole blood. Parenteral hyperalimentation for several days to a week may reverse a negative nitrogen balance in starving patients. It may be required longer than a week preoperatively. If used preoperatively, it should be continued postoperatively until satisfactory gastrointestinal tract function returns. See Chapter 7 for a detailed discussion.

DIABETES

Diabetes should be under control (*e.g.*, a blood sugar level of less then 200 and no significant ketonuria, although a fasting individual without diabetes may normally have some ketonuria) prior to anesthesia and surgery. Once this state is achieved, the patient is fasted appropriately preoperatively, and hypoglycemic agents such as insulin and tolbutamide should be withheld or reduced the day of surgery because the patient is not receiving food. If insulin were to be given without nutriment, dangerous levels of hypoglycemia could occur under anesthesia, and serious brain damage could result. Usually the blood sugar level is measured just prior to operation and in some instances intraoperatively. Some surgeons like to give small amounts of insulin in the intravenous solution. I prefer to let the patient spill sugar during the operation and treat it postoperatively, which is usually easy because the patient receives nothing by mouth and relatively small amounts of glucose intravenously.

HEMATOLOGIC DISORDERS

Blood transports oxygen most efficiently when the hemoglobin is in the range of 14 to 15 g/dl. As the patient becomes anemic, the blood is less viscous and flows through the capillaries faster, but it transports less oxygen. At hemoglobin levels of less then 10 g/dl, the blood carries so little oxygen that there is poor reserve for episodes of decreased cardiac output, hypotension, or hypoxia. Most surgeons and anesthesiologists will proceed with an operation if the hemoglobin is 10 g/dl but prefer to transfuse the patient preoperatively if it is lower.

With very high levels of hemoglobin the blood becomes increasingly viscous, flows slowly through capillaries, and requires more cardiac work to deliver oxygen to the tissues. There is a risk of intravascular thrombosis and the possibility of stroke. An additional difficulty is that the large volume of red cells leaves a relatively small amount of plasma, and blood in the small vessels in the operative field does not clot as quickly as usual but keeps oozing. For patients with hemoglobin levels of greater then 22 g/dl or a hematocrit of 65% (as in certain patients with congenital heart disease), it is wise to perform plasmapheresis to bring the hemoglobin down to a safe level preoperatively.

The importance of good blood coagulation for hemostasis in surgery is clear. Some patients have clotting deficiencies; hemophilia and Christmas disease are obvious examples. Other patients whose blood may not clot properly are those with cirrhosis, obstructive jaundice, malabsorption, thrombocytopenia, or sepsis as well as those who have not been fed for some days. If there is any question of a patient's ability to clot blood, a prothrombin time, partial thromboplastic tissue test, and platelet count should be obtained. If the first two tests are abnormal, they may be corrected by administering 10 mg to 25 mg of vitamin K 24 hr preoperatively. If the clotting factors do not respond to this dose, they will occasionally respond to larger doses. Otherwise, fresh frozen plasma must be administered preoperatively or intraoperatively. Patients with low platelet counts can be helped with platelet transfusions, which are usually given at the beginning of the operation because of the short half-life of platelets. Patients who have had recent shock or sepsis may have disseminated intravascular coagulation, which requires very intensive support.

Patients receiving anticoagulants should usually stop taking the agent (heparin or coumadin) long enough in advance to allow coagulation to return to normal.

Patients whose white blood cell count is very low may tolerate an operation reasonably well but may have a greater likelihood of subsequent infection if the operation requires cutting into or across the alimentary or genitourinary tract. In addition, the method of anesthesia chosen may require inserting an endotracheal tube through the mouth into the trachea, with attendant bacteriologic contamination and subsequent pulmonary infection. Prophylactic antibiotics may be considered in such cases.

CARDIAC DISEASES

Many patients who need surgery have coexisting heart disease. Frequently the condition of the heart can be improved prior to surgery, but in some cases it cannot. The coexistence of heart disease may lead the surgeon to re-evaluate the indication for surgery or to modify the procedure. It may greatly influence the choice and conduct of anesthesia, and it may be reason for more careful intraoperative and postoperative monitoring and support.

Aortic stenosis is a treacherous condition that may be serious but asymptomatic. The diagnosis is suspected by hearing a typical crescendo–decrescendo systolic murmur in the second right interspace that radiates to the neck. The myocardial oxygen demand is great because of the thick myocardium and greatly increased tension–time index. Hypotension and decreased cardiac output are poorly tolerated. Sudden death under anesthesia is well known. Aortic stenosis greatly increases the risk of surgery.

Congestive heart failure should be corrected prior to surgery by the use of salt restriction, diuretics, and digitalis. Subsequent fluid therapy may need to be modified.

Angina pectoris increases the risk of intraoperative or postoperative arrhythmias or myocardial infarction. It may be improved preoperatively by weight reduction, control of hypertension, and the use of propranolol and vasodilators. It may require modification of the planned procedure and the choice of anesthesia, and it calls for more careful support and monitoring.

Recent myocardial infarction is a contraindication to all but the most urgent surgery. Operation should be postponed until at least 6 months from the infarction to minimize the risk of recurrent infarction or arrhythmia under anesthesia.

Patients who have had an old myocardial infarction or a Q wave of undetermined age usually can undergo anesthesia and surgery if appropriate care is taken to avoid hypoxia and hypotension.

Patients with congenital or valvular heart disease who require any kind of surgical procedure, including dental work or endoscopy, should be treated with antibiotics to prevent subsequent endocarditis from a transient bacteremia. The antibiotics are usually aimed at gram-positive cocci and are best started shortly before the procedure.

PULMONARY PROBLEMS

The most common group of postoperative problems affects the pulmonary tree. These complications include atelectasis, pneumonitis, pneumonia, and post-traumatic pulmonary insufficiency. Preoperative preparation is aimed at preventing these postoperative problems, which are more common in patients with chronic obstructive bronchopulmonary disease. Such patients will sometimes have improved pulmonary function if they are treated with expectorants, intermittent positive pressure breathing, postural drainage, and chest percussion preoperatively. Bronchitis may require antibiotic therapy.

Cigarette smoking is widespread and causes great damage to the tracheobronchial tree; the cilia are paralyzed by it, and secretions are greater. If a patient gives up smoking preoperatively, there will be fewer pulmonary complications. There is some benefit in having the patient stop smoking for as short a period as 1 to 3 days preoperatively, although 2 weeks is preferable.

Upper respiratory infections are common, and there is some increased risk of postoperative pneumonia associated with them. Elective procedures should be postponed until 2 or 3 weeks after the cold has cleared. More urgent procedures can be carried out in the presence of such infections.

Pneumonia is a strong contraindication to surgery. It is likely to become more extensive postoperatively, and to proceed with an operation in the presence of pneumonia is hazardous. Elective surgery should be postponed until at least 6 weeks after the pneumonia has cleared.

Many of the factors leading to post-traumatic pulmonary insufficiency cannot be avoided. A few can—for example, avoid overhydration and aspiration and filter blood with a micropore filter in cases requiring massive transfusion. Intrapleural collections of air or fluid displace lung volume and cause varying degrees of atelectasis. Such collections should be drained by needle aspiration or by tube thoracotomy prior to a major operation and general anesthesia. In particular, pneumothorax should be treated with a chest tube prior to anesthesia to avoid development of a tension pneumothorax under the anesthesiologist's positive pressure ventilation.

LIVER

The liver makes serum albumin and clotting factors and performs myriad metabolic jobs. When it functions poorly, a patient's blood may not clot well and may not be improved by vitamin K. In addition, poor liver function is associated with poor wound healing and a higher rate of infection. Patients with acute hepatocellular disease should not undergo operation except in urgent situations. Liver function in patients with cirrhosis may improve if the patients are treated with rest and a high-protein, high-calorie diet for 2 or 3 weeks preoperatively. This is best accomplished in the hospital where it can be supervised and where alcoholic beverages are less readily available.

Ascites related to liver disease may be treated and removed by a similar supportive program in which diuretics are employed judiciously. An abdominal operation on a patient with ascites causes the patient to lose this protein-rich fluid abruptly. It usually re-forms in the postoperative period at the expense of other fluid compartments and must be replaced, which complicates the management of the patient's fluid and electrolyte therapy. In addition, the ascitic fluid may leak out through the wound or through a drain site, leading to infection. If the ascites can be cleared preoperatively, the results are likely to be much better.

OBSTRUCTED HOLLOW VISCERA

In general, if a patient's disease process includes obstruction of one of the hollow viscera such as the bladder, the colon, or the stomach, the surgery is easier and the results are better if the organ can be decompressed prior to definitive surgery; the stomach can be decompressed by nasogastric suction, the colon by colostomy or cecostomy, and the bladder by urethral catheterization or a suprapubic tube if a catheter cannot be passed. The biliary tract can be drained with a percutaneous transhepatic catheter.

THYROID

Hyperthyroidism produces increased oxygen consumption by all tissues, a greater cardiac output, autonomic nervous system imbalance, and central nervous system hypersensitivity. Such patients tolerate fright, pain, hunger, and rage poorly. They are far more prone to fibrillation either of the atrium or of the ventricle. They are very sensitive to adrenergic and anticholinergic drugs. To attempt operation on a patient with even mild hyperthroidism is to risk thyroid storm and ventricular fibrillation. The preoperative preparation of such a patient requires several weeks to bring the thyroid activity under control with such antithyroid medication as propylthiouracil or methimazole. If a patient is sensitive to these, potassium perchlorate may be used. The degree of control achieved should be documented by measurement of circulating levels of thyroid hormone preoperatively. The management of the hyperthyroid patient requiring emergency surgery is more complicated. The reader is referred to the *Manual of Pre-Operative and Post-Operative Care* for a detailed discussion.

The hypothyroid patient is sensitive to many drugs and most anesthetics. The heart tires easily and cannot respond to an added load. For elective surgery, thyroid function is restored to normal by administering thyroid hormones, starting with small doses. In the emergency situation, the minimum surgical procedure that will tide the patient over is chosen. Tri-iodothyronine is administered in small amounts, and all drugs and anesthetic agents are used in drastically reduced amounts.

The elderly and the very young are more sensitive to disturbed thyroid function than are young adults.

URINARY SYSTEM

The kidneys eliminate nitrogenous waste products and control fluid and electrolyte balance. They have a vital role in maintaining hemostasis and the internal milieu. When they function poorly because of a disease process, the internal milieu is distrubed, and many intracellular processes proceed abnormally. Wounds heal poorly. Urinary function may improve with hydration and relief of obstructive uropathy. Optimal improvement in renal function is desirable prior to surgery because there may be additional insults to the kidney related to the operative procedure and associated drugs such as antibiotics. Kidneys that are in the best possible condition preoperatively will withstand the operation better and serve the patient more effectively postoperatively. In patients with severe renal disease, dialysis may be required to bring the BUN and creatinine level low enough to promote good healing. As a rule, if the BUN is over 100, wounds cannot be expected to heal, and it is preferable to have the BUN less than 60.

BIBLIOGRAPHY

American College of Surgeons Committee on Pre- and Post-Operative Care: Manual of Pre-Operative and Post-Operative Care, 2nd ed. Philadelphia, W B Saunders, 1971

BEAL JM, RAFFENSPERGER JG: Diagnosis of Acute Abdominal Disease. Philadelphia, Lea & Febiger, 1979

EISEMAN B, WOTKYNS RS: Surgical Decision Making. Philadelphia, W B Saunders, 1978

GOLDMAN DR: Medical Care of the Surgical Patient. Philadelphia, J B Lippincott, 1982

KYLE J, HARDY JD: Scientific Foundations of Surgery. London, William Heinemann, 1981

ROE BR: Perioperative Management in Cardiothoracic Surgery. Boston, Little, Brown & Co, 1981

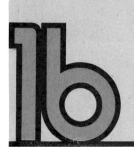

James F. Arens/Joseph C. Gabel

Anesthesia

The term *anesthesia* was first introduced by Oliver Wendell Holmes to describe a state in which a patient suffered no pain. The required effects of an anesthetic are deep sleep, analgesia, and obtundation of reflexes. With the discovery of anesthetic drugs, a continuing cycle was started: better anesthesia allowed performance of more complicated surgery, and more complicated surgical procedures forced the continued advancement of anesthesiology

The inclusion of a chapter concerning anesthesia is appropriate in a textbook of surgery, since at present less than 50% of all anesthetics administered in the United States are administered by anesthesiologists. The rest are administered primarily by nurse anesthetists, who, by state practice acts, work under the direction of the operating surgeon where there is no anesthesiologist in attendance. Thus the surgeon must be knowledgeable in both the principles and the techniques of anesthesia. Also, many significant developments have been brought about in anesthetic practice by surgeons; Harvey Cushing, for example, was responsible for development of the anesthetic record.

PREOPERATIVE PREPARATION OF THE PATIENT

PREOPERATIVE EVALUATION

The preoperative evaluation of the surgical patient is probably the most important procedure in preventive medicine for reducing the postoperative complication rate. This includes the patient's overall condition and specific information about respiratory, cardiovascular, renal, cerebral, and hepatic function, and fluid and electrolyte balance. Screening tests are meaningless unless they are carefully evaluated by attending physicians and consultants before surgery. Separate studies done by Tarhan and Topkins demonstrated that the shorter the interval between a previous myocardial infarction and surgery, the greater the mortality. A thorough preoperative pulmonary evaluation is appropriate for patients with lung disease. Blood urea nitrogen (BUN), creatinine levels, and urine analysis offer a coarse screening procedure for kidney disease, as do liver enzyme studies for the hepatic system. Pay appropriate attention to preoperative evaluation of the patient's airway to ensure maintenance

PREANESTHETIC PATIENT ASSESSMENT
Respiratory function
Cardiac function
Renal function
Hepatic function
Cerebral function
Fluid, electrolyte, blood-volume status
Medication history
Allergies
Transfusion history
Previous anesthesia and problems

of a patent airway throughout the anesthetic course (Fig. 16-1). The ability of the patient to open his mouth, the shape of the mandible, and the state of dental hygiene, including loose teeth, are obvious and necessary considerations. A thorough drug history is essential, because drugs such as beta-blocking agents, steroids, phenothiazines, and enzyme inducers (*e.g.,* phenobarbital and diphenylhydantoin) may significantly alter the anesthetic course. Make a detailed history of previous anesthesia, specifically checking on the types of anesthetics employed as well as any untoward or unusual reactions.

PREMEDICATION

An empathetic preoperative visit is extremely important in allaying the patient's apprehension, fear, and misunderstanding about impending surgery. An appropriate history and physical examination as well as a thorough interview do much to instill confidence in the patient about the team in surgery into whose hands the patient entrusts his life.

Premedication, normally a combination of two or more drugs, must be tailored not only to the patient's chronological age but also to his physiological age. Narcotics, barbiturates, or tranquilizers are used to create psychic sedation in the preoperative patient. In addition, these drugs have been shown to decrease the anesthetic requirements; that is, they lower the minimum alveolar concentration (MAC). Debate continues as to whether narcotics or· barbiturates are the preferred preanesthetic sedative. Some point out that most patients prior to surgery have no pain, and therefore narcotics are unnecessary; others feel that narcotics not only produce sedation but also alter the patient's mood so as to allay apprehension more effectively. One of the disadvantages of narcotic premedication is that it produces respiratory depression with a shift of the carbon dioxide response curve to the right. Many times this respiratory depression extends into the postoperative recovery period; narcotic depression is one of the causes that must be ruled out in postoperative apnea. It has also been noted that with some of the major tranquilizers, most often droperidol, the patient may seem calm while inwardly he is exceedingly apprehensive.

Anticholinergics are also used prior to surgery, for two purposes: to reduce vagal reflex activity and to reduce secretions. There is considerable debate as to whether these parasympatholytic drugs should be given intramuscularly before surgery, intravenously immediately before the induction of anesthesia, or not at all. If the patient is given an anticholinergic drug on the ward, he feels very hot and flushed and often complains of dryness of the mouth. If an anticholinergic such as atropine is given intravenously prior to the start of an anesthetic, the drug alone may produce serious arrhythmias. However, many of the halogenated anesthetic compounds exert a strong parasympathomimetic effect, with the subsequent production of either sinus or nodal bradycardia and hypotension. Because of this, when using halogenated anesthetics, many advise the preanesthetic administration of anticholinergics, most frequently the belladonna alkaloids. Atropine has a much stronger vagolytic action than does scopolamine. On the other hand, scopolamine has a more potent drying action than does atropine. In addition, scopolamine produces depression of the central nervous system (CNS) characterized especially by amnesia. Scopolamine is often used as a premedication before regional anesthesia. Scopolamine delirium may oc-

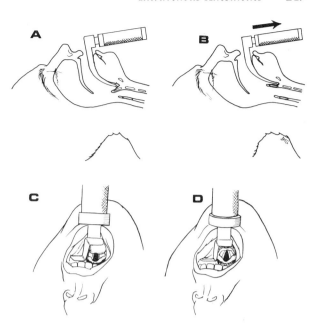

Fig. 16-1. Laryngoscopy with a Macintosh laryngoscope. Facile exposure of the larynx is essential to the smooth induction of endotracheal anesthesia and in many other maneuvers that require secure access to the tracheobronchial tree. (*A*) Laryngoscope placed anterior to epiglottis. (*B*) Laryngoscope advanced and lifting force applied in the direction of handle. (*C*) Epiglottis lifted, exposing posterior half of larynx. (*D*) Epiglottis lifted, exposing entire portion of cords except for the anterior commissure (proper exposure for intubation).

cur, both in the elderly and in obstetrical patients. Physostigmine salicylate, an anticholinesterase compound that crosses the blood-brain barrier, is effective therapy for scopolamine delirium. Glycopyrrolate has recently been introduced as a potent anticholinergic agent. It is used for premedication and, in acute-care medicine, to reduce gastric acidity.

INTRAVENOUS ANESTHETICS

BARBITURATES

The most common of all intravenous anesthetics are the ultrashort-acting barbiturates. Ultrashort-acting barbiturates are used only for the production of unconsciousness in surgery to allow for a smoother, less traumatic induction of surgical anesthesia with one of the inhalational agents. These drugs may also be employed during the course of anesthesia in an attempt to potentiate one of the very weak inhalation agents, such as nitrous oxide, or to produce sedation in a patient who is still apprehensive despite adequate anesthesia following a successful regional block. Antianalgesia has been ascribed to barbiturates. Administration of such a drug to a patient with incomplete regional anesthesia may cause the patient to become uncooperative and unmanageable. Barbiturates do not produce anesthesia as such, because complete abolition of reflex activity does not occur.

The ultrashort-acting barbiturates are capable of producing profound changes in the cardiovascular system by producing direct myocardial depression as well as vasodilatation. Thus, profound hypotension not infrequently results when one of these compounds is administered to a patient with either severe myocardial dysfunction or severe hypovolemia. The uptake and distribution of such compounds are important considerations in clinical practice. For example, the body is classified into four parts; vessel-rich group (VRG); muscle group (MG); fat group (FG); and vessel-poor group (VPG). Although only 9% of the body mass constitutes the vessel-rich group, this portion of the body mass receives 75% of the total cardiac output. Therefore, a large percentage of the administered intravenous dose obviously goes directly to the coronary circulation, thereby producing the myocardial depression, and to the cerebral circulation, producing rapid loss of consciousness. The amount of the drug taken up by any tissue is determined by the tissue solubility and the blood flow to that tissue, as well as the differential between the concentration of the drug in the blood and the concentration in the tissue itself. Thus, very rapidly—within a minute—the vessel-rich group has received a high percentage of the drug. The partition coefficient then reverses, and the drug again begins to reenter the blood. In 5 to 7 minutes the muscle group contains most of the compound, and by 20 minutes the drug is largely contained in the fat group. Thus the patient wakes up following the administration of the ultrashort-acting barbiturates because of redistribution, not because of metabolism. Thiopental is metabolized by the liver at the rate of 10%/hr of the total dose. However, when large doses of thiopental are given over long periods, recovery times may be prolonged. In addition, in patients who are hypovolemic with compensatory vasoconstriction, it is apparent that a smaller dose of thiopental will be required for the production of unconsciousness; it is also apparent that the patient is more susceptible to profound hypotension, because vasodilatation overcomes the vasoconstrictive compensatory response to hypovolemia. A greater percentage of the administered intravenous dose of thiopental, therefore, initially goes to the myocardium and to the cerebral circulation.

Never administer barbiturates to patients with acute intermittent porphyria. The direct intra-arterial injection of thiopental has resulted in tissue necrosis of the upper extremity. The most significant decrease in this complication has resulted from the use of dilute solutions, such as 2.5% solutions and less. If such an injection is given, the needle should be left in place and vasodilators, such as intravenous lidocaine (Xylocaine) and tolazoline (Priscoline), should be administered through the needle or cannula. Additionally, a sympathetic block of the upper extremity should be performed, as well as heparinization of the patient. Etiologically, the reaction was formerly attributed to alkalinity (*p*H of thiopental is 9–11) but it is now felt to be due to the drug itself.

KETAMINE

Ketamine is a phencyclidine derivative recently introduced as an intravenous anesthetic. Ketamine is classified as a dissociative (disconnective) anesthetic that produces profound analgesia with the maintenance of reflex activity. Ketamine does not relieve visceral pain and therefore cannot be used as the sole anesthetic for intra-abdominal or intrathoracic surgery; however, it has been used extensively in burn patients. It has the advantage of producing cardiovascular stimulation, with an increase in both the blood pressure and the pulse rate. In the unconscious state, the patient usually can maintain his airway during ketamine anesthesia. One of the major problems associated with the use of this anesthetic is its simplicity of administration. It has now been well documented that ketamine does not protect the patient against aspiration, even though, theoretically, laryngeal reflex activity is intact. In addition, the airway may become obstructed when ketamine is administered, and the ability to maintain a patent airway is as important here as with any other anesthetic. Ketamine may produce hypotension, especially in the patient who is severely hypovolemic. Therefore, adequate hydration and maintenance of adequate volume status are also important. The major side-effects associated with the use of ketamine are hypertension and recurrent unpleasant dreams, especially in adults. The latter effect may be decreased, although not completely eliminated, by the concomitant administration of sedative drugs such as diazepam or droperidol.

It is essential to administer an anticholinergic compound prior to ketamine because of copious secretions. Very large doses of ketamine are often followed by a prolonged recovery period, and ventilatory insufficiency may occur. Ketamine is generally considered to be contraindicated in patients who have a history of a cerebral vascular accident, significant hypertension, or increased intracranial pressure (because of the additional increased intracranial pressure following ketamine), as well as in psychiatrically disturbed patients, patients with full stomachs, and patients who have visceral pain.

INHALATIONAL ANESTHETICS

A wide variety of inhalational agents have been introduced into anesthesia over the past several decades, but most have been abandoned either because of flammability or toxicity.

NITROUS OXIDE

Nitrous oxide is the most commonly used nonflammable inhalational anesthetic agent today. It is frequently used to potentiate other inhalational agents (*e.g.,* halothane, enflurane) or as a primary agent supplemented by narcotics, barbiturates, or muscle relaxants. This agent is very weak and must be used in high concentrations if amnesia and analgesia are to be produced; borderline oxygen concentrations (21%–30%) may need to be administered. Thus, the use of N_2O in hypoxemic patients is relatively contraindicated. Because nitrous oxide is a weak agent, hypertension may result because of light anesthesia. Be careful to avoid administering an overdose of one of the adjunctive agents in an attempt to provide adequate anesthesia.

Nitrous oxide is 30 times more soluble than nitrogen; therefore, when a nitrous oxide anesthetic is terminated, hypoxia may occur because of nitrous oxide reentering the alveolus from the blood. This phenomenon is referred to as *diffusion anoxia.* The administration of 100% O_2 for 5 minutes at the conclusion of the operation is an effective means of avoiding this problem.

Because of the solubility of nitrous oxide, cavities previously filled with air either increase in size or increase in pressure during nitrous oxide anesthesia. Closed-loop bowel obstruction, pneumothorax, cerebral ventricles filled with air for pneumoencephalography, and air emboli typify the problem.

Since the minimal concentration of nitrous oxide required to produce true anesthesia at standard conditions is 101% MAC, adjunctive agents must be used when adequate oxygen concentrations are administered. On the other hand, a "little nitrous" may render a debilitated patient unconscious; and if the patient has a full stomach, aspiration of gastric contents is a distinct likelihood.

HALOTHANE

Halothane (Fluothane) was introduced into clinical anesthesia in 1956 in England and subsequently studied extensively in the United States by Stephen.

Halothane significantly affects cardiovascular function. It exerts a significant negative inotropic effect on the heart that is intensified with deeper anesthesia. Halothane produces peripheral pooling with decreased venous return because it is a smooth-muscle relaxant. Consequently, profound hypotension may result following halothane anesthesia in patients who are significantly hypovolemic. Parasympathomimetic effects, ganglionic blocking activity, and depression of the vasomotor center are other reasons for hypotension with halothane. Some of the negative inotropic effects can be counteracted by the intravenous administration of either calcium chloride or one of the digitalis preparations. In patients with significant heart disease, the parasympathomimetic effect may cause a nodal rhythm with a decrease in cardiac ouput of 25%. Intravenously administered atropine is an effective antidote. Disturbing ventricular arrhythmias may develop, especially in the presence of hypercarbia. Multifocal PVCs, malignant PVCs (PVCs falling near the upstroke of the T wave), and frequent PVCs (more than 6–7/min) require therapy if adequate alveolar ventilation fails to abolish the arrhythmias. The concomitant use of epinephrine and halothane is still at issue. The dosage schedule and guidelines suggested by Katz are widely quoted.

Halothane depresses respiratory function by decreasing alveolar minute ventilation. Bronchial smooth muscle is relaxed directly by halothane. Therefore, halothane is considered the anesthetic agent of choice for patients who have bronchial asthma. Since halothane does not irritate the respiratory tract, its use results in less secretions. This agent, at present, is considered by many to be the drug of choice for pediatric anesthesia. Little muscle relaxation is produced *per se* by halothane. For major abdominal surgery, muscle relaxants are a required adjunct.

Halothane is considered to be a useful drug in anesthetizing patients in shock because of its ability to improve splanchnic blood flow. However, caution must be exercised in such situations to avoid a relative overdose. Volume replacement can often be guided by the patient's cardiovascular responsiveness under halothane anesthesia.

Several years after the introduction of halothane, reports of liver necrosis began to filter into the literature. Mushin states that the incidence is 1 in 10,000 administrations. Halothane is not a true hepatotoxin, according to Klatskin's criteria. An impurity of halothane manufacture was found to be hepatotoxic and subsequently was removed; however, hepatitis still is seen. Twelve to eighteen percent of absorbed halothane is broken down in the liver to trifluoroacetic acid, which is not hepatotoxic. Cohen suggests that individual variation in enzymatic activity could, in theory, produce a toxic product. Enzyme induction may also play a contributing role. Repeated halothane exposure is reported to cause a higher incidence, since a single halothane administration acts as an enzyme inducer. No hard rule can be given for a safe interval between halothane exposures. In cases of "halothane hepatitis," the Australian antigen is negative. The histopathology of halothane hepatitis is very similar to that seen in acute viral hepatitis. It has been suggested that the hepatitis is a hypersensitivity reaction. This theory seems feasible when cases of recurrent hepatitis related to halothane sensitization in anesthesiologists are reviewed. Certainly a patient who develops unexplained fever or jaundice following administration of halothane should not be given halothane again.

ENFLURANE

Enflurane (Ethrane) is another potent halogenated nonsymmetrical nonflammable ether which has recently been introduced into anesthesia. This drug produces alterations to cardiovascular and respiratory parameters similar to those produced by halothane. The tendency toward arrhythmia production seems less, although nodal rhythm is not infrequent. Muscle relaxation is more profound and necessitates reduction of nondepolarizing muscle-relaxant dosages to one third of the calculated dosages. Increases in blood glucose levels also are noted.

Grand mal seizures have occurred under anesthesia when enflurane was administered in high concentrations and with hyperventilation. Cessation of the agent and reduction of the ventilatory rate and volume often suffice to stop the seizures. If these measures fail, intravenous administration of diazepam, thiopental, or succinylcholine may be required to prevent hypoxemia secondary to the seizures. A small amount of fluoride ion results from enflurane metabolism. Administration of enflurane to patients with significant renal compromise seems unwarranted.

ISOFLURANE

Isoflurane (Forane) has recently been introduced into clinical anesthesia. Isoflurane is only slightly metabolized and up to this time is believed to be devoid of serious renal, hepatic, and CNS side-effects. The respiratory and cardiovascular changes are similar to those produced by enflurane.

MUSCLE RELAXANTS

A muscle relaxant interferes with the passage of impulses from a motor nerve to a skeletal muscle. Muscle relaxants in present clinical use either produce persistent depolarization (depolarizing relaxants) or compete competitively with acetylcholine (nondepolarizing relaxants) by combining with receptor sites usually occupied by acetylcholine.

Depolarizing muscle relaxants (*e.g.,* succinylcholine) initially produce muscle fasciculations followed by a depressed response to both twitch and tetanic stimulation but show no fade with subsequent stimuli and no post-tetanic facilitation. Post-tetanic facilitation refers to the phenomenon where, following a prolonged tetanic stimulation with a subsequent pause, the first twitch stimulus elicits a greater response than that usually produced by a similar degree of twitch stimulus (Fig. 16-2).

Nondepolarizing muscle relaxants do not cause fasciculations but cause a fade with both twitch and tetanic stimuli. In addition, post-tetanic facilitation occurs. Moreover, nondepolarizing relaxants can be reversed effectively by anticholinesterase compounds such as prostigmine.

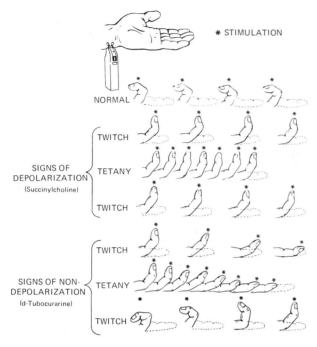

* STIMULATION

NORMAL

SIGNS OF
DEPOLARIZATION
(Succinylcholine)

TWITCH

TETANY

TWITCH

SIGNS OF NON-
DEPOLARIZATION
(d-Tubocurarine)

TWITCH

TETANY

TWITCH

Fig. 16-2. With depolarization block note the diminution in the twitch response, with no fade with subsequent twitches. In the curare-type block there is diminution in twitch response, fade with both twitch and tetanic stimuli, and augmentation of the twitch response after tetany (bottom line). (Reproduced with permission, from Wylie WD, Churchill-Davidson HC: A Practice of Anaesthesia, 3rd ed. London, Lloyd-Luke (Medical Books), 1972)

SUCCINYLCHOLINE

Succinylcholine is the most commonly used muscle relaxant. Because it has a very short duration of action, succinylcholine is the relaxant usually used to facilitate tracheal intubation. For prolonged relaxation a continuous infusion may be used. However, following such an infusion, prolonged muscle relaxation may occur. This may be due to an absolute or a relative overdose or to the development of a dual block (desensitization block) wherein there is evidence of both a depolarizing and a nondepolarizing block. Dual block is managed by ventilatory support and not by administration of anticholinesterase compounds.

In approximately 1 in 3000 patients there is atypical pseudocholinesterase that is incapable of destroying succinylcholine normally broken down by serum pseudocholinesterase. In such patients, administration of succinylcholine produces ventilatory insufficiency for about 4 hours. Ventilatory support is the treatment of choice.

After repeated intravenous doses of succinylcholine, bradycardia may occur especially in children, because of a cholinergic effect. In conditions in which there is muscle damage or wasting—such as trauma, burns, or quadraplegia—succinylcholine may produce hyperkalemia sufficiently severe to cause cardiac arrest. In such patients, nondepolarizing muscle relaxants are a more proper choice, even for intubation. Fasciculations produce an increase in intragastric pressure, which may make aspiration more likely in patients with full stomachs. Pretreatment with a nondepolarizer 3 minutes prior to succinylcholine administration prevents any significant intragastric pressure increase. A rise in intraocular pressure is also noted; consequently, succinylcholine is contraindicated in those patients who have an "open globe" eye injury.

d-TUBOCURARINE

d-Tubocurarine produces muscle relaxation by direct competitive inhibition with acetylcholine and therefore can be reversed effectively by prostigmine, an anticholinesterase, because of the law of mass action. It has an onset of action of 3 minutes, with a 45- to 60-minute duration. Not infrequently, a hypotensive effect occurs following large doses of intravenous tubocurarine because of ganglionic blockade. This side-effect is obviously more pronounced in hypovolemic patients. Bronchoconstriction has been noted following administration of tubocurarine and is thought to be caused by histamine release. Electrolyte imbalance, especially hypokalemia, may markedly potentiate the relaxant effect.

Ether compounds potentiate curare so that only one third the usual dose need be administered if a potent ether compound (*e.g.,* enflurane) is utilized. Up to 80% of curare is excreted unchanged into the urine. However, in the presence of renal failure, curare may be effectively handled by the liver. Thus, curare is felt to be the muscle relaxant of choice for patients with renal failure. Curare has often been said to be contraindicated in patients with myasthenia gravis. Although its effect is markedly exaggerated in such patients, it is still considered the muscle relaxant of choice. However, very small doses are indicated—if, indeed, a muscle relaxant is necessary in such a patient.

PANCURONIUM

Pancuronium was recently introduced because of two properties: the absence of ganglionic blockade and the absence of histamine release. Since it is a nondepolarizing relaxant, it too can be reversed by anticholinesterases. Both the blood pressure and pulse rate are elevated secondary to vagolytic and adrenergic effects. The lack of cardiovascular depression makes pancuronium a useful adjunct for managing the patient in shock. However, such stimulation is not desirable in patients with marked hypertension or those with borderline cardiovascular reserve who tolerate poorly an increase in myocardial oxygen consumption. Prolonged relaxation may occur in patients with renal failure, because pancuronium is partially eliminated by the kidney.

Although muscle relaxants have dramatically changed the practice of anesthesia, complications other than those mentioned in preceding paragraphs are sometimes seen. Ventilatory insufficiency due to residual paralysis does indeed occur. Some simple monitoring techniques aid in detecting this problem. Nerve stimulators (*e.g.,* blockade monitor) are useful to determine the quantity of relaxant required during surgery as well as the degree of residual paralysis at the conclusion of the operative procedure. The ability to sustain the response to tetanic stimulation is a good sign of muscle strength. The patient's ability to hold his head up off the table for 30 seconds is also useful. Ability to generate a vital capacity of three times the estimated tidal volume can be simply measured by a respirometer and is important, in that it represents the degree of muscle activity required to generate an effective cough. The ability to generate 20 cm H_2O negative pressure on inspiration also is a sign of adequate ventilatory muscular mechanics.

Whereas the depolarizing relaxants cannot be readily reversed pharmacologically, the nondepolarizing relaxants can be reversed by anticholinesterase compounds. Neostigmine is most commonly used to allow accumulation of sufficient quantities of acetylcholine to compete effectively for the receptor sites with, for example, curare. Since parasympathomimetic effects are produced, atropine should be given either before or simultaneously with the anticholinesterase. Failure to give atropine will result in copious secretions and marked bradycardia. Neostigmine may be associated with life-threatening arrhythmias if it is administered in the face of severe respiratory acidosis or hypoxemia. Because of the parasympathomimetic effect of neostigmine, it is contraindicated in patients who have bronchial asthma. The administration of more than 5 mg of neostigmine is unwarranted.

REGIONAL ANESTHESIA

SPINAL

Spinal anesthesia is an effective and safe form of anesthesia that has lost popularity primarily because of malpractice fears and a public aware of the bad press associated with spinals. However, to abandon its use is not in the interests of good medicine.

To produce spinal anesthesia, a local anesthetic is injected into the subarachnoid space to block the spinal ganglia and nerve roots (Fig. 16-3). The lumbar puncture is made at L3–4 or L4–5 to avoid the spinal cord itself. If a parasthesia is noted, withdraw the needle and reinsert it to obtain a free flow of fluid in all four quadrants; the spinal fluid should be free of blood. The level of spinal anesthesia is controlled by altering the specific gravity of the mixture to be injected. The specific gravity of cerebrospinal fluid averages 1.007, with the range extending from 1.004 to 1.009. A local anesthetic drug mixed with 10% dextrose and water is heavier than spinal fluid (hyperbaric), and one mixed with sterile water is lighter than spinal fluid (hypobaric). Isobaric solutions are rarely used because of problems in controlling the height of the anesthetic. Since hyperbaric solutions migrate cephalad in the head-down position, the level can be adjusted to the appropriate dermatome. L1 is the dermatome supplying the skin at the pubic crest, T10 the umbilicus, T6 the xiphoid, and T4 the nipple line.

Saddle block refers to spinal anesthesia of the sacral dermatomes only (perineal anesthesia) and is, in fact, rarely attained because of failure to allow sufficient time for the anesthetic to become fixed.

Nerves are blocked in order of their size, with the myelinated fibers being blocked last. Sympathetic nerves are blocked first, followed by pain, touch, deep pressure, and, finally, the motor nerves. The use of differential spinals in pain problems is based on the above phenomenon. Sympathetic paralysis extends about two levels higher than the sensory block; motor paralysis, two levels lower.

The duration of spinal anesthesia depends primarily on the chemical nature of the drug. The agent is removed from the spinal fluid by absorption into the bloodstream. Vasoconstrictors decrease the rate of absorption and thereby prolong anesthesia. Epinephrine, 0.2 mg, prolongs local anesthetic duration by 50%; Neo-synephrine, 5 mg, prolongs it 100%.

A decrease in blood pressure often follows the onset of spinal anesthesia. Such hypotension is due to a decrease in sympathetic tone, with vasodilatation of peripheral arterioles as well as venous capacitance vessels. Venous return is decreased, with a reduction in cardiac output. Initially, the fall in blood pressure is associated with an increase in pulse

rate. The effect is much more pronounced in the face of hypovolemia. After approximately 20 minutes a fall in blood pressure may be associated with a decreased pulse rate in a high spinal because of the block of the thoracolumbar sympathetics. The parasympathetics from the cranial outflow tract predominate. The latter situation readily responds to intravenous atropine. In the former instance, rapid administration of fluids is initially used; if the hypotension persists, ephedrine, 12.5 to 25 mg intravenously, is the drug of choice. Nausea and vomiting following the onset of spinal anesthesia should suggest decreased medullary perfusion secondary to hypotension. Sudden changes in position in patients under spinal anesthesia may produce severe hypotension. Because of the distinct possibility of hypotension, the administration of a spinal anesthetic prior to the placement of an intravenous route is indeed foolhardy.

If the spinal ascends into the thoracic area, intercostal paralysis results. Occasionally, a patient complains of dyspnea because of proprioceptive loss of chest movement. Since the diaphragm normally accounts for up to 60% of the vital capacity, a spinal must cause anesthesia of C3, 4, and 5 (phrenic nerve) before measurable ventilatory inadequacy results. Should this occur, ventilatory support is necessary. It must be remembered that the patient's sensorium is intact throughout resuscitation. Obviously, facilities for ventilatory support must be present whenever a spinal is to be used. Renal function remains adequate as long as an adequate mean arterial blood pressure is maintained.

Many surgeons prefer spinal anesthesia for intestinal work because the gut contracts under spinal anesthesia. However, because of this, the technique is contraindicated in bowel obstruction, not only because of the possibility of aspiration but also because of a potential blowout of the bowel secondary to gut contraction.

The supposed complications following spinal anesthesia have done much to decrease its popularity. Headache is the most common complication and is caused by the leakage of spinal fluid through the arachnoid puncture site. The smaller the needle, the lower the incidence of spinal headache; however, the smaller needle renders the performance of the tap more difficult. The needle sizes most commonly used range from 22- to 25-gauge. Onset of headache occurs 36 to 48 hours following the spinal. The headache is described as dull-aching to throbbing; it is often retro-

Fig. 16-3. Spinal anesthesia represents a very useful technique for the appropriately selected patient.

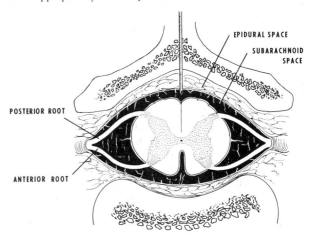

orbital, though it may be in the occipital area; characteristically it becomes more severe when the head is elevated; it is usually self-limited to 5 days but may last for weeks. Treatment consists of reassurance, forced hydration, and appropriate analgesics and then, if such therapy is unsuccessful, the injection of saline into the caudal canal. A volume of saline sufficient to produce meningismus following injection at a slow rate has proved particularly effective. Twenty-five to 75 ml of normal saline is required. Recently, the use of an epidural blood "patch" has been introduced as a successful therapeutic device; this consists of the injection of 5 to 10 ml of the patient's own blood epidurally at the site of the arachnoid puncture.

Septic meningitis is fortunately very rare and often caused by faulty technique. Aseptic or chemical meningitis may develop but usually subsides within 24 hours and requires no therapy.

Other neurologic sequelae have been reported but are very rare. Cauda equina syndrome consists of urinary retention, fecal incontinence, loss of sensation in the perineal area, and impotence. The etiology is not completely understood but may be related to the injection of medications directly into the cord. Adhesive arachnoiditis is a progressive disease exhibiting similar findings. It is believed to result from a toxic effect of the drug on the meninges; the arachnoiditis eventually produces ischemia of the spinal cord. Although the exacerbation of a previously existing neurologic disease can rarely if ever be linked to spinal anesthesia, this anesthesia is best avoided in patients who have or have had neurologic disease. Since neurologic sequelae may follow continuous spinal anesthesia, this technique is used infrequently. The extent of anesthesia is influenced by position, baricity, volume, and rate of injection. Smaller volumes are required in the elderly and in the patient at term pregnancy.

EPIDURAL

Epidural anesthesia is produced by injecting a local anesthetic drug into a vascular space lying between the dura and the periosteum of the spinal canal and extending from S5 to the foramen magnum. If the injection is made at S5 through the sacrococcygeal membrane, the procedure is called caudal anesthesia; if made at L3–5, it is called (lumbar) epidural anesthesia. The degree of hypotension following epidural anesthesia is similar to that following spinal, whereas the degree of motor paralysis is reduced. The major advantages of epidural anesthesia are two:

1. There is no headache, since no subarachnoid puncture is made.
2. Continuous anesthesia for long procedures can be safely performed by insertion of a catheter.

The major disadvantages of epidural anesthesia as compared to spinal anesthesia are the following:

1. The procedure is technically more difficult to perform.
2. Approximately five times more drug is required, thereby increasing the likelihood of a local anesthetic reaction, since the epidural space is highly vascular.
3. If subarachnoid puncture with the large epidural needle does occur, there is the real likelihood of a spinal headache. If the total dose for epidural anesthesia should be injected intrathecally, a total spinal could result.

Epidural anesthesia is a very effective anesthetic technique that does have greater patient acceptance. The continuous technique is particularly useful in lengthy peripheral procedures where the duration of surgery cannot be readily determined.

The following contraindications must be taken into account before selecting either epidural or spinal anesthesia:

1. Preexisting neurologic disease presents a problem (as has already been mentioned).
2. If the patient refuses either modality, the physician subjects himself to assault and battery charges if he should persist.
3. Patients at the extremes of age range are often mentioned. Small children, because of fear, may do poorly under spinal. However, in very elderly patients, regional anesthesia may be the agent of choice, especially for peripheral procedures.
4. Increased intra-abdominal pressure causes higher levels of anesthesia as well as more profound hypotension.
5. Severe hypovolemia must be corrected before administration of the anesthetic. Failure to do so may result in profound hypotension or cardiac arrest.
6. A full stomach contraindicates the use of a regional anesthetic that decreases the patient's ability to cough and to protect himself from aspirating.
7. Patients with coronary artery disease and hypertensive cardiovascular disease tolerate hypotensive levels poorly. In such patients, both the epidural and the spinal forms of regional anesthesia are probably contraindicated.
8. Anticoagulation may be associated with a subarachnoid hemorrhage or with an epidural hematoma if these techniques are employed. Certainly one should avoid a continuous epidural in an anticoagulated patient. The safety of heparinizing a patient after the epidural catheter has been placed has not been established.
9. Insertion of a needle in a patient with septicemia may cause contamination of the space entered and precipitate a catastrophic situation.
10. The use of spinal or epidural anesthesia in patients with significant preexisting pulmonary disease may aggravate the disease process by decreasing the vital capacity and the mean expiratory flow rate.

LOCAL

Ever since Karl Koller produced topical anesthesia in 1884 by instilling cocaine into the conjunctival sac, more effective and less toxic local anesthetic compounds have been sought. No ideal local anesthetic drug has yet been produced. Knowledge of their chemistry, pharmacology, and toxicity must be gained if these drugs are to be used safely and effectively.

The injectable anesthetic compounds, in general, fall into two groups: esters (acid plus alcohol) and amides (acid plus amine). The suffix *caine* refers to the fact that a local anesthetic contains nitrogen. Since almost all local anesthetics do have a nitrogen atom, allergy to "caine" drugs is meaningless.

The chemical group containing the largest number of injectable anesthetics is comprised of the para-aminobenzoic acid ester derivatives. Drugs in this group include procaine (Novocain), tetracaine (Pontocaine), chloroprocaine (Nesacaine), and others. Compounds included in the amide group are lidocaine (Xylocaine), mepivacaine (Carbocaine), and bupivacaine (Marcaine).

Local anesthetics are marketed as salts. However, it is the free-base portion of the drug that is active. Local anesthetics injected into inflamed areas are ineffective not only because of increased absorption but also because the inflamed tissues are acidotic. Commercially prepared epinephrine-containing solutions of local anesthetics are likewise less effective than those without epinephrine because acidic antioxidant stabilizers must be added to prevent epinephrine breakdown. Various types of nerve fibers show differences in susceptibility. It has been noted that the time required for blockade by a particular drug varies inversely with the square of the radius of the nerve. Therefore, autonomic nerves are blocked first, followed by sensory and, finally, motor nerves, which are the largest and are also myelinated.

The duration of action is determined by the chemical nature of the drug itself, the duration of contact, and protein binding. Epinephrine increases duration of contact because of vasoconstriction. Local anesthetics are eventually absorbed into the bloodstream and are either metabolized in the liver or hydrolyzed in the plasma by enzymes. For example, procaine is hydrolyzed by the enzyme procaine esterase, which is identical to pseudocholinesterase, the enzyme response for succinylcholine metabolism. The prolonged action of bupivacaine is believed to result from a high degree of protein binding.

Systemic reactions to local anesthetics are, unfortunately, familiar. Rarely are the reactions caused by an allergic phenomenon, although anaphylaxis or dermatitis can occur. Many of the so-called reactions are caused by the epinephrine in the local anesthetics. The majority of local anesthetic reactions are the result of overdosage. At present, most reactions occur in the bronchoscopy room or in the coronary-care unit, where continuous lidocaine infusions are used to treat arrhythmias. Reactions occur because of high blood levels of local anesthetics, which may result from an excessive dose or rapid absorption. Symptoms of overdosage are manifested in either the vascular system or the CNS. Anxiety and hysteria are often difficult to distinguish from early CNS excitation. Other prodromal signs include somnolence, disorientation, scotomata, and tinnitus. Grand mal seizures may follow. Following the seizure, a postictal state develops which may be manifested by coma, decreased reflexes, and apnea. The depression rarely lasts more than a few minutes. Treatment of the CNS toxicity needs to be directed at preventing hypoxemia secondary to convulsions. Some recommend that a short-acting muscle relaxant (succinylcholine) be given to control convulsions, followed by intubation and ventilation. However, unless personnel are skilled in endotracheal intubation, such therapy may be more hazardous than the problem. In addition to adequate oxygenation, ultrashort-acting barbiturates administered intravenously in small incremental doses will accentuate the postictal depression. Barbiturates administered preoperatively are felt to diminish the risk of seizures. Diazepam also has been used effectively in the prevention, as well as the treatment, of local anesthetic seizures.

Large doses of local anesthetics not only reduce cardiac irritability but also produce direct myocardial depression. Both myocardial depression and vasodilatation may result. Treatment of cardiovascular collapse under these conditions is best effected with drugs possessing primarily beta-stimulating properties.

If overdoses are to be avoided, the following maximum allowable dosages need to be known:

Procaine	1 g
Mepivacaine	500 mg
Lidocaine	500 mg
Bupivacaine	225 mg
Cocaine	160 mg
Tetracaine	100 mg

If the physician injects the smallest volume of the least concentrated solution needed, combines it with a vasoconstrictor to retard absorption, and avoids intravascular injection, reactions will be few. However, the availability of an injectable rapid-acting drug (diazepam or barbiturate) and the capability to provide artifical ventilation are requisites for any physicians using a local anesthetic drug.

Solutions containing epinephrine should not be injected into digits, the penis, or the ear because of the danger of gangrene. Multidose vials of epinephrine should not be used in the operating room because of the danger of injecting 1:1000 epinephrine. Such an injection results in a hypertensive crisis that may produce cardiovascular collapse or a cerebrovascular accident.

Careful attention to detail produces a block that provides excellent anesthesia and a patient who is comfortable and without fear. A poor block produces a very apprehensive patient who requires supplemental anesthesia. Barbiturates are sometimes used to supplement a poor block, and since barbiturates are antialgesics the patient may become wild and unmanageable. Narcotics represent a more appropriate approach pharmacologically. Pride in one's blocking abilities as well as proper patient evaluation do much to assure satisfactory local anesthesia.

TECHNICAL CONSIDERATIONS

Much of the anesthetist's effort should be concerned with avoiding harm to the unconscious patient. There are serious complications and special problems associated with anesthesia. Because a variety of criteria are used to define anesthetic morbidity and mortality, it is difficult to compare the many published series of data. One particular aspect of the problem does shine through the fog of semantics: the vast majority of anesthetic problems are not due to the anesthetic *per se* but to the administration of that anesthetic. There is nothing more dangerous than a complacent anesthetist.

A shocking catalog of misadventures now exists. So that all may recognize and avoid the errors and complications of others, this section summarizes special problems that have been recognized recently and refers to some older ones for reemphasis. Although necessarily incomplete, this review can serve both as impetus to and reference for continued vigilance.

A seriously ill patient in the hands of highly trained and conscientious anesthetists and surgeons is certainly more likely to have a benign course during and after surgery today than in the past. Optimal anesthetic care is predicated on the thorough identification of risk factors. Patients for both elective and emergency surgical procedures should be in optimal condition. Upper-respiratory-tract infections, for example, have been shown to lead to a higher incidence of postoperative respiratory problems. The patient who has allergic rhinitis, on the other hand, carries no particular predilection for respiratory complications. Each clinical situation must be evaluated separately. The decision to proceed is based on the evaluation that the patient is in as near optimal condition as possible. We must make a most diligent effort to restore each organ or system deficiency preoperatively. The attainment of optimal conditions increases the patient's ability to tolerate, compensate for, and recover from the trauma and stress of major surgery.

TRACE ANESTHETIC CONCENTRATIONS IN THE OPERATING ROOM ATMOSPHERE

A national study of occupational disease among operating room personnel indicates that women members in the operating-room–exposed group were subjected to increased risks of spontaneous abortion, congenital abnormalities in their children, cancer, and hepatic and renal disease. No increase in cancer was found among exposed men, but there was an increased incidence of hepatic disease similar to that among women. Furthermore, alterations in cognitive function attendant to relatively short exposures to trace anesthetic concentrations have recently been reported. These potential health hazards, with their subtle and insidious effects, have led the Ad Hoc Committee on the Effect of Trace Anesthetics on the Health of Operating Room Personnel of the American Society of Anesthesiologists to set forth a carefully constructed program of measures to reduce personnel exposure.

PATIENT POSITIONING

The effects of posture on respiration can be offset by the use of an endotracheal tube and assisted or controlled by ventilation. Circulatory effects can be modified significantly by slow and careful movement and positioning of the patient. Although various neurologic deficits have been reported following anesthesia and surgery, postoperative brachial plexus palsy remains one of the most common. Such deficits are entirely avoidable. Most are probably caused by hyperabduction of the arm. The arms should be adducted and placed at the patient's side whenever possible. When the arm must be abducted, it should be elevated above the horizontal plane and pronated.

Pressure injuries caused by only minor malpositioning, as well as the increased incidence of postural hypotension, air embolism, and respiratory obstruction associated with extreme surgical posturing, emphasize the necessity for careful positioning and constant monitoring for evidence of complications.

MONITORING

As surgery has become more extensive and therapeutic approaches more aggressive, intensive physiological monitoring has become an essential part of the anesthetist's armamentarium. To provide dependable information, intensive monitoring must be done routinely. Equipment malfunction and signal artifact are difficult to detect when one is unfamiliar with such aberrations.

Electricity is more than just a hazard in causing explosions. The patient's safety is often unwittingly jeopardized as various monitoring devices are attached. Electrocution occurs when the individual becomes the component that closes the circuit in which lethal currents flow. A review by Bruner clearly and succinctly delineates this problem.

Electrical burns may occur during anesthesia and surgery. Heat produced by an electric current is the product of the current density and the resistance of the circuit. Needle electrodes present an area of high resistance because of the small area of contact. The current from an electrocautery unit may dissipate through monitor leads when a patient is inadequately grounded, thus resulting in high heat production in a small area. The use of needle electrodes for electrocardiographic monitoring should be discouraged.

Much direct physiological monitoring can be accomplished with simple equipment. In addition to the electrocardiogram, radial artery cannulation for arterial blood pressure and blood gas measurements, central venous pressure measurement as an indicator of blood volume and cardiac function, and thermometry are now commonplace. Each technique can bring its own complications, but when it is employed carefully the complications are reduced to a minimum.

The insertion of a cannula into the radial artery carries the possibility of thrombosis or arterial spasm, which, however, is of little significance if the palmar arch is supplied by an ulnar artery. The presence of the ulnar artery can be established by direct palpation or exsanguination of the hand by making a fist to see if the hand flushes (Allen's test). Most other peripheral arteries have from time to time been advocated as sites for placement of arterial cannulas. Other factors appear more important than the site in preventing complications. These include judicious attention so that air and foreign materials are not injected (peripheral embolization), frequent or continuous infusions of a heparinized isotonic solution, and removal of the catheter at first sign of compromised distal circulation.

Placement of the central venous cannula has received extensive treatment in the literature. Aseptic placement of such catheters by whatever chosen route cannot be too strongly emphasized. The value of and problems with right-sided pressure measurements in the evaluation of cardiac function are discussed elsewhere. We are admonished from time to time as to what drugs should or should not be injected centrally. There is little reason why any specific and appropriate pharmacologic agent should not be introduced through a centrally placed catheter as long as sensible precautions as to rapidity of injection and concentration of the solution are observed.

Hyperthermia or severe hypothermia may occur during operation. The need to observe the patient's temperature, particularly during long operations in the very young and in the old, cannot be overemphasized. Again, many techniques are available; the important fact is that temperature must be monitored whenever a patient is anesthetized.

SPECIFIC PROBLEMS ASSOCIATED WITH ANESTHESIA

ASPIRATION PNEUMONITIS

Aspiration of gastric contents remains a major anesthetic problem. There are many causes of regurgitation, and all of them cannot be eliminated. Regurgitation occurs more often than is generally suspected, it may be silent, it often occurs when least expected, and it occasionally proves fatal. No infallible method of prevention has been proposed. Although massive aspiration of gastric contents is frequently a catastrophic event, aspiration of lesser amounts can be occult.

Regional anesthesia should be employed whenever practical in patients with full stomachs. In addition to the obvious history of recent ingestion, other mechanisms may be important in anticipating regurgitation. The most important of these factors for patients undergoing elective surgery are hiatal hernia, obesity, and nervousness. When general anesthesia is necessary in high-risk patients, the placement of a cuffed endotracheal tube is mandatory, preferably while the patient is awake if there is any question of gastric distention. When a rapid induction technique is indicated, several points need to be emphasized. The head-up tilt has proved insufficient to prevent complications, since 9 of 48 patients reported in a series by Dennick died immediately after induction of anesthesia from cardiovascular collapse. Most authorities agree that the head-down tilt, with a rapid sequence of thiopental, oxygen (breathed spontaneously), and succinylcholine, is probably less apt to lead to complications than are other methods. With the use of succinylcholine, preoxygenation by spontaneous breathing of 100% oxygen is sufficient to prevent hypoxia during intubation. The major objection to the use of succinylcholine is that fasciculations and contractions of the abdominal musculature raise intragastric pressure. These complications can be eliminated by the injection of a small (3 mg) dose of d-tubocurarine 3 to 5 minutes prior to the succinylcholine injection. The cricoid pressure method of esophageal compression should be employed during the induction period. The endotracheal tube balloon should be inflated before release of the cricoid pressure.

Other therapeutic measures may have a place in the prophylaxis of aspiration pneumonitis. Taylor and Pryse-Davies have shown the effectiveness of 15 ml of magnesium trisilicate by mouth, with the premedication, in minimizing the severity of pulmonary lesions following aspiration.

Once aspiration has occurred, many therapeutic regimens are advocated. The mainstay of treatment has remained supportive, utilizing bronchodilators, expectorants, steroids, antibiotics, oxygen administration, and if necessary, tracheostomy. Positive pressure ventilation is used frequently in a supportive role, though usually only after respiratory failure has become severe. Such primarily symptomatic treatment has left much to be desired, and the associated mortality remains as high as 70%.

The keynote to success in the treatment of aspiration pneumonitis is prompt, vigorous therapy. Delay and halfhearted treatments have no place in the approach to this disease state. The use of large doses of corticosteroids is not supported by Modell and others; it is at least reasonable to state that steroids may not be the buttress of treatment as was once advocated. Recent studies suggest that mechanical ventilation may play more than a supportive role. Active ventilation of animals immediately after aspiration, but before physiological parameters were affected, was associated with 100% survival in a series reported by Cameron. Early prophylactic positive pressure ventilation is advocated following aspiration of gastric contents.

CARDIAC ARRHYTHMIAS

Arrhythmias may be provoked by numerous factors during the course of anesthesia. The vast majority of arrhythmias are supraventricular and are benign. Should they persist and be associated with a rapid ventricular response, efforts should be made to reverse them. A sudden occurrence of

---

TREATMENT OF CARDIAC DYSRHYTHMIAS

General: Treat hypoxemia and shock; optimize circulating volume and blood oxygenation; treat electrolyte disturbance, especially K^+ and Ca^{++} abnormalities, and acid-base disturbances. EKG monitoring is very important.

Dysrhythmia	Treatment
Sinus tachycardia	Restore circulating volume or treat congestive failure
	Treat pain
	Decrease cardiac accelerator drugs
	Treat hyperthyroidism if present
Premature atrial contractions	Observe and monitor for other arrhythmias
Paroxysmal supraventricular tachycardia	Treat hypoxia; treat digitalis toxicity if present
	Rule out myocardial infarction, congestive failure, or thyrotoxicosis
	If very rapid rate: verapamil, cardioversion, propranolol, digitalis, or phenylephrine
Atrial flutter	Cardioversion or rapid digitalization until ventricular rate is less than 100 beats/min
	Quinidine helpful with digitalis
	Consider verapamil or propranolol
Atrial fibrillation	Cardioversion or digitalization to control rate to less than 100 beats/min
	Quinidine helpful after digitalis
	Consider verapamil or propranolol
Premature ventricular contractions	Observe; rule out digitalis toxicity or myocardial infarction
	Lidocaine, quinidine, Bretylium if very frequent
Ventricular tachycardia	Urgent cardioversion, IV lidocaine
	Suspect MI or digitalis toxicity
	Monitor for impending ventricular fibrillation
Ventricular fibrillation	Cardiac massage immediately
	Urgent cardioversion, IV lidocaine
	Suspect MI, hypoxemia
AV block	Atropine, isoproterenol
	Decrease cardiac-decelerating drugs
	Electrical pacing
AV nodal rhythm	Usually self-limited
Sinoatrial block	Self-limited
	Atropine if refractory
Asystole	Cardiac massage
	Intravenous epinephrine, glucagon, isoproterenol
	Calcium gluconate (or intracardiac administration)

atrial fibrillation or flutter should immediately suggest that the patient is in heart failure (a reentrant mechanism due to stretching of the atrial wall). Ventricular tachycardia is always serious and must be treated. Supraventricular brady-arrhythmias are usually benign. Ventricular bradyarrhythmias, however, are usually associated with heart block and are thus a serious problem. Ventricular escape results in a very slow rate and almost invariably compromises cardiac output. Patients who preoperatively have trifascicular block and a history of Stokes-Adams attacks, angina, or heart failure should have an artificial pacemaker placed. Patients with bifascicular block and the above symptoms are controversial; a Holter apparatus should be used to confirm that the symptoms are provoked by the bifascicular block progressing to a complete heart block. Never look upon arrhythmias as a separate entity. They must be considered as one manifestation of many that may signal an untoward course in cardiac performance.

INADVERTENT HYPOTHERMIA

Normal heat-regulating mechanisms are compromised in anesthetized patients. As a result, potentially dangerous reductions in body temperature can develop insidiously and rapidly. Hypothermia is most commonly caused by the air-conditioned environment in the operating room and the administration of cold fluids and blood. Thermal blankets are recommended for preventing operative heat loss, but their usefulness and safety have been questioned. Morris demonstrated that a single warming blanket covered by two layers of thin cotton blanket was not effective in preventing hypothermia in lightly anesthetized, paralyzed adults in cold operating rooms. Additionally, thermal blanket injuries have been reported. The maintenance of ambient temperatures in the range of 21° C to 24° C appears a salient recommendation as a means of decreasing intraoperative heat loss. Cardiac irregularities occur at a body temperature of about 30° C, although they may be present earlier if there is any CO_2 retention or electrolyte abnormalities. Metabolism of certain anesthetic drugs may not continue at the normothermic rate, and therefore these drugs may exert their effects long into the postoperative period. Decreased respiratory exchange, secondary to residual paralysis or anesthesia and coupled with the increased O_2 requirements caused by shivering in the postoperative period, gives rise to a highly dangerous situation. Dramatic decreases in body temperature *must* be avoided.

MALIGNANT HYPERPYREXIA

Malignant hyperpyrexia, first reported by Denborough in 1962, is characterized by fever, tachycardia, tachypnea, and cyanosis. The overall incidence has been reported to be 1 in 15,000 anesthetics in children and 1 in 50,000 adults. There is a geographic variation to these figures, especially in areas where familial evidence of this syndrome is present. Cases have been reported in patients as young as 2 months and as old as 78 years. Malignant hyperpyrexia may be triggered by a multitude of agents. While halothane or succinylcholine is most often involved, either drug is not invariably part of the picture. Malignant hyperpyrexia has occurred with all general anesthetics. It has been suggested that belladonna derivatives, monamine oxidase inhibitors, chlorpromazine, and other phenothiazines may predispose the patient to the condition or trigger it in susceptible individuals.

Clinically, if active rigidity of the masseter muscles occurs following succinylcholine, a presumptive diagnosis of ma-

lignant hyperpyrexia can be made. The other most consistent early sign is tachycardia. This tachycardia, often associated with other arrhythmias, is accompanied by tachypnea and dark blood in the surgical field. Rigidity may or may not be present. Fever is a late sign, but any rise in body temperature necessarily suggests the diagnosis of malignant hyperpyrexia. As stated previously, routine monitoring of temperature within the operating theater is mandatory. Early laboratory findings include metabolic and respiratory acidosis, hypoxemia, hyperkalemia, hypermagnesemia, myoglobinemia, and elevated lactate and pyruvate levels. Diagnosis is made by the clinical recognition of the sequelae of the severe acidosis and the confirmatory laboratory data mentioned earlier.

Successful treatment of malignant hyperpyrexia requires preparedness, early diagnosis, and vigorous therapy. A supply of iced intravenous fluid and a standardized inventory of therapeutic agents are vital.

Symptomatic therapy includes cessation of anesthesia, hyperventilation with 100% oxygen, intravenous injection of Dantrolene sodium 1–10 mg/kg, administration of sodium bicarbonate, initiation of cooling by utilization of large volumes of iced fluids intravenously, submergence in ice, iced lavage of body cavities and surgical wound, the use of gastric hypothermia or partial cardiopulmonary bypass, administration of diuretics (furosemide and mannitol), and administration of insulin and glucose. Procainamide in large doses (1 g/500 ml) has been shown to be effective in arresting the runaway metabolism and is an important adjunct to be applied as soon as the syndrome is diagnosed. Late complications may include consumption coagulopathy, acute renal failure, inadvertent hypothermia, pulmonary edema, skeletal muscle swelling, and neurologic sequelae.

PATIENT CONSIDERATIONS

RESPIRATORY COMPLICATIONS

Respiratory complications in the elderly patient, especially in patients with preexisting chronic lung disease, remain a difficult problem. It is especially important to emphasize the place of pre- and postoperative chest physiotherapy in this group of patients. Various mechanical devices, such as intermittent positive pressure breathing (IPPB), rebreathing tubes, water bottles, and intratracheal catheters, have been proposed to assist in postoperative respiratory care. The patient who can cough effectively but whose efforts are diminished because of pain or residual anesthesia can indeed be benefited by a wide variety of approaches. The patient who cannot raise his secretions, however, must be attended by active nursing involvement, including endotracheal suctioning and chest physiotherapy; as yet there are no mechanical devices capable of replacing these specific therapeutic modalities.

A frequent cause of postoperative respiratory complications in this group is simply the exacerbation of preexisting disease. However, acute respiratory insufficiency with severe hypoxemia in the postoperative period is not confined to patients with preoperative chronic lung disease. There is an increase in the alveolar–arterial oxygen gradient during general anesthesia regardless of the type of surgery or its magnitude. Levels of oxygenation during general anesthesia are beyond predictability. Aging results essentially in reduction of vital capacity, increase in functional residual capacity, and increase in dead space—changes manifest by small airway closure and V-Q abnormalities. The postoperative additive effects of central depression from the anesthetic agents, neurologic defects from muscle relaxants, thoracic immobility from dressings, and the splinting effect of pain are highly compromising to the respiratory component of this frequently already compromised ventilatory system. Fortunately, mechanical support of ventilation has few limitations and many advantages. Elective short-term IPPB should, therefore, be considered in the geriatric patient after all major operations, and longer term support, 24 to 48 hours or longer, is mandatory for the critically ill.

CARDIAC FUNCTION

Since, with each advancing decade, the incidence of electrocardiographically demonstrable coronary artery disease increases, the chance that the stress of anesthesia and surgery may precipitate cardiac decompensation also increases. The same is true for patients with other types of heart disease. Those with established rheumatic or hypertensive cardiac disease may first experience congestive heart failure during the intra- and postoperative period. Brockner studied 235 patients, 166 of whom were operated on for carcinoma of the stomach; their ages were between 60 and 89 years. Among those with cardiac symptoms, EKG changes suggesting degeneration, and an enlarged heart revealed by x-ray film and to whom no digitalis was given preoperatively, half required postoperative digitalization. Deutsch recommends administering digitalis before any major operation when there is a history of cardiac symptoms or electrocardiographic changes suggestive of degeneration or when enlargement of the heart has been demonstrated radiologically. The importance of recognizing marginal cardiac function in the geriatric patient cannot be overemphasized. The increased margin of cardiac reserve afforded by prophylactic digitalization has recently received added support by studies in animals demonstrating protection against the depression in contractile force caused by both pentobarbital anesthesia and hemorrhagic shock.

A patient with a history of myocardial infarction, even if it occurred many years before, has 50 times the likelihood of reinfarction as does a patient of similar age without a history of infarction who is having the same operation. Although different investigators have reported varying reinfarction and mortality rates, when myocardial infarction is recent the risks of anesthesia and surgery are significantly increased. In a 2-year study from the Mayo Clinic, patients who were operated on within 3 months of infarction had a 37% reinfarction rate. This rate decreased to 16% in patients from 3 to 6 months after infarction, and remained at 4% to 5% when infarction had occurred more than 6 months previously. It is important to note that in this series primary infarction or reinfarction occurring after surgery was highly lethal: 54% of the patients died.

Patients who have had a previous infarction must be monitored intensely throughout the perioperative period. Supplemental oxygen provides significant hemodynamic effects following myocardial infarction and should be administered in the postoperative period. Daily electrocardiograms for comparison with preoperative ones are needed to detect "silent" infarction.

BIBLIOGRAPHY

ARENS JF: General principles of anesthesia. In Hardy JD (ed): Rhoads Textbook of Surgery, 5th ed, p 470. Philadelphia, J B Lippincott, 1977

BOOTH DJ, ZUIDEMA GD, CAMERON JL: Aspiration pneumonia: Pulmonary arteriography after experimental aspiration. J Surg Res 12: 48, 1972

BROCKNER J: The evaluation of surgical patients for preoperative digitalization. Acta Chir Scand 129:1, 1965

BRODY GL, SWEET RB: Halothane anesthesia as a possible cause of massive hepatic necrosis. Anesthesiology 24:29, 1963

BRUCE DL, BACH MJ, ARBIT J: Trace anesthetic effects on perceptual, cognitive and motor skills. Anesthesiology 40:453, 1974

BRUNER JMR: Hazards of electrical apparatus. Anesthesiology 28:396, 1967

CAMERON JL, ANDERSON RP, ZUIDEMA GD: Aspiration pneumonia: Results of treatment by positive-pressure ventilation in dogs. J Surg Res 8:447, 1968

CHURCHILL-DAVIDSON HC, KATZ RL: Dual, phase 1, or densensitization block? Anesthesiology 27:536, 1966

COHEN EN: Metabolism of halothane. Anesthesiology 28:651, 1967

COHEN EN: A report. Occupational diseases among operating room personnel: A national study. Anesthesiology 41:321, 1974

COUSINS MJ, MAZZE RI: Methoxyflurane nephrotoxicity: A study of dose response in man. JAMA 225:1611, 1973

COVINO BG: Comparative clinical pharmacology of local anethestic agents. Anesthesiology 35:158, 1971

CROWELL JW, SMITH EE: Oxygen deficit and irreversible hemorrhagic shock. Am J Physiol 206:313, 1968

DE JONG RH, HEAVNER JE: Diazepam prevents local anesthetic seizures. Anesthesiology 34:523, 1971

DENBOROUGH MA, FORSTER JFA, LOVELL RRH et al: Anaesthetic deaths in a family. Br J Anaesth 34:395, 1962

DENNICK OP: Deaths associated with anaesthesia. Anaesthesia 19:536, 1964

DEUTSCH S, DALEN JE: Indications for prophylactic digitalization. Anesthesiology 30:648, 1969

DOWNS JB, CHAPMAN RL, MODELL JH et al: An elevation of steroid therapy in aspiration pneumonitis. Anesthesiology 40:129, 1974

DRIPPS RD, VANDAM LD: Long-term follow-up of patients who received 10,098 spinal anesthetics. I. Failure to discover major neurological sequelae. JAMA 156:1486, 1954

EGER EI, SAIDMAN LJ: Hazards of nitrous oxide anesthesia in bowel obstruction and pneumothorax. Anesthesiology 26:61, 1965

FARMON JV: Heat loss in infants undergoing surgery in air-conditioned theatres. Br J Anaesth 34:543, 1962

FOLDES FF, MCNALL PG: Myasthenia gravis: A guide for anesthesiologists. Anesthesiology 23:837, 1962

GOLDBERG AH, MALING HM, GAFFNEY TE: The value of prophylactic digitalization in halothane anesthesia. Anesthesiology 23:207, 1962

KATZ RL, MATTEO RS, PAPPER EM: The injection of epinephrine during general anesthesia with halogenated hydrocarbons or cyclopropane in man. 2. Halothane. Anesthesiology 23:597, 1962

KLATSKIN G: Mechanisms of toxic and drug induced hepatic injury. In Fink BR (ed): Toxicity of Anesthetics. Baltimore, Williams & Wilkins, 1968

LITTLE DM JR: Posture and anaesthesia. Can Anaesth Soc J 7:2, 1960

MAUNEY FM JR, EBERT PA, SABISTON DC JR: Postoperative myocardial infarction: A study of predisposing factors, diagnosis and mortality in a high risk group of surgical patients. Ann Surg 172:497, 1970

MORRISA RH, KUMAR MB: The effect of warming blankets on maintenance of body temperature of the anesthetized paralyzed adult patient. Anesthesiology 36:408, 1972

MUSHIN WW, ROSEN M, BOWEN DJ et al: Halothane and liver dysfunction: A retrospective study. Br Med J 2:329, 1964

PANDAY J, NUNN JF: Failure to demonstrate progressive falls of arterial PO₂ during anaesthesia. Anaesthesia 23:38, 1968

PRICE HL: A dynamic concept of the distribution of thiopental in the human body. Anesthesiology 21:40, 1960

RYAN JF: Treatment of acute hyperthermia crisis. In Britt (ed): International Anesthesiology Clinics, vol. 17. Boston, Little, Brown & Co, 1979

SHERLOCK S: Progress report—halothane hepatitis. Gut 12:324, 1967

STEPHEN CR, LAWRENCE JH, FABIAN LW et al: Clinical experience with Fluothane: 1400 cases. Anesthesiology 19:197, 1958

TAYLOR G, PRYSE-DAVIES J: The prophylactic use of antacids in the prevention of the acid-pulmonary-aspiration syndrome (Mendelson's syndrome). Lancet I:288, 1966

TOLMIE JD, JOYCE TH, MITCHELL GD: Succinylcholine danger in the burned patient. Anesthesiology 28:467, 1967

TWO

Specific Organs and Organ Systems

Head and Neck

Robert F. Ryan/Michael P. Vercimak

Lesions of the Mouth, Tongue, Jaws, and Salivary Glands

263

There are many benign inflammatory and congenital lesions of the oral cavity. However, the lesions which involve the surgeon most often are the malignant neoplasias. Although this group of neoplasms makes up a relatively small proportion of all cancer (5% in men and 21% in women), its treatment remains largely surgical and requires, for its efficacy, the skill in nutrition and reconstruction and the critical assessment of results that are fundamental to the field of surgery. In dealing with any lesion, a systematic approach should be followed. The usual classification regarding cause is shown in Fig. 17-1. Such an outline is most helpful in differential diagnosis.

The immunologic interactions of head and neck malignancies and their hosts are receiving increasing attention. It has been noted that T-cell populations are decreased in patients with head and neck malignancies. Anergy—absent or greatly decreased recall sensitivity to common antigens—is noted in many patients with these neoplasms. Return of immune recall after treatment denotes a good prognosis, while persistent anergy seems to be an ominous prognostic sign.

The appropriate approach to oral cavity carcinoma is the subject of a great deal of debate but there are very few prospective randomized studies. It is important, therefore, that the head and neck surgeon be familiar with the methods of classifying these lesions so that lesions of a similar stage can be compared and treatment results evaluated objectively. The classification of the American Joint Committee for Cancer Staging and End-Results Reporting has been widely accepted (see TNM system in Chapter 14, *e.g.,* Table 14-3). It evolved from earlier efforts but still has several shortcomings, such as the fact that it is a clinical system. For this reason it will probably undergo further refinements. Keep an additional data sheet, on which to log a lesion's size, extent of involvement, histological grade, and so on. Note any revisions as a result of surgical removal and pathological exam, in such a way as to distinguish them from the preoperative assessment.

ORAL CAVITY

The following anatomic boundaries of the various areas of the oral cavity, as defined by the American Joint Committee, will be the ones used in this chapter.

The oral cavity extends from the skin-vermillion junction of the lips to the junction of the hard and soft palate above and to the line of circumvallate papilla below and is divided into the following specific areas: lip, buccal mucosa, lower alveolar ridge, upper alveolar ridge, retromolar trigone and floor of mouth, hard palate, and the anterior two thirds of the tongue.

LIP

The lip begins at the junction of the vermillion border with the skin and includes only the vermillion surface or that portion of the lip from the vermillion border to the point of contact of the upper and lower lips.

BENIGN LESIONS

Congenital Lesions

The most important congenital condition of the lips is the cleft; its cosmetic, functional, and surgical implications alone warrant a complete discussion and are handled in Chapter 43. Other congenital conditions include mucous pits, small blind pouches at or below the vermillion border that are treated by meticulous excision, and microstomia, the congenital presence of a small oral opening. This may be significant enough to impair nutrition and therefore may require early correction.

Infectious Conditions

Lip infections may be caused by viral, bacterial, or fungal agents. In most cases these are self-limiting and respond to nonsurgical and supportive measures. Only rarely is biopsy indicated to differentiate them from malignant neoplasms. One exception to this rule is cancrum oris (noma). This is an extremely destructive virulent necrotizing lesion thought to be caused by synergistic interactions of several different species of bacteria under anaerobic conditions in a compromised host. Treatment involves vigorous anaerobic antibiotic therapy, debridement of necrotic tissues, and plastic reconstruction of residual defects.

Trauma

Lacerations are common and frequently involve the entire thickness of the lip. Repair is by meticulous reapproximation of the anatomical layers. Silk or absorbable suture material is used on the mucosal side, and monofilament nonabsorbable material on the skin surface. Exact approximation of the vermillion border is essential for optimal results and should be performed before apposition of the remainder of the skin margin.

Burns

Burns of the lips are seen in little children who bite through the insulation of electrical appliance cords. These burns are often third degree and frequently involve the commissures. Although early excision has been advocated, most authors

Fig. 17-1.   Diagram of diseases of the head and neck region.

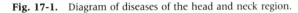

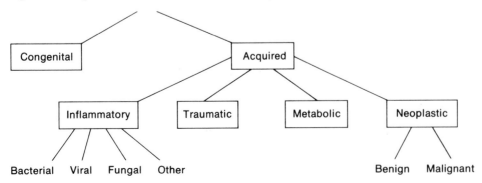

recommend hospitalization of these patients, with careful debridement of the necrotic tissue and observation for hemorrhage from disruption of the labial artery. Reconstructive measures are often required but are done as secondary procedures.

Other Benign Lesions

The skin of the lip is heir to many of the benign lesions that may be found in the skin and subcutaneous tissues elsewhere. A few are unique when they occur in this area and therefore merit special consideration.

Vascular Lesions. Capillary hemangiomas are present at birth and may grow at an alarming rate before undergoing regression. Excision is indicated for bleeding, infection, or functional impairment (Fig. 17-2). Cavernous hemangiomas are composed of large ectatic vessels. These lesions occur in early childhood and gradually enlarge, causing cosmetic and functional impairment. They typically have numerous feeding vessels and are difficult to embolize. Resection and reconstruction give the most consistent results. Telangiectases occur on the lips in the form of venous lakes (venous varix), and port-wine stains (nevus flammeus). They are significant aesthetically, but they neither impair function nor undergo neoplastic degeneration. A third type of telangiectasia occurs as a small scattered blanching lesion over the lip and mucous membranes, is associated with similar lesions in the gastrointestinal tract, and makes up part of the symptom complex of Osler-Weber-Rendu disease.

Pigmented Lesions. Peutz-Jeghers syndrome is characterized by gastrointestinal hamartomatous polyps associated with melanin pigmentation of the lips, buccal mucosa, and digits. The finding of these characteristic lesions denotes a much improved outlook for patients with congenital intestinal polyps.

PREMALIGNANT LESIONS

Hyperkeratosis is a whitish thickening on the lips associated with chronic trauma or sun exposure. It has been given the name leukoplakia because of its clinical appearance, but the designation encompasses a wide variety of lesions from

Fig. 17-2. The capillary hemangioma in the upper lip of this infant is regressing.

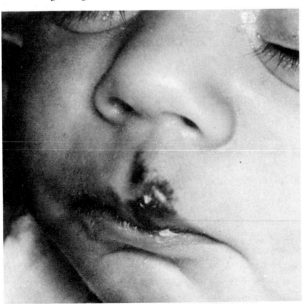

simple keratosis to infiltrating carcinoma. Since there is little association between the clinical appearance of leukoplakic lesions and their degree of invasiveness, all whitish patches on the lips and oral mucosa must be taken seriously. In a large series the probability that a clinical lesion represented a premalignant or malignant lesion was 20%. It can be assumed that there is a high association between this lesion and frank carcinoma, but the exact incidence of malignant degeneration is unknown, with estimates varying from 2% to 70%.

MALIGNANT LESIONS

Carcinoma of the lip is the most common malignancy of the oral cavity, comprising 25% of all cancers of this group. The lower lip is the primary site in 90% of lesions. Actinic exposure is well established as an etiologic factor, with 80% of patients having a clear history of years of exposure to sunlight. Men are affected more commonly, in a ratio of 20:1, and typically have fair skin and a light complexion. The association between lip cancer and smoking is less well defined than for other areas of the oral cavity, and no definite association has been established between pipe smokers and carcinoma of the lip. The peak age of incidence is 60 years, and 80% of patients are 50 or older.

The lesions are generally well differentiated (85%). Key prognostic factors are the late occurrence of neck metastasis and the degree of differentiation. Because of their conspicuous anatomic location, these lesions are characteristically noted when they are small; 80% of patients will present with T1 lesions. This is the primary factor contributing to the overall 5-year survival of 90%. Cancer of the lip is also a less aggressive malignancy than cancers of other areas of the oral cavity, even in the presence of regional metastasis. Several authors could not demonstrate a difference in survival in tumors stages I through III. Patients who develop recurrence at the primary site or have delayed cervical lymph node metastasis appear to have approximately a 50% 5-year survival.

The number of patients who present with clinically positive lymph nodes varies from 6% to 20%. Of those patients with clinically positive nodes, histologic metastasis is confirmed in about 20% of cases. This high rate of false positive node assessments is a major criticism of the TNM system and probably accounts for similar outcomes of the different stages.

With these facts in mind, the best approach to patients with carcinoma of the lip can be determined. For Stage I lesions, simple excision of the lesion with a 1-cm margin of normal tissue is sufficient (Fig. 17-3). Radiation therapy for small lesions has been shown to be equally efficacious in eradicating the tumor but has the disadvantages of a slightly higher local recurrence rate, delayed cosmetic deformity, and a treatment course protracted over several weeks. For patients with clinically positive submental nodes, a suprahyoid dissection is recommended, with frozen section analysis of lymphoid tissue. If histologic confirmation of metastasis is found, the procedure is extended to a formal radical neck dissection; if this area is negative, no further dissection need be carried out.

Surgical salvage of recurrent carcinoma is successful in 50% of cases. All patients with the diagnosis of an epidermoid carcinoma of the lip should be followed closely for several years after resection. In addition, there is approximately a 20% incidence of a second malignancy among patients with carcinoma of the lip. The actual significance

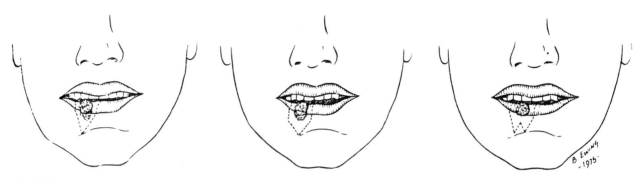

Fig. 17-3. Stage I lesions of the lip. (*Left*) The traditional V excision for small lesions should be avoided because recurrences are too frequent. (*Center*) A shield excision gives wider margins of resection than those obtained with a V excision. (*Right*) A W resection can be modified to obtain a better closure after resection of small lip lesions.

of such a correlation is difficult to assess, however, as many of the reports come from large cancer institutions with a variable amount of interdepartment referrals; and in the peak age of incidence of this lesion, cancer in general accounts for about one third of the general mortality.

BUCCAL MUCOSA

The buccal mucosa includes all the membrane lining of the inner surface of the cheek and lips, from the line of contact of the opposing lips to the line of attachment of mucosa of the alveolar ridge (upper and lower) and the pterygomandibular raphe.

BENIGN LESIONS

Mucocele
A mucocele is a smooth, painless, soft, freely movable mass that contains mucoid material. Mucoceles occur on the inner aspect of the lower lip in 60% of cases and are believed to result primarily from trauma to the excretory apparatus of a minor salivary gland, leading to extravasation of salivary excretion into the surrounding soft tissue.

Fibrous Lesions
Fibrous lesions are caused by various irritative conditions, such as malfitting dentures or nervous biting of the cheek mucosa, or as a response to other chronic irritations arising in the oral mucous membrane of the lip, palate, tongue, and (most commonly) cheek. They appear variously as pedunculated, sessile, hard or soft, smooth or covered with a granular surface. Their clinical course is benign, and treatment consists of correcting the underlying cause and excision.

PREMALIGNANT LESIONS

The cheek is the most common site of leukoplakia in the oral cavity. As noted in the discussion of hyperkeratosis of the lip, leukoplakia should be excised when noted and carefully examined for *in situ* or frankly invasive carcinoma. It is often associated with sites of chronic irritation caused by dentures or snuff dipping.

MALIGNANT LESIONS

Verrucous carcinoma, also found on the gingiva and occasionally in other areas of the upper aerodigestive tract, is the least common of buccal carcinomas. In the buccal mucosa, it commonly occurs in the mandibular-buccal sulcus and appears as a raised papillary mass with a granular surface. This lesion is associated with the chewing of tobacco and the use of snuff. It is regarded as an indolent process occurring slowly over many years of irritation, with metastasis to the regional nodes occurring late. With appropriate treatment, patients with verrucous carcinoma should have 5-year survival rates of from 60% to 75%.

Exophytic and ulceroinfiltrative carcinomas constitute the majority of buccal malignant neoplasms. An exophytic carcinoma presents as a soft white raised area in the midcheek, often without symptoms; the ulceroinfiltrative carcinoma extends into the surrounding buccinator muscle and adjacent tissues early and presents as a painful, firm, ulcerated mass. Both varieties are deeply infiltrative and highly aggressive, often with palpable submandibular nodes. Extension onto the gingiva and anterior tonsillar pillars is common; in the latter case, radical resection is extremely difficult. Overall 5-year survival rates in older series ranged from 30% to 52%. These series may have been misleading because of the inclusion of varieties of verrucous carcinoma. A more recent series using surgery and surgery in combination with radiation therapy reports an absolute cure rate of 34%, with survivals of 77%, 65%, 27%, and 18% for stages I to IV, respectively. Lymph node involvement was the most significant prognostic factor. Failure of therapy occurs in the form of local recurrence (43%) and regional metastasis (37%). Therefore, primary treatment of these lesions consists of wide composite resections with *en bloc* radical neck dissection. In the case of a verrucous carcinoma with no clinical adenopathy, wide excision alone yields acceptable results, but radical excision of the occasionally far-advanced verrucous carcinoma is indicated, as these lesions remain localized even at this stage. The use of radiation therapy preoperatively, postoperatively, or as a primary modality is controversial. There is some evidence that it may lead to significantly lower survival rates and, with the verrucous variety, is associated occasionally with recurrence in the form of a much more virulent lesion. Most radiologists refuse to treat verrucous lesions.

GINGIVA—ALVEOLAR RIDGES AND RETROMOLAR TRIGONE

This area consists of three components:

Lower alveolar ridge. This ridge includes the alveolar process of the mandible and its covering mucosa, which extends from the line of attachment of the mucosa in the buccal gutter to the line of free mucosa of the floor of the mouth. Posteriorly it extends to the ascending ramus of the mandible.

Upper alveolar ridge. The upper ridge is the alveolar process of the maxilla and its covering mucosa, which extends from the line of attachment of mucosa in the upper gingival gutter to the junction of the hard palate. Its posterior margin is the upper end of the pterygopalatine arch.

Retromolar gingiva (retromolar trigone). This is the attached mucosa overlying the ascending ramus of the mandible from the level of the posterior surface of the last molar tooth to the apex superiorly adjacent to the tuberosity of the maxilla.

BENIGN LESIONS

Cysts
Gingival cysts occur in adults and children as a smooth gingival swelling and result from cystic degeneration of rests of dental lamina. Treatment in adults consists of simple excision.

Granulomas
Granuloma pyogenicum is a lesion predominantly of the gingiva but occasionally also occurs on the buccal mucosa, lips, and tongue. The name is somewhat misleading; it is probably not a response to infection but is generally associated with trauma. Microscopically it consists of numerous capillaries with an infiltration of inflammatory cells. It is completely benign, and cure is effected by simple excision for biopsy. *Granuloma gravidarum* is identical in appearance to the pyogenic granuloma. It appears early in pregnancy and disappears near term.

MALIGNANT LESIONS

Again, malignancies of the gingiva are almost exlusively epidermoid carcinoma. They comprise 10% of oral malignancies and are often overlooked or misdiagnosed until they are far advanced. There is a male predominance of 7:1, with the presenting symptoms being malfitting dentures, loose teeth, or (mistakenly) a dental abscess. They infiltrate early, with invasion of bone in half the cases, and rapidly metastasize to the submandibular nodes. Since radiation therapy to tumors infiltrating bones is rarely successful and is often associated with dental degeneration and osteoradionecrosis, treatment of choice is surgical resection. In the lower gingiva this is accomplished by *en bloc* resection of tumor and mandible and radical neck dissection. In the upper gingiva this *en bloc* principle still applies, but neck dissection is reserved for those cases with clinically positive nodes. Defects in the maxilla may be closed by local flaps or special dental prosthesis which obturate nasaloral fistula. Survival figures vary somewhat with reported series, presumably as a result of the high false positive rate of clinical assessment of submandibular nodes. Overall 5-year survival rates on the order of 40% to 50% are reported, with a significantly poorer prognosis if there is histologic evidence of cervical node involvement.

FLOOR OF THE MOUTH

The floor of the mouth is the semilunar space over the mylohyoid and hyoglossus muscles, extending from the inner surface of the lower alveolar ridge to the under surface of the tongue. Its posterior boundary is the base of the anterior pillar of the tonsil. It is divided into two sides by the frenulum of the tongue and contains the ostia of the submaxillary and sublingual salivary glands.

BENIGN LESIONS

Ranula
The term ranula is applied to a cyst obscuring the floor of the mouth produced by a partial obstruction of the salivary duct, usually by a stone. Treatment consists of excision or marsupialization of the cyst. If the process is chronic, the gland may need to be excised.

Dermoid Cyst
A dermoid cyst is a relatively rare lesion, present invariably in the midline, and which often simulates a ranula. Treatment is by complete excision.

MALIGNANT LESIONS

Cancer of the floor of the mouth is of particular significance, as resection in the past led to the most deforming disabilities of all intraoral cancer. Attempts to minimize this deformity by radiation therapy are fraught with difficulties. This cancer comprises 10% to 15% of all oral carcinomas and most often presents as a deceptively normal lesion on the anterior portion of the floor of the mouth. Because the tissues of the floor of the mouth are relatively loose, the lesions infiltrate early along the mandible and posteriorly to the base of the tongue, a clinical finding that denotes an ominous prognosis. Men in their fifth and sixth decades predominate over women, although there is evidence that the incidence in women is increasing.

Treatment plans involving surgery after radiation therapy and combination therapy with and without intra-arterial infusion have been employed. Both surgery and radiation therapy have high complication rates, including salivary fistula, infection, aspiration pneumonia, and carotid hemorrhage. The control rates for small lesions are similar. The incidence of osteomyelitis and sequestration when radiation therapy is used for larger lesions rises in direct proportion to the size of the tumors to 50% for lesions over 4 cm. With improved techniques that have become possible largely due to free flap transfers and composite myocutaneous flaps, the use of surgery as a therapeutic modality is gradually replacing radiation therapy. Survival rates with these new techniques are showing some improvement. Recent series show an 89% survival for T_1 and T_2 (Stage I) lesions and a 56% survival for those with more advanced tumors (T_3 lesions). Radiation therapy rates for similar groups of patients in this same study were 64% and 27%, respectively. These figures may be compared with a study published a decade earlier which showed survival rates of 49% to 69% for earlier lesions, with a disappointing 7% to 24% for advanced lesions. Figure 17-4 illustrates the current treatment with simultaneous reconstruction for a far-advanced cancer of the floor of the mouth involving much of the mandible.

HARD PALATE

The hard palate is the semilunar area between the upper alveolar ridge and the mucous membrane covering the palatine process of the maxillary palatine bones. It extends from the inner surface of the superior alveolar ridge to the posterior edge of the palatine bone.

BENIGN LESIONS

Torus palatinus
Torus palatinus is an exostosis of the paired palatal processes of the maxillae that occurs in the midline (Fig. 17-5). It is

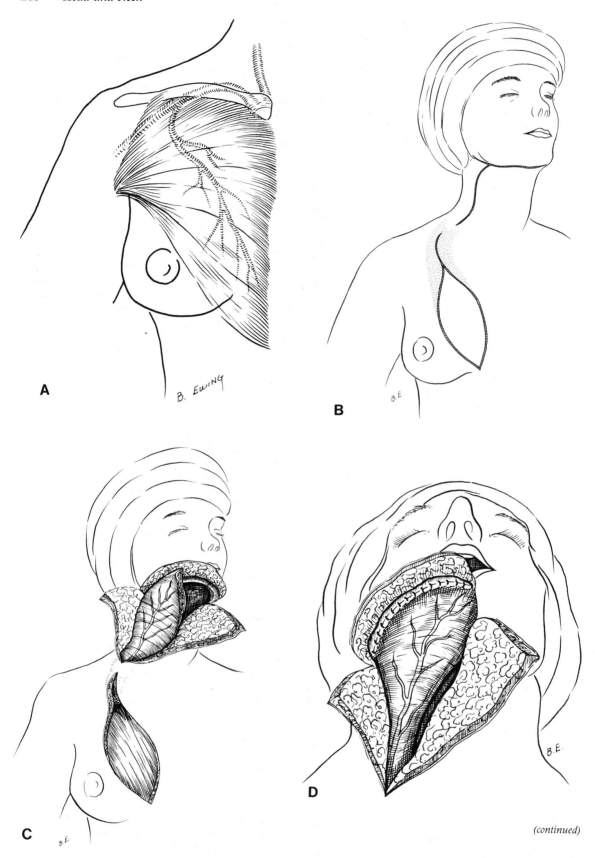

A

B. EWING

B

B.E.

C

B.E.

D

B.E.

(continued)

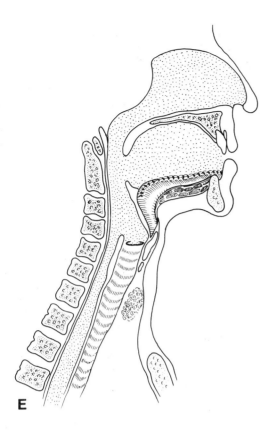

E

Fig. 17-4. Treatment for far-advanced cancer of the floor of the mouth. (*A*) Major arterial supply to the pectoralis major muscle. (*B*) Incision used for neck dissection and glossectomy with musculocutaneous flap. (*C*) Tunneling of musculocutaneous flap to reach to the oral cavity. (*D*) Suturing of the skin from the chest wall to the buccal mucosa after removal of most of tongue and floor of mouth. The flap is sutured in to cover the replaced mandible. (*E*) Chest flap sutured in place from the epiglottis to mucous membrane inside the lip covering the replaced mandible.

symmetrical, covered with mucosa, and rarely becomes a problem except in fitting dentures.

Necrotizing Sialometaplasia

Necrotizing sialometaplasia is an idiopathic necrotizing ulcerative process of the palate characterized microscopically by ischemic necrosis of the minor salivary glands with interstitial release of mucus and subsequent inflammation. It is self-limiting and appears to be a unique response to injury. It is important to differentiate this lesion from carcinoma of the palate.

Fig. 17-5. This large torus palatinus will need to be removed before the patient can be well fitted with dentures.

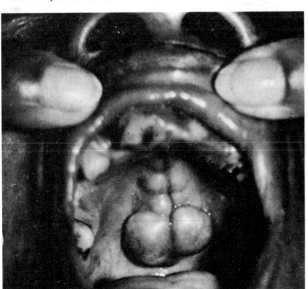

MALIGNANT LESIONS

Salivary Tumors

The palate is unique among the intraoral regions in that it is one area in which the majority of tumors are of minor salivary gland origin rather than epidermoid. This single area accounts for more than 50% of all minor salivary tumors. Further aspects of these malignancies will be developed in the salivary gland discussion.

Squamous Cell Carcinomas

Squamous cell carcinomas make up 20% to 25% of malignancies of this area, except in cultures where there is the habit of smoking tobacco products with the lighted end held in the oral cavity. It primarily occurs in patients over 50 years of age and occurs in men twice as often as in women. Surgery with *en bloc* dissection and radical neck nodal dissection in cases of large lesions with clinically positive nodes is the treatment of choice. Treatment fails in a significant number of cases due to local recurrence and is usually evident within 18 months following primary resection. Prognostic factors of highest significance are size of primary tumors and nodal metastasis. The 5-year survival is 65% for Stage I lesions, decreasing to a survival rate of essentially zero for Stage IV lesions.

ANTERIOR TWO THIRDS OF THE TONGUE (ORAL TONGUE)

The anterior two thirds is a freely mobile portion of the tongue that extends anteriorly from the line of circumvallate papillae to the undersurface of the tongue at the junction of the floor of the mouth. It is composed of four areas: the tip, the lateral borders, the dorsum, and the undersurface (nonvillous surface).

BENIGN LESIONS

Lingual Tonsil

Lingual tonsil refers to the congenital occurrence of lymphoid tissue on the tongue. It produces no mucosal ulceration and requires no therapy.

Lingual Thyroid

Lingual thyroid refers to the presence of functional thyroid tissue on the tongue and represents failure of the thyroid anlage to descend into the neck from its point of origin on the base of the tongue. Evaluation of lesions in this area should include a thyroid scan. Treatment is by thyroid suppression with oral hormone, with excision as required if this treatment fails. Autotransplantation of this tissue may be beneficial.

Glossitis Rhomboidica Medians

Glossitis rhomboidica medians is a congenital anomaly in which the midline portion of the tongue is smooth, raised, and reddish because of the absence of papillae. No treatment is necessary, and there is no malignant degeneration associated with this lesion.

Granular Cell Myoblastoma

Granular cell myoblastoma is a discrete submucosal lesion without overlying ulceration that tends to occur in the upper GI tract, particularly in the tongue. It is entirely benign but should be excised to differentiate it from cancer.

MALIGNANT LESIONS

Squamous cell carcinomas make up 97% of malignancies in this area (Fig. 17-6). The tongue is second only to the lip in total incidence of carcinoma of the oral cavity. Patients are typically male tobacco and alcohol users in their sixth to eighth decades. The lesion may present as a nondescript area of focal thickening and roughness or as clinical leukoplakia. Other forms of presentation are as a painless, superficial ulceration or desquamation. Some are morbidly exophytic, while deeply infiltrative types may have no surface ulceration until late in their course.

Evaluation of patients with this lesion includes thorough physical examination, with special attention to node-bearing areas of the neck and bimanual examination of the tongue. Lesions from the tip of the tongue metastasize to the submental nodes first. Lesions of the lateral aspect of the tongue metastasize to the submandibular nodes first. While these cancers usually occur in older men, they can occur in young women, as shown in Figure 17-6a. This 27-year-old was referred for evaluation and treatment in December 1979. The lesion had been enlarging for at least six months, but its significance had eluded her dentist, who had built a crown for a tooth that was broken and had "irritated" the tongue. The patient was Stage IV, as the lesion was over 4 cm in size and the patient had four clinically positive nodes in the right neck that were later shown to contain metastatic tumor. She had a subtotal glossectomy and right radical neck dissection after sensitization with chemotherapy. The second picture shows the patient two years later free of disease (Fig. 17-6b).

Treatment of these lesions involves surgical resection, resection and node dissection, radiation therapy pre-op, post-op, or alone, and radiation or surgical salvage for recurrent lesions. Unfortunately, adequate controlled, randomized, or prospective studies are lacking to substantiate the advantages of any single or combination therapy over any other. A recent report from a large institution well known for many years of specialized treatment of tumors offers the following suggestion:

Treatment of T_1NO carcinoma of the tongue is equally effective with either intraoral surgical excision or a localized dose of radiation. For T_2 lesions, intraoral excision alone is the proper initial treatment, since local and regional occurrences can be handled adequately in 96% of patients. Surgery

Fig. 17-6. (*A*) A 27-year-old female with a Stage IV squamous cell carcinoma of the lateral surface of the tongue. The patient had four clinically positive nodes. (*B*) The patient 2 years after subtotal glossectomy and right radical neck dissection. The patient had four histologically positive nodes.

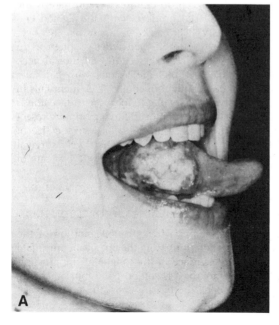
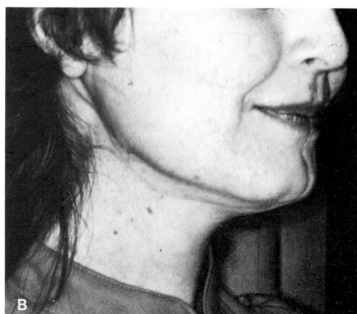

should also be the initial treatment in patients with lesions staged T$_3$ or T$_4$. The surgery should be tailored to adequately remove the gross and microscopic disease. Postoperative radiation is indicated if there is extension of disease into the pterygoid area, involvement of large nerves, or multiple cervical nodes. Gross tumor cut through at the time of surgery, proven microscopic residual disease in small nerves, lingual musculature, or adjacent mucosa after repeated reexcision with frozen section analysis are also criteria for immediate postoperative radiation. Mandible resection is indicated for tumor attached to the periosteum. In T$_2$, T$_3$, or T$_4$ tumors, radiation is contraindicated as initial therapy; the rate of initial failure in the tongue is unacceptably high, and the results of "salvage" therapy of recurrences are discouraging.

Whatever the method used, the previously published 5-year survival rates (overall determinant) are 30% to 40%, with a survival rate of 65% for small lesions with no metastasis. With more attention to building up the patient's own immunologic response before surgery, it is believed that current rates for T$_3$–T$_4$ lesions can be improved.

SALIVARY GLANDS

The salivary system consists of three major components: the parotid, the "lesser" salivary glands—submaxillary and sublingual—and the "minor" salivary glands.

The parotid is the largest, the most thoroughly studied, and the most often involved with disease processes. It is divided into "lobes" by the facial nerve and its branches, the superficial lobe being located external to the facial nerve and the deep lobe below this structure. The division is more one of convenience than of anatomy, however, as no discrete plane or septum is consistently found. In fact, the entire substance of the gland is intertwined around the facial nerve. The technique of dissecting and preserving the nerve with superficial parotidectomy is well described by Beahrs et al.

The submaxillary gland is located below the "lower maxilla" or mandible. It lies deep to the mylohyoid muscle and superficial to the hyoglossus muscle. Its excretory duct (Wharton's duct) travels anteriorly and opens in the midline sublingual caruncula. Tumors of the submaxillary gland are malignant in 60% of cases, as contrasted to the parotid, where the incidence of malignancy is 20% to 30%. Of the benign submaxillary lesions, mixed tumor is reported in over 90% of cases. Of malignant lesions, adenoid cystic carcinoma is the most common cell type, occurring in about 50% of cases. Malignant lesions most often present as a lump only rarely associated with pain. The outlook for these tumors has not improved over the past 15 years. For this reason some authors have advocated a more aggressive approach to the earlier lesions, including wide block dissections with incontinuity neck dissections even for earlier lesions. Survival rates at 5 years are presently a dismal 25% to 30%.

The sublingual gland is the smallest of the lesser salivary glands. Lesions are unusual but are malignant in over 70% of cases. Of the malignant lesions, adenoid cystic carcinoma and mucoepidermoid carcinoma are the most common. Treatment of malignancies of this area may require partial mandibulectomy with radical neck dissection. Survival rates are similar to those for submaxillary malignancies.

Minor salivary glands are similar in structure and function to the rest of the salivary system. They are widely distributed in the mucosa of the lips and cheek, hard and soft palate, uvula, floor of mouth, nasopharynx, larynx, lacrimal glands, trachea, and even skin and breasts. There are estimated to be 400 to 700 of these structures in the oral cavity alone, with the heaviest concentration on the palate. Treatment of malignancies includes *en bloc* resection and radical neck dissection for metastasis. This requires a sophisticated knowledge of reconstructive techniques for reconstruction of the surgical defects. Several reports have suggested beneficial effects when roentgen therapy is combined with surgery of these lesions.

BENIGN LESIONS

Mumps is an acute painful parotitis caused by a strain of paramyxovirus. It most often occurs in younger age groups and is highly communicable. Although usually a mild self-limiting malady, it may be associated with serious sequelae. A vaccine which affords 95% protection is available (Jeryl Lynn strain).

Mikulicz's syndrome is a nonspecific clinical term that refers to bilateral enlargement of the lacrimal and salivary glands caused by a variety of diseases: leukemia, lymphoma, tuberculosis, sarcoidosis.

Sjögren's syndrome is the triad of dry eyes (xerophthalmia), dry mouth (xerostomia), and "dry joints" (chronic arthritis). It is associated with an autoimmune complex of diseases and is manifested histologically by lymphocytic infiltration of the lacrimal and salivary glands. Treatment is symptomatic.

Pyogenic parotitis, which may be diffuse or localized and suppurative, occurs in surgical patients, debilitated patients, and those with severe uncontrolled underlying disease. The parotid glands are swollen and painful and may exude pus from the orifice of Stensen's duct. Inspissation of the saliva from dehydration or lack of dietary stimulation in patients with nasogastric tubes are thought to be etiologic factors. Treatment consists of antibiotics (*Staphylococcus aureus* being the most common organism cultured), rehydration, and the use of secretagogues. If an area of discrete fluctuance develops, dependent drainage is indicated with due regard to the anatomy of the facial nerve.

Warthin's tumor (papillary cystadenolymphomatosum) is an asymptomatic mass typically occurring at the angle of the mandible in older men (average age 56 years). It is thought to arise from inclusions of ductal epithelial elements in the parotid lymph node. Scanning with ^{99m}Tc pertechnetate is useful, as are needle aspirations, in the diagnosis of this lesion. Recurrence is uncommon after complete excision, usually by superficial parotidectomy. The lesion is bilateral in approximately 10% of patients.

Sialolithiasis is almost exclusively a problem of the submandibular gland and often arises in patients with chronic sialadenitis. The stones are often radiopaque. Therefore, diagnosis is by roentgenogram and physical exam. Optimal treatment involves removing the affected gland along with the calculus.

Pleomorphic adenoma (mixed tumor) is the most common neoplasm of salivary tissue, comprising 53% to 71% of these lesions. It presents as a solitary, slowly growing, painless, firm, smooth movable mass without nerve involvement. Diagnosis is by history and histologic exam at the time of surgery and hinges on the finding of both mesenchymal and epithelial elements in the specimen. Treatment is by complete excision of the tumor with a wide margin of normal tissue. Optimally this implies total parotidectomy with preservation of the facial nerve branches, a procedure facilitated by the use of surgical loupes. There is no place for enucleation in the treatment of a mixed tumor. This type of inadequate treatment subjects the patient to an unacceptably high rate of recurrence and the possibility of malignant degeneration.

TRAUMA

The parotid gland is, by virtue of its location, subject to iatrogenic or external trauma. Laceration of Stensen's duct with surrounding branches of the facial nerve requires meticulous reapproximation with microsurgical precision. Failure to recognize such an injury or an ineffective repair may result in salivary fistulas, facial paralysis, and chronic sialadenitis. An interesting sequela of auriculotemporal nerve injury is the development of Frey's syndrome, or gustatory sweating, in which the stimulus to salivation produces sweating over the parotid area. Although rarely disabling, this syndrome may be occasionally confused with a salivary fistula. It can be alleviated by section of Jacobsen's nerve within the middle ear, but reassurance often suffices to allow patients to tolerate this minor disability.

MALIGNANT LESIONS

The treatment of parotid neoplasms requires that the surgeon become familiar with the common histologic types of malignancies, as the biologic behavior and the prognosis vary widely with each. The names given to these variants are similar sounding and often a source of confusion, but their malignant "personalities" are quite unique and bear heavily on three important decisions a surgeon must make when faced with a parotid neoplasm:
1. Subtotal vs. total parotidectomy
2. Disposition of the facial nerve
3. Indication for and timing of neck dissection

The role of adjunctive radiation or chemotherapy at present is undefined. Several encouraging reports have emerged, but until double-blind prospective studies substantiate their efficacy their incorporation into treatment regimens remains empirical.

Malignant mixed tumors (carcinoma ex pleomorphic adenoma) are aggressive malignancies that comprise 1% to 10% of all salivary tumors. Their distinctive feature is the presence of mesenchymal tumor tissue in a malignant tumor also containing epithelial structures. It metastasizes most often to regional lymph nodes and lungs and to a lesser extent to bone and brain. Typically the patient gives a history of rapid growth in a long-standing parotid mass that may be accompanied by pain and facial nerve paralysis. Treatment consists of radical total parotidectomy. Regional or metastatic spread is an extremely ominous prognostic sign and usually signifies death within a year. Nodes with obvious clinical involvement should be removed, but radical neck dissection has not been shown to alter the outcome.

Mucoepidermoid is the name given to salivary malignancies that show "mixed epidermoid and mucus-secreting patterns." They comprise 3% to 9% of all salivary gland tumors. They are unique in that their prognosis is greatly dependent on their histologic grade. Low-grade malignancies have nearly 100% 15-year survival rates, but intermediate and high-grade neoplasms have a correspondingly poor prognosis. Initial spread is to regional lymph nodes, and therefore

radical neck dissection should always accompany total parotidectomy for all the high- to intermediate-grade malignancies. Low-grade malignancies carry such a favorable prognosis that radical neck dissection is not indicated.

Adenoid cystic carcinoma (cylindroma) is a slow-growing malignancy that comprises 4% of all salivary tumors. Its distinguishing characteristic is its tendency to invade peripheral nerves early in its course. It presents with nerve palsy and pain and recurs despite apparently "curative" resections. For this reason, adjunctive radiation therapy holds the most promise for this type of lesion. Its prognosis depends upon its location, the palate and parotid having a much better prognosis than the submandibular gland. Unfortunately, it is the most common malignancy in the submandibular gland.

Acinous cell carcinoma (acinic) comprises 2% to 4% of parotid tumors and carries the best overall prognosis of the parotid malignancies. It is believed to derive from the terminal portions of the salivary duct system and—like its breast counterpart, the lobular carcinoma—has the greatest incidence of bilaterality (3%). Most of these lesions are slow-growing, late to metastasize, and easily resected, but approximately 10% (without any distinguishing histologic characteristics) recur, metastasize, and pursue a very aggressive course. This has led to considerable variation of opinion as to their disposition. However, with the techniques available today for reconstruction and nerve repair, a "Russian roulette" approach to the patient is not warranted and minimum acceptable therapy should consist of total radical parotidectomy.

Adenocarcinoma is the name given to those carcinomas that cannot be categorized into one of the above four groups but that still can be identified as a glandular malignancy. These tumors exhibit a wide range of aggressive tendencies, but certain clues are helpful in tailoring therapy and in prognosis. Histologic staging—that is, local destructive infiltration apparent on microscopic exam—suggests a poor prognosis. Similarly, local recurrence has been associated with a 67% mortality. The implications of regional nodes and distant metastases are similar; therefore, node dissections would appear to be more helpful for staging rather than tumor eradication.

Undifferentiated carcinomas are rare, extremely lethal tumors. Little evidence exists to support the usefulness of any modality of therapy in altering the poor prognosis.

Squamous cell carcinoma is generally considered to be a relatively rare tumor of the salivary glands, comprising only about 3% of malignant lesions. It acts much like squamous cell carcinoma of other areas of the neck, with local recurrence and regional spread being prominent features. Treatment is by total parotidectomy with regional node dissection.

LESIONS OF THE JAW

The elements of the jaw are the upper maxilla and the "lower" maxilla (mandible). Their ectodermal and mesodermal elements give rise to a variety of benign and malignant lesions.

CONGENITAL LESIONS

There is some overlap between congenital lesions and neoplastic lesions of the jaw. The lesions of congenital origin that most often present in adulthood will therefore be considered under other topics, and only those that are apparent at birth will be considered in this section. Clefts of the lip frequently extend into the maxilla and are one of the more common congenital anomalies. They also are covered elsewhere.

Congenital cysts are benign growths that occur most often along lines of embryonic fusion. Treatment is by complete excision of the epithelial sac.

Epignathus is a congenital condition in which vestigial elements of a twin are attached to either maxilla. These tumors are classed as teratomas and occasionally undergo malignant degeneration. In the lesions depicted (Fig. 17-7A, B), the teratomatous portion had what appeared to be limb buds and oral and anal orifices. The lesion was excised at 5 days, and internal fixation was achieved with a Kirschner wire followed by a rib graft at 5 weeks of age.

ACQUIRED LESIONS

TRAUMATIC

Traumatic lesions are covered elsewhere under jaw fractures.

METABOLIC

Metabolic conditions which affect the skeletal system in general similarly affect the jaws.

Fig. 17-7. (*Top*) Epignathus in a 5-day-old infant. This teratoma was attached to the mandible, which was also cleft, as well as the lower lip. (*Bottom*) The child at 3 years, after resection of the teratoma and a rib graft to the mandible.

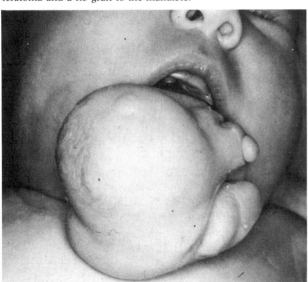

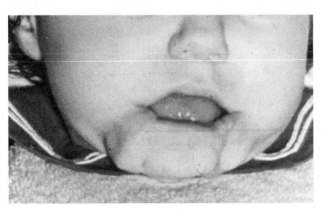

INFLAMMATORY

Inflammatory conditions, especially osteomyelitis and osteoradionecrosis, are common complications of trauma and radiation to the head and neck area. Treatment involves complete excision of the sequestrum and devitalized bone with primary soft tissue coverage and external fixation as necessary. Permanent restoration of bone continuity is undertaken when all signs of infection have resolved, and involves composite flap techniques and microvascular or avascular bone grafting.

BENIGN NEOPLASTIC LESIONS

Nearly all benign lesions have ectodermal and mesodermal elements, so clear separation of tumors according to embryonic origin is not feasible. Division into odontogenic and nonodontogenic categories, however, provides a clear separation between those tumors and cysts that arise from those elements involved with the formation and maintenance of teeth and those that arise from the elements of the jaw not involved in odontogenesis.

Odontogenic Tumors and Cysts

Examples of odontogenic tumors are adenoameloblastoma, ameloblastic fibroma, odontoma, cementoma, and odontogenic myxoma. These lesions contain varying amounts of dentin and cementum and require complete excision to eradicate them and to differentiate them from malignant lesions.

Odontogenic cysts are the result of appendages of epithelium which grow with the teeth in the jaws. Examples of these cysts are the simple follicular or primordal cysts, dentigerous cysts, and periodontal or radicular cysts. Treatment requires excision of the epithelial sac, with preservation of the tooth if one is present.

Nonodontogenic Tumors

Some of the more important and more frequently encountered nonodontogenic lesions of the jaws include fibrous dysplasia, osteomas, and Paget's disease.

Fibrous dysplasia includes a spectrum of diseases that have in common the replacement of normal bony architecture by firm, partially calcified tumors rich in collagen. These lesions occur in the first and second decades of life and become a problem when they cause facial deformity. Occasionally these lesions recur rapidly after incomplete excision, but sculpting of the lesions by curettage and partial excision to reestablish normal bone contour is generally the treatment of choice. There has been a suggested association between malignant degeneration of this lesion and treatment with radiation therapy. Since fibrous dysplasia is otherwise benign, this modality is therefore contraindicated in treatment of this lesion.

Osteoma is a slow-growing lesion most often found in the mandible that contains mature bone. When these lesions are noted in association with multiple soft-tissue tumors, the diagnosis of Gardner's syndrome is suggested. While this is a rare occurrence, the surgeon should always be alert to the possibility of Gardner's syndrome, since the intestinal polyps which also are associated with this malady have a very high incidence of malignant degeneration.

Paget's disease (osteitis deformans) is a common affliction of elderly patients. In patients with any evidence of involvement, the incidence of associated jaw involvement is approximately 20%; symptoms are usually ill-fitting dentures or a nonspecific jaw pain. Operation on or near bones so affected carries an increased risk of osteomyelitis, fistula, and bleeding.

MALIGNANT NEOPLASTIC LESIONS

Ameloblastoma

Ameloblastoma is a tumor of odontogenic origin. It may be cystic or solid and usually presents as a slowly growing submucosal mass in the jaw. Although it is most often benign, it occasionally metastasizes and pursues an aggressive course (Fig. 17-8). Partial excision and curettage is associated with an unacceptably high recurrence rate and is to be condemned. Treatment is by complete excision of the lesion with a margin of normal tissue.

Osteogenic Sarcoma

This sarcoma is a rare malignancy of the facial bones that has distinctly different characteristics from osteogenic sarcoma of other skeletal bones: the presenting symptom is usually a painless mass in the jaws. This lesion is associated with a high degree of local recurrence and poor survival rates, especially for lesions of the maxilla. Several reports have shown survival rates in the 25% to 40% range for 5 years, but a recent report has suggested improved survival may be obtained with early radical surgical extirpation of primary lesions in combination with interstitial preoperative radiation.

Chondrogenic Tumor

Chondrogenic tumors are rare lesions of the jaw with an extremely poor prognosis. Malignant lesions grow rapidly and invade surrounding structures. Lung and bone metastases are frequent.

Fig. 17-8. A 42-year-old woman with a massive ameloblastoma or adamantinoma with extension into the temporal fossa. While the local tumor was resected, the patient later died of pulmonary metastasis.

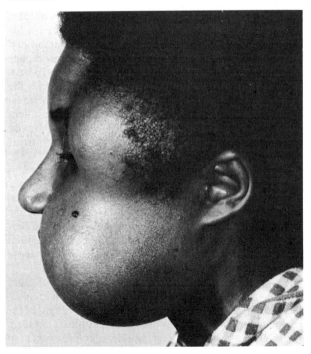

Burkitt's Tumor

Burkitt's tumor is a very malignant neoplasm of undifferentiated lymphoreticular cells that was first recognized in African children. The variety that occurs in the United States, although more uncommon, is more often associated with abdominal tumors and carries a worse prognosis. Favorable responses to chemotherapy (cyclophosphamide) have been noted.

SURGICAL TREATMENT OF HEAD AND NECK TUMORS

There is little doubt that, in most cases where feasible, the best management of cancer is to separate all the tumor from the patient by surgical removal. Effective application of this modality of therapy, however, requires careful selection, planning, and a large measure of surgical judgment. Clinical experience, special training, and research serve as avenues to developing this judgment, but it is not necessary for every surgeon to repeat unsuccessful techniques and experiments in the process of developing expertise. Many unsound practices are clearly recognized and can be summarized as follows:

1. Open biopsy of a lump in the neck before performing a complete head and neck and general physical examination.
2. Inadequate incisional biopsy of an oral cavity lesion.
3. Inadequate excisional biopsy of a suspicious oral cavity lesion.
4. Failure to review previous histopathology slides.
5. Permitting a histopathologic benign diagnosis to override a clinical diagnosis of carcinoma.
6. Biopsy of larynx, hypopharynx, nasopharynx, esophagus, or trachea before radiologic studies, when such studies are indicated to aid in the evaluation of the extent of disease.
7. Lack of multidisciplinary approach, where indicated.
8. Tailoring the scope of surgical resection to the ability of the surgeon rather than to the objective requirement imposed by the lesion.
9. Compromise of the ablative phase of surgery in order to accommodate limited reconstructive skills.
10. Assessing the degree of success or failure of radiation therapy on the basis of the response of the lesion during or immediately on completion of treatment.
11. Prolonged watch-and-wait attitude in the face of an asymptomatic mass.
12. Inadequate search for an occult primary.
13. Abandonment of the patient with neck metastasis from an undetectable primary.
14. Enucleation of tumors of the major salivary glands.
15. Treating a patient with antibiotics for an extended period of time without a biopsy.

INDICATIONS AND TECHNIQUES

Once the diagnosis of malignancy has been made and its extent defined, many surgical techniques are available to eradicate or palliate the disease process. Procedures that involve large *en bloc* resections of various muscle groups, portions of the facial skeleton, and contiguous regional node-bearing tissue are referred to as "commando" operations. These composite procedures are technically challenging but not often indicated, since malignant processes requiring such extensive resections are very often systemic when diagnosed and not amenable to extirpation.

The most enduring and widely applicable operation in this area is the radical neck dissection. The rationale and technique first reported in 1905 and 1906 by Crile, based on Halsted's principles of single block dissection of the primary lesion with resection of the regional lymphatic drainage, remain the basis of modern surgical practice.

In the 1940s, interest in this procedure was reviewed by Hayes Martin. He clearly defined the indications for the procedure as follows:

1. There should be clinical evidence that cancer is present in cervical lymphatics. . . .
2. The primary lesion giving rise to metastasis should have been controlled clinically; or, if it is not controlled, there should be a plan to remove the primary at the same time the neck dissection is performed. . . .
3. There should be a reasonable chance of complete removal of the cervical metastasis. . . .
4. There should be no clinical or roentgenographic evidence of distant metastasis. . . .
5. Neck dissection should offer a more certain cure than radiation therapy.

When this procedure is performed for known disease, it is said to be "therapeutic" as opposed to prophylactic. In the latter case, the procedure is performed for tumors which have a high incidence of metastasis. Much controversy exists as to the indication for prophylactic neck dissection, and the general trend has been away from this practice in the past several years. Several authors now suggest that less extensive procedures may be sufficient in many cases. These modifications spare the sternocleidomastoid muscle, the internal jugular vein, and the spinal accessory nerve and limit nodal dissections in carefully selected cases to portions of node-bearing tissue in the vicinity of the primary lesion.

In the classical radical neck procedure, the plan is to remove all the lymphatics and nodal tissue between the platysma and the deep cervical fascia from the level of the mandible superiorly, the lateral border of the strap muscles medially, the border of the trapezius posteriorly, and the clavicle inferiorly, sparing the marginal mandibular branch of the facial nerve, the vagus, phrenic, and hypoglossal nerves, and the cervical sympathetic chain.

COMPLICATIONS

Common complications of radical neck dissection include flap necrosis, seromas and hematomas, oropharyngeal cutaneous fistulas, carotid rupture, thoracic duct fistula and pneumothorax, swallowing difficulty and postoperative airway obstruction, and shoulder pain.

FLAP NECROSIS

Flap necrosis is reduced by choice of incisions in such a manner as to prevent long narrow pedicles of tissue. The MacFee incision is useful in this regard and is especially indicated if the patient has received preoperative radiation.

SEROMAS AND HEMATOMAS

Seromas and hematomas are avoided by the use of suction drains. Routine pre- and intraoperative antibiotics are recommended whenever large neck flaps are used or the course of dissection involves violation of the integrity of the mucous membranes. In the postoperative period a vigorous program of oral hygiene with pulsatile jet irrigation where feasible is recommended.

FISTULAS

Oropharyngeal cutaneous fistulas have a variety of contributing factors, including tight closures, compromised flaps, or previous irradiation. They dissect under flaps and contribute to tissue disruption, infections, slough, and carotid "blowout." Avoidance of this devastating complication lies in preoperative nutritional rehabilitation and careful attention to basic surgical principles of tissue approximation without tension and dissection techniques that minimize tissue destruction. Once a fistula is established, treatment includes drainage, debridement, nutrition and provision for fistula closure with regional or pedicle flaps to supply oral lining.

CAROTID RUPTURE

Carotid rupture occurs in approximately 3% of all neck dissections and bodes approximately a 30% mortality. It usually represents the culmination of a series of postoperative complications and has a high association with preoperative radiation. Free grafts of dermis have been recommended for those dissections where disruption is likely to occur. Once the carotid artery becomes exposed, however, recommended coverage is by nonirradiated pedicle or myocutaneous flap. Patients who are at high risk for this complication should be kept under close observation. Impending rupture is handled by elective carotid ligation. Vessel repair will not be successful. Rupture is controlled with direct pressure while the patient undergoes volume stabilization. The artery is then ligated above the site of rupture, in uninfected tissue if possible. Reconstruction of the artery by vessel graft or prosthesis usually has not been successful.

THORACIC DUCT FISTULA AND PNEUMOTHORAX

Thoracic duct fistula and pneumothorax are uncommon complications. The former usually abates spontaneously, and the latter is handled with a closed thoracotomy drainage.

SWALLOWING DIFFICULTY AND AIRWAY OBSTRUCTION

Postoperative aspiration of secretions is common because of difficulty in swallowing, edema, loss of tongue mobility, and section of the superior laryngeal nerve which renders the upper larynx anesthetic and negates the stimulus for the cough reflex. Section of the superior pharyngeal constrictor muscle improves swallowing and thereby helps to prevent aspiration.

Airway obstruction occurs because of edema or wound hematoma or secondary to aspiration. Tracheostomy is indicated in composite procedures involving the tongue, resection of a portion of the mandible, and bilateral neck dissections. This last procedure carries a significantly increased mortality when done simultaneously and therefore should be performed as a staged operation.

SHOULDER PAIN

The patient is usually ready for discharge within a week after surgery, with the most permanent disability being a weak shoulder with a variable amount of residual pain. This can be alleviated by sparing the spinal accessory nerve and by physical therapy to strengthen accessory muscle groups.

MORTALITY

The mortality for uncomplicated radical neck dissection is approximately 1%.

BIBLIOGRAPHY

American Joint Committee for Cancer Staging and End Results Reporting. Manual for Staging of Cancer 1977. American Joint Committee, Chicago, 1977

ARIYAN S, CUONO CB: Myocutaneous flaps for head and neck reconstruction. Head & Neck Surg Mar/Apr:321, 1980

BACKSTRON A, JAKOBSSON PA, NATHANSON A et al: Prognosis of squamous cell carcinoma of the gums with cytologically verified cervical lymph node metastasis. J Laryngol 89:391, 1975

BATSAKIS JG: *Tumors of the Head & Neck.* pp. 520–521. Baltimore, Williams & Wilkins Co, 1979

BEAHRS OH, ADSON MA: The surgical anatomy and technique of parotidectomy. Am J Surg 95:885, 1958

BEAHRS OH, WOODS JE: In Hardy JD: Complications in Surgery and Their Management, 4th ed, p. 280. Philadelphia, W B Saunders, 1981

CAWSON RA: Premalignant lesions in the mouth. Br Med Bull 31:164, 1975

CRILE GW: Excision of cancer of the head and neck with special reference to the plane of dissection based on 132 operations. JAMA 47:1780, 1906

EVANS JF, SHAH JP: Epidermoid carcinoma of the palate. Am J Surg 142:451, 1981

FOOTE FW JR, FRAZELL EL: Tumors of the major salivary glands. Cancer 6:1065, 1955

FRABLE MA, FISCHER RA: Granular cell myoblastomas. Laryngoscope 86:36, 1976

FRANKLIN JD, SHACK RB, STORE JD et al: Single-stage reconstruction of mandibular and soft tissue defects using a free osteocutaneous groin flap. Am J Surg 140:492, 1980

GIFFORD GH JR, MARTZ AT, MacCOULLUM DW: The management of electrical mouth burns in children. Pediatrics 47:113, 1971

GUILLAMONDETAL OM, OLIVER B, HAYDEN RF: Cancer of the anterior floor of the mouth—selective choice of treatment and analysis of failures. Am J Surg 140:560, 1980

HELLER KS, STRONG EW: Carotid arterial hemorrhage after radical head and neck surgery. Am J Surg 138:607, 1970

HENDRICLES JL, MEDELSON BC, WOODS JE: Invasive carcinoma of the lower lip. Surg Clin North Am 57:837, 1977

JESSE RH, BALLANTYNE AJ, LARSON D: Radical or modified neck dissection: A therapeutic dilemma. Am J Surg 136:516, 1978

MARTIN HE, DEL VALLE B, EHRLICH H et al: Neck dissection. Cancer 4:441, 1951

POLLOCK WJ, BITSEFF EL, RYAN RF: Rapid transfer of thoracoacromial flaps to the face and neck. Plast Reconstr Surg 50:433, 1972

RUSS JE, JESSE RH: Management of osteosarcoma of the maxilla and mandible. Am J Surg 140:572, 1980

RYAN RF, LITWIN MS, KREMENTZ ET: A new concept in the management of Marjolin's ulcers. Ann Surg 193:598, 1981

SALIBIAN AH, RAPPAPORT I, FURNAS DW et al: Microvascular reconstruction of the mandible. Am J Surg 140:499, 1980

SEHDEV MK, HUVOS AG, STRONG EW et al: Ameloblastoma of maxilla and mandible. Cancer 33:324, 1974

SHAW HJ, HARDINGHAM M: Cancer of the floor of the mouth: Surgical management. J Laryngol 91:489, 1977

SHIFFMAN MA: Familial multiple polyposis associated with soft tissue and hard tissue tumors. JAMA 182:514, 1962

SPIRO RH, STRONG EW: Epidermoid carcinoma of the tongue; treatment by partial glossectomy alone. Am J Surg 122:707, 1971

U.S. Department of H.E.W.: *Management Guidelines of Head and Neck Cancer.* NIH Publication N. 80-2037, Sept., 1979, pp. 1–11

WALDRON CA: Fibro-osseous lesions of the jaws. J Oral Surg 28:58, 1970

WALDRON CA, SHAFER WG: Leukoplakia revisited. A clinicopathologic study of 3256 oral leukoplakias. Cancer 36:1386, 1975

WURMAN LH, ADAMS GL, MEYERHOFF WL: Carcinoma of the lip. Am J Surg 130:470, 1975

Winsor V. Morrison

Ear, Nose, Paranasal Sinuses, Pharynx, and Larynx

This chapter gives a brief outline of the innermost core of otorhinolaryngology. Modern otolaryngology overlaps other surgical specialties in certain areas, such as head and neck surgery, bronchoesophagology, and maxillofacial and reconstructive surgery.

CLINICAL APPROACH

As in all medicine and its specialties, the history is of utmost importance. The examiner, beginning with the chief complaint, seeks out minute details of the disease. Pertinent systems review is carried out as it relates to the chief complaint and suspected disease. Hereditary factors deserve special attention because many genetic syndromes affect structures and functions of the head and neck.

The examination of the otolaryngology patient requires certain special instruments that are common to all physicians, such as the otoscope and other instruments that are usually found in ear, nose, and throat clinics. The nasal speculum, laryngeal mirrors of various sizes, and a good electric head light or a good light source with reflecting head mirror are essential.

Following the history, it is desirable to establish a routine in examination of the otolaryngology patient. This avoids undue attention to one particular area, perhaps at the exclusion of another. It is suggested that the examination begin with the ears and progress to the nose, mouth, pharynx, nasopharynx, larynx, and neck, in that order. Examination of the ear includes tuning-fork tests as a screening method to determine possible hearing loss. If hearing loss is detected, audiologic evaluation is mandatory.

EAR

The ear is composed of several structures within or around the temporal bone. The external ear is the sound collector. It consists of the pinna, the external auditory canal, and the outer surface of the tympanic membrane. The middle ear contains the malleus, incus, and stapes, through which the sound energy gathered by the tympanic membrane is directed into the perilymph at the oval window. The eardrum and ossicles are an impedance-matching system that prevents loss of energy during the air-to-fluid transition of sound energy. With loss of any part of this conductive ossicular chain, there is significant hearing impairment. The inner ear is housed within the petrous portion of the temporal bone and consists of the cochlea and saccule, the auditory part of the inner ear, and the labyrinth, or balance system, consisting of the utricle and three semicircular canals.

DISEASES OF THE EXTERNAL EAR

AURICLE

The auricle (pinna) assists in sound collection and localization. Congenital malformations present in numerous ways, including lop ears, hypoplasia, and total absence (anotia). There are other lesser deformities, such as preauricular cyst and fistulas, and congenital tumors, for example, dermoid cysts and lymphangioma. The presence of these congenital abnormalities should point out the possibility of other genetic syndromes. Their treatment is surgical.

An injury to the auricle may cause a hematoma, which, by lifting off its nourishing perichondrium, destroys cartilage. Prompt treatment with aspiration, drainage, and pressure dressing is necessary to prevent the thickened or shriveled cauliflower ear seen in some wrestlers and boxers. Frostbite of the auricle is frequently seen in cold climates and is treated with gradual warming. Keloid is frequently seen in dark-skinned races. Lacerations of the pinna should be cleansed, débrided, and closed by layers to facilitate prompt healing.

Infections of the auricle may result in perichondritis, a very painful condition of the ear. It usually occurs following trauma or surgery to the external ear. Treatment should be prompt and vigorous, beginning with Burow's solution soaks, administration of antibiotics, and incision and drainage where fluctuation occurs. Erysipelas, a streptococcal infection of the surrounding skin, may also occur.

Dermatologic lesions are numerous. Seborrhea of the head may involve the auricle as an eczematous rash. Facial acne usually does not involve the pinna. Allergic reactions are common and usually are due to contact with cosmetics, eyeglass frames, costume jewelry, and soaps. Elimination of these offenders is the best treatment. Among the neoplasms of the outer ear are sebaceous cysts, hyperkeratosis, cutaneous horns, and basal cell and squamous cell carcinomas. Excision is the treatment of choice, and in large lesions skin transplants may be necessary.

EXTERNAL AUDITORY MEATUS

Atresia

Among congenital abnormalities, atresia of the outer canal, many times associated with a malformed auricle and middle ear, is relatively frequent. Acquired forms of atresia develop as a result of injuries, burns, or chronic infections of the ear canal. Treatment is surgical, and the outcome depends upon the severity of the abnormality.

Foreign Bodies

Insertion of foreign bodies is frequent in children and mental retardates. These objects may be insects, vegetable matter, paper, pencil leads, rubber erasers, or plastic or metal objects. Insects in the canal are most distressing; they should be killed immediately by instillation of alcohol or mineral oil and then removed gently with a forceps. Irrigation with warm water is often satisfactory except with vegetable matter, which may swell and become impacted. In neglected cases, antibiotics and analgesics are necessary. Removal may require anesthesia.

Cerumen

Cerumen, or ear wax, is a yellowish natural substance of varying consistency. It is bacteriostatic and will usually migrate to the outer meatus naturally if left alone. In some

EXTERNAL OTITIS	
Etiology	Bacterial, usually *Pseudomonas*, *Staphylococcus*, or *Proteus*, but may be fungal, especially *Aspergillus niger* or *Candida albicans*; hypersensitivity to many drugs, chemicals, and cosmetics may also occur
Dx	Pain, swelling, tenderness, and moisture involving the external auditory canal or auricle
Rx	Antibiotics and steroids topically; occasionally requires systemic antibiotics

patients, there is insufficient production to prevent atrophy or dryness of the canal skin. These ear canals are more likely to be infected by various organisms. Increased production of cerumen may cause the accumulation of a hard plug that may eventually obstruct the canal during a swim or shower. These hardened masses may be removed by first softening them with ceruminolytic agents such as hydrogen peroxide or sodium bicarbonate solution. The wax plug may then be flushed out with mildly warm tap water, provided a drum perforation is not present or suspected.

External Otitis

External otitis is a common disorder that may be acute or chronic. It may be due to various causes. Acute otitis externa is usually bacterial in origin and is caused most commonly by *Pseudomonas*, *Staphylococcus*, *Proteus*, or *Streptococcus* organisms. The infection may be localized, as in furunculosis, or diffuse, involving the entire ear canal. Acute external otitis may have a sudden onset and be very painful, with fever and general malaise. The skin of the ear canal may be swollen, wet, extremely tender, and erythematous. In the furuncle, the lesion may point at the meatus of the ear canal. Treatment of external otitis may begin with antibiotic–steroid ear drops; severe cases may require a wick soaked in the same solution and inserted into the swollen ear canal. Burow's solution soaks, constantly applied, are also very effective.

Chronic external otitis is frequently seen in the diabetic or immunocompromised patient. The infecting agent may be a fungus, commonly *Aspergillus* or *Candida* species, or a gram-negative coliform-type organism. An extremely severe form of the disease is called malignant external otitis. It is nearly always seen in diabetics and is due to the *Pseudomonas* bacteria. Although not a neoplasm, it may have a fatal outcome.

Another form of dermatitis involving the external ear is herpes zoster oticus (Ramsay Hunt syndrome), in which small vesicles are seen in the external auditory canal or on the auricle early in the course of the disease. Severe pain, facial palsy, hearing loss, tinnitus, and vertigo with nystagmus may be present. The disorder is due to a viral infection of the geniculate ganglion of the facial nerve. Treatment is symptomatic, and most patients recover without sequelae.

Seborrheic dermatitis may be treated with Selsun shampoo or steroid creams. Eczema of the ear may develop as a hypersensitivity reaction to contact with cosmetics or jewelry.

Neoplasms

Among neoplasms found in the external ear is the osteoma, which is a hard enlargement, usually of the anterosuperior or posterosuperior portion of the external auditory canal just lateral to the tympanic membrane. It may be bilateral. Extreme cases may almost obscure the tympanic membrane. These exostoses frequently are found in patients who swim in cold water. Adenomas may be small, benign tumors originating in the cerumen glands. These may become malignant and are then the highly invasive adenocarcinomas of the cerumen glands. Basal cell carcinomas, adenocarcinomas, and squamous cell carcinomas may also occur. The treatment is surgery, sometimes requiring radical temporal-bone excision. Radiation therapy may be required as an adjunct.

DISEASES OF THE MIDDLE EAR

The boundaries of the middle ear are the medial surface of the drum laterally, the eustachian-tube orifice anteriorly, the jugular bulb and carotid artery below, with the cochlear promontory medially, and the tegmen plate above. The malleus, incus, and stapes transmit sound energy from the eardrum to the oval window of the labyrinth. The cochlear fluids are the perilymph in the scala vestibuli and scala tympani and the endolymph in the scala media. The cochlear fluids have access to the vestibular system through the ductus reuniens. Landmarks of the normal eardrum are the lateral (short) process of the malleus; the malleus handle, including the umbo; and the light reflex anterior and inferior to the umbo on the pars tensa. The pars flaccida (Shrapnell's membrane) is the upper fourth of the tympanic membrane. It is flaccid due to the absence of the middle fibrous layer of the drum in that area.

BULLOUS MYRINGITIS

Bullous myringitis of the eardrum is due to the *Mycoplasma* organism. As its name implies, it consists of bullae on the outer surface of the tympanic membrane. It is due to fluid collection beneath the epithelial layer of the drum. One or both ears may be affected, but hearing remains relatively good. These lesions are extremely painful, but when ruptured they may be much more tolerable. Appropriate antibiotics are administered both systemically and topically. Analgesics are required.

DRUM RUPTURE

The tympanic membrane tears easily when compressed air or shock waves of an explosion, a blow to the ear, or a fall into water as in diving or water skiing occurs. Slight pain and bleeding are present, and, upon examination, one may see a small perforation or a large rent in the drum. If due to injuries in water, these perforations may quickly become infected and should have prophylactic antibiotic therapy. Small lacerations heal readily; however, larger tears are best handled by the otolaryngologist using an operating microscope and repositioning and splinting the edges of the drum laceration. In basal skull fractures involving the temporal bone, cerebrospinal fluid otorrhea may be present and can lead to meningitis.

HEMATOTYMPANUM

Blood within the middle ear may appear as a bluish liquid behind the eardrum and may be idiopathic or secondary to trauma (as in basal skull fractures). Tinnitus and conductive hearing loss are frequently present. This condition usually resolves spontaneously, but in protracted cases myringotomy and suction may be desirable.

BAROTITIS

Barotitis is a condition that results from extreme barometric pressure changes, as seen in airplane passengers. It usually occurs in people who have eustachian-tube swelling secondary to allergy or infections. As the airplane passenger ascends, the atmospheric pressure within the middle ear easily escapes down the eustachian tube, causing no discomfort; however, when descent occurs, the swollen eustachian tube does not readily admit the increased air pressure into the middle-ear space. This leads to a negative pressure within the middle ear, which is soon followed by a serous effusion. Treatment consists of the Valsalva maneuver or Politzer inflation of the middle ear, decongestant nose drops, and, occasionally, myringotomy.

OTALGIA

Earaches may be due to many causes, including acute external otitis, acute otitis media, and physical trauma. Referred pain may occur from the distribution along cranial nerves V, VII, IX, and X, as well as the cervical nerves C2 and C3. A small branch of the vagus nerve reaches the external auditory canal and is known as Arnold's nerve. Stimulation of it may reflexly cause a cough. Costen's syndrome, temporomandibular joint arthritis, may result from malocclusion of the teeth, nervous tension, blows to the mandible, and excessive mandibular motion, as in gum chewing and constant speaking. The treatment of this painful condition and its concurrent otalgia depends upon removal of the offending cause.

OTITIS MEDIA

Types

Serous. A serous or mucoid secretion in the middle-ear cavity commonly occurs in children as a result of hypertrophy of the adenoids and in the presence of nasal allergy or viral infections. This effusion may cause a conductive-type hearing loss and, if secondarily infected, produces acute otitis media. In adults, a unilateral effusion may signal a nasopharyngeal carcinoma. Treatment depends on the underlying cause and may involve adenoidectomy with myringotomy and insertion of ventilating tubes (Fig. 17-9).

Acute Suppurative. Bacterial infections of the middle ear result when upper respiratory bacteria invade the middle ear through the eustachian tube. These are often complications following viral infections and occur commonly in childhood diseases. *Streptococcus, Staphylococcus, Pneumococcus,* and *Hemophilus influenzae* are the most common bacterial

Fig. 17-9. Typical sites of myringotomy (left drum).

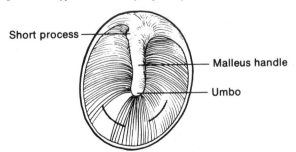

Short process

Malleus handle

Umbo

ACUTE OTITIS MEDIA	
Etiology	Bacterial infections (*Pneumococcus, Streptococcus, H. influenzae*), viral infections, trauma, and eustachian-tube dysfunction secondary to allergy or infection
Dx	Severe otalgia with erythema of tympanic membrane with bulging and absence of normal landmarks. Decreased hearing, roaring, tinnitus, and usually a history of antecedent upper respiratory infection
Rx	Analgesics, systemic antibiotics appropriate for above organisms, and possible myringotomy

agents. Acute mastoiditis may occur in untreated or unresponsive cases and may require a simple mastoidectomy.

Acute Necrotizing. Unusually virulent forms of hemolytic streptococcus sometimes associated with scarlet fever or measles may cause a rapidly progressive and necrotizing destruction of the eardrum, ossicles, and canal wall. Chronic otitis media commonly follows.

Tuberculous. Fortunately, tuberculous otitis media is a relatively rare form of ear infection; it especially occurs in those who drink unpasteurized milk. Characteristically, there are multiple drum perforations and pale granulations.

Chronic. The chronic form occurs in two types: simple mucoid and dangerous bone-invading. The simple mucoid type presents as a continuous or recurrent mucous discharge from a central perforation of the drum without involvement of the anulus tympanicus. Treatment is conservative and includes management of allergic factors, hypertrophic tonsils and adenoids, sinus disease, or nasal obstruction; frequent cleansing of the ear; and instillation of antibiotic drops. Once the ear remains dry, the drum perforation can be closed by simple myringoplasty or by the repeated cautery method as an office procedure.

The dangerous bone-invading type results from a marginal perforation of the eardrum through which the canal skin invades the middle ear. Once inside the middle ear, the squamous stratified epithelium becomes a foreign body, the cholesteatoma that erodes the surrounding bone in any direction. We distinguish several types of cholesteatoma: True, or congenital, cholesteatoma originates from embryonal epithelial remnants; primary acquired cholestea-

CHRONIC OTITIS MEDIA	
Etiology	Inadequately treated or neglected acute infections of the middle ear, traumatic eardrum perforations, and poor eustachian-tube function with secondary cholesteatoma formation
Dx	History of tympanic-membrane perforation, recurrent purulent drainage, hearing loss, and cloudy or sclerotic mastoid x-ray films
Rx	Medical initially, with topical and systemic antibiotics; surgical treatment usually required

toma results from ingrowth of squamous epithelium through Shrapnell's membrane; and secondary acquired cholesteatoma (the one described above) results from ingrowth of squamous canal skin through a marginal antrum perforation. The danger from cholesteatoma is its bone-invading expansion until vital structures are reached and destroyed, leading to intracranial complications. Treatment may require radical mastoidectomy.

Operative Procedures

Mastoidectomy. When an acute otitis media advances to the state of bone destruction within the mastoid, all air cells must be systematically evacuated. This simple mastoidectomy must be as radical as possible and leads to complete healing of the infection, closure of the eardrum, and return of normal hearing (Fig. 17-10). Radical mastoidectomy is reserved for cholesteatoma. Usually, the mastoid is poorly pneumatized in such cases. Nevertheless, all air cells must be removed, all granulation tissue curetted, and all cholesteatoma carefully peeled out. Drum and ossicles are often destroyed. If they can be left intact, a modified radical mastoidectomy has been accomplished for preservation of hearing. The radical mastoidectomy should be as conservative as possible (Fig. 17-11). Most cases can be handled by a combination of disease eradication and reconstructive procedures, called tympanomastoidectomy.

Tympanoplasty. Once the chronic infection in the ear has been controlled or is dry, the eardrum can be grafted or reconstructed using temporalis muscle fascia or vein.

Complications

Both acute and chronic otitis media may spread from the middle ear, causing various complications that are grouped into two types, extracranial and intracranial.

Extracranial. The most frequent extracranial complication is the breakthrough of pus through the cribriform area behind Henle's spine of the mastoid plate: subperiosteal abscess. When the pus breaks through the mastoid tip and spreads beneath the sternomastoid muscle, it produces an indurated swelling in the neck known as Bezold's abscess. Facial paralysis occurs more often in chronic otitis media than in the acute cases. In the former, it is caused by gradual bone erosion by the cholesteatoma; in the latter, it usually

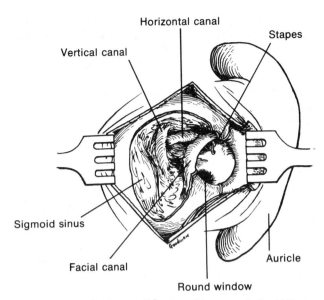

Fig. 17-11. Radical mastoidectomy with removal of middle-ear structures.

results from a congenital dehiscence around the facial canal. Petrositis, or apicitis, produces Gradenigo's syndrome, with copious purulent discharge from the ear canal, lancinating pain behind the ipsilateral eye, and paralysis of the homolateral lateral rectus muscle.

When a cholesteatoma erodes the horizontal semicircular canal, a fistula into its lumen is created. This exposes the membranous canal to pus and toxins, causing serous labyrinthitis. Pressure exerted into the external ear canal produces acute dizziness, a few beats of rapid nystagmus to the same side (typical fistula sign), and Romberg's sign to the opposite side. Hearing is usually decreased from the chronic disease, and tinnitus may have set in, indicating the beginning involvement of the cochlea. Total deafness may occur, plus complete loss of vestibular function. This deterioration usually indicates the progression of the serous stage into purulent labyrinthitis.

Intracranial. The simplest and most common type of intracranial complication, the extradural abscess, is an accumulation of pus between the superior tegmen plate and dura of the middle fossa, or sinus plate and sigmoid sinus (perisinuous abscess), or posterior pyramid and cerebellar dura. Thrombosis of the sigmoid sinus was quite frequent in the preantibiotic era, when a coalescent mastoiditis eroded the sinus plate, causing a perisinuous abscess with subsequent thrombophlebitis of this venous duct. When the thrombosis continues in retrograde fashion into the emissary vein, edema over the mastoid develops, called Griesinger's sign. Although considerably less frequent than before, meningitis is still the relatively most common cause of death from otitis media. Subdural abscess is a local accumulation of pus between the dura and arachnoid. Brain abscess, although not common, is still a dreaded complication of otitis media. It more commonly occurs in long-standing or neglected cases of chronic otitis media.

OTHER MIDDLE-EAR LESIONS

Otosclerosis

A primary disease of the labyrinth capsule, otosclerosis is characterized by foci of new bone formation. It affects only the labyrinth capsule in humans because this portion of the

Fig. 17-10. Simple mastoidectomy.

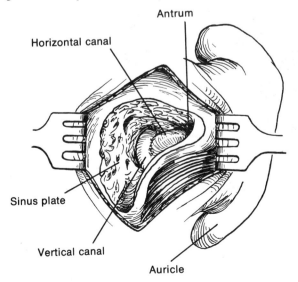

petrous bone remains in embryonal size for life. It affects women twice as often as men and usually is progressive with pregnancy. Characteristically, onset is between the ages of 20 and 30. The site of its predilection is the fissula ante fenestram, the area just anterior to the stapes footplate. Clinically, it causes conductive hearing loss. In some patients, it may involve the cochlear capsule and thereby result in a sensorineural hearing loss. Rarely, a hereditary condition known as van der Hoeve's syndrome (osteogenesis imperfecta, blue scleras, and otosclerosis) is found. Treatment is surgical (Fig. 17-12).

Tympanosclerosis

Also known as adhesive otitis media, tympanosclerosis presents as calcified plaques within the layers of the eardrum and also may involve the middle-ear mucosa. It causes fixation of the ossicles and conductive hearing loss. The usefulness of surgical treatment may be limited because of recurrence of the disease process.

Congenital Malformations

Congenital malformations are often associated with other anomalies, particularly those involving the branchial arches. In essence, parts of the ossicles are missing, the malleus or stapes may be fixed, and so on.

Middle-Ear Injuries

Injuries of the middle ear are of various types, from blast injuries to penetrating wounds. One of the most common is the dislocation or fracture of the incus and stapes as a result of a faulty myringotomy. Penetrating wounds are frequently caused by accidental insertion of hairpins or needles while scratching the ear.

Tumors of the Middle Ear

Benign. Chronic otitis media, especially when associated with cholesteatoma, often causes the formation of polyps that consist of granulation tissue. Granulomas are usually foreign-body reactions to chronic infection, especially cholesteatoma. If they look pink and sluggish, they may be tuberculous.

Glomus Jugulare. This nonchromaffin paraganglioma is related to similar tumors occurring in other areas, such as the carotid body tumor. It is a benign vascular tumor, of unknown etiology, that originates from the jugular bulb in the hypotympanum. If it arises from the promontory, it is called glomus tympanicum. Even though the tumor is histologically benign, its slow growth invades the surrounding structures, very much like the cholesteatoma.

Malignant. Squamous cell carcinoma, adenocarcinoma, sarcoma, metastatic carcinoma, and multiple myeloma are rare lesions of the middle ear and mastoid. Pain, bleeding, and chronic discharge are the early symptoms. Subsequent invasion causes facial palsy, total deafness, and loss of balance, with vertigo.

DISEASES OF THE INNER EAR

The inner ear or labyrinth has two parts: the phylogenetically old (present in fishes) superior portion, consisting of the

Fig. 17-12. Treatment of otosclerosis with stapedectomy. Schema shows the completed procedure, with wire and fat lobule used as the prosthesis.

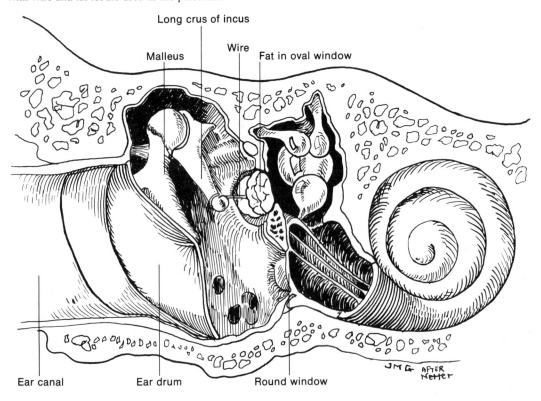

three semicircular canals and the utricle for the sense of balance, and the more recent (developed by amphibians) inferior portion, containing the saccule and cochlea, the latter for hearing. This distinction is of clinical importance, in that the old vestibular labyrinth is more resistant to disease than is the younger cochlear portion. The labyrinth capsule or petrous bone is hollowed out by the labyrinth structures, presenting the bony labyrinth. Within these cavities lined by endosteum, the membranous labyrinth is suspended in the perilymph, a fluid similar to serum with high sodium and low potassium. By contrast, the endolymph inside the membranous labyrinth is similar to endocellular fluid with high potassium and low sodium. This difference in electrolytes produces an electrical charge, the resting potential like that in a battery.

Vestibular function for balance is studied by the disciplines of neurophysiology and neurotology; it is tested by a sophisticated vestibular test battery and objectively recorded by means of electronystagmography, ENG (Fig. 17-13). Cochlear function for hearing is explored by physiological acoustics and audiology; it is tested by refined hearing tests administered by qualified audiologists. Among these tests, objective electrocochleography is also a clinical tool.

SENSORINEURAL HEARING LOSS

Hereditary
Almost 100 specific disease entities or syndromes are known that cause inherited, familial hearing loss. All modes of transmission occur, dominant, recessive, and X-linked mendelian, as well as chromosomal aberrations. Many types are congenital (*i.e.*, present at birth); others emerge gradually in childhood, adolescence, or early adulthood. None is curable, and prevention through eugenic family counseling is the only solution to the problem. In practice, it is important to discover the deaf children at the earliest possible age to

	HEARING LOSS
Etiology	Hereditary deafness, infectious diseases, toxic drugs, trauma, and genetic predisposition
Dx	History of hearing loss, abnormal tuning-fork tests, audiograms
Rx	Surgery or hearing aids

fit them with a suitable hearing aid. If this is not done and usable residual hearing is not used, grave damage to the child's language development and subsequent learning ability will occur.

Prenatal
During pregnancy, various maternal afflictions can cause inborn deafness. Among these are rubella, Rh incompatibility, syphilis, drugs, malnutrition, infectious diseases, and diabetes.

Perinatal
Obstetrical problems include prolonged labor, anoxia, prematurity, and head trauma with convulsion. These high-risk infants must be observed for possible deafness. Various objective hearing test procedures are being elaborated, such as the cribogram, the electrical recording of body movements inside the crib in response to monitored sound stimulation.

Toxic
Numerous drugs are toxic to the the inner ear, producing bilateral, symmetrical, high-tone loss. These drugs include quinine, salicylates, aniline dyes, tobacco, alcohol, aminoglycoside antibiotics, and some diuretics, such as ethacrynic acid and furosemide.

Fig. 17-13. Principle of electronystagmography. The difference in potential between the negatively charged retina and the positively charged cornea makes possible recording of eye movements.

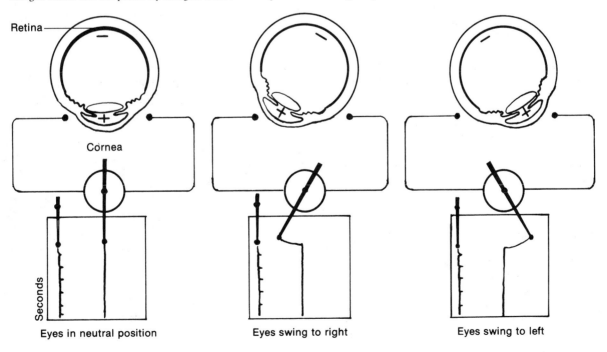

Eyes in neutral position   Eyes swing to right   Eyes swing to left

Infectious

Among the bacterial causes of hearing loss, we find meningitis (usually total and bilateral), encephalitis, tuberculosis, and scarlet fever, the latter two through eroding mastoiditis or necrotizing otitis media, with resulting labyrinthitis. Syphilis, congenital, secondary, or tertiary, may cause sudden or gradual hearing loss and vertigo. Viral infections may cause deafness during the febrile stage of measles, mumps, and influenza, usually unilaterally.

Traumatic

Several types of traumatic hearing loss occur. Head injury often causes temporal-bone fracture. The longitudinal fracture traverses the outer ear canal (with drum rupture) and the middle ear. The hearing loss is usually moderate and of conductive type. The transverse fracture passes through the osseous labyrinth, usually resulting in total permanent deafness, loss of vestibular function, and frequent temporary facial palsy. Concussion of the labyrinth may cause temporary or permanent hearing loss. Blast trauma from a nearby explosion usually ruptures the eardrum; it may fracture or dislocate the ossicles and often causes concussion of the labyrinth. Noise-induced hearing loss has become a major health hazard in industry. Exposure to prolonged loud noises, hunting, or pistol practice at first causes auditory fatigue. With further exposure, the hearing loss becomes permanent. It always begins at the frequencies around 4000 Hz to 6000 Hz and later spreads increasingly to adjacent frequencies. Ear protectors must be used for prevention.

Presbycusis

In analogy to presbyopia, normal hearing begins to decline progressively after age 40. The causes are degenerative changes, from the cochlea to the highest auditory cortex in the temporal lobe. Typically, the hearing loss begins with the bilateral and symmetrical lowering of the upper limit of hearing, which lies at 20,000 Hz in youth. With further advance of age, the upper limit eventually reaches the region of the speech frequencies, between 500 and 2000 Hz, and the hearing loss begins to be noticeable. Correction by a hearing aid becomes increasingly difficult with the prominence of the central factors of involution, as these older people simply can no longer comprehend well.

Sudden

This otologic emergency refers to the sudden onset of severe hearing loss without apparent cause. It usually occurs unilaterally. Any age-group may be afflicted. Viral causes have been mentioned; syphilis is another possibility. Often a vascular lesion is assumed, such as transitory spasm or lasting thrombosis or embolism. A newly discovered cause is rupture of the round window, with escape of perilymph. The usual cause is sudden increase in intracranial pressure from violent vomiting, heavy nose blowing, straining, and the like.

Tinnitus

Ringing or roaring in the ears is a common complaint. Just as one sees "stars" when being hit on the eye, the cochlea reacts to any disturbing irritation by its "adequate" response, the sensation of sound. Ringing is the pain in the cochlea. Tinnitus is mostly subjective, sensed only by the subject. It becomes objective when the examiner can hear it as well, such as with vascular lesions around the ear, palatal myoclonus, and nuchal muscle spasms. Almost any disease of the middle and inner ear can cause subjective ear noises. Many internal diseases, especially the ones with vascular changes, also cause tinnitus. All ototoxic drugs produce tinnitus as an early symptom.

Restoration of Hearing

Conductive hearing losses may be corrected by various forms of surgical procedures. Sensorineural hearing loss may be improved artificially by use of various electrical hearing aids. Under development at the present time, but seldom clinically feasible, is the cochlear implant. This is a miniaturized hearing aid that is implanted under the postauricular skin with two tiny electrodes entering the middle ear and inserted through the round-window membrane. The external receiver transmits its energy through an induction coil to the subcutaneous instrument.

DISORDERS OF BALANCE

Vertigo

Vertigo, the Latin word for dizziness, is used to distinguish true rotary vertigo of vestibular origin from the numerous and vague forms of dizziness from all other causes, usually internal diseases. True vertigo is a sensation of turning exactly as experienced when spinning around. General dizziness means the same as lightheadedness, giddiness, blacking out, and so forth and is devoid of a whirling sensation. True vertigo is accompanied by spontaneous nystagmus; dizziness is not. Vertigo can be caused by many diseases of the ear, as well as by numerous neurologic lesions when they involve the vestibular pathways. It is explored by the vestibular test battery, which is part of the neurotologic examination.

Nystagmus

Nystagmus is an oscillatory movement of the eyeballs. Among the many varieties of nystagmus, we are concerned here only with the vestibular type. It has two phases, a slow phase, which represents the vestibular stimulation, and a fast return of the eyes from cerebral correction. The nystagmographic curve, therefore, has a sawtooth shape. Vestibular nystagmus occurs in three directions: horizontal, vertical, and rotatory. Since the fast phase is the one readily seen by the unaided eye, its direction is used to describe the

DISORDERS OF BALANCE	
Etiology	Distention of the membranous labyrinth (endolymphatic hydrops) of unknown cause, commonly called Meniere's disease. Viral infections, trauma, cerebrovascular disorders, and degenerative neurologic disorders also common
Dx	Recurrent vertigo, tinnitus, hearing loss, and nystagmus may be present. Nausea and vomiting may or may not be present. Audiogram, x-ray film, ENG, and CT scan are required
Rx	Low-salt diet, diuretics, and antivertiginous drugs (*e.g.*, Antivert by mouth or Scopolamine intramuscularly. Neurology consultation advised

nystagmus: right and left for horizontal, up and down for vertical, clockwise and counterclockwise for rotatory.

Objective nystagmography records the velocity of the slow phase in angular degrees of displacement. Five types of vestibular nystagmus are differentiated: Spontaneous, when present without any stimulation; positional, with sudden changes of head position; induced, from performing any of the vestibular test procedures; inverted, when occurring in the direction opposite to that expected (*e.g.*, with fistula symptom); and perverted, when of other type than expected (*e.g.*, rotatory instead of horizontal, usually from central lesions). Vestibular function can be tested by ENG.

Meniere's Disease

Popularly known as "inner-ear trouble" Meniere's disease is produced by endolymphatic hydrops, with distention of the membranous labyrinth. The etiology is unknown. Both sexes are equally affected, and some cases may be hereditary.

The disease begins in early adulthood and lasts usually until late middle age. Vertigo beginning at a later age has another cause, usually a vascular or central lesion. Hydrops occurs in sudden attacks of a few hours' duration and may recur several times a week. Remissions are quite frequent. The attack begins with a sensation of pressure or fullness in the ear, chiefly unilaterally. This is followed by low-frequency tinnitus, sudden increase of the fluctuating hearing loss, and typical spinning vertigo with spontaneous nystagmus, nausea, vomiting, and pallor.

Diagnosis is made from the history and the audiologic findings. Vestibular testing shows spontaneous nystagmus and depressed labyrinth function on the affected side.

Treatment is mainly medical and follows the individual pattern. Nicotine and alcohol use must be forbidden. Many patients are heavy salt users, and a low-sodium diet with potassium chloride is often helpful (Furstenberg diet). Food allergy is quite frequent, requiring an elimination diet. Further general medical measures include correction of hormonal dysfunction (hypothyroidism, glucose tolerance, menstrual cycle), administration of diuretics, and psychotherapy in the cases of excessive work habits. Antivertiginous drugs are numerous and useful for prolonged control. Some patients respond to vasodilators. Severe cases may require hospitalization.

If medical measures fail, surgical therapy may be needed. It includes ultrasound or cryotherapy applied to the horizontal semicircular canal, several types of endolymphatic sac operations with a subarachnoid shunt, sacculotomy through the stapes footplate, and labyrinthectomy as a last resort. This multitude of approaches shows the difficulty of management in some cases.

Labyrinthitis

Inflammation of the labyrinth may be acute or chronic. The acute type may be serous or purulent. Acute serous labyrinthitis may follow stapes surgery. The acute purulent form may be caused by early acute otitis media or erosion by a chronic cholesteatoma. Chronic labyrinthitis can only be serous, such as with fistula symptom, because the purulent form inevitably invades the subdural space, with meningitis or cerebellar abscess, unless promptly arrested. Serous labyrinthitis may be localized to one structure or diffuse when spreading over the entire labyrinth. Symptoms and signs are sudden profound sensorineural hearing loss, roaring tinnitus, spontaneous nystagmus (irritative to the affected side in the reversible serous phase and paralytic to the good

side with the irreversible purulent type), vertigo, depressed vestibular function, positive Romberg and other vestibular test signs, nausea, and vomiting. Treatment is expectant and symptomatic for the serous type; the purulent form requires labyrinthectomy.

Vestibular Neuronitis

Following some acute respiratory infection, presumably of viral origin, a sudden attack of vertigo sets in that lasts continually for about 1 week. The patient is acutely ill and bedridden. Ear examination is normal, and hearing remains good, without tinnitus, but vestibular function is markedly depressed on one or both sides, with nystagmus, falling to one side, nausea, and vomiting. The acute phase gradually subsides during several weeks, with return of complete function within a few months. There are no recurrences.

Benign Paroxysmal Vertigo

Also known as positional vertigo, benign paroxysmal vertigo causes brief episodes of dizziness only with certain positions of the head. It is believed to be due to lesions of the otoliths within the saccule and utricle, often following a head injury. Hearing remains normal. The diagnosis is made by the positional test, which means bringing the head rapidly into various positions. After a brief latency, nystagmus appears and lasts for up to 30 seconds. It is fatigable in that it does not occur with an immediate second test. When there is no latency and fatigability, a central lesion should be suspected and evaluated by neurologic examination. The benign peripheral form is self-limiting, and normal function returns within a few months.

Cerebellopontine Angle Tumor

A new growth in the cerebellopontine angle area is chiefly an acoustic neurinoma (70%–80%); meningioma, Recklinghausen's bilateral neurofibroma, congenital cholesteatoma, and cystic arachnoiditis make up the rest. These slow-growing lesions usually begin with unilateral hearing loss of the retrolabyrinth neural type and tinnitus. Speech discrimination is especially poor. Vertigo and labyrinth depression follow until involvement of cranial nerves V and then VIII indicates the late symptoms. Diagnosis is confirmed by increased spinal fluid protein and radiologic signs of a widened internal auditory meatus, obtained by computed tomography (CT scan), tomographs, or Pantopaque study. Treatment is surgical, either by the supratemporal or transtemporal approach by a properly trained otologist or by the neurosurgical posterior fossa approach for large lesions.

NOSE

The nose is the body's air conditioner in that it filters, warms, and humidifies the air to be inhaled. Exclusion of the nose, such as in laryngectomized "neckbreathers," leads to disagreeable complications, such as potentially obstructive, dry tracheitis, with severe crusting during the winter months when room air is dry.

It is the organ of smell, which is regressing in human beings, who no longer need this sense for survival and procreation. A fair number of healthy persons have a poor sense of smell, and this sense is easily lost from disease (*e.g.*, influenza, carbon monoxide poisoning, head trauma). Parosmia occurs with endocrine imbalances; cacosmia (subjective foul smell) may be due to lesions in the phylogenetically old part of the brain, the uncinate gyrus. The olfactory epithelium extends over the upper part of the nasal dome.

Vocal resonance of the three nasal speech sounds (M, N, and Ng) heard while the palate is relaxed belongs to the articulatory, communicative function of the upper airway and foodways. Lesions of the velopharyngeal sphincter cause excessive nasal resonance of all speech sounds, such as with palatal paralysis (rhinolalia) or cleft palate (rhinoglossia).

The phylogenetically old significance of the nose as a secondary sex characteristic is evidenced by certain rhinopathias during menstruation or pregnancy, by certain psychosexual disorders, and by nose bleeding as vicarious menstruation, typically all in women.

Interest in the nose is shared by several specialties: general practice, dermatology, plastic surgery, rhinology, and, possibly, endocrinology.

DISEASES OF THE EXTERNAL NOSE

MALFORMATIONS

Hereditary or simply congenital malformations of the nose are not frequent. The most typical is the deviation to one side of the entire nose with cleft lip. Otherwise, there occur various median or lateral lesions, such as dimples, clefts, median sulcus with double nose, dermoids, and subcutaneous meningoencephaloceles. All require surgical repair, if feasible. The most serious malformation is choanal atresia, unilateral or bilateral, from persistence of the bucconasal membrane. Neonates, who are obligatory nose breathers, become cyanotic when sucking. Emergency treatment in the bilateral case uses the McGovern nipple, followed by piercing the occlusion with a sharp probe and inserting polyethylene tubes. Definitive transpalatal repair follows at age 6 months.

TRAUMA

Falls, blows, or other blunt trauma to the face frequently include fracture of the nasal skeleton, chiefly the nasal bones. Diagnosis is easy by palpation, which discloses crepitation, confirmed by x-ray film. Closed reduction by internal elevation, with packing and external splinting, usually suffices. Laceration or cuts require débridement and careful suture in layers. A new type of iatrogenic trauma stems from energetic or prolonged pernasal intubation of trachea or stomach. The indwelling tube may cause pressure atrophy of a turbinate or septal ulceration.

DERMATOLOGIC LESIONS

Dermatologic lesions are numerous, frequent, well known, and usually easy to treat. Furuncle of the upper lip or nasal vestibule is an acute infection of a sebaceous cyst or hair follicle by *Staphylococcus aureus*. The lip or nasal tip is red, swollen, and tender. When a fluctuant center develops, it may rupture or may have to be lanced. Local hot packs, administration of analgesics, and intensive antibiotic therapy are mandatory because of the potentially lethal outcome of such lesions. The lip and nasal tip drain through the angular vein, which joins the ophthalmic vein and thus the cavernous sinus. Its thrombosis is manifested by chemosis, proptosis, retrobulbar abscess, and meningitis. If the infection is limited to the hair follicles in the nasal vestibule, it is called vestibulitis, treatment being the same as for furuncle. Its chronic form results from irritation, such as picking the overly dry skin. It is relieved by A and D Ointment.

Erysipelas is an acute infection of the skin and its subcutaneous tissue from *Streptococcus hemolyticus* following a scratch. The slightly raised, deep-red area over the nose is very tender. Intensive antibiotics are in order. Impetigo contagiosa is an acute infection of the superficial epidermis, usually from staphylococcal or streptococcal infection. The initial vesicles around the nares promptly become pustular, with yellow fluid, and then crust. Antibiotic ointment and avoidance of spread control the lesions. Herpes simplex, caused by its specific virus, follows many acute febrile illnesses in herpes-prone patients. Pustular vesicles around the upper lip and nasal tip break, with watery discharge, and heal promptly within 1 or 2 weeks. Manual contagion of the eyes must be avoided.

Acne vulgaris involves the face and back, mostly in adolescents, and is probably due to a combination of allergic, glandular, metabolic, and, possibly, emotional factors. It is a chronic inflammation of sebaceous glands, with formation of papules, pustules, and comedones ("blackheads"). Treatment belongs to the dermatologist. Acne rosacea is a chronic lesion of the nasal skin, with increasing hyperemia until permanent telangiectasia over the nasal tip occurs ("rum nose"). Causes include alcoholism, with secondary malnutrition and, possibly, endocrine complications. Treatment by the dermatologist varies individually. With further progression, the lesion turns into the rhinophyma, an unsightly hypertrophy of the entire skin over the nose, involving the sebaceous glands, connective tissue, and vessels. Treatment is surgical, with excision of all redundant skin, possibly with skin graft.

Lupus vulgaris is a tuberculous lesion of the skin; it may be primary, from infection of a skin defect, or secondary, from a chest focus. Brownish papules on the nose progress into soft tubercles that ulcerate and heal with deforming scars. Systemic chemotherapy is needed as for any other form of tuberculosis. Lupus erythematosus (LE), with its well-known perinasal butterfly-shaped erythema, is a systemic collagen disease, probably from an autoimmune reaction. The reddish, elevated patches progress to atrophic scars with whitish scales. The pathognomonic LE cells in the blood confirm the diagnosis. Treatment is in the province of internal medicine (*e.g.,* steroids).

BENIGN TUMORS

The congenital angioma is the most important of the benign tumors. This blood-vessel tumor occurs in two forms, the small, flat, capillary type and the larger, purple red cavernous type. They may regress, but any increase with the child's age requires surgical treatment. Papilloma is a pedunculated or sessile wartlike lesion in the nasal vestibule; it is excised under local anesthesia. Senile keratosis afflicts fair-skinned people with long exposure to sunlight. It is a brownish, elevated, scaly lesion and should be excised because it is premalignant.

MALIGNANT TUMORS

The tip of the nose is the common site of basal cell carcinoma, which is radiosensitive and rarely metastasizes. It begins as a small papule with central ulceration and crusting. It progresses peripherally with raised, white edges. When completely excised or irradiated, it does not recur. Squamous cell carcinoma is more serious because it tends to metastasize early into the preauricular, parotid, or submandibular nodes. At first, it is a raised induration that soon ulcerates. With further growth, it expands peripherally and invades deep.

Although very small lesions may be removed by excision biopsy, usually a wide excision with plastic repair is needed.

EPISTAXIS

Nosebleed is not a disease but a consequence of numerous abnormalities, local and general. The local causes are chronic atrophic rhinitis, nasal fracture, local or general rhinitis sicca from overly dry environmental air, septal perforation (postoperative or spontaneous), foreign bodies, angioma, or malignant tumors. The systemic causes are even more numerous: various hematologic disorders, including familial hemorrhagic telangiectasia (Weber-Rendu-Osler), the various purpuras, hemophilia and other coagulation defects, leukemias and aplastic anemia, hypertension, arteriosclerosis, nephritis, liver cirrhosis, diabetes, the prodromal stage of the acute infectious diseases, vicarious menstruation, and sudden ascent to high altitudes.

Findings

There is a seasonal predilection in the winter months that points to at least two contributing factors: relative vitamin C deficiency causing capillary fragility and dry room air. All age-groups are afflicted. Children have frequent, mild nosebleeds from picking the nose, anterior crusting in dry air, emotional upsets in school, or heavy nose blowing. Older age-groups are afflicted by the vascular and systemic diseases. A sudden rise in blood pressure in hypertension often causes sudden and severe bleeding from the nose, as if from a safety valve to spare the more important cerebral vessels. The sites of predilection are, in order, the venous network over the anterior septum, known as the area of Kiesselbach or Little, especially in children; the superior bleeding from the anterior ethmoidal artery; and the posterior bleeding from end branches of the internal maxillary artery, including the sphenopalatine artery.

Management

Management is often an ordeal for patient and physician and, therefore, requires gentle caution. While packing of the nose is in progress, initial examinations for determination of the cause should be started (blood pressure, complete blood count and differential, coagulation studies as needed). Sedation is indicated to calm the patient and lower the blood pressure if elevated. Nasal packing proceeds according to precise technique and depends on the site of bleeding. Mild anterior bleeding is easily controlled by compression, topical anesthesia, and cautery (electric, silver nitrate pearl, trichloroacetic acid). High anterior bleeding requires packing of the nose with one of the modern inflatable devices that

are less traumatic than gauze packing. Posterior bleeding requires either a postnasal pack according to several techniques or one of the inflatable devices.

Medicinal Adjuvants

A great variety of drugs have been used for control of the bleeding. Coagulation defects or other hematologic disorders must be suitably corrected. Vitamin K is needed for prothrombin deficiency, vitamin C counteracts capillary fragility, especially during winter, and Premarin seems to be beneficial for diffuse bleeding. Other medical problems must be managed as found and indicated.

Surgical Interventions

If all other measures fail, arterial ligations become necessary. Anterior high bleeding requires ligation of the anterior and posterior ethmoidal arteries, which are end branches of the ophthalmic artery and thus stem from the internal carotid system, as well as the internal maxillary artery through a Caldwell-Luc approach, with opening of the posterior antral wall. Ligation of the external carotid artery in the neck just above the superior thyroid artery is technically easier but does not control bleeding from the two ethmoidal arteries. Repeated anterior bleeding is sometimes controlled by submucous resection of the nasal septum, especially if it is markedly deviated, because the scarring alters the blood supply.

DISEASES OF THE INNER NOSE

FOREIGN BODIES

Foreign bodies are seen frequently in children, who like to stuff anything into the nostrils. They cause unilateral nosebleed or discharge. Following topical anesthesia and vasoconstriction, most of the foreign bodies can be removed promptly with a grasping forceps. Uncooperative or very young children need general anesthesia to avoid additional injury.

RHINOLITH

A nose stone is a calcareous deposit, usually around a foreign body. Extraction requires topical anesthesia and vasoconstriction to shrink the tissues. Extra-large rhinoliths may have to be broken into fragments before they can be removed. Some atrophy of a turbinate from the pressure may persist temporarily.

RHINITIS

Acute

Coryza is caused by a group of filterable viruses with shortlasting immunity, hence the possibility of contracting several colds each year and the poor results of preventive vaccination. In addition to the exposure, predisposing factors determine whether the infection will be contracted. Such factors are sudden cold weather, chilling, getting wet, lowered resistance from fatigue or indigestion, sudden change of climate (as with jet travel), and low humidity. Incubation lasts usually from 1 to 3 days but may be as short as a few hours. The prodromal signs include dry tickle in the epipharynx, sneezing, and perhaps soreness of the tonsillar neck nodes. Low-grade fever and malaise are followed by nasal congestion with watery discharge. If the discharge becomes thicker and purulent, secondary bacterial invasion has occurred that often involves other parts of the

EPISTAXIS	
Etiology	Mucous membrane dryness from a variety of causes, trauma, foreign bodies, hypertension, and neoplasms
Dx	Important to locate the source of bleeding: X-ray films and CT scans important in persistent or recurrent cases
Rx	Cauterization or nasal packing, control of hypertension, and in severe cases, internal maxillary artery and ethmoidal artery ligation

RHINITIS	
Etiology	Bacterial and viral agents are most common. Of the bacterial agents, *Streptococcus*, pneumococcus, and *H. influenzae* predominate. In viral rhinitis, adenoviruses, childhood diseases, and influenza A and B are most common. In allergy, the inhalants (dust, molds, pollens, animal danders, feathers, and smoke) are causative, while the ingestants (eggs, milk, wheat, fish) may be the source.
Dx	History, scratch or intradermal skin tests, sinus films, nasal smears, and culture
Rx	Antihistamine–decongestants, antibiotics when indicated, removal or control of environmental offenders, and, in more severe cases, topical or systemic steroids

airways. Treatment is symptomatic in the proverbial manner: salicylates, rest, sufficient humidity, and fluids. Antibiotics are useless except against a secondary bacterial infection. Full recovery usually occurs within 1 week.

Bacterial

Bacterial rhinitis is usually caused by *Streptococcus, Staphylococcus,* pneumococcus, *hemophilus,* or *Neisseria catarrhalis.* The clinical manifestations resemble viral coryza except that the systemic signs are more toxic. Diagnosis is confirmed by culture, which also indicates the proper antibiotic. Spread to the adjacent airways is frequent.

Specific Forms

Another form of viral rhinitis is the influenzal rhinitis during epidemics. The systemic symptoms are still more severe. Specific vaccines are helpful in susceptible persons. Exanthematous rhinitis precedes the skin rash of the specific childhood diseases. Simultaneous otitis media from the same virus is common. Irritant rhinitis follows exposure to allergenic inhalants. Sneezing and watery discharge are typical, promptly suppressed by antihistaminics.

Chronic

Chronic rhinitis occurs in two forms. The hypertrophic form results from a series of bouts of acute rhinitis that eventually fail to heal because of some complicating factors, such as frequent infections, low general resistance, irritants, unfavorable climate, chronic infection of adjacent structures, and allergy. The chief complaint is nasal obstruction with mouth breathing, which results in dry pharyngitis. The mild headache is popularly labeled "sinus headache." Mucous discharge may be tenacious, hanging into the nasopharynx as it is propelled there by the centripetal undulations of the epithelial cilia—the widely bemoaned "postnasal drip." It is particularly noticeable and disturbing in heavy smokers as their "morning cough," which abates promptly with cessation of smoking. From the constant irritation, the nasal mucosa becomes hypertrophic, looking dark red. It shrinks slowly after spraying with a vasoconstrictor. Treatment aims at elimination of the likely causes. Nose drops are contraindicated because their rebound phenomenon produces increased congestion. Systemic decongestants are more help-

ful. The mulberry-like hypertrophy of the posterior ends of the lower turbinates may have to be snared off. Alkalol is a soothing physiological solution for prolonged use by nasal irrigation.

Atrophic

Atrophic rhinitis leads to inflammatory atrophy and shrinkage of the entire nasal mucosa, with ultimate destruction of its ciliated epithelium and great widening of the nasal cavity with drying and fetid crusting. The disease is common in persons in dusty, dry climates and among workers in dusty, irritant surroundings; it is rare in humid climates. When the dryness is in the foreground, it is called rhinitis sicca. Crusting with foul odor is known as ozena, caused by *Klebsiella ozaenae.* If it follows a specific disease, it is a secondary or specific atrophic rhinitis. Autogenous vaccines have been used with variable success. The best treatment is nasal irrigation with a warm alkaline solution, such as Alkalol. In advanced cases, the nasal air space can be narrowed by submucosal implantation of autogenous bone chips, tantalum mesh, or some inert plastic.

Allergic

Allergic rhinitis, a frequent ailment and the chief cause of sinus headache and postnasal drip, is an atopy because of its familial nature. It may be acute, chronic, seasonal, or perennial. More frequent in warm, humid climates, it is related by history to other types of allergy. It represents a hypersensitivity response of the nasal mucosa to sensitizing allergens. The etiologic agents are differentiated into several offenders. Inhalants are the most frequent. Ingestants are poorly tolerated foods of almost any kind. Contactants include any object that proves irritating. Bacterial allergy means an oversensitivity to some organism present in the patient's own flora. Physical allergy stems from sudden changes in climatic factors. Contributing factors include heredity, endocrine imbalance, any acute infection, emotional imbalance, and weather changes.

Rhinitis Medicamentosa

Rhinitis medicamentosa is a self-inflicted variety of chronic rhinitis, usually of the allergic type. It results from prolonged use of nose drops. It is diagnosed by history, swollen nasal mucosa, and prompt shrinkage with decongestant spray. Another type is the nasal congestion caused by some antihypertensive drugs that dilate the nasal blood vessels. Vasomotor rhinitis is an older term for the allergic phenomena inside the nose, chiefly the physical allergy type such as in patients who cannot tolerate the sun without sneezing, nasal obstruction, and other reactions.

Primary Amebic Meningoencephalitis

A relatively recently discovered disease is caused by a soil ameba of the genus *Naegleria,* which thrives in water contaminated by decaying matter. Persons swimming or bathing in such waters risk having the amebae enter the nose; subsequently, these amebae damage the mucosa, penetrate the cribriform plate along the nerve fibers, and invade the subarachnoid space around the olfactory bulb. The inflammation advances over the entire brain and the amebae spread, with progressive encephalitic destruction. Death occurs promptly within a few days unless the disease is recognized immediately, by the finding of the amebae within the spinal fluid, and treated vigorously with amphotericin B.

DISEASES OF THE NASAL SEPTUM

Septal Deviation
The nasal septum is straight in children unless they break the nose and acquire a traumatic deviation. In adults, the septum is almost always more or less deviated and asymmetrical. More severe degrees of deviation are caused by nasal trauma. Another cause is high arched palate from the maxillary compression with prolonged mouth breathing. The symptom is nasal obstruction, typically and consistently on the side of the major deviation. If a sharp septal spur digs into the opposite turbinate, it may cause Sluder's sphenopalatine neuralgia. It is diagnosed when topical anesthesia of the area stops the pain. Treatment of the neuralgia and nasal obstruction is surgical.

Septal Perforation
A hole in the anterior septum may result from many causes: septal surgery, repeated or deep cauterization, chromium dust exposure, tuberculosis, leprosy, debilitating infections (typhoid), dry rhinitis, or cocaine abuse. The posterior septum is perforated by a syphilitic gumma, leading to the saddle-nose deformity. Many perforations remain asymptomatic. Others may cause bleeding, tickling crusts, or a whistling noise while breathing. Larger holes require plastic repair with a skin graft. The same septal dermoplasty is also used to control repeated nosebleed from hereditary hemorrhagic telangiectasia when it originates from the septum.

Septal Hematoma
Blood may accumulate between the septum cartilage and its mucoperichondrium, lifting it away and cutting off the septal nutrition. If it becomes infected, it turns into a septal abscess. The patient is severely ill and has fever and throbbing pain in the nose, which is very tender. When the nasal mucosa is damaged and opposing denuded areas are produced, they heal by fibrinous exudation that organizes into single or multiple adhesions between these parts: septal synechia.

NASAL GRANULOMAS
Syphilis may afflict the nose as primary chancre, secondary catarrhal rhinitis, tertiary posterior septal ulceration, and congenital snuffles. The rare involvement of the nose by tuberculosis is usually secondary to advanced pulmonary tuberculosis. Rhinoscleroma, caused by Klebsiella rhinoscleromatis, is a granulomatous inflammation producing firm blue-red nodules that heal by stenosing scar formation. Other granulomas include sarcoidosis, the various fungal infections, lethal midline granuloma, and Wegener's granulomatosis. The cause of the latter two is unknown.

NASAL TUMORS

Polyps
These pedunculated, edematous, grayish yellow, grapelike formations are caused by herniation of the mucosa from within the nasal sinuses, usually from long-standing allergy, often with secondary infection. Usually multiple and bilateral, they originate in the ethmoidal labyrinth and extrude from the middle and upper nasal meatus. The single choanal polyp presenting in the nasopharynx always comes from one maxillary antrum. Symptoms are the same as those of allergic rhinitis. Surgical removal uses the nasal snare, which is looped around each polyp. Recurrence is frequent and requires allergy management.

Hemangioma
Hemangioma is a blood-vessel tumor of the capillary or cavernous type; it causes unilateral epistaxis and, possibly, nasal obstruction.

Papilloma
When arising from the respiratory epithelium, papilloma causes bleeding and nasal obstruction and may become malignant. It is removed by wide excision. Inverted papilloma is a cauliflowerlike mass, with proliferation of the superficial epithelium deep into the stroma. It must be widely excised because it tends to recur and may become malignant. Other tumors include lipoma, adenoma, myxoma, osteoma, chondroma, fibroma, lymphangioma, glioma, meningocele, and meningoencephalocele.

Malignant Tumors
The squamous cell carcinoma is the most frequently seen malignant tumor, followed by adenocarcinoma, various sarcomas, and rare lesions such as cylindroma, neuroepithelioma, malignant melanoma, and plasmacytoma. They may originate in the nasal vestibule (melanoma), inside the nose, or within the sinuses. The main sign is the unilateral occurrence of all symptoms, obstruction, swelling, displacement, bleeding, discharge, tearing, and late pain with regional anesthesia (infraorbital nerve). Treatment is difficult because many of these lesions are seen in a late stage. It combines radical surgery, irradiation, and, possibly, chemotherapy.

PARANASAL SINUSES
The accessory sinuses are hollowed-out cavities within the bones of the cranium. There are eight: two frontal sinuses (one or both of which may be absent), two ethmoidal labyrinths, two sphenoids separated by a median septum, and two maxillary antra (Fig. 17-14). They are lined with the same ciliated mucosa as the inner nose, with which they are continuous. They are grouped in two series. The anterior series comprises the antra, frontals, and anterior ethmoidal cells, all of which drain into the middle nasal

Fig. 17-14. Paranasal sinuses.

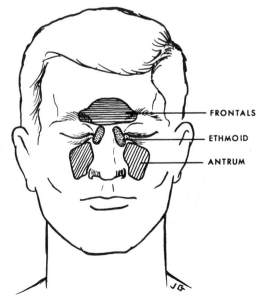

ACUTE SINUSITIS	
Etiology	As in acute rhinitis: pneumococci, *H. influenzae*, *Staphylococcus aureus*, anaerobic streptococci, and *Bacteroides*. Obstruction of the nasal passages or sinus ostia predisposes to infection.
Dx	Face pain, headache, upper dental pain, and nasal congestion, possibly with fever and leukocytosis; confirmed by x-ray film
Rx	Vasoconstrictors, antibiotics, analgesics, and, in resistant cases, surgical drainage

meatus beneath the middle turbinate. The posterior series consists of the posterior ethmoidal cells and the sphenoids. They drain into the superior nasal meatus above the middle turbinate. Finding pus in one or both of these locations indicates which of the sinuses is involved.

ACUTE SINUSITIS

Acute sinusitis is usually caused by acute infection of the respiratory tract when the inflammation extends into the sinuses through their natural ostia. Simultaneous hematogenous infection of the entire respiratory mucosa is likely with the acute systemic infections of childhood, as well as with influenza. The responsible agents are the same as with the common cold, that is, at first viral, then bacterial superinfection.

PREDISPOSING FACTORS

Low resistance to colds also contributes to frequent sinus infection. Among the local factors, any obstruction of the sinus ostia will promote retention of secretion, reduced ventilation, and, thus, entry of infection. In the case of the antrum, dental disease of the premolars and first two molars can cause its infection, especially after extraction with rupture of a root through the antral floor.

SYMPTOMS

Acute sinusitis manifests itself chiefly by general malaise and pain over the involved sinus. Pressure, toothache, and tenderness are found over the antra. Pain from the ethmoidal sinuses extends across the nose and behind the eyes, while involvement of the frontal sinuses causes throbbing pain over the forehead, extending exactly as far as the sinuses are developed (which can be shown by gentle percussion). Pain from sphenoidal sinus infection is felt over the vertex, occiput, or mastoids. Examination shows typical findings. The entire nasal mucosa is red, swollen, and edematous. After decongestion, pus is seen emerging from the specific ostia. The diagnosis is confirmed by history, palpation and percussion, transillumination, and sinus x-ray films.

TREATMENT

The acutely ill patient is treated as if for influenza: bed rest, analgesics, broad-spectrum antibiotics until the culture and sensitivity tests indicate the optimal drug, nasal decongestants to promote drainage, heat over the face, and room humidifier.

It is wise to postpone any surgical procedure in the acutely febrile patient for a few days until the highly acute phase has abated. There are exceptions when the patient, especially with frontal sinusitis, fails to respond promptly; trephination may be necessary to relieve pain and swelling and prevent subsequent complications. For maxillary sinusitis that does not respond to treatment, antral lavage, either through the natural ostium by a special curved cannula or by direct puncture through the inferior meatal wall with a large-bore spinal needle, may be necessary (Fig. 17-15). Proetz displacement is a useful procedure for subacute and chronic cases of ethmoidal and sphenoidal sinusitis. With the patient's head hanging over the edge of the table, a mild vasoconstrictor and antibiotic solution is instilled into the nose. While one nostril is held closed, gentle negative pressure is applied to the other and the procedure is repeated with the untreated nostril.

ACUTE COMPLICATIONS

In the infant without fully developed antra, an infection of the maxillary area may result in acute maxillary osteomyelitis. It must be treated vigorously to avoid fatal progression. Young children easily develop orbital cellulitis from a break of an acute ethmoidal sinusitis through the lamina papyracea. It must be incised and drained. If the diploic veins around the frontal sinus become thrombosed, the infection turns into osteomyelitis of the frontal bone, which does not respect the suture lines. Wide exposure is necessary until healthy bone is reached. Frontal sinusitis may also break through the inner table and cause several intracranial complications. A break into the infratemporal

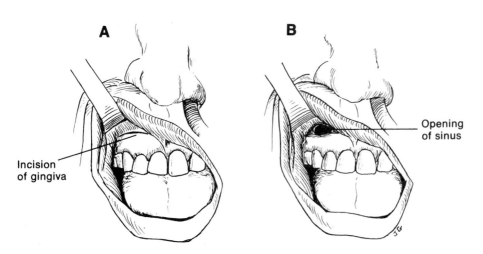

A Incision of gingiva

B Opening of sinus

Fig. 17-15. Caldwell-Luc operation. (*A*) Incision of gingiva. (*B*) Entry through bone of canine fossa.

fossa may produce eye symptoms and mask other complications. A rare complication of sinusitis may be cavernous sinus thrombosis. All these intracranial complications require radical procedures for sinus exenteration, wide exposure, and open drainage, often with the help of the neurosurgeon.

CHRONIC SINUSITIS

The chronic form of sinusitis poses problems quite different from those posed by the acute forms. Sinusitis becomes chronic for various predisposing factors, environmental influences, and a final precipitating cause. Allergic sinusitis is frequent.

SYMPTOMS

When a patient with chronic sinusitis complains of headache, it is more likely a tension headache. The chief complaint is nasal obstruction, chiefly from the swelling of the turbinates or from nasal polyps. Mucus or purulent discharge may be seen at the typical drainage points and in the nasal pharynx. Tenderness is not present unless with a complication. When allergy is in the foreground, the signs of allergic rhinitis are prominent.

DIAGNOSIS

Diagnosis is confirmed by transillumination or radiology. The surgical drainage procedures demonstrate the type of secretion. The presence of polyps invariably points to allergic affliction of the antra and ethmoids. Culture and sensitivity tests may be helpful if a specific infection is causing a bacterial allergy.

COMPLICATIONS

Complications include osteoma of the frontal sinus, frontal mucocele, frontal osteomyelitis with Pott's puffy tumor over the forehead, meningitis, brain abscess, and encephalitis.

SINUS SURGERY

Indications for surgery are twofold. An absolute indication is the presence of any of the complications, acute or chronic. All tumors of the nose and its sinuses, including the allergic polyps, also give absolute indications for surgery. The indications become relative when the conservative treatment fails to bring significant improvement, when the patient is sufficiently plagued by his complaints, and when the diagnostic tests demonstrate irreversible changes of the mucosa.

OTHER SINUS PROBLEMS

NEUROSURGICAL

Trauma to the cribriform plate, tumors in that area, rarely a congenital dehiscence, or intranasal surgery may cause a leak of cerebrospinal fluid from the nose (cerebrospinal rhinorrhea). Transsphenoidal hypophysectomy is another example of intensive collaboration between rhinology and neurosurgery.

TRAUMATIC

Treatment of fractures of the nasal bones, maxilla, antra, frontal sinuses, and the adjacent orbit, zygoma, and mandible is well within the province of rhinology, although many of these patients are traditionally managed by plastic surgery and oral surgery as well.

PHARYNX

NASAL PHARYNX

The epipharynx is the uppermost of the three levels of the upper foodway. It is attached to the base of the skull superiorly and loosely connected to the spine posteriorly. In front, it opens into the nose through the two posterior nares or choanae. It is thus part of the respiratory tract and consequently covered by respiratory ciliated epithelium down to the level of the hard palate. In this area, a transitional epithelium provides the gradual change to the stratified squamous epithelium of the foodways. As elsewhere in the body, transitional epithelium is highly prone to undergo malignant change with chronic irritation, hence the high incidence of the various malignant tumors in the nasopharynx.

The upper dome of the pharynx is formed by the clivus of the occipital bone and the sphenoid body. This area is occupied by the pharyngeal tonsil, commonly known as the adenoid (tissue), which is large in children and atrophies during adolescence. On the two sides we see the torus tubarius, the cartilaginous portion of the opening of the eustachian tubes. Slightly behind lies the fossa of Rosenmüller, also filled with adenoid tissue, the tubal or Gerlach's tonsil. The entire wall is formed by the superior pharyngeal constrictor muscle, which is innervated by the ninth and tenth cranial nerves.

MALFORMATIONS

The nasal pharynx takes part in various congenital malformations. The most frequent is cleft palate. Since the tensor

CHRONIC SINUSITIS	
Etiology	Neglected or inadequately treated acute sinusitis may progress to a chronic state
Dx	Thick, tenacious, mucopurulent nasal discharge; chronic nasal obstruction; and radiographic evidence of thickened or polypoid nasal and sinus mucosa. Pain is infrequent.
Rx	Correction of nasal obstruction and control of allergy and environmental factors. Although a trial of antibiotics and nasal decongestants may be given, surgery is usually necessary.

DISORDERS OF THE PHARYNX	
Etiology	Viral and bacterial infections with secondary hypertrophy of lymphoid tissue (tonsils and adenoids), allergies are contributory. Neoplasms, both benign and malignant, may be present.
Dx	Inspection, culture, and tissue biopsies as appropriate; in lesions of the nasopharynx, x-ray film and CT scans are essential
Rx	According to disease process, but usually antibiotics or surgery

veli palatini originates partly from the tubal cartilage, most palatal malformations also involve the tubal function of ventilating the middle ears. Once this function is disturbed, chronic atelectatic middle-ear disease follows, with all its consequences. In fact, at least 50% of all children with cleft palate also have chronic middle-ear disease of the various types. Further malformations include clefts through the sphenoid body with meningoencephalocele, which must not be mistaken for adenoids.

INFLAMMATION

The acute cold begins as a tickling sensation in the nasopharynx. This is soon followed by watery discharge from the nose. When the viral infection turns to bacterial, the secretion from the sinuses, the entire nasal mucosa, and the nasal pharynx becomes purulent. Allergic secretion tends to be thin, mucoid, or watery. Thick, tenacious exudate is bacterial. The much deplored postnasal drip is either a smoker's pharyngitis or an allergic sign. Since the nasal pharynx is not directly accessible to medication applied by the patient, it must be treated by paying attention to any possible offending cause in the nose and sinuses.

ADENOID HYPERTROPHY

The adenoids are part of the lymph tissue surrounding the pharynx in the form of Waldeyer's ring. Its further components are the lateral tubal tonsils, the palatal or faucial tonsils, and the lingual tonsil. Tonsils and adenoids are large in children because they are part of the immune system. When adenoid hypertrophy becomes obstructive from recurrent infection, the signs of nasal obstruction become obvious. When left uncorrected, chronic adenoiditis also shows purulent discharge coming down from the nasopharynx.

Adenoidectomy has the following indications: nasal obstruction, serous or recurrent purulent otitis media, and visible hypertrophy. It is carried out under general anesthesia with careful exposure of the nasopharynx with a palatal retractor. The hypertrophic tissue is then cut out with ring curettes and punch forceps. As a rule, tonsillectomy is carried out at the same time, unless it is contraindicated in itself. Each case must be observed for the possible presence of a submucous cleft palate or palatal insufficiency, which is a contraindication to adenoidectomy because hypernasal speech would result.

BENIGN NEOPLASMS

The choanal polyp has already been discussed; it always emanates from one antrum. Chordoma is a remnant of the embryonic notochord which grows expansively and causes local destruction. Surgical removal is not rarely followed by recurrence, which then requires radiotherapy. Tornwaldt's cyst means a nasopharyngeal bursitis. It is attached to the occipital bone and presents as a flat cyst with purulent discharge. It is removed by electrocautery. Another nasopharyngeal cyst occurs at the site where the embryonal tissue invaginated as Rathke's pouch to form the epithelial portion of the pituitary. Juvenile angiofibroma is a histologically benign neoplasm that destroys all surrounding structures by invasive growth. Almost without exception it occurs in adolescent boys, begins with nasal hemorrhage and obstruction, and tends to regress with maturity, suggesting a hormonal factor. Diagnosis includes angiography to delineate the feeding vessels for optimal ligation hemostasis. The tumor is extraordinarily vascular, so biopsy must

be carried out in the operating room. Treatment requires radical resection and radiotherapy. Androgens are sometimes helpful.

MALIGNANT TUMORS

By far the most frequent tumor in the nasopharynx is the squamous cell carcinoma. Other epithelial tumors include the lymphoepithelioma, adenocarcinoma, and transitional cell carcinoma. It is not known why these tumors are many times more frequent in the Chinese race, even when American-born. In the reticuloendothelial group we find the reticulosarcoma, lymphosarcoma, and plasmacytoma. Connective tissue tumors include sarcoma, fibrosarcoma, and chondrosarcoma. Diagnosis becomes obvious when Trotter's syndrome is present: unilateral serous otitis, unilateral nasal obstruction and bleeding, and ipsilateral lymph node metastasis in the posterior cervical triangle. Treatment is limited to external irradiation because the base of the skull cannot be removed surgically. Cranial nerve paralysis is a late sign, indicating the intracranial spread. If the primary lesion can be controlled by irradiation, the cervical metastasis may be removed by radical neck dissection.

OROPHARYNX

The mesopharynx extends approximately as far as seen with a tongue depressor (*i.e.*, from the soft palate to the level of the epiglottis). Together with the oral cavity, it serves the ingestion, chewing, and swallowing of food. Oral breathing is normal only for great physical exertion and speaking (or singing). Since time immemorial the physician has scrutinized the tongue and oral cavity because, indeed, the vast majority of all diseases, somatic and psychogenic, lead to typical changes in the oral mucosa. Their discussion fills a textbook of stomatology. Consequently, the entire field of medicine, general and almost all specialties, is interested in the oral cavity for diagnostic cues. The treatment of oropharyngeal lesions likewise is shared by many disciplines: all dental subspecialties, stomatology, oral surgery, plastic surgery, and otolaryngology.

MALFORMATIONS

The most frequent malformations include the various types of cleft lip and palate, alone, or as part of syndromes. Glossoptosis with Pierre Robin syndrome, bifid tongue, ankyloglossia, macroglossia and microglossia, rare asymmetries of the palatal arches, congenital fibromas between tongue and palate, and congenital palatal insufficiency are further examples. They are important to the laryngologist when scheduling tonsil surgery because an overlooked velopharyngeal incompetence, for various reasons, causes postoperative hypernasal speech. Malformation of the tongue may cause articulatory speech disorders, but such relationship must be carefully evaluated by a team of specialists.

TONSILS

Being part of Waldeyer's ring, the palatal or faucial tonsils serve an important function in lymphopoiesis and immune-body formation. They are therefore large and active in children. During middle age, they gradually atrophy until they may be barely visible in old people. In general, they should not be removed until age 4, unless for compelling reasons.

Follicular Tonsillitis

When a viral tonsillitis becomes secondarily infected, or when it is part of a communicable bacterial infection, chiefly in children, the exudative form develops. It is usually caused by hemolytic streptococcus and begins with a sudden sore throat accompanied by systemic toxicity, fever, chills, and malaise. The swollen and reddened tonsils are covered by a whitish follicular exudate, which may coalesce to a nonadherent membrane. Its chief difference from diphtheria is the lack of spread beyond the tonsils. To avoid the not infrequent complications of streptococcal tonsillitis (such as rheumatic fever or nephritis), adequate antibiotics must be given for up to 10 days.

Peritonsillar Abscess

Quinsy is a frequent complication of many attacks of acute tonsillitis. Caused by hemolytic streptococcus, pneumococcus, or staphylococcus, it begins as another bout of tonsillitis but does not get better despite treatment. Unilateral pain is followed by increasing dysphagia and trismus with drooling. The patient is acutely ill with high fever, toxic, dehydrated, and prostrate. A marked swelling and edema is seen around one tonsil, with the uvula being pushed to the opposite side. The abscess is incised following topical anesthesia. The optimal point is halfway between the uvula and the last molar. In a sitting position, the patient spits out the pus that squirts from the incision. If not promptly found, the pus may be located by spreading the incision with a hemostat. Massive antibiotics are given, and intravenous fluids may be necessary. A peritonsillar abscess is an absolute indication for tonsillectomy because each subsequent bout becomes more serious (Fig. 17-16).

Chronic Tonsillitis

Chronic inflammation or infection of the tonsils is not easily diagnosed except by a postoperative pathological section, which demonstrates three types: lacunar infection of the crypts, parenchymatous increase in number and size of germinal centers, and interstitial fibrosis and atrophy. The most reliable clinical signs, especially following longer observation, are the following: repeated attacks of tonsillitis or cervical adenopathy; irregular scarring, asymmetry, and deep crypts, often with expressible detritus of bad odor; a discrete circumtonsillar erythema of the palatal arches;

Fig. 17-16. Peritonsillar abscess on right side.

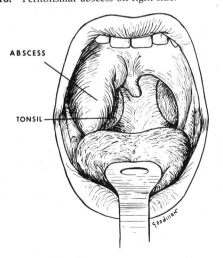

tender cervical lymph nodes; frequent malaise, with slight fever; bacteriologic demonstration of pathogenic bacteria from the crypts; and evidence of a true focal infection, with exacerbation of distant lesions with each tonsillitis. Chronic tonsillitis may even persist in small tonsil remnants left behind during a tonsillectomy.

Tonsillectomy

Indications. Indications have been discussed above and comprise marked hypertrophy, with dyspnea and dysphagia; repeated attacks of tonsillitis, with frequent morbidity; serous otitis media; peritonsillar abscess; persistent cervical adenopathy, particularly with abscess formation; true chronic tonsillitis in the adult; and a focal infection from bacterial allergy. If present in the professional singer, these indications carry even more weight because the operation should be performed early in the career. Once a singer has established his vocal technique over the years, he finds it increasingly difficult to adjust his movements of tone placement to the altered anatomical situation of a tonsillectomized throat with the inevitable scarring. Some middle-aged singers have lost their careers after successful tonsillectomies for vital indications.

Contraindications. Contraindications are numerous and include all blood dyscrasias unless corrected; tuberculosis; uncontrolled diabetes; cardiac problems; palatal malformations, including submucous cleft and palatal shortness or paralysis (but not bifid uvula alone); uncontrolled hypertension; marked unilateral hypertrophy without prior biopsy, because this may be a lymphoma or other tumor; acute illness with leukocytosis over 10,000; and surgery in professional singers around middle age, unless to preserve life.

Technique. The procedure has varied greatly over the years. The partial tonsillotomies with various guillotinelike instruments in vogue during the past century are now rightfully condemned. In fact, great care must be exercised to take the tonsils out completely to the base of the tongue; otherwise, they regrow partially. Sluder's ingenious technique with his special gliding blade is adequate only for simple hypertrophy in young children. Otherwise, surgical dissection within the tonsil capsule is now the universally preferred method. It is being done in various ways: in Rose's position or lying flat, with the surgeon to one side of the patient, both with general intubation anesthesia, or sitting, with local anesthesia for adults, as generally done in Europe (Fig. 17-17).

Hemorrhage. Hemostasis is the most important detail of a proper tonsil operation. In the absence of bleeding tendency, with careful technique, and without major scarred adhesions, bleeding is usually mild and easily controlled. Many different techniques have evolved in the course of years. Primary hemostasis is now achieved in various ways. Some still like the sliding Coakley knot applied with two hemostats. Figure-of-eight sutures are effective but may be difficult in a child's small mouth; on occasion, a curved needle has broken off and then had to be retrieved with a metal detector. Since the introduction of the nonflammable agents, diathermic cautery has become widely used, except for an unusually brisk arterial bleeder. The patient must leave the table with dry fossae.

Two types of postoperative hemorrhage are distinguished, primary and secondary. Primary hemorrhage occurs on the first day for several reasons: incomplete hemostasis at surgery; slipping of a ligature, especially a sliding knot;

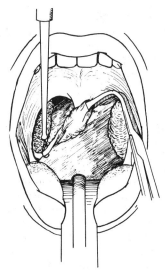

Fig. 17-17. Tonsillectomy. Note incision of the mucosa; the tonsil has been dissected from its capsule and is now ready to be snared off.

opening of a thrombosed vessel; or vasodilatation following local anesthesia in adults. It is a serious condition in a child who may have swallowed large amounts of blood before the hemorrhage is detected. Warning signs are frequent swallowing, rise in pulse rate, or vomiting of blood. Immediate hemostasis in the operating room is mandatory because coagulant medications are useless. Primary hemorrhage is the principal cause of postoperative mortality, fortunately lower than 1:10,000. Secondary or late hemorrhage occurs around the seventh day, when the white fibrin coating sloughs off and a blood vessel may open. This is also the time when the pain or earache (the glossopharyngeal nerve and its connection with the tympanic plexus) may recur for the same reason.

Tonsil Tumors

Benign. Since the large number and great variety of oral neoplasms had to be excluded from this presentation, only a few typical lesions need to be mentioned. Papilloma is a squamous epithelial tumor that may occur anywhere in the oral cavity but quite typically is found on the palatal margins, around the uvula and tonsils. It is locally excised. Lingual thyroid means a nondescended gland that remained at the foramen cecum where it developed. It is treated according to the rules of thyroid surgery. Leukoplakia around the tonsil is a premalignant lesion and must be widely excised. There is a general rule that malignancies are the more dangerous, the deeper they are located in the oral cavity, lip lesions being the relatively least harmful.

Malignant. The most frequent tonsil tumor is the squamous cell carcinoma, occurring typically in heavy smokers and drinkers. Tobacco chewing is associated with buccal carcinoma. Treatment depends on the size of the lesion, stage of disease, and presence of metastasis. In general, treatment is surgical, the extent of which depends upon the staging and extent of metastasis of the disease. Postoperative radiation therapy is advised approximately 4 weeks following the operation. Chemotherapy is a helpful adjunct in large lesions. Lymphoepithelioma is quite radiosensitive and is treated with irradiation. It is important not to mistakenly diagnose a marked unilateral tonsil enlargement as a simple hypertrophy, because it may be a tumor.

PHARYNGITIS

Acute
Acute pharyngitis may be caused by various infections—viral pharyngitis (herpangina, pharyngoconjunctival fever, influenza, mononucleosis); bacterial forms (strep throat, scarlet fever, diphtheria, tuberculosis); the three stages of syphilis; fungal types (thrush, actinomycosis)—and by trauma (caustic uvulitis, palatal burns).

Chronic
Chronic pharyngitis also is a group of diseases of various etiology: hypertrophic pharyngitis from a constitutional weakness (granular pharyngitis, lateral bands, lymphomas); atrophic forms from constitutional, climatic, or environmental causes; and pharyngeal pain from an elongated styloid process (Eagle's syndrome).

NEUROLOGIC PATHOLOGY OF THE PHARYNX

Palatopharyngeal Paralysis
The palate is innervated by cranial nerves V and X and the pharynx by nerves IX and X. Their paralysis at the base of the skull produces the foramen jugulare syndrome. Progressive weakness of the muscles about the head and neck is caused by myasthenia gravis. The nerves afflicted by bulbar paralysis (V, VII, IX, X, XI, XII) are also examined by the laryngologist.

Glossopharyngeal Neuralgia
Although rare, glossopharyngeal neuralgia is a distressing pain around the tonsil or below it. The sudden, brief attacks are triggered by some local movement. Nothing abnormal can be seen in the area of the nerve, but local or topical anesthesia temporarily relieves the pain, which is also diagnostic.

HYPOPHARYNX

The laryngopharynx forms the lower portion of the pharynx. Somewhat funnel shaped, it surrounds the laryngeal vestibule. Anteriorly, it begins with the two valleculae between the base of the tongue and the epiglottis. On each side, it descends into the conical recess of the piriform sinus, which borders on the larynx at the aryepiglottic folds. Posteriorly, the cricoid plate is surrounded by the cricopharyngeus muscle, which closes the esophageal inlet. The entire hypopharynx is covered by stratified squamous epithelium, which borders on the transitional zone before becoming respiratory epithelium slightly inside the laryngeal vestibule where the mechanical forces of all laryngeal reflexes cease to stress the mucosa.

FOREIGN BODIES

Pointed objects may easily get stuck in the hypopharynx. Sites of predilection are the lingual tonsil, valleculae, piriform sinuses, and cricopharyngeal sphincter. Some of these objects are not radiopaque and therefore elude detection on x-ray films. When carefully searched for with mirror and palpating finger, they should be found promptly and extracted with a suitably bent forceps.

LINGUAL TONSILLITIS

Some persons develop a more or less marked hypertrophy of the lymph follicles at the base of the tongue behind the V-shaped row of circumvallate papillae. This may happen following tonsillectomy but may occur without it. One then sees an irregular lumpy appearance of the tongue base, sometimes even with follicular exudate. This hypertrophic lymph tissue may become infected in exactly the same way as all the other tonsil tissue. Acute infection may be unilateral, with ipsilateral cervical lymph nodes. Chronic infection is very similar to chronic tonsillitis in general. Sometimes a localized abscess may form that needs to be incised.

PARAPHARYNGEAL ABSCESS

The parapharyngeal space is bounded by the superior pharyngeal constrictor medially and the internal pterygoid muscle laterally. It ends superiorly at the base of the skull and opens inferiorly into the mediastinum. It is traversed by the carotid artery and jugular vein, which adds to the potential dangers that can emanate from this area. Infection of this space may occur from a simple tonsillitis, peritonsillar abscess, pharyngeal lesion, dental extraction, or deep injection for tonsillectomy. The offending bacteria are the same that cause the original infection. The patient is acutely ill with fever, unilateral sore throat and swollen neck, dysphagia, trismus, even dyspnea. The lateral wall of the pharynx is swollen and bulging on one side, and the tonsil protrudes without being abscessed. Treatment comprises massive doses of antibiotics, intravenous fluids, and surgical drainage by lateral pharyngotomy.

Complications include septicemia from internal jugular vein thrombosis, pharyngeal hemorrhage from erosion of the carotid artery or one of its branches, descending mediastinitis, or ascending invasion of the base of the skull, with meningitis. Aggressive surgical intervention then uses appropriate vessel ligations and wide exposure of the abscess.

RETROPHARYNGEAL ABSCESS

The posterior pharyngeal muscle wall is loosely connected to the prevertebral fascia, and this space is occupied by the prevertebral lymph nodes. Two types of abscesses may develop in this prevertebral space: the acute abscess, usually in children, and the cold abscess, from tuberculosis of the cervical spine. The acute abscess is usually caused by streptococci and staphylococci spreading from an acute upper respiratory infection (tonsil, adenoids, pharynx). The young child becomes acutely ill with fever, dysphagia, cervical adenopathy, stiff neck, and moderate dyspnea. Inspection and palpation shows fullness of the posterior pharynx, with pooling of secretions in the piriform sinuses. Lateral x-ray films may demonstrate the extent of the abscess. They also may be misleading, because children usually have a wider retropharyngeal space than do adults. The cold abscess is chiefly an orthopaedic problem. Although a large, fluctuating pharyngeal abscess may be evacuated transorally, the definitive treatment is by the lateral cervical approach, with subsequent application of collar, traction, and so forth.

TUMORS

The chief neoplasm of the hypopharynx is the squamous cell carcinoma. Typically occurring in heavy smokers and drinkers with poor eating habits, the lesion often escapes detection for several reasons: It afflicts ''silent'' areas that do not give rise to subjective symptoms until pain sets in from ulceration; it does not cause dysphagia until reaching a larger size or, again, ulcerating; and addicted persons neglect their personal hygiene and pay no attention to slowly enlarging lumps in the neck. Treatment depends on the stage and size of the lesion. Partial pharyngectomy, laryngectomy, hemimandibulectomy, and radical neck dissection may have to be carried out in various combinations. Defects are covered by flaps (forehead, pectoral). Small lesions may respond to radiotherapy, alone or combined with surgery. The cure rates are not favorable. Other neoplasms include hemangioma, neuroma, neurofibroma, cysts around the epiglottis, and some rare sarcomas.

PARALYSIS

The hypopharynx is innervated by the pharyngeal plexus of nerves IX and X, as well as by the recurrent laryngeal nerve. Vagus paralysis reduces the motility of the esophagus, so its peristaltic action is diminished. As a result, frothy mucus and saliva accumulate in the piriform sinus on the afflicted side. This pooling of saliva is an important sign of motor paralysis of the vagus system. If hypoesthesia is also present, aspiration and choking complicate the condition. For differential diagnosis, it is important to investigate the esophagus, where a neoplasm may cause the same pooling of saliva.

GLOBUS SENSATION

The subjective complaint about a lump in the throat was frequent at times when conversion reactions were more common than at present. It was then called globus hystericus. The patient, usually a nervous female, complains vividly about some obstruction that will not go down with swallowing. It feels like the tight throat when one is on the verge of tears and has the same cause, spasm of the cricothyroid muscle. On the basis of neurovegetative imbalance, some emotional conflict causes overcontraction of the esophageal inlet. The diagnosis is made by exclusion of organic disease through careful examination, possibly including esophagogram or esophagoscopy. A wide variety of lesions may cause similar types of dysphagia.

LARYNX

The larynx is an extremely complicated organ whose exquisitely coordinated function is still far from well understood. Its skeleton is made up of several cartilages: thyroid wing, cricoid ring, two arytenoids with their sesamoids (corniculate and cuneiform), and epiglottis. These cartilages are interconnected by joints and ligaments and attached by membranes to the hyoid bone above and the trachea below. Several muscles form three groups: one pair of abductors, the posterior cricoarytenoids for respiration; a group of adductors for vocal cord approximation (for phonation and reflex glottal closure); and the two external tensors, the cricothyroid muscles. The supraglottic larynx develops from the fourth branchial arch, and the infraglottic larynx develops from the sixth. Hence, all details of blood supply, lymph flow, innervation, and anatomical compartmentalization follow the same embryonic arrangements. This is also the reason for the strange course of the inferior laryngeal nerve, which is recurrent around the aortic arch on the left

DISORDERS OF THE LARYNX	
Etiology	Congenital malformations, infections, trauma, and neoplasms
Dx	Hoarseness, stridor, airway obstruction, cough, and hemoptysis; laryngoscopy, both indirect and direct, fiberoptic endoscopy radiographs (plain film, laryngograms, and CT scan)
Rx	Based on etiology, but usually antibiotics, steroids, or surgery. Irradiation may be used in small neoplasms or as an adjunct to surgery in larger ones. Speech therapy in laryngeal lesions secondary to voice abuse or trauma

and the subclavian artery on the right. The subglottic larynx extends from the edge of the vocal cords along the elastic cone down to the first tracheal ring. The entire inner larynx is covered by ciliated respiratory epithelium, except for the vocal cords, whose mechanically stressed function requires squamous stratified epithelium. The intervening transitional epithelium is cancer prone, as usual. A lesion extending throughout the upper ventricular folds, the vocal cords, and the infraglottic cone is termed transglottic (Fig. 17-18).

PHYSIOLOGY

The functions of the larynx are manifold. Primarily, it serves as a safety valve to prevent intrusion of anything except air into the larynx. Once some fluid or particle has been aspirated, it is expelled by the cough reflex which further serves to clear the lungs. Glottal closure is also necessary for intrathoracic pressure during physical exertion and for intra-abdominal pressure for bearing down. Phonation is a superimposed function of lesser vital importance. In animals, voice serves various purposes of communication for mating, family life, defense of territory, and aggression. In human beings, the additional learned behavior of vocal communication through speech presents the highest achievement

of cultural life. The laryngeal functions may thus be summarized as respiration, protection, fixation, and phonation.

MALFORMATIONS

CONGENITAL STENOSIS

The vocal cords develop from a horizontal primordial membrane that splits in the midline to form the glottis. Failure to separate produces various degrees of glottal stenosis, from an anterior web to total atresia of the glottis. The degree of dyspnea and dysphonia depends on the size of the web.

LARYNGEAL CLEFT

In a rare malformation, the cricoid plate is split open by a vertical cleft of variable length. Similar to a tracheoesophageal fistula, this causes constant aspiration, with resulting pneumonitis. Diagnosed with direct laryngoscopy, the cleft is repaired by plastic closure of muscle and mucosa.

LARYNGOMALACIA

Congenital laryngeal stridor from laryngomalacia represents a laryngeal immaturity with overly flaccid cartilages. The inspiratory stridor is worse in the prone position. Laryngoscopy with an anesthesia blade reveals an otherwise normal larynx. Bronchoscopy may be added to rule out subglottic obstruction. Reassurance suffices, because the infants outgrow the stridor by the second year.

SUBGLOTTIC HEMANGIOMA

Usually associated with skin hemangioma, subglottic hemangioma causes stridor but no hoarseness. The soft, blue, compressible tumor is seen with direct laryngoscopy and on lateral x-ray films. Following tracheotomy, the lesion may be removed by cryotherapy, laser, or electrodesiccation. Biopsy is contraindicated, because the hemorrhage could be fatal.

CONGENITAL SUBGLOTTIC STENOSIS

Although narrowing of the subglottic elastic cone is often due to postnatal infection with subsequent scarring, a truly inborn type exists also. A fibrous stenosis can be gradually dilated, following an urgent tracheotomy. Administration of steroids appears to be helpful.

LARYNGOCELE

Two types of laryngeal diverticulum occur as an abnormal enlargement of the saccule of the laryngeal ventricle: internal and external. The internal laryngocele is a herniation of the saccule that expands inside the thyrohyoid membrane, causing a bulging of one ventricular fold on phonation. The expansion of the ventricular fold then covers the true vocal cord, producing hoarseness by this dampening effect. Small internal laryngoceles are best treated by voice therapy to avoid excessive vocal pressure. External laryngocele is more common. It penetrates the thyrohyoid membrane and dissects into the neck. The swelling expands on coughing or with Valsalva's maneuver. Diagnosis is confirmed by laminagraphic x-ray films. Surgical excision proceeds by the lateral cervical approach.

VOCAL CORD SULCUS

Abnormalities of the vocal cords cause congenital or dysplastic dysphonia but no dyspnea. The most typical (though rare) defect is the vocal cord sulcus (of Citelli), a horizontal,

Fig. 17-18. Mirror laryngoscopy. The cords begin to abduct for respiration.

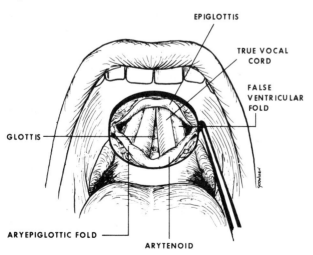

EPIGLOTTIS

TRUE VOCAL CORD

FALSE VENTRICULAR FOLD

GLOTTIS

ARYEPIGLOTTIC FOLD

ARYTENOID

shallow furrow along the medial edge of one or both cords. This gives the appearance of double vocal cords. The resulting voice disorder has a peculiar dissonant sound quality, somewhat like a broken pot. Voice therapy is useless.

CONGENITAL GLOTTAL HYPOPLASIA

Underdevelopment of the vocalis muscle, usually bilaterally, often accompanies the congenital sulcus. In that case, the glottis is bowing to various degrees. This glottal deficiency causes reduced glottal resistance with air leak, audible as vocal breathiness. Teflon injection may be tried with caution in carefully selected cases. The congenital dysplasia afflicts young persons. The same atrophy with glottal bowing may develop in older age as a sign of general involution.

CROSSED ARYTENOIDS

A rare finding in an otherwise normal larynx is a peculiar crossing of unusually elongated arytenoids. This visible abnormality cannot cause dyspnea or dysphonia in itself, just as a bifid uvula alone does not cause hypernasal speech. Yet, this typical malformation may be an alerting sign that something else may be maldeveloped inside such a larynx. (Although at least one world-famous tenor was known to have had this malformation, which did not disturb him in the least, the presence of any of these congenital abnormalities may be grounds to dissuade aspiring students from a vocal career if the slightest additional vocal difficulty is present.)

Other lesions include the congenital cyst, which usually occurs in the supraglottic area. Producing stridor, it should first be aspirated and then removed endoscopically. Cri du chat (cat's cry) syndrome is due to a chromosomal anomaly. The larynx is abnormally small, with a rhomboid glottis, causing the thin, catlike voice.

TRAUMA

LACERATIONS

The "cut throat" injury by assault or suicidal attempt leaves a more or less horizontal gaping wound at various levels of the larynx. The lacerations injure the larynx in many ways. Immediate repair, following tracheotomy, by suturing in layers with or without stenting often preserves satisfactory function. Some victims of shotgun blast have the entire larynx blown away, leaving a big hole in the neck. The great vessels are not always injured. With such survival, nothing can be done except to complete the laryngectomy and close the pharynx.

FRACTURE

Laryngeal fracture is now frequently seen following an automobile accident. In young females with a soft cartilaginous larynx, the elastic tissues are splayed apart, causing massive lacerations within the larynx and of the posterior pharyngeal wall by the shearing force of the thyroid wings. In older males, with an ossified larynx, the bones simply break in various directions, causing varied types of closed or open fractures. Laryngeal injury is recognized by several typical signs: pain in the throat, the spitting of blood, loss of voice, dyspnea, and crepitation on palpation if fractured. Surgical repair uses open reduction, wiring, and splinting, always with tracheostomy. The impact may dislocate one or both arytenoids or the cricothyroid joints. Diagnosis is made by direct laryngoscopy, which shows that the arytenoid can be repositioned and will then move again. Rupture of the trachea is sutured, taking care not to injure the recurrent nerves as they course upward between the trachea and esophagus. If they are torn, nerve suture may be attempted but often is not successful.

HEMATOMA

Bleeding inside the larynx is a frequent finding. One sees a bluish swelling, often with glottal obstruction. It must be evacuated, preferably through a window cut in the thyroid cartilage. Otherwise, the shrinkage during organization causes much scarring and glottal obstruction. Even a relatively minor injury, such as a blow during contact sports, may damage the larynx by contusion. There may be a minor internal hemorrhage, a tear in the mucosa, or a strain on muscles or ligaments. Symptoms are correspondingly mild, except that the voice usually suffers to various degrees.

INTUBATION GRANULOMA

In the early days of intubation anesthesia with less perfect equipment and technique, quite often the tube rubbed against the cord edges and produced a large, pink granuloma on one or both cords. This was easily removed by direct laryngoscopy and did not recur, and there was full recovery of the voice. Prolonged tracheal intubation now produces another lesion. The inflated cuff causes ischemia and mucosal necrosis of the trachea, with subsequent severe stenosis. This difficult problem of tracheal resection and reanastomosis is outside the scope of this chapter. Some persons, often singers, develop a spontaneous vocal cord hemorrhage. This is the same as the spontaneous hemorrhage beneath the conjunctiva of an eye, perhaps following overexertion. Treatment by voice rest leads to complete recovery. Recurrences should be avoided by treating the underlying causes.

HORMONAL LARYNGOPATHIAS

Laryngopathia gravidarum causes distressing dryness and crusting of the larynx and trachea during some pregnancies. Treatment is symptomatic, with inhalations, humidification, and expectorants. Complete recovery follows delivery. Some women, especially singers, develop a circumscribed swelling and reddening of only one vocal cord, called vasomotor monochorditis. This usually happens at the time of menstruation. It causes moderate degrees of hoarseness and must be treated by the gynecologist following exact hormone assay. Tuberculosis, syphilis, and cancer must be excluded.

Male hormonal deficiency prevents normal male maturation, including the larynx, which retains the puerile or feminine size, causing the voice to remain high and effeminate, the eunuchoid voice. Early castration has the same effect, as previously done to obtain harem eunuchs and castrato singers. Treatment of male hypogonadism is successful only if begun early. Female virilization is the female opposite of male underdevelopment. The causes are manifold: adrenal hyperfunction, certain ovarian tumors, hermaphroditic malformations, and, lately, certain iatrogenic side-effects. In Europe, it was fashionable for a while to give anabolic steroids for various purposes. The female larynx became virilized, with corresponding lowering of the voice to a booming baritone. The same may happen with hormone substitutes following hysterectomy, if they contain androgens. Virilizing tendencies have also been noted with some birth control pills, which must then be carefully selected by the gynecologist.

Hypothyroidism produces various general deficiencies all

over the body. One of them is a chronic edema of the vocal cords, which might be mistaken for allergy or chronic laryngitis. Thyroid supplementation relieves this type of hoarseness. All factors that accompany aging afflict also the larynx, causing laryngeal senescence; the voice ages with us. If the cords become plumper from inflammation and congestion, the voice is lowered. If their atrophy is in the foreground, the voice becomes high and thin. Individual differences are great, and the female voice changes somewhat earlier than the male.

HABITUAL LARYNGOPATHIAS

The cigarette smoker's throat is unmistakable. The pharynx is red and the mucosa has a whitish sheen and may look wrinkled like cigarette paper. The cords are red, plump, swollen, and uneven, and may show the various precancerous lesions of chronic irritation as proved by biopsy. Smoking is unquestionably one of the chief causes of laryngeal cancer. It is aggravated by alcohol, which removes inhibitions, which then increases the smoking and talking. Vocal nodules represent a tissue reaction to prolonged mechanical irritation, exactly like a callus on the hand or a corn on the toe. The cause is vocal abuse. The epithelium becomes thickened through hyperkeratosis and is raised into a more or less broad-based node. When vocal abuse continues, a node will grow into a larger polyp. Eventually it becomes pedunculated and may flop up and down with breathing. Histologically, it is similar to a node, except that it is more edematous. It must be excised by microlaryngoscopy. With the passage of time, the smoking, alcohol, and vocal abuse damage the entire cordal mucosa to such an extent that the submucosal space becomes filled with Reinke's edema. The cords look greatly swollen and edematous and are covered by a flabby yellowish mucosa. The voice is extremely low, harsh, and raucous, especially in women.

The contact ulcer granuloma, first described by Virchow a century ago, is frequent in metropolitan areas of the United States but quite rare in Europe. The personality type is characteristic: driving, oversensitive, self-demanding, compulsive, and perfectionistic. The complaint is a vague pain in the neck, perhaps slight huskiness. Laryngoscopy shows a gray, soft, smooth granuloma over the vocal process of one arytenoid and a shallow ulcer or similar granuloma on the other. Removal of the granuloma or cautery of the ulcer is inevitably followed by recurrence. The best treatment is explanation of the problem and psychotherapeutic guidance.

Phonasthenia means the functional weakness of the voice in professional voice users. Jackson described it as myasthenia laryngis. It must not be confused with myasthenia gravis. Phonasthenia afflicts nervous, insecure, tense, perhaps neurotic persons who strain their voices during their vocal occupations. While the complaints are lively, little is seen in the larynx. Treatment comprises much psychotherapy, voice therapy, and reassurance.

Phonation with the ventricular folds is called ventricular dysphonia. It occurs in several forms: vicarious, paralytic, habitual, cerebellar, and psychogenic. Treatment depends on the underlying cause. Psychogenic (previously hysterical) dysphonia and aphonia occur in two subtypes. In the hyperkinetic type, glottal closure is excessive and the voice is extremely hoarse and harsh. In the hypokinetic type, there is a psychological regression to the primary function of the larynx as a breathing organ. The glottis remains open during attempts at phonation and only a faint whisper is heard. Spastic dysphonia differs from the psychogenic dysphonias in many ways. It comes on gradually, afflicts chiefly persons who must talk much on their jobs, and is characterized by a choked, tense, strained manner of phonation that divides the vowels into two portions: "I-i go-o ho-ome." Hence, it has been called stuttering with the vocal cords. Treatment is quite difficult and in some cases may require sectioning of one recurrent nerve (Fig. 17-19).

LARYNGITIS

ACUTE

Acute epiglottitis afflicts children chiefly. It is caused by the respiratory pathogens, predominantly *H. influenzae*. The onset is sudden, progression is rapid, and symptoms are serious. The child is restless from hypoxia, and the epiglottis is fiery red and swollen, as seen with a tongue blade. In adults, the laryngeal mirror confirms the condition. Treatment must be prompt and vigorous, with antibiotics, humid oxygen tent, steroids, and, possibly, tracheostomy or endotracheal tube.

Acute infectious laryngitis may be part of any acute upper respiratory tract infection; therefore, one encounters, for instance, acute pharyngolaryngitis, laryngotracheitis, and rhinolaryngobronchitis. The acutely ill patient may have fever, sore throat (especially when trying to talk), a painful cough, variable hoarseness, and the other signs of acute infection.

Acute specific laryngitis includes all acute, general infections that involve the upper airways: influenza, scarlet fever, measles, whooping cough, diphtheria, Vincent's angina. The treatment is directed toward the primary disease, with all its special requirements. Acute edematous laryngitis may accompany any acute local infection, such as strep throat, peritonsillar abscess, and parapharyngeal abscess. Moreover, the acute laryngeal edema may be of allergic nature, such as angioneurotic edema. Treatment is the same as for anaphylactic shock.

Acute laryngotracheobronchitis (croup) is an acute infection of the subglottic larynx and trachea in young children, usually boys, chiefly by *H. influenzae*. The disease

Fig. 17-19. Arytenoidectomy by suspension laryngoscope for bilateral recurrent nerve paralysis.

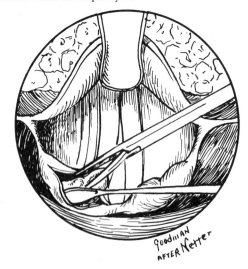

progresses very rapidly from a mild rhinitis to fever, barking "croupy" cough, inspiratory stridor, retraction, cyanosis, and death if not promptly recognized. Although the upper airways may show relatively little pathology, the loose tissue of the subglottic cone is swollen to almost airtight closure. Immediate treatment includes the following: high-humidity croupette with racemic epinephrine added to the inhalation fluid; broad-spectrum antibiotics until specifically selected by the culture results; steroids; and *no sedatives.*

Acute traumatic laryngitis is caused by exposure to smoke, chemical fumes, pesticide mists, and similar irritants that produce thermal or chemical burns of the upper airways. These produce acute inflammatory signs, with red swelling of the larynx and trachea with acute exposure. Pale allergic swelling predominates in the cases of chronic exposure. Treatment includes removal from the offending agents, antihistaminics, voice rest, and inhalations.

CHRONIC

Hypertrophic

The causes of chronic laryngitis are numerous. The climate plays a role. Irreparable tissue changes may result from repeated attacks of acute laryngitis. Chronic infections within the upper airways may sustain a chronic infection of the larynx. Without doubt, all the irritants of an unfavorable environment, such as dry air, dust, fumes, and chemical irritants, are contributing factors. The vocal cords are swollen from chronic edema, round-cell infiltration, perhaps hemosiderin deposits from old hemorrhages, hyaline degeneration, and other signs of chronic tissue inflammation. The epithelium is changed by the various types of epithelial metaplasia, as discussed before. As a result of the physical changes within the cords, the voice is hoarse and raucous to various degrees, which is aggravated by the patient's habitual vocal abuse and his attempts at clearing his voice through forcing it. The condition is progressive unless corrected and inevitably leads to the precancerous changes that eventually become malignant. Treatment begins with elimination of all offending agents, circumstances, and habits. Microsurgery may be necessary to correct epithelial hypertrophies by decortication, ablation of polyps, and so forth. Biopsy is imperative in all suspicious cases with leukoplakia and similar metaplasias. Inhalations, with or without ethereal oils, are always helpful.

Pachydermia is frequent in central Europe but relatively rare in the United States. Caused by the various chronic irritations, a verrucous hyperplasia develops at the posterior commissure. The vocal processes of the arytenoids may be similarly afflicted. The voice is usually hoarse because the vocal cords are diseased from the same causes. Biopsy is indicated, because even the most benign-looking lesion may harbor malignant changes.

Atrophic laryngitis occurs when a long-standing chronic laryngitis undergoes atrophic changes from shrinking fibrosis and scarring. The muscles are damaged by the interstitial edema and round-cell infiltration and become atrophic. This results in bowing of the glottis on phonation, causing a weak, breathy, husky voice.

Specific

The most important form of specific laryngitis is tuberculous laryngitis. Secondary to tuberculosis of the lungs, chiefly by hematogenous spread, tubercles form first over the posterior larynx, including the posterior commissure. Later, the gran-ulomas may appear all over the entire larynx. The symptoms depend on location of the lesions: hoarseness when the cords become involved, and painful dysphagia from ulcerations around the laryngeal vestibule, especially the epiglottis. Perichondritis and cartilage necrosis are late complications. Treatment is the same as for tuberculosis in general.

Syphilitic laryngitis occurs when the larynx becomes involved in the secondary stage. Typical mucous patches develop, as elsewhere in the oral cavity or pharynx. The tertiary form develops as a gumma, usually within one vocal cord. At first there appears a diffuse redness, followed by thickening and induration. Later, the lesion ulcerates, involves the joints and cartilages, and heals with contracting fibrosis.

Other specific forms of laryngitis include mycotic diseases (moniliasis, histoplasmosis, actinomycosis); rare bacterial diseases, such as laryngeal rhinoscleroma; or systemic diseases, such as sarcoidosis, pemphigus, Wegener's lethal midline granulomatosis, and primary and secondary amyloidosis. The diagnosis requires careful investigation of the upper airways, including biopsies, and medical consultation until the underlying condition can be ascertained. Treatment is then carried out jointly with the consulting internist.

ARTHRITIS

ACUTE

Involvement of the two pairs of laryngeal joints is usually part of generalized rheumatoid arthritis. The chief complaint is pain during talking and swallowing, localized around the area of the afflicted joint. The cricothyroid joint feels tender on palpation and may be swollen. If the cricoarytenoid joint is involved, it feels tender on moving the larynx, such as with swallowing, and it looks red, swollen, and somewhat immobilized. Hoarseness appears only if the cords are involved by the swelling. Treatment follows the rules of rheumatology (salicylates, steroids).

CHRONIC

Involvement of the cricothyroid joints may remain asymptomatic, except that the rigidity of the joints may interfere with the vocal cord tension by the cricothyroid muscles, causing loss of the high tones, especially worrisome in singers. When the cricoarytenoid joints become thickened and fixed, the signs are determined by the type of fixation. Immobilization near the midline, especially if bilateral, causes dyspnea. If the joints are fixed in a more abducted position, various degrees of hoarseness are in the foreground. Differential diagnosis from laryngeal paralysis is achieved with the passive motility test, which shows whether an arytenoid can be moved with a forceps. Bilateral median fixation requires tracheotomy or arytenoidectomy, as for bilateral laryngeal paralysis.

PARALYSIS

SUPERIOR LARYNGEAL NERVE

External Branch

One of the two branches of the superior laryngeal nerve, the external, is motor to the cricothyroid muscle, the only intrinsic laryngeal muscle not innervated by the inferior laryngeal nerve. This muscle stretches the vocal cords and is therefore the external tensor, which regulates the modulations of pitch. Its paralysis causes loss of the high register, which disturbs women because their voices then acquire a malelike quality. In the unilateral case, laryngoscopy shows an oblique glottis with the posterior commissure deviated to the side of the paralysis. The gross movements of adduction and abduction remain intact. The afflicted cord appears shorter, flaccid, and lower than the good cord. The usual causes are thyroidectomy, neuritis, such as from diphtheria, and trauma with contusion of the nerve.

Internal Branch

The inner branch of the superior laryngeal nerve is purely sensory and parasympathetic. It supplies the sensation and the mucous glands of the supraglottic larynx to the level of the cords. It enters the larynx together with the superior laryngeal vessels at the posterior end of the thyrohyoid membrane. This is the point where it may be anesthetized for the relief of dysphagia. Its paralysis produces laryngeal anesthesia, unilateral or bilateral, which, in turn, causes aspiration and choking. The causes may be central, with laryngospasm and involvement of the external branch. Peripheral causes include neuritis and trauma. There is no treatment, except of some underlying lesion.

INFERIOR LARYNGEAL NERVE

Also known as the recurrent nerve, the inferior laryngeal originates on the left side below the aortic arch, curves around it, and runs upward in the tracheoesophageal groove to enter the larynx behind the cricothyroid joint. On the left side, it leaves the vagus below the subclavian artery, curves around it, and then follows the same course upward as on the left side. This embryologically explained long course exposes both nerves to a multitude of lesions; including central lesions, lesions at the jugular foramen, lesions in the neck, lesions from thyroidectomy; cardiac lesions on the left, lung cancer on both sides, and scarring tuberculosis in the right lung apex. If no cause can be found, a viral neuritis is assumed and the paralysis is called idiopathic. For the same reasons, the left nerve is more often involved. On both sides, the nerves split into several branches when entering the larynx.

Pure Abductor Paralysis

According to Semon's law, the abducting posterior cricoarytenoid muscle has the greater proclivity to be the first to be paralyzed from a slowly progressive disease. Conversely, it recovers last when a lesion can regress. Abduction is a dual process. At first, the abducted cord relaxes passively to the intermediate line; then it is actively abducted to the lateral position. Adduction follows the reverse sequence: passive relaxation from the lateral to the intermediate line, then active adduction to the median line. With pure abductor paralysis, the afflicted cord is limited to the movement between median and intermediate; all that is lost is full abduction to the lateral line. The cause is either a slowly progressive lesion anywhere along the course of the nerve or the last stage of recovery in a reparable lesion. As long as glottal closure remains complete, the voice is clear, sometimes even in singers. Dyspnea may be noticed only on grave exertion.

Recurrent Nerve Paralysis

The inferior laryngeal nerve has two main branches: a ventral motor group for all intrinsic laryngeal muscles (except the cricothyroid) and a dorsal sensory group for sensory and parasympathetic innervation of the infraglottic larynx. Unilateral paralysis immobilizes the cord near the median or paramedian position because all intrinsic muscles are afflicted. In slowly progressive lesions, glottal closure with the help of the good cord may remain adequate and no vocal disturbance is noted. Moderate dyspnea may occur with exertion. This is seen, for example, with syringobulbia, which is promptly diagnosed from the combination of laryngeal hemiparalysis and rotatory nystagmus. If dysphonia is heard with a cord in the midline position, it must be of nonorganic, psychogenic origin. When the cord is immobilized in the paramedian position, glottal closure becomes inadequate. In addition to the adducting external cricothyroid muscle, the two parts of the single interarytenoid muscle (straight and oblique) have a double innervation from both sides and therefore remain partially active on the paralyzed side. The glottal deficiency from the paramedian position causes moderate to marked dysphonia with air waste and hollow cough. Some dyspnea is felt because the short-winded speaking effort causes increased inspirations.

The causes are the same as indicated previously. Unilateral paralysis following thyroidectomy may recover in at least one third of the patients or become compensated by the good cord. Viral neuropathies may subside within several months. This good prognosis in many cases should be reinforced through voice therapy. If vocal disability persists for more than 6 to 9 months, or if the lesion is bound to be permanent, such as with pneumonectomy, augmentation of the paralyzed cord with injection of silicone or Teflon brings dramatic improvement of voice and cough, with lasting results.

Bilateral Midline Paralysis

Bilateral midline paralysis was previously referred to as bilateral abductor paralysis. When both recurrent nerves are paralyzed, both cords are immobilized at the paramedian lines. Usually some residual motility remains so that the cords meet in the midline for practically normal phonation and can relax to the paramedian lines for severely limited respiration. The dyspnea may not be distressing at rest but becomes worse, with loud inspiratory stridor, with exertion.

The causes are again manifold, ranging from congenital nuclear aplasia and forceps birth injury to viral neuropathies. Repeated thyroidectomy is a typical cause for two reasons. The second operation is usually more difficult because, for example, of the previous scarring, so both nerves may be injured inadvertently. It has also been observed that at the time of the first thyroidectomy one nerve may be permanently damaged, with temporary dysphonia. During the second (or third) procedure, the other nerve may become paralyzed, with immediate severe dyspnea, requiring tracheotomy. This is one reason why every thyroidectomy candidate should have a preoperative laryngoscopy.

Treatment is surgical. A permanent tracheostomy can be performed, inserting a valved tube that allows respiration and phonation. The more modern procedures are various types of laterofixation of one arytenoid through lateral cervical (Woodman) or peroral (Thornell) approaches. The problem with these is the dilemma of the permanent loss of the laryngeal valve. The wider one makes the paralyzed glottis, the better the breathing, but the poorer the voice, and vice versa. Reinnervation has been tried many times but usually does not succeed, because the fibers do not find the proper connections, which results in aimless movements.

VAGUS NERVE

Combined Laryngeal Paralysis

When one vagus nerve is paralyzed anywhere from its somatomotor nucleus ambiguus down into the chest, all its fibers become involved in the paralysis. This includes the following: palatal hemiparalysis with deviation to the good side, pharyngeal hemiparalysis, loss of gag reflex on that side, paralysis of both laryngeal nerves, and hemiparalysis of the upper esophagus, with pooling in the piriform sinus. The functional losses therefore include slightly hypernasal speech, perhaps nasal regurgitation, choking and aspiration, and severe dysphonia or aphonia because the paralyzed cord is now in the intermediate position. This is the result of the combined paralysis of both laryngeal nerves on that side, the superior and the inferior. Loss of cricothyroid muscle function lets the paralyzed cord relax to the intermediate position, where it remains immobilized by the loss of all other intrinsic laryngeal muscles. The gaping glottis prevents closure for phonation, causing severe dysphonia. If dyspnea is complained of, it is subjective; speaking causes such air waste that the patient feels out of breath. Teflon augmentation, perhaps in several sessions, provides excellent improvement of voice, cough, and aspiration.

Bilateral Vagus Paralysis

Bilateral vagus paralysis is rare and usually is due to a bulbar lesion or other cerebral pathology. In addition to the aspiration through the widely open glottis, such unfortunate patients also have additional deficits, such as anarthria, dysphagia, and paralysis. Unilateral Teflon augmentation may be considered to make the glottis smaller by half, but this is usually of little help.

TUMORS

BENIGN

Infantile Laryngeal Papillomatosis

Increasing evidence indicates that a filterable papovavirus causes the endemic disease juvenile papillomatosis, which is rather frequent in the Mississippi Valley and quite rare in other areas (Fig. 17-20). Multiple papillary epithelial tumors with a vascular core develop all over the larynx. Histologically, these papillomas are identical with papillomas else-

Fig. 17-20. Juvenile papillomatosis (laryngoscopic view).

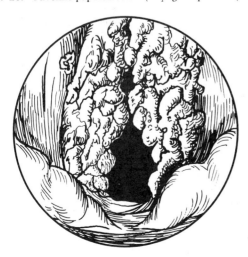

where in the body. Often, the patient has cutaneous warts from which the virus may be cultivated. The usual onset is around age 2, except when the mother had vaginal warts at the time of delivery, which causes the onset as early as 6 months. Increasing dysphonia and dyspnea are the typical symptoms. If neglected, an acute cold may precipitate sudden suffocation. Numerous treatments have been proposed in the past, but only the surgical techniques have survived. With microlaryngoscopy, the multiple wartlike lesions are carefully excised down to, but not into, the normal tissue. Several modifications include CO_2 laser vaporization, cryosurgery, and ultrasound irradiation. The lesions recur inevitably, sometimes at a rapid rate necessitating repeat laryngoscopies every few months. There is a marked tendency for spontaneous regression at puberty, or at least in late adolescence. Some cases continue for life, turning into the adult papilloma. Several authors have reported improved results with the use of autogenous vaccine prepared from the excised papilloma, in addition to the surgical management.

Adult Papilloma

There are two varieties of papilloma in the adult. One continues on from the infantile papillomatosis and may last until death. The other develops for the first time in middle age and tends to remain a single lesion limited to one cord. The two adult forms may change into squamous cell carcinoma. It has been suspected that some of these malignant changes occurred in patients who had prior radiotherapy. The histologic picture resembles the infantile type. The growth rate and recurrence are much slower than in children. Dysphonia is the main symptom, but dyspnea does not occur except in neglected cases. Surgical treatment is the same as in children, except that tracheotomy is almost never needed.

Other Lesions

The congenital subglottic hemangioma has already been discussed. Cysts may be congenital or acquired later. They are filled with mucus and occur around the epiglottis or on the vocal cords. Unless they occupy the cords, they are asymptomatic and may be left alone. Excision by direct laryngoscopy is optional. Among the rare lesions are the neurofibroma anywhere within or around the larynx, the adenoma around the ventricles, the myxoma, which resembles a polyp, the fibroma, and the chondroma, which arises from one of the cartilages. All of these lesions are treated surgically, either by thyrotomy, direct laryngoscopy, or the lateral cervical approach.

MALIGNANT

Squamous Cell Carcinoma

Laryngeal carcinoma is among the more frequently occurring tumors. It used to predominate greatly in men, with a ratio of 15:1, until mid century. Recently, the ratio is becoming smaller, seemingly because women in the cancer age have been smoking for several decades. The chief cause is undoubtedly overuse of tobacco, alcohol, and the voice. As discussed previously, the numerous environmental and habitual irritants produce the various forms of premalignant epithelial changes that comprise the groups of chronic laryngitis. The symptoms begin with hoarseness. The middle-aged man who remains hoarse for several weeks needs a careful laryngoscopy, especially if he smokes, drinks, and talks much. With progression of a neglected malignancy, the advanced symptoms include pain in the throat, referred earache, cough, dysphagia, increasing dyspnea, hemoptysis, cervical adenopathy, weight loss, and other signs of cachexia. The findings depend on the stage of the disease, which is classified according to the TNM system. Early lesions may resemble leukoplakia or present as irregular, grayish, nodular patches anywhere in the larynx. They are intrinsic if within the laryngeal vestibule and extrinsic if outside, the latter with a poorer prognosis because of the richer lymphatic supply. With increasing growth, the lesion spreads in any direction. Cervical metastasis appears at different rates: early with extrinsic lesions and relatively late with cordal lesions. Examination includes direct laryngoscopy for biopsy and delineation of the extent of the lesion, contrast laryngogram for demonstration of subglottic extensions, x-ray studies for observation of metastases, and additional studies in advanced cases.

Treatment of Laryngeal Cancer

Therapy depends on the stage of the lesion. In general, three modes of treatment are in use: surgery, radiotherapy, and chemotherapy. An early lesion is confined to the midportion of one vocal cord, leaving motility intact. The voice is moderately hoarse, and there is no dyspnea or dysphagia and no cervical adenopathy. The best treatment is a modern form of radiotherapy, which effects a complete cure, with return of normal appearance and function of the cord and, therefore, an almost perfectly normal voice. Smoking must be forbidden, and the patient returns for regular office examinations. Chordectomy through a frontal laryngofissure (thyrotomy) has an equally good prognosis, with over 90% 5-year cure rate, but it leaves the patient with a severe dysphonia. It may be preferable in the unreliable patient who will not stop smoking and who will not return regularly. A small supraglottic lesion strictly above the vocal cords is amenable to horizontal supraglottic hemilaryngectomy. The cords and arytenoids are left intact. Because of the inevitable severe dysphagia and aspiration, the patient needs a nasogastric feeding tube for several weeks until he can relearn to swallow without the protective mechanism of the upper larynx.

When a cord lesion reaches the anterior commissure but not the arytenoid with good cord movement, and when it does not extend too far subglottically, it is suitable for vertical hemilaryngectomy. In this procedure, the thyroid wing is excised with the lesion. The defect is covered with a skin graft and the laryngeal lumen kept open with a stent. The great advantage of this procedure is that it leaves the chief laryngeal functions intact: normal respiration, good swallowing, and some sort of gruff voice by means of a horizontal scar band opposite the good cord. As soon as the afflicted cord becomes fixed, the cricoarytenoid joint has been invaded and the lesion requires total laryngectomy (Fig. 17-21). Whenever cervical adenopathy has developed, or in extrinsic, hypopharyngeal lesions with an early incidence of metastasis, radical neck dissection is added to the laryngectomy. Bilateral neck dissection must be staged because the simultaneous ligation of both internal jugular veins is poorly tolerated. Metastatic disease or recurrences following irradiation are treated with chemotherapy with various combinations of antimetabolic and antineoplastic drugs. The results are variable and not always encouraging.

Other Tumors

Among the rare malignant lesions of the larynx are the adenocarcinoma, the synovial sarcoma, and other rare types of sarcomas. Some of these highly malignant lesions have occurred in young children or adolescents. Some are amenable to radiotherapy, alone or with subsequent surgery. Others require laryngectomy, possibly with neck dissection.

Alaryngeal Voice

Following laryngectomy, the patient is totally aphonic and speechless, a grave psychological burden. For a long time, efforts have been made by both laryngologists and speech pathologists to rehabilitate these patients for a productive life. The oldest and optimal method is esophageal voice. The patient learns to aspirate air into the upper third of the esophagus which he then belches out through vibration of the intact cricopharyngeus sphincter. This low, gruff voice then activates the articulating oral structures to a serviceable speech. About one third of the patients are unable to learn esophageal voice for various reasons. They are then given an electrolarynx as a vocal prosthesis. Several surgeons have attempted various surgical procedures for the purpose of rechanneling the tracheal air into the upper esophagus. These artificial tracheoesophageal air fistulas lead the normal

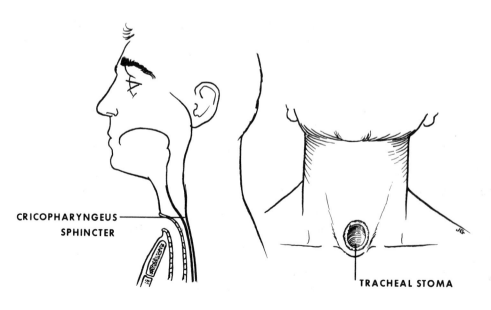

Fig. 17-21. Total laryngectomy. The patient becomes a neck breather and learns to phonate within the cricopharyngeus sphincter.

CRICOPHARYNGEUS SPHINCTER

TRACHEAL STOMA

expiratory airstream into the esophagus, where it activates the vicarious glottis. Another American method uses a plastic valve that connects the tracheal air to a surgical tract into the pharynx. If successful, these tracheoesophageal voices are superior to esophageal phonation.

Drs. Godfrey E. Arnold and Myron W. Lockey developed material which has been drawn upon extensively in the formulation of this chapter.

BIBLIOGRAPHY

ARNOLD GE: Physiology (and pathology) of speech. Encyclopaedia Britannica, 15th ed, vol 17, p 477. Chicago, 1974

BALLENGER JJ: Diseases of the Nose, Throat, and Ear, 12th ed. Philadelphia, Lea & Febiger, 1977

BONE RC, RYAN AF: Intracochlear microprobe analysis. Laryngoscope 92, No. 4:385, April 1982

BULL TR: Color Atlas of E.N.T. Diagnosis. Chicago, Year Book Medical Publishers, 1974

BURKET LW: Oral Medicine, 6th ed. Philadelphia, J B Lippincott, 1971

DAVIS H, SILVERMAN SR: Hearing and Deafness, 3rd ed. Titusville, NJ, Holt, Rinehart & Winston, 1970

DeWEESE DD, SAUNDERS WH: Textbook of Otolaryngology, 4th ed. St. Louis, C V Mosby, 1973

ELLIS M: Ear, Nose and Throat. Clinical surgery series No. 11. Philadelphia, J B Lippincott, 1966

FAIRBANKS DN: Antimicrobial Therapy in Otolaryngology. Washington, DC, American Council of Otolaryngology—Head and Neck Surgery, 1980

FARB SN: Otolaryngology. Medical outline series. Garden City, NY, Medical Examination Publishing, 1970

GOODHILL V: Ear Diseases, Deafness, and Dizziness. Hagerstown, Harper & Row, 1979

HALL IS, COLMAN BH: Diseases of the Nose, Throat and Ear, 10th ed. Baltimore, Williams & Wilkins, 1973

HOLLENDER AR: The Pharynx. Chicago, Year Book Medical Publishers, 1953

HOUSE WF, BERLINER KI: Cochlear implants: Progress and perspectives. Ann Otol Rhinol Laryngol (Suppl 91) 91:11, 1982

JACKSON C, JACKSON CL: Diseases of the Nose, Throat and Ear, 2nd ed. Philadelphia, W B Saunders, 1959

JAZBI B: Pediatric Otorhinolaryngology: A Review of Ear, Nose and Throat Problems in Children. New York, Appleton-Century-Crofts, 1980

LEDERER FL, HOLLENDER AR: Basic Otolaryngology, 4th ed. Philadelphia, F A Davis, 1956

LEE KJ: Essential Otolaryngology, 2nd ed. Garden City, NY, Medical Examination Publishing, 1977

LUCHSINGER R, ARNOLD GE: Voice, Speech, Language: Clinical Communicology. Belmont, CA, Wadsworth, 1965

MAWSON SR: Diseases of the Ear, 2nd ed. Baltimore, Williams & Wilkins, 1967

MONTGOMERY WW: Atlas of Head and Neck Surgery, 2 vols. Philadelphia, Lea & Febiger, 1971

MYERSON MC: The Human Larynx. Springfield, IL, Charles C Thomas, 1964

NEWBY HA: Audiology, 3rd ed. New York, Appleton-Century-Crofts, 1972

PAPARELLA MM, SHUMRICK DA: Otolaryngology, vols 1–3. Philadelphia, W B Saunders, 1980

PROCTOR DF: The Nose, Paranasal Sinuses and Ears in Childhood. Springfield, IL, Charles C Thomas, 1963

RYAN RE, OGURA JH, BILLER HF et al: Synopsis of Ear, Nose and Throat Diseases, 3rd ed. St. Louis, C V Mosby, 1970

SATALOFF J: Hearing Loss. Philadelphia, J B Lippincott, 1966

SAUNDERS WH, PAPARELLA MM: Atlas of Ear Surgery, 2nd ed. St. Louis, C V Mosby, 1971

SCHUKNECHT HF: Otosclerosis. Boston, Little, Brown & Co, 1962

SCHULTZ RL, MORRISON WV: Short-term intubation in children with acute epiglottitis. South Med J 75, No. 2: 1, 1982

SCOTT-BROWN WG, BALLANTYNE J, GROVES J: Diseases of the Ear, Nose and Throat, 2nd ed. vols 1–2. London, Buttersworth & Co, 1965

SENTURIA BH, MARCUS MM, LUCENTE FE: Diseases of the External Ear, 2nd ed. New York, Grune & Stratton, 1980

SHAMBAUGH GE, JR: Surgery of the Ear, 3rd ed. Philadelphia, W B Saunders, 1980

SOBOL SM, WOOD BG, CONOYER MC: Glossopharyngeal neuralgia: Asystole syndrome secondary to parapharyngeal space lesions. Head Neck Surg 90, No. 1: 16, 1982

WOLFSON RJ: The Vestibular System and Its Diseases. Philadelphia, University of Pennsylvania Press, 1966

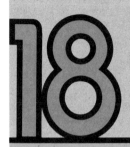

The Skin and Subcutaneous Tissues: Melanoma and Other Lesions

Charles M. Balch

Cutaneous Melanoma

Melanoma is an important malignancy for surgeons to know about, since it can be cured with surgery if it is diagnosed and treated at an early stage. The frequency of melanoma is highest in the southeastern and southwestern parts of the United States. It is likely that the higher incidence of melanoma in these locations is related to increased exposure to ultraviolet irradiation and a genetically susceptible population. Individuals at increased risks for developing melanoma are generally those with fair skin who have a tendency to sunburn rather than tan after sunlight exposure. Melanoma occurs in all adult age groups (median age: 38 years), it has an equal sex distribution, and it can arise in the skin anywhere on the body. The lower legs are the most common site in women, while the back is the most common site in men.

Although melanoma is relatively infrequent, comprising 1% to 2% of all malignancies, its incidence is increasing at a faster rate than almost any other cancer. In most studies, the incidence of melanoma is doubling every 6 to 10 years. Fortunately, the natural history of melanoma appears to have changed during the past few decades, for the typical melanomas are now thinner, less invasive, and more curable.

Most current staging systems divide melanoma patients into three stages: localized disease (Stage I), regional metastases (Stage II), and distant metastases (Stage III). However, since about 80% of patients do not have metastatic melanoma at the time of initial diagnosis, the American Joint Committee for Cancer Staging has recently proposed a four-stage system: Stage I patients under the new staging system include those with low risk for metastatic disease (*i.e.*, <1.5 mm in tumor thickness), Stage II patients have localized melanomas with a higher risk for occult metastatic disease (>1.5 mm thickness), Stage III patients have limited regional node metastases, and Stage IV patients have advanced regional metastases or distant metastases.

DIAGNOSIS AND PATHOLOGY

A change in a mole is the most important characteristic that should warrant a biopsy. This includes any changes in its size, contour, configuration, or color (Fig. 18-1). Some of the typical clinical features of a cutaneous melanoma include: variegation in color, irregular raised surface, an irregular perimeter with indentation, and ulceration of the surface epithelium. Occasionally, patients will complain of a burning or itching sensation within the mole. All physicians should be liberal in their biopsy policy of any pigmented lesions that undergo changes in their physical characteristics.

BIOPSY PROCEDURE

A simple elliptical excision of the pigmented lesion with a narrow rim of normal skin is the optimal procedure for most routine biopsies. Shave biopsies or curette biopsies for

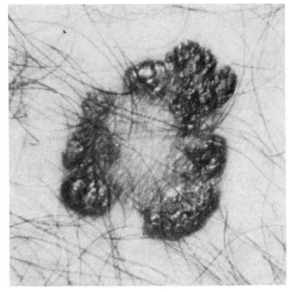

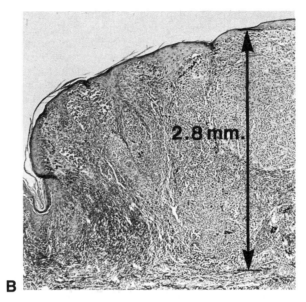

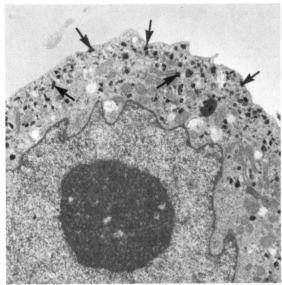

Fig. 18-1. Characteristic features of melanoma. (*A*) Typical melanoma on a male chest. The lesion is multicolored with a raised irregular surface and notched perimeter. (*B*) By light microscopy, the tumor invades through the papillary dermis. The thickness measures 2.8 mm (Breslow microstaging) using an ocular micrometer. It is important to measure the total vertical height of the melanoma. (*C*) Ultrastructural examination of a melanoma by electron microscopy demonstrates melanosomes (arrows) in the cytoplasm that distinguish melanoma from other malignant tumors.

suspicious melanomas are contraindicated, for they preclude the microstaging of the tumor (thickness and level of invasion) that is critical for prognosis and also for deciding about appropriate surgical treatment. An alternative, but less ideal, biopsy method is to perform either a punch biopsy or an incisional biopsy. These limited biopsies, however, must penetrate the entire dermis to include the subcutaneous tissues in order to perform microstaging.

PATHOLOGY

Cutaneous melanoma generally arises as a tumor comprised of atypical melanocytes at the dermal–epidermal interface. When invading the dermis, the melanoma cells tend to destroy preexisting structures and form a tumor mass. Angiogenesis is an early pathological feature of melanoma. Wallace Clark defined vertical and radial (horizontal) growth phases of melanomas and found that the vertical growth phase had a direct correlation with survival, while the radial growth did not. Superficial (lateral) spreading growth patterns have more of a radial growth phase, while the nodular form of melanoma has a predominantly vertical growth

phase. Recently, pathologists have recognized with increasing frequency a noninvasive precursor lesion that has been termed either "melanoma *in situ*," "atypical melanocytic hyperplasia," or "Clark's level I melanoma." This entity is not associated with any risk of metastases and should not be categorized as a malignant lesion. Pathological diagnosis of metastatic melanoma is generally straightforward. In problem cases, ultrastructural examination by electron microscopy is helpful, for the presence of melanosomes in the cytoplasm of metastatic tumor cells is a hallmark of melanoma (see Fig. 18-1).

MICROSTAGING

Microstaging is now an integral part in the pathological diagnosis and the clinical management of melanoma. Two methods have been proposed. The Breslow microstaging method measures the thickness of the lesion using an ocular micrometer to measure the total vertical height (not just the depth) of the melanoma, from the granular layer to the area of deepest penetration (see Fig. 18-1). The Clark microstaging method categorizes different levels of invasion that reflect increasing depth of penetration into the dermal layers or the subcutaneous fat (*i.e.,* levels II, III, IV, or V). Significant regression of the tumor invalidates the prognostic value of these microstaging methods. While both the tumor thickness and the level of invasion can predict the risk of metastases, data from several institutions have clearly demonstrated that tumor thickness is a relatively more accurate and reproducible prognostic parameter than interpreting the level of invasion.

TUMOR THICKNESS

One of the most important features about measuring tumor thickness in patients with localized melanoma is that it can distinguish patient populations at risk for occult metastatic disease in regional nodes alone from those with high risk and distant metastases as well. Melanomas can thus be classified into three categories based upon the measured tumor thickness: thin, intermediate thickness, and thick melanomas (Fig. 18-2). *Thin melanomas,* those that are less than 0.76 mm in vertical height, have an extremely low risk of developing any metastatic disease. The estimated metastatic risk is about 1% to 5%, assuming there is no evidence of regression in the lesion. *Intermediate thickness melanomas* (0.76 to 3.99 mm) have an increasing risk (up to 50% or 60%) of having regional node micrometastases but still have a low risk of distant metastatic disease (about 10% to 20%). The majority of patients with *thick melanomas* (>4 mm) die within 5 years because of the high risk (greater than 60% to 80%) of distant metastatic disease, even though it was undetectable at the time of initial diagnosis. It should be noted that tumor thickness no longer predicts the patient's clinical course once metastatic melanoma becomes evident, either in the regional lymph nodes or at distant sites.

Fig. 18-2. Estimated risk for patients with clinically localized melanomas that microscopic metastases will become clinically evident in regional nodes (within 3 years) and at distant sites (within 5 years) for melanomas subgrouped by thickness categories. (Balch CM: Surgical management of regional nodes in cutaneous melanomas. J Am Acad Dermatol 3:511, 1980)

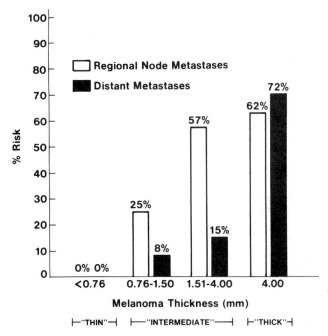

LEVEL OF INVASION

The different levels of invasion can clearly delineate different risk categories for metastatic melanoma. However, several inherent problems with this technique have become evident since it was first proposed. First, the Clark microstaging method requires an interpretation as to the exact level of penetration into the dermis. Because this judgment is sometimes difficult, the method is not reproducible with a high degree of accuracy among all pathologists. A second problem with the level of invasion is that it does not account for tumor growth above the epidermis. This is an important consideration for some lesions, particularly those of the polypoid or pedunculated variety that may not invade deeply into the skin. A third limitation is the wide variation in the thickness of melanomas having the same level of invasion. It is now clear that when there is a discrepancy between these two measurements (such as a "thin" level IV melanoma or a "thick" level III lesion), the actual measurement by an ocular micrometer reflects the risk of metastases more accurately.

MELANOMA ULCERATION

Ulceration of a melanoma is an important histopathological feature that reflects a more biologically aggressive tumor. This parameter is now being used increasingly to help predict the risk of metastatic disease. In fact, ulceration is the only histologic feature of melanoma that predicts the clinical course both for patients with localized melanoma and for those with nodal metastases. Ulceration is best defined as a disruption of the epithelium overlying the melanoma as seen on microscopic slides.

METASTATIC EVALUATION

The most frequent site of metastases in melanoma is to the regional lymph nodes. In a minority of patients (5% to 8%), nodal metastases can arise from an unknown primary site. Presumably the primary melanoma completely regressed.

Once the disease is disseminated to distant sites, it is found most often in lung, liver, bone, and brain. Melanoma is uniquely able to metastasize to virtually any organ, including such unusual sites as the intestinal tract and the heart.

A careful history and physical examination is the most important part of the metastatic evaluation. This includes careful attention to any enlargement of lymph nodes. Chest roentgenograms and liver function tests are also appropriate screening tests for occult metastatic disease. There is some evidence that an elevated lactate dehydrogenase (LDH) is also indicative of metastatic melanoma. In the absence of signs and symptoms of metastases after this initial screening evaluation, further roentgenograms or scans are neither warranted nor cost effective because of the low yield of occult metastatic disease in patients with clinically localized melanoma or with nodal metastases. Thus there is probably little place for bone scans, liver scans, and brain scans in these patients unless there are abnormalities in the screening evaluation that would suggest metastases in these areas.

SURGICAL MANAGEMENT OF THE PRIMARY MELANOMA

Local control of the primary melanoma consists of a wide excision of the primary tumor with a margin of normal-appearing skin around the melanoma or the biopsy site.

CUTANEOUS MELANOMA

Diagnosis: A change in a mole (variegation in color, irregular perimeter or surface, ulceration).

Biopsy: Full thickness to enable microstaging.

Microstaging: Measured thickness is more accurate and predictive than the level of invasion. Three categories are defined: *thin* (<0.76 mm), *intermediate thickness* (0.76–4 mm), and *thick* (>4 mm).

Primary melanoma treatment: Surgical excision of the mole or biopsy site with a minimum margin of 2 cm of normal skin for thin melanomas and a minimum of 3 cm margin for intermediate and thick lesions.

Regional nodes: A lymphadenectomy is indicated for enlarged, firm nodes suspected of containing metastatic melanoma and in selected patients with normal-appearing nodes who have intermediate thickness melanoma (0.76 to 4 mm).

Prognostic factors: Tumor thickness, ulceration, gender, and site are the dominant predictive factors for patients with localized melanoma; number of metastatic nodes and ulceration are most predictive for patients with regional node metastases; number and site of metastases are most predictive for distant disease.

Other treatments: Radiation therapy (high dose–low fraction) is effective for skin and soft tissue metastases, as well as for bone and brain disease. Results with chemotherapy and immunotherapy have been suboptimal.

Until recently, the routine surgical approach was to remove the primary melanoma with a 3- to 6-cm margin and apply a split thickness skin graft to the defect. However, it has become increasingly clear that the risk for local recurrence correlates more with the tumor thickness than the margins of surgical excision. It therefore seems more rational to excise melanomas using surgical margins that vary according to risk for local recurrence (Table 18-1).

TABLE 18-1 SURGICAL MANAGEMENT OF STAGE I MELANOMA*

MELANOMA THICKNESS (mm)	PRIMARY MELANOMA EXCISION (MINIMAL MARGIN)	ELECTIVE REGIONAL NODE DISSECTION
In situ	1 cm	No
<0.76 mm	2 cm	No
0.76–1.5 mm	3–4 cm	Selected patients (especially men)
1.5–4 mm	3–4 cm	Yes
>4 mm	3–4 cm	No (unless for staging)

*Patients with clinically enlarged nodes suspected of metastases should have a therapeutic node dissection and excision of the primary melanoma with a 3- to 4-cm margin.

The earliest lesion is a melanoma *in situ.* This is a noninvasive tumor that is not malignant but is a precursor of melanoma. Multiple sections through the lesion are necessary to be certain there are no areas of microinvasion into the dermis. Although the natural history of these noninvasive lesions is not completely understood, there is a risk of local recurrence (either as *in situ* or invasive melanoma) if they are not reexcised after biopsy. It is therefore recommended that the biopsy site of an *in situ* melanoma be excised with a 1-cm margin of skin.

For thin melanomas (measuring <0.76 mm in thickness), there is only a minimal risk of a local recurrence in all reported patient series, despite wide variations in the surgical margins of excision. The recommended surgical management of these lesions is wide excision of the melanoma with about a 2-cm minimal margin. This is generally performed as a generous elliptical incision and a primary skin closure.

For intermediate and thick melanomas (those exceeding 0.76 mm in thickness), a 3- to 4-cm margin is routinely employed because of an increasing risk of local recurrence (up to 10% to 20% for thick melanomas). Oftentimes, even radical excisions can be closed with mobilization of skin flaps or with rotational flaps. If this is not possible, a split thickness skin graft is used to cover the defect. The underlying fascia is generally incorporated into the surgical resection, although the evidence for documenting the need of a subfascial dissection is sparse.

Melanomas located around the hands, feet, and face generally do not lend themselves to a wide surgical excision because of their anatomic location. In these circumstances, the surgeon must use his best judgment to excise the lesion as widely as possible within the constraints of the surrounding structures. Melanomas of the ear are generally excised with a hemiauriculectomy or a wedge excision of the lesion. Melanomas arising beneath the fingernails (subungual melanomas) are generally treated with a digital amputation just below the distal interphalangeal joint.

SURGICAL MANAGEMENT OF REGIONAL METASTASES

Regional lymph nodes are the most frequent sites of metastases in patients with cutaneous melanomas. Metastatic melanoma may occur clinically as enlarged, firm lymph nodes or it may present as microscopic metastases in the lymph nodes that are clinically occult. These two settings require different types of clinical assessment and surgical judgment requiring lymph node management.

CLINICALLY EVIDENT NODAL METASTASES

In patients with clinically evident nodal metastases, the treatment approach is straightforward, consisting of a radical excision of the regional lymph node basin. Since a palpable tumor measuring 1 cm in diameter already contains approximately one billion cells, the tumor burden in these patients is quite large and the results of surgical treatment alone poor. In fact, melanoma patients with nodal metastases have a high risk (about 85%) of harboring microscopic metastases at *distant* sites when metastases become clinically detectable in the regional lymph nodes. Nevertheless, these patients are a heterogeneous group, with some patients who are cured with surgery and others who have different clinical courses after developing metastatic disease.

A radical lymphadenectomy is the treatment of choice for patients with suspected or proven nodal metastases. A partial lymph node dissection or simple excision of nodal metastases is not sufficient treatment for patients with metastatic melanoma. In two thirds or more of these patients, metastatic disease was present in other lymph nodes. Since the surgeon's ability to detect nodal metastases by clinical criteria is not optimal, a philosophy of limited excision for only clinically detectable nodes will often compromise both the palliative and curative goals of surgical treatment.

IN-TRANSIT METASTASES

In-transit or satellite metastases are a regional form of metastasis that arise in the lymphatics or soft tissues between the primary melanoma and the regional lymph nodes. The optimal treatment for these lesions located on an extremity is whole limb perfusion with chemotherapy and hyperthermia. In patients with one or a few cutaneous or subcutaneous lesions, surgical excision of these lesions may also be effective. Other alternative treatment approaches include irradiation therapy or immunotherapy using intralesional injections of BCG vaccine.

MANAGEMENT OF CLINICALLY NORMAL REGIONAL LYMPH NODES

Decisions regarding management of suspected nodal metastases are more difficult in patients with normal regional lymph nodes by physical examination. The central question in this decision revolves around the timing of any operation to excise regional lymph nodes. The surgeon has two options. First, he can perform an elective (immediate) regional node dissection to remove suspected microscopic or clinically occult metastatic tumor. The second option would be to defer this procedure until any nodal metastases have grown sufficiently large for clinical detection by palpation. A therapeutic (delayed) regional node dissection is then performed.

The efficacy of elective lymph node dissection for melanoma is still controversial. Since it is clear that all melanoma patients do not benefit from this procedure, the debate centers around defining the subgroups of patients who have improved survival rates with elective lymphadenectomy compared to those whose initial management of the lymph nodes is observation only.

Since the cure rate for a delayed therapeutic node dissection is so poor (about 10% to 20%), many surgeons have favored an immediate excision of regional lymph nodes in an effort to remove nodal micrometastases before they can disseminate to more distant sites. Thus, the primary justification for elective lymphadenectomy is to improve survival rates in patients at risk for harboring regional node micrometastases. In this setting, the surgical logic depends upon a biologic rationale for predicting which patients are at high risk for metastatic melanoma.

Tumor thickness can provide a quantitative estimate of the risk for occult metastatic melanoma, both at regional and distant sites (see Fig. 18-2). This parameter is thus a useful guide for selecting patients who might benefit from elective lymph node dissection (see Table 18-1). In addition, the presence or absence of ulceration, the patient's gender and age, the location of the lesions, and the operative risk should also be considered.

Thin melanomas (<0.76 mm) are associated with localized disease and virtually a 100% cure rate. A lymphadenectomy would provide no therapeutic benefit in such patients. Intermediate thickness melanomas (0.76 to 4 mm) have an increasing risk (up to 70%) of harboring occult regional metastases, but a relatively low risk (<10% to 20%) of distant metastases. Patients with these lesions might therefore benefit from an elective lymph node dissection. Thick melanomas (>4 mm) not only have a high risk of regional node micrometastases (>60%); they also are associated with a high risk (>70%) of occult distant metastases at the time of initial presentation. These patients do poorly, since the distant metastases negate the benefit of a surgical procedure on the lymph nodes in most instances. The goal of treatment for thick melanomas is palliative, so a lymphadenectomy can be deferred until any nodal metastases have become clinically evident. Alternatively, an immediate lymphadenectomy might be justified as a staging procedure in patients with thick melanomas so as to document the pathologic status of the lymph nodes prior to entry into adjuvant therapy trials.

Melanomas located on the trunk can have ambiguous lymphatic drainage that makes it difficult for the surgeon to assess accurately which nodal basins are at risk for harboring microscopic metastases. In these circumstances, a radionuclide cutaneous scan is an accurate and reproducible test for determining the lymphatic drainage of trunk melanomas (Fig. 18-3).

TREATMENT OF DISTANT METASTASES

CHEMOTHERAPY

The results with chemotherapy for metastatic melanoma have been very disappointing. Dacarbazine (DTIC-Dome) is the most active agent available, but this has a relatively low partial response rate (15–20%), a short duration of response (1–3 months), and a high incidence of toxicity (especially nausea and vomiting). Complete remissions with this drug are unusual. At the present time, drug combinations that include DTIC-Dome are the mainstay of treatment for metastatic melanoma. More active and less toxic drugs are needed.

RADIATION THERAPY

Melanoma can no longer be considered as radioresistant, even though the response rates are poor with conventional dose fraction schedules. *In vitro* studies and clinical trials suggest that there is a large shoulder in the radiation survival curve of melanoma cells. It has been shown that higher dose fractions with longer intervals between treatment provide excellent palliation for metastatic melanoma in the skin, soft tissue, and lymph nodes. One recommended dose schedule is 600 rads twice a week for three weeks. Radiation therapy can also be very effective palliation for symptomatic metastases located in bone and frequently is effective in relieving symptoms of metastatic brain disease.

IMMUNOTHERAPY

Immunologic responses to tumor antigens have been demonstrated in patients with melanoma more than in those

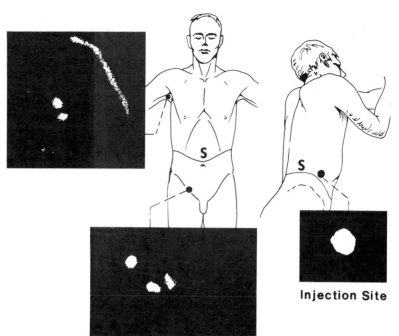

Fig. 18-3. Technetium-99m sulfur colloid cutaneous scan of a melanoma located just above the iliac crest. The lesion is below the lymphatic watershed (Sappey's line), so the lymphatics from this melanoma should drain only to the inguinal nodes. However, the lymphatic drainage in this patient was bidirectional, with migration of the tracer both to the inguinal nodes (*lower left image*) and to the axillary nodes (*upper image*). A scan over the perilesion injection is shown in the lower right image. (Meyer et al: Technetium-99m sulfur colloid cutaneous lymphoscintigraphy in the management of truncal melanoma. Radiology 131:205, 1979)

with any other type of tumor. Both cellular and humoral immune responses to melanoma antigens have been demonstrated, and there are significant abnormalities of immune competence in these patients. Because of these implications, there has been considerable research involving immunotherapy. A variety of techniques and agents have been attempted, but unfortunately the impact on survival rates has been minimal. Nonspecific immunotherapy reagents, such as BCG or C Parvum, have had little impact on survival rates of melanoma patients overall, but there are probably some subgroups of patients where this form of immunotherapy may be slightly better than surgical treatment alone. New approaches, such as monoclonal antibodies, modulation of immune regulatory cells (helper and suppressor cells), and melanoma-specific immunotherapeutic agents, will no doubt lead to more sophisticated attempts at immune manipulation in the future.

PROGNOSTIC FACTORS AND RESULTS

A prognostic factors analysis of melanoma patients provides useful information for evaluating results of surgical treatment and for clinical research trials involving adjuvant systemic therapy, such as chemotherapy or immunotherapy. When evaluating these treatments, it is important to identify those predictive factors that can accurately separate patients into different groups for metastatic disease. Otherwise, differences (or lack of differences) between treatment regimens being compared may not be due to the therapy itself but may only reflect imbalances of prognostic factors. The dominant prognostic variables for each stage of melanoma are shown in Tables 18-2 and 18-3. These factors were identified from a multifactorial (multivariate) analysis of 13 clinical and pathological variables from a combined series of over 2000 melanoma patients treated at the University of Alabama in Birmingham and at the University of Sydney (Australia) over a 25-year period (1955–1980). The survival rates for certain subgroups of these 2000 melanoma patients

are shown in Figure 18-4. They demonstrate that melanoma is a very heterogeneous disease that encompasses an extraordinary diversity of biological behavior, ranging from highly curable to incurable.

TABLE 18-2   PRIMARY PROGNOSTIC FACTORS THAT PREDICT THE CLINICAL COURSE OF MELANOMA PATIENTS

	UNFAVORABLE CATEGORY
Stage I (localized melanoma)	
Tumor thickness	>1.5 mm
Ulceration	present
Sex	male
Location	trunk
Stage II (regional metastases)	
Number of metastatic nodes	>one
Ulceration	present
Sex	male
Stage III (distant metastases)	
Location	visceral
Number	> one

TABLE 18-3   A CLASSIFICATION OF STAGE I MELANOMA BY TUMOR THICKNESS

CATEGORY	RISK OF OCCULT REGIONAL METASTASES	RISK OF OCCULT DISTANT METASTASES
Thin (<0.76 mm)	low	low
Intermediate thickness (0.76 to 3.99 mm)	high	low
Thick (>4 mm)	high	high

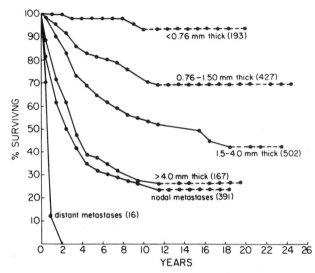

Fig. 18-4. Twenty-five-year survival curves for melanoma patients presenting with different stages of disease. The upper four curves are the results in patients with clinically localized melanomas of varying thickness. The lower two curves are the results in patients presenting with metastatic disease in regional nodes or at distant sites. These 1696 cases represent a combined series of melanoma patients treated at the University of Alabama in Birmingham and the University of Sydney (Australia). The number of patients in each group is shown in parentheses.

BIBLIOGRAPHY

BALCH CM, MURAD TM, SOONG S et al: A multifactorial analysis of melanoma: I. Prognostic histopathological features comparing Clark's and Breslow's staging methods. Ann Surg 188:732, 1978

BALCH CM, MURAD TM, SOONG S et al: Tumor thickness as a guide to surgical management of clinical Stage I melanoma patients. Cancer 43:883, 1979

BALCH CM, SOONG S, MILTON GW et al: Changing trends in cutaneous melanoma over a quarter century in Alabama, USA, and New South Wales, Australia. Cancer (in press)

BALCH CM, SOONG S, MILTON GW et al: A comparison of prognostic factors and surgical results in 1,786 patients with localized (Stage I) melanoma treated in Alabama, USA, and New South Wales, Australia. Ann Surg (in press)

BALCH CM, SOONG SJ, MURAD TM et al: A multifactorial analysis of melanoma. II. Prognostic factors in patients with Stage I (localized) melanoma. Surgery 86:343, 1979

BALCH CM, SOONG SJ, MURAD TM et al: A multifactorial analysis of melanoma. III. Prognostic factors in melanoma patients with lymph node metastases (Stage II). Ann Surg 193:377, 1981

BALCH CM, WILKERSON JA, MURAD TM et al: The prognostic significance of ulceration of cutaneous melanoma. Cancer 45:3012, 1980

BRESLOW A: Prognosis in cutaneous melanoma: Tumor thickness as a guide to treatment. Pathol Annu 15:1, 1980

BRESLOW A, CASCINELLI N, VAN DER ESCH EP et al: Stage I melanoma of the limbs: Assessment of prognosis by levels of invasion and maximum thickness. Tumori 64:373, 1978

BRESLOW A, MACHT SD: Optimal size of resection margin for thin cutaneous melanoma. Surg Gynecol Obstet 145:691, 1977

CLARK W, GOLDMAN L, MASTRANGELO M: Human Malignant Melanoma. New York, Grune & Stratton, 1979

DAS GUPTA TK: Results of treatment of 269 patients with primary cutaneous melanoma: A five-year prospective study. Ann Surg 186:201, 1977

DAY CL JR, MIHM MC JR, SOBER AJ et al: Narrower margins for clinical Stage I malignant melanoma. N Engl J Med 306:479, 1982

DAY CL JR, SOBER AJ, KOPF AW et al: A prognostic model for clinical Stage I melanoma of the upper extremity: The importance of anatomic subsites in predicting recurrent disease. Ann Surg 193:436, 1981

ELDH J, BOERYD B, PETERSON LE: Prognostic factors in cutaneous malignant melanoma in Stage I. Scand J Plast Reconstr Surg 12:243, 1978

ELWOOD JM, LEE JH: Recent data on the epidemiology of malignant melanoma. Semin Oncol 2:149, 1975

EVANS RA, BLAND KI, MCMURTREY MJ et al: Radionuclide scans not indicated for clinical Stage I melanoma. Surg Gynecol Obstet 150:532, 1980

FEE HJ, ROBINSON DS, SAMPLE WF et al: The determination of lymph shed by colloidal gold scanning in patients with malignant melanoma: A preliminary study. Surgery 84:626, 1978

GUILIANO AE, MOSELEY H, MORTON DL: Clinical aspects of unknown primary melanoma. Ann Surg 191:98, 1980

HABERMALZ H, FISCHER J: Radiation therapy of malignant melanoma: Experience with high individual treatment doses. Cancer 38:2258, 1976

HOLMES EC, MOSELEY HS, MORTON DL et al: A rational approach to the surgical management of melanoma. Ann Surg 186:481, 1977

KREMENTZ ET, CARTER RD, SUTHERLAND CM et al: The use of regional chemotherapy in the management of malignant melanoma. World J Surg 3:289, 1979

MCGOVERN VJ: Pigmented cutaneous lesions: The difficult case. Pathol Annu 13:415, 1978

MEYER CM, LECKLITNER ML, LOGIC JR et al: Technetium 99m sulfur-colloid cutaneous lymphoscintigraphy in the management of truncal melanoma. Radiology 131:205, 1979

MEYER JE, STOLBACH L: Pretreatment radiographic evaluation of patients with malignant melanoma. Cancer 42:125, 1978

MIHM MC JR, CLARK WH JR, REED RJ: The clinical diagnosis of malignant melanoma. Semin Oncol 2:105, 1975

MILTON GW: Malignant Melanoma of the Skin and Mucous Membrane. New York, Churchill Livingstone, 1977

MILTON GW, SHAW HM, FARAGO GA et al: Tumour thickness and the site and time of first recurrence in cutaneous malignant melanoma (Stage I). Br J Surg 67:543, 1980

MOSELEY HS, GIULIANO AE, STORM FK et al: Multiple primary melanoma. Cancer 43:939, 1979

SHAW HM, MCGOVERN VJ, MILTON GW et al: Histologic features of tumors and the female superiority in survival from malignant melanoma. Cancer 45:1604, 1980

VERONESI U, ADAMUS J, BANDIERA DC et al: Delayed regional lymph node dissection in Stage I melanoma of the skin of the lower extremities. Cancer 49:2420, 1982

WANEBO HJ, FORTNER JG, WOODRUFF et al: Selection of the optimum surgical treatment of Stage I melanoma by depth of microinvasion: Use of the combined microstage technique (Clark-Breslow). Ann Surg 182:302, 1975

Anatolio B. Cruz, Jr./J. Bradley Aust

Lesions of the Skin and Subcutaneous Tissue

The skin, the largest organ in the human body, has a total surface area of 1 sq m to 2 sq m in adults. It is an integral part of the body organism and not only covers vital structures but also has special independent functions, performing numerous complex physiological functions essential to survival.

The skin is often involved in and affected by a multitude of pathologic processes, most of which are not within the scope of this chapter. We, therefore, have chosen to emphasize pathologic entities of the skin that the surgeon may encounter in the practice of his specialty.

ANATOMY AND HISTOLOGY OF THE SKIN

The skin is a complex, elastic fibrostructure that encases all the living tissues and organs of the human body and maintains a close relationship with the organs that it covers through the connective tissues, blood vessels, nerves, and lymphatics (Fig. 18-5). The skin consists of two layers: the epidermis and the dermis.

EPIDERMIS

The epidermis is composed of cells called keratinocytes (malpighian cells, Langerhans' cells, and melanocytes). Each group of cells maintains its own integrity and is not connected by any structures; the groups are simply in contact with one another.

The epidermis is the outermost layer of the skin and is composed of stratified squamous epithelium. The epidermis may be divided into layers. Starting from the outermost layer, the stratum corneum or horny layer is thickest in the palmar and plantar areas and is composed of dead epithelial cells that have become horny or keratinized. This is the

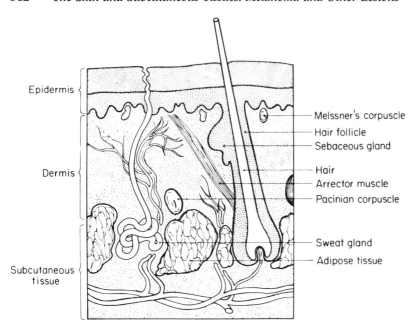

Epidermis {
Dermis {
Subcutaneous tissue {

— Melssner's corpuscle
— Hair follicle
— Sebaceous gland
— Hair
— Arrector muscle
— Pacinian corpuscle

— Sweat gland
— Adipose tissue

Fig. 18-5.   Cross section of skin.

material that is desquamated. These cells are flattened, are dry, and have no nucleus, and the cellular outlines are lost and have been replaced by keratin.

The stratum lucidum is only seen in the thicker skins of the palms and the soles. The stratum granulosum, the stratum malpighii (or prickle cell), and the stratum germinativum (or basal cell) comprise the remaining layers of the epidermis. The basal-cell layer consists of three types of cells—the basal cell (keratinocytes), the Langerhans' cell, and the melanocytes—and gives origin to all the other layers, progressing in the opposite direction. Melanocytes are derived from the neural crest and migrate during early embryonic life to the stratum germinativum. Pigments are transferred from the melanocytes to the keratinocytes. Langerhans' cells resemble melanocytes and are found in the upper layers of the malpighian layer. They do not, however, stain for melanin with dopa, and their functions are not known.

DERMIS

The dermis, also known as the corium, is a dense fibrous layer immediately beneath the epidermis. It gives tensile strength and elasticity to the skin. The dermis contains the blood vessels, lymph vessels, nerve endings (for touch and sensation), hair follicles, muscle elements, and extension of fatty tissue. The surface of the dermis, called the papillary layer, is characterized by numerous papillary structures. The deep layer is named the reticular layer. The papillae contain the terminal sensory nerve and capillaries and interdigitate with the overlying epidermis. Papillae vary in height and are arranged parallel to one another.

The connective tissue is composed of two different fibers, collagenous and elastic. The collagenous fibers appear as bundles of wavy white fibrous tissue and are held together by a semifluid material called the ground substance, which is produced by fibroblasts. Elastic fibers are arranged either parallel or obliquely to the collagenous fibers and, in addition, are intertwined among them. These fibers are abundant in the head and neck areas.

EPIDERMAL APPENDAGES

Epidermal appendages include hair, nails, eccrine and apocrine sweat glands, and sebaceous glands. Associated with the hair are small, nonstriated muscles called arrectores pilorum, which are attached obliquely to the hair follicles. Contraction of these muscles causes hair erection.

ECCRINE SWEAT GLANDS

In humans, eccrine glands are numerous, and distribution is heaviest in the face, neck, palms, and soles. The main function of the eccrine sweat gland is to assist in the regulation of body temperature through the evaporation of the water produced. Eccrine sweat glands are long tubules with the lower end coiled spherically in the reticular layer, where the secretory portion of the glands is located. The upper end is the duct, and the walls of the coil are formed by a single layer of two types of cells, the dark cells containing mucopolysaccharides, and the clear cells containing a small amount of the same substance, plus glycogen, the latter disappearing when sweat is produced. The sweat glands are innervated by sympathetic nerve fibers that are cholinergic.

APOCRINE GLANDS

The large coiled apocrine glands are closely associated with the hair follicles into which they empty. They are located mainly in the axilla, groin, genitalia, and perianal areas. The ceruminous glands in the external auditory canal and Moll's glands in the eyelids are modified apocrine glands. These glands secrete a milky fluid that is odorless unless infected. It may be light or dark and is stimulated by rubbing, by emotional stimuli, and by certain pharmacologic agents. The apocrine glands are innervated by adrenergic nerve fibers.

SEBACEOUS GLANDS

The sebaceous glands are small saccular glands that are frequently branched and are present in every part of the body except the palms and the soles. The ducts open into the hair follicles and directly out of the skin from the glabrous surfaces bordering the lips, labia minora, and prepuce. These glands are classified as holocrines because their secretions are produced by decomposition of cells of the inner layer that mix in the lumen of the duct with degenerated cells and other debris, producing an oily substance called sebum, which prevents dryness of hair and skin.

BASIC PHYSIOLOGICAL FUNCTIONS OF THE SKIN

TEMPERATURE REGULATION

The skin provides a major function in body thermal regulation by producing sweat, which in turn is cooled by evaporation. Sweating is brought about by muscular exercise, heat, and reaction to emotional stimuli. Furthermore, the circulatory system, particularly the arteriovenous shunts, is involved in the regulatory mechanism of the body temperature.

PROTECTIVE COVERING

Not only does the skin serve to contain the proteins, fluids, electrolytes, lipids, and so forth to prevent their loss, but the skin also serves as a protective covering in that it prevents the entry of pathogenic organisms into the body. In addition, this is where the nerve endings are located for sensation, pain, touch, and temperature, all of which are important in activities for daily living and survival. Percutaneous absorption or permeability also allows the passage of certain substances from the outside into the body.

Some of the substances that pass through the skin with some ease are lipid-soluble substances (*e.g.*, steroids and other hormones) and also toxic substances such as arsenicals. The skin is also permeable to certain vitamins. Another of the skin's important functions is the production of a greasy mixture of sebum, sweat, and exfoliated epidermal cells that forms a surface film over the total area of the skin. This film contains urea, uric acid, amino acids, ammonia, triglycerides, free fatty acids, wax, alcohols, sterols, phospholipids, and many other substances. These complex materials and the *p*H also serve as defense mechanisms against infection, provide lubrication to help maintain the physical integrity of the skin, and promote proper hydration of the corneum.

MICROBIOLOGY OF THE SKIN

Bacteria commonly found on the skin reside mainly in the keratin layer in the opening of the hair follicles and the sweat glands. Although the skin is considered to be one single continuous organ, the type of bacterial population varies from one anatomical area to another. For example, the skin in the perianal and genital areas largely reflects the organisms found in the lower gastrointestinal tract. By and large, the most common organisms found on the skin are staphylococci, streptococci (both viridans and *Streptococcus faecalis*), and some mycobacteria. In addition, *Neisseria*, corynebacteria, clostridia, enteric bacilli, bacteroides, spirochetes, and mycoplasms are found elsewhere in the body, particularly in the perianal area. It is the action of some of these organisms, particularly gram-positive organisms acting

on the secretions of the different sweat glands, to produce the typical body odor.

The natural *p*H of the skin tends to control and retard the growth of many bacteria. Despite vigorous mechanical cleansing and the use of bactericidal agents, the skin cannot be completely sterilized; however, the number of bacteria can be drastically reduced, as in preoperative preparation allowing surgical procedures to be done with minimum chances of postoperative infection. However, in burns and traumatic amputation, the skin is naturally grossly contaminated with its bacterial flora, and the presence of devitalized tissue invites and fosters sepsis.

VIRAL LESIONS

VERRUCA VULGARIS

Verruca vulgaris is the most common viral lesion observed in the skin and may appear in any part of the body and in varying forms. It usually occurs on the hand, initially as a shiny, translucent, pinhead-sized, discrete hyperkeratosis and progressing later to a circumscribed tumor, elevated, with a rough surface. When found in the plantar surface of the foot, where it may cause substantial pain to the patient if located in an area where there is much pressure, the lesion is referred to as a plantar wart. When the keratotic surface is shaved off, a soft and pulpy core surrounded by a firm horny ring is revealed. The plantar wart is treated with simple excision or curettage.

VERRUCA PLANA

Verruca plana is a flat wart, usually multiple and numerous, commonly found on the face, neck, and dorsum of the hand. More specifically, verruca plana warts are most commonly located on the forehead, nose, cheeks, and around the mouth. Treatment usually consists in electrodesiccation, freezing, surgical excision, or chemotherapy using 25% glutaraldehyde. There is a high incidence of recurrence in verruca plana with formation of daughter warts, but in many cases these lesions spontaneously regress.

CONDYLOMA ACUMINATUM

Sometimes called a venereal wart, condyloma acuminatum is principally found around the perianal–vulval area and the glans penis. It frequently starts as a small, pointed projection, which multiplies, forming large vegetating clusters. These lesions are characterized by hyperkeratosis, acanthosis, and papillomatosis. Treatment of a few scattered lesions consists in local application of 25% podophyllin or surgical excision with electrocautery of the base. When the lesions are extensive and confluent, often involving the anal canal, substantial surgical excision may be required. The rate of recurrence is fairly high, and it is not unusual for the patient to undergo repeated treatments. In those lesions with florid acanthosis, differentiation from squamous cell carcinoma may be somewhat difficult.

MOLLUSCUM CONTAGIOSUM

Molluscum contagiosum begins as a single or multiple, rounded, dome-shaped, pink, waxy papule, 2 mm to 5 mm in diameter, with a slight central depression that is umbilicated with a central core containing keratinous material. The lesions extend into the dermis, where they are sharply delineated by a connective-tissue capsule, and consist of a mass of proliferating epidermis. Within the mass are cells whose cytoplasm is filled with eosinophilic inclusion particles, the so-called molluscum bodies, from which the responsible virus has been isolated. Rupture of the molluscum papule into the dermis may cause an intense inflammatory dermal reaction. Treatment is either with curettage, electrodesiccation, topical cantharidin, a strong iodine solution, or adequate local excision.

BACTERIAL INFECTIONS

TUBERCULOSIS

Cutaneous tuberculosis is relatively uncommon in the United States; however, it is encountered in several forms depending on whether or not the patient has had prior exposure and depending on the adequacy of host response. Primary cutaneous tuberculosis usually occurs in areas of minor trauma, and, if host response is adequate, a cutaneous Ghon complex is formed within approximately 6 weeks. If host resistance is poor, hematogenous miliary spread may occur. The four cutaneous manifestations of tuberculosis are as follows:

Lupus vulgaris. This lesion is characterized by reddish brown patches of nodules that coalesce to form plaques that show a tendency to heal in one area as progression occurs in a different site. It also has a tendency to form ulcerations that, upon healing, leave deforming scars. Lupus vulgaris is frequently seen on the face and other exposed parts of the body. It follows an indolent, slow-growing, and protracted course. Tubercle bacilli may be difficult to demonstrate, and culture is necessary for its identification.

Tuberculosis verrucosa cutis. This lesion presents as a verrucous nodule with or without suppuration. The nodule may be described as a hyperkeratotic, dull-red lesion that demonstrates very little growth. It is found in such people as prosectors and meat handlers, in whom infected material may be mechanically introduced into the skin. It is frequently located in the dorsum of the fingers, hands, ankles, and buttocks.

Scrofuloderma. This is a cutaneous tubercular lesion manifesting a direct invasion to the skin through lymphatic channels or areas adjacent to progressive diseases of bone or lymph nodes. Clinically, the lesions have a reddish granulation with edema and exudation, crusting, small sinuses, or ulceration with undermined edges.

Tuberculosis cutis orificialis. This form of tuberculosis is also known as tuberculosis ulcerosa and is frequently found at the mucocutaneous borders of the mouth, nose, anus, and genitalia and on the mucous membranes of the mouth and the skin immediately surrounding the orifices. This lesion is usually found in very sick patients with extensive visceral tuberculosis in whom host resistance is so poor that the oral or mucocutaneous areas are seeded with organisms from the pulmonary or gastrointestinal tracts.

Treatment is chemotherapy, namely, isoniazid, streptomycin, para-aminosalicylic acid (PAS), and ethambutol. Surgical excision may be employed for very small tuberculosis verrucosa cutis lesions. Systemically ill patients require adequate supportive care; complete bed rest is mandatory.

LEPROSY

Leprosy is an extremely uncommon disease in the United States; however, it has been reported that there are over 1000 known and registered cases of leprosy within the continental United States. In general, there are three clinical forms of this disease: tuberculoid leprosy, borderline leprosy (with two subsidiary forms on either side of this manifestation), and lepromatous leprosy, these forms being in the order of decreasing resistance or immunocompetence of the patient.

The typical tuberculoid leprosy lesion is a large erythematous plaque with sharp outer margins fading centrally to a flattened clear zone that is rough, anhidrotic, hairless, hypopigmented, and anesthetic. In this lesion, the bacilli are difficult to find and may be limited to no more than one or two nerves in the related skin areas. The only way to differentiate the noncontagious granulomatous reaction from sarcoidosis is to find neural involvement.

Borderline leprosy patients present with smaller, more numerous, and less sharply marginated skin lesions. Low-grade bacteremia may be present; granulomas are present in the lymph nodes, liver, and testicles.

In lepromatous leprosy, the lepra cells, filled with acid-fast bacilli, are plentiful. The early lesions are multiple erythematous, ill-defined macules and papules, which progress to loss of normal anatomical structures, resulting in significant deformities. The lepromin skin test or Mitsuda antigen is an immunologic test indicative of host resistance to *Mycobacterium leprae;* it is not a diagnostic test, but it is useful in estimating the patient's resistance to the disease and his immune status (*i.e.,* in the patient known to have leprosy, a positive lepromin skin test is diagnostic of tuberculoid leprosy and a negative skin test indicates the poor prognosis of lepromatous leprosy if the patient is not treated). Treatment of leprosy mainly involves chemotherapy employing dapsone, long-acting sulfonamides, clofazimine, rifampicin, and ethionamide. The surgical treatment is usually reconstructive, to correct deformities and improve function. This is followed by rehabilitation, which may include the use of appliances to augment the functions of disabled extremities.

CLOSTRIDIAL INFECTION

Clostridial infection is caused by members of the anaerobic clostridia organisms, most commonly *Clostridium welchii.* These are spore-forming gram-positive bacilli that are found in abundance in the environment. The infection usually follows a penetrating wound, dirty laceration, or open fracture. Subcutaneous crepitation may develop, and x-ray films of the extremities usually demonstrate gas bubbles in the tissue. The process usually spreads rapidly, and necrosis of soft tissue, fascia, and skin may occur. There is a gray to reddish brown discharge from the wound, and the patient may complain about pain in the areas immediately surrounding the wound (Fig. 18-6).

Treatment consists in immediate, thorough, and aggressive débridement of the wounds, generous incisions, and elevation of flaps. Massive doses of antibiotics (usually penicillin, 1 million to 4 million units, intravenously every 4 hours) and adjuvant hyperbaric oxygen therapy may be

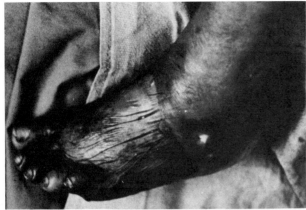

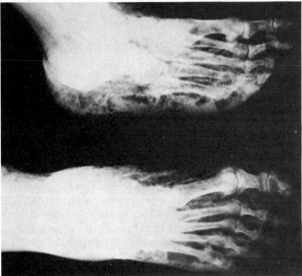

Fig. 18-6. (*Top*) Gas gangrene involves the left foot; extensive bullae have become confluent and are surrounded by an area of cellulitis. Note the advancing line of bulla formation on the anterior aspect of the ankle joint. (*Bottom*) Roentgenograms of the same foot clearly demonstrate gas formation in both the superficial and the deep tissues. This is a useful adjunct in demonstrating and delineating the areas of involvement in gas gangrene.

employed. In mixed infection, combination appropriate antibiotic therapy should be administered and the patient should also receive tetanus toxoid and tetanus immune human globulin. Vigorous supportive therapy in the form of intravenous fluids, electrolytes, and colloids is imperative.

NECROTIZING FASCIITIS

Necrotizing fasciitis is a serious fulminating surgical infection usually caused by group A β-hemolytic streptococci alone or in combination with staphylococci, the latter sometimes being the predominant organism. Occasionally, gram-negative organisms such as *Pseudomonas aeruginosa* and *Escherichia coli* have also been reported. In most cases, the initiating injury is minor and may not even have been detected by the patient. Predisposing factors are those conditions or diseases that cause debility and reduce host resistance to infection, such as diabetes, cancer, and chemotherapy. However, normal, healthy people are by no means immune to this devastating infection. Infection may follow standard surgical procedures such as appendectomy, gas-

trectomy, or cholecystectomy. The essential feature of this necrotizing fasciitis is a fulminating streptococcal or staphylococcal infection of the superficial and deep fasciae and subcutaneous tissue. This results in thrombosis of the subcutaneous vessels, with subsequent gangrene of the overlying skin.

Systemic manifestations are prominent in the forms of extreme prostration, toxicity, and disorientation. Both pulse rate and temperature are usually elevated. In the early stages, the affected area becomes swollen, red, painful, and warm, and the process can be observed spreading in all directions with alarming speed. Approximately 36 hours after the onset, dusty blue gray patches become manifest, with bullae that initially contain a reddish fluid, progressing later to black. Eventually, as the process progresses, the underlying skin becomes necrotic, extensively undermining the skin and subcutaneous tissue down to the deep fascia.

Treatment is immediate and adequate surgical débridement of involved skin and underlying tissue. Existing undermining of skin may require generous separate counterincisions to facilitate drainage. Local wound care consists in diligent, mechanical cleansing and the application of loose packs or gauze soaked with various topical agents (*e.g.*, Dakin's solution, zinc oxide, zinc peroxide, hydrogen peroxide, povidone–iodine, and normal saline solutions). Penicillin, given systemically in massive doses, is the antibiotic of choice. This may be combined with other appropriate antibiotics when a mixed infection exists. General supportive management to correct extracellular fluid volume deficiencies, including electrolyte imbalance, is of utmost importance. In addition, because of severe hemolysis, multiple blood transfusions become necessary.

SYNERGISTIC BACTERIAL GANGRENE

Synergistic bacterial gangrene is caused by a combination of microaerophilic nonhemolytic streptococcus and aerobic hemolytic *Staphylococcus aureus*. Other organisms, such as *Escherichia coli* and many of the *proteus* species, have also been found in combination with streptococcus. Infection may begin in a manner indistinguishable from usual postoperative infections, including puncture wounds from unsterile hypodermic injection. After about a week, however, the gross characteristics of synergistic bacterial gangrene become evident. Skin edges separate and are surrounded by a zone of erythema; with progression, the edges become purplish, raised, and undermined and surround an area of necrotic granulation tissue. The purplish areas become gangrenous in a few days, and the skin changes to a dirty, grayish brown with a dull-appearing surface similar to suede. The process, which may last for weeks or months unless intensive and definitive therapy is instituted early, spreads rapidly in all directions. Intense pain, together with the rapidly advancing gangrenous process, results in severe deterioration of the patient's general condition.

Treatment is adequate and wide débridement and the use of appropriate antibiotics. Adjuvant hyperbaric oxygen therapy may be considered in some of the more refractory cases.

HIDRADENITIS SUPPURATIVA

Hidradenitis suppurativa is an infection of the apocrine gland and its surrounding tissue usually caused by staphylococci or streptococci. The characteristic clinical course is one of chronicity and recurrent acute exacerbations, with the formation of sinuses and fistulas. Since most of the apocrine glands in the body are concentrated in the axilla, perineum, and perianal areas, these areas are most frequently involved in hidradenitis suppurativa (Fig. 18-7). With increasing chronicity, severe scar formation and deformity can result.

Treatment of the acute exacerbation of the disease is usually conservative and consists in draining the abscess, applying local heat, and administering antibiotics as indicated. We have emphasized an early and aggressive definitive therapy in the form of wide local excision with primary closure or skin grafts, or wide excision followed with advancement or rotation of skin flaps once the acute inflammatory process has subsided.

FURUNCULOSIS

A furuncle or boil is an acute, painful, round, localized reddish swelling; it is initially firm, eventually becomes fluctuant, and ends in suppuration. The lesion, which begins as an infection around a hair follicle, is usually caused by *Staphylococcus aureus.* Multiple lesions often develop and may continue on to chronicity. The most commonly affected areas are the axillae, back of the neck, and buttocks, but furunculosis can occur anywhere in the body. Predisposing factors are poor hygiene, irritation by scratching, and friction (particularly in persons with compromised immune systems, such as malnourished persons, alcoholics, diabetics, and others with medical conditions that would tend to lower resistance).

Fig. 18-7. Hidradenitis suppurativa of the right axilla. The skin of the entire axilla was excised and replaced immediately with split grafts. This cured the disease without cicatrix. (A.G., 52-4228)

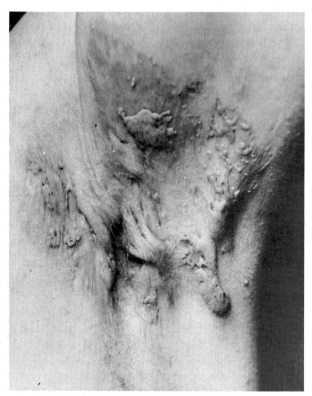

CARBUNCULOSIS

A carbuncle is a lesion composed of a number of furuncles in a localized area. The abscesses initially appear as multiple points, which progress to suppuration; therefore, the area involved may have multiple draining sinuses. Significant tissue loss occurs with resulting shallow and deep ulcer formation. The etiologic factor again is *Staphylococcus aureus.* Carbuncles are common in diabetics and in patients with other conditions that compromise the resistance.

Carbunculosis is treated with aggressive surgical débridement, employing grid and cruciate incisions and removing all necrotic tissue. Local wound care is important; there should be frequent changes of packing in combination with topical antibiotics, Dakin's solution, or povidone–iodine solution. Appropriate systemic antibiotics are given in most cases, and correction of the predisposing factors should be undertaken (*e.g.,* control of diabetes mellitus, improved nutrition, and alleviation of other debilitating conditions).

FUNGAL INFECTIONS

PHYCOMYCOSIS

Phycomycosis (mucormycosis) is an infection produced by fungi belonging to the order Phycomycetes. Although these fungi are found extensively in nature and are generally saprophytes, they are opportunistic and become pathogenic. This is particularly true in persons debilitated from conditions such as poorly controlled diabetes mellitus, leukemia, malignancies, burns, aggressive chemotherapy, or immunosuppressive therapy, all of which result in decreased host resistance. The lesions produced are similar to those of necrotizing fasciitis. Biopsy of the lesion usually reveals the typical nonseptate branching hyphae amidst necrotic tissue.

Treatment consists in early and adequate débridement, combined with aggressive supportive therapy and control or amelioration of the underlying primary disease responsible for the lowered host resistance. Chemotherapy in the form of amphotericin B, despite its toxicity, is the treatment of choice.

CHROMOMYCOSIS

Chromomycosis is a chronic indolent cutaneous disease caused by two genera of dematiacious fungi. Four species of *Phialophora* and *Cladosporium carrioni* are usually the etiologic agents, but a few aberrant and closely related species have been reported. Infection of the skin with *Cladosporium trichoides* has been noted on occasion; however, most of the lesions are in the form of brain abscesses. The cutaneous manifestation is usually misdiagnosed clinically as carcinoma, but on histologic examination, the typical brown fungus spores are found and their color and crosswall usually establish the diagnosis.

Treatment is systemic administration of amphotericin B or 5-fluorocytosine, the latter being preferred because of its lack of systemic toxicity and its proved effectiveness both *in vivo* and *in vitro.*

NORTH AMERICAN BLASTOMYCOSIS

Cutaneous involvement in blastomycosis is usually secondary to pneumonic blastomycosis. The etiologic agent is

Blastomyces dermatitidis, and the skin lesions are in the form of multiple enlarging verrucous plaques with numerous microabscesses (Fig. 18-8). The skin lesion has been grossly mistaken for epidermoid carcinoma. Diagnosis is easily established by demonstration of the organisms in giant cells on biopsy; smears and cultures should also confirm the diagnosis. Treatment is chemotherapy, preferably employing dihydroxystilbamidine and amphotericin B.

CYSTS

EPIDERMOID CYST

Epidermoid inclusion cysts develop when elements of the epithelium become entrapped subcutaneously as a result of traumatic inoculations. These cysts are lined by epithelium that cornifies similarly to interfollicular epidermis in the upper third of the external root sheath. These lesions are often located in the upper extremity, particularly in the hand. Treatment is complete surgical excision.

SEBACEOUS CYST

Sebaceous cysts result from duct obstruction of the sebaceous glands located in the hair follicles. The benign cyst is regarded by some as a form of epidermoid inclusion cyst that includes the hair follicle. It is considered a myth as opposed to being a distinct entity. Treatment is complete surgical excision, which should result in complete cure. Often, however, the cyst becomes infected and has to be incised and drained much like an ordinary abscess. For permanent cure, surgical

Fig. 18-8. Blastomycosis of the skin, with central healing and scarring.

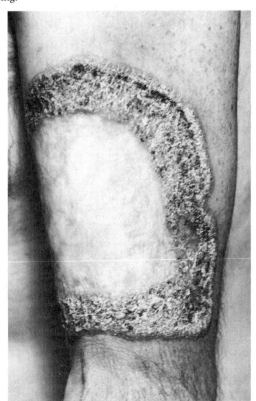

excision should be carried out when the inflammatory reaction has subsided completely.

DERMOID CYST

Dermoid cysts are congenital keratinous cysts generally found along the lines of embryonic closure, particularly on the face, scalp, occiput, and sacral areas. The cyst is soft and is not usually fixed to the skin. It contains various epidermal structures (*i.e.,* hair, sebum, and a lining of stratified squamous epithelium). Treatment is surgical excision. Care must be taken in the treatment of this lesion, particularly if it is located in the head, where it may have an intracranial communication or extension. Appropriate preoperative workup is indicated. The operative procedure should be done under general anesthesia, with adequate provisions for the surgeon to have full control of any problems that may be encountered during the dissection.

PILONIDAL CYST AND SINUS

Pilonidal cysts are considered inclusion cysts of the body, and sinuses appear as small openings commonly found in the intergluteal fold of the so-called natal cleft in the sacrococcygeal area, about 3 cm to 5 cm posterior and superior to the anal orifice. Hair is found in approximately 25% to 40% of the cases. It is thought that the majority of cases result from hairs penetrating root-end first into the dermis and eliciting a foreign-body reaction, but some have maintained that this condition is congenital in origin and have presented evidence by demonstrating epithelium-lined spaces in skin and subcutaneous specimens excised randomly from intergluteal folds of infants and children at autopsy. A high incidence of pilonidal cysts and sinuses is found in siblings (5.7%–13%), which favors, at least in part, the congenital cyst theory.

Pilonidal cysts and sinuses have been described in other areas, such as the umbilicus, axilla, and female genital organs, where the skin folds are prominent. This supports the theory of acquired origin in the pathogenesis of these lesions. Furthermore, there have been numerous reports that barbers develop lesions in their hands, particularly in the interdigital folds, that are similar or indistinguishable from pilonidal sinuses occurring elsewhere.

For acutely inflamed lesions, particularly those that have obvious abscess formation, conservative treatment consisting of incision and drainage of abscess and application of local heat is recommended until the acute inflammatory process has resolved. In quiescent, noninflamed cases, the treatment of choice is that of adequate surgical excision, including margins of normal skin and subcutaneous tissue down to the presacral fascia. Primary closure has been used by many with excellent results comparable to those obtained with primary excision and leaving the wound open to granulate and heal by secondary intention or suturing the edges of the skin to the presacral fascia, leaving only a narrow strip of open wound. The advantage of primary closure is a shorter convalescent time. A large, gaping wound allowed to heal by granulation and secondary intention obviously takes a longer time to heal, although this technique is perfectly acceptable, especially for cases that present some doubt in regard to contamination and infection.

It is recommended that the elliptical incision be oriented along an oblique axis about 45° in relation to the vertical axis of the body so that when primary closure is effected it eliminates the anal cleft. This reduces the propensity of that area for recurrence resulting from repeated reimplantation of hair into the dermis in clefts or skin folds. Being so oriented, the closure is subjected to less lateral tension and will not tend to gape. A Z-plasty closure technique may also be used to advantage.

The incidence of recurrence has been reported to be 5% to 25%, and this may be a reflection of an incomplete excision of the primary lesion or a lesion *de novo,* resulting from reimplantation of hair, particularly in a situation in which the natal cleft has not been obliterated.

KERATOSES

ACTINIC KERATOSIS

Actinic or solar keratosis occurs in that portion of the epidermis exposed to excessive sunlight. It is seen often in older persons with fair skin who have been farmers, sailors, or ranchers—those who are typically exposed to excessive sunlight. The epidermis develops atrophic atypical dysplastic and hyperplastic changes usually involving the interfollicular epidermis, with the stratum corneum being replaced by a parakeratotic scale. Accumulation of this scale leads to the formation of cutaneous horns. This lesion is considered precancerous and should be treated as such.

Treatment consisting of excision, freezing, or curettage has been successful, and more recently, antineoplastic agents such as 5% to 10% 5-fluorouracil cream have been used with great success. As a preventive measure, it is important that a person predisposed to develop this lesion be advised to protect the skin against excessive exposure to sunlight.

SEBORRHEIC KERATOSIS

Seborrheic keratosis is a wartlike lesion that appears in middle-aged people and usually occurs on the trunk and face. It varies from gray brown to black and has a somewhat greasy surface. Sometimes the lesion may be so markedly pigmented that it is mistaken for melanoma and subsequently excised.

In treating solitary seborrheic keratosis, currettage or simple surgical excision is adequate. Any sign such as an increase in size, bleeding, irritation, or itching should be taken as indication for excision.

KERATOACANTHOMA

Keratoacanthoma is a lesion that arises from the wall of the upper portion of the hair follicle. It is often confused with epidermoid carcinoma; however, there are some distinctive characteristics that differentiate keratoacanthoma from squamous cell carcinoma: It has been observed to arise in previously undiseased skin with no antecedent actinic keratosis, it has a rapid growth of 2 to 6 weeks followed by a stationary period of another 2 to 6 weeks, and it undergoes spontaneous regression over a period of several weeks, leaving a slightly depressed scar (Fig. 18-9).

It may be impossible for biopsies to distinguish this lesion from a well-differentiated epidermoid carcinoma, or vice versa. A feature favoring the diagnosis of epidermoid carcinoma is the presence of a desmoplastic tumor stroma.

This is not, however, encountered in all cases of squamous cell carcinoma. Histologically, a cross section featuring craters, a flasklike configuration, a red color, cytoplasmic eosinophilia, mild atypia, and less than three typical and one atypical mitoses per high-power field should support a diagnosis of keratoacanthoma.

Treatment is total excision for definitive diagnosis and cure. Fulguration has also been employed with good results, and x-ray therapy has been used for giant keratoacanthomas when surgical incision or electrosurgical methods were not feasible.

BENIGN PIGMENTED LESIONS

JUNCTIONAL NEVUS

Junctional nevus is a light to dark brown or black pigmented lesion varying in size from a few millimeters to several centimeters. It has a flat, smooth, and hairless surface with an irregular edge, and the proliferation of melanoblast originates in the basal layer of the epidermis and extends down into the dermis. These lesions are found most often on the upper and lower extremities, particularly the soles, palms, nail beds, mucous membranes, and, occasionally, genitalia. This lesion may evolve into melanoma.

Fig. 18-9. Multiple keratoacanthoma of the skin. These lesions may be mistaken for epidermoid carcinoma, clinically and microscopically.

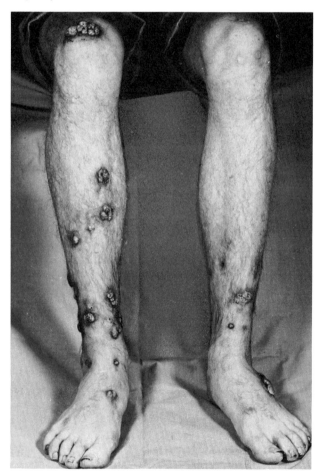

COMPOUND NEVUS

Compound nevus is composed of junctional and intradermal components. The surface is often elevated and nodular and may have a macular ring around the periphery. Hairs may be present, and this type of nevus may also develop into melanoma.

INTRADERMAL NEVUS

Intradermal nevus is usually less than 1 cm and may be warty, flat, sessile, or pedunculated with an irregular edge. The nevus cells are predominantly or entirely within the dermis and may have few junctional components.

GIANT PIGMENTED NEVUS

The giant pigmented nevus is histologically similar to the intradermal nevus and involves large areas of the body. Often it is called the bathing trunk nevus. This type of nevus has predominantly dermal components, but junctional elements have also been observed. The problem is not only cosmetic, because melanoma develops in 10% to 17% of patients.

Treatment is total excision, preferably in stages if the lesion is large. Plastic reconstructive procedures of skin grafting and flap rotation should be employed.

BLUE NEVUS

The blue nevus is intensely blue or blue black and is small, usually 1 cm or less. The edge is sharp and well defined, and melanocytes with heavy pigmentation are situated in the dermis. Some reports indicate that the blue nevus may cause pigmentation of the draining lymph nodes, but this in no way constitutes malignancy.

JUVENILE MELANOMA

Juvenile melanoma is a pigmented lesion quite indistinguishable from melanoma found in adults. This lesion is encountered in prepubertal children and is considered benign. Wide local excision usually results in cure.

HUTCHINSON'S MELANOTIC FRECKLE

Hutchinson's melanotic freckle is a pigmented lesion usually presenting as a brown macule on the face of middle-aged persons. Although its growth is normally slow, it can be unpredictable. Color is uneven, ranging from brown to black with interspersed pale areas. The surface has been described as being plaquelike to modular. There is proliferation of atypical melanocytes in the junctional zone. Over 50% of these lesions develop into melanoma.

Treatment of Hutchinson's freckle is surgical excision. In regard to other pigmented lesions, any change in size, color, or pigment distribution, bleeding, itching, crusting or ulceration, and development of satellite or daughter nodules should be clear indications for excision biopsies to rule out melanoma.

BENIGN TUMORS

KELOID

Keloid is a benign tumor composed of dense fibrous tissue of the skin that develops following injury. It may be in the form of surgical incision, lacerations, burns, vaccinations, or other trauma that results in a break of the skin. The tumor not only extends above the surface of the skin but, by lateral contiguity, may involve the surrounding areas. The usual areas of predilection are the head and neck and the deltoid and presternal areas; nonetheless, it may occur anywhere in the body.

The black race and other dark-skinned people, even black-haired whites, have a greater propensity for keloid formation. The appearance of the lesion ranges from a raised, flat, thickened area in the skin to a pedunculated and multilobed structure. There is a strong tendency for these people to have a recurrence of keloids following surgical excision.

Cryotherapy for small lesions has been used with success, although this technique has also been applied, in stages, to lesions larger than 5 cm, treating only a small portion of the lesion each time. For keloids that are approximately 4 to 6 months old, x-ray treatments have been beneficial, particularly when combined with surgical excision, in which case a dose is also given postoperatively to the area. Intralesional injection of triamcinolone suspension mixed with 2% lidocaine, using a small 26-gauge needle, into various portions of the lesion has also produced some excellent results.

When the keloid covers an extensive area, wide excision well into the area of normal tissue should be made, preferably under local anesthesia mixed with equal parts of triamcinolone suspension. After the excision, intralesional injection should be repeated at weekly intervals and adjuvant x-ray therapy should be considered. If primary reapproximation of wound edges cannot be attained, split-thickness skin grafting should be carried out. Careful and meticulous surgical techniques should be observed. Trauma should be held to a minimum and leaving irritating sutures in the subcutaneous and subcuticular areas should be avoided. In planning operative procedures, particularly in known keloid formers, the incision should be made along the natural anatomical skin creases.

LIPOMA

Lipoma is a benign fatty tumor that can arise in any location of the body where fat is present. It is found most commonly in the upper half of the body, particularly the head and neck, shoulders, and back. It varies in diameter from a few millimeters to many centimeters. Histologically, lipoma is composed of lobules of fat enclosed by a thick, fibrous capsule. The lobules themselves are separated by a thin fibrous stroma that may extend to the corium of the skin, giving rise to the dimpled appearance of overlying skin whenever the area is pinched. The deeper lipomas have a tendency to infiltrate between fascial planes, particularly in the posterior neck, where there is an abundance of fibrous tissue separating fatty lobules.

There is a low incidence of this tumor containing sarcomatous elements in the ratio of approximately 100:1. Although the incidence is low, it would seem appropriate to excise all of what appears clinically to be lipoma, especially a rapidly growing lesion, to rule out liposarcoma. Lipomas may be single or multiple, and it has been observed that patients with neurofibromatosis, multiple endocrine abnormalities, or adenomatosis have an increasing incidence of multiple lipomas.

In treating lipoma, we have observed that the usual way of enucleating the fatty tumor may be impossible in the posterior neck, precipitating incomplete excision and recurrence. In this particular region of the body, sharp *en bloc* dissection should be carried out with an adequate margin of normal tissue to prevent recurrence. Complete surgical excision should result in definitive cure.

LYMPHANGIOMA

Lymphangiomas are congenital benign tumors composed of spaces filled with lymph and separated from one another by thin, fibrous septa with no communications with the rest of the lymphatic vascular network. It is felt that during embryonic development, lymphangiomas were lymphatic buds that became isolated from the rest of the lymphatic vascular system. There are three forms observed clinically: capillary, cavernous, and cystic. The cystic and cavernous lymphangiomas have certain characteristics similar to some of the hemangiomas. These tumors are often found in the areas of the head, neck, axilla, and groin. They start out as small, lymph-filled lymphatic buds but may continue to grow, encroaching on neighboring structures. Cystic hygromas may be a form of the latter stage of cavernous lymphangiomas.

Treatment is complete surgical excision, which usually results in definitive cure.

HEMANGIOMAS

CAPILLARY (PORT-WINE) HEMANGIOMA

Capillary hemangioma is a benign lesion presenting as a reddish or purplish patch in the skin; its growth parallels that of the host child. The histologic picture shows packed, dilated normal capillaries in the dermal and subdermal regions or layers of the skin, and it is found most commonly in the head and neck area and thorax. As it grows, the lesion eventually becomes nodular and soft.

Treatment has been disappointing; the lesion is resistant to x-ray therapy and other modalities of topical treatment. Tattooing with skin-colored pigments has been tried; however, it is not only painful but also gives less than satisfactory results. Wide excision with skin grafting or flap advancement may be carried out, but the results may also be less than satisfactory. Small lesions may be excised with primary closure.

IMMATURE HEMANGIOMA (STRAWBERRY TYPE)

Strawberry hemangioma, usually observed at birth, grows rapidly during the first few months of life. It appears as a dome-shaped lesion that is usually dull red. It is composed of closely packed epithelial cells with very small vascular spaces. It has no cavernous components and can contain, on closer microscopic examination, several mitotic figures. The color is red to crimson, and the lesion may become tense. The surface becomes smooth when the infant cries or strains. As the child grows older, at approximately 1 year of age, the hemangioma becomes flaccid and pale blue and may eventually disappear.

Treatment consists primarily in reassuring parents that the lesion will most probably disappear as the child grows older. Small lesions may be treated with cryotherapy, especially if they are inconspicuously located.

CAVERNOUS HEMANGIOMA

Cavernous hemangioma is usually rounded or flat, bright red or deep purple, and spongy. Consistency varies and is affected by the amount of fibrous connective tissue in the lesion. This lesion, which usually occurs in the head and neck areas (but may be found elsewhere), consists mainly of numerous mature blood vessels, including many arteriovenous communications, and usually involves deeper tissues such as the central nervous system. These large hemangiomas have been reported to undergo thrombosis, ulceration, or infection, in which case prognosis becomes poor. Other abnormalities, thrombocytopenia for example, are sometimes observed.

In rare instances, hemangiomas may be composed mainly of veins or of a combination of arteries and veins, the latter being called cirsoid hemangiomas or aneurysms. In the Klippel-Trenaunay syndrome, there is an association of varicose veins, soft-tissue and bone hypertrophy, and cutaneous hemangioma. Cases of multifocal hemangiomatosis associated with the involvement of internal organs have also been described.

Treatment is wide surgical excision, but sometimes it may be impossible to excise completely the fingerlike projections or sacs. Muscle or silicone-sphere embolization has been employed to treat the large, disfiguring, and unresectable lesion; this has resulted in significant amelioration. Small doses of x-rays expedite the spontaneous involution and are recommended in patients in whom trauma can produce ulceration. Careful shielding is mandatory, and lesions in the thyroid and genital areas should not be treated by this modality.

SWEAT GLAND TUMORS

ECCRINE SWEAT GLAND

There are several histologic types of benign eccrine sweat gland tumors, including poroma, porosyringoma, mixed tumors, cylindroma, spiradenoma, and syringoadenoma, which usually appear as nodules in the skin and occasionally become ulcerated. These lesions are excised usually with clinical impressions of leiomyoma, neuroma, or a glomus tumor. Light microscopy, aided by data provided by histochemical testing techniques and ultrastructural methodology, generally confirms a diagnosis of eccrine sweat gland tumor.

Treatment with electrodesiccation, cryotherapy, or surgical excision has been successful, depending upon the size and number of the lesions.

APOCRINE SWEAT GLAND

Benign apocrine sweat gland tumors are normally found in the areas of the labia and perineum and are mostly papillary hidradenoma. Those apocrine sweat gland tumors found mainly on the face are termed hidrocystoma or cystadenoma. Another group of adenomas derived from the apocrine glands in the external auditory canal is called ceruminoma or ceruminous adenoma, but they do not produce cerumen. Cystadenoma is often misdiagnosed as a basal cell epithelioma or as a nevus, especially when it presents as a bluish, cutaneous lesion. Adequate excision is the definitive treatment.

GLOMUS TUMORS

Glomus tumors are rare, benign, excruciatingly painful small tumors of the skin and subcutaneous tissue. They are usually found in the extremities, particularly in the hands and feet, with the majority of the latter being in the subungual area;

they may also occur in other parts of the body. This tumor is derived from a normal glomus, which is an end-organ apparatus consisting of an arteriovenous anastomosis. It plays a role in the regulation of blood flow in the extremity and is involved indirectly in thermal regulation.

This tumor is usually single but may be multiple on rare occasions and measures an average 0.5 cm to 2 cm. Those located in the terminal phalanges may erode the bone, which is the result of the pulsation of the tumor. The color of the tumor varies from deep red to purple or blue, the latter being more common. With changes in temperature, the color of the tumor changes, becoming bluer with colder temperatures. It is most common in the fifth decade of life but may be found in patients of all ages. This tumor is usually extremely sensitive and produces excruciating and lancinating pain. With minimal stimulation, a series of paroxysms of pain radiates from the area of the tumor to the entire extremity. Attacks of pain may come on spontaneously and may be associated with exposure to cold. The pain of the glomus tumor may be associated with various sympathetic vasomotor disturbances, such as localized sweating or Horner's syndrome. However, nontender glomus tumors are encountered. Treatment involving total excision of the tumor results in complete cure of the condition.

DESMOID TUMORS

Desmoid tumors, composed of firm and fibrous tissue, can be found in various areas of the body, especially in the abdominal wall. A benign tumor may be locally invasive, increasing the likelihood of incomplete excision, which may give rise to recurrence. On occasion, the tumor may grow to such proportions that it may produce marked symptoms secondary to encroachment and pressure on structures such as large nerves. Treatment requires complete and adequate excision; on rare occasions, because of size and anatomical location, more radical surgical procedures, such as amputation or hemipelvectomy, are necessitated.

NEUROFIBROMA

Neurofibroma is a benign tumor of the peripheral nerves that is distinct from schwannomas, including the gross electron microscopic characteristics and its clinical course. Neurofibromas contain all the elements of the peripheral nerve, mainly the neurites, fibroblasts, Schwann cells, and perineural cells. This tumor can be solitary or multiple, the latter being observed in a condition known as neurofibromatosis or von Recklinghausen's disease, and may occur in any part of the body. Neurofibromatosis is associated with lesions of multiple pigmented areas in the skin, called café au lait spots.

Approximately 3% to 15% of patients with neurofibromatosis will develop malignant degeneration. This degeneration is confined to the lesion that arises from large nerve trunks. Neurofibromatosis has also been observed to be associated with medullary carcinoma of the thyroid, pheochromocytoma, mucosal neuromas, and other neoplasms, including cutaneous soft-tissue sarcomas and malignancies of the skin and gastrointestinal tract.

Treatment is surgical excision of the bulkier lesions, particularly those that are symptomatic and those that have undergone a rapid increase in size. Should the lesion become sarcomatous, it should be treated with aggressiveness, employing wide excision and, if necessary, forequarter or hindquarter amputation to achieve control of the primary lesion.

NEURILEMOMA

Neurilemoma is a benign encapsulated tumor of the peripheral nerves that arises from the sheath cells of Schwann and thus is also known by the name of schwannoma. Electron microscopic examination of schwannomas easily reveals the origin and differentiates this entity from neurofibroma, the other benign tumor of peripheral nerves. The most common locations are in the extremities (particularly the flexor surface), mediastinum, posterior spinal roots, head and neck, and cerebellopontine angle. The nerve bundles are observed to be splayed and flattened in the capsule by the tumor mass and are not incorporated in the substance of the tumor. Neurilemoma is treated with complete excision with preservation of the nerve bundles.

MALIGNANT TUMORS

CARCINOMA

CARCINOMA *IN SITU*

Carcinoma *in situ* is characterized by flat, scaly lesions that may be difficult to differentiate grossly from actinic keratosis. The lesion will show full-thickness involvement of the epidermis by dyskeratosis or frankly neoplastic squamous cells. There may also be some surface maturation and keratinization. This form of skin tumor is found in areas that are exposed to actinic radiation. It is also frequently confused with Bowen's disease, which characteristically occurs in nonexposed areas. Treatment begins with biopsy, which is necessary to establish the diagnosis. Surgical excision or application of 5% fluorouracil cream has been found to be effective. Cryosurgery and electrodesiccation likewise have been used with success.

BOWEN'S DISEASE

Bowen's disease presents as scaly, erythematous plaques that occur in areas of the skin that are not normally exposed to sunlight. The histologic picture is difficult to distinguish from that of carcinoma *in situ;* therefore, diagnosis may be impossible on the basis of histologic appearance alone. Diagnosis is often based on its indolent course, distribution, and morphological pattern.

It is reported that Bowen's disease is associated with a high incidence of primary cancer elsewhere, often in the viscera. It behooves the surgeon to search carefully for other possible primary sites of cancer elsewhere in the body when Bowen's disease is diagnosed.

The treatment of choice is adequate surgical excision; however, this may be impractical, especially in patients with multiple lesions. Our experience is that the skin manifestation can be managed adequately with topical application of 5% fluorouracil cream. Fulguration and curettage are also effective.

SQUAMOUS CELL CARCINOMA

Squamous cell carcinoma, or epidermoid carcinoma, occurs frequently in areas of the body exposed to actinic radiation. The type of patient prone to this cutaneous malignancy is the so-called fair-skinned, blue-eyed blonde or those with thin and dry skin and ruddy cheeks who spend most of their time outdoors (*e.g.,* farmers, sailors, ranchers, and fishermen). Men patients predominate over women in a ratio of approximately 3:1. A review of associated literature reveals that there is a higher incidence of squamous cell carcinoma in people living in the southern latitudes of the United States and in other countries that receive substantial sunlight, as in Australia.

Squamous cell carcinoma may develop in areas of the skin that have received ionizing radiation and in areas of draining sinuses, chronic osteomyelitis, ulcers, or old burn scars. The lesion starts as a slightly indurated nodule with central ulceration. The central portion of the lesion gradually becomes a larger ulcer marked by an irregular base often covered by crusts. The margins of the lesion tend to be raised and present a rolled appearance. The spread is progressive both laterally and downward into the deeper tissues. Lymph node metastasis does occur, but it is quite rare, occurring in about 5% of all cases. The majority of this involves the regional lymph nodes.

Wide surgical excision followed by primary closure, skin grafting, or flap rotation or advancement has been the treatment of choice. Regional lymph nodes should be inspected carefully, and node dissection should be carried out if there are suspicious lesions in the nodal areas. All of the margins of the resected specimen should be properly marked for correct orientation so that the pathologist may examine it for adequacy of excision. Radiation therapy is also used in combination with definitive surgical treatment, especially in large lesions. Mohs' chemosurgery has also been used successfully in the treatment of both early and moderately advanced squamous cell carcinoma. We have employed 5% fluorouracil cream effectively in early lesions; in large lesions of the head and neck, we have had considerable success using a combination of intra-arterial or systemic multidrug chemotherapy, simultaneous or sequential x-ray therapy, and definitive surgical procedure.

BASAL CELL CARCINOMA

Basal cell carcinoma is a malignant tumor of the skin that grows slowly and arises from the basal cells of the epidermis and the follicles. It is the most frequent form of skin cancer and occurs in those areas exposed to the sun. It is also related to the number of pilosebaceous units present. As is true in people with squamous cell carcinoma, fair-skinned, blue-eyed people who stay outdoors for long periods have a higher incidence of basal cell carcinoma. The male/female ratio is about 2:1, slightly less than that of squamous cell carcinoma.

Although this is a slow-growing tumor, if neglected it can erode into deeper structures such as cartilage, bone, orbit, and brain and can eventually cause the death of the patient. Distant metastasis is very rare, and only a few reported cases are from a primary basal cell carcinoma of the skin.

The appearance of basal cell carcinoma may vary. It may be nodular, deeply ulcerative, superficial, erythematous, multicentric, sclerosing, or morpheaform, the latter presenting as a wide, flat lesion with a central scarred area; extensions may be serpiginous. Biopsy should always be performed to establish dignosis. In rare cases, the presence of keratinocytic differentiation on histologic examination gives rise to such terminology as basosquamous cell carci-

noma; however, these tumors behave just like basal cell carcinoma.

Curettage, electrodesiccation, and cryosurgery have been used with success, particularly in smaller lesions and by experienced physicians. Chemosurgery using Mohs' technique has also met with considerable success, and a similar treatment using topical chemotherapeutic agents such as 5% fluorouracil cream has been found to be likewise successful, particularly in the superficial ulcerated forms. We strongly favor surgical excision whenever feasible, with primary plastic reconstruction, be it skin grafting, flap advancement, or flap rotation in the larger lesions.

Use of a combination of modalities, such as regional or systemic chemotherapy combined with simultaneous or sequential x-ray therapy and definitive surgical excision where indicated, has met with a high degree of success. Surgical excision must be done with precision, with the lines of resection being marked with ink or methylene blue. The specimen should also be marked with suture materials so that proper orientation is possible, particularly when the tumor is found at the line of resection. In this manner, the surgeon may be able to reexcise the area where he initially cut through the tumor. A high cure rate of 90% or more should be possible.

SWEAT GLAND CARCINOMA

Sweat gland carcinomas are rare tumors. They demonstrate a variable clinical course, often starting as a slow-growing cutaneous nodule. Then they suddenly exhibit a dramatic increase in the rate of growth and widespread metastases.

Before stringent criteria were established for the proper diagnosis of sweat gland carcinoma, the term was loosely applied to different tumors of the skin, many of which were not truly sweat gland in origin. Since the work of Stout and Cooley, Gates and associates, Berg and co-workers, Miller and colleagues, and the authors' own review, it has been possible to cull from the literature cases of true sweat gland carcinoma that satisfy the criteria set forth by these authors.

As an adjunct to the proper diagnosis of sweat gland carcinoma, histochemical methods have been applied. These have proved useful in determining if the tumor is of sweat gland origin and whether or not it is derived from the eccrine or apocrine sweat glands.

Most of these tumors are encountered in the middle-aged group; however, they have been known to occur in adolescents, usually as single lesions. Nevertheless, multiple primary sweat gland carcinomas have been reported.

Because of its potential for aggressive local invasion and distant metastases, the cure rate has been less than satisfactory. In view of its penchant for local recurrence and distant metastasis, primarily to the regional lymph nodes and eventually to distant organs, treatment calls for initial aggressive surgical excision, including regional lymph node dissection. Chemotherapy may be tried for palliation of widespread disease.

ADENOACANTHOMA

Adenoacanthoma (pseudoglandular squamous cell carcinoma) was first described as adenoacanthoma of the sweat glands and then as pseudoglandular carcinoma. It has also been called adenoid squamous cell carcinoma. The tumor is considered an epidermoid carcinoma, which is usually found in sun-exposed areas, face and ears. Initially, this rapidly growing lesion presents a verrucous surface, then follows by ulceration with crusting.

The lesion may resemble a keratoacanthoma and should be differentiated from rodent ulcer; it has very little tendency to metastasize or invade deeper tissue. Adequate surgical excision is the treatment of choice; however, radiation therapy has been used with good results.

MYCOSIS FUNGOIDES

Mycosis fungoides is a malignant skin condition in the form of raised scaly plaques or nodules, microscopically similar to lymphoma. Its clinical course is protracted. It tends to be multicentric and may present as bright red or brown. The lesion has been classified into three stages: premycotic, mycotic, and tumorous. The terminal picture of mycosis fungoides is associated with the development of distant foci of malignant lymphoma in about 30% of the patients. This occurs equally in both sexes and in adults between the ages of 30 and 70.

Mycosis fungoides is sensitive to radiation therapy, particularly the electron beam, because of the superficial nature of the cutaneous lesion. Topical nitrogen mustard and combination systemic chemotherapy of cyclophosphamide, methotrexate, vincristine, prednisone, and bleomycin, in conjunction with radiation therapy, have produced long-term remission.

SOFT-TISSUE SARCOMA

The term *soft tissue* customarily includes the structures that envelop the body and fill in the interstices of the retroperitoneum, mediastinum, and orbit. The soft tissues we are concerned with in this chapter are the connective tissues, the blood and lymphatic vessels, and the smooth and striated muscles located in the skin and subcutaneous tissues, which are all derived from the primitive mesenchyme. Malignant tumors derived from the neuroectoderm are also included, since they are intermingled with the structures mentioned above and behave similarly. The word *sarcoma* is derived from the Greek, meaning fleshy tumor.

In more recent times, the term has been applied chiefly to the malignant tumors derived from the mesenchyme, fleshy or not. Soft-tissue sarcomas account for approximately 1.2% of all malignancies. Little is known about their etiology, although occasionally fibrosarcoma can arise in scar tissue from burns and excessive irradiation. Proportionately, children are somewhat more prone to suffer from this tumor than are adults. Sarcomas found in children under 15 years of age account for about 4% of all juvenile malignant tumors. The lower extremity is the primary location in 40% of patients, the upper extremity in 20%, the trunk in 20%, the head and neck area in 10%, and the retroperitoneal region in 10%.

Most, if not all, of these tumors are usually treated with aggressive radical surgical extirpation. Often, the tumor appears localized when it is actually pseudoencapsulated; there is a proclivity for the tumor cells to spread along musculofascial planes. It would dictate, therefore, wide radical surgical excision, including 4 cm to 5 cm of normal tissue as margin, and groups of muscles will often have to be excised from their origins to their insertion. Furthermore, in many cases, especially with the involvement of important neurovascular structures and a small size or area to preclude wide excision, amputation becomes the only effective sur-

gical primary procedure. Amputation is usually carried out one joint level above the location of the primary, which would mean hemipelvectomy or forequarter amputation for lesions in the proximal thigh and upper arm, respectively. Although the mode of distant spread is usually hematogenous, the excision of regional lymph nodes should be part of the planned surgical therapy, since 5% to 20% of patients with soft-tissue sarcoma have lymph node involvement. Overall treatment with surgery alone of the different soft-tissue sarcomas produces an average 5-year survival rate of 45%.

Combined-modality therapy of soft-tissue sarcoma, particularly in the extremities, using combination chemotherapy, irradiation, and surgery, has been attempted. For example, for sarcomas of suitable size in the extremities, the so-called limb-salvage multidisciplinary therapeutic approach has been advocated (*e.g.,* preoperative chemotherapy involving intra-arterial Adriamycin, followed by radiotherapy), and wide local excision has been attempted by a few investigators. The local regional treatment has been followed by high-dose methotrexate with citrovorum-factor rescue to deal with the micrometastases that may be present at the time of treatment; although this approach results in major disfigurement of the limb, the proponents claim good local regional control of the disease, with preservation of significant limb function.

Systemic chemotherapy consisting of combinations (*e.g.,* Adriamycin, actinomycin D, dimethyltriazeno imidazole carboxamide, vincristine, cyclophosphamide, and methotrexate) has been used in the treatment of disseminated soft-tissue sarcoma. Among these are liposarcoma, angiosarcoma, chondrosarcoma, rhabdomyosarcoma, synovial cell sarcoma, and fibrosarcoma. Response (partial and complete) of greater than 50%, lasting a median duration of 3½ to 5 months, has been noted in 40% of these patients. Rhabdomyosarcoma, specifically the embryonal variety, has shown a significant response to a combination of radiotherapy, surgery, and a chemotherapeutic regimen of vincristine, actinomycin D, and cyclophosphamide, which had resulted in a high response rate and approximately a 65% survival rate with no evidence of disease beyond 5 years.

FIBROSARCOMA

Fibrosarcoma, as the name implies, is comprised of fibrous connective tissue. These tumors are generally classified as differentiated or undifferentiated, depending upon the potential for distant spread. In general, grades I and II of Broders' histologic classification are considered differentiated, while grades III and IV are considered undifferentiated. Histologically, in the differentiated group, reticulum fibers are mixed with malignant spindle cells, while the undifferentiated varieties are characterized by an increased number of mitotic figures, pleomorphism, and a lack of reticulum fibers. The cause is unknown, although there are a few reports of fibrosarcoma arising in burn scars or at the site of a chronic draining sinus tract. Cutaneous lesions are usually slow to metastasize; most fibrosarcomas tend to be well differentiated. Grossly, they are firm, large, round or elliptical-shaped masses that are usually painless. The differentiated forms occur most commonly in the trunk (44%) and extremities (41%), while the undifferentiated forms occur in the extremities (70%), especially the lower extremities (54%) and the trunk (20%).

Effective therapy must embody the principles of wide

local excision. The local recurrence rate in most series is about 60%. If there is tumor recurrence, particularly in the undifferentiated variety, then amputation should be strongly considered if technically feasible.

In one series of 50 soft-tissue sarcomas, there were 17 cases of fibrosarcoma, 16 of which were treated for cure. In this group of 16, 10 had local excision and 6 required radical amputations. There was local recurrence in nine of ten having wide local excision and in only one of six in the amputation group.

Principles of management for fibrosarcoma include biopsy, wide local excision with a margin of at least 4 cm on all sides (if muscles are involved, their origins and insertions should be excised), and radical amputation if local or regional recurrence is observed of any sarcoma other than grade I fibrosarcoma. Depending on the grade of the tumor, there is a high survival rate in the more differentiated varieties. Overall, there is a 40% to 50% 5-year survival rate.

DERMATOFIBROSARCOMA PROTUBERANS

Dermatofibrosarcoma protuberans is a nodular neoplasm usually found in the dermis. It is composed of fibrocytes arranged in radial whorls. Often, although it remains localized for a number of years, it may undergo a phase of rapid growth, with the formation of multiple nodules. Distant metastases have been known to occur, although rarely, and lymph node metastasis is likewise rare. Histologically, this lesion cannot be distinguished from low-grade fibrosarcoma.

Aggressive wide local excision is recommended for cure. With this type of treatment, the recurrence rate should be less than 50% and the long-term cure rate at least 80%.

MALIGNANT FIBROUS HISTIOCYTOMA

Malignant fibrous histiocytoma is probably the most common soft-tissue sarcoma to occur in older patients, although we have observed this tumor in younger patients. It occurs most frequently in the thigh, followed by the chest wall, shoulder region, and retroperitoneum. In most patients, these tumors are deep seated, nodular, and between 5 cm and 10 cm in diameter. Small superficially located tumors in the dermis or subcutaneous layer do occur and appear to have a more favorable prognosis. Malignant fibrous histiocytoma is characterized by a wide variety of cellular compositions in pattern, not only from tumor to tumor but also in different portions of the same tumor. The least pleomorphic form of the neoplasm has a distinct whorl pattern similar to that found in dermatofibrosarcoma protuberans. With increasing pleomorphism, this pattern disappears and is replaced by a giant-celled picture with eosinophilic cytoplasm and one or more hyperchromatic nuclei with a bizarre appearance, which makes differentiation from pleomorphic rhabdomyosarcoma somewhat difficult.

By and large, malignant fibrous histiocytomas are composed of several types of cells: plump, fibroblastlike spindle cells; round or oval mononuclear cells resembling histiocytes; and giant cells with one or more nuclei. Often, there are foamy histiocytes and cells with hemosiderin in them. The three main variants of malignant fibrous histiocytomas are giant cell, xanthomatous, and myxoid.

Treatment includes aggressive surgical extirpation with adequate margins of normal tissue. A tumor confined to the subcutaneous layer without invasion of deeper structures

has a local recurrence rate of 60%, and distant metastasis occurs in slightly over 20% of patients. Overall, the rate of distant metastasis is over 40%, and in 18% of the patients the tumor recurs locally before distant metastases become manifest. The most common sites of distant metastases are the lung (82%), lymph nodes (28%), liver (18%), and bone (15%). Five-year survival rates are between 41% and 60%.

LIPOSARCOMA

Liposarcoma is derived from fatty tissue and is malignant from the onset of its growth. There are differentiated and undifferentiated varieties, and although they have a relatively slow growth rate, they can become large. Satellite nodules may be observed around the main mass, and multicentric lesions have also been reported. Microscopic pictures range from the characteristic signet-ring lipoblast with a lobulated pattern to a highly undifferentiated lesion composed of small cells. Approximately 40% to 50% of tumors will metastasize to the lung, and about 60% recur following local excision. The extremities are usually involved in 60% of patients, the retroperitoneal space in 15%, and the subcutaneous trunk in 15%. These are the most common of the sarcomas, comprising approximately 20% of the total group of soft-tissue sarcomas.

The treatment of choice is radical extirpation. Because of its slow rate of growth and late metastasis, reexcision with cure is possible on many occasions. Liposarcoma responds poorly to radiation therapy. The 5-year survival rate in treated liposarcoma is 35% to 40%.

LEIOMYOSARCOMA

Leiomyosarcoma of the skin is an extremely rare lesion. It is slow to grow and metastasizes late. Grossly, the tumors are solid and may appear circumscribed. Microscopically, the cells have blunt-ended nuclei with interlacing cellular bundles and much anaplasia; bizarre cells with multiple nuclei are seen, as well as frequent mitoses of up to one to ten per high-power field.

Leiomyosarcoma should be treated with radical wide excision. Prognosis is intermediate among sarcomas, with a 5-year survival rate of 40% to 45%.

RHABDOMYOSARCOMA

Rhabdomyosarcomas arise from striated muscles and are divided into four groups: embryonal rhabdomyosarcoma and sarcoma botryoides (which occur in children), alveolar rhabdomyosarcoma (which occurs in young adults), and pleomorphic rhabdomyosarcoma (which also occurs in adults). As has been described earlier, the combined-modality treatment of embryonal rhabdomyosarcoma in children has tremendously improved the outlook of this disease. Pleomorphic rhabdomyosarcoma is locally invasive, and at the time of diagnosis, 30% of patients have already had evidence of pulmonary metastases (Fig. 18-10). Metastases to regional lymph nodes occur in approximately 15%. This tumor is most commonly found in the extremities, 50% in the lower extremities, 15% in the upper extremities, and 10% in the head and neck area. Therapy should be wide surgical excision or amputation. The local recurrence rate is over 50%, and the 5-year survival rate is approximately 35%.

Alveolar rhabdomyosarcoma is characterized microscopically by its pseudoalveolar appearance. Myofibrils and striations are more difficult to find. These tumors are highly anaplastic, exhibiting a tremendous growth rate and a poor

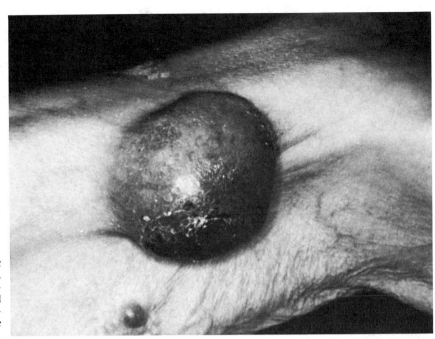

Fig. 18-10. Grossly, this pleomorphic rhabdomyosarcoma appeared as a large, elevated, purplish red lesion with a daughter satellite in the lateral aspect of the distal right thigh of a 65-year-old man. Pulmonary metastases were already present at the time of diagnosis.

prognosis. At the time of diagnosis, 75% of patients already have pulmonary metastases and regional node metastases. This tumor affects adults in their twenties and tends to develop more often in the upper extremities. Treatment is radical amputation, including the regional lymph nodes. The prognosis is dismal, with a 5-year cure rate of only 2%.

In general, the rhabdomyosarcomas are locally aggressive, with a high incidence for hematogenous spread to the lungs and to the regional lymph nodes. Because of this, serious consideration should be given to adjuvant therapy.

MALIGNANT HEMANGIOENDOTHELIOMA

Malignant hemangioendothelioma is the malignant form of hemangioma and is often found in the head and neck area. It pursues a rapid clinical course, starting as a small tumor and relentlessly spreading to involve the whole scalp or face or both. Grossly, this is a very vascular tumor and tends to involve the deeper tissues. Histologically, it is composed of malignant endothelial cells and large vascular spaces. Endothelioblasts are readily detached and carried away to the lung by the bloodstream. Radical wide surgical excision is the course of treatment. Prognosis is generally poor because metastases to the lungs occur early.

LYMPHANGIOSARCOMA

Lymphangiosarcoma is extremely rare, usually developing in patients who have had long-standing lymphedema of the arm secondary to radical mastectomy (Fig. 18-11). The lymphangiosarcoma has often been known to develop in the lower extremities, also associated with chronic lymphedema. The skin appears edematous, with bluish or purplish elevations; lesions are frequently multiple. In later stages, the lesions coalesce to present huge hemorrhagic masses. This is a tumor that usually develops in the sixth decade, an average of 10 or more years after radical mastectomy. Microscopically, the lymphatic cells composing the tumor often assume a striking papillary pattern, with numerous islands connected by cords of tissue and surrounded by one or several layers of malignant cells. Sometimes the tumor assumes a medullary pattern that could be mistaken for undifferentiated metastatic adenocarcinoma. On rare occasions, the tumor cells may assume a spindle shape. The tumor metastasizes early by way of the bloodstream to the lungs.

Forequarter or hindquarter amputation is usually the necessary treatment to control the lesion; however, the prognosis is poor, with a 5-year survival rate of less than 10%. This tumor is not responsive or sensitive to chemotherapy or radiation therapy.

KAPOSI'S SARCOMA

Kaposi's sarcoma is a relatively rare disease in the United States, but it is quite common in certain parts of continental Africa, accounting for over 10% of all malignant neoplasms. This tumor occurs most commonly in men of Jewish, Italian, and black extraction, and the ratio of men to women is 3:1. Although the peak incidence occurs at about 50 to 55 years of age, the disease has also been found in younger persons.

The lesion of Kaposi's sarcoma usually manifests initially as multiple blue dermal nodules or plaquelike structures usually on the feet, legs, and hands and progressing proximally (Fig. 18-12). The lesion may become pedunculated, not unlike that of pyogenic granulomas. Lesions that are not in the cutaneous layer may be identified in the subcutaneous layer by angiographic techniques. The clinical course of Kaposi's sarcoma is extremely variable and, as a rule, prolonged, although instances of rapid and fatal progressions have been reported. Four major clinical types of Kaposi's sarcoma have been identified: nodular, florid, infiltrative, and lymphadenopathic. The nodular form is indolent and benign, while the other forms are clinically aggressive, tending to spread systemically early while concurrently involving distant organs. Its spread and dissemination is through the bloodstream and lymphatic system.

Treatment with wide surgical excision may be employed in a localized form of the disease, but most often excision is used to establish the diagnosis. More disseminated stages of the disease have been treated with some degree of success using combination chemotherapeutic agents (*e.g.*, actinomycin D and vincristine), with response rates ranging from

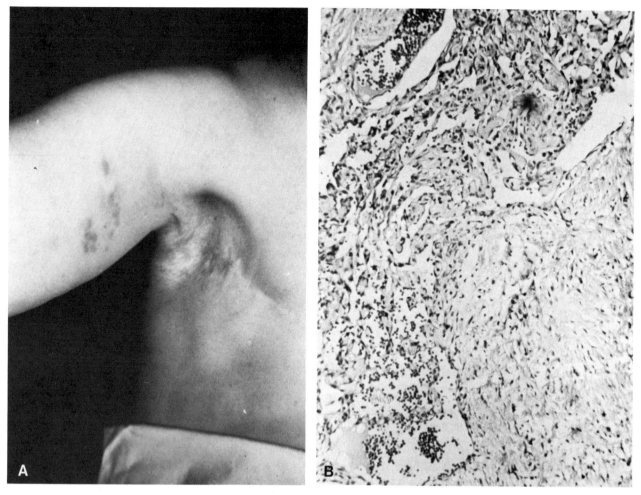

Fig. 18-11.   Postmastectomy lymphangiosarcoma. (*A*) Note the raised lesions on the inner aspect of the arm; these are bluish purple. (*B*) Microscopically, there are an abundance of islands of lymphoblasts and a tendency to form a papillary pattern and interspersed lymph vascular channels. (H&E, × 150)

25% to 65%. The nitrosoureas (CCNU and BCNU combined with DTIC) have also produced significant responses. Radiation therapy has been employed to a limited degree with varying degrees of success. The 5-year survival rate is approximately 40%, and about half of these survivors have no evidence of disease.

MALIGNANT HEMANGIOPERICYTOMA

Malignant hemangiopericytomas occur on the skin or in the subcutaneous tissues in any part of the body. The nodule is firm and may grow as large as 10 cm in diameter. It is composed of endothelium-lined tubes and sprouts that are filled with blood and surrounded by cells with oval or spindle-shaped nuclei; they are believed to be classic pericytes. Histologically, these are very similar to glomus tumors; however, hemangiopericytomas are rarely painful. The tumor has variable growth characteristics, from lying dormant for a long time to exhibiting a very accelerated and aggressive clinical course at other times. It has the potential to metastasize to the lung, and this occurs in about half of the patients.

Treatment is wide local excision. The incidence of local recurrence is approximately 50%. The tumor frequently has a prolonged course, and the 5-year survival rate is approximately 50%.

MALIGNANT SCHWANNOMA

Malignant schwannoma originates from the nerve sheath and demonstrates local invasion and also the potential for metastatic dissemination by way of the bloodstream. The tumors are highly cellular and have a microscopic appearance of whorls of spindle-shaped cells in a pattern of interlacing bundles with frequent mitotic figures. Approximately half of all patients with malignant schwannomas are also found to have von Recklinghausen's disease.

When malignant schwannoma is found in extremities, treatment demands radical amputation, since the local recurrence following wide local excision exceeds 60%. The overall 5-year survival rate is about 20%.

GRANULAR CELL MYOBLASTOMA

Granular cell myoblastoma is a relatively rare tumor. It is histologically distinct, being composed of compactly arranged cells, each with an abundance of cytoplasm containing many eosinophilic granules. Electron microscopic studies suggest that it is most likely of Schwann cell origin. Its clinical behavior lies between the benign and malignant characteristics of tumors, and wide local excision results in cure for most patients.

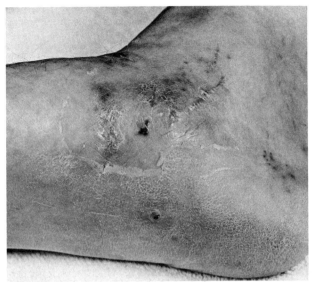
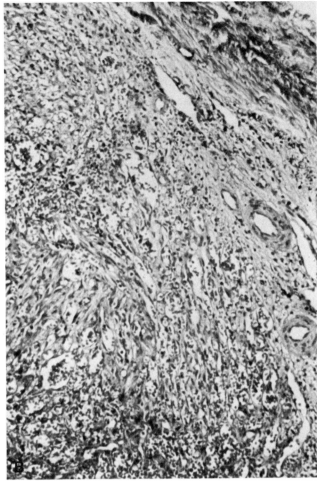

Fig. 18-12. (*A*) Multiple black nodules of Kaposi's sarcoma involving the foot. Such lesions mimic melanocarcinoma. (*B*) Microscopically, there are numerous interlacing spindle-shaped cells in between the slitlike vascular spaces. (H&E, × 150)

ALVEOLAR SOFT PART SARCOMA

Alveolar soft part sarcoma is another rare tumor of undetermined histogenesis. The most popular theory is that the tumor arises in nonchromaffin paraganglionic tissue. In any event, the tumor has a classic histologic appearance, showing pseudoalveolar structure in a glomerular pattern. It has a peculiar predilection for the right side of the body and the extremities. It occurs more commonly in women.

Treatment is wide local excision. This is attended with a 25% incidence of local recurrence; however, two thirds of the patients will have distant metastases, and lymph node involvement is found in about 10%. The overall survival rate is about 60% for 5 years and 50% for 10 years. It has a prolonged, but inexorable, course, and patients with known metastases have been known to survive 20 years.

DECUBITUS ULCERS (BED SORES, PRESSURE SORES)

Necrosis and loss of skin and soft tissue usually result from prolonged pressure, particularly over bony prominences such as the greater trochanter, ischial tuberosities, and sacrum, in debilitated, unconscious, and paralyzed patients. Good nursing care, adequate equipment that provides for the frequent turning of patients, and use of special air mattresses, foam rubber, and sheepskin should help prevent the occurrence of this very frustrating complication.

When dealing with this problem, the best treatment is prevention. It usually involves the concerted effort of the surgical and nursing teams to render excellent wound care in preparation for coverage of the defect, usually with a pedicle flap or rotation of a musculocutaneous flap. The wound preparation usually includes resection of underlying necrotic and infected bursae, ligaments, fascia, and bone. The donor site, likewise, will require special attention in that it will have to be covered with skin graft and protected from breaking down. Last but not least, the nutritional status of the patient should be maintained at optimal levels by adequate alimentation through intravenous or enteral routes.

BIBLIOGRAPHY

ALDAY ES: Pilonidal cyst and sinus: Radical excision and primary closure. Surg Clin North Am 53:559, 1973

ALTEMEIER WA, FURSTE WL: Gas gangrene. Surg Gynecol Obstet 84:507, 1947

ANDREWS EC, ROCKWOOD CA, CRUZ AB JR: Unusual surgical infections: Gas gangrene, necrotizing fasciitis, phycomycosis, synergistic bacterial gangrene. Tex Med 65:44, 1969

AUST JB: Soft tissue sarcomas. In Horton J, Hill GJ (eds): Clinical Oncology. Philadelphia, W B Saunders, 1977

BERG TW, McDIVITT RW: Pathology of sweat gland carcinoma. Pathol Annu 3:123, 1968

CARABELL SC, GOODMAN RL: Radiation therapy for soft tissue sarcoma. Semin Oncol 8:201, 1981

DAS GUPTA TK: Management of soft tissue sarcomas. Surg Gynecol Obstet 137:1012, 1973

DRUTZ J: Leprosy: An infectious disease. In Hoeprich PD (ed): A Guide to the Understanding and Management of Infectious Processes. Hagerstown, Harper & Row, 1972

ENZINGER FM: Recent developments in the classification of soft tissue sarcomas. In Management of Primary Bone and Soft Tissue Tumors. The University of Texas M.D. Anderson Hospital and Tumor Institute. Chicago, Year Book Medical Publishers, 1977

GRAHAM JH, HELWIG EB: Bowen's disease and its relationship to systemic cancer. Arch Dermatol 83:738, 1961

HERRMANN JB: Lymphangiosarcoma of the chronically edematous extremity. Surg Gynecol Obstet 121:1107, 1965

LINDBERG RD, MARTIN RG, ROMSDAHL MM: Surgery and postoperative radiotherapy in the treatment of soft tissue sarcomas in adults. Am J Roentgenol 123:123, 1975

LITWIN MS, RYAN RF, REED RJ et al: Topical chemotherapy of advanced cutaneous malignancy with 5% fluorouracil cream. J Surg Oncol 3:351, 1971

LONG JC, MIHM MC: Mycosis fungoides with extracutaneous dissemination: A distinct clinicopathologic entity. Cancer 34:1745, 1974

MITTS DL, SMITH MT, RUSSELL L et al: Sweat gland carcinomas: A clinicopathological reappraisal. J Surg Oncol 8:23, 1976

MOHS FE: Chemosurgery for the microscopically controlled excision of skin cancer. J Surg Oncol 3:257, 1971

MORTON DL, EILBER FR, TOWNSEND CM JR et al: Limb salvage from a multidisciplinary approach for skeletal and soft tissue sarcomas of the extremity. Ann Surg 184:268, 1976

ROSENBERG SA, GLATSTEIN EJ: Perspective on the role of surgery and radiation therapy in the treatment of soft tissue sarcomas of the extremities. Semin Oncol 8:190, 1981

SHIU MH, HAJDU SI: Management of soft tissue sarcoma of the extremity. Semin Oncol 8:172, 1981

SMITH BL, FRANZ JL, MIRA JG et al: Simultaneous combination radiotherapy and multidrug chemotherapy for Stage III and Stage IV squamous cell carcinoma of the head and neck. J Surg Oncol 15:91, 1980

STOUT AP: Liposarcoma: The malignant tumor of lipoblasts. Ann Surg 119:86, 1944

STOUT AP: Fibrosarcoma: The malignant tumor of fibroblast. Cancer 1:30, 1948

STOUT AP: Hemangiopericytoma: A study of twenty-five new cases. Cancer 2:1027, 1949

STOUT AP: Sarcomas of the soft tissues. Cancer 11:210, 1961

STOUT AP, TATTES R: Tumors of the soft tissues. In Atlas of Tumor Pathology, Second Series, Fascicle I. Washington DC, Armed Forces Institute of Pathology, 1966

SUTOW WW, MAURER HM: Chemotherapy of sarcomas: A perspective. Semin Oncol 8:207, 1981

19

The Breast

Arthur J. Donovan

Whilst the changes for the reproduction of the species are proceeding in the uterus, Nature is not unmindful or regardless of the wants of the offspring so soon as it shall be born; but in all the classes of Mammalia, she has provided glands to supply bountifully, by the secretion of milk, that nourishment which the young animal will require soon after it begins to breathe. The Breasts, or Mammae, are formed for this purpose.

—SIR ASHLEY COOPER

EMBRYOLOGY
DEVELOPMENT
ANATOMY
  Arterial Supply
  Venous Drainage
  Lymphatic Drainage
FUNCTION
DIAGNOSIS OF BREAST DISEASE
  History
  Physical Examination
  Diagnostic Radiology
  Histology
    Cytology of Fluid
    Needle Aspiration (Solid Mass)
    Needle Biopsy
    Open Biopsy
  Sex Steroid Binding
  Other Tests
PATHOPHYSIOLOGIC DISTURBANCES
      (NON-NEOPLASTIC)
  Gynecomastia
  Chronic Cystic Mastitis
  Mammary Duct Ectasia
  Fat Necrosis
BENIGN NEOPLASMS
  Fibroadenoma
  Cystosarcoma Phyllodes (usually benign)
  Intraductal Papilloma
  Other Benign Neoplasms
INFLAMMATORY PROCESSES
NIPPLE DISCHARGE
CANCER OF THE BREAST
  Epidemiology and Etiology
    Hereditary
    Biologic

    Environmental
  Natural History
    Pattern of Growth
    Hormone Sensitivity
  Pathology
    Paget's Disease
    Duct Cell Origin
    Lobular Carcinoma
    Sarcoma
    Bilateral Cancer
    Pregnancy
    Occurrence in Males
    Inflammatory Cancer
  Classification: Staging
  Pretreatment Evaluation
  Treatment Modalities
    Surgery
    Radiation Therapy
    Chemotherapy
    Hormonal Manipulation
  Recommendations for Therapy
SPECIAL PROBLEMS
  Hypercalcemia
  Pleural Effusion
  Visceral Metastasis
  Prognosis
  Rehabilitation

The breast is a modified sweat gland that produces milk under hormonal influence.

Carcinoma is the most significant disease of the breast because it is the most frequently occurring cancer in American women. Careful evaluation of the common features of breast disease (*i.e.,* pain, nipple discharge, or a mass) is required to exclude malignancy. Findings of physical examination, needle aspiration, mammography, and biopsy will usually establish a correct diagnosis. As breast self-examination is performed by more women there will likely be an increase in early detections of breast cancer.

Carcinoma of the breast is best treated by appropriate surgical resection whenever possible. Metastatic tumor may exhibit hormonal responsiveness, radiation sensitivity, or response to systemic chemotherapy. Ductal carcinoma is the most common breast cancer and metastasizes to regional lymph nodes by hematogenous routes or by recurrence at the site of a treated primary tumor. At least 50% of breast cancers confined to the breast and regional nodes may be cured at 10 years with appropriate surgical and adjunctive chemotherapy. Appropriate clinical staging of breast carcinoma allows optimum choice of treatment modalities to maximize cure, survival, and palliation.

Benign conditions of the breast are important because of the discomfort they produce and because of their frequent confusion with neoplastic disease. Gynecomastia, chronic cystic mastitis (CCM), mammary ductal ectasia, fat necrosis, fibroadenoma, cystosarcoma phylloides, intraductal papilloma, and breast abscess are all benign conditions that must be differentiated from breast cancer.

EMBRYOLOGY

In some mammals, several pairs of breasts develop in the "milk line" that extends from the axilla to the groin. In the human, one pair of pectoral breasts develop. The remainder of the "milk line" disappears. Supernumerary nipples or accessory mammary tissue may occur at any point along the embryonic "milk line," most frequently in the axilla. One or both breasts may be congenitally absent (amastia), one or both nipples may be absent (athelia), or supernumerary nipples may be present (polythelia). The nipples may be inverted.

DEVELOPMENT

Ducts, rudimentary acini, and the nipple are distinctive features during the last trimester of pregnancy. The breast remains a dormant organ during infancy. In the male, this dormancy persists. In the female, hormonal stimulation by estrogenic and progestational steroids during puberty causes ductal and acinar proliferation. Deficiency of ovarian function can delay development; precocious puberty can result in early development of the breast. Such early development is occasionally caused by a functioning ovarian tumor. One breast may develop more rapidly than the other. The breasts, for unknown reasons, may continue to grow and attain gigantic size. Spontaneous regression of such virginal hypertrophy will not occur. Reduction mammoplasty is indicated.

ANATOMY

The breast, a modified sweat gland, is suspended between the superficial and deep layers of the superficial fascia and lies on the pectoralis major fascia. It extends from the second to the sixth or seventh rib and from the lateral edge of the sternum to at least the anterior axillary line. An elongation of mammary tissue regularly extends on the pectoralis major muscle toward the axilla (*i.e.,* the axillary tail of Spence). Anterior and posterior suspensory ligaments of connective tissue suspend the breast to the skin and underlying pectoral fascia.

The fully developed breast is one of a pair of symmetrical organs that are conical in shape. The nipple projects slightly laterally and superiorly, an orientation that facilitates suckling. The nipple is everted and surrounded by the deeply pigmented areola.

The acini of the breast are lined by cuboidal epithelium and enveloped by a sheath of collagen. The acini are connected to an alveolar duct that drains into a lobular duct. The lobule is the basic unit of the breast. The lobular

ducts join lobar ducts, which number approximately 20. A layer of myoepithelial cells is arranged in a spiral fashion about the ductal system. The lobar duct enters a milk sinus that is located just beneath the nipple and is drained by a very short excretory duct lying within the nipple. Selected features of mammary anatomy are shown in Figure 19-1.

The nipple contains smooth muscle that when contracted causes the nipple to become erect. The skin of the more deeply pigmented areola contains both sweat glands and modified sebaceous glands. The latter, which may be slightly elevated above the surface, are known as the glands of Montgomery.

ARTERIAL SUPPLY

The principal sources of arterial supply to the breast are shown in Figure 19-2, *A.*

VENOUS DRAINAGE

The superficial veins of the breast drain into the internal mammary vein. The veins that drain the deeper portions of the breast may communicate with the intercostal veins that drain into the vertebral venous system, a fact that may be significant in metastasis from the breast.

LYMPHATIC DRAINAGE

The dominant pathway for lymphatic drainage of the entire breast is to the axilla. Drainage can also occur to the internal mammary lymph nodes, a particularly important route if the axillary lymphatics are blocked and in drainage from the areola and medial quadrants.

A circumareolar lymphatic plexus drains the superficial portions of the breast, and lymph passes from this plexus through subcutaneous channels to the axilla. Lymph originating about the mammary lobules may enter the circumareolar plexus or may pass deeply and then laterally to the axilla. Large lymphatic channels traverse the retromammary space, lying on the pectoral fascia. Lymphatics from the

Fig. 19-1. Cross section of the breast, showing selected features of mammary anatomy.

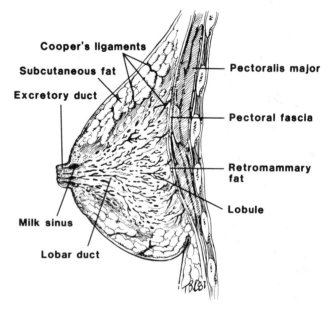

Cooper's ligaments
Subcutaneous fat
Excretory duct
Milk sinus
Lobar duct
Pectoralis major
Pectoral fascia
Retromammary fat
Lobule

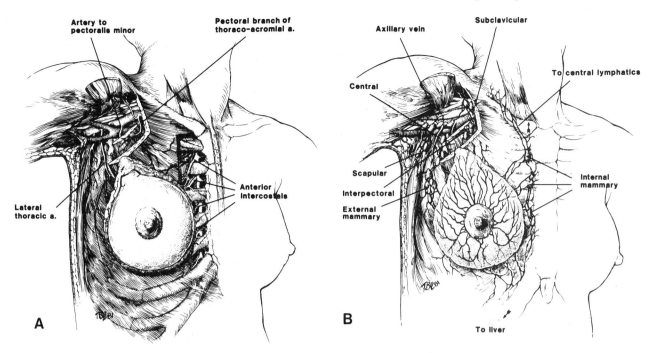

Fig. 19-2. The arterial supply of the breast (*A*) and the lymphatic drainage (*B*). The various groups of nodes are as shown.

breast penetrate the pectoral fascia and pectoralis major muscle to gain access to lymph nodes lying between the pectoralis major and minor muscles, which are known as Rotter's nodes.

Both axillary and internal mammary lymphatic channels drain to nodes above the clavicle. The inferior portion of the internal mammary chain is in continuity with the lymphatic plexus in the liver.

The axillary nodes normally number 35 to 50; the internal mammary nodes, 5 to 10. The identity and locations of the various groups of nodes to which the breast drains are shown in Figure 19-2, *B*.

FUNCTION

During each menstrual cycle, the breast is prepared to assume its lactational function should an ovum be fertilized. Following menstruation and under estrogenic and subsequent progestational stimulation, the breast hypertrophies due to edema in the connective tissue and the formation of new acini. These changes reach a peak prior to menstruation. Thereafter, involution is rapid.

Should impregnation occur, further profound changes occur consequent to continued hormonal stimulation, both placental and pituitary in origin. There is extensive branching of the ductal system and formation of new acini. The nipple and areola darken, as occurs in all hyperestrogenic states. Montgomery's glands become more prominent.

Following delivery and with abrupt ablation of placental secretion, secretion of prolactin by the pituitary gland increases. Granules form in the acinar cells, which discharge milk. The passage of the milk through the ductal system is enhanced by the action of the spirally placed myoepithelial cells, probably stimulated by oxytocin. Lactation ensues and persists if breast feeding is initiated. Afferent neurogenic impulses stimulated by suckling probably act through the hypothalamus to provide for continued release of prolactin

and oxytocin. If suckling is not established, or when breast feeding ceases, there is rapid involution of the proliferative changes evoked by pregnancy. The breast resumes its resting state. Estrogenic steroids inhibit secretion of prolactin, and administration of estrogen will hasten involution. Certain hormonal stimuli of the breast are shown in Figure 19-3.

Following the menopause and with cessation of ovulation the breast is no longer subjected to cyclic hormonal stimulation. Glandular elements atrophy, the relative proportion of fat increases, and the breast becomes a functionless organ.

DIAGNOSIS OF BREAST DISEASE

Three complaints, alone or in combination, are the usual reason that individuals seek attention for disease of the breast: pain, discharge from the nipple, or a mass. A known or suspected mass is the complaint in at least three fourths of cases. The distribution of mass lesions as to type is shown in Figure 19-4.

HISTORY

A sense of fullness and pain in the breast that increases prior to the menstrual period and declines thereafter is a frequent complaint and is referred to as mastodynia. Occasionally quite distressing, it reflects proliferative changes and edema in the breast that are preparatory, should conception occur. Mastodynia is common in CCM, which is also called cystic disease.

The hormonal environment in which mammary pathology develops is established with the taking of a thorough history, which includes age of menarche and menopause, natural or artificial menopause, age at first pregnancy, number of pregnancies, nursing history, and use of estrogen or progesterone as the Pill or as treatment of the menopausal syndrome. History of familial breast disease, of prior breast disease, or of trauma may be relevant. Information is sought

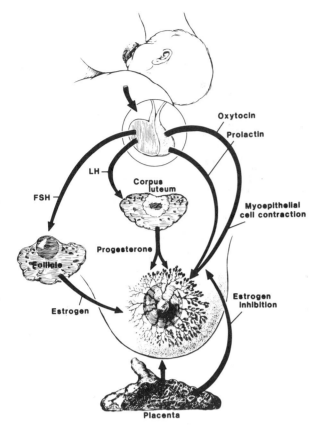

Fig. 19-3. Hormonal influences: the effect of estrogens on ductal proliferation, of progesterone on acinar proliferation, and of prolactin and oxytocin on lactation.

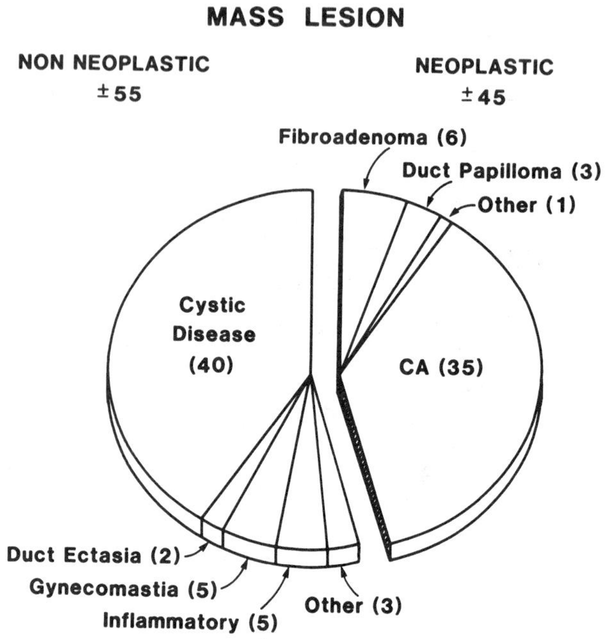

concerning any change observed in a mass lesion and as to the site, the nature, and the frequency of any nipple discharge.

PHYSICAL EXAMINATION

Key elements in physical examination of the breast are inspection and palpation. Inspection is best performed with the patient sitting; palpation is best performed with the patient supine. Only a large tumor will cause a visible bulge; a smaller cancer may cause contraction with elevation of the breast and nipple and inversion of the nipple or both. A more advanced cancer can retract the overlying skin by contraction of Cooper's ligaments (*i.e.,* skin dimpling). Skin dimpling is, on rare occasion, caused by fat necrosis, mammary duct ectasia, plasma cell mastitis, sclerosing adenosis, or granular cell myoblastoma, all of which are

THE BREAST LUMP	
Etiology	The lump may be a cyst or neoplasm and may be benign or malignant.
Dx	History (including age) and physical examination, mammograms, and biopsy (aspiration of cyst or tumor, or open biopsy) are required.
Rx	Benign lesions are excised, and mastectomy with or without radiation therapy or chemotherapy for malignancy is performed.

MASS LESION

NON NEOPLASTIC
±55

NEOPLASTIC
±45

Fibroadenoma (6)
Duct Papilloma (3)
Other (1)

Cystic Disease (40)

CA (35)

Duct Ectasia (2)
Gynecomastia (5)
Inflammatory (5)
Other (3)

Fig. 19-4. Incidence of breast mass lesions.

benign diseases. Crusting of the nipple suggests Paget's disease, a form of breast cancer. Lymphedema of the skin, usually due to lymphatic obstruction by cancer, causes the skin to be pitted and to resemble an orange peel (peau d'orange). Pitting is due to dermal fixation by rete pegs.

Diffuse redness of the skin over the breast with a sharp margin comparable to erysipelas may occur with streptococcal cellulitis or "inflammatory cancer." In inflammatory cancer, the dermal lymphatics are invaded by cancer cells. A localized area of rubor can be caused by a cancer that is directly invading the skin or a cancer may ulcerate.

The patient is instructed to hyperextend the shoulders. This tenses the pectoral fascia and places tension on Cooper's ligaments. The breast normally elevates. If cancer is present the elevation may not be symmetrical or the smooth contour of the breast may be broken and a mass noted as a localized bulge. Skin dimpling may become apparent. The breasts are also examined while the patient's arms are raised over the head and while leaning forward so that the upper torso is flexed at the waist to about 90°. The above actions may elicit changes in contour similar to those evoked by hyperextension of the shoulders.

The patient is allowed to recline in a comfortable position. A small pillow beneath the scapula may elevate the breast slightly and facilitate the examination. The breasts are inspected to detect any change in contour, either confirmatory or on observation with the patient sitting or only detected in recumbency.

The balls of the terminal digits, and not the fingertips, are the proper agents for palpation of the breast. Reduction of friction between the fingers and the skin with oil or soap facilitates palpation. The fingers should be rolled over the breast and the glandular tissue flattened between the skin and chest wall. Each quadrant should be examined sequentially. If a mass is felt, is it smooth as a cyst, irregular and stony hard as a cancer, or rubbery and almost balottable as a fibroadenoma? Transillumination in a dark room may establish that a mass is a cyst. A saucerlike depression will

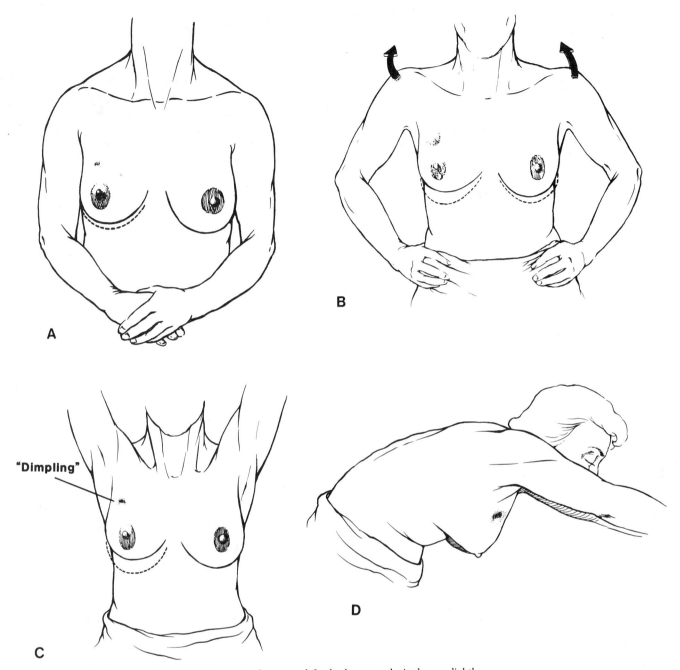

A

B

"Dimpling"

C

D

Fig. 19-5. Physical examination of the breast. In the upper left, the breast and nipple are slightly elevated. The other positions elicit more subtle findings.

be felt beneath the nipple. A ridge of fibrous tissue is usually present in the intramammary fold. A mass palpated while the patient is supine should also be felt with the patient in a sitting position.

Fixation of a mass to the skin may not be obvious. If the thumb and the forefinger are placed 4 cm to 6 cm apart over the mass and slowly and gently approximated by compression of the skin like an accordion, subtle skin fixation may be detected. Normally, the skin will form a progressively convex surface. A concavity may develop as a very early sign of fixation of anterior Cooper's ligaments. Haagensen believes that subtle skin changes may be detected in most cases of breast cancer, including minor contour changes, nipple displacement, or skin fixation.

Examination of the breast that is the site of aggressive CCM is difficult. A small cancer may be missed. Differentiation of a neoplasm from an area of CCM in a "lumpy" breast is a challenge to even the most experienced physician. Three-dimensional lesions palpated in the "lumpy" breast of CCM should be evaluated at both the mid and the end point of the menstrual cycle. Following menstruation, a mass may regress or, conversely, reduction in breast density may make a neoplasm more easily definable. Repeated examinations by the same physician over a period of time are essential.

The examination for regional lymph nodes may be done with the patient supine, erect, or both. The right axilla is examined with the left hand; the left, with the right. When

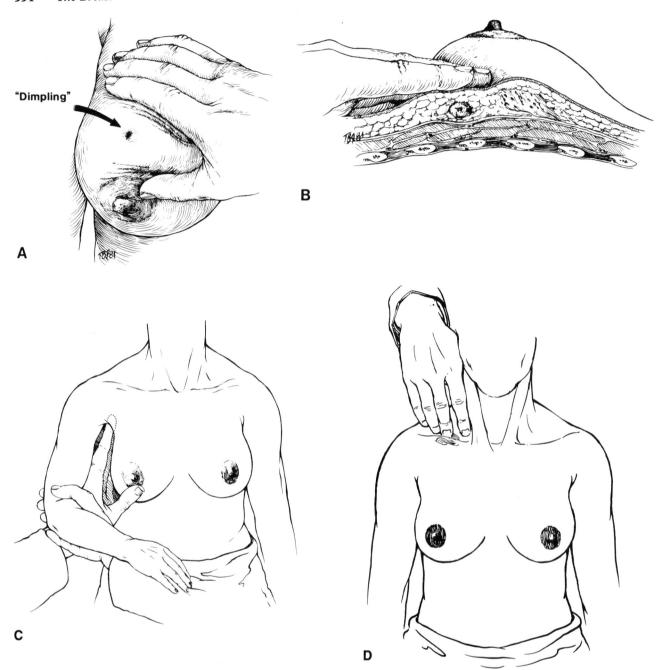

Fig. 19-6. Physical examination of the breast, the axilla, and the supraclavicular fossa. In the upper left, the use of the flat of the fingers and not the tips is emphasized.

sitting, the forearm on the side of the axilla to be examined is allowed to rest comfortably on the examiner's opposite forearm. This permits relaxation of muscles in the shoulder girdle. The fingers of the examining hand are slid into the apex of the axilla and swept downward against the chest wall. The supraclavicular fossa is best examined by standing behind the patient so that the fingertips can be inserted deeply behind the clavicle. The techniques for examination of the breast and axilla are shown in Figures 19-5 and 19-6.

When the complaint is nipple discharge, the physician should attempt to determine whether it is serous, lactiferous, or bloody, from single or multiple sites, and unilateral or bilateral (Fig. 19-7).

Following the completion of the breast examination, the physician should record his findings including size and location of any three-dimensional lesion. An example of a form that can be used for this purpose is shown in Figure 19-8. All lesions should be measured with a caliper and ruler. A change in the size of a mass on serial examination can only be established if one has precisely identified and recorded the size on a prior examination.

The American Cancer Society has supported an aggressive campaign of self-examination of the breast by all women for the purpose of the "early" detection of breast cancer. Inspection can be carried out before a mirror. Palpation is facilitated by examination while showering, when deceased friction between the fingers and the breast is maximized by

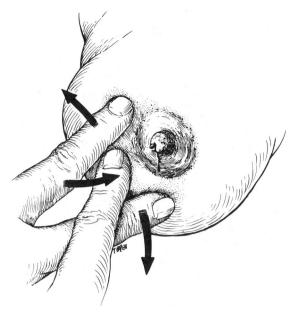

Fig. 19-7. The technique for examination of the breast to elicit nipple discharge. This maneuver is carried out in a circumferential fashion.

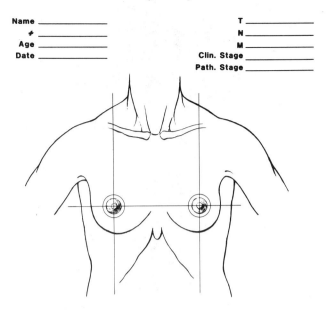

Fig. 19-8. This form is utilized to document findings on examination of the breast and of the regional lymphatic drainage areas.

the use of soap. Women should be strongly encouraged to examine the breasts at least monthly and to seek medical attention if a mass is felt or an alteration is detected.

DIAGNOSTIC RADIOLOGY

Mammography is performed with either standard radiographs or the Xerox technique. The latter employs an aluminum plate, subsequently transferred to a radiograph. To the neophyte, the details of intramammary anatomy are more apparent on the xerograph. For the experienced radiologist, the diagnostic accuracy of the two techniques is comparable. Two views of the breast are taken: a craniocaudal view and a mediolateral view. Mammography can reveal features classic of either benign breast disease or cancer (Fig. 19-9).

The critical question concerning mammography in a woman with a breast mass is its accuracy in the diagnosis of cancer. When mammograms are obtained of a breast with a mass that is cancer, the mass will not be diagnosed as cancer by the radiograph in well over 10% of cases. A false-positive diagnosis of cancer is far less frequent. Depending on the radiologist, a diagnosis of "cannot exclude cancer" can be common. This report is not of diagnostic value. The incidence of false-negative and of equivocal reports is too high to make mammography a reliable technique for exclusion of the diagnosis of cancer, when a mass lesion is palpable. The small breast that does not project off the chest wall and the dense breast of CCM may particularly limit the accuracy of mammography.

Mammography has been studied extensively as a screening technique for early detection of breast cancer. The studies of the Health Insurance Plan (HIP) of New York are a basic source of knowledge in these regards. Two cohorts were studied: one with routine annual physical examination and one with physical examination and mammography. These studies demonstrate that breast cancer can be detected by mammography at a preclinical stage, that is, when the

tumor is not palpable. A cancer detected by mammography has about a 20% likelihood of nodal metastasis, is generally less than 2 cm in size, and has greater than 90% five-year survival following definitive treatment. Among 100 asymptomatic women screened and found to have cancer, the tumor will be detected only on physical examination in about 40% of cases, only by mammography in another approximate 40%, and by both techniques in about 20% of cases. A modification of a table from the publications of HIP is presented in Table 19-1.

Concern has arisen as to the potential carcinogenic effect of the radiation received coincidental to screening mammography, and a recommendation has been made that mammographic screening be limited to postmenopausal women. The dose of radiation to which the patient is exposed has been reduced since the early experience with mammography and is currently less than 1 roentgen. The advisability of routine screening of premenopausal women is again under discussion.

The National Cancer Institute and the American Cancer Society have jointly sponsored a multi-institutional study of mammography. This study has confirmed that mammography can detect breast cancer before it is palpable. It is hoped that follow-up of the patients entered into this study will provide reliable data on the impact of mammographic screening on survival in a large cohort of women with breast cancer.*

In the light of current knowledge, mammography is suggested in several circumstances:

Examination of the opposite breast in a case with a suspicious mass or a proved cancer in one breast. The goals are the detection of a synchronous covert cancer and as a baseline study for future follow-up.

* The results of the NCI-ACS Breast Cancer Demonstration Project have been published and show that, among 3557 cases of proven cancer, 41.6% were detected by mammography alone, 47.3% by mammography and physical examination, 8.7% by physical examination only, and 2.4% by unknown means. (CA—A Cancer Journal for Clinicians 32:217, 1982)

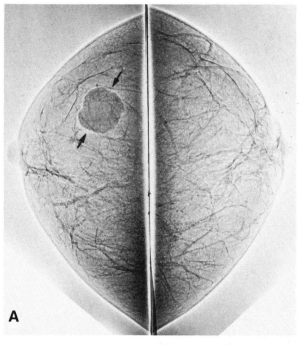

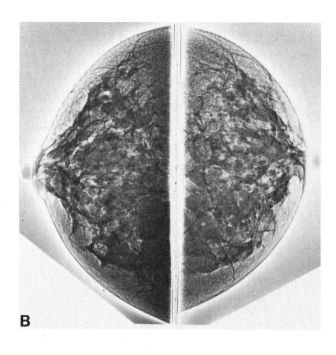

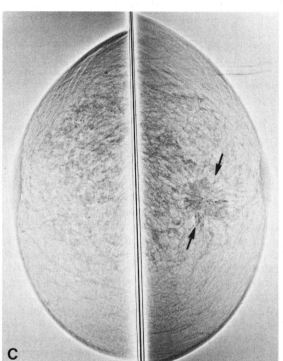

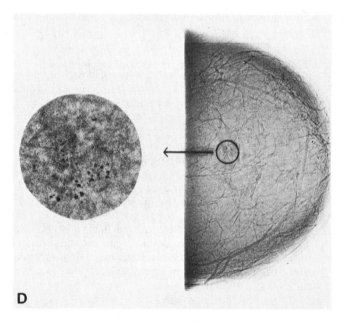

Fig. 19-9. Typical findings on mammography: (A) a fibroadenoma, (B) diffuse chronic cystic disease, (C) overt cancer, and (D) cancer detected only by stipled calcifications on mammography.

	TABLE 19-1	BREAST CANCERS DETECTED IN 132 PATIENTS ON SCREENING BY AGE GROUP AND MODALITY

		AGE AT DIAGNOSIS (%)†		
MODALITY*	Total	40–49	50–59	60 or Older
Mammography only	44 (33.3)	6 (19.4)	27 (41.5)	11 (30.6)
Clinical only	59 (44.7)	19 (61.3)	26 (40.0)	14 (38.9)
Clinical and mammography	29 (22.0)	6 (19.4)	12 (18.5)	11 (30.6)

*Initial evidence for biopsy recommendation made independently by the two modalities.
† Percentages may not add to 100 due to rounding.
(Shapiro S: Evidence on screening for breast cancer from a randomized trial. Cancer 39:2776, 1977)

Annual follow-up of cases treated for breast cancer for detection of dysynchronous cancer of the opposite breast. *In situ* lobular neoplasias are included.

Strong family history of breast cancer. An annual mammogram is indicated.

Follow-up study of cases with florid chronic cystic mastitis. Serial studies seek to detect changes that are not recognized by palpation.

Nipple discharge without a palpable mass. An occult tumor is sought.

The above indications for mammography are not meant to be exclusive.

Mammography does not provide a definitive diagnosis. Too often, a patient with a mass in the breast and a mammography report of "negative," "indeterminate," or of benign disease is reassured only to return with a more advanced breast cancer. The pathologic nature of a discrete mass in the breast must be established by histologic examination irrespective of the result of a mammogram.

HISTOLOGY

A histologic diagnosis must be established for every solid mass in the breast. Only thus can the diagnosis, including that of cancer, be established and proper treatment instituted. Several techniques exist by which material can be obtained for histologic examination.

CYTOLOGY OF FLUID

Cytologic examination can be performed on fluid aspirated from a cyst or draining from the nipple. Cyst fluid is centrifuged, and a slide is prepared from the sediment. The study is specifically indicated if the fluid that is aspirated is bloody or is from a recurrent cyst. Nipple discharge is placed on a slide and fixed as for a Papanicolaou smear. The diagnosis of cancer is rarely made by cytology, reflecting the rarity of cyst cancer and the infrequency of nipple discharge as a reflection of cancer.

NEEDLE ASPIRATION (SOLID MASS)

A No. 21 or smaller needle can be inserted into a mass in the breast with the patient under local anesthesia. A 2-ml syringe is attached to the needle, and suction is applied as the needle is withdrawn. A cyst may be aspirated. If the mass is solid, the "fluid" in the needle is expressed onto one or more slides and immediately fixed by a commercial hair spray. The preparation is stained with hematoxylin and eosin and examined. In at least 60% of cases of cancer the diagnosis is established, if the cytologist is experienced with the technique. False-positive reports are almost unknown. The larger the cancer, the more likely a positive diagnosis can be made. The high failure rate in the diagnosis of cancer does not negate the value of this simple procedure when results are positive.

NEEDLE BIOPSY

Rather than needle aspiration, a needle biopsy may be performed on a solid mass in the breast. The Trucut or Menghini needle is used. The core of tissue is fixed for routine sections. The accuracy is high: a false-positive diagnosis of cancer is almost unheard of and the diagnosis of cancer is established in 75% or more of the cases of

cancer so biopsied and studied by an experienced pathologist. The diagnosis of malignancy is more likely to be established with a larger cancer.

Needle biopsy is unwise if the mass is situated deeply in the breast and on the pectoral fascia. Should the needle penetrate through the tumor and into the fascia, tumor cells may be inoculated into the pectoral muscle. The possible implantation of tumor cells in the tract between the skin and the tumor is not a cause for serious concern. This tract will be excised with the tumor during subsequent treatment or will be included in the field if radiation therapy is the primary therapy. The site for insertion of the needle should be selected with these thoughts in mind.

Needle biopsy, when the result is positive, is an excellent means to diagnose breast cancer. Indeed, needle biopsy may be less likely to disseminate tumor cells than an incisional or excisional biopsy. Needle biopsy or aspiration may establish the diagnosis of cancer or of another specific process for which definitive treatment will be instituted. A diagnosis of "breast tissue," "indeterminate," "benign," or CCM by one name or another by needle biopsy is not adequate to exclude a diagnosis of cancer when a mass is present in the breast. An open biopsy must be performed. Needle aspiration and biopsy each have too high an incidence of false-negative results to be used as a means to exclude a diagnosis of cancer.

OPEN BIOPSY

Open biopsy of a mass in the breast may be excisional or incisional. Both false-positive or false-negative reports are extremely rare. Excisional biopsy may be both diagnostic and therapeutic in the case of a benign tumor. Excision is recommended for a presumed fibroadenoma, in a case of nipple discharge believed due to a ductal papilloma, or with a lesion that on exploration of the breast proves to be a previously unrecognized cyst or a solid lesion less than 3 cm in diameter. If the mass lesion is greater than 3 cm in diameter, or located deeply in the breast, an incisional biopsy by knife or biopsy forceps is performed. Depending on frozen section and final diagnosis, the surgeon will determine if further tissue should be removed for biopsy and what treatment is needed. Resection of a large amount of tissue is to be avoided with a benign process such as CCM, because of the resultant cosmetic deformity. Excisional biopsy of a cancer greater than 3 cm in diameter will almost certainly traverse microscopic areas of tumor extension. If the operative site is inadvertently entered during subsequent surgery, the operative field will be contaminated with tumor cells. In reference to breast cancer Halsted wrote:

"I believe that we should never cut through cancerous tissues, when operating, if it is possible to avoid doing so. The wound might become infected with cancer either by the knife which has passed through the diseased tissue, and perhaps carries everywhere the cancer-producing agents, or by the simple liberation of the cancer cells from their alveoli, or from the lymphatic vessels. The division of one lymphatic vessel and the liberation of one cell may be enough to start a new cancer."

A circumareolar incision is ideal for subsequent cosmesis and preferred if the lesion is so located as to be accessible by this route. If the biopsy site must be located elsewhere on the breast, a circular incision consistent with Langer's lines will result in a more cosmetic scar than will a radial incision. One must select the site while recognizing that if the tumor is malignant, the resultant tract must be excised with a wide margin in subsequent surgery.

Special strategy is required for biopsy of a lesion that is detected on mammography but not palpable. A needle can be passed into the area of the tumor and the location of the needle adjacent to the "tumor" confirmed by radiograph. Less than 0.1 ml of methylene blue is injected through the needle. If the dye is diluted 2:1 with diatrizoate meglumine and diatrizoate sodium (Renografin), a radiograph can be obtained immediately thereafter to confirm the location of the injection in relation to the suspicious lesion. The patient is transferred directly to the operating room, the breast is explored, and the area where methylene blue was deposited is excised. If calcification was present, the specimen is sent to radiology for specimen radiography to ensure that the area of calcification was removed.

SEX STEROID BINDING

The ability of tumor cells to bind sex steroids, both estrogen and progesterone, should be established in all cases of malignancy. This information may be important in selection of subsequent therapy. Fresh tissue is necessary for the study. A portion of tissue measuring 1×1 cm and weighing 1 g is desirable. It is frozen in liquid nitrogen or dry ice. Either a biopsy specimen may be studied or a portion of tumor may be removed from the breast immediately after its resection. Inordinate delay may cause a decrease in the level of binding and a spurious result.

A strategy must be established to ensure that data on binding will be obtained in all cases of cancer. When an incisional biopsy is performed and a frozen section reveals cancer, a portion of the tissue can be frozen and used for studies of sex steroid binding. When an excisional biopsy is performed, the pathologist should be the individual to determine whether a frozen section is indicated. Should gross examination lead to the conclusion of benign disease and a frozen section is not performed but the final sections reveal cancer, the opportunity to establish the level of sex steroid binding will have been lost. If the diagnosis of cancer was established by needle aspiration or biopsy, binding can be studied on tissue removed during resectional surgery.

Interest has developed regarding clonogenic assays of tumor tissue. Tumor cells are grown in tissue culture and the resultant clone of cells is exposed to a variety of chemotherapeutic agents to determine which agents inhibit proliferation of the tumor. The clinical value of the clonogenic assay is not established. If the technique becomes a clinical routine, tissue required for the study can be obtained as for estrogen binding.

OTHER TESTS

Cannulation of the ducts through the papilla for ductograms or to obtain cells for cytology is painful for the patient, is of unproved diagnostic accuracy, and has not been widely employed. Ultrasound of the breast can diagnose a cyst but is not precise in distinguishing benign from malignant solid lesions. Neoplasms generate heat, but thermography has not proved to be particularly useful because of poor sensitivity and specificity.

PATHOPHYSIOLOGIC DISTURBANCES (NON-NEOPLASTIC)

GYNECOMASTIA

Gynecomastia is enlargement of the breast in the male, which is most often a proliferative response of rudimentary mammary tissue to the evolving hormonal milieu of the adolescent. The enlargement is central and may be unilateral or bilateral. The mechanism leading to a unilateral response to systemic stimulus has not been identified. Spontaneous regression usually occurs. If the degree of enlargement causes serious embarrassment, plastic reconstruction is justified. Comparable transient mammary enlargement, associated with the male menopause and termed *senescent gynecomastia,* may be observed in older males.

Gynecomastia may occur with primary Klinefelter's syndrome (testicular atrophy), secondary Klinefelter's syndrome of advanced hepatic disease, certain genetic disorders of abnormal sexual development, the hyperestrogenic state (endogenous or exogenous), any disease leading to testicular atrophy, or as a response to drugs such as digitalis and marijuana.

CHRONIC CYSTIC MASTITIS (C.C.M.)

A variety of pathologic processes may develop in the breast consequent to the cyclic hormonal stimulation that occurs during the years of active ovarian function. Referred to as CCM, these changes probably reflect repeated hypertrophy followed by incomplete involution. Most students believe that the process reflects an imbalance in the mammary response to stimulation by estrogens, progestins, and prolactin. More recently, unproved claims have been made that caffeine induces CCM.

Both epithelial and stromal proliferation occur in CCM. Cysts may form that vary from 1 mm to 2 mm to several centimeters in diameter. Multiple microcysts are referred to as Schimmelbusch's disease. Larger cysts may appear blue on visual examination (*i.e.,* the blue-domed cyst of Bloodgood). When epithelial proliferation predominates, the term *sclerosing adenosis* is employed. This process may be difficult to distinguish histologically from carcinoma. Predominant stromal proliferation is referred to as *fibrous dysplasia.* Proliferation of ducts without acini is termed *blunt duct adenosis.* Apocrine metaplasia of ductal epithelium may occur.

The term *chronic cystic mastitis* is not truly descriptive of this wide diversity of pathology. Although the disease is chronic, cystic manifestations may not be predominant and the disease is certainly not inflammatory. Despite these disclaimers, the term is understood and has been used for decades. Physicians generally understand the pathology that is under discussion when one refers to "chronic cystic mastitis" or "cystic disease." The clinical manifestations of CCM are seen almost exclusively in the menstruating female and are most unusual after the menopause. Mastodynia may be severe.

Physical examination of the breasts of women with CCM usually reveals a feeling of fullness and diffuse nodularity, (*i.e.,* a "lumpy" breast). A predominant mass may be noted. If the mass is a cyst, it is usually well demarcated, smooth, and movable. The proper treatment of a cyst is aspiration

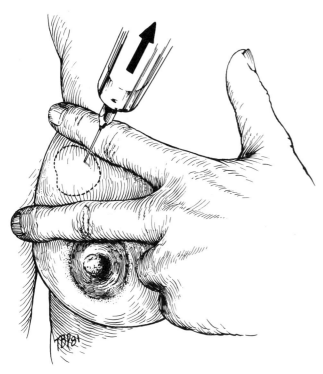

Fig. 19-10. A cyst is fixed between the fingers and aspirated.

(Fig. 19-10). The cyst fluid is straw colored in cystic mastopathy. Cytologic examination of the aspirated cyst fluid is rarely of diagnostic benefit. If the aspirate is bloody, should the cyst recur within days of aspiration or the mass lesion not disappear completely after aspiration, a suspicion of cyst cancer must arise. Excision with histologic confirmation of the nature of the mass is then necessary.

Unresolved controversy exists regarding the relationship of CCM and mammary cancer. This cannot be settled on the basis of the histologic identification of the simultaneous presence of both diseases. Histologic evidence of CCM may be present in about three fourths of women, even those over the age of 70. Therefore, histologically, CCM and cancer occur simultaneously in the vast majority of cases. A clinical approach would be the determination of the incidence of cancer in patients previously treated for CCM. Haagensen found this incidence to be increased by a factor of four among 1,693 patients who had been treated for CCM.

Detection of cancer can be difficult in the patient with diffuse CCM and "lumpy breasts." The results of mammography may not be reliable. A solid mass lesion that persists unchanged throughout the menstrual cycle is suspect and requires a precise histologic diagnosis. The selection of patients with CCM for breast biopsy can be difficult. If at least one fourth of patients who submit to open biopsy do not have a neoplasm, the physician is not discriminating enough in his selection of cases for biopsy.

Mastodynia is usually controlled by analgesics. Androgenic steroids may relieve pain, but their use cannot be justified because of resultant masculinization and increased libido. Danazol, a synthetic androgen that suppresses both luteinizing hormone and follicle-stimulating hormone, has become popular in treatment of mastodynia. It is only mildly androgenic. Danazol is recommended not only to relieve

mastodynia but also to induce regression of CCM. The latter action has not been proven.

MAMMARY DUCT ECTASIA

Mammary duct ectasia is a disease of the involuting breast. The collecting ducts in the subareolar area are dilated and are filled with cellular debris. The contents of the ducts gain access to the periductal tissues and initiate an intense response that is quite comparable to plasma cell mastitis. Mammary duct ectasia is associated with pain and tenderness. Nipple inversion and dermal fixation can occur. Breakdown of tissue can result in small cystic cavities. Therapy is excisional. At the time of excision, variable numbers of dilated ducts are encountered. These are filled with sebaceous-appearing material that oozes from transected ducts like toothpaste.

In the nursing woman, a ductal opening may become obstructed and a galactocele may form.

FAT NECROSIS

An area of fat necrosis may occur anywhere in the breast as a mass lesion. An ecchymosis, presumed to be a reflection of the trauma that produced the necrosis, may be present. A history of trauma is obtained in only about one half of the cases. The histologic picture is quite comparable to that of advanced stages of mammary duct ectasia and of plasma cell mastitis. The exact interrelationship between trauma causing fat necrosis, advanced stages of mammary duct ectasia, and plasma cell mastitis is not precisely defined. Each can cause skin dimpling and all are very firm lesions that can masquerade clinically as a cancer.

USUALLY BENIGN NEOPLASMS

FIBROADENOMA

Fibroadenoma is the most common mammary neoplasm in women under 25 years of age. It rarely is diagnosed following menopause. The tumor has some degree of hormonal dependence, as evidenced by reports of more rapid growth during pregnancy and of epithelial proliferation in fibroadenomas excised from women taking oral contraceptives. The tumor may be multiple and bilateral. The fibroadenoma is rubbery, firm, and nonencapsulated. Sharply demarcated from surrounding mammary tissue, the cut surface bulges when hemisectioned. There is a varying preponderance of connective tissue and epithelial elements. When detected, the tumor is usually 2 to 4 cm in diameter. Treatment consists of enucleation.

On occasion, a fibroadenoma attains great size and is termed a *giant* fibroadenoma. The precise size that warrants this description is not defined.

CYSTOSARCOMA PHYLLODES

Cystosarcoma phyllodes (leaflike) is a term applied to a tumor that is not necessarily cystic and in the majority of cases is not malignant. It may represent progression from a preexisting fibroadenoma and has epithelial and stromal elements.

The diagnosis of cystosarcoma phyllodes is based primarily on a high degree of cellularity of the stroma with hyperchromatic nuclei and some mitoses, a pattern not seen in a giant fibroadenoma. The peak incidence of cystosarcoma phyllodes is near the menopause. The tumor may measure less than 5 cm in diameter but frequently attains great size (20 cm to 30 cm in diameter).

A cystosarcoma phyllodes is not encapsulated, and microscopic projections of tumor penetrate the surrounding breast. Thus, enucleation may lead to recurrence. The tumor should always be removed with a rim of surrounding breast tissue. In the very large tumors, this will usually require a simple mastectomy. If the tumor lies on the pectoral fascia, at the least the fascia should be removed. The distinction between a fibroadenoma and cystoadenoma phyllodes cannot be made on gross examination. An incisional biopsy of a tumor greater than 3 cm in diameter may distinguish the two on frozen section and lead to enucleation of the former and wide excision of the latter.

Cystosarcoma phyllodes may manifest a malignant behavior. Metastases occur in about 10% of cases; local invasion is considered evidence of malignancy. The metastases are almost invariably of the mesothelial elements and are blood borne. A histologic pattern that assures identification of the tumor that is capable of metastasizing does not exist. Lymph nodes are not involved, and regional node dissections are not indicated.

INTRADUCTAL PAPILLOMA

Intraductal papilloma occurs in one of the major ducts, generally in the juxta-areolar area of the premenopausal or juxtamenopausal patient. The tumor is usually only 1 mm to 2 mm in diameter, soft, and friable and bleeds easily. The hallmark of intraductal papilloma is serous or bloody discharge from the nipple. If the tumor is as large as 3 mm to 4 mm, it may be palpable beneath the areola. Rarely, a diffuse process defined as papillomatosis of the ducts occurs. The incidence of malignancy is increased.

OTHER BENIGN NEOPLASMS

Benign tumors may arise from any of the mesodermal cells present in the breast. Apocrine gland tumors may occur. Granular cell myoblastoma occurs on rare occasion. When epithelial proliferation predominates, the term *sclerosing adenosis* frequently is employed by pathologists. Islands of glandular cells exist amid extensive fibrous tissue and can easily be confused with cancer.

INFLAMMATORY PROCESSES

Acute infections of the breast (acute mastitis) are most often related to lactation. The offending organism probably enters the breast through a crack in the nipple. Diffuse streptococcal cellulitis may occur, or an abscess may form, most frequently due to staphylococcal infection. The abscess tends to be deep within the breast substance and multilocular. It may extend into the retromammary space, and accurate diagnosis can be hard to make initially.

Appropriate antibiotic therapy is indicated in the treatment of bacterial infections of the breast. Inadequate drainage can follow simple incision into the surface presentation of a multilocular mammary abscess. General anesthesia is

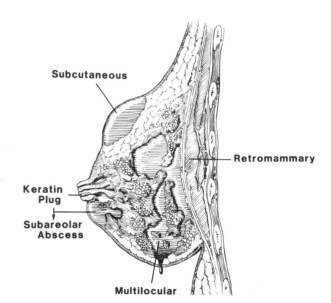

Fig. 19-11. Breast abscess. The keratin plug blocks the excretory duct in a case of recurrent subareolar abscess. The multilocular nature of breast abscess is emphasized.

required to break down adequately the septums that separate loculations of the abscess and to establish drainage.

Recurrent subareolar abscess (Fig. 19-11) occurs most commonly in younger women. One or more milk sinuses located just beneath the nipple undergo squamous metaplasia and become plugged with keratin. There is tissue breakdown and abscess formation. A sinus may form following either spontaneous or surgical drainage. Recurrence is the rule. Definitive treatment consists of excision of the involved sinus and the excretory duct through a circumareolar incision. Salient features concerning breast abscesses are shown in Figure 19-11.

Thrombophlebitis of the superficial thoracoepigastric vein is known as Mondor's disease. The thoracoepigastric vein extends from the hypochondrium upward on the lateral aspect of the breast to the anterior axillary line. The etiology of Mondor's disease is not known. The process is usually self-limited.

NIPPLE DISCHARGE

Serous nipple discharge is due to duct papilloma in about three fourths of cases and to the use of oral contraceptives, to CCM and, rarely, to malignancy in the remainder.

Blood in nipple discharge is due to duct papilloma in over three fourths of cases, but it may be seen during pregnancy and is occasionally due to cancer.

In addition to the postpartum state, trauma to the chest wall and breast manipulation may cause lactorrhea. Drugs (phenothiazines, methyldopa, and oral contraceptives), hypothyroidism, and pituitary necrosis can also be associated with lactorrhea. The galactorrhea/amenorrhea syndrome accounts for about one fourth of cases of nonpuerpural galactorrhea and is due to a prolactin-secreting tumor of the pituitary gland. The pituitary adenoma may be chromophilic or acidophilic. The diagnosis can be confirmed by documentation of elevated serum prolactin by radioimmunoassay, by tomographic demonstration of a pituitary tumor, or by both measures. The tumor is usually a microadenoma.

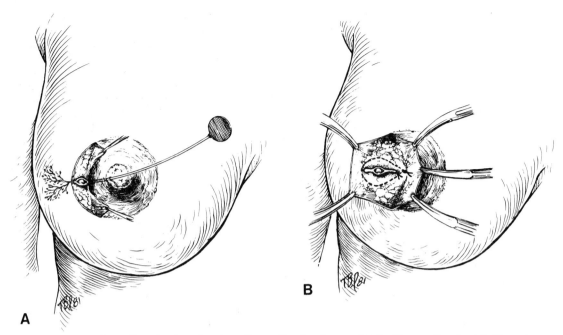

Fig. 19-12. Surgical excision of an intraductal papilloma. The duct is cannulated with a small probe (*A*). Through a circumareolar incision, the duct containing the papilloma and immediately surrounding tissue is excised (*B*).

The breast is examined to detect the site of nipple discharge (see Fig. 19-7). If a mass is not palpable, a mammogram is obtained to identify a covert tumor. The technique of duct exploration for intraductal papilloma, the most common cause of serous or bloody discharge from a duct, is shown in Figure 19-12. Only the duct containing the papilloma needs to be excised and not the entire plica of ducts or a large wedge of breast.

CANCER OF THE BREAST

EPIDEMIOLOGY AND ETIOLOGY

The breast is the most frequent site of cancer among women. The diagnosis will be made in approximately 1 of 10 women now alive, about one half of whom will ultimately die of the disease. In actual numbers, approximately 90,000 new cases of breast cancer are diagnosed annually in the United States and almost 40,000 women die of breast cancer each year. Despite intense efforts to achieve diagnosis at an early biologic stage of the disease and to provide optimal treatment, the age-adjusted death rate has not changed greatly in the past 50 years. Cancer of the breast is more likely in white than in black women and is more often seen in the Western culture.

The etiology of breast cancer is unknown, but a number of factors—hereditary, biologic, and environmental—are either known or suspected to be related to its occurrence.

HEREDITARY

A woman with a strong family history of breast cancer is at markedly increased risk. A strong family history is one wherein multiple members of the same or preceding generations have had breast cancer. Under such circumstances, the likelihood of the development of breast cancer is certainly more than doubled. A sporadic case of breast cancer within a family does not significantly increase risk.

BIOLOGIC

The known biologic events that affect the incidence of breast cancer are largely hormonal in nature. Breast cancer is more frequent in nulliparous females, women with menarche before age 12, or with late menopause. This observation suggests that a longer duration of hormonal stimulation is deleterious. Conversely, the incidence of breast cancer may be decreased with early menopause or in the woman who has lactated. A woman who has less than three pregnancies or whose first child is born after she has reached the age of 30 has a somewhat greater risk for the development of breast cancer. The frequency of breast cancer may be somewhat higher in women who have cancer of the ovary or uterine corpus. The most common precursor of breast cancer is breast cancer. The incidence of bilateral clinically overt breast cancer is about 14%—7% synchronous and 7% developing subsequent to the initial diagnosis.

The relationship between CCM and breast cancer is unclear. Occasionally the pathologist will identify such a degree of dysplasia and cellular atypia on a portion of breast removed as a biopsy and diagnosed as CCM that he is concerned about malignancy, either synchronous or as a subsequent event. He may recommend, at the least, extremely careful follow-up or, at the most, prophylactic mastectomy.

The role of endogenous estrogens and progestational agents in the genesis of breast cancer has been studied extensively in the animal laboratory and in larger population groups. These studies are important because of the use of the Pill for contraception and the widespread administration of estrogen steroids in the treatment of the menopausal syndrome. Some evidence exists that the Pill may reduce the incidence of CCM and of epithelial atypia. In laboratory animals, large doses of estrogens can promote the development of mammary cancer. A similar relationship has not been proven in humans. The fact that estrogenic hormones can deleteriously affect the behavior of established breast cancer has focused attention, perhaps inappropriately, on their role in genesis of the disease.

ENVIRONMENTAL

Few environmental factors are known to increase or decrease the risk of breast cancer. Several studies have suggested that administration of reserpine increases the likelihood of breast cancer, but this has not been proven. Trauma has also not been shown to result in the development of breast cancer.

NATURAL HISTORY

PATTERN OF GROWTH

Cancer of the breast is protean in its manifestation and extraordinarily variable in course. The disease is not identical in any two cases. The terms *early* and *late* can be imprecise. *Early* usually refers to a small tumor of the breast, perhaps called "minimal" if less than 1 cm in diameter and without demonstrable metastases; *late* refers to tumor disseminated to either regional lymph nodes or distant organs and less often to extensive mammary tumor. In fact, tumors less than 1 cm in size may be overtly disseminated, whereas a large tumor of the breast may have invaded skin and chest wall without, as yet, regional or distant metastases. The concept of slow doubling times suggests that a tumor has been present for several years before becoming overt. The rate of growth may vary at different times in the course of the disease.

The traditional concept of progression of breast cancer was that the tumor developed in the breast and spread first to involve regional lymph nodes, either by lymphatic permeation or embolization. Hematogenous dissemination was considered a late manifestation, with involvement of solid viscera, such as liver, lungs, brain, or bone. Most authorities now acknowledge that this conceptualization of the spread of breast cancer is an oversimplification. Lymph nodes may be involved by direct extension, but, alternatively, viable tumor cells entering the lymphatics may be shunted into venous channels and the lymph nodes may be seeded by cells arriving through the arterial blood supply. The exact role of the regional lymph nodes has not been established: are the nodes a mechanical filter or an immunologically protective barrier or both? Are the nodes deficient and in some instances preferentially seeded? Lymph node metastasis may be the only overt sign of spread of breast cancer.

The nodes in the axilla may not be invaded by breast cancer in a stepwise fashion, beginning with the external mammary nodes and progressing to the central nodes and into the apex of the axilla. Most often, the central nodes are involved first. Invasion of the internal mammary nodes usually occurs after the tumor has spread to the axillary nodes. Only about 15% of cancers located in the medial quadrants with negative axillary nodes have tumor in the internal mammary nodes; about one third of such patients with tumor in the axillary nodes will have tumor in the internal mammary nodes. When the internal mammary nodes contain cancer, the tumor may invade the medial intercostal space and be observed as a parasternal mass.

The axillary nodes are conveniently described as being at level I, lateral to the lateral border of the pectoralis minor muscle; level II, between the lateral and medial borders of the muscle; and level III, between the medial border of the pectoralis minor and the apex of the axilla. Auchincloss, many years ago, reported that apical (level III) and interpectoral (level II) nodes may be involved without involvement of level I nodes.

Warwich established that breast tissue can project into the pectoral fascia. Lymphatics may pass through the muscle. Tumor cells are not found in lymphatic channels within the pectoralis major muscle. If the muscle is not removed during treatment of breast cancer, recurrence that can be attributed to failure to remove intramuscular lymph channels is essentially unrecognized. The nodes between the pectoralis major and minor muscles (*i.e.*, Rotter's nodes) receive lymph both by the transpectoral route and from lymphatics that pass around the lateral border of the pectoralis major muscle. Thus, their impregnation by breast cancer does not always mean that transpectoral spread has occurred.

Hematogenous dissemination of tumor may occur early in the course of the disease. The current popular theory conceptualizes that breast cancer is systemic in most cases by the time the tumor is palpable. This is certainly true in those cases in which disseminated disease becomes apparent only after a free interval during which local therapy has successfully controlled local disease.

The appearance of distal metastases or the local recrudescence of cancer may be delayed for weeks, months, years, or decades following treatment of the primary tumor, a highly variable "free interval." Proliferation of covertly disseminated tumor or of microscopic foci of cancer in the mammary area is delayed by unrecognized host factors generally accepted to be immune in nature and referred to as "host resistance." The behavior of the tumor reflects the balance between biologic aggressiveness of the tumor and this immune response. One example of disruption of the delicate balance between host and tumor is the rapid progression of previously covert cancer that can be observed in a pregnant woman. The alteration in hormonal environment during pregnancy may disrupt the delicate balance between tumor and host.

Breast cancer may manifest an inexorable progression. MacDonald wrote extensively with respect to "biological predeterminism." Carried to its ultimate conclusion, the Calvinistic concept of biologic predeterminism states that when a patient develops breast cancer, the disease's course is already determined; the tumor may never be fully eradicated, although therapy may alter the course of the disease. This course may be highly varied and protracted; the patient may die of another cause before the cancer progresses, but if life were prolonged enough, the cancer would still be present.

Despite wide acceptance of the concept of early dissemination of breast cancer and of biologic predeterminism, the local treatment of tumor overtly localized to the breast and regional lymph nodes is, in approximately one-half of patients, followed by prolonged survival without breast cancer. Death results from some other disease. Survival declines in direct relationship to the extent of axillary node involvement as reflected in Table 19-2. One must be careful not to be so mesmerized with the concept of early dissemination and of predeterminism that one ignores the achievements of the past century in local treatment of breast cancer. These conjectures must not become the basis for therapeutic nihilism. Some of the results of numerous excellent clinical trials are reflected in Table 19-3 and have also been summarized by Fisher.

The course of disease that is progressive is highly variable.

TABLE 19-2   SURVIVAL OF PATIENTS WITH BREAST CANCER RELATIVE TO CLINICAL AND HISTOLOGIC STAGE

CLINICAL STAGING (AMERICAN JOINT COMMITTEE)	CRUDE 5-YR SURVIVAL (%)	RANGE OF SURVIVAL (%)
Stage I	85	82–94
Tumor <2 cm in diameter		
Nodes, if present, not felt to contain metastases		
Without distant metastases		
Stage II	66	47–74
Tumors <5 cm in diameter		
Nodes, if palpable, not fixed		
Without distant metastases		
Stage III	41	7–80
Tumor >5 cm or,		
Tumor any size with invasion of skin or attached to chest wall		
Nodes in supraclavicular area		
Without distant metastases		
Stage IV	10	
With distant metastases		

HISTOLOGIC STAGING (NSABP)	CRUDE SURVIVAL (%) 5 Yr	CRUDE SURVIVAL (%) 10 Yr	5-YR DISEASE-FREE SURVIVAL (%)
All patients	63.5	45.9	60.3
Negative axillary lymph nodes	78.1	64.9	82.3
Positive axillary lymph nodes	46.5	24.9	34.9
1–3 positive axillary lymph nodes	62.2	37.5	50.0
>4 positive axillary lymph nodes	32.0	13.4	21.1

NSABP, National Surgical Adjuvant Breast Project
(Henderson IC, Canellos GP: Cancer of the breast: The past decade: I. N Engl J Med 302:18, 1980)

TABLE 19-3   A COMPARISON OF SURVIVAL RELATIVE TO TREATMENT METHOD AMONG PATIENTS COMPARATIVELY STAGED

STUDY	TREATMENT REGIMEN	CRUDE SURVIVAL AT 10 YR (%) Stage A Patients	Stage B Patients
Miller	Simple mastectomy + 1000 rads	40	26
Handley	Conservative radical mastectomy	61	25
Butcher	Radical mastectomy ± radiotherapy*	56	30
Haagensen	Radical mastectomy ± radiotherapy*	70	40
Dahl-Iverson	Extended radical mastectomy ± radiotherapy*	57	24
Kaae	Simple mastectomy + 4200 rads	50	32
		Axillary Node Negative	Axillary Node Positive
Handley	Conservative radical mastectomy	75	35
Haagensen	Radical mastectomy ± radiotherapy	75	38

* Radiotherapy for selected patients
(Henderson IC, Canellos GP: Cancer of the breast: The past decade: I. N Engl J Med 302:22, 1980)

In some cases, the disease always remains regional in its clinical manifestations. Tumor that is initially not resectable or recurs following surgery may invade the chest wall, extend into the pleural space, become apparent in regional nodes, or spread to involve the opposite breast, or all of the above may occur. Diffuse nodules, referred to as lenticular metastases, may develop on the skin of the ipsilateral chest, contralateral breast, and chest wall, both anterior and posterior. Recurrence of tumor in the scar from a mastectomy almost always means that tumor was transected and tumor cells were seeded into the wound during the operation. Too often, it reflects ill-advised surgery. Extension around the entire circumference of the chest (en cuirasse tumor) may rarely occur. Ulceration, necrosis, and bleeding are the hallmarks of these forms of locally invasive disease. In other cases, local control has been achieved and visceral dissemination to the liver, lungs, and brain may be the dominant pattern. Osseous metastasis is the dominant course in a third group, often with local control. Permutations of all of the above can be seen. The majority of patients with breast cancer will ultimately manifest progressive cancer, if one considers those with advanced disease when first seen and those with disease recrudescent at a variable interval following primary treatment.

HORMONE SENSITIVITY

Beeston, in 1893, observed that removal of the ovaries resulted in regression of breast cancer. Subsequent experience with hormonal manipulation in patients with breast cancer has established that in about one third of cases the tumor is hormone dependent, that is, regression of cancer occurs consequent to alteration in the hormonal environment. In the past, methods did not exist to identify the tumors that were hormone dependent. The development of techniques to determine the ability of mammary cancer to bind estrogen and progestins has greatly facilitated the identification of the patient with a hormonally dependent tumor. Exactly why some tumors bind sex steroid is not known but such binding and its relationship to tumor behavior are believed to be related to receptors on the cytoplasmic membrane of the tumor which will bind steroids. Binding occurs in normal mammary cells. When malignant transformation occurs, some tumors retain this ability to bind hormones and others do not. If the ability to bind is retained, the tumor may respond as would the normal cell to hormonal stimulation.

The level of binding which is considered positive and negative is arbitrarily selected based on the levels of binding observed in patients whose tumors have been determined to be hormonally dependent by observation of their response to empirically selected hormonal therapy. The level can be expressed as femtimoles per gram of wet tissue or of cytosol protein. Currently, binding for estrogen is considered positive at most laboratories at a level of 5 fmol/mg cytosol protein whereas the level of positivity for progestin is in many instances considered to be 10 fmol/mg of cytosol protein. About two thirds of cases of breast cancer are positive for estrogen binding (ER +) and the majority of these will also bind progestins (PR +). Most of the remaining third of cases will not bind either estrogen (ER −) or progestin (PR −). A very small number of cases are ER − and PR +.

Correlation of sex steroid binding and response to hormonal therapy applies to surgical or pharmacologic suppression of estrogens, administration of estrogens to postmeno-pausal females, and administration of androgens and progestins. About two thirds of cases that bind both estrogen and progestin (ER +, PR +) have a cancer that will respond favorably to hormonal manipulation, whereas slightly less than one half of cases are hormone dependent if estrogen receptor positive and progestin receptor negative (ER +; PR −). The likelihood of hormone dependence in ER − patients is less than 10%. Evidence suggests that the majority of these responders are the small group that is ER −, PR +. Thus, determination of progestin receptors may help to identify a small group of cases that are estrogen receptor negative and hormone dependent. This may be the greatest usefulness of determination of progestin receptors. Evidence exists to suggest that cases that are estrogen receptor negative may have a generally poorer prognosis.

Administration of estrogens may accelerate the rate of growth of breast cancer in the premenopausal patient. For that reason estrogens are not administered to a patient who has been treated for breast cancer until after at least 5 years of disease-free survival. The same prohibition should be applied to pregnancy. Lifelong avoidance of endogenous estrogen is preferred.

PATHOLOGY

Cancer of the breast may arise from cells lining the ducts, including the myoepithelial layer, or from cells in the breast lobule. The tumor is located in the upper outer quadrant in almost one half of cases and in the juxta-areolar area in another one fourth. The final one fourth of cases are randomly distributed in the remainder of the breast. An accepted pathologic classification of adenocarcinoma of the breast that is based on both the cellular origin of the tumor and its morphology is as follows:

  I. Paget's Disease of the Nipple
  II. Duct Origin
    A. In situ (noninfiltrating, intraductal)
    B. Infiltrating
      1. Scirrhous
      2. Medullary
      3. Comedo
      4. Papillary
      5. Colloid
      6. Tubular
  III. Lobular Origin
    A. In situ
    B. Infiltrating

PAGET'S DISEASE

Adenocarcinoma of the breast in which the tumor cells invade the nipple is called Paget's disease. The tumor grows out from the excretory ducts onto the nipple to produce a lesion resembling eczema. The underlying cancer may not be palpable in many cases but is always present. Biopsy of the nipple will reveal Paget cells, which are large with clear cytoplasm and small dark nuclei. When these vacuolated cells are seen, the diagnosis of Paget's disease is established, irrespective of whether the underlying tumor is felt. The prognosis is better in patients without a palpable mass.

DUCT CELL ORIGIN

About 75% of cases of breast cancer are infiltrating lesions arising from the duct cell, perhaps the myoepithelial layer. A scirrhous pattern predominates. The tumor provokes a proliferative fibrous reaction and is gritty and gray, with white chalk streaks reflecting desmoplastic areas. On cut surface, tentacles extending into the surrounding breast are noted. Such an infiltrating, rather than pushing, margin is associated with a poorer prognosis. Anaplastic tumors and those with vascular invasion also have a poorer prognosis. Microscopic invasion of the nipple can occur, even with more peripheral tumors. Medullary, comedo, papillary, colloid, and tubular cancers, all of duct cell origin, are less common, and each has a more favorable prognosis than the usual scirrhous cancer. Medullary cancer has diffuse lymphocytic infiltration. In comedocarcinoma, the ducts are plugged with cellular debris, which on cut surface protrudes from the ducts and resembles comedones ("blackheads").

LOBULAR CARCINOMA

Lobular carcinoma is often *in situ,* and the infiltrating variant has a more favorable prognosis than cancer of duct cell origin. Haagensen prefers the term *lobular neoplasia* to lobular carcinoma *in situ* for the noninfiltrating lesion because of its very low biologic potential. Lobular neoplasms, particularly the *in situ* lesions, may be diagnosed at the time of breast biopsy for another purpose, such as a suspicious lesion in CCM. In cases of lobular neoplasms, it has become customary to perform a mirror image biopsy of the opposite breast. This will reveal a lobular carcinoma *in situ* in about three fourths of patients. The biologic significance of the *in situ* lesions, identified serendipitously during biopsy for another purpose or on biopsy of the opposite breast, has not been proven. These may be dominantly "pathologists' cancers," which will rarely attain clinical significance.

Therapy as aggressive as bilateral mastectomy has been recommended by some for a case of lobular neoplasm documented in both breasts whether infiltrating or *in situ.* Haagensen, who is hardly recognized as a conservative in the advocacy of resectional therapy of breast cancer, considers this to be far too aggressive therapy. Rather, he recommends repeated examinations of the breast with an *in situ* neoplasm as well as annual mammography. Infiltrating cancer will become manifest in about 15% of patients and is as likely to be in one breast as the other. An infiltrating lobular cancer should be treated like any other cancer.

SARCOMA

Sarcoma of the breast is rare. The most common sarcoma is the malignant form of cystosarcoma phyllodes.

BILATERAL CANCER

The incidence of bilaterality of breast cancer must be considered both in terms of clinical manifestation and pathologic diagnosis. As noted previously, overt cancer develops in the opposite breast of a woman with breast cancer in about 14% of cases; 7% is synchronous with the initial diagnosis and 7% occurs during subsequent follow-up. If one performs serial whole organ sections of the opposite breast in a patient with proved breast cancer, a small foci that will justify a pathologic diagnosis of cancer will be found in almost all patients, not only those with lobular carcinoma. These lesions are generally "pathologists' cancer" and will never attain clinical significance in the patient's lifetime. The incidence of clinical bilaterality is not high enough to warrant routine bilateral mastectomy in the treatment of breast cancer. The opposite breast should be followed closely.

PREGNANCY

Breast cancer that develops during pregnancy may be overlooked because of the already profound changes taking place in the breasts. Any solid mass detected in the breast during a pregnancy must be promptly biopsied. More cases of cancer will be at an advanced stage at the time of diagnosis, and the prognosis for the group as a whole is poor. For the few fortunate cases without lymph node involvement, the prognosis is comparable to that for the nonpregnant patient at the same stage of disease. For cases with dissemination, including lymph node metastasis, the hormonal environment of pregnancy and lactation is provocative of aggressive tumor growth. Lactation should be promptly suppressed in the postpartum patient with breast cancer.

OCCURRENCE IN MALES

Less than 1% of breast cancer occurs in males. It carries a poor prognosis consequent to a high incidence of local invasion when first seen and a high incidence of lymph node metastasis. The tumors are hormone dependent in a higher percentage of cases than in the female. Orchiectomy and estrogenic steroids may induce remission, either alone or in combination.

INFLAMMATORY CANCER

An inflammatory cancer of the breast is a specific type of tumor which is highly aggressive and invades the dermal lymphatics. The skin appearance is that of a streptococcal cellulitis. The process is painful. Surgery promotes the spread of inflammatory cancer. This lesion is to be distinguished from direct extension of a tumor into the skin, which may create an area of redness, from necrosis of tumor with secondary infection, from "peau d'orange," or from the rare instance of breast abscess developing behind an obstructive cancer of the ducts.

CLASSIFICATION: STAGING

Several systems have been developed for the clinical staging of breast cancer. The T, N, and M system adopted by the American Joint Committee on Staging in 1977 has become the standard system (see Chapter 14). The varying combinations of T, N, and M are grouped into stages I through IV in a functionally useful fashion. The Columbia Clinical Classification was formerly quite widely employed and its stages A through D are quite similar to the stages I through IV of the Joint Commission schema.

Any clinical system for staging for breast cancer carries an inherent error of major importance. In about one third of cases of breast cancer in which clinical examination of the axilla by an experienced examiner fails to reveal palpable lymph nodes, tumor will be found in the nodes when they are examined microscopically. Conversely, in about one fourth of cases in which nodes are palpable in the axilla, and the clinical staging is Stage II, the palpable nodes when examined by the pathologist will not be found to contain tumor. Thus, comparison of cases of breast cancer cases staged clinically with another cohort staged by pathologic examination carries an enormous inherent error and renders comparison of small groups highly suspect. Furthermore, comparison of two groups, both staged clinically, will be suspect if the groups are small. Inaccuracy of staging is magnified with an inexperienced examiner.

PRETREATMENT EVALUATION

The patient must be evaluated to determine as accurately as possible the clinical stage of the disease before therapeutic recommendations are made. In addition to physical examination, mammography of the opposite breast is performed in a search for occult contralateral tumor. A chest radiograph is essential. The serum alkaline phosphatase level is determined. Neither radiographs nor radioisotope scans of bone, liver, or brain are performed routinely. Should the patient complain of bone pain, an isotope scan of the skeleton is performed. Abnormal results of liver function tests, particularly an elevation of the level of alkaline phosphatase, are an indication for liver scan. A brain scan is performed if the findings of the history or physical examination arouse any suspicion of brain metastases. These are the usual routine procedures for clinical staging for Stage I, II, and III breast cancer. If, for any reason, the disease is suspected to be Stage IV when first seen or is recurrent following initial therapy, bone and liver scans are performed routinely. Standard chest radiographs and at least a bone scan are obtained before any major new direction in therapy is undertaken. The role of computed tomography in staging is not yet defined and CT scans are employed selectively.

Radioisotope scans are more frequently performed for identification of osseous metastases than are standard radiographs. Areas of increased activity on isotope scan should be confirmed as lytic or blastic metastases by radiograph. Areas of inflammation, such as arthritis, may show increased activity by isotope scan. The isotope scan has the advantage of screening the entire skeleton. Radiographs are usually taken of only the skull, ribs, spine, and pelvis. Other bones are not examined in the absence of symptoms. An area of persistent osseous pain with a negative isotope scan should be examined by standard radiographs. A metastasis is on rare occasion visible on the radiograph that was not seen by isotope scan.

TREATMENT MODALITIES

In the past, the treatment of a woman with a mass in the breast suggestive of cancer, and without overt dissemination, most often consisted of open biopsy under general anesthesia, frozen section examination, and a form of mastectomy if cancer was diagnosed. Several reports demonstrated that a delay of 2 weeks or more between biopsy and surgery did not alter the prognosis. Increasingly in recent years, the patient wishes to know the exact diagnosis and to discuss therapeutic options before definitive therapy is initiated. In some states, including Massachusetts and California, the physician must by law discuss these options with the patient. Increasingly, the practice is to establish the diagnosis by one of the biopsy techniques previously described. Therapy is then discussed with the patient and her family.

Four forms of therapy are employed in the treatment of breast cancer: (1) surgery, (2) radiation therapy, (3) chemotherapy, and (4) hormonal manipulation. The former two are local therapy; the latter two are systemic in effect. Immunotherapy has not been established as an efficacious therapy. The vast majority of cases of breast cancer will receive multiple forms of therapy during the course of the disease. Formerly, surgery was the preeminent form of therapy for disease overtly limited to the breast and ipsilateral axilla. Currently, the advantages of all forms of therapy are considered and therapy is often multimodal. When multi-

modal initial therapy is employed, the practice has been to consider surgery primary and other therapy adjunctive. The term *conjunctive* for all forms of therapy is probably more appropriate.

SURGERY

Extirpation is a traditional form of therapy for a tumor of the breast. It was employed in ancient Egypt and Rome, and the modern era in surgical treatment of breast cancer dates from the end of the 19th century when Drs. William Stewart Halsted and Herbert Willy Meyer reported on the results of radical mastectomy in the treatment of breast cancer. This "complete" operation consists of elevation of thin skin flaps and removal of the entire breast, the underlying pectoral fascia and muscles, and the ipsilateral axillary contents (Fig. 19-13). The operation was based on a meticulous study of the lymphatic extension of breast cancer. Resection of muscles was advised to remove a potential site of local extension and to permit a more complete axillary dissection. Prior to the adoption of radical mastectomy, local failure occurred in the majority of cases following initial treatment of breast cancer. Halsted's early cases had at least Stage II and in most instances Stage III disease with a 100% incidence of axillary node metastasis. The Halsted radical mastectomy resulted in a survival at 3 years of approximately one half of patients selected for the operation, with local failure in a small minority. This record in local control of the disease was a monumental achievement. Radical mastectomy became the standard form of therapy for breast cancer.

Latter-day critics of Halsted and radical mastectomy often ignore the fact that Halsted never heard of a mammogram and would never have seen what is commonly referred to today as "minimal" breast cancer. Radiation therapy and chemotherapy were unknown modalities. That Halsted's knowledge of the mechanism of lymphatic permeation and of systemic dissemination may be incomplete in the light of later research does not negate the magnitude of his accomplishments. Halsted himself discussed modifications of therapy relating to stage of disease. Had he worked in an era in which patients were seen with "minimal" disease and had the option of multimodality therapy been available to him, his therapeutic recommendations might have varied. As inappropriate as are polemics that ignore the fact that Halsted had limited therapeutic options available for patients with advanced disease is blind adherence to his precepts that ignore the differing stages in which patients are currently seen and the variety of therapeutic options now available. The record achieved with radical mastectomy is the base from which modifications in therapy must be measured. Adoption of new forms of therapy and abandonment of radical mastectomy require assurance that the results will at least equal the record for the Halsted mastectomy.

Radical mastectomy has been modified through the years in a variety of ways. Haagensen attempted to identify more precisely those patients who were suitable for this procedure. At one time, he performed a triple biopsy of the breast—the lymph nodes in the first, second, and third intercostal spaces and the node in the apex of the axilla. If any of these nodes contained cancer, he did not perform the radical mastectomy. His results with radical mastectomy were greatly improved in that he excluded from surgery the patients least likely to benefit, but the triple biopsy was never widely adopted.

Haagensen also identified certain criteria that he consid-

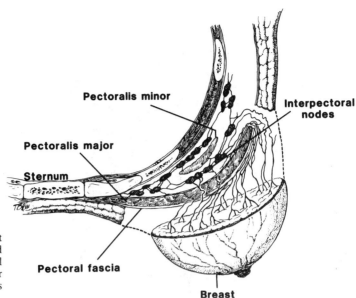

Fig. 19-13. The components involved in surgical treatment of breast cancer: breast, pectoral fascia, pectoralis major and minor muscles, and axillary lymph nodes. Level I is lateral to the pectoralis minor, level II anterior (interpectoral) or posterior to the muscle, and level III medial to the pectoralis minor muscle.

ered to reflect inoperability insofar as radical mastectomy is concerned:

1. Any two of the following grave signs:
   a. Skin edema: < one third of breast
   b. Ulceration
   c. Fixation to chest wall
   d. Axillary node(s) > 2.5 cm in diameter
   e. Fixation axillary nodes
2. Skin edema: > one third of breast
3. Satellite skin nodules
4. "Inflammatory" cancer
5. Supraclavicular and internal mammary metastases
6. Edema ipsilateral arm
7. Distant metastasis
8. Pregnancy

This list was subsequently modified and the criteria are not absolute. For example, breast cancer developing during pregnancy is not considered inoperable.

Extension of radical mastectomy beyond the removal of the breast, pectoral muscles, and axillary contents was attempted by Halsted, who dissected the supraclavicular nodes. This did not achieve additional long-term survival. Urban has recommended extension of the operation to include the internal mammary nodes. Extended radical mastectomy is particularly recommended by him for patients with medial or subareolar lesions and axillary nodes positive for cancer. The incidence of positive internal mammary nodes would be highest in these cases. This operation has not been widely adopted.

The most widely adopted modification of the mastectomy performed in cases of breast cancer is that which preserves the pectoral muscles (Fig. 19-14). The modified radical mastectomy provides a more favorable cosmetic result and facilitates breast reconstruction, should the patient wish to pursue that option. Stage I and II breast cancer, which comprise the majority of patients, rarely invades the pectoral fascia, which acts as a barrier to penetration of the muscle by tumor. The plane for resection of the breast in a modified radical mastectomy should be beneath the fascia that is thus removed with the breast. Irrespective of size, when the tumor is situated deeply in the breast and near the fascia, at the least that portion of pectoralis major beneath the

tumor is removed with the specimen. Patey has recommended resection of the pectoralis minor muscle to facilitate axillary dissection; Auchincloss does not believe that this is necessary. Modified radical mastectomy, removing the breast, pectoral fascia, and axillary contents in continuity, has become the standard operation in the treatment of the majority of women with breast cancer.

More recently, surgical therapy consisting of less than total mastectomy has been suggested. Such therapy would consist of either resection of a quadrant of a breast or removal of only the tumor itself (*i.e.*, tylectomy). Based on current knowledge, these operations must be considered without proof of efficacy for control of the tumor within the breast. If performed, tumoricidal radiation therapy to the breast should be employed and should, under these circumstances, be considered the primary therapy insofar as the breast is concerned.

Complete axillary dissection has been a standard component of surgical therapy of infiltrating breast cancer. In addition to the perceived therapeutic benefit of removal of lymph nodes containing cancer, an accurate pathologic staging of the cancer is possible. The inaccuracy of clinical staging of the axilla has already been discussed. If the axillary nodes contain cancer, current practice is to administer postoperative chemotherapy. An advantage to a partial axillary dissection or "sampling" for purposes of staging is difficult to perceive. A "sampling" of only the external mammary or level I nodes may occasionally be negative when higher nodes contain tumor. The difference in morbidity with a complete rather than a partial axillary dissection is minimal. The cosmetic result is the same. Neither carries major risk of lymphedema. Biologic cost in relation to subsequent tumor behavior has not been established. If the axilla is not dissected or only "sampled" at the time of mastectomy, the question of therapeutic radiation to the axilla will arise if positive nodes are present on the "sampling." Radiation therapy is not more effective than surgery in control of axillary tumor and does not produce a better cosmetic result; the fee for radiation therapy will be considerably greater than the small difference between the surgeon's fee for a partial rather than complete axillary dissection.

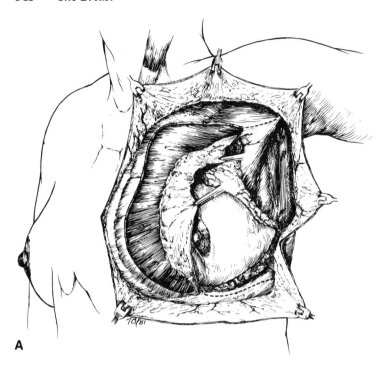

A

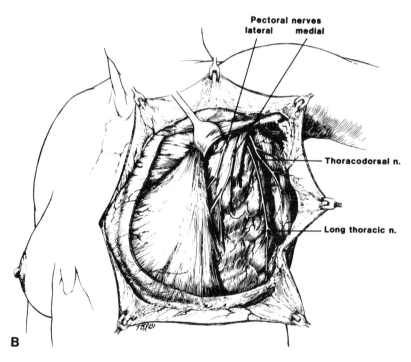

B

Pectoral nerves
lateral   medial

Thoracodorsal n.

Long thoracic n.

Fig. 19-14. Modified radical mastectomy. (*A*) Skin flaps have been elevated. The breast, together with the pectoral fascia, is being dissected from the pectoral muscles. (*B*) The mastectomy has been completed, preserving the nerves as shown. The designation of medial and lateral for pectoral nerves relates to the cord of origin from the brachial plexus. The pectoralis major is retracted and the relationship of the pectoral nerves to the pectoralis minor is depicted.

The studies of the National Surgical Adjuvant Breast Project (NSABP) reveal that in those instances in which the axilla is not dissected, only about one half of the one third of patients who might be predicted on the basis of empirical evidence to be likely to develop lymph node metastases will do so. This observation does not negate the above advantages of complete axillary dissection.

Complications of mastectomy and axillary dissection include loss of a portion of the skin flaps and collection of lymph and serum beneath the skin flaps and in the axilla. Injury to the pectoral, thoracodorsal, or long thoracic nerves can result in paralysis and atrophy of the pectoral, latissimus dorsi, and serratus anterior muscles, respectively. The prin-

cipal late complication of mastectomy is lymphedema of the arm. This is rarely seen following modified radical mastectomy. Wound infection and radiation therapy in conjunction with surgery appear to increase the likelihood of chronic lymphedema. Trivial infections of the extremity, such as a paronychia, that occur in a patient who has undergone axillary dissection may result in delayed appearance of lymphedema. Lymphangiosarcoma very rarely develops in a severely lymphedematous arm. Elevation and compression may reduce the degree of lymphedema but usually do not eliminate the problem.

The above considerations relate to the case of breast cancer overtly limited to the breast and ipsilateral axilla—

Stages I, II and III. Surgery has a very limited role in "debulking" or for "toilet" in Stage IV breast cancer. The transection of tumor during the course of the resection of breast cancer is a serious error in judgment and will almost certainly ensure local recurrence. "Debulking" which transects a tumor is contraindicated. The therapies available are inadequate to control recurrence on the chest wall. Fungating tumor is the usual result.

RADIATION THERAPY

Ionizing radiation directed to the breast and the axilla can destroy cancer and result in long-term local control of tumor. Increasing experience is now being reported with the use of an external beam of radiation therapy in a dose of approximately 5000 roentgens to the breast and axilla for the treatment of breast cancer overtly localized to the breast and ipsilateral axilla. With larger tumors, the external beam therapy may be supplemented with interstitial irradiation. Criteria for selection of patients for this therapy are not clear. Most reports consist of small numbers of highly selected cases followed for brief periods. In patients with Stage I disease, the evidence is accumulating that radiation therapy is effective. For patients with Stage II or III disease, the record in radiation therapy is confusing. Calle's experience is frequently cited with regard to radiation therapy as primary treatment. In this study, tumors greater than 3 cm were biopsied and treated with radiation therapy by external beam whereas tumors less than 3 cm were excised with subsequent radiation. Over one half of those with biopsy and radiation required subsequent mastectomy (Table 19-4). This incidence of local failure far exceeds that of surgery. Wound complications in subsequent surgery are greatly increased by prior radiation therapy. In patients with tumors less than 3 cm that were excised prior to irradiation, 16 of 120 had local recurrences and 14 of the 16 underwent surgery. These results are certainly not reassuring. Additionally, the breast may be scarred by radiation and the cosmetic result may be less than desired. The role of radiation therapy as the dominant therapy of breast cancer overtly limited to the breast and ipsilateral axilla is yet to be established.

Radiation therapy was formerly widely employed in conjunction with mastectomy in cases with positive axillary nodes. Radiation therapy was directed postoperatively to the chest wall and axilla, as well as to the supraclavicular and internal mammary nodes. In that the majority of these cases would never develop local recurrence, this prophylactic radiotherapy was needless in most cases. The overall incidence of recurrent tumor on the chest wall was reduced from 12 to 14% to 6 to 8%. Several studies, including a randomized study by the NSABP, failed to demonstrate improved survival. Thus, most authorities today do not routinely employ postoperative radiation therapy. In those cases in which regional recurrence develops, radiation therapy is probably as effective as palliative therapy is when used "prophylactically."

In cases with Stage IV breast cancer, radiation therapy may arrest progression and control local disease. Radiation therapy will be successful in the control of a regional recurrence that develops following surgical treatment in at least one half of such cases. Local control of cancer is not to be equated with survival of the patient, who may succumb to disseminated cancer. Radiation therapy is highly effective in control of pain from osseous metastasis. Radiation therapy is a local form of therapy and is particularly applicable to patients with recurrent localized disease whether it be on the chest wall, in regional lymph nodes, or in bone.

CHEMOTHERAPY

The introduction of chemotherapy after World War II, first as nitrogen mustard, provided the physician with a form of systemic therapy of breast cancer. Chemotherapeutic agents destroy tumor cells. Depending on the pharmacokinetics of the agent employed, destruction may occur at different stages in the cycle of cell growth. In that all cells in the tumor do not divide synchronously, only a certain percentage of the total population of tumor cells may be destroyed during a given course of therapy with a certain agent. To be effective, repeated courses are needed.

Since the introduction of chemotherapy, interest has developed in the use of early systemic chemotherapy as a component of multimodal therapy of breast cancer overtly limited to the breast and ipsilateral axilla. Covert dissemination of cancer or microscopic residua of cancer in the mammary region are present at the time of the treatment in over one half of these cases. Such foci will ultimately become overt in patients who will die of breast cancer. The low tumor burden in patients with such covert disease suggests that chemotherapy might permanently eradicate these foci, in contrast to the experience with chemotherapy

TABLE 19-4   RESULTS AT 5 YEARS OF PATIENTS TREATED BY EXCLUSIVE IRRADIATION

STAGE	NUMBER OF CASES	ABSOLUTE SURVIVAL NED*	ALIVE NED* WITH BREASTS PRESERVED		WITH SECONDARY MASTECTOMY
			Irradiation alone	Secondary limited surgery	
T2 N0 N1a	136	112 (82%)	45/112	6	61
T2 N1b	67	44 (65%)	18/44	2	24
T3 N0 N1a	86	56 (64%)	24/56	1	31
T3 N1b	105	56 (53%)	22/56	2	32
	394	268 (68%)	109/268 (41%)	11/268 (4%)	148/268 (55%)

* NED, No evidence of disease
(Calle R, Pilleron JP, Schlienger P et al: Conservative management of operable breast cancer: Ten years' experience at the Foundation Curie. Cancer 42:2049, 1978)

TABLE 19-5 **RESULTS OF EARLY SYSTEMIC THERAPY WITH CMF ADJUVANT PROGRAM (MILAN), ANALYZED 4 YEARS AFTER MASTECTOMY**

	RELAPSE RATE (%)	
	Mastectomy only	Mastectomy plus CMF
All patients	53	34*
Premenopausal patients	59	25*
Postmenopausal patients	48	44
Premenopausal patients with		
1 positive node	51	17*
2 or 3 positive nodes	52	12*
4 or more positive nodes	77	49*
Survival (%)		
All patients	74	83*
Premenopausal patients	72	90*

* Statistically significant differences when compared with mastectomy only (P < 0.05).
CMF: cyclophosphamide, methotrexate, 5-fluorouracil
(Henderson IC, Canellos GP: Cancer of the breast: The past decade. II. N Engl J Med 302:86, 1980)

in cases with overtly disseminated, recurrent, or locally advanced breast cancer.

Extensive studies of chemotherapy have been carried out by the NSABP and the Tumor Institute in Milan, Italy. These studies, using phenylalanine mustard (NSABP) or Cytoxan, methotrexate, and 5-fluorouracil (Milan), have established that repeated courses of chemotherapy over a period of 1 or 2 years in conjunction with surgical treatment of overtly localized cancer may improve disease-free interval. These results are most impressive in premenopausal women with fewer than four positive axillary nodes. The results from Milan are summarized in Table 19-5. The fact that chemotherapy may induce amenorrhea has raised the question of whether conjunctive chemotherapy is a chemical oophorectomy. Studies of ovarian function following conjunctive chemotherapy do not support this hypothesis. The group from Milan reported that if conjunctive chemotherapy in postmenopausal women is carried to full recommended dosage, these women also benefit. Benefit of conjunctive chemotherapy for women without positive nodes has not been established. Because of the short- and possible long-term morbidity of chemotherapy, including oncogenesis, it is not recommended for such patients. Results to date with the use of conjunctive chemotherapy relate dominantly to an increased disease-free interval. Final data on survival are awaited. The word "cure" is used when chemotherapy is employed in conjunction with surgery. When only surgery is employed, the surgeon has customarily referred to "five-year survival." This use of the word "cure" reflects the belief that conjunctive chemotherapy eradicates covert disseminated disease. That such is true remains to be proved.

When breast cancer is locally advanced (T4), overtly disseminated, or regionally recurrent, chemotherapy is a palliative form of therapy. Tumor may regress either partially or totally; recrudescence with ultimate progressive disease is the rule. A combination of chemotherapeutic agents may induce a higher incidence of remission, without cumulative toxicity. The combination of cyclophosphamide, methotrexate, 5-fluorouracil, vincristine, and prednisone was de-

scribed by Cooper as efficacious. Vincristine contributes disproportionally to toxicity in this combination of chemotherapy. Although initial reports indicated an incidence of remission of cancer in over 70% of cases, subsequent experience with combination chemotherapy reveals that regression of at least 50% of tumor mass occurs in about one half of cases, with complete regression in less than 20% of cases. The duration of remission is often distressingly brief, a mean duration of 8 to 10 months. Whether incidence and duration of remission is greater when drugs are administered in combination or sequentially is unproved. Adriamycin and cyclophosphamide are both effective as single agents. Data from the report of Canellos and Henderson that indicate results with single agents are provided in Table 19-6, and the results with combination chemotherapy in treatment of advanced or Stage IV breast cancer are shown in Table 19-7. A predictive test for responsiveness to chemotherapy does not currently exist. The clonogenic assay may have potential in this regard. Patients who are estrogen-receptor positive may be more likely to respond favorably to chemotherapy, although the evidence is conflicting in this regard.

HORMONAL MANIPULATION

There is extensive past experience with oophorectomy in conjunction with mastectomy. These studies established that a prolonged "free interval" might follow "prophylactic oophorectomy" in premenopausal women but that ultimate survival was not affected. Recent studies of the antiestrogen tamoxifen as a conjunct to surgery and chemotherapy suggest that it might increase the disease-free interval in postmenopausal women who are estrogen receptor positive.

In the treatment of advanced breast cancer, hormonal therapy consists of withdrawal of estrogens either surgically or through pharmacologic means, the administration of estrogens to the postmenopausal patient, and the use of androgens or progestins. Techniques for surgical ablation of estrogens include oophorectomy, adrenalectomy, and hypophysectomy, the last being an indirect technique. Because of immediate effect, surgical ablation of the ovaries is preferred to radiation castration. Postmenopausal women rarely respond favorably to hormonal ablation. Tamoxifen is effective in reducing estrogen levels and for inexplicable reasons may be efficacious in both premenopausal and postmenopausal women. Aminoglutethimide suppresses adrenal secretion of estrogens. Postmenopausal women who undergo regression of breast cancer with administration of estrogen in the form of diethylstilbestrol or estradiol, and whose disease has subsequently progressed, may experience further regression when estrogen is withdrawn.

Androgenic steroids may result in regression of breast cancer in premenopausal women. The side-effects of testosterone (*i.e.,* hirsutism, increased libido, and masculinization) far exceed therapeutic benefit. Synthetic androgens with limited side-effects are not particularly efficacious. Adrenocortical steroids may on occasion be beneficial in the treatment of breast cancer, if only consequent to the euphoria and increased appetite that result. They can be employed as a last resort when all other therapy has failed. Hormonal manipulation is more effective in the treatment of soft tissue cancer, of nodular pulmonary metastasis, and of bone metastasis. Other visceral metastases, such as liver and brain, respond poorly to hormonal therapy. The duration of regression of breast cancer when such occurs with hormonal manipulation is about 18 months. The patient

TABLE 19-6   ACTIVITY OF THE SINGLE AGENTS MOST COMMONLY USED TO TREAT BREAST CANCER*

AGENT	NO. OF PATIENTS	NO. OF LITERATURE SERIES	OBJECTIVE RESPONSE RATE (%)
Doxorubicin (Adriamycin) (A)	193	6	35
Cyclophosphamide (C)	529	13	34
Methotrexate (M)	356	14	34
Thiotepa	162	4	30
5-Fluorouracil (F)	1263	15	26
Phenylalanine mustard (L-PAM)	177	3	22
Chlorambucil	54	2	20
Vincristine (V or O)	226	5	21

* Modified from Carter, 1976
(Henderson IC, Canellos GP: Cancer of the breast: The past decade. N Engl J Med 302:79, 1980)

TABLE 19-7   RESPONSE TO DRUG COMBINATIONS COMMONLY USED TO TREAT BREAST CANCER

STUDY	REGIMEN*	NO. OF PATIENTS	RESPONSE RATE (%) Complete Plus Partial Responses†	RESPONSE RATE (%) Complete Responses	MEDIAN DURATION (MONTH) Response	MEDIAN DURATION (MONTH) Survival
Swiss Group for Clinical Cancer Research (SAKK), 1975	CMP	78	43	4	7.3	15.4
	CMF-VP	91	49‡	7‡	8.0	16.0
Milan, 1976	CMF	53	57	11	8.0	17.5
	AC→→CMF	52	52‡	15‡	8.6‡	22.5‡
Houston, 1976	FAC	44	73	14	8.0	15.0
	FAC-BCG§	45	76	31	12.0	22.0‖
Eastern Cooperative Oncology Group, 1977	CMF	90	48	15	5.3	14.8
	CMFP	88	63‖	25‖	8.5‡	18.05‡
	AV	178	53‡	18‡	8.0‡	13.0‡
Southwest Oncology Group, 1978	AF	105	42	10	5.5	16.0
	AFC	103	43‡	14‡	8.3‡	15.3‡
	AFCM	105	49‡	11‡	8.8‡	16.3‡
National Cancer Institute, 1978	CMF	40	62	7.5	6.0	17.0
	CAF	38	82‡	18‖	10.4‡	27.2‡
Bowman-Gray, 1978	CMF-VP	72	57	11	13.0	20.2
	CAF-VP	76	58‡	13‡	15.8‡	33.0‡

* Randomized trials; for abbreviations, see Table 19-6 (P = Prednisone)
† Objective regressions of >50% of measurable tumor volume
‡ Difference from value on line above not considered statistically significant
§ Single nonrandomized trial included
‖ Difference from value on line above considered significant, P < 0.05
(Henderson IC, Canellos GP: Cancer of the breast: The past decade. II. N Engl J Med 302:80, 1980)

who responds favorably to one type of hormonal manipulation is more likely to experience regression with other forms of hormonal therapy. As has already been discussed, the ability of the tumor to bind sex steroids is the most important criterion in selection of cases for hormonal manipulation.

RECOMMENDATIONS FOR THERAPY

The selection of therapy for the individual with breast cancer is currently in a state of chaos. Advocates of various viewpoints and "authorities" often generate more heat than light on the subject. The "authorities" include physicians, consumer specialists, and the patients themselves. The area of greatest controversy relates to the selection of surgery or radiation therapy, alone or in combination, as initial therapy. Recommendations all too frequently are based on preliminary reports concerning small numbers of highly selected patients followed for a brief period, with disease-free interval the base and few long-term survival figures. In the sections that follow, specific recommendations will be made with respect to selection of therapy for patients with Stage I, II,

III, and IV disease. All cases of disease recurrent following initial therapy will be considered as Stage IV. The recommendations for therapy for Stage I, II, and III disease are based on clinical staging. When the pathologic staging becomes known, additional therapeutic modifications may be made. In Stage IV disease, both clinical and pathologic staging are likely to be known when initial therapy is chosen. In each instance, recommendations will be made with respect to surgery, radiation therapy, chemotherapy, and hormonal therapy. In a disease as varied as breast cancer, all possible options cannot be considered in a chapter of finite length but broad guidelines will be sketched.

STAGE I

Surgery

In situ carcinoma may be treated by wide local excision and careful follow-up of both breasts with routine physical examinations and mammography. For infiltrating adenocarcinoma of the breast, a modified radical mastectomy is recommended. Even in the so-called minimal breast cancers, detected only on mammography, the incidence of positive axillary nodes is at least 20%. The disadvantages of a "sampling" or a partial axillary dissection or less than total mastectomy have already been discussed.

Radiation Therapy

Radiation therapy to the breast is an alternative to modified radical mastectomy in initial therapy for the breast itself when an infiltrating Stage I breast cancer has been diagnosed by biopsy, tylectomy, or quadrant resection. The patient should be informed that conclusive evidence does not exist that this therapy is as effective as surgery and that subsequent mastectomy may be necessary. The breast having been preserved, the axilla can be treated by surgery or radiation. Positive axillary nodes are present in clinical Stage I breast cancer in at least one third of cases. A distinct disadvantage of radiation therapy to the axilla is failure to identify precisely cases of covert axillary node metastasis that might benefit from conjunctive chemotherapy. For this and the other reasons previously stated, axillary dissection is preferable to radiation therapy to the axilla, even when the breast itself is treated with radiation.

Chemotherapy

Chemotherapy is not recommended for patients with clinical Stage I disease determined on the basis of axillary dissection to be pathologically Stage I. If positive lymph nodes are detected in the axilla, conjunctive chemotherapy in the form of Cytoxan, methotrexate, and 5-fluorouracil over a period of 12 to 18 months is recommended for premenopausal patients. Chemotherapy is optional and usually recommended in postmenopausal patients with positive nodes.

Hormonal Therapy

Hormonal therapy is currently not recommended as a component of the primary treatment of patients with Stage I disease, irrespective of the pathologic status of the axillary lymph nodes.

STAGE II

The majority of patients with breast cancer will be first seen with Stage II disease. These are patients with tumors variable in size who, in over 50% of instances, will ultimately prove to harbor tumor in the axillary lymph nodes.

Surgery

A modified radical mastectomy is the treatment of choice for patients with Stage II breast cancer.

Radiation Therapy

Radiation therapy is not yet acceptable as the primary treatment for Stage II disease. The incidence of local failure is not well enough established and initial reports are not reassuring. Radiation therapy to regional lymph nodes, in conjunction with surgical therapy, has not been found in controlled studies to prolong survival. In patients with medial quadrant or subareolar cancer, conjunctive radiation therapy to the internal mammary nodes following mastectomy is still recommended by many serious students of breast cancer. This recommendation is based on the greater likelihood of invasion of these nodes in such cases, particularly if axillary nodes contain cancer.

Chemotherapy

Conjunctive chemotherapy is recommended as for patients with Stage I disease.

Hormonal Therapy

Hormonal therapy is not currently recommended as conjunctive therapy of patients with Stage II disease, alone or with chemotherapy.

STAGE III

Surgery

The tumor should be surgically resected with a wide margin. A resection of underlying muscle is usually indicated with a T3 tumor. If axillary nodes are not fixed to other structures, an axillary dissection is performed—a standard radical mastectomy. A skin graft may be necessary.

Radiation Therapy

Radiation therapy is preferable to excision in initial therapy of a large tumor of the breast which cannot be clearly circumscribed surgically. Axillary nodes fixed to other structures are irradiated. Depending on response to initial radiation, surgical resection may be considered subsequently. Radiation therapy to the regional nodal areas and to the postoperative surgical wound may be desirable in cases with initial surgical resection. Each case of Stage III breast cancer is individualized. The combination of surgery and radiation therapy thought most likely to achieve local control is selected.

Chemotherapy

Chemotherapy may be employed as a conjunctive therapy following initial surgery or radiation therapy, or both, in patients with Stage III disease, both cases with and without positive nodes. Its use as initial therapy to be followed by surgery or radiation therapy is experimental.

Hormonal Therapy

Hormonal therapy is not usually recommended as a component of initial therapy of Stage III disease.

STAGE IV

Therapy for Stage IV or recurrent breast cancer is undertaken with the understanding that the goal is palliation, that is, relief of symptoms without hope of "cure." In selecting therapy, the following eight principles should be considered:

1. Local therapy is most appropriate for local cancer (*i.e.*, surgery, irradiation).
2. Disseminated tumor is usually treated with systemic therapy (*i.e.*, chemotherapy, hormonal manipulation).
3. The morbidity of therapy should be balanced against the probability of benefit. As an example, oophorectomy, which carries a rather low morbidity, may be justified even in an estrogen-receptor–negative patient because of the possibility that up to 10% of patients might respond and that the response would be of long duration.
4. Sequential therapy is preferred. One type of therapy at a time is employed (chemotherapy, hormonal manipulation, radiation therapy). Morbidity of therapy should be less with sequential therapy. Exceptions are combinations of agents for chemotherapy, radiation to a local area such as painful osseous metastases combined with systemic therapy for other disseminated tumor, and combined modality therapy for very rapidly progressive cancer. Examples of the latter are inflammatory cancer or lymphangitic pulmonary metastasis. It is not known whether the incidence of remission and duration of life after the cumulative favorable responses to several therapies exceed that with a "shotgun" approach, where incidence of initial remission may be higher. The physician should jealously ration therapies available to the patient with a fatal disease. This is best achieved with sequential therapy.
5. Visceral metastases respond less well to any therapy, and chemotherapy is more efficacious for hepatic metastases than is hormonal manipulation.
6. First reliance for systemic therapy is hormonal therapy for cases that are positive for estrogen binding and chemotherapy for cases negative for estrogen binding.
7. The onset of regression is more rapid with chemotherapy than hormonal therapy. If regression has not occurred within 6 weeks, it is unlikely with chemotherapy; a regression consequent to hormonal therapy may not be seen for up to 3 months.
8. Disease may behave in three general fashions following initiation of the course of palliative therapy: (a) progression, (b) regression, or (c) static disease. Regression is usually not declared significant unless measurable disease decreases by 50%, new disease does not appear, and duration of regression is at least 3 months. Such objective regression is not necessarily palliation. For palliation to occur symptoms must improve. Static disease is not a negligible result with palliative therapy of rapidly progressive disease. A period of stability may persist for months or years. Osseous metastases may never recalcify but not progress or be symptomatic. The Karnofsky scale of behavior is an attempt to qualify subjective response (see Chapter 14).

Surgery

Surgery has a very minor role to play in the treatment of Stage IV disease. "Debulking" may be desirable if tumor is not transected. A rare patient with a chest wall recurrence, and without evidence of metastatic spread, may be treated by wide local excision. On only an extraordinarily rare occasion will long-term survival result.

Radiation Therapy

Radiation therapy is most important in the control of inoperable cancer in the breast, of regionally recurrent disease, for brain metastasis, and in the control of bone pain.

Chemotherapy

Multi-agent chemotherapy is usually employed for patients with Stage IV disease who are estrogen-receptor negative or receptor positive with progressive tumor after a trial of hormonal therapy.

Hormonal Therapy

In the premenopausal patient, surgical oophorectomy is the first choice in hormone therapy. In the case of the postmenopausal patient, either tamoxifen or exogenous estrogens are administered. The use of tamoxifen and aminoglutethimide has largely eliminated adrenalectomy and hypophysectomy in the treatment of breast cancer.

SPECIAL PROBLEMS

HYPERCALCEMIA

Hypercalcemia is a cause of death in as many as 15% of cases of breast cancer. It is usually associated with extensive osseous metastasis. A patient with osseous metastasis with lethargy and anorexia may be judged terminal when, indeed, the patient's clinical deterioration is due to hypercalcemia. The administration of cortisone, hydration, and saline diuresis will usually control the hypercalcemia. Mithramycin is also effective. Its duration of action is brief, but if hypercalcemia is controlled, either chemotherapy or hormonal therapy can be instituted.

PLEURAL EFFUSION

Malignant pleural effusion can be a particularly difficult problem. The fluid should be removed from the chest either by thoracocentesis or by insertion of a tube for continuous drainage. Instillation of radioisotopes in the pleural space to control tumor by local radiation has not been particularly efficacious. The use of chemotherapeutic agents, such as 5-fluorouracil and nitrogen mustard, may be effective in controlling pleural effusion, as may be locally infused atabrine or tetracycline.

VISCERAL METASTASIS

Patients with cerebral metastasis from breast cancer should initially receive cortisone to decrease edema, followed by total cerebral irradiation. Chemotherapy is preferable to hormonal therapy for hepatic metastasis or rapidly progressive pulmonary metastasis of the lymphangitic type.

Some breast carcinomas secrete mucus and at times it may be difficult to be certain that a biopsied metastasis arose from the breast or from some other gland-forming organ.

PROGNOSIS

Approximately one half of patients with the diagnosis of breast cancer will survive without disease for 5 years. The survival for various stages of the disease is summarized in

Table 19-2. The untreated patient has about the same prognosis as Stage IV disease, that is, about a 10% five-year survival.

REHABILITATION

The American Cancer Society conducts an active program for rehabilitation of the patient who has undergone mastectomy called "Reach for Recovery." Early postoperative motion and physiotherapy are important in arm and shoulder function. The patient deserves psychological support in adjustment. Plastic surgery can be considered in selected cases.

There is considerable interest in breast reconstruction following surgical resection for treatment of breast cancer. Such considerations are dominantly related to patients with pathologic Stage I disease or, at the most, Stage II disease. Because of the incidence of nipple invasion by cancer, attempts at nipple preservation are to be condemned. If reconstruction is to be attempted, a transverse incision for mastectomy is preferable and a modified rather than radical mastectomy. The patient who is to undergo plastic reconstruction must be cognizant that multiple procedures may be required. Reconstruction of the opposite breast may be necessary for symmetry.

Bilateral subcutaneous mastectomy may be considered in selected instances. These include a very strong history of breast cancer and florid fibrocystic disease in a patient with fear of cancer to the point of significant mental distress.

BIBLIOGRAPHY

AUCHINCLOSS H: Significance of location and number of axillary metastases in carcinoma of the breast: A justification for conservative operation. Ann Surg 158:37, 1963

BONADONNA G, ROSSI A., VALAGUSSA P, BANFI A, VERONESI U: The CMF program for operable breast cancer with positive axillary nodes. Cancer 39:2904, 1977

BONADONNA G, VALAGUSSA P: Dose-response effect of adjuvant chemotherapy in breast cancer. N Engl J Med 304:10, 1981

CALLE R, PILLERON JP, SCHLIENGER P et al: Conservative management of operable breast cancer: Ten years experience at the Foundation Curie. Cancer 42:2045, 1978

COOPER A: Anatomy and Diseases of the Breast. Philadelphia, Lee and Blanchard, 1845

COOPER RG: Combination chemotherapy in hormonal resistant breast cancer. Proc Am Assoc Cancer Res 10:15, 1969

FISHER B: Cooperative clinical trials in primary breast cancer: A critical appraisal. Cancer 31:1271, 1973

FISHER B, GLASS A, REDMOND C, FISHER ER, BARTON B, SUCH E, CARBONE P, ECONOMOU S, FOSTER R, FRELICK R, LERNER H, LEVITT M, MARGOLESE R, MACFARLANE J, PLOTKIN D, SHIBATA H, VOLK H: L-phenylalanine mustard (L-PAM) in the management of primary breast cancer. Cancer 39:2883, 1977

HAAGENSEN CD: Disease of the Breast, 2nd ed. Philadelphia, W B Saunders, 1971

HALSTED WS: The results of operations for the cure of cancer of the breast performed at the Johns Hopkins Hospital from June, 1889, to January, 1894. Ann Surg 20:497, 1894

HENDERSON IC, CANELLOS GP: Cancer of the breast: The past decade, N Engl J Med 302:17, 78, 1980

MACDONALD I: Biological predeterminism in human cancer. Surg Gynecol Obstet 92:443, 1951

MOXLEY JH, ALLEGRA JC, HENNEY J, MUGGIA F: Treatment of primary breast cancer: Summary of the National Institutes of Health Consensus Development Conference. JAMA 244:797, 1980

PATEY DH, DYSON WH: The prognosis of carcinoma of the breast in relation to the type of operation performed. Br J Cancer 2:7, 1948

RHOADS JE (ed): Proceedings of an NIH Consensus Conference on Steroid Receptors. Cancer 46:2759, 1980

RHOADS JE (ed): Proceedings of the 1979 Conference on Breast Cancer. Cancer 46:859, 1980

SHAPIRO S: Evidence on screening for breast cancer from a randomized trial. Cancer 39:2772, 1977

SHERMAN BM, SCHLECHTE J, HALMI NS, CHAPLER FK, HARRIS CE, DUELLO TM, VANGILDER J, GRANNER DK: Pathogenesis of prolactin-secreting pituitary adenomas. Lancet 2:1019, 1978

TURNER-WARWICK RT: The lymphatics of the breast. Br J Surg 46:574, 1959

URBAN JA: Surgical excision of internal mammary nodes for breast cancer. Br J Surg 51:209, 1964

URBAN JA: Management of operable breast cancer: The surgeon's view. Cancer 42:2066, 1978

Endocrine System

20

Stanley R. Friesen

Overview

Endocrinopathies, ranging pathologically from cellular hyperplasia to metastatic malignancies, produce symptoms because of their hypersecretion of protein or steroid hormones, which act on specific end-organs and result in an exaggeration of their biologic functions.

A distinguishing feature of most neuroendocrine tumors is that systemic manifestations result from even small functioning endocrine dysplasias. A galaxy of syndromes occurs as a consequence of the autonomous tumor elaboration of humoral substances that overwhelm the normal homeostatic mechanisms of physiologic neuroendocrine control. The full-blown clinical pictures that accompany neuroendocrine hypersecretion depend upon several intermediary steps in endocrine pathophysiology, beginning with the nature of the instigating pathologic process; the degree of synthesis and storage of amines, polypeptides, and steroids in neurosecretory granules; the presence of stimulation or suppression of their secretion and release across the cellular membrane, permitted by the calcium ion or inhibited by such substances as somatostatin (SST); the characterization and molecular size of the circulating polypeptides; and, finally, the responsiveness of unblocked membrane receptors on the specific end-organs. An interruption in this endocrine chain may abrogate the expected systemic syndrome and give rise to so-called nonfunctioning endocrine tumors. Nonfunctioning tumors may simply represent a failure to identify the humoral substance or to recognize a subtle clinical picture.

SYNOPSIS

Neuroendocrine system The dimensions of our understanding of the neural and the endocrine system have increased by virtue of intense investigations in both basic and clinical sciences. Specialized cells secrete three types of hormones: amines and polypeptides (APUD system of neuroectodermal origin) and steroids (of mesodermal origin). These interdependently regulate metabolic function and produce homeostasis by their control of their specific end-organs.

Pathogenetic types Endocrinopathies may be sporadic or genetic (familial) in origin; the latter are characterized by multiplicity of cellular changes in multiple organs in multiple members of families. Endocrine tumors may also function entopically (hormones native to the organ) or ectopically, in which the tumor may elaborate any of the precursor polypeptides.

Clinical considerations Recent advances in diagnosis and therapy include quantitative assays of circulating hormones, their responses to stimulation and suppression testing, and the combined modalities of surgical and chemotherapeutic treatment, as well as palliative receptor blockers.

As is the case in most clinical situations, the diagnosis and management of patients are best accomplished when the pathogenesis is understood. There has occurred a remarkable proliferation of information in both basic and clinical sciences that has tended to expand the dimensions of the neuroendocrine system. An integration of the basic and the clinical observations should lead to better understanding of the pathogenesis of endocrinopathies and their treatment.

NEUROENDOCRINE SYSTEM

DIMENSIONS

The functional integrity of living beings is almost miraculously maintained by a complex internal communication system involving both the endocrine and the autonomic nervous systems. In health, the regulation of physiological responses to external and internal environment is mediated by humoral substances having endocrine and paracrine actions and by neurotransmitters, also having both distant and local actions. The interdependence of the neural and the humoral controlling systems has prompted a return to a single designation for the neuroendocrine system. Even in disease, manifestations resulting from abnormal activity in both components are frequently observed in the same clinical syndrome.

As early as 1910, Pavlov, in his experiments on gastric secretion in animals, proposed that the regulation of various organs in the body was mediated by the nervous system; just prior to that, in 1902, Bayliss and Starling had developed evidence of a humoral regulatory mechanism such as the duodenal secretin influence on the exocrine pancreas. Shortly thereafter, Edkins, in 1905, found that there was a gastric secretagogue in the antrum that also regulated acid secretion without neural connections; he called this humoral substance gastric secretin, which has since been contracted to gastrin. Each of these early investigators understood and acknowledged the presence of the so-called opposing mechanisms, but the closeness with which the neural and humoral regulatory mechanisms function has been appreciated only recently.

Within the past 2 decades, the immensity of the neuroendocrine system has been realized by the identification of a large body of regulatory cells in the gastrointestinal tract, including the endocrine pancreas, so that now the dimensions range from the hypothalamus, pituitary, and pineal in the brain, through the pharyngeal endocrine system, lungs, gastrointestinal tract, adrenals, gonads, and even placenta, when present. The autonomic nervous system, including the adrenal medulla and the gastrointestinal ganglion cells, is closely implicated in function with the traditional endocrine system (Fig. 20-1).

The central hypothalamic–pituitary component is related to the peripheral component of the system in a number of ways, including functionally, by their trophic actions and feedback controls; embryologically, by the similar origins of many of the cells from the neuroectoderm; by the similar ancestral capabilities of amine storage and peptide synthesis; by the notable observations of the same polypeptides in both the hypothalamus and the gastrointestinal tract; and by the more recent and revolutionary finding that there is a common neuron-specific enolase, an enzyme, present in both neural and endocrine cells and their tumors but not in non-neuroendocrine tumors.

Within the traditional endocrine axis, consisting of the pituitary-thyroid-adrenal-gonadal glands, the internal secretions from the pituitary and thyroid consist of peptides and amines, while from the adrenal cortex and gonads, the humoral substances are steroids. The difference is accountable to the contrasting origins embryologically (neuroectoderm for the first two and mesoderm for the latter two). It is now recognized that the endocrine cells in the gastrointestinal tract, including the pancreas, comprise an endocrine "organ" of such magnitude that in size and complexity it tends to overshadow the remainder of the endocrine system. The clear cells of the gastrointestinal tract were described first in 1932 by Feyrter, who considered them to be a "diffuse endocrine epithelial organ." His additional use of the term *paracrine* has come to denote the diffuse system of cells that secrete hormones that have a local effect on neighboring cells. These so-called paracrine cells, situated as they are among and near potential target organs, constitute a large body of interacting and intercommunicating cells within another axis, the enteroinsular axis. For the most part, the stimulation and suppression of secretion and the response of the target cells all occur in a localized region, but these paracrine cells seem also to have an endocrine (humoral) action, such as the duodenal secretin action on the pancreas and the effect of insulin and glucagon on the liver.

NEUROENDOCRINE CELLS

APUD CONCEPT

The embryologic derivation of many of the central and peripheral neuroendocrine cells to a large extent determines their humoral capacities. The peripheral steroid-secreting endocrine tissues of the adrenal cortex and the gonads differentiate from mesodermal origins, and the humoral products act generally on cytoplasmic (rather than membrane) receptors, influencing the necessary biologic functions in protein synthesis. On the other hand, the larger part of the neuroendocrine system, including the gastroenteropancreatic system, which secretes the peptide and amine hormones, is of neuroectodermal origin. All of the cells of neuroectodermal origin, including the neural crest, have common cytochemical characteristics; this observation has led to the development of the APUD concept and has clarified many aspects of identification of neuroendocrine cells and their functional capabilities. The acronym refers only to a few of the many common characteristics of these cells, namely, *A*mine *P*recursor *U*ptake and *D*ecarboxylation, leading to amine and polypeptide synthesis. The ability of these cells to take up precursor amines, store amines, and synthesize peptides is basic to their normal and abnormal potentialities. The charter members of the APUD cell system, those first having been shown to be derived from the neural crest part of the neuroectoderm, are the C cells of the thyroid and the medullary cells of the adrenal; both, in disease, are associated in the syndrome of multiple endocrine adenopathy, type II. The parathyroid cells have not been shown to have APUD cytochemical characteristics, but they are presumed to be of neuroectodermal origin because comparative embryologic studies suggest their origins from neural placodes adjacent to pharyngeal pouches. This origin is similar to that of the pituitary and hypothalamus. In

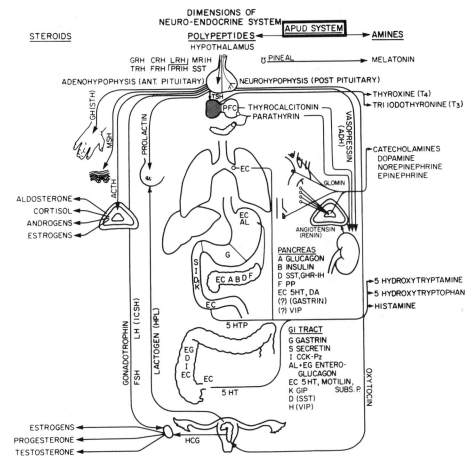

Fig. 20-1. The endocrine system elaborates amines, polypeptides, and steroids. The protein humoral substances are secreted by cells having common neuroectodermal embryologic origin and APUD cytochemical characteristics, while the steroids arise from the mesoderm. All three components are interdependent in function. (Friesen SR: Current dimensions of the endocrine system. In Longmire WP Jr et al [eds]: Advances in Surgery, vol 10. Chicago, Year Book Medical Publishers, 1976)

Figure 20-1, it can be observed that the amine- and polypeptide-secreting cells (APUD cells) constitute a larger proportion of the neuroendocrine system than the smaller, steroid-secreting group. The functional integrity of each group is dependent upon the other; cortisol is necessary for APUD cell synthesis of proteins, and the steroid cells are dependent and responsive to the central trophic polypeptides of the hypothalamus and pituitary gland.

APUD CELL FUNCTION

Just as most tissues of the body are regulated by neural and humoral influences, so the neuroendocrine cells themselves are controlled by at least four types of environmental influences (Fig. 20-2). The endocrine cell may be "closed" or "open," with microvilli with which to "sensor" the luminal environment. An example of the open cell is the gastrin (G) cell of the antral mucosa, which is responsive to both chemical (*p*H) and physical (distention) influences. Other cells are presumed to be closed but are responsive, nevertheless, to tissue-fluid osmolarity and to chemical stimuli that diffuse into the cell; an example of a closed cell is the beta islet cell, in which the concentration of glucose influences the secretion or storage of insulin. Hormonal and chemical influences regulate the endocrine cell predominantly by means of feedback mechanisms within the neuroendocrine system. Neural and physical influences also

affect endocrine cell function. Examples of neural influences even from remote instigation might be the central nervous system stimulation through the autonomic vagus nerves that affect the G cells of the antrum at the sight of the food, or the adrenal release of epinephrine, triggered by the sight of danger. An example of a physical stimulus is the renal influence on circulating osmolarity of the blood, which in turn physically affects the posterior pituitary release of antidiuretic hormone.

The rate and direction of the endocrine cell functions of synthesis, storage, and secretion in either direction depend upon whether the cells' environment is stimulating or suppressing its action. Normal and hyperplastic endocrine cells are capable, generally, of responding to both stimulation and suppression, whereas autonomous cells usually are not; these responses are useful as diagnostic tests. Functioning neoplastic cells, on the other hand, may respond to stimulation in a paradoxical way; examples of such unexplained responses include the calcium or secretin stimulation of pancreatic gastrinomas and the calcium or pentagastrin stimulation of medullary carcinoma of the thyroid, tumors that release calcitonin.

The synthesis of the hormone in the endocrine cells is carried out by intracellular enzymes. The storage of the hormone within the secretory granules in the cytoplasm of the cells is variable, depending upon whether the cell is

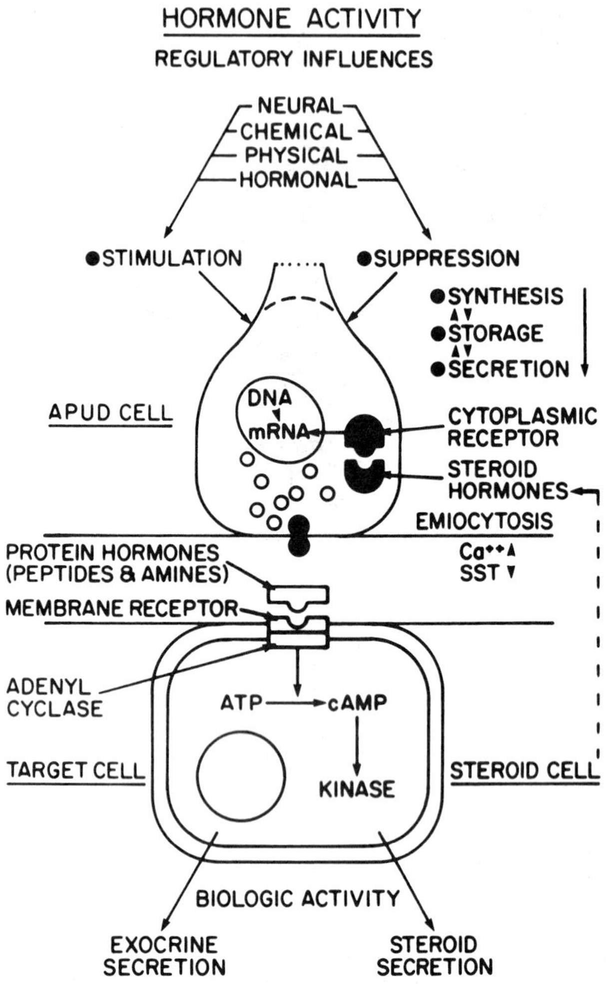

HORMONE ACTIVITY

REGULATORY INFLUENCES

Fig. 20-2. The physiologic activity between the neuroendocrine APUD cells and their target organs of either exocrine cells or endocrine steroid cells is specific, and their relationship is interdependent. The APUD cell is capable of synthesis, storage, and secretion and depends on its degree of stimulation and suppression and also on the presence of the steroid cortisol. The liberated amine or peptide, by its specific attraction to the membrane receptor, activates the biologic activity of the target cell. The steroid hormone, in turn, activates the intracellular cytoplasmic receptor of the APUD cell.

being stimulated or suppressed. The secretion of the humoral product from the endocrine cell appears to be influenced not only by its environment but also by the calcium-ion concentration at its membrane. Hormone release can also be inhibited specifically by another polypeptide, SST; this is true of the release of growth hormone (somatotropin), gastrin, insulin, glucagon, and perhaps other polypeptides except thyrocalcitonin and parathyrin.

HUMORAL PRODUCTS

Historically, the first humoral substance to be recognized (1894) as having a messenger function was an amine, epinephrine. The first use of the word *hormone* (Gr. *hormaein*—to excite or to arouse) was by Bayliss and Starling in 1902 to describe the action of secretin in an extract of duodenal mucosa on the exocrine pancreas. This latter hormone was later identified as a polypeptide. Thus, the first two hormones, an amine and a polypeptide, are not

only representative of APUD-cell secretory products but were identified originally by their function of provoking a physiological action, a biologic phenomenon. Many additional humoral products have been identified by their function, physiological or pharmacologic, before their molecular composition was determined. The prototype of the third type of hormone, the steroids, is cortisol (hydrocortisone), which was isolated as recently as 1937; its importance is suggested by the fact that it is the only steroid hormone that is essential to life.

Whereas most hormonal substances have been identified with specific endocrine cells and specific physiological actions on the target cells, some seem only to function as markers without a known purpose; human pancreatic polypeptide (hPP) is such a circulating polypeptide. It does have pharmacologic and physiological actions that are antithetical to cholecystokinin–pancreozymin (CCK–PZ) and has been reported to be increased in about 50% of tumors and in the blood of patients with endocrine neoplasms of the pancreas, such as insulinomas, gastrinomas, vipomas, and glucagonomas. However, its chief importance is its role in the detection of the pancreatic component of multiple endocrine adenopathy, type I.

There are other humoral substances that sometimes circulate in association with normal hormones which themselves have strong physiological actions, such as the various prostaglandins and the kinins, which are present in excess in patients with the carcinoid syndromes, pancreatic cholera, and medullary carcinoma of the thyroid gland. The significance of these "extrahormonal" substances is still unknown.

It is important to think of the circulating hormones not only in terms of their chemical composition (amines, polypeptides, and steroids) but also in terms of their functional interrelationships. For instance, insulin and glucagon have opposing actions and share the natural responsibility for carbohydrate metabolism with growth hormone, thyroxine, epinephrine, cortisol, and SST; parathyrin and thyrocalcitonin are antithetically involved in the divalent-ion metabolism of calcium and phosphorus, and they share one of their end-organs (the renal tubules) with another hormone, aldosterone, which is involved in the mineral metabolism of sodium and chloride. Gastrin and secretin provide opposing acidity or alkalinity for luminal digestion of food. Another and more useful categorization of hormones is to consider their metabolic function in terms of being anabolic or catabolic. Those humoral agents with a general anabolic purpose are insulin, gastrin, growth hormone, and the androgens; the remainder are generally catabolic, particularly glucagon, SST, thyroxine, and the secretinlike humoral agents, which include vasoactive intestinal peptide (VIP), CCK–PZ, and gastric inhibitory peptide (GIP).

The measurement of elevated levels of circulating hormones in the blood must take into account the normal diurnal variations due to the inherent circadian rhythm, particularly the pituitary and adrenocortical elaboration, and also whether environmental factors such as fasting, feeding, and basal or active states are influential at the time.

Although a hormone that is normally released from normal endocrine cells may be the same small molecular structure as when elaborated from a hyperplastic or tumorous cell, it is a general rule that when a malignancy of the endocrine cells elaborates that humoral product, the hormone is usually of a larger molecular size, a precursor peptide displaying altered biologic and immunologic capabilities. Some of these tumor products are the larger pro-hormones, such as proinsulin.

TARGET CELLS AND RECEPTOR MECHANISMS

Circulating hormones produce their effect by their action upon their specific and responsive target cells, which, in turn, produce their biologic effect (see Fig. 20-2). The target cells may be specific glands, such as that part of the adrenal cortex that is responsive to the trophic polypeptide corticotropin (ACTH), or they may be diffusely scattered cells, as in response to growth hormone and thyroxine. A target cell may respond to more than one stimulus by virtue of the fact that it may possess more than one type of receptor; for instance, there are three separate receptors on the gastric parietal cell: one for gastrin, one for acetylcholine, and one for histamine. Receptors for at least 12 of the polypeptide hormones have now been identified, and these receptors form an integral part of the target-cell membrane. When the hormone, the "first messenger," combines with its specific membrane receptor, the enzyme adenylcyclase is activated to catalyze the conversion of adenosine triphosphate (ATP) to cyclic adenosine monophosphate (cAMP), the "second messenger"; cAMP, together with its kinase, then initiates the primary biologic function of that cell. Such membrane receptors can be blocked pharmacologically, for example with cimetidine blockade of the H_2 receptor, or the membrane receptor can be occupied by a competing polypeptide, such as CCK, which has a competitive attraction for the gastrin receptor. The activity of the cAMP receptor mechanism can be measured; an important biologic function of the polypeptides VIP and parathyroid hormone is the stimulation of increased measurable cAMP receptor activity.

Steroid hormones, on the other hand, combine with intracellular cytoplasmic receptors after diffusion through the target-cell membrane. The steroid hormone receptor complex is than transferred into the nucleus of the target cell where gene transcription occurs and deoxyribonucleic acid (DNA) is converted to messenger ribonucleic acid (RNA); in this way, specific proteins, including the polypeptides, are synthesized.

NEUROHUMORAL HOMEOSTASIS

NORMAL

When all the mechanisms of the regulation of endocrine cell function and target cell response are in balance, a remarkable normal homeostasis is evident, not only for the efficient use and metabolism of energy, food, water, and minerals but also for the preservation of life by neurovascular responses and, indeed, the preservation of the species by steroid hormone influences between the adrenals, the gonads, the placenta, and the brain. The simple act of contemplating and consuming a meal initiates a series of neurohumoral transmissions, beginning with vagal stimulation of acid, antral release of gastrin, duodenal secretin inhibition of gastric secretion, and stimulation of pancreatic bicarbonate secretion. Insulin, glucagon, hPP, and CCK–PZ release occurs after absorption of glucose, proteins, and fats. After temporary fluctuations, the concentrations of the polypeptides and exocrine products in the blood return almost immediately to stable basal levels. The rapidity of the fluctuations is fastest with the amines, followed by the polypeptides, while the steroid changes in activity are more

sluggish. The rather strong challenge of 100 g glucose during an oral glucose tolerance test in a normal person is handled so that homeostasis with normal glucose and insulin values is attained within 2 hours. When there is a prolonged stimulation, as in some abnormal disease states, compensatory regulation within normal bounds is a rule, at least for a time. It appears that compensatory reactions to a prolonged abnormal environment are possible chiefly by the development of a reactive hyperplasia. It is not known what it is that disrupts the balance of homeostasis to the point of decompensation of neuroendocrine control, but the theoretical possibilities include the development of reactive hyperplasia in compensation for or in response to a chronic abnormal environment and the development of hyperplasia or dysplasia upon genetic instigation or some unknown instigation toward neoplasia *de novo*.

DECOMPENSATED

The normal balance of the internal milieu is easily decompensated by the autonomous hypersecretion of humoral substances from neoplastic tumors. Within the wide spectrum of clinical syndromes due to functional endocrinopathies, there are hyperfunctioning hyperplasias due to genetic instigation, such as the familial multiple endocrine adenopathies; other syndromes, however, may not have a pathogenetic basis except to result, possibly, from abnormal environmental influences. Among the latter group are increasing numbers of endocrinopathies that are based histologically on hyperplasia and include the parathyroid hyperplasias resulting from thiazide, glucocorticoid administration, or irradiation. Included also are the adrenocortical hyperplasias associated with abnormal cholesterol metabolism in the adrenogenital syndrome and, possibly, the islet cell hyperplasias of nesidioblastosis, which is present in the hypoglycemia of infancy.

It is not known whether dysfunction precedes the development of hyperplasia. Conversely, hyperplasia of endocrine cells may lead to endocrine dysfunction. There is some evidence that hyperplasia may proceed to neoplasia. The association of more than one type of histologic pattern in the same gland or in the same patient suggests a progression toward neoplasia in patients who are at risk for hereditary medullary thyroid carcinoma and who have progressive increase in serum thyrocalcitonin levels in response to calcium infusion. Hyperplasia of the thyroid C cells has been observed to precede the development of medullary carcinoma. At the other end of the spectrum of endocrinopathies are the frequently observed remissions and exacerbations. Even spontaneous regressions of metastatic endocrine tumors are sporadically reported.

PATHOGENETIC TYPES OF ENDOCRINOPATHIES

SPORADIC AND GENETIC

When endocrine tumors were first recognized, it was considered that the sporadic pathologic process was usually an adenoma, largely because early reports described a single lesion of insulinoma, gastrinoma, parathyroid adenoma, and pituitary adenoma. Soon, however, islet hyperplasias were observed, either as the sole abnormality or in association with tumors in the same gland. When the genetic familial multiple endocrine adenopathies were recognized as being distinct from the sporadic occurrences, the concept of hyperplasias and multiple tumors became challenges in diagnosis and therapy. Islet hyperplasia, consisting of an increase in the number of islet cells and consequently enlarged islets, is distinguished by some from nesidioblastosis. The latter term, coined by Laidlaw for "islet building" and reported by Vance as being pathogenetic in genetic multiple endocrine adenopathy, type I, is histologically described as transformation of epithelial acinar cells into islet cells.

It is not unusual for islet cell tumors to be designated histologically as carcinoid tumors. This microscopic description, particularly in foregut endocrine tumors, should not deter the clinician from a search for associated functional secretion of polypeptides in addition to the possible elaboration of the amine serotonin. A diagnosis of malignancies involving the neuroendocrine cells is difficult histologically and is usually defined as demonstrating tumor invasion or the presence of metastases.

ENTOPIC AND ECTOPIC

APUD cell tumors may excessively release their humoral substances in either entopic or ectopic fashion. Pancreatic islet tumors serve as useful examples for both entopic and ectopic release of amine and polypeptide hormones. At the present time, tumors have been identified as arising from each of the five known types of islet cells. These orthoendocrine tumors elaborate humoral substances that are native to the islets. This entopic release includes the polypeptides (glucagon from the alpha cells, insulin from the beta cells, SST from the delta cells, hPP from the F cells) and the amine serotonin from the enterochromaffin cells. Some of the clinical pictures may be relatively silent, as with those that secrete SST and hPP. Other pancreatic islet tumors may just as commonly elaborate polypeptides that are not normally native to that organ; such ectopically functioning tumors include the relatively common gastrinoma, the vipoma, the corticotrophinoma, the parathyrinoma, and other rarer entities. Although gastrin-containing islet cells have been found in the fetal pancreas, most cytologists have not identified those cells in the normal adult pancreas. Ectopic humoral output of polypeptides may be multiple and mixed, in which one clinical picture may predominate. The majority of these ectopically functioning tumors are potentially malignant, and their secretory product is disproportionately that of prohormones, large and heterogenous precursor molecules of the polypeptides with variable biologic activity. The normal mature APUD cell contains hormone-processing enzymes, peptidases that cleave large prohormone molecules into the smaller polypeptides for that cell's normal singular function, thus repressing all other functions. The theory of ectopia involves the idea that the precursors of the APUD cell have a totipotential capability of synthesizing and secreting any of the polypeptides. When or if the APUD cells become malignant by any instigation, the cells revert to the primitive precursor state, lose the hormone-processing polypeptidase ability, derepress, and elaborate large-molecular prohormones having the activity of any of the potential polypeptides, an ectopic phenomenon. Ectopic tumors may be associated also with APUD cell hyperplasia. Even malignant tumors of cells that are not usually considered to be endocrine APUD cells may elaborate protein or polypeptide substances excessively; when polypeptide hormones are secreted, the malignant cell is con-

sidered by some to have disdifferentiated to assume APUD functional characteristics for the release of polypeptides. The syndromes that arise from these nonendocrine tumors are designated as paraendocrine syndromes.

The pathogenetic types of syndromes therefore involve determining sporadic or genetic etiology, entopic or ectopic function, and, finally, hyperplastic or neoplastic process. Some of these differentiations can be made by family history, evidence of multiplicity, and localization studies. Stimulation and suppression tests generally produce normal responses in hyperplasias but not in autonomous neoplasias.

CLINICAL CONSIDERATIONS

DIAGNOSTIC ADVANCES

The development of quantitative radioimmunoassay measurements of circulating polypeptides has paved the way for accurate and earlier diagnoses of neuroendocrine tumors. Prior to that important accomplishment, only qualitative bioassays were possible. A new era in diagnoses came with Yalow and Berson's methodology for quantitative determinations of immunoreactive insulin (IRI) in 1959. At the same time, Gregory and Tracy biochemically elucidated the constituency and properties of the gastrin molecules in antral mucosa and in gastrinomas. Their identification and the subsequent synthesis of the active terminal pentapeptide led the way to immunochemical identification of the gastrin cells by McGuigan and radioimmunoassay of gastrin in serum by Stremple and Meade. The production of antibodies to synthetic protein segments has made assays possible for more candidate hormones than there are recognized clinical syndromes.

Although basal fasting levels of circulating polypeptides are usually diagnostic as tumor markers, the more recent development of stimulation and suppression tests has made diagnoses more secure in terms of the underlying pathologic abnormality and the detection of genetic predisposition. Virtually all normal or hyperplastic endocrine cells respond appropriately to their environment; neoplastic cells, however, either are autonomous or respond in a paradoxical manner. An example of this phenomenon is that the hypersecretion due to antral G cell hyperplasia with hypergastrinism responds to a standard test meal but not to intravenous secretin stimulation; on the other hand, a neoplastic pancreatic gastrinoma does not respond excessively to a standard test meal but does respond to intravenous secretin stimulation.

TUMOR LOCALIZATION

Because neuroendocrine tumors are usually small and soft, the more common techniques for localization are often fruitless. Physical examination, palpation, and radioisotopic and computed tomography tests do not fare very well in localization of tumors. Because many of these tumors are hypervascular, angiographic demonstration is possible in from 50% to 90% of patients; this technique, however, is too often not helpful. More recently, tumor localization has been possible by selective assays of the suspect humoral product in the venous blood draining from the suspected site of tumor. Intravenous catheterization and selective venous assays are becoming more and more applicable, but the technique requires sophisticated equipment and technical expertise. The newest of these techniques is the percutaneous transhepatic–transportal venous assay of blood draining the pancreas and gastrointestinal tract for the presence of serotonin, gastrin, insulin, and other humoral products. Selective venous assays are also used for the localization of persistent parathyroid tumors after unsuccessful operative exploration and also for lateral localization of adrenal tumors by catheterization of the adrenal or renal veins. The primary indication for the preoperative use of selective venous assays is failure of localization of small (less than 1 cm) or multiple lesions by computed tomography or arterial angiography.

NEW THERAPEUTIC MODALITIES

The premier role of surgical excision of resectable endocrine tumors has been undisputed since the first documentation of satisfactory results in patients with insulin-secreting adenomas or parathyroid adenomas. Its effectiveness persists even in patients who have developed malignant lesions with limited local lymph node metastases and in patients with hyperfunctioning endocrine hyperplasias who respond to subtotal excisions. The characteristically chronic rate of growth of most endocrine tumors, particularly of the entopic variety, favors surgical intervention, even for palliation. Because of the functional nature of the tumors, both primary and metastatic, surgical excision of the primary and even the metastatic lesions has been advocated; moreover, surgical excision of the target organ is frequently of clinical benefit, particularly in patients with metastatic pancreatic gastrinomas and in patients who have adrenocortical hyperplasia secondary to ACTH-secreting tumors. An unexpected but rare benefit of total gastrectomy for metastatic pancreatic gastrinomas has been the occasional (eight patients in the United States) observation of regression of metastases following excision of the end-organ by total gastrectomy. It is in patients with diffusely metastatic lesions accountable to late diagnoses or in patients with the genetic manifestations of multiple neoplastic lesions that surgical treatment directed at the tumor may ultimately fail. It is precisely these clinical situations that have prompted the development and use of specific chemotherapeutic agents for the tumor and the palliative application of receptor blockade of the biologic effect of the tumor polypeptide. Hormonal therapy, such as with the inhibitory SST, has demonstrated a palliative role in hyperinsulinism and hyperglucagonism.

Among recent therapeutic advances, the development of receptor blockers such as cimetidine has been the most exciting and universally applied palliative measure for the Zollinger-Ellison syndrome. Its blockade of the H_2 receptor also interrupts the effect of the gastrin and acetylcholine receptors on the gastric parietal cell, effectively decreasing its acid secretory capacity. It has been hoped that this receptor blocker might have an effect on the tumor itself or its hormonal release, similar to that sometimes observed after total gastrectomy for the Zollinger-Ellison syndrome; however, such an effect has not been forthcoming. On the other hand, actual progression of tumor has been observed in patients while receiving cimetidine treatment, and rising serum gastrin values have been observed. Prolonged administration of cimetidine requires continuous patient compliance, and its long-term effectiveness is not known. The chief indication for its use in the Zollinger-Ellison syndrome is for control of gastric-acid hypersecretion in three groups of patients: those patients with nonresectable gastrinomas metastatic to the liver who have not had total gastrectomy or in whom specific chemotherapy has failed; those patients, with and without multiple endocrine adenopathy, type I, who present with acute ulcer manifestations, including hypercalcemic crises, during which cimetidine provides time for confirmation of the diagnosis and preparation of the patient for appropriate surgical treatment; and those patients who have refused surgical intervention, usually because cimetidine treatment has resulted in a false sense of security.

Therapeutic measures that offer more hope of benefit or cure for patients with nonresectable metastases from any of the apudomas, in particular of the pancreas, consist of newly developing specific chemotherapeutic agents that can be administered intra-arterially or intravenously. Streptozotocin drugs, which were first used experimentally to produce diabetes by the destruction of beta insulin-secreting cells, have produced complete tumor remission in some patients and are generally effective in approximately 50% of a variety of metastatic apudomas of the pancreas.

RECOGNITION OF CLINICAL SYNDROMES

The remarkable advances in conceptual, technical, diagnostic, and therapeutic modalities have materially influenced the clinical detection and management of the old and the newer endocrine syndromes. Just as early clinical descriptions of endocrinopathies spurred advances in basic endocrine research, clinicians with the added advantage of studying at first hand have, in turn, applied and adapted that information to the care of their patients.

Considering the universality of the neuroendocrine system, particularly in light of the common embryology and cytochemical characteristics, it is remarkable that the clinical syndromes produced by hyperfunctioning tumors should be so varied and bizarre. The spectrum of clinical pictures ranges from minimal symptomatology, associated with so-called nonfunctioning or asymptomatic tumors, to the fulminating clinical crises, associated with hypercalcemia, perforated jejunal ulcer, and profound hypoglycemia.

The mechanism of the production of symptoms may differ among various endocrinopathies. Whereas most tumors produce their symptoms by virtue of excessive elaboration of the humoral products that act on specific exocrine end-organs, some polypeptides act on other endocrine end-organs. An example of the endocrine-to-endocrine mechanism is the effect of corticotropin on the adrenal cortex, as is seen in the pituitary type of Cushing's disease and in the ectopic elaboration of ACTH from pulmonary and pancreatic tumors. The effect of SST-secreting tumors is also an example in which this inhibitory hormone affects the cells that secrete insulin, glucagon, and growth hormone. More commonly, however, the effect is on the exocrine end-organs, which is exemplified by the pancreatic gastrinoma effect on the stomach; the parathyroid adenoma influence on the renal tubules, the bones, and the brain; and the effect of insulin and glucagon on the liver.

Symptoms can also be due to pressure effects of expanding endocrine tumors on surrounding endocrine cells; pituitary tumors in this way produce manifestations of hypofunction, such as hypogonadism.

Endocrinopathies may come to mind purely by their association with other clinical states; for instance, somatostatinomas have been found serendipitously in the pancreas at the time of cholecystectomy for cholecystolithiasis.

Endocrine tumors have been detected in completely asymptomatic patients by the laboratory screening of patients who demonstrate chemical abnormalities such as hypercalcemia, hyperglycemia, or hypoglycemia.

Finally, patients with a positive family history of endocrinopathies prompt further elucidation of genetic forms by means of prospective screening of the relatives at risk for multiple endocrinopathies. In this regard, assays for hPP are particularly useful in the detection of the pancreatic component in such patients and their families.

There are certain types of symptoms in a clinical situation that may initiate the discovery of hidden endocrinopathies. Gastrointestinal ulceration due to hypersecretion of acid is a notable example in which the pathogenesis requires differentiation; such ulceration could be due to neurogenic vagal influence or antral G cell hyperfunction or pancreaticoduodenal gastrinomas. The presence of diarrhea after exclusion of more common causes may lead to the diagnosis of secretory diarrhea due to elaboration of VIP or GIP, medullary carcinoma of the thyroid, carcinoid tumors, or the Zollinger-Ellison syndrome. The presence of hypertension may, during diagnostic differentiation, call attention to the presence of Cushing's syndrome, pheochromocytomas, or aldosteronomas. The presence of gallstones and diabetes might suggest a diagnosis of somatostatinoma of the pancreas. The symptomatology mnemonically referred to as "stones, bones, moans, and groans" may call attention to the possibility of hyperparathyroidism. Finally, the mere presence of a mass such as a palpably enlarged cervical lymph node may be the only clue to the presence of medullary carcinoma of the thyroid gland.

Clinicians are becoming increasingly aware of the need for differentiation between similar endocrinopathies by means of venous assays for the circulating humoral substances, using both basal and provocative testing. Notable among the stimulation tests is the intravenous calcium stimulation for pancreatic gastrinomas, insulinomas, and carcinoid tumors. Intravenous secretin stimulation, as has been mentioned, is extremely useful in the detection of pancreatic gastrinomas in the Zollinger-Ellison syndrome and for its failure to detect excessive gastrin response from the antral mucosa in the pseudo-Zollinger-Ellison syndrome. In the latter instance, the standard test meal is useful in corroborating antral G cell hyperplasia. The standard test meal is also used to stimulate the release of pancreatic polypeptide from the pancreatic component in asymptomatic patients with the multiple endocrinopathy, type I. The stimulation tests for medullary carcinoma of the thyroid and C cell hyperplasia include the use of pentagastrin, calcium, and even alcohol. The most notable of the suppression tests includes the dexamethasone suppression test to identify the nature of a patient's hypercortisolism.

BIBLIOGRAPHY

BAYLIN SB, MENDELSOHN G: Ectopic (inappropriate) hormone production by tumors: Mechanisms involved and the biological and clinical implications. Endocr Rev 1:45, 1980

BAYLISS WM, STARLING EH: The mechanism of pancreatic secretion. J Physiol 28:325, 1902

DAVIS CE, VANSANT JH: Zollinger-Ellison syndrome: Spontaneous regression of advanced intra-abdominal metastases with 20-year survival. Ann Surg 189:620, 1979

DEVENEY CW, DEVENEY KS, JAFFE BM et al: Use of calcium and secretin in the diagnosis of gastrinoma (Zollinger-Ellison syndrome). Ann Intern Med 87:680, 1977

EDKINS JS: On the chemical mechanism of gastric secretion. Proc R Soc Lond 76:376, 1905

FEYRTER F: Uber die Pathologie peripherer vegatativer Regulationen am Beispiel des Karzinoids und des Karzinoidsyndrom. In Handbuch der Allgemainen Pathologie. Berlin, Springer-Verlag, 8:2, 1966

FRIESEN SR: APUD tumors of the gastrointestinal tract. In Hickey RC (ed): Current Problems in Cancer. Chicago, Year Book Medical Publishers, 1976

FRIESEN SR: Treatment of the Zollinger-Ellison syndrome: A twenty-five-year assessment. Am J Surg 143:331, 1982

FRIESEN SR, BOLINGER RE (eds): Surgical Endocrinology, Clinical Syndromes. Philadelphia, J B Lippincott, 1978

FRIESEN SR, KIMMEL JR, TOMITA T: Pancreatic polypeptide as screening marker for pancreatic polypeptide apudomas in multiple endocrinopathies. Am J Surg 139:61, 1980

FRIESEN SR, SCHIMKE RN, PEARSE AGE: Genetic aspects of the Z-E syndrome: Prospective studies in two kindred; antral gastrin cell hyperplasia. Ann Surg 176:370, 1972

GREGORY RA, TRACY HJ: Constitution and properties of two gastrins extracted from hog antral mucosa. J Physiol 169:18, 1963

GREGORY RA, TRACY HJ, FRENCH JM et al: Extraction of a gastrin-like substance from a pancreatic tumor in a case of Zollinger-Ellison syndrome. Lancet I:1045, 1960

INGEMANSSON S, LARSSON LI, LUNDERQUIST A et al: Pancreatic vein catheterization with gastrin assay in normal patients and in patients with the Zollinger-Ellison syndrome. Am J Surg 134:558, 1977

KAPLAN EL, JAFFE BM, PESKIN GW: A new provocative test for the diagnosis of the carcinoid syndrome. Am J Surg 123:173, 1972

KAPLAN EL, RUBENSTEIN AH, EVANS R et al: Calcium infusion: A new provocative test for insulinomas. Ann Surg 190:501, 1979

KIMMEL JR, HAYDEN LJ, POLLOCK HG: Isolation and characterization of a new pancreatic polypeptide hormone. J Biol Chem 250:9369, 1975

LAIDLAW GW: Nesidioblastoma, the islet tumor of the pancreas. Am J Pathol 14:125, 1938

LIPS CJM, VAN DER SLUYS VEER J, VAN DER DONK JA et al: Common precursor molecule as origin for the ectopic-hormone-producing-tumour syndrome. Lancet 1:16, 1978

MCCARTHY DM: The place of surgery in the Zollinger-Ellison syndrome. N Engl J Med 302:1344, 1980

MCGUIGAN JE: Gastric mucosal intracellular localization of gastrin by immunofluorescence. Gastroenterology 55:315, 1968

MCGUIGAN JE, TRUDEAU WL: Immunochemical measurement of elevated levels of gastrin in the serum of patients with pancreatic tumors of the Zollinger-Ellison variety. N Engl J Med 278:1308, 1968

PAVLOV IP: The Work of the Digestive Glands. Thompson WH (trans): London, Charles Griffin & Co, 1910

PEARSE AGE: The diffuse neuroendocrine system and the APUD concept: Related »endocrine« peptides in brain, intestine, pituitary, placenta, and anuran cutaneous glands. Med Biol 55:115, 1977

STREMPLE JF, MEADE RC: Production of antibodies to synthetic human gastrin I and radioimmunoassay of gastrin in the serum of patients with the Zollinger-Ellison syndrome. Surgery 64:165, 1968

TAPIA FJ, BARBOSA AJA, MARANGOS PJ et al: Neuron-specific enolase is produced by neuroendocrine tumours. Lancet I:808, 1981

UNGER RH: Somatostatinoma. N Engl J Med 296:998, 1977

VANCE FE, STOLL RW, KITABCHI AE et al: Familial nesidioblastosis as the predominant manifestation of multiple endocrine adenomatosis. Am J Med 52:211, 1972

YALOW RS, BERSON SA: Assay of plasma insulin in human subjects by immunologic methods. Nature 184:1648, 1959

ZOLLINGER RM, ELLISON EH: Primary peptic ulceration of the jejunum associated with islet cell tumors of the pancreas. Ann Surg 142:709, 1955

Jules Hardy/Gérard Mohr

The Pituitary

EMBRYOLOGY, ANATOMY, BLOOD SUPPLY, AND NORMAL HISTOLOGY

The pituitary gland, or "hypophysis cerebri," hangs at the base of the brain, attached to the hypothalamus by the pituitary stalk and encased in a depression of the sphenoid bone, the sella turcica. Its major role in endocrinologic and metabolic control rests upon its dual functional relationship to the diencephalon—the adenohypophysis secretes trophic hormones that are controlled by hypothalamic factors, and the neurohypophysis secretes ADH (antidiuretic hormone, or vasopressin), oxytocin, and some other derivates called neurophysins that are mediated by the neurosecretion of the hypothalamic nuclei.

EMBRYOLOGY

This functional duality between the glandular portion and the neural portion of the pituitary is explained by their different origins during early embryonic life. The upward growth and progressive invagination of the ectoderm of the primitive buccal cavity called Rathke's pouch or the craniopharyngeal canal forms the adenohypophysis. The neurohypophysis results from a downward protrusion of the floor of the diencephalon (Fig. 20-3).

ANATOMY

The pituitary gland is a yellow ovoid-shaped structure that measures about 12 mm in its transverse, 8 mm in its anteroposterior, and 6 mm in its vertical axis. Its weight varies between 0.5 g and 0.6 g in adult males; it is slightly heavier in women and may increase by 20% or more during pregnancy. The anterior lobe of the pituitary gland is divided into three parts: the pars distalis (pars glandularis), which is the major secretory portion; the pars tuberalis, which is a thin strip of tissue wrapped around the base of the neural stalk; and the pars intermedia, which is formed by the posterior part of the gland and the cleft, a thin cavity between the two lobes. The posterior lobe also consists of three parts: the infundibular process (neural lobe, or pars nervosa), which is the main part; the infundibular stem (neural stalk), which is the nervous part of the stalk; and the infundibulum (median eminence of the tuber cinereum), which is the upper end of the stalk attached to the hypothalamus. The close connections of the pituitary gland with the median eminence of the hypothalamus consist of two parts: a direct neural connection through the infundibular process and neural lobe and an indirect vascular connection through the blood vessels of the portal system. These pathways form the anatomic basis for neuroendocrine control of the pituitary gland by the central nervous system.

The pituitary fossa is a depression of the body of the sphenoid bone, limited anteriorly by the tuberculum sellae turcicae and posteriorly by the posterior clinoid processes. The lateral and superior limits of the sella turcica are formed by dural expansions, the medial walls of the cavernous sinuses, and the diaphragma sellae. The cavernous sinuses contain the carotid arteries and the sixth cranial nerve, whereas the lateral wall of the cavernous sinus contains the third and fourth cranial nerves and the first and second divisions of the fifth nerve. The diaphragma sellae is a membranous dural expansion with a central opening through which passes the pituitary stalk; it varies in size, allowing in some cases an arachnoidal prolapse of the chiasmatic cistern into the sella turcica.

Immediately above the diaphragma sellae lie the optic

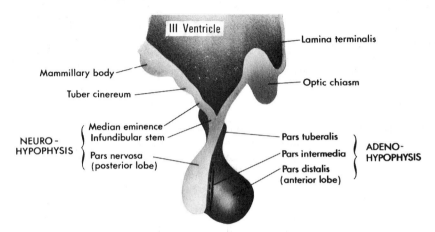

Fig. 20-3. Schematic anatomy of the hypothalamo-hypophyseal region.

nerves and the optic chiasm, the latter containing cross-fibers for both temporal fields (nasal retina) and uncross-fibers for both nasal fields (temporal retina). Variations in the position of the optic chiasm are encountered. In some cases with a prefixed chiasm, visual symptoms may appear early in the growth of a pituitary neoplasm, whereas in a postfixed chiasm, the tumor may reach considerable size before visual impairment becomes evident.

Behind and above the optic chiasm the pentagon-shaped optochiasmatic cistern is bounded anteriorly by the frontal lobe, laterally by the temporal unci, and posteriorly by the brain stem and the anterior wall of the third ventricle.

BLOOD SUPPLY

There are three major arterial supplies to the hypothalamo-neurohypophyseal axis: The superior hypophyseal artery provides vascular support to the infundibulum, the middle hypophyseal artery to the pituitary stalk, and the inferior hypophyseal artery to the neurohypophysis. There is a capillary network linking the neurohypophysis to the hypothalamus.

The venous drainage linking the hypothalamus to the anterior hypophysis is composed of large portal veins with both a downward and an upward flow. There are also short portal veins between the anterior and posterior hypophyses. The main venous drainage runs through hypophyseal veins from the neurohypophysis into the cavernous sinus. This recent finding of an upgoing flow through the venous portal system to the hypothalamus supports a new concept that the brain is also a target endocrine organ.

NORMAL HISTOLOGY

When a midhorizontal section is performed through the pituitary gland, three different areas are recognized in the anterior region. A central "mucoid wedge" contains abundant cells with PAS and lead-hematoxylin reactivity. On each side are the lateral "acidophil" wings where the majority of acidophil cells are localized. By combining the techniques of immunocytochemistry, histologic stains, and electron microscopy, six different cell types can be recognized: (1) growth hormone or somatotropic cells, (2) prolactin or lactotropic cells, which are located mainly in the lateral portions of the gland, (3) adrenocorticotropic hormone (ACTH) or corticolipotropic cells, which are located mainly in the central mucoid wedge close to the posterior

lobe, (4) gonadotropic cells, which consist of both follicle-stimulating hormone (FSH) and luteinizing hormone (LH) cells, are located mainly in the central wedge but are also found in the lateral wings, (5) thyroid-stimulating hormone (TSH) or thyrotropic cells, which are located mainly in the anterior subcapsular area of the median wedge, and (6) chromophobe cells, which are diffusely distributed within the pituitary parenchyma (Fig. 20-4).

The posterior lobe consists of nerve fibers and terminal ramifications of the hypothalamo-hypophyseal tract and of "pituicytes," glial cells that are intimately associated with sinusoid capillaries.

This topographic distribution of nuclei or pools of cells secreting the various hormones of the pituitary constitutes an anatomic basis for the selective distribution of hypersecreting pituitary microadenomas.

ENDOCRINE FUNCTIONS OF THE PITUITARY GLAND

Once believed to be the "conductor" of the endocrine system, the pituitary gland now appears to be part of a highly sophisticated neuroendocrine system, which, originating within the central nervous system, acts upon the hypothalamus through neurotransmitters such as dopamine and norepinephrine.

Of the many hypothalamic regulatory substances so far postulated, only three have been isolated and structurally determined and their physiological activity demonstrated: thyrotropin-releasing hormone (TRH), luteinizing hormone–releasing hormone (LH–RH); growth hormone–releasing inhibiting hormone (GH–RIH, or somatostatin). The chemical nature of the others is still unknown. A prolactin-inhibiting factor (PIF) has not been isolated yet but may be a dopaminergic agent (DA).

ADENOHYPOPHYSEAL HORMONES

There are seven main hormones secreted by the anterior pituitary that have a distinct function:
1. ACTH, which stimulates the adrenal cortex to the biosynthesis of cortisol and has been named the "stress hormone"
2. Melanotropin (β-melanophore-stimulating hormone [MSH]), which controls the skin pigmentation

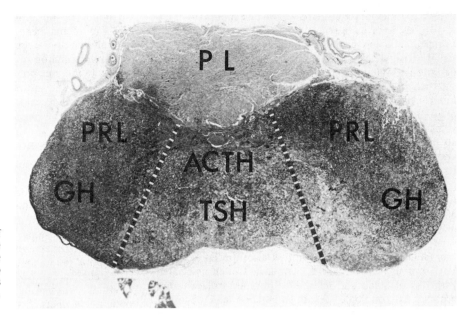

Fig. 20-4. Midhorizontal section of a normal hypophysis showing the three main zones: a central mucoid zone containing ACTH and TSH cells; two lateral wings containing nuclei or pools of cells. *PRL,* posterior; *GH,* anterior. (*PL* = posterior lobe)

3. Lipotropins (β-LPH, γ-LPH), which are responsible for fat-mobilizing activity; β-LPH is the prohormone for endorphins (endogenous morphine-like substances)
4. TSH, which stimulates the thyroid gland to produce thyroid hormones
5. Gonadotropins (FSH, LH), which influence the male and female germinal organs and affect reproduction
6. Somatotropin (growth hormone), which affects body growth and has also a diabetogenic anti-insulin action on glucose metabolism
7. Prolactin (PRL), which promotes the development of the mammary gland and the activation of lactation

All these anterior pituitary hormones can be measured directly with high accuracy by radioimmunoassay.

NEUROHYPOPHYSEAL HORMONES

1. Vasopressin (ADH) plays a major role in salt and water metabolism by regulating the volume and osmolarity of the plasma.
2. Oxytocin plays a significant role in contraction of the uterus during labor and has a secondary role in lactation.

3. Neurophysins are derivates of vasopressin and oxytocin; their exact action is unknown, but current research has already shown important applications because this biologic activity is easily measurable.

PITUITARY TUMORS	
Etiology	Adenoma, craniopharyngioma
Dx	Headache; visual disturbances; hypo- or hyperpituitarism; pituitary hormone–specific syndromes; elevated serum prolactin, ACTH, TSH, GH, and MSH; CT scan
Rx	Transsphenoidal resection, intracranial resection

CLINICAL MANIFESTATIONS OF PITUITARY TUMORS

The majority of pituitary tumors are represented by adenomas, epithelial neoplasms arising from the adenohypophyseal tissue and accounting for 8% of all primary intracranial tumors. Craniopharyngiomas, arising from epithelial rests of Rathke's pouch, occur in two thirds of the cases in childhood and adolescence and are manifested as pituitary hypofunction or visual impairment. In rare instances, primary tumors such as meningiomas, chordomas, gliomas, epidermoid and dermoid cysts, germinomas, and teratomas may arise in or near the sella. Primary intrasellar cysts are known as Rathke's cleft cysts.

ENDOCRINE PITUITARY SYNDROMES

Pituitary dysfunction of tumor origin results in certain decreased or increased endocrine functions, sometimes together.

HYPOPITUITARISM

In children and adolescents pituitary hypofunction results in growth retardation called pituitary dwarfism, as well as reduced basal metabolism, arterial hypotension, decreased skin pigmentation, and delayed or absent puberty. It is usually seen with craniopharyngiomas. Recently, chromophobe pituitary microadenomas causing growth failure in children have been reported. In adults hypopituitarism may be partial, accounting for decreased libido, impotence–frigidity and amenorrhea in gonadotropin deficiency, and increased fatigue and hypotension in corticotropin deficiency. Panhypopituitarism is usually found in large nonsecreting adenomas in advanced stages.

HYPERPITUITARISM

Selective overproduction of pituitary hormones is characteristic of hypersecreting pituitary adenomas (endocrine active adenomas).

Growth Hormone–Secreting Adenomas

In adults these eosinophilic adenomas produce the well-known acromegaly with increased development of soft tissues and membranous bones of the face and extremities. Headaches, joint pain, paresthesias in the hands, and nocturnal diaphoresis are also common symptoms. Diabetes mellitus or glucose intolerance and visceromegaly are frequently associated. Gigantism occurs in children and youngsters when growth hormone–secreting adenomas arise before closure of the epiphyses. In both instances, the disease may evolve for many years before a tumor has reached sufficient size to produce visual symptoms. Frequently there are mixed growth hormone– and prolactin-secreting adenomas.

Prolactin-Secreting Adenomas

Since the introduction of radioimmunoassay measurements of prolactin, prolactinomas have emerged as the most frequent pituitary adenomas. They are characterized by the syndrome of amenorrhea–galactorrhea, which may occur spontaneously after withdrawal of oral contraceptive medication or in the postpartum period. It is often associated with loss of libido and infertility. In males prolactinomas produce loss of libido, sexual impotence, and oligo- or azoospermia. Gynecomastia or galactorrhea may also be encountered in males. Biologically these tumors are diagnosed early by the significant elevation of serum prolactin levels. Microadenomas as small as 4 mm in diameter were found to cause these clinical pictures.

ACTH-LPH/MSH–Producing Adenomas

The classic clinical picture of Cushing's disease is characterized by truncal obesity, plethoric face, buffalo hump, hirsutism, and varicosities, in combination with other systemic and metabolic disorders such as hypertension, muscle weakness, menstrual disorders, mental disorders, and osteoporosis. It is due to hypercortisolism, in which a tripartite entity described as Cushing's syndrome may be produced from ectopic, adrenal, or pituitary origin. It is now recognized that a pituitary basophilic adenoma accounts for the cause of hypercortisolism in over 80% of cases. ACTH microadenomas may be present long before gross sellar enlargement becomes evident on skull roentgenograms.

Nelson's syndrome occurs after bilateral adrenalectomy for treatment of Cushing's disease, resulting in the development of the undetected primary pituitary adenoma. It is mainly associated with hyperpigmentation.

Thyrotropin-secreting adenoma produces a rare syndrome that simulates Graves' disease of hyperthyroidism and exophthalmos; it is due to autonomous oversecretion of TSH.

Gonadotropin (FSH, LH)-secreting adenomas are also rare entities that may be associated with polycystic ovaries.

PITUITARY APOPLEXY

In rare instances, pituitary adenomas may undergo acute degeneration with either massive intra-adenomatous hemorrhage or autonecrosis, resulting in a dramatic picture of acute headaches, loss of consciousness, subarachnoid hemorrhage, sudden blindness, and compression of both cavernous sinuses. If not treated, this catastrophic event may rapidly lead to death.

HEADACHES

Constant retro-orbital headache is encountered in approximately 50% of patients with an enclosed tumor due to the stretching of the aponeural sheet of the sella turcica and the diaphragma sellae. However, even with small adenomas, migrainous or intermittent headaches are often associated with oversecretion of growth hormone and PRL, probably owing to the metabolic effect on the water retention mechanism.

OPHTHALMOLOGIC SYMPTOMS

CHIASMAL SYNDROMES

In tumors with suprasellar extension, early chiasmatic compression can be detected only by specific clinical examination of the visual fields by confrontation using colors and by specific visual field assessment: Quadrantanopic defects for red color can be detected clinically, and campimetry will show upper quadrantanopic defects for the central isopters. With extensive suprasellar expansion, complete bitemporal hemianopia follows.

Parallel to the visual field defects, progressive decrease of visual acuity results from stretching of the chiasmatic and optic nerve fibers, heralded by pallor of the optic discs at fundoscopy. In the late stage, optic atrophy and progressive blindness occur.

EXTRAOCULAR MUSCLE DISTURBANCES

Large pituitary tumors may compress the lateral wall of the sella turcica and stretch the nerve fibers of the extraocular muscles in the cavernous sinus wall. The most frequent extraocular palsy involves the sixth cranial nerve, sometimes bilaterally.

ENDOCRINE EVALUATION OF PITUITARY DISORDERS

Most pituitary hormones and even some hypothalamic-releasing hormones (TRH and LH–RH) are currently measurable by radioimmunoassay. Preoperative endocrinologic assessment has two major goals: first, the recognition of specific hypersecretion in secreting adenomas such as growth hormone, PRL, and ACTH-LPH and, second, the diagnosis of latent or overt pituitary insufficiency.

NONSECRETING ADENOMAS

Static tests measure base hormone levels of plasma cortisol (compound F) and urinary cortisol for adrenocortical function; plasma T_3 and T_4 as well as TSH for thyroid function; and plasma testosterone, LH, and FSH for the pituitary gonadal axis.

DYNAMIC TESTS

Induced hypoglycemia following insulin administration normally stimulates growth hormone (GH), PRL, and ACTH secretion. Adequate elevation of basal levels demonstrates a sufficient anterior pituitary reserve of these hormones.

TRH TEST AND LH–RH TEST

Intravenous administration of these releasing hormones allows evaluation of the pituitary reserve of thyrotropin and PRL (TRH test) and gonadotropin (LH–RH test).

When the ACTH reserve is decreased, adequate pre- and postoperative coverage with steroids is mandatory. Thyroid and gonadal substitution, although less vital, is still important.

HYPERSECRETING ADENOMAS

Basically, hypersecreting adenomas can be detected by radioimmunoassay of the specific hormones involved. In borderline cases, additional dynamic tests will sometimes allow differentiation between tumoral and nontumoral hypersecretion.

GH ADENOMAS

In acromegaly, elevated GH levels above 5 ng/ml are found. Following oral hyperglycemia, GH levels fail to drop below 5 ng/ml. Paradoxical elevation of GH after TRH administration confirms the presence of active acromegaly.

PROLACTINOMAS

Elevated PRL levels above 20 ng/ml are suggestive of PRL-secreting adenomas. Absence of PRL response to TRH administration is usually observed. A suppression test using bromocriptine (a dopamine receptor–blocking agent) can also be used. Chlorpromazine administration has been utilized to assess PRL reserve; in adenomas, this reserve seems to be decreased compared with nontumoral hyperprolactinemia.

ACTH–LPH ADENOMAS

(See also The Adrenal Glands, later in this chapter.)
Urinary free cortisol is usually higher than 150 μg/24 hr. Plasma cortisol levels are elevated throughout the day in Cushing's disease. A suppression test using dexamethasone allows differentiation between pituitary and adrenal hyperadrenocorticism. In pituitary Cushing's disease, urinary free cortisol should decrease by 50% after dexamethasone (8 mg/day for 2 consecutive days). Stimulation tests using metyrapone and ACTH are followed by large increases of urinary 17-OH steroids and urinary cortisol in Cushing's disease.

RADIOLOGIC EVALUATION AND CLASSIFICATION OF PITUITARY TUMORS

RADIOLOGIC EVALUATION

The radiologic examination of the sellar region plays a major role in the diagnosis of pituitary tumors.

PLAIN SKULL FILMS

Plain skull films and stereoscopic sellar x-rays will show gross modification of the sella turcica caused by large tumors. Small tumors are readily detected by asymmetrical enlargement of the sella, producing a double floor contour.

POLYTOMOGRAPHY

Polytomography of the sella turcica is particularly useful in patients with a small or normal-appearing sella. The triad of thinning, ballooning, and concavity of the sellar floor is typical. On frontal tomograms, asymmetrical lowering of the floor is highly suggestive of a microadenoma in GH- and PRL-secreting pituitary syndromes, whereas a central depression is more frequently encountered in ACTH microadenomas.

COMPUTED TOMOGRAPHY

CT scanning has revolutionized the diagnosis of pituitary tumors. It allows a search for suprasellar masses in a noninvasive fashion and has largely replaced pneumoencephalography. The star-shaped optochiasmatic cistern can be scrutinized for tumor expansions above the diaphragma sellae, and various degrees of suprasellar expansions can be recognized according to the degree of filling of the cisternal pentagon. Possibly associated hydrocephalus is also easily detected by CT scanning. More recently, high resolution scanning associated with frontal cuts permits the positive diagnosis of intrasellar microadenomas.

CEREBRAL ANGIOGRAPHY

The role of cerebral angiography in the preoperative diagnosis is presently restricted mainly to the differential diagnosis of intra- or parasellar vascular lesions such as intracavernous aneurysms or meningiomas of the tuberculum or diaphragma sellae. In large adenomas with suprasellar expansion, both proximal portions of the anterior cerebral arteries are elevated.

RADIOLOGIC CLASSIFICATION OF PITUITARY ADENOMAS

This classification results from combined grading of bony modifications of the sella and the degree of suprasellar expansion if present (Fig. 20-5).

CLASSIFICATION ACCORDING TO THE BONY SELLA

The study of polytomograms of the sella allows a distinction to be made between "enclosed" adenomas with intact, although modified, sellar floor (grades 0, I, and II) and "invasive" adenomas with local or diffuse destruction of the sella (grades III and IV).

Fig. 20-5. Radiologic classification of the sella turcica and pituitary tumors. (*SSE* = suprasellar expansion)

ADENOMAS	ENCLOSED	GR. 0	NORMAL	
		GR. I <10 mm	MICRO-ADENOMA	
		GR. II >10 mm	NO SSE	
			SSE	
	INVASIVES	GR. III LOCALIZED	NO SSE	
			SSE	
		GR. IV DIFFUSE	NO SSE	
			SSE	

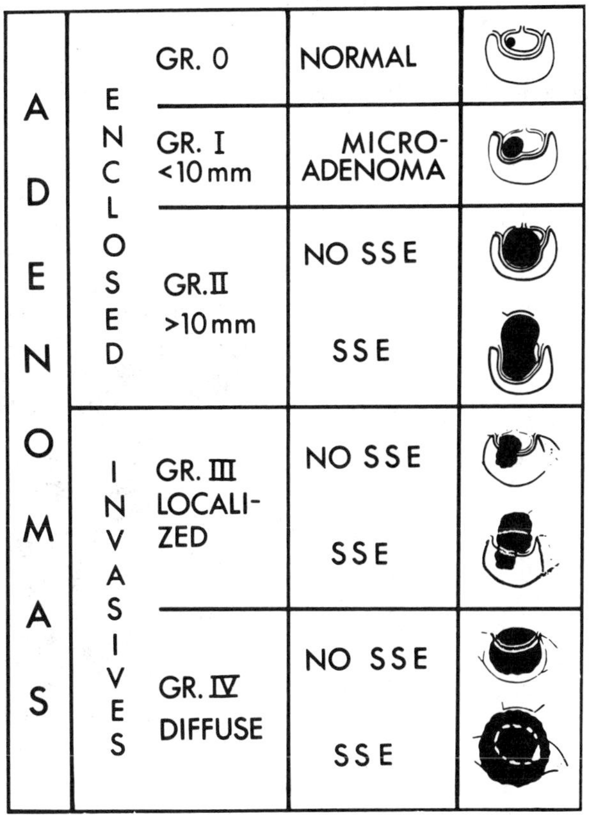

Grade 0: Normal-sized sella with horizontal and homogeneous floor (normal vertical and anterior–posterior diameter not exceeding 16 mm × 13 mm).

Grade I: Normal-sized sella, but the sellar floor shows local thinning and lateral lowering. This is typical for microadenomas measuring less than 10 mm in diameter.

Grade II: Global asymmetrical widening of the sella with thinning of the dorsum sellae and anterior clinoid processes.

Grade III: The widened sellar floor shows local erosion indicative of local invasion of the dural and bony elements.

Grade IV: The sellar boundaries are completely invisible on roentgenograms ("phantom sella"). In these cases, the tumor has largely infiltrated the dura and bone and fills most of the sphenoid sinus. These adenomas are not cancerous as such but their total surgical removal is impossible.

CLASSIFICATION OF SUPRASELLAR EXPANSION

Type A: The suprasellar expansion bulges into the chiasmatic cistern as much as 10 mm above the diaphragma sellae. There is an encroachment of the infundibular and supraoptic recesses of the third ventricle. On CT-scanning, there is less than 25% filling of the optochiasmatic cistern by the tumor.

Type B: The tumor reaches 20 mm above the diaphragma sellae and fills out the anterior portion of the third ventricle. On CT scan, 50% to 75% of the optochiasmatic cistern is filled.

Type C: A voluminous suprasellar expansion fills the third ventricle as much as 30 mm above the diaphragma sellae, reaching the foramina of Munro. Obstructive hydrocephalus may be present. On CT scan, the optochiasmatic cistern is no longer visible.

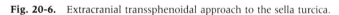

TREATMENT OF PITUITARY TUMORS

There are three main goals of therapy for pituitary tumors: first, effective chiasmal decompression to restore vision or stop visual compromise; second, total selective removal of the tumor for biologic cure; and third, preservation of proper function of the pituitary gland by sparing the normal pituitary tissue and avoiding any substitutional therapy.

These goals may be achieved by medical treatment, surgery, or radiotherapy. Surgical treatment, however, has become the cornerstone in the management of pituitary tumors, particularly since the major technical refinements owing to the use of microsurgical techniques have become common.

SURGICAL METHODS

INTRACRANIAL SUBFRONTAL APPROACH

Indications for craniotomy are largely restricted to meningiomas, craniopharyngiomas of the suprasellar type, or other lesions with small sellae. In pituitary adenomas, an endocranial approach is only necessary in patients with voluminous suprasellar expansion or asymmetrical tumor growth in the frontal or temporal fossa. The intracranial approach ("pterional" approach) consists of a lateral frontal craniotomy reaching the pterion; the ridge of the smaller sphenoid wing is followed and leads directly to the anterior clinoid process. Minimal elevation of the frontal lobe using cerebral relaxation techniques such as lumbar spinal drainage and mannitol allows exposure of the right optic nerve, which is then followed to the optic chiasm. The tumor expansion in front of the chiasm is usually readily accessible. Total removal is achieved by intracapsular excision of the tumor tissue. Particular care must be taken when dissecting the capsule from the pituitary stalk and the hypothalamus.

Fig. 20-6. Extracranial transsphenoidal approach to the sella turcica.

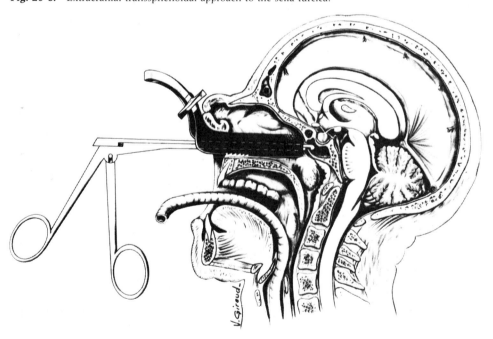

EXTRACRANIAL TRANSSPHENOIDAL APPROACH

Rapid and safe access to the sella turcica is achieved by entering the sphenoid sinus through the nose. More than 60 years ago, Harvey Cushing introduced the sublabial transseptal transsphenoidal approach to the pituitary but discontinued the use of this technique in the late 1920s, probably because of the high incidence of recurrence owing to blind operative maneuvers, which resulted in incomplete tumor removal in the majority of cases. After 30 years of universal use of the transfrontal operation, the extracranial transsphenoidal approach was reintroduced by Guiot. In the early 1960s, Hardy refined the transsphenoidal technique by adding the use of the operating microscope, monitoring by televised fluoroscopy, and microsurgical techniques of dissection, which allow precise differentiation between pathologic and normal tissue. This transsphenoidal microsurgical procedure (Fig. 20-6) has now become the standard modern technique for pituitary adenomas.

Fig. 20-7. Microsurgical removal of a 6-mm prolactin-secreting microadenoma in the posterior–inferior region of the lateral wing of the gland (*A*). Intraoperative radiographic outline of the tumor bed with barium sulfate solution (*B*) shows the position and size of the cavity.

DESCRIPTION OF TRANSSPHENOIDAL ADENOMECTOMY

APPROACH TO THE SELLA

After a horizontal sublabial incision, the nasal mucosa is separated from the nasal septum and elevated posteriorly until the floor of the sphenoid sinus on one side and the nasal septum on the opposite side is deflected. However, when a septum deviation is present, the inferior third of the cartilaginous portion is resected, and a bilateral submucosal dissection is achieved. A specially devised bivalve speculum is introduced, thus producing a newly formed cavity. The vomer bone and the sphenoid floor are removed, and the sphenoid sinus is entered. The sellar floor is visualized and its position confirmed by fluoroscopy. The operating microscope is moved into place, and the sellar floor is entered, using a blunt instrument and a punch rongeur, creating a rectangular opening.

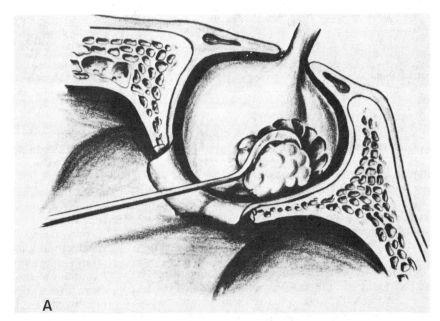

A

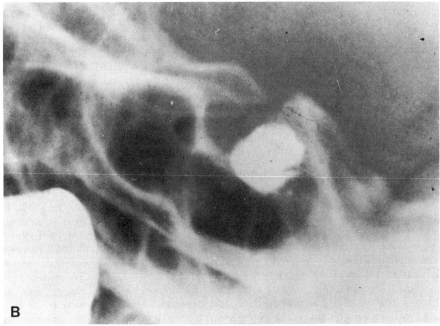

B

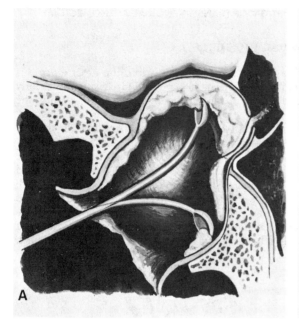
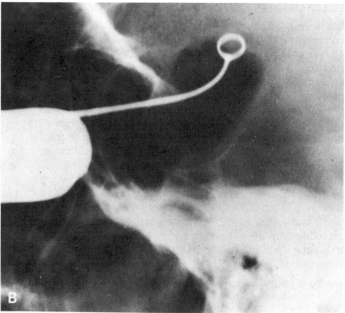

Fig. 20-8. Transsphenoidal removal of a large pituitary adenoma with suprasellar expansion. (*A*) After the tumor cavity is emptied, the suprasellar expansion collapses into the sellar cavity. The normal gland is identified located posteriorly. (*B*) Intraoperative fluoroscopy showing the position of the curette in the suprasellar region. After tumor removal, the suprasellar region is outlined by air projecting into the cistern.

INTRASELLAR PROCEDURE

Removal of Microadenomas

The dura is opened in a cruciate fashion; in prolactinomas or GH adenomas, the tumor is readily visible at the anterior–lateral aspect of the gland, sometimes herniating spontaneously through the dural opening. When the anterior surface of the gland appears normal, incision is necessary. Microcurettes are then used to enucleate the adenoma (Fig. 20-7). If the adenoma has not yet been found, a wedge-shaped resection of the pituitary wing is performed to create more exposure. Using higher magnification, the normal and pathologic tissues can be distinguished by their differences in color and consistency.

When the lesions are smaller than the pituitary gland, the microadenomas in the various secreting disorders have specific localizations. In Cushing's disease, microadenomas are most often found far posteriorly in the central mucoid zone, in contact with the neural posterior lobe. GH microadenomas are most often found in the anterior part of the lateral wing, and PRL microadenomas are found in the posterior inferior portion of the lateral wing. The removal of the adenoma is completed by aspiration, using low power suction. Absolute alcohol may be used in some cases for additional tumor bed sterilization. In doubtful cases, intraoperative frozen section biopsies may help achieve more radical excision.

Removal of Large Adenomas with Suprasellar Expansion

Using a lumbar subarachnoid catheter, air is introduced immediately before the positioning of the patient on the operating table, ensuring an adequate pneumoencephalogram outlining the suprasellar expansion. Once the floor of the sphenoid sinus has been opened, this cavity is usually partially filled by a bulging of the enlarged sellar floor. It is usually so thin that it is easily entered by a blunt probe. A large window is created, and transdural puncture is performed as a first step in aspirating a possible cystic or hemorrhagic adenoma. The dura is incised in a cruciate fashion, and the gelatinous gray-purple tissue of the tumor herniates spontaneously into the sphenoid sinus. Using suction, malleable spoons, and curettes, the tumor is progressively debulked (Fig. 20-8). Particular care must be taken during curettage of the lateral wall to avoid bleeding from the cavernous sinuses. In very large tumors, the use of an angled mirror can help remove more tissue in the hidden corners laterally and superiorly. The suprasellar expansion now collapses spontaneously into the sella, and the tumor tissue is removed until the slightly translucid and pulsating diaphragma sellae appears. Total removal of the suprasellar expansion is achieved when the diaphragma sellae is well collapsed within the sella. This can be confirmed on fluoroscopy by the presence of air projecting into the sella.

CLOSURE

In rare cases with persistent oozing from the tumor bed, the sella is left open, and the tumor cavity is drained for 24 hr, using a rubber French catheter. Otherwise, the sella is usually closed, using a piece of cartilage from the nasal septum. If some cerebrospinal fluid leakage is observed owing to an opening in the arachnoid membrane, a duroplasty is carried out using a piece of fascia and muscle from the patient's thigh to achieve a watertight closure. Antibiotic powder is dusted into the sphenoid sinus. The nasal mucosa is reapproximated with endonasal packs. Nasopharyngeal tubes are introduced into each nostril to ensure comfortable free nasal airways in the postoperative period. A few loose catgut sutures are placed on the gingival mucosa.

Because of the relatively benign procedure, patients are usually ambulatory on the night of surgery. Nasal packs are removed after 48 hr, and patients are usually discharged from the hospital on the fifth postoperative day. Patients with preoperative endocrine deficits are given necessary replacement hormones. If cortisone is given, it is tapered down within 5 days. Incidental transient diabetes insipidus is controlled with intramuscular Pitressin-tannate injections or desmopressin acetate (DDAVP) in nasal drops.

BIBLIOGRAPHY

CUSHING H: The Pituitary Body and Its Disorders: Clinical States Produced by Disorders of the Hypophysis Cerebri. The Classics of Medicine Library, p 301, 1910–1979

GUIOT G et al: Adénomes Hypophysaires, p 216. Paris, Masson et Cie, 1958

HARDY J: Transsphenoidal microsurgery of the normal and pathological pituitary. Clin Neurosurg 16:185, 1969

HARDY J: Transsphenoidal hypophysectomy. Neurosurgical techniques. J Neurosurg 34:581, 1971

HARDY J: Transsphenoidal surgery of hypersecreting pituitary tumors. Diagnosis and treatment of pituitary tumors. In Proceedings of a Conference Held in Bethesda, Maryland, pp 180–194. Amsterdam, Excerpta Medica, 1973

HARDY J: Microsurgery of the hypophysis: Subnasal transsphenoidal approach with television magnification and televised radiofluoroscopic control. In Rand RW (ed): Microneurosurgery, 2nd ed, pp 87–103. St. Louis, CV Mosby, 1978

HARDY J: Transsphenoidal microsurgical treatment of pituitary tumors. In Recent management of acromegaly. Results in 82 patients treated between 1972 and 1977. J Neurosurg 50:454, 1979

HARDY J: Ten years after the recognition of pituitary microadenomas. In Faglia G, Giovanelli MA, MacLeod RM (eds): Pituitary Microadenomas, pp 7–14. New York, Academic Press, 1980

HARDY J, VEZINA JL: Transsphenoidal neurosurgery of intracranial neoplasms. Adv Neurol 261, 1976

KRIEGER DT, HUGHES JC: Neuroendocrinology. Sunderland, Sinauer Associates, 1980

MARTIN JB, REICHLIN S, BROWN GM: Clinical Neuroendocrinology, Contemporary Series. Philadelphia, F A Davis, 1977

WILSON CB, DEMPSEY LC: Transsphenoidal microsurgical removal of 250 pituitary adenomas. J Neurosurg 48:13, 1978

Colin G. Thomas, Jr.

The Thyroid

The extirpation of the thyroid gland for goiter typifies better than any operation, the supreme triumph of the surgeon's art. A feat which today can be accomplished by any reasonably competent operator without danger of mishap and which was conceived more than 1,000 years ago might appear an unlikely competitor for a place in surgery so exalted.

—HALSTED*

* Halsted WS: The Operative Story of Goiter. Baltimore, Johns Hopkins Press, 1919.

The thyroid gland was described by Galen (160–200 AD) in his *De Voce* and more completely by Vesalius in 1543 (*The Fabrica*). Wharton (1656) contributed the name "thyroid" or "oblong shield". Enlargement of the thyroid has been known from the earliest history, incantations against goiter being found in Hindu records (2000 BC). The thyroid is the most common endocrine gland to be disturbed by changes in size and function; goiter is worldwide in distribution. The function of the thyroid was interpreted primarily from associated diseases; for example, goiter associated with cretinism, myxedema following thyroid extirpation (Kocher, 1883), and goiter accompanying hyperthyroidism (Perry, 1786; Graves, 1835; Von Basedow, 1840). Von Basedow is credited with emphasizing the triad of goiter, exophthalmos, and palpitation. Gull reported a cretinoid state (myxedema) in adult women in 1874. Murray was the first to use thyroid extract in the treatment of myxedema (1891). More explicit understanding of thyroid hormone depended upon Kendall's crystallization of thyroxine (1915), the definition of its chemical structure (Harrington, 1926), and the identification of L-triiodothyronine as the active hormone by Gross and Pitt-Rivers (1954). When the cause of goiter or hyperthyroidism was unknown, management of these diseases was empirical, with thyroidectomy being the only known effective treatment for large obstructing goiters or hyperthyroidism. Albucasis, a bold Bagdad surgeon, carried out the first successful thyroidectomy about 1000 AD. The first subtotal thyroidectomy for hyperthyroidism was performed by Rehn in 1884. It remained for Kocher to develop the technique of thyroidectomy, and his studies of the physiology of goiter earned him the Nobel Prize in 1909.

Surgery remained the principal mode of therapy for all types of goiter until the demonstration by Marine (1917) of the role of iodine deficiency in the genesis of goiter. With the introduction of iodized salt there was an associated reduction in the incidence of goiter. Iodine was used by Plummer (1923) as a means of ameliorating thyrotoxicosis and reducing the mortality from thyroidectomy for toxic goiter from approximately 20% to less than 1%.

Riedel described a rare form of chronic thyroiditis in 1896, and the most common form of thyroiditis (struma lymphomatosa) was recognized by Hashimoto in 1912. Subacute (granulomatous) thyroiditis was reported by de Quervain in 1904.

Calcitonin, a calcium-lowering hormone arising from parafollicular C cells in the thyroid, was discovered by Copp and colleagues in 1962.

The frequency of thyromegaly and surgical treatment for it are reflected by the role of thyroidectomy in the establishment of many of the great clinics in this country, such as the Lahey, Crile, Mayo, and Hertzler clinics—all of which established reputations for excellence in thyroid surgery. Surgery now plays a lesser role than in the past. The change in indications for thyroidectomy reflects (1) greater understanding of the causes and differing biologic behavior of various types of goiter; (2) the availability of effective medical therapy for many goiters, such as radioiodide (1936) and antithyroid drugs (1943); (3) the development of methods for identifying the etiology of goiter without an open operation; and (4) the effectiveness of surgery in the treatment of most varieties of thyroid cancer.

ANATOMY AND ANOMALIES

The thyroid gland (oblong shield) is a bi-lobed structure connected by an isthmus, weighing approximately 0.3 g/kg body weight (Fig. 20-9). It is intimately attached to the trachea and larynx, which it partially surrounds. A pyramidal lobe commonly extends as a narrow projection superiorly from the isthmus to the region of the thyroid cartilage. The blood supply is derived from the superior and inferior thyroid arteries. The superior thyroid artery arises at the level of the hyoid bone and passes caudally in proximity with the superior laryngeal nerve to divide into medial, lateral, and posterior branches, which enter the superior pole of the thyroid gland. The inferior thyroid artery, a branch of the thyrocervical trunk, usually enters the gland in its midlateral aspect with the recurrent laryngeal nerve lying anterior to, posterior to, or between its branches. An accessory artery, the thyroid ima, may be present, arising from the aortic arch and entering the thyroid from its inferior aspect. An extensive capillary plexus lies in proximity with the follicular basement membranes. On the surface of the gland a rich venous plexus drains into the superior, middle, and inferior thyroid veins. A lymph capillary network envelops all thyroid follicles and drains into a superficial subcapsular lymph plexus. Collecting trunks from this network drain to a first echelon of lymph nodes located in the

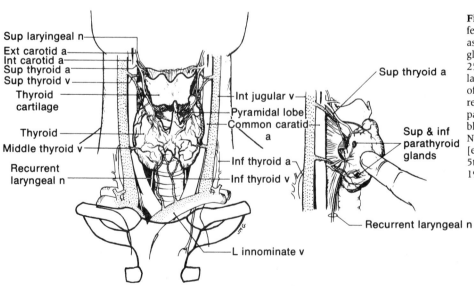

Sup laryngeal n
Ext carotid a
Int carotid a
Sup thyroid a
Sup thyroid v
Thyroid cartilage
Thyroid
Middle thyroid v
Recurrent laryngeal n

Int jugular v
Pyramidal lobe
Common caratid a
Inf thyroid a
Inf thyroid v

L innominate v

Sup thryoid a
Sup & inf parathyroid glands
Recurrent laryngeal n

Fig. 20-9. The principal anatomic features of the thyroid gland and associated structures. The normal gland weighs approximately 20 g–25 g, and the right lobe is slightly larger than the left. The proximity of the superior laryngeal nerves, the recurrent laryngeal nerves, and the parathyroids to the thyroid and its blood supply are depicted. (Nelson NC: Thyrotoxicosis. In Hardy JD [ed]: Rhoads Textbook of Surgery, 5th ed. Philadelphia, J B Lippincott, 1977)

paracapsular region, pretracheal area, jugular vein, and along the recurrent laryngeal nerve. A prelaryngeal node (Delphian node) presages the underlying cause of associated thyromegaly. Innervation of the thyroid is from the sympathetic and parasympathetic divisions of the autonomic nervous system. Arising from the vagus are the parasympathetic fibers, which reach the gland through branches of the laryngeal nerves. Sympathetic fibers arising chiefly from the cervical ganglion parallel the blood supply of the gland.

The functional unit is the follicle, supported by a vascular system, nerves, connective tissue, and a capsule. Each follicle is a spheroid structure of a single layer of cuboidal epithelium surrounding a lumen containing colloid. The apical surface of the cell is relatively complicated, marked by pseudopods and microvilli, whereas the internal structure is comparable to that of other cells. Structurally, the gland is composed of thyroid lobules consisting of 2 to 40 follicles bound together by connective tissue and supplied by a single artery and vein. Within the lobule an arterial twig supplies each follicle with a plexus of capillaries. This type of blood supply with arteriovenous anastomoses permits a highly dynamic blood flow influenced by vasohumoral mechanisms and may account for the altered sensitivity of follicular epithelium to thyrotropic stimuli. The location of adenomatous changes in general corresponds to the blood supply of the lobules. Parafollicular C cells constitute a second type of cell population. These cells are derivatives of the ultimobranchial bodies and secrete calcitonin.

Intimately associated with the thyroid are the recurrent laryngeal nerves. Branches of the vagus nerve, these "recurrent" nerves are usually located in the tracheoesophageal sulcus and lie in proximity to the branches of the inferior artery before entering the larynx at the cricothyroid articulation (Fig. 20–9). It is not unusual for the recurrent nerve to divide into one or more branches prior to entering the larynx. In approximately 1% to 2% of individuals, because of the absence of the right fourth branchial arch and the origin of the right subclavian artery from the sixth branchial arch, the larynx may be innervated directly from the vagus nerve, usually at the level of the cricothyroid articulation.

The external branch of the superior laryngeal nerve (nerve of Galli-Curci) courses along the superior thyroid artery and supplies the cricothyroid muscle (Fig. 20-9). The intimate association of this nerve with the branches of the superior thyroid artery places it at risk when these vessels are ligated during thyroidectomy (see Fig. 20-19*B*). Loss of function of the cricothyroid is associated with difficulty in modulating the "tone" of the voice. The career of Almelita Galli-Curci, an internationally known soprano of the 1920s, was abbreviated following thyroidectomy and the presumed functional loss of her cricothyroid muscle.

Anomalies of the thyroid are not uncommon and are related to the thyroid's embryologic origin from entoderm (foramen cecum) and its descent early in embryonic life by way of the thyroglossal duct to its ultimate location anterior to the second and third tracheal rings. The thyroglossal duct eventually becomes attenuated and usually disintegrates. Persistence of thyroid epithelium along this tract may account for lingual or other thyroid tissue, which is subject to the same pathologic alterations that occur in the thyroid proper. Failure of resorption of the tract may be manifest by a midline *thyroglossal duct cyst* (with or without associated thyroid epithelia). *Ectopic thyroid* has also been described lateral and caudal to the inferior lobes and in the superior and posterior mediastinum. Most of these intrathoracic

lesions represent extensions of an adenomatous goiter, which may have only a tenuous connection to the parent gland (see Fig. 20-15). *Lingual thyroid* or other ectopic thyroid presents as a mass at the base of the tongue. Its avidity for radioiodine should identify its thyroidal origin. Management by thyroid-stimulating hormone (TSH) suppression is appropriate in the absence of continuing enlargement or change in the physical characteristics suggestive of neoplasm. Absence of one lobe of the thyroid has been described. Cervical masses lateral to the sternocleidomastoid muscle may be composed of normal-appearing thyroid follicles. Although initially thought to be benign lateral aberrant thyroid tissue, they must be considered metastases of papillary-follicular carcinoma. The finding of lymphatic tissue at the margin of such masses constitutes proof of metastatic disease. Non-neoplastic ectopic thyroid follicles are occasionally seen in cervical lymph nodes. Characteristically, these follicles vary in number from a few to a hundred, in contrast to metastatic carcinoma, which usually assumes a more globular form and contains a greater number of follicles. Ectopic thyroid tissue may be seen in ovarian teratomas and rarely produces hyperthyroidism.

PHYSIOLOGY

Thyroid hormone (TH), as thyroxine (T_4) and triiodothyronine (T_3), is secreted by the thyroid gland as modulated by the blood level of TSH by means of a feedback mechanism between TH and TSH that regulates the secretion of TSH by thyrotropic cells in the anterior pituitary. Thyrotropin-releasing hormone (TRH) modulates the secretion of TSH (Fig. 20-10). Thyroid hormone synthesis and secretion are further influenced by the iodide pool, inherent metabolic defects, and drugs. Iodide is absorbed from the gastrointestinal tract into the circulatory system, with the kidney and thyroid competing for this iodide pool. Iodide is trapped and oxidized by the thyroid cell through the action of a peroxidase and hydrogen peroxide (H_2O_2), forming compounds with the iodine atom bound to tyrosine in thyroglobulin. Coupling of iodinated tyrosine molecules in follicular thyroglobulin results in the formation of iodothyronines (T_3 and T_4). The protein thyroglobulin is synthesized in the ribosomes of the thyroid cell and transported into colloid; iodination of tyrosine occurs within thyroglobulin at the interface between cell and colloid. Secretion of thyroid hormone occurs when thyroglobulin re-enters the cells and is degraded by proteolytic enzymes and proteases, releasing iodothyronines (T_4, T_3) into the blood. Both hormones pass freely in both directions between blood and peripheral tissues such as liver, kidney, and muscle mass, where they are metabolized and exert their hormonal effects. Liver and kidney most actively convert a large part of T_4 to T_3 by monodeiodination. Approximately two thirds of all circulating T_3 is derived by monodeiodination of T_4, and the remaining third is derived from thyroid secretion. The thyroid synthesizes and secretes much more T_4 than T_3; the T_4/T_3 ratio of serum concentrations of bound hormone is approximately 100:1 and that of free or dialyzable hormone is 10:1. T_4 is largely an extracellular and T_3 an intracellular hormone. There are specific nuclear binding sites for T_3 but not for T_4. Approximately 60 μg of T_4 and 30 μg of T_3 are metabolized daily.

The uptake of iodide by the thyroid as measured by radioiodine uptake is a reflection of the amount of iodide ingested daily and that required for hormone synthesis—

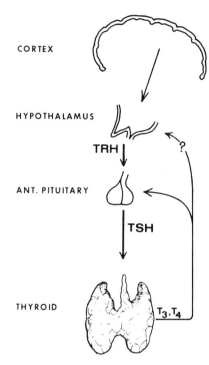

Fig. 20-10. Diagram of extrathyroidal regulatory factors that affect the thyroid. The concentration of the free triiodothyronine (T₃) and thyroxine (T₄) in the blood inhibits or enhances the secretion of thyroid-stimulating hormone (TSH) from the anterior pituitary in a negative feedback relationship. TSH-releasing hormone (TRH) from the hypothalamus enhances the release of TSH, and the concentration of TRH to which the pituitary is exposed modulates the threshold at which the T_3, T_4–TSH negative feedback system operates. The control of TRH secretion includes higher central nervous system factors and probably a positive feedback–stimulating effect by T_3 and T_4. (Nelson NC: Thyrotoxicosis. In Hardy JD [ed]: Rhoads Textbook of Surgery, 5th ed. Philadelphia, J B Lippincott, 1977)

for example, if 500 μg is ingested and 70 μg is needed for hormone synthesis, there is a 14% uptake. Iodide uptake is not a reliable index of thyroid function or metabolic status or of hyper- or hypothyroidism.

The synthesis and secretion of TH are affected not only by TSH but also by pharmacologic agents that may affect either hormone or both. $KClO_4$ competes with iodide trapping within the cell, causes a release of trapped and unbound iodide, and controls secretion by depleting the availability of iodide. Its toxicity limits its therapeutic use. Thioamides (propylthiouracil and methimazole) prevent hormone synthesis by inhibiting the binding of iodide to tyrosine. Propylthiouracil has the added action of constraining the peripheral conversion of T_4 to T_3. Iodide in pharmacologic amounts (greater than 10 mg/day) inhibits the formation of TH as well as its release. Lithium has an action similar to that of iodide. Upon release from the gland, T_4 is bound primarily to thyroxine-binding globulin (a protein carrier), with about 0.04% remaining free. The amount of free hormone depends upon the equilibrium between the hormone available and the level of binding proteins. The level of thyroxine-binding globulin synthesized in the liver is influenced by estrogens (which increase it) and androgens (which decrease it), malnutrition (decrease), and a number of drugs that affect liver function. Propranolol, in addition to its role as a beta-blocker, also inhibits the conversion of T_4 to T_3 in the periphery.

T_4 has a biologic half-life of 7 days and T_3 of 1 day. T_4 is in part metabolized in the peripheral tissues by deiodination to triiodothyronine and, to a lesser extent, to the inactive stereoisomer r-triiodothyronine.

LABORATORY FINDINGS AND TESTS OF THYROID FUNCTION

Laboratory tests of thyroid function complement the clinical evaluation of the patient's metabolic status. They are designed to provide biochemical documentation of suspected thyroid dysfunction, the clinical manifestations of which may be subtle and nonspecific. The basal metabolic rate (BMR) as measured by oxygen consumption is the oldest means of evaluating metabolic rate but has been replaced by more sophisticated tests (Table 20-1).

1. Total serum hormone concentration of T_4 is measured by radioimmunoassay (T_4 RAI) and expressed as micrograms per deciliter. Free hormone concentration may be measured (FT_4).

2. The T_3 resin uptake (T_3U) measures the unsaturated thyroxine-binding sites on thyroxine-binding globulin.

3. Serum L-triiodothyronine is measured by radioimmunoassay (T_3 RAI).

4. The free thyroxine index estimates the free hormone concentration and is calculated after determining the triiodothyronine uptake (T_3U) and the total serum T_4.

5. TSH is measured by radioimmunoassay, which is more reliable in detecting elevated concentrations (thyroid hypofunction) than reduced concentrations (hyperthyroidism, suppressive treatment).

6. Thyroid autoantibodies can be detected against various antigens arising within the thyroid, for instance, thyroglobulin, microsomal antigen, nuclear component, thyroid-stimulating immunoglobulins, and colloid component other than thyroglobulin. Thyroid autoantibodies to thyroglobulin and microsomal antigen are most useful in identifying autoimmune (Hashimoto's) thyroiditis. These antibodies also may be present, although in somewhat lower titers, in subacute thyroiditis, Graves' disease, and adenomatous goiter.

7. Radioiodine uptake at 6 hr to 24 hr measures the avidity of the thyroid gland for iodide and is a reflection of the rate of synthesis of T_4: T_3 and the available iodide ingested daily. This test does not appraise the patient's metabolic status but provides critical information in planning treatment with radioactive iodine and in the diagnosis of certain entities: that is, subacute thyroiditis and iatrogenic hyperthyroidism.

8. The TRH–TSH test evaluates the TSH content of the adenohypophysis by stimulating release of TSH through the action of TRH (Fig. 20-11). By measuring the increase in serum TSH, a differentiation can be made between pituitary (absent response) and hypothalamic (normal response) hypothyroidism. The test is useful in identifying TSH suppression due to Graves' disease, hyperfunctioning thyroid nodules, and exogenous TH. It replaces the T_3 suppression test formerly used to determine thyroid autonomy. The adequacy of TSH suppressive treatment may be evaluated by this test.

9. Thyroglobulin (Tg RAI) is measured as μg/dl. The intrathyroidal glycoprotein in which iodothyronines are synthesized and stored circulates in small amounts in the normal subject and may be useful in assessing persistent or recurrent thyroid carcinoma after total thyroidectomy.

TABLE 20-1   COMMON CURRENT THYROID FUNCTION TESTS

TEST ASSESSMENT	DESCRIPTION	NORMAL RANGE[a]
T_4	Measures total serum T_4; screening test of choice	5–12 μg/dl
T_3U	A test of serum-binding avidity for T_4 and T_3—not a test of serum T_3	0.85–1.15
FTI (T_7)	Product of $T_4 \times T_3U$, usually indicating FT_4 and FT_3; misleading in ill patients	5–12
FT_4	Direct measurement of FT_4	
T_3 (T_3 RIA)	Measures total serum T_3; elevated in thyrotoxicosis	60–200 ng/dl
TSH	Measures circulating pituitary TSH; elevated in actual or impending thyroid failure	0–5 μU/ml
ATA	Antithyroglobulin and antithyroid microsomal antibodies; characteristically high in	<1:10
AMA	lymphocytic thyroiditis	<1:100
RIU	*In vivo*-thyroid radioiodine uptake; low diagnostic value	9%–30%/24 hr
TRH test	Measures pituitary response to TRH—enhanced in primary thyroid failure, decreased in thyrotoxicosis. Distinguishes primary, secondary, and tertiary hypothyroidism	TSH two to three times baseline at 30 min

[a] Varies with laboratory
(After Levy RP; Workshop on the Thyroid. American Thyroid Association, 1979)

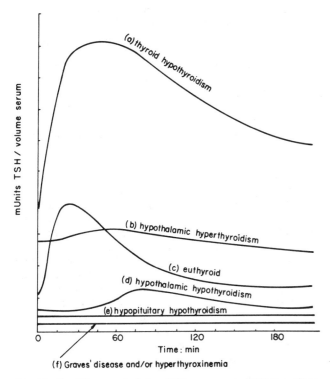

Fig. 20-11. Diagram depicting TSH response to TRH in various types of thyroid disorders. (Bartuska DG, Dratman MB: Evolving concepts of thyroid function. Med Clin North Am 57:1117, 1973)

HYPERTHYROIDISM

GRAVES' DISEASE

Almost 200 years have elapsed since Caleb Hilliery Parry (1755–1822) saw his first case of exophthalmic goiter in 1786. "A 37-year-old woman, the first patient, caught cold 'lying in.' 'Rheumatic fever' followed with violent palpitations of the heart. Three months after delivery the thyroid began to enlarge and became enormous. The carotid arteries on each side were greatly distended, the eyes were protruded from the socket, and the countenance exhibited an appearance of agitation and distress, especially on any muscular exertion. She suffered no pain in her head but was frequently affected with giddiness. Each systole of the heart shook the whole trunk of the body." This classic description of Graves' disease was published posthumously by Parry's son in 1825. A third component, namely, pretibial myxedema, was described later by Dore (1901).

Graves' disease is of unknown etiology but is most likely an autoimmune disorder in which antibodies to the human TSH receptor (thyroid-stimulating immunoglobulin), liberated by lymphocytes, bind to TSH receptor sites in the thyroid, stimulating the gland to produce T_4 and T_3 beyond the amount required for normal homeostasis. The hyperthyroxinemia results in characteristic effects on the entire organism through the cellular action of T_4 and T_3, primarily in regulating and speeding synthetic processes within the cells. The normal feedback mechanism between TSH, T_4, and T_3 is not operative, and the severity of the hypermetabolism is related to the serum level of T_4 and T_3. The initial stimulus for the generation and liberation of human thyroid-stimulating immunoglobulins (HTSI) is unknown. It may be present as a trait in families with Graves' disease and in euthyroid ophthalmic Graves' disease and is almost certainly responsible for the hyperthyroidism of that disorder. Originally, this activity was detected using an *in vivo* guinea pig bioassay, and because of the prolonged time course necessary it was given the name long-acting thyroid stimulator (LATS). Treatment of Graves' disease reduces the

HYPERTHYROIDISM	
Etiology	Endogenous thyroid stimulator, autonomous thyroid adenoma, excess TSH (rare)
Dx	Tachycardia, nervousness, insomnia, sweating, heat intolerance, weight loss, exophthalmos, diarrhea, hyperactive reflexes, thin hair, increased free thyroxine index and T_3, increased TSH (rare)
Rx	Propranolol, thioamides, iodine, radioiodine thyroid ablation, subtotal thyroidectomy

incidence of HTSI from virtually 100% to less than 50% in those managed with antithyroid drugs or radioiodide. Subtotal thyroidectomy has a dramatic effect on circulating HTSI levels, reducing them to approximately 15%. The relation of ophthalmopathy and dermopathy to HTSI is poorly defined because these entities may run courses that are completely independent of thyromegaly and hyperthyroidism.

The natural course of the disease is unclear, since some form of definitive therapy is received by essentially all patients. Satler (1911) reported that approximately 20% of patients died, and approximately 40% followed a course of remissions and exacerbations with continuing thyrocardiac disability. In the remaining 40% spontaneous remissions occurred, with recovery usually requiring several years; a few of these patients developed hypothyroidism.

Graves' disease has an estimated incidence of 19.8 per 100,000 population. Although it may occur at any age, it is more common in the third and fourth decades and predominates in women. It is familial and overlaps with other autoimmune diseases such as Hashimoto's thyroiditis, pernicious anemia, and immunologic thrombocytopenic purpura.

The clinical manifestations are characterized by a history of increasing nervousness, emotional lability, irritability, weight loss despite an increased appetite, intolerance of heat, excessive sweating, and consciousness of an increased pulse and cardiac activity. These symptoms may be accompanied by easy fatigability, muscle weakness (particularly of the proximal muscle groups), and diarrhea. Cardiovascular symptoms predominate in children and older patients. Clinical findings include eye changes, hyperkinesia, wide pulse pressure, tachycardia, increased precordial activity, hyperactive reflexes, smooth, warm, moist skin, fine hair, and onycholysis. Diffuse thyromegaly (two to four times the normal size) with thrill or bruit is frequent. Auricular fibrillation or cardiac failure may be present in older patients. Pretibial myxedema is unusual. Ocular changes are common and are more frequent in adults than in children. They include stare, lid lag, lid retraction, proptosis, and occasionally minor degrees of conjunctival edema. These are not specific and may remit with control of the disease. Infiltrative ophthalmopathy ("malignant exophthalmos"), specific for Graves' disease, may be concurrent or a late development. These findings are more severe, consisting of chemosis, lid and soft tissue edema, limitation of extraocular movements, corneal involvement, and, rarely, optic nerve involvement (sight loss). Exophthalmos may be symmetrical or asymmetrical. Unilateral exophthalmos is not rare.

The differential diagnosis includes other causes of hypermetabolism (*e.g.*, pheochromocytoma, factitious hyperthyroidism, anxiety states, or cancer). The clinical diagnosis is confirmed by thyroid function studies, primarily the free thyroxine index (Table 20-1). T_3 RAI, the most sensitive test, is usually the first to be elevated and the last to fall within normal limits.

Treatment of Graves' disease is directed toward (1) reducing the functioning mass of hyperplastic thyroid by destruction with radioiodide, subtotal resection, or control of thyroid secretion by agents blocking hormone synthesis (thioamides); (2) inhibiting T_4 release (by iodides); (3) modulating the peripheral conversion of T_4 to T_3 (by propylthiouracil or propranolol); or (4) blockade of β-adrenergic receptors (propranolol). Propranolol modulates many of the manifestations of the disease (tachycardia, cardiac overactivity, hyperkinesia, muscle weakness) but does not change the underlying hypermetabolism caused by the hyperthyroxinemia. Propranolol is contraindicated in patients with antibodies to β-adrenergic receptors (*e.g.*, allergic asthma, cystic fibrosis) and in patients with α-adrenergic and cholinergic sensitivity, chronic obstructive pulmonary disease, congestive heart failure, or hypoglycemia. Also excluded are patients on quinidine or psychotropic drugs. Occasionally a patient may be completely unresponsive to propranolol.

Radioactive iodine is preferred by some for virtually all patients with thyrotoxicosis except neonates and those who are pregnant or when it is precluded by a low iodine uptake. Treatment failures are rare, although hypothyroidism usually results. Except for potential hypothyroidism there have been no untoward effects, such as thyroid cancer or congenital anomalies in offspring, but there is still some reluctance to treat children and women of childbearing age (potential mothers) with radioiodide.

Antithyroid drugs are used primarily in patients in the younger age groups with a small goiter, maintaining a euthyroid state for 18 to 24 months while awaiting a spontaneous remission. Problems with this approach are those of patient compliance and a low but definite incidence of toxicity (*e.g.*, skin rash, neutropenia, alteration in liver function). Even with prolonged therapy remissions are unlikely to be sustained in more than 40% to 50% of patients. Propranolol has not been effective as a sole means of therapy.

Indications for subtotal thyroidectomy in Graves' disease are patients under the age of 20 who, because of a large goiter, are unlikely to undergo remission with antithyroid drugs; who develop drug reactions to thioamides; who, because of personality or social environment, cannot be relied upon to follow a medical regimen; or who do not experience remission with thioamide drugs as indicated by persistent thyromegaly or the need to continue medication beyond 1 or 2 years. In addition, operation is recommended for women in the childbearing age who are potential mothers. The potential hazards of radiation exposure and transmissible genetic damage associated with radioiodine therapy are avoided. Thyroidectomy is preferred in patients in whom the findings suggest the possibility of a coexistent neoplasm. Surgical treatment is contraindicated in patients who have recurrent thyrotoxicosis after subtotal thyroidectomy, who have existing recurrent nerve paralysis, and who, despite being rendered euthyroid, remain poor surgical risks.

PLUMMER'S DISEASE (TOXIC NODULAR GOITER)

Plummer in 1913 described a form of hyperthyroidism that occurred in patients with long-standing multinodular goiter. He considered it an inevitable consequence of nodular goiter, often requiring 15 years to develop after onset. The manifestations are due to the associated hyperthyroxinemia and are usually more mild than those of Graves' disease. The cardiovascular manifestations are more prominent but have a subtle onset associated with tachycardia, increased pulse pressure, hyperkinesia, and skin changes; eye signs, dermopathy, muscle weakness, and emotional lability are absent. The causative mechanism is unknown, although it is postulated that autonomy of function is achieved after years of thyroid stimulation, ultimately resulting in hyperthyroidism.

GOITER	
Etiology	Goitrogens, enzyme defect, iodine deficiency (rare in U.S.)
Dx	Palpable thyromegaly, thyroid scan, exclude solitary nodule
Rx	Thyroid suppression, subtotal thyroidectomy for (1) airway obstruction, (2) dysphagia, (3) cosmetic improvement, (4) suspicion of malignancy

Treatment is similar to that for Graves' disease, with the option of long-term antithyroid drugs, radioiodide, or subtotal thyroidectomy. Because of the size of the goiter and the relatively low uptake of iodide, radioiodine is frequently ineffective. Subtotal thyroidectomy is preferred because it achieves prompt control of the hyperthyroidism as well as correction of the goiter. Unless the patient is severely toxic, preparation for surgery can usually be achieved with propranolol. Iodides are not usually advised because of the possibility of enhancement of thyrotoxicosis.

TOXIC ADENOMA

A variant of Plummer's disease is the hyperfunctioning or toxic thyroid adenoma. Most hyperfunctioning thyroid lesions (Fig. 20-12E, F) do not produce hyperthyroidism until they become a mass 3 cm or more in diameter. The "adenoma" may produce primarily L-triiodothyronine, "T_3 thyrotoxicosis."

Treatment can consist of radioiodide administration or thyroidectomy. Because of the unpredictability of the dose required and exposure of the remaining gland to low-dose radiation, lobectomy with complete excision of the lesion is preferred. The remaining "normal" parenchyma is usually sufficient to maintain euthyroidism. Although carcinoma has been reported in hyperfunctioning adenomas, it is sufficiently infrequent not to constitute an indication for thyroidectomy.

Most hyperfunctioning nodules (autonomously functioning thyroid lesions) are not associated with hyperthyroidism, and many such "nodules" are observed. Indications for treatment are related to the size of the lesion and the propensity of the patient to develop hyperthyroidism. Other considerations are the life expectancy of the patient and the practicability of periodic observation. In general, the larger the mass and the younger the patient, the more warranted is surgical treatment. Euthyroid patients in the older age group with small nodules (less than 2 cm) may be observed. The same objections to the use of radioiodine apply as in the management of toxic nodules. Lobectomy is the operation of choice.

OTHER CAUSES OF HYPERTHYROXINEMIA

Hyperthyroidism has been reported with TSH-producing tumors of the pituitary, the critical finding being an inappropriately elevated TSH level. Thyroid hyperfunction may also accompany hydatidiform molar pregnancy and trophoblastic tumors in both males and females. The hyperthyroidism appears to be caused by an abnormal thyroid stimulator that is most likely human chorionic gonadotropin.

Hyperthyroidism may be a consequence of the factitious

Fig. 20-12. Radionuclide scans in various thyroid disorders. (*A*) Normal silhouette. (*B*) Minimal thyromegaly. Heterogeneous uptake compatible with but not diagnostic of Hashimoto's thyroiditis. (*C*) Enlarged gland with normal configuration consistent with diffuse toxic goiter (Graves' disease). (*D*) Thyromegaly with variable uptake (areas of hyper- and hypofunction) consistent with adenomatous goiter. (*E*) Hyperfunctioning area in right lobe consistent with autonomously functioning thyroid lesion and minimal TSH suppression. (*F*) Hyperfunctioning area in right lobe consistent with autonomously functioning thyroid lesion and complete TSH suppression (essential absence of uptake in left lobe). Compare with (*E*). (*G*) Hypofunctioning area, lateral aspect of right lobe, consistent with adenomatous goiter or carcinoma. (*H*) Palpable mass involving left lower pole, nonfunctioning, consistent with cyst or neoplasm. (*I*) Ectopic functioning thyroid in region of thyroglossal duct cyst, absence of uptake in region of normal thyroid gland.

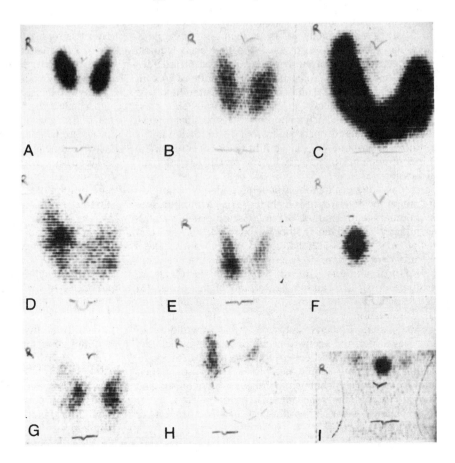

or iatrogenic ingestion of excessive amounts of TH. Iatrogenic hyperthyroidism is most commonly associated with the management of nontoxic nodular goiter in older patients without recognizing that 25% to 30% of these may be autonomous.

SURGICAL TREATMENT OF THYROTOXICOSIS

The objective of surgical treatment of hyperthyroidism is to remove a sufficient amount of the diffuse hyperfunctioning thyroid (as in Graves' disease) or all of the hyperfunctioning nodules (as in Plummer's disease) to render the patient euthyroid. Permanent control of the hyperthyroidism is accomplished in approximately 95% to 97% of patients. The advantage of thyroidectomy is the immediacy of the control of hyperthyroidism with a predictable result. The need for prolonged drug therapy as well as the theoretical genetic hazards associated with radioiodine therapy are avoided. The disadvantages are the risks associated with any major surgical procedure and those peculiar to partial thyroidectomy, that is, recurrent laryngeal nerve injury, hypoparathyroidism, and permanent hypothyroidism.

PREOPERATIVE PREPARATION

Subtotal thyroidectomy is an elective operation, and the patient's thyrotoxicosis should be controlled preoperatively by thioamide drugs. Restoration of euthyroidism improves nutritional status and provides the patient with normal homeostatic mechanisms and responses to the stresses of anesthesia and surgery. Preparation of the patient with Lugol's solution alone is less acceptable and is associated with greater risk. However, the vascularity of the diffuse toxic goiter of Graves' disease as well as the severity of the hyperthyroxinemia can be reduced by preoperative administration of Lugol's solution. Beta-adrenergic blockade (propranolol) is used chiefly as an adjuvant to thioamides, particularly if large doses of the latter have been required or if the patient is not euthyroid at the time of intended thyroidectomy. Propranolol may be used alone or in conjunction with Lugol's solution in the preparation of the patient who is intolerant of antithyroid drugs or who is noncompliant. With such an approach it is possible to have the patient undergo operation within 10 to 14 days. The last dose of propranolol is given 2 hr before operation, and it is continued postoperatively for several days in gradually decreasing doses.

Preoperative evaluation of patients undergoing surgical treatment for thyrotoxicosis includes (1) a technetium scan in nodular goiter and in Graves' disease when there is asymmetry of the gland or other reason to suspect coexistent neoplasm (1% to 2%); (2) indirect laryngoscopy for appraisal of vocal cord function; (3) determination of serum calcium, phosphorus, and total protein; (4) chest roentgenogram to evaluate possible mediastinal extension of the goiter; (5) determination of circulating thyroglobulin antibodies; and (6) examination for the presence of Chvostek's sign.

The patient rendered euthyroid by antithyroid drugs tolerates any of the agents utilized for general anesthesia. If propranolol has been employed, myocardial depressants such as halothane should not be used because of their additive action; anticholinergic drugs are antagonistic and should not ordinarily be administered preoperatively or intraoperatively. For technical aspects of this operation see Figure 20-19 *A, B, D.*

RESULTS OF SURGICAL TREATMENT

Subtotal thyroidectomy is a highly effective means of controlling thyrotoxicosis. The incidence of recurrent disease, estimated to be in the range of 1% to 5%, is inversely related to the incidence of hypothyroidism. Recurrence after thyroidectomy for Plummer's disease is essentially nil.

Hypothyroidism develops in 5% to 50% of patients, usually within 1 to 2 years. In subsequent years there is usually a slight further increase (*e.g.,* 1.5%/year). The incidence of hypothyroidism has little relation to the initial total gland mass but can be related to the estimated weight of the thyroid remnant, for example, the incidence is 45% to 70% with a remnant weight of approximately 2 g to 4 g compared with an incidence of less than 20% when a remnant of 8 g to 10 g is left. The autoimmune nature of the disease also influences the overall rate of hypothyroidism. Patients with lymphocytic infiltration are more likely to develop hypothyroidism. It should be emphasized that postoperative recurrence is a far more serious complication than hypothyroidism.

The mortality of the surgical treatment of thyrotoxicosis after appropriate preoperative preparation using modern anesthetic agents and performed by an experienced thyroid surgeon is nil. The associated morbidity, estimated to be 0.5% to 4%, is related primarily to damage to the recurrent laryngeal nerves and parathyroid glands. There is no good information concerning the incidence of damage to the external branch of the superior laryngeal nerve. The usual hospital stay following subtotal thyroidectomy is 2 to 4 days.

SPECIAL PROBLEMS

PREGNANCY

Hyperthyroidism complicates pregnancy in approximately 0.1% of patients, creating an increased risk to the fetus (*e.g.,* abortion, prematurity, and perinatal death). The diagnosis may be overlooked because many of the symptoms of thyrotoxicosis occur in early pregnancy. Management must reflect the fact that drugs may cross the placenta and affect the fetus and fetal thyroid–pituitary axis. Antithyroid drugs are usually advised when the disease is mild. Radioactive iodine is contraindicated. More severe thyrotoxicosis is best treated with subtotal thyroidectomy performed during the second trimester with preparation by antithyroid drugs and propranolol. Since HTSI crosses the placenta, neonatal thyrotoxicosis may occur but is usually self-limited.

MALIGNANT EXOPHTHALMOS

Whereas most ocular changes associated with thyrotoxicosis improve with time and treatment, infiltrative exophthalmopathy may be severe, threatening sight. Most critical is the need to avoid hypothyroidism. Other measures that have been employed are corticosteroids, x-ray therapy, lateral tarsorrhaphy, and surgical decompression of the orbits. Total thyroidectomy has been recommended but without good supporting data.

THYROID STORM/CRISIS

Thyroid storm/crisis should be suspected in any patient with untreated or partially treated thyrotoxicosis in whom fever, vomiting, agitation or delirium, and tachycardia appear suddenly or become worse. This complication, previously associated with thyroidectomy in the thyrotoxic patient, is infrequent but still occurs and is usually precipitated by acute stress (*e.g.,* infection, operative procedure). It requires emergency treatment with large doses of antithyroid drugs (*e.g.,* propylthiouracil [250 mg every 6 hr], iodides, propranol, or pharmacologic doses of hydrocortisone) and general supportive measures (parenteral fluids, glucose, physical cooling) as indicated. If these measures are ineffective, plasmapheresis or peritoneal dialysis may be required.

APATHETIC HYPERTHYROIDISM

Hyperthyroidism may be present in the elderly without the usual overt manifestations of tremor, anxiety, and hyperkinesia. The onset may be insidious with tachycardia, auricular fibrillation, cardiac failure, muscle weakness, and weight loss. A goiter is usually present but without eye signs. The diagnosis of "masked" hyperthyroidism of the elderly can be confirmed by the usual thyroid function studies including a T_3 RAI. Treatment is the same as that for Graves' disease with a preference for radioactive iodine.

THYROIDITIS

STRUMA LYMPHOMATOSA (HASHIMOTO'S THYROIDITIS)

Chronic lymphocytic (Hashimoto's) thyroiditis is one of the more common causes of diffuse thyromegaly in both children and adults; it has an incidence of 2% at autopsy examination. The frequency of the disease appears to have increased during the past several decades. The disease predominates in the female. It is considered an autoimmune disease because a variety of antithyroid antibodies, including microsomal and thyroglobulin antibodies, have been detected in the patients' serum. It is not established that these antibodies are cytodestructive. Both humoral and cell-mediated immunity are probably involved in the production of the inflammatory response. The tendency for Hashimoto's thyroiditis (and Graves' disease) to occur in members of the same family is well recognized.

Hashimoto's thyroiditis is characterized by defective hormone synthesis, manifested as a lack of organification of trapped iodide. Accompanying the reduction in the functional capacity of the thyroid there is an increase in TSH secretion and development of a goiter. Associated fibrosis may accentuate the lobulations of the thyroid, creating asymmetry and simulating a nodular goiter or neoplasm. Antithyroglobulin and antimicrosomal antibodies are usually present when an assay of sufficient sensitivity is used. These titers may fall in long-standing disease. Other disorders (*e.g.,* subacute thyroiditis, Graves' disease, thyroid cancer, and adenomatous goiter) may be associated with some increase in thyroid antibody titers. The presence of very high antibody titers is characteristic of Hashimoto's thyroiditis. Thyroid scans using technetium-99m or radioiodide characteristically demonstrate a heterogeneous uptake. Because of the defect in organification of trapped iodide, there may be discordant imaging when comparing scans using technetium-99m, which measures the trapping ability of the epithelial cell, and radioiodide, which measures both trapping and organification.

Characteristic pathologic findings include small follicles depleted of thyroglobulin; distorted, enlarged epithelial cells with large nuclei and eosinophilic cytoplasm (Askanazy cells); and varying degrees of fibrosis. Accompanying these changes is a diffuse lymphocytic infiltration with germinal centers.

The clinical manifestations are those of a diffuse and slowly progressive goiter. The goiter is usually asymptomatic unless it is accompanied by local pressure symptoms or the insidious development of mild hypothyroidism. The physical findings are those of diffuse goiter—firm and rubbery with a somewhat bosselated surface, maintaining the configuration of the normal gland. The enlargement may be asymmetrical, simulating a neoplasm or adenomatous goiter. Characteristic thyroid function studies include a normal or slightly decreased free thyroxine index, an increased TSH level, positive tests for antithyroglobulin or antinuclear antibodies, and a thyroid scan demonstrating heterogeneous uptake of the radionuclide. The clinical and laboratory findings are usually sufficiently characteristic for diagnosis. In patients with asymmetrical enlargement of the thyroid gland, nodular thyroiditis, or incomplete regression on suppressive therapy, a cutting needle biopsy or aspiration biopsy for cytologic examination may be necessary to confirm the clinical diagnosis. Since thyromegaly is in part secondary to TSH stimulation, suppressive treatment with thyroid hormone (0.15 mg–0.2 mg of thyroxine daily) usually results in regression of the goiter. The degree of regression will depend upon the relative components of lymphoid infiltration, compensatory thyroid hyperplasia, and fibrosis. Regression may never be complete. However, partial thyroidectomy is rarely needed for relief of compressive symptoms associated with failure of regression.

Hashimoto's thyroiditis may coexist with benign (adenomatous) goiter or malignant thyroid disease. There does not appear to be an increased incidence of well-differentiated carcinoma. Thyroidectomy in Hashimoto's thyroiditis is indicated to identify coexistent neoplasia in the presence of (1) a dominant mass with incomplete regression on suppressive therapy; (2) progression of thyromegaly despite suppressive therapy; (3) physical findings suggesting malignancy, and (4) indeterminant findings on needle biopsy (*e.g.,* lymphoma versus thyroiditis). Although there is an increased incidence of lymphoma in Hashimoto's disease, it is of insufficient frequency to warrant thyroidectomy on this basis.

Hashimoto's thyroiditis may be associated with mild thyroxinemia ("Hashitoxicosis"). This entity can be distinguished from Graves' disease by a low iodine uptake or by biopsy. Eye signs have been described. The hyperthyroidism is usually self-limited and can be managed symptomatically with antithyroid drugs or propranolol.

Thyroiditis also occurs following irradiation in infancy and childhood. It is the second most frequent histologic change following focal hyperplasia. The pathogenesis is thought to be related to cell damage and destruction secondary to ionizing radiation. The release of thyroglobulin and altered epithelial cell microsomes acting as antigens elicits a cellular and humoral response. The histologic findings are those of chronic lymphocytic thyroiditis.

RIEDEL'S STRUMA

In 1896 Riedel described three cases of goiter characterized by a woody or fibrous component with involvement of adjacent strap muscles. Riedel's thyroiditis, if a true entity, is rare. Clinically, the findings are similar to those of an infiltrating cancer, from which Riedel's thyroiditis can be differentiated only by repeated biopsies. The disease is believed to be self-limited, although occasionally it requires tracheostomy because of the constriction of the trachea.

SUBACUTE (GRANULOMATOUS, DE QUERVAIN'S) THYROIDITIS

Subacute thyroiditis is considered a viral infection, usually occurring in young women several weeks following an upper respiratory or other viral infection. It is manifested as pain either in the region of the thyroid or referred to the ear or angle of the jaw. There may be systemic manifestations of loss of feeling of well-being and easy fatigability as well as those associated with mild hyperthyroxinemia. The thyroid is exquisitely tender in part or entirely. Characteristic laboratory findings include an elevated serum T_4 level and suppressed radioiodide uptake.

The clinical picture is usually sufficiently characteristic that the diagnosis can be made on the clinical features alone. Occasionally, if there has been an insidious onset and the inflammatory process is confined to one lobe, the physical findings may simulate cancer—namely, a hard, firm mass that may be only slightly tender with maintenance of the topography of the lobe. The disease is usually self-limited to a few weeks, during which symptomatic relief can be achieved with salicylates. With severe symptoms corticosteroids may be required and usually provide prompt relief. They can be discontinued over a period of a month. Rarely, the disease undergoes exacerbation or recurs and persists for several months. Recovery is associated with restoration of normal thyroid function.

ACUTE SUPPURATIVE THYROIDITIS

Acute suppurative thyroiditis usually occurs in association with bacteremia or bacterial infection in the region of the head or neck. Clinical signs of an infection and an enlarged, firm, exquisitely tender mass in the thyroid in the absence of pathognomonic (laboratory) findings of subacute thyroiditis are characteristic of suppurative thyroiditis. Ultrasound may be helpful in identifying tissue necrosis. The diagnosis may be substantiated by needle aspiration. Staphylococci, streptococci, and pneumococci are the most common organisms. Because of the dense fascial planes of the neck, surgical drainage should not await the development of fluctuation. When the inflammatory process is intralobar, complete excision of the abscess by lobectomy is the treatment of choice, with appropriate antibiotic coverage. Recurring abscess indicates an underlying lesion that may require lobectomy.

NONTOXIC ADENOMATOUS (NODULAR) GOITER

Goiter is an enlargement of the thyroid gland, implying a weight in excess of 30 g or a "thyroid gland whose lateral lobes have a volume greater than the terminal phalanges of the thumb of the person being examined."* Benign goiter is further categorized as diffuse or nodular by morphologic status, functioning or nonfunctioning by radionuclide scan,

---

* Stansbury JB, Ermans AM, Hetzel BS et al: Endemic goitre and cretinism: Public health significance and prevention. WHO Chron 28:220, 1974.

toxic or nontoxic on clinical grounds, and according to histopathologic characteristics. Although benign goiters may be further classified according to presumed etiology (*e.g.,* endemic [iodine deficiency], familial, or sporadic), this is of limited value in the United States, where the addition of iodine to foodstuffs has essentially eliminated iodine-deficient goiter.

The development of an adenomatous (nodular) goiter is considered the response of the thyroid to continuous stimulation by thyrotropin as a consequence of a relative deficiency of T_4. The natural history of the disease is that of a diffuse goiter of childhood and adolescence followed by development of a nodular goiter (see Fig. 20-16). Unless there is a severe deficit in TH synthesis (goitrous hypothyroidism), the patient will remain euthyroid.

The nodule(s) may represent one or more of the entities comprising adenomatous goiter, for example, localized colloid nodule, cellular nonfunctioning adenoma, cyst (reflecting degenerative changes in a colloid nodule), and relatively acellular hyperfunctioning nodules (autonomously functioning thyroid lesions). Focal (lobular) areas of hyperplasia may enlarge and, with progressive growth, persist as an adenoma. Such an adenoma may be of varying size and histologic appearance (follicular adenoma, fetal adenoma, Hurthle cell adenoma). Why some individuals develop a solitary nodule (follicular adenoma) and others a hyperfunctioning nodule or, more commonly, multiple colloid nodules is not clear. Although the solitary nodule occurs most often in the third and fourth decades and the multinodular goiter in later years, solitary nodules may become manifest only late in life, and occasionally multinodular goiter is observed during early adulthood.

Adenomatous goiter is insidious in development and is usually asymptomatic until there is visible enlargement or asymmetry of the neck or an incidental finding on physical examination. With continuing growth, the goiter may become unsightly, or there may be associated pressure symptoms (local discomfort, dysphagia, dyspnea, or hoarseness). Owing to their relatively slow growth and ease of displacement of other structures, they may be relatively large yet remain asymptomatic. Substernal goiters, presumably because of their confinement within the thoracic inlet, are more likely to be evidenced by local pressure, cough, dysphagia, or dyspnea due to compression of the trachea and esophagus; sometimes they are associated with engorgement of the cervical veins. The incidence of thyrotoxicosis in nodular goiter is low.

The clinical incidence of nodular goiter in adults is approximately 4%, and there is a marked predilection for the female. Autopsy figures give an incidence of nearer 50%, with approximately three fourths of the nodules in the older age group being multinodular.

DIAGNOSIS AND MANAGEMENT OF THE SOLITARY THYROID NODULE

The problem of the nontoxic nodular goiter consists in its differentiation from thyroid cancer and the disposition of those patients who have symptoms because of the size, location, and occasional hyperfunction of the goiter.

HISTORY

Accurate information is obtained about the duration of the thyromegaly, recent enlargement of an existing goiter, and past history of hypo- or hyperthyroidism and, in particular,

SOLITARY "COLD" THYROID NODULES	
Etiology	Cyst, adenoma, carcinoma, thyroiditis
Dx	Palpable thyroid nodule, cold nodule on scan, ultrasonogram of thyroid or CT scan
Rx	Response to thyroid suppression, needle biopsy, thyroid lobectomy, appropriate resection if necessitated by carcinoma or radioiodine therapy

external irradiation to the head or neck. A family history of goiter or thyroid cancer is also important.

PHYSICAL EXAMINATION

Physical examination helps to differentiate the solitary nodule from asymmetrical enlargement of one lobe or other conditions simulating a thyroid mass. Inspection will reveal the overall configuration of the thyroid and the mobility of an associated mass on deglutition. Bidigital palpation is required to provide a three-dimensional concept of the size of the mass, its physical characteristics, and the topography of the involved lobe. Careful appraisal will differentiate the solitary mass from those that are multiple or present in both lobes. A smooth, firm globular mass is consistent with a cyst. Adenomas may seem cystic. Hardness is characteristic of cancer but is also present in long-standing goiters that have undergone fibrosis or calcification. Palpation for enlarged cervical lymph nodes in the anterior neck and along the jugular chain completes the examination. Any change in quality of the voice requires evaluation of vocal cord function by indirect laryngoscopy.

THYROID FUNCTION STUDIES

Most patients are euthyroid. Confirmation can be made by determining the free thyroxine index. When the laboratory studies are not consistent with the clinical impression, determination of the serum TSH and RAI T$_3$ may identify the patient with associated hypothyroidism or the rare patient with "apathetic hyperthyroidism" or T$_3$ thyrotoxicosis (see Table 20-1).

THYROID IMAGING

The functional image of the thyroid gland can be portrayed by a thyroid scan following the administration of short-lived radionuclides (^{99m}Tc, ^{123}I). Scanning permits definition of the size and configuration of the thyroid as well as determination of function of macroscopic areas within the gland. Areas of abnormal function must be carefully correlated with the clinical findings. A "nodule" is a clinical, not a radiologic, finding (Fig. 20-12).

Scanning with ^{99m}Tc measures the "trapping" function of the thyroid epithelium, whereas radioiodide (^{123}I, ^{131}I) measures trapping (at 2 hr) and organification (2–6 hr) and organification and hormone release (24 hr). Disparate imaging occurs when defects in hormone synthesis result in trapping but no organification, as seen in some thyroid tumors and forms of thyroiditis (peroxidase defects).

Scans are helpful in differentiating benign from malignant lesions. Thyroid adenomas, malignant tumors, and cysts are invariably nonfunctioning or "cold" on scan. Adenomatous nodules characteristically demonstrate hypofunction; how-

ever, degenerative changes, hemorrhage, fibrosis, and cyst formation may cause them to be nonfunctional. Scans are of limited value because they are unable to differentiate between the intrinsic activity of a nodule and that resulting from normally functioning overlying thyroid parenchyma.

Thyroid scanning is also of value in identifying residual functioning tissue after thyroidectomy, aberrant thyroid, or functioning thyroid cancer that has metastasized to bone, lymph nodes, or lung.

ULTRASONOGRAPHY

Ultrasonography using the B mode is of value in determining the cellularity of tissue in response to a high-frequency pulse. The technique is complementary to imaging (scanning) and is of chief value in defining hypofunctioning or nonfunctioning thyroid nodules as solid (Fig. 20-13), cystic (Fig. 20-14), or mixed with solid components. Solid lesions are most likely to be adenomas, carcinomas, or adenomatoid nodules. Sequential measurements of the nodule are helpful in evaluating growth or response to hormonal suppression. Cystic lesions usually represent degenerated adenomatoid nodules but may also be present in well-differentiated thyroid cancer. Mixed cysts are associated with a higher incidence of cancer than "pure" cysts. Lesions that are less than 1 cm in diameter, are broad or flat, or substernal in location are difficult to assess by this technique. The size and configuration of substernal or intrathoracic goiters are best evaluated by CT scan (Fig. 20-15).

THYROID BIOPSY AND DIFFERENTIAL DIAGNOSIS

Histopathologic characteristics of the thyroid gland can be studied using a cutting needle (Vim-Silverman or Tru-Cut) biopsy technique with removal of a core of tissue for routine microscopy, or by aspiration of cells through a fine or large bore needle (No. 22–No. 19) and examined for their cytologic characteristics. Both techniques are useful in the differentiation of adenomatous goiter, cyst, thyroiditis, and papillary, undifferentiated, and medullary cancer. Follicular

Fig. 20-13. Ultrasonogram demonstrating a sonodense adenoma (*AD*). (*TR* = trachea; *TH* = right lobe of thyroid; *V* = internal jugular vein)

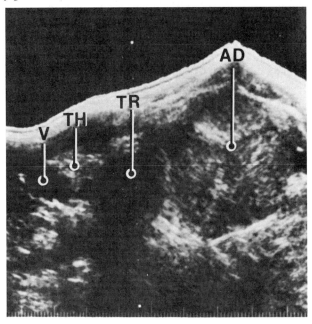

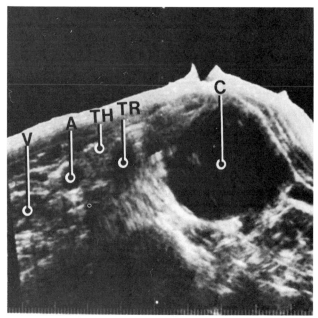

Fig. 20-14. Ultrasonogram demonstrating a sonolucent cyst of the left lobe of the thyroid (*C*). (*TR* = trachea; *TH* = thyroid; *A* = carotid artery; *V* = internal jugular vein)

adenoma cannot be differentiated from follicular adenocarcinoma. Biopsies may be performed as outpatient procedures; the morbidity of a cutting needle biopsy is higher than that of an aspiration biopsy.

The limitations of these techniques are related to the procurement of a representative sample of the thyroid lesion (small and substernally located nodules are constraints) and appropriate interpretation. False-negative (about 4%) and false-positive (about 1%) results may occur. The overall diagnostic accuracy of needle aspiration (aspiration biopsy cytology) is estimated to be greater than 90% by experienced cytopathologists. The test is most helpful when smears are read as malignant, indeterminate, or benign. The first usually represents papillary carcinoma or, less frequently, medullary or anaplastic carcinoma or lymphoma. Indeterminate smears will be encountered with cellular follicular adenomas and follicular adenocarcinomas. Benign findings are usually associated with a cyst, adenomatous nodule, or thyroiditis. An inadequate specimen is procured in approximately 10% of patients and requires reaspiration.

Thyroid biopsy plays a complementary role in the diagnosis of thyroid nodules and in differentiating those that can be managed by observation and suppression and those requiring excision for diagnosis or treatment. A final decision must be based on all factors including the clinical findings. For those patients considered to have a benign nodule and observed or placed upon suppressive therapy, needle aspiration can be repeated at 6- to 12-month intervals depending on the clinical course. The fear of implantation of tumor cells by these techniques has been alleviated by the scarcity of case reports.

SUPPRESSIVE THERAPY

Treatment with exogenous thyroid hormone is reasonable in patients who have an elevated TSH level or who have adenomatous goiters (by cytopathologic examination) that are hypofunctioning as opposed to nonfunctioning. The ability to establish a cytopathologic diagnosis in most in-

stances has placed less emphasis on suppressive therapy to differentiate thyrotropin-dependent and (presumably) benign nodules from thyroid cancer. Clinical data from prior experience indicate that nodules most likely to regress were hypofunctioning, solid, and less than 2 cm in diameter, occurred in women with a median age of 45, and had a relatively short history. In selected patients approximately 20% demonstrated complete regression of the nodule, and an additional 20% demonstrated partial regression. There are no data on the histologic characteristics of adenomatous nodules that regress with suppressive therapy.

The history and physical findings, in conjunction with one or more of the above laboratory studies, should permit the diagnosis of autonomously functioning thyroid lesions, thyroid cysts, chronic thyroiditis, adenomatous (nodular) goiter, and thyroid cancer. There will be some patients in whom the diagnosis is still indeterminate. Selection of surgical treatment in these patients is based upon identification of those at greatest risk (Table 20-2). The highest incidence of cancer occurs in children, males, women below the age of 40, and those with a prior history of irradiation to the head or neck or family history of medullary carcinoma. Older patients with a mass of recent origin also fall into this category.

Common thyroid disorders that may present as solitary nodules, in order of their relative incidence, are as follows:
1. Adenomatous goiter
2. Adenoma
3. Chronic (Hashimoto's) thyroiditis
4. Hyperfunctioning adenoma (autonomously functioning thyroid lesion)
5. Cysts, usually a manifestation of adenomatous goiter
6. Well-differentiated carcinomas

Infrequent causes of unilobular thyromegaly include the following:
1. Poorly differentiated cancers
2. Medullary carcinoma
3. Subacute (de Quervain's) thyroiditis
4. Lymphoma
5. Metastatic cancer
6. Suppurative thyroiditis
7. Congenital absence of one lobe of the thyroid, with compensatory enlargement of the remaining lobe

Nonthyroid disorders that may simulate a solitary nodule and can usually be differentiated by the history and physical findings are lymphadenitis, thyroglossal duct cyst, cancer metastatic to the cervical lymph nodes, Hodgkin's disease, midline cervical dermoid, cystic hygroma, lipoma, parathyroid adenoma or cyst, cervical–thymic cysts, neurogenic tumors or cysts, carcinoma or sarcoma of the cervical esophagus, and sternocleidomastoid fibrosis.

In patients in whom differentiation between a benign and a malignant lesion cannot be established, a total lobectomy is advised in order to make a histologic diagnosis. Other indications for operation on the solitary thyroid nodule are related to disfigurement, recurrence of a cyst after failure to control it by aspiration and suppressive treatment, and the potential for development of hyperthyroidism in young persons with an autonomously functioning lesion. (See previous discussion, Toxic Adenoma.)

MULTINODULAR GOITER

Surgical removal of a nontoxic multinodular goiter is performed primarily for the relief of pressure symptoms, respiratory tract obstruction, dysphagia, or disfigurement. Less frequently, multinodular goiter is removed because of its potential for carcinoma or for producing hyperthyroidism. During the past few decades there has been a marked reduction in the incidence of multinodular goiter, and huge goiters are relatively uncommon. Owing to the goiter's gradual encroachment upon the airway, symptoms may develop rather insidiously, and considerable compromise may exist by the time the patient seeks medical consultation. The ensuing narrowing of the trachea may interfere with pulmonary drainage, predisposing the patient to retention of bronchial secretions and intercurrent respiratory tract infections. Most of these individuals have goiters of many years' duration with pathologic changes consisting of colloid nodules, hyperfunctioning nodules, follicular adenomas, degenerating nodules, and cysts, as well as fibrosis and calcification. Many of the changes represent the end result

of this long-term TSH stimulation. As a consequence, suppressive treatment with TH is notoriously unsuccessful in causing regression of goiters of long duration (Fig. 20-16).

The clinical diagnosis of multinodular goiter may be confirmed by studies with radioiodine, which characteristically exhibit a normal or low uptake and an irregular and heterogeneous pattern on scintiscan (see Fig. 20-13*D*). X-rays of the neck may demonstrate calcification in both nodular goiter and cancer.

Extension of a nodular goiter to the anterior mediastinum is not an uncommon finding and may be associated with symptoms of dysphagia or respiratory tract obstruction. Confirmation of an anterior mediastinal mass as a goiter can usually be achieved by scintiscan. In some circumstances, however, the degenerative changes are such that there is little or no uptake of radioiodine. Usually the

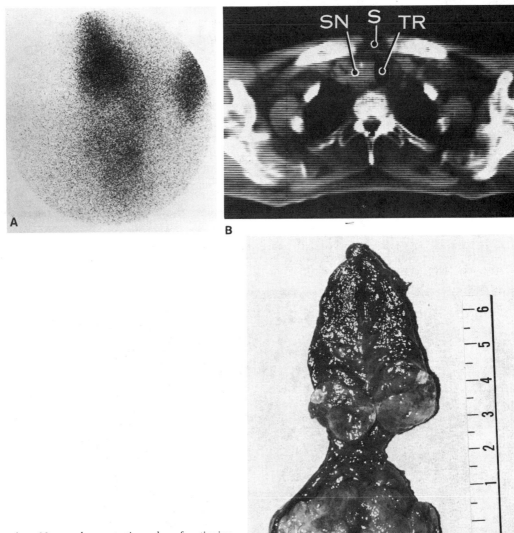

Fig. 20-15. (*A*) Technetium-99 scan demonstrating a hypofunctioning area in the region of a palpable nodule in the right lower pole of the thyroid and decreased uptake in an impalpable "sequestered nodule" caudad to the right lobe. (*B*) CT scan demonstrating the sequestered nodule (*SN*) at the thoracic inlet with displacement and compression of the trachea (*TR*). Note the focal calcification within the nodule. (*S* = sternal notch) (*C*) Bisected surgical specimen of right lobe of thyroid depicting the hypofunctioning adenomatous nodule and the sequestered nodule lying in the thoracic inlet.

associated enlargement of the thyroid gland is readily palpable in the neck. Continuity of an intrathoracic mass with a cervical shadow is evidence of thyroid origin (Fig. 20-15). Failure to outline the thyroid tissue in the mediastinum by scintiscan does not exclude the presence of a poorly functioning colloid nodule. Surgical removal of a mediastinal goiter can almost always be achieved through cervical exposure and rarely requires mediastinotomy. Mediastinal goiters projecting posterior to the subclavian artery or aortic arch present special problems and may require a combined cervicothoracic or entirely thoracic approach. The differential diagnosis of a mediastinal goiter includes aneurysms of the innominate artery and the aortic arch and primary or secondary tumors of the upper mediastinum (*e.g.*, thymoma, lymphoma, dermoid, and carcinoma of the lung).

CANCERS OF THE THYROID

Cancer of the thyroid is not a single entity but a spectrum of neoplasms with differing biologic characteristics and behavior that are reflected in their classification (see following list).

TABLE 20-2   CHARACTERISTICS OF BENIGN AND MALIGNANT THYROID NODULES

	MALIGNANT	BENIGN
Age at onset	Under 40 years	Over 40 years
Sex	Male	Female
Nodule(s)	Solitary	Multiple
Duration	Recent origin	Long-standing
Suppressive therapy	Progressive	Regression
Image	Nonfunctioning with ^{99m}TC or radioiodide	Functioning or hypofunctioning by scan
Sonodensity	Solid on B-mode ultrasonography	Cystic on B-mode ultrasonography
Other	History of irradiation to head or neck Cervical adenopathy	

Fig. 20-16.   Gross findings in a multinodular goiter from a woman after 3 years of suppressive therapy. The normal thyroid parenchyma had regressed with persistence of the goiter. Follicular adenoma, cyst formation, and degenerative changes are evident.

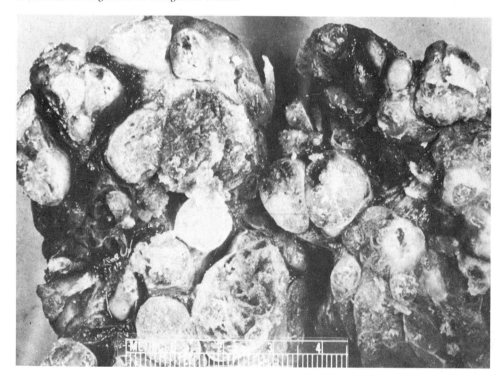

CLASSIFICATION OF THYROID NEOPLASMS

Well-differentiated carcinomas
    Papillary, including papillary–follicular
        Occult multicentric or minimal thyroid cancer (<1 cm)
        Invasive
    Follicular
        Encapsulated
        Invasive
Medullary with amyloid stroma
Undifferentiated (anaplastic, spindle cell, giant cell)
Lymphoma
Other (epidermoid, sarcoma, metastatic)

Thyroid cancer is an infrequent disease and an uncommon cause of death. In the United States malignancies of the thyroid are estimated to be responsible for 0.5% to 1% of all clinical cancers and to have an incidence of 25 per 1,000,000 population per year, accounting for approximately 1150 deaths annually. Much of the interest in thyroid cancer is created by the frequency of nodular goiter and other relatively common benign lesions of the thyroid, from which thyroid cancer should be differentiated. There is considerable diversity of opinion about methods of diagnosis, surgical treatment, and the role of adjuvant therapy in the management of these neoplasms. The variability of biologic behavior, the long natural history, and the lack of controlled observations of the results of treatment are responsible for these conflicting views. In routine autopsies the incidence approximates 0.8%. When special techniques are used, the frequency varies with the number of sections procured and with geography, for instance, 5.7%, 13%, and 28%. Most of these cancers, however, have little clinical significance. In areas with a high incidence of occult cancer there is no increase in deaths from thyroid cancer. In patients undergoing operation to differentiate nodular goiter from thyroid cancer, the incidence of carcinoma varies between 15% and 40%. The incidence of well-differentiated carcinoma in patients undergoing subtotal thyroidectomy for Graves' disease approximates 1%.

ETIOLOGY

Studies of etiologic mechanisms in human beings and experimental animals suggest that TSH, radiation injury, and other environmental factors are important. Neoplasms of the thyroid occur spontaneously in a number of species, and TSH stimulation increases the incidence of experimental thyroid tumors. Genetic predisposition, carcinogens, and prolonged goitrogenic stimulus result in neoplasms that vary in time of genesis, functional status, and growth potential. Iodine deficiency, thiourea, and radioiodine (^{131}I), alone or in combination, have all induced thyroid neoplasms in animals. These neoplasms initially are dependent upon TSH for growth. With continued stimulation and with retransplants into other hosts, they may become autonomous. The common denominator in the development of thyroid neoplasms in the experimental animal is persistent stimulus by TSH.

An analysis of conditions under which thyroid neoplasms are known to occur in human beings discloses that a history of radiation is common. Exposure of the thyroid to 100 to 700 rads during the first few years of life is associated with a 1% to 7% incidence of thyroid malignancy, which may occur from 10 to 30 years later. Radiation exposure later in life for treatment of acne or cervical arthritis has also been implicated; the average interval between radiation injury and development of well-differentiated cancer is 12.3 years. Data from a study of Hiroshima survivors indicate that thyroid carcinoma is more prevalent among those who were exposed to ionizing radiation. Somewhat paradoxically, there is no evidence to date that ^{131}I as used in the therapy of hyperthyroidism is associated with an increased incidence of thyroid cancer. Probably the radiation dosage required to control hyperthyroidism is also sufficient to prevent cell replication.

A stimulus for thyroid neoplasia may be furnished by iodine deficiency or congenital defects in TH synthesis. The role of iodine deficiency in the development of thyroid cancer in humans is seen in areas of endemic goiter. The incidence of thyroid cancer in these areas is several times that in other parts of the world. Several decades of iodine administration for reduction of the incidence of goiter have been associated with a decrease in age-specific mortality rates from thyroid cancer. However, iodine prophylaxis of goiter in endemic regions has not eliminated malignant neoplasms of the thyroid.

The transition of well-differentiated to poorly differentiated thyroid cancer, characterized by increased degrees of autonomous and aggressive behavior of the neoplasm, occurs in approximately 5% of patients. Progression appears to be enhanced by a combination of irradiation and hypothyroidism, the latter providing stimulation by way of the TSH feedback mechanism. Progression may be, but is not always, arrested by the administration of TH.

BIOLOGIC BEHAVIOR

WELL-DIFFERENTIATED NEOPLASMS

The diagnosis, treatment, and prognosis of malignant neoplasms of the thyroid should be directly related to their morphology. About 75% of thyroid carcinomas are well differentiated. The most common presenting finding is an asymptomatic solitary mass in the thyroid gland of a euthyroid patient. The primary lesion in the thyroid gland may be so small that it cannot be identified on physical examination. An enlarged cervical lymph node due to metastatic spread from an occult primary lesion is occasionally the presenting finding. Well-differentiated thyroid neoplasms are twice as common in women as in men. The mean age of these patients at the time of diagnosis is about 45 years.

Well-differentiated carcinomas consist of epithelial cells similar to those of the normal thyroid gland. The cells tend to form follicles or acini, which may contain colloid. The cytologic features characteristic of most malignancies—cellular atypia, anaplasia, nuclear hyperchromatism, and mitotic figures—are conspicuous by their infrequency. The biologic behavior of well-differentiated carcinomas is indolent and is characterized by slow progression over a period of years with extension to regional lymph nodes and late and infrequent metastasis to distant sites.

Papillary (Papillary–Follicular) Carcinoma

Papillary carcinoma is the most common of the well-differentiated neoplasms. Grossly, the lesion appears to infiltrate the adjacent thyroid parenchyma but may be encapsulated (5% to 10%), simulating an adenoma. Histopathologically, the tumor consists of papillary formations, each having a fibrovascular core (Fig. 20-17). The nuclei of

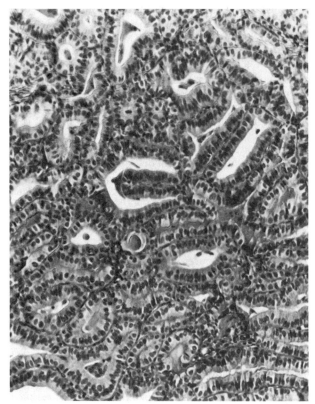

Fig. 20-17. Papillary carcinoma. (Hematoxylin and eosin stain; original magnification × 130)

the cells of this tumor have a characteristic ground-glass vesicular appearance. Psammoma bodies are frequent, and multicentricity by microscopic criteria is common. Approximately 25% of these tumors are composed of papillary elements alone; the remainder contain neoplastic thyroid follicles and are classified as mixed papillary–follicular carcinomas.

The frequency of cervical lymph node metastasis is highly variable. It is present in pretracheal (Delphian), paracapsular lymph nodes and in nodes accompanying the recurrent laryngeal nerve in the tracheoesophageal sulcus. More advanced disease is characterized by extension to nodes along the internal jugular vein, in the posterocervical triangle, and in the superior mediastinum. The most common distant metastases occur in the lung and are frequently miliary in appearance (see Fig. 20-18); they may be sufficiently occult to be identified only by radionuclide scan. Metastases may also present as nodular masses.

Radiation-associated thyroid cancer is usually papillary and is commonly multifocal (50%); approximately the same percentage have associated lymph node metastases. In general, these cancers are biologically similar to sporadic papillary carcinomas except for the higher incidence of multicentricity and lymph node metastasis.

Follicular Carcinoma

Follicular adenocarcinoma constitutes approximately 15% to 20% of thyroid cancers. Macroscopically, the tumor may appear as an encapsulated adenoma or it may be diffusely infiltrating. Microscopically, it most closely resembles the normal thyroid follicles, varying in size and sometimes containing colloid. The absence of a capsule, extension into the normal thyroid parenchyma, and vascular and lymphatic invasion, which may be absent, are the criteria for diagnosis. The encapsulated follicular adenocarcinoma is difficult to differentiate from a benign follicular adenoma without having the entire lesion available for histologic examination. Hurthle (oxyphilic) cell and clear cell carcinoma are variants of this tumor. Extension to distant organ systems is infrequent and usually occurs years after the primary lesion becomes manifest. Lungs and bones are the most common sites of distant metastasis. Cervical lymph nodes are less frequently involved than with papillary carcinomas. Since follicular carcinomas most closely resemble normal thyroid tissue, they have the greatest avidity of all thyroid cancer for radioiodine. The more differentiated the neoplasm and the more colloid it forms, the more likely it is to take up ^{131}I.

Medullary Carcinoma

Medullary carcinoma, described by Hazard et al. (1959) constitutes 4% to 8% of malignant thyroid neoplasms. It typically presents as small asymmetrical masses in the thyroid or, rarely, as cervical lymph node metastases. Twice as common in women as in men, it has the highest clinical incidence during the sixth decade of life. Medullary cancer may be sporadic or familial (in a ratio of 4:1); if familial, it may be a component of one of the multiple endocrine adenopathies (MEA IIa or MEA IIb). A familial medullary carcinoma without associated endocrinopathy has also been described. MEA IIa comprises medullary carcinoma, pheochromocytoma(s), and parathyroid hyperplasia. It is inherited as an autosomal dominant trait with complete penetrance but variable expressivity. All patients have medullary carcinoma, 60% have multiglandular parathyroid hyperplasia, and 40% have pheochromocytoma(s). MEA IIb consists of medullary carcinoma, pheochromocytoma(s), a Marfanoid habitus, characteristic facies, multiple mucosal neuromas, and ganglioneuromatosis. This carcinoma is more aggressive than that in MEA IIa. Medullary carcinomas are characterized histologically by solid sheets of polyhedral and spindle-shaped cells, with a large amount of hyalinized stroma interposed between the interlacing masses of cells. These neoplasms arise from the parafollicular C cell that originates in the embryonic neural crest tissue and migrates to a position within the thyroid and, to some extent, the parathyroid and thymus in early fetal life. These cells, like others arising from the neural crest, have a biosynthetic ability characterized by *a*mine *p*recursor *u*ptake and *d*ecarboxylation (APUD). The calcitonin secreted by these cells constitutes a tumor marker that may be a key to early diagnosis and prognosis. The neoplasm demonstrates mitotic activity, and vascular and lymphatic involvement is common. Extension into normal thyroid is present without evidence of encapsulation. Medullary carcinoma frequently metastasizes to lymph nodes and may also involve the lung, liver, bone, and the central nervous system. Intractable diarrhea may be a consequence of a large volume of tumor. Nutmeg by mouth may provide relief.

All patients should be screened for the possibility of associated pheochromocytoma(s), and treatment for such tumors has priority over thyroidectomy. The accompanying parathyroid hyperplasia correlates poorly with elevated parathormone levels in peripheral blood and does not require routine subtotal parathyroidectomy. The clinical diagnosis of hyperparathyroidism warrants the excision of grossly enlarged parathyroid glands with preservation of parathyroid function. Treatment of medullary carcinoma

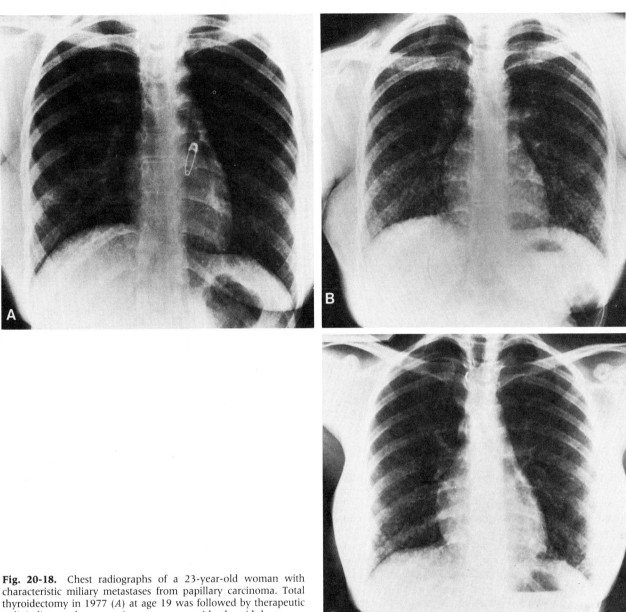

Fig. 20-18. Chest radiographs of a 23-year-old woman with characteristic miliary metastases from papillary carcinoma. Total thyroidectomy in 1977 (*A*) at age 19 was followed by therapeutic radioiodine and suppressive treatment with thyroid hormone. Follow-up radiographs taken (*B*) in 1979 and (*C*) in 1981.

consists of total thyroidectomy with excision of the regional lymphatic drainage of the thyroid (see later discussion of Surgical Treatment).

Pretesting families with potential disease is recommended because the prognosis after total thyroidectomy, when the tumor is confined to the thyroid gland, is good.

All patients should be followed postoperatively by periodic evaluation of calcitonin levels. This is a very sensitive test, and in some circumstances the levels have remained elevated without clinical evidence of recurrent disease. Radiation therapy is relatively ineffective. Chemotherapy, with the exception of adriamycin, has not proved helpful.

UNDIFFERENTIATED CARCINOMAS

Approximately 15% of malignant thyroid neoplasms are classified as undifferentiated (*e.g.*, giant cell and spindle cell carcinomas). They are twice as common in women as in men, with a mean age of 60 years at diagnosis. Usually there is a short history of a rapidly enlarging, conspicuous, hard mass in the thyroid gland. It may be unilateral or bilateral. Hoarseness, dysphagia, or dyspnea are frequent presenting symptoms. Macroscopically, the neoplasms are diffusely infiltrating, extending into and beyond the thyroid parenchyma. Microscopically, they consist of sheets or masses of atypical, anaplastic, and hyperchromatic epithelial cells with numerous mitotic figures. The biologic behavior of these neoplasms contrasts sharply with that of well-differentiated thyroid carcinomas. Rapid progression occurs with early metastatic spread to lymph nodes and other organ systems. The aggressiveness of these neoplasms is indicated by the invasion or compression of the recurrent laryngeal nerves, the esophagus, and the trachea; such compression is frequently present at diagnosis. The interval from the time a mass is first noted in the neck until death ensues from distant metastatic disease or local extension of the neoplasm in the neck may be as short as 3 months.

Because of the aggressiveness of the neoplasm, complete surgical excision of the primary lesion is usually not possible. Distant metastatic disease at the time of diagnosis is not uncommon. Metastasis may develop in the lungs, bones, gastrointestinal tract, urinary tract, and central nervous and other organ systems.

LYMPHOMA

Lymphomas of the thyroid, formerly considered small cell neoplasms, constitute 2% to 4% of thyroid malignancies. The sex incidence and presenting findings are similar to those of undifferentiated carcinoma. The mean age of the patients at diagnosis is about 55 years. These tumors are characterized by homogeneous sheets and masses of relatively uniform small cells. There is usually no encapsulation, the neoplasm invading adjacent normal thyroid and sometimes extrathyroidal soft tissues. Lymph node extension and extranodal spread in the neck may be present. These lesions are less aggressive than anaplastic malignancies and are usually responsive to radiation therapy.

OTHER NEOPLASMS

Other rare neoplasms that have been described as occurring in the thyroid gland include adenoacanthoma, squamous cell carcinoma, and fibrosarcoma. These all may be variants of anaplastic carcinoma. Metastatic spread to the thyroid gland from other primary sites of malignancy (primarily the breast and lung) occurs but is rare.

DIAGNOSIS

The symptoms and physical findings correlate well with the biologic characteristics of the histologic type of thyroid malignancy. A long history of goiter is more often present with poorly differentiated than with well-differentiated neoplasms. A well-differentiated cancer grows slowly and commonly presents as an asymptomatic mass confined to one lobe or the isthmus of the thyroid gland. Rarely is the mass of sufficient size to produce tracheal compression, dysphagia, or local pressure symptoms. Rapidly growing, poorly differentiated neoplasms are invasive and are more frequently associated with local symptoms, such as cervical discomfort or fullness, tightness, pain referred to the ear or angle of the jaw, dysphagia, dyspnea, stridor (rarely), and hoarseness. Hoarseness is usually secondary to invasion of the recurrent laryngeal nerve. Indirect laryngoscopy confirms loss of vocal cord function in patients who are hoarse or are symptomatic. Half of the patients with medullary cancer and more than 70% of those with undifferentiated cancer are symptomatic.

The physical findings are related to the type of neoplasm. Well-circumscribed, encapsulated, papillary–follicular or follicular carcinoma is soft to firm in consistency and one to several centimeters in diameter. Invasive and infiltrating papillary or follicular carcinoma is frequently hard and is more often poorly defined or irregular. The latter are frequently associated with one or more enlarged cervical lymph nodes near the internal jugular vein. Occasionally, the primary cancer is diffuse and is manifested only by an increase in the size and consistency of one lobe. Cervical lymph node metastases may be the chief manifestation of papillary and follicular lesions. Advanced disease is characterized by more extensive metastases involving the lymph nodes of the deep jugular chain, posterior cervical triangle,

and contralateral side of the neck. Undifferentiated neoplasms frequently infiltrate the strap muscles and soft tissue. A bruit is uncommon over the primary tumor. However, metastatic follicular carcinoma involving bone or soft tissue is sometimes associated with a thrill or bruit. Metastatic renal carcinoma is the only other cancer that produces similar physical findings.

Radiographs of the neck may show tracheal compression or displacement, depending upon the size of the mass. Focal calcification, more common in long-standing nodular goiter, may also be seen with thyroid cancer owing to the presence of psammoma bodies. Well-differentiated thyroid cancer usually remains localized to the neck. In patients dying from thyroid cancer, extensive local disease with invasion of the trachea is common.

The clinical studies permitting a more precise diagnosis of thyroid cancer are outlined in the earlier section on Diagnosis and Management of the Solitary Thyroid Nodule.

SURGICAL TREATMENT

The primary method of treatment of all thyroid malignancies is surgical excision. Differences of opinion exist about the amount of thyroid gland to be excised and the role of lymph node resection in management. The broad spectrum of biologic behavior of thyroid neoplasms has important implications for treatment.

PARTIAL THYROIDECTOMY

Partial thyroidectomy (resection of part of one lobe or a portion of both lobes) has no place in the management of any malignant thyroid neoplasm. The high incidence of residual and recurrent disease and a morbidity that is similar to that of lobectomy contraindicate this approach.

LOBECTOMY

Lobectomy is the operation of choice in well-differentiated carcinomas that are grossly limited to one lobe and are less than 2 cm in diameter. If the lesion is located near the isthmus, the isthmus should be excised. The recurrent laryngeal nerve is identified but not manipulated before the lobe is excised. An effort is made to identify and preserve the parathyroid glands. Paracapsular lymph nodes, including an enlarged Delphian node, should be included with the surgical specimen. After the lobe containing the gross lesion is excised, a frozen section is made to establish the diagnosis. The diagnosis is the joint responsibility of the pathologist and the surgeon. Because of striking biologic and clinical differences, it is important to determine the histologic type of the neoplasm and the presence of lymphatic spread on the basis of frozen section examination. Grossly encapsulated follicular carcinoma should be distinguished from well-differentiated cancers that are diffusely infiltrative.

TOTAL AND NEAR-TOTAL THYROIDECTOMY

Total and near-total thyroidectomy is indicated for large and diffusely infiltrating well-differentiated carcinomas, for those with gross involvement of the isthmus and the contralateral lobe, for all tumors with lymph node metastasis, for medullary carcinoma, and for poorly differentiated carcinoma in selected patients. Near-total thyroidectomy consists of a complete lobectomy on the side of the primary lesion. The posterior capsule and a shell of thyroid tissue (1 g–2 g in weight) are preserved on the contralateral side to protect the recurrent laryngeal nerve and the blood supply to the parathyroid glands. The multifocal character of many well-differentiated carcinomas and the possible need for subsequent radioiodine therapy make total thyroidectomy a reasonable choice. However, complete excision of the grossly uninvolved lobe should not be carried out at the risk of injury to the intact remaining recurrent nerve and parathyroid glands. Total thyroidectomy increases the incidence of postoperative hypoparathyroidism and vocal cord paresis and does not seem to result in a significant improvement in survivorship. It is requisite for complete removal of all gross carcinoma and for patients who because of distant metastases are candidates for radioiodine therapy.

CERVICAL LYMPH NODE EXCISION

Cervical lymph node excision in well-differentiated and medullary carcinoma is indicated by histologically confirmed metastases in lymph nodes. The type of operation depends upon the pathologic findings. Particular attention should be paid to the routes of lymphatic flow peculiar to the thyroid, that is, adjacent to the thyroid capsule, along the recurrent laryngeal nerve, in the pretracheal areolar tissue, and along the internal jugular vein. Because of the anatomy of the neck, it is impossible to excise the lymph nodes in continuity with the primary neoplasm. Lymph node metastases may be manifest only by a firmer consistency of a node with little change in size. This is particularly true for nodes along the recurrent laryngeal nerve. All firm or enlarged nodes (ipsilateral and contralateral) should be excised by a modified type of anterior neck dissection. It is usually unnecessary to sacrifice the internal jugular vein. However, with extensive lymph node involvement (*i.e.,* nodes along the internal jugular vein, in the posterior cervical triangle, and in the upper part of the neck) a more radical neck dissection is indicated with removal of the internal jugular vein. Unless involved by direct extension (rare), the sternocleidomastoid muscle is preserved and reconstructed at the end of the operation. Involved superior mediastinal lymph nodes can usually be removed through a cervical incision. Rarely is a sternum-splitting incision indicated.

There is no convincing evidence of increased survival in patients undergoing "prophylactic" lymph node resection. Because of the prolonged indolent course characterizing well-differentiated thyroid carcinomas, lymph node metastases appearing later may be removed without jeopardizing survival. For the same reason, there is no need to perform a radical neck dissection in a patient with minimal lymph node involvement.

TRACHEAL SURGERY

Partial tracheotomy is indicated to remove local areas of invasion less than 2 cm in diameter. Resection of a circumferential section of trachea in an effort to cure the patient is rarely indicated. Tracheostomy may be necessary in the patient who has an advanced, bulky, poorly differentiated carcinoma in order to maintain an airway. This occurs less often with well-differentiated carcinomas. Tracheostomy may be required in anticipation of the severe laryngeal edema sometimes associated with removal of laryngeal lymphatics accompanying extensive neck dissections and total thyroidectomy. Similarly, injury to both recurrent laryngeal nerves (either neuropraxia or neurotmesis) in association with extensive resections for advanced disease constitutes an indication for a tracheostomy.

THYROIDECTOMY—TECHNICAL CONSIDERATIONS

The success of surgical treatment depends upon excision of the disease process by lobectomy, subtotal thyroidectomy (Graves' disease), or near-total or total thyroidectomy and preservation of the external branch of the superior laryngeal nerve(s), the recurrent laryngeal nerve(s), and the parathyroid glands. The operation is best performed under general endotracheal anesthesia with the patient in a semi-Fowler's position and the neck hyperextended. Exposure of the thyroid gland is achieved by a transverse collar incision placed 3 cm above the sternal notch (Fig. 20-19*A*). Skin flaps in the subplatysmal fascial plane are developed superiorly to the thyroid cartilage and inferiorly to the manubrium. Separation of the strap muscles in the midline provides adequate access to the underlying thyroid gland in most circumstances. Transection of the strap muscles (high to maintain innervation) may be required for exposure of large nodular or neoplastic goiters. Ligation and division of the middle thyroid vein(s) will permit rotation of the gland medially to expose the inferior thyroid artery, inferior thyroid veins, and parathyroid glands. Incision of the suspensory ligaments of the superior pole of the thyroid facilitates identification of the external branch of the superior laryngeal nerve as it emerges medially from its association with the superior thyroid artery prior to entering the cricothyroid muscle (Fig. 20-19*B*). Avoidance of injury is accomplished by dissection and individual ligation of the lateral, anterior, and posterior branches of the superior thyroid artery as they enter the thyroid gland. The recurrent laryngeal nerve is most readily identified in the avascular plane caudad to the inferior pole of the thyroid in the tracheoesophageal sulcus. The recurrent nerve on the right may lie in a slightly more oblique location than that on the left. The nerve commonly divides into two or more branches. Injury is most likely when the nerve is in an aberrant location because of displacement by a nodular goiter or neoplasm or when achieving hemostasis from vessels near the nerve. Injury is best avoided by locating the nerve caudad to the inferior pole of the thyroid and, in subtotal resection, by tracing it to the region of the inferior thyroid artery. In lobectomy for suspected neoplasms, the nerve should be dissected along its medial aspect until it enters the larynx (Fig. 20-19*C*). Particular care should be taken to identify and ligate in advance those small branches of the inferior thyroid artery that will require division to separate the thyroid gland from the overlying nerve. The right recurrent nerve is "nonrecurrent" in about 1% to 2% of patients owing to the anomalous origin of the right subclavian artery from the sixth rather than the fourth branchial arch. Under these circumstances, the nerve arises directly from the vagus at the level of the cricothyroid articulation.

Preservation of parathyroid function requires identification of the inferior and superior parathyroid glands in paracapsular areolar tissue, most commonly on the posterolateral aspect of the thyroid. The main trunk of the inferior thyroid artery should not be ligated. By maintaining a plane of dissection between the thyroid capsule and the parathyroid glands, the individual branches of the inferior thyroid artery can be ligated as they enter the gland. With this approach the parathyroids can usually be preserved with an intact blood supply. This is usually more readily achieved for the inferior than for the superior parathyroid glands. Should the parathyroid be deprived of its blood supply, it should be cut into 1 mm to 2 mm fragments and placed in

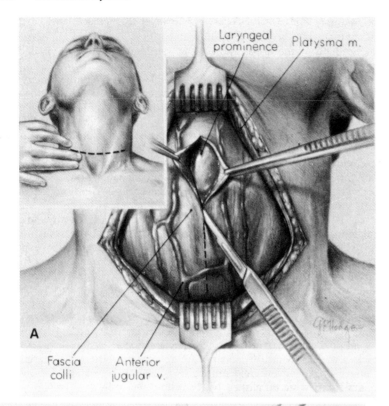

Fascia colli   Anterior jugular v.

Laryngeal prominence   Platysma m.

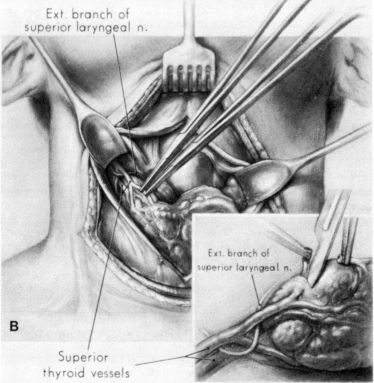

Ext. branch of superior laryngeal n.

Ext. branch of superior laryngeal n.

Superior thyroid vessels

Fig. 20-19. Technique for thyroidectomy.

(*A*) A transverse collar incision is placed approximately 3 cm cephalad to the sternal notch. After elevation of the platysma superiorly to the thyroid cartilage and inferiorly to the clavicles, the cervical fascia is divided in the midline, and strap muscles are retracted to expose the underlying thyroid gland.

(*B*) Following division of the suspensory ligament at the level of the thyroid cartilage, the superior pole of the thyroid is retracted laterally to expose the superior pole vessels and the external branch of the superior laryngeal nerve. The superior thyroid vessels are divided after they branch in order to avoid injury to the external branch of the superior laryngeal nerve.

individual muscle pockets in the sternocleidomastoid in patients with benign disease and in the pectoralis major through a separate incision in patients with malignant disease.

The cervical sympathetic chain lying on the anterior scalene muscles may be exposed in patients undergoing dissection for lateral cervical lymph node metastases. It needs to be preserved from injury, as does the inferior cervical ganglion, which may be mistaken for an enlarged lymph node.

The common carotid artery should also be protected from prolonged retraction, particularly in individuals with associated atherosclerosis. It may be severely distorted by a large adenomatous goiter.

(*C*) In the performance of a lobectomy, the terminal branches of the inferior thyroid artery are divided individually on the thyroid capsule. The recurrent nerve is identified and traced to its entrance into the cricothyroid articulation by "unroofing" the overlying thyroid gland. Note the proximity of the ligament of Berry to the nerve.

(*D*) In subtotal thyroidectomy for hyperthyroidism, approximately 1 g to 2 g of thyroid in the region of the posterior capsule is left bilaterally. The lateral portion of the capsule is not sutured to the trachea. (Thompson NW, Olsen WR, Hoffman GL: The continuing development of the technique of thyroidectomy. Surgery 73:913, 1973)

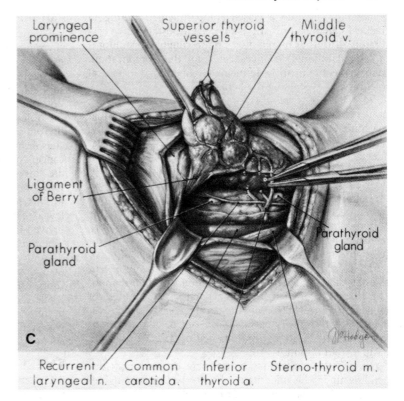

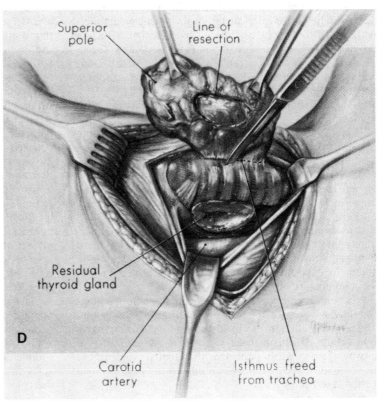

COMPLICATIONS OF THYROIDECTOMY AND POSTOPERATIVE MANAGEMENT

Complications unique to thyroidectomy include primarily hypoparathyroidism and airway obstruction (*e.g.*, postoperative bleeding, injury to recurrent laryngeal nerves, and laryngeal edema). Rarely is there damage to the cervical sympathetics, phrenic nerve, or thoracic duct, nor is there development of pneumomediastinum or pneumothorax. Damage to the external branch of the superior laryngeal nerve may alter the tone of the voice but does not compromise the airway.

Postoperative hemorrhage may be arterial or venous in origin. The former is more life-threatening because it involves bleeding into a closed compartment, resulting in tracheal compression. Any patient with postoperative respiratory distress as manifest by stridor, cough, or symptoms of hypoxia should be investigated for this complication. Management consists of immediately opening the cervical incision and evacuating the hematoma.

Recurrent nerve paralysis—temporary (neuropraxia) or permanent (neurotmesis)—may follow direct (cutting, crushing, stretching) or indirect (ischemic) injury to the recurrent laryngeal nerves. In the absence of laryngeal edema, *unilateral* recurrent nerve paralysis is well tolerated and may be manifest only by a "brassy" cough, slight hoarseness, or compromise of the airway with air hunger on exercise. The diagnosis can be positively established only by indirect or direct laryngoscopy in the postoperative period. Usually within a few months there is compensatory medial movement of the remaining normal vocal cord with re-establishment of a more functional voice. *Bilateral* nerve paralysis is incompatible with an adequate airway except as established by tracheostomy or endotracheal intubation. The diagnosis of bilateral nerve paralysis constitutes an indication for tracheostomy, the permanency of which will depend upon recovery of function of one or both recurrent laryngeal nerves. Recovery from neuropraxia will usually occur within 6 months.

Hypoparathyroidism may be transient or permanent depending upon the quantitative loss of parathyroid tissue. Owing to the short half-life of the biologically active parathormone, complete loss of parathyroid function, whether due to ischemia or surgical removal, is usually manifest within 6 hr to 8 hr by a positive Chvostek sign (which is positive in 10% of the normal population), positive Trousseau sign, symptoms of paresthesias, cramping of the hands and feet, and, if untreated, frank tetany. The hypocalcemia may be more insidious in onset, developing for 2 to 3 days, and is usually indicative of less severe hypoparathyroidism. Immediate management of hypocalcemia is accomplished by administering intravenous calcium gluconate, restoring calcium to the lower limits of normal, and administering the biologically active $1,25,(OH)_2$ vitamin D. Calcium carbonate (1 g daily) is administered by mouth on resumption of oral feeding. In long-term management without renal impairment, chronic hypoparathyroidism is managed by calciferol and calcium carbonate by mouth.

Laryngeal edema sometimes occurs after extensive operations for thyroid cancer and interference with laryngeal lymphatics owing to skeletalization of the larynx. Laryngeal edema in association with unilateral recurrent nerve paralysis may require tracheostomy.

Tracheal collapse may follow tracheomalacia from a long-standing goiter with tracheal deviation and compression. This is most likely to occur in association with laryngeal obstruction. Tracheomalacia alone is rarely the cause of airway obstruction. In patients with potential problems the use of a soft cuffed endotracheal tube in the postoperative period is indicated.

ADJUVANT MEASURES IN THYROID CANCER

Adjuvant measures in the management of thyroid cancer consist of thyroid hormone for TSH suppression, radioactive iodine, external irradiation, and chemotherapy. The selection of these measures will depend upon the type of neoplasm, its extent, the age and sex of the patient, and residual or recurrent disease.

TSH SUPPRESSION

All patients with thyroid cancer should be placed upon thyroid hormone for life. Although TSH suppression has its greatest application in well-differentiated cancers, there are anecdotal reports of poorly differentiated tumors responding to it. The rationale for TSH suppression is based upon the documented dependency of some thyroid cancers on TSH, the role of TSH as a promoting factor in experimental thyroid cancer in animals, and the presence of TSH receptor sites in most benign tumors and well-differentiated thyroid cancers. Clinical findings also suggest that recurrence rates are lower and survivorship better in patients on thyroid hormone. It should also be recognized, however, that many tumors recur despite TSH suppression. Further, increased levels of TSH are reportedly associated with transformation of well-differentiated thyroid carcinomas to more poorly differentiated types. Finally, following total thyroidectomy, thyroid hormone is essential to maintain euthyroidism. T_4 in a dosage of 0.2 mg to 0.25 mg will cause adequate suppression of TSH in most patients. Serum TSH and T_4 levels should be measured to evaluate the dosage and to monitor compliance. In patients with known recurrent or persistent disease, a TRH–TSH test is recommended to ensure adequacy of dosage.

RADIOIODINE

Radioactive iodine has been used both prophylactically and therapeutically in the management of well-differentiated cancers. Its value prophylactically is not well documented, and without controlled studies the evidence is only suggestive that it reduces the incidence of recurrent disease. Its use prophylactically would seem justified in older patients with well-differentiated carcinomas who are likely to have more aggressive disease. Radioiodine is clearly indicated therapeutically in patients with residual or recurrent cervical neoplasms not amenable to surgical excision and in patients with distant metastases, primarily to lung or bone. It is particularly valuable in controlling pulmonary metastases detected only by pulmonary scanning. Patients older than 40 years of age with well-differentiated cancer and those with bony metastasis from papillary carcinoma are less likely to respond to radioactive iodine therapy. Treatment is repeated at yearly intervals until there is no longer uptake by the neoplasm, avoiding pulmonary fibrosis and bone marrow damage. Serum thyroglobulin also serves as a useful marker of thyroid cancer, and in the absence of any normal thyroid tissue it can be used as an index of persistent or recurrent disease demonstrating the need for further radioiodine therapy. Radioiodine therapy has no place in the management of medullary or poorly differentiated carcinomas.

Suppressive therapy with T_4 and the use of radioactive iodine are not mutually exclusive but should be considered complementary. Suppressive therapy is usually discontinued approximately 3 to 4 weeks prior to radioactive iodine therapy to permit endogenous TSH to rise. Suppressive therapy is resumed following treatment with radioiodine.

EXTERNAL IRRADIATION

External beam therapy given by megavoltage x-rays, cobalt (^{60}Co) gamma rays, or high-energy electrons is indicated primarily for lymphomas, undifferentiated carcinomas, and those well-differentiated tumors not amenable to surgical excision, thyrotropin suppression, or radioiodide therapy. Radiation therapy is complementary to the surgical excision of well-circumscribed lymphomas. For extensively infiltrating lymphomas, radiotherapy is the treatment of choice after confirmation of the diagnosis by open biopsy.

CHEMOTHERAPY

There has been very limited success in the management of undifferentiated carcinomas with chemotherapy. It has been used primarily as an adjunct to radiation therapy. Somewhat encouraging results have followed the use of adriamycin. It has no role in the treatment of well-differentiated neoplasms.

PROGNOSIS IN THYROID CANCER

Prognosis in thyroid cancer (Fig. 20-20) is related to a number of factors, the most important of which are the histologic classification of the tumor and the age of the patient. Perhaps in no other malignant disease does youth have such a favorable influence on survivorship. Other factors that influence prognosis are sex, tumor size, encapsulation, extrathyroidal extension, lymph node and systemic metastases, and treatment. A history of prior irradiation

Fig. 20-20. Note the long survival (years) with the differentiated papillary and follicular and medullary carcinomas, as compared to the short survival (months) with undifferentiated carcinoma. (Beahrs OH, Pasternak BM: Cancer of the Thyroid Gland. In Ravitch MM et al [eds]: Current Problems in Surgery. Chicago, Year Book Medical Publishers, 1969)

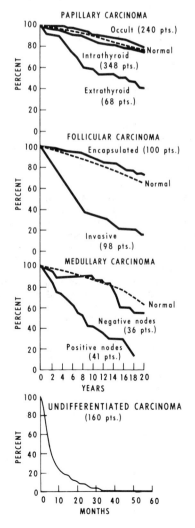

increases tumor multicentricity and the incidence of lymph node metastasis but does not change the aggressiveness of the tumor.

Papillary carcinoma, including tumors with a follicular component, has the best prognosis. The clinical course is usually long, with an overall mortality varying between 10% and 20% depending upon the risk factors. In patients under 21 years, the disease appears to be almost benign. Factors that favor a normal survivorship are youth (less than 21 years), female sex, tumors less than 1.0 cm (occult), confinement within the thyroid gland, and a single focus of disease. Involvement of the regional lymph nodes is associated with a higher incidence of local recurrence but has little effect on prognosis. Factors associated with more aggressive tumors and a shorter survival include size (more than 1.5 cm in diameter), capsular invasion, age (over 40), and sex (male). Multicentric tumors, particularly when the initial treatment is partial as opposed to near-total or total thyroidectomy, are prone to local recurrence. The poorest prognosis occurs in the older age group (over 40 years) with existing pulmonary or bony metastases at the time of diagnosis.

Follicular carcinoma is also a slowly growing neoplasm whose malignant nature is indicated by blood vessel or capsular invasion. Well-encapsulated tumors with minimal vascular invasion are associated with an essentially "normal" survival (Fig. 20-20). Those with extensive vascular or parenchymal invasion have a poorer survival. The size of the tumor seems to have less influence than it does in papillary cancers. Follicular carcinomas are more aggressive in patients over 40 years with distant metastases, particularly to bone, and are associated with a shortened survival.

Patients with *medullary carcinoma* have a prognosis intermediate between that for well-differentiated and that for undifferentiated thyroid cancers. Survival is correlated with the stage of the disease and whether the diagnosis was made on the basis of clinical findings (usually representing more advanced disease) or by provocative tests. The calcitonin response to provocative testing provides an index to tumor volume and extent of disease (metastasis) and overall prognosis. Patients with MEA IIb who have mucosal neuromas in addition to parathyroid disease have a more aggressive neoplasm and consequently a poorer prognosis.

Undifferentiated (anaplastic, giant cell, spindle cell) *cancers* are biologically very aggressive tumors; death due to local invasion occurs within 1 to 2 years of diagnosis. Exceptions occur in patients in whom these tumors are small and confined within the thyroid, are identified with a well-differentiated component, and are treated by radical surgery with external irradiation.

Lymphomas (previously classified as small cell carcinomas) are associated with a very good survival depending upon the stage of the disease and the response to irradiation.

BIBLIOGRAPHY

General

CLARK OH: TSH suppression in management of thyroid nodules and thyroid cancer. World J Surg 5:39, 1981

DeGROOT LJ, FROHMAN LJ, KAPLAN EL et al (eds): Radiation Associated Thyroid Carcinoma. New York, Grune & Stratton, 1977

DE VISSCHER M: The Thyroid Gland. New York, Raven Press, 1980

THOMPSON NW, OLSEN WR, HOFFMAN GL: The continuing development of the technique of thyroidectomy. Surgery 73:913, 1973

WERNER SC, INGBAR SH: The Thyroid: A Fundamental and Clinical Text. Hagerstown, Harper & Row, 1978

Anatomy and Physiology

BARTUSKA DG, DRATMAN MB: Evolving concepts of thyroid function. Med Clin N Am 57:1117, 1973

BRENNAN MD: Thyroid hormone. Mayo Clin Proc 55:33, 1980

HUNT S, POOLE M, REEVE TS: A reappraisal of the surgical anatomy of the thyroid and parathyroid glands. Brit J Surg 55:63, 1968

LARSEN PR: Thyroid-pituitary interaction: Feedback regulation of thyrotropin secretion by thyroid hormones. New Engl J Med 306:23, 1982

SCHWARTZ HL, Oppenheimer JH: Physiologic and biochemical actions of thyroid hormone. Pharmacol Ther 3:349, 1978

VAN HERLE AJ, VASSART G, DUMONT J: Control of thyroglobulin synthesis and secretion. New Engl J Med 301:307, 1979

Diagnostic Procedures and Tests of Thyroid Function

ASHCRAFT MW, VAN HERLE AJ: Management of thyroid nodules: II. Scanning techniques, thyroid suppressive therapy and fine needle aspiration. Head Neck Surg 3:297, 1981

LOWHAGEN T, WILLEMS S, LUNDELL G et al: Aspiration biopsy cytology in diagnosis of thyroid cancer. World J Surg 5:61, 1981

PATTON JA, HOLLIFIELD JW, BRILL AB et al: Differentiation between malignant and benign solitary nodules by fluorescent scanning, J Nucl Med 17:17, 1976

ROSEN IB: Diagnostic studies of thyroid cancer. J Surg Oncol 16:233, 1981

ROSEN IB, WALLACE C, STRAWBRIDGE HG, et al: Reevaluation of needle aspiration cytology in detection of thyroid cancer. Surgery 90:747, 1981

THOMAS CG JR, BUCKWALTER JA, STAAB EV et al: Evaluation of dominant thyroid masses. Ann Surg 183:463, 1976

VAN HERLE AJ, ULLER R: Elevated serum thyroglobulin marker of metastases in differentiated thyroid carcinomas. J Clin Invest 56:272, 1975

WELLS S, BAYLIS S, MARSTON L et al: Provocative agents in the diagnosis of medullary carcinoma of the thyroid gland. Ann Surg 188:139, 1978

Hyperthyroidism and Thyroiditis

BARNES HV, GANN DS: Choosing thyroidectomy in hyperthyroidism. Surg Clin N Am 54:389, 1974

CLARK OH, GREENSPAN FS, DUNPHY JE: Hashimoto's thyroiditis in thyroid cancer: Indications for operation. Am J Surg 140:665, 1980

HAIBACH H, AVIOLI LV: Hyperthyroidism in Graves' disease: Current trends in management and diagnosis. Arch Int Med 136:725, 1976

LEE TC, COFFEY RJ, CURRIER B, CANARY J: Propranolol and thyroidectomy in the treatment of thyrotoxicosis. Ann Surg 195:766, 1982

SOLOMON DH, BEALL GN, TERASAKI PI et al: Autoimmune thyroid diseases: Graves' and Hashimoto's. Ann Int Med 88:379, 1978

THOMAS CG JR, RUTLEDGE RG: Surgical intervention in chronic (Hashimoto's) thyroiditis. Ann Surg 193:769, 1981

VOLPE R: The role of autoimmunity in hypoendocrine and hyperendocrine function. Ann Int Med 87:86, 1977

Adenomatous Goiter

BECKERS C: Non toxic goiter. In deVisscher M (ed); The Thyroid Gland. New York, Raven Press, 1980

DOBYNS BN: Goiter. Curr Prob Surg 6:2, 1969

HAMBURGER JI: Solitary autonomously functioning lesions. Am J Med 58:740, 1975

JENNY H, BLOCK MA, HORN RC et al: Recurrence following surgery for benign thyroid nodules. Arch Surg 92:525, 1965

Thyroid Cancer

ALDINGER KA, SAMAAN NA, IBANEZ M et al: Anaplastic carcinoma of the thyroid: A review of 84 cases of spindle and giant cell carcinoma of the thyroid. Cancer 41:2267, 1978

BLOCK MA: Management of carcinoma of the thyroid. Ann Surg 185:133, 1977

BUCKWALTER JA, GURL NJ, THOMAS CG JR: Cancer of the thyroid in youth. World J Surg 5:15, 1981

BUCKWALTER JA, THOMAS CG JR: Selection of surgical treatment for well differentiated thyroid carcinomas. Ann Surg 176:565, 1972

CADY B: Surgery of thyroid cancer. World J Surg 5:3, 1981

CADY B, SEDGWICK CE, MEISSNER NS et al: Risk factor analysis in differentiated thyroid cancer. Cancer 43:810, 1979

CLARK OH, CASTNER BJ: Thyrotropin "receptors" in normal and neoplastic human thyroid tissue. Surgery 85:624, 1979

CLARK OH, OKERLUND MD, CAVALIERI RS et al: Diagnosis and treatment of thyroid, parathyroid and thyroglossal duct cyst. J Clin Endocrinol Metab 48:983, 1979

DEVINE RM, EDIS AJ, BANKS PM: Primary lymphoma of the thyroid: A review of the Mayo Clinic experience through 1978. World J Surg 5:33, 1981

FAVUS MJ, SCHNEIDER AB, STACHURA ME et al: Thyroid cancer occurring as a late consequence of head and neck irradiation: Evaluation of 1056 patients. New Engl J Med 294:1019, 1976

FUKUNAGA FH, YATANI R: Geographic pathology of occult thyroid carcinomas. Cancer 36:1095, 1975

GOTTLIEB J, HILL C: Chemotherapy of thyroid cancer with Adriamycin. New Engl J Med 290:193, 1974

LYNN J, GAMBROS OI, TAYLOR S: Medullary carcinoma of the thyroid. World J Surg 5:27, 1981

MAZZAFERRI EL: Papillary and follicular thyroid cancer: Selective therapy. Compr Ther 7:6, 1981

MAZZAFERRI EL, YOUNG RL, OERTEL JE et al: Papillary thyroid carcinoma: The impact of therapy in 576 patients. Medicine 56:171, 1977

SILVERBERG SG, HUTTER RVT, FOOTE FW JR: Fatal carcinoma of the thyroid: Histology, metastases and causes of death. Cancer 25:792, 1970

SIROTA DK, SEGAL RL: Primary lymphomas of the thyroid gland. JAMA 242:1743, 1979

THOMAS CG JR, BUCKWALTER JA: Poorly differentiated neoplasms of the thyroid. Ann Surg 177:732, 1973

THOMPSON NW, DUNN EL, BATSAKIS JG et al: Hurthle cell lesions of the thyroid gland. Surg Gynecol Obstet 139:555, 1974

THOMPSON NW, NISHIYAMA RH, HARNESS JK: Thyroid carcinoma: Current controversies. Curr Probl Surg 15:1, 1978

TUBIANA M: External radiotherapy and radioiodine in the treatment of thyroid cancer. World J Surg 5:75, 1981

WELLS SA, DALE JK, BAYLIS SB et al: The importance of early diagnosis in patients with hereditary medullary thyroid carcinoma. Ann Surg (in press)

WOOLNER LB, BEAHRS OH, BLACK BM et al: Thyroid carcinoma: General considerations and follow-up data on 1181 cases. In Proceedings of the Second Imperial Cancer Research Fund Symposium: Thyroid Neoplasia. London, Academic Press, 1968

Norman C. Nelson

The Parathyroids

HISTORY

While still a medical student in 1877, Ivar Sandstrom discovered the parathyroid glands in a dog dissection and within the next 2 years had confirmed the presence of these glands in cats, oxen, horses, rabbits, and humans. His classic and beautifully illustrated publication of 1880, in which he reported his work, was entitled *On a New Gland in Man and Several Mammals* and was the first well-documented observation of the parathyroid glands. Earlier publications by Remark (1858) and Virchow (1860) had separately commented on the discovery of parathyroid glands. Sandstrom's publication was in Swedish and was not well known for some years. Accordingly, other reports of parathyroid gland discovery were subsequently published by Baber (1881), Gley (1891), and Kohn (1895).

In 1908, MacCallum and Voegtlin ascribed the tetany following parathyroidectomy to the rapid fall in the plasma calcium level that resulted. In 1915, a Viennese pathologist, Schlagenhaufer, recounted several autopsy reports revealing parathyroid tumors in patients with von Recklinghausen's disease and recommended that parathyroidectomy be used as treatment for this condition. In 1925, Mandl, an assistant in the Department of Surgery in Vienna, finally removed a parathyroid tumor from a patient with von Recklinghausen's disease. In 1926, Dubois, in New York, unaware of the Vienna experience, recommended that one of his patients undergo parathyroid exploration. His patient had "brittle bones," together with hypercalcemia, hypercalciuria, and a negative calcium balance. Dubois postulated that such a condition might by brought about by excessive parathyroid hormone (PTH) and thus believed that a parathyroid abnormality might be present.

Following the first operations for parathyroid disease in Austria and in the United States, experience with primary hyperparathyroidism developed at a fairly rapid pace with the work of Albright (1934), Rogers and Keating (1947), Cope (1957), and others.

Until the 1960s, the detection of patients with primary hyperparathyroidism was related in large part to a search for this possibility in patients who had bone disease, renal lithiasis, peptic ulcer, pancreatitis, or a few other conditions that were known to be associated. In the mid 1960s, however, automated multiple biochemical blood analyses became a commonplace diagnostic screening procedure, and many patients without characteristically associated diseases were found to have hypercalcemia due to primary hyperparathyroidism. Since that time, the vast majority of patients with primary hyperparathyroidism have the condition detected when high serum calcium values are found in routine biochemical screening analyses. A large proportion of these patients are relatively asymptomatic, and many do not have complaints or associated medical problems that might specifically point to the diagnosis of primary hyperparathyroidism.

EMBRYOLOGY

The parathyroid glands arise from the third and fourth branchial pouches and are first recognizable in the 8-mm to 9-mm human embryo. The parathyroid glands that arise from the third pouch appear with the thymus as bilobed bodies that move caudally as the heart descends into the thorax. The parathyroid component usually separates from the thymus at about the level of the lower poles of the thyroid gland, and thus it is the lower parathyroid glands that arise from the third branchial pouch.

Although the characteristic location of the lower parathyroid glands is at or near the lower poles of the thyroid, it is not uncommon for these glands to remain anatomically associated with the thymus and, in many instances, to actually lie within the thymic capsule. As a consequence, the lower parathyroid glands may be located low in the neck or in the anterior mediastinum as far caudad as the pericardium. Occasionally, a lower parathyroid gland will even be in the posterior mediastinum. Rarely, it may be located above the upper pole or lateral to the midportion of the thyroid gland as a result of the arrested normal embryologic descent of third branchial pouch elements.

The parathyroid glands that arise from the fourth branchial pouch do so as bilobed structures with the ultimobranchial bodies. The ultimobranchial bodies, or so-called lateral anlage of the thyroid, join the lateral lobes of the thyroid and become separate from the associated parathyroid glands. The fourth branchial pouch–derived parathyroid glands are usually more medial than the glands that arise from the third pouch and are located posterior to the upper thyroid poles at about the level of the cricoid cartilage. It is, therefore, the upper parathyroid glands that come from the fourth branchial pouch.

The upper parathyroid glands tend to occur in their characteristic location more consistently than the lower glands. Variations do occur, with upper glands being positioned higher, lower, or more laterally than might be expected. Because of the close association during embryogenesis of the upper glands with the ultimobranchial bodies, the rarely encountered intrathyroidal parathyroid is most often an upper gland.

ANATOMY

There are usually two upper and two lower parathyroid glands. It is uncommon for supernumerary glands to be present, but this has been the case in 2% to 5% of anatomic dissections. As a rule, when supernumerary glands are identified, they are smaller than normal. The total number of parathyroid glands is seldom more than five, although as many as eight have been detected.

The average weight of each normal gland is between 30 mg and 40 mg, with a range of 10 mg to 70 mg. It is usually observed that the lower glands are a bit larger than the upper ones. The glands are covered by a thin, colorless capsule and are yellowish to orange tan. Color, in large part, is dependent upon the amount of fat they contain. There is great variation in gland shapes because they are not supported internally by a rigid stroma and are soft and compressible, thus often assuming a configuration dictated by molding from firmer surrounding structures; they have been described as oval, spherical, teardrop shaped, pancake shaped, and bean shaped. Glands from adults measure 3 mm to 6 mm in length, 2 mm to 4 mm in width, and 0.5 mm to 2 mm in thickness. Each gland has a clearly defined vascular pedicle, and it is generally stated that the inferior thyroid artery usually provides the blood supply to all four. In fact, the parent feeding vessel is often from a branch of the superior thyroid artery, and ectopically located glands may receive their blood supply from a variety of adjacent arteries.

The usual location of the parathyroid glands is illustrated in Figure 20-21. As commented upon in the description of parathyroid embryology, ectopic locations are not rare but the lower glands have greater variability (Fig. 20-22). Since there is no firm pedicle that fixes parathyroid glands to a particular spot, it also is noteworthy that as an abnormal gland enlarges, it may migrate or extend from its normal location by virtue of its increased weight and the force of gravity. The negative pressure in the thorax may also cause caudal movement of an enlarged gland, bringing it more toward or into the mediastinum.

PHYSIOLOGY AND PATHOPHYSIOLOGY

PARATHYROID HORMONE

PTH is a polypeptide made up of 84 amino acids with a molecular weight of 9500. Intracellular precursors to this hormone of larger molecular weight have been identified, but it is currently thought that under normal circumstances only PTH itself is released into the circulation. Recently, however, by radioimmunoassay analysis of the effluent venous blood from parathyroid adenomas, an apparent fragment of PTH with a molecular weight of approximately 6000 has been identified as making up a significant proportion of secreted hormone. The amount of this fragment that is secreted is determined by antiserums that measure the carboxy-terminal portion of the polypeptide sequence.

After secretion of PTH, it is apparent that significant proteolysis occurs, and smaller immunoreactive fragments of the hormone are readily measured in serum. Generally, a carboxy-terminal fragment with a molecular weight of about 6000 and an amino-terminal fragment with a molecular size of 4500 may be found. The carboxy-terminal species is most often significantly elevated in patients with primary hyperparathyroidism, and immunoassays that detect this fragment are diagnostically most helpful in patient assessments. Although postsecretory proteolysis of PTH is considered to be the principal source of both carboxy-terminal and amino-terminal fragments, it also now appears, as previously noted, that fragments of smaller molecular weight are at least in some circumstances directly secreted by parathyroid cells.

CONTROL OF SECRETION

The control of PTH secretion relates, for the most part, to the level of plasma calcium. It is generally agreed that the ionized portion is responsible for the effect on the parathy-

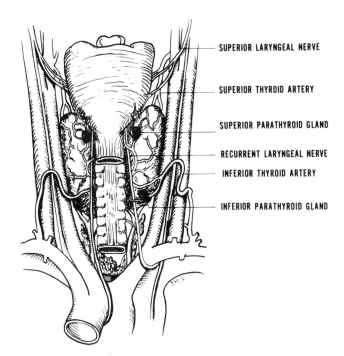

SUPERIOR LARYNGEAL NERVE

SUPERIOR THYROID ARTERY

SUPERIOR PARATHYROID GLAND

RECURRENT LARYNGEAL NERVE

INFERIOR THYROID ARTERY

INFERIOR PARATHYROID GLAND

Fig. 20-21. Posterior view of the thyroid gland and pharynx shows parathyroid glands and related structures in their normal positions.

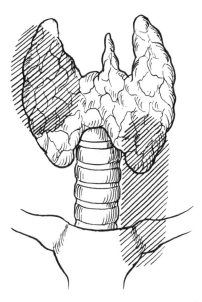

Fig. 20-22. View of the thyroid. Shaded areas indicate usual boundaries wherein upper (*left*) and lower (*right*) parathyroid glands may be located. The parathyroids are posterior or lateral to the lobes of the thyroid gland.

roids, although most clinical assessments and experiments report values in terms of total plasma or serum calcium concentration. A negative feedback mechanism operates wherein higher calcium levels suppress and lower calcium levels stimulate secretion. This system normally functions to maintain total serum calcium values in a relatively narrow range, between 9.0 and 10.5 mg/dl. One other divalent cation, magnesium, appears to affect PTH secretion in a fashion similar to that of calcium but to a much less

significant degree. It should also be noted that chronic magnesium deficiency impairs PTH secretion.

It has been known for some time that an occasional patient with a pheochromocytoma would have hypercalcemia that would be corrected when the pheochromocytoma was removed. This is apparently due to an epinephrine β-adrenergic receptor–activated stimulation of the parathyroid cells to secrete PTH. β-Adrenergic receptor blocking agents such as propranolol abolish this effect. More recently, it has been observed that the histamine receptor blocking agent cimetidine will occasionally lower PTH secretion in patients with both primary and secondary hyperparathyroidism. Although this effect has not been consistently documented and does not seem to be quantitatively of great significance, it does point to a role for histamine as a possible mediator for PTH secretion.

From what has been cited, it can be seen that the control of PTH secretion is more complex than merely a negative feedback system between the parathyroid glands and the plasma calcium concentration. However, despite the involvement of other substances affecting PTH secretion, it is important to appreciate that the regulatory role of plasma calcium remains predominant.

ACTION

Parathyroid hormone has a number of different actions at different sites in the body, all of which to a greater or lesser extent preserve plasma calcium values within normal limits. The three anatomical locations where PTH exerts its principal direct and indirect effects are the skeleton, the kidneys, and the gastrointestinal tract. In the skeleton, PTH enhances bone resorption when plasma calcium values fall by stimulating both osteocytic and osteoclastic osteolysis. In addition, PTH inhibits the flow of osteoclasts to osteoblasts and activates osteoprogenitor cells to preosteoclasts, thus increasing the population of bone-resorbing osteoclasts. Its most profound effect is to increase rapidly (within minutes) the movement of calcium ions into the extracellular fluid from the osteocyte–osteoblast cell complex of compact bone.

In the kidney, PTH increases the tubular reabsorption of calcium and also enhances reabsorption of magnesium and ammonium. Parathyroid hormone additionally diminishes tubular reabsorption of phosphate and causes an increased urinary phosphate loss. The urinary excretion of potassium, sodium, bicarbonate, and amino acids also is increased by the effect of PTH. One additional action of PTH in the kidney that affects calcium metabolism is that of catalyzing the formation of the vitamin D metabolite 1,25-dihydroxycholecalciferol (1,25[OH]$_2$D$_3$, or calcitriol) from 25-hydroxycholecalciferol (25[OH]D$_3$). This former substance, calcitriol, is very potent in increasing calcium absorption from the gastrointestinal tract. It is now accepted that the principal effect of PTH on the gastrointestinal tract to increase calcium absorption is not a direct one but rather one of enhancing the formation of calcitriol in the kidney.

By virtue of its different actions on calcium metabolism in the skeleton, kidneys, and gastrointestinal tract, a chronic exposure of the body to abnormally high PTH values will ordinarily lead to hypercalcemia. This occurs despite possible compensatory changes in the endocrine system or in calcium excretion. Loss of parathyroid function, as in removal of the parathyroid glands, will cause hypocalcemia that usually requires active treatment. Both hyperparathyroidism and hypoparathyroidism are discussed later in greater detail.

CALCITONIN

Calcitonin is a straight-chain polypeptide having 32 amino acids and secreted by the parafollicular or C cells of the thyroid. These parafollicular cells are embryologically derived from the ultimobranchial bodies and are mainly clustered at about the juncture of the upper and middle third of the central portion of the lateral thyroid lobes.

CONTROL OF SECRETION

Both calcium and various gastrointestinal hormones affect the secretion of calcitonin. Supraphysiologic plasma calcium levels will stimulate calcitonin secretion, as will the hormones gastrin, pancreozymin, and glucagon.

ACTION

Calcitonin acts to decrease plasma calcium values, and in this respect its effects are principally upon bone. In somewhat the opposite fashion of PTH, calcitonin diminishes bone-resorptive osteoclast function and inhibits the flux of calcium into the blood and extracellular fluid from the osteocyte–osteoblast cell complex of compact bone. This latter effect occurs rapidly and accounts for the major hypocalcemic action of calcitonin.

Calcitonin also causes hypophosphatemia when given in large doses. It was formerly thought that this was mostly the result of a phosphaturic effect, but it is now believed that the main reason is the movement of phosphate out of the extracellular space and into the intracellular fluid compartment. The principal tissue involved in this intracellular phosphate movement has not been identified beyond doubt, although it is likely bone.

In contradistinction to the situation in which a chronic excess of PTH ordinarily leads to hypercalcemia, continuing high plasma values of calcitonin do not cause hypocalcemia. Patients who have tumors, such as medullary carcinoma of the thyroid, that may secrete large amounts of calcitonin will have normal plasma calcium values unless some additional problem coexists.. It should also be noted that removal of all thyroid tissue, and thus the source of calcitonin, will not change plasma calcium levels.

D VITAMINS

In humans, vitamin D is produced normally in the skin by ultraviolet light from the sun irradiating its precursor 7-dehydrocholesterol. The substance formed is cholecalciferol, or vitamin $D_3(D_3)$. In warm climates, it is possible for all human vitamin D requirements to be met by more or less year-round sun exposure. However, in temperate and colder climates, it is generally necessary for oral vitamin D supplements to be provided, especially in the winter months. This is usually accomplished by providing added dietary vitamin D.

After vitamin D is either formed in the skin or provided in food, it rapidly accumulates in the liver, where it undergoes 25-hydroxylation and is converted to 25-hydroxycholecalciferol. This substance, in what might be regarded as physiologic levels, has no appreciable function and must be further metabolized to be active. This takes place in the kidney, where, under the influence of $25(OH)D_3$-1-α-hydroxylase, the physiologically active metabolite 1,25-dihydroxycholecalciferol, or calcitriol, is formed.

As mentioned previously, PTH stimulates the biosynthesis of calcitriol, and it is this latter substance, itself now properly designated as a hormone, that most directly affects calcium metabolism. In the gastrointestinal tract, calcitriol causes an increase in calcium absorption regardless of whether or not PTH is present. This effect is not blocked by actinomycin D. Calcitriol is also a potent mobilizer of calcium from bone. However, in this circumstance, PTH must be present and actinomycin D will abolish its action. The mechanism by which calcitriol mobilizes calcium from bone is somewhat obscure but probably involves increased production of calcium-mobilizing proteins.

Calcitriol additionally affects phosphate metabolism by stimulating intestinal absorption and possibly causing renal conservation of this anion. The net effect of vitamin D acting in concert with PTH is to maintain normal, physiologically functional calcium–phosphate metabolism.

Deprivation of vitamin D, together with insufficient calcium intake, may lead to hypocalcemic tetany, and if there is chronic vitamin D deficiency and phosphate depletion, osteomalacia will result. Vitamin D in great excess for long periods of time may lead to hypercalcemia and demineralization of the skeleton, with the possibility that ectopic soft-tissue calcifications may develop.

OVERVIEW OF INTERACTIONS OF PARATHYROID HORMONE, CALCITONIN, AND VITAMIN D

Parathyroid hormone is clearly the most potent single substance that affects calcium metabolism, with its direct effects on bone predominating. By PTH causing bone resorption, it modulates the flux of calcium out of osseous tissue in response to a hypocalcemic stimulus. As plasma calcium values become normal, the fall of PTH in the blood tends to stop bone resorption. In the kidney, PTH action conserves calcium by increasing tubular reabsorption, but this is not as significant in maintaining normal plasma calcium values as is its effect on bone or its other indirect effect of supporting intestinal absorption of calcium by stimulating the formation of calcitriol in the kidney. The vitamin D metabolite calcitriol is a potent substance that enhances calcium absorption from the gut, as well as mobilizes bone calcium; thus, PTH and calcitriol are the most important hormones involved in calcium homeostasis.

The role of calcitonin in critically influencing human calcium metabolism is not well established. Although calcitonin clearly acts to decrease bone resorption and causes hypophosphatemia, neither a long-standing excess nor a long-standing absence of this hormone causes any profound change in calcium or phosphate metabolism in persons who are otherwise normal.

PRIMARY HYPERPARATHYROIDISM

Primary hyperparathyroidism is a disease of unknown etiology that results from the chronic exposure of the body to excessive amounts of PTH derived from autonomous overfunction of one or more abnormal parathyroid glands. It is important to differentiate primary hyperparathyroidism from secondary hyperparathyroidism. In the latter condition, overactivity of the parathyroid glands is the consequence of a specifically detectable stimulus, such as the calcium and phosphate metabolic aberrations that result from chronic renal failure. Secondary hyperparathyroidism is discussed in greater detail in a subsequent section.

Because of the overproduction of PTH, patients with

PRIMARY HYPERPARATHYROIDISM

This disease has nonspecific symptoms and signs; is often characterized by weakness, fatigue, and lassitude; and is frequently associated with kidney stones, peptic ulcer disease, and varying degrees of bone involvement.

Etiology

Most often due to a single parathyroid adenoma (80%–85%) with almost all remaining cases caused by primary chief-cell hyperplasia of all four glands. Multiple adenomas and functioning carcinoma are very rare (2%–3%).

Dx

Demonstrated hypercalcemia due to no other cause and substantiated by inappropriately elevated levels of serum immunoreactive PTH.

Rx

Parathyroid exploration with identification of all four parathyroid glands to establish pathologic change. If a parathyroid adenoma is found, removal is curative. Chief-cell hyperplasia will require subtotal parathyroidectomy; usually 3½ glands need to be removed.

primary hyperparathyroidism characteristically have hypercalcemia and hypophosphatemia. Almost all have excess phosphate in the urine, and many also are found to have hypercalciuria. Other less consistent or diagnostically helpful blood and urine changes are discussed in the section on diagnostic methods.

INCIDENCE

It has been estimated that primary hyperparathyroidism is present in approximately 1 of every 1000 ambulatory adults in the United States. The disease is uncommon in children and young adults but becomes increasingly prevalent from the third decade of life onward. The incidence of the disease is two to three times higher in women than in men. Recent studies tend to indicate that the increased prevalence in women is especially remarkable in older people, with one report showing primary hyperparathyroidism to be seven times more common in women than men in the age-group over 70 years.

PATHOLOGY

Primary hyperparathyroidism is due most commonly to a single adenoma in one of the four parathyroid glands. In most series, such cases make up 80% to 85% of all patients. The next most common cause is primary chief-cell hyperplasia in all four glands. Except for the occasional patient with water-clear-cell hyperplasia or carcinoma, it constitutes the pathologic change in the remaining cases. A much higher percentage of hyperplasia has been cited by some authors, but their criteria used to assign this diagnosis have been questioned.

Parathyroid adenomas vary greatly in size; some tumors are no larger than 0.5 cm in diameter, and others are ten times that size or larger. Similarly, the tumors vary in weight from as little as 50 mg to over 50 g; the average, however, is somewhat less than 1 g. Adenomas are encapsulated, yellowish tan to orange brown, and somewhat soft and pliable. They are usually ovoid, but many variations in configuration are encountered. These tumors are usually made up of sheets of chief cells with a varying admixture of clusters of oxyphils and water-clear cells. Occasionally, an adenoma will be composed predominantly of oxyphils or water-clear cells; more rarely, it will be composed of fat cells, with relatively few chief cells or other cell types. This latter situation has led to the term *lipoadenoma*. Most adenomas, however, contain very few if any fat cells.

A parathyroid adenoma is almost impossible to differentiate from an enlarged hyperplastic parathyroid gland made up principally of chief cells. Obviously, if all four glands are enlarged and hypercellular, a diagnosis of hyperplasia is appropriate even though the individual enlarged glands may all have a histologic pattern that is indistinguishable from an adenoma. Some hyperplastic glands present a nodular appearance, with irregular clusters of chief or oxyphil cells packed together, or separated, by varying amounts of fat. This histologic pattern has been designated nodular hyperplasia. In any given case of hyperplasia, it is noteworthy that the involved parathyroid glands may differ in size. One or two of the affected glands may even be near normal while the others are unequally enlarged.

It has long been held than an adenoma may be classified as such if there is an identifiable rim of apparently normal parathyroid gland just outside the tumor capsule. Although this is helpful in differentiating adenoma from hyperplasia, such a finding is not always present with adenomas. It fact, some hyperplastic glands appear to present this same picture. It is unfortunate that both ultrastructural and histochemical characteristics are similar in adenomas and hyperplastic glands and therefore cannot be used to tell one from the other. In general, patients who have more than one parathyroid gland involved in what could be either adenomatous or hyperplastic change should probably be classified as having hyperplasia. It is possible for someone to have two adenomas, of course, but this is rare.

Recently, a histochemical technique has been used to distinguish between normal and abnormal parathyroid glands. Fat stains applied to normal parathyroid tissue in patients with adenomas generally reveal abundant large fat granules in the cytoplasm of the suppressed chief cells. Such stains show only sparse and spotty distribution of fat in the chief cells of either adenomas or hyperplastic glands. This technique can be applied to either permanent or frozen-section tissue specimens.

Water-clear-cell (wasserhelle-cell) hyperplasia is seldom encountered; in fact, relatively large series of patients with primary hyperparathyroidism rarely contain a single case. Characteristically, all four glands are enlarged and brown to chocolate in color. Although they are encapsulated, there is a tendency for greater lobulation than seen with adenomas or chief-cell hyperplasia. Histologically, only large water-clear cells are present within the thin capsule. This condition was described well before chief-cell hyperplasia, and several cases were found from 1934 to 1960, but it is now extremely uncommon to find patients with this problem. The reason for this is obscure.

Parathyroid carcinoma is rare and presents in no more than 2% or 3% of patients with primary hyperparathyroidism. Grossly, a carcinoma tends to be a ligher gray tan than an adenoma and is firm to hard. It also is common for a parathyroid carcinoma to adhere to or infiltrate adjacent tissues and have a poorly defined capsule. Histologically, blood vessel invasion and bizarre nuclear forms and mitoses are seen, and the tumor's locally invasive behavior often can be appreciated. Not every parathyroid carcinoma has all of these characteristics, but it is usually not too difficult to make an accurate diagnosis.

SYMPTOMS AND SIGNS

The symptoms of primary hyperparathyroidism are, for the most part, nonspecific and characteristically involve multiple organ systems, including the genitourinary tract and the skeletal, gastrointestinal, and neuromuscular systems. It is noteworthy, however, that many patients with primary hyperparathyroidism will have minimal complaints or be essentially asymptomatic.

Patients with this disease often complain of weakness, lassitude, easy fatigability, loss of memory, bone and arthritislike pains, and constipation. If hypercalcemia is moderately severe, nausea and vomiting can occur; at very high plasma calcium values, in the range above 15 mg/dl, confusion, somnolence, and coma may occur. Many patients have polyuria and compensatory polydipsia. The polyuria is the result of an increased loss of phosphate and, often, calcium in the urine and also because hypercalcemia, *per se,* interferes with the ability of the kidneys to concentrate urine. It also is not uncommon for patients to complain of vague abdominal aches and pains with no detectable specific gastrointestinal disease or dysfunction.

ASSOCIATED SIGNS AND ILLNESSES

Primary hyperparathyroidism causes and is associated with a group of diseases and conditions that bear special comment.

SKELETAL SYSTEM

Historically, hyperparathyroidism was first recognized because of the effect of excessive PTH on bone, causing osteitis fibrosa cystica generalisata, or von Recklinghausen's disease of bone. This condition is histologically characterized by a decrease in the number of bone trabeculae and an increase in multinucleated osteoclasts seen in scalloped areas on their surfaces. There is also a marked replacement of normal cellular and marrow elements by fibrovascular tissue. Brown cell tumors or osteoclastomas, which are microscopically giant cell tumors, may occur, and these appear roentgenographically as radiolucent, sharply defined, bony lesions that cannot be differentiated from the bone cysts that are also occasionally present in von Recklinghausen's disease. There is additionally a diffuse osteopenia, which resembles osteoporosis. Because of this, as well as the brown cell tumors and bone cysts, pathologic fractures may occur. Subperiosteal bone resorption also occurs and is actually the most specifically characteristic skeletal change that can be detected on x-ray film. It is most often seen along the radial side of the middle phalanges in posteroanterior views of the hand. Additionally, subperiosteal bone resorption may be seen in the skull, at the distal ends of the clavicles, and at the insertions of the hamstring muscles on the inferior rami of the pubes.

The incidence of generalized osteitis fibrosa cystica associated with primary hyperparathyroidism has decreased dramatically since the disease was first recognized. From 1930 through 1950, slightly over 50% of patients with primary hyperparathyroidism were so affected, but during the next 2 decades, the incidence decreased to approximately 20%. More current reported series indicate that only about 10% of patients with primary hyperparathyroidism can be classified as having von Recklinghausen's disease of bone.

The reason for this change in incidence is not completely clear. At first, a general dietary increase in calcium in the population was postulated, but this has been questioned. The possibility that earlier diagnoses are being made before the ravages of severe bone disease can develop also has been considered. Additionally, it is possible that pathologic changes associated with primary hyperparathyroidism are somehow expressed differently depending upon an individual patient's susceptibility. This susceptibility may be affected by genetic or environmental factors or by matters relating to nutrition or coexisting illness. If this selective susceptibility premise is correct, it might be further postulated that in a large population of patients with primary hyperparathyroidism, relatively few would ever develop generalized osteitis fibrosa cystica. The apparent high incidence of generalized osteitis in the earlier years of our awareness of primary hyperparathyroidism may have come about because we were looking at a relatively small segment of all patients with this disease. More recently, an increased knowledge of other conditions caused by or associated with primary hyperparathyroidism and vastly improved diagnostic methods have allowed us to make evaluations on what might now be more properly defined as the total population of patients with this condition.

KIDNEY

Patients with primary hyperparathyroidism have a greatly increased incidence of kidney stones. Nephrocalcinosis, although much less common, also is found with increased frequency in primary hyperparathyroidism, but it is uncommon to find both renal lithiasis and nephrocalcinosis in the same patient. Until routine screening automated blood biochemical analyses became prevalent in the 1960s, approximately 70% of all cases of primary hyperparathyroidism were detected because this possibility was considered in patients with kidney stones. Although only 1% to 3% of patients with calcium-containing kidney stones have primary hyperparathyroidism as the etiology for their renal lithiasis, it has nevertheless been quite productive to consider the possibility so that a potentially correctable cause for the condition could be found. Despite the fact that current diagnostic procedures and methods yield many essentially asymptomatic patients with primary hyperparathyroidism, the incidence of radiographically detectable nephrolithiasis in this group is still approximately 30%.

As might be expected, a considerable proportion of the morbidity and even mortality from primary hyperparathyroidism relates to nephrolithiasis and nephrocalcinosis. Renal colic from stone passage, obstructive uropathy, and destroyed renal function can all result. Correction of primary hyperparathyroidism in the patient with renal lithiasis usually prevents formation of additional stones unless there is a coexisting and continuing infection in the kidney. In some patients who still harbor renal stones when their parathyroid disease is effectively treated, these stones will grow smaller, fragment, and pass spontaneously. In addition, many of the effects of hyperparathyroidism on kidney function, such as impaired renal concentrating ability and tubular acidification mechanisms, are reversible. However, once renal function has been seriously damaged by the effects of primary hyperparathyroidism, it is unusual for there to be any significant improvement, even if the parathyroid disease is corrected. At best, no additional renal functional loss will occur. However, in some cases, particularly with continuing genitourinary tract infection, further renal compromise may ensue.

GASTROINTESTINAL TRACT

It is not unusual for patients with primary hyperparathyroidism to complain of vague abdominal pain for which no particular cause can be found. There is an increased incidence of coexisting peptic ulcer disease, however, and probably of pancreatitis as well. Peptic ulcer disease occurs in about 15% of patients with primary hyperparathyroidism, in contrast to an occurrence in the general population of approximately 5%. The most attractive theory as to this causal relationship is that hypercalcemia stimulates the release of gastrin, which subsequently leads to increased gastric acid production. Thus, increased gastric acid secretion is not a direct effect of PTH; rather, it is the hypercalcemia resulting from PTH excess that causes hypergastrinemia and excessive acid production.

The relationship of pancreatitis to primary hyperparathyroidism is not quite as well established as that of peptic ulcer disease. Most reports indicate that patients with primary hyperparathyroidism display an increased incidence of pancreatitis that is greater than might be expected from chance alone. The basis for this relationship is not clear, and several different types of pancreatitis have been noted. Although acute edematous and acute hemorrhagic pancreatitis have been observed, the most commonly noted association is with chronic pancreatitis. In any event, it is well to remember that pancreatitis may be a clue to an otherwise unsuspected case of primary hyperparathyroidism. It should also be borne in mind that serum calcium values may be depressed in either acute or chronic pancreatitis and that this possibility must be considered when evaluating laboratory studies.

NEUROMUSCULAR AND NEUROPSYCHIATRIC MANIFESTATIONS

Many patients with primary hyperparathyroidism experience muscular weakness. In some, it is a relatively minor manifestation of the disease, but in others, the degree of associated disability is profound. Symptomatically, the proximal muscles of the extremities are usually most affected, and patients report difficulty with stair climbing or even standing erect from a seated position. Any activity that requires holding the arms upward, such as hanging up wash on a clothesline, also may be difficult. Recent studies have demonstrated a specific lesion in the type II cells of the noncardiac striated muscles of patients with primary hyperparathyroidism. This change, which is reversible following correction of the hyperparathyroid state, is thought to be related to the symptom of weakness.

It is not unusual for patients with primary hyperparathyroidism to complain not only of fatigue, lassitude, and weakness but also of forgetfulness, mild depression, and psychomotor retardation. Occasionally, the patient will display an overt psychosis, which may improve after successful parathyroidectomy. Some patients, especially those with more severe hypercalcemia (in the range of 15 mg/dl and higher), may appear confused or disoriented and display symptoms suggestive of an organic brain syndrome. Older people seem to be particularly prone to this latter problem,

which most often is corrected when the primary hyperparathyroidism is cured.

MULTIPLE ENDOCRINE ADENOPATHY SYNDROMES

Primary hyperparathyroidism is associated with two well-recognized multiple endocrine adenopathy (MEA) syndromes, each of which is characterized by an autosomal dominant pattern of inheritance. The MEA type I syndrome consists primarily of tumors of the pituitary, parathyroids, and pancreas, and the MEA type II syndrome is characterized by medullary carcinoma of the thyroid, pheochromocytoma, and tumors of the parathyroids. It is important to realize that in neither syndrome do all of the endocrinopathies necessarily occur synchronously but that each endocrine abnormality may become manifest many years apart from another.

THYROID CANCER

An increased incidence of nonmedullary thyroid cancer has been reported in patients with primary hyperparathyroidism when compared with the general population. As many as 2.5% of patients with primary hyperparathyroidism in one large, recently reported series also had nonmedullary thyroid cancer. Histopathologically, the thyroid neoplasia is most commonly papillary adenocarcinoma, although a few cases of pure follicular adenocarcinoma have been reported.

There has been speculation that the increased incidence of thyroid cancer in patients with primary hyperparathyroidism results from a common etiologic stimulus. In this regard, it has been proposed that low-dose irradiation to the head and neck area during infancy and childhood, a well-documented etiologic factor in thyroid cancer, may also influence the development of parathyroid tumors.

HYPERTENSION

High blood pressure is common in patients with primary hyperparathyroidism. Since essential hypertension itself is also very common, it is obvious that high blood pressure as such is not a particularly significant indicator of possible hyperparathyroidism. It is apparent, however, that hypercalcemia may aggravate or actually lead to increased blood pressure. This is probably brought about by high plasma calcium values increasing the sensitivity of vascular smooth muscle to endogenous catecholamines. It is possible, of course, for renal damage resulting from primary hyperparathyroidism to cause hypertension, but this seems uncommon. Recent studies have documented a significant fall in blood pressure in hypertensive patients with primary hyperparathyroidism following correction of their parathyroid disease.

MISCELLANEOUS ASSOCIATIONS

Hyperuricemia and gout have been noted with increased frequency in patients with primary hyperparathyroidism. The reason for this relationship is unknown. There have been periodic literature citations that gallstones occur more commonly in association with primary hyperparathyroidism, but there is no reliable substantiation of this possible relationship. Idiopathic hypertrophic subaortic stenosis apparently becomes symptomatic earlier in patients with primary hyperparathyroidism, and the diagnosis of the heart problem should be a clue to look for coexisting parathyroid disease.

One ocular manifestation of hypercalcemia at least bears mention. Hypercalcemia from any cause may lead to the deposition of calcium about the limbus of the cornea, which can be visible on inspection. This band keratopathy, as it is known, resembles arcus senilis or Kayser–Fleischer rings and can be determined accurately to be deposited calcium only by slit lamp microscopy. Band keratopathy has no diagnostic specificity for primary hyperparathyroidism but is only an indicator of hypercalcemia, present or past, from any cause.

DIAGNOSTIC METHODS

Hypercalcemia is the hallmark of primary hyperparathyroidism. In fact, without substantiation that hypercalcemia is or has been present, the diagnosis is open to question. However, the plasma calcium values vary considerably from time to time and in a significant number of these patients periods of normocalcemia occur. Unfortunately, most diagnostic studies to detect possible primary hyperparathyroidism in normocalcemic patients lack specificity and cannot be relied upon. The measurement of plasma immunoreactive PTH of course is a potential specific measure of parathyroid function, but even here there are pitfalls, which will be discussed. In general terms, one might recall the gastroenterologists' dictum of "no acid, no ulcer" and substitute "no hypercalcemia, no primary hyperparathyroidism."

The normal range for total serum calcium in most laboratories is from 8.8 mg to 10.5 mg/dl. The values for men are about 0.1 mg to 0.2 mg/dl higher than those for women in the same age-group, with the elderly having normal values as much as 0.3 mg/dl lower than young adults. Although the ionized fraction of total serum calcium more accurately reflects parathyroid function, most laboratories report results as total serum calcium. Therefore, whenever plasma calcium values are evaluated, it also is mandatory to measure the serum protein and, additionally, to quantify the albumin and globulin values. Approximately 46% of blood calcium is bound to protein and almost all of this to the albumin fraction. Thus, a significant dysproteinemia characterized by either hypoalbuminemia or hyperalbuminemia may incorrectly point to no parathyroid disease or to primary hyperparathyroidism. A rough guide to correct for serum protein abnormalities is to adjust total serum calcium upward or downward by 0.8 mg/dl for each gram per deciliter of serum protein below or above normal, respectively. It also is important to be aware that venous stasis caused by prolonged tourniquet time prior to drawing a blood sample may spuriously increase total serum calcium by causing hemoconcentration and an increase in the fraction of calcium bound to protein.

Most patients with primary hyperparathyroidism have hypophosphatemia and hyperchloremia. These findings are not invariable, however. Because of the often-noted hypophosphatemia together with hyperchloremia, a diagnostic discriminant value of the ratio of chloride to phosphate has been proposed. The vast majority of patients with a chloride/phosphate ratio above 33 have been noted to have hyperparathyroidism, while those with ratios in the range of 17 to 32 usually do not. It is necessary to inject the cautionary note that an evaluation of the chloride/phosphate ratio in itself will not allow one to either make or disprove the diagnosis of primary hyperparathyroidism.

Patients who have significant bone disease associated with hyperparathyroidism characteristically will have an elevated serum alkaline phosphatase level. In fact, such a finding even without roentgenographic evidence of generalized osteitis should be a clue to the surgeon that these patients may have a more dramatic fall in plasma calcium value than is usual after operative correction of primary hyperparathyroidism, as the "hungry" bones reclaim their depleted calcium stores. In some of these patients, calcium values may fall below normal and lead to symptoms of tetany.

Following the first description of radioimmunoassay of PTH in 1963, numerous modifications and refinements of this procedure led to its current use as a very helpful clinical diagnostic test in evaluating parathyroid function. Native PTH and its amino- and carboxy-terminal fragments may be measured by somewhat different specific immunoassays. In general terms, a radioimmunoassay that is specific for the carboxy-terminal region of the parathyroid molecule has proved to be most effective as a diagnostic tool. In many laboratories, however, approximately 10% of patients with primary hyperparathyroidism will have immunoreactive PTH values below what might be expected. In other patients, because of ectopic or pseudohyperparathyroidism (to be discussed subsequently), the values for immunoreactive PTH may be somewhat elevated. In any event, when considering radioimmunoassay test results, it is well to bear in mind that any serum PTH value must be evaluated together with the simultaneously determined serum calcium value.

Urinalyses of phosphate, calcium, nephrogenous cyclic adenosine monophosphate (AMP), and hydroxyproline have been used to evaluate patients suspected of having primary hyperparathyroidism. With parathyroid overactivity, phosphate is usually excreted in great excess in the urine, but such a finding is not specific enough to have real diagnostic significance. In the 1960s, it was common to calculate such things as the tubular reabsorption of phosphate (TRP) and the phosphate excretion index (PEI) as a measure of possible hyperparathyroidism. Characteristically, in primary hyperparathyroidism, the TRP would be low and the PEI above normal. These tests had a wide margin of error, however, with many false-positives and false-negatives, and have now been generally abandoned.

Despite the fact that patients with primary hyperparathyroidism have an increased tubular reabsorption of calcium in the kidney, the increased amount of calcium in the glomerular filtrate will in many cases lead to hypercalciuria. An increased urinary excretion of calcium is thus indicative of, but not diagnostic for, primary hyperparathyroidism. It also should be remembered that idiopathic hypercalciuria is not rare, and other diseases, such as sarcoidosis and cancer, can cause excess calcium loss in the urine. Women with abnormally high calcium losses in the urine are far more likely than men to have parathyroid disease as the cause. The reason for this is unknown.

An increased amount of nephrogenous cyclic AMP in the urine has been cited as indicative of primary hyperparathyroidism. This also seems to be the case with hydroxyproline, but these diagnostic studies have not found general usefulness as yet.

The cortisone-suppression test has been proposed as a means to separate parathyroid from nonparathyroid hypercalcemia. Cortisone acetate, 200 mg/day, or an equivalent dose of hydrocortisone is given for 10 days, with serum calcium values determined before, during, and at the conclusion of the test. In most cases of nonparathyroid hypercalcemia, the serum calcium values will become normal or be significantly suppressed. Such is the case usually in sarcoidosis, vitamin D intoxication, hyperthyroidism, Addison's disease, and many patients with cancer. Unfortunately, false-negative and false-positive results will occur, and thus the test is rarely used today.

DIFFERENTIAL DIAGNOSIS

Before radioimmunoassay of PTH became readily available, the diagnosis of primary hyperparathyroidism was made usually by excluding all other possible causes of hypercalcemia, leaving only autonomous parathyroid hypersecretion as the etiology. In general, other causes of hypercalcemia either were easily detectable or could be ruled out without great difficulty. Unfortunately, there were always some troublesome cases in which this was not so. Certainly, the addition of PTH immunoassay to the diagnostic tests used to evaluate patients with hypercalcemia has helped a great deal, but, as might be expected, there remain a few troublesome cases that can be difficult to assess. It is of the utmost importance to emphasize that the result and diagnostic inference of a PTH immunoassay should not be substituted for an evaluation of all possible etiologies for hypercalcemia, since immunoassay findings can be misleading.

Although there are many reasons for hypercalcemia, by far the two most common are malignant disease and primary hyperparathyroidism. The nonparathyroid causes for hypercalcemia are listed in Table 20-3, and each is discussed.

MALIGNANCY

Cancer in its various forms probably is responsible for hypercalcemia as often as, if not more than, primary hyperparathyroidism. Solid tumors with associated osteolytic metastases are a leading cause, with breast cancer being the most common by far. Many other visceral cancers with lytic bone metastases fall into this group, including lung, thyroid, gastrointestinal, and kidney. Certain hematologic malignancies with skeletal involvement, such as multiple myeloma, can lead to hypercalcemia, and other cancers, without associated osseous metastases, can produce humoral

substances that cause hypercalcemia. Most prominent in this latter group are primary cancers of the lung, kidney, pancreas, and bladder, although others have been identified.

The elevated plasma calcium values that are seen in patients with osteolytic metastases may logically be attributed to localized bone destruction and the liberation of excessive amounts of calcium into the extracellular space, with in some instances a combined effect of some humoral substance that is produced by the cancer. Breast cancer with its possible production of prostaglandins is an example. In the case of multiple myeloma, it is believed that a lymphokine, osteoclast-activating factor, is produced to enhance bone resorption and add to the hypercalcemic effect of the locally destructive myeloma cells infiltrating the skelton.

Lung cancer is the most common of the nonparathyroid malignant tumors that may produce a humoral substance causing hypercalcemia. It is thought that lung, pancreatic, kidney, and bladder cancers all may make a PTH-like polypeptide that can give rise to an increase in plasma calcium values. This has been termed pseudohyperparathyroidism, and other substances such as prostaglandins may be involved as well.

The hypercalcemia of malignancy is frequently accompanied by additional signs of cancer, such as tumor, pain, weight loss, and other organ-specific indications of disease. Obviously, chest x-ray films, intravenous pyelography, gastrointestinal contrast studies, and other diagnostic tests may be helpful in detecting primary or metastatic cancer.

In patients with ectopic production of PTH, or pseudohyperparathyroidism, serum calcium values tend to be quite high, 14 mg/dl or above, and corresponding immunoassay values for PTH are usually low to normal or only slightly elevated. If a humoral substance not measured by the parathyroid immunoassay is responsible for the hypercalcemia, or if a nonhumoral mechanism is the cause for the high plasma calcium values, immunoreactive PTH will be low or unmeasurable, since the hypercalcemia will suppress normal PTH secretion.

SARCOIDOSIS AND OTHER GRANULOMATOUS DISEASES

A significant number of patients with Boeck's sarcoid will have hypercalcemia at some time during the course of their illness. The reported incidence varies greatly from one series to the next but averages about 20%, and it is believed that hypercalcemia results from an increased sensitivity to vitamin D. In most patients with sarcoidosis and hypercalcemia, serum immunoreactive PTH values will be undetectable or low, but this is not an invariable finding. Hypergammaglobulinemia is often seen in sarcoidosis but not in primary hyperparathyroidism. If chest films and pulmonary function studies are not suggestive of sarcoidosis, it may be helpful to have an ophthalmologic evaluation to look for evidence of old or active uveitis. Finally, the high plasma calcium values seen in sarcoidosis almost always will be suppressed to or toward normal by a cortisone-suppression test.

Other chronic granulomatous diseases besides sarcoidosis have been associated with hypercalcemia, although only rarely so. Tuberculosis and berylliosis are examples, and it is presumed that the pathogenesis is similar.

HYPERTHYROIDISM

A mild degree of hypercalcemia is not rare in thyrotoxicosis and has been reported in as many as 20% of one series of hyperthyroid patients. It apparently is due to slightly in-

---

TABLE 20-3 **CAUSES FOR HYPERCALCEMIA OTHER THAN PRIMARY HYPERPARATHYROIDISM**

Malignancy
Solid tumors with bone metastases: breast, lung, thyroid
Hematologic tumors involving bone: multiple myeloma, leukemia, lymphoma
Tumors secreting humoral factors
PTH-like substance: lung, kidney, pancreas
Other: lung, breast, bladder

Sarcoidosis and Other Granulomatous Diseases (Tuberculosis, Berylliosis)
Hyperthyroidism
Milk-alkali syndrome
Vitamin D or A intoxication
Adrenal insufficiency
Prolonged immobilization
Thiazide diuretics
Familial benign hypercalcemia
Pheochromocytoma
Idiopathic hypercalcemia of infancy
Hypophosphatasia

creased bone turnover, which may be caused by an increase in PTH secretion due to a heightened sensitivity to catecholamines. β-adrenergic receptor blocking agents such as propranolol will normalize plasma calcium values in patients with thyrotoxicosis. Hypercalcemia also disappears with correction of hyperthyroidism.

MILK-ALKALI SYNDROME

Years ago, it was not uncommon to treat acid–peptic disease with milk and soluble antacids such as sodium carbonate or bicarbonate. This combination could lead to an increased absorption of calcium with resultant hypercalcemia and hypercalciuria. Now that nonabsorbable antacids have generally replaced sodium carbonate or bicarbonate, the syndrome has almost disappeared. There is a present-day counterpart to the milk-alkali syndrome, however, since some patients with symptoms of peptic ulcer will treat themselves by drinking large quantities of milk and by taking one of the commercially available, over-the-counter antacid preparations containing calcium carbonate. This can produce hypercalcemia, but there is a rapid return to normal when the calcium carbonate is withdrawn.

VITAMIN D INTOXICATION, VITAMIN A INTOXICATION

Large doses of vitamin D, in the range of 50,000 or 100,000 units daily for several weeks or months, can cause hypercalcemia. The mechanism involves an increased absorption of calcium from the gut, as well as increased bone resorption. The patient's medical history will usually lead to the diagnosis of vitamin D intoxication. The observed hypercalcemia is quickly corrected with large doses of cortisone.

Vitamin A intoxication also can lead rarely to hypercalcemia. The usual dose required is 50,000 units to 100,000 units daily. The diagnosis can be established by history and by finding increased vitamin A levels in the serum. Treatment with cortisone will rapidly bring serum calcium values to normal.

ADRENAL INSUFFICIENCY

Patients with untreated Addison's disease may have hypercalcemia, probably caused by the hemoconcentration and hyperproteinemia that those patients display. High plasma calcium values rapidly revert to normal with appropriate steroid treatment.

PROLONGED IMMOBILIZATION

Although prolonged immobilization seldom leads to hypercalcemia, this can occur if someone with a high rate of bone turnover is abruptly placed at bed rest (*e.g.*, patients with active Paget's disease or vigorously active adolescents or young adults). The resulting hypercalcemia can be quite severe but very quickly disappears with ambulation.

ADMINISTRATION OF THIAZIDE DIURETICS

The use of thiazide diuretics can slightly, although significantly, increase plasma calcium concentrations in normal persons, but this effect is ordinarily transient. If thiazides are given to someone with primary hyperparathyroidism, however, the hypercalcemic effect is exaggerated, and some have even suggested their use to unmask subclinical cases of parathyroid disease. The pathogenesis of thiazide-induced hypercalcemia probably involves a contraction of the extracellular space with some hemoconcentration, in addition to an effect on both kidney and bone. With initiation of thiazide treatment, there is an early increased loss of both sodium and calcium in the urine; with long-term therapy, renal conservation of both cations occurs. It also is likely that there is an increased skeletal turnover of calcium that is caused by thiazides and that this is exaggerated in the presence of excess PTH. Thus, thiazides may cause a transient slight increase in serum calcium in normal persons, but this should present no special problems in the differential diagnosis of primary hyperparathyroidism.

FAMILIAL BENIGN HYPERCALCEMIA

Familial benign hypercalcemia, or familial hypocalciuric hypercalcemia, was first described in 1972 and appears to be an autosomal dominant disorder with full penetrance. Patients are characteristically asymptomatic and have mild hypercalcemia with a strikingly low urinary excretion of calcium. Serum immunoreactive PTH values are usually normal, and serum phosphate is often low normal. These patients may be thought to have primary hyperparathyroidism, and a few have been operated upon on that premise. Fortunately, the condition is uncommon and at present is best suspected because of family history, mild asymptomatic hypercalcemia with normal serum PTH values, and marked hypocalciuria.

PHEOCHROMOCYTOMA

Occasionally, the patient with pheochromocytoma will have hypercalcemia. In such circumstances, one should always remember the possibility of a MEA type II syndrome and the possibility that primary hyperparathyroidism may coexist with pheochromocytoma. In patients with pheochromocytoma and without hyperparathyroidism, the hypercalcemia is a direct effect of the epinephrine increasing PTH secretion. This effect of epinephrine is mediated by β-receptor-site activation and is blocked by drugs such as propranolol. In these patients, treatment with propranolol will eliminate hypercalcemia.

IDIOPATHIC HYPERCALCEMIA OF INFANCY

Idiopathic hypercalcemia of infancy is a rare condition often seen in association with multiple congenital cardiovascular and facial lesions. Although the cause for the hypercalcemia is obscure, it may relate to an increased sensitivity to vitamin D.

HYPOPHOSPHATASIA

Congenital hypophosphatasia is an extremely uncommon illness characterized by a lack of alkaline phosphatase in bone, plasma, and leukocytes and by the excretion of phosphoethanolamine in the urine. Bone x-ray films demonstrate changes characteristic of rickets. Plasma calcium and phosphate values are usually normal, although hypercalcemia can occur. The features of the disorder other than hypercalcemia allow it to be easily distinguished from primary hyperparathyroidism.

PREOPERATIVE TUMOR LOCALIZATION

Although most parathyroid tumors are not especially difficult to find at operation, one of the altogether too common and frustrating problems the surgeon may encounter is an abnormally located and elusive adenoma or hyperplastic gland (Figs. 20-23 and 20-24). Because of this, it has seemed appropriate that some special effort be made toward preoperative localization of abnormal tissue if this is reasonably

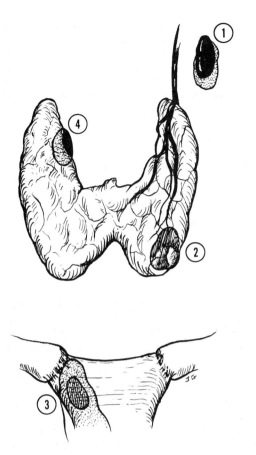

Fig. 20-23. Ectopic locations where parathyroid glands and tumors are occasionally found. (*1*) A tumor above and lateral to the upper pole of the thyroid lobe. This is an undescended lower parathyroid, and the tissue about it is associated thymus. (*2*) A lower parathyroid tumor has enlarged by encroaching upon the adjacent thyroid and appears to be almost intrathyroidal. (*3*) A lower parathyroid tumor is within the thymic capsule in the anterior upper mediastinum. (*4*) An upper parathyroid tumor is medial to the upper pole of the thyroid.

Fig. 20-24. Additional ectopic locations for parathyroid glands or tumors. True intrathyroidal parathyroids are almost always upper glands. Most retroesophageal parathyroid tumors also arise in upper glands.

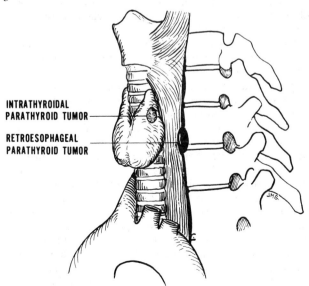

INTRATHYROIDAL PARATHYROID TUMOR

RETROESOPHAGEAL PARATHYROID TUMOR

possible. A large number of different studies and tests have been used in an attempt to accomplish this goal, but unfortunately none is uniformly successful.

Simple physical examination of the neck and thyroid area is seldom helpful in locating parathyroid tumors. Most parathyroid tumors, because of their size, consistency, and location, cannot be felt; only 2% or 3% actually may be palpable.

Plain x-ray films of the chest or neck area also are seldom helpful. Only occasionally will a large upper mediastinal tumor be detected, and it is very uncommon for a parathyroid tumor to be large or firm enough to cause deviation of the tracheal air column. Esophageal barium contrast studies have been more successful in locating parathyroid tumors than have plain x-ray films.

Scans of the thyroid area using radioactive selenomethionine have been used to locate parathyroid abnormalities. This type of study, however, produces only a low degree of success in locating smaller tumors and is rarely used today.

Sonography often is a helpful preoperative study in locating parathyroid tumors. The usually performed gray-scale sonography has been reported by some to be successful in over 80% of cases. Recently improved high-resolution real-time sonography has been cited as being even more accurate in finding tumors, but such high success rates have not, as yet, been experienced in most centers.

Computed tomography (CT scanning) also may be of assistance in locating larger tumors and especially those in the mediastinum. Although this technique is of limited value at this time, improved results may come as the resolution limits of CT scanning are increased.

Because parathyroid tumors are metabolically active lesions, thermography has been used as a localization method. Thus far, however, this technique has lacked both specificity and sufficient accuracy to be very useful.

Thyroidography also has been used in an attempt to localize parathyroid tumors. In this procedure, radiopaque water-soluble contrast material is injected into the thyroid gland. The contrast material outlines the thyroid itself, and an immediately adjacent nonopaque parathyroid tumor may be seen distorting the normal thyroid contour. So far, this method of identifying parathyroid tumors has had limited usefulness.

Selective arteriography has been extensively studied and used as a means of locating parathyroid tumors. The technique involves selectively injecting radiopaque contrast material into the inferior or superior thyroid artery, the internal mammary artery, or all of these vessels. In experienced hands, a vascular tumor blush can be found by this method in over 90% of cases. Because of the incidence of central nervous system complications in some patients, selective arteriography is probably best reserved for special cases, such as those with previously unsuccessful neck explorations for parathyroid disease.

Selective catheterization of the different thyroid veins and analysis of immunoreactive PTH in the various blood samples obtained have been used to locate overactive parathyroid glands. Higher than normal PTH levels in blood samples obtained from the veins draining either the right or the left lobe of the thyroid can localize a parathyroid tumor to the side from which the higher values are obtained. Additionally, very high values of immunoreactive PTH obtained from both sides may point to multiple-gland involvement and indicate parathyroid hyperplasia instead of an adenoma as the cause for primary hyperparathyroidism. It should be emphasized that this is a very exacting procedure that is both time-consuming and costly and that extensive experience with the technique is necessary to achieve consistently reliable results. Thus, selective venous sampling procedures should be reserved for special problem cases.

The parathyroid squeeze test has been used to determine which side of the neck contains a parathyroid tumor. In this test, a blood sample is drawn from a peripheral vein; immediately thereafter, one side of the neck, adjacent to the trachea from the level of the upper border of the thyroid cartilage to the clavicle, is vigorously massaged for 10 to 20 seconds. One minute after the massage is completed, an additional blood sample is obtained. Two hours later, the same procedure is repeated, massaging the *opposite* side of the neck. An analysis of premassage and postmassage blood samples for immunoreactive PTH often reveals a significant increase immediately following massage on the side that contains the parathyroid tumor. This squeeze test has a high degree of success in lateralizing parathyroid abnormalities.

None of the tests or techniques described is a substitute for a careful and meticulous parathyroid exploration performed by an experienced surgeon. In fact, many surgeons do not rely upon any of these special studies in the uncomplicated patient and reserve their use for special problem cases.

ADDITIONAL DIAGNOSTIC COMMENT: PREOPERATIVE BLOOD BIOCHEMICAL VALUES OF SPECIAL SIGNIFICANCE

First and foremost as a point of emphasis, any patient about to undergo an operation for primary hyperparathyroidism should have been determined to have hypercalcemia. It is worth repeating that without documented hypercalcemia, the diagnosis is open to question. The values for serum calcium obtained prior to operation also will provide the surgeon with additional information concerning the size of the patient's parathyroid tumor or tumors. In general, the size of adenomatous or hyperplastic parathyroid glands is proportional to the level of serum calcium; thus, high calcium values usually are found with larger tumors. Although this is not always the case, it can serve as an indication of what may be encountered.

If patients with primary hyperparathyroidism have an elevated serum alkaline phosphatase level, they may be presumed to have significant osteitis with depleted bone mineral stores. Following correction of their disease by successful parathyroidectomy, and presumably as bone remineralization occurs, plasma calcium values may fall below normal and give rise to symptoms of tetany. For this reason, a preoperative elevation of serum alkaline phosphatase is a clue to an increased likelihood of postoperative tetany.

Chronic exposure to excessive amounts of PTH often leads to an increased loss of potassium in the urine. Some patients with primary hyperparathyroidism, therefore, will be hypokalemic and need to have potassium supplements prior to operation. Potassium-depleted patients are particularly prone to develop life-threatening cardiac arrhythmias and are unduly sensitive to nondepolarizing muscle relaxants. Thus, it is important for the surgeon to be aware of the increased incidence of hypokalemia in patients with primary hyperparathyroidism.

As has been previously noted, patients with primary hyperparathyroidism have an increased incidence of both hyperuricemia and clinical gout. Any patient with gout who has an operation has an increased risk of an attack of acute gouty arthritis postoperatively. Hyperuricemia should alert the surgeon to this possibility and prepare him to initiate prompt treatment at the first sign of joint involvement to abort a severe attack.

TREATMENT

The optimal treatment for primary hyperparathyroidism is operation to find and remove all, or nearly all, abnormal parathyroid tissue. Nonoperative treatment presently leaves much to be desired, and a discussion of this form of therapy is found in the section on special problems.

OPERATION

Operations to correct primary hyperparathyroidism should be performed only by surgeons who are well versed in the anatomy of the area involved and who have been trained to recognize the variable appearances of both normal and abnormal parathyroid glands. The operation itself should be meticulously carried out to avoid bloodstaining of the tissues so that normal color variations in fat lobules, lymph nodes, thymic tissue, and parathyroid glands are not obscured. The accompanying illustrations depict the areas where parathyroid tumors are usually found, as well as some of their more common ectopic locations (see Figs. 20-21 through 20-24).

Because of the possibility of pluriglandular involvement, it is important to find all four parathyroid glands, if possible. In the usual patient, one gland will be represented by an adenoma and the other three will be more or less normal. In these cases, the adenoma should be removed and a biopsy taken of one of the remaining glands to confirm its identity and evaluate its histology. More extensive removal of parathyroid tissue is not necessary when an adenoma is the cause of primary hyperparathyroidism. Some advocate the routine removal of the adenoma and 2½ of the remaining glands. The thought here is that a high percentage of all patients with primary hyperparathyroidism have occult hyperplasia in their apparently grossly normal parathyroid glands. However, it should be emphasized that this is a minority opinion.

If all four parathyroid glands are involved in a hyperplastic process, it is best to remove three glands entirely and a portion of the fourth, leaving behind what is estimated to be 60 mg to 75 mg of parathyroid tissue on an intact vascular pedicle. The remnant should be approximately the size of two normal glands.

During the operation, in *all* cases, it is important to establish the nature of tissue removed by frozen-section histology. Both normal and abnormal parathyroid glands have been mistaken grossly for lymph nodes, fat lobules, thymic tissue, and thyroid nodules. These misperceptions need to be clarified before an operation is concluded, so that proper treatment can be carried out at that time and a second operation avoided. It is especially important to emphasize that the first, and, one hopes, only, parathyroid operation represents the prime opportunity to evaluate correctly and to treat primary hyperparathyroidism. Any subsequent neck operation to cope with continuing or recurrent disease will be technically difficult and much less likely to be successful. All possible sites for ectopic glands, therefore, should be carefully explored; this includes even the removal and serial section of a lobe of the thyroid if a missing tumor might be contained therein.

Occasionally, but in no more than 1% or 2% of patients, a parathyroid tumor will not be in reach of the usual neck exploration. These adenomas or hyperplastic glands will be in the mediastinum. Although most mediastinal parathyroid tumors can be removed through the usual neck incision, some will not be accessible by this approach. If such is the case, a sternal splitting incision will be necessary. Most surgeons prefer not to add a formal mediastinal exploration to the patient's initial neck operation but to defer that to another time. It is, of course, extremely important to terminate the neck exploration only after an extensive search leaves one convinced that a parathyroid tumor has not been overlooked.

POSTOPERATIVE CARE

The usual patient recovering from a successful operation for primary hyperparathyroidism requires no special care. Plasma calcium values usually return to normal during the first postoperative day with no attendant significant symptoms. In a few patients, however, and especially in those who have preoperative high serum alkaline phosphatase values associated with active osteitis, the plasma calcium values will fall below normal and lead to symptoms of tetany. If this is the case, patients will complain of tingling sensations in the toes and fingers and of circumoral paresthesias. Occasionally, they will experience muscle cramps, but this is not common. Chvostek's sign and Trousseau's sign may be present, but it is well to remember that Chvostek's sign can be elicited in about 25% of normal persons. These symptoms and signs are usually mild and transient, and no treatment other than reassurance is necessary. More severe tetany may be treated with oral calcium supplementation, and only rarely will parenteral medication be needed.

If added oral calcium is required, it is best to use calcium carbonate powder and to avoid calcium lactate or gluconate tablets or powder. Tablets of the latter preparations may be poorly absorbed, and neither has as much available calcium as does calcium carbonate on a weight-comparison basis.

In rare instances, where severe postoperative tetany seems to respond poorly to calcium alone, it may be well to add magnesium to the patient's treatment protocol. Some patients apparently are also magnesium depleted, and addition of this ion is necessary before calcium therapy can be as effective as it should be.

Vitamin D, dihydrotachysterol, or calcitriol should not be used to treat the early postoperative symptoms of tetany. These and other such preparations should be reserved for patients who are ultimately shown to have permanent hypoparathyroidism.

PROGNOSIS

The long-term cure rate of patients who have successful removal of a solitary parathyroid adenoma has been over 95%. Patients who have subtotal parathyroidectomy to correct primary chief-cell hyperplasia do less well but seem to have permanent good results between 85% and 90% of the time.

About half of the patients with functioning parathyroid carcinomas die of their disease. Carcinoma tends to recur locally in the neck and to metastasize to regional lymph nodes, as well as to the lungs, liver, and bones. Most deaths are due to the complications of hypercalcemia and not to organ replacement by tumor.

SPECIAL PROBLEMS IN PRIMARY HYPERPARATHYROIDISM

Ordinarily, patients with primary hyperparathyroidism present no particular difficulty with either diagnosis or treatment. Periodically, however, some present with unusual problems that require special attention. A few of the more important ones are described and commented upon.

SEVERE HYPERCALCEMIA

Severe hypercalcemia to the degree of 16 mg/dl or higher may be a life-threatening emergency. It occurs infrequently in patients with primary hyperparathyroidism but often enough so that the possibility should never be ignored. It has been said that the etiology of severe hypercalcemia is usually malignant disease and that such an occurrence or complication in primary hyperparathyroidism is so uncommon that it almost excludes the possibility of this diagnosis. Unfortunately, the idea that they are probably dealing with terminal malignant disease has caused some physicians to be less than vigorous in their diagnostic assessment of severely hypercalcemic patients. This preconceived notion may be much to the patient's detriment, because it delays recognition of a highly curable cause for a potentially fatal problem.

Most patients with severe hypercalcemia due to primary hyperparathyroidism have large parathyroid tumors, many of which are palpable. Certainly, a mass in the thyroid region of the patient with severe hypercalcemia should focus one's attention on the possibility of parathyroid disease. It also should be stressed that the most effective treatment for parathyroid-caused severe hypercalcemia is the correction of the hyperparathyroidism by operation as soon as it is safe to do so. Undue delay awaiting possible long-term amelioration of the condition by nonoperative therapy is usually not wise. It is proper, however, not to operate upon patients until plasma calcium values have been brought to as near normal as possible by hydration and appropriate drug therapy.

Rehydration is the first treatment that should be used in the patient who has severe hypercalcemia associated with primary hyperparathyroidism. Almost all these patients have sustained significant fluid losses and are hemoconcentrated. Unless there is some reason to restrict sodium, rehydration should be carried out with intravenous normal saline solution so that natriuresis will be encouraged. It is well known that renal sodium and calcium excretion directly parallel one another, and a diuresis initiated by sodium-containing solutions will increase urinary calcium losses. Often, simply rehydrating these patients and establishing a good urine flow will bring their plasma calcium values into a range where they may be safely treated by operation.

If simple rehydration does not have the desired effect, it often is helpful to enhance urinary calcium losses by increasing the amount of intravenous saline given and adding the diuretic furosemide. As much as 6 liters of isotonic saline may be given daily, and up to 100 mg furosemide every 2 hours may be used. With such a treatment program, it is important to monitor carefully serum potassium and magnesium levels and to provide appropriate supplementation of these ions as necessary.

As an alternative to forced diuresis or if vigorous fluid and diuretic therapy is not effective, mithramycin may be used. Mithramycin is a cytotoxic substance that rapidly and profoundly inhibits bone resorption. The dose is 25 µg/kg in 500 ml to 1000 ml normal saline infused over a 4- to 8-

hour period. Plasma calcium values almost always fall significantly within 24 to 48 hours, often to normal levels. If circumstances indicate, another dose of mithramycin may be given 24 hours after the first and repeated as often as every 24 to 48 hours, if necessary.

There are other methods to deal with severe hypercalcemia, but they are either potentially too dangerous or will not predictably lower PTH-induced high plasma calcium values. Intravenous phosphate solutions will lower plasma calcium values no matter what the etiology. This is brought about by the intravascular precipitation of calcium phosphate complexes. Renal failure and other undesirable consequences may occur, however, and therefore such treatment is seldom indicated.

Large doses of cortisone will favorably affect hypercalcemia caused by vitamin D intoxication, sarcoidosis, multiple myeloma, and many other malignant diseases but seldom will be helpful in patients with primary hyperparathyroidism. Unfortunately, calcitonin usually will not be materially beneficial in severe hypercalcemia caused by parathyroid disease.

NONOPERATIVE MANAGEMENT

Although operative treatment is the best therapy for primary hyperparathyroidism, this occasionally will not be possible. Patients with repeated unsuccessful parathyroid explorations, those with illnesses that preclude operation, and those who refuse surgery are in this category. These patients should be approached in an entirely different fashion from those previously described who have severe, life-endangering hypercalcemia.

It is best to strive for elimination of symptoms and for a urinary calcium excretion of no more than 300 mg/day. This usually requires a maintenance of plasma calcium values between 11 mg and 12 mg/dl. Values for plasma calcium below this actually may be harmful, since even adenomas are responsive to hypocalcemia, and the resulting increased PTH secretion may aggravate bone resorption.

The best course of treatment for these patients is usually that of oral phosphate supplementation. Most patients with primary hyperparathyroidism are phosphate depleted because of the increased renal phosphate loss caused by excess PTH. Thus, added phosphate will not only depress serum calcium values but may well rebuild depleted osseous stores of this anion. Several oral preparations of phosphate are available, including Neutra-Phos, Phos-Tabs, and Fleet's Phospho-Soda. The dosage must be titrated to suit individual patient needs.

ASYMPTOMATIC PRIMARY HYPERPARATHYROIDISM

As has been previously discussed, the advent of automated blood biochemical screening in the 1960s led to the diagnosis of primary hyperparathyroidism in many patients who did not have symptoms specifically suggestive of this disease. In fact, a rather significant number of these patients were asymptomatic and had only a slight elevation in serum calcium. There arose the obvious question of whether or not operative treatment was indicated.

In 1968, the Mayo Clinic initiated a prospective evaluation of such patients. They excluded from the study patients with serum calcium values 1 mg/dl or higher above normal, for whom operation was recommended. Over a 10-year period of periodic continuing evaluations, 23% of an original group of 142 patients underwent neck explorations. The indications most commonly cited were an increase in serum calcium values, decreased renal function, and active renal stone disease. It became apparent that a significant proportion of the original asymptomatic group would either demonstrate worsening hypercalcemia or become overtly symptomatic. It also was obvious that the majority would not.

With such a data base, it might seem logical to recommend a management program of repeated periodic evaluations and resort to operation only upon the appearance of symptoms or more severe hypercalcemia. This course of action, however, ignores problems of patient noncompliance and the difficulty of securing repeated assessments. There also remain the unanswered questions of just what may be the long-term added risks of minimal hypercalcemia to the skeletal and the cardiovascular systems. When one considers the increased incidence of hypertension with hypercalcemia and the possible aggravation of postmenopausal osteoporosis by even mild hyperparathyroidism, these are obvious legitimate concerns. For these and other reasons, it is difficult to be dogmatic about how asymptomatic patients with primary hyperparathyroidism and minimal hypercalcemia should be managed. For the present, if a properly trained experienced surgeon is available, it is probably best to recommend operative treatment in most such cases.

REOPERATION FOR CONTINUING OR RECURRENT DISEASE

As emphasized previously, the best chance the surgeon has to correct primary hyperparathyroidism is at the first operation. Reexploration of the neck is a difficult procedure at best, because of scarring and the obliteration of normal tissue planes. As a result of the added technical problems, there is an increased risk of damaging recurrent laryngeal nerves or the remaining normal parathyroid tissue. Also, difficulties with dissection will make previously undetected parathyroid tumors more difficult to locate.

In the majority of instances in which an operation to correct primary hyperparathyroidism has been unsuccessful, the offending abnormal tissue remains in the neck or in the upper mediastinum and is potentially accessible through a neck approach. Obviously, in some cases, adenomatous or hyperplastic parathyroid glands will be deep in the mediastinum, and a sternal splitting incision will be necessary for their removal. In either instance, it is desirable to make special efforts at preoperative tumor localization before a second exploration. If skilled personnel are available, either selective angiography or determination of serum immunoreactive PTH values from veins draining the thyroid area may be particularly helpful. Other localizing techniques, such as sonography, CT scanning, or selenomethionine scanning, may be attempted, but these are not as likely to be of assistance.

ASSOCIATED ENDOCRINOPATHIES

Thyroid disease is the most commonly associated endocrine problem in patients with primary hyperparathyroidism. Statistically, thyroid adenomas or adenomatous goiter is most common. Nonmedullary thyroid cancer is also a possibility, and all such problems may be dealt with at the same time the parathyroid disease is treated.

If an MEA syndrome is suspected, the possibility of coexisting pituitary and pancreatic lesions (MEA type I) or of medullary thyroid carcinoma and pheochromocytoma (MEA type II) should be considered. Skull films, visual-field testing, and obvious signs or symptoms of pituitary dysfunction, along with symptoms of either gastric acid hypersecretion or hyperinsulinism, may indicate problems related to the MEA type I syndrome and would dictate more specific diagnostic testing. If an MEA type II syndrome is suspected, pentagastrin stimulation with measurement of serum immunoreactive calcitonin almost always will detect medullary carcinomas, and urinary determinations of vanillylmandelic acid, the metanephrines, or the catecholamines themselves will help with the diagnosis of possible pheochromocytoma.

Patients who have one of the MEA syndromes present two special problems in management. First, it is important for the surgeon to be aware that primary hyperparathyroidism in association with MEA syndromes is due much more frequently to chief-cell hyperplasia than are sporadically occurring cases. In fact, 50% or more of all patients will have this pathologic basis for their parathyroid disease, and at operation this possibility must be diligently pursued.

Another potential problem relates to the priority for treatment in simultaneously occurring endocrinopathies. Obviously, patients with both medullary thyroid carcinoma and parathyroid disease can have their problems dealt with at the same operation. Other patients with hyperparathyroidism and a virulent ulcer diathesis (Zollinger-Ellison syndrome) or a pheochromocytoma may need to have surgical treatment for these latter conditions before parathyroidectomy. An individual judgment will have to be made in these cases. The surgeon must bear in mind that although pharmacologic control of gastric hypersecretion or hypertension is possible, it is usually not difficult to cope with mild hypercalcemia if the parathyroid problem is deferred to a second operation.

DISEASE DURING PREGNANCY

Primary hyperparathyroidism is not often a complication of pregnancy. The relatively young age at which most pregnancies occur, of course, is the most important factor in this low incidence. Symptoms and signs may reflect any of the changes brought about by parathyroid overactivity, but most reported cases have had slight or moderate hypercalcemia without overt bone disease. Untreated primary hyperparathyroidism during pregnancy results in a significantly increased risk of spontaneous abortion and fetal mortality.

Ionized calcium readily crosses the placental barrier and may lead to suppression of parathyroid tissue in the fetus if the pregnant woman has hypercalcemia. Shortly after birth, the infant may have hypocalcemic tetany. Initially, the newborn's suppressed parathyroid glands may not be able to respond efficiently to the fall in plasma calcium values that occurs during the neonatal period. For this reason, neonatal hypocalcemic tetany can be a clue to previously undiagnosed primary hyperparathyroidism in the mother.

Operation and, depending on the pathology encountered, removal of an adenoma or most of the hyperplastic parathyroid tissue is the treatment of choice. This is best done during the second trimester, since maternal and fetal complications are less likely during this period.

DISEASE DURING CHILDHOOD

The most important feature of childhood primary hyperparathyroidism is the fact that it is so uncommon. Because of this, the diagnosis may not be suspected when symptoms occur that might be due to hypercalcemia or some of the complications of hyperparathyroidism. Children with primary hyperparathyroidism often complain of lassitude and easy fatigability; arthritislike joint pains are surprisingly frequent, although clinical osteitis is otherwise uncommon. Renal complications, such as stone disease or nephrocalcinosis, are rare.

The proper treatment for these patients is operative removal of either the offending adenoma or an appropriate amount of hyperplastic parathyroid tissue.

SECONDARY HYPERPARATHYROIDISM

Secondary hyperparathyroidism may be defined as an adaptive response of the parathyroid glands to secrete increased amounts of PTH because of a detectable abnormality that is external to the glands themselves. In all cases, the common denominator is a reduction in plasma ionized calcium caused by the different extraparathyroidal abnormalities. This hypocalcemia leads to hypersecretion of PTH in an effort to adapt to the abnormality and maintain normal plasma calcium values. Characteristically, patients with secondary hyperparathyroidism will have either normal or slightly depressed plasma calcium levels, depending upon the degree of successful adaptation.

ETIOLOGY

Many different diseases may cause secondary hyperparathyroidism. These include Vitamin D deficiency, hereditary vitamin D dependency, vitamin D–resistant rickets, pseudohypoparathyroidism, hypomagnesemia, and chronic renal failure. In this group of disorders, only chronic renal failure is likely to require operative treatment directed at the parathyroid glands, so it will be the only problem discussed in any detail here.

Chronic renal failure may lead to severe secondary hyperparathyroidism, which can cause renal osteodystrophy, soft-tissue calcifications, severe intractable itching, progressive muscular weakness, severe lassitude, and depression. The osteodystrophy is characterized by both osteitis fibrosa and osteomalacia and can result in bone pain and pathologic fractures. Soft-tissue calcification may occur in the skin, in the blood vessels, and especially about the joints.

PATHOPHYSIOLOGY

The pathogenesis of secondary hyperparathyroidism in chronic renal failure relates to impaired renal phosphate excretion, disordered vitamin D metabolism, and decreased end-organ sensitivity to PTH. As renal failure progresses, there is decreased glomerular filtration with resultant phosphate retention. As plasma phosphate increases, there is a reciprocal fall in plasma ionized calcium, which results in an increased secretion of PTH. A decrease in tubular reabsorption of phosphate in the remaining nephrons, and thus an increase in renal phosphate loss, occurs under the influence of an increase in PTH secretion. This form of compensation to reduce plasma phosphate values will gradually deteriorate with progressive renal failure until chronic hyperphosphatemia ensues. This, of course, results in a continuing hypocalcemic stimulus for PTH secretion.

As renal failure becomes more pronounced, abnormalities in vitamin D metabolism play an important role in aggravating secondary hyperparathyroidism. The kidney is the only site where $1\text{-}\alpha$-hydroxylation of 25-hydroxycholecalciferol takes place to form 1,25-dihydroxycholecalci-ferol (1,25 [OH]$_2$D$_3$, or calcitriol). In the later stages of renal failure, 1-α-hydroxylase activity decreases and the formation of calcitriol is inhibited. Intestinal malabsorption of calcium results, since calcitriol is the principal hormone that positively influences the absorption of this cation. Thus, at this stage, both malabsorption of calcium and the effect of hyperphosphatemia act together to intensify the hypocalcemic stimulus for PTH secretion.

Renal failure also blunts the effect of PTH on bone. Despite high circulating PTH levels due to secondary hyperparathyroidism, the degree of osseous resorptive response is disproportionately low, even though destructive osteitis fibrosa and osteomalacia may ultimately result. The reason for this change in osseous-tissue response is not known, but it possibly is related to the altered vitamin D metabolism that occurs in renal failure.

Although this brief description of changes leading to secondary hyperparathyroidism in renal failure highlights well-documented abnormalities that obviously have etiologic significance, there are undoubtedly other more complex mechanisms also at work. In particular, the interactions of PTH and vitamin D metabolites need better clarification.

PATHOLOGY

The chronic hypocalcemic stimulus that leads to secondary hyperparathyroidism is presumably responsible for the increase in the mass of functioning parathyroid tissue that occurs. Hyperplastic parathyroid glands show an increase in both absolute and relative numbers of chief cells and either an absence or a marked decrease in fat cells. Gross, microscopic, and ultrastructural appearances in involved glands are simular to those seen in primary chief-cell hyperplasia. In some cases of longstanding renal failure, the masses of hyperplastic tissue take on a nodular pattern.

TREATMENT

Many patients with mild or moderate secondary hyperparathyroidism associated with renal failure can be successfully treated with dietary restriction of phosphate and oral supplements of absorbable calcium. It also is usually desirable to add phosphate-binding antacids to decrease absorption of this anion. In many patients, this will lower plasma immunoreactive PTH values. In some, it will even lead to improvement of established osteodystrophy. Calcitriol also may be given to increase intestinal absorption of calcium, but its use must be carefully monitored to avoid hypercalcemia. It is important in patients who are being treated with hemodialysis not to aggravate a negative calcium balance by using dialysate with calcium concentrations below 5.7 mg/dl. Dialysate calcium concentrations between 6.5 and 8.0 mg/dl may even be used to help produce a positive calcium balance.

Despite active therapy, certain cases of secondary hyperparathyroidism due to renal failure will become severe and intractable. Bone pain, pathologic fractures, soft-tissue calcifications, uncontrollable pruritus, and marked lassitude and depression may develop. Such patients are best treated with parathyroidectomy.

The most commonly performed operation in these cases is subtotal parathyroidectomy, much as would be done to treat primary chief-cell hyperplasia. Unfortunately, this is not as successful in patients with secondary hyperparathy-

roidism, and recurrence of the problem is not uncommon. For this reason, some have used total parathyroidectomy with autotransplantation of a portion of the resected parathyroid tissue into the forearm musculature or simply total parathyroidectomy without autotransplantation.

If the latter operation is performed, it will be necessary, of course, to treat the patient with oral calcium supplements and probably either dihydrotachysterol or calcitriol to maintain normal plasma calcium levels. On the other hand, autotransplantation of parathyroid tissue to the forearm has a twofold attraction. First, in most cases the transplanted tissue will function and temper the need for treatment with calcium and vitamin D. Second, if the transplanted tissue becomes overactive and an additional resection is required, the operation can be done relatively easily, even under local anesthesia.

It might seem appropriate in some severe cases of renal hyperparathyroidism to defer parathyroidectomy and plan for a subsequent kidney transplant to ameliorate the hyperparathyroid state. This is probably not the best course for most patients when one considers the unpredictable availability of donor kidneys and the fact that renal transplantation, in many instances, will not correct hyperparathyroidism. It also should be noted that the postoperative care of kidney transplant patients with uncorrected severe secondary hyperparathyroidism can be complicated by significant hypercalcemia and difficulty in controlling mineral metabolism.

TERTIARY HYPERPARATHYROIDISM

Occasionally, patients with secondary hyperparathyroidism will develop hypercalcemia with or without renal transplantation. It has been thought that this is caused by an autonomously functioning adenoma that has developed in one of the hyperplastic parathyroid glands. The newly arisen, nonsuppressible adenoma thus is responsible for the hypercalcemia. Although this may seem to be a plausible explanation, it is probably not often the case. In most such patients at operation, parathyroid hyperplasia, not adenoma, is found. This merely points up the fact that secondary hyperplasia may fail to involute despite removal of the original hypocalcemic stimulus and indeed may become nonsuppressible.

HYPOPARATHYROIDISM

ETIOLOGY

Parathyroid hormone–deficient hypoparathyroidism traditionally has been classified as either postsurgical or idiopathic. The so-called idiopathic type contains many variants, including congenital absence of the parathyroid glands, branchial dysembryogenesis, the multiple endocrine deficiency–autoimmune–candidiasis syndrome, and isolated late-onset hypoparathyroidism. The conditions included in the idiopathic hypoparathyroidism group do not require specific surgical care related to the parathyroid abnormality and therefore are not discussed.

Surgical hypoparathyroidism is by far the most common form of PTH-deficient hypoparathyroidism. All other forms of acquired hypoparathyroidism are extremely rare and are mentioned only for completeness' sake. In this latter category are cases that occur following radioactive iodine treatment for hyperthyroidism, with hemosiderosis, and following neoplastic infiltration of the parathyroid glands.

Permanent hypoparathyroidism resulting from operations on the thyroid gland has been reported with varying frequency. It depends upon the type of operation performed, as well as the skill and experience of the surgeons involved. Operations for Graves' disease have had this complication noted in from 0 to 4%, depending upon the series. Total thyroidectomy for thyroid cancer with or without a concomitant lymphadenectomy has a higher incidence of associated hypoparathyroidism. Figures in the range of 5% to 10% or even higher have been cited.

Occasionally, the patient operated upon for primary hyperparathyroidism will develop hypoparathyroidism. This usually occurs in patients who have had a subtotal parathyroidectomy for chief-cell hyperplasia and in whom the remaining parathyroid tissue either has been infarcted or is insufficient in amount to maintain normal function. Of course, hypoparathyroidism is the desired result of total parathyroidectomy done for certain patients with secondary hyperparathyroidism and is not a misadventure of the treatment.

SYMPTOMS AND SIGNS

Acquired, permanent hypoparathyroidism is characterized by symptoms of tetany accompanied by hypocalcemia, hyperphosphatemia, and unmeasurable or lower than would be expected values for serum immunoreactive PTH. Manifestations of tetany vary considerably in severity. They may consist merely of tingling sensations in the fingers or toes, or there may be severe muscle spasms in the face and extremities. An attack often begins with tingling in the fingers and toes and around the mouth. This sensation spreads proximally in the limbs and across the face and may be replaced with numbness. A tenseness of muscles in the hands and forearms and in the feet and legs may occur next, followed by muscle spasms in these same areas. Spasm of intrinsic laryngeal muscles may occur and lead to stridor, but this is very uncommon. Although the symptoms and signs of tetany are alarming, the condition is seldom life-endangering.

Incipient or latent tetany may be detected by eliciting Chvostek's or Trousseau's signs. Chvostek's sign may be detected in up to 25% of normal persons and thus is not as reliable an indicator of latent tetany as is Trousseau's sign.

There are a variety of other findings that occur with hypoparathyroidism. At any time after the onset of the problem, patients with preexisting epilepsy are more prone to seizures. Since standard anticonvulsants may have an anti–vitamin D effect, it is important to monitor these patients very closely and maintain normal plasma calcium values at all times.

Cataracts are the most common complication of chronic hypocalcemia, but it usually takes from 5 to 10 years before they interfere with vision. Effective treatment will either prevent their occurrence or arrest progression.

Basal-ganglia calcifications also develop in chronic hypoparathyroidism. This is generally a late complication with an average interval of 17 years between the onset of hypoparathyroidism and radiographically detectable basal-ganglia lesions. This complication may be accompanied by signs of extrapyramidal disease, such as parkinsonism, but that is far from universal. Many patients are asymptomatic.

Some patients with long-standing hypoparathyroidism will complain of dry, scaly skin; brittle nails; and dry, coarse hair. Atopic eczema and psoriasis may also become manifest after the onset of hypoparathyroidism. Treatment that is effective in controlling hypocalcemia will usually correct or improve these problems.

A number of less common complications can occur, and all seem due to chronic hypocalcemia. These include asymptomatic papilledema, intestinal malabsorption and steatorrhea, congestive heart failure, and some psychiatric disorders. All of these tend to improve with restoration of normal plasma calcium values.

TREATMENT

Acquired hypoparathyroidism occurs in varying degrees of severity. Some patients have no symptoms and need no therapy; others are committed to lifelong medication. Most of the time, this problem will respond well to treatment, and the results should be comparable to those that can be achieved with replacement therapy for other endocrine deficiencies.

Patients with acute symptoms of hypocalcemic tetany that occur shortly after thyroidectomy or parathyroidectomy often need treatment with parenteral calcium, although oral supplementation may be all that is required. Calcium gluconate as a 10% solution can be given intravenously if immediate relief of symptoms is necessary. The dose for adults is 10 ml to 20 ml, and it should not be given any more rapidly than 1 ml/minute. Parenteral calcium should be given with great care to patients who are taking digitalis and probably only with electrocardiographic monitoring. Oral calcium carbonate may be used instead of, or as a supplement to, intravenous calcium gluconate. One gram every 2 to 3 hours while the patient is awake is often sufficient, but larger amounts may be needed. If continued parenteral medication is needed, 10 ml of 10% calcium gluconate may be added to 500 ml intravenous solution and infused over a 6-hour period.

Permanent hypoparathyroidism with significant hypocalcemia will require lifelong treatment. In most cases, some form of vitamin D is all that is needed, but an occasional patient will need supplemental oral calcium as well. A low phosphate diet is of obvious advantage in treating hypoparathyroidism. In practice, however, this is hard to achieve. The best that can be hoped for usually is avoidance of high-phosphate foods such as milk and other dairy products.

Calcitriol is now commercially available, and ultimately it should prove to be the best vitamin D preparation used to treat hypoparathyroidism. There has not been extensive experience with the use of calcitriol in the treatment of this condition to date, however, and it remains very expensive. Most often, ergocalciferol, or vitamin D_2, is relied upon for long-term treatment. Vitamin D_2, just as all vitamin D preparations or their analogues, is a potentially dangerous drug that can cause hypercalcemia and hypercalciuria with resultant renal damage. The dose that is selected must be carefully evaluated in this regard, and it is best to start with a relatively small amount and wait until the potential maximum effect has taken place before any incremental change. The main disadvantages of vitamin D_2 are the length of time it takes to reach its maximum effect (4–12 weeks) and the time it takes for the effects of a toxic dose that has caused hypercalcemia to subside.

The goal of treatment should be to maintain plasma calcium values in the lower half of the normal range. The ultimate daily dose of vitamin D_2 that will accomplish this is usually between 1.25 and 3.75 mg (50,000 units–150,000 units). The vitamin D analogue dihydrotachysterol may be used instead of ergocalciferol. It has the advantage of a shorter latent period to reach its maximum effect, but the drug is rather expensive. The usual daily maintenance dose of dihydrotachysterol is 0.3 mg to 1.0 mg.

PSEUDOHYPOPARATHYROIDISM

Pseudohypoparathyroidism is a rare, hereditary disorder characterized by the symptoms and signs of hypoparathyroidism, together with distinctive skeletal and developmental defects. Presently, it is believed that pseudohypoparathyroidism has a sex-linked dominant inheritance.

The mineral metabolic abnormality is due to end-organ unresponsiveness to PTH. The degree of unresponsiveness in different patients varies, but the prototypical case will display lack of effect of PTH on bone and kidney. Specifically, bone resorption is defective, and there is increased loss of calcium in the urine, as well as phosphate retention. In addition, the renal hydroxylation of 25-hydroxycholecalciferol to form calcitriol is defective, and the intestinal absorption of calcium is impaired as a consequence. These changes result in hypocalcemia and hyperphosphatemia.

There is no apparent defect in PTH synthesis; the chronic hypocalcemic state leads to hyperplasia of the parathyroid glands. Operative treatment for parathyroid hyperplasia is not indicated.

These patients usually become symptomatic at about 8 years of age, when tetany occurs. This can range from slight tingling sensations to convulsions. It is not uncommon to detect mental retardation, which apparently is not due to hypocalcemia. Multiple soft-tissue calcifications are common and are present in the basal ganglia in about 50% of patients.

The associated skeletal and developmental abnormalities often include short stature; round face; short neck; thick, stocky body build; and multiple discrete anomalies of individual bones. The skeletal changes are characterized by shortened metacarpal and metatarsal bones and multiple exostoses. Classically, it is the fourth and fifth metacarpals or metatarsals that are involved, and the defect may be unilateral. If only one digit is involved, it is invariably the fourth.

Treatment is the same as for patients with acquired hypoparathyroidism. Vitamin D almost always is required, and oral calcium supplements also may be necessary.

PSEUDOPSEUDOHYPOPARATHYROIDISM

Pseudopseudohypoparathyroidism has been applied to patients who have the same spectrum of distinctive developmental and skeletal abnormalities as those with pseudohypoparathyroidism but who do not have evidence of hypoparathyroidism.

PARATHYROID CYSTS

Parathyroid cysts are rare; fewer than 150 cases have been reported. The vast majority of these have not been associated with primary hyperparathyroidism. It is not unusual for either parathyroid adenomas or hyperplastic glands to undergo partial cystic degeneration, and it is likely that this is the reason that some patients who have so-called parathyroid cysts also have hyperparathyroidism.

It has been suggested that nonfunctioning parathyroid cysts are simply retention cysts derived from the normal glands, but their etiology is unknown.

These lesions vary in diameter from 2.0 cm to 25 cm and usually contain clear serous fluid. The cyst wall is often gray white and translucent. Microscopically, small clusters of parathyroid cells are seen intermingled with the fibrous tissue of the cyst wall.

Parathyroid cysts generally are found in the lower part of the neck and are often confused with thyroid tumors on physical examination. Their cystic nature becomes apparent with either aspiration or sonography. In some cases, the aspirated cyst fluid contains a high titer of PTH. These cysts tend to refill following aspiration. Appropriate treatment consists in operative removal.

BIBLIOGRAPHY

Austin LA, Heath H: Calcitonin: Physiology and pathophysiology. N Engl J Med 304:269, 1981

Avioli LV: The therapeutic approach to hypoparathyroidism. Am J Med 57:34, 1974

Bess MA, Edis AJ, van Heerden JA: Hyperparathyroidism and pancreatitis: Chance or a causal association? JAMA 243:246, 1980

Bruining HA, van Houten H, Juttmann Jr et al: Results of operative treatment of 615 patients with primary hyperparathyroidism. World J Surg 5:85, 1981

Castleman B, Roth SI: Tumors of the Parathyroid Glands, Fascicle 14, Atlas of Tumor Pathology. Washington, DC, Armed Forces Institute of Pathology, 1978

Cope O: Hyperparathyroidism: Diagnosis and management. Am J Surg 99:394, 1960

Cope O: The story of hyperparathyroidism at the Massachusetts General Hospital. N Engl J Med 274:1174, 1966

Cope O: Hyperparathyroidism: Too little, too much surgery? N Engl J Med 295:100, 1976

Doppman JL: Parathyroid localization arteriography and venous sampling. Radiol Clin North Am 14:163, 1976

Goldsmith RS, Johnson WJ, Arnold CD: The hyperparathyroidism of renal failure: Pathophysiology and treatment. Clin Endocrinol 3:305, 1974

Juler GL, Kutas A, Skowsky WR: Primary hyperparathyroidism: A pleomorphic disease. Am Surg 47:483, 1981

Martin KJ, Hruska KA, Freitag JJ et al: The peripheral metabolism of parathyroid hormone. N Engl J Med 301:1092, 1979

Mundy GR, Cove DH, Fisken R: Primary hyperparathyroidism: Changes in the pattern of clinical presentation. Lancet 1:1317, 1980

Nainby-Luxmoore JC, Langford HG, Nelson NC et al: A case-comparison study of hypertension and hyperparathyroidism. J Clin Endocrinol Metab 55:303, 1982

Parfitt AM: Surgical, idiopathic, and other varieties of parathyroid hormone-deficient hypoparathyroidism. In DeGroot LJ, Cahill GF, Martini L et al (eds): Endocrinology, p 755. New York, Grune & Stratton, 1979

Paterson CR, Gunn A: Familial benign hypercalcemia. Lancet 2:61, 1981

Purnell DC, Scholz DA, Smith LH: Diagnosis of primary hyperparathyroidism. Surg Clin North Am 57:543, 1977

Rosenberg J, Orlando R, Ludwig M et al: Parathyroid cysts. Am J Surg 143:473, 1982

Scheible W, Deutsch AL, Leopold GR: Parathyroid adenoma: Accuracy of preoperative localization by high-resolution real-time sonography. J Clin Ultrasound 9:325, 1981

Scholz DA, Purnell DC: Asymptomatic primary hyperparathyroidism. Mayo Clin Proc 56:473, 1981

SEIPEL CM: An English translation of Sandstrom's *Glandulae Para-thyroideae.* Bull Inst Hist Med 6:179, 1938

SHANE E, BARQUIRAN DC, BILEZIKIAN JP: Effects of dichloromethylene diphosphonate on serum and urinary calcium in primary hy-perparathyroidism. Ann Intern Med 95:23, 1981

VAN HEERDEN JA, BEAHRS OH, WOOLNER LB: The pathology and

surgical management of primary hyperparathyroidism. Surg Clin North Am 57:557, 1977

WANG CA: The anatomic basis of parathyroid surgery. Ann Surg 183:271, 1976

WANG CA, GUYTON SW: Hyperparathyroid crisis: Clinical and path-ologic studies of 14 patients. Ann Surg 190:782, 1979

James D. Hardy

The Adrenal Glands

ANATOMY

An adrenal gland represents four organs in one: There are the three zones of the adrenal cortex, which have largely different functions, and the adrenal medulla. The adrenal cortex and the medulla have separate embryologic origins. The medullary portion is derived from the chromaffin ectodermal cells of the neural crest. These cells split off and eventually form the sympathetic ganglion cells that come to lie adjacent and ventrolateral to the aorta, where they form the paraganglia. However, the larger mass of these cells gradually becomes associated with the mesodermal cells that will become the adrenal cortex. Eventually, a specific mass of chromaffin cells derived from the ectoderm becomes enclosed within the mesodermal cells of the cortex, and this specific mass forms the adrenal medulla. Because the sympathetic ganglia ultimately extend all the way from the neck to the urinary bladder, a paraganglioma may be found at any site along this chain, although such tumors are more likely to be found near the level of the kidney or along the lower aorta at the level of the organs of Zucker-kandl. The term *pheochromocytoma* is used both as a generic term embracing all tumors involving the chromaffin issue wherever found and for tumors arising in the adrenal medulla; the term *paraganglioma* is applied to such chro-maffin tumors arising elsewhere. Most often, however, the term pheochromocytoma is used in the broadest sense and denotes all tumors of chromaffin tissue found anywhere along the sympathetic chain.

Like chromaffin tissue, which has widespread distribu-tion, adrenocortical rests may be found outside the adrenal gland proper, although they are usually adjacent to the kidney or in the ovary or even in the testes.

The gross anatomy of the adrenal glands is depicted in Figure 20-25. The left adrenal gland is situated just adjacent to and medial to the upper pole of the kidney and adjacent to the aorta. Venous drainage is largely through the central

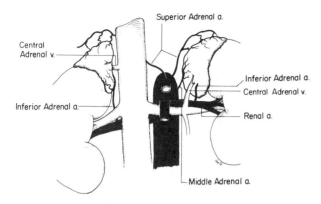

Fig. 20-25. Topographic anatomy and blood supply of the adrenal gland. (Hardy JD: Cushing's syndrome. In Hardy JD [ed]: Rhoads Textbook of Surgery, 5th ed. Philadelphia, J B Lippincott, 1977)

adrenal vein, which drains into the left renal vein, but there are other smaller venous channels if the central vein becomes occluded. The arterial supply, in contrast, is variable and is represented by relatively small vessels. There is usually a branch from the aorta and one from the renal artery. Even so, the central vein is the major vascular structure encountered in removing the adrenal gland; the arteries are simply ligated in the course of exposing and mobilizing the adrenal. At operation the adrenal glands may be exposed from an anterior transverse incision. The left adrenal is approached by dividing the gastrocolic omentum and then dividing the peritoneum along the inferior margin of the pancreas and retracting the pancreas anteriorly and cephalad. The gland can also be approached using a standard loin or kidney incision. Other approaches include use of a thoracoabdominal incision, especially when a large tumor is present, or a posterior approach with the patient lying in the prone position. The anterior abdominal approach is perhaps most widely used.

The right adrenal gland also lies along the medial aspect of the upper pole of the right kidney, and its blood supply is similar to that of the left adrenal. However, in the right adrenal gland, the central adrenal vein, its largest vascular structure, is short and enters directly into the inferior vena cava beneath the liver. Therefore, although it is usually a simple matter to excise the left adrenal in the absence of major enlargement from a tumor, excision of the right adrenal can result in avulsion of the central adrenal vein from the vena cava, leading to serious hemorrhage if it is not identified and managed appropriately. The right adrenal gland is approached by freeing the duodenum and reflecting it medially, exposing the inferior vena cava, which is then followed upward beneath the liver. The right adrenal gland is identified lying between the inferior vena cava and the kidney, adjacent to the diaphragm.

PHYSIOLOGY

The microscopic anatomy of the adrenal cortex is of particular functional interest. Three zones can be readily identified: (1) the outer zone, or zona glomerulosa, which secretes aldosterone; (2) the middle zone, or zona fasciculata, which secretes cortisol; and (3) the inner zone, or zona reticularis, which secretes androgens and estrogens. These three zones are distinct microscopically, and their hormonal secretions are likewise characteristic of each zone. There is, however,

some cross-over in the actual metabolic effects of the hormones, especially cortisol, which is secreted by the zona fasciculata and has sufficient mineral effects to replace completely the need for aldosterone most of the time. Again, there is some overlap betweeen the secretory capacities of the zona fasciculata and the zona reticularis, and perhaps even the zona glomerulosa as well.

There is a very sensitive feedback mechanism between the anterior pituitary, which secretes adrenocorticotrophic hormone (ACTH), and the adrenocortical secretion of cortisol. As the blood level of cortisol rises, the release of ACTH by the anterior pituitary declines and vice versa (Fig. 20-26). The stimulus for the release of ACTH is the neural hormone corticotropin-releasing factor (CRF), which is produced by the hypothalamus. The sensitivity of this feedback mechanism is somewhat altered after trauma to permit development of a higher blood level of cortisol. The rate of release of CRF and ACTH not only is normally regulated by the plasma level of cortisol but may actually be increased by circumstances in which psychic stress results in impulses descending from the cerebral cortex. Usually, however, the release of CRF and ACTH to stimulate the secretion of cortisol by the zona fasciculata is governed by the plasma level of cortisol. One aspect of the rate of cortisol secretion is important in the diagnosis of hyperfunction of the adrenal cortex. Normal people exhibit "sleep–wake" or *diurnal variation* (circadian rhythm) with regard to the rate of secretion of cortisol, the plasma level being highest just as night is ending and declining thereafter to reach its lowest level during the next night. This diurnal variation is lost in patients with Cushing's syndrome, although the cause may vary. The syndrome may be due to abnormalities such as a small functioning pituitary adenoma with increased elaboration of ACTH, or ACTH increase may be derived from an ectopic source such as an oat cell carcinoma of the lung; alternatively, the increased cortisol level may be caused by a functioning tumor of the adrenal cortex itself. The lack of this diurnal variation, which establishes abnormal function of the adrenal cortex, and appropriate other tests for the identification of hyperadrenocorticism will be described later. By means of these tests, the precise cause of the loss of diurnal variation in Cushing's syndrome can be identified and appropriately treated.

The adrenal medulla may elaborate a variety of catecholamine substances. Normally, the adrenal medulla elaborates both epinephrine and norepinephrine, but primarily epinephrine. However, the adrenal medulla can also, in certain instances, elaborate less mature cortical amines such as dopamine. In general, if the secretion of epinephrine in the urine is substantial, and if there is a similar increase in the excretion of norepinephrine, the functioning adrenal chromaffin tumor will be found in the adrenal gland itself. In contrast, if the tumor is elaborating almost entirely norepinephrine, with little or no increase in epinephrine, the tumor may represent a paraganglioma or extra-adrenal tumor that may be located anywhere from the neck to the urinary bladder along the sympathetic chain, although it will be found in the abdomen most of the time.

The surgeon becomes involved primarily with patients who have adrenocortical or adrenomedullary hyperfunction. Nonetheless, as will be seen later, adrenocortical insufficiency may be a definite risk in a given patient, and appropriate therapy for acute or chronic adrenocortical insufficiency may be required before operation.

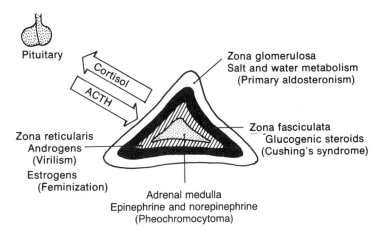

Fig. 20-26. The adrenal gland. (Hardy JD: Pathophysiology in Surgery. Baltimore, Williams & Wilkins, 1958)

DISORDERS OF THE ADRENAL CORTEX

PRIMARY HYPERALDOSTERONISM

The term *primary hyperaldosteronism* (primary aldosteronism) is applied to the excessive production of aldosterone by the adrenal cortex, mainly the zona glomerulosa. Primary hyperaldosteronism, or "low-renin" aldosteronism, connotes hypersecretion arising from disease in the adrenal cortex itself, usually a benign adenoma. Secondary hyperaldosteronism, on the other hand, is essentially due to renal disease and is commonly accompanied by a measurable increase in the elaboration of renin by the kidney. Adrenal surgery is not indicated in secondary hyperaldosteronism.

PRIMARY HYPERALDOSTERONISM	
Etiology	Solitary adrenocortical benign tumor of zona glomerulosa in 85%–90% of cases, secreting excess aldosterone.
Dx	Hypertension or hypokalemia, or both, leads to measurement of plasma renin and aldosterone secretion in urine on a normal sodium diet. Aldosterone is increased and renin is normal or low. Radiologic methods (CT scan especially) disclose tumor.
Rx	Resection for unilateral tumor. Recurrence is rare. Prognosis is good to excellent except in rare instances of bilateral adrenocortical hyperplasia or malignancy.

In 1954 it had been apparent for some time that, when all known adrenocortical steroids had been identified in the urine, there remained behind in the "amorphous fraction" or residue some substance that had a powerful effect on water and electrolyte metabolism. In that year aldosterone was isolated by Simpson and associates. In 1955 Conn reported on a patient whose clinical features were termed primary aldosteronism. The findings consisted of hypertension, muscle weakness, hypokalemia, and an increased excretion of a sodium-retaining hormone in the urine; this clinical picture was subsequently named Conn's syndrome. It is most often found in women between the ages of 30 and 50, but it also occurs in males and has been reported at all ages.

PATHOLOGY

Primary hyperaldosteronism is caused by a benign adenoma in 85% of patients and by bilateral nodular adrenocortical hyperplasia in most of the others, but occasionally it results from a functioning adrenocortical malignancy. These chromate-yellow, 1 cm to 2 cm tumors are almost always unilateral. Because they may be small and soft, they can be missed at operation, and it is important to mobilize the adrenal glands to permit careful inspection not only of the anterior surface but also of the posterior surface. Recurrences following removal of an adenoma are rare.

CLINICAL FACTORS

Basically, the clinical findings that initiate eventual laboratory demonstration of excessive aldosterone production are hypertension and hypokalemia. Metabolic alkalosis and a high-normal or elevated serum sodium level are commonly present. Signs and symptoms experienced by the patient are caused by hypertension and sodium retention (headache, cardiac enlargement, heart failure), hypokalemia and general potassium deficit (muscle weakness and even paralysis, paresthesias, and muscle cramps), hypokalemic renal damage (polyuria, polydipsia), and hypernatremia (with increased blood volume).

DIAGNOSIS

The diagnosis of hyperaldosteronism is established on the basis of clinical findings that lead to the measurement of aldosterone excretion in the urine. The patient should be placed on a normal sodium diet, and thus any low-sodium diet or chlorothiazide diuretics should be stopped at least a month before measuring the rate of aldosterone excretion in the urine. The normal level of excretion is about 10 μg/24 hr. In hyperaldosteronism, the level may rise to as much as 40 μg per day. Once hyperaldosteronism has been established, the next step is to determine whether it is due to primary aldosteronism or secondary aldosteronism, because renal disease may be present in both instances. This determination is made primarily by measuring plasma renin levels in the supine position with the patient on a normal sodium intake. If primary hyperaldosteronism is present, the plasma renin level will be normal or low; in secondary hyperaldosteronism the level will be high. Thus, the two basic laboratory measurements in the diagnosis of suspected

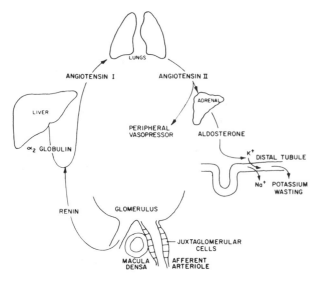

Fig. 20-27. The renin-angiotensin-aldosterone system. Aldosterone production follows the release of renin from the juxtaglomerular cells in the normal individual. (Carey LC, Anderson GW: Primary aldosteronism. In Hardy, JD [ed]: Rhoads Textbook of Surgery, 5th ed. Philadelphia, J B Lippincott, 1977)

primary hyperaldosteronism are the determination of the urinary excretion of aldosterone and the plasma renin levels under appropriately controlled conditions. The normal renin–angiotensin–aldosterone system is shown in Figure 20-27.

In addition, a number of supportive functional tests have been employed in the diagnosis of hyperaldosteronism. These include administration of Pitressin to attempt to increase the specific gravity of the characteristically large volumes of urine; there will be no increase if the patient has hyperaldosteronism. Also, a therapeutic test with spironolactone may be employed. Spironolactone is an antagonist of aldosterone at the level of the kidney tubule. It does not reduce the secretion of aldosterone, but it will diminish the water and electrolyte abnormalities and symptomatology of primary hyperaldosteronism.

LATERALIZATION OF THE TUMOR

Once the diagnosis of primary hyperaldosteronism has been established, it is important to lateralize the usually unilateral benign adenoma. This may be done by measuring renal or central adrenal vein blood aldosterone levels or occasionally by selective venous angiograms or arteriograms of the adrenal glands. However, noninvasive methods such as iodocholesterol (radioactive) adrenal scan, ultrasonography, or computed tomography (CT) scan are preferable. Of course, in the approximately 10% of patients with primary aldosteronism due to bilateral adrenocortical hyperplasia no cortical adenoma will be demonstrated.

PREOPERATIVE PREPARATION FOR SURGICAL THERAPY

The mainstay of nonoperative or medical therapy is spironolactone. However, since 85% to 90% of cases of primary aldosteronism are caused by a unilateral benign cortical adenoma, surgical excision of the tumor remains at present the treatment of choice. The principal preoperative preparation consists of liberal potassium therapy and sodium restriction to bring the serum potassium level up to normal. A low potassium level predisposes to serious cardiac ar-

rhythmias during operation. Preoperative preparation is usually not difficult, but if chronic hypertension and secondary renal damage have led to heart failure, more careful and more prolonged preoperative measures will be required.

OPERATION

At operation we prefer an upper abdominal transverse incision (Fig. 20-28). If preoperative studies have succeeded in identifying the tumor on one side or the other, some surgeons prefer the posterior approach through the bed of the 12th rib, or else the loin or kidney incision on the side involved. They feel that the presence of a well-localized tumor on one side virtually excludes, on a percentage basis, the need to explore the other adrenal.

Once an abdominal incision has been made in the usually thin and usually female patient, the involved adrenal is explored and carefully mobilized, preserving the blood supply but permitting inspection of both its anterior and posterior surfaces. These tumors may be only 2 mm to 3 mm in diameter but are usually about 1 cm to 2 cm in size and are a vivid yellow. They are often soft and barely palpable. We have had the experience of being unable to see or to palpate a tumor on the anterior surface of the gland, only to visualize it readily once the posterior surface

Fig. 20-28. Surgical approach to the adrenal glands. (Hardy JD: Cushing's syndrome. In Hardy JD [ed]: Rhoads Textbook of Surgery, 5th ed. Philadelphia, J B Lippincott, 1977)

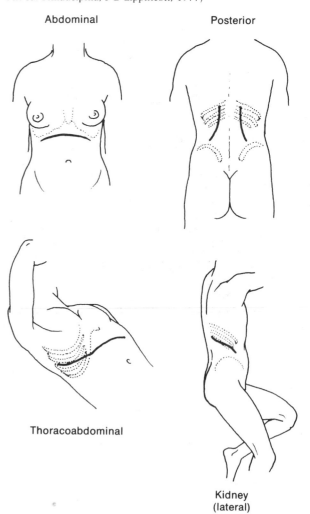

Abdominal

Posterior

Thoracoabdominal

Kidney
(lateral)

of the gland could be inspected. If it is possible to remove the tumor with the distal or cephalad one half or two thirds of the gland while preserving the portion adjacent to the renal vein, we do so. If this is not possible, the entire gland on that side is removed. If no tumor can be identified despite secure preoperative lateralization on that side, the other adrenal should be explored. If no tumor is found on the other side, attention is redirected to the first side, and the entire gland is removed. Some of these tumors are very small and may be found only on careful sectioning in the laboratory. If only adrenal hyperplasia is found, spironolactone therapy may be employed postoperatively.

Postoperative complications are usually not serious, but of course may include any of the usual possible complications of laparotomy. Sodium supplementation may be needed. Adrenocortical (cortisol) insufficiency following unilateral adrenalectomy for primary aldosteronism should be rare if the blood supply to an explored opposite adrenal was preserved. Occasionally, the remaining adrenal zona glomerulosa may have been so suppressed by the functioning tumor on the opposite side that aldosterone secretion is subnormal for a time. In such uncommon instances fludrocortisone therapy (0.1 mg/day orally) should be employed until the remaining gland has regained its normal ability to secrete aldosterone.

Failure to diagnose primary hyperaldosteronism—and the presence of this insidious and variable disease can often go unsuspected—and failure to achieve timely and effective treatment may result in the usual complications of hypertension, including stroke, heart failure, and renal failure.

PROGNOSIS

The prognosis is excellent if a benign adenoma is found and removed before chronic primary hyperaldosteronism with hypertension has produced cardiac and renal damage.

HYPERADRENOCORTICISM (CUSHING'S SYNDROME AND CUSHING'S DISEASE)	
Etiology	Cushing's *syndrome* may be due to excessive adrenocortical production of cortisol (zona fasciculata), to pituitary ACTH excess (Cushing's *disease*), to ectopic ACTH production (*e.g.*, oat cell carcinoma of lung), or to other causes such as adrenal corticosteroid therapy. Diffuse metabolic and physical changes are present.
Dx	Clinical evidence is the basis for diagnosis. Laboratory measurements of cortisol in plasma and urine and ACTH in plasma are needed. Roentgenographic localization of pituitary, adrenal, or ectopic tumor is useful (CT scan very useful).
Rx	Excision of pituitary tumor or bilateral adrenalectomy in Cushing's disease is performed. Resection of an adrenocortical tumor or appropriate management of ectopic ACTH focus such as lung carcinoma may be needed. Radiation, o,p'-DDD, bromocriptine, or other drug therapy is palliative only. Prognosis is good if there is no malignancy.

Symptoms of headache and nocturia are relieved, and the blood pressure can be expected to return to normal in days or weeks. If primary hyperaldosteronism is due to hyperplasia, one cannot expect that unilateral adrenalectomy will effect a complete cure, and spironolactone therapy may be indicated. In the rare instance when hyperaldosteronism is due to adrenocortical malignancy, the patient will not often be cured of the malignancy.

CUSHING'S SYNDROME (HYPERADRENOCORTICISM)

The term *Cushing's syndrome* is applied to a group of clinical findings that are produced by an excessive amount of circulating cortisol. The syndrome may be caused either by excessive production of glucocorticoids by the adrenal cortex or by the administration of excessive amounts of glucocorticoids in the treatment of arthritis, hepatitis, renal disease, or numerous other conditions. The production of excessive amounts of glucocorticoids by the adrenal cortex may be stimulated by excessive secretion of ACTH by the anterior pituitary gland, or it may be due to a tumor of the adrenal cortex that is autonomous and does not depend on the ACTH stimulus. The syndrome may also be caused by ectopic production of ACTH—for example, by a variety of malignant tumors, most notably undifferentiated bronchial carcinoma. Therefore, because the constellation of clinical findings that characterize Cushing's syndrome may be caused by a wide variety of factors, the term *Cushing's disease* is reserved for circumstances in which excessive production of ACTH by the pituitary gland itself results in excessive stimulation of the zona fasciculata of the adrenal cortex to produce excessive amounts of cortisol, whereas the term Cushing's syndrome embraces the cushingoid features produced by excessive cortisol no matter what the mechanism.

HISTORICAL NOTE

In 1912 Cushing published a monograph, The Pituitary Body and Its Disorders, in which he described five patients with a symptom complex that came to be known as Cushing's syndrome (Fig. 20-29). He later included additional cases, and it was his belief that a small basophilic adenoma of the pituitary caused the disease by elaborating a substance that had a stimulative effect upon the adrenal cortex. In detail and accuracy his early description still includes the essential features of the syndrome (Table 20-4). However, as has been seen, in the ensuing years the possible causes of Cushing's syndrome have been shown to be multiple, both intra-adrenal and extra-adrenal, and the accurate differential diagnosis of Cushing's syndrome now requires somewhat sophisticated laboratory studies.

PATHOPHYSIOLOGY

As noted previously, Cushing's syndrome is caused by excessive secretion of cortisol, whether by a functioning adrenocortical tumor representing largely the zona fasciculata, or by excessive ACTH production by the pituitary gland itself (usually from a small basophilic adenoma), or by ectopic ACTH secretion (as by an oat cell carcinoma of the lung). Of course, the syndrome may also be produced by cortisone therapy used for various medical conditions. It has been seen that normally the amount of ACTH released by the anterior lobe of the pituitary gland is regulated by CRF, which is released by the hypothalamus. CRF brings about the release of ACTH, which in turn stimulates the

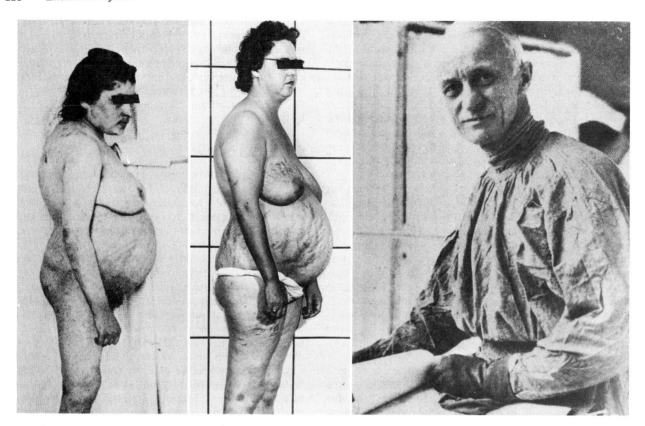

Fig. 20-29. (*Left*) Cushing's original case. (Cushing H: The basophil adenomas of the pituitary body and their clinical manifestations [pituitary basophilism]. Bull Johns Hopkins Hosp, 50:137, 1932) (*Middle*) Patient with Cushing's syndrome, showing marked striae of breasts, abdomen, buttocks, and upper thighs. (*Right*) Harvey Cushing, pioneer neurosurgeon and clinical physiologist who first clearly described Cushing's syndrome. (Fulton JF: Harvey Cushing, A Biography. Springfield, IL, Charles C Thomas, 1946)

adrenal cortex to produce cortisol. Within the adrenal cortex, it is believed that cyclic AMP (cAMP) is the intracellular mediator of the steroidogenic action of ACTH. The rate of cortisol secretion is determined by the amount of ACTH reaching the adrenal cortex, and cortisol in turn acts through

TABLE 20-4 FREQUENCY OF SIGNS AND SYMPTOMS IN CUSHING'S SYNDROME

SIGN OR SYMPTOM	OCCURRENCE (%)
Obesity (truncal)	95
Hypertension	85
Glycosuria and decreased glucose tolerance	80
Hirsutism (usually nonsexual)	75
Menstrual and sexual dysfunction	75
Purple striae	65
Weakness	65
Plethoric, moon face	60
Easy bruisability	55
Osteoporosis	55
Psychiatric disturbances	50
Acne	50
Edema	50
Poor wound healing	40
Polyuria, polydipsia	20

a feedback mechanism to diminish the rate of release of ACTH by the anterior pituitary as the plasma level of cortisol rises. This feedback mechanism is normally subject to a marked diurnal variation (Fig. 20-30). This diurnal variation is lost in the patient with Cushing's syndrome, because excessive production of ACTH (either by the anterior pituitary itself or by an ectopic source such as a malignant tumor) may continuously stimulate the adrenal cortex, or a tumor of the adrenal cortex itself may continuously secrete cortisol independent of any influence by ACTH secretion. Therefore, the presence or absence of the diurnal variation (sleep–wake cycle), as determined by measurement of plasma and urine cortisol excretion, is an important element in the accurate diagnosis of the presence of Cushing's syndrome or Cushing's disease. Normally, the highest plasma levels of ACTH (and thus the highest levels of cortisol) are observed at the time of awakening, and the lowest levels occur at approximately the time the individual ordinarily goes to sleep. The normal plasma cortisol level is approximately 10 µg to 25 µg/dl in the morning and 5 µg to 10 µg/dl in the evening. In addition to the feedback mechanism and the sleep–wake cycle, a third factor in the regulation of ACTH secretion is stress. Major surgical trauma or infection can produce an increase in ACTH secretion, and this stimulus may override the normal diurnal rhythm. The normal morning plasma cortisol level is approximately 20 µg/dl, and this level may rise readily to 30 µg to 50 µg/dl following a major operation. It has been shown that ACTH levels rise during laparotomy even if sufficient cortisol is

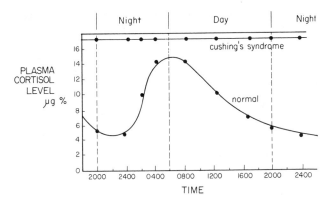

Fig. 20-30. Normal diurnal variations in plasma cortisol levels, compared with straight-line level in Cushing's syndrome. (After Hume)

concurrently infused to maintain a plasma concentration of from 100 μg to 500 μg/dl.

CLASSIFICATION OF CAUSES

The causes of Cushing's syndrome may be classified as ACTH-dependent or ACTH-independent. In approximately 75% of patients Cushing's syndrome is due to excessive release of ACTH by the pituitary gland. It is becoming increasingly apparent that most such patients have a tumor of the anterior lobe of the pituitary, although this tumor may be only 1 mm to 2 mm in size (Salassa et al; Wilson and Dempsey). The patient is characteristically a woman 25 to 45 years old. An ectopic ACTH focus such as oat cell carcinoma, malignant carcinoid of the lung, or a neoplasm elsewhere is responsible for about 1% to 2% of all cases of Cushing's syndrome, and exogenous ACTH or corticosteroid therapy may produce the same effect.

ACTH-independent causes of Cushing's syndrome consist largely of adenoma of the adrenal cortex (10%) and adrenocortical carcinoma (10%). Adrenocortical nodular hyperplasia may become independent of ACTH, and, rarely, adrenocortical tumors may occur elsewhere (*e.g.,* from adrenal rests in the ovary). Of course, the most common single cause of cushingoid changes is exogenous glucocorticoid therapy for medical conditions.

Cushing's syndrome is usually distinct from the adrenogenital syndrome (virilism), but at times mixed syndromes occur in which the patient with Cushing's syndrome exhibits evidence of virilism as well, especially when adrenocortical carcinoma exists, producing an excess of both corticosteroids and androgens.

DIAGNOSIS

The diagnosis of Cushing's syndrome can be a simple matter when all or most of the clinical features of this condition are present, but it can be difficult when there are only one or two of the common clinical findings. Moreover, the changes may be subtle and may have developed slowly over a period of many years. It can be very helpful to compare a photograph of the patient made 10 years previously with the patient's present appearance. In contrast, a patient may occasionally develop the most florid picture of Cushing's disease over a relatively short span of weeks. A high index of suspicion is necessary to achieve early diagnosis in the patient whose physical changes are minimal.

Clinical Findings

The clinical findings in Cushing's syndrome are presented in Table 20-4. The individual patient may have only some of these signs or virtually all of them if the metabolic changes have been severe.

Obesity (Truncal). Obesity with weight gain is the most common and usually the most prominent finding in 95% of patients (see Fig. 20-29). The weight gain represents an absolute increase in fat because the patient usually undergoes concomitant lean tissue loss. Obesity appears to be limited largely to the trunk, but this is due in part to the fact that the extremities appear smaller owing to muscle wasting. A cervicodorsal accumulation of fat, the "buffalo hump," is useful diagnostically but is not invariably present; moreover, it may be present in persons who do not have Cushing's syndrome. It is important to distinguish the patient who has Cushing's syndrome from those who are simply fat.

Moon Face. A rounding of the face ("moon face") is a prominent feature of Cushing's syndrome in most patients.

Hypertension. Approximately 85% of patients with Cushing's syndrome have hypertension. It is not often severe, usually in the range of 150 to 180 mm Hg systolic and perhaps 90 to 100 mm Hg diastolic. This hypertension is rarely associated with papilledema. Cardiomegaly may develop. Hypokalemia is common because the high amount of circulating cortisol results in excessive loss of potassium in the urine.

Other Clinical Findings. Glycosuria and decreased glucose tolerance are found in approximately 80% of patients with Cushing's syndrome. This "steroid diabetes" rarely leads to ketosis and acidosis. The diabetic state returns to normal when the presence of excessive circulating cortisol has been abolished.

Menstrual and sexual dysfunction are common. Amenorrhea or other abnormalities of menstrual function occur in about 75% of premenopausal women. Most women are sterile during the active stage of Cushing's syndrome, but Cushing's syndrome may develop during pregnancy. In males, Cushing's syndrome usually results in reduced libido, and such patients may show testicular softening and true or pseudogynecomastia.

Hirsutism, an increase in body hair growth, is present in about 75% of patients with Cushing's syndrome. When cortisol is secreted excessively, the increase in body hair is somatic in distribution rather than sexual, as in virilism produced by androgens. Thus, in Cushing's syndrome the increased hair growth appears on the sides of the face, the forehead, the limbs, and the trunk. This hair is generally soft and not as bristly as that caused by excess androgen. In mixed syndromes, such as those in adrenocortical carcinoma, an increase in both somatic and sexual hair may be seen.

Acne and seborrhea are common in patients with Cushing's syndrome, especially when the patient is also secreting significant amounts of androgen.

Purple striae are second only to obesity in incidence, and this feature is very prominent in most physicians' concept of Cushing's syndrome. However, well-defined striae are present in only about 65% of these patients. Striae may be purplish or reddish purple and may appear over most of the trunk (both anteriorly and posteriorly), on the breasts, and on the buttocks. They should be distinguished from striae gravidarum, which are white, and from simple obese striae, which develop in fat people and are also usually white but may be pink. Cushing's striae are due to the thinness of the skin caused by loss of protein secondary to the catabolic effects of cortisol. In Cushing's syndrome the striae are usually wide, whereas in obesity and pregnancy they are generally narrower.

Weakness is a common complaint of patients with Cushing's syndrome. It is especially annoying to the patient, and friends find it hard to understand how a person who appears so fat and apparently healthy can be so weak—the "weak fat person" of Cushing's syndrome. The weakness is due primarily to muscle wasting, but intracellular potassium deficit may also exist even when the serum potassium level is normal.

Purpura, ecchymoses, and a tendency to bruise easily may be the only complaints early in the course of disease. Although the patient may not show other physical signs of Cushing's syndrome, appropriate tests of ACTH and cortisol levels will disclose the presence of Cushing's disease or syndrome. Ecchymoses are due to increased capillary fragility. Blood coagulability is usually normal.

Osteoporosis, psychiatric disturbances, polyuria with polydipsia, and poor wound healing are also features of Cushing's syndrome. Osteoporosis occurs in about half of the patients and may cause back pain and even collapse of the vertebrae with resulting neurologic deficits. Bone resorption is due to loss of protein matrix. Pathologic fractures of the long bones may also occur. Psychiatric disturbances are prominent in some patients with Cushing's syndrome and not infrequently have resulted in admission to psychiatric institutions. About half of the patients with Cushing's syndrome show edema, and some have polyuria and polydipsia. Poor wound healing and poor healing of accidental scars have long been recognized as features of this disease.

On physical examination a tumor may be palpated, but this is rare. Other clinical findings may include retinopathy, renal stones, and peptic ulceration. If one bears in mind the wide variety of side-effects of adrenal steroid therapy, it will be appreciated that the diffuse metabolic effects of these corticosteroids may result in dysfunction of many or most organ systems and tissues on occasion.

Routine Laboratory Values

The blood count may show leukocytosis and an increased hematocrit value. In fact, the polycythemia observed in some patients has long been accepted as one of the features of Cushing's syndrome. Plasma electrolytes may not be significantly altered, but it is not uncommon to find a diminished plasma potassium level, a moderately decreased chloride level, and a metabolic alkalosis. Abnormalities of glucose metabolism have been mentioned earlier. Metabolic studies will show that these patients have a negative nitrogen and potassium balance, one of the effects of excessive cortisol. Rarely, the curious water–electrolyte disturbance in the brain known as pseudotumor cerebri may develop. This condition may be related to hyperosmolar coma.

Differential Diagnosis

Accurate diagnosis and subsequent differential diagnosis of Cushing's syndrome follow a logical series of steps. First, the possible presence of Cushing's syndrome must be suspected from the various clinical findings outlined earlier. Again, only one or two of these findings may be present in a given patient, and the physical changes in the patient may be very subtle. For example, we have had two patients whose only complaint was a tendency to bruise easily and

resulting ecchymoses; otherwise they gave little physical evidence of Cushing's syndrome. Nonetheless, both of these patients proved to have excessive secretion of cortisol when the appropriate laboratory hormonal measurements had been completed. Therefore, the first problem is to suspect the presence of this endocrine abnormality.

The next step is to determine by laboratory methods that there is an excessive secretion of cortisol. Thus, the measurement of cortisol levels in the plasma and urine represents the first definitive laboratory step.

The third step is identification of the primary site of pathology. If this is the anterior pituitary gland, the disease is usually due to a small adenoma that causes excessive elaboration of ACTH. There may be an ectopic focus of excessive ACTH secretion, such as that caused by an oat cell carcinoma of the lung, or there may be normal or subnormal plasma levels of ACTH, in which case tumor of the adrenal cortex itself must be suspected. These various conclusions are reached through appropriate measurements of plasma ACTH levels and plasma and urinary cortisol levels.

To begin with, the patient with Cushing's syndrome will usually have lost the characteristic normal diurnal or sleep–wake rhythm (Fig. 20-30). This loss establishes the presence of continuously elevated cortisol secretion. Next, the patient is given dexamethasone 0.5 mg every 6 hr for 48 hr, and the cortisol levels are determined serially (Fig. 20-31). This dosage of dexamethasone, a highly active steroid that in small doses replaces the need for cortisol, will suppress the pituitary secretion of ACTH and the urinary excretion of cortisol in the normal person, but not in Cushing's syndrome, due to an excess of pituitary ACTH (Cushing's disease). An increase in the dose of dexamethasone from 0.5 mg/6 hr/day to 1.0 mg/6 hr/day will suppress both the plasma ACTH level and the urinary corticosteroid secretion in

Fig. 20-31. Dexamethasone suppression test. (After Hume)

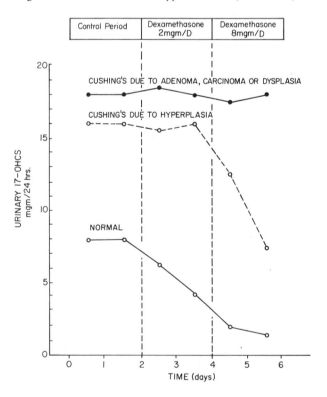

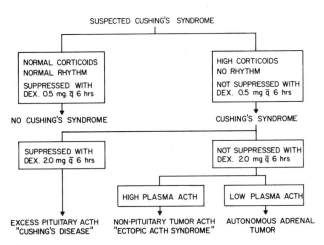

SUSPECTED CUSHING'S SYNDROME

NORMAL CORTICOIDS
NORMAL RHYTHM
SUPPRESSED WITH
DEX. 0.5 mg. q̄ 6 hrs

HIGH CORTICOIDS
NO RHYTHM
NOT SUPPRESSED WITH
DEX. 0.5 mg q̄ 6 hrs

NO CUSHING'S SYNDROME

CUSHING'S SYNDROME

SUPPRESSED WITH
DEX. 2.0 mg q̄ 6 hrs

NOT SUPPRESSED WITH
DEX. 2.0 mg q̄ 6 hrs

HIGH PLASMA ACTH

LOW PLASMA ACTH

EXCESS PITUITARY ACTH
"CUSHING'S DISEASE"

NON-PITUITARY TUMOR ACTH
"ECTOPIC ACTH SYNDROME"

AUTONOMOUS ADRENAL
TUMOR

Fig. 20-32. Protocol for evaluation of patients with suspected Cushing's syndrome. (Scott HW Jr, Foster JH, Rhamy RK et al: Ann Surg 173:892, 1971)

Cushing's disease. If the excessive secretion of ACTH is not due to a pituitary abnormality, the administration of dexamethasone will not suppress the elaboration of ACTH or the secretion of cortisol. If the increased cortisol secretion is due to an adenoma or carcinoma or to dysplasia of the adrenal gland itself, the ACTH level will be normal or subnormal initially and would not be expected to decline further with dexamethasone therapy. In this case dexamethasone in doses of even 2 mg/6 hr/day will not diminish the plasma level of cortisol. Again, when an elevated plasma ACTH is found, it must be due either to increased secretion of ACTH by the pituitary itself or to some ectopic focus such as an oat cell carcinoma of the lung. If the administration of dexamethasone does not result in suppression of the elevated plasma ACTH level, one must conclude that the source of the excessive plasma levels of ACTH lies in an ectopic focus such as oat cell carcinoma of the lung.

Using these logical steps, the diagnosis of hypercortisolism producing Cushing's syndrome and the probable cause of the excessive cortisol production can usually be identified. A schematic representation of the steps necessary for the diagnosis and differential diagnosis of Cushing's syndrome is shown in Figure 20-32.

Radiologic Studies

Radiologic techniques useful in the diagnosis of Cushing's syndrome continue to become more and more sophisticated. These techniques include the basic ones of visualization of an enlarged or eroded sella turcica caused by a pituitary tumor; demonstration of an adrenal gland tumor; and identification of the ectopic source of ACTH (*e.g.*, oat cell bronchial carcinoma or tumor elsewhere). In addition to these fairly gross changes, which may be variously identified with conventional roentgenograms, ultrasonography, or, most important, CT scans, recent advances in the quality of arteriography have made possible the demonstration of very small pituitary tumors no more than 1 mm to 2 mm in diameter by the use of arteriography and image intensification. Using such highly effective arteriographic methods, it has become increasingly apparent that Cushing's disease due to increased ACTH secretion by the anterior pituitary is almost always due to a tumor of the anterior pituitary that can be large but is often small. The CT scan has become one of the most important diagnostic techniques for iden-

tification of the presence of, and for lateralization of, an adrenal tumor, as well as for the identification of small ectopic foci of ACTH secretion such as an oat cell carcinoma of the lung. At present most instances of Cushing's syndrome that are not iatrogenic are caused by a tumor somewhere, either a small tumor in the pituitary gland, a tumor acting as an ectopic focus of ACTH secretion, or a tumor of the adrenal gland itself. The various roentgenographic procedures just mentioned, plus arteriography and venography of the adrenal glands, permit lateralization of the adrenal tumor when the tumor is actually in one of the adrenal glands. If the venogram is employed, the concentration of steroids in the adrenal vein blood flow can be sampled with a catheter on both sides. However, CT scans are increasingly effective, and invasive techniques are on the decline.

MANAGEMENT

Nonoperative Treatment

The management of Cushing's syndrome is usually surgical, but both pituitary irradiation and the insecticide chemical *o,p'*-DDD have been used. Unfortunately, radiation therapy to the pituitary has proved unsatisfactory in approximately half of the patients so treated, and it has never gained widespread acceptance. More recently, bromocriptine (Spark et al.) has been employed to suppress continued elevation of ACTH secretion by the pituitary after surgery or radiation has failed to bring ACTH levels down to normal for a sustained period of time. If the increased elaboration of ACTH is derived not from the pituitary but from some ectopic source such as an oat cell carcinoma of the lung, treatment should be directed toward the primary problem of the lung cancer. Often this cannot be controlled adequately, and the ACTH secretion continues. The patient's clinical signs and symptoms can be improved by administering the drug aminoglutethimide, which prevents the conversion in the adrenal cortex of cholesterol to Δ-5-pregnenolone. This reduces the secretion of cortisol, and the signs and symptoms of Cushing's syndrome decline, even though the plasma ACTH level remains high. The drug *o,p'*-DDD attacks the zona fasciculata and the zona reticularis of the adrenal cortex but tends to spare the zona glomerulosa, which secretes aldosterone. This drug has been used especially for adrenal tumors that could not otherwise be resected but also occasionally in patients with "routine" Cushing's disease caused by a pituitary tumor. In effect, this treatment represents a type of "medical adrenalectomy."

Surgical Management

Surgery remains the mainstay for the management of most patients with Cushing's syndrome and for virtually all patients with Cushing's disease due to excessive secretion of ACTH by the anterior pituitary. Benign tumors of the adrenal cortex should be resected, and the results are generally excellent. Malignant tumors are usually not cured, and the disease must be treated as effectively as possible with radiation or with aminoglutethimide. As noted earlier, when ectopic secretion of ACTH by malignant tumor is present, therapy must be directed toward the primary malignant disease, with drug palliation when feasible.

Most of the time, however, Cushing's syndrome is due to Cushing's disease caused by excessive secretion of ACTH by the anterior pituitary, and thus surgical therapy will be directed toward either the pituitary gland itself or toward ablation of the adrenal glands, the target organ of ACTH. It will be recalled that Cushing originally suggested that Cushing's disease was usually due to a pituitary tumor, although this could not always be demonstrated. Now, however, with CT scans and imaging intensification arteriography, even very small tumors in the pituitary gland are being found in most patients with Cushing's disease. Thus, in surgical centers where there is appropriate experience with pituitary surgery, there is a strong trend toward operating upon the pituitary gland for Cushing's disease. When sophisticated pituitary neurologic surgery is not available, bilateral total adrenalectomy, with or without autotransplantation of slices of the adrenal gland to a rectus or sartorius muscle, is still commonly performed.

Preoperative Preparation for Adrenalectomy. The most important feature of preoperative preparation is, in a sense, the accurate differential diagnosis of Cushing's syndrome. This is accomplished by the methods previously outlined. If the patient has a significant potassium deficit, it should be corrected prior to operation. Otherwise, bilateral total intra-abdominal adrenalectomy is performed in much the same manner as described for the exposure of the adrenal gland for excision of an aldosterone-secreting tumor (Fig. 20-28). Because the patient is rendered totally dependent upon adrenal cortical replacement therapy by excision of both adrenal glands, the anesthesiologist and the surgeon must begin an intravenous drip of hydrocortisone at the beginning of the operation regardless of whether or not any adrenal tissue is implanted in a muscle as an autotransplant. We have found the intravenous administration of hydrocortisone 100 mg/6 hr for the first 48 hr to be satisfactory. A scheme for this drug therapy is presented in Table 20-5.

Postoperative Management. The transoperative and postoperative administration of hydrocortisone intravenously and cortisone intramuscularly should be scrupulously executed. If steroid replacement therapy is not adequate, acute adrenocortical insufficiency, which is reflected by tachycardia, hypotension, hyperthermia at times, reduced urine output, and disorientation, may develop. A suggested dosage schedule for steroid therapy is given in Table 20-5.

Although total adrenalectomy with appropriate steroid maintenance therapy thereafter generally does manage the clinical signs and symptoms of Cushing's syndrome satis-

TABLE 20-5 **RECOMMENDED DRUG DOSAGES IN SURGICAL TREATMENT OF CUSHING'S SYNDROME**

Transoperative	Hydrocortisone 100 mg IV Cortisone 50 mg IM
Immediate postoperative period (first 48 hr)	Hydrocortisone drip, 100 mg IV q 6 hr Cortisone 50 mg IM q 6 hr
Postoperative day	
3	Cortisone 50 mg IM q 6 hr Cortisone 50 mg IM + 50 mg cortisone orally
4	
5	Same
Chronic maintenance	25–37 mg cortisone per day (1 to 1½ pills) or hydrocortisone 20–30 mg/day (1 to 1½ pills) + 9 α-fluorohydrocortisone (Florinef) 0.1 mg/day (1 pill)

factorily, various aspects of pituitary function may not be normal for months or even years afterward. After months or years, Nelson's syndrome may develop owing to enlargement of a pituitary tumor, which may be a chromophobe adenoma; this may impinge upon the optic chiasm, causing various degrees of defects in the visual fields. These pituitary tumors usually develop about 3 years after adrenalectomy or later. Some surgeons routinely administer 4000 rads of radiation to the pituitary after bilateral adrenalectomy for Cushing's disease to diminish the risk of hyperpigmentation if the patient has not had pituitary irradiation prior to adrenalectomy. We have not employed radiation in this manner. Once a tumor has developed it must be treated either by radiation or by surgical removal or, more recently, by experimental bromocriptine. The question still remains whether these late pituitary tumors are enlargements of tumors that were present originally or represent the development of a new tumor secondary to excision of the adrenal glands.

Adrenocortical Atrophy

If Cushing's syndrome is due to a functioning adrenal cortical tumor on one side, the other adrenal may have become atrophic owing to the prolonged elevation of plasma cortisol. Careful replacement therapy must be given in these patients until it is certain that the remaining adrenal is able to provide the amount of cortisol necessary for health. Malignant tumors secreting ACTH ectopically are not often cured by any means available at the present time.

VIRILISM, FEMINIZATION, AND OTHER ADRENOCORTICAL DISORDERS

To recapitulate, the outer zone of the adrenal cortex, the zona glomerulosa, secretes primarily aldosterone. The middle zone, the zona fasciculata, secretes cortisol, and the inner zone, the zona reticularis, secretes both androgens and estrogens. There may be overlap between the secretory capacities of the three layers, but predominantly they secrete the hormones as indicated.

VIRILISM (ADRENOGENITAL SYNDROME AND MASCULINIZATION)

Excessive secretion of androgens by the zona reticularis causes masculinization.

Virilism in Children

The onset of virilism may occur in intrauterine life, at birth, or at any time later in life. In men, of course, such changes are hardly noticeable, but in females the changes can be very striking. If the condition begins in childhood, it is usually but not always due to adrenocortical hyperplasia with excessive secretion of androgens. If the condition begins in adult life, it is commonly due to a tumor, often malignant.

The child with ambiguous genitalia is seen frequently in pediatric practice. It is a most difficult problem to manage clinically because of its etiologic complexity and because the assignment of gender role depends on the outcome of the clinical studies. The diagnostic evidence is usually obtained in an atmosphere charged with emotion, and few clinical situations are more taxing on the total skills of a physician than this one. He must establish the optimal biologic and psychological sex of rearing for the child, make decisions under the duress of parental pressure for immediate action, and allay the apprehensions, guilt, and shame of the parents while counseling them to avoid situations that might later embarrass the child.

It is not safe to diagnose the underlying cause of ambiguity or predict the biologic suitability of a given gender role solely on the basis of the medical history and the appearance of the genitalia, nor is it advisable to hasten gender assignment by means of "emergency" laparotomy prior to adequate laboratory investigation because surgery can be hazardous in some cases (*e.g.*, salt-losing congenital adrenocortical hyperplasia).

The physician can make a working diagnosis in most cases after completion of the medical history, physical examination, and sex chromatin analysis of cells from the buccal epithelium. The newborn with ambiguous genitalia who has a positive buccal sex chromatin smear must be considered to have congenital adrenocortical hyperplasia until proved otherwise, and the possibility of a sodium-losing crisis should be anticipated. Most commonly, the infant with a positive sex chromatin finding will be female, but in rare circumstances it may be a male, and it is now more appropriate to search for a Y chromosome as well. For comparison, two children, one with virilism and the other with Cushing's syndrome, are presented in Figure 20-33. The difference between the two syndromes is striking in the fully developed case.

There are four clinical types of virilism: (1) simple virilism; (2) virilism and sodium loss; (3) virilism and hypertension; and (4) the 3-β-hydroxysteroid dehydrogenase defect. In all cases the main characteristic of the disorder is an excessive production of adrenal androgens. This is due to defects in various enzymes, and the effect of the enzyme deficiency is a reduction in the secretion of cortisol. In a compensatory attempt to supply the physiological requirements for cortisol, the pituitary secretes large amounts of ACTH. The resulting overstimulation of the adrenal cortex causes an excessive production of androgens with consequent virilization. In turn, this can cause incomplete differentiation of the external genitalia in the female fetus (hermaphrodism) and, after birth, progressive virilization in both sexes (Fig. 20-34). This is a complex problem and requires a team approach. Nonetheless, the administration of adequate amounts of cortisone will supply the need for cortisol, and it will abolish the excessive secretion of ACTH by the anterior pituitary, resulting in regression of masculinization. However, the pre-existing changes in the external genitalia, including enlargement of the clitoris, may not regress completely and will usually require surgical intervention eventually. Again, it is most important to study the individual child carefully and to decide on the basis of the facts which gender assignment will be most appropriate for that child. The female child with ambiguous external genitalia may have a normal uterus, tubes, and ovaries.

Genetics of Virilizing Adrenocortical Hyperplasia

Virilizing adrenocortical hyperplasia occurs frequently in siblings, the female showing pseudohermaphrodism and the male macrogenitosomia praecox (Fig. 20-34). It appears that the enzymatic defect in congenital adrenocortical hyperplasia is a familial autosomal recessive hereditary disease. When two heterozygous carriers of the trait marry, as is the case with parents of affected patients, the chances that their offspring will be affected are 1:3.

Virilism in Adults

In contrast to the virilization in the newborn and older children, which is usually due to adrenocortical hyperplasia but occasionally to a tumor that may be malignant, the onset of virilization in adult life is usually caused by functioning adrenocortical tumor, often malignant. Again the basic problem is excessive production of androgens by the adrenal or, rarely, by an adrenal rest in the ovary; at times the culprit is a true ovarian tumor, the arrhenoblastoma. Appropriate investigation is directed toward identification of the nature of the pathologic lesion causing excessive production of androgens. The investigative studies are the same as those described for Cushing's syndrome; of these, CT scans are becoming perhaps the leading single radiologic investigative method. When there is no neoplasia, virilism is compatible with essentially normal longevity, in contrast to Cushing's syndrome, but most often a neoplasm represents the primary lesion. Once a nonmalignant neoplasm is removed surgically, most of the masculinizing features will regress, including enlargement of the clitoris to some extent, absence of female fat distribution, balding, facial hair, and other features. Unfortunately, if a deep voice has been well established, it may not return completely to normal. Curiously, the appearance of a masculinizing tumor in males has been very rare in our experience. Of course, the physical signs would not be as apparent in the adult man, but the presence of a malignant tumor certainly should have been noted. Nonetheless, adult men do have malignant adrenocortical tumors, and these tumors do at times secrete excessive amounts of androgen as well as estrogen and cortisol.

Fig. 20-33. (*Left*) Virilism due to increased androgen secretion in young girl. Note enlarged clitoris. (*Right*) Cushing's disease due to excessive corticoids in young girl. In contrast to late developing congenital virilism, which may be compatible with normal longevity, Cushing's disease represents a diffuse metabolic disorder that commonly may ultimately cause death unless adequately treated. (Albright F: Cushing's syndrome. Harvey Lect, 38:123, 1942-1943)

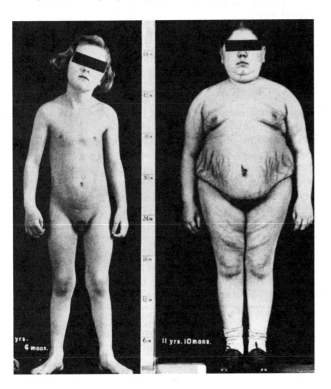

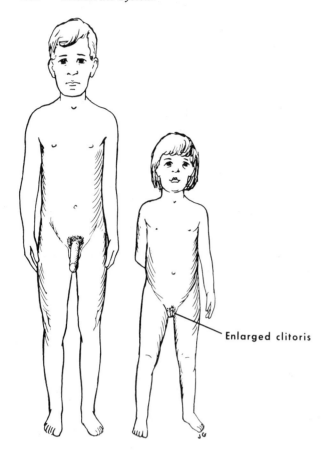

Enlarged clitoris

Fig. 20-34. Siblings, ages 6 and 4 years, with congenital adrenal hyperplasia. (Moynihan PC: Virilism and feminization in children. In Hardy JD [ed]: Rhoads Textbook of Surgery, 5th ed. Philadelphia, J B Lippincott, 1977)

FEMINIZATION

Feminization in a young girl could be due to a feminizing true tumor of the ovary, the granulosa cell tumor. Feminizing tumors of the adrenal cortex are rare. These tumors, when seen, almost always occur in males, although they sometimes occur in young females. A feminizing tumor in an adult woman would not of course present the same striking changes that would be observed with development of a feminizing tumor in a man, and thus some benign tumors in women may escape detection. One of the best surveys of feminizing adrenocortical tumors in the male was that of Gabrilove et al., who reviewed 52 patients from the literature. Gynecomastia was present in 98%, a palpable tumor in 58%, atrophy of the testes in 52%, and additional evidence of feminization in various other frequencies (Table 20-6).

The differential diagnosis consists of identifying and excluding the various possible causes of gynecomastia in the adult man. Urinary estrogen levels are usually markedly elevated and are higher in patients with carcinoma than in those with a benign adenoma. Although the tumors reported were mainly feminizing tumors, a mixed clinical picture was also observed in some patients, including aspects of Cushing's syndrome (Gabrilove et al.). The cells most often resemble those of the zona reticularis, as would be expected.

Surgical removal of a benign tumor is followed by a good prognosis. Unfortunately, most of these tumors are

TABLE 20-6 FEMINIZING ADRENOCORTICAL TUMORS IN THE MALE: CLINICAL FINDINGS IN 52 PATIENTS

SIGN OR SYMPTOM	%
Gynecomastia	98
Palpable tumor	58
Atrophy of testis	52
Diminished libido and/or potency	48
Pain at site of tumor	44
Tenderness of breast	42
Pigmentation of areolae	27
Obesity	27
Feminizing hair change	23
Atrophy of the penis	20
Hypertension	16
Increasing skin pigmentation	12

(Gabrilove JL, Sharma DC, Wotiz HH et al: Feminizing adrenocortical tumors in the male. Medicine 44:37, 1965. [Modified from Scott HW JR, Rhamy RK: The pituitary and adrenals. In Sabiston DC Jr (ed): Davis-Christopher Textbook of Surgery, 2nd ed. Philadelphia, W B Saunders, 1972])

malignant, and distant metastases are common by the time the diagnosis has been established.

ADRENOCORTICAL TUMORS AND CYSTS: FURTHER COMMENT

It has been pointed out that adrenocortical tumors, especially carcinomas, may secrete several different types of hormones, thus producing a mixed clinical picture. In addition, some adrenocortical tumors have little or no function. It is probable that most adrenocortical tumors do function to some extent but at so low a level that it is not clinically detectable, especially in males. In fact, some adrenocortical tumors are found unexpectedly at operation, and this is also true of the rare adrenal cysts. Among the nonfunctioning adrenocortical tumors is the curious myelolipoma of the adrenal gland.

Adrenocortical tumors should be excised; if they are benign, the prognosis is excellent. Otherwise, a combination of surgery, radiation, and chemotherapy is indicated, but the outlook in such cases is often poor.

ADRENOCORTICAL INSUFFICIENCY

Acute Insufficiency

A variety of circumstances may give rise to acute adrenocortical insufficiency. These include hemorrhage into the adrenals, trauma, overwhelming sepsis, operative stress on adrenals largely replaced by a metastatic tumor, and, of course, operation on the adrenal glands. The condition is often not recognized, but it should be considered in the differential diagnosis of refractory hypotension, confusion, tachycardia, hyperthermia, and reduced urine output. If acute adrenocortical insufficiency is even suspected, a therapeutic trial of hydrocortisone IV drip (100 mg/6 hr) together with sodium chloride solution and dextrose, should be started immediately. To wait for a chemical diagnosis could be too late, and there are no lasting effects from short-term steroid dosage of 24 hr to 48 hr.

Chronic Insufficiency (Addison's Disease)

Chronic adrenocortical insufficiency is most often caused by prolonged autoimmune disease with resulting adreno-

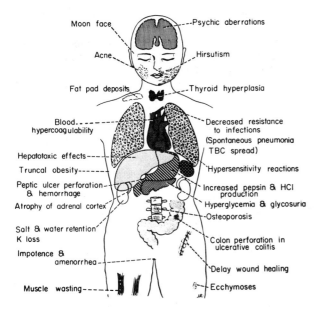

Fig. 20-35. Undesirable side-effects of prolonged steroid therapy. Side-effects of corticosteroid therapy usually present excessive manifestations of normal potentialities. (Hardy JD, Meena AL: Hazards and safeguards in steroid therapy. Surg Clin North Am 37:1425, 1957)

cortical atrophy but may also be due to corticosteroid therapy, metastatic tumor, pituitary (ACTH) insufficiency, or infections (including tuberculosis). Actually, this condition is seldom seen in surgical practice, but this fact makes its occurrence even more hazardous, because it may be entirely unsuspected preoperatively and may result in all the manifestations of acute adrenocortical insufficiency when the stress of anesthesia and operation is imposed.

An appropriate plan of management should be followed after the condition is suspected. A drip of 100 mg of hydrocortisone in 500 ml of dextrose–saline is begun intravenously empirically at once, and this dosage, along with other supportive measures, is continued for 6-hr periods

until the acute emergency situation has passed. Then more accurate laboratory diagnosis should be carried out and the patient placed on appropriate long-term adrenocortical replacement therapy.

Complications of Adrenocortical Therapy

As indicated previously, there are few if any lasting side-effects from 24 hr to 72 hr of acute corticosteroid therapy, but chronic therapy, representing hypercortisol dosage, will produce the undesirable side-effects of Cushing's syndrome (Fig. 20-35). Therapy should be limited to actual need.

DISORDERS OF ADRENAL MEDULLA AND OTHER CHROMAFFIN TISSUE

PHEOCHROMOCYTOMA

The term pheochromocytoma is commonly given to a functioning tumor that secretes catecholamines. The tumor may lie within an adrenal gland or it may arise from the sympathetic chain anywhere from the neck to the wall of the urinary bladder. Tumors arising in the adrenal gland usually secrete both epinephrine and norepinephrine, whereas those lying along the sympathetic chains secrete primarily norepinephrine. Some tumors with more immature cells, such as neuroblastoma, may secrete preponderantly dopamine (Fig. 20-36). Therefore, there is some advantage in reserving the term pheochromocytoma for tumors that arise in the adrenal gland and produce increased secretion of both norepinephrine and epinephrine; the term paraganglioma is applied to tumors that arise outside the adrenal gland and secrete primarily norepinephrine. A "nonchromaffin" paraganglioma that may be nonfunctioning may occur also. In the subsequent discussion the term pheochromocytoma will be used throughout.

Pheochromocytoma in the adult is usually benign; it is more often malignant in children. In children, the adrenal neuroblastoma, which also secretes catecholamines, is usually malignant. Not all pheochromocytomas secrete catecholamines.

Fig. 20-36. Synthesis of catecholamines. (Hume DM: Pheochromocytoma. In Astwood CB, Cassidy CE (eds): Clinical Endocrinology. II. New York, Grune & Stratton, 1968)

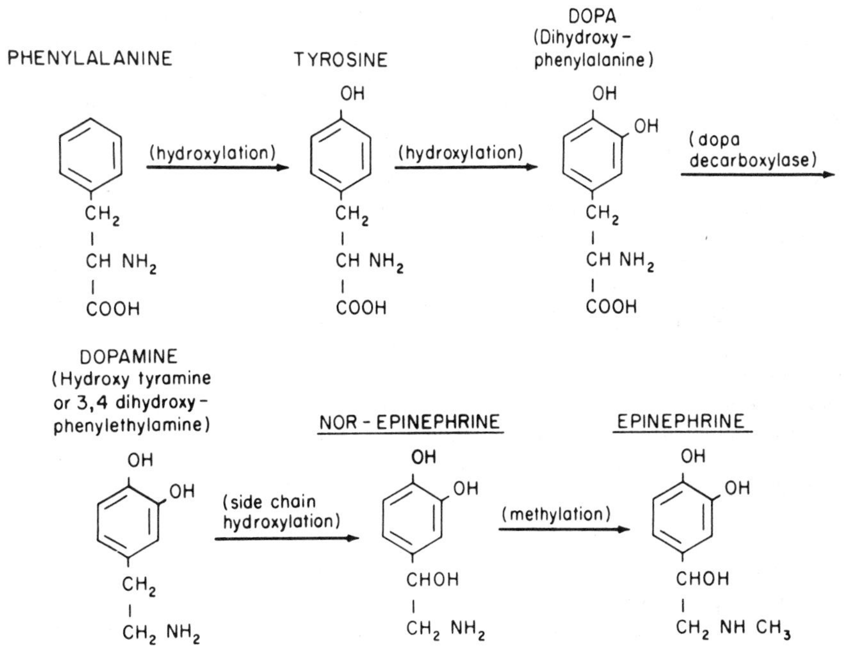

PHENYLALANINE $\xrightarrow{\text{(hydroxylation)}}$ TYROSINE $\xrightarrow{\text{(hydroxylation)}}$ DOPA (Dihydroxy–phenylalanine) $\xrightarrow{\text{(dopa decarboxylase)}}$

DOPAMINE (Hydroxy tyramine or 3,4 dihydroxy–phenylethylamine) $\xrightarrow{\text{(side chain hydroxylation)}}$ NOR-EPINEPHRINE $\xrightarrow{\text{(methylation)}}$ EPINEPHRINE

PHEOCHROMOCYTOMA

Etiology	Excessive catecholamine production by chromaffin tumor either in the adrenal medulla or anywhere along the sympathetic chain from the neck to the urinary bladder
Dx	Paroxysmal or sustained hypertension Varied symptoms of nervousness, tremor, sweating, and so on Measurement of metanephrine and normetanephrine and VMA in urine Localization of tumor by CT scan
Rx	Excision of tumor after 7 to 14 days treatment with up to 50 mg phenoxybenzamine (Dibenzyline) orally every 6 hr to dilate previously constricted vasculature and allow repletion of plasma volume. Prognosis good in absence of malignancy

PATHOLOGY AND PATHOPHYSIOLOGY

Pathology

Historical Notes. As early as 1893, Manasse and others had described certain characteristics of pheochromocytomas, but it was not until 1922 that Labbe, Tinel, and Doumer recorded the first complete study of a classic case. They published a report of a woman, 28 years of age, who suffered from violent attacks of vomiting associated with tremor, chilliness, and palpitation. The blood pressure was highly variable but usually elevated. The patient died of acute pulmonary edema, and autopsy revealed a tumor just above the left adrenal gland. The first case of paroxysmal hypertension diagnosed during life was that reported by Vaquez, Donzelot, and Gerandel in 1929. In 1927, Charles Mayo explored the abdomen of a 30-year-old woman who had attacks of paroxysmal hypertension associated with dyspnea, headache, tachycardia, and vomiting. A tumor intimately associated with the left adrenal gland was removed, and the patient was cured. In 1937, Beer, King, and Prinzmetal demonstrated preoperatively in an animal preparation a pressor substance that appeared in a patient's blood during crises. Following adrenalectomy with removal of the tumor, this effect was abolished.

Malignant Potential. Pheochromocytomas have often been characterized as physiologically malignant but (usually) histologically benign. In adult patients only about 10% of these tumors are histologically malignant and thus may metastasize. In adults malignant pheochromocytoma is more commonly found in males, whereas in children it is more common in females. Many pheochromocytomas appear malignant histologically, even showing venous invasion at times, without ever subsequently demonstrating a true malignant potential by metastasizing. We have treated such a patient who had tumor extension into the veins of Batson along the spinal column. However, this patient has survived, with only mild hypertension, for years. Thus, the only fully acceptable criterion of malignancy with this tumor is definite evidence of metastasis to sites unusual for adrenal tissue, such as the liver or lung. In addition, the identification of such distant metastases is essential for the definitive diagnosis of malignancy because these tumors may be bilateral or multifocal, and a tumor of chromaffin tissue at another site along the sympathetic chain could represent another primary tumor and not a metastasis.

Recurrence of a functioning tumor following its excision can usually be identified by serial measurement of the catecholamines and their metabolites in the urine. Following excision of the original tumor, the urinary catecholamine values may have declined to normal, only to rise again with recurrence or the development and growth of metastases elsewhere. The metastases may represent more primitive cell types than the primary tumor and may now produce the metabolic products of dopamine in addition to those of epinephrine and norepinephrine.

In contrast to Cushing's syndrome, for which adrenocortical hyperplasia is the most common etiology, hyperplasia of the adrenal medulla causing a catecholamine excess occurs with extreme rarity, to our knowledge; abnormal hyperfunction is virtually always due to a tumor.

Location. Approximately 85% of pheochromocytomas are found in the adrenal glands themselves, with the right adrenal involved somewhat more often than the left. Both adrenals are involved in approximately 10% of cases, with a somewhat higher incidence of bilaterality in children. The extra-adrenal sites along the sympathetic chains include the neck (2%), thorax (12%), upper abdomen (43%), the organs of Zuckerkandl in the region of the inferior mesenteric artery (29%), the more distal regions of the posterior abdominal wall and pelvis (2%), and the urinary bladder (12%). A striking feature of pheochromocytoma in the wall of the bladder is that a paroxysmal attack may be set off by micturition. Pheochromocytoma has even been found inside the pericardium, and hibernoma has masqueraded as pheochromocytoma.

Familial Incidence and Neurocutaneous Syndromes. The pheochromocytoma is now recognized as a prominent participant in the continuously expanding complex of genetically determined or at least genetically influenced polyglandular syndromes, otherwise characterized as "multiple endocrine adenopathy" (MEA) or "multiple endocrine neoplasia" (MEN). Perhaps the two most striking familial circumstances are those seen in the patient with von Recklinghausen's neurofibromatosis (approximately 5% of these patients also have pheochromocytoma) and MEA II (Sipple's syndrome), in which medullary carcinoma of the thyroid, pheochromocytoma, and, at times, parathyroid adenoma may all be present. When there is a strong familial relationship, pheochromocytoma is inherited by simple mendelian dominance with varying but usually high penetrance. Familial pheochromocytomas are different from sporadic pheochromocytomas in that they are more apt to be bilateral or multiple, and are somewhat more likely to be extra-adrenal or even extra-abdominal. Familial pheochromocytomas affect children more often than adults, and there is a definite predilection for the organs of Zuckerkandl in familial cases. Familial adrenal pheochromocytomas are more apt to be on the left, whereas sporadic adrenal pheochromocytomas are more apt to be on the right, as noted previously.

In addition to Sipple's syndrome (MEA II) and von Recklinghausen's multiple neurofibromatosis, pheochromocytoma may be associated with cafe-au-lait spots, tuberous sclerosis (Bourneville's disease), meningofacial angiomatosis (Sturge-Weber's disease), and still other conditions.

Pheochromocytomas Associated With Other Endocrine Tumors. It has been noted that pheochromocytoma may be associated with functioning tumors of other endocrine organs. The relationship to Sipple's syndrome has been cited, wherein pheochromocytoma and medullary thyroid carcinoma are associated, often with a functioning parathyroid tumor. The C-cells of the thyroid, which secrete calcitonin, and the adrenal medulla are derived from the ectoderm, whereas the rest of the thyroid and the adrenal cortex are derived from the entoderm. In Sipple's syndrome the pheochromocytomas are frequently bilateral (about 65%), and there is a strong familial history of pheochromocytoma (35%) and of medullary carcinoma of the thyroid (35%). The inclusion of parathyroid adenoma in Sipple's syndrome has come into fairly general use. Finally, pheochromocytomas have been reported occasionally in association with most of the commonly recognized endocrine organs.

Pathophysiology

The pathophysiology of pheochromocytoma is produced by the excessive secretion of catecholamines. Norepinephrine is the hormonal mediator of sympathetic neurovascular tone, whereas acetylcholine is liberated at the ends of parasympathetic nerve fibers.

Metabolism of Catecholamines. The three catecholamines that are found in normal human tissues are dopamine, norepinephrine, and epinephrine (see Fig. 20-36). Epinephrine and norepinephrine are more germane to this discussion of pheochromocytoma. Again, epinephrine is elaborated principally in the adrenal gland, with norepinephrine (and dopamine) being released at the ends of the postganglionic fibers of the sympathetic nervous system and in the central nervous system as well.

Norepinephrine is a relatively pure α stimulator, though in large amounts it can also produce certain β effects. Epinephrine has a mixed effect, but it is a much more potent α stimulus than is norepinephrine, though it does have strong β stimulation as well. Dopamine, widely used recently in the clinical management of various postoperative hypotensive states and thus threatened oliguria, produces a strong cardiac β stimulation and at the same time a specific renal vasodilatation to increase urine output. Thus, whether the tumor is producing epinephrine or norepinephrine or both, as is commonly the case when the adrenal medulla is involved, the clinical findings are similar. All three primary catecholamines are found in the chromaffin tissue of the sympathetic nervous system, which includes the adrenal medulla.

Hypermetabolism. The patient with pheochromocytoma frequently exhibits evidence of hypermetabolism, including a significant elevation of the basal metabolic rate (BMR) (Table 20-7). This is true whether the principal hormone being overproduced is norepinephrine or the more metabolically active epinephrine. In earlier times, when the BMR was the principal test performed in determining hyperthyroidism, patients with pheochromocytoma at times underwent thyroidectomy with the mistaken diagnosis of hyperthyroidism. At present, the modern laboratory tests of thyroid function should prevent this potentially disastrous mistake in diagnosis. Death may occur when a patient with pheochromocytoma is subjected to an unrelated operation. The patient with chronic pheochromocytoma is usually thin because of the increased metabolism stimulated by the elevated level of circulating catecholamines.

The functioning pheochromocytoma can also produce hyperglycemia, glycosuria, and other suggestive evidence of diabetes mellitus. Thus, pheochromocytoma should be

TABLE 20-7   SYMPTOMS AND SIGNS OF PHEOCHROMOCYTOMA

	% (APPROXIMATE)	
	Adult	Child
Symptoms		
Persistent hypertension	65	92
Paroxysmal hypertension	30	8
Headache	80	81
Sweating	70	68
Palpitation, nervousness	60	34
Pallor of face	40	27
Tremor	40	
Nausea	30	56
Weakness, fatigue	25	27
Weight loss	15	44
Abdominal or chest pain	15	35
Dyspnea	15	16
Visual changes	10	44
Constipation	5	8
Raynaud's phenomenon	5	
Convulsions	3	23
Polydipsia, polyuria		25
Puffy, red, cyanotic hands		11
Signs		
BMR over +20%	50	83
Fasting blood sugar over 120 mg/100 ml	40	40
Glycosuria	10	3
Eyeground changes	30	77

(Hume DM: Pheochromocytoma. *In* Astwood EB, Cassidy CE (eds): Clinical Endocrinology, II. New York, Grune & Stratton, 1968)

considered in the patient who appears to have atypical hyperthyroidism or atypical diabetes mellitus.

Hypertension. An elevated arterial blood pressure, either paroxysmal or sustained, is perhaps the most common clinical finding that leads ultimately to the diagnosis of functioning pheochromocytoma (Table 20-7). Approximately 90% of patients with a functioning pheochromocytoma will have an elevated blood pressure at one time or another. The most dramatic type is that in which the patient periodically experiences hypertension, precipitated by a wide variety of stimuli including palpation of the abdomen, defecation, micturition, certain positional movements, and many other even relatively minor stimuli. The hypertension is accompanied by any or most of the symptoms shown in Table 20-7. Particularly prominent, in our experience, have been headache, sweating, palpitation, nervousness, circumoral pallor, and tremor. The severe attack may produce dyspnea due to pulmonary edema secondary to acute left ventricular failure. The patient may actually die in such an attack, from a stroke or acute left ventricular failure. Paroxysmal attacks usually last only a few minutes but may last several hours.

If the tumor persists long enough, the hypertension may eventually become chronic and continuously sustained, owing in part to renal damage. The patient may then no longer have the paroxysmal attacks, although paroxysmal attacks can be mounted upon an already chronically elevated blood pressure. Hypertension may be produced whether the patient is secreting an excess of norepinephrine or epinephrine, or both, and the signs and symptoms shown by the patient in an acute attack closely resemble those produced by an epinephrine or norepinephrine drip.

There are other conditions that may produce paroxysmal hypertension. These include anxiety states, eclampsia, and malignant carcinoid crisis. Hemorrhage into the pheochromocytoma may occur, the so-called adrenal apoplexy, and can produce a severe hypertension that may be followed by shock and sudden death. A pheochromocytoma may also present as an acute intra-abdominal emergency.

Pheochromocytoma During Pregnancy. The occurrence of pheochromocytoma during pregnancy poses special problems. At one time the incidence of death for both the mother and the fetus at the time of delivery was reported to be as high as 50%. However, with current methods of α and β adrenergic receptor blockade through delivery and the early postpartum period, the mortality rate for both fetus and mother should be vastly reduced. With this type of drug management it should now be possible to allow delivery and then to remove the pheochromocytoma electively in the late postpartum period. On the other hand, if the presence of the pheochromocytoma is established early in pregnancy, the wisest course would be to prepare the patient with phenoxybenzamine (Dibenzyline) and then remove the tumor, preferably in the middle trimester.

The symptoms shown by the pregnant patient with pheochromocytoma are not particularly different from those shown by other patients. However, the presence of hypertension may lead to a diagnosis of pre-eclampsia or eclampsia unless the urine is carefully screened for the increased metabolites of catecholamines. The time of delivery is particularly hazardous.

DIAGNOSIS

History

The major elements of the history have already been given and are summarized in Tables 20-7 and 20-8. Basically, the patient has hypertension either paroxysmally or chronically, as well as other symptoms already outlined that suggest the possibility of a functioning chromaffin tumor.

Physical Examination

The physical examination may present few if any remarkable features. Of course, should the physician see the patient during an attack, the striking signs and symptoms should be virtually diagnostic, though there are other conditions that can produce such attacks including carcinoid crises. The history of attacks in a patient with von Recklinghausen's neurofibromatosis should always suggest the possibility of a catecholamine-secreting tumor. As stated previously, the patient with pheochromocytoma is usually thin. If rarely the patient with a pheochromocytoma is obese, the hypertension and other metabolic evidence of catecholamine excess will usually prove to have been paroxysmal. Another physical finding of some value is the fact that rarely will the veins of the back of the hand be dilated and distended in a patient who has a functioning pheochromocytoma. This chronic venous constriction results in a contracted blood volume. The reduced blood volume may permit the development of hypotension following resection of a functioning tumor because the previously constricted vascular bed will now be dilated. This hypovolemia can be corrected

TABLE 20-8	SYMPTOM COMPLEXES OF PHEOCHROMOCYTOMA

1. Symptom-free patients, with pheochromocytoma an incidental or accidental finding
2. Symptom-free patients who die suddenly after minor trauma
3. Patients with typical attacks
4. Patients with sustained hypertension indistinguishable clinically from essential or renal vascular hypertension
5. "Diabetics," with or without hypertension
6. Patients with headaches, fever, and nausea, or the metabolic changes of pheochromocytoma, without either sustained or paroxysmal hypertension
7. Patients who present with "hyperthyroidism," especially if BMR does not fall with treatment. RAI and PBI are normal, and patient has hypertension
8. Patients with unexplained shock during anesthesia or minor trauma
9. Patients with cardiac irregularities, tachycardia, or arrest with induction of anesthesia or beginning of operation
10. Patients whose symptoms simulate an acute anxiety attack
11. Patients who have attacks when voiding (occasionally occurs with pheochromocytoma in bladder)

(Hume DM: Pheochromocytoma in the adult and in the child. Am J Surg 99:458, 1960)

preoperatively by preparing the patient with phenoxybenzamine over a period of days to relieve the vasoconstriction and allow the blood volume to expand spontaneously.

Rarely, the pheochromocytoma can be palpated, which may set off a paroxysmal attack. Because abdominal palpation may precipitate an attack even though no tumor may actually be palpated, this maneuver should be exercised with caution. Should an attack be precipitated, it will usually respond promptly to an intravenous drip of phentolamine (Regitine).

Diagnostic Studies

Roentgenographic Procedures. Various roentgen examinations can be useful in the localization of a pheochromocytoma, whether in the adrenal gland itself or elsewhere along the sympathetic chain from the neck to the urinary bladder (Fig. 20-37). A mass may be demonstrated in the chest or in the region of the adrenal gland, using both plain films and tomograms. An intravenous pyelogram may show displacement of the kidney by a pheochromocytoma within the adrenal gland itself, or it may show displacement of the ureter. Other procedures include aortography and transcaval venography.

More recently, however, the CT scan has virtually replaced the invasive studies. Van Heerden and colleagues have reported recent experience at the Mayo Clinic. These authors analyzed 106 patients who had undergone operation for pheochromocytoma from 1971 through 1980. Twelve patients had a pheochromocytoma as a manifestation of the MEA II syndrome. Twenty patients were found to have

PHEOCHROMOCYTOMA

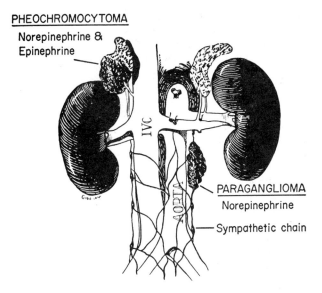

Norepinephrine &
Epinephrine

PARAGANGLIOMA
Norepinephrine

Sympathetic chain

Fig. 20-37. Pheochromocytoma located in an adrenal gland commonly results in increased urinary excretion of both epinephrine and norepinephrine. The extra-adrenal pheochromocytoma (sometimes characterized as a paraganglioma) elaborates a preponderance of norepinephrine, often with little or no epinephrine. These facts can be of some assistance in determining the possible location of a functioning catechol-secreting tumor. (Hardy JD: Tumors of the adrenal glands. Surg Clin North Am 42:545, 1962)

extra-adrenal paraganglioma. Fifteen patients had malignant tumors, and eight of these tumors were encountered in a group with extra-adrenal lesions. The authors reported that in recent years nephrotomography, selective angiography, and venous sampling had been essentially abandoned in favor of CT scan. With an accuracy of more than 90%, the CT scan represented the major step forward in the overall management of pheochromocytoma patients during the past decade. Incidentally, with a positive CT scan and measurement of urinary metanephrines and vanillylmandelic acid (VMA), which had accuracy rates of 95% and 89% respectively, they found that little else was needed for the effective diagnosis and lateralization of these functioning tumors. Adrenal medullary scanning is also becoming more useful.

Laboratory Studies

Whereas the first step in the diagnosis of a pheochromocytoma is to suspect that the lesion may exist, the next step is to demonstrate conclusively by plasma and urinary measurements of catecholamines and their metabolic products that the secretion of these substances is elevated. The third step is to identify the location of the tumor, whether in the adrenal glands or at some other position along the sympathetic chain from the neck to the urinary bladder. As indicated earlier, if the hormone being secreted in excess amounts is largely norepinephrine, the tumor is somewhat more likely to be found in an extra-adrenal location, whereas if both epinephrine and norephinephrine excretion are substantially elevated, the tumor is, in our experience, likely to be found in the adrenal gland itself. Again, the determination of the urinary metanephrines and VMA are the most commonly used and sensitive diagnostic aids. Fractionation of the urinary and plasma catecholamine levels will further increase the diagnostic accuracy for pheochromocytoma. Normal levels of urinary excretion of these

substances are presented in Table 20-9. We have yet to encounter a patient with a functioning pheochromocytoma whose urinary excretion of catecholamines and their metabolic products was not elevated in a 24-hr urine sample.

Various other laboratory studies may be performed, but these are the most important ones used at present. Functioning neuroblastomas other than pheochromocytoma may also secrete small amounts of catecholamines, as may the many small neurogenic tumors of the patient with extensive von Recklinghausen's neurofibromatosis or the child with a neuroblastoma, which may show renewed catecholamine secretion in the urine upon the recurrence of a malignant tumor or from unresected metastases. However, these non-pheochromocytoma neurogenic tumors rarely secrete catecholamines to the extent that the pheochromocytoma can and frequently does achieve.

In an emergency situation, measurement of either plasma catecholamine levels or the rate of urinary catecholamine secretion over a period of just a few hours may be sufficient to afford the diagnosis of a functioning catecholamine tumor. The differential diagnosis of pheochromocytoma consists of the exclusion of other conditions that can cause hypertension such as coarctation of the aorta, renal ischemia, primary aldosteronism, Cushing's disease, and hyperthyroidism. Essential hypertension comprises the largest segment of patients with hypertension, and this hypertension probably has some renal basis in most of these patients. Massive retroperitoneal hemorrhage or peptic ulceration may occasionally present with pheochromocytoma. As mentioned previously, other causes of confusing diagnoses in patients with a functioning pheochromocytoma include diagnosed hyperthyroidism, due to the excessive metabolic rate; diabetes mellitus, due to glycosuria; some type of malignancy because of extensive weight loss; and pre-eclampsia or eclampsia in the pregnant woman.

MANAGEMENT OF PHEOCHROMOCYTOMA

The definitive management of pheochromocytoma is surgical resection, but it is important to prepare the patient adequately for operation. In earlier times the diagnosis of pheochromocytoma was considered a major emergency, and the operation was performed as quickly as possible. However, with the present availability of phentolamine (Regitine) and propranolol for emergencies and phenoxybenzamine (Dibenzyline) for more long-term preparation, operation should be delayed until the phenoxybenzamine has been administered by mouth for approximately 1 week to 10 days. This preoperative preparation will achieve adequate dilatation of the previously constricted vasculature and subsequent repletion of the previously contracted plasma volume by the normal physiological processes and will avoid the need for blood tranfusion at operation.

TABLE 20-9 APPROXIMATE NORMAL LEVELS OF URINARY CATECHOLAMINES AND THEIR METABOLITES

METABOLITE	NORMAL EXCRETION RATE
Epinephrine	0–20 µg/24 hr
Norepinephrine	10–70 µg/24 hr
Metanephrine Normetanephrine }	<1.3 mg/24 hr
Vanillylmandelic acid (VMA)	1.8–7.0 mg/24 hr

α-ADRENERGIC RECEPTOR BLOCKADE

Both phentolamine and phenoxybenzamine have been used orally for prolonged or chronic management of pheochromocytoma. In acute emergencies, intravenous phentolamine can be very useful, although it does have certain hazards. The oral dosage of phenoxybenzamine may reach approximately 50 mg every 6 hr, beginning initially with 10 mg every 6 hr. Even larger doses may be used if they are well tolerated, but the patient's condition must be followed carefully. Although many symptoms are relieved, blood pressure may not be satisfactorily controlled. Oral administration of phentolamine is not always effective owing to erratic absorption and transient action, but it has proved useful in some instances when other therapy has failed. Phenoxybenzamine has been found by us and others to be very useful in achieving a chronic reduction in blood pressure in patients with unresectable pheochromocytoma.

It is important to give phenoxybenzamine in divided doses each day for about 7 to 10 days prior to operation. It will be recalled that approximately 25% of blood volume is in the arterial tree, whereas perhaps 75% of blood volume is in the venous system and capillaries. These have been chronically constricted by catecholamines from the tumor, but vasoconstriction is slowly relaxed by Dibenzyline, permitting restoration of a normal effective blood volume before operation. Preoperative preparation with phenoxybenzamine has also diminished the incidence of hypotension immediately following resection of pheochromocytoma.

β-ADRENERGIC RECEPTOR BLOCKADE

Further, the β receptor blocking agent propranolol may be used before, during, and following operation for management of β effects, particularly tachycardia and arrhythmias. However, this drug has certain hazards, especially when the dosage is excessive. The dosage recommended for effective preoperative adrenergic receptor blockade is approximately 20 mg to 50 mg per day by mouth in several divided doses and increased as tolerated.

Again, for emergency management of acute paroxysmal attacks, an infusion of phentolamine is very useful, although occasionally complications have accompanied its use. It is a sympatholytic agent.

THE OPERATION

Anesthetic Management

The potentially serious complications of a pheochromocytoma crisis during operation are now largely avoided by preoperative treatment with phenoxybenzamine and the use of a phentolamine drip during surgery if needed. Although arrhythmias may be controlled with propranolol, we have usually employed a lidocaine drip for this purpose. If propranolol is used, it should be administered only after an α blockade has been established, either with several days of phenoxybenzamine therapy preoperatively or with a phentolamine drip at operation.

The anesthetic agent to be employed will depend upon the preference of the anesthesiologist. We have used halothane without difficulty. Diazepam (Valium) and narcotics such as morphine have proved useful and safe, with succinylcholine for relaxation.

Operative Technique and Problems

The major problems met during and immediately following the operation are precipitation of a paroxysmal hypertensive attack when the tumor is manipulated during operation, and development of severe hypotension following removal of the tumor. Fortunately, both of these complications have now been essentially eliminated by the use of phenoxybenzamine for 7 to 10 days preoperatively. If marked hypertension should occur during manipulation of the tumor, a phentolamine drip should be instituted, and this will usually prove effective in controlling the blood pressure. The postoperative hypotension that was once a puzzling and serious problem has been largely abolished with preoperative drug therapy that dilates the vasculature, especially the veins, and allows the body to restore a normal effective circulating blood volume.

The actual technical removal of a pheochromocytoma usually presents little difficulty, especially if it is located on the left side. The general approaches to the adrenal glands were outlined earlier (see Anatomy). If the pheochromocytoma is on the right side, as it more frequently is in adults, and if a large tumor is involved, especially if it is malignant with surrounding invasion and is wedged between the right renal vessels and the vena cava just below the diaphragm, there can be a considerable hazard of blood loss from the vena cava if care is not exercised throughout the procedure. In this instance, much mobilization of the tumor must be achieved before its main blood supply, the short central vein entering the inferior vena cava beneath the liver, can be visualized and securely ligated and divided.

MANAGEMENT OF PHEOCHROMOCYTOMA IN PREGNANCY AND OF FUNCTIONING METASTASES

Pheochromocytoma in Pregnancy

The presence of pheochromocytoma during pregnancy, especially near term, constitutes a very serious risk to both the mother and the fetus at the time of delivery. Unfortunately, an erroneous diagnosis of pre-eclampsia is frequently made in these patients because eclampsia is more common obstetrically than is the rare pheochromocytoma. Nonetheless, several such patients have been referred to us from our obstetrical service over the years. The patient should be adequately treated with phenoxybenzamine and then operated upon prior to delivery. Preferably in some circumstances, the patient may be placed on phenoxybenzamine therapy and carried through labor and then operated upon later for the functioning adrenomedullary tumor.

Management of Functioning Metastases

From time to time a patient will be encountered who has distant metastases from a malignant pheochromocytoma. These metastases secrete catecholamines, often somewhat more immature in chemical structure than epinephrine and norephinephrine; at times dopamine is secreted. These patients may be managed satisfactorily with long-term phenoxybenzamine therapy, but if this proves ineffective or gradually less and less effective, phentolamine has proved helpful, with or without propranolol therapy, for the control of cardiac arrhythmias. α-Methyltyrosine may be helpful.

CONCLUDING COMMENT

Although it is a rare tumor, the pheochromocytoma has always been a subject of much interest because of the pervasive metabolic effects of the catecholamines that are secreted in excess by these tumors. Furthermore, because they are most frequently benign histologically, accurate diagnosis and removal of these lesions will usually restore the individual to health. Failure to discover the tumor may well lead to death from the complications of hypertension such as stroke, myocardial infarction, acute pulmonary edema, or renal failure.

BIBLIOGRAPHY

Adrenal Cortex

NELSON DH: The Adrenal Cortex: Physiological Function and Disease (Major Problems in Internal Medicine, Vol 18). Philadelphia, W B Saunders, 1980

Primary Aldosteronism

BARTTER FC, LIDDLE GW, DUNCAN LE et al: The regulation of aldosterone secretion in man: The role of fluid volume. J Clin Invest 35:1306, 1957

CONN JW: Primary aldosteronism, a new clinical syndrome. J Lab Clin Med 45:3, 1955

CONN JW: Plasma renin activity in primary aldosteronism. JAMA 190:222, 1964

GRUNDY HM, SIMPSON SA, TAIT UF: Isolation of a highly active mineralocorticoid from beef adrenal extract. Nature (London) 169:793, 1952

JAVADPOUR N, WOLTERING EA, BRENNAN MF: Adrenal neoplasms. Curr Probl Surg 17:1, 1980

MACKETT MC, CRANE ME, SMITH LL: Surgical management of aldosterone-producing adrenal adenomas: A review of 16 patients. Am J Surg 142:89, 1981

MELBY JC, SPARK RF, DOLE SL et al: Diagnosis and localization of aldosterone producing adenomas by adrenal vein catheterization. N Engl J Med 277:1050, 1967

SIMPSON SA, TAIT UF, WETTSTEIN A et al: Isolierung eines neuen kristallizierten Hormons aus Nebennieren mit besonders höher Wirksamkeit auf den Mineralstoffwechsel. Experientia 9:333, 1953

Cushing's Syndrome

CUSHING H: The basophil adenomas of the pituitary body and their clinical manifestations (pituitary basophilism). Bull Johns Hopkins Hosp 50:137, 1932

FELDMAN JM: Cushing's disease: Editorial: A hypothalamic flush. N Engl J Med 293:930, 1975

FRANKSSON C, BIRKE G, PLANTIN L-O: Adrenal autotransplantation in Cushing's syndrome. Acta Chir Scand 117:409, 1959

GIFFORD S, GUNDERSON JC: Cushing's disease as a psychosomatic disorder. A report of ten cases. Medicine 49:397, 1970

HARDY JD: Autotransplantation of adrenal remnant to thigh in Cushing's disease; preserving residual cortical activity while avoiding laparotomy. JAMA 185:134, 1963

HARDY JD: Surgical management of Cushing's syndrome with emphasis on adrenal autotransplantation. Ann Surg 188:290, 1978

ISAWA T et al: Cushing's syndrome caused by recurrent malignant bronchial carcinoid. Case report after 12 years' observation. Am Rev Resp Dis 108:1200, 1973

KANDALL-TAYLOR P: Hyperosmolar coma in Cushing's disease. Lancet 1:409, 1974

NELSON DH, SPRUNT JG: Pituitary Tumors Postadrenalectomy for Cushing's Syndrome. Proceedings of the Second International Congress of Endocrinology, London, 1964, p. 1053. (International Congress, Series 83). Excerpta Medica, 1965

ROBERTS AK, PYE IF: Acute Cushing's syndrome associated with thymic carcinoma. J R Coll Surg (Edinburgh) 19:32, 1974

SALASSA RM, LAWS ER JR, CARPENTER PC et al: Transsphenoidal removal of pituitary microadenomata in Cushing's disease. Mayo Clin Proc 53:24, 1978

SCOTT HW JR, FOSTER JH, RHAMY RK et al: Surgical management of adrenocortical tumors with Cushing's syndrome. Ann Surg 173:892, 1971

SPARK RF, BAKER R, BIENFANG DC et al: Bromocriptine reduces pituitary tumor size and hypersecretion. Requiem for pituitary surgery? JAMA 247:311, 1982

TEMPLE TE, JONED DJ JR, LIDDLE GW et al: Treatment of Cushing's disease. Correction of hypercortisolism by *o,p'*-DDD without induction of aldosterone deficiency. N Engl J Med 281:801, 1969

WILSON CB, DEMPSEY LC: Transsphenoidal microsurgical removal of 250 pituitary adenomas. J Neurosurg 48:13, 1978

YOUNG HH: A technique for simultaneous exposure and operation on the adrenals. Surg Gynecol Obstet 54:179, 1936

Virilism, Feminization, and Other Adrenocortical Disorders

BONGIOVANNI AM: Unusual steroid pattern in congenital adrenal hyperplasia: Deficiency of 3-β-hydroxy-dehydrogenase. J Clin Endocrinol 21:860, 1961

DOHAN FC, ROSE E, EIMAN JW et al: Increased urinary estrogen excretion associated with adrenal tumors: Report of four cases. J Clin Endocrinol 13:415, 1953

GABRILOVE JL, SHARMA DC, WOTIZ HH et al: Feminizing adrenocortical tumors in males: Review of 52 cases including case report. Medicine 44:37, 1965

JAILER JW: Virilism. Bull NY Acad Med 29:377, 1953

MATTOX VR, HAYLES AB, SALASSA RM et al: Urinary steroid patterns and loss of salt in congenital adrenal hyperplasia. J Clin Endocrinol 24:517, 1964

MOSIER HD, GOODWIN WE: Feminizing adrenal adenoma in a seven-year-old boy. Pediatrics 27:1016, 1961

SMITH AH: A case of feminizing adrenal tumor in a girl. J Clin Endocrinol 18:318, 1958

WILKINS L: A feminizing adrenal tumor causing gynecomastia in a boy of five years contrasted with a virilizing tumor in a five-year-old girl. Classification of seventy cases of adrenal tumor in children according to their hormonal manifestations and a review of eleven cases of feminizing tumor in adults. J Clin Endocrinol 8:111, 1948

Pheochromocytoma

BEER E, KING FH, PRINZMETAL M: Pheochromocytoma with demonstration of pressor (adrenalin) substance in blood preoperatively and during crisis. Ann Surg 106:85, 1937

BLAIR RG: Phaeochromotytoma and pregnancy: Report of a case and review of 51 cases. J Obstet Gynecol Br Commonwealth 70:110, 1963

BRENNAN MF, KEISER HR: Persistent and recurrent pheochromocytoma: The role of surgery. World J Surg 6:397, 1982

FRED HL, ALLRED DP, GARBER HE et al: Pheochromocytoma masquerading as overwhelming infection. Am Heart J 73:149, 1967

HARDY JD, McPHAIL JL, GALLAGHER WB JR: Pheochromocytoma: Shock following resection. Notes on mechanism with catecholamine measurements in case during pregnancy. JAMA 179:107, 1962

HARRISON TS, SEATON JD, CERNY JC et al: Localization of pheochromocytoma by caval catheterization. Arch Surg 95:339, 1967

van HEERDEN JA, SHEPS SG, HAMBERGER B et al: Pheochromocytoma: Current status and changing trends. Surgery 91:367, 1982

HUME DM: Pheochromocytoma in the adult and in the child. Am J Surg 99:458, 1960

ISAACS H, MEDALIE M, POLITZER WM: Noradrenaline-secreting neuroblastomata. Br Med J 1:401, 1959

JELLIFFE RS: Phaeochromocytoma presenting as a cardiac and abdominal catastrophe. Br Med J 2:76, 1952

LABBE MJ, TINEL J, DOUMER E: Crises solaires et hypertension paroxystique en rapport avec un tumeur surrenale. Bull Mem Soc Med Paris 46:982, 1922

LI FP, MELVIN KEW, TASHJIAN AH JR et al: Familial medullary thyroid carcinoma and pheochromocytoma: Epidemiologic investigations. J Nat Cancer Inst 52:285, 1974

LIEPHART CJ, NADELMAN EJ: Hibernoma masquerading as pheochromocytoma. Radiology 95:659, 1970

MANASSE P: Ueber die hyperplastichen Tumoren der Nebennieren. Virchows Arch Pathol Anat 133:391, 1893

MANNING PC JR, WOOLNER GD, BLACK BM et al: Pheochromocytoma, hyperparathyroidism and thyroid carcinoma occurring coincidentally. N Engl J Med 268:68, 1963

MAYO CH: Paroxysmal hypertension with tumor of retroperitoneal nerve: Report of a case. JAMA 89:1047, 1927

MEANY TF, BUONOCORE E: Selective arteriography as a localizing and provocative test in the diagnosis of pheochromocytoma. Radiology 87:309, 1966

MITTY HA et al: Adrenal venography: Clinical-roentgenographic correlation in 80 patients. Am J Roentgenol 119:564, 1973

OLSON JR, ABELL MR: Non-functional, nonchromaffin paragangliomas of the retroperitoneum. Cancer 23:1358, 1969

PINCOFFS MC: A case of paroxysmal hypertension associated with suprarenal tumor. Trans Assoc Am Physicians 44:295, 1929

PRADALIER A, LEBRAS PH, THOMAS M et al: Pheochromocytoma of the bladder. Ann Med Int (Paris) 125:39, 1974

ROTH GM, HIGHTOWER N, BARKER NW et al: Familial pheochromocytoma. Report on three siblings with bilateral tumors. Arch Surg 67:100, 1953

SHARP WV, PLATT RL: Familial pheochromocytoma: Association with von Hippel-Lindau's disease. Angiology 22:141, 1971

SIPPLE JH: The association of pheochromocytoma with carcinoma of the thyroid gland. Am J Med 31:163, 1961

SIZEMORE GW, GO VLW, KAPLAN EL et al: Relations of calcitonin and gastrin in the Zollinger-Ellison syndrome and medullary carcinoma of the thyroid. N Engl J Med 288:641, 1973

SPIEGEL HE: Catecholamine measurements in pheochromocytoma and neuroblastoma. Ann Clin Lab Sci 4:174, 1974

STEINER AL, GOODMAN AD, POWERS SR: Study of a kindred with pheochromocytoma, medullary thyroid carcinoma, hyperparathyroidism and Cushing's disease: Multiple endocrine neoplasia, type 2. Medicine 47:371, 1968

THOMPSON NW: Comment on "Persistent and recurrent pheochromocytoma: The role of surgery," Brennan MF, and Keiser HR. World J Surg 6:397, 1982

VAN WAY CW, SCOTT HW JR, PAGE DL et al: Pheochromocytoma. Curr Probl Surg, June, 1974

VAQUEZ H, DONZELOT E, GERANDEL E: Les crises d'hypertension arterielle paroxystique. Presse Med 34:1529, 1926

WERMER P: Endocrine adenomatosis and peptic ulcer in a large kindred. Am J Med 35:205, 1963

WILLIAMS, ED: A review of 17 cases of carcinoma of the thyroid and phaeochromocytoma. J Clin Pathol 18:288, 1965

John S. Kukora

Gastrointestinal Hormones

THE GUT AS AN ENDOCRINE ORGAN

The gastrointestinal tract and related organs are now recognized as the largest endocrine system of the body, containing not only the largest mass of endocrine cells but also the largest number of distinct hormones. An explosion of new information in the past two decades related to gastrointestinal hormonal physiology has yet to be accompanied by a similar abundance of clinical applications, but much clinically relevant progress appears imminent. Despite current intensive work in the study of gastrointestinal hormones, there are many gaps in our understanding of the multiple, variable, and subtle effects of most known hormones and their mutual interactions, and many other hormones remain to be identified. New organizational concepts have afforded a much simpler overview of this complex system than was previously possible, and the current prolific research interest centered on gastrointestinal hormones should enhance future understanding of this endocrine system in health and disease.

HISTORICAL REVIEW

The concept of a blood-borne chemical messenger or hormone was proposed in 1902 by Bayliss and Starling to describe the stimulation of pancreatic exocrine secretion by secretin, thus initiating the subsequent study of the entire field of endocrinology. In 1922, Banting and Best concentrated insulin from pancreatic extracts, the only known gastrointestinal hormone that is essential for life. Graham in 1927 first resected an insulin-secreting tumor, or insulinoma, and Whipple in 1935 described the clinical features of hyperinsulinism. The existence of the hormone gastrin was postulated by Edkins as early as 1905. In 1955, Zollinger and Ellison described their syndrome of severe hyperchlorhydria, peptic ulceration, and diarrhea associated with a pancreatic islet tumor. Gregory and Tracy purified and characterized gastrin by 1964. Coons perfected an immunologic tissue stain in 1955 that allowed cellular localization of specific chemicals, and in 1959 Yalow and Berson developed the technique of radioimmunoassay for insulin. Both of these powerful techniques have been applied extensively in the study of the localization and quantitative release of most other gastrointestinal hormones. A diffuse endocrine system was proposed by Feyrter as early as 1938, and the APUD concept (*Amine Precursor Uptake and Decarboxylation*) was elaborated by Pearse in 1966. These have provided a unifying concept of gastrointestinal endocrinology in the perspective of other hormonal and central nervous system regulatory processes.

THE APUD CONCEPT AND GASTROINTESTINAL HORMONE-PRODUCING CELLS

The endocrine cells of the gastrointestinal tract are located diffusely throughout the alimentary organs such as the stomach, pancreas, and intestines, and their secretory products are called gastrointestinal hormones or gastroenteropancreatic hormones. These cells are members of the family of APUD cells, their name indicating their cellular capacity for synthesis and storage of bioactive amines and peptide hormones. Thus, gastrointestinal endocrine cells are related to other widely dispersed APUD cells such as the C cells of the thyroid, parathyroid, adrenal medulla, carotid body,

Fig. 20-38. An electron photomicrograph shows the cytoplasm of an enterochromaffin cell containing dense ovoid, round, and dumbbell-shaped secretory granules. The nucleus occupies the right upper corner of the field. (Courtesy of Dr Virginia Lockard)

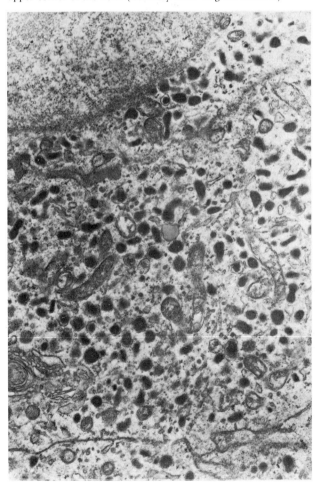

TABLE 20-10   CLASSIFICATION OF CURRENTLY IDENTIFIED GASTROINTESTINAL ENDOCRINE CELLS*

CELL TYPE	HORMONAL PRODUCT
P	Bombesin and bombesinlike
EC	5-HT, substance P, motilin
D_1	VIP
PP	Pancreatic polypeptide
D	Somatostatin
B	Insulin
A	Glucagon
X	Unknown
ECL	Unknown
G	Gastrin
S	Secretin
I	Cholecystokinin
K	GIP
N	Neurotensin
L	GLI

* Adopted by convention at Lausanne, Switzerland, in 1977

and the melanoblasts of the skin, among others. All these cells are embryologic derivatives of neuroectoderm, and the cells are characterized by specific histologic features including the staining characteristics of argyrophilia and masked metachromasia. The cells contain high levels of nonspecific esterases, cholinesterases, and mitochondrial α-glycerophosphate dehydrogenase. Electron micrographs show that these cells contain characteristic secretory granules that allow recognition of cells producing particular hormones by the size, shape, and electron density of the granules, especially when combined with immunocytochemical staining (Fig. 20-38). As new hormones are identified and isolated, the list of characterized gastrointestinal endocrine cells continues to grow (Table 20-10).

PHYSIOLOGY AND BIOCHEMISTRY OF GASTROINTESTINAL HORMONES

Endocrine cells of the gastrointestinal tract differ from endocrine cells of other organs because they are dispersed among nonendocrine cells throughout the length of the gut and pancreas instead of forming discrete glandular organs. The apex of many gastrointestinal endocrine cells contacts the intestinal lumen, allowing physiological regulation of the cells' hormonal secretion by the luminal content—for example, the stimulation of secretin and repression of gastrin by acidic duodenal content.

The endocrine cells of the pancreas form clusters, the islets of Langerhans, distributed throughout the exocrine parenchyma of the gland. The juxtaposition of these cells is thought to allow secretory regulation of differing islet cells among each other as well as modulation of the function of the exocrine pancreatic acinar cells.

Most gastrointestinal hormones are secreted into the blood and produce systemic effects, a classic endocrine response. The systemic effects of insulin release on glucose metabolism is a typical *endocrine* response. Other gastrointestinal hormones are released locally near the cells of origin and are thought to effect a *paracrine* response on local target cells. No definite proof of such a method of action has yet been conclusively shown, although the mechanism appears highly probable for several hormones. Some hormones are known to be released in the circulation, but no physiologically certain evidence of endocrine activity is yet established. These are termed *hemocrine* substances, an example of which is pancreatic polypeptide. Neurocrine hormones are those identified in storage granules of neurons or neuronal plexuses; when such substances are released into the circulation and have an observable effect, the substance is designated *neuroendocrine*. Certain hormones such as gastrin appear to be secreted into the gut lumen (as well as into the circulation), an observation that is currently of unknown significance.

The presence of identical polypeptide hormones in central nervous system peptidergic neurons and gastrointestinal endocrine cells, the so-called brain–gut peptides, implies another physiological mechanism of brain–gut–somatic interaction in addition to the classic voluntary and autonomic nervous systems. The intimate association of autonomic nerve fibers and APUD cells of the gut and other organs and the prevalence of many identical brain–gut peptides imply the presence of a much more complicated gastrointestinal regulatory physiological mechanism than the autonomic and humoral mechanisms emphasized heretofore.

The biochemistry and physiology of gut hormones have been partially clarified through several modern research developments. The use of the radioimmunoassay (Fig. 20-39) has permitted reproducible measurement of physiological quantities of specific hormones in picogram/milliliter concentrations. Improvements in protein purification and sequencing have facilitated the isolation and characterization of many peptide hormones. In several cases the hormone's amino acid sequence, cell of origin, secretory stimuli, and response patterns have been determined, and a number of hormonally mediated physiological effects have been observed without clarification of the major role of the hormone in normal physiological processes. For many hormones a great deal of information is available about effects on gut motility, secretion, absorption, vascular permeability, membrane uptake, and other biochemical processes, but the role of the hormone in health or disease is uncertain. For other hormones, notably gastrin, glucagon, and insulin, the role of the hormone in physiological control has been well elucidated, and excess or deficiency states have been correlated with distinct clinical syndromes.

Biochemically, the majority of recognized gut hormones are peptides; however, some are amines (serotonin, histamine, melatonin) or sterols (25-hydroxycholecalciferol).

The peptide hormones that are well characterized biochemically show a great deal of heterogeneity of molecular size in blood and tissue samples of functionally and immunologically identical peptides (Table 20-11). This heterogeneity appears to be related to the mechanism of synthesis of the hormone, which involves a high molecular weight prohormone, a secreted form, and a number of breakdown metabolites of the hormone. Although heterogeneity allows careful study of the mechanisms of hormonal biosynthesis, release, and degradation, it has complicated study of many hormones by introducing wide variability in radioimmunoassay techniques among different laboratories and created *in vivo* differences of biologic activity in different preparations of purified hormones.

Despite this heterogeneity of weight among forms of the same peptide, many similar or identical amino acid sequences are shared by families of gastrointestinal hormones. These similarities probably reflect the evolution of several

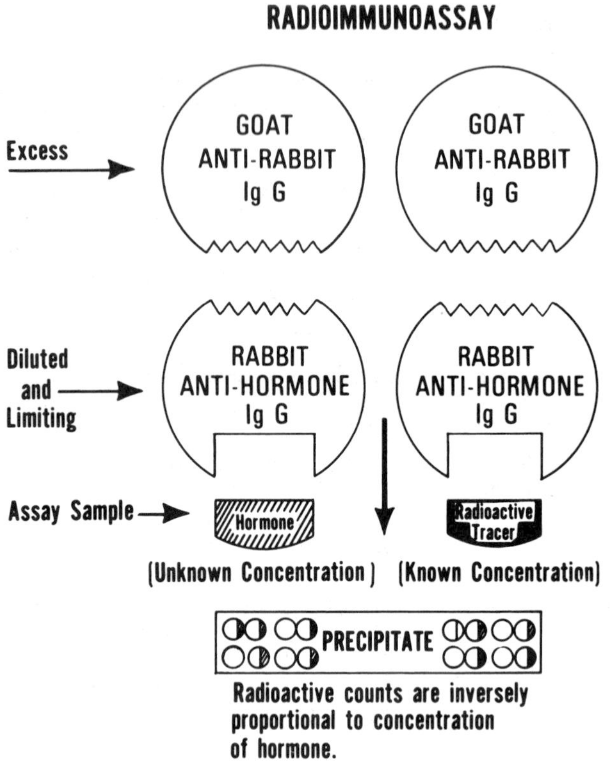

RADIOIMMUNOASSAY

Radioactive counts are inversely proportional to concentration of hormone.

Fig. 20-39. A typical radioimmunoassay scheme for a gastrointestinal hormone is depicted. A sample of fluid with unknown hormone concentration in incubated in the presence of a tracer (a known amount of the hormone to which is coupled a radioactive atom, usually ^{125}I) and a limited quantity of specific antibody to the hormone and tracer. A competition between the unknown hormone and the tracer for binding sites on the limiting antibody is established. A second antibody is used to precipitate the first antibody, and unbound tracer and hormone in the supernatant is decanted. The amount of radioactivity in the precipitate is inversely proportional to the concentration of hormone in the sample and is measured from standardized curves based on known concentration of hormones in the radioimmunoassay.

peptides from a common ancestral precursor molecule. Two families of gastroenteropancreatic hormones based on structural similarity are recognized. The *gastrin family* includes cholecystokinin, (met)-enkephalin, motilin, and somatostatin. The *secretin family* includes secretin, glucagon, vasoactive intestinal peptide (VIP), gastric inhibitory polypeptide (GIP), and bombesin.

THE PEPTIDE HORMONES

The following descriptions attempt to summarize the current understanding of a number of gastrointestinal hormones. The list of hormones is not complete but includes those of recognized clinical importance as well as a number of different hormones under current investigation.

ACTH AND ENDOGENOUS OPIATES

ACTH (adrenocorticotropic hormone) is derived from a larger precursor molecule that also serves as a precursor for the family of chemicals called endorphins (for *end*ogenous *morphin*es). Both ACTH and endorphins share a common peptide sequence, and the related two enkephalins are pentapeptides differing in a single amino acid. ACTH and

TABLE 20-11   HETEROGENEITY OF GASTRIN*

GASTRIN RESIDUES PER MOLECULE		ALTERNATE NAMES	TYPE I NONSULFATED	TYPE II SULFATED
Gastrin	?	Component I		
Gastrin	34	Big gastrin, component II		
Gastrin	17	Little gastrin, component III	(gastrin I) Nonsulfated	(gastrin II) Sulfated
Gastrin	14	Mini gastrin, component IV		
Gastrin	5	Pentagastrin		
Gastrin	4	Tetragastrin		

* Larger gastrins that have a tyrosine residue located 6 residues from the C-terminal end appear to exist *in vivo* either with a sulfate residue on the tyrosine side chain (type II) or lacking the sulfate (type I). The first gastrin characterized was gastrin-17, which is also the most biologically active. Sephadex filtration separates gastrin into components I–IV. Component I may be circulating progastrin or an artifact such as big-big gastrin.

other endorphins are found in multiple locations in central nervous system neurons as well as in G and other endocrine cells of the stomach, duodenum, and pancreas. Both exhibit morphinelike effects of pain modulation in the central nervous system and decreased gastric acid secretion and motility in the gut. ACTH in the pancreas may have a role in insulin release.

BOMBESIN

Bombesin is a 14-amino acid peptide that was originally isolated from frog skin but has been localized in the mammalian brain (hypothalamus) and also in the gastrointestinal tract and lung. Several other related amphibian peptides have been identified in mammalian neuroendocrine cells. In the brain bombesin appears to be involved in regulation of hypothalamic–pituitary function in a manner similar to endorphins. In the gut bombesin enhances gastrin, gastric inhibitory polypeptide, and cholecystokinin–pancreozymin release. It also inhibits vasoactive intestinal peptide secretion and gut motility.

CHOLECYSTOKININ–PANCREOZYMIN (CCK–PZ)

Cholecystokinin–pancreozymin is secreted by I cells in the duodenum and proximal jejunum and is also found in the brain. Initially thought to be separate hormones because of differing physiological effects, cholecystokinin and pancreozymin were shown to be the same 33–amino acid peptide in 1966. The major physiological effects of CCK–PZ are the promotion of gallbladder contraction and the stimulation of exocrine enzyme secretion by the pancreas. The hormone also causes relaxation of the sphincter of Oddi and weakly stimulates gastric acid secretion, probably by binding to gastrin receptors. The stimuli for CCK–PZ release includes amino acids, peptides, fat, and acid in the duodenal lumen.

GASTRIC INHIBITORY POLYPEPTIDE (GIP)

Gastric inhibitory polypeptide is a 43–amino acid polypeptide produced by K cells of the duodenum and proximal jejunum. Among other effects, the hormone was named because of its ability to suppress gastric secretion and motility. Its major physiological effect, however, appears to be stimulation of insulin release from the islets of Langerhans

in the presence of a modest or high serum glucose concentration. For this effect the hormone is also denoted as *g*lucose-dependent *i*nsulin-releasing *p*olypeptide. Its actions suggest the existence of an enterohumoral mechanism for stimulation of insulin production. Excessive GIP release and hyperinsulinemia have been documented in obese individuals and may be implicated in the pathogenesis of adult-onset diabetes mellitus.

GASTRIN

Gastrin is secreted by G cells in the gastric antrum, duodenum, and jejunum. Its major physiological action is the stimulation of gastric parietal cell hydrogen ion secretion. In addition, it is a weak stimulant of pancreatic exocrine secretion, bile flow, gallbladder contraction, and intestinal motility. The stimuli to gastrin release are high antral *p*H, antral distention, vagal stimulation of the stomach, and high luminal protein or amino acid content. Gastrin is found normally in the fetal pancreas but not in the adult pancreas. Gastrin-secreting tumors of the pancreas cause the pathologic state of hyperchlorhydria and diarrhea described by Zollinger and Ellison.

The large number of differing but biologically active gastrin molecules has been alluded to earlier in discussing heterogeneity; these molecules include big gastrin (G34$_I$, G34$_{II}$), little gastrin (G17$_I$, G17$_{II}$), and mini gastrin (G14$_I$, G14$_{II}$). The subscripts I and II denote the presence (G$_{II}$) or absence (G$_I$) of a sulfate residue on a particular tyrosine side chain. A big-big gastrin was identified but later shown to be an artifact. Other higher molecular weight gastrins (particularly component I gastrin) are noted that may be gastrin precursors. Each has a different half-life and biologic activity that collectively may represent different stages in the synthesis and breakdown of the hormone. Pentagastrin is a synthetic pentapeptide containing the biologic active site of the larger gastrin molecules and is used clinically to stimulate gastric acid production.

GLUCAGON

Glucagon is synthesized and secreted as a 29–amino acid peptide by the A or α cell of the pancreatic islets. It functions as an insulin antagonist and causes carbohydrate release from intracellular stores in response to a decrease in blood glucose. Various peptides of differing higher molecular weights that react immunologically with antisera against pancreatic glucagon have been isolated from the intestine and are referred to as enteroglucagons or, more correctly, as glucagonlike immunoreactivity (GLI). The physiological role of GLI is not yet clearly established but may be related to an enteric control mechanism for insulin secretion. GLI also may be a repressor of gastrointestinal motility.

INSULIN

Insulin is a peptide hormone secreted by the B or β cells of the pancreatic islets of Langerhans. A higher molecular weight prohormone, proinsulin, which is larger than the 51–amino acid insulin molecule, is recognized intracellularly and in the serum of patients with insulin-secreting tumors. Insulin stimulates glucose uptake by the liver and peripheral muscle and other somatic cells, lowers the circulating blood glucose, and stimulates fat and protein synthesis. Serum glucose and amino acid increases are the major stimuli to insulin release, although a number of other gastrointestinal and other hormones may modulate the response (notably gastrin, secretin, CCK–PZ, GIP, somatostatin, catecholamines, and others). Deficiency of insulin production or impairment of its cellular receptor sites results in the hyperglycemia of diabetes mellitus.

MOTILIN

Motilin is a 22–amino acid peptide purified after the observation that a humoral substance elaborated after alkaline stimulation of the duodenum was able to produce strong gastric contractions. The hormone is found only in the mucosa of the upper small intestine and is localized to enterochromaffin cells, which may also store serotonin. Food substances in the intestine tend to stimulate motilin release, which through its effect on smooth muscle in the stomach and intestine augments gastric motility and emptying along with intestinal transit.

NEUROTENSIN

Neurotensin is a 13–amino acid peptide first isolated as a byproduct during the purification of substance P from cattle hypothalami. Relatively large amounts of the hormone have been localized to the ileal mucosa in so-called NT cells. In pharmacologic doses neurotensin acts as a kinin, causing vasodilation and enhanced vascular permeability. In smaller doses the hormone promotes glucagon release and hyperglycemia and inhibits gastric acid production. Neurotensin rises postprandially in proportion to the size of the meal, but its underlying physiological role is poorly understood. High postprandial levels have been observed in patients with dumping syndrome.

PANCREATIC POLYPEPTIDE

Pancreatic polypeptide consists of 36–amino acid residues. It appears to be present only in the pancreas in a number of different animal species and is not only located in the peripheral cells of the islets of Langerhans but also appears to be dispersed among the exocrine cells of the gland. Cells containing pancreatic polypeptide are designated PP cells, and a much larger number of such cells is located in the duodenal end of the pancreas than in its tail. Pancreatic polypeptide levels rise in the serum after ingestion of any food substance, a response mediated in part by gastric distention, the vagus nerve, and cholinergic nonvagal pathways, probably in conjunction with another humoral gastrointestinal messenger. In mammals the substance does not seem to vary with insulin and glucagon production but does increase with β- and decrease with α-adrenergic stimulation. At physiological levels pancreatic polypeptide decreases pancreatic enzyme, fluid, and bicarbonate output and increases gastrointestinal motility while decreasing bile flow into the duodenum. The finding of markedly elevated levels of serum pancreatic polypeptide in many patients with APUDomas of the pancreas or carcinoid tumors of the gastrointestinal tract is clinically important and serves as a very useful biologic tumor marker.

SECRETIN

Secretin is a 27–amino acid peptide secreted by the S cells of the duodenum and jejunum. Its major action is the stimulation of water and bicarbonate secretion into the exocrine pancreatic fluid, which neutralizes gastric acid entering the duodenum. The stimulus to the S cell is an acid *p*H in the duodenum and jejunum. The hormone also tends to inhibit gastric acid secretion, stimulates bile flow from the liver, and augments the activity of CCK–PZ.

SUBSTANCE P

Substance P is located in many sites in the central, peripheral, and autonomic nervous system. In the gastrointestinal tract, substance P is found in close association with serotonin in the enterochromaffin (EC) cells located diffusely throughout the esophagus, stomach, small intestine, and colon. In the nervous system, the 11–amino acid substance appears to act as a neuromodulator in the transmission of sensory impulses and exhibits a similarity to endorphins. In the gut, substance P probably acts in a paracrine fashion to regulate motility. In pharmacologic doses the substance behaves as a tachykinin and causes intense intestinal cramping, vasodilation, hypertension, and facial flushing, which suggests that it may be partly responsible for the symptoms of the malignant carcinoid syndrome.

SOMATOSTATIN

Somatostatin is a 14–amino acid peptide first discovered in the hypothalamus as the inhibitor of growth hormone release. The hormone has also been localized to D cells of the stomach, duodenum, and pancreatic islets. The substance is an inhibitor of secretion of numerous other substances, including insulin, glucagon, growth hormone, thyrotropin, VIP, gastrin, CCK–PZ, secretin, motilin, GIP, pancreatic polypeptide, and others. Because of its rapid inactivation in plasma the role of somatostatin appears to be that of a paracrine modulator of other peptide hormones. The hormone also directly inhibits gastric acid production, gastric emptying, pancreatic (exocrine) secretion, gallbladder contraction, and visceral blood flow. The clinical administration of somatostatinlike agents has decreased peptide secretion from functional APUDomas.

VASOACTIVE INTESTINAL PEPTIDE (VIP)

Vasoactive intestinal peptide (VIP) was isolated as a byproduct during preparation of cholecystokinin and consists of 28 amino acids. VIP has been localized to the D_1 cells of the small intestinal mucosa as well as the pancreatic islets and may function as a neurotransmitter in the autonomic nervous system. In pharmacologic doses it acts as a smooth muscle relaxant, a strong inhibitor of gastric acid production, and a stimulator of pancreatic bicarbonate and water secretion. It also tends to stimulate hepatic glycogenolysis and enteric secretion and to cause vasodilation and diarrhea. The hormone may function physiologically as a paracrine substance because the hormone appears to stimulate strongly the release of glucagon by the islets of Langerhans in the pancreas and to a lesser extent the production of insulin. It may act in combination with somatostatin as a paracrine regulator of the insulin–glucagon system. VIP has been postulated to be an agent responsible for diarrhea in the watery-diarrhea-hypokalemia-achlorhydria (WDHA) syndrome (Verner-Morrison syndrome).

AMINE HORMONES

5-HYDROXYTRYPTAMINE (SEROTONIN)

5-Hydroxytryptamine (5-HT), or serotonin, is an amine hormone produced by hydroxylation of tryptophan and subsequent decarboxylation of the amino acid. The hormone is produced by the enterochromaffin (EC) cells of the intestine along with motilin and substance P and other humoral substances. Other APUD cells widely dispersed through the body can also produce this amine. The substance stimulates smooth muscle contractions and affects gut motility, causes peripheral vasodilation, and is a bronchial constrictor. 5-HT is rapidly degraded from the circulation by monoamine oxidase in the lungs and liver and is excreted through the urine as 5-hydroxyindoleacetic acid (5-HIAA). Excess production of the hormone may be responsible for some of the manifestations of the carcinoid syndrome.

PATHOLOGY RELATED TO GASTROINTESTINAL HORMONES

Endocrine disease is usually distinguished by the effects of hormonal excess or deficiency and this feature characterizes the known syndromes in which gastrointestinal hormones are implicated in the pathogenesis.

DEFICIENCY STATES

The most common gastrointestinal hormone deficiency disease is diabetes mellitus, which in the juvenile-onset variety is due to the deficient production of insulin by the pancreatic β cells. In juvenile diabetics (type I) there is a reduction in the total number of β cells in the pancreatic islets that may be secondary to a viral, chemical, or autoimmune-induced necrosis of these cells. In the adult-onset form of diabetes (type II) there is defective receptor sensitivity to insulin, although some insulin is secreted. The metabolic effects of diabetes include hyperglycemia, osmotic diuresis, and a tendency to systemic ketoacidosis. Although the diagnosis and treatment of diabetes is not in the specific domain of surgery, the ever-increasing number of patients with diabetes who require surgery either because of complications of their disease or for other reasons necessitates a clear understanding of the therapy of diabetic patients

during anesthesia and the perioperative period by all surgeons.

Although no other syndromes of gastrointestinal hormonal deficiency states are as clearly defined as diabetes, there are indications that certain gastrointestinal problems may be related in part to impaired secretion or action of some hormones. An example of such a condition is celiac disease, which is characterized by decreased gut motility and malabsorption of lipids and has been related to impaired release of cholecystokinin and secretin, resulting in deficient pancreatic exocrine secretion and gallbladder contraction. Other candidate diseases in which deficient hormonal activity has been suggested, although not conclusively demonstrated, include gastroesophageal reflux, duodenal ulcer, spastic colitis, and severe obesity.

HYPERSECRETORY STATES

APUDOMA AND PATHOLOGY

Syndromes of gastrointestinal hormonal excess are relatively better characterized than are those of deficiency. These clinical states are usually caused by excessive production of single or multiple hormones by neoplasms of the APUD cells of the gastrointestinal tract and associated organs, which are commonly designated as APUDomas. Histologically, these neoplasms resemble their APUD cells of origin in that they have secretory granules and other ultrastructural characteristics of gastrointestinal endocrine cells, yet they often show the hyperchromatic and disordered nuclei characteristic of neoplastic cells. Such APUDomas exist as solitary benign adenomas or, more commonly, as carcinomas when lymphatic, hepatic, and other bloodborne metastases are present or when perineural or perivascular invasion is observed. In other hypersecretory states, particularly in patients with familial endocrinopathy, a widespread hyperplasia of APUD cells is observed, usually in the pancreas, where there is an increase in the total number of islets and the number of cells in each islet. This observation of hyperplasia suggests an unidentified stimulant or absent repressor of APUD cell proliferation in these patients. An APUDoma is fully characterized when the secretory products within its granules have been identified. The APUDoma is then referred to by its hormone product followed by the suffix ''-oma,'' for example, gastrinoma, VIPoma, insulinoma. A substantial number of gastrointestinal APUDomas appear to be nonfunctional at the time of diagnosis, a finding that may represent true endocrinologic nonfunction or that may be due to an inability to characterize biochemically and recognize its secretory products.

DIAGNOSIS AND TREATMENT

The recognition of a hypersecretory gastrointestinal APUDoma usually depends on the clinical manifestations of the hormone produced in excess. These manifestations are often initially subtle and are frequently confused by more likely explanations for their cause than a functional APUDoma. Early detection of malignant APUDomas is essential, especially if cure is to be effected. Unfortunately, the majority of APUD carcinomas are discovered only when they are so far advanced that curative surgical resection is precluded, by advanced signs of intestinal obstruction, abdominal pain from involvement of the mesenteric and celiac axes, or signs of hepatic metastases. The screening of high-risk individuals with a known familial endocrinopathy is likely to afford higher proportions of early detection and cure, but the

CLINICAL SIGNS AND SYMPTOMS OF FUNCTIONAL GASTROINTESTINAL ENDOCRINE NEOPLASMS

Peptic ulcer	Gastrinoma
Diarrhea Cramping	Carcinoid tumor Gastrinoma VIPoma
Wheezing Flushing	Carcinoid tumor
Hyperglycemia	Glucagonoma Corticotrophinoma
Skin rash and hyperglycemia	Glucagonoma
Hypoglycemia	Insulinoma
Hypokalemia	VIPoma

majority of patients with sporadic presentations must depend on acute clinical awareness of the possibility of an APUDoma when they first seek medical treatment. Signs and symptoms of diarrhea, flushing, wheezing, cramping, hyperglycemia, skin rash, hypoglycemia, hypokalemia, and peptic ulcer should always raise the suspicion of a functional endocrine neoplasm.

Once an APUDoma has been suspected its presence is generally confirmed by measurement of elevated levels of its secretory products in blood or of hormonal metabolites in urine. Certain stimulation tests have been developed to detect the secretion of some hormones—for example, a calcium- or secretin-stimulated gastrin determination, a leucine- or glucagon-stimulated insulin determination, and a pentagastrin-stimulated calcitonin determination.

After confirmation of the presence of an APUDoma is obtained, it should be localized by one of numerous modalities. Many of these tumors are rather small (less than 2 cm) and may evade detection by the usual barium contrast examinations of the gastrointestinal tract and other organs. Overall, the visceral arteriogram is most likely to demonstrate an intra-abdominal APUDoma because these tumors are usually highly vascular and demonstrate a "tumor blush" owing to early venous filling in the tumor. With careful selective and subselective angiography, tumors as small as 1 cm have been identified reliably within the pancreas, liver, or small intestine (Fig. 20-40). The computed tomographic (CT) scan has shown increasing usefulness in localizing pancreatic APUDomas as well as hepatic metastases. In certain cases, selective mesenteric, splenic, and portal venous hormone samples may be obtained to localize the relative position of a functional tumor that otherwise eludes localization (Fig. 20-41). A high step-up of the particular hormone product of the tumor suggests its relative localization.

Surgical removal of APUD neoplasms offers the best likelihood of cure, especially when the tumor is surgically accessible without distant metastasis. Celiotomy is justified to search for an occult tumor if all attempts at nonoperative localization are unsuccessful. Careful search is made for small palpable lesions in and about the pancreas, celiac axis, liver, stomach, duodenum, small bowel and its mesentery, and the colon and mesocolon. Resection should always contain a margin of normal tissue if possible because of the tendency for local invasion even in tumors that otherwise appear benign.

Unfortunately, many tumors at the time of celiotomy

will be unresectable for cure either because of widespread metastases or because of invasion of contiguous structures such as the mesenteric vessels that cannot be sacrificed. In these instances an attempt to debulk as much of the neoplasm as possible is justified to decrease the amount of hypersecreting tissue and hence palliate the symptoms of hypersecretion. Chemotherapeutic agents offer some benefit in controlling the growth of some of these tumors, especially combination chemotherapy using streptozotocin. Survivals of 20 years or longer have been reported with metastatic gastrointestinal APUDomas, and survival of 10 years or longer occurs commonly because of the intrinsically slow growth rate of many of these tumors.

RECOGNIZED SYNDROMES

In this section five specific syndromes of gastrointestinal hormonal excess will be discussed. These are the best characterized and most commonly recognized syndromes and include the hypersecretory states associated with gastrinoma, insulinoma, glucagonoma, carcinoid tumor, and VIPoma. The familial multiple endocrine adenopathy syndromes are rare neuroectodermal disorders that include several pancreatic APUDomas.

Gastrinoma

The clinical manifestations of gastrin-secreting tumors are related to the consequences of gastric acid hypersecretion. Gastrinoma patients have severe, atypically located, multiple and unrelenting duodenal and jejunal peptic ulcerations that often recur promptly after conventional medical or surgical treatment. Hemorrhage, perforation, and obstruction are common, and most patients have severe diarrhea caused by large quantities of gastric acid entering the duodenum that may inactivate pancreatic digestive enzymes, irritate the small bowel mucosa, or stimulate other motility-enhancing factors in the gut.

Gastrin is normally produced by the G cells of the antral mucosa and duodenum, but the majority of gastrinomas are usually derived from pancreatic islet cells that normally contain no gastrin in the adult. Other gastrinomas have been described in the wall of the duodenum, stomach, or intestine or in the liver. Approximately 75% of gastrinomas are malignant or multifocal within the pancreas, and 25% are associated with other features of the multiple endocrine adenopathy type I (MEA I) syndrome.

The diagnosis is suspected because of unusual severity of peptic ulcer disease, a family history of ulcer disease, atypical or multiple locations of ulcers in the distal duodenum or jejunum, associated diarrhea, or hypertrophic

GASTRINOMA

Etiology	Gastrin-secreting pancreatic or duodenal APUDoma; MEA I
Dx	Severe peptic ulcer diathesis Recurrent ulcer, hyperchlorhydria, diarrhea Elevated fasting serum gastrin level Secretin-stimulated gastrin assay
Rx	Cimetidine APUDoma resection Total gastrectomy

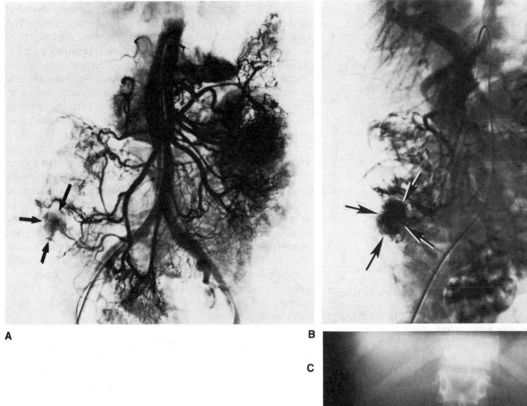

A

B

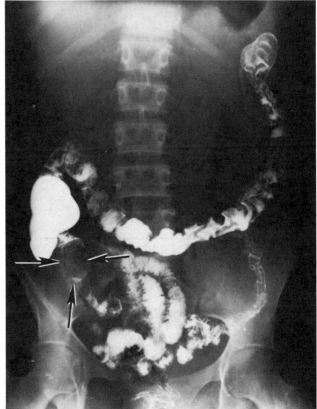

C

Fig. 20-40. An arteriogram of the superior mesenteric artery (*A*) shows a hypervascular tumor in the region of the terminal ileum. The venous phase angiogram (*B*) shows the venous blush and portal drainage of the tumor. The barium enema (*C*) shows the corresponding luminal defect. At celiotomy, a 3 cm carcinoid tumor of the ileum was found. Hypervascularity and early venous filling characterize gastrointestinal APUDomas and allow localization of most tumors greater than 1 cm in diameter.

gastric folds. Barium flocculation caused by excessive gastric acid is noted on upper gastrointestinal roentgenograms. An elevated fasting serum gastrin determination (greater than 200 pg/ml) is strong supportive evidence for the syndrome. Because of the low cost and wide availability of the gastrin radioimmunoassay, a basal fasting gastrin determination appears to be a wise precaution in all patients about to undergo surgery for peptic ulcer, since most of these patients usually represent severe failures of medical therapy or have

a serious complication of their ulcer diathesis and are a group at risk for harboring a gastrinoma.

Patients with atrophic gastritis, pernicious anemia, retained gastric antrum in the duodenal stump of a Billroth II gastrectomy, chronic gastric outlet obstruction, impaired renal function with decreased renal clearance of gastrin, or the rare syndrome of antral G-cell hyperplasia may also demonstrate elevated plasma gastrin levels. Patients with a functional gastrinoma can usually be differentiated from

TRANSHEPATIC PANCREATIC VENOUS CATHETERIZATION

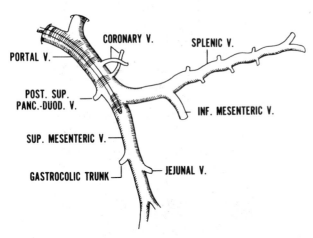

Fig. 20-41. A catheter is passed into the portal vein over a needle placed percutaneously in the right lobe of the liver; the needle penetrates a smaller portal venous radicle. Blood samples are taken at the time of fluoroscopy for measurement of hormone concentrations. A step-up of hormone levels in one area of the portal, splenic, or superior mesenteric veins suggests the relative location of a functional APUDoma.

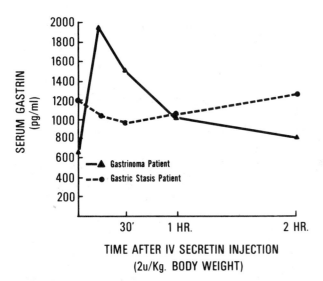

Fig. 20-42. A rise in serum gastrin levels greater than 200 pg/ml distinguishes a patient with gastrinoma (*solid line*) from a patient with gastric stasis due to pyloric scarring (*broken line*) after infusion of secretin (2 units/kg body weight).

these others by use of a calcium- or secretin-stimulated plasma gastrin determination. An increase of gastrin secretion by 100% or greater, or 200 pg/ml from basal levels following secretin stimulation, is reliably diagnostic of a gastrinoma (Fig. 20-42). Other tests suggesting a gastrinoma, although not as reliable as the secretin-stimulated gastrin assay, include the measurement of basal gastric acid secretion, which usually exceeds 15 mEq/hr, and a ratio of basal to maximal stimulated histalog acid output of 0.6 or greater. Temporary improvement of the gastric acid hypersecretion is often noted after resection of the parathyroid adenomas of MEA I patients with a gastrinoma because the lower serum calcium levels decrease the gastrin output from the gastrinoma.

The traditional therapy of gastrinoma has been resection of the tumor whenever possible and total gastrectomy. The rationale for total gastrectomy is the removal of all acid-secreting cells to prevent recurrent peptic ulceration, because most gastrinomas are found to be multicentric or incurably metastatic at the time of the initial operation. Recently, the prolonged use of cimetidine to block parietal cell acid secretion has been advocated to delay or replace surgery or to decrease the extent of surgery to a vagotomy and pyloroplasty or partial gastrectomy with the hope of avoiding the nutritional complications of total gastrectomy. Although cimetidine with or without limited gastric surgery will enable the patient to maintain better gastric reservoir capacity, its long-term effectiveness is unproven. All attempts to remove the gastrinoma if possible should be made at the time of diagnosis to ensure the best outcome for the 11% to 20% of patients in most reported series who are resectable for potential cure. Total gastrectomy is still the treatment of choice for most patients, especially those with poor response to cimetidine. Patients with metastatic gastrinoma frequently exhibit tumor responsiveness to streptozotocin and other agents, and 3- to 10-year survivals with metastatic disease have been reported.

Carcinoid Tumors and the Carcinoid Syndrome

Carcinoid tumors are the most common gastrointestinal APUDomas and are derived from the enterochromaffin cells of the gastrointestinal tract and its embryologically derived structures. The term *carcinoid* implies literally "resembling a carcinoma" because of early uncertainty about its metastatic potential. Current knowledge suggests that all carcinoid tumors should be considered potentially malignant neoplasms with the possible exception of small tumors of the appendix. The neuroectodermally derived enterochromaffin cells of origin are located throughout the gastrointestinal tract, gallbladder, pancreas, bronchial tree, and urogenital tract, and carcinoid tumors of the bronchi, esophagus, stomach, duodenum, gallbladder, pancreas, small and large intestines, appendix, rectum, ovary, testis, and urethra have been described. The most common site of origin of carcinoid tumors is the appendix, followed in order by the small intestine, rectum, and bronchial tree. Carcinoid tumors are the most common tumor of the small intestine.

Many carcinoids are clinically asymptomatic and are discovered incidentally at celiotomy. The majority of small appendiceal carcinoids are found incidentally within the appendix at the time of appendectomy for appendicitis. Other carcinoids may present with signs of bleeding or obstruction in the gastrointestinal tract or bronchi. A group

CARCINOID	
Etiology	Enterochromaffin APUDoma Serotonin, histamine, bradykinin, and other hormonal hypersecretion
Dx	Flushing, cramping, diarrhea Incidental finding at appendectomy Bowel or bronchial obstruction or hemorrhage Urinary 5-HIAA
Rx	Resection with involved nodes Pharmacologic blockade Chemotherapy

of patients with functional carcinoid tumors secreting into the nonportal venous system may exhibit the carcinoid syndrome, characterized by flushing, diarrhea, and occasional wheezing or other symptoms. This syndrome occurs when the hormone products of the tumor are not inactivated by passage through the liver.

Carcinoid tumors tend to be multicentric in origin and are often associated with other malignant diseases either endocrine or nonendocrine in nature. A small percentage of carcinoid tumors are found in patients with the MEA I and MEA II syndromes. Carcinoid tumors metastasize by way of the blood, lymphatics, or direct extension in the manner of most gastrointestinal adenocarcinomas. Lymph node and hepatic metastases are seen most commonly, but lung, brain, and bone metastases can occur with advanced disease. Carcinoid tumors can synthesize a number of biologically active substances, such as serotonin, histamine, bradykinin, prostaglandins, calcitonin, ACTH, substance P, motilin, growth hormone, parathormone, insulin, and glucagon, among others. The symptoms of excess amounts of any of these hormones may be the characterizing feature of a particular carcinoid tumor.

The carcinoid syndrome is thought to be produced primarily by serotonin that gains access to the systemic circulation, implying a functional tumor located away from portal venous drainage or the presence of hepatic metastasis. Serotonin released exclusively into the portal circulation is normally converted on initial passage through the liver into the inactive metabolite 5-hydroxyindoleacetic acid (5-HIAA), which is excreted in the urine. Other bioactive substances, particularly bradykinins, prostaglandins, histamine, motilin, or 5-hydroxytryptophan may be responsible for some features of the syndrome. Attacks of severe facial flushing with associated diarrhea and cramping occur regularly in the majority of patients with the malignant carcinoid syndrome. Facial venous telangiectasia, tricuspid and pulmonic valve fibrosis, bronchoconstriction, hypotension, peripheral edema, and a pellagralike skin rash (due to a relative niacin deficiency because of increased usage of tryptophan by the tumor) occur less frequently. Alcohol or food ingestion may provoke the flushing attacks, which may also be evoked clinically by calcium or epinephrine infusion. Elevated levels of urinary 5-HIAA are the most reliable evidence of the presence of a functional carcinoid tumor. Increased urinary levels of 5-hydroxytryptophan are occasionally seen without elevated 5-HIAA levels in certain "foregut" carcinoid tumors. Hepatomegaly due to extensive metastatic tumor will be noted in the majority of patients with the carcinoid syndrome caused by a primary gastrointestinal carcinoid.

Radical surgical removal of the primary tumor, involved regional nodes, and accessible metastases remains the treatment of choice for carcinoid tumors. In the case of appendiceal carcinoids less than 1 cm in diameter, a resection of the appendix itself will suffice because the incidence of metastases from small appendiceal carcinoids is very low. Rectal carcinoids, if small, are generally treated by local resection, reserving abdominoperineal resection for tumors larger than 2 cm or for those demonstrating local invasiveness after transanal excision. Bronchial carcinoids are treated by tracheal or bronchial resection, lobectomy, or pneumonectomy, depending on their location. Attempts to debulk metastatic or incurable carcinoid tumors whenever possible are indicated to decrease the secretory mass of the tumor; this may alleviate or delay the onset of the carcinoid syndrome and improve the quality of the patient's life.

Pharmacologic attempts to control the carcinoid syndrome are variably successful. It is important to recognize and treat promptly carcinoid crisis, which may follow surgical manipulation of a carcinoid tumor under anesthesia, producing acute severe hypotension, bronchoconstriction, pulmonary edema, and severe loss of circulating fluid into extravascular spaces. The use of corticosteroids, aspirin, indomethacin, phenoxybenzamine, propranolol, ϵ-aminocaproic acid, cyproheptadine, antihistamines, aprotonin (Trasylol), dopamine, α-methyldopa, phenothiazines, and methysergide as well as the experimental agents parachlorophenylalanine and 5-fluorotryptophan have all been reported useful in the treatment of carcinoid syndrome or crisis.

Treatment of patients with unresectable metastatic carcinoid tumors has been improved by chemotherapy with multiple agents such as adriamycin, cyclophosphamide, 5-fluorouracil, methotrexate, and streptozotocin.

Collected 5-year survival rates are as follows:

Localized disease	95%
Regional nodal spread	65%
Distant spread	20%

The overall 5-year survival for patients with resectable tumors is about 65%.

Insulinoma

Hypoglycemia is the physiological result of excessive or inappropriate insulin release by insulinomas derived from pancreatic islet β cells. Insulinomas are evenly distributed among all racial, sexual, and age groups, and about 10% of them are associated with the MEA I syndrome.

Clinical manifestations include alterations of mental status, confusion, unusual behavior, weakness, amnesia, coma, or seizure, all due to neuroglycopenia. Blurred vision, diplopia, and signs of secondary catecholamine release such as tachycardia, palpitations, and sweating are frequently present. Often such patients are mistakenly diagnosed as suffering from a primary psychological or neurologic disorder. Symptoms typically appear many hours after the last food ingestion. Whipple's triad is observed in about 75% of insulinoma patients after a 24-hr fast. Persistent neurologic injury may result from severe prolonged attacks, particularly in children.

Repeated glucose determinations and simultaneous serum insulin measurement by radioimmunoassay during a prolonged fast of up to 72 hr monitored carefully in the hospital will confirm the characteristic abnormally low serum glucose levels with high serum insulin levels. Elevated serum insulin

INSULINOMA	
Etiology	Insulin-secreting APUDoma
Dx	Altered CNS function
	Fasting hypoglycemia
	Elevated serum insulin/glucose ratio
	Pancreatic arteriography, CT scan
	Selective venous hormone sampling
Rx	Pancreatic exploration
	Resection of APUDoma or debulking
	Streptozotocin and diazoxide for metastases

WHIPPLE'S TRIAD

1. Symptoms of glucose deficiency after fasting or exercise
2. Documented blood glucose less than 50 mg/dl
3. Prompt relief of symptoms after exogenous glucose administration.

Central nervous symptoms of neuroglycopenia that occur with fasting or exercise should be investigated by repeated blood sugar determinations after a carefully monitored fast.

to serum glucose ratios are reliably diagnostic of insulinoma. In some cases use of an intravenous tolbutamide infusion with measurement of serum insulin and glucagon may assist in confirming the diagnosis. The differential diagnosis of hypoglycemia includes functional hypoglycemia, exogenous insulin or hypoglycemic agent administration, liver failure, hypothalamic–pituitary abnormality, and certain neoplasms such as large sarcomas that may produce hypoglycemia.

After the diagnosis is established, every attempt should be made to localize the tumor within the pancreas before surgery. The most useful studies are selective and subselective angiography, CT scan of the abdomen, and selective portal, splenic, and mesenteric vein insulin measurements. Most tumors more than 5 mm in diameter can be localized by arteriography alone owing to their hypervascularity (Fig. 20-43).

The majority of insulinomas are single benign tumors. About 10% are malignant based on evidence of local invasiveness or metastasis, and about 10% of the malignant tumors have hepatic metastasis at the time of diagnosis. Another 10% of patients with insulinoma will have two or more discrete adenomas or microadenomatosis with hypercellularity or increased numbers of islets throughout the pancreas.

Careful intraoperative observation and palpation of the pancreas followed by resection of the tumor and surrounding pancreas if necessary is the treatment of choice. Enucleation of the tumor, distal pancreatic resection, and (rarely) a pancreaticoduodenectomy may be performed depending on the location and characteristics of the tumor. Near total pancreatectomy (85%–95%) may be required if diffuse microadenomatosis or nesidioblastosis is present. The latter is a diffuse pancreatic islet cell hyperplasia in which the islet cells appear as ribbons rather than as discrete islets; it is associated with hypoglycemia, usually in children under the age of 2 years. If the tumor cannot be localized prior to or at surgery, progressive pancreatic resection with cutting of the specimen and monitoring of blood glucose levels may be preferable to blind total resection of the head or tail of the gland. When the tumor cannot be located or completely removed, the drug diazoxide is effective at inhibiting tumor insulin release. Streptozotocin in combination with other chemotherapeutic agents may inhibit metastatic tumor.

Glucagonoma

Glucagonomas are rare APUDomas originating from α cells of the pancreatic islets. They produce a characteristic skin rash and mild diabetes. Stomatitis, anemia, diarrhea, weight loss, and venous thrombosis may be associated.

The tumors characteristically contain A cells and secrete pancreatic glucagon; however, other cell types are occasionally seen within the tumors, and higher molecular weight glucagons or proglucagon may be elaborated.

The diagnosis depends on recognition of the characteristic severe necrolyzing bullae of the trunk (Fig. 20-44), which move from place to place and are therefore described as migratory necrolytic erythema, usually associated with mild diabetes mellitus. Confirmation of the disease depends on measurement of elevated serum glucagon levels by radioimmunoassay.

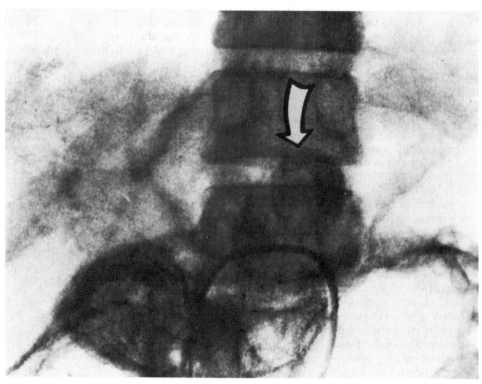

Fig. 20-43. A 2 cm insulinoma of the body of the pancreas is seen overlying the lumbar spine on subtraction angiography. (Courtesy of Dr James D Hardy)

GLUCAGONOMA	
Etiology	Glucagon-secreting APUDoma
Dx	Diabetes mellitus
	Necrolyzing skin rash
	Elevated serum glucagon levels
	Pancreatic arteriography
Rx	Pancreatic exploration
	Tumor resection and debulking if metastasis is present

These tumors may be localized by arteriography, abdominal CT scan, or selective venous hormone sampling. Surgical removal of the tumor and debulking of the metastases is the initial treatment of choice.

Unfortunately, about 60% of glucagonomas are malignant and have metastasized at the time of celiotomy. Nonetheless, with debulking of metastatic tumor masses survivals of more than 10 years are reported owing to the slow growth of glucagonomas. Streptozotocin appears to be of less value in treating metastatic glucagonoma than in treatment of other metastatic APUDomas.

VIPoma

A rare syndrome characterized by severe watery diarrhea, potassium loss, and decreased gastric acid production has been described in association with certain pancreatic, adrenal, or sympathetic chain APUDomas. This syndrome is often referred to as the "watery diarrhea, hypokalemia,

Fig. 20-44. The skin rash of glucagonoma is shown in a 55-year-old male patient (*A*). The rash involves the lower trunk more than the upper trunk or the extremities and produces severe bullae with secondary infection. Improvement of the rash after debulking of a large metastatic glucagonoma is evident in (*B*). (Courtesy of Dr Norman W Thompson)

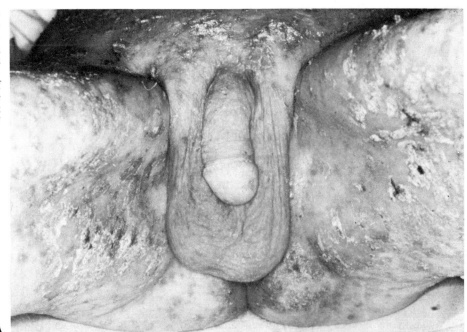

A

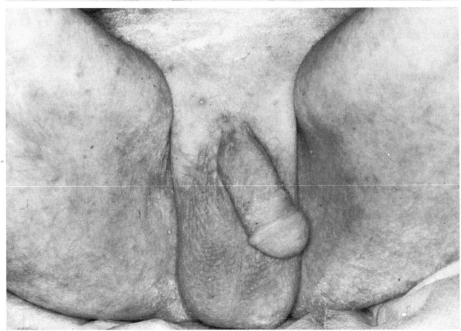

B

VIPoma	
Etiology	VIP-secreting APUDoma ? other endocrine agonists
Dx	Watery diarrhea with elevated potassium Hypokalemia Hypochlorhydria Pancreatic arteriogram and CT scan Elevated serum VIP levels
Rx	Pancreatic exploration APUDoma resection or debulking Streptozotocin, indomethacia

achlorhydria" (WDHA) syndrome, the "pancreatic cholera" syndrome, or Verner-Morrison syndrome.

Most patients with the syndrome suffer from profound diarrhea, with stool volumes of up to 5 liters per day and 10 to 20 bowel movements daily. The stool is very thin and watery and contains a high concentration of electrolytes, particularly potassium and bicarbonate. Stomach acid is very low or absent, and there is surprisingly little steatorrhea or evidence of gastrointestinal malabsorption.

The pathophysiology of the syndrome appears to be related in many cases to excessive secretion of VIP, which is thought to produce a hypersecretion of electrolyte-rich small intestinal fluid through a cyclic AMP mechanism that overwhelms the colonic capacity to reabsorb the fluid. The achlorhydria is ascribed to an inhibitory substance produced by the tumor that may also be VIP. Prostaglandins, pancreatic polypeptides, and other unknown substances have also been implicated as potential agonists in the mediation of the syndrome.

Differential diagnosis includes laxative abuse, villous adenoma of the colon, celiac disease, gastrinoma, and carcinoid tumor as well as medullary carcinoma of the thyroid, all of which may be associated with severe diarrhea. The measurement of elevated VIP levels affords strong substantiation of the diagnosis, but normal levels do not exclude the possibility of an APUDoma. Low gastric acid levels distinguish the syndrome from gastrinoma.

Pancreatic angiography and abdominal CT scans are helpful in localizing these tumors. Complete resection or debulking of metastases will provide the best relief from the incapacitating diarrhea, which is usually refractory to pharmacologic therapy. About 60% of these tumors are metastatic at the time of diagnosis. Streptozotocin may be helpful in chemotherapy of these tumors, and the diarrhea may be helped in some cases by administration of steroids or prostaglandin inhibitors such as indomethacin.

MULTIPLE ENDOCRINE ADENOPATHY

The term multiple endocrine adenopathy (MEA) describes several genetically determined syndromes of hyperfunction of more than two types of APUD cell in a single patient. Other terms used to describe the syndromes include pluriglandular syndrome, multiple endocrine adenomatosis, familial endocrinopathy, and multiple endocrine neoplasia syndrome. The particular APUD cell systems involved in the MEA syndromes allow a convenient grouping into two categories designated the MEA I and MEA II syndromes. Each of these rare syndromes may occur sporadically, but more commonly each is familially transmitted by an autosomal dominant mode of inheritance with high penetrance and variable expressivity.

MEA I

The MEA I syndrome consists of the occurrence of any two or more of the following endocrine abnormalities in a patient: a pancreatic APUDoma, parathyroid hyperplasia or adenoma, pituitary adenoma, adrenal cortical hyperfunction, or thyroid adenoma. Only very rarely will all the endocrine systems noted be involved. The most common pancreatic APUDomas observed in the syndrome are, in order of decreasing frequency: gastrinoma, insulinoma, VIPoma. The most common clinical manifestation of the syndrome is the association of a gastrinoma with hyperparathyroidism. Treatment of the syndrome consists of the usual surgical resection of the involved endocrine tissues. Unfortunately, there tends to be a somewhat higher incidence of malignancy among pancreatic APUDomas of the MEA I syndrome than among sporadic cases.

MEA II

The MEA II syndrome consists of a familial association between medullary carcinoma of the thyroid and pheochromocytoma in the same patient. A subgroup, MEA IIb, consists of medullary carcinoma of the thyroid and pheochromocytoma in association with multiple mucosal neuromas of the tongue, lips, and conjunctiva and a marfanoid habitus. Diarrhea is the usual manifestation of the medullary thyroid carcinoma. Early diagnosis of medullary thyroid carcinoma is essential to allow an opportunity for surgical resection and cure. For kindred at risk the use of the pentagastrin-stimulated thyrocalcitonin determination affords early detection of the disease in infancy.

BIBLIOGRAPHY

Basso N, Grossman M, Lezoche E et al (eds): Gastrointestinal hormones and pathology of the digestive system. Adv Exp Med Biol 106:1, 1978

Buchanan KD: Gastrointestinal hormones. Clin Endocrinol Metab 8:249, 1979

Edis AJ, McIlrath DC, Van Heerden JA et al: Insulinoma—current diagnosis and surgical management. Curr Probl Surg 13:5, 1976

Friesen SR: Surgical Endocrinology: Clinical Syndromes. Philadelphia, J B Lippincott, 1978

Hanssen LE, Myren J, Schrumpf E et al (eds): The 2nd International Symposium on Gastrointestinal Hormones. Scand J Gastroenterol 13 (Suppl 49): 1978

Modlin IM: Endocrine tumors of the pancreas. Surg Gynecol Obstet 149:751, 1979

Modlin IM, Albert D, Sank A: Current aspects of gut hormones. J Surg Res 30:602, 1981

Rehfeld JF: Gastrointestinal hormones. In Crane RK (ed): International Review of Physiology. Gastrointestinal Physiology III. Baltimore, University Park Press, 1979

Thompson JC (ed): Gastrointestinal Hormones. A Symposium. Austin, University of Texas Press, 1975

Thompson JC (ed): Symposium on gastrointestinal hormones. World progress in surgery. World J Surg 3:389, 523, 1979

Laurence Y. Cheung/Walter F. Ballinger

Manifestations and Diagnosis of Gastrointestinal Diseases

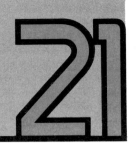

Cardinal symptoms and signs of gastrointestinal diseases are discussed as a unit in this chapter rather than in sections specific to a particular disease or disorder, since they may represent a manifestation of more than one organ of the gastrointestinal tract or may even be caused by an extraintestinal disorder. For example, jaundice may occur from hemolytic causes, hepatocellular diseases, or diseases of the biliary system and pancreas. Vomiting can result from psychological factors, diseases of the central nervous system, or diseases of the gastrointestinal tract. The intent of this chapter is to describe the etiology, pathophysiology, and clinical evaluation of each of the major manifestations of the gastrointestinal diseases.

MANIFESTATIONS AND DIAGNOSIS OF GASTROINTESTINAL DISEASES

The evaluation of complaints and signs of intra-abdominal disease depends upon thorough and thoughtful integration of the patient's history, the physical examination, and the interpretation of laboratory and diagnostic studies. Recognition of the "acute" or "surgical" abdomen is of paramount importance to any physician attending patients with intra-abdominal problems. Understanding of normal intra-abdominal anatomy and physiology along with the pathophysiology of diseases that present as abdominal pain, dysphagia, anorexia, nausea, vomiting, constipation, diarrhea, intestinal obstruction or ileus, gastrointestinal bleeding, or jaundice is essential in arriving at an accurate diagnosis. Recognition of patterns of symptoms and signs occurring with intra-abdominal diseases can often simplify formidable diagnostic problems.

ABDOMINAL PAIN

The word *pain* is derived from the Greek *poine,* which means penalty or punishment. However, pain in the modern sense is the stimulus that brings the ailing patient to the physician, and therefore its characterization is of great importance to the physician. The knowledge of pain mechanisms is essential for the diagnosis and location of the disease process within the abdominal cavities. Therefore, a careful analysis of abdominal pain may help the physician to determine its cause and to outline appropriate treatment. In general, pain should be relieved by medication once it is no longer serving its useful purpose for the diagnosis of the disease. On the other hand, premature treatment of pain, *per se,* may mask the diagnosis and be dangerous to the patient and misleading to the physician.

ANATOMY AND PHYSIOLOGY

Transmission of pain in the peripheral nervous system is served by two specific sets of peripheral nerve fibers, each differentially sensitive to destructive stimuli. Small, myelinated A-delta fibers, 3μ to 4μ in diameter, are distributed principally to skin and muscle. A-delta fibers transmit fast, pricking, or "first" pain. The other specific set of unmyelinated C fibers, 0.4μ to 1.2μ in diameter, are found in muscle, peritoneum, parietal peritoneum, and viscera. They transmit slow, burning, or "second" pain. The sensory afferents that transmit interperitoneal abdominal pain are of the latter type. Sensation transmitted by these C fibers tends to be slow, dull, poorly localized, and of longer duration.

The receptors for pain and the other sensory modalities present in the viscera are similar to those in skin, but there are marked differences in their distribution. There are no proprioceptors in the viscera and few temperature and touch sense organs. Therefore, if the abdominal wall is infiltrated with a local anesthetic, the surgeon can make an incision over the intestine in a patient who is awake without causing significant pain. Pain receptors are present in the viscera, although they are more sparsely distributed than in somatic structures. Certain types of stimuli may cause diffuse stimulation of pain nerve endings throughout an organ, resulting in severe pain. For example, occluding the blood supply to a large area of intestine can result in such extreme pain.

Afferent fibers from visceral structures reach the central nervous system by way of sympathetic or parasympathetic pathways (Fig. 21-1). Visceral afferent fibers from most abdominal organs mediating pain travel with the sympathetic nerves except for those of the upper esophagus and those of the pelvic organs, which follow the parasympathetics of the pelvic nerve. Their cell bodies are located in the dorsal roots and the homologous cranial-nerve ganglia. Visceral sensation travels along the same pathway as somatic sensation, in the spinal thalamic tracts and thalamic radiations. The cortical receiving areas for visceral sensation are intermixed with the somatic receiving areas in the postcentral gyri. The vagi do not transmit pain from the gut despite the fact that 90% of their nerve fibers are sensory. Therefore, the ability to feel pain from the abdominal viscera is unaltered after vagotomy. Most of the mechanoreceptors and chemoreceptors from the vagus nerve are concerned with reflux regulation of gastrointestinal motility and secretion.

Where spinal nerves overlie the abdomen, pain fibers penetrate inward to innervate the parietal peritoneum. Therefore, the parietal peritoneum is exquisitely sensitive, and light mechanical stimuli cause severe pain in conscious humans. For example, where the inflamed appendix touches the parietal peritoneum, pain impulses emanate from the parietal peritoneum and pass directly through the spinal nerve to the spinal cord at a level of approximately L1 or L2. The source is perceived directly over the irritated peritoneum in the right lower quadrant of the abdomen and is of the sharp type, since the impulses are mediated by myelinated A-delta fibers in the abdominal wall.

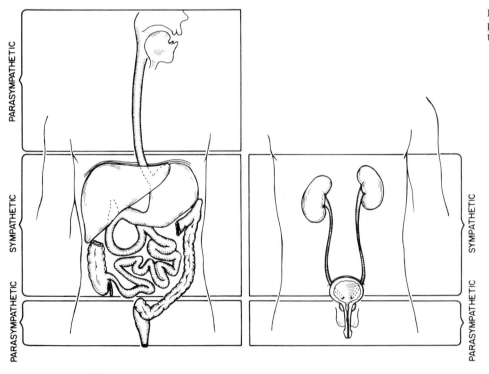

Fig. 21-1. Sympathetic and parasympathetic pain innervation of the abdominal viscera.

TYPES

There are three types of abdominal pain: visceral, parietal, and referred. True visceral pain is usually caused by disordered motility, as in the case of intestinal or biliary tract obstruction. Parietal pain derives from inflammation of the parietal peritoneum. Any slight movement of the peritoneum may aggravate it. For this reason, patients with peritonitis tend to lie perfectly still and are sensitive to any movement that jiggles the peritoneum or anything touching it. In contrast, the patient with true visceral pain frequently moves around in an attempt to find a more comfortable position. Finally, pain may be referred from visceral organs or parietal surfaces by direct involvement of afferent nerve roots. Referral is along dermatome routes, which share different neurons from a distant site. Referred pain may be felt in the skin or other deeper organs. For example, gallbladder pain is referred classically to the interscapular regions.

VISCERAL

In general, abdominal viscera have sensory receptors for no other modalities of sensation besides pain, and visceral pain differs from surface pain in many important aspects. One such difference between surface pain and visceral pain is that highly localized areas of damage to the viscera rarely cause severe pain. On the other hand, stimuli that cause diffuse stimulation of pain nerve endings throughout a viscus cause severe pain. Principal forces to which visceral fibers are sensitive are stretching or tension, such as in the wall of the gut. This can be the result of distention of a hollow viscus or forceful muscular contractions. Nerve endings of pain fibers in the hollow viscera are located in the muscular wall. In the solid viscera, such as the liver and kidney, they are located in the capsule. Thus, stretching of the capsule from parenchymal swelling may cause pain.

Ischemia

Ischemia causes visceral pain in perhaps the same way as it does in other tissues, presumably because of accumulation of acidic metabolic end products or products such as bradykinin or serotonin that stimulate the pain nerve endings. It may also lower the threshold to other noxious stimuli.

Inflammation

As noted, bacterial or chemical inflammation may produce visceral pain. Inflammation sensitizes the nerve endings and lowers the threshold to pain from other stimuli. The mechanism by which inflammation itself produces visceral pain is not clear. It has been suggested that the release of bradykinin, serotonin, histamine, or prostaglandin may mediate the pain caused by inflammation.

Spasm of a Hollow Viscus

Spasm of a hollow viscus such as the gallbladder, bile duct, ureter, or intestine can produce pain exactly the same way that spasm of skeletal muscle causes pain. This presumably results from diminished blood flow to the muscle combined with increased metabolic needs of the muscle for nutrients. Pain from a spastic viscus often occurs in the form of rhythmic cycles. It increases to a high degree of severity and then subsides. The rhythmic cycles result from rhythmic contraction of smooth muscles. For example, each time a peristaltic wave travels along an overly excitable spastic gut, a cramp occurs.

Overdistention of a Hollow Viscus

Overdistention of a hollow viscus also produces pain, perhaps because of overstretch of the tissue itself. Overdistention may also compromise the blood supply to the organ by compression of the blood vessel, thereby perhaps promoting ischemic pain.

PARIETAL

The parietal surface of the visceral cavities is supplied mainly by spinal nerve fibers that penetrate from the surface of the body inward. When a disease affects a viscus, it often spreads to the parietal wall of the visceral cavity. This wall, like the skin, is supplied with extensive innervation, including the fast A-delta fibers, which are different from the fibers in the true visceral pain pathway of sympathetic nerves. Pain from the parietal wall of a visceral cavity is frequently very sharp and pricking, although it can also be burning and aching. Therefore, a knife incision through the peritoneum is very painful even though a similar cut through an organ such as the intestine is not.

REFERRED

Referred pain is felt in areas supplied by the same neurosegment as the diseased organ and is due to the existence of a shared central pathway for afferent neurons from different sites. Therefore, a patient may feel pain in a part of his body that is considerably distant from the tissue causing the pain. Frequently, it is initiated in one of the visceral organs and is referred to an area of the body surface although occasionally pain can even be referred from one surface area of the body to another. Pain may also originate from a viscus and be referred to another deep area of the body not exactly coinciding with the location of the viscus producing the pain.

The most widely accepted mechanism of referred pain is illustrated in Figure 21-2. Visceral pain fibers are shown to synapse in the spinal cord with some of the same second-order neurons that received pain fibers from the skin. When visceral fibers are stimulated, the stimulus may spread into some of the neurons that normally conduct pain sensation only from the skin. Therefore, the patient may feel that the sensation actually originates in the skin itself. Because the visceral afferent sympathetic or parasympathetic pain fibers are responsible for transmitting sensations of pain referred

Fig. 21-2. Mechanism of referred pain. Branches of visceral pain fibers synapse in the spinal cord with pain fibers from the skin.

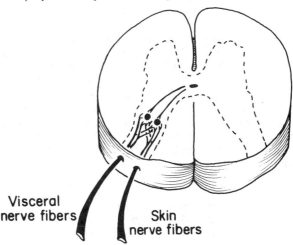

Visceral nerve fibers

Skin nerve fibers

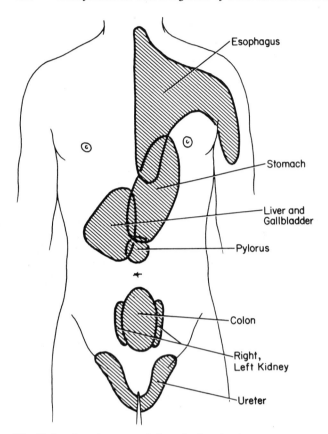

Fig. 21-3. Anterior areas of visceral referred pain.

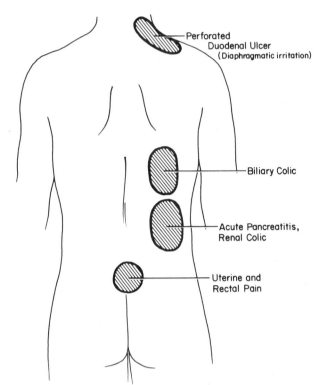

Fig. 21-4. Posterior areas of visceral referred pain.

from a specific visceral site, the location of referred pain on the surface of the body is in the dermatome of the segment from which the visceral organ was originally derived in the embryo. Some of the areas of referred pain on the surface of the body are shown in Figures 21-3 and 21-4.

VISCERAL AND REFERRED PAIN FROM ABDOMINAL ORGANS

The following section describes some generalizations regarding the location and quality of pain from a specific organ.

ESOPHAGUS

Esophageal pain is usually referred to the pharynx and lower neck and is usually felt as substernal discomfort near the site of the disease. Distention with balloons placed at various levels has demonstrated that the subject is able to indicate accurately the site of the stimulus in this organ. Thus, a stimulus from the upper esophagus produces pain in the neck, whereas a stimulus from the lower third of the esophagus is usually felt near the xiphoid process. Irritation of the distal esophagus may cause chest pain similar to that produced by ischemic heart disease, although the pain has nothing whatsoever to do with the heart. Pain from the esophagus may be caused by spasm due to chemical or bacterial inflammatory irritation, especially noted during reflux of gastric contents into the distal esophagus.

STOMACH AND DUODENUM

Pain from the stomach and duodenum may be referred to the anterior surface of the chest or upper abdomen in the midline of the epigastrium. It is frequently characterized as

burning pain. Disease of the duodenal bulb, such as duodenal ulcer, may produce discomfort somewhat to the right of the epigastrium. Most peptic ulcers occur within 1 or 2 inches on the duodenal or gastric site of the pylorus, and pain from such ulcers is usually referred to a surface point approximately midway between the umbilicus and the xiphoid process. The origin of ulcer pain is perhaps chemical irritation from the acidity of the gastric content; therefore, it is usually relieved by neutralization of the luminal acid by antacid. This pain is characteristically burning.

SMALL INTESTINE

Pain originating from the jejunum to the proximal ileum is usually referred to the midabdomen around the umbilicus. Disease or other stimuli from the distal ileum usually causes referred pain to the periumbilical area but occasionally may be felt in the lower abdomen or to the right of the midline. An example of this is Crohn's disease of the terminal ileum, which may mimic acute appendicitis.

COLON

Pain from the colon may be localized to the lower midabdomen. Irritation from the rectum may create local discomfort or cause pain to be referred posteriorly over the sacrum.

GALLBLADDER AND COMMON BILE DUCT

Pain originating from the gallbladder or the common bile duct is usually localized to the right upper quadrant or the mid epigastrium. Therefore, it may be similar to the pain caused by peptic ulcer disease. The pain may be burning, which would make it difficult to distinguish from peptic ulcer disease, although colicky pain often occurs in gallbladder and common bile duct disease, due to repeated spasms of these structures in response to inflammation or, especially, stones. Referred pain from the gallbladder is usually localized between the scapulae or to the right upper quadrant of the abdomen. The biliary system is supplied by fibers from T6 to T10, but most originate from the T9 dermatome.

PANCREAS

Inflammation of the pancreas results in intense pain in areas both anterior to and behind the pancreas. Therefore, it is usually felt in the midline or to the left side of the epigastrium. It is often referred to the back, in the upper lumbar and lower dorsal areas. Inflammatory processes in the tail of the pancreas may irritate the left diaphragm, which will be felt in the left shoulder.

KIDNEYS

The kidneys and ureters are all retroperitoneal structures and receive most of their pain fibers directly from the skeletal nerves. Therefore, pain is usually felt directly behind the diseased structure. Occasionally, pain is referred through visceral afferents to the anterior abdominal wall below the umbilicus on both sides. Pain from the urinary bladder is felt directly over the bladder, presumably because the bladder is well innervated by parietal pain fibers. Pain from the ureters may be referred to the groin and testicles because afferent nerve fibers synapse in the cord with fibers from the genital areas.

UTERUS

Both parietal and visceral afferent fibers may be transmitted from the uterus. Therefore, the low-abdominal crampy pain of dysmenorrhea may be mediated through the sympathetic afferents. On the other hand, lesions of the uterus may cause parietal pain in the lower back or side. This pain is conducted over parietal nerve fibers and is usually sharper than that associated with dysmenorrhea. Like other hollow viscera, the uterus becomes painful in response to obstruction, distention, or severe contraction.

OVARIES

The ovary is insensitive to most stimuli because it does not have a capsule. Ovarian inflammation or tumors are usually asymptomatic unless there is strangulation by torsion or rupture of a cyst, which may irritate the overlying parietal peritoneum.

CLINICAL EVALUATION

Abdominal pain may be caused by a great variety of gastrointestinal and intraperitoneal diseases (Table 21-1). It may occasionally be caused by the following extra-abdominal diseases:

Pneumonia

Pleurisy

Pericarditis (acute and chronic)

Coronary artery disease

Diabetic ketosis

Hyperparathyroidism

Acute porphyrinuria

Lead intoxication

Herpes zoster

Tabes dorsalis

Hemochromatosis

TABLE 21-1   COMMON CAUSES OF ABDOMINAL PAIN

Inflammation
  Peptic ulcers: esophagus, stomach, duodenum, jejunum
  Acute gastritis
  Regional enteritis (inflammation alone is rarely an indication for operation)
  Acute cholecystitis
  Acute pancreatitis (inflammation alone is rarely an indication for operation)
  Acute appendicitis
  Peritonitis, including localized abscess

Obstruction
  Congenital: atresia, stenosis, volvulus, bands, cysts
  Inflammatory: enteritis, granulomas, diverticulitis, peritonitis
  Neoplastic: primary or metastatic
  Obturative: gallstones, bezoars, meconium, parasites, foreign bodies
  Other: hernia, adhesions, volvulus, intussusception, irradiation, endometriosis

Perforation
  Peptic ulcer: esophagus, stomach, duodenum, jejunum
  External trauma, including iatrogenic perforation due to instrumentation
  Intraluminal foreign body
  Neoplasm
  Ulcerative colitis
  Acute appendicitis, diverticulitis, cholecystitis

Hemorrhage
  Esophageal varices, Mallory–Weiss lacerations
  Peptic ulcer: esophagus, stomach, duodenum, jejunum
  Acute hemorrhagic gastritis
  Trauma: penetrating or nonpenetrating
  Neoplasm
  Diverticulitis

(Ballinger WF, Zuidema GD: The acute abdomen. In Paulson M et al [eds]: Gastroenterologic Medicine, p 556. Philadelphia, Lea & Febiger, 1969)

Benign paroxysmal peritonitis

Epilepsy

Psychiatric causes

Henoch-Schönlein purpura

Essential hyperlipemia

Spider bites

Drug addiction

Drugs (*e.g.*, aspirin, Butazolidin)

Infectious mononucleosis

In most patients, a careful history, physical examination, and laboratory findings generally result in a correct diagnosis. In some cases, however, the etiology of recurrent or persistent abdominal pain may present diagnostic difficulties.

When a patient presents with a major complaint of abdominal pain, the acuteness of the pain is a major factor in determining the clinical approach to the patient. Evaluation may be slow and deliberate if symptoms have been present for a long time without recent exacerbation. It would be important to achieve an exact diagnosis in such patients. On the other hand, the principal goal in patients with acute illness is to determine whether prompt operation is required. Complete and exact diagnosis in such patients may delay the operation. An indication for surgery is usually determined by severe localized or diffuse peritoneal irritation or intestinal obstruction. An orderly approach to patients with acute abdominal pain should be taken, such as obtaining history, performing a physical examination, and obtaining laboratory data. Such an orderly approach can usually be completed within an hour or two and should not be abandoned in most patients who present with an acute abdomen. There are only a few abdominal conditions that require urgent operative intervention without complete work up. An example is exsanguinating hemorrhage from a ruptured abdominal aortic aneurysm; in such a case, the patient must be rushed to the operating room immediately. Fortunately, this type of situation is relatively rare, and even in such instances a few minutes are required to assess the critical nature of the problem and establish a probable diagnosis.

HISTORY

The history of abdominal pain is extremely important in making the differential diagnosis. Therefore, the patient must be questioned carefully regarding the following aspects of a complaint of abdominal pain:

1. Location. The site of the pain and the extent to which it is localized must be determined. Although visceral pain tends to be poorly localized, the pain produced by irritation of the parietal peritoneum is usually confined to the area involved by the disease. Familiarity of the location of referred pain may be of great help in the diagnosis of abdominal pain. For example, pain in the shoulder may signify diaphragmatic irritation from diseases such as ruptured duodenal ulcer. A pain derived from biliary and pancreatic disease is often referred to the back.
2. Character. Some diseases produce pain with a distinct quality. For example, pain resulting from disordered motility is usually crampy except when ileus is present, in which case the pain may become constant. Other well-known examples are the burning or gnawing pain of duodenal ulcer or the substernal heartburn of esophagitis.
3. Intensity. Severity of pain is loosely related to the magnitude of the noxious stimuli. A perforated viscus or mesenteric occlusion, for example, produces excruciating pain. The former is often followed by a period of relative relief before peritoneal signs occur. The more severe the pain, the more likely it is to be referred. On the other hand, the severity of the pain may not be a reliable indication of the degree of irritation in some patients because of the interaction of various factors that determine the response.
4. Duration and frequency. Severe acute pain persisting for more than 6 hours often implies a surgical problem, such as perforation, obstruction, or strangulation of a hollow viscus. Intestinal obstruction is usually associated with episodes of crampy pain with pain-free intervals. Steady and severe pain in the presence of intestinal obstruction is indicative of ischemia from strangulation. Chronic pain of duodenal ulcer, on the other hand, rarely occurs immediately after meals but appears later in the interprandial period.

5. Aggravating or alleviating factors. Aggravation by anxiety and tension points to functional disorders such as irritable bowel syndrome. Relief by eating or taking antacids implies duodenal ulcer disease, whereas aggravation upon eating suggests an obstructive component. Association with drugs such as aspirin or alcohol suggests gastric or duodenal inflammatory ulceration. Diffuse abdominal pain appearing 30 minutes to an hour after meals suggests the possibility of intestinal angina. Aggravation by positional factors such as bending or straining is noted in gastroesophageal reflux. A history of previous ulcer operation may suggest dumping syndrome, afferent loop syndrome, or adhesions. Passage of a gallstone may be characterized by intense and progressive pain in the right upper quadrant with abrupt relief leaving a dull aching sensation in the area.

PHYSICAL EXAMINATION

Thorough physical examination is essential in the diagnosis of acute abdominal pain. It may uncover unsuspected abnormalities as well as attest to a specific hypothesis formed from the history. Examination begins with a general inspection. The general physical appearance may indicate shock with a perforated viscus, peritonitis, or strangulation. On occasion, the facial expression of the patient will provide valuable evidence of the serious nature of the pain. The importance of repeated surveillance of facial expression as a reflection of the severity of pain, as well as of the attitude to illness, the surgeon, and the hospital, cannot be overemphasized. The position in bed is noteworthy. Immobility and dislike of movement are suggestive of localized or generalized peritonitis, whereas restlessness is indicative of severe crampy pain from a hollow viscus due to obstruction. In patients with localized or generalized peritonitis, the knees are frequently drawn up to relax tension of the abdominal wall. The patient with pure visceral pain may change position frequently. The abdomen should be inspected for any local or generalized distention. All the hernia orifices must be examined as a routine, and special attention must be directed to the femoral canal because a femoral hernia is easily missed in an obese patient. The respiratory movement of the abdominal wall should be carefully noted; any limitation indicates some rigidity of the diaphragm or abdominal muscle.

Auscultation may reveal evidence of paralytic ileus, with absent bowel sounds secondary to an inflammatory condition. Generalized peritonitis causes decreased or absent peristalsis. Hyperperistalsis suggests an intestinal obstruction. Vascular bruits may be clues to an aortic or splanchnic artery aneurysm.

Palpation of the abdomen should be especially gentle at first and started at a part of the abdomen farthest removed from the point of maximum pain. A rough and painful examination is not only difficult for the patient but may be misleading to the physician. Palpation will suggest the extent and the intensity of muscular rigidity; it will locate any tender area or hyperesthetic area. It is our preference to have the patient's thigh flexed while palpating the abdomen and to reassure the patient during the examination, to reduce voluntary guarding as much as possible.

Percussion of the abdomen must also be carried out with the greatest of gentleness. The purpose of percussion is to estimate the amount of distention of the intestine, determine abnormal liver dullness, and exclude the presence of a distended urinary bladder. It also is perhaps the best way to elicit peritoneal irritation (Fig. 21-5). Light percussion over the tender area may confirm the presence of peritonitis of the parietal peritoneum, and it is suggested that this be done before heavier palpation, since the former is more sensitive in localizing areas of tenderness.

When tenderness is present, it is important to determine whether it is localized or diffuse. Diffuse tenderness indicates generalized peritonitis. Localized tenderness suggests an early, uncomplicated stage of the disease, diseases such as acute cholecystitis, acute appendicitis, or diverticulitis. Mild tenderness without peritoneal irritation is more compatible with acute gastroenteritis or some other nonsurgical conditions.

Rebound tenderness is produced by pressing slowly and deeply over a tender area and then suddenly releasing the hand. It is essentially a rough examination, and the patient may experience sudden and severe pain on the rebound. Rebound tenderness merely confirms the presence of peritoneal irritation of the parietal peritoneum over the area. Since the same information may be obtained by light percussion, demonstration of rebound tenderness is not necessary in most patients.

Abdominal rigidity is the result of the highly protective contraction of the abdominal muscles in some patients with generalized peritonitis. On the other hand, its absence does not exclude the possibility of generalized peritonitis, since ''boardlike'' rigidity is less frequent than generally believed and muscular rigidity and resistance may be slight even in the presence of serious peritonitis. In elderly or feeble patients, muscular rigidity is less noticeable, as is the case also in patients in whom the abdominal wall is very fat and flabby and the muscles are thin and weak.

Hyperesthesia

Hyperesthesia in response to gentle touch or to pen stroke over the skin may appear in the dermatome affected by

Fig. 21-5. Light percussion elicits peritoneal irritation without undue discomfort to the patient.

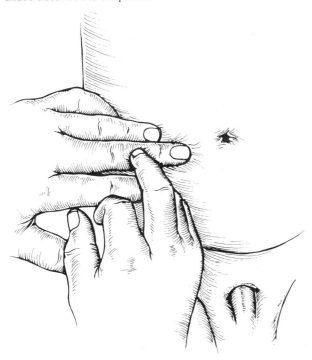

intraperitoneal parietal pain. Although its presence might be helpful, it is often absent even though significant localized peritonitis exists.

Psoas Muscle Rigidity

If there is an inflamed focus in relation to the psoas muscle, the corresponding thigh is often flexed by the patient to relieve the pain. Often, a lesser degree of such contraction can be determined by making the patient lie on the opposite side and extending the thigh on the affected side to full extent. Pain will be caused by this maneuver if the psoas muscle is rigid from either reflex or direct irritation. The value of this test is significant, particularly in the diagnosis of appendicitis if the appendix is located in the retrocecal position.

Genital, rectal, and pelvic examinations are an essential part of the evaluation in every patient with abdominal pain. Rectal examination is extremely important and informative. Pressing forward, backward, upward, and laterally, the whole lower pelvis can be explored. Pelvic examination will determine the presence and the position of any pelvic tumor or swelling. Acute pelvic inflammatory disease or a twisted ovarian cyst or uterine fibroid also may be found.

LABORATORY TESTS

A complete blood count with specific interest in the white blood cell count is important to define the presence of an inflammatory process. Hematocrit determinations will suggest hemoconcentration or anemia. Urinalysis is directed toward evaluating urinary tract infection, diabetes, or hematuria. Red blood cells in the urine may suggest calculi as a cause of abdominal pain. The elevation of serum or urine amylase is most frequently associated wih acute pancreatitis. However, it is not specific, since many other intra-abdominal diseases, such as perforated duodenal ulcer, cholecystitis, and intestinal obstruction, may also produce an elevated serum amylase level. An upright film of the abdomen may often demonstrate areas of ileus or intestinal obstruction. Upright or lateral decubitus films are frequently helpful in determining the presence of air within the intestinal lumen or free air within the peritoneal cavity. A chest film is useful, particularly in patients over the age of 40 and in children with upper abdominal pain, because pneumonia may occasionally cause upper abdominal pain. Paracentesis may be helpful, particularly in injured patients who are obtunded and who are difficult to evaluate for the presence or absence of peritoneal irritation. Ultrasonography may be a useful test in the early evaluation of patients with suspected acute cholecystitis or pseudocyst of the pancreas, although cholecystography may be needed to demonstrate gallstones in patients whose acute episode of pain is resolved. In patients suspected of chronic abdominal angina, mesenteric angiography may reveal mesenteric arterial stenosis. It is to be emphasized that laparotomy itself may constitute an important and necessary tool in the diagnosis of acute abdominal pain, paticularly in the presence of localized or diffuse peritoneal signs.

Chronic recurrent undiagnosed abdominal pain is a significant clinical problem and often has led to repeated laparotomies. Usually the patient has had many recurrent attacks for years without developing weight loss. Barium x-ray studies of the upper and lower gastrointestinal tract may demonstrate normal findings or questionably abnormal findings. Many of these patients are psychologically unstable, and follow-up examinations usually fail to reveal an organic source of the symptoms. In some patients, functional disturbances characterized by spasm of the gut are responsible for pain. In perplexing cases, the question arises as to the value of diagnostic laparotomy in those patients with chronic abdominal pain. If there are no objective findings, such as fever, jaundice, or abnormalities on x-ray film, laparotomy is usually negative. On the other hand, in the presence of at least one objective finding, diagnostic laparotomy frequently leads to a specific diagnosis that may explain the pain.

DYSPHAGIA

Dysphagia connotes difficulty in swallowing and is usually described by the patient as "the food just won't go down right" or "the food sticks." Dysphagia usually indicates esophageal disease or malfunction.

The act of normal swallowing is customarily divided into oral, pharyngeal, and esophageal phases. The first two phases of swallowing, oral and pharyngeal, take place in less than a second. In the first phase, the bolus of food or liquid is moved into the pharynx by contraction of the mylohyoid muscle. Aspiration into respiratory passages is prevented by closure of the soft palate, glottis, and epiglottis. In the second phase, the material is transported through the pharynx by contraction of the pharyngeal muscle, which is accompanied by synchronous relaxation of the upper esophageal constrictor muscle. This establishes a pressure gradient that propels the material into the upper esophagus.

The esophageal phase of swallowing moves the bolus through the esophagus into the stomach. A peristaltic wave sweeps material down the esophagus, traversing the lower esophageal sphincter, which is simultaneously relaxed, permitting material to enter the stomach. These reflexes are controlled by the fifth, seventh, ninth, tenth, and eleventh cranial nerves, which innervate the striated muscles of the oropharynx and upper third of the esophagus, as well as the smooth muscle comprising the lower two thirds of the esophagus. The motor innervation of the smooth muscle portion of the esophagus is cholinergic.

Transport of the bolus through the esophagus is dependent upon the pressure gradient produced by the primary peristaltic contraction plus the effect of gravity. The propulsion of the bolus from the esophagus into the stomach is also dependent upon relaxation of the inferior esophageal sphincter, which reacts autonomously in response to pressure or peristalsis in the lower esophagus.

Secondary peristalsis is exactly the same as primary peristalsis except that the initiating event is introduction of a bolus directly into the esophagus rather than a swallow. Secondary peristaltic contractions occur when an esophageal segment is distended by a solid bolus of food.

Tertiary esophageal contractions are localized, nonpropulsive, simultaneous contractions that may be spontaneous or induced by swallowing. The most important feature of tertiary contractions is that they are nonperistaltic. They occasionally occur in the normal esophagus but are more common in pathologic states and with aging.

ETIOLOGY

Dysphagia may be caused by oral, pharyngeal, or esophageal abnormalities. The first two include disorders of the mouth, upper respiratory tract, and pharynx (from such painful lesions of the mouth or tongue as tonsillitis or oropharyngeal

carcinoma) and neurologic lesions, typified by poliomyelitis or myasthenia gravis.

Esophageal dysphagia is usually caused by two basic abnormalities of the esophagus: mechanical narrowing of the lumen, either intrinsic or extrinsic, and a motor disorder, such as achalasia or scleroderma (Table 21-2). The specific characteristics of dysphagia can be of some help in differentiating between these two categories.

Achalasia and diffuse esophageal spasm are the two major forms of esophageal motor dysfunction that lead to dysphagia. Achalasia is a disease characterized by dysphagia to liquids and solids, weight loss, occasionally sharp retrosternal chest pain, and, less commonly, nocturnal regurgitation and aspiration. It has been well established histopathologically that the esophagus in patients with achalasia has lost its intrinsic autonomic innervation. There is an absolute decrease to complete absence of Auerbach's plexus, especially in the distal half of the esophagus. This abnormality results in failure of relaxation of the lower esophageal sphincter with swallowing and an absence of peristalsis in the body of the esophagus. Diffuse esophageal spasm is a syndrome also characterized by dysphagia to liquids and solids and nonspecific chest pain. In patients with diffuse esophageal spasm, tertiary esophageal contractions predominate as the major esophageal motor abnormality. Esophageal spasm may be primary (idiopathic or presbyesophagus of the elderly), or it may be secondary to other conditions in the esophagus, such as scleroderma, diabetic neuropathy, esophagitis, and obstructive lesions.

Mechanical obstruction may be due to benign strictures or carcinoma of the esophagus. The most common type of benign stricture causing mechanical obstruction is reflux esophagitis. Other benign strictures include lower esophageal ring (web or Schatzki's ring), corrosive ingestion, and trauma. Malignant lesions of the esophagus are usually squamous cell carcinoma of the esophagus but also may occur with upward invasion of adenocarcinoma of the stomach. Squamous cell carcinoma of the esophagus may occur at any level of the esophagus but is most commonly seen in the distal third. Adenocarcinoma is usually limited to the distal esophagus, particularly at the gastroesophageal junction.

CLINICAL EVALUATION

A well-taken history may give clues as to whether the dysphagia is caused by mechanical obstruction or motility disorders. A complete description of the symptom with particular reference to the duration, location, and timing in relation to ingestion of food may suggest a more specific

TABLE 21-2   CAUSES OF ESOPHAGEAL DYSPHAGIA

	MECHANICAL NARROWING	MOTOR DISORDER
Progression	Often	Usually not
Type of Bolus	Solids (unless high-grade obstruction)	Solids or liquids
Temperature Dependent	No	Worse with cold liquids

etiology within these two categories of dysphagia. For example, malignant lesions should be suspected if the caliber of solid food that is able to be swallowed decreases over a period of several months. Association of heartburn and regurgitation might point to a stricture secondary to esophagitis. The temperature of the material that arrests in the esophagus may also help in investigation of the cause of dysphagia. Increase in dysphagia after ingestion of cold liquids and alleviation by warm liquids point to a motor disorder. It may also be of help to know the method by which the patient seeks relief from an obstructing bolus. Dysphagia from mechanical narrowing of the lumen often is relieved only by self-induced vomiting or regurgitation. However, in motor disorders of the esophagus, it may be possible to dislodge the solid bolus by repeated swallowing of liquids. Therefore, careful analysis of the patient's symptoms and of the characteristics and the nature of the dysphagia alone may provide diagnostic accuracy in approximately 80% of patients. During physical examination, particular attention should be paid to the detection of cervical lymph nodes, suggesting mediastinal or esophageal lesions. The stigmata of scleroderma may be found by careful inspection of the patient's fingers. Barium study of the esophagus is frequently diagnostic for obstructing lesions. Esophagoscopy with biopsies will further confirm the nature and the pathology of the obstructing lesion. The use of cineesophagography or manometric motility studies is particularly helpful in determining disorders of motility.

ANOREXIA, NAUSEA, AND VOMITING

ANOREXIA

Anorexia is a significant decrease in the desire to eat despite all the physiological stimuli that would normally produce hunger. Most organic diseases of the gastrointestinal tract, for example, acute appendicitis, esophageal carcinoma, and peptic ulcer disease, may lead to anorexia. It should be emphasized that nondigestive diseases such as heart disease and pneumonia may also produce anorexia. Therefore, it is an important but nonspecific symptom. Other associated symptoms and signs, such as abdominal pain, vomiting, or diarrhea, are necessary to implicate a gastrointestinal etiology. The absence of anorexia in the presence of other gastrointestinal symptoms may help to rule out acute inflammatory processes such as appendicitis.

Anorexia nervosa results from severe psychological disturbance that relates to normal intake of food. It should be suspected if a patient has severe weight loss but no evidence of malabsorption. The disease is several times more common in adolescent girls and young women than in men. It is characterized by severe weight loss, amenorrhea, and a specific psychopathology. The onset occurs around the time of puberty, and the patient expresses a fear of becoming fat and resorts to an abnormal behavior of food refusal or excessive exercise or both.

NAUSEA AND VOMITING

Nausea, retching, and vomiting are three stages, usually, but not always, expressed sequentially. Characteristic changes in gastrointestinal motility have been recognized for each of these stages.

Nausea is a distress of the stomach, a distaste for food, and, often, an urge to vomit. Although a variety of stimuli may produce nausea, the neuropathways mediating nausea are not well understood. During nausea, gastric tone is reduced and peristalsis in the stomach is diminished or absent. In contrast, the tone of the duodenum and proximal small intestine tends to be increased and duodenal contents may reflux into the stomach.

Retching consists in spasmodic and abortive respiratory movements with the glottis closed. During this stage, gastric compression results from increased intra-abdominal pressure due to sudden respiratory inspiration, forceful descent of the diaphragm, and contraction of the extra-abdominal musculature. The pyloric end of the stomach contracts, but the proximal stomach and the esophagogastric junction are relaxed.

Vomiting refers to the forceful expulsion of stomach contents through the esophagus and mouth. This usually occurs by a forceful sustained contraction of the abdominal muscles at the time when the cardia of the stomach is raised and open and the pylorus is contracted.

Experimental studies suggest that all emetic responses are mediated through reflex arcs that pass through a vomiting center, regardless of whether these responses are initiated at peripheral or central sites. There are two anatomically and functionally separate units in the brain concerned with the act of vomiting, a vomiting center in the reticular formation, which is excited directly by visceral afferent impulses arising from the gastrointestinal tract, and a chemoreceptor trigger zone in the floor of the fourth ventricle. The trigger zone is implicated in drug-induced emesis and also in the vomiting associated with uremia, infections, motion sickness, and diabetic ketoacidosis. However, the chemoreceptor trigger zone is not able to cause vomiting without the mediation of an intact vomiting center. Whether the vomiting center is under the control of higher cortical or brain stem structure is not certain.

Afferent pathways to the vomiting center arise from almost all sites in the body. Irritation of the mucosa of the upper gastrointestinal tract causes vomiting. Impulses are relayed from the mucosa to the vomiting center over visceral afferent pathways in the sympathetic nerves and vagi. Although neither vagotomy nor sympathectomy alone abolishes the vomiting of gastrointestinal origin, the vagus is considered the more important afferent pathway from this stimulus. The efferent pathways are mainly somatic, presumably in the vagi, sympathetics, and phrenics and in the cranial supply to pharyngeal muscles. It involves the phrenic nerves to the diaphragm, spinal nerves to the abdominal and intercostal muscles, and efferent visceral fibers along the vagi and sympathetic nerves to the intestine and muscles of the pharynx and larynx. Vomiting is probably an integrated somatovisceral process. The act of vomiting requires the coordinated closure of the glottis, contraction and fixation of the diaphragm in inspiratory position, closure of the pylorus, and relaxation of the proximal stomach and gastroesophageal junction. This is followed by forceful contraction of the abdominal, diaphragmatic, and intercostal muscles, which increases the intra-abdominal pressure and causes regurgitation.

CLINICAL EVALUATION

Vomiting may be the first indication of a surgical emergency such as intestinal obstruction, peritonitis, or cholecystitis. Vomiting can be an early manifestation in patients with carcinoma of the stomach or gastric outlet obstruction secondary to duodenal ulcer. Therefore, a careful description of vomiting in the history may provide clues as to the underlying disease that causes vomiting.

The timing of vomiting in relation to meals may suggest different underlying causes. Vomiting soon after a meal is common in patients with peptic ulcer near the pyloric channel, presumably because of irritation, edema, and spasm of the pylorus. Delayed vomiting (more than 1 hour after a meal) is also characteristic of gastric outlet obstruction or a motility disorder of the stomach. Vomitus containing food eaten 12 hours earlier is rarely seen in patients with psychoneurotic vomiting and is strong evidence for outlet obstruction. Vomiting in the early morning before breakfast is characteristic of pregnancy. Vomiting often relieves pain caused by peptic ulcer disease but not pain caused by pancreatitis or biliary tract disease.

The content of the vomitus should be investigated. Blood or coffee-ground material in the vomitus indicates upper gastrointestinal tract bleeding. The presence of bile indicates an open connection between the proximal duodenum and the stomach. Even with partial obstruction at the gastric outlet, it is unusual to find bile in the vomitus. The odor of vomitus may also be important. A fecal odor suggests intestinal obstruction of long duration, gastrocolic fistula, or, occasionally, bacterial overgrowth in the proximal small intestine, such as in patients with blind loop syndrome. Examination of patients who have been vomiting should be directed especially to the presence or absence of weight loss, abdominal mass, abdominal distention, visible intestinal peristalsis, umbilical or inguinal hernia, abdominal scar indicating previous operation, jaundice, or the signs of peritonitis. Prolonged vomiting may produce metabolic abnormalities such as hypovolemia, hypokalemia, and metabolic alkalosis. Metabolic alkalosis develops primarily in gastric outlet obstruction because of the loss of H^+ in the vomitus and secondarily because of contraction of the extracellular fluid without a concomitant loss of bicarbonate and because of a shift of H^+ into the cell as a result of potassium deficiency. Hypokalemia usually results from decreased intake of potassium, from the loss of potassium in the vomitus, and, most importantly, from renal potassium waste. Sodium depletion also develops because of the loss of sodium in the vomitus and in some cases because of renal sodium loss in association with bicarbonate excretion. The clinical presentation of sodium depletion may include hyponatremia, hypotension, decreased blood volume, and hemoconcentration. Therefore, therapy should be instituted early to correct the electrolyte and fluid deficiency and systemic acid–base balance. The underlying cause must be treated whenever this is known.

Symptomatic therapy to control vomiting, like that to control pain, should be used with caution and, if possible, should not mask diagnosis of serious or life-threatening import, such as intestinal obstruction. Medications such as the antihistamine dimenhydrinate (Dramamine) and the antiemetic (and psychotropic) agent chlorpromazine appear to act on several areas, including the chemoreceptor zone, whereas trimethobenzamide (Tigan) acts strictly on the chemoreceptor zone. Prochlorperazine (Compazine) seems to be more effective than many of the other medications but carries with it the danger of producing significant side-effects. In general, antiemetic drugs are more effective for prophylaxis than for treatment. The choice of agent usually depends upon the cause of vomiting. Antihistamines are recommended for motion sickness or vomiting caused by other vestibular disturbances. Chlorpromazine or prochlorperazine is preferred for vomiting caused by drugs or irradiation and for postoperative vomiting. All these agents may have significant side-effects; therefore, they should be administered with caution.

CONSTIPATION

Constipation may imply that the stool occurs with relative infrequency or that the stools are too small, too hard, or too difficult to expel. These symptoms are difficult to quantify. Frequency of stool is variable in the normal population. Several studies of stool frequency show that normal subjects pass at least three stools per week. These data do not differ whether they were obtained by questionnaire or by stool collections. However, it is oversimplifying the problem to define constipation simply on the basis of stool frequency and to ignore the other aspects of constipation, such as small stools, feeling of incomplete evacuation, hard stools, and difficulty at expulsion. It is one of the symptoms that has been frequently, but incorrectly, self-diagnosed by patients. One of the reasons for the frequent misdiagnosis and confusion is that the range of normality is extremely broad. In a healthy population, stool frequency may vary between three times a day and two or three times a week without symptoms or associated ill effects.

COLONIC MOTILITY

Colonic movements are well organized, and patterns of flow are consistent with three important functions of the colon. The first function is the absorption of water. Second, the colon maintains an abundant intraluminal bacterial population. Third, colonic movements control the delivery of feces. In the proximal colon, annular contractions of the colonic wall are associated with rhythmic antiperistalsis. It drives the colonic content toward the cecum, where it is retained for long periods. In the middle part of the colon, the major activities constitute annular contractions that divide the fecal mass and tend to move the feces very slowly toward the rectum. In the most distal part of the colon, there are strong contractions oriented to move the fecal mass distally. Excitation of these contractions results from stimulation of the pelvic nerves. It has been stated that the fecal bolus normally does not pass beyond the sigmoid into the rectum until defecation is about to occur. This view is not consistent with common clinical experience that fecal material does present in the rectum in the interdefecatory period and is normally found during digital examination of the rectum. In addition, radiologic studies have shown that in some subjects, at least, the entire left side of the colon from the splenic flexure downward may be emptied in defecation.

Continence includes sphincteric continence and rectal continence as two separate functions. Sphincteric continence refers to the complex actions and properties of the internal and external sphincters and of the anal canal. Rectal continence refers to the capacity of the rectum to act as a reservoir. The rectum has the ability to allow an increase in volume within its lumen without a corresponding increase in pressure. However, when the rectum is distended beyond a certain degree, it then initiates afferent nervous impulses conducted by the hypogastric and pelvic nerves to the sacral cord, where efferent impulses are discharged. The process of defecation may be entirely involuntary, but it is usually assisted by voluntary contractions of the muscles of the abdomen and diaphragm and the voluntary relaxation of the external anal sphincter. All of these well-coordinated actions increase the colonic pressure and force the stool through the relaxed internal and external sphincters.

ETIOLOGY

Constipation is not a disease but a symptom of many diseases. The diseases that cause constipation may be grouped as systemic or gastrointestinal in origin (Table 21-3).

SYSTEMIC CAUSES

One of the most common forms of constipation is based on public misconception, often enhanced by advertisement emphasizing the virtues of "regularity." This misconception (one stool per day) leads to a secondary form of constipation resulting from abuse of laxatives to achieve this imaginary goal. Laxative abuse results in excessive emptying of the colon with a consequent delay in sufficient intraluminal distention to produce an urge. This desensitization may in turn increase laxative requirement.

Metabolic disorders such as diabetes, porphyria, uremia, and hypokalemia may induce constipation. Endocrine disorders such as hyperthyroidism, hypercalcemia, hyperparathyroidism, and pregnancy may also cause constipation. Constipation may be the primary complaint in some patients suffering from these metabolic disorders.

Other factors have been said to result in constipation. However, there is not sufficient evidence to support the cause–effect relationship between these factors and constipation. For example, lack of exercise and traveling long distances may be associated with constipation. It is not known if exercise has any effect on colonic function. Constipation may become an increasing problem with aging. However, geriatric pathology is not sufficiently understood to explain the mechanisms of constipation in these patients.

GASTROINTESTINAL CAUSES

Abnormalities of the colon, rectum, and anus may lead to constipation. It may be due to failure of propulsion along the colon, failure of passage through the anal canal, or excessive mucosal absorption in the large intestine. Failure of propulsion along the colon may be caused by disorders of innervation (neurogenic) or muscular abnormalities. The common causes of neurogenic constipation include aganglionosis, intestinal pseudo-obstruction, Chagas' disease,

spinal cord abnormalities such as in multiple sclerosis and tabes dorsalis, and cerebral abnormalities such as Parkinson's disease or cerebral tumors. Muscular abnormalities may be caused by an irritable colon syndrome, diverticular disease, and other conditions. Constipation may also result from distal colonic obstruction due to extraluminal or intraluminal tumors, strictures, sigmoid volvulus, hernias, prolapse of the rectum, stricture resulting from an inflammatory process, or ischemic colitis.

The presence of painful anal conditions such as fissures may establish a vicious cycle consisting of painful sphincter spasm leading to constipation, which in turn leads to further fissuring and further pain. Constipation may also develop from faulty habits resulting from frequently suppressing the need to defecate because of time constraints.

CLINICAL EVALUATION

HISTORY

History plays an important role in the evaluation of patients complaining of constipation. Early onset in life may lead to a diagnosis of a congenital cause. Congenital causes of constipation, such as Hirschsprung's disease, may become manifest at any time during the first decade of life. However, the cause of the disease may progress slowly, and therefore the patient may not consult the physician until years later.

Primary local symptoms of constipation are the infrequent and often painful passage of hard stools. With excessive retention and abnormal abdominal distention, crampy pain may ensue. Associated symptoms accompanying constipation may be related to mechanical obstruction, which will lead to nausea and vomiting. Reflex symptoms may include back pain or hip pain and, occasionally, headache. Fever is sometimes reported after an extremely long period of retention. Direct questioning of the patient is indicated, concerning the color, consistency, and caliber of the stool, as well as the presence of melena (blood) or undigested food.

PHYSICAL EXAMINATION

Digital examination, anoscopy, and proctosigmoidoscopy are necessary to rule out the presence of anal fissures, ulcers, or hemorrhoids, as well as rectal tumors and strictures. Digital examination may also reveal abnormalities in anal sphincter tone, and the consistency of the stool as well as the presence or absence of blood or mucus in the stool should be noted. Cutaneous sensations should be checked and may be deficient in neurogenic disorders. The abdominal examination may reveal increased bowel sounds suggestive of obstruction or palpable masses in the descending and sigmoid colon.

BARIUM ENEMA AND COLONOSCOPY

The use of barium enema is mainly limited to diagnosing organic constipation of colorectal origin. In constipation of recent origin, the barium enema is mandatory to rule out any organic disease that may cause mechanical obstruction. However, its value may be limited in patients with chronic constipation. Colonoscopy may provide further help if a specific organic disease is suspected.

MOTILITY TESTS

Rectal sphincteric manometric tests are useful in differentiating idiopathic megacolon from aganglionic megacolon (Hirschsprung's disease). Colonic motility studies may help

---

TABLE 21-3   COMMON CAUSES OF CONSTIPATION

Systemic Causes
   Drug-induced: analgesics, anticholinergics, antacids
   Metabolic disorders: diabetic neuropathy, hypothyroidism, hypokalemics

Gastrointestinal Causes
   Neurogenic: aganglionosis (Hirschsprung's disease), intestinal pseudo-obstruction, Chagas' disease
   Colonic obstruction: neoplasms, diverticulitis, strictures
   Colonic functional disorders: diverticular disease, irritable colon
   Anal disorders: stenosis, fissures, fistulas

differentiate atonic from spastic constipation by measuring compliance of the colon. It must always be remembered that results obtained in patients should be compared with those obtained in normal subjects under similar conditions.

OTHER DIAGNOSTIC TESTS

Many patients who complain of constipation simply do not eat enough residual fiber. In these patients, the first positive step is to prescribe a diet containing an adequate amount of crude fibers. It is also essential to instruct the patient to stop taking drugs if he can, particularly laxatives, and not to use enemas. The ideal duration of this dietary treatment probably should be a month. Those who still complain of constipation and who have an abnormal pattern of defecation may require further studies of colonic transit times. Radiopaque markers, easily cut from a radiopaque Levin tube, are ingested. The patient continues to eat a high-residual diet. The markers can be followed by plain abdominal films for 7 days after ingestion. This test permits one to objectify the complaint of constipation, confirming the results of the history. It also permits the detection of those patients who give an inaccurate or unreliable history of their bowel habits.

DIARRHEA

Diarrhea is defined as the excessively frequent passage of loose stools. As with constipation, it is a symptom of many diseases. Most acute diarrhea is of infectious origin or is caused by dietary and toxic factors. When diarrhea is chronic or recurrent, it is more likely a symptom of more serious gastrointestinal disease.

ETIOLOGY

Diarrhea may be caused by four major mechanisms: the presence of an excessive amount of poorly absorbable but osmotically active substances in the gut lumen (osmotic diarrhea), excessive intestinal secretion (secretory diarrhea), an abnormal absorptive process, and deranged intestinal motility.

OSMOTIC DIARRHEA

Diarrhea may be a result of the accumulation of poorly absorbable solutes in the lumen of the intestine. This is usually caused by ingestion of some laxatives or maldigestion of ingested food. When the poorly absorbable solutes in the lumen cause higher osmotic pressure of the luminal content than of plasma, this osmotic pressure gradient causes water secretion into the lumen. Osmotic diarrhea is best represented by that produced by postgastrectomy syndromes (dumping syndrome), saline cathartics, or undigested lactose caused by lactase deficiency. Clinically, osmotic diarrhea is distinguished by the fact that diarrhea stops when the patient fasts.

SECRETORY DIARRHEA

Most secretory diarrhea originates in the small intestine or colon. In contrast to osmotic diarrhea, secretory diarrhea persists in the fasting state. In secretory diarrhea, the effect of osmotic pressure of the luminal content is the same as that of plasma. Increased secretion into the lumen generally is a response to infectious organisms (such as cholera and pathogenic coliform organisms), vasoactive intestinal polypeptides, prostaglandins, and peptide hormone–producing tumors such as medullary carcinoma of the thyroid and islet cell tumors. Many of these diseases may result in increased intestinal propulsion or altered motility, in addition to or caused by the hypersecretion. Colonic hypersecretion can be induced by bile acids within the colon when a significant portion of the terminal ileum has been resected, interfering with ileal reabsorption of bile acid. Other inflammatory bowel diseases, such as Crohn's disease and ulcerative colitis, may also be the cause of secretory diarrhea. Secretory diarrhea is usually voluminous. Most of the time the stool volume is greater than 1 liter/day. Stool osmolarity is almost entirely accounted for by sodium, potassium, and their anions, and thus severe metabolic abnormalities may result. This is in contrast to osmotic diarrhea, in which the concentration of normal electrolytes is much less than the osmolarity of fecal fluid.

ABNORMAL ABSORPTIVE MECHANISM

Diarrhea may be a result of an abnormal anion absorptive mechanism. The classic example is congenital chloridorrhea. In this disease, the patient is unable to absorb chloride actively, that is, the ileal and colonic mucosae are not able to transport chloride and bicarbonate against their respective electrochemical gradients. The result of this defect is a reduced rate of fluid absorption, acidification of the luminal contents, and a high chloride concentration in the fluid remaining in the lumen of the ileum and colon. This is expressed clinically by diarrhea, with a chloride concentration greater than the sum of the sodium and potassium concentration. Other examples of this type of diarrhea are bile acid or fatty acid malabsorption. Clinically, the diarrhea will either disappear or be greatly reduced when patients fast. However, there is no osmotic gap in fecal fluid, and therefore electrolytes in the fecal content account for all or nearly all of the fecal osmolarity. Lastly, ionic makeup of fecal fluid is abnormal, indicating malabsorption of some specific ion.

DERANGED INTESTINAL MOTILITY

Motor disturbance alone may result in small-volume diarrhea. Abnormalities of absorption or secretion, or both, must be present to account for large-volume diarrhea. Rapid colonic transit may be due to increased propulsive activity and is most commonly seen in irritable bowel syndrome. Antibiotic-associated diarrhea is caused by local mucosal inflammation. Serotonin found in malignant carcinoid syndrome can produce hyperperistalsis of the small intestine and atony of the colon, resulting in diarrhea. Partial intestinal obstruction may lead to compensatory hyperactive propulsive movements with intermittent diarrhea. Radiation proctitis and, occasionally, diverticulitis or ischemic proctitis may account for small-volume diarrhea. In this group of patients, urgency and frequency of stools may represent the prominent complaint rather than large-volume loose stools. Emotional disorders are commonly associated with chronic diarrhea of small volume. The exact mechanism has not been defined.

CONSEQUENCES

The consequences of diarrhea are dependent on the intensity and duration of the symptom. Severe or prolonged diarrhea may result in salt and water depletion, potassium depletion, and abnormal acid–base balance.

SALT AND WATER DEPLETION

When salt and water are lost in isotonic proportions, a contraction of the extracellular fluid compartment occurs and hemoconcentration develops. At this stage, the serum sodium is normal and the intracellular compartment is not significantly altered. These patients usually take salt-poor fluid orally, so that hyponatremia commonly results. In osmotic diarrhea, water loss is proportionately greater than that of sodium. Therefore, dehydration with hypernatremia may occur. Thus, diarrhea with water and salt depletion may be associated with a normal, low, or high serum sodium concentration, depending upon the type of fluid ingested and the nature of the diarrhea.

POTASSIUM DEPLETION

Potassium depletion may occur in association with salt and water depletion but occasionally may be an isolated finding. Isolated potassium depletion is most likely to occur in long-standing mild diarrheal states, such as chronic laxative abuse. It may be a result of nearly complete reabsorption of filtered sodium by the kidney in these patients, whereas renal potassium loss is usually continued even after potassium depletion has developed.

ACID–BASE DISTURBANCES

Metabolic acidosis may result from high bicarbonate content in the stool, production of acid due to starvation, or compromised renal function. Stool *p*H and direct measurement of bicarbonate concentration in fecal fluid, however, are of no help in determining the effect of diarrhea on acid–base balance. For instance, organic acids of bacterial origin may react with the bicarbonate of intestinal content to form CO_2, which would disappear from stool. Thus, diarrhea stools may have low bicarbonate concentration and low *p*H, but the patient may be sustaining a net loss of base from the body and may develop systemic acidosis. In addition to the primary effect of stool losses of base, secondary effects, such as hypokalemia, starvation, shock, and impairment of renal function, may also contribute to acidosis.

CLINICAL EVALUATION

HISTORY

A careful history is of significant help to the physician in establishing the diagnosis of the underlying disease that causes or is associated with diarrhea. It may also provide useful information about the nature of the disease or disease process. Passage of blood indicates an inflammatory, infectious, or neoplastic disease. Passage of pus in the stool indicates inflammation or infection. In addition to the character of the stools, the presence or absence of abdominal pain and its location should be determined. The physician should distinguish large-volume from small-volume diarrhea. When the stools are consistently large, the underlying disorders of the disease are likely to be in the small intestine or the proximal colon. In small-volume diarrhea, the patient has frequent urges to defecate but passes small quantities of feces. This syndrome is likely to be associated with disease or disorders of the left colon and rectum. Intermittent diarrhea and constipation suggests an irritable colon syndrome or diabetic autonomic neuropathy. Diarrhea that persists during fasting and is voluminous suggests a secretory cause. Diarrhea that stops when the patient fasts suggests

osmotic diarrhea. Diarrhea at night favors organic disease over the irritable bowel syndrome.

The family history of any diarrheal disease may also be helpful. Hereditary pancreatitis, multiple endocrine adenopathy, ulcerative colitis, and regional enteritis may have a high incidence within a family.

Any correlation with diet, especially milk intolerance, should be noted. The possibility of exposure to infectious agents should be estimated. The association of diarrhea with an emotional conflict should be searched for. The association of nausea and vomiting is more characteristic of intestinal malignancy, ulcerative colitis, or amebic dysentery.

PHYSICAL EXAMINATION

Stools are examined for infectious agents, ova and parasites, pus, and food particles, and cultures should be taken. Every patient with diarrhea should have his stool examined for fat droplets.

A complete physical examination should also reveal important clues to the causes of diarrhea. Important findings include, for example, an abdominal mass, abdominal tenderness, a perianal fistula or abscess, fever, edema, liver enlargement, ascites, intestinal distention, and fecal impaction. Arthritis is particularly common in patients with ulcerative colitis and regional enteritis or Whipple's disease. The nutritional status of the patient and evidence of fluid and electrolyte depletion should be carefully noted.

PROCTOSIGMOIDOSCOPY

In the initial work-up of the patient with diarrhea, it is important that the proctosigmoidoscopy be done without a cleansing enema, which may wash away mucosal exudates and actually alter the appearance of the mucosa itself. In most instances, the small amount of fecal matter can be avoided easily, and since most abnormalities are diffuse, diarrheal fecal matter does not greatly interfere with proctosigmoidoscopy. The presence or absence of pus on the rectosigmoid mucosa is extremely important. Pus is encountered in inflammatory bowel disease and infectious colitis but not in the irritable colon syndrome. The rectal and sigmoid mucosae should be carefully examined for ulcerations, friability, polyps, and tumors. The anal region should also be visualized during proctosigmoidoscopy.

LABORATORY STUDIES

The complete blood count and serum electrolytes will indicate some of the consequences of diarrhea, such as anemia, salt and water depletion, potassium depletion, and systemic acid–base imbalance. The correction of these abnormalities may be of more importance initially than reaching a specific diagnosis.

After the history and the physical, proctoscopic, and stool examinations, the clinician has some idea of the nature of the problem and a plan for additional studies is formulated to reach a specific diagnosis as rapidly as possible. If irritable colon syndrome seems most likely, a barium enema may be necessary to rule out organic disease, particularly in older patients, before the diagnosis can be accepted. In young adults, x-ray studies may not be required for the diagnosis of irritable bowel syndrome; however, it may be advisable in some of these patients, in that a negative x-ray examination affords added reassurance that organic disease is not present. If an infectious cause for the diarrhea seems most likely, the initial effort should be directed toward examination and culture of the stool, mucosal exudate, or blood.

Barium contrast studies should be delayed until these are completed because the barium enema interferes with identification of parasites for a period of several weeks. If drug-induced colitis is suspected, proctosigmoidoscopy and, occasionally, barium enema examination may be diagnostic. If neoplasm is suspected, barium contrast x-ray films are used initially to confirm the diagnosis and to determine the extent and the location of the disease in the small or large intestine. In patients suspected of inflammatory bowel disease following proctoscopy, the radiologist should be warned and the air-contrast portion of the barium study either should not be used or should be used only with great caution because of the danger of perforation. As a rule, with few exceptions, barium enema should not be done for about 1 week following a rectal biopsy.

LAPAROTOMY

Rarely, laparotomy or, to a lesser degree, laparoscopy may be considered as a diagnostic procedure. Usually these procedures are resorted to when tissue is required to establish a diagnosis. For example, a full-thickness small-bowel biopsy may be indicated in the differential diagnosis of malabsorption, lymphoma, or Whipple's disease. However, this should be considered only when other nonoperative methods fail to establish a correct diagnosis.

INTESTINAL OBSTRUCTION

Intestinal obstruction refers to interference of cephalocaudad transit of intestinal contents. It may be produced by mechanical obstruction of the bowel lumen or by paralysis of the intestinal muscle. Strictly speaking, the term *ileus* is synonymous with obstruction of the bowel; in practice, however, it usually refers to an adynamic or paralytic state of the intrinsic intestinal musculature.

ETIOLOGY

MECHANICAL OBSTRUCTION

There are three categories of abnormalities responsible for mechanical intestinal obstruction (Table 21-4).

Obturation of the Lumen

Obturation obstruction may be caused by several diseases, such as polypoid tumor of the bowel; gallstone, which can enter the intestinal lumen by way of a cholecystoenteric fistula; intussusception; and others (Figs. 21-6 and 21-7). Intussusception of the intestine is usually caused in the adult by an abnormality within the bowel wall, such as a tumor. Foreign bodies, feces, or bezoars may also obstruct the lumen of the intestine.

Intrinsic Bowel Lesions

The common intrinsic bowel lesions producing intestinal obstruction are neoplasms and inflammatory processes, such as in Crohn's disease. Rarely, strictures of the intestine may result from an intestinal anastomosis or radiation therapy. In small children or infants, intrinsic bowel lesions that produce intestinal obstruction are often congenital, as in atresia or stenosis.

Extrinsic Bowel Lesions

Occlusion of the small intestine by adhesions from a previous operation is the leading cause of obstruction of the small intestine. Adhesions may produce obstruction by a band of

tissue that compresses the bowel or by kinking and angulation. Extrinsic masses, such as annular pancreas, anomalous vessels, abscesses, hematomas, and neoplasms, may cause mechanical bowel obstruction. External hernias, such as inguinal, femoral, umbilical, and incisional hernias, are also important causes of mechanical obstruction of the small intestine. More rarely, internal hernias into congenital fossae or mesenteric defects may occur. The most common cause of colonic obstruction is due to neoplasm. Volvulus is a result of an abnormal rotation of a portion of the alimentary canal, which twists about itself. This abnormality usually results in kinking of the gut, producing mechanical obstruction. Some underlying abnormalities are usually present. Cecal volvulus may occur when the cecum or the right colon is intraperitoneal with a mesentery, rather than retroperitoneal. An abnormally long or redundant sigmoid colon may result in sigmoid volvulus. Closed-loop obstruc-

---

TABLE 21-4 COMMON CAUSES OF INTESTINAL OBSTRUCTION

I. Mechanical causes
  A. Obturation obstructions: gallstones, foreign bodies, bezoars, meconium, parasites such as ascaris, tapeworms
  B. Intrinsic bowel lesions
    1. Congenital: atresias, stenosis, malrotations, cysts and reduplications, Meckel's diverticulum, malformations of anus and rectum
    2. Inflammatory
      a. Small bowel: regional enteritis, tuberculosis, actinomycosis
      b. Large bowel: diverticulitis, ulcerative colitis, lymphopathia with rectal stricture
      c. Granulomas: tuberculosis, actinomycosis
    3. Small bowel: benign tumors, malignant tumors, carcinoid
    4. Large bowel: benign tumors, malignant tumors, carcinoid
    5. Miscellaneous: intussusception, traumatic strictures, endometriosis, irradiation strictures
  C. Extrinsic bowel lesions
    1. Adhesions
    2. Hernia
      a. External: inguinal, femoral, umbilical, ventral, Richter's, Littre's, epigastric
      b. Internal: hiatal, through a mesenteric or omental defect, lesser sac
    3. Obstruction due to compression by intra-abdominal, extraintestinal mass: abscess, tumor (carcinomatosis, pelvic mass), pregnancy, annular pancreas or pressure by superior mesenteric vessels
II. Adynamic ileus
  A. Intra-abdominal causes: peritonitis, prolonged simple obstruction
  B. Extraperitoneal irritation: retroperitoneal hematoma, infarction, nerve injury
  C. Extra-abdominal causes
    1. Toxic: pneumonia, empyema, uremia, generalized infection
    2. Metabolic: Electrolyte imbalance, porphyria
    3. Neurogenic: Spinal cord lesion, fractures of spine or ribs involving nerve roots
III. Idiopathic intestinal pseudo-obstruction

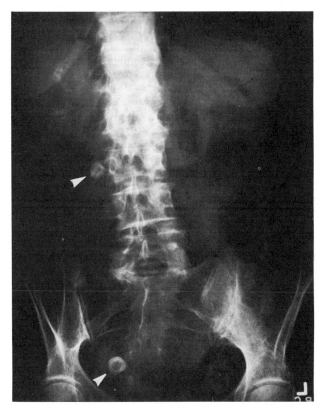

Fig. 21-6. Flat film of the abdomen in a patient with gallstone ileus. Note the air-filled dilated small intestines and two radiopaque gallstones (*arrows*).

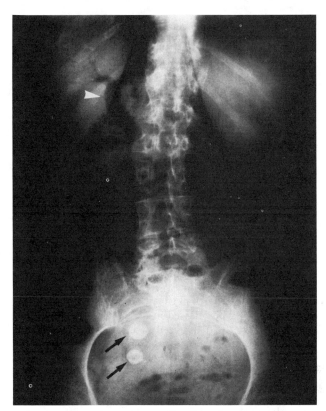

Fig. 21-7. Upright film of the abdomen in the same patient as shown in Figure 21-6. The light arrow indicates the biliary tract outlined by air (aerobilia); the dark arrows indicate stones.

tion results when both limbs of the loop are obstructed so that neither aboral progression nor regurgitation is possible.

PARALYTIC (ADYNAMIC) ILEUS

Paralytic ileus occurs most commonly after operations or abdominal trauma but may also result from electrolyte disturbances, such as hypokalemia; vascular insufficiency; and chemical irritants, such as blood, bile, and bacteria. It may also be caused by neural or humoral factors. Since there are reflexes that inhibit intestinal motility, it is commonly seen in patients following major trauma, especially spinal fractures. Retroperitoneal hemorrhage may produce an adynamic state of the bowel. Ischemia of the intestine also inhibits motility.

IDIOPATHIC INTESTINAL PSEUDO-OBSTRUCTION

Although most patients with gaseous distention of the intestine have either mechanical intestinal obstruction or paralytic ileus, patients may have recurring intestinal obstruction without demonstrable mechanical occlusion of the bowel nor ileus; this can be ascribed to peritonitis, metabolic disturbances, or drugs. *Idiopathic intestinal pseudo-obstruction* is defined as a chronic illness characterized by symptoms of recurring intestinal obstruction of unknown etiology. There is a controversy over whether the disease is caused primarily by abnormalities of the intramural nerve plexus or by abnormalities of the intestinal smooth muscle. The principal manifestations are crampy abdominal pain, vomiting, distention, and in some patients, diarrhea. Symptoms are experienced early in life by most patients with this disease. Physical examination usually reveals abdominal distention with mild tenderness. Radiologic studies show nonspecific

distended small and large intestines. The transit time is prolonged when barium is swallowed and followed through the small intestine. Barium enema demonstrates distention of the colon, but no site of obstruction is demonstrated. The treatment of severe attacks of idiopathic intestinal pseudo-obstruction may require nasogastric suction and intravenous fluids. Surgical procedures should be avoided if the diagnosis can be established with certainty.

PATHOPHYSIOLOGY

SIMPLE MECHANICAL OBSTRUCTION OF THE SMALL INTESTINE

Mechanical obstruction of the small intestine results in accumulation of fluid and gas proximal to the site of obstruction. Distention of the intestine proximal to the obstruction is initiated by ingested fluid, digestive secretion, and intestinal gas. Accumulation of large quantities of fluid above an obstruction is striking and progressive. It has been suggested that obstruction causes hypersecretion of digestive juices. On the other hand, some investigators feel that the principal defect is not hypersecretion of digestive juices but rather the inability of obstructed bowel to absorb water and electrolytes at the normal rate. Current available evidence from animal experiments does not indicate clearly which mechanism is responsible for the accumulation of fluid within the lumen in intestinal obstruction. The bowel immediately above the obstruction is the most affected initially. It becomes distended with fluid and electrolytes, and circulation is impaired. When obstruction is present for a long time, the proximal portion of the intestine also loses the ability to handle fluid and electrolytes, and the entire bowel proximal to the obstruction becomes distended. The loss of fluid and electrolytes may be further perpetuated by vomiting. Another route of fluid and electrolyte loss is into the wall of the involved bowel. Some of this fluid may also exude from the serosal surface of the bowel, resulting in free peritoneal fluid. The extent of fluid and electrolyte loss into both the bowel wall and the peritoneal cavity depends on the extent of bowel involved in venous congestion and edema and the length of time before the obstruction is relieved. All of these sources of fluid and electrolytes deplete the extracellular fluid space, which in turn results in hemoconcentration, hypovolemia, renal insufficiency, shock, and death, unless replacement of the fluid and electrolytes lost is prompt and accurate.

Swallowed air is probably the most important source of gas in intestinal obstruction, because swallowed air has a high nitrogen content and nitrogen is not absorbed by the intestinal mucosa. Therefore, the intestinal gas proximal to obstruction is predominantly nitrogen. Other gases include oxygen, hydrogen, CO_2, and methane. These five gases comprise 99% of intestinal gas in normal persons. Carbon dioxide may also be released in the upper intestine when hydrochloric acid is neutralized by bicarbonate. Therefore, CO_2 represents the predominant duodenal gas. Most of the CO_2 is rapidly absorbed by the bowel and does not appear in large quantity in the distal intestine. Intestinal bacteria, which produce hydrogen and methane, are normally limited to the colon. However, it is possible that abnormal flora in the small bowel during intestinal obstruction produces some hydrogen or methane that contributes to the distention. Increased intramural pressure from fluid and gas may further compromise mucosal blood flow, leading to necrosis and subsequent exudation of blood and plasma into the lumen while bacterial invasion and transport of toxins occur across the damaged mucosa.

STRANGULATION OBSTRUCTION

Strangulation of the intestine occurs when the circulation of the obstructed portion is impaired. Strangulation is more frequently seen in closed-loop obstruction, since interference with blood supply may occur either from the same mechanism that produced obstruction of the intestine, such as a twist of the bowel on its mesentery, an extrinsic band, or from distention of the obstructed loop. The secretory pressure in the closed loop quite rapidly reaches a level sufficient to interfere with venous return from the loop. In strangulation obstruction, the patient may suffer all the ill effects of simple obstruction in addition to the effects of strangulation. Strangulation thus causes loss of blood and plasma both into the lumen of the strangulated segment and into the peritoneal cavity. Shock eventually ensues, particularly if the patient is already dehydrated. As venous congestion increases, the arterial supply is eventually cut off. Strangulation may progress to gangrene of the intestine; rupture or perforation of the strangulated segment occurs and is a devastating complication, leading to generalized peritonitis. In addition to the loss of blood and plasma, an important factor in strangulation obstruction is the release of toxic material from the strangulated intestine into the peritoneum and then into the circulation. The toxic material may be absorbed from the peritoneal cavity, producing systemic effects, especially gram-negative or endotoxin shock, complicating that due to hypovolemia.

It is extremely important to recognize the clinical features suggesting strangulation in the patient with intestinal obstruction. The findings of severe and constant pain, tachycardia, leukocytosis, tenderness, and guarding should alert the clinician to the possibility of strangulation.

COLONIC OBSTRUCTION

In general, there are fewer ill effects in patients with colonic obstruction than in those with obstruction of the small intestine. First, obstruction of the colon, with the exception of volvulus, usually does not strangulate. In addition, fluid and electrolyte loss progresses more slowly in colonic obstruction than in obstruction of the small intestine, since the colon is principally a storage organ, whereas the small intestine has an important absorptive and secretory function. The degree of distention of the small intestine in colonic obstruction depends on the competency of the ileocecal valve. In patients who have a competent ileocecal valve, there may be little or no small-bowel distention. However, colonic obstruction and distention in these patients may behave as a closed-loop obstruction. When the colon is massively distended by gas, it may perforate. The cecum is the most common site for perforation because of its spherical shape, relatively thin wall, and large diameter.

CLINICAL EVALUATION

The initial symptoms of intestinal obstruction include crampy abdominal pain, vomiting, distention, and failure to pass flatus. The severity of each of these symptoms depends largely on the site, degree, and duration of the obstruction. In patients with proximal obstruction, vomiting may be profuse and unassociated with abdominal distention. In distal obstruction, the vomiting will be less frequent and may become feculent because of the large bacterial population of intestinal contents during obstruction. Obstipation and failure to pass gas from the rectum are characteristic of complete obstruction but are evident only after the bowel distal to the obstruction has been evacuated. The pain in mechanical obstruction of the small intestine is usually crampy, occurring at 4- to 5-minute intervals in proximal obstruction and less frequently in distal obstruction. The crampy abdominal pain may subside in chronic obstruction because motility may be inhibited by bowel distention. Severe, constant abdominal pain may suggest strangulation. Particular attention should also be paid to systemic effects of intestinal obstruction. Tachycardia and, later, hypotension may indicate severe dehydration, peritonitis, or both. Fever may suggest the possibility of strangulation. It is important to determine whether the abdominal distention is due to a distended, gas-filled intestine or to ascites. Ascites is usually characterized by a fluid wave, shifting dullness, and fullness in the flanks. Abdominal tenderness is a frequent finding in patients with intestinal obstruction. Severe peritoneal irritation may suggest strangulation and peritonitis. Palpation may reveal muscle guarding. Auscultation is of significant value. In simple mechanical obstruction, the abdomen is quiet except during attacks of colic, at which time the sounds become loud, high-pitched, and metallic. In paralytic ileus, an occasional isolated bowel sound is heard. Acute intestinal obstruction can usually be diagnosed on the basis of history and physical examination. Any patient having crampy abdominal pain, vomiting, abdominal distention, and tenderness should be considered to have intestinal obstruction unless the diagnosis can be confidently excluded.

LABORATORY FINDINGS

The loss of large amounts of fluid and electrolytes by vomiting or by accumulation within the intestine is principally responsible for the laboratory findings in simple mechanical obstruction. In the early phases, hemoconcentration due to fluid loss will be indicated by a rise in the hematocrit. There may or may not be changes in the concentration of sodium, potassium, and chloride in the plasma, especially if the losses of fluid and electrolytes have not been corrected. Fluid loss is initially compensated by antidiuresis, so these patients may not be able to produce a urine specimen until after intravenous fluid therapy has been started. High urine specific gravity is usually present.

In the untreated patient, there is a gradual reduction of the plasma sodium and chloride concentration, because sodium-free water, derived from oxidation of fat, tends to restore the loss of extracellular fluid but not the electrolytes. Metabolic acidosis may be noted due to the combined effect of dehydration, starvation, ketosis, and loss of alkaline secretion in most cases. Metabolic alkalosis may occur and is usually due to loss of acidic gastric juice from vomiting. The white blood cell count is usually slightly to moderately elevated. A very high white blood cell count strongly suggests strangulation obstruction or mesenteric vascular occlusion. The serum amylase level may be elevated in intestinal obstruction; this may be due to peritoneal absorption after leakage from the compromised intestinal wall.

RADIOLOGIC EXAMINATIONS

Radiologic examination of the abdomen is vital to the diagnosis. Plain recumbent, upright, and lateral decubitus films are vital in determining whether the obstruction is located in the small or the large intestine. Furthermore, an upright chest film will demonstrate elevation of the diaphragm, as well as free air under the diaphragm if perforation is present. Air–fluid levels may be seen in the obstructed bowel in the upright and lateral decubitus positions. Typically, the small bowel occupies the more central portion of the abdomen and the colonic shadow is on the periphery of the abdominal film or in the pelvis. Patients with complete mechanical obstruction of the small intestine usually have minimal colonic gas or none at all. Small-bowel obstruction results in stepladder distribution of the loops of intestine. Jejunal obstruction is characterized by prominent valvulae conniventes; ileal obstruction is not. Plain films may show distended haustra in colonic obstruction. Valvulae conniventes can often be distinguished from haustra because the valvulae traverse the entire lumen as a straight line or as a coiled-spring appearance, whereas haustra are asymmetrical and do not extend across the entire lumen from one side to another. Patients who have colonic obstruction with a competent ileocecal valve may show colonic distention but little small-bowel gas. On the other hand, patients with colonic obstruction and an incompetent ileocecal valve usually have radiographic evidence of small-bowel and colonic obstruction. Occasionally, plain films fail to distinguish colonic from small-bowel obstruction. The safest and quickest way to distinguish colonic from small-bowel obstruction in these patients is by a carefully performed barium enema. Barium contrast studies by mouth should be avoided if colonic obstruction is not ruled out. Paralytic ileus is usually characterized by irregular gas distention of the stomach, small intestine, and colon. Sometimes it can be difficult to distinguish paralytic ileus from mechanical obstruction by radiographic findings. In such cases, barium studies may be of help in distinguishing between ileus and mechanical obstruction (Fig. 21-8).

TREATMENT

Although the clinical signs of strangulation must be sought, there is no infallible method of detecting strangulation preoperatively. For that reason, most patients with intestinal obstruction should be managed operatively to prevent the development of serious complications and to avoid overlooking undetected instances of strangulation. The overlapping sequence of events in managing patients with intestinal obstruction should be proper diagnosis, replacement of fluid and electrolytes lost, decompression of the bowel, and timely surgical intervention. Patients with intestinal obstruction are likely to be depleted of water, sodium, chloride, and potassium. Intravenous therapy usually should begin with isotonic sodium chloride solution. After adequate urine output is observed, potassium chloride should be added to the solution. Sufficient fluid should be given to elevate and maintain urine output and restore to normal the vital signs. The decision when to operate depends upon the duration of obstruction and its consequent abnormalities in fluid, electrolyte, and acid–base balance; improvement of vital organ function or correction of concomitant cardiopulmonary disorders and other vital organ functions; and consideration of the risk of strangulation.

Fig. 21-8. Contrast study of a patient with obstruction of the small intestine. Note the dilated upper small intestines. Plain abdominal films of this patient did not show distended loops of small intestine because they were filled with fluid.

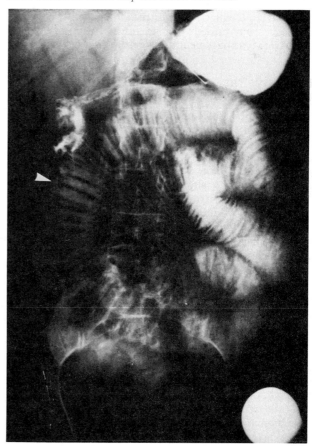

In addition to fluid and electrolyte therapy, nasogastric suction with a Levin tube will empty the stomach, thereby reducing the hazard of pulmonary aspiration of vomitus, reducing any elevation of the left hemidiaphragm, and minimizing further intestinal distention from swallowed air during the preoperative period. Some surgeons prefer to use an intestinal tube, such as the Miller–Abbott tube, to decompress the distended small intestine. It is usually necessary to position these long intestinal tubes fluoroscopically, and in some patients, intubation of the small intestine may be difficult even with fluoroscopic manipulation. Compression of the distended small intestine may facilitate the technical aspect of an operation for small-bowel obstruction and is therefore very desirable. However, the use of a long intestinal tube in small-bowel obstruction should not delay operative treatment of almost certain complete acute mechanical obstruction. Essentially, all patients with mechanical intestinal obstruction should be operated upon once the patient is properly prepared for surgery and the diagnosis is properly made. In occasional circumstances, a period of decompression may be warranted before an operation is considered. For example, in patients with gastric outlet obstruction, the operation can be safely delayed until fluid and electrolyte imbalance is corrected. Patients who developed intestinal obstruction immediately after an abdominal operation may require a period of decompression following which air and fluid may pass freely through. In patients with obstruction caused by disseminated intra-abdominal cancer, it may be difficult to determine whether operation will provide significant palliation. Patients with obstruction of the colon due to sigmoid volvulus may be decompressed by sigmoidoscopy or colonoscopy. Elective operation can then be performed to prevent recurrent volvulus. Finally, the obstruction caused by Crohn's disease, usually incomplete, may respond with a period of conservative management using nasogastric suction.

OPERATIVE TREATMENT OF INTESTINAL OBSTRUCTION

Several surgical procedures can be used for the relief of intestinal obstruction. In simple mechanical obstruction, lysis of adhesions or reduction of an intussusception or incarcerated hernia may relieve the obstruction. Enterotomy is necessary for removal of obturation, such as gallstones or bezoars. Occasionally, intestinal bypass may be used for an obstructing lesion. More frequently, the lesion is excised and intestinal continuity is restored after excision. The approach to colonic obstruction is somewhat different from that of small-bowel obstruction. The classic method of treating obstruction of a left colonic lesion includes three separate operative stages: (1) relief of distention by colostomy proximal to the obstruction, (2) removal of the diseased segment of colon and anastomosis, and (3) closure of the colostomy when healing of the anastomosis is complete, often weeks later. Staged procedures are performed because intestinal obstruction and its sequelae are significant and life-threatening and therefore should be relieved as quickly and simply as possible and because surgical anastomosis of a distended colon with its compromised blood supply can be hazardous. However, it is now understood that colonic resection can be done safely in most instances at the first operation. If this is the case, we prefer two stages: resection of the diseased segment, leaving a proximal colostomy and distal mucous fistula, and later closure of the colostomy.

Obstructive lesions of the cecum and right colon are managed differently from those of the left colon. Right colectomy can usually be done safely in patients with an obstructing lesion because the obstructed colon can be removed and dilated distal small bowel can usually be sutured safely to the normal transverse colon. Some surgeons may elect a bypass operation, such as an ileotransverse colostomy, to relieve the obstruction in the cecum, with a later elective resection of the right colon. We prefer to reserve the bypass operation only for patients in whom the resection is technically difficult or hazardous.

TREATMENT OF PARALYTIC ILEUS

Paralytic ileus can usually be treated with nasogastric suction and intravenous fluid administration. In some cases of paralytic ileus, particularly those with extreme distention in the distal small intestine, passage of a long small-intestinal tube such as a Miller–Abbott tube into the intestine may be helpful. If the intestinal tube can be passed successfully, it provides intestinal decompression superior to that achieved with a nasogastric tube. Parasympathomimetic drugs or sympathetic blocking agents may be of value to stimulate small bowel motility in occasional patients. However, these drugs should not be used unless mechanical obstruction and intra-abdominal sepsis are excluded with certainty. When ileus persists or appears without obvious underlying causes, one should continue to look for causes of mechanical obstruction, intra-abdominal sepsis, or peritonitis. In occasional patients, a laparotomy may be necessary to exclude these factors with confidence.

GASTROINTESTINAL BLEEDING

Gastrointestinal bleeding is a common and serious problem. Mortality rates associated with gastrointestinal bleeding range from 5% to 50%, depending upon the underlying cause of bleeding. Early recognition and proper treatment of gastrointestinal bleeding may result in lower morbidity and mortality. The advent of endoscopy and arteriography not only has significantly improved the diagnostic accuracy but also has provided therapeutic alternatives.

Bleeding may be manifested by hematemesis, melena, or hematochezia. Hematemesis refers to vomiting of blood, either bright red or brown and precipitated, resembling coffee grounds. Hematemesis strongly suggests a bleeding site above the ligament of Treitz. Rarely, hematemesis may be due to lesions in the proximal small intestine. Melena is defined by the passage of tarry, black stools. Melena usually means that bleeding is from a site above the ileocecal valve and is related to the effect of digestive and bacterial processes on intraluminal blood. Often, bleeding lesions in the right colon present as melena, due to stasis of blood in that area. The tarry color is usually attributable to the production of acid hematin by the action of gastric acid on hemoglobin. Melena without hematemesis generally indicates a lesion distal to the pylorus but has been associated with slower bleeding proximal to the pylorus. Hematochezia is defined by the passage of fresh red blood from the rectum. Hematochezia is usually a result of colonic bleeding; it does not, of course, eliminate the upper gastrointestinal tract as the source of blood loss. Occult bleeding may occur in some patients, stools appear normal but are shown on chemical determination to contain blood.

SYSTEMIC EFFECTS

CARDIOVASCULAR RESPONSES

The patient's cardiovascular responses to gastrointestinal blood loss depend upon the rate and extent of blood loss. They are also influenced by the capacity of the patient to respond to volume depletion. In general, in an otherwise healthy person, a series of nonspecific cardiovascular responses occur after a significant hemorrhage (*i.e.,* over 25% of the intravascular volume within a period of a few minutes to several hours). As blood volume falls, cardiac output and systolic blood pressure decrease, followed by a decrease in diastolic blood pressure and an increased pulse. This is associated with an increase in peripheral vascular resistance. Blood pressure responses occur first in the form of orthostatic hypotension. With continued blood loss, the venous and arterial beds constrict in an attempt to maintain the central circulation. Clinically, these changes may be manifested by skin pallor and peripheral cyanosis. This may be followed by decreased blood flow to the splanchnic and renal circulation with progressive reduction of urine output. Ultimately, complete anuria or acute tubular necrosis results. Rarely, prolonged mesenteric vascular insufficiency produces ischemic changes in the intestine. Continued blood loss may also compromise blood flow to the brain and myocardium. Compromised cerebral circulation results in mental confusion; ischemia of the myocardium is reflected in the electrocardiogram, which may show ST-segment depression and T-wave inversion. These changes may be reversible if the blood loss is replaced rapidly. On the other hand, inadequate volume replacement may result in the secondary effects of prolonged shock, such as anoxia, cellular dysfunction, and acidosis, and may eventually result in death.

HORMONAL RESPONSES

Other more gradual compensatory physiological responses include the release of antidiuretic hormone and aldosterone acting to reestablish volume at the expense of extravascular fluid and urine flow. These fluid shifts may be manifested by a progressive dilution of plasma proteins and reduction in the hematocrit and hemoglobin concentration. Clinically, considerable individual variation in this compensatory response is noted, depending upon the state of hydration, age, ability to reabsorb the fluid loss into the gut, and rate of fluid ingestion by infusion. Therefore, the lowest hemoglobin level may not be noted for 48 to 72 hours in some patients.

UPPER GASTROINTESTINAL TRACT BLEEDING

ETIOLOGY

Although a great number of lesions above the ligament of Treitz may be the source of upper gastrointestinal tract bleeding, the common causes are peptic ulcer disease (duodenal and gastric ulcers), acute erosive diseases of the stomach (gastritis and stress ulcers), esophageal varices, and the Mallory-Weiss syndrome (Table 21-5). Considerable variations can be expected in their relative incidence, depending on the patient population from which the data are collected. The use of endoscopy as a diagnostic measure indicates that the incidence of gastritis as a cause of bleeding is higher than previously reported. Other less common

TABLE 21-5   SOURCES OF GASTROINTESTINAL HEMORRHAGE

I. Upper gastrointestinal tract bleeding
  A. Inflammatory
    1. Duodenal ulcer
    2. Gastritis
    3. Gastric ulcer
    4. Esophagitis
    5. Stress ulcer
    6. Pancreatitis
  B. Mechanical
    1. Hiatus hernia
    2. Mallory-Weiss syndrome
    3. Hematobilia
  C. Vascular
    1. Esophageal or gastric varices
    2. Aortointestinal fistula
    3. Hemangioma
    4. Rendu-Osler-Weber syndrome
    5. Mesenteric vascular occlusion
    6. Blue nevus bleb
  D. Systemic
    1. Blood dyscrasias
    2. Collagen diseases
    3. Uremia
  E. Neoplasms
    1. Carcinoma
    2. Polyps (single, multiple, Peutz-Jeghers syndrome)
    3. Leiomyoma
    4. Carcinoid
    5. Leukemia
    6. Sarcoma
II. Lower gastrointestinal tract bleeding
  A. Inflammatory
    1. Ulcerative colitis
    2. Diverticulitis
    3. Enterocolitis, regional (Crohn's disease)
    4. Enterocolitis, tuberculous
    5. Enterocolitis, irradiation
    6. Enterocolitis, bacterial
    7. Enterocolitis, toxic
  B. Mechanical (diverticulosis)
  C. Neoplasms
    1. Carcinoma
    2. Polyps (adenomatous and villous, familial polyposis, Peutz-Jeghers syndrome)
    3. Leiomyoma
    4. Sarcoma
    5. Lipoma
    6. Metastatic (melanoma)
  D. Anomalies (Meckel's diverticulum)
  E. Vascular
    1. Hemorrhoids
    2. Aortoduodenal fistula
    3. Aortic aneurysm
    4. Hemangioma
    5. Mesenteric thrombosis
    6. Hereditary hemorrhagic telangiectasia
    7. Blue nevus bleb
  F. Systemic
    1. Blood dyscrasias
    2. Collagen diseases
    3. Uremia

(Ballinger WF, Zuidema GD: The acute abdomen. In Paulson M et al [eds]: Gastroenterologic Medicine, p 227. Philadelphia, Lea & Febiger, 1969)

causes of upper gastrointestinal tract hemorrhage include gastric neoplasm, esophagitis, hematobilia, and duodenal diverticulum.

Peptic ulceration is a common cause of massive upper gastrointestinal tract hemorrhage, accounting for approximately one third to one half of all cases. Approximately 20% of patients with peptic ulcer will experience this complication, which is responsible for one third to one half of the deaths from peptic ulcer. The bleeding is generally caused by the inflammatory process eroding into a regional artery. In the case of duodenal ulcers, the gastroduodenal artery is usually eroded. Therefore, those ulcers in the duodenum that bleed significantly are usually located in the posterior surface of the duodenal bulb. Since no major blood vessel lies on the anterior surface of the duodenal bulb, ulcerations in the anterior surface are not as prone to massive bleeding as to perforation. Patients with concomitant bleeding and perforation may have two ulcers, a bleeding posterior ulcer and a perforated anterior one. In some patients, the bleeding is sudden and massive. In others, chronic anemia and weakness as a result of slow blood loss may be the only findings. The diagnosis is often suggested by a history of typical ulcer pain. However, previous ulcer symptoms may not be present. In the case of gastric ulcers, the left and right gastric arteries and their branches are most frequently involved and eroded by the ulcers.

The next most common cause of upper gastrointestinal tract bleeding is a group of superficial lesions that can best be defined as acute erosive diseases of the stomach. This includes drug-induced gastritis and stress ulcerations. A number of drugs are known to be injurious to the gastric mucosa. Salicylates and salicylatelike compounds are known to be ulcerogenic. It is estimated that 20 billion such compounds are consumed annually. Alcohol is also known to be injurious to the gastric mucosa, and in the United States, the annual consumption of alcohol is in excess of 30 billion dollars. Nonsteroidal, nonsalicylate anti-inflammatory compounds such as indomethacin and naproxen and corticosteroids are also associated with erosive injury of the gastric mucosa. Drug-induced erosions are usually associated with mild superficial erosions. However, these erosions can occasionally result in significant hemorrhage. Even though the initial episode of bleeding may be life-threatening, aggressive nonoperative treatment usually suffices. Only a few patients require operation, and the necessity for such treatment seems to be decreasing. Stress ulcer bleeding in patients with severe burn, massive trauma, hypovolemic shock, renal failure, respiratory failure, and severe sepsis presents a serious clinical challenge. Endoscopic studies have established that acute mucosal erosions are common in patients who have suffered massive burns and other major physical trauma, with a net incidence of over 90%. However, such lesions bleed only rarely, and one must therefore conclude that erosions are common after specific types of physical injury but that bleeding, the clinical hallmark of the disease, is uncommon. Multiple factors may be involved in the development of acute stress erosions in the stomach. Of these, mucosal ischemia is thought to be the primary etiologic factor. Mucosal ischemia reduces the mucosal ability to buffer the H^+ entering the tissue from the lumen and therefore renders the mucosa more susceptible to acid injury. Hypersecretion of acid is usually seen in patients following head injury; however, it is not a uniform finding in patients with sepsis or trauma. Disruption of the gastric mucosal barrier to back diffusion (lumen to cell) of acid has previously been implicated as a cause of stress ulceration. Recent studies have indicated that stress ulceration is usually the result of compromised capacity of the mucosa to withstand or buffer the influxing H^+ rather than a consequence of an increase in the amount of back diffusion of acid. Acute ulcers associated with central nervous system tumors or injuries (Cushing's ulcer) differ from stress ulcers because they are associated with elevated levels of serum gastrin and increased gastric acid secretion. Morphologically, they are similar to ordinary gastric or duodenal peptic ulcers. Cushing's ulcers are more prone to perforate than are other kinds of stress ulcers.

Esophageal or gastric varices account for approximately 10% of all cases of upper gastrointestinal tract bleeding. However, it is the most common cause of bleeding in patients with cirrhosis or extrahepatic obstruction of the portal vein. On the other hand, it is important to remember that only about 50% of patients who are known to have esophageal varices and who are bleeding will be bleeding from the varices. The remainder bleed from other lesions, such as gastritis, peptic ulcers, esophagitis, or the Mallory-Weiss syndrome. Once variceal bleeding is endoscopically confirmed, it must be understood that the prognosis is much worse than for almost any other cause of gastrointestinal bleeding. Approximately 40% to 50% of patients with bleeding varices will rebleed, and the mortality rate from each bleeding episode is between 30% and 40%. Esophageal or gastric variceal bleeding is nearly always associated with hematemesis and is generally very profuse. The Mallory-Weiss syndrome is probably responsible for about 10% of patients with acute upper gastrointestinal tract bleeding. This lesion consists of a tear several centimeters long in the gastric mucosa near the esophagogastric junction. It is usually, but not always, preceded by forceful retching. The tear extends through the mucosa and submucosa but not into the muscularis mucosa. Most of these lesions are confined to the stomach and occasionally may extend into the distal esophagus. Two thirds of the patients with the Mallory-Weiss syndrome may have an associated hiatus hernia. A variety of miscellaneous bleeding accounts for up to 5% to 10% of upper gastrointestinal tract bleeding. Neoplasms less commonly result in active bleeding. Bleeding associated with gastric carcinoma is caused by erosion of the tumor into the underlying vessels. The bleeding is usually of mild to moderate degree. Other tumors, such as leiomyoma or leiomyosarcoma of the stomach, may be manifested by profuse bleeding, often from a pinpoint erosion through the mucosa into the deeper tumor. Polyps, either single or multiple, may also cause bleeding.

DIAGNOSIS

History

The history usually gives a clue to the level and the lesion of the gastrointestinal tract that is bleeding. Past gastrointestinal symptoms, such as peptic ulcer disease, the findings of previous radiologic studies, and the use of alcohol, aspirin, or other ulcerogenic drugs are often helpful. The presence of pain may suggest a gastrointestinal lesion disrupting the mucosa, such as peptic ulceration, gastritis, or esophagitis. Bleeding from a Mallory-Weiss tear or from esophageal varices is generally painless. Vomiting immediately preceding the onset of gastrointestinal bleeding suggests the possibility of a Mallory-Weiss tear; however, approximately 50% of patients with this lesion will not give the classic history of vomiting and retching prior to hematemesis.

The history of previous gastrointestinal bleeding from a known lesion increases the possibility that the patient may be bleeding from the same lesion again. However, it must be emphasized that patients that have bled from one lesion may also have an increased risk of bleeding from another. Therefore, the plan to establish the diagnosis must not be altered on this account only. A careful drug history is extremely important, and this must include not only prescription drugs but also easily obtained over-the-counter drugs, such as aspirin. Since the history of abuse of alcohol may not be accurate, clinical indicators of alcohol abuse should be sought and corroboration of history by the family should be obtained. History of dysphagia suggests esophageal lesions, such as reflux esophagitis, possibly with ulceration, or carcinoma of the esophagus, which also bleeds occasionally.

Physical Examination

It is difficult to estimate the amount of blood lost in either the vomitus or the stool, and, as mentioned, the hematocrit and hemoglobin levels are unreliable initially. Thus, it is extremely important to assess the extent of blood loss with particular reference to careful evaluation of pulse and blood pressure (lying and sitting), skin color and diaphoresis. In addition, examination of the patient with upper gastrointestinal tract bleeding is directed toward finding the stigmas of the various diseases considered in the etiology. For example, patients with chronic alcoholism may demonstrate spider angiomas, facial flushing, abdominal venous distention, liver palms (palmar erythema), peripheral edema, jaundice, and muscle wasting. The presence of abdominal tenderness may suggest the possibility of acute inflammatory bowel disease or penetrating duodenal ulcer. The mucous membrane should be investigated for melanin spots of the Peutz-Jeghers syndrome. Erythema nodosum may indicate the presence of inflammatory bowel disease. Petechiae and ecchymoses may also suggest a hemorrhagic diathesis in the patient. A careful ear, nose, and throat examination should be performed, particularly in patients with no obvious cause of bleeding, to rule out the possibility of swallowed blood from nasopharyngeal bleeding.

Laboratory Tests

Blood should be drawn for initial laboratory studies at the time of insertion of the intravenous line. This must be accomplished in many patients before or during the taking of the history, since restoration of intravascular volume and measurement of laboratory values, as well as typing and crossmatching of blood for early replacement, are lifesaving in many of these patients. The extent of anemia may be assessed by the hematocrit level. However, the fall in hematocrit level will depend upon the rate and type of fluid replacement, and the hematocrit may be normal or only slightly low before equilibration occurs. Repeated hematocrit readings taken at 4- to 6-hour intervals are more meaningful. Elevation of the white blood cell count is common.

Coagulation studies should be assessed as soon as possible in all patients with gastrointestinal bleeding, particularly those who continue to bleed following apparent adequate blood replacement. The initial blood smear should provide an estimate of the number of platelets. Inadequate replacement of clotting factors and platelets during massive transfusions may also enhance the extent of the gastrointestinal bleeding. Clinical chemistries are also directed toward determining the presence of hepatocellular dysfunction. Elevation of blood urea nitrogen (BUN) in an otherwise normal patient occurs because the products of digested blood in the gastrointestinal tract are absorbed, the metabolic breakdown of which is reflected in the BUN level. Cessation of bleeding is accompanied by rapid fall of the BUN. Therefore, sequential determination of the BUN can be important in the management of the patient.

Specific Diagnostic Techniques

Rarely, bleeding is so rapid that immediate operation without preoperative diagnostic procedure is necessary to save the patient's life. More commonly, transfusion can easily allow time for accurate diagnosis and preparation of the patient for surgery. The initial management can often be made within 1 or 2 hours after the acutely bleeding patient has entered the hospital. In most instances, this aggressive approach will result in a patient whose bleeding is at least temporarily under control, whose blood volume has been restored to approximately normal, and who has been adequately monitored so that recurrent bleeding can be detected quickly. When this stage is reached, additional specific diagnostic tests should be performed. The decision concerning the timing and sequence of specific diagnostic procedures depends on the information obtained from the history and physical examination and the relative skill of immediately available personnel. These procedures include endoscopy, angiography, barium x-ray studies, and, possibly, scanning techniques. In most cases, the first diagnostic measure is endoscopic examination of the upper gastrointestinal tract. Studies should be conducted as soon as the patient's condition has stabilized; thus, the source can be identified while bleeding is still active. Endoscopy has been shown to be more accurate than x-ray film in demonstrating bleeding from peptic ulcers, acute gastritis, Mallory-Weiss tear, and esophagitis. Although barium radiography is equally accurate in demonstrating esophageal varices, endoscopy is more likely to indicate whether the varices present are actually responsible for the bleeding episodes. When skilled endoscopists are available, over 80% of the bleeding lesions are demonstrated. This figure is reduced to only 20% to 50% in patients studied by barium contrast radiography. It must be stressed that an optimal examination by endoscopy requires a clean lumen and a cooperative patient. This objective is best accomplished when the patient is clinically stable. In occasional patients, repeat endoscopy often will confirm the initial diagnosis and contribute valuable follow-up information and is particularly helpful if the first endoscopic examination is nondiagnostic.

Selective angiography has been used for both diagnostic and therapeutic purposes. For diagnosis, it is most helpful when other studies fail to demonstrate a cause of bleeding. This is particularly the case in patients whose profound bleeding obscures endoscopic visualization. Angiography may provide two findings for identification of bleeding sites. First, contrast medium escapes from the vasculature into the lumen of the involved segment and can be readily recognized. This requires a moderate rate of bleeding, and it has been demonstrated that the rate of blood loss must be in excess of 0.5 ml/minute to visualize contrast in the gastrointestinal lumen by angiography. Second, an actual lesion may be identified by visualizing an arteriovenous malformation, the vascular blush of tumor, a vessel displaced by tumor, or a visceral aneurysm. Angiography must be performed before upper gastrointestinal tract barium x-ray study, because the latter will obscure the field.

Selective arterial catheterization can also be used for therapy in demonstrated gastrointestinal bleeding. After the bleeding point is identified, a small catheter is guided into the artery supplying the bleeding area and a vasoconstricting agent, usually vasopressin, is infused at the rate of 0.1 unit to 0.4 unit/minute. In esophageal variceal bleeding, the superior mesenteric artery is infused to reduce splanchnic blood flow and thus decrease portal venous flow and pressure. In many patients, the bleeding is controlled by arterial infusion of vasopressin. In some patients, bleeding is only temporarily controlled or partially controlled. However, it will allow time for an operation to be performed under more optimal circumstances. Regional vasoconstrictive therapy should be used only in patients in whom the potential benefit justifies the risks, since complications are not infrequent from such therapy.

Until recently, barium contrast studies were the mainstay of diagnosis in patients with acute hemorrhage from the upper gastrointestinal tract. A major disadvantage has been the inability of the examiner to determine whether the abnormalities seen in barium studies were, in fact, the actual bleeding sites. For example, 20% to 50% of the patients with demonstrated esophageal varices are bleeding from another lesion. Another disadvantage is that some superficial lesions, such as erosions and tears, are not readily identifiable by radiographic contrast studies. The use of double or air contrast studies of the gastrointestinal tract, recently popularized in Japan, has been shown to be more accurate in detecting superficial lesions. This procedure is accomplished by using a small amount of highly concentrated contrast mixture and a source of gas or air. Higher diagnostic yields of small and superficial erosions are reported, and some signs of active bleeding are recognized. This technique may gain increasing use as radiologists become familiar with it.

LOWER GASTROINTESTINAL TRACT BLEEDING

Bleeding distal to the ligament of Treitz is usually occult or heralded by melena or hematochezia and is usually not accompanied by hematemesis (see Table 21-5).

SMALL INTESTINE

Bleeding from the small intestine frequently presents even greater diagnostic difficulty than that from lesions in the esophagus, stomach, or duodenum. Peptic ulceration in a Meckel's diverticulum may bleed when ectopic gastric mucosa is present. In such cases, the bleeding may be preceded by ulcerlike pain located in the periumbilical area or right lower quadrant of the abdomen. Inflammatory bowel disease is a common cause of intestinal bleeding. Ileocecal intussusception is a lesion of childhood occurring most commonly before the age of 2. It may present as lower gastrointestinal tract bleeding by passage of dark clots or "currant jelly" stool. Although tumors of the small intestine are rare, a good number of them may be accompanied by bleeding. These neoplasms include leiomyomas and polyps, either single or multiple, as in familial polyposis. Carcinomas, sarcomas, lymphomas, and leukemia have all been reported to be associated with bleeding. Carcinoid tumors rarely may cause bleeding. Hemangiomas and hereditary telangiectasias within the wall of the intestine may also be the source of bleeding from the small intestine.

In bleeding from the small intestine, the nasogastric aspirate is usually negative and endoscopic examination is of little use beyond the ligament of Treitz. One must,

therefore, use angiography or barium studies. The patient with active severe bleeding from an area suspected to be distal to the ligament of Treitz should be investigated initially with selective angiography, if available. If bleeding appears active but is not demonstrated by angiography, passage of a long tube into the intestine will permit intermittent aspiration every 15 or 20 cm. When blood is obtained from the tube, the tube should be secured and barium may then be instilled through the tube to visualize the involved segment. It may be necessary to withdraw the tube a few inches to be well upstream from the lesion.

COLON

Massive hemorrhage from lesions distal to the ileocecal valve is much less common than from the upper gastrointestinal tract. As noted previously, an upper gastrointestinal tract source must always be considered, even in patients who present with rectal bleeding, because massive bleeding from the duodenum or even the stomach may induce rapid intestinal transit and present as grossly bloody stools. Massive colonic bleeding in adults is usually caused by diverticular disease, vascular abnormalities, ulcers, ulcerative colitis, ischemic colitis, or other less common lesions. Benign or malignant neoplasms rarely cause massive bleeding but do bleed slowly. Vascular abnormalities such as arteriovenous fistula are more common than was thought before the use of endoscopy and are probably responsible for much right colon bleeding. Selective angiography is by far the most accurate method of diagnosis, provided the bleeding is at the rate of at least 0.5 ml to 1.0 ml/minute at the time of the examination. The examination of the right colon and small intestine is by catheterization of branches of the superior mesenteric artery. Examination of the left colon is sometimes more difficult because the inferior mesenteric artery may be more difficult to catheterize. Active bleeding lesions may be demonstrated by a collection of contrast media within the lumen of the bowel adjacent to the bleeding site. In patients who have stopped bleeding, there is still some opportunity to visualize colonic lesions of vascular origin. Arteriovenous malformation of the right colon has been found to be a major source for recurring lower gastrointestinal tract hemorrhage of obscure origin. Once an active bleeding site is demonstrated during arteriography, pharmacologic treatment with intra-arterial infusion of vasoconstrictor can be attempted. This often results in at least temporary control of the bleeding so that consideration and preparation of the patient for operation, if indicated, may be carried out.

Barium enema is preferable in less acute situations and may well demonstrate colonic neoplasm, diverticular disease of the colon, ischemic colitis, or inflammatory bowel disease. Air contrast studies are much more likely to visualize smaller polypoid lesions. Colonoscopy is not helpful in acutely bleeding patients because of technical difficulties associated with the unprepared bowel filled with blood. However, colonoscopy provides a valuable supplement to proctoscopy and barium enema for evaluation of nonactive colonic bleeding sites. In skilled hands, high diagnostic accuracy has been reported in detecting a wide spectrum of colonic lesions by colonoscopic examination.

RECTUM AND ANUS

Rectal and anal bleeding is usually manifested by rectal bleeding when the blood is not well mixed with stool or is on the surface of the stool. It may be caused by hemorrhoidal disease, anal fissures or ulcers, and proctitis. A rectal examination and proctosigmoidoscopy should be done to search for the presence of these diseases as well as anorectal tumors. The rectal mucosa should be adequately visualized for ulcers, strictures, edema, friability, inflammation, and other active bleeding sites. The coating of mucus should be wiped away with a cotton swab to evaluate the underlying mucosa for granularity or friability, suggestive of ulcerative colitis or proctitis.

Mortality from massive lower gastrointestinal tract hemorrhage at least equals or probably exceeds that of upper gastrointestinal tract bleeding. In spite of recent innovative diagnostic and therapeutic developments, gastrointestinal tract hemorrhage continues to present the clinician a major challenge in both diagnosis and therapy. A logical approach to the problem involves resuscitation and stabilization of the patient, a critical choice of the variety of new diagnostic techniques, and then selection of specific therapy based on the diagnostic findings. The correct management of the patient is enhanced by close and continuing cooperation among primary care physicians, surgeons, gastroenterologists, and radiologists.

JAUNDICE

The terms *jaundice* and *icterus* are synonymous and refer to a yellow color of the serum and often of the sclerae of the eyes, skin, and mucous membranes. This yellowness is the result of accumulation of free or conjugated bilirubin in these tissues. It is usually detectable when the total plasma bilirubin is greater than 3 mg/dl of serum. Hyperbilirubinemia may be due to excess production of bilirubin, decreased uptake of bilirubin into the hepatic cells, disturbed intracellular protein binding or conjugation of bilirubin, disturbed secretion of bilirubin into the bile canaliculi, or intrahepatic or extrahepatic bile duct obstruction. Therefore, the knowledge of bilirubin metabolism and excretion is essential in the differential diagnosis and management of patients with jaundice. Normal bilirubin metabolism and the evaluation of the jaundiced patient are discussed in the evaluation of liver disease in Chapter 27.

BIBLIOGRAPHY

Abdominal Pain

BOTSFORD TW, WILSON RE: The Acute Abdomen, 2nd ed. Philadelphia, W B Saunders, 1977

BREWER RJ, GOLDEN GT, HITCH DC et al: Abdominal pain: An analysis of 1,000 consecutive cases in a university hospital emergency room. Am J Surg 131:219, 1976

COPE Z: The Early Diagnosis of Acute Abdomen, 15th ed. London, Oxford Universty Press, 1979

GUILLEMIN R: Endorphins: Brain peptides act like opiates. N Engl J Med 296:226, 1977

HILL OW, BLENDIS L: Physical and psychological evaluation of "nonorganic" abdominal pain. Gut 8:221, 1967

LIM RKS: Pain. Ann Rev Physiol 32:269, 1970

MELZACK R, WALL PD: Pain mechanisms: A new theory. Science 150:971, 1965

MENACKER GJ: The physiology and mechanism of acute abdominal pain. Surg Clin North Am 42:241, 1962

WAY LW: Abdominal pain and the acute abdomen. In Sleisenger MH, Fordtran JS (eds): Gastrointestinal Disease: Pathophysiology, Diagnosis and Management, 2nd ed, chap 20, pp. 394–404. Philadelphia, W B Saunders, 1978

Dysphagia

BENNETT JR, HENDRIX TR: Diffuse esophageal spasm: A disorder with more than one cause. Gastroenterology 59:273, 1970

DAVENPORT HW: Physiology of the Digestive Tract, 3rd ed. Chicago, Year Book Medical Publishers, 1971

EDWARDS DAW: Flow charts, diagnostic keys, and algorithms in the diagnosis of dysphagia. Scott Med J 15:378, 1970

EDWARDS DAW: Discriminative information in the diagnosis of dysphagia. J R Coll Physicians Lond 9:257, 1975

HIGHTOWER NC: Swallowing and esophageal motility. Am J Dig Dis 3:562, 1958

INGELFINGER FJ: Esophageal motility. Physiol Rev 38:533, 1971

Anorexia, Nausea, and Vomiting

DAVENPORT HW: Physiology of the Digestive Tract, 3rd ed. Chicago, Year Book Medical Publishers, 1971

FELDMAN M, FORDTRAN JS: Vomiting. In Sleisenger MH, Fordtran JS (eds.): Gastrointestinal Disease: Pathophysiology, Diagnosis and Management, 2nd ed, chap 10, pp. 200–216. Philadelphia, W B Saunders, 1978

GREGORY RA: Changes in intestinal tone and motility associated with nausea and vomiting. J Physiol (Lond) 105:58, 1946

HAWKINS C: Anorexia and loss of weight. Br Med J 2:1373, 1976

HILL OW: Psychogenic vomiting. Gut 9:348, 1968

LUMSDEN K, HOLDEN WS: The act of vomiting in man. Gut 10:173, 1969

McGUIGAN JE: Anorexia, nausea, and vomiting. In MacBryde CM, Blacklow RS (eds): Signs and Symptoms, 5th ed. Philadelphia, J B Lippincott, 1970

PINDER RM, BROGDEN RN, SAWYER PR et al: Metoclopramide: A review of its pharmacological properties and clinical use. Drugs 12:81, 1976

Constipation

BURKITT DP, WALKER ARP, PAINTER NS: Effect of dietary fibre on stools and transit times, and its role in the causation of disease. Lancet 2:1408, 1972

CONNELL AM, HILTON C, IRVINE G et al: Variation of bowel habit in two population samples. Br Med J 2:1095, 1965

DEVROEDE G: Constipation: Mechanisms and management. In Sleisenger MH, Fordtran JS (eds): Gastrointestinal Disease: Pathophysiology, Diagnosis and Management, 2nd ed, chap 18, pp. 368–386. Philadelphia, W B Saunders, 1978

EDWARDS DAW, BECK ER: Movement of radiopacified feces during defecation. Am J Dig Dis 16:709, 1971

Diarrhea

BINDER HJ: Pharmacology of laxatives. Ann Rev Pharmacol Toxicol 17:355, 1977

DONOWITZ M, BINDER HJ: Jejunal fluid and electrolyte secretion in carcinoid syndrome. Am J Dig Dis 20:1115, 1975

EVANSON JM, STANBURY SW: Congenital chloridorrhea or so-called congenital alkalosis with diarrhea. Gut 6:29, 1965

FIELD M: Intestinal secretion. Gastroenterology 66:1063, 1974

FORDTRAN JS: Speculations on the pathogenesis of diarrhea. Fed Proc 26:1405, 1967

LOW-BEER TS, READ AE: Diarrhoea: Mechanisms of treatment. Gut 12:1021, 1971

PHILLIPS SF: Diarrhea. Postgrad Med 57, No. 1:65, 1975

Intestinal Obstruction

CARMICHAEL MJ, WEISBRODT NW, COPELAND EM: Effect of abdominal surgery on intestinal myoelectric activity in the dog. Am J Surg 133:34, 1977

ELLIS H: Collective review: The cause and prevention of postoperative intraperitoneal adhesions. Surg Gynecol Obstet 133:497, 1971

HEIMBACH DM, CROUT JR: Treatment of paralytic ileus with adrenergic neuronal blocking agents. Surgery 69:582, 1971

JONES RS: Intestinal obstruction: Pseudo-obstruction and ileus. In Sleisenger MH, Fordtran JS (eds): Gastrointestinal Disease: Pathophysiology, Diagnosis and Management, 2nd ed, chap 22, pp. 425–436. Philadelphia, W B Saunders, 1978

SCHUFFLER MD, LOWE MC, BILL AH: Studies of idiopathic intestinal pseudo-obstruction. Gastroenterology 73:327, 1977

SMITH J, KELLY KA, WEINSHILBOUM RM: Pathophysiology of postoperative ileus. Arch Surg 112:203, 1977

SULLIVAN MA, SNAPE WJ, MATARAZZO SA et al: Gastrointestinal

myoelectrical activity in idiopathic intestinal pseudo-obstruction. N Engl J Med 297:233, 1977

WRIGHT HK, O'BRIEN JJ, TILSON MD: Water absorption in experimental closed segment obstruction of the ileum in man. Am J Surg 121:96, 1971

Gastrointestinal Bleeding

BAUM S, NUSBAUM M: The control of gastrointestinal hemorrhage by selective mesenteric arterial infusion of vasopressin. Radiology 98:497, 1971

BAUM S, NUSBAUM M, CLEARFIELD HR et al: Angiography in the diagnosis of gastrointestinal bleeding. Arch Intern Med 119:16, 1967

BEHRINGER GE, ALBRIGHT NL: Diverticular disease of the colon: A frequent cause of massive rectal bleeding. Am J Surg 125:419, 1973

CHEUNG LY: Treatment of established stress ulcer disease. World J Surg 5:235, 1981

CONN HO, RAMSBY GR, STORER EH et al: Intra-arterial vasopressin in the treatment of upper gastrointestinal hemorrhage: A prospective, controlled clinical trial. Gastroenterology 68:211, 1975

KATON RM: Experimental control of gastrointestinal hemorrhage via the endoscope: A new era dawns. Gastroenterology 70:272, 1976

KATON RM, SMITH FW: Panendoscopy in the early diagnosis of acute upper gastrointestinal bleeding. Gastroenterology 65:728, 1973

KELLER RT, LOGAN GM JR: Comparison of emergent endoscopy and upper gastrointestinal series radiography in acute upper gastrointestinal haemorrhage. Gut 17:180, 1976

KNAUER CM: Mallory-Weiss syndrome. Gastroenterology 71:5, 1976

LAUFER I: Assessment of the accuracy of double contrast gastroduodenal radiology. Gastroenterology 71:874, 1976

MALT RA: Control of massive upper gastrointestinal hemorrhage. N Engl J Med 286:1043, 1972

MOODY FG: Rectal bleeding. N Engl J Med 290:839, 1974

MOODY FG, CHEUNG LY: Stress ulcers: Their pathogenesis, diagnosis, and treatment. Surg Clin North Am 56:1469, 1976

MOSS G: Cause of azotemia after gastrointestinal hemorrhage: Examining an old wives' tale. Am J Surg 130:269, 1975

NUSBAUM M, CONN HO: Arterial vasopressin infusions: Science or seance? Gastroenterology 69:263, 1975

POUNDER RE, WILLIAMS JG, MILTON-THOMPSON GJ et al: Effect of cimetidine on 24-hour intragastric acidity in normal subjects. Gut 17:133, 1976

RITCHIE WP, JR: Bile acids, the "barrier," and reflux-related clinical disorders of the gastric mucosa. Surgery 82:192, 1977

SILEN W: New concepts of the gastric mucosal barrier. Am J Surg 133:8, 1977

SILVERSTEIN FE, AUTH DC, RUBIN CE et al: High-power argon laser treatment via standard endoscopes: 1. A preliminary study of efficacy in control of experimental erosive bleeding. Gastroenterology 71:558, 1976

Frank G. Moody/William C. DeVries

The Esophagus and Diaphragmatic Hernias

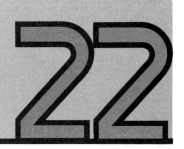

HISTORICAL ASPECTS OF ESOPHAGEAL DISEASE

The anatomical inaccessibility of the esophagus has contributed to a delay in an understanding and treatment of its diseases relative to other organs of the digestive system. A variety of pathologic conditions of the esophagus, however, are now recognized, and newer diagnostic modalities are contributing to improved therapies at an exponential rate. Traumatic lesions of the cervical esophagus were identified in ancient times, and survivals were observed when the cervical esophagus sealed to the skin, allowing the wound to heal gradually by secondary intention. There is also inferential evidence that benign as well as neoplastic strictures of the esophagus were treated by dilation at this time, but there is little documentation that this was done with success. The anatomical dissections during the Renaissance provided a systematic way to study the consequences of esophageal injury and stricture so that by the middle of the 18th century techniques had been developed to remove foreign bodies and dilate strictures of the cervical esophagus. By the mid 19th century, strictures were being approached by internal as well as external myotomies with some success but with what would be considered today a prohibitive death rate. Major advances in esophageal surgery awaited the imaging potential of radiography and endoscopy, which occurred in the early part of the 20th century. Successful major operations on the intrathoracic esophagus were enhanced by the development of endotracheal anesthesia, antibiotics, and blood transfusions during World War II. The time sequence of these historical events is recorded in Table 22-1.

TABLE 22-1   HISTORY OF DIAGNOSIS AND TREATMENT OF ESOPHAGEAL DISEASE

THERAPEUTIC TECHNIQUE	RESEARCHER	DATE
Dilatation (achalasia)	Willis	1670
Resection (cervical)	Czerny	1877
Endoscopy	Jackson	1890
Barium swallow	Bachem, Gunter	1910
Myotomy	Heller	1913
Resection (body)	Thorek	1913
Manometry	Code	1962
Hiatal hernia repair	Allison	1951
	Belsey	1953
	Nissen	1956
	Hill	1961

FUNCTIONAL ANATOMY

The esophagus is an epithelial-lined muscular tube that in humans extends from the lower end of the pharynx at the cricoid cartilage to the upper end of the stomach within the peritoneal cavity. This elongated course within three major areas of the body (*i.e.,* neck, thorax, and abdomen) provides a variety of unique relationships to other organs (*i.e.,* tracheobronchial tree and lungs, the heart and great vessels, the phrenic and vagus nerves, and the thyroid, parathyroid, and thymus glands) and a vulnerability to numerous pathologic abnormalities (Fig. 22-1). The anatomical relationships and functional characteristics of the esophagus are critical to its normal function. The esophagus is also influenced by its relationship to the mouth and pharynx above and to the stomach below.

The primary function of the esophagus is to transport ingestants from the mouth to the stomach. A thick muscular coat, which consists of an external longitudinal and an inner circular layer, is well suited for this purpose. Both muscle layers are striated in their upper third and gradually become exclusively composed of smooth muscle in their lower half. This arrangement makes sense, because it is important to have voluntary control of the inlet to the esophagus and involuntary control of its outlet. A stout circular band of striated muscle, the cricopharyngeus, forms a high pressure zone (HPZ) at the upper end of the esophagus. The activities of this sphincter are coordinated with the movements of the larynx, pharynx, and uvula to prevent aspiration into the tracheobronchial tree during eating or regurgitation of gastric contents.

The lower end of the esophagus does not have a true anatomical sphincter but does demonstrate an HPZ on manometric examination. This HPZ is called the lower esophageal sphincter (LES). The LES is of critical importance in preventing reflux of gastric contents into the esophagus, which, because of its location within the posterior mediastinum of the thorax, has a pressure that is 5 torr below atmospheric pressure and 10 torr below pressures generated within the stomach (Fig. 22-2). It is self-evident that a pressure in excess of 10 torr is required to prevent the backward movement of gastric contents. Furthermore, the LES must relax during deglutition in order for ingestants to pass into the stomach (Fig. 22-3).

The esophagus is lined by stratified squamous epithelium, a tough integument that is well designed to withstand the physical and chemical stresses of what is placed in the mouth. Mucous glands, which lie in the submucosa, play an important role in lubricating the epithelium and providing it with a protective layer when irritants are ingested.

Normal esophageal function requires the orderly passage of liquids and solids from the mouth to the stomach and their containment within the stomach during digestion. The

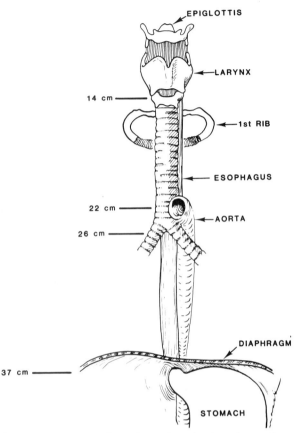

Fig. 22-1. Anatomic relationships. The pathophysiology and manifestation of esophageal disease are influenced by the anatomic relationship of the esophagus to adjacent organs. Of special importance is its contiguity with the pharynx and stomach and its proximity to the respiratory passages.

Fig. 22-2. Esophagogastric pressures. The pressure within the lower esophageal segment (LES) provides a barrier to the regurgitation of gastric contents into the esophagus. Note the intra-abdominal position of the terminal 4 cm to 5 cm of esophagus, which contributes in part to this high-pressure zone (HPZ), which is well above the subatmospheric pressures within the body of the esophagus.

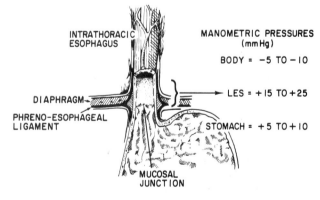

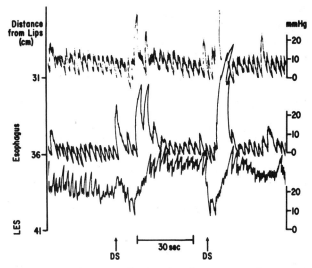

Fig. 22-3. Relaxation of LES. This demonstrates the pressure profile within the distal esophagus and the LES following a dry swallow (DS). Note the contraction waves at 31 cm and 36 cm from the incisors, followed by a relaxation of the LES in the lowest tracing.

importance of the upper esophageal sphincter, the cricopharyngeus, and the HPZ within the LES has already been alluded to. Ordinarily, liquids and well-chewed solids pass very quickly (2 to 3 seconds) from the pharynx to the stomach by gravity. The activity of the upper and lower sphincters is coordinated by a swallow to relax and contract at precisely the right time. A peristaltic wave is not required, except when large chunks of food gain entrance to the body of the esophagus. Three wave forms, however, can be identified within the body of the esophagus: primary waves follow swallowing and are presumed to represent sequential contraction of the circular muscle; secondary waves occur after the ingestant has passed into the stomach and serve to strip the esophagus of any remaining material after the initial evacuation; and tertiary contractions appear to serve no useful purpose in the process of deglutition and are, in some instances, a sign of disturbed esophageal function.

The neurohormonal control of esophageal function is poorly understood. The vagus nerve appears to play a supplemental or permissive role in esophageal function. Central vagal denervation does not produce a measurable defect in esophageal motility or function of the LES. In situations in which the LES pressures are decreased, administration of stable esters of acetylcholine will cause an increase in the LES. Furthermore, intact vagal innervation will enhance the weak agonist action of gastrin. Metoclopramide, an agonist for smooth muscle contraction, also has a more profound effect on pressures within the LES when a background of a vagomimetic agent is provided. It is now clear that gastrin by itself does not play an important role in maintaining LES tone. Cholecystokinin, a polypeptide that has a close structural relationship to gastrin, however, may contribute to the pressure within the LES, since it has been found to be a stronger agonist than gastrin when studied in an in-vitro preparation of isolated esophageal smooth muscle. Studies have clearly shown that the mechanism for progression of contractions within the esophagus lies within its muscular wall and most likely involves the myenteric plexus. Inhibitory nerves are thought to play an important role in the process of contraction, since a period

of relaxation is required prior to a contraction and spontaneous contractions are not a characteristic of esophageal smooth muscle. LES function depends critically on coordinated relaxation as ingestants approach the lower end of the esophagus. The manometric equivalents of pressure waves within the lower end of the esophagus are shown in Figure 22-3.

DISEASES OF THE ESOPHAGUS

The esophagus is the site of many diseases that have profound effects on esophageal function and in many instances the survival of those afflicted. These abnormalities are listed below:

   I. Congenital Anomalies
      Esophageal atresia
      Tracheoesophageal fistula
      Vascular ring
      Duplication
      Esophageal webs
  II. Diverticula
      Zenker's
      Mid-esophageal
      Epiphrenic
 III. Inflammatory lesions
      Acid reflux
      Alkaline reflux
      Caustic ingestion
      Barrett's epithelium
      Candidiasis
      Crohn's disease
  IV. Benign Tumors
      Leiomyoma
      Fibrous polyp
      Lipoma
      Hemangioma
      Lymphangioma
      Glomus tumor
      Neurofibroma
   V. Malignant tumors
      Carcinoma
      Leiomyosarcoma
      Fibrosarcoma
      Malignant melanoma
  VI. Motor Abnormalities
      Achalasia
      Primary spasm
      Diabetes
      Scleroderma
      Poliomyelitis
      Posterior inferior cerebellar artery occlusion
      Amyotrophic lateral sclerosis
      Huntington's chorea
      Multiple sclerosis
      Dermatomyositis
      Myotonic dystrophy
 VII. Miscellaneous
      Foreign body
      Cartilaginous spur
      Presbyesophagus
      Acquired esophageal web (Plummer-Vinson syndrome)

The most common congenital anomalies are esophageal atresia, which presents at the time of birth as an inability to take oral feedings, and pulmonary dysfunction as a consequence of a tracheoesophageal fistula. Vascular rings and esophageal webs are uncommon and often do not become manifest until later in life when they cause obstruction to the ingestion of solid foods. Diverticula of the esophagus occur in association with motor abnormalities of the upper (Zenker's) or lower (epiphrenic) end of the esophagus or in its midaspect when inflammatory diseases external to the esophageal wall, such as tuberculous lymphadenitis, cause distortion by traction.

The most common inflammatory lesions of the lumen of the esophagus are related to esophageal reflux of gastric (acid) or duodenal (alkaline) contents. Lye ingestion used to be a common and serious form of esophageal injury prior to a major health campaign to advise mothers to keep lye well outside the reach of their children. Barrett's esophagitis is thought to be a variant of an acquired replacement of the injured squamous epithelium of the lower end of the esophagus in patients with advanced reflux esophagitis. It is possible that some individuals might be born with a columnar type of epithelium of the lower end of the esophagus that is quite sensitive to acid reflux. This question has not as yet been resolved. *Candida* has become a fairly common infectious cause of esophagitis, usually occurring in debilitated patients who are being treated for a serious illness. Crohn's disease, while unusual in the upper gastrointestinal tract, has been reported within the pharnyx as well as the esophagus and must be kept in mind whenever an inflammatory stricture of the esophagus is encountered in a patient who has the disease in other parts of the lower intestinal tract.

The most common benign tumor, leiomyoma, may cause difficulty with swallowing, but usually its presence is unsuspected until a barium roentgenogram is taken of the esophagus. Benign polyps, lipomas, lymphangiomas, and glomus tumors are all rare lesions of the esophagus. Hemangiomas are relatively common and must be thought of when patients present with bleeding from the upper gastrointestinal tract.

Squamous cell carcinoma is by far the most common malignant tumor of the esophagus. This is unfortunate, since it is an aggressive biologic neoplasm that usually kills in a short period of time. Lymphomas, leiomyosarcomas, fibrosarcomas, adenocarcinomas, and malignant melanomas also can occur in the esophagus and must be thought of when a patient presents with esophageal obstruction.

Motor abnormalities of the esophagus are not only very common but also are poorly understood. The most common motor abnormality is called achalasia, a condition in which the LES fails to relax on deglutition. Primary spasm of the esophagus is also common and is a most distressing problem, since it presents as severe substernal chest pain. A variety of systemic illnesses have a profound effect on esophageal motility. Patients with diabetes, scleroderma, and dermatomyositis, as well as a variety of neural and muscular abnormalities, will present with symptoms of esophageal dysfunction.

The proximity of the esophagus to the mouth makes it vulnerable for the ingestion of a variety of foreign objects. Safety pins, coins, chicken bones, and other objects can become lodged in the esophagus and lead to inflammation within its wall, perforation into the chest or mediastinum, or obstruction to its lumen. The esophagus can also be obstructed by conditions within adjacent structures, such as cartilaginous spurs on the spine, aneurysms of the thoracic

aorta, cancers within the lung, and lymphoma within the lymph nodes of the mediastinum. The esophagus is also vulnerable to injury by penetrating objects, such as bullets and knives, and occasionally can suffer disruption from vigorous vomiting or extreme blunt trauma.

CLINICAL FEATURES

The normal esophagus provides for the rapid and efficient movement of ingestants from the pharynx to the stomach without sensation or other perception of the occurrence. This indeed is a remarkable event, since foodstuffs are often of a large size as they leave the mouth, especially in those individuals who fail to or cannot chew their food. Furthermore, it is well known that very large objects can be accommodated by the esophagus, whose distensibility appears to be extraordinary without producing pain. Unfortunately, the epithelium is quite sensitive to marked changes in *p*H. The ingestion of strong alkaline substances (*e.g.,* lye) or the regurgitation of gastric acid, digestive enzymes, or bile causes an inflammation of the epithelial lining and its submucosa termed *esophagitis*. When esophagitis is severe and prolonged, the lumen of the esophagus becomes fixed and narrowed by fibrous tissues and a stricture results. Distensibility is an important mechanical characteristic of the esophagus. Loss of distensibility by stricture formation leads to a significant delay in the passage of ingestants from the mouth to the stomach.

Neurologic disorders that affect the pharyngeal nerves have a profound effect on deglutition. For example, cerebrovascular lesions that involve the origins of the glossopharyngeal nerve may lead to an inability of the cricopharyngeus to relax (cricopharyngeal achalasia). The muscular tone of the body of the esophagus may be influenced by systemic illnesses such as diabetes or collagen vascular diseases that affect neuromuscular transmission within the myenteric plexus, which lies between the muscle layers of the esophagus. There are two primary motility disturbances of the esophagus: achalasia and primary spasm. Achalasia is characterized by a failure of relaxation of the LES following a swallow and simultaneous low pressure contractions within the body of the esophagus. Patients with primary spasm have a normal LES but simultaneous and prolonged high pressure waves within the body of the esophagus upon swallowing.

ESOPHAGEAL PAIN

Heartburn is one of the most common symptoms of esophageal dysfunction (Table 22-2). The burning discomfort occurs beneath the sternum and characteristically is diffuse and confined to the midline. In fact, its occurrence is so common that it cannot be considered an indication of a diseased esophagus but rather is a manifestation of the reflux of gastric contents into the esophageal lumen. The pain has been primarily associated with acid reflux, although it is known that patients who have had their stomachs removed may also experience heartburn when the refluxed material clearly is alkaline in *p*H. Patients who complain of heartburn may, in fact, have little or no evidence of inflammation of the mucosal lining of the lower esophagus. Some patients with heartburn may have morphologic evidence of severe esophagitis by gross inspection of the epithelium as well as by histologic examination of biopsy specimens. These symptoms, when mild, and associated with the ingestion of alcohol or large meals, do not require

TABLE 22-2	**SYMPTOMS OF ESOPHAGEAL DISEASE**

SYMPTOM	DISEASE
Heartburn	Esophagitis
Substernal pain	Primary spasm
Odynophagia	Esophageal ulcer, candidal esophagitis
Dysphagia	Stricture, cancer, achalasia
Regurgitation	Stricture, reflux

extensive medical evaluation. Their persistence, however, in the face of dietary counseling and antacid therapy, requires a comprehensive evaluation, as will be described below in the discussion of the treatment of reflux esophagitis.

Ulceration of the lining of the esophagus in the presence of severe esophagitis leads to a constant severe pain beneath the lower sternum or xiphoid that is exacerbated by eating (odynophagia). This pain is so intense that it forces the patient to seek medical advice. Hospitalization is usually required, since simple measures of antacid therapy usually do not provide relief and the patient is unable to sustain nutrition. The pain is usually so severe that narcotic analgesics are required for relief.

A third type of pain is that associated with primary spasm of the esophagus. This pain is also intense but can be distinguished from the esophageal pain of ulceration by its suddenness in onset and its location beneath the middle and upper part of the sternum, with radiation into the neck or either shoulder. This pain is not exacerbated or relieved by eating nor is it relieved by the ingestion of antacids. Often patients with the initial episode of this type of pain are thought to have had a myocardial infarction. Fortunately, the painful episode subsides spontaneously within several moments only to return following an unspecified period of time. Primary spasm usually occurs in tense individuals and often is precipitated by a period of anxiety, frustration, or anger. It is difficult to make a specific diagnosis of primary spasm, since it is necessary to perform esophageal manometry at the time that the spasm occurs and such an opportunity rarely is present.

Curiously, neoplasms of the esophagus are usually not associated with pain. Carcinoma of the esophagus may produce a deep aching discomfort when it invades adjacent organs, but otherwise it usually does not betray its presence by discomfort. This is unfortunate, since patients with carcinoma of the esophagus usually do not know that they have a serious illness until the lesion is far advanced.

DYSPHAGIA

Dysphagia is a generic term for the sensation that food, following its ingestion, has stopped at some point in the esophagus. It may occur as an inability to swallow or as merely a transient sensation of the food sticking at some point after it has been swallowed. This sticking sensation may occur at the level of the point of holdup of the passage of the food, such as at the level of the xiphoid if the hangup is in the lower end of the esophagus. Occasionally, the sticking sensation may refer to the upper sternum or to the level of the cricoid, even though the hangup is in the lower end of the esophagus. Patients with cricopharyngeal abnormalities refer the sensation of sticking to the level of the cricoid. Dysphagia in and of itself is not a painful sensation, although it is associated with a fear of choking. In addition,

it usually inhibits the further ingestion of food, although in some conditions (*e.g.,* achalasia) the patient learns to wash the food through with the swallowing of liquids, thereby relieving the sensation and allowing the further ingestion of food. Patients with benign strictures of the esophagus may present with dysphagia to solids but not to liquids. In fact, they may sustain themselves for many years by the ingestion of pureed foods and liquids. Patients with cancer of the esophagus, on the other hand, have a progressive type of dysphagia initially to solids and then to liquids. A characteristic of patients with motor abnormalities is that they may have dysphagia to both liquids and solids. Furthermore, such patients usually do not lose weight, since they learn early in their disease to take in large volumes of liquids in order to encourage esophageal emptying by gravity.

The importance of a single episode of dysphagia, especially in middle-aged or older people, cannot be minimized. It may be the first sign of cancer of the esophagus and, therefore, must be investigated vigorously, as will be described below.

REGURGITATION

When ingestants fail to pass from the esophagus, or are refluxed back into the esophagus from the stomach, they may return to the mouth and be expectorated or aspirated into the tracheobronchial tree. This symptom is called regurgitation. Regurgitation is a symptom that accompanies reflux esophagitis and benign or malignant strictures of the esophagus. In addition, it may be a manifestation of a large Zenker's or epiphrenic diverticulum. The effects of regurgitation and aspiration on the lung may be subtle. Patients with a hiatal hernia with reflux and recurrent episodes of pneumonia should be evaluated for the possibility of reflux regurgitation and aspiration. A common manifestation of reflux and regurgitation is that which occurs on the movement of materials from the stomach and esophagus into the mouth on reclining or during stooping. It is the latter symptom that on occasion will bring the patient with free reflux to the attention of the physician. This symptom requires a diagnostic workup because of its potential for causing aspiration pneumonia.

DIAGNOSIS

PHYSICAL EXAMINATION

The esophagus is well shielded from the examiner's fingers for most of its length and therefore rarely offers palpable findings when diseased. An exception is a large Zenker's diverticulum that may present with extraneous sounds on eating or as a mass in the neck. Infants with tracheoesophageal fistula characteristically regurgitate saliva and have an excessive amount of air within the gastrointestinal tract. Occasionally, adults with esophageal cancer will have a large lymph node palpable within the left (Virchow's node) or right subclavicular region that is evidence of advanced disease. Diagnosis of esophageal abnormalities, therefore, usually requires radiography, endoscopy, and, in selected cases, manometry.

RADIOGRAPHIC EXAMINATION

Frontal and lateral chest roentgenograms may provide useful information regarding esophageal disease. In fact, they represent almost a definitive way to make the specific diagnosis of tracheoesophageal fistula at birth. In the adult, they may reveal the presence of a hiatal hernia, the enlarged esophagus of achalasia, or the mediastinitis or pleural effusion associated with a perforation of the esophagus spontaneously (Boerhaave's syndrome) or by a foreign body. In addition, they usually identify the presence of a foreign body lodged within the esophagus, since these are usually radiopaque.

Most esophageal diseases, however, are more subtle than the above disorders and require a contrast material in order to identify the specific pathologic process. Barium is usually the opaque medium of choice, since it provides rather stark detail of the intraluminal course of the esophagus. Water-soluble agents such as Gastrografin are used when it is suspected that a perforation has occurred, since barium within the pleural or abdominal cavity causes a dense inflammatory reaction. On the contrary, the water-soluble materials are much more offensive to the tracheobronchial tree; therefore, when obstruction of the esophagus is suspected, barium is the agent of choice. The barium esophagogram can help not only to identify the location of the lesion but also to provide precise information as to its etiology. Figure 22-4 is a composite of a series of characteristic lesions that can be identified by a barium esophagogram. Negative results of a barium esophagogram, in a patient with dysphagia, do not exclude significant esophageal disease. For example, a small neoplasm of the esophagus might be missed by this technique. In addition, it usually does not provide information on motility disturbances of the esophagus other than achalasia. The typical beaklike appearance of achalasia is shown in Figure 22-5. Tertiary contractions (Figure 22-6) may be an indication of a primary motor disorder of the esophagus, but in the elderly, it is a normal finding. When motility disturbances of the esophagus are suspected, a dynamic radiographic study called a cinefluorogram should be obtained. This in essence is a time/motion study of the passage of contrast media through the esophagus. It is surprising that even this elegant study often does not reveal the presence of abnormalities such as primary spasm or even achalasia in its early form.

RADIONUCLIDE IMAGING

The esophageal emptying of a radiolabeled meal may be of some help in identifying subtle esophageal diseases. For example, it provides the best means for studying esophageal function during the ingestion of solid foods. In addition, it allows an estimation of the length of time that materials may reside within the esophagus after their ingestion and supposed passage into the stomach. There is some early work to suggest that radionuclide imaging may help to identify those patients who have esophagitis on the basis of poor stripping of the esophagus by secondary contraction waves. This modality is only in its early phase of evaluation and awaits further clinical trials.

ENDOSCOPY

The lumen of the esophagus can be readily and safely examined with the flexible fiberoptic endoscope. The standard end-viewing scope used in this procedure can be passed easily and safely through the cricopharyngeus to provide a full view of the esophagus from its orad to its caudad end. In addition, the instrument can be passed on into the stomach and duodenum in order to look for associated acid-peptic or neoplastic disease. There are two lumens within the scope, one for instilling and recovering irrigating fluids and a second for taking biopsies at points of interest. The flexible fiberoptic bundles provide a means for careful examination of the full extent of the epithelial lining of the esophagus. A smaller version called a pediatric endoscope with a diameter of 9 mm allows examination of areas of narrowing of the esophagus and, in addition, the passage of the instrument through strictures for biopsies within or below the lesion. This technology has offered a very precise way to make a tissue diagnosis of epithelial lesions of the esophagus. Hiatal hernia, diverticula, esophageal varices, and other intraluminal abnormalities can also be identified by this technique. The endoscope, however, usually does not provide an opportunity to diagnose motility disturbances of the esophagus. For example, it can readily be passed through an area of apparent narrowing at the lower end of the esophagus in patients with achalasia.

Biopsies of the epithelial lining of the esophagus are obtained when visual lesions are encountered. This is an important study for the specific diagnosis of esophagitis and cancer. It is especially important to take biopsies in the region of suspected Barrett's epithelium, since the latter may be associated with metaplastic changes indicating an early carcinoma. Lesions within the wall of the esophagus such as a leiomyoma are not biopsied since the disruption of the mucosa in the region may make subsequent enucleation both difficult and dangerous. Lesions of this type can usually be diagnosed by the barium roentgenogram. Endoscopy is always indicated in patients who present with upper gastrointestinal bleeding or dysphagia. Cancers of the esophagus occasionally can be missed by endoscopy if areas of stricture are not negotiated in order to take the biopsies within the middle aspect of the lesion. In this situation, it is possible to take brushings of the area and to subject the recovered material to cytologic examination.

MANOMETRY

The motor activity of the esophagus can best be characterized by measuring pressure profiles within its lumen. This is accomplished by the passage of an array of three small polyethylene catheters into the lumen of the stomach. Each catheter has a small hole 5 cm from its tip and the holes are arranged so that they are at 5-cm intervals. The catheters are perfused slowly with a constant flow of saline in order to prevent occlusion by mucus. As the array of catheters are withdrawn through the LES, they provide a pressure profile as is seen in Figure 22-7. The static measurement of the LES pressure can be supplemented by positioning the catheters so that a pressure can be obtained within the body of the esophagus as well as within the LES. This therefore provides evidence of peristaltic progression of a pressure wave within the body of the esophagus and relaxation of the LES on deglutition. In achalasia, there is a lack of peristaltic progression as well as relaxation of the LES. Primary spasm of the esophagus provides extremely high simultaneous pressure waves.

Manometry is especially helpful in the precise identification of the pressure relationships between the body of the esophagus and the stomach in hiatal hernia and reflux esophagitis. It provides a quantitative estimate of the pressure within the LES. Pressures below 10 torr are consistent with a low LES pressure and are an indication that the HPZ within this area has been lost. Low LES pressures are associated with and may be the cause of reflux esophagitis.

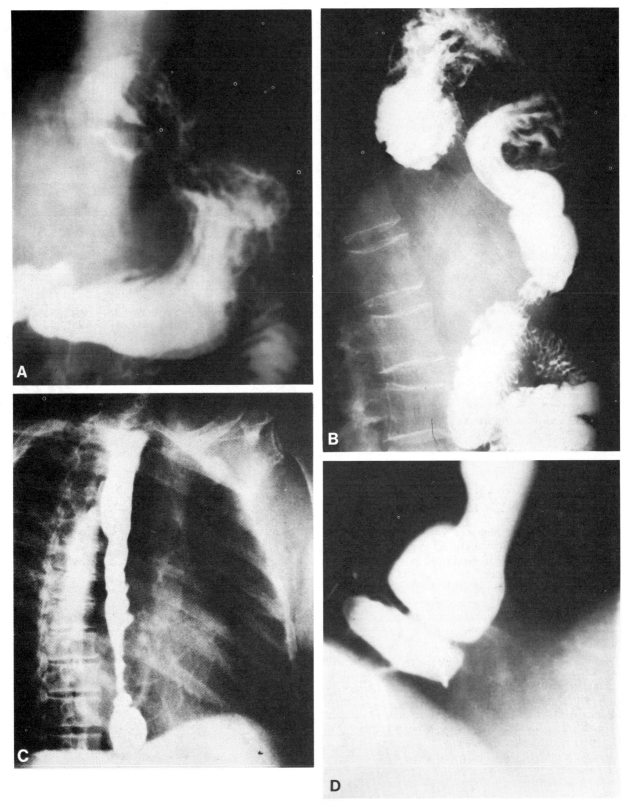

Fig. 22-4. Characteristic lesions on barium esophagogram. Lesions of the esophagus can be identified by barium roentgenogram. Definitive diagnosis, however, requires endoscopic visualization and biopsy when neoplastic or inflammatory lesions are suspected. (*A*) Direct (sliding) hiatal hernia; (*B*) paraesophageal hiatal hernia; (*C*) benign stricture in association with a hiatal hernia; (*D*) lower esophageal (Schatzki's) ring.

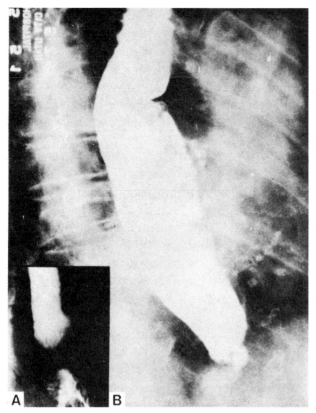

Fig. 22-5. Early achalasia. Barium roentgenogram of early achalasia (*B*), in which the esophagus is moderately increased in diameter and its lower end reveals a typical beaklike deformity (*A*).

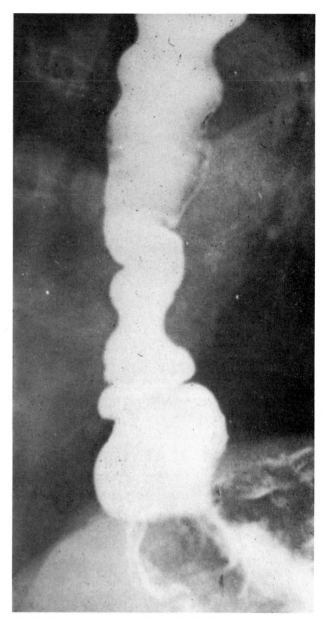

Fig. 22-6. Tertiary contractions. This barium esophagogram reveals tertiary contractions, which may occur without symptoms in the older patient (presbyesophagus) or be a manifestation of primary esophageal spasm.

A *p*H electrode can be attached to the manometric apparatus so that it can be drawn from the stomach into the esophagus following the measurement of the pressure in the lower esophageal sphincter. With one of the openings in the manometric device still within the stomach, acid can be instilled and the *p*H within the body of the stomach measured. The *p*H in the body of the stomach is usually greater than 4. A decrement in *p*H below 4 following instillation of acid and an increase in intra-abdominal pressure by leg raising or Valsalva maneuver is further proof that esophagitis may be on the basis of gastric acid reflux. In some instances, it is of value to instill hydrochloric acid into the esophagus to see if indeed a patient's pain or presumed reflux esophagitis can be reproduced in this manner (Bernstein's test). This is done in a blind fashion with neutral solutions as well as acid solutions, since many patients with reflux esophagitis are extremely sensitive to the passage of any fluid across their esophageal mucosa. The precision of reflux manometry and endoscopic biopsy has rendered this test obsolete, except in situations in which the former techniques are not readily available.

TREATMENT

CONGENITAL ANOMALIES

Vascular Rings

Vascular rings usually do not manifest difficulties during infancy but become apparent during early adult life as a source of obstruction to the esophagus. Patients usually present in their teens with high dysphagia. Barium esophagography reveals a typical constriction of the esophagus of the area, and angiography will usually show which vessels are involved. The definitive treatment, if dysphagia is persistent or progressive, is to divide the vascular ring by a transthoracic procedure. The results are excellent in the hands of an expert thoracic or pediatric surgeon.

Webs, Cysts, and Duplications

Esophageal webs of a congenital nature are rare lesions that may reveal their presence by inability to feed and regurgitation during infancy. Some do not manifest symptoms until adulthood. Symptomatic webs may be disrupted by endoscopy or peroral bougienage, thereby avoiding a formal operation on the esophagus. Occasionally, stout rings within the body of the esophagus require resection by a transthoracic route. Other congenital anomalies of the esophagus, such as duplications and esophageal cysts, often will require

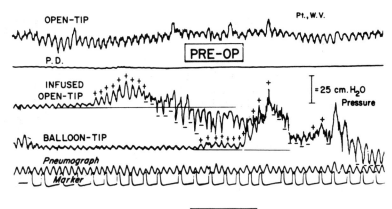

OPEN-TIP · Pt., W.V.

P.D.

PRE-OP

INFUSED OPEN-TIP

= 25 cm. H₂O Pressure

BALLOON-TIP

Pneumograph

Marker

POST-OP

OPEN-TIP

P.D.

INFUSED OPEN-TIP

BALLOON-TIP

Pneumograph

Marker

Fig. 22-7. Pressure profile, LES. A direct (sliding) hiatal hernia can be identified by its manometric profile. As polyethylene tubes are slowly pulled through the lower esophageal sphincter, the pressure is noted to be low in amplitude. Furthermore, respiratory reversal occurs within the high-pressure zone as a manifestation of its location within the mediastinum. This is corrected by replacing the LES into the abdomen by a Hill repair.

surgical intervention because of the uncertainty of their origins. Furthermore, lesions of this type may lead to chronic dysphagia. Their treatment usually consists of simple excision, which almost always can be accomplished without entering the lumen of the esophagus.

ESOPHAGEAL DIVERTICULA

Pharyngoesophageal (Zenker's) Diverticula

Protrusion of the mucosal lining of the upper esophagus between the cricopharyngeus muscle below and the thyropharyngeus portion of the inferior constrictor of the pharynx above can lead to a pharyngoesophageal diverticulum. The incomplete fusion of the muscle bundles provides a point of weakness in the area. The cricopharyngeus is a stout, powerful sling lying between the rami of the cricoid cartilage, and in this strategic position it provides a gateway to the esophagus. The mechanism of formation of a diverticulum in the area is thought to be related to excessive pressures generated by the cricopharyngeus. It is for this reason that they are called "pulsion" diverticuli. While they originate posteriorly, they usually present as a compressable mass in either side of the neck as they enlarge. They may be associated with gurgling sounds during eating, dysphagia when they become fully distended and compress the esophagus, and regurgitation and aspiration when they discharge their contents. The natural history of such lesions has not been well studied. It is clear, however, that when small, they are asymptomatic. It is thought that the history is one of progressive increase in size as a consequence of a primary motor disturbance within the cricopharyngeus. Surgical treatment at an early stage consists of division of the cricopharyngeus, an operation that is simple, safe, and effective. Large pharyngoesophageal diverticula can also be treated effectively in this manner, although the traditional, standard approach has been excision of the diverticulum as shown schematically in Figure 22-8, with or without division of the cricopharyngeus.

Fig. 22-8. A Zenker's diverticulum, when large, is best managed by excision (*A*). A complementary division of the cricopharyngeus (myotomy) will reduce the chance of recurrence or postoperative dysphagia (*B*).

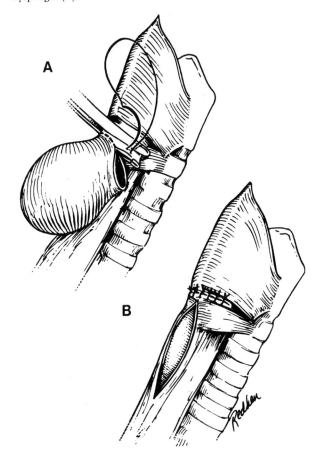

The operation is performed through an incision that parallels the anterior border of the sternocleidomastoid muscle. Elevation of the left lobe of the thyroid with care to avoid the left recurrent laryngeal nerve provides direct access to the cricopharyngeus, which is divided in its middle aspect. If a diverticulectomy is to be performed, the diverticulum is mobilized and clamped at a distance of at least 2 cm from its point of origin in order to avoid constriction at the point where its neck is closed with an inner row of absorbable and an outer inverting row of nonabsorbable sutures. Suspension of the sac of a diverticulum to the inferior sphincter above is an acceptable and probably preferred alternative for moderate-sized diverticula.

Epiphrenic Diverticula

Pulsion diverticula can occur at any point within the body of the esophagus, but except for those that occur at the lower end, they usually are small and without symptoms. Those that occur just above the esophagogastric junction (epiphrenic) do so in conjunction with primary motility disturbances of the esophagus, or hiatal hernia disease. They often are large and associated not only with the symptoms of the underlying motility disturbance but also with dysphagia from mechanical compression of the lower end of the esophagus or with pain and bleeding from stasis ulceration. One of the common but often overlooked signs of their presence is recurrent bouts of regurgitation pneumonitis.

The diagnosis of epiphrenic diverticulum is usually made by roentgenography (Fig. 22-9). Manometry should also be performed in order to identify the specific motor abnormality present. Endoscopy can also be accomplished safely, once being aware that the scope may easily pass into the diverticulum. Inspection of the esophagus and the diverticulum must be carried out with caution. Cancer has been reported on a few occasions in patients with long-standing diverticula.

The surgical treatment consists of the same principles as described above for phrenoesophageal diverticulum: myotomy and excision of the diverticulum. In this instance, the myotomy is tailored to the disease: a short myotomy away from the diverticulum when associated with achalasia and a long myotomy when primary spasm is present.

Traction Diverticula

Inflammatory lesions within the mediastinum may distract the wall of the esophagus away from its lumen, leading to a true "traction" diverticulum in contrast to the pseudodiverticulum of the "pulsion" lesions described above. The "traction" diverticula can be distinguished by their small size and conical, often irregular, appearance. They usually are not associated with symptoms and should not be excised, since the risk of esophageal leak is prohibitively high.

ESOPHAGEAL WEBS

Thin, membranous areas of narrowing within the lumen of the esophagus are called webs because of their filamentous nature. Webs consist of atrophic mucosal folds that extend partially or fully around the lumen of the esophagus. In the latter case, the opening through the web may be within its center (concentric) or its margin (eccentric). These distinctions are trivial, but the location of the web along the longitudinal axis of the esophagus is of prime clinical importance. While most webs are acquired and thereby manifest their presence in adult life, some are congenital

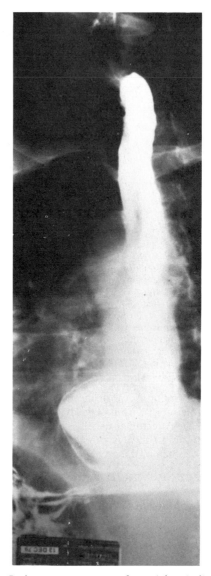

Fig. 22-9. Barium roentgenogram of an epiphrenic diverticulum. This is usually a sign of disturbed motility within the lower end of the esophagus. Treatment consists of excision and a myotomy on the contralateral side of the esophagus.

and present symptoms at birth. Congenital webs are rare but should be suspected when a newborn regurgitates or fails to take feedings. Webs in the adult must be distinguished from muscular contraction rings. The differential features will be discussed below.

Upper Esophageal Webs (Plummer-Vinson Syndrome)

Webs that occur within the upper or cervical esophagus in the adult are often associated with fissured lips (cheilosis), dry skin, smooth tongue, flat brittle nails (koilonychia), weight loss, dysphagia, and iron deficiency anemia. This cluster of signs and symptoms is called the Plummer-Vinson syndrome in the United States and the Paterson-Kelly syndrome in Europe, thereby identifying the individuals who described the manifestations of the disease. Iron deficiency anemia plays a key role in the development of the web by a mechanism as yet unknown. Surprisingly, the web disappears in most cases when the anemia has been corrected.

The syndrome has a predilection for Anglo-Saxon women (85%) in their middle to late age. It is a rare condition in countries in which iron supplements are added to bread. There is an association between the syndrome and carcinoma of the cervical esophagus, a coincidence that can be favorably influenced by early treatment of the anemia.

The diagnosis is usually made by recognition of the multiple signs described above in an anemic female with dysphagia. A thick barium swallow with cineradiography will usually demonstrate the presence of one or more fine indentations on the barium column within the esophageal lumen. The mucosal webs never extend below the arch of the aorta. Fiberoptic endoscopy should be done with caution in order to identify the fine, veil-like web, which can usually be disrupted with ease by passage of the endoscope. This maneuver may cure the dysphagia, but more importantly, it is essential for exclusion of an early cancer.

Treatment of the iron deficiency anemia by administration of ferrous lactate or gluconate (1 gm) three times a day will relieve the dysphagia when hemoglobin levels have reached 70% of normal. Bougienage offers an even quicker way to disrupt the web if endoscopy has failed to do so.

Midesophageal Webs

Webs that occur in the midesophagus may be of congenital origin or may be acquired as a consequence of esophagitis in association with a Barrett's epithelium. The latter can be easily distinguished from a true membranous web, since patients with Barrett's esophagitis usually present with a long-standing history of heartburn and dysphagia. Furthermore, the barium roentgenogram of the esophagus will demonstrate a short stricture in the midesophagus often in association with a hiatal hernia. Endoscopy reveals esophagitis, rather than a membranous rim of esophageal mucosa.

Lower Esophageal Webs (Schatzki's Ring)

Congenital webs can also occur within the lower end of the esophagus, but they are rare compared with a Schatzki's ring, which is a common roentgenographic finding. There has been considerable controversy as to whether a Schatzki's ring is a consequence of reflux esophagitis, a normal configuration of the esophagogastric junction, or radiographic evidence of a hiatal hernia. All three are likely. Esophagitis may make a ring more prominent because of edema within its submucosal tissues. The presence of a type I hiatal hernia may accentuate the presence of a ring, and the ring itself delineates the merging of the epithelial linings of the esophagus and stomach. Rings are only of importance when they reduce the diameter of the esophageal outlet to a critical level (10 mm to 20 mm in diameter). Patients with a small diameter ring without esophagitis usually complain of intermittent dysphagia, especially to solids. In fact, they soon learn to chew their food well, for failing to do so may require a trip to an emergency room for removal of an undigested morsel by endoscopy.

Symptomatic rings can be seen by endoscopy as a white membrane with a concentric opening. They can also be easily visualized on the barium esophagogram, especially when intra-abdominal pressure is increased by the Valsalva maneuver following passage of the barium into the stomach. Lower esophageal rings can be dilated by progressive esophageal dilatation by the passage of mercury-weighted bougies. It is best to perform a series of dilatations in order to gain passage of up to a 50-F bougie. Rings can also be safely incised by electrocautery through the endoscope or ruptured by balloon tamponade. Rarely do they require surgical incision. In fact, they can easily be fractured by the insertion of a finger through a high gastrotomy at the time of hiatal hernia repair for reflux esophagitis. Rings in this situation may be thicker than in the nonesophagitis case and usually can best be dilated by intraoperative transoral passage of progressively larger mercury-weighted bougies.

CAUSTIC INJURY

Concentrated solutions of sodium hydroxide (lye) and hydrochloric acid are commonly used as cleaning agents within the home and therefore are readily available to unsuspecting children. Lye ingestion is by far the most common form of caustic injury, especially when the material is taken in its liquid form. The ingestion of acid is infrequently encountered and usually is the consequence of an attempted suicide. The extent of injury that follows the ingestion of caustic materials depends on the concentration of the material ingested and whether it is taken in liquid or solid form. The secretory status of the stomach contributes to the extent of gastric injury at the time of lye ingestion. The highest percentage of lye ingestions is in children under 5 years of age. However, only approximately 30% of these patients with suspected cases will show objective evidence of injury. On the contrary, while adults represent only approximately 40% of patients admitted for lye ingestion in most series, approximately 80% will demonstrate rather extensive corrosive injury. The reason for this is that children likely take a small mouthful of either the crystal or liquid form of lye and expectorate, whereas adults who ingest the material are intent on taking a large amount in order to kill themselves. Usually the ingestion of a large amount of lye by either a child or an adult is associated with burns around the mouth and in the pharynx. In some cases, however, an injurious amount of lye can be ingested with almost no evidence of external injury. Attempts to develop appropriate packaging and warning on bottles that contain caustic materials may well lead to a marked reduction of this unfortunate and preventable injury in the future.

Early Management

Patients who are suspected of having ingested a caustic material should be brought immediately to an emergency facility for evaluation and therapy. Both acid and alkali can lead to airway obstruction by pharyngeal edema. Therefore, assessment of ventilation as well as pharyngeal injury should be made early in the course of the examination. In addition, both materials can cause perforation of either the esophagus or the stomach. Acid is more likely to contribute to the latter, although alkali perforations occur in about 10% of cases in which a large amount of liquid lye has been ingested.

Early diagnostic maneuvers should include a careful examination of the mouth and pharynx, lungs, and abdomen. A chest roentgenogram and flat and upright films of the abdomen should be taken as a baseline to which subsequent roentgenograms can be compared. No attempt should be made to induce retching or provide for lavage of the stomach. Usually the damage has already been done by the time the patient reaches the hospital. Barium roentgenograms are of no value in assessing the extent of caustic injury. Rather, at an appropriate time in the patient's course following resuscitation and stabilization, a careful fiberoptic endoscopy should be performed. This usually can be carried out safely within the first 24 to 48 hours, or even earlier if there is no evidence of oral or pharyngeal injury. The purpose of endoscopy is to assess whether there has been significant injury to the esophagus or stomach. The endoscopy, therefore, is carried out to a point where penetrating injury of the mucosa is demonstrated. It is not necessary to go below this point, where the risk of injury to the ulcerated, friable esophagus is high. It is convenient to grade the gross evidence of injury on a scale from 1 to 4, since it has been well established that with only mild injury, aggressive and prolonged therapy is not necessary. When there are ulcerations within the esophagus with exudates and granulation tissue, then the chance for subsequent fibrosis and stricture formation is high. Strictures almost always occur in situations in which there is evidence of severe mucosal ulceration; they almost never occur in the absence of mucosal ulceration.

The natural history of moderate to severe injury from lye ingestion is one of healing and repair over a 4- to 5-week period. The patient may initially experience substernal discomfort, but this usually subsides within a period of a few days. With moderate injury, the patient may be able to ingest liquids without difficulty. In severe injury, however, it is best to pass a small nasogastric tube that can be used for enteral feedings during the period of complete repair. There is no documentation that a nasogastric tube may prevent subsequent stricture formation; therefore, it is probably best to use a small nasogastric tube in order to reduce the pharyngeal discomfort associated with the larger, rigid tubes. Antibiotics should be provided in cases of severe injury in order to reduce the possibilities of septic mediastinitis. A cephalosporin, or ampicillin, given over a period of 5 to 7 days will suffice for this purpose. There continues to be controversy as to whether corticosteroids help to reduce the incidence of stricture formation. They certainly should not be used in cases of mild injury, since such cases never go on to stricture formation. Furthermore, they have not been found to be efficacious in cases of severe injury, and they may serve to mask the early manifestations of severe penetrating or perforating lesions. They may be of value in cases of moderate injury in which there are multiple superficial ulcerations of the mucosal lining of the esophagus.

Late Management

Patients with moderate to severe caustic injury should be managed in the hospital during the early phases of their recovery. It is important to maintain a high level of nutrition in order to enhance the process of repair. In patients who are ill from their injury, it is possible to provide full nutritional support by parenteral hyperalimentation. Enteral feedings, however, are preferable because they can be carried out in the home once the period of acute concern has passed. Moderate to severe injury may require hospitalization for a week or longer. It is surprising, however, that many individuals even with severe injury can tolerate progressive oral feedings a few days after injury. This clinically quiescent period can induce a false sense that all is well, when in fact the esophagus during its repair is going on to progressive stenosis. It therefore is important to provide close follow-up for each patient so that the evidence of early fibrosis can be ascertained and treated by sequential bougienage. A barium swallow should be taken 10 to 14 days after the initial injury, at biweekly intervals for the next 6 weeks, and then each month for the next 3 months. This will bring the patient through the maximum period of

risk for esophageal stenosis and avoid the unfortunate circumstance in which the patient returns with malnutrition and total closure of the esophageal lumen.

Conservative Management of Caustic Stricture

Patients who present with signs of early stricture formation, either as evidenced clinically by dysphagia, or roentgenographically by a stricture on barium swallow, are candidates for esophageal dilatation by bougienage (Fig. 22-10). This is a procedure that can be carried out most simply by having the patient swallow graded, tapered, mercury-weighted bougies of the Maloney or Hurst type. If the fibrotic process is identified early, then one can start usually with a 24- to 26-F size and progressively dilate up to a size 40 F. It is not recommended to go beyond this level of dilatation, since excessive stretching will lead to further injury followed by fibrosis in the process of repair. If the stricture is identified at a time when a bougie cannot be passed, then it will be necessary for the patient to undergo endoscopy so that the stricture can be dilated through the endoscope with small filiform catheters until such time as a string can be passed through the opening into the stomach. The availability of the string will then allow progressive dilatation over the string with the rigid Plummer dilators until such time as the tapered, mercury-weighted bougies can be tolerated. Occasionally, the patient will require retrograde dilatation with Tucker dilators, which requires an operative procedure whereby a small ureteral catheter is passed from the stomach to the mouth through a gastrostomy. A string is attached and drawn into the stomach. The Tucker dilators are then drawn progressively in a retrograde fashion through the stricture until an adequate opening is obtained. This is the safest way to dilate a tight, mature stricture. A gastrostomy tube and string is left in place for subsequent retrograde dilatations until antegrade bougienage can be accomplished.

In patients with advanced injury, it is best to leave a large nasogastric tube in place because it is anticipated that there will be progressive stenosis of the esophagus in the early postinjury period. It is possible to begin dilatation during the early phase of repair so that an adequate channel is ensured. Patients can be taught to swallow an appropriate size bougie, and therefore it is possible for them to carry out the care of an aggressive fibrotic esophagitis at home once trained to do so.

Late Management of Caustic Stricture

Patients who have a full-thickness injury to the esophagus from caustic ingestion over a long extent of the esophagus require frequent bougienage. A point may come in the management of such patients that esophageal replacement is a desired alternative. Patients who require this aggressive form of therapy usually have an extensive length of the esophagus involved. It may therefore be necessary to provide an esophageal substitute by colonic or jejunal interposition. It is also advisable to remove the diseased portion of the esophagus, since the incidence of subsequent carcinoma following lye injury is significant. Patients who respond to bougienage and eventually go on to normal alimentation without dysphagia should be followed carefully over the years, since the esophagus injured in this way has been rendered an oncogenic insult that may not manifest a frank cancer for 30 or 40 years. Unfortunately, there is no simple way to identify such a cancer early except to advise the patient to come for an examination whenever esophageal symptoms intervene. Furthermore, it probably would be in

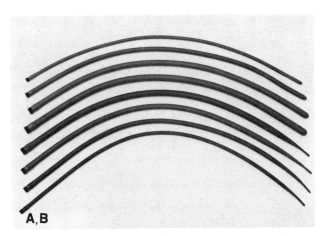
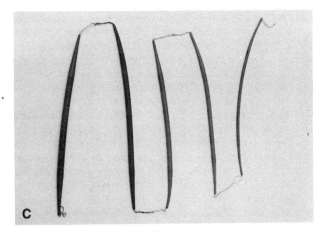
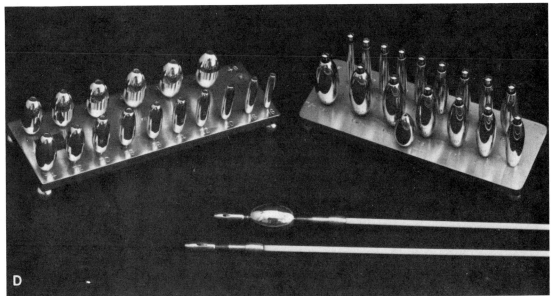

Fig. 22-10. Bougies are rigid instruments employed to dilate esophageal strictures. The Hurst and Maloney (*A* and *B*) dilators are weighted with mercury in order to help their passage by gravity. Tucker dilators (*C*) are used when the stricture is refractory to dilatation from above, and it is necessary to perform the dilatation in a retrograde fashion. Plummer dilators (*D*) are used when rubber bougies cannot be passed through the stricture. They can be passed over a string that has been drawn into the stomach by a small lead weight. The string provides a guide for the rigid dilator, thereby preventing esophageal rupture.

the patient's best interest to be seen annually if indeed severe esophageal injury has been incurred.

PRIMARY MOTILITY DISTURBANCES

Achalasia

Pattern Recognition. Most diseases can be identified by their natural history and the symptoms they produce. Achalasia is no exception. In fact, the diagnosis can be made with a high degree of accuracy if the clinical features of the disease are kept in mind. Achalasia is usually a disease of middle age, but it is occasionally seen in children. It occurs in about equal incidence for either sex. Occurrence of associated symptoms is infrequent. Therefore, dysphagia appears to be the major symptom of concern and forms the focus for diagnostic workup. In the early stages of achalasia the patient senses a sticking sensation, usually at the level of the xiphoid, after the ingestion of liquids or solids. Liquids, especially when cold, initiate this symptom more frequently

than solids. Dysphagia in the early phases of the disease is infrequent and is well tolerated for many years. Weight loss is uncommon, and pain is unusual. As a consequence, patients with achalasia do not seek medical attention until the symptom of dysphagia interferes with their life-style or

ACHALASIA	
Etiology	Decreased number of myenteric ganglion cells LES relaxation failure on swallowing
Dx	Dysphagia with sensation of sticking food Upper gastrointestinal studies show dilated esophagus to LES Manometry shows high LES pressures
Rx	Balloon dilatation LES myotomy

enjoyment of a meal. In fact, it is of great interest to observe the tricks that such patients develop to evacuate the esophagus. The most common consists of washing foods through with a large volume of liquid. In the later stages of the disease, they learn that various positions, twists, and compression will help to relieve the sticking sensation that now they have come to expect with each meal.

Some patients with achalasia do have pain, and they indeed represent a difficult variant of the disease. The pain is usually severe and is localized to the substernal area. It occurs as a spasm that may last from a few to several minutes. This pain is so bothersome that patients usually seek medical advice shortly after its onset, rather than rely on self-treatment. Heartburn is rare in achalasia for reasons that will be elucidated below. Regurgitation of undigested food is common as the disease progresses. The patient rarely complains of regurgitating a bitter (bile) or sweet (gastric juice) tasting material. Bad breath may become a problem, but its occurrence is so commonplace that it hardly serves as a diagnostic sign.

Etiologic Considerations. Although the pathophysiology of achalasia is not understood, there is a small body of investigative work that is worthy of discussion. First, the parasympathetic ganglion cells within the myenteric plexus between the longitudinal and circular muscle layers of the esophagus are markedly reduced in number. Initially this was thought to be the result of stretching of the muscular wall of the dilated esophagus; however, it is now known that ganglion cells are sparse or absent in the nondilated LES of most patients. Second, patients with parasitic infestation of the myenteric plexus by *Trypanosoma cruzi* develop signs and symptoms of achalasia. This disease is common in South America, but it is rare in other countries and is not thought to be the cause of achalasia in the United States. Third, and a point of extreme interest, a decrease in cells within the area of the dorsal motor nucleus of the vagus has been found at autopsy. Achalasialike manometric changes have also been produced in dogs by ablation of the supranodosal ganglion. Finally, injury to the esophageal myenteric plexus by cold, heat, chemicals, or excision will lead to the characteristic manometric signs of the disease. Although these are indirect pieces of evidence, they do serve to implicate the autonomic nervous system in the disease. A point of special interest and importance in diagnosis is the fact that the body of the esophagus is very sensitive to parasympathetic stimulation and responds to parasympathomimetic agents such as methacholine chloride (Mecholyl) with vigorous, simultaneous, repetitive contractions, as will be discussed below. This response is consistent with Cannon's law that denervated organs are supersensitive to the humoral agents that control their function.

Diagnosis. The definitive diagnosis of achalasia requires manometric evaluation of the pressure characteristics of the body of the esophagus and the LES. Manometric changes found typically with this disease may be compared with the normal picture as shown in Figure 22-3. Note the high pressures within the LES (usually about 40 torr) and, more important, failure of the sphincter to relax below pressures found within the stomach. It is important to keep in mind that the sphincter may relax in part but not enough to allow the passage of ingested foodstuffs. The postmyotomy study serves to illustrate the tertiary, nonpropulsive nature of the contractions within the body of the esophagus (Fig. 22-11). A profound decrease in resting pressures of the LES, which still demonstrates an inability to relax on swallowing, is

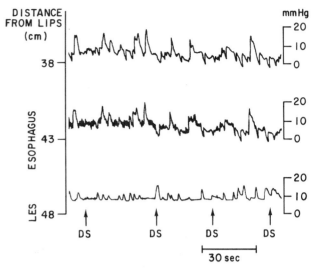

Fig. 22-11. Postmyotomy manometry. This manometric tracing demonstrates pressure characteristics of the LES and lower esophagus after a modified Heller myotomy. Note the relatively feeble contractions within the body of the esophagus following deglutition and the low pressures within the LES. There is an absence of either relaxation or contraction within the latter zone. The beneficial results from disruption of circular muscle by either surgical or medical means are related to this marked reduction in pressure within the LES. Unfortunately, a favorable manometric result in this case was accompanied by symptomatic reflux esophagitis.

also seen. Fortunately, the pressure is now low enough to allow food to pass readily into the stomach. On occasion, this pressure may be so low that gastric contents reflux into the esophagus, as was the case in this example. As mentioned above, a pathognomonic finding in achalasia is an accentuated response to parasympathetic stimulation. Such a response is demonstrated manometrically in Figure 22-11, in which vigorous simultaneous contractions accompany a modest increase in pressure within the body of the esophagus following administration of 3.0 mg methacholine chloride. The normal esophagus would not respond in this way to a dose even three times as great.

Unfortunately, manometry is not available in all medical communities, and the diagnosis must rest on conventional diagnostic techniques.

Treatment. The definitive treatment of achalasia requires disruption of the circular layer of smooth muscle within the LES area. This can be accomplished by vigorous dilatation of this area by a balloon, which is rapidly inflated with air or water to a pressure of 300 torr for 15 seconds (Fig. 22-12). The balloon is positioned within the LES under fluoroscopic control. Patients undergoing this treatment usually feel a severe subxiphoid pain; therefore premedication with an analgesic and a tranquilizer should be employed. The results from forceful dilatation in this way are fair to good, with 60% of patients receiving complete relief of symptoms after one treatment and an additional 10% responding to a second treatment. Most gastroenterologists prefer this form of therapy. (However, rarely, the esophagus may be perforated.)

An alternative therapeutic modality consists of division of the circular muscle of the lower end of the esophagus by surgical means. This undoubtedly offers a precise and less traumatic way of dividing the circular muscle layer of the lower esophagus. In addition, results (75% to 85% good results) are superior to those reported for hydrostatic rupture,

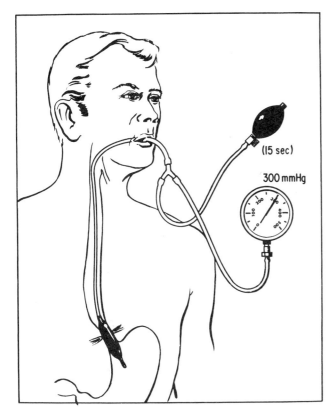

Fig. 22-12. Schematic representation of forceful dilatation by hydrostatic bougienage. The balloon is positioned within the lower esophageal sphincter under fluoroscopic control and then rapidly expanded to a pressure of 300 torr by a hand bulb for 15 seconds.

(15 sec)

300 mmHg

TABLE 22-3   THERAPEUTIC ALTERNATIVES FOR TREATMENT OF ACHALASIA

FACTOR	PROCEDURE		
	Simple Dilatation	Hydrostatic Rupture	Heller Myotomy
Convenience	1+	2+	3+
Risk	0	<0.1%	<0.5%
Result	3+	2+	1+
Cost*	$60	$150	$600

1+ = Best.
* Utah prices, 1975.

and the mortality is low. The major disadvantages are the need for hospitalization and thoracotomy and a low but finite incidence of reflux esophagitis (3%). It is curious that this complication has not been reported for hydrostatic rupture. Possibly this relates to the fact that patients who fail to respond to bougienage, or have problems subsequent to the procedure, are referred for surgical therapy and are thereby included in the 30% who have less than optimal results. The relative advantages and disadvantages of each procedure are listed in Table 22-3. Although cost factors in the past have not been a major concern in treatment programs, there is growing awareness that they will be in future years. A reasonable therapeutic program, therefore, appears to be one or two attempts at forceful dilatation by hydrostatic bougienage, performed in a hospital setting by a professional who has had extensive experience with this technique. If this fails to provide complete relief of symptoms, then esophagomyotomy should be performed after time has been allowed for resolution of the injury received by forceful dilatation (about 6 weeks).

Unfortunately, there is no way at present to treat achalasia by pharmacologic means or by invasive techniques less drastic than hydrostatic rupture or esophagomyotomy. Various types of anticholinergic and antispasmodic drugs have been tried but without success. Simple bougienage with mercury-weighted tubes (Hurst or Maloney dilators) has led to only temporary relief of symptoms even when tubes up to a diameter of 50 F (about 1.6 cm) have been passed through the LES. Earlier treatment programs included vigorous passage of a whale bone through the spastic sphincter, an effective maneuver because of the shape, rigidity, and diameter of this unique object. Some gastroenterologists still employ passage of metal dilators (usually guided by a string) through the lower esophagus into the stomach. Metal dilators that can be suddenly expanded with the LES (Stark dilator) have also been extensively used in the past, but the trend is toward balloon disruption or surgical division of the LES.

Esophagomyotomy is a simple surgical procedure that has been well standardized. The steps of the operation as performed at the Mayo clinic, an institution that has pioneered the treatment of achalasia, are shown in Figure 22-13. The lower esophagus is approached through a left thoracotomy at the level of the bed of the eighth rib. The pleural reflection is incised and the esophagus is mobilized, with careful preservation of the vagus nerves. In addition, the esophagogastric junction is mobilized from the esophageal hiatus to allow visualization of 1 cm to 2 cm of stomach. The esophagus is kept under tension by a soft rubber drain that encircles the esophagus. A linear incision is made through the circular muscle layer for a distance of 5 cm to 8 cm, with care being taken to bring the incision onto the stomach for a distance of only 3 mm to 5 mm. It is important to divide all circular muscle fibers. Entrance into the lumen of the esophagus can be avoided with careful dissection. Separation of the muscularis from the submucosa at the margin of the incision is an important maneuver to ensure that the divided layers do not reapproximate as healing occurs. The borders of the right crus should be approximated if a small hiatus hernia is encountered. There is increasing interest in performing a more definitive repair of the hiatal defect in order to prevent subsequent reflux esophagitis. Our preference is to perform a Belsey Mark IV hiatal hernia repair when a defect exists at the esophageal hiatus. This provides a partial fundoplasty and patch over the esophagomyotomy yet does not completely occlude the lower end of the esophagus. A Nissen fundoplasty, in which the stomach is wrapped around the lower esophagus, has the potential disadvantage of offering too much resistance to the passage of food through an esophagus, the contractility of which has become attenuated.

The treatment of achalasia with associated primary spasm presents a difficult challenge. A long esophagomyotomy that extends from the stomach to the aortic arch appears to offer the best chance for symptomatic relief. The results are far from ideal, with only about half of such patients gaining full relief from dysphagia. Possibly, resection of the esophagus with colonic reconstruction will provide an answer for the most advanced cases of this disorder. Resection of the distal esophagus with esophagogastric anastomosis, how-

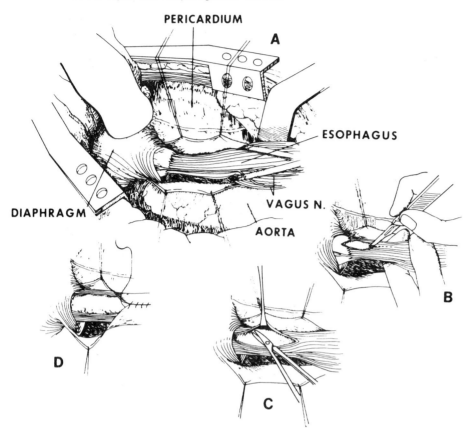

Fig. 22-13. Schematic sequence of a modified Heller myotomy. (*A*) The lower end of the esophagus is approached through the bed of the left eighth rib. A tape for purposes of traction is passed around the esophagus. (*B*) An incision, about 5 cm in length, is made through the circular muscle to the underlying muscularis at a point equidistant between the vagi, which are carefully preserved during the dissection. (*C*) The muscularis is dissected away from the margins of the incision to prevent reapproximation by a fibrous bridge. (*D*) The pleural reflection is closed over the lower mediastinum to reconstruct the anatomy of the area.

ever, has not been a very successful procedure for the treatment of achalasia.

Primary Spasm

Distinguishing Features. Patients with primary spasm complain of a deep severe substernal pain that may radiate into either the shoulder or the neck. Dysphagia is also a frequent complaint but characteristically is episodic and not progressive as in achalasia. The differential features that distinguish primary spasm are compared in Table 22-4.

Diagnosis. Manometry is the key to the diagnosis of primary spasm. Unfortunately, the patient's esophagus may not reveal the characteristic sign of the syndrome—high pressure waves within the body of the esophagus at the time of manometric study. In fact, several such studies may be required in order to by chance capture such an event. LES pressures and relaxation to a swallow are usually normal. Barium roentgenogram may reveal tertiary contractions,

which provides support for the diagnosis when the patient presents with the episodic substernal chest pain so typical of the disease.

Treatment. The initial treatment of primary spasm is medical. The patient should be encouraged to abstain from alcohol, tobacco, tea, and coffee. Administration of a mild sedative such as diazepam (Valium) may be helpful, since attacks are often stress related. Nitroglycerin has been reported to be helpful in some cases, as is the calcium antagonist nifedipine. Unfortunately, few patients ever become totally symptom free; yet they do not suffer nutritional consequences from the disease. The progression of an occasional case to achalasia has suggested the possibility that primary spasm and achalasia are a spectrum of the same disease. Some cases of primary spasm respond to a long esophagomyotomy in which the muscular coat of the esophagus is split from the esophagogastric junction to at or above the aortic arch. A controversy exists as to whether the LES should be divided in this procedure, which of necessity must be done through the left chest. Most surgeons agree, however, that an antireflux procedure should be included if reflux esophagitis is to be avoided.

ACQUIRED TRACHEOESOPHAGEAL FISTULA

Acquired communications between the esophagus and tracheobronchial tree occur at points within the neck or thorax where the two organ systems are contiguous. They usually originate as a consequence of neoplasm, infection, or trauma. Etiologic factors are listed below:

1. Cancer
   a. Esophagus
   b. Lung
   c. Trachea

TABLE 22-4	DIFFERENTIAL CHARACTERISTICS OF ACHALASIA AND PRIMARY SPASM	
	ACHALASIA	**PRIMARY SPASM**
Dysphagia	Common	Rare
Pain	Rare	Common
Barium esophagogram	Abnormal	Normal
Endoscopy	Normal	Normal
Motility	Nonrelaxing LES	Hypertonic contractions

2. Trauma
   a. Blunt (external)
   b. Endoscopy
   c. Operation
   d. Endotracheal tube
   e. Foreign body
3. Infection
   a. Tuberculosis
   b. Syphilis
   c. Histoplasmosis
4. Chemical
   a. Lye
   b. Acid

ESOPHAGEAL PERFORATION	
Etiology	Penetrating injury (gunshot, stab wound) Iatrogenic Spontaneous (i.e., distention, Boerhaave's syndrome)
Dx	Pain, crepitus of neck, fever Chest x-ray (Mediastinal air, hydrothorax) Esophagogram
Rx	Hydration, antibiotics Prompt surgical drainage and closure

Patients with such lesions often complain of symptoms associated with the underlying disease that contributed to the fistula. For example, those with tuberculosis, in which inflamed carinal nodes have led to the problem, will present with weight loss, fever, and cough. Those who have their lesion as a consequence of cancer of the esophagus will describe progressive dysphagia, regurgitation, and weight loss. A distinctive feature of tracheoesophageal fistula is cough after swallowing, which is usually worse with liquids.

The diagnosis of a fistula is most easily made by a barium esophagogram which demonstrates the tracheobronchial tree. Esophagoscopy may not reveal a small inflammatory fistula but is definitive when the lesion is secondary to a cancer arising within the esophageal mucosa. Bronchoscopy is an essential component of the workup, because it will reveal the extent of involvement to the trachea or bronchus and will establish the diagnosis if the etiology derives from this area.

Therapy is directed toward prevention of the passage of ingestants and saliva from the esophagus into the trachea. Nasogastric intubation with tube feedings often is sufficient in esophageal cancer, since tracheoesophageal fistula in this disease is usually a terminal event. An esophageal tube (*e.g.,* Celestin, Mousseau-Barbin) may also be placed, but they are associated with the complication of further erosion by pressure necrosis. Cervical esophagostomy can be used in severely symptomatic patients. Even colonic or jejunal bypass, with or without esophagectomy, has been tried with some success for this purpose. Radiotherapy rarely contributes to fistula closure.

Traumatic fistula from blunt or penetrating trauma provides a more promising therapeutic challenge. Most such lesions occur within the upper portion of the chest and are available though a right thoracotomy for surgical repair. Attention should first be paid toward nutritional repletion by parenteral hyperalimentation. Those patients with a fistula caused by infection should have specific antibiotic therapy. A traumatic fistula from endotracheal tube or cuff erosion or from blunt or penetrating injury may be approached more directly without delay. The operation consists of separation of the esophagus from the trachea and of suture of each viscus with nonabsorbable sutures. The suture lines are separated by an interposed leaf of pleura. Nearly 90% of benign fistulas can be successfully treated in this way.

PERFORATION OF THE ESOPHAGUS

Traumatic Rupture

The esophagus, although well shielded by the sternum and thorax, is nonetheless subject to blunt penetrating injury from without and within. The mechanisms of perforation depend on the offending vector. For example, a stab wound to the neck or chest may lead to a simple and clean laceration, while a bullet wound, depending on the caliber, may be associated with an extensive area of esophageal necrosis around the wound of entrance and exit. Instrumental perforations of the body of the esophagus usually occur at points of stricture or weakness within the esophageal wall caused by diverticula. The cervical esophagus just beyond the cricopharyngeus also used to be a point of occasional perforation when the use of the rigid esophagoscope was common. This instrument has for the most part been supplanted by the flexible fiberoptic scope, the use of which has remarkably reduced this complication.

Esophageal perforation is associated with the leakage of air and esophageal contents into the neck or mediastinum, depending on the level of injury. Pain and the signs of infection may occur early as bacteria multiply within the periesophageal area. Perforations of the cervical and thoracic esophagus may be associated with crepitus at the base of the neck. Diagnosis is best obtained by a water-soluble contrast study. This study should be done whenever perforation is suspected.

Esophageal perforations require prompt surgical therapy after diagnosis. Preoperative preparation includes nasogastric intubation, broad-spectrum antibiotic therapy, and intravenous alimentation. Cervical perforations are best treated by suture of the opening and drainage of the neck when identified early. Small perforations in this area recognized late (48 hrs to 72 hrs) can be treated conservatively and drained if resolution of the signs of inflammation are not prompt. Thoracic perforations require immediate exploration, which is accomplished through the right chest for high lesions and through the left for those within its lower third. The procedure used is dictated by what is found. A distal laceration at the point of erosive esophagitis and narrow stricture can be effectively treated by division of the stricture to the point of laceration and repair by sewing the anterior surface of the stomach to the margins of the esophagus. Perforations above neoplastic strictures should be treated by esophageal resection and appropriate reconstruction depending on the level of the lesion. Simple lacerations in the body are closed with a double row of nonabsorbable sutures. Lesions of this type at the esophagogastric junction should be covered by a proximal gastric wrap as employed for a Nissen fundoplication. Perforations that are encountered late in their course should be initially treated by drainage of the mediastinum through the chest cavity that reveals contamination by esophageal contents or leakage of contrast material. Contamination can be reduced by performing a cervical esophagostomy and a gastrostomy. Esophageal reconstruction is then carried out at a later date when the patient is improved.

Patients with complex perforations should be placed on parenteral hyperalimentation if gastrostomy has not been performed. Antibiotics should be continued for at least 10 days, and removal of drains, which in thoracic level injuries is a chest tube, should not be done until closure has been demonstrated by a water-soluble contrast study. The patient should not be fed until this has been accomplished, which usually occurs between the fifth to eighth day post-injury.

Spontaneous Perforation (Boerhaave's Syndrome)

Esophageal perforation may occur following sudden increases in intra-abdominal pressure. Coughing, retching, heavy lifting, or even parturition may lead to a dramatic increase in intraesophageal pressure when gastric contents are vigorously refluxed into the esophagus against a closed cricopharyngeus. Tears in this situation usually occur in the left posterior aspect of the lower esophagus. Males experience this complication five times more frequently than females. Obviously, the event is associated with the sudden onset of retrosternal or left chest or shoulder pain following an episode of retching. Baron John van Wassenaer, Grand Admiral of Holland, was the first patient described to have suffered such an event. The Dutch physician Boerhaave discovered that the baron had a perforated esophagus and surmised in his report in 1724 that retching 18 hours previously had caused the esophageal perforation that he found at autopsy.

The diagnosis should be suspected when a critically ill dyspneic patient presents with air in the mediastinum or with fluid within the left hemithorax. Water-soluble contrast barium roentgenography helps to confirm the diagnosis.

Treatment is directed toward fluid resuscitation, control of sepsis, operative drainage of the mediastinum and pleural cavity, and suture repair of the esophagus. Unfortunately, many cases are delayed in diagnosis, contributing to a friable and necrotic esophagus at the point of suture. These cases are best managed by drainage of the chest by tube thoracostomy, cervical esophagostomy, and gastrostomy. An acceptable approach would include a gastric patch of the tear if its margins were unsatisfactory for suture. Postoperative care consists, as in other perforations, in control of infection, in enteral or parenteral hyperalimentation, and in nonfeeding until healing of the tear is demonstrated by barium swallow.

BENIGN TUMORS

Benign tumors of the esophagus are rare disorders. Most of them are of mesothelial origin (leiomyoma). Benign epithelial neoplasms are uncommon, yet they are important to consider when ruling out malignancy and may be responsible for esophageal-related symptoms. In contrast to carcinoma, the prognosis is very good for successful treatment.

Leiomyomas

Leiomyomas of the esophagus are the most common benign tumors of the esophagus and account for more than 60% of reported lesions of this type. These smooth muscle tumors occur mainly in the thoracic portion of the esophagus (greater than 90%), but they are only occasionally found in the cervical portion (7%) because of a lack of involuntary muscle in that area. They are also frequently found in the stomach, small bowel, and colon. Occasionally these tumors are found in multiple sites along the body of the esophagus. Most leiomyomas measure from 1 cm to 17 cm in diameter (usually 5 cm to 8 cm) and are solitary and well encapsulated. Resected leiomyomas have been reported to weigh up to 5,000 g. They are thought to originate in the muscularis mucosa, muscularis propria, or muscular component of blood vessels or as aberrant embryonic cell rests. Approximately two thirds of all leiomyomas occur in men, who are usually 20 to 50 years of age. When they occur in women, they frequently arise in the sixth decade. No known etiologic factors have been implicated.

Dysphagia presents as the initial symptom in approximately 48% of patients. There may also be weight loss, pain, or bleeding. The barium esophagogram reveals a smooth-walled filling defect with sharp borders where the tumor meets the normal esophageal wall. The diagnosis is established by the observation, by endoscopy, of a firm intramural mass bulging into the lumen. The mucosa is usually not involved and the mass is freely movable. The esophagoscope can easily be passed beyond the lesion. Any lesion fitting the above criteria should not be biopsied for fear of destroying tissue planes required for effective enucleation at thoracotomy, which is the treatment of a leiomyoma of the body of the esophagus. The tumor is usually lodged in the muscular layers of the esophagus with an intact mucosa. It should be biopsied at the time of surgery by frozen section because malignant degeneration has been described. Esophageal resection is rarely required for benign lesions.

Polyps of the Esophagus

Polyps of the esophagus (20% of benign tumors) are intraluminal lesions that may cause dysphagia or even be regurgitated into the larynx with asphyxiation if they reach a large size. They are composed of a fibroblastic core and usually are covered with a normal epithelium. Occasionally small tumors can be removed by esophagoscopy, but most require excisional therapy. These tumors occur almost exclusively in the cervical area.

Other Benign Tumors

Lipomas, vascular tumors, and neurofibromas occur extremely rarely and are only mentioned for brief consideration. These are located throughout the body of the esophagus, and attention is directed toward these lesions by the symptoms of dysphagia, bleeding, or pain.

ESOPHAGEAL CANCER	
Etiology	Squamous cell and adenocarcinoma (lower one third)
	Smoking, alcohol, carcinogens, chronic inflammation
Dx	Dysphagia
	Esophagogram
	Esophagoscopy and biopsy
	Staging evaluation (CT, liver scan)
Rx	Surgical resection or palliative bypass
	Radiotherapy and chemotherapy

MALIGNANT TUMORS

Carcinoma of the esophagus is an uncommon disease in the United States. Except in unusual circumstances, it is incurable; most patients die within 2 years regardless of therapy. While dysphagia associated with carcinoma of the esophagus was noted in the early Middle Ages, it was not until the turn of the century when Janeway designed a safe esophagoscope that the surgical correction of the disorder could be introduced. Resectional and bypass therapy for this disorder have evolved over the past 50 years to the point at which acceptable forms of palliation are now available.

Incidence

Cancer of the esophagus in the United States is a disease most commonly affecting older men (7 per 100,000 males per year). The male-to-female ratio is 4:1. The average age at onset is approximately 62 years, with women generally affected at an earlier age. Blacks are affected more often than whites. Carcinoma of the esophagus is mostly of the squamous cell type. Its occurrence is evenly distributed throughout the esophagus. Distal esophageal carcinomas are equally divided between the squamous epithelial and the adenocarcinoma cell type. Adenocarcinoma of the distal esophagus is thought to be gastric in origin, but whether this is from glandular cells congenitally present in the distal esophagus or acquired as a result of recurrent esophagitis is disputed.

There is a remarkable geographic distribution of carcinoma of the esophagus in the world. Carcinoma of the esophagus in Iran has an incidence of 115 per 100,000 in men and 130 per 100,000 in women. In Ceylon, the disease is primarily a disease of females. In South Africa among the Bantu people the disease is epidemic with an equal incidence of male to female distribution. Several interesting studies have been reported from North China. In Fansien Province, the incidence is approximately 23.7 per 100,000 per year. In the neighboring Linhsien Province, there is a reported incidence of 109 per 100,000 per year among both men and women. In this province high levels of nitrosamines have been identified in pickled vegetables preserved in earthen jars. Many of these jars contained high amounts of the fungus *Geotrichum candidum*. Also in Linhsien Province, domestic fowls are affected by various types of pharyngeal carcinomas. In these areas of high incidence of the disease, mass screening clinics have been effective in finding early cases of esophageal carcinoma. These areas in China report high curative rates with surgical therapy. Among 170 cases reported from North China, 90.3% of the patients had survived.

In addition to age, sex, race, and geography, four high-risk factors have been identified:

1. Age, sex, race, and genetic factors
2. Carcinogens: alcohol, hot food, cigarette smoking, irradiation, nitrosamines, nitrates, zinc
3. Nutrition: malnutrition, poor oral hygiene, vitamin and trace element deficiency, iron deficiency
4. Miscellaneous: Barrett's esophagus, caustic injury of esophagus, alcoholism, reflux esophagitis, leiomyoma leukoplakia, scleroderma, hiatal hernia, and diverticula

Many patients with squamous cell carcinomas of the esophagus have a nutritional history of iron deficiency, hypovitaminosis A and C, malnutrition, and deficiencies of trace elements such as molybdenum, manganese, barium, magnesium, and copper. A group of carcinogens has also been postulated. There is a higher incidence of carcinoma of the esophagus among those patients who consume alcohol, tobacco, hot tea, and spices. A higher incidence than normal is also reported in people ingesting a diet high in nitrates, nitrosamines, and zinc. Among the Bantu, there is a high incidence of carcinoma implicated among those patients chewing betel nuts. Most irritative diseases of the esophagus have been implicated in a higher incidence of carcinoma of the esophagus than usual (*i.e.,* esophageal diverticula, gastroesophageal reflux, diaphragmatic hernias, Barrett's esophagus, lye burns, and alcoholism). For unknown reasons, gastrectomy and poor dental hygiene have also been implicated.

Pathology

Carcinoma of the esophagus usually presents with symptoms of obstruction from a fungating lesion that protrudes into its lumen. The studies from North China suggest that the time period from the carcinoma *in situ* to the time of full obstruction is generally 2½ years. While squamous cell carcinoma is the most common, other forms of malignancy of the esophagus are also identified such as mucoepidermoid carcinoma, carcinosarcoma, adenocarcinoma, lymphoma, and leiomyosarcoma.

Since the disease is usually discovered late, most tumors at the time of diagnosis have significant invasion and metastasis. Carcinoma in the middle portion of the esophagus may metastasize to lymph nodes in the immediate vicinity but often may already be at a distant nodule site at the time of detection. Metastases to the lung, liver, pancreas, and kidney are not unusual at the time of detection of the primary. Lower third esophageal cancers usually spread to the cardiac portion of the stomach, celiac axis, aortic nodes, and liver. Carcinomas in the cervical region frequently metastasize to the lateral neck. Carcinomas in the thoracic portion of the esophagus frequently invade by local means to the tracheobronchial tree (usually left membranous portion of the tracheal left main stem). Invasion to the aorta as well as to the vena cava and pulmonary veins is not unusual. Frequently, the carcinoma will extend in a submucosal fashion down the thoracic esophagus before spreading to the local lymph nodes. Since the esophagus does not contain a serosal layer, the tumor can easily spread to contiguous structures. Furthermore, lymphatic drainage is frequently unpredictable and spread by vascular means is usually rapid.

Diagnosis

Ninety-five percent of the patients with esophageal carcinoma have dysphagia as the earliest symptom. Esophageal pain, regurgitation, anorexia, hematemesis, and hoarseness are unusual as presenting symptoms. In most patients, dysphagia begins initially as an inability to swallow solid foods and progresses within several months to intolerance to liquids also. Postlethwait reports that in 107 patients studied, the majority of the patients were admitted to the hospital after having symptoms for a period of 1 to 3 months. It is believed that the symptoms of dysphagia do not occur until the lumen is highly occluded. By this time most of the patients have significant systemic abnormalities present. Most patients are profoundly immunologically deficient and have a weight loss of 10 to 30 pounds.

Laboratory Examinations

The diagnosis of esophageal carcinoma is made by a barium esophagogram. The characteristic signs of carcinoma of the esophagus are narrowing and irregularity of the lumen of the esophagus (see Fig. 22-4). Frequently the edge of the lesion is shown as an abrupt shelf. Occasionally, esophageal cancer presents as a tapered narrowing, making the differential diagnosis from benign esophageal stricture difficult.

Visualization of the stomach by barium roentgenography is also important since the roentgenogram may later be used in the formation of a gastric tube. Computed tomography (CT) may be helpful in diagnosing the extent of the lesion and may delineate invasion of contiguous structures. Endoscopic examination by esophagoscopy as well as by bronchoscopy is critical in diagnosing the lesion as well as in determining its extent of spread. Currently, it is controversial as to whether rigid or flexible esophagoscopy should be performed. Rigid esophagoscopy is useful in obtaining an adequate biopsy as well as in evaluating fixation of the tumor.

Assessment of liver function is also important. Elevation of the alkaline phosphatase or serum glutamic oxaloacetic transaminase (SGOT) should be followed by a CT or radioisotopic scan. Brain scans, as well as bone scans, should be used only if involvement is suggested by the history or findings on physical examination.

Esophageal cytology has been used by Chinese physicians as a method of screening patients with early stages of the disease. This is not practical in the United States, where the incidence of the disease is low. Cytologic examination may be valuable during esophagoscopy or during passage of a sound or tube through the obstructed esophagus, when biopsy is not possible or negative. Biopsy of supraclavicular nodes, when palpable, may help to make a diagnosis and stage the extent of the disease.

Treatment

Since carcinoma of the esophagus is usually an incurable disease, palliation is the goal of therapy in most cases. Radiotherapy has emerged as one of the more popular treatments for carcinoma of the esophagus. Unfortunately, the sensitivity of the tumor to radiation is frequently low and sometimes unresponsive. Radiotherapy, when effective, offers a nonoperative treatment that will relieve the esophageal stenosis and allow symptomatic improvement. There is general agreement that radiation therapy is the preferred treatment for upper third esophageal lesions. Surgical resection of lesions in this area has generally been disappointing. The effectiveness of surgical versus radiation therapy remains controversial in middle third esophageal lesions. If surgical resection can be carried out with an acceptable mortality (<10%) and morbidity, this form of therapy is preferable. Most authors agree that radiation therapy offers little advantage over surgery for treatment of carcinoma of the lower third of the esophagus. Preoperative radiation therapy has been offered as a method of extending survival after resection. The results of this approach, however, remain inconclusive. Chemotherapy has also not shown efficacy, but studies employing bleomycin and BCG have provided encouraging results.

Operative Therapy

Operability for cancer of the esophagus is approximately 58%, and resectability is 39%. Operative therapy generally consists of one of four methods: (1) dilatation and intubation, (2) gastrostomy and esophagostomy, (3) resection, and (4) bypass.

Several endoesophageal tubes have been suggested for palliative treatment. These tubes are generally a soft rubber or plastic with reinforced wire loops. The selected tube is placed under rigid esophagoscopy through the obstructive lesions, thus allowing saliva and food to pass passively through the tumor. Many of these tubes have been employed in patients in the large series in South Africa. The advantages of these tubes are that they are easy to place and require only a short hospitalization. However, several complications have been described with these tubes. Perforation has occurred in many of these patients. Tube dislodgements with asphyxiation have been described as well as tube obstruction and bleeding. Kairaluoma, in 1977, described a 16% mortality with placement of this tube. Most surgeons in the United States have been discouraged from using these intraluminal tubes and prefer to use either resection or bypass.

Gastrostomy and cervical esophagostomy have been used in a large series of patients who were too ill to undergo resection. In this form of palliation, the cervical esophagostomy is brought out in the low neck and feeding gastrostomy performed. Most physicians feel that this is poor palliation and patients frequently choose not to use the feeding gastrostomy. A cervical esophagostomy is also a highly undesirable and unattractive mode of therapy. Esophageal resection and replacement appears to be the safest and the most reliable way of treating a patient with carcinoma of the middle or lower portion of the esophagus. The most common operation performed is esophagogastrectomy (Fig. 22-14). This may be done with or without resection of the tumor. It entails mobilizing the stomach with its vasculature and elevating it into the chest where it is anastomosed to the esophagus. This operation may be performed through a left thoracotomy, a left thoracoabdominal approach, or a midline abdominal incision, freeing up the stomach, and a right thoracotomy to resect the tumor and anastomose the esophagus.

Bypass procedures are highly effective as palliative therapy and may have the advantage of being easier operations for seriously ill patients to tolerate (Fig. 22-15). The entire stomach may be used after mobilizing it through abdominal incision as a bypass. Greater curvature gastric tubes may also be used to bypass the lesion. These gastric tubes may be anastomosed into the high cervical region without a thoracotomy. Colon interposition has also been shown to be highly successful in bypassing either resected lesions or as palliative therapy. The right transverse or left colon may be used as an esophageal substitution with excellent results. A segment of jejunum may also be used for bypass. However, the blood supply to the jejunum is frequently not as reliable as that of the colon and allows for only short segments. Semirigid tubes may also be placed through the obstructing lesion for short-term palliation.

Mortality figures are generally governed by the choice of the operation as well as by the ability and experience of the operating surgeon. Centers in the United States that are doing high-volume esophageal surgery have reported mortalities with the esophageal resection in the range of 5% to 10%. These centers emphasize the necessity of vigorous preoperative preparation. When one is considering modes of therapy for a palliative operation, the mortality and morbidity of the procedure must be carefully considered before one therapy is chosen over another. Postoperative

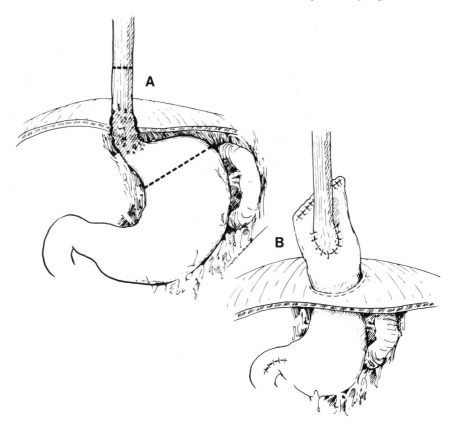

Fig. 22-14. Esophagogastrectomy. After removing the lesion, the mobilized stomach is brought up in the chest and anastomosed to the esophagus.

complications of bypass and resection procedures include anastomotic leaks, respiratory failure, sepsis, hemorrhage, and pneumonia.

Results of Treatment

Postlethwait, in his collected series of 16,000 cases, reported a 5-year survival of approximately 8% with resections and a 5-year survival of 3% for all patients. Mean survival for 701 patients with various forms of carcinoma was approximately 4 months when no therapy was given, approximately 5 to 6 months with gastrostomy and bypass, 7 months with palliative resection, and 25 to 35 months with curative resection.

Carcinoma of the esophagus is an extremely dismal disease, with most patients dying within several months after diagnosis, regardless of the form of therapy. Palliation is the most reasonable goal of the therapy, whether it be radiation therapy or operation. Radiation therapy, although controversial, is effective in relieving the obstruction in many high-risk patients. Resective or palliative bypass appears to be the most common and often the simplest form of therapy, allowing the patient to leave the hospital rapidly and resume an acceptable life-style.

HIATAL HERNIAS AND REFLUX ESOPHAGITIS

A hiatal hernia is a condition in which a portion or all of the stomach extends into the mediastinum through the esophageal hiatus of the diaphragm. It can be identified by radiographic (see Fig. 22-4), manometric, or endoscopic means. There is still controversy as to whether the radiographic demonstration of a Schatzki's ring is indicative of a hiatal hernia in all instances. We do not believe so, since it can be commonly demonstrated on routine barium gastrointestinal series in patients without symptoms of esoph-

agogastric disease. There is also confusion as to whether a hiatal hernia is truly a disease.

Two types of hiatal hernias can be distinguished by barium meal (Fig. 22-16). Type I is the more common and is identified by the direct passage of the cardia of the stomach through the esophageal hiatus. In this so-called direct or sliding hernia, the esophagogastric junction moves cephalad into the mediastinum as a unit. A type II hiatal hernia is shown in Figure 22-4. In this abnormality, the esophagogastric junction remains within the abdomen and the cardia and occasionally the entire body of the stomach rolls into the mediastinum between the tethered fibers of the right crus of the diaphragm. The definition of a type I or type II hiatal hernia is more than semantic, since each has its peculiar characteristics. For example, a type I hernia may be associated with reflux esophagitis, while a type II hernia rarely is so affected. The latter, however, may undergo torsion and infarction, while the type I almost never does so. There are two other types of diaphragmatic hernias that will be discussed below, one congenital and the other traumatic. The congenital diaphragmatic hernia will be discussed in the section on anatomical considerations, since it occurs through defects at points of fusion of the diaphragm.

Intra-abdominal viscera may also herniate through areas of mechanical disruption of the diaphragm by blunt or sharp injury. Such lesions are termed *traumatic hernias* and are to be distinguished from hiatal hernias since they may involve the stomach as well as other viscera and do not occur through the esophageal hiatus.

Anatomic Considerations

The intrathoracic and intra-abdominal viscera are maintained within their respective cavities by the diaphragm, a fibromuscular septum that derives from the primordial

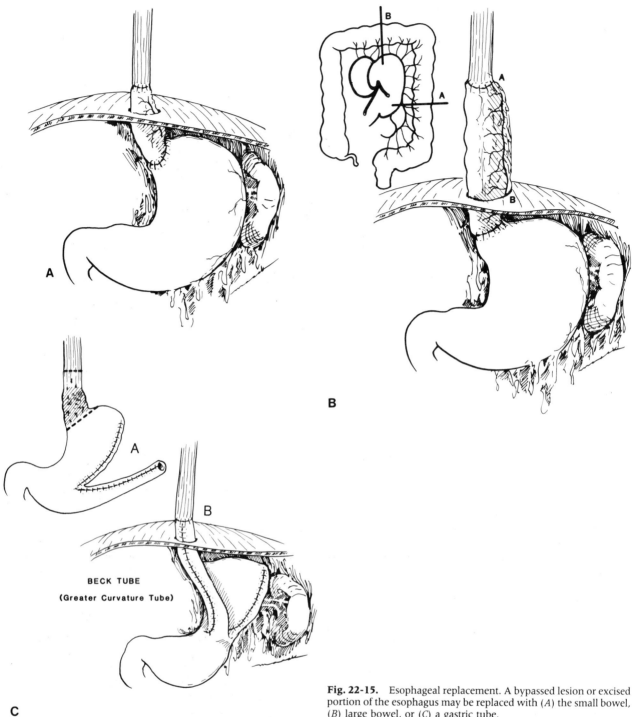

Fig. 22-15.   Esophageal replacement. A bypassed lesion or excised portion of the esophagus may be replaced with (*A*) the small bowel, (*B*) large bowel, or (*C*) a gastric tube.

septum transversum. The abdominal and thoracic cavities as well as the mediastinum are delineated by the eighth week of gestation as the septum transversum fuses with the pleuropericardial and pleuroperitoneal membranes. Congenital hernias occur at points where various components of the diaphragm fail to fuse to each other or the body wall (Fig. 22-17). A Bochdalek hernia occurs through the posterior pleuroperitoneal canal that fails to obliterate during gestation. This is to be distinguished from an anterior diaphragmatic hernia through the foramen of Morgagni, which occurs at a point of malfusion of the diaphragm between the sternal and costal margins.

Hiatal hernias occur through the esophageal hiatus, which is circumscribed by the fibers of the right crus. It is not known whether the enlargement of the esophageal hiatus that accompanies large hiatal hernias is secondary to chronic protrusion of the stomach into the mediastinum or is primary in the genesis of the lesion. The phrenoesophageal ligament or membrane is an important structure in this regard, since it is attenuated in both types of hiatal hernias and is thought by some to be a factor in their genesis. The phrenoesophageal membrane represents a fusion of the mediastinal and diaphragmatic pleura with the peritoneum and transversalis fascia as it straddles the esophagogastric

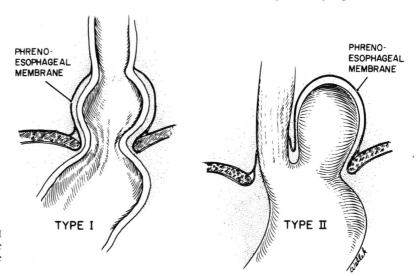

Fig. 22-16. Schematic of type I and type II hernias. The two major types of hiatal hernia are the type I, sliding, or axial hernia (*left*), and the type II, rolling, or paraesophageal hernia (*right*).

junction. This membrane is usually quite well developed posteriorly, thereby providing a tether for the abdominal esophagus to the base of the right crus at the level of the first lumbar vertebra. The ligament has an anterior and posterior leaf that attaches, respectively, a few centimeters above and below the mucosal junction of the esophagogastric junction. It envelops a prominent pad of fat whose purpose has not yet been elucidated. This arrangement allows for a remarkable vertical movement of the esophagogastric junction and thereby may provide protection to this area during forceful emesis or rapid increases in intra-abdominal pressure. There is no evidence that the phreno-esophageal ligament plays a primary role in the function of the LES, except that in type I hiatal hernia it provides for transmission of intra-abdominal pressure into the mediastinum as a consequence of the hernia sac that develops as the esophagogastric junction moves caudad.

Type I Hiatal Hernia (Sliding or Direct)
Pathophysiologic Basis for Symptoms. As described above, a type I hiatal hernia is one in which the esophagogastric junction has passed caudad through the esophageal hiatus. This event can be demonstrated in 90% of individuals on

Fig. 22-17. Congenital points of herniation: (*A*) esophageal hiatus, (*B*) posterolateral Bochdalek's defect, (*C*) mid-diaphragmatic-pericardial Bochdalek's defect, (*D*) retrosternal foramen of Morgagni.

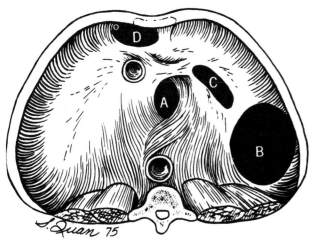

the barium esophagogram during maneuvers that increase intra-abdominal pressure. It therefore must be considered a normal finding. Symptoms, however, may arise when a large portion of the stomach resides within the mediastinum, or when the LES pressures are low, allowing reflux of gastric contents into the esophagus. There is now ample evidence to show that the majority of patients with hiatal hernia have normal LES pressures, even when large portions of the stomach pass into the mediastinum. On the contrary, the majority of patients with reflux esophagitis usually have a moderate to large size type I hernia. Furthermore, episodes of reflux are less frequent in patients with long abdominal esophageal segments. Even gastric tubes or intestinal substitutes for the lower esophagus require an intra-abdominal segment of greater than 3 cm if reflux is to be prevented.

Intra-abdominal pressure apparently helps to supplement the intrinsic barrier of the LES during periods of increased intragastric pressure. On the other hand, the LES remains competent even when in the mediastinum in many patients with type I hernias. This suggests that the intra-abdominal position is not critical when LES pressures are normal. When LES pressures are low, however, a return to the intra-abdominal position is a desirable goal and a rationale for all current methods of surgical treatment of reflux esophagitis.

Esophagitis is a major consequence of esophagogastric reflux. Curiously, not all patients with esophagitis have symptoms. Most, however, complain of "heartburn," a burning discomfort behind the sternum. Endoscopic visualization of the esophagus at this stage may reveal a normal-appearing mucosa or mild erythema. Long-standing heartburn usually is associated with an advanced form of erosive esophagitis, characterized by ulcerations, exudates, and a friable, hemorrhagic mucosa. Deep ulcerations are usually associated with persistent severe pain that is aggravated by eating. Fibrosis and stricture are the final stage of uncontrolled chronic acid-peptic esophagitis. Some patients, especially in the older age-group, will present with dysphagia as a consequence of stricture without ever having experienced heartburn. It is also surprising to see patients with severe untreated heartburn for many years with normal barium roentgenograms and only mild mucosal inflammation. Patients with heartburn and mild esophagitis may complain of dysphagia and yet the esophagus appears normal on the barium esophagogram. These patients should have esophageal manometry, since they may harbor an underlying primary motility disorder. It is known, however, that patients with esophagitis have disturbed esophageal motor function that interferes with secondary contractions responsible for stripping the esophagus of regurgitated material. Possibly this minor motility disturbance is responsible for the esophagitis that occurs in patients with low LES pressures.

Regurgitation of gastric contents is a frank sign of free reflux and usually occurs when a patient is supine or bends over. Aspiration pneumonitis can be a subtle consequence of nocturnal regurgitation and is a definite hazard for the older patient whose pulmonary function may be already compromised by years of reflux and tracheobronchial aspiration.

Esophagitis may also be a source of gastrointestinal bleeding; usually this is slow and associated with a low-grade anemia. Patients with portal hypertension, however, may present with massive hematemesis as a consequence of erosion into the submucosal varix. Bleeding may also occur from ulcerations within the upper part of the stomach that is trapped within the hernia complex. It is otherwise rare for there to be symptoms from the portion of the stomach that lies between the LES above and the esophageal crus below. Possibly some of the nonspecific symptoms presented by patients with hiatal hernias, without demonstrable esophagitis, are on this basis.

Management of Reflux Esophagitis. The initial therapy of esophagitis is directed toward the reduction of esophagogastric reflux. It is presumed that acid-peptic digestion plays a primary role in the symptoms of esophagitis, since antacid therapy either by ingestion of buffer or by acid secretory inhibition by cimetidine leads to relief of heartburn. Coffee and alcohol should be eliminated from the diet, and an effort toward abstinence from tobacco should be encouraged. Nocturnal reflux can be reduced by elevating the head of the bed on "building blocks," which usually are eight inches in height. Patients are advised to eat small meals (usually six) frequently during the day and to avoid a large meal in the evening or a snack before retiring. Trials are currently underway to establish the efficacy of metoclopramide and cholinomimetic agents that are known to increase pressures within the LES. It is likely that drugs that increase the barrier function of the LES will be important adjuncts to

medical therapy in the future. Weight reduction is also an important component of medical therapy. Obese patients with reflux esophagitis should be placed on a 1200-calorie, carefully supervised diet. Unfortunately, compliance is difficult to obtain over the length of time required to gain significant weight reduction.

The usual indication for surgical therapy is failure of medical therapy. Most patients with reflux esophagitis will respond to medical therapy; only a few require an operation. Unfortunately, these cannot be easily identified. Patients who present with advanced esophagitis and peptic ulcer disease of the duodenum almost always require surgical therapy directed toward both diseases. In addition, reflux esophagitis with stricture should be managed by an early operation. Patients with a Barrett's esophagitis usually fall into this category.

It is important for the surgeon to establish that a patient's symptoms are from reflux esophagitis. All surgical candidates therefore should have endoscopy and biopsy if the esophagitis is not grossly obvious. In addition, the surgeon should establish that the patient has had a proper course of medical management. Success of surgical therapy depends critically on proper selection of the patient as well as the operation.

Operations for reflux esophagitis are appropriately called antireflux procedures. Three operations remain popular after many years of usage: (1) Nissen fundoplication, (2) Hill posterior gastropexy, and (3) Belsey Mark IV repair. Each of these operations prevents reflux by wrapping all or a portion of the cardia around the lower end of the esophagus and attempting to return and contain the lower end of the esophagus within the abdominal cavity. Details of the three operations are shown in Figure 22-18. The Hill and Nissen operations can be accomplished through the abdomen, thereby providing for the opportunity to attend to other problems such as gallstones or pyloric obstruction. The Belsey operation can only be performed through the chest, but a Nissen fundoplication can be performed by either route. The thoracic route is desirable when a peptic stricture is present, since it offers an opportunity to gain full mobilization of the lower esophagus. Failure to fully mobilize the esophagus could lead to a wrap of the stomach around itself with no relief of the esophagitis.

The results of the three operations are comparable, with possibly a small advantage accruing to the Nissen fundoplication as regards relief of heartburn. Naturally, there are vocal advocates of each procedure. The issue, however, is selection of the procedure that can best be performed by the surgeon and tolerated by the patient. Possibly in the future the partial Nissen fundoplication and posterior anchoring of the esophagogastric junction as currently advocated by Hill will become the standard abdominal procedure and the Belsey operation (with further refinements to decrease the 5% to 15% recurrence rate) the preferred transthoracic approach. The recurrence rate for each procedure appears to be in the range of 10% over a 5-year follow-up, with increments of about 2% per year thereafter. The Nissen fundoplication must be done loosely if a peculiar syndrome called "gas-bloat" is to be avoided. Some patients after this procedure cannot belch. In addition, they develop aerophagia and progressive distention of their stomach and small intestine. A loose wrap tends to minimize this distressing complication, which is associated with crampy abdominal pain and numerous nonspecific complaints from the patient.

Newer surgical approaches are directed toward increasing

GASTROESOPHAGEAL REFLUX	
Etiology	Decreased LES pressure
	Hiatal hernia (type I)
	Esophagitis secondary to acid reflux
	Complications: Ulcer, bleeding, stricture
Dx	Heartburn, regurgitation, aspiration
	Substernal pain, G-I bleeding
	Upper G-I radiograms
	Esophagoscopy, biopsy for carcinoma
	Manometric and acid reflux studies
Rx	Antacids, cimetidine
	Weight reduction
	Six small meals—pre-bedtime fast
	Surgery (antireflux procedure) for complications or intractability (Nissen, Hill, Belsey)

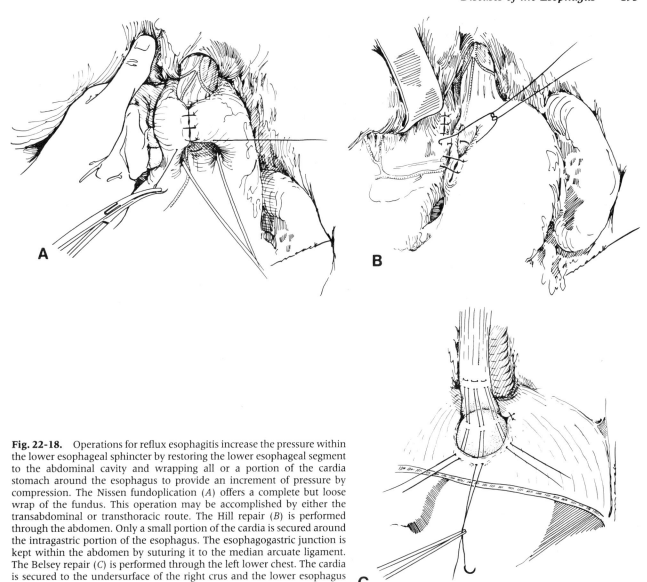

Fig. 22-18. Operations for reflux esophagitis increase the pressure within the lower esophageal sphincter by restoring the lower esophageal segment to the abdominal cavity and wrapping all or a portion of the cardia stomach around the esophagus to provide an increment of pressure by compression. The Nissen fundoplication (*A*) offers a complete but loose wrap of the fundus. This operation may be accomplished by either the transabdominal or transthoracic route. The Hill repair (*B*) is performed through the abdomen. Only a small portion of the cardia is secured around the intragastric portion of the esophagus. The esophagogastric junction is kept within the abdomen by suturing it to the median arcuate ligament. The Belsey repair (*C*) is performed through the left lower chest. The cardia is secured to the undersurface of the right crus and the lower esophagus for two thirds of its circumference.

the barrier function of the LES by placing prosthetic and biologic materials around it. This approach is so new that its efficacy has not as yet been established. The antireflux procedures currently in use as described above are relatively safe and effective and will provide a standard against which the newer approaches must be evaluated by controlled trials.

Management of Peptic Strictures. Strictures associated with reflux esophagitis require dilatation for relief of dysphagia and aggressive antacid therapy if recurrence is to be prevented. Medical therapy of strictures usually fails, and for this reason an antireflux operation should be performed after the peptic nature of the stricture has been ascertained. Short strictures low in the esophagus can be managed by the transabdominal route. In this operation, the strictured esophagus is fully mobilized from the mediastinum and the stricture is dilated by the passage of soft mercury-weighted rubber dilators (Maloney) from above, with the operator's hand around the stricture to monitor the passage of the dilator. It is not necessary to gain full dilatation at this point. Passage of a 38-F or 40-F dilator is usually sufficient. Overdilatation may lead to injury and subsequent further

fibrosis with repair. It is best to delay full dilatation to a time when the esophagitis subsides following the performance of an antireflux procedure of the Hill or Nissen type. Long strictures are best approached through the left chest, with mobilization of the esophagus and dilatations of the esophagus as described above. Reflux in this approach is controlled by either the Nissen or Belsey operation. Strictures with marked shortening of the esophagus can be managed by developing a gastric tube of the upper end of the stomach. This is accomplished by vertical stapling and division of the upper stomach along the left side of the esophagus from the angle of His. This operation, called a Collis gastroplasty, is completed by wrapping the fundus of the stomach around the newly constructed gastric tube, thereby providing a high pressure zone within the intra-abdominal portion of the neoesophagus. Advanced strictures that fail to dilate are best treated by a modification of the Thal procedure as described by Woodward. In this operation, the stricture is divided, and the opening is closed by the advancement of the anterior surface of the stomach that is covered with a split-thickness skin graft. The operation is completed by a

Nissen fundoplication in order to control reflux. Replacement of the lower esophagus by a segment of small or large intestine offers a satisfactory but more complex alternative to the problem. Advanced strictures of this type are difficult to manage, and surgical results with even aggressive therapy are not optimum. It is for this reason that reflux esophagitis should be identified and treated vigorously at an early stage. An antireflux operation should be used promptly when medical therapy fails.

Management of Barrett's Esophagitis. Barrett's esophagitis represents a rare but important form of the disease in which the squamous epithelial lining of the lower esophagus is replaced by columnar epithelium. There continues to be some debate as to whether this disease is inherited or acquired. It is generally agreed that the columnar lined esophagus has a high potential for malignant change, and for this reason the epithelial lining of the esophagus of patients with Barrett's epithelium must be carefully monitored by endoscopy and biopsy. While initial therapy is medical and directed toward control of the esophagitis by antacids, most patients progress to ulcerative esophagitis and stricture unless an antireflux procedure is performed. Control of reflux will allow the lower esophagus to be relined by squamous epithelium. In addition, the symptoms of reflux subside and strictures resolve. Therefore, patients with Barrett's esophagitis should undergo an antireflux procedure when the disease is identified. It is not yet known whether control of the reflux esophagitis will decrease the malignant potential of the disease, but the observation that the metaplastic change is reversed suggests that such may be the case.

Surgical Management of Type II Hernia (Paraesophageal)

The esophageal junction of patients with type II hernia resides within the abdomen and the LES is usually normal. Patients with this abnormality rarely complain of heartburn or have evidence of esophagitis. They present with three problems, all related to anatomical distortions associated with having a portion or all of the stomach within the chest. First, they may have duodenal ulcer disease as a consequence of the antrum lying above the fundus of the "upside down" stomach, thereby losing the normal negative feedback of acid control. This is an unusual but serious complication, expecially if perforation of a duodenal ulcer should occur high in the upper abdomen or mediastinum. A second and more frequent complication is associated with trapping of food or air within the herniated stomach. This may lead to severe pain in the lower chest or upper abdomen, vomiting, and stasis ulceration within the lining of the stomach. The most serious complication, and one that has led to the idea that all type II hernias require surgical repair, is gastric infarction due to torsion and compromise of the blood supply to the stomach.

The surgical repair of a type II hernia consists of returning the stomach to the abdominal cavity and closure of the rent within the esophageal hiatus. Occasionally the operation is difficult because of adhesions between the gastric wall, the hernia sac, and the mediastinal pleura. The opening into the mediastinum is large and lax, and therefore it is always possible to accomplish the reduction and repair by the transabdominal route. Steps in the procedure are shown in Figure 22-18. In cases where there is established reflux esophagitis (*i.e.*, a so-called mixed hernia) an antireflux

procedure is added to the operation. Associated duodenal or gastric ulcer disease is treated by a highly selective vagotomy.

Congenital Hernias

Congenital herniation through the posterolateral foramen (Bochdalek hernia) usually manifests itself at birth as respiratory distress. This is a consequence of failure of the lung to develop within the involved hemithorax. Furthermore, function of the opposite lung is compromised by compression from the mediastinum created by the herniated intra-abdominal viscera. The diaphragmatic defect usually is on the left side, since the right side of the diaphragm is shared by the bulk of the liver. Therapy is directed toward respiratory support and correction of the severe respiratory acidosis, which is often present. Surgical repair consists of reduction of herniated viscera (which may include stomach, large and small intestine, liver, spleen, or a kidney), and suture of the opening in the diaphragm. Adhesive bands that accompany the associated malrotation are divided. The fascial layers of the abdomen are frequently left unapproximated in order to allow room for replacement of intra-abdominal viscera. In this case, only the skin of the abdomen is closed, thus creating a large ventral hernia.

Anterior diaphragmatic hernias (Morgagni), also of congenital origin, often do not become manifest until adulthood. These openings behind the sternoxiphoid are small and only become symptomatic when a loop of transverse colon chances to find its way into a well-defined sac in the area. Most herniations of this type occur on the right side (90%). Patients may complain of intermittent episodes of large bowel obstruction. Diagnosis can be made on a chest roentgenogram and confirmed by a barium enema. Treatment is surgical and consists of reducing the herniated viscus, excising the sac, and closing the vent in the diaphragm.

Traumatic Hernia

Traumatic rupture of the diaphragm with herniation of the gastrointestinal tract may follow blunt or penetrating injury. The latter is most frequently the result of a stab wound to the abdomen or chest, a shotgun blast at close range, or another high-velocity gunshot wound, all of which may cause an extensive laceration of the diaphragm. Penetrating disruptions are usually on the left side, since most assailants with a knife are right-handed and are aiming for the heart. Blunt disruptions are also on the left and usually posterior. It is possible that right-sided injuries are equally common, but evisceration of abdominal contents into the right hemithorax is prevented by the liver. Traumatic herniation often goes unrecognized unless the patient is carefully evaluated or is operated on at the time of injury. Over half of the traumatic diaphragmatic hernias are recognized at a time remote from the causative trauma and in many instances are merely an incidental finding on a chest film. The remaining traumatic hernias are shown roentgenographically at the time of injury or during abdominal or thoracic exploration for associated problems. Treatment consists of surgical repair of the diaphragm after return of the herniated viscera and attention to associated injuries. Chronic herniation should also be treated surgically, even when it is asymptomatic, since pulmonary function is compromised by the contents of the hernia, and obstruction within the intrathoracic intestine could be a lethal event.

BIBLIOGRAPHY

ANGELCHIK JP, COHEN R: A new surgical procedure for the treatment of gastroesophageal reflux and hiatal hernia. Surg Gynecol Obstet 143:246, 1979

APPELQVIST P, SALMO M: Lye corrosion carcinoma of the esophagus: A review of 63 cases. Cancer 45:2655, 1980

APPELQVIST P, SILVO J, RISSANEN P: The results of surgery and radiotherapy in the treatment of small carcinomas of the thoracic oesophagus. Ann Clin Res 11:184, 1979

BEHAR J, SHEAHAN DG, BIANCANI P et al: Medical and surgical management of reflux esophagitis: A 38-month report of a prospective clinical trial. N Engl J Med 293:263, 1975

BELSEY RH: Gastroesophageal reflux. Am J Surg 139:775, 1980

BENJAMIN SB, GERHARDT DC, CASTELL DO: High amplitude, peristaltic esophageal contractions associated with chest pain and/or dysphagia. Gastroenterology 77:478, 1979

BERNSTEIN JM, JULER GL: Colon interposition versus esophagogastrostomy for esophageal carcinoma. Am Surg 46:216, 1980

BORTOLOTTI M, LABO G: Clinical and manometric effects of nifedipine in patients with esophageal achalasia. Gastroenterology 80:39, 1981

BOSCH A, FRIAS Z, CALDWELL WL: Adenocarcinoma of the esophagus. Cancer 43:1557, 1979

BREWER LA III: History of surgery of the esophagus. Am J Surg 139:730, 1980

BRUGGEMAN LL, SEMAN WB: Epiphrenic diverticula: An analysis of 80 cases. Am J Roentgenol 119:266, 1973

BURRINGTON JD, RAFFENSPERGER JG: Surgical management of tracheoesophageal fistula complicating caustic ingestion. Surgery 84:329, 1978

CAMPBELL GS, BURNETT HF, RANSOM JM et al: Treatment of corrosive burns of the esophagus. Arch Surg 112:495, 1977

CSENDES A, VELASCO N, BRAGHETTO I et al: A prospective randomized study comparing forceful dilatation and esophagomyotomy in patients with achalasia of the esophagus. Gastroenterology 80:789, 1981

CURCI JJ, HORMAN MJ: Boerhaave's syndrome: The importance of early diagnosis and treatment. Ann Surg 183:401, 1976

DEMEESTER TR, WANG CI, WERNLY JA et al: Technique, indications, and clinical use of 24-hour esophageal pH monitoring. J Thorac Cardiovasc Surg 79:656, 1980

ECKARDT VF, ADAMI B, HUCKER H et al: The esophagogastric junction in patients with asymptomatic lower esophageal mucosal rings. Gastroenterology 79:426, 1980

EIN SH, SHANDLING B, SIMPSON JS et al: Fourteen years of gastric tubes. J Pediatr Surg 13:638, 1978

ELLIS FH JR: Pharyngo-esophageal diverticula and cricopharyngeal incoordination. Mod Treat 7:1098, 1970

ELLIS FH JR: Esophagogastrectomy for carcinoma: Technical considerations based on anatomic location of lesion. Surg Clin North Am 60:265, 1980

ELLIS FH JR, GIBB SP: Reoperation after esophagomyotomy for achalasia of the esophagus. Am J Surg 129:407, 1975

ELLIS FH JR, GIBB SP: Esophagogastrectomy for carcinoma: Current hospital mortality and morbidity rates. Ann Surg 190:699, 1979

ELLIS FH JR, GIBB SP, CROZIER RE: Esophagomyotomy for achalasia of the esophagus. Ann Surg 192:157, 1980

EVANGELIST FA, TAYLOR FH, ALFORD JD: The modified Collis-Nissen operation for control of gastroesophageal reflux. Ann Thorac Surg 26:107, 1979

EZDINLI EZ, GELBER R, DESAI DV et al: Chemotherapy of advanced esophageal carcinoma: Eastern Cooperative Oncology Group experience. Cancer 46:2149, 1980

FELDMAN M, IBEN AB, HURLEY EJ: Corrosive injury to oro-pharynx and esophagus. Eighty-five consecutive cases. Calif Med 118:6, 1973

FERGUSON R, DRONFIELD MW, ATKINSON M: Cimetidine in treatment of reflux oesophagitis with peptic stricture. Br Med J 2:472, 1979

GATZINSKY P, BERGH NP, LOF BA: Hiatal hernia complicated by oesophageal stricture: Surgical treatment and results: A follow-up study. Acta Chir Scand 145:149, 1979

GIULI R, GIGNOUX M: Treatment of carcinoma of the esophagus. Retrospective study of 2,400 patients. Ann Surg 192:44, 1980

GRIFFITH JL, DAVID JT: A twenty-year experience with surgical management of carcinoma of the esophagus and gastric cardia. J Thorac Cardiovasc Surg 79:447, 1980

HANSEN JB, JAGT T, GUNDTOFT P et al: Pharyngo-oesophageal diverticula—a clinical and cineradiographic follow-up study of 23 cases treated by diverticulectomy. Scand J Thorac Cardiovasc Surg 7:81, 1973

HAWKINS DB, DEMETER MJ, BARNETT TE: Caustic ingestion: Controversies in management: A review of 214 cases. Laryngoscope 90:98, 1980

HENDERSON RD: Nissen hiatal hernia repair: Problems of recurrence and continued symptoms. Ann Thorac Surg 28:587, 1979

HENDERSON RD, PEARSON FG: Preoperative assessment of esophageal pathology. J Thorac Cardiovasc Surg 72:512, 1976

HICKS LM, MANSFIELD PB: Esophageal atresia and tracheoesophageal fistula: Review of thirteen years' experience. J Thorac Cardiovasc Surg 81:358, 1981

HIEBERT CA, O'MARA CS: The Belsey operation for hiatal hernia: A twenty-year experience. Am J Surg 137:532, 1979

HILL LD: Intraoperative measurement of lower esophageal sphincter pressure. J Thorac Cardiovasc Surg 75:378, 1978

HO CS, RODRIGUES PR: Lower esophageal strictures, benign or malignant. J Can Assoc Radiol 31:110, 1980

HUBBARD SG, TODD EP, DILLON ML et al: Palliation for esophageal carcinoma. Ann Thorac Surg 29:551, 1980

JALUNDHWALA JM, SHAH RC: Epiphrenic esophageal diverticulum. Chest 57:97, 1970

JARA FM, TOLEDO-PEREYA LH, LEWIS JW et al: Long-term results of esophagomyotomy for achalasia of esophagus. Arch Surg 114:935, 1979

JOHNSON DG, HERBST JJ, OLIVEROS MA et al: Evaluation of gastroesophageal reflux surgery in children. Pediatrics 59:62, 1977

JORDAN PH JR: Parietal cell vagotomy facilitates fundoplication in the treatment of reflux esophagitis. Surg Gynecol Obstet 147:593, 1978

KASAI M, MORI S, WATANABE T: Follow-up results after resection of thoracic esophageal carcinoma. World J Surg 2:543, 1978

KIRSH MM, PETERSON A, BROWN JW et al: Treatment of caustic injuries of the esophagus: A ten-year experience. Ann Surg 188:675, 1978

KIRSH MM, RITTER F: Caustic ingestion and subsequent damage to the oropharyngeal and digestive passages. Ann Thorac Surg 21:74, 1976

KOOP CE, SCHNAUFER L, BROENNIE AM: Esophageal atresia and tracheoesophageal fistula: Supportive measures that affect survival. Pediatrics 54:558, 1974

LANDING BH: Syndromes of congenital heart disease with tracheobronchial anomalies. Am J Roentgenol 123:679, 1975

LANZA FL, GRAHAM DY: Bougienage is effective therapy for most benign esophageal strictures. JAMA 249:844, 1978

LEONARDI HK, SHEA JA, CROZIER RE et al: Diffuse spasm of the esophagus. Clinical, manometric, and surgical considerations. J Thorac Cardiovasc Surg 74:736, 1977

LICHTER I: Motor disorder in pharyngoesophageal pouch. J Thorac Cardiovasc Surg 76:272, 1978

LITTLE AG, DEMEESTER TR, KIRCHNER PT et al: Pathogenesis of esophagitis in patients with gastroesophageal reflux. Surgery 88:101, 1980

LONDON RL, TROTMAN BW, DIMARINO AJ JR et al: Dilatation of severe esophageal strictures by an inflatable balloon catheter. Gastroenterology 80:173, 1981

MANNELL A, PLANT M: Total oesophagectomy in black patients with cancer of the oesophagus. S Afr Med J 58:285, 1980

MAULL KI, SCHER LA, GREENFIELD LJ: Surgical implications of acid ingestion. Surg Gynecol Obstet 148:895, 1979

MESSIAN RA, HERMOS JA, ROBBINS AH et al: Barrett's esophagus: Clinical review of 26 cases. Am J Gastroenterol 69:458, 1978

MOLINA JE, LAWTON BR, AVANCE D: Use of circumferential stapler in reconstruction following resections for carcinoma of the cardia. Ann Thorac Surg 31:325, 1981

NAEF AP, SAVARY M, OZZELLO L: Columnar-lined lower esophagus: An acquired lesion with malignant predisposition: Report on 140 cases of Barrett's esophagus with 12 adenocarcinomas. J Thorac Cardiovasc Surg 70:826, 1975

OKIKE N, PAYNE WS, NEUFIELD DM et al: Esophagomyotomy versus forceful dilation for achalasia of the esophagus: Results in 899 patients. Ann Thorac Surg 28:119, 1979

ONG GB, LAM KH, LAM PH et al: Resection for carcinoma of the superior mediastinal segment of the esophagus. World J Surg 2:497, 1978

OTTINGER LW, WILKINS EW JR: Late results in patients with Schatzki rings undergoing destruction of the ring and hiatus herniorrhaphy. Am J Surg 139:591, 1980

PATTON AS, LAWSON DW, SHANNON JM et al: Reevaluation of the Boerhaave syndrome: A review of 14 cases. Am J Surg 137:560, 1979

PEARSON FG, HENDERSON RD: Long-term follow-up of peptic strictures managed by dilatation, modified Collis gastroplasty, and Belsey hiatus hernia repair. Surgery 80:396, 1976

PETTERSSON GB, BOMBECK CT, NYHUS LM: Influence of hiatal hernia on lower esophageal sphincter function. Ann Surg 193:214, 1981

POLK HC JR: Fundoplication for reflux esophagitis: Misadventures with the operation of choice. Ann Surg 183: 645, 1976

POLK HC JR: Indications for, technique of, and results of fundoplication for complicated reflux esophagitis. Am Surg 44:620, 1978

POPOVSKY J: Esophagogastrostomy in continuity for carcinoma of the esophagus: Its use for unresectable tumors of the lower third of the esophagus and cardia. Arch Surg 115:637, 1980

POSTLETHWAIT RW: Surgery of the Esophagus. New York, Appleton-Century-Crofts, 1979

POSTLETHWAIT RW: Technique for isoperistaltic gastric tube for esophageal bypass. Ann Surg 189:673, 1979

RADIGAN LR, GLOVER JL, SHIPLEY FE et al: Barrett esophagus. Arch Surg 112:486, 1977

RAY JF III, MYERS WO, LAWTON BR et al: The natural history of liquid lye ingestion (rationale for aggressive surgical approach). Arch Surg 109:436, 1974

SAUNDERS NR: The celestin tube in the palliation of carcinoma of the oesophagus and cardia. Br J Surg 66:419, 1979

SAWYERS JL, LANE CE, FOSTER JH et al: Esophageal perforation: An increasing challenge. Ann Thorac Surg 19:233, 1975

SIEBER AM, SIEBER WK: Colon transplants as esophageal replacement: Cineradiographic and manometric evaluation in children. Ann Surg 168:116, 1968

SILLIN LF, CONDON RE, WILSON SD et al: Effective surgical therapy of esophagitis: Experience with Belsey, Hill, and Nissen operations. Arch Surg 114:536, 1979

STEIGER Z, FRANKLIN R, WILSON RF et al: Complete eradication of squamous cell carcinoma of the esophagus with combined chemotherapy and radiotherapy. Am Surg 47:95, 1981

SYMBAS PN, HATCHER CR JR, HARLAFTIS N: Spontaneous rupture of the esophagus. Ann Surg 187:634, 1978

URSCHEL HC JR, RAZZUK MA: Collis-Belsey: Fundoplication for uncomplicated hiatal hernia and gastroesophageal reflux. Ann Thorac Surg 27:564, 1979

URSCHEL HC JR, RAZZUK MA, WOOD RE et al: Improved management of esophageal perforation: Exclusion and diversion in continuity. Ann Surg 179:587, 1974.

VANTRAPPEN G, JANSSENS J, HELLEMANS J et al: Achalasia, diffuse esophageal spasm, and related motility disorders. Gastroenterology 76:450, 1979

WATERSTON D: Colonic replacement of esophagus (intrathoracic). Surg Clin North Am 44:1441, 1964

WEBB WR, KOUTRAS P, ECKER RR et al: An evaluation of steroids and antibiotics in caustic burns of the esophagus. Ann Thorac Surg 9:95, 1970

WELCH RW, LUCKMANN K, RICKS P et al: Lower esophageal sphincter pressure in histologic esophagitis. Dig Dis Sci 25:420, 1980

WELSH GF, PAYNE WS: The present status of one-stage pharyngoesophageal diverticulectomy. Surg Clin North Am 53:953, 1973

WESDORP E, BARTELSMAN J, PAPE K et al: Oral cimetidine in reflux esophagitis: A double-blind controlled trial. Gastroenterology 74:821, 1978

WICHERN WA JR: Perforation of the esophagus. Am J Surg 119:534, 1970

WILSON RF, SARVER EJ, ARBULU A et al: Spontaneous perforation of the esophagus. Ann Thorac Surg 12:291, 1971

WOLLOCH Y, DINTSMAN M: Iatrogenic perforations of the esophagus: Therapeutic considerations. Arch Surg 108:357, 1974

WOODWARD ER: Surgical treatment of gastroesophageal reflux and its complications. World J Surg 1:453, 1977

WU YK, CHEN PT, FANG JP et al: Surgical treatment of esophageal carcinoma. Am J Surg 139:805, 1980

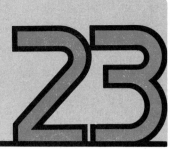
The stomach, lying transversely in the upper abdomen, is an expansile organ whose major function is to provide a receptacle for ingested food and fluids. While food is in the stomach, preparation for its digestion is initiated by the chemical action of acid and pepsin and by the mechanical grinding action of the antrum. When the gastric chyme develops the proper consistency, it is metered in small aliquots through the pylorus into the duodenum. Here the chyme is further mixed by the to-and-fro motor activity of the duodenum with the digestive juices of the pancreas and liver before being moved along into the intestine by peristalsis.

ANATOMY

The following is not an exhaustive discussion of the anatomy of the stomach but is intended to describe some aspects of surgical significance. For a more detailed discussion of gastric anatomy the reader is referred to the text by Griffith.

The different parts of the stomach have been variously named by anatomists, histologists, and physiologists. In this chapter, the proximal two thirds of the stomach, which has a thin muscular wall and a mucosal lining that is characterized grossly by longitudinal folds, will be called the *fundic gland area* of the stomach. The *pyloric gland area* denotes the distal one third of the stomach, which is characterized by a thick muscular wall and an absence of mucosal folds (Fig. 23-1). The duodenum, separated from the stomach by the muscular pyloric sphincter, consists of four portions, although there are no sharp lines of demarcation between the different parts. The first portion extends from the pyloric sphincter to the apex of the duodenal bulb and is also devoid of mucosal folds. It is characterized microscopically by submucosal Brunner's glands that secrete a clear viscous alkaline material (*p*H 8–9). Throughout the remainder of the duodenum the mucosal folds are circular. The second portion or the descending limb of the duodenum contains the ampulla of Vater, into which the common bile duct and pancreatic duct empty. The third or the transverse portion of the duodenum lies anterior to the spine and is crossed on its ventral surface by the superior mesenteric artery and vein. This is the most common portion of the duodenum ruptured by blunt trauma. The fourth portion of the duodenum is the ascending limb. It ends at the ligament of Treitz, which is also the beginning of the jejunum.

The wall of the stomach is composed of three closely fused *muscular layers,* consisting of the inner oblique muscle fibers that create a sling around the esophagogastric junction, an outer layer of longitudinal muscular fibers, and a middle layer of circular muscle fibers. The oblique fibers are said to contribute to the competency of the esophagogastric junction and aid in the prevention of esophageal reflux. The muscular wall of the fundic gland area is thin compared with the pyloric gland area and has the capacity to distend

in order to accommodate a full meal. The thick wall of the antrum, on the other hand, acts as a triturating organ to begin the digestive process by homogenizing the gastric contents. The pyloric sphincter musculature separates the stomach and duodenum. It is usually evident by palpation, and in some patients, adults as well as infants, it may be so hypertrophic as to require that it be sectioned to prevent gastric outlet obstruction. The duodenum consists of an outer longitudinal and an inner circular muscular coat throughout. This configuration is interrupted only by the sphincter of Oddi which controls the evacuation of the ampulla of Vater.

The *mucosa* of the fundic gland area is convoluted and consists of oxyntic or parietal cells, zymogen or chief cells, and mucus cells, which produce acid and intrinsic factor, pepsin, and mucus, respectively. The acid-stimulating hormone gastrin and mucus are produced by the gastrin (G) cells and mucus cells of the pyloric gland area.

If one looks at the surface of the gastric mucosa in the fundic gland area with the scanning electron microscope, there are folds surrounding gastric pits. The surface of the folds is covered with columnar mucus epithelial cells (Fig. 23-2). These cells extend into the foveola down to the neck area where several gastric glands join together. Parietal cells are most numerous in the midportion of the glands, and chief cells are densest in the deepest portion of the glands. The surface epithelial cells appear to have their origin from undifferentiated cells in the deepest portion of the foveola and neck. These cells migrate to the surface of the pits and

Fig. 23-2. Diagrammatic representation of gastric glands in the fundic gland area of the stomach. These glands are confluent at the neck. Their contents empty into the gastric lumen through the gastric pit.

Fig. 23-1. The stomach is divided on the basis of its physiological functions into two main portions. The proximal two thirds, the fundic gland area, acts as a receptacle for ingested food and secretes acid and pepsin. The distal third, the pyloric gland area, mixes and propels food into the duodenum and produces the hormone gastrin.

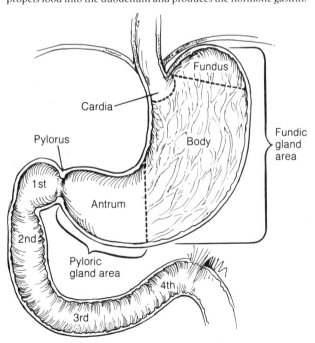

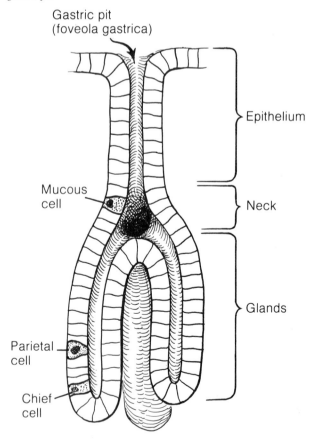

in humans cause a complete renewal of the surface epithelium every 4 to 8 days.

The glands of the pyloric gland area are similar, but the foveola are deeper and the glands are more coiled. The cells in the glands appear similar to those in the Brunner's glands in the duodenum. There are argentaffin and argyrophil endocrine cells as well as gastrin-producing endocrine cells. The duodenum contains specialized endocrine cells that produce a variety of gastrointestinal hormones. These cells decrease progressively in number from the proximal to the distal portion of the duodenum.

The *blood supply* of the stomach is generous (Fig. 23-3). The right gastric artery, a branch of the hepatic artery, and the left gastric artery, a direct branch from the celiac artery, form an arcade along the lesser curvature. On the greater curvature, the right gastroepiploic artery from the gastroduodenal artery and the left gastroepiploic artery, a branch of the splenic artery, form a second arcade that supplies the distal two thirds of the greater curvature. The proximal third of the greater curvature receives its blood supply from the short gastric vessels that come from either the left gastroepiploic or the splenic artery. The most proximal portion of the stomach receives additional blood supply from the esophagus and the inferior phrenic artery. The blood supply of the duodenum is derived primarily from the anterior and posterior pancreaticoduodenal arteries, which arise from the gastroduodenal and superior mesenteric arteries, respectively.

The submucosal blood supply of the stomach is quite rich, but during periods of shock and temporarily following vagotomy blood is shunted from the mucosa to the muscular wall. Because the blood supply of the stomach is so extensive, any one of its four major vessels is capable of maintaining gastric viability. In very high gastric resections in which all four major sources of blood are ligated, there is a risk of necrosis of the small gastric pouch. The blood supply to the duodenum is more critical than that to the stomach. The duodenum cannot be preserved, for example, when performing resection of the head of the pancreas without putting the viability of the duodenum in almost certain

jeopardy. Venous drainage of the stomach and duodenum is primarily through the portal system by way of the short gastric vessels, the gastroepiploic, splenic, and coronary veins. These veins come into great clinical prominence in patients with portal hypertension when blood flow through them is reversed.

The *parasympathetic and sympathetic nerves* contribute a dual innervation of the stomach. The sympathetic innervation provides the route for pain perception. The parasympathetic system by way of the vagi has been more extensively studied with respect to its effect on gastric physiology. The vagus nerves are composed of mainly (90%) afferent fibers and only a few (10%) efferent fibers. The function of the afferent fibers is largely unknown, but they are important in transmitting long vagovagal reflexes from stomach to the stomach and other visceral organs. The efferent fibers of the vagus nerves are related to acid secretion and gastric motility.

The left vagus nerve passes through the esophageal hiatus anterior to the esophagus. It divides into the hepatic branches and those supplying the stomach. The right vagus lies posterior to the esophagus closely adherent to the adventitia surrounding the aorta. It divides into the celiac branch that supplies the small bowel and pancreas. Its other branches supply the posterior wall of the stomach. The main vagal branches to the stomach are the anterior and posterior nerves of Latarjet, which are derived from the anterior and posterior vagal trunks, respectively. They lie along the lesser curvature of the stomach. They give off branches to the fundic gland area and then terminate in the pyloric gland area (Fig. 23-4).

PHYSIOLOGY

PRODUCTION OF HYDROCHLORIC ACID

Gastric juice consists of hydrochloric acid, pepsin, mucus, and intrinsic factor. Acid secretion is formed by parietal cells of which there are approximately 1 billion. Their average maximal secretory rate is 22 mEq of acid per hour in the

Fig. 23-3. The stomach's blood supply is primarily from branches of the celiac artery. The duodenum has a dual blood supply, from branches of the celiac and the superior mesenteric artery.

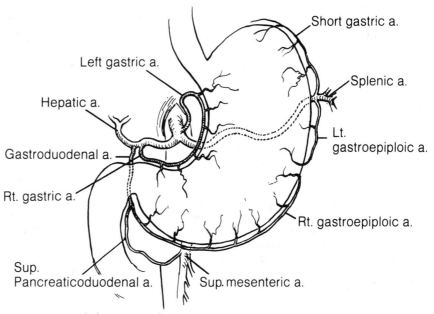

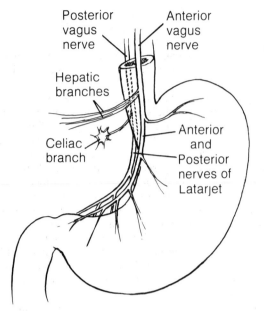

Fig. 23-4. Distribution of the anterior and posterior vagus nerve trunks. In addition to the gastric branches, the anterior vagus gives off the hepatic nerves and the posterior vagus sends branches to the celiac plexus.

adult. For each hydrogen ion secreted, a molecule of CO_2 derived from arterial blood or from mucosal metabolism is converted to bicarbonate and ultimately enters the interstitial fluid. This conversion in the parietal cells is catalyzed by a high concentration of the enzyme carbonic anhydrase. The amount of bicarbonate entering the blood is directly proportional to the amount of acid secreted. It is responsible for the metabolic alkalosis or the "alkaline tide" that results from hypersecretion.

Gastric epithelium also transports bicarbonate into the gastric lumen by a mechanism that is probably under cholinergic control. It has been suggested that the transport of bicarbonate to the gastric lumen protects the mucosa from damage by intraluminal acid. One theory holds that hydrochloric acid and potassium are secreted by the parietal cells and that sodium and bicarbonate are secreted by other than parietal cells. Variations in the composition of gastric juice depend on the proportion of parietal and nonparietal secretion. At low rates of secretion the nonparietal components constitute the major fraction of gastric juice whereas at high rates of secretion the parietal components increase, resulting in higher concentrations of hydrogen, potassium, and chloride. More detailed information regarding the biochemical aspects of acid secretion is available elsewhere.

STIMULATION OF ACID SECRETION

Gastric secretion in humans is primarily under the control of the vagus nerves. This is true for the so-called cephalic phase as well as for the gastric phase of gastric secretion. The gastric phase and the intestinal phases are also under hormonal control. While it has been useful to divide acid secretion into three phases, this is an oversimplification of the physiological process. The interrelationship between these phases of acid secretion was first enunciated by Grossman.

THE CEPHALIC PHASE

The major physiological stimulant to acid secretion in humans is eating. The cephalic phase is mediated by the vagus nerves in response to the sight, taste, and smell of food. If food is eaten but not permitted to enter the stomach (sham feeding), the cephalic phase can be isolated from the effects of the other phases on gastric secretion. The vagal center can also be stimulated by glucopenia. Therefore the cephalic phase can be activated by drugs such as insulin, tolbutamide, and 2-deoxyglucose, which deprive the brain of glucose by decreasing its supply or interfering with its utilization. Vagotomy abolishes or reduces the acid response to insulin. It is assumed that any response of acid secretion to insulin after vagotomy is due to incomplete vagotomy. There is no proof, however, that acid secretion in response to insulin is solely via the vagus nerve.

The cephalic or vagal phase of acid secretion is a neurohumoral mechanism that influences gastric secretion in several ways. First, there is a direct cholinergic stimulation of parietal cells; second, gastrin which stimulates the parietal cells is released from the antrum and duodenal mucosa by vagal stimulation; and third, vagal innervation sensitizes the parietal cells to all stimuli. The peak acid response to sham feeding is about 50% of the maximal response to pentagastrin. Acidification or resection of the antrum and duodenal bulb will reduce the response to sham feeding by about 50%. In humans the normal response to sham feeding is not restored after acidification or resection of the antrum by a threshold dose of gastrin as it is in dogs. The exact mechanism for reduction of the cephalic phase of acid secretion in humans by antrectomy is unclear. In humans the gastrin component of the cephalic phase of gastric secretion is small, the peak serum gastrin level after sham feeding being only 50% of that with a protein meal. In Fordtran's opinion, this contributes unimportantly to the cephalic phase of acid secretion. It appears that in humans direct vagal stimulation of the parietal cells is the most important factor in the cephalic phase of acid secretion, whereas in dogs direct vagal release of gastrin and the maintenance of parietal cell sensitivity are the more important aspects of cephalic stimulation.

THE GASTRIC PHASE

The gastric phase is activated by mechanical distention or chemical stimulation of the fundic and pyloric gland areas. It is mediated both by local release of gastrin and by local cholinergic stimulation of parietal cells. The responses to these stimuli in dogs are somewhat different from those observed in humans. It has not been demonstrated in humans as in dogs that short intramural cholinergic reflexes are responsible for gastrin release. In the normal human, antral distention does not cause an increase in acid secretion, although it does in patients with an active duodenal ulcer. Distention of the fundic gland area causes an increased acid secretion in the normal human and in those with duodenal ulcer. Since acid secretion in response to distention is unaccompanied by an increase in serum gastrin but is abolished by atropine, it is assumed to be mediated by cholinergic, long vagovagal reflexes and short intramural reflexes that stimulate the parietal cells (Fig. 23-5).

The chemicals in food known to stimulate acid secretion when placed in the stomach are primarily the amino acids phenylalanine, tryptophan, and cysteine. The principal mechanism by which these substances stimulate acid secre-

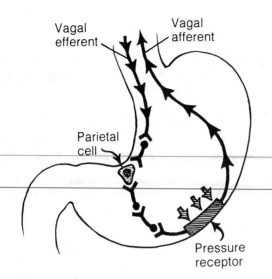

Fig. 23-5. The gastric phase of gastric secretion is in part operative by long and short vagal reflexes that occur in response to gastric distention.

tion is the release of gastrin. Most likely the chemical stimulants for gastrin release in the gastric lumen act directly on the exposed portion of the gastrin cells. Acidification (less than pH 2.5) of the pyloric gland area will block gastrin release in response to these stimuli.

THE INTESTINAL PHASE

Food in the upper small intestine stimulates gastric acid secretion by the release of duodenal gastrin. It is thought that the intestinal phase of acid secretion is also mediated by an unidentified hormone called entero-oxyntin, which is not duodenal gastrin. In humans, portal venous shunts cause an exaggerated intestinal phase, suggesting that the unidentified entero-oxyntin is inactivated by the liver. Absorbed amino acids are thought to account for an appreciable portion of the acid secretion of the intestinal phase. Although the identity of the hormonal agent responsible for the intestinal phase of acid secretion is unknown, it is clear that the mediator is not gastrin even though it is potentiated by gastrin in dogs.

INHIBITION OF GASTRIC SECRETION

Vagal and local release of antral gastrin is pH dependent and is blocked at pH 2.5 or lower with the hydrogen ion exerting its inhibitory effect directly on the gastrin cell. Acid, fat, and hypertonic solutions in the duodenum inhibit acid secretion. Secretin is one of the inhibitors released by acid but other hormones and nervous mechanisms are also likely involved. Inhibition of acid secretion by duodenal bulb acidification requires a duodenal pH of around 4. Cholecystokinin released by fat in the duodenum inhibits gastrin-stimulated secretion, as well as acid secretion in response to all stimuli. Additional peptides, VIP, GIP, somatostatin, and perhaps other hormones released from the upper intestine and pyloric gland area inhibit acid secretion. The physiological significance of VIP and GIP, both structurally related to secretin, is unknown, although the inhibition of acid secretion by GIP is considered pharmacologic. Massive resection of the small bowel sometimes causes hypergastrinemia and hypersecretion. The mechanism is unknown, but

it is thought to be related to the removal of intestinal humoral factors that suppress antral gastrin release or in some other way inhibit acid secretion.

Failure of the inhibitory mechanisms to function properly may contribute to duodenal ulcer in humans. Studies have indicated that acid inhibition of gastrin release from the pyloric gland area is less in duodenal ulcer patients than in nonulcer patients. It has also been demonstrated that parietal cell sensitivity to gastrin is higher in duodenal ulcer patients than in normals. The increased sensitivity is possibly due to increased vagal tone, a decreased inhibition at the parietal cell, or a prolonged action of released gastrin.

BACK DIFFUSION OF ACID IN THE STOMACH

Under normal circumstances, acid in the gastric lumen diffuses back through the mucosa very slowly. The normal barrier to back diffusion can be injured by a variety of agents, including bile acids, alcohol, and salicylates. If the agent is ionizable, it must be in its un-ionized lipid-soluble form to enter the mucosa to injure the barrier. Once the barrier has been injured, greatly increased amounts of acid can back-diffuse through the gastric mucosa. Identification of a broken barrier is suggested by an increased bidirectional permeability to sodium, permitting an increased accumulation of sodium in the gastric lumen. The increased backward movement of acid through the mucosa causes additional mucosal damage that leads to ulceration and bleeding. The nature of the gastric barrier is not well understood. It resides in the cell membranes and in the tight junctions. It is composed of lipids and proteins. Why it appears to be more vulnerable to injury than a barrier in the duodenum is unknown.

GASTRIC MOTILITY

To accommodate an ingested meal, receptive relaxation of the stomach occurs. This is a vagal response to swallowing that inhibits the tonic contraction of the proximal stomach. Dilatation of the stomach begins with the initiation of swallowing and is completed by the presence of ingested contents within the stomach.

Electrical impulses known as the electrical slow wave, gastric pacesetter potential, pacemaking potential, or basic electrical rhythm originate in the gastric pacesetter high along the greater curvature. These potentials occur with great regularity every 20 seconds and progress distally over the stomach. The function of this electrical system is to integrate the movements of the pyloric gland area. The pacesetter potentials spread from the pacesetter toward the pyloric gland area (antrum). Whether the antrum contracts depends on a second electrical signal that occurs in the antrum. It occurs with greater rapidity than the slow waves and is called the action potential or spike potential. This proceeds and indeed appears to initiate the contractions of the antrum. The contraction wave moves with progressive acceleration and depth to the pylorus, ending in simultaneous contraction of the terminal antrum and pylorus.

Most of the material pushed into the antrum by the peristaltic wave is repelled backward as the distal antrum continues to contract against a closed pylorus. A small amount of gastric contents is metered into the duodenum just prior to the terminal contraction of the antrum and closure of the pylorus. The initiation and effectiveness of peristalsis are dependent on the integrity of the vagus nerves.

The consistency and the volume of gastric contents govern the rate of gastric emptying. Duodenal receptors in response to various products of digestion inhibit gastric emptying by hormonal and reflex mechanisms that are not entirely understood.

The secretion of acid and pepsin and the highly integrated motor activity of the pyloric gland area permit the initiation of digestion and the mechanical grinding of gastric contents so that its osmolality is acceptable to the duodenum. Nearly all operations on the stomach interfere in some way with the important and highly integrated activity that controls gastric emptying. Many of the undesirable and serious sequelae of gastric surgery result from the loss of the metering action that the pylorus and antrum exert on gastric emptying.

GASTRIC ANALYSIS

Measurement of gastric acid secretion became popular when Dragstedt measured the overnight acid secretion in his patients with duodenal ulcer. This test was discarded in favor of a 1- or 2-hour collection under basal condition. The mean secretion will vary with age and sex but the mean in a duodenal ulcer patient is approximately 4 mEq/hr. This is twice the amount produced by a normal patient, although the overlap between the two groups is significant. In order to obtain greater separation between patients with and without ulcers, Kay introduced the concept of measuring the maximal acid output achieved in response to a stimulus such as histamine, betazole, or pentagastrin. This test also failed to provide a sharp separation between normal patients and those with duodenal ulcer.

Gastric analysis does have clinical value. Achlorhydria is incompatible with the presence of a benign ulcer for the axiom "no acid, no ulcer" is still true. A truly achlorhydric patient in whom the gastric roentgenogram demonstrates an ulcer most likely has a cancer. On the other hand, the presence of gastric acid does not exclude the possibility of a gastric cancer.

If the basal acid output is greater than 10 mEq/hr, a Zollinger-Ellison tumor (gastrinoma) should be considered. This diagnosis is more likely if the basal acid output approaches the maximal acid output and the ratio of these two tests is 0.6 or greater. Confirmation of a gastrinoma is facilitated by the increase in serum gastrin and acid secretion in response to secretin administration.

The Hollander insulin acid secretory test was originally proposed to test for the completeness of vagotomy. It is based on the hypothesis that hypoglycemia will stimulate the vagal centers. If the vagi have been completely severed, there should be no acid secretion in response to insulin hypoglycemia. There is no proof, however, that acid secretion in response to hypoglycemia is mediated solely by the vagus nerves. Hypoglycemia activates adrenergic as well as cholinergic mechanisms, and the former may be involved in gastrin release and acid secretion after insulin administration. There is poor correlation between the Hollander test and recurrent ulcer. Therefore, the test appears to have little clinical usefulness and should probably be abandoned in view of its potential hazard.

CHRONIC GASTRIC ULCER

The onset of chronic gastric ulcer occurs with greater frequency in older patients while the onset of duodenal ulcer is more common during the second and third decades

GASTRIC ULCER	
ETIOLOGY	Uncertain causes: normo-, hypo-, or hyperchlorhydria; carcinoma with ulceration; drug- or stress-related ulcers
Dx	Epigastric pain, variable vomiting, anemia Upper GI series for ulcer crater Gastroscopy and biopsy to establish if carcinoma
Rx	Avoid ulcer-promoting factors Use antacids Reassess for healing at 6 to 8 weeks If ulcer not healed, repeat gastroscopy and biopsy Proceed to celiotomy and gastric resection to remove ulcer or carcinoma

of life. For convenience, gastric ulcers can be divided into three types. Type I ulcers occur along the lesser curvature usually on the antral side near the antral-fundic border. Type II ulcers occur at or just proximal to the pylorus, and type III ulcers occur in various other areas of the stomach and are frequently drug related.

Type I ulcers were thought to occur in patients who had gastric stasis, poor gastric emptying, and low acid secretion. These patients do not have poor gastric emptying unless there is a concomitant duodenal ulcer and an element of obstruction. Acid secretion in patients with gastric ulcers tends to be lower than in patients with duodenal ulcers, but the overlap between the two groups is so great that this cannot be used as a distinguishing feature. The pathogenesis of type I ulcers is unclear. A current popular theory is that duodenal contents reflux into the stomach, injuring the gastric mucosa along the lesser curvature, which is the area of greatest exposure. Back diffusion of acid through the injured mucosa results in peptic acid ulceration. Loss of acid from the gastric lumen by back diffusion makes the low acid secretion based on secretory testing more apparent than real.

Type II (prepyloric) ulcers are those 1 cm to 2 cm proximal to the pylorus. This is purely arbitrary. Thus it is difficult to characterize this type of ulcer accurately. Type II ulcers appear clinically related to duodenal ulcers and respond to surgical treatment in a manner similar to duodenal ulcers. Patients with a pyloric or prepyloric ulcer treated by antrectomy and Billroth I anastomosis without vagotomy, will have a recurrence rate in the vicinity of 30%. This is similar to the recurrence rate for patients with duodenal ulcer treated by this means. Type II ulcers should therefore be treated as duodenal ulcers.

Type III ulcers occur in various other locations of the stomach. These ulcers are frequently multiple and occur in association with stress, particularly sepsis and shock, and with the use of ulcerogenic drugs. (Salicylates are the most prevalent but by no means the only drugs.) Antirheumatic steroidal and nonsteroidal drugs seem to share this common bond. The etiology of ulcers associated with drugs is most likely due to injury of the mucosal barrier, making the mucosa more susceptible to ulceration by acid. Ulceration associated with the stress of shock is most likely the result of decreased mucosal blood flow, making the mucosa more susceptible to injury and ulceration.

CLINICAL MANIFESTATIONS AND DIAGNOSIS

Patients with a gastric ulcer complain of epigastric pain relieved by eating or antacids. Sometimes eating actually makes the pain worse. This is particularly true in patients with pyloric channel ulcers with an element of obstruction. The diagnostic studies in patients with such symptoms include roentgenographic examination, gastroscopy, and biopsy. There is no constellation of symptoms that allows the diagnosis of gastric ulcer on clinical grounds. Opinions differ as to whether gastroscopy should be the first study performed. In my opinion, gastroscopy and radiologic studies are complementary and not mutually exclusive; however, I am inclined to favor gastroscopy as the initial procedure. This procedure is safe, accurate, and, along with biopsy and gastric washings, provides definitive diagnosis. Even with these diagnostic aids, the diagnosis of cancer will be overlooked in perhaps 5% of patients with a diagnosis of benign gastric ulcer. Whether a benign gastric ulcer becomes malignant is still a question that may never be settled. Most share the view that malignancies ulcerate but that benign gastric ulcer rarely, if ever, becomes malignant. Both benign and malignant lesions are most common in the pyloric gland area. The correct diagnosis should be more readily made in this area than in some of the more obscure areas of the stomach where it is difficult to see and obtain a biopsy specimen.

MEDICAL TREATMENT

Medical treatment of gastric ulcers consists of antacid therapy. Results of studies have demonstrated that the current generation of histamine H_2-receptor antagonists offers no advantages in the treatment of benign gastric ulcers.

Seventy percent of gastric ulcers heal in 6 weeks. Forty percent of those that heal recur in 2 years. The high failure rate with respect to healing, the high recurrence rate, and a significant incidence of unsuspected and undiagnosed cancer have caused many surgeons to recommend operation whenever the diagnosis of a type I or type II chronic gastric ulcer is rendered. Type III chronic ulcers due to chronic salicylate abuse do not respond well to withdrawal of the drug and are also best treated by surgery and abstinence from further use of the drug.

Type III acute gastric ulcer associated with the use of drugs, sepsis, burns, or head injuries becomes manifest by upper gastrointestinal bleeding. These patients are best treated by removing the offending drugs and appropriate treatment of their trauma or sepsis. Additional supportive and therapeutic methods including adequate intravenous nutritional supplementation, antacid therapy, H_2-blockers, and pitressin are used. With the proper management of shock and infection, bleeding from a stress ulcer may stop spontaneously. Thus it is difficult to know which of the therapeutic modalities used are responsible for cessation of bleeding. It bears repeating that the most important aspects of the treatment of stress or drug-related ulcers consist of adequate treatment of shock and sepsis and withdrawal of drugs.

OPERATIVE TREATMENT

Operative treatment for type I chronic gastric ulcer has varied with one's perception of its pathogenesis. Believing that gastric ulcers are caused by gastric stasis and resulting antral hyperfunction, some authors attempted to prevent antral hyperfunction by performing drainage procedures alone. The results were universally bad and the operation was abandoned. The most frequent operation performed for treatment of gastric ulcer is antrectomy: Billroth I anastomosis with or without vagotomy. The recurrence rates reported have ranged from 0 to 4.4%. The operation has the disadvantage that removal of the pyloric sphincter and pyloric gland area destroys the regulatory mechanism for controlled gastric emptying. Pyloroplasty combined with vagotomy constitutes the second most popular operation for type I gastric ulcer. The recurrence rate with this operation has been reported to range from 0 to 14%. It has the further disadvantages that the function of the pyloric sphincter and pyloric gland area are interfered with and that the ulcer is not removed for pathologic study. Its advantage is that in some cases it may be a safer operation than resection.

Believing that injury to gastric mucosa by duodenal contents makes the mucosa more susceptible to ulceration by acid has caused some to study the use of parietal cell vagotomy combined with intraluminal excision of the ulcer. This procedure does not facilitate reflux of duodenal contents into the stomach, gastric emptying remains nearly normal, acid secretion is reduced, and the entire ulcer is submitted for pathologic study. The entire stomach and pylorus are preserved. If the assumptions on which this operation was devised are correct, one might expect the early favorable results that have been reported to continue.

Type II ulcer should be treated as an ordinary duodenal ulcer, which will be discussed below. Chronic type II ulcers related to drug ingestion are best treated surgically as type II ulcers even though the offending drug has been withdrawn. Acute type III ulcers and erosive gastritis due to stress have been treated by a variety of surgical procedures. Pyloroplasty, truncal vagotomy, and oversewing of the bleeding points are occasionally satisfactory if the bleeding is from a few discrete areas. Usually for the severely bleeding patient with generalized bleeding, who would be unlikely to withstand a second operation, near total gastrectomy in order to guarantee no further bleeding is done. For the less seriously ill and for the majority of patients requiring operation, distal gastrectomy and vagotomy is recommended.

CHRONIC DUODENAL ULCER

DIAGNOSIS

Chronic duodenal ulcer produces symptoms that may be indistinguishable from those produced by gastric ulcer. However, the diagnosis of a duodenal ulcer can be made much more reliably by history than can diagnosis of a gastric ulcer. The first symptoms of a duodenal ulcer occur at a younger age than those of a gastric ulcer. Males are affected with greater frequency than females. The characteristics of duodenal ulcer are that their symptoms occur rhythmically, periodically, and frequently at certain times of the year. The symptoms are worse prior to eating and may be relieved by eating or the use of antacids. The patient's symptoms may be progressive and eventually interfere with his sleep, requiring that medications be taken during the night. The symptoms may be misinterpreted because the examiner fails to communicate in terms that the patient understands and relates to. The physician may

DUODENAL ULCER	
Etiology	Mucosal injury by gastric acid pepsin; exacerbated by nicotine, caffeine, alcohol, salicylates
Dx	Epigastric pain, relieved by food, antacids Upper GI series shows crater or deformity Ulcer seen on esophagogastroduodenoscopy
Rx	Avoid ulcer-promoting factors Use antacids and cimetidine Surgery: vagotomy and drainage, vagotomy and resection for intractable pain, or parietal cell vagotomy

inquire about the presence of epigastric distress, which the patient vehemently denies having, whereas he is adamant about the presence of heartburn, indigestion, or gas that is relieved by Tums, Rolaids, Alka Seltzer, or some other over-the-counter preparation that he takes regularly in large amounts. The symptoms of ulcer are sufficiently nonspecific that other conditions such as reflux esophagitis, biliary tract, or pancreatic diseases must be excluded.

The diagnosis of an ulcer is best confirmed by upper gastrointestinal endoscopy, although many still prefer to use radiologic techniques as the primary mode of investigation. Gastric analysis has been used in the study of patients with duodenal ulcer, but it has a limited role in diagnosis and even less in the treatment of duodenal ulcer. The absence of acid in the presence of an ulcerating gastric lesion suggests the presence of gastric carcinoma. Anacidity may alert the clinician to pernicious anemia, and basal hyperacidity that approaches the level of secretion obtained with maximal stimulation with Histalog or pentagastrin suggests the existence of a gastrinoma.

The hope that the level of gastric secretion would discriminate between gastric and duodenal ulcers or that the level of acid secretion would aid in the selection of the optimal type of operation to be performed in a given patient has not materialized. There are conflicting opinions regarding the validity of using the acid secretory rate as the basis for selection of patients who are at greater risk of developing recurrent ulcer if parietal cell vagotomy is performed. In general, acid studies are primarily of research value and are of limited clinical value.

MEDICAL TREATMENT

The majority of patients with duodenal ulcer are candidates for medical treatment, which consists of abstinence from ulcerogenic agents such as nicotine, caffeine, alcohol, salicylates, and corticosteroids. It was long held that specific diets were important in treatment of an ulcer, but this concept now has a low priority in the treatment regimen. Anticholinergic drugs were once popular therapeutic agents for treatment of duodenal ulcer. Their role now is unclear. They have no role as the primary treatment but they may be useful as adjunctive therapy in patients who have failed on other medical treatments. Anticholinergic drugs together with H_2- antagonists may prove efficacious in certain patients with high secretory rates. Newer anticholinergic drugs may be more specific for the parietal cell, causing fewer of the

unpleasant side-effects when given in therapeutic doses. Currently histamine H_2- receptor antagonists and antacids consisting of magnesium oxide and aluminum hydroxide are the most popular forms of medical therapy for duodenal ulcer. Prospective studies indicate that both of these forms of therapy are equally effective if taken in the prescribed dosage. The disconcerting fact is that placebo therapy has been reported nearly as effective as drug therapy in treatment of duodenal ulcer. The significance of these observations is unknown.

The results of treatment show that about 25% of duodenal ulcers cannot be brought to complete healing and of those that do come to complete healing 30% will recur when treatment is discontinued. Patients become elective surgical candidates when medical treatment fails to heal the ulcer and relieve symptoms. Under these circumstances the patient's ulcer is said to be intractable. Operation is also indicated when patients are tired of recurring episodes of ulcer distress taking their annual toll in pain, disability, lost time from work, and the need for intermittent medical treatment. Under these circumstances an ulcer cannot be said to be truly intractable; yet the time comes when many patients desire a better way of life than that afforded by treatment of their ulcer several times a year—year after year—with medication. These people should not be denied the option of treatment by operation. Other indications for operation besides intractability include bleeding, perforation, and obstruction.

OPERATIVE TREATMENT

Gastroenterostomy alone was once an operation widely used for the treatment of duodenal ulcer. This operation was associated with a high recurrent ulcer rate and is seldom used now. On the other hand, for a patient who, for medical reasons, is a poor operative candidate and who has pyloric obstruction, simple gastroenterostomy may be a viable option to solve the problem temporarily with as little surgery as is possible.

A distal two-thirds to three-fourths partial gastrectomy without vagotomy is the first operation for duodenal ulcer to withstand the test of time and which is still used (Table 23-1). After resection, gastrointestinal continuity can be restored by gastroduodenostomy (Billroth I) or by gastrojejunostomy (Billroth II). The high rate (30%) of recurrent ulcers after gastroduodenostomy led to the abandonment of this procedure in favor of the Billroth II. The reason for the unsatisfactory results after Billroth I anastomosis is unclear, but a possible explanation is that the residual parietal cells remain innervated and therefore sensitive to all stimuli including gastrin, which is released in greater amounts from the duodenum after gastroduodenostomy than from the jejunum after gastrojejunostomy. The different types of common resective procedures used for treatment of duodenal ulcer are seen in Figure 23-6.

When performing a Billroth II anastomosis the jejunum can be brought behind the colon or in front of the colon. It can be anastomosed to the gastric stump in either an isoperistaltic or antiperistaltic fashion. Each technique is satisfactory, and none has a distinct advantage over the others, although each surgeon may feel strongly that one way is better than another. There is evidence that the afferent limb should be short to reduce the possibility of recurrent ulcer, and that the transected stomach should be partially closed from the lesser curvature rather than making

TABLE 23-1   COMMONLY PERFORMED OPERATIONS FOR DUODENAL ULCER

OPERATION	MORTALITY (%)	RECURRENCE RATE (%)	ADVANTAGE(S)	DISADVANTAGE(S)
Two-thirds to three-fourths distal gastrectomy	~1 elective	5–15 (higher if B₁)	None	Small gastric reservoir, dumping
Vagotomy and drainage	<1	5–10	Technically facile procedure, maintains gastric reservoir	Dumping, diarrhea, recurrence
Vagotomy and distal gastrectomy	~1	2–3	Lowest recurrence rate	Dumping, diarrhea, moderate gastric reservoir
Parietal cell vagotomy	0–<1	5–25	Lowest rate of diarrhea and dumping, maintains gastric reservoir	Technically difficult, high recurrence rate

Fig. 23-6. Diagrammatic representation of distal partial gastrectomy, with gastrointestinal continuity being restored by gastroduodenostomy (Billroth I) and gastrojejunostomy (Billroth II), with and without truncal vagotomy. (Sleisenger MH, Fordtran JS [eds]: Gastrointestinal Disease, 2nd ed. Philadelphia, W B Saunders, 1978)

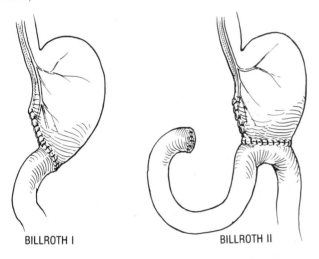

BILLROTH I   BILLROTH II

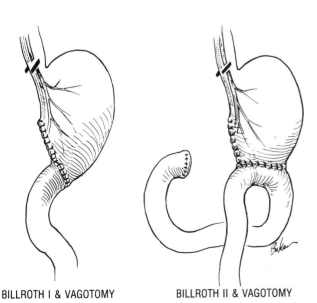

BILLROTH I & VAGOTOMY   BILLROTH II & VAGOTOMY

an anastomosis with the entire cut end of the stomach to the jejunum (Polya anastomosis). Narrowing the outlet of the stomach in this way may slow gastric emptying and diminish symptoms of dumping.

There are other important technical points. If it is impossible to obtain a secure closure of the duodenal stump, the duodenum should be closed around a large tube and a controlled duodenal fistula should be established. Care must be taken to avoid injury of the pancreas and the common duct.

Technical complications may include pancreatitis, which is associated with any operation that includes resection of the distal stomach and may be related to injury of the pancreas at the time of resection. Acute pancreatitis may occur also in patients with afferent loop obstruction if distention within the duodenal loop is sufficiently great to cause reflux of duodenal contents into the pancreatic duct. Pancreatitis may be mild or sufficiently acute and fulminating to result in death.

Common duct injury at the time of resection is most likely to occur if the duodenum is foreshortened and the common duct is drawn up into an inflammatory mass surrounding the ulcer. In this circumstance, a T-tube should be placed into the common duct to aid in its identification and in the prevention of its injury. Injuries of the common duct are also likely to occur when the ulcer is at the apex of the bulb or in the postbulbar area of the duodenum, particularly if the indication for surgery is a bleeding postbulbar ulcer. Bleeding ulcers in this area can cause such serious technical problems at operation that I believe that any ulcer located in this position is an indication for elective operation.

Undesirable sequelae after gastric resection occur with increased frequency as greater amounts of the stomach are removed to reduce the higher rate of recurrent ulcers associated with resections of lesser magnitude. Although the acceptance of distal two-thirds to three-fourths partial gastrectomy has diminished, the only controlled evaluation of this operation demonstrated that its clinical results were equally as good as those obtained with the other operations tested. The use of distal gastric resection without vagotomy has decreased due to the logical arguments that it is desirable to preserve as much gastric reservoir as possible and that there is little to recommend distal partial gastrectomy over vagotomy and antrectomy, which appear to be safer procedures in most surgeons' hands.

Some of the immediate postoperative complications after distal partial gastrectomy and gastrojejunostomy are shown in Figure 23-7. These include mechanical obstruction of the efferent or afferent limbs of the anastomosis caused by angulation of the limbs, a twist of the jejunum anastomosed to the stomach, inflammatory processes secondary to an anastomotic leak, and idiopathic fat necrosis. An afferent limb obstruction if complete is a closed loop obstruction with its attendant complication of bowel necrosis. The increased pressure that occurs within the duodenum if the afferent loop is partially obstructed enhances the chance for disruption of the duodenal stump closure. Leakage from an insecurely closed duodenal stump is a potential complication even though there is no distal obstruction. If the duodenal closure appears compromised at the time of operation, it can be drained with a tube as mentioned previously. The controlled fistula that results will heal after the tube is removed.

Postoperative hemorrhage may occur from a bleeding suture line or from the base of a bleeding ulcer not secured properly at the time of operation. Neither of these complications occurs frequently, but when it is evident that the patient has lost 1 or 2 units of blood in a brief period and blood continues to be present in the nasogastric tube, limits should be set on the amount of blood loss that will be tolerated before the patient undergoes reoperation.

Some of these complications do not occur after a Billroth I type of anastomosis because there are no efferent or afferent limbs to obstruct. However, the high recurrent ulcer rate that occurs following the Billroth I anastomosis precludes its use unless vagotomy is also done. Nevertheless, this method of reconstruction has its own complications, which include obstruction or leakage at the anastomosis. Leakage of a Billroth I anastomosis, unless the entire anastomosis has broken down, is easier to manage and less lethal than an uncontrolled duodenal fistula. Sometimes a difficult Billroth I anastomosis can be simplified if, instead

of attempting to resect a posterior ulcer, the anastomosis is performed using the bed of the ulcer. The use of interrupted sutures will be helpful in preventing anastomotic obstruction caused by the pursestringing effect of a continuous suture. *Truncal vagotomy and drainage procedures* became the next operation to receive wide acceptance for the treatment of chronic duodenal ulcer (see Table 23-1). Vagotomy has two specific effects on acid secretion: (1) it removes the direct effect of vagal stimulation of the parietal cells and (2) it reduces the sensitivity of parietal cells to gastrin or any other stimulus. Persuaded that extensive subtotal gastric resection was associated with many undesirable complications as well as a high mortality, Dragstedt and Owens introduced transthoracic vagotomy in 1943. Postoperative gastric stasis and the occurrence of gastric ulcers because of gastric stasis led these investigators to combine transabdominal truncal vagotomy with gastroenterostomy and, ultimately, vagotomy with pyloroplasty. The various types of drainage procedures that have been used are demonstrated in Figure 23-8. Just as with subtotal gastric resection, these procedures are associated with technical complications.

A leaking pyloroplasty or gastroenterostomy is a major complication that can lead to stomal obstruction, fistula, and abscess. Peritonitis and death may be the ultimate outcome. Obstruction of the drainage procedure can lead to gastric stasis and gastric ulcer. Delayed gastric emptying after vagotomy may also be due to loss of gastric motility. Metoclopramide may be useful in the treatment of this condition. Differentiation between gastroparesis and stomal obstruction can be made by gastroscopic examination. Placement of a gastroenterostomy too high on the greater curvature of the stomach may cause the duodenal contents to reenter the stomach through the gastroenterostomy stoma. Recirculation of gastric and duodenal contents by this means will increase antral stimulation, acid hypersecretion, and the possibility of marginal ulcer. Complications including dumping, diarrhea, and recurrent ulcers that are common to all gastric operations are discussed under the section on complications after gastric surgery.

Truncal vagotomy combined with a distal gastrectomy of the pyloric gland area and a Billroth I or II type of anastomosis is currently the most common operation used for treatment of duodenal ulcer (see Table 23-1). Because of its profound effect on the reduction of acid secretion, the recurrent ulcer rate (2% to 3%) is lower than after any other operation. The disadvantages of the operation are the sequelae of dumping, diarrhea, and bilious vomiting which are not uncommon. As with all types of resection, the need to dissect in the area of an inflammatory mass surrounding the duodenum increases the mortality, which should be an unacceptable complication for elective surgical treatment of a benign disease.

I showed in a prospective randomized study that vagotomy and antrectomy can be performed under elective conditions for treatment of duodenal ulcer with an operative mortality and clinical results equivalent to or better than those obtained with vagotomy and drainage if the operation is withheld from patients with severe inflammation surrounding the duodenum. Therefore, there is no need to subject all patients to the higher risk of recurrent ulcer and the possible need for reoperation by performing vagotomy and drainage when there is no clear advantage of this operation except in those patients in whom it would be difficult to operate on because of an inflammatory process surrounding the duodenum. The choice between these two

Fig. 23-7. Diagrammatic representation of some complications that occur after gastric surgery.

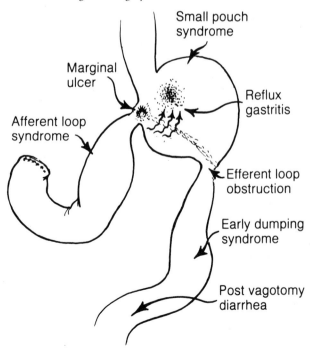

Small pouch syndrome

Marginal ulcer

Reflux gastritis

Afferent loop syndrome

Efferent loop obstruction

Early dumping syndrome

Post vagotomy diarrhea

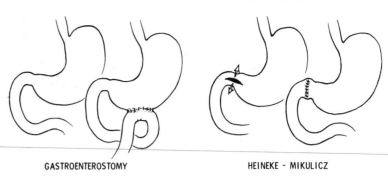

GASTROENTEROSTOMY   HEINEKE - MIKULICZ

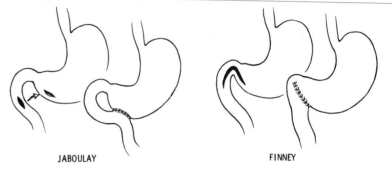

JABOULAY   FINNEY

Fig. 23-8. Four drainage procedures used to improve gastric emptying after truncal or selective vagotomy. (Sleisenger MH, Fordtran JS [eds]: Gastrointestinal Disease, 2nd ed. Philadelphia, W B Saunders, 1978)

most commonly used operations is best made at the operating table on the basis of the potential problems perceived by the surgeon. The risk of recurrence after vagotomy and drainage is more acceptable than the risk of death in a patient in whom the technical problems surrounding a resection appear to be great.

Selective vagotomy rather than truncal vagotomy has been combined with drainage and resection procedures. The different types of vagotomy are depicted in Figure 23-9. Since selective vagotomy does not denervate any of the abdominal viscera other than the stomach, it seemed a highly logical operation. Nevertheless, it was not widely accepted because it was more difficult to perform and it was difficult to prove that sparing the hepatic and celiac branches of the left and right vagus nerves, respectively, permitted more normal functioning of the organs that remain innervated.

There is evidence now that sacrifice of the extragastric vagi adversely affects small bowel function and increases bile lithogenicity. Retention of the extragastric vagi is credited with preventing or reducing the problem of postvagotomy diarrhea. In dogs, there are several lines of evidence to suggest that the extragastric branches of the vagi are responsible for inhibition of acid secretion and that this mechanism is preserved by selective vagotomy. Whether this is true in humans is unknown. It has been shown that the secretory response time of the pancreas to secretagogues in the lumen of the small bowel is of shorter duration than is the response time to cholecystokinin administered into the portal vein. This is due to a cholinergic mechanism that is lost by truncal vagotomy but presumably is preserved by selective vagotomy.

The degree of gastric denervation by selective vagotomy is equal, if not superior, to that obtained with truncal vagotomy. Improvement in the rate of complete gastric vagotomy after selective vagotomy is attributed to greater anatomical precision required to perform this operation. There are no complications unique to selective vagotomy.

The use of selective vagotomy does not obviate the necessity to perform a complementary resection or drainage procedure. Although this has been attempted, it has been condemned by those who have tried it because of the stomach's failure to empty.

Parietal cell vagotomy without a drainage procedure is a further effort to improve the results of gastric surgery for duodenal ulcer (see Table 23-1). This newest concept of vagotomy consists of cutting only the vagal branches supplying the fundic gland area of the stomach. This operation not only preserves all of the extragastric branches of the vagi, as in the case of selective vagotomy, but it preserves the branches of the pyloric gland area as well (see Fig. 23-9).

Conservation of the innervation to the pyloric gland area preserves its motility, making it unnecessary to resect, destroy, or bypass the pylorus to ensure satisfactory gastric emptying. The operations that destroy or bypass the pyloroantral pump—antrectomy, pyloroplasty, and gastroenterostomy—are responsible for gastric incontinence and the dumping syndrome. The cause for vagotomy diarrhea is unknown, but it is considered by some to be due to intestinal hurry following small bowel denervation. The diarrhea resulting from loss of the pylorus is associated with unregulated gastric emptying. It was expected, therefore, that preservation of the pylorus associated with parietal cell vagotomy would reduce dumping and diarrhea by permitting near-normal gastric emptying and that preservation of the extragastric vagi would reduce vagotomy diarrhea. Most investigators have, in fact, found that the frequency of diarrhea and dumping are in the range of 5%, significantly lower than with other gastric operations.

Because parietal cell vagotomy does not require opening of the stomach or the creation of a suture line, the immediate morbidity and mortality have been less than with any other form of gastric operation. The absence of an anastomosis eliminates complications such as anastomotic leaks and afferent and efferent loop syndromes. The mortality in

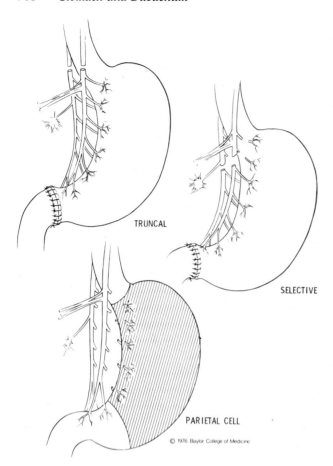

TRUNCAL

SELECTIVE

PARIETAL CELL

© 1976 Baylor College of Medicine

Fig. 23-9. Three types of vagotomy: truncal or total intra-abdominal vagotomy, selective or total gastric vagotomy, and parietal cell vagotomy or vagotomy of the fundic gland area of the stomach. (Sleisenger MH Fordtran JS [eds]: Gastrointestinal Disease, 2nd ed. Philadelphia, W B Saunders, 1978)

several large series has been zero and in one collected series involving 40 different surgeons it was 0.26%.

The possibility that gastric stasis might occur with parietal cell vagotomy as it had following truncal vagotomy without drainage was a concern initially. In reality when the pylorus is of adequate caliber and the pyloric gland area is not excessively denervated, gastric stasis is less of a problem after parietal cell vagotomy than after selective vagotomy, antrectomy and a Billroth I anastomosis. Fear that retention of an innervated antrum might release excessive gastrin was another unfounded concern that delayed acceptance of parietal cell vagotomy. The basal gastrin levels after parietal cell vagotomy have been no greater than after selective or truncal vagotomy. Reduction in acid secretory rates including the response to a test meal has been as great after parietal cell vagotomy as that obtained after selective or truncal vagotomy and drainage. A retained innervated antrum, therefore, is not a liability in the duodenal ulcer patient provided it is well drained and is in continuity with the acid-secreting portion of the stomach.

The operation has been extensively studied and widely used for 12 years. The recurrence rate has been generally reported between 5% and 10%, although there are reports both higher and lower. There is a learning curve for every surgeon, and during this period the recurrence rate may be as high as 25%. One of the most important technical aspects for the satisfactory performance of parietal cell vagotomy

as well as the other two types of vagotomy is that the distal esophagus be sufficiently mobilized so that all vagal branches going to the fundic gland area of the stomach be identified and cut. While some surgeons are of the opinion that the ultimate recurrent ulcer rate after parietal cell vagotomy is unknown, it is reasonable to suggest that the eventual recurrence rate should be the same or better than the rate incurred after truncal vagotomy and pyloroplasty. Accepting this assumption, the benefits derived from the operation so outweigh the advantage of a lower recurrence rate achieved with vagotomy and antrectomy that it has become the operation of choice in many centers.

COMPLICATIONS OF PEPTIC ULCERS

PERFORATION

A perforated ulcer may be either of the duodenum or stomach, but perforated duodenal ulcers are more common. Perforations usually occur anteriorly into the free peritoneal cavity but a gastric perforation can be posteriorly into the lesser sac. Although the presentation of a perforation may be slow and insidious the usual presentation of a perforated ulcer is one of sudden onset of severe abdominal pain that is referred to the shoulder. The pain is so severe that the patients usually come to the hospital within a few hours. An individual with a perforated ulcer may or may not give a history of previous ulcer disease. The antecedent symptoms may have been minor and have preceded perforation by only a few days. Frequently the patient is in such distress from his recent perforation that previous symptoms pale into insignificance not to be recalled until after operation.

The most striking physical finding is the rigidity of the abdomen due to peritoneal soilage and chemical peritonitis. The course following perforation depends on the size of the perforation and the amount of peritoneal soilage. If the perforation quickly becomes walled off by surrounding structures and contamination is minimal, a perforated ulcer may be overlooked and the patient may go on to recovery without complications. On the other hand, patients with perforated ulcers treated by nonoperative means, namely nasogastric suction, will have a high complication rate.

The distribution of gastric contents within the abdomen

GASTRODUODENAL ULCER COMPLICATIONS: PERFORATION	
Etiology	Intraperitoneal leakage of duodenal fluid from transmural duodenal ulcer
Dx	Acute onset (severe abdominal pain, hypotension, tachycardia), rigid "boardlike" abdomen, absent bowel sounds; abdominal radiogram shows pneumoperitoneum in more than half the patients; radiographs using Gastrografin; leukocytosis and hyperamylasemia
Rx	Intravenous hydration, antibiotics, electrolyte correction, nasogastric decompression, prompt celiotomy, and closure of perforated ulcer with or without definitive ulcer operation preferred in most patients

will affect the presentation. Usually an acute, perforated ulcer is readily recognized but it can mimic almost any inflammatory process in the abdomen. While the following list is not all inclusive, the features of a perforated peptic ulcer can be confused with the clinical presentation of pancreatitis, gangrenous bowel, appendicitis, cholecystitis, diverticulitis, and, in the female, ruptured or bleeding ovarian cyst or tubal pregnancy.

Laboratory findings include a mild leukocytosis that increases as bacterial contamination intervenes. A mild elevation of serum amylase occurs secondary to its absorption from the peritoneal cavity. The most important finding is air in the abdominal cavity seen on roentgenographic studies. This finding may be absent in 20% of patients with perforated ulcer, and when present it may be due to causes other than perforated peptic ulcer. Radiographs to demonstrate free air are taken in the upright or left lateral decubitus position. For these to be of greatest value the technician must allow sufficient time to permit air, if present, to gravitate and collect so that it can be demonstrated. Occasionally, diagnostic procedures such as peritoneal lavage and roentgenographic studies with contrast material are used to establish the correct diagnosis of the acute abdominal condition.

MEDICAL TREATMENT

Usually the diagnosis of a perforated ulcer is easily made and supportive treatment is begun. These measures consist of initiating nasogastric suction, correcting intravascular fluid and electrolyte levels, establishing a good urinary output, and administering a wide-spectrum antibiotic.

Treatment in some countries still consists, preferentially, of nonoperative measures, with the above measures constituting the entire treatment. This technique, while it has been effective, is complicated by a high rate of intra-abdominal sepsis and it is rarely used in the United States except in patients who are inordinately poor operative risks or who were seen many hours after their perforation.

OPERATIVE TREATMENT

Operative therapy is the treatment of choice but should be preceded by the resuscitative measures outlined above. The urine output and the central venous pressure should be monitored to ensure satisfactory fluid levels. The type of operation may be either simple closure of the ulcer by an omental patch or one of the definitive operations already discussed for the elective treatment of duodenal ulcer.

Simple closure consists of approximation of the opening with sutures and a reinforcement of the closure with an omental patch. When bringing a piece of omentum over the duodenum to cover the ulcer, caution is required that the piece of omentum is long enough that it will reach easily without causing rotation and obstruction of the duodenum. It is important that nonabsorbable sutures are used and that they are not placed into the lumen of the gut where they can act as a continuous focus for inflammation and erosion. When simple closure is used to treat a perforated ulcer, precautions must be taken to ensure that there is an adequate lumen to prevent gastric outlet obstruction, that there is no secondary posterior bleeding ulcer, and that there is no malignancy present in a gastric ulcer. Infection is an uncommon complication of perforated ulcer if operation is performed promptly, if an adequate cleansing of the peritoneal cavity is performed, and if the patient is given a broad-spectrum antibiotic.

Patients who have an obstructing as well as a perforated ulcer require an emptying procedure in addition to closure of the perforation. Approximately 2% of patients with an anterior perforated ulcer also have a posterior bleeding ulcer, which if unrecognized may require a second operation unnecessarily.

The mortality rate for simple closure of all perforated ulcers is approximately 15%. The high mortality rate is a reflection of the poor condition and the associated illnesses that so many of these patients have rather than the inadequacies of the operation.

While simple closure is still the most commonly used operation for treatment of a perforated duodenal ulcer, gastric surgeons are performing more frequently a definitive ulcer operation at the time the patient is operated for perforated ulcer. Of those patients who give a history of ulcer symptoms or in whom a chronic ulcer is found at operation, perhaps three fourths will continue to have symptoms or require subsequent ulcer surgery if nothing more than a simple closure is performed at the time of perforation. The difficulty at operation is our inability to know precisely which individual will or will not continue to have further difficulty if only a simple closure is performed. For this reason, there is an increasing tendency for surgeons to perform a definitive ulcer operation at the time of perforation if the patient is in good health and has not been in shock and if peritoneal soilage is not excessive.

Truncal vagotomy and antrectomy or pyloroplasty have been the definitive procedures most commonly used. More recently, fixation of an omental patch over the perforation combined with parietal cell vagotomy has been recommended. This procedure is attractive because it provides protection against further ulcer complications for patients who would otherwise have had further ulcer problems if definitive surgery were not performed. At the same time it does not cause any serious morbidity for those patients who might not have had any further ulcer complications had no definitive operation been performed. This is an important consideration for those favoring definitive operation because the selection of patients who will have further difficulty if untreated from those who will not is not infallible.

Those who advocate definitive operation may claim that it is as safe a procedure as simple closure, but it must be recognized that those performing definitive operation relegate the poor risk patients to the simpler operation so that the comparison is not valid.

HEMORRHAGE

Bleeding is a common complication of peptic ulcers that must be distinguished from other causes of upper gastrointestinal bleeding. These other common causes include esophageal varices, erosive gastritis, Mallory-Weiss tears, and gastric carcinoma. Patients presenting with peptic ulcer bleeding may have an antecedent history of ulcer or they may present with no history of peptic ulcer, so-called silent bleeding. Instead of being due to chronic ulcer disease, silent bleeding may be due to the ingestion of a drug such as a salicylate.

Bleeding from a peptic ulcer can vary in intensity from a mild chronic blood loss to a torrential life-threatening hemorrhage. In general, hemorrhage from a gastric ulcer is greater than that from a duodenal ulcer and bleeding from the latter is more likely to stop than that from the former. In a high percentage of patients (70% to 80%), bleeding

---

GASTRODUODENAL ULCER COMPLICATIONS: HEMORRHAGE

Etiology	Ulcer erosion into adjacent artery (frequently gastroduodenal artery)
Dx	Hematemesis, melena, shock, hypotension, anemia
	Esophagogastroduodenoscopy
	Celiac arteriography
Rx	Intravenous hydration, transfusion, nasogastric tube decompression, and lavage
	Cimetidine and antacids if stable
	Surgery: Oversewing ulcer and definitive ulcer operation for massive hemorrhage or medical failure to control hemorrhage
	Possible nonoperative interventions: Vasopressin infusion, selective arterial transcatheter embolization, endoscopic ulcer coagulation, or laser treatment

---

from a duodenal ulcer will stop without surgical intervention. The ulcers that bleed greatest and are most likely to require emergency operative intervention are those that occur posteriorly and erode the gastroduodenal artery.

DIAGNOSIS OF BLEEDING SOURCE

The diagnosis of the cause of upper gastrointestinal bleeding can best be made by upper gastrointestinal endoscopy. There is a difference of opinion among medical endoscopists and surgeons as to whether the diagnosis of the cause of bleeding alters the management or outcome of the patient. If the hemorrhage does not warrant emergency surgery, emergency endoscopy will not have been needed. The problem is that if emergency surgery is not required at the time or shortly after the patient's admission to the hospital, it may become necessary during the next few days when rebleeding occurs. This eventuality is unpredictable. In the event of continued or recurrent bleeding an accurate preoperative diagnosis of the source of bleeding is very valuable to the surgeon. This is particularly true when the patient has more than one lesion capable of bleeding. For example, 20% of patients with esophageal varices will have a concomitant duodenal ulcer that might be the source of bleeding. The literature leaves no doubt that endoscopy is the most accurate method of documenting the source of bleeding. Although endoscopy does not have first priority in a bleeding patient, it is reasonable and safe to recommend endoscopy for patients with upper gastrointestinal bleeding at a convenient time soon after they have been stabilized while there is still the possibility to determine the cause for bleeding.

MEDICAL TREATMENT

The initial management of peptic ulcer bleeding consists of correcting intravascular volume by the intravenous administration of a crystalloid solution (usually NaCl). Immediate and subsequent hemoglobin and hematocrit determinations are performed as the severity of bleeding dictates. Blood should be administered as required to maintain a normal blood volume. With the use of a large bore gastric tube, the stomach should be aspirated of clots and subsequently irrigated with saline. Usually bleeding will cease. Older patients are less likely to stop bleeding than younger patients and they tolerate continued bleeding or repeated bleeding less well because their cardiovascular system is less accommodating and the effects of hypotention on vital organs are more injurious. Older patients, particularly if they are known to have significant cardiovascular involvement, must be given consideration for surgery at an earlier time than a younger person with an equivalent blood loss. Older patients should not be permitted to have repeated hemorrhagic insults requiring large volumes of blood before making a decision to operate.

OPERATIVE TREATMENT

The decision whether to perform an operation will depend on multiple factors including age, amount of blood loss, rate of continued bleeding, existence of chronic diseases, ingestion of ulcerogenic agents, and whether the patient has had previous bleeding episodes. If the patient has bled from a gastric ulcer, operation should be given high priority because of the poor response without surgery.

The safest operation that will at the same time stop bleeding and have the lowest rate of recurrent bleeding is a subject of disagreement. The two most frequently used operations are (1) truncal vagotomy and pyloroplasty with suture ligation of the bleeding ulcer and (2) truncal vagotomy, antrectomy, control of the bleeding, and reconstitution of gastrointestinal continuity. The first operation has been said by some to be less effective in controlling bleeding than is the second. Yet truncal vagotomy, oversewing of the ulcer, and pyloroplasty is perhaps the most commonly used of the two operations for bleeding. To be effective, multiple nonabsorbable sutures must be used. They must be placed in different planes and deeply enough in the tissue surrounding the bleeding point that the underlying vessel or vessels will be securely ligated. Sutures placed superficially in the duodenal wall will be inadequate to stop bleeding. When the ulcer is in the usual location, that is, just distal to the pylorus, this is a safe technique. If, however, the ulcer is in the postbulbar area, in the vicinity of the ampulla of Vater, the risk of injury to the underlying common duct or pancreatic duct is greater. For this reason, a postbulbar ulcer is best treated by elective surgery whenever the diagnosis is established rather than risk the complication likely to occur if the patient is operated on under emergency conditions.

The recurrence of bleeding is a major complication of the surgical treatment of a bleeding duodenal ulcer. The rate of rebleeding after truncal vagotomy, pyloroplasty, and oversewing of the ulcer is no higher and the mortality is lower than that which occurs after vagotomy and resection. On the other hand, under certain circumstances when the ulcer is too large or calloused or inappropriately located for satisfactory treatment by vagotomy and pyloroplasty, gastric resection in spite of its greater risks may be required.

Wound infection, while uncommon after elective surgery for duodenal ulcer, occurs with greater frequency in patients operated on for major bleeding in which large clots present in the stomach provide a perfect culture medium for contamination of the peritoneal cavity and the wound. In addition to the use of antibiotics, copious irrigations with several liters of saline are crucial for the prevention of this complication.

PYLORIC OBSTRUCTION

CAUSES FOR OBSTRUCTION

Gastric outlet obstruction may result from a duodenal, a pyloric, or a prepyloric ulcer. These causes must be distinguished from polyps, antral webs, and other benign causes of gastric outlet obstruction as well as from carcinoma of the stomach. Usually, patients with obstruction have had a long ulcer history but, being more stoic than most ulcer patients, have tolerated their symptoms until the obstruction has become high grade with gastric retention and dilatation manifested by anorexia, vomiting, and malnutrition. When these patients eventually undergo operation, the degree of stenosis may be so great that one cannot conceive that it was possible for anything to pass from the stomach into the duodenum.

Patients with obstruction due to pylorospasm secondary to an ulcer may be indistinguishable from those in whom the obstruction is due to cicatricial stenosis. The differentiation is important because the former may be expected to improve with medical management, while no amount of medical therapy will improve the compromised gastric outlet of the latter. The most direct method to distinguish between gastric obstruction due to spasm and that due to fibrosis is to attempt passage of the gastroduodenoscope into the duodenum. Roentgenograms can be notoriously misleading in trying to make this differentiation. In both cases an air fluid level may be seen in the stomach on the plain abdominal films and marked barium retention is evident in the stomach during the upper gastrointestinal series.

Gastric outlet obstruction in patients who have a high gastric secretory rate can cause severe fluid and electrolyte imbalance as a result of vomiting. The loss of large amounts of HCl causes a rise in extracellular HCO_3^-. $NaHCO_3$ is lost in the urine, but ultimately the kidney attempts to conserve further loss of Na^+ by substituting K^+ for Na^+. The resulting electrolyte disturbance, hypokalemic alkalosis accompanied by hypochloremia and hyponatremia, is characteristic for gastric outlet obstruction. The accompanying intravascular volume depletion leads to a fall in the glomerular filtration rate and prerenal azotemia.

PREPARATION REQUIRED FOR OPERATION

Treatment of gastric outlet obstruction must begin with correction of the fluid and electrolyte imbalance and renal

---

GASTRODUODENAL ULCER COMPLICATIONS: OBSTRUCTION	
Etiology	Pyloric channel narrowing from ulcer-associated edema and fibrosis
Dx	History of ulcer symptoms, nonbilious vomiting, weight loss, hypokalemic alkalosis Upper GI series shows barium retention, gastric dilatation Gastroscopy to rule out neoplasm
Rx	Intravenous hydration, electrolyte and acid-base correction Nasogastric tube decompression Nutritional assessment and therapy Surgery: Vagotomy plus resection or drainage

---

dysfunction. The stomach should be thoroughly cleansed with a large bore tube which should then be substituted for a Levin tube that is connected to intermittent suction. Antacid therapy plays little role in therapy of the obstructed stomach. Use of histamine H_2-antagonists is more practical therapeutically because they conserve fluids and electrolytes rather than wasting them into the lumen of the stomach. If the obstruction is functional, time should be given for the edema and spasm to subside. The stomach's ability to regain its capacity to empty can be gauged by placing 500 to 700 ml of saline into the stomach. If the residual after 30 minutes is greater than half of the volume administered, obstruction still persists. Similar information can be obtained by intermittently clamping the nasogastric tube and determining the amount of gastric juice that accumulates in a given period of time. If the gastric residual is less than 100 ml after 4 hours of no suction for several successive periods, a diet can be started and progressed as tolerated by the patient.

If the obstruction is due to fibrosis and stricture, the same preliminary medical measures are necessary to prepare the patient for surgery. A period of gastric decompression of 3 to 5 days is desirable to give the stomach an opportunity to recover from its muscular decompensation and regain its tone following a long period of dilatation.

OPERATIVE TREATMENT

Any of the operative procedures used for the elective treatment of duodenal ulcer is suitable in the obstructed patient. The most frequently used procedure is vagotomy and antrectomy. Our concern that poor gastric emptying would occur after vagotomy and pyloroplasty because of muscular decompensation after long-standing obstruction has not been substantiated. Vagotomy and pyloroplasty is a perfectly acceptable operation if the stomach is properly decompressed preoperatively. Even enthusiasts of parietal cell vagotomy without drainage have recommended that this operation is suitable in obstructed patients if the pylorus can be dilated. In my experience this is true if dilatation is confined to patients with obstruction due to edema and spasm, but for patients with anatomical obstruction when it is necessary to disrupt the pylorus by forceful dilatation it is best not to use this operation.

STRESS ULCERATION

CAUSES OF STRESS ULCERS

Stress ulcers are superficial ulcers usually confined to the fundic gland area of the stomach. They are usually not associated with pain and are manifested by bleeding. These lesions occur most frequently in association with trauma, shock, burns, sepsis, and many serious illnesses. An excellent symposium on this subject has been edited by Ritchie.

A similar type of lesion also occurs with ingestion of certain drugs such as alcohol and salicylates. The clinical course of drug-induced gastritis is less severe than that encountered with stress ulceration in postoperative, traumatized, or severely ill patients.

In patients severely traumatized by multiple organ injuries, multiple gastric erosions are found endoscopically in nearly all patients within three days of their injury. Stress ulcers can develop also within 72 hours in patients with a 50% body burn. While most of these lesions bleed microscopically, a small percent bleed significantly. The pathogenesis of these lesions is not precisely known. The current theory suggests that the gastric barrier to the back diffusion of acid is broken by a number of factors including ischemia (shock), bile, or other duodenal contents that reflux into the stomach, decreased cellular energy content of the mucosa, histamine, or some other unidentified factors that decrease the cytoprotection of the gastric mucosa. If the gastric barrier is broken and the metabolic processes of the mucosa are depressed, the permeability of the gastric mucosa to hydrogen ions is increased and the ability of the tissue to buffer diffusing acid is impaired, leading to further tissue injury.

The stress ulcers associated with intracranial trauma (Cushing's ulcer) are deeper, more penetrating, and are not associated with increased mucosal permeability and bleeding unless accompanied by shock, sepsis, or other serious complication. Gastric secretion and serum gastrin levels are increased in patients with Cushing's ulcer compared with stress ulcers, although there is no relationship between the level of serum gastrin and the development of ulcer in these patients.

Endoscopy is the best method of diagnosing the cause for bleeding in the seriously ill patient. Other methods are unsatisfactory for revealing the superficial stress ulcer. Endoscopy should not be withheld because the patient is too ill to withstand the procedure. There are no contraindications to endoscopy, because patients in intensive care units can be given whatever support is necessary to permit this examination.

PROPHYLAXIS

The first stage of treatment of stress ulcers is their prevention. Those critically ill patients at high risk for developing a stress ulcer should be aggressively treated prophylactically with antacids. Histamine H_2- receptor antagonists are widely used, but their efficacy in the prevention of stress ulcers in the critically ill patient is not established except in patients with head and thermal injuries.

TREATMENT

If stress ulceration develops, aggressive antacid therapy should be initiated if it has not already been used. Histamine H_2- antagonists and pitressin are also used without documentation that they contribute to the cessation of bleeding from a stress ulcer. The most important aspects of treatment are the control of sepsis (drainage of abscesses and antibiotics) and the correction of metabolic derangements.

If bleeding becomes life-threatening, surgery is the last resort. If the number of bleeding areas is discrete, vagotomy and pyloroplasty with oversewing of the bleeding points through a separate gastrotomy can be performed. The rebleeding rate following this operation is high. Vagotomy and pyloroplasty are best suited for treatment of drug-related ulcers. If the bleeding can be encompassed by a subtotal gastric resection, this operation combined with vagotomy is the operation of choice. In those patients in whom the bleeding is massive, in whom it originates in the upper stomach, and in whom continued or rebleeding will certainly be fatal, total gastrectomy should be performed.

COMPLICATIONS OF GASTRIC SURGERY

MORTALITY

Death is the most serious of all complications following elective gastric surgery for peptic ulcer. Through the years the objective of gastric surgeons has been to make gastric surgery safer. Timing of an operation is a critical factor. An elective operation in an ultra high-risk patient should be avoided if the indication for operation is intractability. On the other hand, poor-risk patients requiring operation for emergent or urgent conditions should be brought to the best possible preoperative condition and operated on before their condition deteriorates beyond the point that operation has little opportunity of being successful.

The simplest or most effective operation that will handle the problem requiring operation should be performed. The following are several examples. A patient who has general peritonitis and septic shock after perforation of an ulcer should undergo simple closure and not a definitive operation. A patient over 50 who has had a previous myocardial infarction should not be permitted to bleed multiple units of blood within a few hours without plans having been made for operation. At operation the simplest procedure known to control peptic ulcer bleeding, that is, suture ligation of a bleeding ulcer, truncal vagotomy, and a pyloroplasty, is recommended. If the ulcer is so large and calloused that one cannot depend on suture ligation to stop bleeding, gastric resection may be the procedure of choice. In case of extensive bleeding from erosive gastritis, the patient's chance of survival may be greatest by electing total gastrectomy rather than a simpler but less definitive operation, even though this means selection of the operation with the highest morbidity and mortality for the most critically ill patient.

The mortality following gastric operations is primarily related to the complication of sepsis due to leaking suture lines. In an effort to reduce mortality, Dragstedt developed truncal vagotomy for the treatment of ulcers. Presently the mortality of truncal vagotomy combined with either gastrectomy or a drainage procedure is extremely low and nearly equal. There are numerous series of cases where the mortality is zero after both types of procedures when done under elective conditions. More realistically, the mortality is 2% for truncal vagotomy and resection and 1% for truncal vagotomy and drainage. The mortality following parietal cell vagotomy without drainage in many large series has been zero and is 0.26% in a collected series of nearly 5,000 patients. The mortality for operations done under emergency conditions is quite different. It may be 10% to 15% overall in patients with perforated ulcer treated by simple closure and as high as 30% in patients operated on for bleeding peptic ulcer.

RECURRENT ULCERS

A recurrent ulcer is usually the price one pays for selecting an operation with fewer complications and a lower mortality rate rather than an operation that has a more profound effect on lowering acid secretion. Recurrent ulcers after treatment of duodenal ulcers are due to continued high acid secretion. Causes for continued increased acid secretion include incomplete vagotomy or inadequate gastric resection, gastric stasis following an unsatisfactory drainage procedure, retained antrum out of continuity with the acid stream following resection and Billroth II anastomosis, or an unsuspected Zollinger-Ellison tumor. The role of G-cell hyperfunction is not clearly delineated.

Patients with recurrent ulcer usually present with pain or bleeding, sometimes with obstruction or perforation. The type of pain is similar to that presented initially; however, it may be located more to the left side if the patient has had a Billroth II type of anastomosis. The interval between the initial operation and the recurrence of symptoms may be a few weeks to many years.

Patients suspected of recurrent ulcer should have a serum gastrin determination performed. They should undergo endoscopy as a first diagnostic procedure since interpretation of roentgenographic studies is unreliable because of distortion and artifacts created by previous operation. Gastric secretory studies are of limited value except in the diagnosis of a Zollinger-Ellison tumor. They may be useful in determining the completeness of vagotomy.

Medical therapy of a recurrent ulcer is difficult after all operations except parietal cell vagotomy. After parietal cell vagotomy, a recurrent ulcer lends itself to medical therapy as if it were a *de novo* ulcer. Treatment is successful in approximately 80% of patients. In my opinion the high rate of healing of recurrent ulcers by medical therapy after parietal cell vagotomy is because the small bowel is not abnormally exposed to acid secretion by the creation of an artificial stomal opening between the stomach and small bowel.

Patients not responding to medical management require reoperation. Patients with a prepyloric ulcer have an ulcer diathesis similar to that of a patient with a duodenal ulcer. Recurrence following antrectomy alone in such a patient can successfully be treated by vagotomy. Recognizing the potential for development of a recurrent ulcer, I do not treat type II gastric ulcers with antrectomy without vagotomy.

Patients who have recurrent ulcer after vagotomy, antrectomy, and Billroth II anastomosis should have their duodenal stump examined and biopsied for retained antrum. In the presence of extensive duodenal inflammation at the original operation it is understandable that the antrum may have been transected rather than the duodenum. As a consequence a small piece of antrum attached to the duodenum is in an alkaline environment which may cause hypergastrinemia and a recurrent ulcer.

For patients with recurrent ulcer after a previous two-thirds to three-fourths gastric resection, we prefer to perform vagotomy or revagotomy if this appears to have been attempted but is incomplete. Reoperation is performed through the abdomen because this approach not only permits vagotomy but it also permits examination of the duodenal stump for retained antrum. The abdomen may be examined for pancreatic tumor and other unexpected abdominal pathology which can be appropriately dealt with. The abdominal route also allows for reresection of the stomach if this is the indicated method of treatment.

Patients previously treated by vagotomy and a drainage procedure may be treated by revagotomy if a major trunk was initially overlooked. This possibility is highly likely if the patient secretes 10 mEq of HCl or more per hour in response to maximal stimulation with Histalog, pentagastrin, or insulin. The posterior nerve trunk is the one most likely to have been missed. It is the largest of the two nerves lying in the adventitia between the esophagus and aorta, yet it is the more difficult of the two nerves to find. In this event, revagotomy may be successful treatment. If a virgin nerve trunk is not found, the patient should undergo antrectomy.

Patients with recurrent ulcer after parietal cell vagotomy who do not respond to medical therapy can best be treated by antrectomy alone or antrectomy and revagotomy if secretory testing suggests that the previous vagotomy was completely inadequate.

The role of G-cell hyperfunction in the formation of a recurrent ulcer after vagotomy and drainage is unclear. How to recognize these patients before their original operation as patients requiring antrectomy is under investigation. A basal hypergastrinemia and an enhanced gastrin response to food may help to identify these patients. Evidence that the condition probably exists is suggested by the fact that many patients with recurrent ulcer after vagotomy and drainage can be treated successfully by antrectomy. Patients suspected of harboring a Zollinger-Ellison tumor will be discussed later, but it should be emphasized that whenever a patient has a recurrent ulcer the possibility of a gastrinoma should be kept in mind and appropriate studies performed.

GASTROJEJUNOCOLIC FISTULA

Gastrojejunocolic fistula represents a special type of recurrent ulcer that occurs after a gastrectomy and a Billroth II anastomosis. The recurrent ulcer at the gastrojejunostomy lies in close proximity to the transverse colon which it ultimately erodes, resulting in a fistula between the colon, jejunum, and the stomach. Such a lesion is best demonstrated by a barium enema rather than the upper gastrointestinal roentgenogram because the preferred direction of flow is from the colon through the fistula and into the stomach rather than in the reverse direction.

The fecal contamination of the upper gastrointestinal tract by this circular flow leads to the formation of deconjugated and dehydroxylated bile acids, which are damaging to the intestinal mucosa and cause severe malabsorption. There is also a competition between the host and intestinal bacteria for B_{12} absorption that leads to anemia.

Gastrojejunocolic fistulas have become uncommon with the use of vagotomy combined with resection and with fewer Billroth II anastomoses being done. There is no medical treatment for this condition, and the operative risk in the debilitated patient is substantial. It is now less than in the past because of greater opportunity to improve the patient's nutritional status with total parenteral alimentation. Operative treatment includes the resection of those segments of transverse colon, jejunum, and stomach involved with the ulcer and reestablishing gastrointestinal continuity either by a Billroth I or Billroth II anastomosis. A vagotomy should also accompany the operation if it has not already been done.

POSTGASTRECTOMY SYNDROMES

DUMPING

The dumping syndrome refers to any combination of the following symptoms: weakness, faintness, dizziness, tachycardia, diaphoresis, and the need to assume the reclining position. These symptoms begin while a patient is eating or shortly thereafter. The patient may have a feeling of early satiety and nausea but will rarely vomit. Sometimes peristaltic cramps occur followed by an explosive bowel movement. Patients in whom the syndrome is most severe will have symptoms following ingestion of any type or amount of food. Symptoms are worse when liquids are ingested with the meal. Patients with severe symptoms become malnourished because they avoid eating to prevent having the syndrome.

The pathogenesis of early postprandial dumping is uncertain. It is a complex physiological response to the alteration by surgery of the stomach's ability to meter small aliquots of properly prepared gastric contents into the small bowel. The physiological alterations that occur in response to the inappropriate presentation of gastric chyme to the intestine are undoubtedly multifactorial depending on composition, consistency, and speed with which the gastric contents enter the intestine. Dumping has been attributed to movement of fluid into the jejunum in response to the presence of hyperosmolar solutions. This results in a reduction in plasma volume and sympathetic stimulation. This can be further exacerbated by an inappropriate distribution of the residual blood volume to the periphery. The early dumping syndrome has been attributed also to the release of various humoral agents from the gut, including bradykinin and serotonin. However, antiserotonin drugs have been ineffective in preventing or treating the syndrome. Dumping symptoms that occur a few hours after eating (late dumping) are due to inappropriate insulin release in response to high concentrations of glucose entering the small bowel soon after eating.

Patients who have undergone any type of gastric surgery, but particularly those in whom a new stoma is constructed between the stomach and small bowel, are prone to have the dumping syndrome. Gradually, as surgery has become less ablative—with the use of smaller gastric resections, the substitution of selective vagotomy for truncal vagotomy, and more recently the avoidance of any type of drainage procedure by the use of parietal cell vagotomy—the frequency and severity of the dumping syndrome have diminished.

With current operative techniques, patients inclined to have dumping learn that their symptoms can be eliminated or diminished to an acceptable degree by avoidance of overeating or the reduction in the amount of carbohydrates, dairy products, or some other specific food that they eat. Some degree of milk intolerance is a frequent complaint that is common to all types of gastric surgery, including parietal cell vagotomy. Since liquids leave the stomach more rapidly than normal even after parietal cell vagotomy, we believe the fullness, nausea, intestinal cramps, and diarrhea that sometimes occur after drinking milk is a syndrome due to relative lactose deficiency.

Treatment of dumping begins with its prevention, and this is accomplished by using smaller resections, smaller anastomoses when resection is indicated, and parietal cell vagotomy, which preserves the motor function of the antrum and spares the pyloroantral mechanism. When dumping does occur after taking the above precautions, its treatment is almost exclusively dietary. The patient should eat multiple small meals rather than one large meal per day. He should eliminate liquids with the meal, reduce carbohydrate intake, and avoid any particular foods known to precipitate an attack. Drugs are of little or no help.

In a small number of patients, symptoms may be uncontrolled by the above measures and may be sufficiently disabling that reconstructive surgery is indicated. Before considering patients as candidates for reconstructive operations they are challenged with a cocktail of 150 ml of 50% glucose and 100 ml of one-half milk and one-half cream. This is administered through a tube without the patient's knowledge at the conclusion of a gastric analysis. The patient is closely monitored for clinical findings of dumping. If these are not apparent, it is unlikely that he is a candidate for operation.

There are several operative procedures to be considered in the treatment of dumping. If the patient previously had a vagotomy and gastroenterostomy, the gastroenterostomy is taken down. Since the elapsed time between the original and remedial operations will have been adequate for the stomach to regain its intrinsic motility pattern, no further drainage procedure need be done in the absence of pyloric stenosis. Restoration of the pylorus after a Heineke-Mikulicz pyloroplasty by reversing the pyloroplasty can be done by opening the pylorus transversely and suturing it longitudinally. Patients with a large Billroth II anastomosis may benefit by converting this to a smaller Billroth I type of anastomosis (Fig. 23-10). If this proves unsatisfactory, a 10-cm segment of jejunum can be reversed and placed between the gastric remnant and the duodenum. This is an effective operation, but occasionally reflux of duodenal contents will cause gastritis or esophagitis. In that event the reversed segment can be transected to the duodenojejunal anastomosis, the duodenal stump closed, and a Roux-en-Y anastomosis performed to the reversed jejunal segment. The success of this operation has caused some surgeons to suggest that it should be the first reconstructive operation performed for dumping after gastric resection. Vogel and co-workers suggested that the Roux-en-Y gastrojejunostomy without the reversed segment illustrated in Figure 23-11 may be effective in the treatment of dumping because of the delayed emptying observed after this operation. If

Fig. 23-10. Procedures used to correct the gastrointestinal and vasomotor symptoms of dumping after a Billroth II gastrectomy (*A*) include conversion to a Billroth I anastomosis (*B*), insertion of an antiperistaltic limb of jejunum between stomach and duodenum (*C*), and conversion to a Roux-en-Y jejunojejunostomy (*D*).

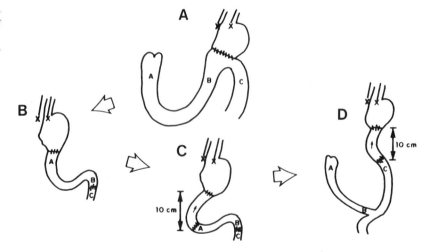

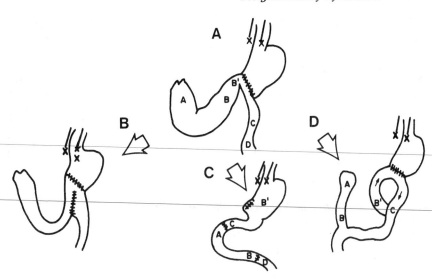

Fig. 23-11. Procedures used to correct the afferent loop syndrome (*A*) include side-to-side jejunojejunostomy (*B*), Henley loop with jejunal interposition between stomach and duodenum (*C*), and Tanner 19 (*D*).

vagotomy was not previously performed, it should be part of the reconstructive operations in order to prevent the occurrence of recurrent ulcers in these otherwise ulcerogenic procedures.

DIARRHEA

Diarrhea after gastric surgery is of two types, that which is a part of the dumping syndrome and that which is related to the performance of vagotomy. Diarrhea associated with dumping usually improves as the dumping improves and as the patient develops more discriminating eating habits. The cause of diarrhea associated with vagotomy is unknown. It occurs intermittently. The patient may have several watery bowel movements a day for several days and then have normal bowel movements until the cycle repeats itself. The occasional patient with severe diarrhea may have multiple watery bowel movements daily or intermittently. They may be explosive, coming without warning, and causing the patient to soil his clothes.

Like dumping, severe postoperative diarrhea associated with dumping has decreased with the use of more conservative operations. Postvagotomy diarrhea has virtually been eliminated by the use of selective and parietal cell vagotomy rather than truncal vagotomy. Patients with the diarrhea of dumping can almost always be managed by dietary means. Patients with postvagotomy diarrhea can be placed on dietary restrictions and treated with antispasmodics, antidiarrheal drugs, and, in severe cases, cholestyramine. If all medical therapy fails and diarrhea is severe enough to warrant an operation, an antiperistaltic 10-cm segment of jejunum may be reversed 100 cm distal to the ligament of Treitz. If vagotomy diarrhea and dumping both exist, an occasional patient may require two reversed jejunal segments, one at the outlet of the stomach and a second 100 cm distal to the ligament of Treitz.

AFFERENT LOOP SYNDROME

The afferent loop syndrome (obstruction) may occur as an acute complication in the early postoperative period as discussed previously. It may occur in the late postoperative period as a chronic problem. Obstruction can result from sharp angulation or kink at the gastrojejunostomy, inflammation secondary to an anastomotic leak, fat necrosis, or recurrent ulcer. If the transected edge of the stomach is sewn to the jejunum on a line that is not parallel to the antimesenteric border of the jejunum, the anastomosis is likely to twist and obstruct.

After eating, bile and pancreatic juices distend the partially obstructed afferent limb. The resulting discomfort is overcome by explosive vomiting of duodenal contents. The meal itself is usually not lost because it enters the efferent limb without difficulty. Overgrowth of bacteria, another complication of stasis in the afferent limb, may cause the blind loop syndrome, resulting in malabsorption and anemia.

The diagnosis is aided by the roentgenographic appearance: little barium enters the afferent limb and that which does demonstrates dilatation of the limb. Provocative tests have been devised using fatty meal or injections of cholecystokinin and secretin to stimulate biliary and pancreatic secretions. Endoscopy is important in eliminating other causes of the symptoms, particularly alkaline gastritis.

All patients with this syndrome should undergo operation. There are several surgical alternatives. The afferent and efferent limbs may be anastomosed side to side. A Billroth II anastomosis can be converted to a Billroth I anastomosis or a Roux-en-Y gastrojejunostomy. There are various modifications of these procedures that can be performed as different technical problems present themselves. These include the Tanner 19 procedure and the Henley loop procedure (anastomosis of the efferent limb into the duodenum and an end-to-end anastomosis of the afferent limb to the distal efferent limb) (see Fig. 23-11).

EFFERENT LOOP SYNDROME

Obstruction of the efferent limb of a gastrojejunostomy may be due to the same causes responsible for the afferent limb syndrome. In addition, obstruction of the efferent limb may be due to herniation of small bowel through the space behind the gastrojejunostomy unless this space is obliterated. If the anastomosis is a Billroth II made anterior to the colon, nothing can be done to obliterate the space. If the anastomosis is retrocolic, careful suturing of the afferent limb to the posterior peritoneum will obliterate the space and prevent the small bowel from herniating behind the anastomosis. Intussusception of the jejunum into the stomach, either antegrade or retrograde, may also occur.

ALKALINE GASTRITIS

Alkaline gastritis occurs after gastric surgery. It is manifested by hyperemia and erosions of the stomach that can extend into the esophagus. The microscopic examination reveals decreased or absent parietal and chief cells, superficial mucosal ulceration, hemorrhage, atrophy, and finally intestinalization of the gastric wall. The condition results from reflux of duodenal contents into the stomach and is manifested by bilious vomiting, weight loss, and epigastric pain made worse by eating.

Alkaline gastritis can easily be confused with acid and alkaline reflux esophagitis clinically and it is important from the standpoint of therapy to separate and identify these different entities. Duodenal contents reflux into a normal stomach but in increasing amounts after pyloroplasty and Billroth I and Billoth II anastomoses, in that order. The material in duodenal secretions responsible for the pathologic changes in the gastric mucosa is not well identified. Bile acids, pancreatic enzymes, lysolecithin, or some combination of these agents have been suggested. Bile acids in the form of deconjugated bile acids have been particularly incriminated and may be the most damaging. The conversion of conjugated to deconjugated bile acids is by bacteria. The risk and extent of alkaline gastritis are directly related to the number of bacteria that increases as the degree of acidity decreases. In fact, histamine-fast achlorhydria is commonly seen and correlates well with the microscopic presence of gastritis.

Medical therapy consistently fails in this condition. Therefore, patients who truly have alkaline gastritis should undergo operation. Use of a 10-cm to 12-cm isoperistaltic segment of jejunum, interposed between the gastric pouch and the duodenum to provide a physiological barrier or valve to prevent reflux, has not been universally successful. A higher success rate is achieved with the Roux-en-Y gastrojejunostomy. It is important to perform the jejunojejunostomy sufficiently distal to the gastrojejunostomy (40 cm) so that reflux of duodenal contents into the gastric pouch will not occur. This procedure is also more effective in the treatment of the afferent loop syndrome than is conversion of a Billroth II to a Billroth I anastomosis because it prevents the possible development of alkaline gastritis. Wider use of parietal cell vagotomy will decrease the frequency of alkaline reflux gastritis as a complication of gastric surgery because the pylorus, which acts as a barrier to duodenal reflux, is preserved.

Bile reflux and gastritis are common after gastric operations; yet there is not a high correlation between these findings and the presence of symptoms. It is not certain, therefore, that bile reflux and the presence of gastritis have anything to do with the clinical manifestations except that the symptoms improve with diversion of duodenal contents from the stomach. It may be that the gastric mucosa in some patients is more sensitive to the noxious agent than in others.

WEIGHT LOSS

Weight loss after gastric surgery is related to the size of gastric resection, the type of vagotomy performed, and whether the pylorus is preserved. Although malabsorption of fat and proteins occurs, decreased food intake is the most common cause of weight loss after gastric surgery. A small gastric pouch may cause early satiety. Food intake may consciously or unconsciously be restricted by the patient in an effort to avoid the various unpleasant postcibal syndromes. The increased 15% to 20% loss of fat and protein that occurs in the stool could be compensated for by increasing the dietary intake. Patients with significant weight loss fail to compensate for these losses because of the postcibal symptoms that result from increased dietary intake.

Rapid gastric emptying results in pancreatic and biliary secretions being out of phase with the passage of the meal through the duodenum. This temporal dissociation prevents ideal mixing and contributes to maldigestion, malabsorption, and weight loss. This effect is accentuated after a Billroth II anastomosis because food passes from the stomach into the efferent limb before pancreatic and biliary secretions reach the efferent limb. Malabsorption also occurs after various operative procedures because pancreatic secretions are decreased, bile acids are diluted below the critical micellar level, and bacterial colonization in the afferent limb causes a blind loop syndrome.

ANEMIA

Anemia after gastric resection, if not due to blood loss, is due to a nutritional deficiency of iron, vitamin B_{12} or folate. Iron deficiency plays the most important role in the development of chronic anemia, but anemia may be the result of any combination of iron, B_{12}, and folate deficiencies. Patients deficient in these substances consume adequate amounts of these nutrients despite a lowered food intake. After gastric resection, iron deficiency anemia in the absence of chronic blood loss results from malabsorption of organic or food-bound iron. Deficiency in B_{12} is also a malabsorption problem due to decreased intrinsic factor or to malabsorption of food-bound B_{12}. In patients with a blind loop syndrome and bacterial overgrowth, B_{12} deficiency my be due to its more effective absorption by bacteria than the intestinal mucosa.

BONE DISEASE

Osteomalacia and osteoporosis may be preexisting conditions that are exacerbated by gastric operations or they may be long-term complications following gastric operations. They are more commonly observed in women than men and occur less commonly after vagotomy and pyloroplasty than after gastric resection. Malabsorption of vitamin D or calcium rather than their decreased dietary intake is responsible for these postoperative bone diseases. Patients with and without osteomalacia consume approximately the same amount of calcium and vitamin D and exhibit the same degree of steatorrhea after gastric surgery. Whether a patient develops bone disease as a long-term complication of gastric operation may depend on the patient's being subjected simultaneously to a secondary cause for calcium demineralization. This may account for its occurring with greater frequency in the postmenopausal female.

ZOLLINGER-ELLISON SYNDROME

Zollinger-Ellison syndrome is due to a malignant, well-differentiated slow-growing non-β islet cell tumor (gastrinoma). It arises primarily in the pancreas, but may occur in the submucosa of the duodenal wall and rarely in the antrum. These tumors produce large amounts of gastrin, causing hypergastrinemia and hypersecretion of acid (>10 mEq/hr) that ultimately lead to peptic ulcer or diarrhea. Patients with a gastrinoma have an increased number of parietal cells that secrete in response to hypergastrinemia at near maximal capacity in the basal state. As a guide, acid secretion in response to further stimulation by Histalog, histamine, or pentagastrin is less than twice the basal level in hypersecretors who have a gastrinoma. The clinical manifestations may be diarrhea alone, but there are usually peptic symptoms associated with virulent ulcers frequently found in unusual locations. Peptic symptoms, in the absence of an ulcer, can be due to duodenitis that precedes the development of an ulcer. The absence of ulcer or ulcer symptoms suggests that the gastroduodenal mucosa of some patients has a uniquely powerful cytoprotective mechanism.

Diarrhea in patients with a gastrinoma is related to the high acid concentration in the duodenum causing inactivation of the pancreatic enzymes and maldigestion. Diarrhea in this syndrome must be distinguished from the diarrhea in the WDHA syndrome where there is *w*atery *d*iarrhea associated with *h*ypokalemia and *a*chlorhydria secondary to a non-β islet cell tumor making an as yet unknown peptide or an unknown combination of known peptides.

The Zollinger-Ellison tumor may be a part of a multiple endocrine adenomatosis syndrome (MEA-I) in which there may be additional adenomas in the parathyroid or pituitary glands. Contrary to a previously held view, evidence does not support an association between hyperparathyroid and peptic ulcer disease unless the parathyroid disease is a part of the MEA-I syndrome. Parathyroid disease is present in excess of 25% of patients with a gastrinoma. Removal of the parathyroid disease may have an ameliorating effect on the gastrinoma.

An interesting aspect of the secretory characteristics of a patient with a gastrinoma is the paradoxical response secretin exerts on acid secretion and the serum gastrin level. Rather than causing their inhibition as occurs in a normal individual, secretin increases serum gastrin and acid secretion. These responses to secretin and similar responses to the infusion of calcium contribute to the diagnosis of a gastrinoma, especially in patients in whom the serum gastrin levels are borderline elevated.

The therapy for a gastrinoma can be separated into the periods before and after the introduction of histamine H_2-antagonists. Prior to these drugs, the tumor was resected if sufficiently localized to do so without performing a total pancreatectomy. Unfortunately approximately 60% of gastrinomas are malignant and have metastasized by the time the patients are explored. Under these conditions it was thought that anything less than total gastrectomy was inadequate because of the unacceptably high rates of recurrent ulcer and mortality associated with lesser operations. Since the advent of histamine H_2-antagonists, there are many whose opinion regarding the operative treatment remains unchanged. There is growing support, however, for a less radical form of treatment of gastrinomas which consists of the use of H_2-blockers alone or H_2-blockers combined with parietal cell vagotomy or selective vagotomy and antrectomy. This is a particularly good solution for the problem patient who has signs of a gastrinoma but no tumor can be found. The actual role of H_2-blocking agents has not been completely defined, but they have aided in the preoperative preparation of patients with gastrinomas and may have an expanding role in their long-term management, making total gastrectomy unnecessary.

MALIGNANCIES OF THE STOMACH

GASTRIC CARCINOMA

There is a wide variation from one country to another in the number of patients who have carcinoma of the stomach. In the United States the frequency has steadily fallen in the past 30 years, yet in some countries including Japan, China and the USSR the rate of gastric cancer is high and essentially unchanged. The explanation for these differences is unknown but it is thought to be related to dietary and not genetic factors.

CLINICAL MANIFESTATIONS

Clinical features produced by carcinomas of the distal third of the stomach include pain, bleeding, and obstruction. Carcinoma of the middle and upper thirds of the stomach is a treacherous disease. Because of the stomach's capacious environment, cancer in these locations often causes no symptoms until it has become large and has metastasized.

Unfortunately the earliest clinical symptoms are vague and no different from those that the patient may have experienced intermittently in the past. Anorexia and weight loss are striking findings and sometimes may be related to dysphagia in patients with cancer at the gastric cardia extending into the esophagus. Paulino reported that gastric cancers were silent in 50% of his cases until extensive invasion of the gastric wall had occurred. Fifty percent of gastric cancers discovered by mass survey have no symptoms at all. The 5-year survival from gastric carcinoma has not improved in 30 years, mainly because of delayed diagnosis.

DIAGNOSIS

The diagnosis of gastric cancer can be confirmed by roentgenographic studies, endoscopy and multiple biopsies, or cytologic specimens obtained by brushing. With these techniques the diagnostic accuracy of gastric cancer should be nearly 100%; however, the error in diagnosis may still range from 5% to 10% in various institutions. These errors occur in ulcers that appear benign but have a small focus of carcinoma present. It is in asymptomatic patients with small ulcerating lesions and a small focus of cancer that the diagnostic accuracy is lowest. Yet it is with these patients

GASTRIC CANCER	
Etiology	Predominantly, types of adenocarcinoma: ulcerating, polypoid, superficial spreading, or linitis plastica Associated factors: diet, alcohol, achlorhydria
Dx	Epigastric pain, vomiting, weight loss, hematemesis, melena, dysphagia Upper GI series shows fixed deformity, mass, or ulceration Gastroscopy and biopsy CT scan for staging
Rx	Surgery: Radical gastrectomy (extent based on location of tumor and associated organ involvement) or palliative gastric bypass Chemotherapy: for nonresectable disease

that we have the greatest opportunity to improve the results of treatment of gastric cancer by earlier recognition and earlier treatment.

CLASSIFICATION

Gastric carcinomas can be divided into four morphological subdivisions: (1) ulcerating, (2) polypoid, (3) superficial spreading, and (4) linitis plastica (Figure 23-12). The prognosis of gastric cancer is related to size, location, the extent of its spread, and its degree of differentiation; the less differentiated, the greater is the likelihood of spread. The good results obtained by surgery in Japan are in part due to the prevalence of the superficial spreading cancer in that population. Gastric carcinomas can be categorized according to the TNM classification (see Chapter 14 and Table 14-3). The survival of patients with gastric cancer can be related to their TNM classification.

Sixty percent of gastric cancers originate in the distal half of the stomach and 40% in the pyloric gland area. The majority of patients have developed metastases by the time they are operated on. A mass may be felt within the abdomen, and metastatic disease may be palpated in the left supraclavicular area (Virchow's node) or in the pelvis on rectal examination (Blumer's shelf) in advanced cases. Other metastatic disease may be discovered by liver scans, ultrasonography, or body or brain CT scans. Metastatic disease can be confirmed by needle biopsies of these various areas performed under CT scan control. If there are no compelling reasons for operation such as bleeding or obstruction, patients with far advanced cancer may be spared an operation by this means.

Half of the patients with gastric cancer are anemic and have guaiac positive stools. From 20% to 30% of patients with adenocarcinoma of the stomach are achlorhydric, a finding that excludes the diagnosis of a benign gastric ulcer. On the other hand, the presence of acid in the stomach does not exclude the possibility that a lesion is malignant.

RESULTS OF OPERATIVE TREATMENT

The only possible cure for gastric cancer is surgery. Cohn in a large series of patients at Charity Hospital in New Orleans found the operability rate was 82% and the resectability rate was 48%. In a private clinic in the same city the operability rate was 82% and the resectability rate was 33%. The overall 5-year survival, however, in the two institutions was a dismal 7.0% and 5.5%, respectively.

In patients who undergo resection, efforts are made to remove the involved stomach, regional lymph nodes, and involved adjacent organs. To accomplish this for lesions in the proximal and middle thirds of the stomach, esophagogastrectomy or a total gastrectomy may be required. Because of reflux esophagitis in survivors, Paulino recommended jejunal interposition after resection. This may be done through a thoracic or combined thoracoabdominal incision. There are virtually no 5-year survivors regardless of the type of operation performed for patients with stage III and IV cancers in the cardia. The 5-year survival for resected stage I cancers in the cardia at the Memorial Sloan-Kettering Cancer Center approached 50%. Results were best with extended total gastrectomy, which might be expected if one considers the potential node metastases from such a lesion (Fig. 23-13).

Results of operation for cancer in the middle and distal thirds of the stomach are also poor for stage III and IV cancers. Areas of lymph node metastases are similar to those for lesions in the cardia. Results are best with an extended subtotal or total gastrectomy, including removal of lymph nodes along the hepatoduodenal ligament, the perigastric

Fig. 23-12. Macroscopic classification of stomach carcinomas: (*A*) polypoid or fungating, (*B*) ulcerated, (*C*) infiltrating (linitis plastica), (*D*) superficial spreading. (Courtesy of Dr. Fernando Paulino)

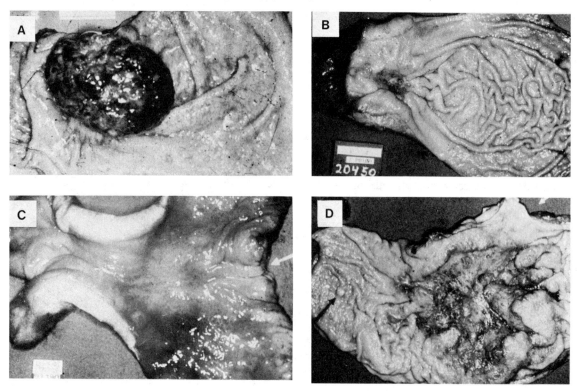

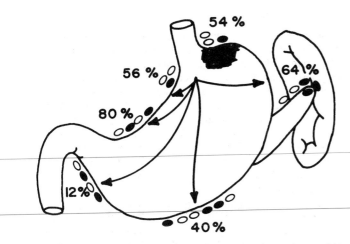

Fig. 23-13. Regional lymph node metastases in patients with adenocarcinoma of the cardia. (After McNeer and Pack)

lymph nodes including the left gastric artery, the majority of the lesser curvature, the greater omentum, spleen, and distal two thirds of the pancreas. Operative mortality is approximately 10%. The overall 5-year survival of those resected at Memorial Sloan-Kettering Cancer Center was 10% to 19%. The median survival of all cases, however, was three months. There has been little improvement in these statistics in 25 to 30 years. Yet there are some encouraging statistics when operation is for early gastric cancer. The cure rate in patients operated on for benign ulcer and found to have an unsuspected cancer in the ulcer is 80%. This demonstrates the need for early diagnosis of gastric cancer if the survival rate is to be improved.

Patients undergoing total gastrectomy can have their gastrointestinal continuity restored by constructing various types of pouches from the jejunum with the objective of providing increased storage and improved nutrition. In this regard, pouches have not been more successful than a Roux-en-Y esophagojejunostomy or the interposition of colon or small bowel between the esophagus and duodenum. After total gastrectomy many patients, but certainly not all, do well nutritionally, but others are bothered to various degrees by dumping, diarrhea, reflux esophagitis, and weight loss. After distal subtotal gastrectomy, continuity is usually reconstructed with an antecolic Polya type gastrojejunostomy. The opportunity for obstruction by recurrent tumor is less with a wide anastomosis performed remote from the area of the duodenum. After proximal subtotal gastrectomy, continuity is restored by an end-to-side esophagogastrectomy. A pyloroplasty is done to prevent stasis after the inevitable vagotomy that accompanies this type of resection.

LYMPHOMAS

Lymphosarcoma of the stomach is an infrequent lesion in comparison with adenocarcinoma. The symptomatology and the diagnostic procedures used are similar to those for adenocarcinoma. Lymphomas assume the gross characteristics of a carcinoma. The histologic patterns are similar to lymphomas in other organs. Treatment of choice consists of resection and radiation therapy if the lesion is localized and chemotherapy if the lesion is disseminated. For those patients resected there is approximately a 50% 5-year survival rate.

LEIOMYOMA AND LEIOMYOSARCOMA

Leiomyomas and leiomyosarcomas are submucosal. They contribute to vague gastrointestinal symptoms but are usually discovered because of gastrointestinal bleeding or because their size impinges on the stomach limiting its capacity. The lesions can extend into the lumen of the stomach, may be confined to the wall of the stomach, or may extend primarily into the abdominal cavity. The diagnosis is made by a characteristic roentgenographic appearance of a circumferential defect with an ulcerated area in the center. Large ulcerated tumors are often complicated by severe bleeding. Treatment is by resection of the stomach since the lesions are resistant to radiotherapy. Prognosis is guarded because it is often difficult to distinguish between benign and malignant lesions microscopically.

OTHER GASTRIC MALIGNANCIES

Other tumors of the stomach are exceedingly rare and include carcinoid tumors, plasmacytoma, glomus tumor, rhabdomyoma and rhabdomyosarcoma, and teratoma.

PREMALIGNANT GASTRIC CONDITIONS

ADENOMATOUS POLYPS

Adenomatous polyps of the stomach may be multiple or single. The hyperplastic adenomatous polyps are the most common. They are usually less than 2 cm, are composed almost entirely of mucus cells, and are benign. Papillary adenomas are like villous adenomas of the colon. They are usually larger than 2 cm, and malignancy has been observed in 25% to 75%. Whether a benign polyp grows and ultimately becomes malignant is an unsettled issue. Polyps occur with greater frequency in areas of chronic gastritis and intestinal metaplasia. Single polyps that are not too large may be removed through the gastroscope. Papillary polyps are more sinister, and an operative approach should be used in their treatment. Multiple polyps involving a local area in the stomach can be removed by a limited resection of the gastric wall. If the entire stomach is involved in multiple polyposis, the large polyps can be removed and the small polyps can be observed, or a total gastrectomy (a rarely indicated procedure) can be done. The indicated course depends on age, medical condition of the patient, complications resulting from the polyps, extent of polyp involvement, and the presence or absence of cancer.

A hyperplastic polyp on a long stalk and near the pylorus may prolapse through the pylorus and cause intermittent gastric obstruction. This requires removal of the polyp either endoscopically or by operation.

CHRONIC GASTRITIS

Chronic gastritis, well described by Chatterjee, embraces a variety of lesions involving the fundic gland area of the stomach and is a separate entity from antral gastritis. Chronic gastritis and achlorhydria may occur with or without the presence of antibodies to parietal cells and intrinsic factor and with or without pernicious anemia. The low acidity in the lumen of patients with chronic gastritis is the result of a reduced parietal cell mass, back diffusion of hydrogen ions through a defective mucosal barrier, and dilution of hydrogen ions in the gastric lumen by a nonparietal cell secretion. Gastritis of the pyloric gland area is more common than gastritis of the fundic gland area, but the frequency of both types of gastritis is greater in patients with gastric than duodenal ulcers. Chronic gastritis is common after gastric operations, yet the frequency of gastric ulcers is not increased in these patients. On the other hand, gastric carcinoma is a recognized late complication (15 to 20 years) of gastric resection. Whether chronic gastritis causes diseases such as gastric ulcer, pernicious anemia, and carcinoma of the stomach or is simply associated with these diseases is unknown.

MISCELLANEOUS GASTRIC AND DUODENAL PATHOLOGY

GASTRIC DIVERTICULA

Gastric diverticula are pulsion type diverticula and are located near the esophagogastric junction, usually on the lesser curvature. They must not be confused with a gastric ulcer. They are usually an incidental finding and are almost always asymptomatic.

GASTRIC BEZOAR

Gastric bezoar may be composed of matted hair (trichobezoars) in mentally deranged patients who eat their hair or of vegetable fibers (phytobezoars). The latter are not uncommon in patients who have had a gastric resection. Bezoars can cause gastric outlet obstruction, pressure necrosis, and bleeding. Although they may be broken up by the use of an endoscope or by the ingestion of a proteolytic agent, they may require surgical removal. Gastroenterologists have broadened the term *bezoar* to include a collection of food in the stomach or residual stomach pouch. They make the diagnosis with increased frequency and have had increasing success with endoscopic treatment.

MENETRIER'S DISEASE

In Menetrier's disease the gastric rugae are very large and are recognized as being abnormally large on roentgenographic studies or at endoscopy. Acid secretion is normal or below normal, but protein loss can be so great as to cause hypoproteinemia. Blood loss may also be a problem. If protein or blood loss is sufficiently great, high subtotal or even total gastrectomy may be the indicated treatment since there is no satisfactory medical management.

MALLORY-WEISS SYNDROME

Mallory-Weiss syndrome is characterized by upper gastrointestinal bleeding following vomiting and forceful retching. On endoscopic examination a linear tear through the mucosa and submucosa for a distance of 1 to 3 cm will be seen in the area of the esophagogastric junction. Almost all of these lesions will stop bleeding spontaneously or with the infusion of intravenous pitressin. For the few that do not stop, a generous longitudinal gastrotomy near the esophagogastric junction is necessary for exposure of the lesion so that it may be oversewn.

GASTRIC VOLVULUS

Gastric volvulus may be in the long axis or the transverse axis of the stomach. In the former, the tethering mechanisms of the stomach (*i.e.*, the gastrocolic, gastrohepatic, or gastrosplenic ligaments) are lax. Volvulus in the transverse axis of the stomach is usually associated with a paraesophageal hiatal hernia or an eventration of the diaphragm. Acute volvulus with obstruction or vascular compromise of the stomach is associated with a 50% mortality and therefore represents a surgical emergency. Chronic volvulus or torsion may be unrecognized because of the absence of symptoms. It also may be unrecognized for many years because the symptoms of pain, bloating, eructation, and pyrosis are so nonspecific. The diagnosis is made by roentgenographic and endoscopic studies. Treatment of this condition is surgical and consists of restoring the stomach to its normal position, anterior gastropexy, and repair of any diaphragmatic defects present.

DUODENAL DIVERTICULA

Duodenal diverticula are common and occur along the medial side of the duodenum. They occur most commonly in the vicinity of the ampulla of Vater and extend into the head of the pancreas. They are to be distinguished from the pseudodiverticula associated with duodenal ulcer disease. It is dangerous to ascribe symptoms of abdominal pain or dyspepsia to these lesions for lack of any other pathology to which symptoms can be attributed. Hemorrhage, perforation, pancreatitis, and biliary obstruction have all been reported to occur in association with duodenal diverticula; however, duodenal diverticula rarely cause symptoms and almost never require operative treatment. If surgery is indicated, identification of the common bile duct is essential to prevent its injury. Whether the diverticulum is treated by resection or inversion into the duodenum will depend on the existing anatomical and pathologic conditions.

MALIGNANT DUODENAL TUMORS

Malignant tumors of the duodenum besides those of the ampulla of Vater are rare. They are either adenocarcinoma, leiomyosarcoma, or lymphomas. The presenting symptoms are pain, bleeding, or obstruction, and they can be diagnosed by roentgenographic studies or endoscopy. A common area for cancer is at the duodenojejunal junction. This area requires close scrutiny by the radiologist because it lies behind the stomach and can be easily overlooked. Treatment of these lesions is best accomplished by pancreaticoduodenal resection if they are sufficiently localized. Lymphoma is the one lesion sensitive to radiation therapy.

BENIGN DUODENAL TUMORS

Benign tumors of the duodenum include pancreatic rests, lipomas, fibromas, and leiomyomas. More likely to cause symptoms are duodenal carcinoids, non-β islet cell tumors of the duodenum producing the Zollinger-Ellison syndrome, and Brunner's gland adenomas. The last lesion can cause duodenal and biliary obstruction and will require pancreaticoduodenectomy. Gastrinomas of the duodenum are quite small and are frequently found incidentally at the time of gastric resection. They are capable of producing the complete Zollinger-Ellison syndrome including metastases, but they do not possess the same malignant potential as comparable pancreatic lesions.

REGIONAL ENTERITIS

Regional enteritis occurs more commonly in the duodenum than in the stomach but it is uncommon in both locations. Complications of Crohn's disease of the duodenum include bleeding, fistula, and obstruction. Roentgenograms of the duodenum show mucosal changes and stenosis not unlike those seen when this disease occurs in the small bowel. The differential diagnosis of Crohn's disease of the duodenum as in the small bowel includes lymphoma. The diagnosis can usually be confirmed by its endoscopic appearance and biopsy. The medical treatment for Crohn's disease of the duodenum is nonspecific and similar to that for the small bowel. Surgery is indicated only for treatment of complications. Bypass gastrojejunostomy is the simplest operation with the prospect of providing symptomatic relief of pain and obstruction.

SUPERIOR MESENTERIC ARTERY SYNDROME

The superior mesenteric artery syndrome is obstruction of the third portion of the duodenum as it passes through the acute angle created by the superior mesenteric artery and the aorta. The poor therapeutic results that occurred from the overdiagnosis of this syndrome resulted in considerable skepticism regarding its actual existence. The diagnosis should be avoided as the explanation for symptoms in the nervous, dyspeptic patient with emesis. The syndrome has been well documented in burn patients who have had rapid weight loss. The acute loss of mesenteric fat during periods of malnutrition is thought to permit the artery to drop posteriorly, causing the duodenum to obstruct. The condition can usually be treated by having the patient eat in the prone position. As his nutrition is restored the syndrome will disappear. Only rarely should it be necessary to perform duodenojejunostomy to bypass the obstruction.

BIBLIOGRAPHY

CHATTERJEE D: Idiopathic chronic gastritis. Surg Gynecol Obstet 143:986, 1976

DAVENPORT HW: Physiological structure of the gastric mucosa. In Code CF (ed): Handbook of Physiology, Alimentary Canal, vol 2, p 759. Washington, DC: American Physiological Society, 1967

GOLIGER JC, DE DOMBAL FT, DUTHIE HL et al: Five to eight year results of Leeds-York controlled trial of elective surgery for duodenal ulcer. Br Med J 2:781, 1968

GRIFFITH CA: Surgery of the stomach and duodenum. In Nyhus LM, Wastell C (eds): Surgery of the Stomach and Duodenum, 3rd ed, pp 41–65. Boston, Little, Brown & Co, 1977

GROSSMAN MI: Integration of neural and hormonal control of gastric secretion. Physiologist 6:349, 1963

HUNT JN, STUBBS DF: The volume and energy content of meals as determinants of gastric emptying. J Physiol (London) 245:209, 1975

JORDAN PH JR: A follow-up report of a prospective evaluation of vagotomy-pyloroplasty and vagotomy-antrectomy for treatment of duodenal ulcer. Ann Surg 180:259, 1974

JORDAN PH JR: Current status of parietal cell vagotomy. Ann Surg 184:659, 1976

KELLY KA, CODE CF: Canine gastric pacemaker. Am J Physiol 220:112, 1971

LITTMAN A (ed): The Veterans Administration Cooperative Study on Gastric Ulcer. Gastroenterology, vol 61, no. 4, part 2. Baltimore, Williams & Wilkins, 1971

McNEER G, PACK GT: Neoplasms of the Stomach. Philadelphia, J B Lippincott, 1967

OBRINK KJ, FLEMSTROM G (eds): Gastric Ion Transport. Acta Physiol Scand Special Supplement, Uppsala, Almquist and Wiksell, 1978

RICHARDSON CT, FELDMAN M, McCLELLAND RN et al: Effect of vagotomy in Zollinger-Ellison syndrome. Gastroenterology 77:682, 1979

RITCHIE WP JR (ed): Stress ulcer and erosive gastritis. World J Surg 5:135, 1981

VOGEL SB, HOCKING M, FELASCA C et al: Delayed gastric emptying of liquids and solids following Roux-en-Y biliary diversion. Ann Surg 194:494, 1981

WAY LW, CAIRNS DW, DEVENEY CW: The intestinal phase of gastric secretion: A pharmacological profile of entero-oxyntin. Surgery 77:841, 1975

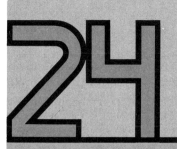

The Mesenteric Small Bowel

G. Robert Mason

Anatomy and Physiology

ANATOMY

GROSS

The mesenteric small bowel is approximately 20 feet in length; however, variations of plus or minus 5 feet are not uncommon. The intestine is a muscular tube lined with a mucous membrane which itself has mucosal folds; in the duodenum these are described as the valves of Kerckring and more distally as plicae circulares or valvulae conniventes. Each of these folds is covered with fingerlike projections of intestinal mucosal cells called villi (Fig. 24-1). Each of the intestinal mucosal cells has a convoluted luminal margin called a brush border. These anatomical structures serve to increase the absorptive area of the small bowel and to give further exposure for active enzymatic activity and passive transport of intestinal contents across the mucosa. Although it is not always apparent at which point the jejunum ends and the ileum begins, one may gain some assistance from the fact that *jejunum* is derived from the Greek *jejune*, "empty," and is often thought to be the proximal two fifths of mesenteric small bowel. Customarily, this portion of the small bowel is flaccid and without obvious intestinal content, as opposed to the ileum, which may contain some fluid content. The word *ileum* is derived from Latin for "coils or twists," perhaps thought to relate to the customary appearance of this portion of the distal small intestine.

MESENTERY

The mesentery of the small bowel centers upon its blood supply from the superior mesenteric artery and courses in a generally triangular form around the superior mesenteric artery and vein, going more to the right than to the left at the base of the mesocolon. Variations in mesenteric attachment to the left may on occasion form small indentations or peritoneal pockets, which have been described to contain portions of internally herniated small intestine. The mesenteric small bowel lies free and is mobile in the abdomen, save for the last few inches of terminal ileum, which is fixed with the cecum to the posterior abdominal wall.

BLOOD SUPPLY

As described above, the blood supply of the small intestine derives from the superior mesenteric artery; however, anastomoses are present, providing collateral circulation through the inferior pancreaticoduodenal artery anastomosing with the superior pancreaticoduodenal branch of the celiac artery and through the marginal artery of Drummond (arch of Riolan) anastomosing with the branches of the inferior mesenteric artery. Venous drainage of the small intestine is through the superior mesenteric vein, which joins the splenic vein and its tributary, the inferior mesenteric vein, to form the portal vein. This latter vein commonly commences just below the inferior margin of the surgical neck of the pancreas. At this point, the superior mesenteric vein is in

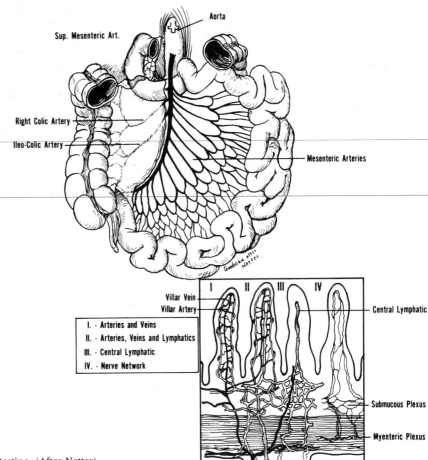

Fig. 24-1. Vascular supply of the small intestine. (After Netter)

relatively close proximity to the inferior vena cava, providing opportunities for anastomoses for relief of portal hypertension. The blood supply of the upper small intestine (jejunum) is primarily through a series of three or four long arcades that may be readily observed if the mesentery is held up to the light. These long arcades of arteries and veins make it possible to use loops of jejunum as drainage conduits or substitutes for esophagus or stomach. Because of the inherent curvature of the mesenteric loops, the jejunum customarily does not reach higher than the pulmonary hilus. Interposition of segments of jejunum, however, will reach to this point as a substitute for esophagus or as a substitute gastric pouch. More distally in the ileum, the branching of the terminal portion of the superior mesenteric artery is more treelike, with longer direct branches and communications of these vessels along the margin of the intestine. Throughout the bowel, there are small muscular branches to the longitudinal and circular coats of the small intestine penetrating the muscular wall at a somewhat oblique angle (rectal arteries). Branches then form a submucosal plexus that contains numerous arteriovenous shunts. Branches are sent from this submucosal plexus into the villi of the small intestine, forming arteriovenous loops within the villi. This provides the physiological basis for a countercurrent exchange mechanism within the villi, thus providing a dampening effect on the absorptive or secretory activity of the intestinal mucosa. Control of blood flow within the mucosa may depend on a variety of humoral agents, such as acetylcholine, prostaglandins, catecholamines, gastrin, serotonin, and other postulated transmitters. These agents may act directly on vessels throughout the mucosa but also may act on a precapillary sphincter mechanism. Exogenous drugs, such as digitalis, vasopressin, and analogues of naturally occurring substances, may also affect mucosal circulation.

LYMPHATICS

In general, the lymphatics of the small intestine follow the arterial supply. Beginning with central lacteals in the villi, leading to a submucosal lymphatic plexus, then exiting the muscular wall, the arcades of the arteries will customarily have clusters of lymph nodes gathered about them. There are also areas of lymphoid tissue in the wall of the distal half of the ileum. These Peyer's patches may be as long as an inch or more and are customarily found on the antimesenteric border of the distal half of the ileum; as a rule they are not found more proximally. Peyer's patches, as other lymphoid tissues in the body, are more prominent in young persons and less apparent in the aged. The lymphatic vessels drain into the main intestinal lymphatic trunk and then to the cisterna chyli. The lymphatics are the major transport route for absorbed lipid.

MUCOSA

The mucous membrane of the proximal small intestine is marked by plicae circulares, which are folds of the submucosa covered by a full thickness of mucous membrane. Toward the distal half of the small intestine, these plicae diminish in size and become less obvious and are not seen at all in the distal portions of the ileum.

INNERVATION

The parasympathetic and sympathetic outflow of the autonomic nervous system supplies the innervation of the mesenteric small bowel. The parasympathetic portion is mediated primarily through the vagus nerve (the tenth cranial nerve), which is distributed to the small intestine from celiac branches in the area of the diaphragmatic hiatus. Other vagal fibers may run separately through the sympathetic nervous system and will find their way through ganglia of the sympathetic nervous system to the small intestine. The sympathetic nervous system innervates the small intestine primarily through the ganglia found at the celiac and superior mesenteric arteries and derives largely from the distal dorsal vertebral roots. The preganglionic fibers of the parasympathetic nervous system travel to the myenteric and submucous plexus of the small intestine, where they form their first ganglia. Conversely, the ganglia of the sympathetic nervous system are located some distance from the small intestine on the aorta and form secondary ganglia within the wall of the small intestine and in the submucosa. Although the action of the parasympathetic nervous system is primarily to lower the threshold for mechanical activity and to enhance motility, the sympathetic nervous system acts in the reverse fashion, elevating the threshold for transmission of the basic electric rhythm (BER) to mechanical activity. There is yet a third modality for influence on intestinal activity. This third modality has been described as a nonadrenergic/noncholinergic nervous system and is described by some as the "purinergic" nervous system. The neurotransmitter substances in this third nervous system have not yet been sufficiently identified to describe in this text. In addition to the above standard types of innervation, there exists also a paracrine system, which consists of the substances described above related to the description of the control of blood flow within the mucosa; this system may also affect intestinal motility and secretion. These substances may be released by local factors such as mechanical stimulation, may be absorbed as a result of intraintestinal content acting upon the intestinal wall, or may be released by neural factors as a local phenomenon.

MICROSCOPIC

The outermost layer of the small intestine is the serosa. This is a single layer of flattened mesothelial cells overlying the longitudinal muscle layer and a small amount of loose connective tissue. The muscular wall of the intestine is composed of two layers of smooth muscle. The outer layer lies in the longitudinal axis of the intestinal tract and overlies an inner circular layer of muscle whose muscle cells are aligned in a perpendicular fashion to the axis of the small intestine. Between the longitudinal muscle layer and the circular muscle layer is a plexus of nerves called the myenteric plexus of Auerbach. Beneath the circular muscle is a second neural plexus called Meissner's plexus.

The submucosa contains a complex lymphatic drainage system and vascular network, as well as ganglion cells and nerve fibers going to the mucous membranes. The myenteric plexus of Auerbach and the submucous plexus of Meissner are interconnected intimately by numerous short nerve fibers. There appear to be connections also between the adrenergic and cholinergic nervous systems through these plexuses. In addition to its physiological function as a major pathway for the circulation and nervous system, the sub-

mucosa is the layer of greatest structural integrity in the wall of the small intestine. This layer is the layer of choice for strength in performing an intestinal anastomosis.

The intestinal mucosa has its own muscular layer, a muscularis mucosa, which is also composed of smooth-muscle cells separating the mucous membrane from the submucosa. The lamina propria is a connective tissue space lying between the muscularis mucosa and the true intestinal epithelium. The crypts in the mucosa of the small intestine (crypts of Lieberkühn) penetrate the lamina propria. In the lamina propria are also found many representatives of the white blood cell series, including eosinophils, mast cells, plasma cells, and lymphocytes. It has been postulated that this white blood cell layer may serve as a primary line of defense against invading bacteria. The lamina propria also contains collagenous, reticular, and elastic fibers. The mucosa then projects in needlelike fashion into the lumen of the intestine as villi. Each villus is surrounded by a relatively flat area of intestinal mucosa called the vestibule. At the base of each vestibule lie numerous crypts of Lieberkühn.

The crypts form a complex endocrine system composed of four different cell types, including Paneth's cells, goblet cells, enterochromaffin cells, and undifferentiated cells. Paneth's cells have been found to contain substances such as lysozyme, IgA, and IgG. The enterochromaffin cells have been divided into two groups, argentaffin and argyrophilic cells. The argentaffin cells have been associated with secretion of serotonin and bradykinin and with the carcinoid tumors. The argyrophilic cells are thought to be primarily related to the amine precursor uptake and decarboxylation (APUD) cells, which produce the various peptide hormones, such as gastrin, secretin, and cholecystokinin. The goblet cells produce mucus, which is said to protect and lubricate the intestinal mucous membrane. It is thought that the undifferentiated crypt cells form the base of the constant renewal of the intestinal epithelium. These cells divide very actively and migrate up to the tip of the villus with loss into the intestinal lumen in as rapidly as 1 to 3 days. Differentiation occurs as these cells migrate toward the tip of the villus, during which time they become mature absorptive intestinal cells with formation of microvilli or a brush border on their tip and apparently develop the active and passive transport mechanisms necessary for normal absorption. Although the major cell population of the villus is composed of absorptive cells, there are also goblet cells and some endocrine cells, which apparently also migrate up to the tip of the villi and are shed. In addition to the structural considerations of the mucous membrane, there is a glycoprotein coat, which is found to be applied directly to the brush border of the small intestine. The chemical composition of this glycoprotein is somewhat different from goblet-cell mucus. It is firmly attached to the brush border as long as the viability of the absorptive cells continues. This has been called by some the "fuzzy" layer of the mucous membrane.

PHYSIOLOGY

DIGESTION AND ABSORPTION

CARBOHYDRATE

Carbohydrate is broken down initially by α-amylases found in the salivary glands (ptyalin). This process is continued by pancreatic secretion of amylases that act upon starch and glycogen to form oligosaccharides. These oligosaccharides are then hydrolyzed by enzymes located on the absorptive surface of the small intestine. The breakdown products of simple sugars such as glucose, galactose, and fructose are derived from lactose and sucrose. They are carried across the intestinal epithelium by specific transport processes related in some cases to the presence of sodium on a mutual carrier protein. Some pentoses may be absorbed by diffusion; however, galactose and glucose are absorbed through active transport processes primarily in the upper and middle small intestine.

PROTEIN–IMMUNOLOGIC FUNCTION

Proteins are cleaved from complex structures to polypeptides beginning in the stomach with the enzyme pepsin, which has a *p*H optimum of 1.6 to 3.2. In the small intestine, the polypeptides are attacked by trypsin, which is derived from its precursor trypsinogen in pancreatic secretion. This precursor is activated by the enzyme enterokinase found in the duodenal mucosa. Trypsin then converts chymotrypsinogen into chymotrypsin and other procarboxypeptidases into carboxypeptidases. In addition, in the intestinal wall, there are aminopeptidases and dipeptidases to break down these proteins to small peptides and free amino acids. Some of the shorter peptides have active transport mechanisms into the intestinal cells, where they are hydrolyzed intracellularly. As a rule, there are active transport mechanisms for levo–amino acids, but dextro–amino acids are absorbed by passive diffusion. One active transport mechanism is available for neutral amino acids, one for basic amino acids, and another for such compounds as proline and hydroxyproline. Amino acids are absorbed throughout the length of the small intestine, perhaps in somewhat greater quantity in the middle small intestine. Here again, like sugar transport, this may be augmented by a high sodium concentration on the mucosal side of the intestinal epithelial cells. Once transported into the mucosal cells, the amino acids seem to diffuse in a passive way into the bloodstream. The protein content of the absorbed proteins comes approximately 50% from food ingestion, 25% from proteins in digestive juices, and 25% from shed mucosal cells. It is possible that some proteins may enter the circulation intact and may in this fashion form an antigenic stimulus for the intestinal lymphatic system to produce antibodies. Manifestations of interest include food allergies and the specific enteric resistance to certain bacterial infections such as cholera.

FAT

Fat is broken down by pancreatic lipase in the duodenum into monoglycerides and diglycerides. These are then emulsified by the detergent action of bile salts, which combine with monoglycerides and fatty acids to form aggregates called micelles. These lipids, in the form of monoglycerides and fatty acids, are absorbed through the intestinal mucosal cells; the short-chain fatty acids cross the cell and enter the portal vein directly, whereas the long-chain fatty acids become esterified to triglycerides within the cell and are then transported into the lymphatics as chylomicrons. The bile salts are carried in the lumen of the small intestine to the ileum, where they are reabsorbed for reexcretion in the bile. Fat absorption takes place primarily in the proximal small intestine; however, some absorption takes place throughout the small intestine. Normal excretion of fecal fat should not exceed 5% of that ingested.

WATER AND ELECTROLYTES

As chyme enters the small intestine, it is often hyperosmotic. This elicits the transfer of water from the wall of the small intestine to its lumen to approach isosmolal concentrations as the meal enters the jejunum. As osmotically active particles produced by digestion are absorbed across the mucous membrane, water is moved passively into the enteric circulation along the osmotic gradient created by transport mechanisms across the intestine. Water thus moves along an osmotic gradient into the intestinal circulation. There is an active transport mechanism associated with ions such as sodium and calcium. The carrier for calcium is located primarily in the upper small intestine. Its formation may be facilitated by high concentrations of vitamin D (1,25-dihydroxycholecalciferol). Iron absorption takes place in the ferrous state (Fe^{2+}), which is facilitated by the presence of ascorbic acid and other reducing substances in the diet. Iron is absorbed actively in the proximal portion of the small intestine. Iron passes into the bloodstream bound to a protein called apoferritin, which is then deposited in tissues in a complex with the protein ferritin. Vitamins such as A, D, E, and K (the fatty acid vitamins) are absorbed primarily in the proximal small intestine. Vitamin B_{12}, however, is complexed with intrinsic factor, a secretion of the parietal cells, and is absorbed almost exclusively in the distal ileum. It is thought that the complex of vitamin B_{12} (cyanocobalamin) is absorbed through the mechanism of pinocytosis.

MOTILITY

REGULATION OF THE MOTILITY OF THE SMALL INTESTINE

The smooth muscle of the wall of the intestine is characterized by an electrical slow wave with a characteristic rhythm or cycle that is peculiar to the intersphincteric portion of the intestinal tract. This slow-wave activity or BER is always present in viable smooth muscle. Mechanical activity or contraction may or may not be present but if present will be at the same rate as the BER for that area of the intestine. Mechanical activity is associated with superimposed spike activity on the BER. The presence of spike activity is augmented by the presence of nervous activity and circulating or local release of neurohumoral-type agents such as acetylcholine. Conversely, the inhibition of spike activity and mechanical activity is associated with circulating levels of neurohumors such as catecholamines. Other substances, such as prostaglandins, gastrin, cholecystokinin, and insulin, tend to stimulate contractions, while secretin and glucagon tend to inhibit them. It can be surmised that the increased outflow of catecholamines surrounding the trauma of anesthesia and surgery will tend to produce a period when mechanical activity of the small intestine is reduced. This is often seen as the postoperative ileus after abdominal operations.

SEGMENTARY CONTRACTION

When contractions occur in the normal state, they are usually in strictly localized areas of 4 cm to 10 cm of the intestinal tract. If food substances are present in the lumen at the time, this contraction may tend to move them either forward or backward and will tend to mix the contents with whatever digestive enzymes are present.

PENDULAR MOVEMENTS

If contractions are present at the same time in several different areas, they may tend to move the intestinal content back and forth in a pendular motion to assist in the above actions and give better exposure to the mucous membrane for absorptive purposes.

PERISTALSIS

From time to time, there will appear more highly coordinated contractile activity which is propulsive in an aboral direction. This has been commonly termed *peristaltic activity*. In general, these peristaltic rushes will occur over a larger area of intestine than the pendular motions but will not pass through the entire mesenteric small bowel. As a reflex within the intestinal tract, contractions are elicited by a bolus of material in the lumen; this contraction occurs on the oral side of the bolus, with relaxation distally. This is known as "Starling's law of the intestine." As this bolus passes distally, further reflexes are established that tend to propel the material through the length of the small intestine. From time to time, contractions will occur in the mesenteric small intestine which will pass the entire length of the small intestine. These "housekeeping waves" are most commonly seen in the interdigestive phase.

There are some substances that have been used for the purpose of radiologic study that tend to augment the peristaltic activity of the intestine and shorten the time required for small-bowel series. Such drugs as cholecystokinin and metoclopramide are currently commercially available for this purpose.

BIBLIOGRAPHY

CIBA Foundation Symposium No. 46: Immunology of the Gut. New York, Elsevier-Dutton, 1977

GLASS GBJ (ed): Gastrointestinal Hormones. New York, Raven Press, 1980

The Secretory Immunologic System. Washington, DC, US Government Printing Office, 1969

G. Robert Mason

Small Bowel Obstruction

Intestinal obstruction is a surgical problem which must be treated with expedition and judgment. The usual causes of mechanical obstruction are adhesions, external hernias, and malignancy. Customary therapy is oriented toward hydration, decompression, and operation.

HISTORY

The recognition of bowel obstruction as a lethal problem dates back many years in medical history. Operations for relief of strangulated hernia causing obstruction are described in standard surgical texts of the early 1800s. Successful relief of intra-abdominal obstruction was delayed until the advent of anesthetic agents in the middle years of the nineteenth century. The techniques of intestinal anastomosis were not available for successful use until the latter years of the nineteenth century. Operations were advised for intestinal obstruction during this period; however, mortality rates were extraordinarily high for a variety of reasons related to the late onset of antiseptic and aseptic technique. The delays inherent in operating on such patients, the knowledge that the outcome was extraordinarily poor, and the hope that enemas and supportive therapy might be helpful were also important factors. Osler in his textbook of medicine advises, among other things, elevating the patient by the feet in order to attempt to shift the bowel about inside the abdomen and relieve the obstruction. As late as the 1930s, it was advised that, in cases of intestinal obstruction, no resection or anastomosis be performed. Knowledge of bacterial content of the bowel and frequent culture of *Clostridium perfringens* (once called *Bacillus welchii*) led to the concept that the dilated small intestine filled with bacteria represented a form of potential sepsis and should be drained. Recommendations of enterotomy to remove the bacterial content were common in this period. The use of rubber tubes for gastric drainage was described by numerous authors in the early years of the twentieth century; however, routine use of nasogastric drainage was popularized by such individuals as Wangensteen and Levin in the early 1930s. Shortly thereafter, longer intestinal tubes were popularized by Miller and Abbott, Cantor, and others. Knowledge of fluid and electrolyte management, although recognized in the early years of the century, grew rapidly during the late 1930s and 1940s with routine use of intravenous infusions to aid in the resuscitation of these patients. The introduction of various antibiotics during and after the 1940s also assisted greatly in reduction of mortality. In spite of these many advances, the mortality rate for bowel obstruction still remains in the area of 8% overall, with elevations in cases of strangulation obstruction to as high as 20% to 30%.

ETIOLOGY

MECHANICAL OBSTRUCTION

The small intestine may be mechanically obstructed by obturation, intrinsic lesions, or extrinsic causes. *Obturation obstruction* is a term applied to internal masses such as polyps, gallstones, or intussusception. Intrinsic lesions may include atresia, congenital stenosis, and strictures from benign or malignant causes. Extrinsic causes include adhesions, anomalies of rotation, extrinsic malignancies, hernias, and volvulus.

PARALYTIC ILEUS

Normally, following operative procedures, a period of time exists where mechanical contractions of the intestine are not observed. This is related to hormonal changes and release of catecholamines following laparotomy or anesthetic agents. In most patients, the recovery from this ileus requires only hours to days. Injuries to the retroperitoneum such as inflammatory lesions, hemorrhage, or trauma may also cause ileus. It is thought that the mechanism involves the outflow of the sympathetic nervous system. Here again, the resolution of the inciting problem will lead to resumption of normal mechanical activity.

NORMAL FLUID FLUX OF THE INTESTINE

The upper gastrointestinal tract is the site of secretion of various digestive enzymes and of the preliminary stages of digestion. These secretions vary in volume but are generally described as in Table 24-1. The active secretion of intestinal juices (succus entericus) has been questioned. However, secretions may be elicited by hyperosmotic substances in the intestinal lumen. The more distal intestine and colon are primarily the sites of absorption of fluid and partially digested foodstuff. Thus, it may be anticipated that obstruction of the upper intestine will be accompanied by symptoms of nausea in the early stages because of bowel dilatation from unabsorbed secretions and ingesta. Later stages are characterized by vomiting of this material, with subsequent dehydration and electrolyte imbalance. The electrolyte contents of the juices listed in Table 24-1 are described in Table 24-2.

CHANGES DUE TO OBSTRUCTION

Obstruction at the pylorus thus results in a major loss of hydrogen and chloride ions, with resultant hypochloremic

TABLE 24-1 GASTROINTESTINAL SECRETIONS PER 24 HOURS

Salivary	1500 ml
Gastric	1000 ml
Pancreatic	2000 ml
Biliary	500 ml

TABLE 24-2 AVERAGE ELECTROLYTE CONTENT OF GASTROINTESTINAL SECRETIONS (IN mEq PER LITER)

	Na^+	K^+	Cl^-	HCO_3^-
Salivary	182	5	40	80
Gastric	140	6	120	25
Pancreatic	160	5	30	120
Biliary	145	5	40	50

Content varies with rate

alkalosis. Obstruction below the ampulla of Vater results in loss of Na^+, K^+ and HCO_3^-, resulting in generalized electrolyte depletion and dehydration and variable gaseous distention (Fig. 24-2). In contrast, an obstruction at the ileocecal valve may not involve external fluid loss and, in the absence of ingested air, may not even result in distention, although this is not usually the case. Mid small-intestinal obstruction is more likely to be associated with distention, particularly when excess air or exogenous fluids are swallowed.

As the bowel distends, contractile activity is stimulated, resulting in cramplike abdominal pain. The frequency of painful contraction of a partially or fully obstructed bowel is greater proximally than distally. Thus, an obstructed jejunum may give symptoms every 3 to 5 minutes, whereas the distal ileum may give symptoms only every 10 minutes or even less frequently. When air and fluid are present in the gut, the vigorous gut contractions will force jets of intestinal content into tense-walled but dilated loops of adjacent bowel, resulting in the high-pitched bowel sounds associated with bowel obstruction. Distention of the small intestine is felt initially as periumbilical pain. Pressure on dilated intestine from the examiner's fingers will cause further pain and guarding.

In situations where a segment of bowel has both ingress

	BOWEL OBSTRUCTION	
Etiology	Many causes	
	Small bowel: Adhesions, hernia, neoplastic, inflammatory, others	
	Large bowel: Neoplasm, volvulus, diverticular disease, and occasionally others	
Dx	Vomiting, crampy abdominal pain, distention, dehydration, surgical scar or palpable hernia, high-pitched bowel sounds	
	Abdominal x-ray film: Air-fluid levels in distended bowel; barium enema.	
	Variable electrolyte disorders	
	Peritonitis; sepsis if gangrenous bowel present	
Rx	Nasogastric suction	
	Intravenous hydration, Na^+ and K^+ replacement	
	Surgery: Herniorrhaphy and reduction	
	Celiotomy: adhesion lysis to bowel resection, colostomy, or other indicated procedures	

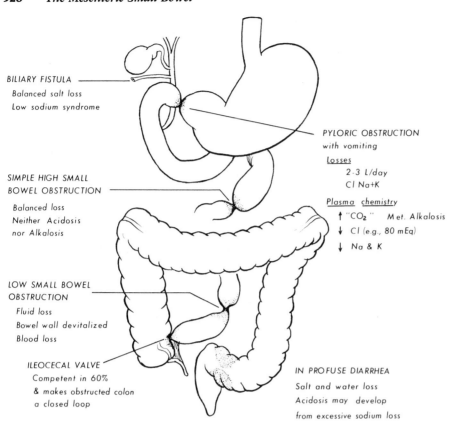

BILIARY FISTULA
Balanced salt loss
Low sodium syndrome

PYLORIC OBSTRUCTION
with vomiting
Losses
2-3 L/day
Cl Na+K
Plasma chemistry
↑ "CO₂"   Met. Alkalosis
↓ Cl (e.g., 80 mEq)
↓ Na & K

SIMPLE HIGH SMALL
BOWEL OBSTRUCTION
Balanced loss
Neither Acidosis
nor Alkalosis

LOW SMALL BOWEL
OBSTRUCTION
Fluid loss
Bowel wall devitalized
Blood loss

ILEOCECAL VALVE
Competent in 60%
& makes obstructed colon
a closed loop

IN PROFUSE DIARRHEA
Salt and water loss
Acidosis may develop
from excessive sodium loss

Fig. 24-2. Physiological derangements in alimentary obstruction. The fluid and electrolyte losses in alimentary tract obstruction are related to the level of the obstruction. The major clinical findings are cramping abdominal pain, distention, and hyperactive peristalsis. These, supported by appropriate radiological studies, are usually diagnostic.

and egress blocked, a so-called closed loop obstruction exists and will cause varying degrees of vascular obstruction. If only the venous drainage is blocked, the venular pressure in the countercurrent perfusion of intestinal villi gradually rises and favors secretion into the lumen until the intraluminal pressure equals that of the arteriolar supply. At this point, stagnation of the circulation occurs, and anoxic changes lead to gangrene of the intestinal wall, with resultant bacterial diffusion into the general cavity and peritonitis. The early inflammatory changes of anoxia lead to edema of the gut wall and often cause corresponding inflammatory changes ("neighborhood inflammation") in the parietes, resulting in localization of pain in that particular somatic dermatome. Hence, periumbilical pain in early appendicitis migrates to later localization in the right lower quadrant. Physicians must be aware of the possibility that such signs as white count elevation, fever and pain progression and localization are not present in as many as 15% of patients with acute inflammatory changes in the bowel. If the history and the physical findings are suggestive of closed loop bowel obstruction, it is often better to explore the abdomen than await more definitive signs of perforation and peritonitis.

CAUSES OF INTESTINAL OBSTRUCTION

Numerous reports in the literature document the changing pattern of causes of intestinal obstruction with the age of the patient and with the passage of time. In the very young, a different pattern is present from that in the adult (compare Tables 24-3 and 24-4). Increases in intervention by surgeons for various intra-abdominal diseases may have led to the relative importance of adhesions as a cause of intestinal obstruction early in life, compared with the rapid rise of

importance of hernia in middle and later years and the more gradual increase in importance of cancer in the later years. Changes in relative importance of the three major causes of intestinal obstruction in adults may be related to the development of better techniques of herniorrhaphy and the tendency to repair hernia whenever feasible. Comparing surveys of causes of obstruction since the late 1800s, hernia has dropped from its leading position as a cause of obstruction, above both adhesions and cancer, to yield to adhesions. Cancer has dropped to third place with the passage of time, originally being more common than adhesions. Patterns of intestinal obstruction by cause also vary with geographic location. Causes such as abdominal tuberculosis and vol-

TABLE 24-3 INTESTINAL OBSTRUCTION IN 110 CHILDREN*

CAUSE	NUMBER	PERCENT
Hernia	42	38
Pyloric stenosis	17	15
Ileocecal intussusception	16	15
Anomalies of rotation	6	5
Adhesions	8	7
Congenital atresia or stenosis	6	5
Imperforate anus	6	5
Annular pancreas	4	4
Meckel's diverticulum	2	2
Hirschsprung's disease	2	2
Colonocolic intussusception	1	1

*Wilson H, Hardy JD, Farringer JL: Intestinal obstruction. I. Causes and management in infants and children. Ann Surg 141:788, 1955

TABLE 24-4   SUMMARY OF CAUSES OF INTESTINAL OBSTRUCTION IN THIRTEEN STUDIES (11,697 ADULT PATIENTS)

CAUSE	NUMBER	PERCENT
Hernia	5222*	
Adhesions	3707	
Cancer	1211	97
Intussusception	481	
Volvulus	480	
Malrotation atresia	234	
Gallstones	107	
Vascular	70	
Meckel's diverticulum	63	
Foreign body	25	
Fecal impaction	21	
Tuberculosis	19	3
Appendiceal abscess	19	
Pelvic abscess	12	
Ileus	10	
Crohn's disease	9	
Mesenteric cyst	3	
Endometriosis	3	

* A number of recent reports indicate that adhesions now exceed external hernias as the commonest cause of small bowel obstruction in the United States.—ED.

vulus are more common in India, according to one report; in Ibadan, Africa, Ascaris infestation and ileocecal perforation such as from *Salmonella hyphora* assume greater importance as causes of obstruction. Institutions dealing with chronic mental diseases may find a high incidence of fecal impaction and volvulus as causes of obstruction.

In our experience, patients with prolonged fluid loss from vomiting or diarrhea, or with malnutrition, may also have ileus from depletion of such ions as calcium and magnesium. Serum levels of these ions should be obtained in such cases prior to reoperation for suspected obstruction.

DIAGNOSTIC AIDS

HISTORY

A history of previous operations or injuries or of known hernias or symptoms suggestive of neoplasm or inflammatory or anticoagulant treatment may be indicative of the cause and site of obstruction.

PHYSICAL EXAMINATION

Physical examination may reveal the signs indicated above under Changes Due to Obstruction.

RADIOLOGIC EXAMINATION

Radiologic studies may show dilated loops of intestine or perhaps the ladder sign, in which fluid levels in the distal segment of the visible loop are higher than the proximal segment. This sign is said to be indicative of mechanical obstruction. The presence of gas patterns throughout the small and large bowel should raise the suspicion of ileus.

If the diagnosis is unclear, an oral dose of radiopaque material such as Gastrografin may show the site of obstruction or may illustrate patency. Although barium is far better for intestinal mucosal detail, this information may not be necessary in all cases.

LABORATORY TESTS

Laboratory studies may show elevation of the white cell count, depending upon the stage of disease; however, in a reported series of 50 patients with strangulation of the small intestine, no leukocytosis was noted in 42%. Similarly, although elevation of temperature may serve as an indicator of gangrenous change, in the same series no temperature elevation was noted in 70% of cases. Electrolyte and hydration aberrations may occur as noted above under Changes Due to Obstruction. These aberrations may indicate the level of obstruction and must be detected and corrected, preferably preoperatively. Urine examination may show evidence of dehydration but, more importantly, may also reveal pyuria from urinary tract infection or from adjacent inflammatory disease. These may produce symptoms indistinguishable from intestinal obstruction.

TREATMENT OF INTESTINAL OBSTRUCTION

Initial efforts at therapy must be oriented toward replacement of fluid and electrolytes and administration of necessary medications such as digitalis and steroids. The excellent contributions of Wangensteen, Cantor, and others in regard to the use of long tubes to decompress the dilated intestine have often focused the attention of house staff and attending surgeons on the passage of a mercury-filled bag rather than on the underlying problem. Nonetheless, the removal of gastrointestinal secretions by a Levin or a longer tube will aid in prevention of tracheal aspiration of these secretions, as anesthesia is induced, and may buy time for diagnostic or therapeutic efforts. However, as Cantor has stated, "Intestinal intubation and decompression of the GI tract should never be considered as a substitute for surgery."

In contrasting nonoperative management of intestinal obstruction with operative management, the risks of unrecognized gangrene must be compared to operative risk. In Smith's study of 447 patients managed 24 hours or longer by nasogastric suction, 16 developed gangrene, an incidence of 3.6%. Four died; the consequent mortality rate was 25%. This is comparable to immediate operation for recognized gangrene in 41 patients with 9 deaths, a mortality of 22%, and should be contrasted with a mortality rate of less than 1% for laparotomy for bowel obstruction without gangrene. It should not be assumed that nasogastric suction will obviate intervention, however, since 79.6% of 716 patients with small bowel obstruction in this series required operations. The treatment of intestinal obstruction can be summarized in three words: decompression, hydration, and surgery.

INITIAL THERAPY

A general recommendation is to place a nasogastric tube in all patients thought to have intestinal obstruction. After replacement of necessary fluids and electrolytes, patients with grave abdominal and physical signs are taken to the operating room. Because patients vary, a strict formula cannot be given; however, grave signs include localized abdominal tenderness and rigidity with leukocytosis (10,000$^+$) and fever. Patients over 65 years of age, mental patients, and neonates tend to be placed in the urgent surgery category. Neonates are included because of the incidence of congenital lesions requiring surgical correction. Older patients tolerate infection less well than those younger and, like mental patients, often do not have the classic abdominal symptoms and physical signs of intestinal gangrene.

The remaining or nonemergency group of patients may be more safely treated by intubation, preferably with a long mercury-weighted tube such as the Cantor tube. Careful reevaluation is necessary for signs of intestinal necrosis. There are several diagnostic entities in which more careful evaluation may benefit the patient. First, in approximately 20% of patients with small bowel obstruction, primarily that resulting from adhesions, the obstruction may resolve and the patient escape operation and further adhesions. The temptation to follow this therapy is stronger in patients with a history of multiple prior operations for obstruction due to adhesions. A second group includes problems such as colon malignancy and diverticulitis. With reduction of fecal passage, the edema and inflammation may subside and allow more accurate diagnosis and thorough bowel preparation. This is particularly true with diverticulitis. A third entity includes radiation enteritis and regional enteritis. Here a more accurate estimate of extent of severity of disease will allow for more rational therapy and long-range benefit to the patient. The last problem, fecal impaction, is found primarily in mentally ill patients but is not uncommon in the elderly. Rectal examination and abdominal x-ray films usually are diagnostic. The condition can produce serious hemorrhage from stercoraceous ulcer and peritonitis or death from perforation. Vigorous but gentle efforts with manual extraction, enemas, and cathartics usually alleviate the problem.

Because of the frequent insecurity relative to presence or absence of gangrenous bowel, it is advisable to consider administration of prophylactic antibiotics. The literature on prophylactic antibiotics is voluminous and will serve as a source of continuing discussion for some time. As a general rule, a broad-spectrum antibiotic such as ampicillin administered in doses of one gram preoperatively may serve as adequate prophylaxis. Other drugs of the cephalosporin group may also be considered.

OPERATIVE THERAPY

APPROACHES AND PROCEDURES

In general, we advocate the use of a general anesthetic with airway control through endotracheal intubation. A midline incision is customary. If previous scars are present, it is often wise to approach the midline through a previously uninvolved area, if possible.

The operative procedure itself should be accompanied by a thorough abdominal examination and a complete examination of the intestinal tract to make sure that not only will an obvious obstructive area be treated but other possible areas of obstruction will also be recognized and treated appropriately. In cases where numerous operations for adhesions have been performed and recurrent obstruction due to adhesions has been the presenting problem, a long tube has been placed as a stent throughout the entire length of the intestine in an effort to prevent further recurrence. This tube serves the dual purpose of stenting the bowel and decompressing it. It has been our feeling that various forms of intestinal plication are not useful and are often dangerous and should not be performed.

POSTOPERATIVE CARE

The electrolyte balance of patients with third space sequestration is often the first major consideration in management of this group of patients. A second major consideration has to do with respiratory problems. Distended bowel placed back into the abdominal cavity will press the diaphragm upward and lead to increased atelectasis and pneumonia. The rationale of decompression to promote ease of closure and easier respiratory management must be balanced by the risks of bacterial contamination from the open bowel. Wound infection rates rise precipitously when aspiration is performed. Also, it has been noted by some that a moderate degree of distention is often associated with a more rapid return of peristaltic activity than in the totally decompressed bowel. Wound infections and fistulas are common in patients with previous obstructions relative to leakage of intestinal content secondary to bowel wall damage.

MORTALITY

In the patient with a single focus of obstruction such as a fibrous band, which is easily lysed without intestinal distension or necrosis, mortality should be that of a routine laparotomy for such patients and usually will be under 1%. At the other end of the scale, a patient with necrotic bowel may have a mortality rate approaching 20% to 30%. Other complicating features (such as those described above with infection, respiratory embarrassment, and fistulas) will lead to similarly increased mortality rates.

ILEUS

Paralytic ileus may be thought of in physiologic terms as the loss of mechanical activity of the small bowel. This is a normal postoperative phenomenon and customarily lasts from three to five days after a major operation, less than two days after a more minor procedure. In some cases, the stomach or colon may be subject to prolonged periods of atony or ileus, particularly in the distended stomach that has been subjected to vagotomy, or in the colon as in Ogilvie's syndrome, which is associated with catastrophic events elsewhere in the body not necessarily related to the gastrointestinal tract, such as myocardial infarction or pneumonia. The customary treatment of postoperative ileus is nasogastric intubation and intestinal decompression.

In otherwise uncomplicated procedures, ileus lasting beyond five days should be suspected of being obstructive in nature, and mechanical obstruction should be ruled out by the methods described earlier. Terms such as *gallstone ileus* have been used to describe the obturation of the small intestine, usually the ileum, by a gallstone that has passed through a cholecystoduodenal or cholecystoenteric fistula into the intestinal tract to a point where it obstructs the bowel lumen. These patients can sometimes be identified by the fact that they are almost always elderly, may have a visible stone of visible opacity usually in the right lower quadrant of the abdomen, and, more important, may have visible air in the biliary tract. Customary treatment for gallstone ileus is to milk the stone back to a relatively normal portion of bowel and remove the stone. Because of attendant problems of age and metabolic problems related to the bowel obstruction, it is often not advisable to proceed to a cholecystectomy, biliary reconstruction, or treatment of a cholecystoduodenal fistula at the time of removal of the biliary stone.

Ileus may also occur in a more drastic sense with a vascular necrosis of the bowel wall or with adjacent inflammation or with such retroperitoneal problems as infection or hemorrhage. Perforation of the gastrointestinal tract with leakage of irritant substances such as acid or bile or formation of abscess will also cause regional or generalized ileus. The treatment of these forms of ileus is inherent in the diagnosis and treatment or the underlying problem. Various forms of pharmacologic therapy have been thought to be efficacious in the treatment of ileus. Drugs such as bethanechol or Urecholine have been advocated. Others have thought that adrenergic blockade might be effective. In general, the use of these drugs as cholinergic stimulants has not been sufficiently effective to warrant their routine use. Conversely, the side-effects associated with adrenergic blocking agents have made them equally undesirable. The use of electrical stimulation for the gut in the postoperative period has been advocated by some but, again, has not been sufficiently efficacious to warrant its routine use.

BIBLIOGRAPHY

AGARWAL SL, SINGH RP: A review of intestinal obstruction. Int Surg 46:113, 1966

BECKER SF: Intestinal obstruction: An analysis of 1007 cases. South Med J 48:41, 1955

CANTOR MO, REYNOLDS RP: Gastrointestinal Obstruction. Baltimore, Williams & Wilkins, 1957

COHN I JR: Intestinal Antisepsis. Springfield, IL, Charles C Thomas, 1968

COLCOCK BP, BRAASCH JW: Surgery of the small intestine in the adult. In Dunphy JE (ed): Major Problems in Clinical Surgery, VII. Philadelphia, W B Saunders, 1968

COLE GJ: A review of 436 cases of intestinal obstruction in Ibadan. Gut 6:151, 1965

GIBSON CL: A study of one thousand operations for acute intestinal obstruction and gangrenous hernia. Ann Surg 32:486, 1900

GILL SS, EGGLESTON FC: Acute intestinal obstruction. Arch Surg 91:589, 1965

KEEN WW: Surgery. Philadelphia, W B Saunders, 1907

LEE PWR: The leucocyte count in acute appendicitis. Brit J Surg 60:618, 1973

LEFFALL LD, QUANDER J, SUPHAX B: Strangulation intestinal obstruction. Arch Surg 91:592, 1965

MASON GR, DIETRICH P, FRIEDLAND GR et al: The radiological findings in radiation induced enteritis and colitis. Clin Radiol 21:232, 1970

MASON GR, GUERNSEY JM, HANKS GE et al: Surgical therapy for radiation enteritis. Oncology 22:241, 1968

MISHRA NK, APPERT HE, HOWARD JM: The effects of distention and obstruction on the accumulation of fluid in the lumen of small bowel of dogs. Ann Surg 180:791, 1974

PANCOAST J: Operative Surgery. Philadelphia, Carey and Hart, 1844

SMITH GA, PERRY JE, YOEHIRO EG: Mechanical intestinal obstructions: A study of 1252 cases. Surg Gynecol Obstet 100:651, 1955

TENDLER MJ, STREETER AN, CARTWRIGHT RS: Acute intestinal obstruction. Southern Surgeon 13:551, 1947

VICK RM: Statistics of acute intestinal obstruction. Br Med 2:546, 1932

WALDRON GW, HAMPTON JM: Intestinal obstruction, a half century comparative analysis. Ann Surg 153:839, 1961

WANGENSTEEN OH: Early diagnosis of acute intestinal obstruction with comments on pathology and treatment with report of successful decompression of three cases of mechanical bowel obstruction by nasal catheter suction siphonage. Western J Surg 40:1, 1932

WELCH CE: Intestinal Obstruction. Chicago, Year Book Medical Publishers, 1958

WICKSTROM P, HAGLIN JJ, HITCHCOCK CR: Intraoperative decompression of the obstructed small bowel. Surgery 73:212, 1973

WILSON H, HARDY JD, FARRINGER JL: Intestinal obstruction. I. Causes and management in infants and children. Ann Surg 141:788, 1955

James D. Hardy

Small Bowel Trauma, Fistula, and Radiation Injury

SMALL BOWEL TRAUMA

CAUSES AND PATHOLOGY

Trauma to the mesenteric small bowel is common. The most frequent cause in most civilian hospitals is probably gunshot wounds, either with shotgun pellets or with bullets from pistols and rifles. However, the relative incidence of gunshot injuries compared with, for example, blunt trauma from motor vehicle accidents will vary with the population served by the given hospital. At the extremes, gunshot wounds may be expected to be penetrating or perforating injuries that may leave multiple holes in the intestine, whereas blunt trauma may "mash" a segment of the small bowel against the spine and cause a partial laceration or even a complete division of the gut at that point, with varying degrees of injury to the mesentery and its vasculature (Fig. 24-3). Complete division of the duodenum in its retroperitoneal position may occur, and signs and symptoms of it may not appear for many hours. However, a gunshot at close range can do just as much blast damage as blunt trauma, and the severity of the pathologic findings at operation tends to be basically similar for both types of injury, except that the gunshot injury will often involve more loops of bowel and perhaps greater overall damage. Knife wounds may not have penetrated the intestine, but the possibility of such injury cannot be ignored and must be excluded before the patient is discharged. There are of course many other possible mechanisms of traumatic injury to the small intestine, but penetrating and blunt trauma are the most common causes.

Peritonitis and continuing small bowel leakage will ensue and usually cause death of the patient if the gut injury is not repaired. However, some small perforations, especially from shotgun pellets fired at a distance of 40 to 50 yards, may not leak sufficiently to produce significant small bowel leakage and fatal peritonitis.

DIAGNOSIS

The general approach to the diagnosis and management of small bowel trauma is presented in Chapter 10, and only a few points of diagnosis need be emphasized here. First, virtually all penetrating gunshot wounds of the abdomen must be explored by laparotomy. Occasionally, by dissecting along the tract and making use of support by peritoneal lavage, it can be determined that the bullet or knife did not enter the peritoneal cavity. If so, formal laparotomy is not required. However, if the knife or missile did penetrate the abdominal wall, it is safer to explore. Prompt operation generally allows effective repair without the hazard of fully developed peritonitis and the resultant potential complications entailed by late repair. A major hazard of late operation is subsequent breakdown of intestinal anastomoses or of vascular anastomoses performed at the first operation, often with fatal results.

At times, an experienced surgeon can, by means of the history, physical examination, roentgenographic studies, and other measures, determine that it is safer to place the patient under close observation and defer any operation. This is acceptable provided that an experienced observer examines the patient at frequent intervals to look for changes in the vital signs, the abdomen, and the white blood cell count. Blunt trauma to the intestine may be initially overlooked in a patient with multiple other injuries unless hemorrhage from the mesentery, spleen, or liver prompts exploratory laparotomy for this hidden blood loss. Moreover, blunt trauma may not be manifested until long afterward;

Fig. 24-3. Common types of injury to the small intestine. Extensive injury or gangrene will require resection. It may be feasible to close small perforations without resection.

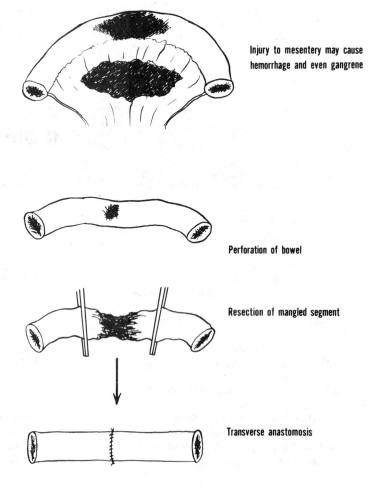

Injury to mesentery may cause hemorrhage and even gangrene

Perforation of bowel

Resection of mangled segment

Transverse anastomosis

for example, an old seatbelt injury may result in stenosis and obstruction.

MANAGEMENT

The important first step is to determine that prompt exploratory laparotomy is indicated. As a rule, injury to the small bowel alone does not produce shock immediately unless there is severance of major mesenteric vessels, and the preoperative preparation usually need not be extensive.

The small bowel should be examined from the ligament of Treitz to the cecum (and the stomach, duodenum, and colon as well). Small perforations from shotgun pellets can be simply inverted with silk sutures. Larger bullet wounds should be debrided and then inverted transversely with an inner row of continuous catgut and an outer row of interrupted silk sutures. Major lacerations may at times be closed transversely, but if the adjacent mesentery is injured as well, it may represent better judgment to resect the involved segment of bowel, carrying the debridement 1 cm to 2 cm back from the margins of injury to excise gut injured by the blast effect. The small bowel is rarely exteriorized at an initial operation because of the fluid and electrolyte and nutritional losses entailed by such a small bowel fistula. However, it is at times very difficult to decide, in the presence of already developed peritonitis, whether to risk subsequent breakdown of a small bowel anastomosis or to exteriorize the small bowel at that point temporarily. If the aorta or some other major intra-abdominal artery has also been injured, this decision becomes even more difficult. In contrast, exteriorization of the colon is readily tolerated.

Other associated intra-abdominal injuries are managed as indicated. We usually place a solution of a broad-spectrum antibiotic (often cephalothin) in the peritoneal cavity and commonly insert Penrose drains, which are brought out through a stab wound in a lower quadrant of the abdomen. If three drains are used, one might extend into the pelvis, one to the subhepatic space (on the right), and the third adjacent to the site of major gut injury. The purpose of the drains is basically threefold: (1) to minimize the pooling of contaminated fluid in the usual sump drainage areas, (2) to identify continued oozing and the probable necessity for transfusion on occasion, and (3) to diagnose and drain early any small bowel fistula that might develop from a bowel injury overlooked at operation (as for example in many-pellet shotgun wounds), or from leakage at a site of simple gut perforation closure, or from an anastomosis. A well-drained small bowel fistula can usually be expected to close under conservative management using antibiotics, intravenous alimentation, and nasogastric suction. In stark contrast, however, an undrained small bowel fistula can prove fatal.

SMALL BOWEL FISTULA

The high-output small bowel fistula can still represent one of the more formidable complications in surgical practice. *It usually develops as a result of a surgical operation,* and thus the incidence can be reduced by careful dissection. However, even with the greatest care during operation, an external or cutaneous small bowel fistula will still develop in some patients. Experienced clinical judgment, unremitting search for effective supportive measures, and appropriate surgical intervention when indicated are all required to save the life of the patient in many instances.

SMALL BOWEL FISTULA	
Etiology	Most often follows a laparotomy; otherwise, external trauma, neoplasm, inflammation, etc.
	May cause dehydration, infection, malnutrition, skin maceration
Dx	Physical findings including escape of gas
	Ingested charcoal or indigo carmine may emerge; roentgenograms
Rx	Nonoperative usually successful: antibiotics, intravenous fluids and nutrition, general support
	Surgery late, or early to achieve good drainage
Prognosis	Generally good

ETIOLOGY AND TYPES OF SMALL BOWEL FISTULAS

In usual practice, the term *fistula* is applied to a communication between one hollow viscus and (1) another hollow viscus (an internal fistula), (2) the surrounding tissues, or (3) the outside (an external fistula). Technically, a communication between a hollow viscus and surrounding tissues might be considered to be simply a sinus; however, a leak from the duodenum into the right upper quadrant of the abdomen, for example, is generally referred to as a duodenal fistula. Thus a fistula may develop between two loops of small bowel, between the small bowel and the colon, or between the small bowel and a portion of the urinary tract, the biliary tract, the cisterni chyli, or the aorta. Although, as noted, most fistulas result from operative trauma, other possible causes include inflammatory lesions such as regional enteritis, blunt or penetrating trauma to the abdomen, neoplasm, foreign body, and radiation damage.

Almost any operative maneuver within the abdomen may give rise to a small bowel fistula, but perhaps the most common circumstance is when the bowel is injured during the course of dissection in an operation performed for small bowel obstruction. In other circumstances, gut that may have been denuded or inadvertently opened leaks following closure, or an anastomosis that had been made may leak postoperatively. Virtually any possible source of trauma to the small intestine has occasionally produced a fistula.

This discussion will deal only with the external (cutaneous) small bowel fistula. A fistula that drains more than 500 ml of fluid to the outside during a 24-hr period is referred to as a *high-output* fistula, whereas a fistula that drains less than 500 ml is referred to as a *low-output* fistula. This arbitrary delineation has practical clinical importance, since the greater the output from the fistula, the worse the prognosis, other factors being equal. However, a fistula that drains only 500 ml does not represent a serious nutritional threat. In general, high-output fistulas are located relatively high in the alimentary tract and are usually more difficult to manage from both nutritional and operative standpoints.

DIAGNOSIS

The diagnosis of small bowel fistula should be suspected whenever a patient who has undergone an abdominal

TABLE 24-5 **DIAGNOSTIC CRITERIA IN ENTEROCUTANEOUS FISTULA**

Character of drainage (early and late)
History of a recent abdominal operation or trauma
Fever, pain, tenderness and rigidity, leukocytosis
Indigo carmine or charcoal marker
Roentgen studies with radiopaque medium
Passage of gas through drainage tract

operation exhibits evidence of excessive intra-abdominal inflammation or drainage (Table 24-5). In general, the patient who has had a routine laparotomy (*e.g.*, for the lysis of small bowel adhesions that may or may not have been producing simple gut obstruction) should not have significant spontaneous abdominal pain after the first 24 hr to 48 hr. Furthermore, he should not have more than the low-grade fever that is a response to the stress of anesthesia and operation, and he should not have marked tenderness or rigidity of the abdominal wall. Of course, the incision itself will remain tender, but the abdomen at a distance from the wound should not be particularly tender, and leukocytosis and tachycardia should not be excessive. If any of these abdominal and systemic signs develop, the possibility of intra-abdominal sepsis should be considered. Moreover, the most likely cause of intraperitoneal sepsis, assuming that significant spillage of small bowel contents did not occur at the time of operation, might well be a small bowel fistula. This may not be immediately apparent, but presently bile stained material will appear at the drain site, if drains were placed, or the material may eventually be extruded between the skin sutures onto the abdominal wall, ultimately causing the wound to become infected and to break down in many instances (Fig. 24-4).

A small bowel fistula is frequently mistaken initially for a simple wound infection, since the material that first emerges from a wound or drain site may well be purulent, rather than the color of bile, which characterizes drainage from the upper small bowel, or the more yellowish appearance of drainage from the lower small bowel. Within 24 hr to 72 hr the initial purulent drainage is usually replaced by material that clearly represents small bowel contents. At times, the intestinal drainage is not sufficient to be completely identifiable, and the presence of a small bowel fistula may remain in doubt. Under these circumstances the fistula may be demonstrated in several ways: The patient may be given indigo carmine or charcoal by mouth and the drainage site inspected to see if this bluish material emerges on the abdominal wall; or the patient may be given a radiopaque medium such as barium and the site of leakage from the small bowel identified on x-ray films. If these methods have failed, at times it may be possible to introduce a catheter into the external drainage tract and inject a radiopaque medium such as Gastrografin; the mucosal markings of the small bowel may thus be demonstrated radiographically. Also, the patient may state that gas has escaped through the drainage site.

GENERAL ASSESSMENT OF THE PROBLEM

The surgeon often first sees the referred patient with a small bowel high-output fistula after the fistula has been present for some time, if the patient is not one whom the surgeon operated upon himself. At the outset it is important to

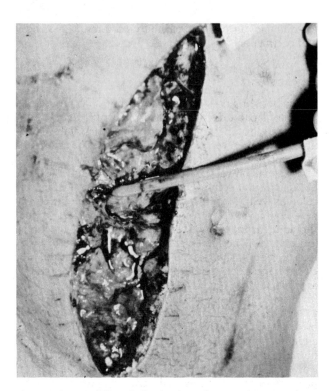

Fig. 24-4. Small-bowel fistula through operative wound. As occurs frequently, the development of a small-bowel fistula resulted in infection and wound separation. Catheter suction was employed for skin protection, since a disposable ileostomy bag could not be properly sealed in this instance.

determine the level of the fistula, whether high-output or low-output, the extent of associated infection, and the degree of nutritional depletion (Table 24-6).

Major factors that enter into the prognosis are the age of the patient, level of the fistula, magnitude of fluid and nutritional losses, presence of intraperitoneal and other infection, presence or absence of distal obstruction of the small bowel, and the presence of associated disease such as cancer or impairment of heart, lung, liver, or kidney function. If a fistula has persisted for weeks, it is less likely to close in the immediate future than is a fresh fistula of only a few days' duration. If the patient is passing flatus and bowel movements per rectum, reflecting alimentary tract patency, one may assume that the hole in the bowel is relatively small, and the prognosis is more favorable than

TABLE 24-6 **PRELIMINARY EVALUATION OF ENTEROCUTANEOUS FISTULA**

General State of Patient
    Age?
    Dehydrated?
    Nutrition: Overall assessment
    Obvious peritonitis?

Nature of Fistula
    High output?
    Well drained?
    Level?
    Distal obstruction?
    Duration?

TABLE 24-7 COMPLICATIONS OF EXTERNAL SMALL BOWEL FISTULA

Water and salt depletion
Peritonitis and sepsis
Nutritional depletion
Skin maceration
Intestinal obstruction
(Pneumonitis)
(Wound complications, plus others)

TABLE 24-8 MANAGEMENT OF EXTERNAL SMALL BOWEL FISTULA

Prevention
Adequate external drainage
Nutritional maintenance
   Water and electrolytes
   Calories and protein
      IV dextrose and amino acid solutions
      Pass tube beyond fistula (for feeding): Hyperalimentation preferred
      Use gut above fistula (?)
      Feeding jejunostomy below fistula (?)
      Blood, plasma, albumin IV (?)
Management of fistulous site
   Collection and measurement of drainage
   Protection of skin
      Collect drainage—tube suction or bag
      Heat lamp to dry
      Cover skin—dermatome glue, ileostomy glue, or other adhesive
      Split mattress
      Karaya gum powder, aluminum hydroxide gel, or aluminum paste to protect skin
Management of infection
   Adequate external drainage
   Antibiotics (sensitivities)
   Excise pyogenic granulomas (not often necessary)
   Drain intra-abdominal abscesses
Operative intervention
   When necessary (less often than before IV feeding)
   Timing
   Technical maneuvers

it might be otherwise. The extent of erosion of the skin surrounding the fistula is an important consideration, for this digestive action of intestinal juice can cause major discomfort to the patient. Moreover, a fistula that produces significant skin erosion is more likely to be a high fistula than a lower one. The presence of significant fever suggests that intra-abdominal sepsis exists and that further operative drainage may be required. The major complications of small bowel fistula are shown in Table 24-7.

Failure of a fistula to close may be due to obstruction of the gut distally, surrounding sepsis, associated cancer, epithelialization of the tract, granulomatous inflammation of the bowel, or a foreign body such as a retained sponge.

MANAGEMENT

The major therapeutic requirements are nutritional therapy, control of infection, care of the skin surrounding the fistula, and operative intervention upon occasion (Table 24-8). The majority of fistulas will close spontaneously, and operation is usually elected only after a significant period of nonoperative support.

NUTRITIONAL MAINTENANCE

Nutritional maintenance must include water, electrolytes, calories, protein, and vitamins.

Water and Electrolytes

The patient with a high-output small bowel fistula may lose from 4 to 6 liters of fluid each day into the collection bottle, sometimes even more. Since he will also require approximately 1500 ml of water for urine formation and perhaps a liter for insensible fluid loss through the lungs and skin, in rare circumstances as much as 8 liters of fluid replacement may be required each day, usually by the intravenous route. Heavy sweating associated with sepsis increases the insensible loss. Thus fluid losses vary greatly from one patient to another and even in the same patient from day to day. Adequate water and salt replacement is achieved by measuring urine volume and fistulous drainage, weighing the patient twice a day if necessary, and noting the clinical evidence of hydration or dehydration, particularly central venous pressure and pulmonary arterial wedge pressures, plus frequent measurements of the plasma electrolyte levels. These data will indicate the types and volume of fluid replacement required. In general, body fluid losses by any route must be replaced with electrolyte solutions. Massive fluid losses require massive fluid replacement, and constant vigilance is required to avoid volume deficits or deficits in specific ions such as sodium, potassium, chloride, calcium, and magnesium.

Calories and Protein

As soon as the immediate water and electrolyte requirements have been determined and this aspect of management has been stabilized, prompt attention must be turned to the administration of calories and protein by every route available. The most important advance in the management of small bowel fistula has been the realization that, if adequate nutritional intake is provided (see Chapter 7), many or most fistulas will close spontaneously, or at least the patient will be rendered a better risk for operative intervention if required.

It is essential to keep in mind always that the fistula may not close for weeks or even months, and that the ultimate major cause of death may be malnutrition or sepsis, or both.

Nutrition may be provided through the alimentary tract—either orally, by tube feeding, gastrostomy, or jejunostomy, or by vein. When the fistula is low in the ileum the drainage may not be excessive and it may be useful to administer nutrients by mouth; whole foodstuffs were thus employed for many years, but recently the value of the elemental diet has been demonstrated by a number of workers. In essence, this diet consists of amino acids and other essential nutrients, has virtually no residue, and hopefully is almost completely absorbed by the time it has reached the level of the low small bowel fistula. In such an instance the losses from the fistula will be much less than if the patient were taking whole foodstuffs that have to be digested. If the patient with a low fistula is unable to take food by mouth because of anorexia or other problems, it may be useful to pass a feeding tube into the stomach and to treat the patient in this way. If the level of the fistula is in the duodenum or high jejunum, it is occasionally possible to pass an oral feeding tube to a point beyond the fistula and thus feed the patient. Unfortunately, small bowel obstruction often precludes successful use of the alimentary tract. Occasionally a feeding jejunostomy can be constructed distal to the fistula. The results with this maneuver are usually not outstanding, though it is at times valuable, and there is some risk that an additional fistula may occur at the site of the jejunostomy through which the feeding tube has been introduced.

The most recent nutritional advance has been the widespread use of intravenous alimentation, or hyperalimentation, performed by introducing a catheter into the superior vena cava and administering a hypertonic solution made up commonly of 50% dextrose and 5% amino acid solution in dextrose (see Chapter 7). A properly mixed solution will contain adequate electrolytes and vitamins and approximately 1 calorie per milliliter. Thus by giving 3 liters of this solution slowly and continuously throughout the 24-hr period, one can administer to the patient the required electrolytes, calories, and nitrogen in a volume of 3000 ml to 4000 ml of solution. If additional fluid supplementation for fistulous losses is required, it is of course given. The average adult patient lying quietly in bed without fever will require about 1500 to 1800 calories and approximately 1 g of protein per kg per day. With intravenous alimentation this level of nutrition can be easily met and even exceeded. Furthermore, both intravenous and oral routes may be used when feasible. As much as 5000 to 6000 calories or even more can be given per day, but in our experience it is relatively difficult to achieve a very high nutritional intake intravenously over a long period of time. Furthermore, unless care is taken, there is always the risk of producing serious metabolic disturbances, one of the most formidable of which is hyperosmolar nonketotic diabetic coma.

It has been shown in both animals and humans that total intravenous maintenance will reduce the volume of fluid loss through the fistula as well as the amount of calories and nitrogen that are lost by this route and that the use of the elemental diet is also associated with smaller volume and nutritional losses than those associated with a regular diet (Fig. 24-5). Intravenous alimentation, an important therapeutic tool in the overall management of small bowel fistula, has its own hazards and complications, and at times it is not fully available to the patient (see Chapter 7).

MANAGEMENT OF THE SKIN AT THE FISTULOUS SITE

Collection of Drainage

It is important to collect all drainage to the extent feasible. It is usually possible to devise some type of catheter or nipple suction arrangement or disposable ileostomy bag by means of which the fluid draining from the fistula can be collected and thus prevented from excoriating the skin of the surrounding abdominal wall. A wide variety of ingenious devices have been designed for this, but in recent years the most satisfactory method has been the initial improvement of the skin surrounding the fistulous opening and then the application of a temporary ileostomy bag utilizing the additional protection of karaya gum powder. However, when the fistula drains into an unusual place—for example, from the small bowel into the vagina—these modalities for collection of the fluid are not efficient, and catheter suction may be necessary. Even so, by appropriate

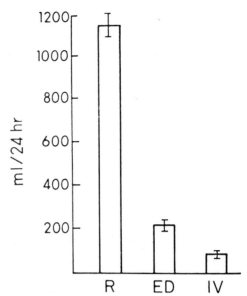

Fig. 24-5. Relative volumes lost through experimental small-bowel fistula in dogs. Comparison of regular diet (*R*), elemental diet (*ED*), and intravenous alimentation (*IV*). Note that the volume of loss through the fistula was vastly less with the *ED* as compared with the *R* dog chow diet, and still less with the *IV* feeding. (Wolfe BM, Keltner RM, Willman VL: Intestinal fistula output in regular, elemental, and intravenous alimentation. Am J Surg 124:803, 1972)

and continuous attention to the collection of the fistulous drainage much skin protection can be afforded.

Further Protection of the Skin

In addition to the collection of fluid with appropriate suction or gravity drainage, a variety of materials and maneuvers are available for the further protection of the skin from the erosive effect of the digestive enzymes in the small bowel contents. These measures include the use of a heat lamp to dry the skin surrounding the site at which the fistulous drainage is being removed by suction, covering the skin with dermatome glue or ileostomy glue or adhesive cellophane, or perhaps the use of a split mattress to allow the drainage to fall directly into a pan beneath the bed until the condition of the skin has improved to the extent that an ileostomy bag can be securely applied. As an alternative to karaya gum powder, either aluminum hydroxide gel or aluminum paste affords considerable protection of the skin.

The objective of all these measures is to improve the condition of the skin to the point that a disposable ileostomy bag can be securely fitted, following which the skin will usually remain protected (Fig. 24-6). Continuous attention to these measures by physicians and nurses is required to achieve maximal success.

MANAGEMENT OF INFECTION

Although the appropriate management of fluid balance and of the site of the fistulous drainage take immediate priority, ultimately it is malnutrition and sepsis that cause most deaths.

In the management of infection, the first requirement is to ensure that the fistula is well drained. If the fistulous drainage from the intestine can emerge easily to the outside through an adequate drainage tract, peritoneal contamination may be minimal and a well walled-off tract may soon

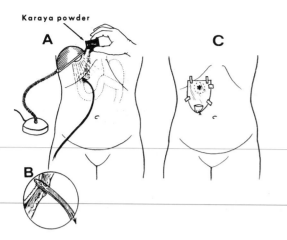

Fig. 24-6. Management of skin. (*A*) Use of heat lamp and karaya powder with catheter suction to improve skin condition prior to application of ileostomy bag. (*B*) Catheter suction at site of fistula. To be effective, this technique requires frequent inspection and readjustment. (*C*) Ileostomy bag applied to healthy skin.

develop. This reduces the risk of widespread peritonitis, multiple abscesses, and bloodstream invasion with septicemia.

If drainage is not adequate, and certainly if no drainage was provided at a preceding operation, prompt operative intervention is essential to make certain that immediate egress of the bowel leakage is possible. Otherwise, the small bowel drainage can spread widely throughout the abdomen and possibly may produce a fatal peritonitis. At the same time that adequate drainage is being established by whatever measures are required, broad-spectrum antibiotics should be administered on an empirical basis until specific organisms have been cultured and antibiotic sensitivities determined. Simple suture of the hole in the intestine is rarely successful owing to surrounding infection. Localized abscesses in the abdomen should be suspected if the patient continues to run a spiking fever after good external drainage has been provided, and major purulent collections will usually require surgical drainage. Sonography and computerized tomography (CT scan) have markedly extended the value of radiologic diagnostic techniques in these cases. Finally, pyogenic granulomas surrounding the fistulous site at the skin surface may require excision or drainage upon occasion. In the presence of spiking fever, especially with chills, the possibility of bloodstream invasion should be considered, and multiple blood cultures should be taken to determine the specific organisms and their antibiotic sensitivities.

Additional serious complications of small bowel fistula include intestinal obstruction distal to the fistula, wound infection and even evisceration, and, not uncommonly, pulmonary infection, which constitutes a leading cause of death in patients with peritonitis.

METHODS FOR ACHIEVING CLOSURE OF THE FISTULA

Spontaneous Closure

The majority of small bowel fistulas will close spontaneously if the requirements for water and electrolyte replacement, nutritional maintenance, and control of infection are met. When one realizes that new tissue must grow at the site of intestinal leakage that is inevitably infected and bathed by digestive enzymes and that the patient is often malnourished, it is manifestly unrealistic to expect most fistulas to close overnight, though some fistulas do close rather abruptly after only a few days. In general, however, it must be assumed that a high-output fistula may not close for days or weeks or even months, and that from the onset every effort must be made to maintain unremittingly the patient's general metabolic reserves as effectively as possible. We treated two patients whose fistulas drained for almost a year, through many operations and vicissitudes, before they were finally successfully healed. Many fistulas—and even the majority—will heal spontaneously if adequate time is made available through vigorous general support of the patient.

Unfortunately, some high-output fistulas deplete the nutritional reserves of the patient so rapidly that it is apparent the patient will not survive the dire circumstances unless successful operative intervention of some type can retard the rate of metabolic deterioration. This is particularly true of duodenal or high jejunal fistulas. Few circumstances in surgical practice require more judgment that deciding when and how to operate on a patient with a severe small bowel fistula, with the knowledge that he represents a considerable operative risk and that the operation itself may not prove successful in closing the fistula. There is a high incidence of breakdown of any type of anastomosis performed in the presence of surrounding infection associated with starvation. Even so, the surgeon will at times perceive that the patient is not likely to survive without an operation that will afford better physiological control of the situation. Again, failure of the fistula to close may be due to obstruction distal to the fistula, granulomatous disease, local infection, epithelialization of the tract, foreign body, or neoplasm (Table 24-9). The presence of one or more of these, plus prolonged massive daily fluid loss through the fistula, may force operative intervention. To repeat, the now uncommon operative intervention is required more often with high small bowel fistulas that are draining profusely than with low small bowel fistulas in which the drainage may not be particularly excessive and the upper reaches of the gut are available for nutritional therapy using an elemental diet.

The timing of any operation is very important, for one wishes both to give the fistula every opportunity to close spontaneously and, at the same time, to resort to operation before the patient is so gravely ill that he cannot survive the metabolic assault of the operation itself.

Local Maneuvers Short of Formal Exploratory Laparotomy

A wide variety of ingenious maneuvers and appliances have been employed in an effort to close the drainage tract of small bowel fistulas. It is not appropriate to review these in detail here; it is enough to say that only limited success has

TABLE 24-9 CAUSES OF FAILURE OF FISTULA TO CLOSE
Distal obstruction
Neoplastic disease
Granulomatous disease
Local infection
Epithelialization of tract
Foreign body

been achieved in this way, and usually the results have been disappointing. In recent years, however, some skin protection and some temporary improvement in the patient's general condition, due to diminished volume of nutritional and fluid loss, have at times been achieved by blocking or plugging the tract, most notably with the acrylic solidifying adhesives. However, we do not use them.

Operations Available for Closing the Fistula

The surgical operations that have been often employed for closing small bowel fistulas are almost as numerous as the prostheses that have been devised for plugging or otherwise occluding the fistulas without operation. After general disappointment with actual occlusion of the fistula at the skin level, three operative approaches came into widespread use: (1) bypassing of the fistula with a side-to-side intestinal anastomosis, performed through a clean operative field, to improve nutrition and general stability for later excision of the fistula itself; (2) division of the bowel just proximal to the fistula, closure of the distal stump, and anastomosis of the proximal end to the transverse colon; and (3) bold excision of the fistula with primary end-to-end anastomosis of the intestine. Actually, various combinations of these may be employed in the same patient, for often several operations are required to rehabilitate the rare patient whose fistula or fistulas will not close under other management.

At the present time, bypass of the fistula is used less than enterocolic anastomosis, though simple bypassing of the fistula may reduce the fluid losses markedly, allowing for improvement in the patient's condition and for eventual operative excision of the fistula if indicated. We prefer bold excision of the fistula if peritonitis and sepsis have cleared and the risk of anastomotic dehiscence is minimal. Such conditions exist when the hole in the gut is adherent to the abdominal wall at the site of external drainage, the rest of the peritoneal cavity being clear of infection. However, primary excision of the fistula is often not feasible and division of the gut proximal to the fistula, with enterocolic anastomosis, may serve very well. If as much as 3 feet of jejunum are available for the enterocolic anastomosis, fluid and nutritional losses are vastly reduced, nutritional stability can be achieved, and infection will eventually clear up in most patients. The excluded bowel may never need to be restored to functional continuity, even when the level of small bowel division was relatively high; however, restoration is readily achieved, if necessary, after intraperitoneal infection has cleared. Operative intervention is assisted by the presence of a long tube in the small bowel to facilitate identification of proximal versus distal bowel relative to the fistula.

Unfortunately, when the fistula is in the duodenum or high in the jejunum, the fluid losses may be huge, and available operative approaches are limited. The hole in the duodenum or the very high jejunum cannot be exteriorized technically. A duodenal stump fistula following a Billroth II distal subtotal gastrectomy will usually close if infection is managed with adequate external drainage, plus other measures. In this case, the patient can often be fed by mouth, and food passes into the intestine through the gastrojejunostomy. The duodenal side fistula represents a more serious problem and, although occasionally managed by distal gastrectomy with gastrojejunostomy, nonoperative therapy, including intravenous alimentation, is usually employed with success. Direct operative attack upon the duodenal fistula itself rarely achieves closure.

PROGNOSIS OF SMALL BOWEL FISTULA

The mortality of small bowel fistula varies considerably in reports from different hospitals. By and large, most observers now report a mortality of less than 20% for high-output small bowel fistulas. The problem with comparing figures from different clinics is that the types and severity of the fistulas cannot be assessed, nor can the quality of the supportive therapy. For example, MacFayden, Dudrick, and Ruberg reported 62 patients with 78 fistulas that had a spontaneous closure rate of 70.5% and an overall mortality of 6.45%. This is by all odds the most favorable report we have seen. However, while acknowledging that this particular group has long experience in the use of intravenous hyperalimentation and general nutritional maintenance, one must assume that many of their patients had relatively mild fistulas without associated neoplasm, peritonitis, or distal obstruction. Even so, the outlook for the patient with a high-output small bowel fistula has been substantially improved in recent years by the advent of more effective intravenous alimentation and better overall management.

RADIATION INJURY TO THE SMALL BOWEL

Radiation injury to the small intestine is not a problem for which the surgeon is consulted frequently, but it can present a variety of challenges upon occasion. High-frequency radiation from any source can produce pervasive cellular damage in any tissue, but the fragile intestine and some other organs are particularly sensitive to radiation damage. This injury most often follows high-dose radiation to an intra-abdominal and usually a pelvic malignancy, such as uterine or prostatic carcinoma. The effects of such radiation can be acute (diarrhea) or chronic (stricture and even perforation and fistula–abscess formation). A remote late effect of the irradiation of tissue is malignant change, such as occurs in thyroid irradiation with the appearance of cancer 10 to 20 years later.

ACUTE EFFECTS OF RADIATION INJURY

The acute effects of radiation on the intestine may result in nausea and vomiting or diarrhea, or both. These acute effects can be expected to subside with conservative therapy in most patients, and not to progress to the late complications for which operation may be required. Even so, bleeding and even perforation can rarely occur in acute cases, as can small bowel obstruction.

LATE EFFECTS OF RADIATION INJURY

It is for the late effects that surgical intervention may be required. These complications may simply be the final stage of continuing symptoms that the patient has had since the original radiation treatment, but often the patient has been free of significant symptoms for many months or years, only to develop small bowel obstruction from chronic cicatrix formation or adhesions. In addition to radiation changes in the gut, the urinary tract can also be injured with at times a distressing radiation cystitis.

Thus the late effects of small bowel injury include diarrhea, malabsorption, bleeding, obstruction, perforation with or without abscess formation, and even enteroarterial fistula. Unfortunately, the patient is apt to attribute any abdominal symptoms to the original tumor, and the surgeon may be hard put to convince either the patient or himself that the symptoms are not due to tumor recurrence. In the case of gut lymphoma, which may itself produce diarrhea–malabsorption, the differential diagnosis between malignancy and radiation effects can become even more difficult.

SURGICAL TREATMENT OF COMPLICATIONS

The surgical measures required will depend upon the specific complication involved. With optimal perioperative supportive therapy, laparotomy will be required for small bowel obstruction, for perforation with peritonitis, and occasionally for otherwise uncontrollable bleeding from a segment of gut ideally identified preoperatively with selective arteriography or barium studies. However, at times many loops of gut are involved, and dense adhesions found at laparotomy can render proper identification and resection of the offending segment very difficult.

Abscesses of significance must be drained. The diagnosis of such collections has been much improved by sonography and CT scan. However, the onset of an abscess, amid radiation-damaged and often densely adherent loops of small bowel, can be quite insidious and may not even be suspected until late. In recent years advances in invasive radiologic techniques have sometimes permitted nonoperative percutaneous insertion of a tube for abscess drainage, using fluoroscopic control. However, because there is always the hazard of perforation of the colon or small bowel, closed tube drainage is generally approached cautiously at the present time, and open laparotomy is still preferred by many or most surgeons.

Finally, the uninitiated might suppose that it would be a simple matter just to perform laparotomy and resect all the diseased small bowel (or colon). Unfortunately, the dense late changes in the friable and densely adherent, matted small bowel can be so severe that complete excision is manifestly impossible without incurring the high risk of a small bowel fistula that might not heal because of radiation damage.

In general, however, most intestinal complications due to radiation injury can be managed with reasonable success by one means or another.

BIBLIOGRAPHY

Bowlin JW, Hardy JD, Conn JH: External alimentary fistulas: Analysis of seventy-nine cases with notes on management. Am J Surg 103:6, 1962

Bury KD, Stephens RV, Randall HT: Use of chemically defined diet for nutritional management of fistulas of alimentary tract. Am J Surg 121:174, 1971

Dudrick SJ, Wilmore DW, Steiger E et al: Spantaneous closure of traumatic pancreatoduodenal fistulas with total intravenous nutrition. J Trauma 10:542, 1970

Hamilton RF, German JD, Stephenson DV Jr et al: The management of high enterocutaneous fistulas. Nebr Med J 56:382, 1971

MacFayden BV Jr, Dudrick SJ, Ruberg RL: Management of gastrointestinal fistulas with parenteral hyperalimentation. Surgery 74:100, 1973

Schmitt EH III, Symmonds RE: Surgical treatment of radiation induced injuries of the intestine. Surg Gynecol Obstet 153:896, 1981

Sheldon GF, Gardiner BN, Dunphy JE: Progress in the management of intestinal fistulae. Rev Surg 27:452, 1970

Soeters PB, Efeid AM, Fischer JE: Review of 404 patients with gastrointestinal fistulas. Impact of parenteral nutrition. Ann Surg 190:189, 1979

Wolfe BM, Keltner RM, Willman VL: Intestinal fistula output in regular, elemental and intravenous alimentation, Am J Surg 124:803, 1972

Moreye Nusbaum

Small Bowel Tumors, Inflammatory Lesions, and Hemorrhage

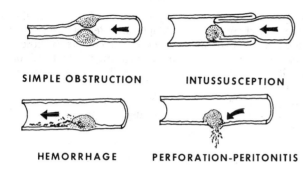

SIMPLE OBSTRUCTION   INTUSSUSCEPTION

HEMORRHAGE   PERFORATION-PERITONITIS

Fig. 24-7. Complications of small-bowel tumors. (Peskin GW: Small bowel tumors including carcinoid. In Hardy JD [ed]: Rhoads Textbook of Surgery. Philadelphia, J B Lippincott, 1977)

SMALL BOWEL TUMORS

CLINICAL MANIFESTATIONS

Symptoms are nonspecific and frequently ignored for long periods of time. A high index of suspicion is important for early diagnosis. Recurrent partial or complete small bowel obstruction is the most common presenting symptom but is frequently dismissed as secondary adhesions. Intussusception led by an intraluminal growth is another cause of obstructive symptoms (Fig. 24-7).

DIAGNOSTIC TECHNIQUES

Despite advances in diagnostic techniques less than 50% of small bowel tumors are recognized preoperatively. Barium examination of the small intestine using the standard delayed small intestinal film is diagnostic in less than 10% of cases. Recent use of small bowel enema with introduction of methylcellulose and barium through a tube placed below the ligament of Treitz will undoubtedly increase the accuracy of this diagnostic method. Mesenteric arteriography, although most helpful in recognizing an acutely bleeding lesion, may on occasion reveal the hypervascularity of a leiomyoma (Fig. 24-8) or carcinoid tumor, or the distortion of the small vessels of an adenocarcinoma. Case reports are frequent, but the exact value of arteriography will be known only with greater utilization of this technique. Computerized tomography (CT scanning) may also be helpful in diagnosing solid tumors of the small bowel as further experience is accumulated with this technique. The most frequent diag-

nostic technique remains exploratory laparotomy for small bowel obstruction unrelieved by tube decompression or for recurrent unexplained episodes of partial or intermittent complete small bowel obstruction. A high index of suspicion will lead to earlier laparotomy in these cases and will enhance the chance of cure in patients with malignant tumors.

BENIGN TUMORS

Benign tumors are found mostly in the ileum (55%), jejunum (25%), and duodenum (20%), and are mostly asymptomatic until obstruction or bleeding ensues. Most common are adenomatous polyps (35%), lipomas (15%), leiomyomas (15%), and hemangiomas (10%). Less common tumors include villous adenoma, Brunner's adenoma, pseudolymphomas, fibromas, neurilemmomas, lymphangiomas, and a variety of hamartomas.

MALIGNANT TUMORS

Malignant tumors are mostly found in the ileum (50%), with 25% in the jejunum and 25% in the duodenum. They present most frequently as nonspecific symptoms such as weight loss or abdominal pain and less frequently as obstruction, bleeding, and perforation. The most common malignant tumors are adenocarcinoma (40%), carcinoids (30%), lymphomas (20%), and leiomyosarcomas (10%). Less common are liposarcomas, fibrosarcomas, malignant schwannomas, metastatic lesions, and angiosarcomas.

SURGICAL THERAPY

The primary and only curative therapy for small bowel tumors is surgery. Simple resection is all that is required for benign small bowel tumors. Occasionally, polypectomy and diverticulectomy without resection may be accomplished. Larger amounts of small bowel may need to be resected if there is mesenteric damage due to an intussusception or gangrene secondary to obstruction.

Malignant tumors should be removed with adequate margins of approximately 6 inches proximal and distal to the lesion and as wide a resection as possible of the mesentery, including all palpable nodes. Care must be taken not to sacrifice the blood supply to the remaining small intestine during the mesenteric resection. Exceptions to this rule include widespread lymphomas when full-thickness biopsy and postoperative radiotherapy and chemotherapy are preferred to massive small bowel resection. Careful inspection by palpation of the small intestine must be done to rule out multiple primary lesions. Despite an aggressive surgical approach 5-year survival rates for adenocarcinoma of the small bowel are only 20% to 30%. Early diagnosis and surgery will undoubtedly improve this statistic.

SPECIAL CLINICAL SYNDROMES

PEUTZ-JEGHERS SYNDROME

Intestinal polyposis associated with abnormal pigmentation of the oral mucosa, lips, and digits are the important features of Peutz-Jeghers syndrome. This syndrome is marked by simple mendelian dominance with a high degree of penetrance; a single pleiotrophic gene is responsible for both the polyps and the pigmentation. The multiple polyps are

SMALL BOWEL TUMORS	
Etiology	Uncommon (0.4% of all sites), presenting as obstruction or occasionally with bleeding or perforation
Dx	Clinical suspicion, barium studies, arteriography, exploratory laparotomy
Rx	Surgical resection: Curative for benign lesions; for malignant lesions, frequently palliative because metastasis requires multiple reoperations and chemotherapy, as in lymphomas and malignant carcinoids

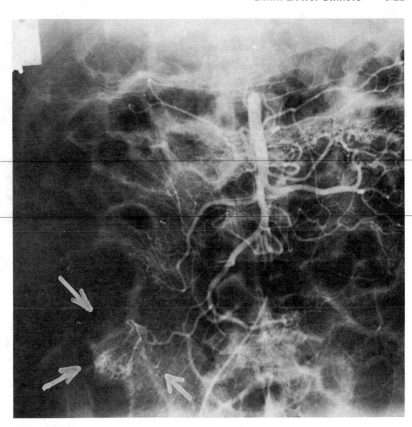

Fig. 24-8. Selective superior mesenteric arteriogram in a patient with a leiomyoma of the distal ileum. Note the characteristic hypervascularity in this small-bowel tumor.

actually hamartomas and are benign, occurring most frequently in the jejunum. In approximately 4% of patients with this syndrome a concomitant malignancy of the gastrointestinal tract is found. In women ovarian lesions are associated with this syndrome. Patients present with intestinal bleeding or intermittent obstruction, usually from intussusception. Surgical therapy is conservative, removing symptomatic lesions only rather than performing multiple or extensive resections of the small bowel.

GARDNER'S SYNDROME

Gardner's syndrome is a variant of familial polyposis in which osteomas and soft tissue tumors are associated with small bowel polyps. Two cases of small bowel adenocarcinoma have been reported in patients with Gardner's syndrome, suggesting a premalignant potential.

MALIGNANT CARCINOID SYNDROME

Carcinoid tumors (see also Chapter 20) are the second most common primary intestinal neoplasm, with approximate frequencies as follows: appendix (40%), small intestine (30%), rectum (15%), bronchus (5%), colon (5%), stomach (4%), and ovary (1%). Occasionally they may occur in the pancreas, biliary tract, and thyroid gland. Carcinoid tumors arise from the enterochromaffin cells of the gastrointestinal tract. They are referred to as argentaffinomas because of the affinity of cytoplasmic granules for silver salts. Grossly these tumors are orange-yellow in color because of their cholesterol content. First described by Lubarsch in 1888, Oberndorfer introduced the term "karzinoid" in 1907 to distinguish them from adenocarcinoma.

Malignant potential is related to size rather than to histology. Less than 2% of lesions less than 1 cm in diameter will metastasize. A coincidental neoplasm can occur in 45% to 50% of patients with carcinoid tumors. Metastasis occurs initially to the regional nodes and then to the liver by way of the portal venous system. These tumors are associated with a desmoplastic reaction related to the stimulation of fibrous tissue by 5-hydroxytryptamine. About 30% of extra-appendiceal carcinoids are malignant. These produce serotonin (5-hydroxytryptamine) and can produce a typical syndrome characterized by episodic attacks of flushing of the skin of the upper torso and head, abdominal pain, hyperperistalsis, diarrhea, bronchospasm, edema, vasomotor instability, cutaneous lesions of pellagra, and endocardial fibrosis of the right ventricle with pulmonary and tricuspid stenosis or insufficiency.

Thirty percent of patients with liver metastases have an associated carcinoid syndrome (Fig. 24-9). Carcinoids arise from neurocrest tissue and are a component of the APUD system of endocrine active lesions.

A variety of vasoactive amines and peptides are produced in the foregut and midgut but virtually none in the hindgut. Serotonin, elaborated in the midgut carcinoid syndrome, is derived from ingested tryptophan, and when a functioning carcinoid tumor is present, tryptophan deficiency and clinical manifestations of pellagra are common. Serotonin is deaminated by monamine oxidase in the liver and lungs and forms 5-hydroxyindoleacetic acid (5-HIAA), which is excreted in the urine. Elevated blood serotonin levels and urinary 5-HIAA levels are diagnostic of carcinoid tumors. Serotonin is no longer considered the sole mediator of the carcinoid syndrome. Release of kinins, histamine, and other vasoactive peptides have been described.

Treatment is primarily surgical, with resection of the primary lesion, metastatic lymph nodes, and as much of the liver metastatic disease as possible. Ligation of the hepatic artery or dearterialization of the liver has been

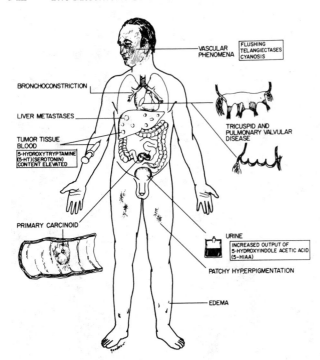

Fig. 24-9. Malignant carcinoid syndrome. (Peskin GW: Small bowel tumors including carcinoid. In Hardy JD [ed]: Rhoads Textbook of Surgery. Philadelphia, J B Lippincott, 1977)

helpful when combined with selective infusions of chemotherapeutic agents. Drug therapy with serotonin antagonists has been disappointing, but combination chemotherapy with such agents as streptozotocin and 5-fluorouracil has been helpful.

Special care in management of anesthesia is required, and avoidance of catecholamine release and premedication with antihistamine-type agents can be helpful.

Prognosis is good. Five-year survival rates vary from 45% to 65% in patients without metastases at surgery to 21% with metastatic disease at the time of surgery.

INFLAMMATORY LESIONS OF THE SMALL INTESTINE

REGIONAL ENTERITIS

ETIOLOGY AND PATHOLOGY

The etiology of regional enteritis is unknown. Numerous theories of lymphatic obstruction, bacterial infections, and hypersensitivity reactions have been discounted. There is evidence of a transmissible agent in experimental animal models but not in humans. Immunologic aspects of the disease have received increasing attention in recent years, and the participation of humoral and cellular immune mechanisms in the etiology or maintenance of this disease has been suggested. The therapeutic use of azathioprine and 6-mercaptopurine has received clinical trials. Various studies suggest that coliform organisms, their metabolic products, the immunologic response of the bowel wall, intestinal T and B lymphocytes, and the reticuloendothelial system all play a role in the etiology and pathologic mechanisms of this disease.

	REGIONAL ENTERITIS
Etiology	Unknown; transmural inflammation with granuloma formation in 50% of cases
Dx	Symptoms: Abdominal cramps, diarrhea, malnutrition, fever
	Signs: Abdominal tenderness, distention, mass, rigidity, and rebound if perforation or abscess present
	Roentgenograms demonstrate signs of complete or partial obstruction or the typical barium findings of mucosal ulcerations and partial obstruction
Rx	Initially medical
	Surgery reserved for complications; a high recurrence rate is recognized

The dominant gross pathologic finding in regional enteritis is submucosal and subserosal fibrosis that produces varied degrees of stenosis. The associated inflammation is marked by edema and round cell infiltration, mostly lymphocytes and occasional eosinophils. Noncaseating granulomas have been reported in 50% to 60% of patients; however, in our series they occurred in only 36% of cases. Small mucosal ulcerations are found early with gross ulcerations in severely diseased bowel.

Crohn's disease is a transmural inflammation involving the mucosa, submucosa, muscularis, and serosa. Grossly there is thickening of the wall and narrowing of the lumen with a leathery or granular serosal surface. There is thickening of the mesenteric bowel angle with overriding of antimesenteric fat. Associated edema and adenopathy is almost always present. The mucosa is coarsely nodular and irregular with ulcerations. The terminal ileum is most frequently involved, but proximal skip areas as well as colonic involvement are frequent. Perianal inflammation and suppuration is frequent. Microscopically there is chronic, edematous, sclerosing inflammation with atrophic mucosal ulcers and round cell infiltration. The submucosa is fibrotic, thick, and edematous. The muscle shows evidence of fistulization, and the serosa is thickened and inflamed. Granulomas are most frequently found in the subserosa but can occur in the mesentery, lymph nodes, and subserosa.

DIAGNOSIS

Regional enteritis may involve any part of the gastrointestinal tract. The diagnosis is made by the clinical presentation, which can be subtle, but usually diarrhea, abdominal pain, partial obstruction, and a palpable abdominal mass suggest the diagnosis. Confirmation is made by barium studies including barium enema and an upper gastrointestinal series with a delayed small intestinal detail film demonstrating acute or chronic obstruction of the small intestine, mucosal ulcerations, and distortions. With air-contrast barium enema and small bowel enema techniques, small ulcerations and fissures can be demonstrated. Mesenteric masses can displace bowel loops. Skip areas can be shown as well as the general extent of the disease. When the terminal ileum is involved, changes along the medial border of the cecum produce a concave impression secondary to the swelling of the terminal ileum and its mesentery and strongly suggest the diagnosis.

Mesenteric arteriography demonstrates changes in the vascularity of the small bowel but does not add to the diagnostic techniques already in use.

CLINICAL PRESENTATION

Local Complications

Obstruction. More than 75% of patients present with some form of obstruction, either because of edema and inflammation of the bowel wall, which encroaches upon the lumen or produces a paralytic ileus owing to swelling and inflammatory reaction, or because of a late finding of fibrosis producing an unrelenting fixed stenosis.

Abscess and fistulas. Abscess can develop within the leaves of the mesentery secondary to fistulization from the lumen or in the parietes or by spread along retroperitoneal spaces, such as the psoas muscle, fixed scars, or pre-existing adhesions. Fistulas can develop between loops of bowel, between the bowel and the skin, or between loops of bowel and the bladder, urethra, uterus, tubes, or vagina.

Perforation. Perforation is rare in Crohn's disease but can occur when an abscess or fistula is not walled off; it is more frequently seen when patients are on steroid therapy.

Bleeding. Occult blood in the stools is frequently found. Only occasionally is bleeding so brisk that it is in itself a major medical or surgical problem.

Perianal disease. In one third of cases there is involvement of the anal canal in Crohn's disease, which presents with fistulas-in-ano and perianal abscesses.

Appendicitis. Acute or chronic enteritis may present with signs and symptoms of acute appendicitis. Occasionally the appendix itself shows the pathologic signs of Crohn's disease.

Systemic Complications

Anemia. Anemia is usually hypochromic and microcytic in nature owing to blood loss and chronic infection. A hyperchromic macrocytic anemia of a megaloblastic variety may develop owing to poor absorption and utilization of vitamin B_{12} and folic acid.

Malnutrition. Malnutrition has varied causes, including poor appetite, rapid transit, reduced absorptive surfaces and malabsorption, partial obstruction, bacterial overgrowth, and excessive bile salts reaching the colon.

Retardation of growth and delayed maturation. Growth retardation is frequently found when the onset of disease occurs before puberty and is frequently associated with chronic malnutrition.

Polyarthritis. Polyarthritis is migratory in nature, involving mostly the extremities and their small joints. Occasionally the spine may be involved as in ulcerative colitis.

Erythema nodosum. The raised indurated skin nodules of erythema nodosum occur infrequently but are similar to those appearing in patients with ulcerative colitis.

Pyoderma gangrenosum. Pyoderma gangrenosum is an infrequent finding in Crohn's disease compared with ulcerative colitis but has been reported.

MEDICAL MANAGEMENT

Initially all patients are placed on a medical program to combat diarrhea and abdominal cramps and improve nutrition. Mild sedatives, antispasmodics, antidiarrheal agents (*e.g.,* Lomotil), bland low-residue diets with nutritional supplements, and hydrophilic agents are all effective in mild disease. In more advanced disease the use of salicylazosulfapyridine (Azulfidine) has been helpful in stabilizing disease or maintaining remissions. Steroids are frequently administered but are reserved for more persistent disease because of associated complications and catabolic effects. Recent trials with 6-mercaptopurine and azathioprine have shown some promise in controlling active disease and diminishing steroid dosage. Some authors have recommended the judicial use of external radiation in refractory cases with extensive disease. Bacille Calmette-Guerin (BCG) injections have resulted in remissions in a small percentage of patients so treated. The disease may be controlled satisfactorily for long periods of time until eventual complications force surgical intervention.

SURGICAL MANAGEMENT

General principles. Surgery for Crohn's disease is reserved for complications of the disease. Limiting the extent of resection is stressed because of the failure of surgery to cure this disease, the high recurrence rate, and the eventual loss of excessive amounts of small bowel through subsequent operations. Many investigators, including Marshak, point out that the disease infrequently extends longitudinally in the small bowel from its presenting pathologic focus unless surgical intervention ensues. Recurrences frequently occur at and proximal to the new anastomosis. The site of resection is based on the gross extent of the disease. Frozen section is not reliable at the margins and leads to needless extension of resection and further loss of small bowel. The presence of mesenteric adenopathy is not a valid indication for extending the amount of resection in the mesentery or for increasing the amount of bowel removed. As suggested by Turnbull, the point of proximal and distal resection should be selected where the mesenteric bowel angle is thin and sharp. This will ensure removal of gross disease including areas of antimesenteric fat wrapping. The mucosa should appear grossly normal, but small, sparsely located mucosal ulcerations should be ignored and not used as a reason to extend the length of resection. If only the terminal ileum is involved, the ascending colon should be preserved and only the cecum removed. If multiple skip areas are involved, only those producing symptoms are resected.

Indications for Surgery

Obstruction. Obstruction may be acute or secondary to edema or swelling of diseased areas, or a loop of bowel may be adherent or kinked to an area of disease. Most often these episodes will subside with intubation and medical therapy, but occasionally lysis of adhesions or resection of diseased bowel may become a necessity. More often obstruction is chronic with pain and distention after each meal due to fibrotic fixed narrowing of the lumen of bowel in the area of disease. Resection is indicated to restore adequate bowel function.

Fistulization. Abnormal communications between loops of bowel or between other viscera and skin require surgical resection with interruption of the fistula. Intravenous nutrition may be successful in closing fistulas, thus delaying the need for surgical resection.

Abscess. Confined and walled-off perforations into the mesentery or retroperitoneum or abdominal wall result in purulent collections with pain, fever, and a tender abdominal mass. Surgical drainage in a single stage with concomitant resection is recommended when possible, although occasionally prior drainage of the abscess may be necessary. However, prior drainage frequently results in the production of an external fistula.

Perforation. Free perforation with peritonitis occurs infrequently but is an urgent indication for surgery. Resection of the area of perforation is required, with either primary anastomosis or construction of a temporary stoma and mucous fistula; the choice depends on the local findings and on the experience of the surgeon.

Intractability. Persistence of active disease requiring frequent hospitalizations with inability to work or to have normal home and social experiences is an indication for resection of diseased intestine. Surgery will frequently allow rehabilitation of the individual and make medical management more successful in the postoperative period. Parenteral nutrition with a prolonged period of bowel rest should precede a surgical approach to intractable disease. In adolescence failure to grow or to develop sexually is an additional indication for surgical resection.

Hemorrhage. Chronic blood loss requiring multiple transfusions and lack of response to a program of bowel rest with parenteral nutrition are indications to proceed with elective resection. Occasionally major hemorrhage ensues, forcing emergency surgical resection to stem blood loss.

Perianal disease. Perianal disease may cause the primary discomfort and complications in a patient with small intestinal Crohn's disease presenting with perianal abscess, fistulas-in-ano, anal ulcers, and deep penetrating fistulas from areas of small bowel disease extending through to the perineum. There is a 30% incidence of this annoying complication. Conservative local surgical therapy with preservation of the sphincter is indicated. Occasionally symptoms may be so severe and persistent that elective resection of the small bowel disease is indicated. This may ameliorate the perianal problems for long periods of time.

Carcinoma. Cancer of the small bowel does occur in Crohn's disease. Approximately 50 cases have been reported in the literature. Forty percent of these were found in surgically excluded loops of diseased bowel. The symptoms are no different from those of underlying disease. Therefore, a high mortality (82%) has been reported from this dire complication despite aggressive surgical therapy. An increase in extra-intestinal cancers in Crohn's disease has also been noted. Extra-intestinal cancers were more frequent in these patients than in those with ulcerative colitis. However, there was less correlation with increasing duration of disease in extra-intestinal cancers than in cancers of the small bowel. It is of interest that an increased incidence of small bowel cancers remote from the site of active Crohn's disease has been reported. The risk of cancer in Crohn's disease increased with time as in universal ulcerative colitis. Patients with long-standing Crohn's disease and surgically bypassed loops are at greatest risk for developing carcinoma. Means of preventing this complication include avoidance of construction of excluded loops and resection of previously excluded loops after 5 years whenever possible.

Surgical Procedures

Resection of gross areas of disease with end-to-end anastomosis is the procedure of choice.

Exclusion procedures are reserved for masses of bowel that are nonresectable owing to acute and chronic inflammation and concomitant dangers of resection at the time of surgery. The exclusion procedure was commonly applied in the early days of surgery for Crohn's disease, but it is now rarely used. The proximal bowel is divided just above the diseased area, the distal end is closed, and the proximal end is anastomosed to the ascending colon or transverse colon to completely exclude the diseased segment.

Bypass procedures are not used except for an occasional burned-out obstructive process in a poor-risk patient in whom a side-to-side ileotransverse colostomy might be used.

Appendectomy. When the disease presents with signs and symptoms of acute appendicitis and exploration reveals Crohn's disease, the appendix is removed only if the cecum is free of edema at its base and will safely hold sutures, thus avoiding postoperative fistulization from incidental appendectomy. Otherwise the appendix is left, and the abdomen is closed without resection unless other indications for resection of the diseased area are present. Occasionally a form of acute enteritis presents in this fashion, and subsequent follow-up fails to demonstrate the clinical development of chronic Crohn's disease.

Recurrence

The recurrence rate for Crohn's disease after surgery is high. In our series of patients, 53% demonstrated recurrence within 5 years. Recurrence rates were more frequent in patients under 30 years of age (62%), in patients with extensive disease with skip areas and colon involvement (67%), and in patients with previous recurrences after surgery (69%). All patients with extensive mesenteric adenopathy suffered recurrences within 5 years. Despite the high recurrence rate after surgery, satisfactory rehabilitation was achieved in 80% of patients with combined surgical and medical therapy. Patients refractory to medical therapy prior to surgery were more easily managed postoperatively. A combination of surgical therapy, medical therapy, and parenteral nutrition requires experienced clinical judgment but can result in rehabilitation from this chronic debilitating disease in most patients.

ROLE OF PARENTERAL NUTRITION IN CROHN'S DISEASE

Techniques of intravenous hyperalimentation by means of a central venous catheter permit a period of complete bowel rest free of oral intake that supplies sufficient calories to restore deficits and permit weight gain. Should surgery become necessary it can be accomplished with lower morbidity and mortality and occasionally can result in prolonged remissions from active disease. Dudrick reported a series of 52 patients with inflammatory bowel disease in which remission occurred more frequently in Crohn's disease than in ulcerative colitis. This has been confirmed in our own experience with a similar series of patients in which approximately 60% of patients with Crohn's disease achieved remission with a program of intravenous nutrition and medical therapy. About 20% had surgery for persistent obstruction, fistulas, or abscess formation, and 20% continued with intractable disease that required surgery. Steinberg, in a study of 42 external fistulas, found that excision of the fistula and the diseased small bowel resulted in success in 84% with a 6% mortality. Dudrick reported a series of patients with intestinal fistulas in Crohn's disease who were treated with intravenous nutrition; 75% of these small bowel fistulas closed spontaneously. The other patients required surgical therapy but were nutritionally replete at the time of surgery and had no mortality and a markedly reduced morbidity. Recently, techniques for home hyperalimentation with in-dwelling Hickman-Broviac catheters have been utilized in the management of patients with short bowel syndrome resulting from multiple resections and in patients with diffuse Crohn's disease. These patients can achieve satisfactory nutritional maintenance and rehabilitation at home.

BACTERIAL, FUNGAL, TUBERCULOUS, VIRAL, AND NONSPECIFIC INFLAMMATORY LESIONS

A wide spectrum of inflammatory lesions may involve the small bowel and is important in the differential diagnosis of Crohn's disease. Specific antifungal and antituberculous drug therapy is indicated when the diagnosis of such lesions is made. Resection of obstructing lesions with subsequent long-term chemotherapy is indicated.

Tuberculous enteritis is the most frequently seen and most important of these miscellaneous inflammatory lesions of the small bowel. The ileum is most frequently involved, followed by the jejunum. The cecum is the portion of the colon most commonly involved. Symptoms are nonspecific and include anorexia, abdominal pain, and diarrhea. If these occur in a patient with pulmonary tuberculosis, the possibility of tuberculous enteritis must be considered. When ileocolonic tuberculosis presents as obstruction, resectional surgery with postoperative antituberculous chemotherapy is indicated.

SMALL BOWEL HEMORRHAGE

DEFINITION AND ETIOLOGY

Small bowel hemorrhage consists of bleeding arising from the mesenteric small bowel from the ligament of Treitz to the ileocecal valve. Lesions of the small bowel that may bleed are numerous and varied. These include primarily congenital lesions such as hemangiomas, telangiectasias, vascular malformations, duplications, and Meckel's and simple diverticula of the small intestine; inflammatory lesions such as regional enteritis, diverticulitis, ulcerations, and erosions; tumors such as leiomyomas, carcinomas, lymphomas, polyps, and lipomas; ectopic mucosal lesions such as aortojejunal fistulas, marginal jejunal ulcerations from Zollinger-Ellison tumors, and hemorrhage from jejunal and ileal varices associated with portal hypertension; and various other lesions such as nonocclusive mesenteric in-

farction and disseminated intravascular coagulation with intestinal microthrombi, among others.

DIAGNOSIS

CLINICAL MANIFESTATIONS

Patients may present with anemia and occasionally occult blood in the stool or with melena. Occasionally bleeding in association with hypotension and bright red or cherry-colored stools by rectum can be massive. There is no blood in the stomach upon passage of a nasogastric tube or upper gastrointestinal endoscopy.

The diagnostic and therapeutic challenge is to localize the site of hemorrhage so that definitive therapy can be instituted. Frequently this is not possible, particularly with the initial episode of bleeding.

BARIUM STUDIES

Barium studies have been only occasionally helpful because conventional delayed detail films and retrograde enemas are rarely diagnostic. The recent development of a new technique of small bowel enema appears promising. This technique involves the passage of a tube into the stomach through the pylorus and past the ligament of Treitz and the insertion through it of barium and methylcellulose. Small mucosal detail is possible with this technique.

SELECTIVE MESENTERIC ARTERIOGRAPHY

Selective superior mesenteric arteriography has been successful in diagnosing a wide variety of small intestinal lesions that are either actively bleeding or potential sources of hemorrhage, such as arterial malformations and vascular ectasias (Figs. 24-10, 24-11). Magnification techniques have been helpful in this diagnosis.

TECHNETIUM SCAN

A technetium scan is capable of detecting 0.1 ml of blood per minute in bleeding from the gastrointestinal tract. Its greatest value has been in identifying distal small bowel and colonic bleeding, and it has become a routine screening technique for active bleeding prior to mesenteric arteriography.

MANAGEMENT

SURGICAL

Exploratory laparotomy with resection of persistently bleeding lesions, particularly tumors, is indicated. If the source of bleeding is unknown, it is advantageous to explore the patient during the time of acute hemorrhage. Occasionally blind resections are indicated, with resection of small bowel commencing 6 inches proximal to the level of blood in the intestine. Intraoperative techniques such as transillumination and fluorescein dye injection are occasionally helpful.

VASOCONSTRICTIVE THERAPY

When bleeding results from arteriovenous malformations, vascular ectasias, or telangiectasias and is diagnosed by arteriography, the continuous infusion of vasopressin into the superior mesenteric arterial catheter can result in temporary control of hemorrhage in most cases, and permanent control in some.

SMALL BOWEL HEMORRHAGE	
Etiology	Relatively rare condition with multiple causes
Dx	Barium studies occasionally helpful Selective arteriography frequently helpful in diagnosis and treatment
Rx	Vasoconstrictive therapy using selective superior mesenteric arterial catheter infusions for temporary (and occasionally complete) control of bleeding Surgical exploration and resection indicated for identified sources of hemorrhage or for undiagnosed bleeding at the time of rebleeding

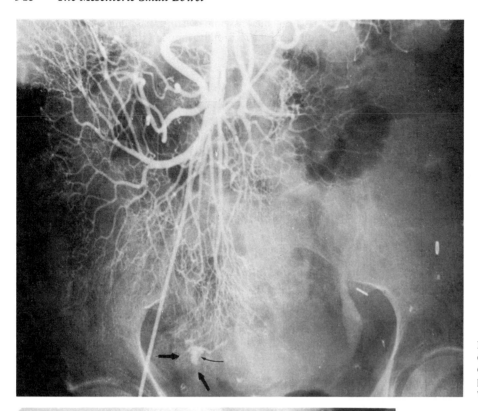

Fig. 24-10. Selective superior mesenteric arteriogram demonstrating extravasation of contrast agent in a patient with bleeding Meckel's diverticulum of the distal ileum.

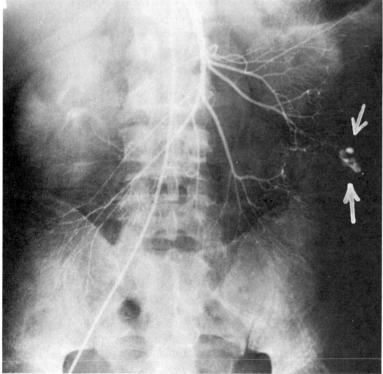

Fig. 24-11. Selective superior mesenteric arteriogram in a patient with active bleeding from a lymphoma of the upper jejunum.

BIBLIOGRAPHY

Small Bowel Tumors

AWRICH AE, IRISH CE, VETTO RM et al: A twenty-five year experience with primary malignant tumors of the small intestine. Surg Gynecol Obstet 151:9, 1980

GARVIN PJ, HERRMAN U, KAMINSKI DL et al: Benign and malignant tumors of the small intestine. Curr Probl Can III:9, 1979

McPEAK CJ: Malignant tumors of the small intestine. Am J Surg 114:402, 1967

WILSON JM, MELVIN DG, GRAY GF et al: Benign small bowel tumors. Ann Surg 181:247, 1974

Inflammatory Lesions of the Small Intestine

FAULKNER RL JR: Tuberculosis as a surgical disease of the abdomen. Ann Surg 160:806, 1964

GREENSTEIN AJ, SACHAR DB, SMITH H et al: Patterns of neoplasia in Crohn's disease and ulcerative colitis. Cancer 46:403, 1980

KIRSNER JB: Observations on the etiology and pathogenesis of inflammatory bowel disease. In Bockus HL: Gastroenterology, 3rd ed, Vol. 2. Philadelphia, W B Saunders, 1976

MACFAYDEN BV, DUDRICK SJ, RUTBERG RL: The management of gastrointestinal fistulae with parenteral nutrition. Surgery 74:100, 1973

STEINBERG DM, COOKE WT, WILLIAMS AJ: Abscess and fistulae in Crohn's disease. Gut 14:865, 1973

THOMAS JH, MACARTHUR RI, PIERCE GE et al: Hickman-Broviac catheters. Indications and results. Am J Surg 140:791, 1980

VALDES-DAPENA AM, STEIN GN: Morphologic Pathology of the Alimentary Canal. Philadelphia, W B Saunders, 1970

Small Bowel Hemorrhage

ALAVI A, DANN RW, BAUM S et al: Scintigraphic detection of acute gastrointestinal bleeding. Nucl Med 124:753, 1977

BAUM S, ATHANASOULIS CA, WALTMAN AC et al: Angiographic diagnosis and control. In Hardy JD, Zollinger RM (eds): Advances in Surgery, Vol. 7. Chicago, Year Book Medical Publishers, 1973

NUSBAUM M, BAUM S, KURODA E et al: Direct serial magnification arteriography as an adjuvant in the diagnosis of surgical lesions of the alimentary tract. Am J Surg 117:170, 1969

George L. Jordan, Jr.

Malabsorption Syndromes

PHYSIOLOGY OF DIGESTION AND ABSORPTION
CAUSES OF MALABSORPTION
CLINICAL MANIFESTATIONS
DIAGNOSIS
SPECIFIC LESIONS OF IMPORTANCE TO THE SURGEON
  Gastric Resection
  Vagotomy
  Gastroileostomy
  Gastrocolic Fistula
  Gastrointestinal Fistulas
  Pancreatic Insufficiency
  Non-β Islet Cell Tumors
  Diseases of the Liver and Biliary Tract
  Enzyme Deficiency in the Small Bowel
  Inflammatory Bowel Disease
  Blind Loop Syndrome
  Vascular Insufficiency
  Small Bowel Resection

PHYSIOLOGY OF DIGESTION AND ABSORPTION

Digestion begins in the mouth, with mastication and the action of salivary enzymes. It continues in the stomach, through the churning action of this organ and the action of hydrochloric acid and pepsin. A mild lipase also is found in the stomach, but its action is relatively unimportant. Further digestion occurs in the duodenum with mixture of the potent proteolytic and lipolytic enzymes from the pancreas as well as the addition of bile, and it is completed in the small bowel. Although alcohol may be absorbed in the stomach, the major absorptive process does not begin until the stomach contents enter the duodenum, where absorption of iron is of special significance. Simple sugars are absorbed rapidly in the upper small intestine, and a normal glucose tolerance test may be recorded in patients who have only a short bowel segment. Protein and fat are absorbed throughout the entire small bowel, whereas the distal ileum preferentially absorbs certain of the fat-soluble vitamins, cholesterol, bile acids for recirculation, and water.

The primary activity in the colon is absorption of fluid and electrolytes. Approximately 800 ml of fluid is secreted into the gastrointestinal tract each day and is absorbed in the small and large intestines, in addition to ingested fluid and fluid contained in solid food. Although the colon has the ability to absorb simple proteins to some degree, in the normal state this is not of great significance.

CAUSES OF MALABSORPTION

Malabsorption may occur as a result of a number of factors (Table 24-10). These include defects of digestion, specific defects of absorption, disturbances in intestinal motility, loss of absorptive surfaces, endocrinopathies, and a number of miscellaneous conditions. Consequently, the diagnosis and treatment of malabsorption syndromes require delineation of the specific etiologic factors, with medical or surgical interventions to correct these defects.

Elsewhere in this volume there are discussions of abnormalities of fluid and electrolyte balance, and other texts discuss primary intestinal mucosal diseases in more detail. This chapter is concerned with malabsorption syndromes that are of primary interest to the surgeon.

CLINICAL MANIFESTATIONS

The clinical manifestations of fat malabsorption include diarrhea, steatorrhea, weight loss, anorexia, and bloating. Although abdominal pain may occur in some syndromes, it is not specifically related to malabsorption. The stools are typically light in color and tend to float on the water when there is increased stool fat. Hypoproteinemia, which may result from a deficiency of protein absorption, may produce edema. The symptoms of carbohydrate malabsorption include watery diarrhea, cramps, and excessive flatus. Steatorrhea is not present. Tetany may result from failure of absorption of calcium or vitamin D. Calcium malabsorption may also produce osteomalacia, with bone pain and pathologic fractures. Anemia may result from a number of absorptive defects, including defective absorption of iron, folic acid, and vitamin B_{12}. Malabsorption of the latter substance also may produce peripheral neuropathy. Other vitamin deficiencies may also produce symptoms.

Many patients do not have classic symptoms but may have a variety of less diagnostic complaints such as abdominal discomfort or symptoms related to a specific deficiency syndrome.

TABLE 24-10 FACTORS RELATED TO MALABSORPTION

DEFECTS OF DIGESTION

Gastric diseases
  Loss of digestive enzymes
Gastric resection
  Loss of digestive enzymes
  Loss of reservoir function
Pancreatic insufficiency
  Cystic fibrosis
  Inflammatory lesions (chronic pancreatitis)
  Pancreatic lithiasis
  Pancreatic fistula
  Neoplastic disease
  Pancreatic resection
Hepatic and biliary disease
  Intrahepatic disease
    Hepatic cellular disease
    Diseases of intrahepatic biliary ducts
  Diseases of extrahepatic biliary ducts
    Stones
    Stricture
    Neoplasms
Deficiency of small bowel enzymes
  Lactase deficiency
  Sucrase-isomaltase deficiency

DEFECTS OF ABSORPTION

Primary intestinal mucosal disease
  Sprue
  Gluten-induced enteropathy
Inflammatory small bowel disease
  Regional enteritis
  Eosinophilic gastroenteritis
  Cytomegalovirus infection
  Tuberculosis
  Parasitic infestations
  Postantibiotic disease

Inflammatory large bowel disease
  Ulcerative colitis
  Crohn's disease of the colon
  Radiation enteritis
Reduced absorptive surface
  Small bowel resection
  Intestinal fistulas
  Gastroileostomy
  Gastrocolic fistula
  Ileal bypass for obesity
Vascular insufficiency
Chronic partial intestinal obstruction
Small bowel involvement in systemic disease
  Lymphoma
  Whipple's disease
  Amyloidosis
  Scleroderma
  Carcinoid syndrome
  Pneumatosis cystoides intestinalis
  Agammaglobulinemia

DISTURBANCES IN INTESTINAL MOTILITY

Certain postgastrectomy syndromes
Non β-cell islet tumors
Special problems resulting from surgical procedures
  Blind loop syndrome
  Postvagotomy diarrhea

ENDOCRINOPATHY

Diabetes mellitus
Hypoparathyroidism
Hyperparathyroidism

MISCELLANEOUS

Congestive heart failure
Protein-losing enteropathy

DIAGNOSIS

When clinical manifestations suggest the possibility of malabsorption, a variety of tests may be indicated. These include the following:

1. *Gross and microscopic examination of the stool.* In the presence of steatorrhea, the gross appearance of the stool is usually fairly typical. The stool is bulky and sticky. The weight of the stools per day significantly exceeds normal. Microscopic examination will demonstrate fat droplets. In patients with protein malabsorption, microscopic examination may disclose an excessive number of striated muscle fibers in the stool.

2. *Chemical determination of stool content.* The fat content of the stool may be determined chemically and reported as grams of fat or percent of dry weight of stool. The amount of fat in the stool is remarkably constant, varying from 5 g to 7 g per day in patients whose dietary intake of fat ranges from 50 g to 150 g per day. Fat should not constitute more than 6% of the dry weight of the stool.

   Severe fat malabsorption with fecal fat values of 40

g per day or more occurs almost exclusively in patients with pancreatic disease or defects in mucosal uptake. Mild steatorrhea may be produced by many lesions.

Chemical determinations of protein loss in the stool can be made in a similar fashion, after placing the patient on a special diet with known protein composition. With a protein intake of 100 g to 120 g per day, normal values of stool protein are approximately 2.5 g per 24 hr. Values above 3 g in 24 hr are considered definitely abnormal. Abnormal enteric protein loss may be documented also by measuring the excretion of chromium-labeled albumin in the stools after intravenous injection. The normal value is less than 1% excretion in 4 days, whereas patients with protein-losing enteropathy have values exceeding 2%.

3. D-*xylose absorption.* D-xylose is a pentose sugar. Measurement of its excretion in the urine following administration of a 25-g dose dissolved in water is one of the best biochemical tests of malabsorption. It is abnormal in the majority of patients whose steatorrhea is of intestinal origin and thus is a relatively specific test for

evidence of small bowel disease. Excretion of 4.5 g in a 5-hr urine specimen after ingestion is considered normal, while excretion of 3 g or less is definitely abnormal.

4. *Carbohydrate absorption.* The measurement of carbohydrate absorption is classically determined by a 3-hr or 5-hr glucose tolerance test. Absorption of starch in young infants can be determined by the use of a breath hydrogen test, which measures the amount of hydrogen produced from unabsorbed sugar present in the large intestine, or by measuring breath $^{13}CO_2$ and stool ^{13}C by mass spectrometry.

When the diagnosis of malabsorption is made, investigations that may aid in delineation of the etiology include the following:

1. *Detailed symptoms and previous history of surgical procedures*
2. *Specific tests for postgastrectomy symptoms*
3. *Plain roentgenograms of the abdomen* The most significant abnormality is pancreatic calcification due to alcoholic chronic pancreatitis.
4. *Roentgenographic studies with barium* These studies are important to diagnose fistulas, primary disease processes such as Crohn's disease, small bowel diverticula, and other abnormalities of motility and configuration.
5. *Mucosal biopsy* Many of the lesions listed in Table 24-10 have characteristic histologic abnormalities of the intestinal mucosa. Thus, the diagnosis can be substantiated by small bowel mucosal biopsy with appropriate histologic examinations, including, when necessary, special stains and electron microscopy. Assay of biopsy material for disaccharidases may provide a specific diagnosis.

SPECIFIC LESIONS OF IMPORTANCE TO THE SURGEON

GASTRIC RESECTION

Partial gastric resection produces a decrease in the reservoir function of the stomach, a decrease of digestion within the stomach remnant, rapid passage of food into the small intestine, and, if a gastrojejunostomy is used for reconstruction, decreased secretion of cholecystokinin, which impairs stimulation of both hepatic and pancreatic secretions. Furthermore, the bypass of the duodenum decreases the absorption of iron, which may produce hypochromic anemia. All of these factors may impair digestion and absorption with resulting diarrhea and weight loss. In most patients, however, the ability of the intestinal tract to accommodate these changes prevents the appearance of symptoms. Gastrectomy with or without vagotomy may be associated with development of certain syndromes that interfere with the absorption of food. These postgastrectomy problems are discussed in Chapter 23).

Total gastrectomy completely eliminates the reservoir and digestive functions of the stomach. The reservoir function can be compensated for to some degree by creation of a jejunal pouch.

VAGOTOMY

Diarrhea may be a complication of truncal vagotomy. Some authors have reported a relatively high incidence, but the incidence is lower following gastric vagotomy or parietal cell vagotomy. The exact cause of the diarrhea is not known. Simple conservative management with antispasmodics and dietary modification results in relief in most patients. Occasionally, surgical reversal of a 10-cm segment of jejunum, producing an antiperistaltic segment, is required. The success rate of this procedure is approximately 80%.

GASTROILEOSTOMY

When a portion of the stomach is removed, gastrointestinal continuity is established by an anastomosis between the gastric remnant and the duodenum (Billroth I) or between the gastric remnant and the jejunum (Billroth II). Rarely, an anastomosis has been made inadvertently between the gastric remnant and the ileum rather than the jejunum. This technical error results in a bypass of most of the small intestine with resulting rapid transit time and decrease in absorptive surface. Severe diarrhea results, and abnormal losses of vitamins, minerals, protein, fat, and fluid occur. The patients lose weight rapidly, and if correction of the defect is not accomplished, any of the malabsorption syndromes may appear.

The treatment is surgical, with take-down of the gastroileal anastomosis and construction of an appropriate gastroduodenal or gastrojejunal anastomosis.

GASTROCOLIC FISTULA

The most commonly reported abnormal communication between the stomach and the colon is a gastrojejunocolic fistula—a complication of marginal ulcer following gastrectomy. These fistulas have become increasingly rare because of the infrequency of marginal ulcer. Fistulas may also result from perforation of benign or malignant gastric ulcers directly into the colon. Although malabsorption may occur because gastric contents pass directly into the colon, bypassing the entire small bowel, the usual mechanism is reflux of colon contents into the stomach, producing continuing bacterial contamination of the entire gastrointestinal tract. Thus, these patients have a bacterial gastroenteritis that produces severe diarrhea. Treatment of the problem is surgical with resection of the lesion and closure of the abnormal opening in the colon.

GASTROINTESTINAL FISTULAS

Fistulas between portions of the gastrointestinal tract and the skin may result from primary disease processes such as Crohn's disease, as a complication of external trauma, or as a complication of surgical procedures upon the gastrointestinal tract. The nature and volume of gastrointestinal losses through the fistulous tract will depend upon the location of the fistula and its size. Thus, a fistula between the common bile duct and the skin will result only in the loss of bile, whereas a fistula between the side of the duodenum and the skin is more serious because there will be loss of gastrointestinal secretions as well as ingested fluid and food. Small fistulas in which the loss amounts to only 200 ml to 300 ml per day may cause no measurable malabsorption because the patient can easily ingest enough to compensate. When the fistulous discharge exceeds 1000 ml per day, however, a severe malabsorption syndrome exists. Furthermore, many fistulas may be complicated by infection. Seeding of the gastrointestinal tract with bacteria may cause diarrhea, which further complicates the malabsorption syndrome. Gastric, biliary, pancreatic, and colonic fistulas usually heal spontaneously in 3 to 6 weeks, and if the fistula is small, no special therapy may be necessary except protection of the skin to prevent digestion by the intestinal contents. In other patients, enteral alimentation may be accomplished through a tube placed beyond the fistulous opening so that absorption of fluid and nutrients may progress normally, even though there is some loss of upper gastrointestinal secretions. When enteral alimentation is not possible, treatment consists of total parenteral nutrition. Anticholinergic drugs may occasionally be used to decrease further the loss through the fistulous opening. With this program, many fistulas will heal spontaneously. Surgical closure is required for the remainder.

PANCREATIC INSUFFICIENCY

Pancreatic external secretion contains the most potent lipase found in the human body as well as potent amylase and proteases. Any disease or surgical procedure that decreases the secretion of pancreatic juice may result in malabsorption. The common diseases that produce this deficiency include pancreatic fistula, chronic pancreatitis, cystic fibrosis, pancreatolithiasis, and obstruction of the pancreatic duct due to inflammatory or neoplastic disease. Surgical procedures that decrease pancreatic secretion include gastric resection with a Billroth II anastomosis and pancreatic resection. Because the pancreas has considerable reserve capacity, a significant decrease in total volume of secretion may occur without producing symptoms. A marked decrease in pancreatic secretion, however, will produce measurable losses of fat and protein in the stool. Clinical manifestations will vary from patient to patient, depending upon the ability of the remainder of the gastrointestinal tract to compensate for this deficiency. Symptoms can usually be controlled by administration of oral enzymes even after total pancreatectomy. When deficiencies are due to pancreatic ductal obstruction or to a pancreatic fistula, surgical correction will cure the malabsorption syndrome. (See also Chapter 28.)

NON-β ISLET CELL TUMORS

Diarrhea may result from gastric hypersecretion caused by gastrin-secreting tumors of the pancreatic islets. In the past, treatment of this problem consisted of total gastrectomy with an attack upon the pancreatic tumor as indicated. More recently, more conservative gastric operations plus cimetidine have reduced the volume of gastric secretion.

Islet cell tumors may secrete other substances such as vasoactive intestinal peptide (VIP) that cause diarrhea through their direct action on the gastrointestinal tract. Treatment consists of excision of the pancreatic tumor. These tumors may be found in the wall of the duodenum, and thus, careful examination of the duodenum is important when surgical exploration is undertaken. (See also Chapters 20 and 23.)

DISEASES OF THE LIVER AND BILIARY TRACT

Bile salts are required for micelle formation and normal absorption of fat and are also important in activation of pancreatic enzymes. Thus, absence of bile from the intestinal tract may result in steatorrhea. Deficiencies of bile result from primary hepatocellular disease such as hepatitis and cirrhosis; from mechanical obstruction of bile flow by stone, tumor, or stricture; and from intestinal resection that impairs the enterohepatic circulation of bile. Mechanical obstructions are treated by surgical intervention. (Bowel resection is discussed later in this chapter.)

ENZYME DEFICIENCY IN THE SMALL BOWEL

Enzyme deficiency in the small bowel may result in symptomatic diarrhea from gastric resection and the loss of the digestive capacity of the stomach. The rapid entrance of food into the small bowel may significantly aggravate these symptoms. Mild deficiencies may become apparent clinically only after gastric resection.

INFLAMMATORY BOWEL DISEASE

The typical symptoms of inflammatory bowel disease, such as regional enteritis, radiation enteritis, and ulcerative colitis, include diarrhea and abdominal pain regardless of the extent of involvement of the intestinal tract. All of these diseases may produce internal or external fistulas. In many patients, symptoms are mild and can be controlled nonoperatively. Severe ulcerative colitis requires total colectomy. When regional enteritis or radiation enteritis is localized to a relatively short segment of bowel, complete relief of symptoms may occur following bowel resection. The portion of the bowel most commonly involved is the ileum, and therefore, following resection, diarrhea may continue owing to the loss of this portion of the intestinal tract. In such cases, cholestyramine may relieve the symptoms.

BLIND LOOP SYNDROME

Following many surgical procedures, a portion of the duodenum or small bowel is excluded from the normal flow of gastrointestinal contents. Most such excluded segments cause no difficulty, but occasionally stasis occurs with bacterial overgrowth, resulting in chronic inflammation and diarrhea. These bacteria may also utilize or inhibit absorption of vitamin B_{12}, resulting in megaloblastic anemia. They may deconjugate bile salts, producing steatorrhea. Conservative treatment with antibiotics and parenteral administration of vitamin B_{12} may result in improvement, but the treatment of choice is surgical removal of the blind loop.

VASCULAR INSUFFICIENCY

Occlusion of two or more of the major vessels supplying the gastrointestinal tract may reduce blood flow to the bowel sufficiently to impair normal motility and digestion of food. The most common symptom is postprandial pain, described as intestinal angina. In some patients, however, decreased vascularity results in failure of absorption and development of diarrhea.

Treatment consists in removal of the occluding lesion or a vascular bypass from the aorta to the superior mesenteric artery. The results of surgical treatment have been excellent (Fig. 24-12).

SMALL BOWEL RESECTION

The length of the small intestine from the ligament of Treitz to the ileocecal valve is approximately 10 feet. Most indi-

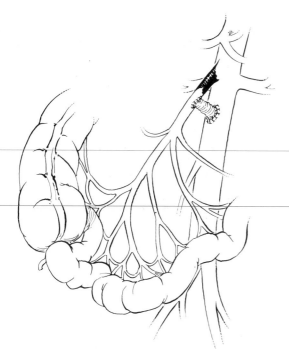

Fig. 24-12. Illustration of the bypass principle utilizing a graft between the aorta and the superior mesenteric artery to improve circulation to the bowel in a patient with occlusion of the superior mesenteric artery.

viduals will tolerate resection of at least half of this length and still retain the ability to maintain satisfactory absorption of protein, fat, and carbohydrates. When less than 4 feet of small bowel remain, however, some individuals will develop a malabsorption syndrome characterized by diarrhea and excessive loss of protein and fat in the stool, although absorption of carbohydrate ingested as simple sugars is usually maintained at normal levels. The ability of the small bowel to absorb is variable, and the occasional patient will be able to maintain good nutrition and have no significant diarrhea with only 1 or 2 feet of small bowel remaining. The shortest portion of tubular intestinal tract in which the patient was able to maintain nutrition by the oral route, although poorly, included the stomach, the duodenum, and the transverse and left colon. This patient had a severe malabsorption syndrome but was able to survive by ingesting large quantities of predigested food.

Following resection of the small intestine, the most severe malabsorption problems occur in the early postoperative period. With the passage of time, there is a significant increase in the absorptive capacity of the remaining bowel. An actual increase in the number of cells has been reported, as well as an increase in the length of the villi, thus producing a significant increase in absorptive surface. There are also reports of actual lengthening of the bowel. Thus, if the patient survives the early postoperative period, improvement in absorption will occur.

Resection of the terminal ileum produces special problems because of its absorption of water, bile salts, and vitamin B_{12}. Hepatic synthesis of bile salts must be increased because of the failure of absorption of bile salts and interruption of the normal enterohepatic circulation. Resections of the ileum (less than 100 cm) rarely cause diarrhea because increased hepatic synthesis of bile salts can compensate for the increased fecal loss. With extensive resection, hepatic synthesis is maximally increased but cannot com-

pensate for these large fecal losses, resulting in a reduction in jejunal bile acid concentration. Micelle formation is inadequate, and absorption of fat is decreased. Furthermore, the presence of unabsorbed bile acids in the colon may cause secretion of salt and water, thereby producing diarrhea. Oral administration of cholestyramine may aid in the reduction of this form of diarrhea. Inadequate bile salt absorption has also been reported to increase the formation of gallstones owing to failure of cholesterol to remain in emulsion in the biliary tract.

Lack of absorption of vitamin B_{12} may result in anemia. This defect, however, can be corrected by appropriate administration of this vitamin by the parenteral route.

Cholesterol is also absorbed preferentially in the distal small bowel, and bypass of the ileum has been utilized as a mechanism to control hypercholesterolemia. This has successfully reduced the cholesterol level in patients with severe hypercholesterolemia, but whether or not it can result in the improvement of atherosclerosis is not yet documented.

When the remaining small bowel measures less than 3 feet in length, the patient is best sustained on total intravenous alimentation for the first 2 to 3 weeks postoperatively. This will allow administration of adequate calories, protein, and vitamins to promote normal healing and maintain good nutrition. If prompt healing of the suture line does not occur, the stimulation of peristalsis and flow of digestive juices may result in a leaking anastomosis that could have been prevented if the bowel was kept at rest. After healing is assured, oral feedings should be instituted slowly with a gradual decrease in parenteral nutrition as tolerance of oral alimentation is gained.

In many of these patients, resumption of normal oral alimentation will be possible, but in others extensive modification of the diet will be necessary. A number of alterations in the diet may be useful. These include the following:
1. A simple increase in total caloric content, because a portion of all food ingested will be absorbed
2. Enzymatic supplements, which may be used to increase the rapidity of digestion and absorption
3. Utilization of antiperistaltic drugs to increase the time of contact of food with the mucosa
4. Dietary supplements, including (a) predigested or elemental diets; (b) liquid vitamins and iron; (c) vitamins or iron (or both) by injection; (d) use of surgical procedures to slow passage of food through the intestinal tract. Four of these procedures will be described.
   (1) Vagotomy and pyloroplasty
       After resection of the small bowel, gastric hypersecretion may occur owing to loss of an inhibiting effect on gastric secretion. This may increase the speed of gastrointestinal transit and produce diarrhea. Vagotomy and pyloroplasty has resulted in the improvement of this type of diarrhea in some patients. Because vagotomy and pyloroplasty may produce diarrhea in otherwise normal individuals, however, this technique has not received widespread utilization.
   (2) Creation of circular loop of small bowel
       This technique is intended to increase the time of contact of food with the absorptive surface by recirculating the food over the same portion of the bowel. In practice, however, it has not proved highly successful, because a major portion of the food enters the colon on the first passage, and reflux from the

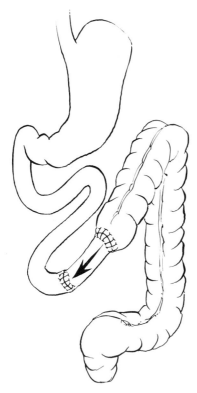

Fig. 24-13. The use of a reversed segment in the management of diarrhea following massive small-bowel resection. In this patient the right colon also had been removed.

colon may result in bacterial contamination that may aggravate the malabsorption problem.

(3) Reversed intestinal segment

This is the most effective technique for improving absorption in patients with the short bowel syndrome. An antiperistaltic segment is produced by reversing a 10 cm to 15 cm segment of the most distal portion of the remaining small bowel, creating a valve action that slows passage through the gastrointestinal tract and increases the time of contact between the intestinal contents and the small bowel mucosa. This technique has been used successfully in a number of patients (Fig. 24-13).

(4) Transplantation of the small bowel

Transplantation of the small bowel would appear to be the most appropriate way to remedy defects caused by bowel resection. Although this technique has been performed experimentally, it has not yet been sufficiently successful clinically to warrant uncontrolled clinical application.

Until a few years ago, if none of the techniques noted above were successful in providing adequate absorption of orally ingested food, the patient was doomed to die. With the advent of home intravenous hyperalimentation, however, there are now many patients who maintain good nutrition through the intravenous route. Depending upon the degree of malabsorption, intravenous feeding may be required only occasionally. In patients with severe problems, total intravenous nutrition is possible, and the patient may carry on most normal activities during the day with the nutritional requirements administered during the evening. A number of patients have survived for several years in this manner.

BIBLIOGRAPHY

ABER GM, ASHTON F, CARMALT MHB et al: Gastric hypersecretion following massive small bowel resection in man. Am J Dig Dis 12:785, 1967

ALTMAN DP, ELLISON EH: Massive intestinal resection: Inadequacies of the recirculating loop. Surg Forum 16:365, 1965

BAER AN, BAYLESS TM, YARDLEY JH: Intestinal ulceration and malabsorption syndromes. Gastroenterology 79:754, 1980

BALLINGER WF II, CHRISTY MG, ASHBY WB: Auto-transplantation of the small intestine; the effect of denervation. Surgery 52:151, 1962

BEJOR J, BROITMAN SA, ZAMCHECK N: Effect of vagotomy on the small intestine. Gut 9:87, 1968

BOCKUS HL: Gastroenterology, 3rd ed, Vol 2. Philadelphia, W B Saunders, 1976

BROIDO PW, GORBACH SL, NYHUS LM: Microflora of the gastrointestinal tract and the surgical malabsorption syndromes. Surg Gynecol Obstet 135:449, 1972

BURY KD, STEPHENS RV, RANDALL HT: Use of a chemically defined liquid elemental diet for nutritional management of fistulas of the alimentary tract. Am J Surg 121:174, 1971

DOBBINS WO III: Electron microscopy of intestinal fat absorption under normal conditions and in malabsorptive states. In Glass GBJ (ed): Progress in Gastroenterology. New York, Grune & Stratton, 1967

DUDRICK JS, LONG JM, STEIGER E et al: Intravenous hyperalimentation, Med Clin North Am 54:577, 1970

FREDERICK PL, SIZER JS, OSBORNE MP: Relation of massive bowel resection to gastric secretion. N Engl J Med 272:509, 1965

FREEMAN HG, KIM YS, SLEISENGER MH: Protein digestion and absorption in man: Normal mechanisms and protein-energy malnutrition. Am J Med 67:1030, 1979

GANGL A, OCKNER RK: Intestinal metabolism of lipids and lipoproteins. Gastroenterology 68:167, 1975

GIBSON LD, CARTER R, HINSHAW DB: Segmental reversal of small intestine after massive bowel resection. JAMA 182:952, 1962

GOLDSTEIN F: Mechanisms of malabsorption and malnutrition in the blind loop syndrome. Gastroenterology 61:780, 1971

HOFMANN AF, POLEY JR: Role of bile acid malabsorption in pathogenesis of diarrhea and steatorrhea in patients with ileal resection. Gastroenterology 62:918, 1972

JORDAN GL JR: Surgical approach to nutritional problems. Adv Surg 8:85, 1974

KINGHAM JG, LEVISON DA, FAIRCLOUGH PD et al: Diarrhoea and reversible enteropathy in Zollinger-Ellison syndrome. Lancet I:610, 1981

KINNEY JM, GOLWIN RM, BARR JF et al: Loss of entire jejunum and ileum and ascending colon: Management of patient. JAMA 179:529, 1962

LAUTERBURG PH, NEWCOMER AD, HOFMANN AF: Clinical value of the bile acid breath test: Evaluation of the Mayo Clinic experience. Mayo Clin Proc 53:227, 1978

LEVINE JM: Nutritional support in gastrointestinal disease. Surg Clin North Am 61:701, 1981

LOSOWSKY MS, WALKER BE, KELLEHER J: Malabsorption in Clinical Practice. New York, Churchill Livingstone, 1974

METZ G, GASSULL MA, DRASAR BS et al: Breath hydrogen test for small intestinal bacterial colonization. Lancet I:6, 1976

OSBORNE MP, FREDERICK PL, SIZER JS et al: Mechanism of gastric hypersecretion following massive intestinal resection: Clinical and experimental observations. Ann Surg 164:622, 1966

PORUS RL: Epithelial hyperplasia following massive small bowel resection in man. Gastroenterology 48:753, 1965

ROWE GG: Control of tenesmus and diarrhea by cholestyramine administration. Gastroenterology 53:1006, 1967

RUBIN CE, DOBBINS WO III: Peroral biopsy of the small intestine. A review of its diagnostic usefulness. Gastroenterology 49:676, 1965

SCRIBNER BH, COLE JJ, CHRISTOPHER TG et al: Long-term total parenteral nutrition: The concept of an artificial gut. JAMA 212:457, 1970

SHEEHY TW, FLOCH MH: The Small Intestine: Its Function and Disease. New York, Harper & Row, 1964

SHELDON GF, GARDINER BN, WAY LW et al: Management of gastrointestinal fistulas. Surg Gynecol Obstet 133:385, 1971

SLEISENGER MH, GLICKMAN RM: Symposium on malabsorption. Am J Med 67:979, 1979

THOMAS JE, JORDAN GL JR: Massive resection of small bowel and total colectomy: Use of reversed segment. Arch Surg 90:781, 1965

TOSKES PP, DAREN JJ: Vitamin B-12 absorption and malabsorption. Gastroenterology 65:662, 1973

WELSH JD, SHAW RW, WALKER A: Isolated lactase deficiency producing postgastrectomy milk intolerance. Ann Intern Med 64:1252, 1966

WILSON FA, DIETSCHY JM: Approach to the malabsorption syndromes as associated with disordered bile acid metabolism. Arch Intern Med 130:584, 1972

WOODWARD ER: The Postgastrectomy Syndromes. Springfield, IL, Charles C Thomas, 1963

ZURIER RB, CAMPBELL RG, HASHIM SA et al: Use of medium-chain triglycerides in management of patients with massive resection of the small intestine. N Engl J Med 274:490, 1966

James D. Hardy

Miscellaneous Other Small Bowel Disorders

DIVERTICULA OF THE SMALL BOWEL
LOCALIZED ULCER OF THE SMALL BOWEL
PNEUMATOSIS CYSTOIDES INTESTINALIS
INGESTED FOREIGN BODIES AND BEZOARS
   Ingested Foreign Bodies
   Bezoars
ASCARIS INFESTATIONS WITH SURGICAL
       COMPLICATIONS
INFECTIVE ENTERITIS

DIVERTICULA OF THE SMALL BOWEL

Diverticula occur infrequently in the jejunum and ileum and are present in 0.1% to 0.5% of small-bowel barium studies (Fig. 24-14). Susceptibility to the formation of diverticula decreases proportionately from the second portion of the duodenum to the terminal ileum. Again, the incidence of colonic diverticula increases from the cecum through the sigmoid colon. The rectum below the peritoneal reflection rarely exhibits diverticula. The incidence of jejunal diverticula in autopsy series ranged from a low of 0.06% to a high of 1.3% when a special effort was made to demonstrate diverticula. Most diverticula in the mesenteric portion of the small bowel are found in the upper portion of the jejunum, usually within a few feet of the ligament of Treitz.

There are two types of diverticula of the small intestine: congenital and acquired. Congenital diverticula are situated on the antimesenteric margin of the intestine and are true diverticula in that they consist of all layers of the intestinal wall. Meckel's diverticulum is the classic example of the true congenital type. The congenital diverticulum is usually solitary.

Acquired diverticula occur on the mesenteric margin of the bowel, where the blood vessels penetrate the bowel wall. They are hernias of the mucous membrane penetrating through the muscular wall at the point of entrance of the vessels. They are pulsion diverticula caused by increased intraluminal pressure. The thin muscular coat pushes out as the diverticula increase in size, and, ordinarily, only a few fibers of the muscularis mucosa are found in the wall of the sac. Acquired diverticula are much more numerous in the jejunum than in the ileum. They are most often multiple, sometimes solitary, and are often associated with diverticula of the colon or duodenum. Acquired small-bowel diverticula have been found almost exclusively in persons over 40 years of age and are seen nearly twice as often in men as in women.

Diverticula of the small intestine are usually asymptomatic and are found incidentally in the course of an x-ray examination or at autopsy. However, serious complications, such as acute inflammation, intestinal obstruction, perforation, and hemorrhage, may rarely occur with the diverticula and require surgical intervention.

Acute diverticulitis usually results from food particles or parasites becoming trapped in a pouch. The symptoms may simulate those of appendicitis. Intestinal obstruction may occur by volvulus, by compression from an inflammatory tumor, or, rarely, by intussusception. Perforation of the diverticulum is usually caused by a foreign body, such as a chicken bone, that has entered the pouch. Perforation may occur into the free abdominal cavity, into the mesentery, or into another intestinal loop, resulting in generalized peritonitis, walled-off abscess, or intestinal fistula. A few cases are recorded in which either aberrant pancreatic tissue or benign or malignant tumors were located in an intestinal diverticulum.

Fig. 24-14. Small-bowel diverticula.

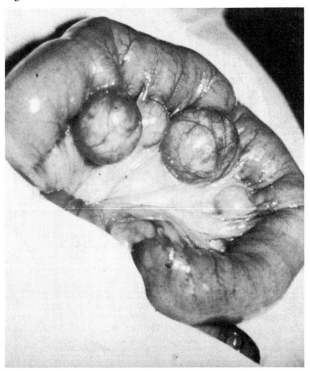

Rarely, diverticulosis of the jejunum may be a significant source of gastrointestinal hemorrhage, which may be chronic or acute; 36 cases of gastrointestinal bleeding caused by jejunal diverticulosis have been reported, and surely many others have not been reported. Inflation of segments of the jejunum by passing gas through a Miller–Abbott tube or by injection of air into isolated segments of the jejunum has been required at times to demonstrate the diverticula. If other more common sources of gastrointestinal bleeding can be excluded, resection of the involved segment and end-to-end anastomosis may be curative. A definite bleeding point in resected jejunal diverticula has been identified only five times in 36 cases. This is in agreement with the experience in bleeding from colonic diverticulosis. Nevertheless, arteriographic and isotopic identification of the site of gastrointestinal bleeding is improving steadily.

A massive diverticulosis of the small bowel may interfere seriously with the absorptive function of the bowel and may be responsible for the occurrence of steatorrhea, megaloblastic anemia, and other symptoms that characterize the malabsorption syndrome.

LOCALIZED ULCER OF THE SMALL BOWEL

Ulcer of the small bowel of unknown cause was first described by Baillie in 1795. A total of 76 cases were reported in the literature between 1936 and 1955. Perforation was the most common complication; stenosis occurred in 32%.

Circumferential primary small-bowel ulcers were then reported with increasing frequency until the introduction of soluble potassium preparations, which replaced the use of enteric-coated potassium tablets. These tablets given to monkeys in a dosage of 100 mg to 1000 mg once or twice daily for 1 or more days induced in most animals severe ulceration in the small bowel. Thiazides had been implicated in the etiology of these lesions; however, thiazides alone did not cause any reaction in the gastrointestinal tract.

Several patients have had two separate small-bowel ulcers. Visceral vascular disease is not a universal feature of these ulcers. In December of 1964, Berg reported 140 cases of stenosing ulcers of the small bowel, associated with ingestion of enteric-coated potassium. Four patients died as a result of this lesion. The stenotic, circumferential nature of these ulcers produced chiefly obstructive symptoms (Fig. 24-15). The duration of therapy and the dosage of potassium chloride did not correlate with the development of the lesions. Boley, in discussing the 140 cases reported to the small-bowel registry, stated that some patients develop small-bowel ulcers after one or two doses and others after several years of medication.

If an enteric-coated irritant such as potassium lies stationary in the bowel while the coating dissolves, the necrotizing properties concentrate on the adjacent mucosa and cause muscle spasm. This brings the mucosa in contact with the irritant and results in circumferential mucosal injury. If the spasm lasts until the the next dose, a barrier has been created and a second application causes extension of the necrosis with eventual stricture and obstruction, very rarely with perforation.

The surgical treatment for this lesion is resection of the involved segment of small bowel and end-to-end anastomosis. No subsequent intestinal symptoms have occurred

Fig. 24-15. Small-bowel ulcer, probably due to enteric-coated potassium, causing cicatricial stenosis and intestinal obstruction. (*A*) Appearance at operation. Note the chronically distended proximal small bowel and collapsed bowel distal to the stricture (*arrow*). (*B*) Appearance of ulcer in excised gut.

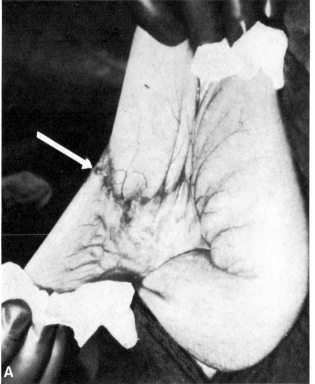
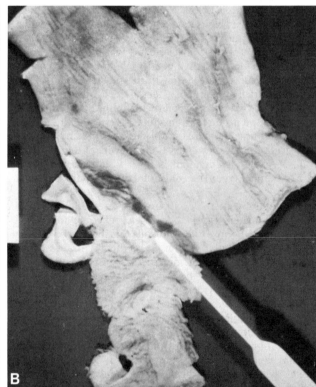

in those patients who had the involved segment of the ileum resected and anastomosed end to end.

Although not all small-bowel ulcers are due to enteric-coated potassium salts, this was the etiologic factor in the great increase in incidence noted in the 2 decades preceding the development of soluble potassium preparations. The avoidance of enteric-coated potassium salts has greatly reduced the incidence of small-bowel ulcers.

PNEUMATOSIS CYSTOIDES INTESTINALIS

Intestinal pneumatosis, also variously called bullous emphysema of the intestine, abdominal gas cyst, and pneumatosis cystoides intestinalis, is an uncommon condition of the intestines characterized by one or more gas-filled cysts in one or more layers of the intestinal wall. Approximately 300 cases were recorded in the literature up to 1962.

The gas cysts vary in size from very minute bubbles to cystlike collections up to 10 cm in diameter. The gas cysts may be single, but they occur usually as multiple clusters, not unlike soap bubbles or clusters of grapes in appearance. The cysts are most commonly located in the lower ileum. They collapse if punctured with a needle, and their contents are usually sterile. Spontaneous rupture gives rise to pneumoperitoneum.

The mechanism of their development is not known, but patients with pulmonary disease with severe cough may rupture their alveoli and air may dissect retroperitoneally and along perivascular routes to the bowel wall.

The symptoms are nonspecific. In 85% of cases, the gas cysts are associated with other lesions of the gastrointestinal tract. The diagnosis is usually made roentgenographically. No treatment is necessary unless one of the rare complications supervenes, such as rectal bleeding, cyst-induced volvulus, or tension pneumoperitoneum. The prognosis in most cases is that of the underlying disease. The cysts may disappear spontaneously or may persist for prolonged periods without serious symptoms.

INGESTED FOREIGN BODIES AND BEZOARS

INGESTED FOREIGN BODIES

The ingestion of sharp foreign bodies is not a rare occurrence, and in the majority of patients, the object proceeds uneventfully through the intestinal tract. In 17% of cases, however, the foreign body becomes lodged in some portion of the intestinal tract, and sooner or later a perforation may occur.

The ingestion of the foreign body is usually unknown to the patient. Fish or meat bones are the usual etiologic agents. In 50% of the cases complicated by perforation of the intestine, patients are in the first 3 decades of life. There is an increased risk of swallowing foreign bodies in patients who wear dentures. In mental institutions and in geriatric patients, the index of suspicion of foreign bodies as a cause of peritonitis, abscess, or fistula should be high.

There are different clinical situations, depending on the time of perforation. Some patients present with acute pain and vomiting, with signs of peritonitis. Other patients have long histories, extending from a few weeks to many years, with late abscesses or fistulas requiring surgery. Jejunal diverticula perforated by a fish bone have sometimes simulated a perforated duodenal ulcer. At surgery, the site of

perforation in the jejunal diverticulum can prove difficult to find.

The great preponderance of perforations in the lower ileal and cecal regions is striking. The appendix and Meckel's diverticulum are predisposed by their shape to perforation by sharp foreign bodies. The foreign body has been reported to perforate a loop of gut while it lay incarcerated in a hernial sac.

The indications for surgery are usually signs relating to perforation, such as peritonitis, abscess, or fistula, which may be evident on x-ray studies. Occasionally, a particularly large foreign body will obstruct the small bowel. The prognosis relates to peritoneal contamination and to the general condition of the patient at the time of surgery.

BEZOARS

Bezoars have long been of interest. In humans, these masses are generally composed of densely entangled vegetable fibers (phytobezoars) or hair (trichobezoars). They occur most frequently in the stomach.

Although in recent years the obstructing bolus in the small bowel has been composed of orange segments in approximately 90% of cases, other vegetable foodstuffs that have been involved are figs, apples, grapefruit, coconuts, beans, brussels sprouts, potato peel, berries, and cabbage. It is of interest that in the comprehensive review by Ward-McQuaid in 1950, the orange was the offending food in only 11% of the cases.

When the patient presents with the findings of acute small-bowel obstruction, emergency laparotomy must be performed. An attempt should be made to fragment or to squeeze the bezoar gently into the cecum. According to Vernon, this procedure is successful in 38% of cases. Removal of the bezoar by enterotomy should be performed if these measures fail. Occasionally, volvulus associated with the bezoar may require a small-bowel resection.

The treatment of the bezoar in the stomach is considered elsewhere. This is not an emergency surgical procedure, and a variety of enzymes, with lavage and endoscopic techniques, are employed to dislodge and remove the gastric bezoar.

Patients who have had a gastrectomy should be advised to avoid fibrous foods, especially oranges, unless these foods can be chewed very thoroughly or can be mechanically minced to fineness prior to ingestion. The incidence of small-bowel obstruction from phytobezoar would be greatly reduced by this precaution.

ASCARIS INFESTATIONS WITH SURGICAL COMPLICATIONS

Ascaris lumbricoides is the parasite most commonly infesting human beings, who are the only susceptible host. Distribution of the worm is worldwide, and the native populations of the Far East show infestation rates as high as 90%. Where raw human feces is used as fertilizer, ascaris infestation is extremely common, and life-threatening surgical complications present frequently.

The adult ascaris preferentially inhabits the jejunum, and fertilized eggs are passed in the stools. The fertilized female may lay up to 200,000 eggs per day. Up to 5000 ascarids have been found in the small intestine of patients with no apparent symptoms.

Inoculation of the small intestine occurs in 99% of

patients on oral ingestion of the ova. The jejunum contains eight times as many worms as does the ileum. Ascarids die in the colon because they are unable to nourish themselves on the contents of the colon. Once ingested, the eggs quickly become larvae, penetrate the intestinal mucosa, and enter lymphatics and vascular channels. The larvae travel to the liver and the lungs through the portal system. In the lungs, the ascarids penetrate the alveolar walls, are coughed up to the hypopharynx, and are swallowed again. Intrajejunal maturation requires 70 days. The adult worms are the largest nematodes infective to humans. On the average, the worms are 20 cm (but may be as much as 35 cm) in length and 6 mm in diameter. The usual adult life span is 1 year. Ova may be found in the stool or in the sputum.

The serious complications of ascarid infestation arise from three sources: the obstructive potential of the parasite in the small bowel, the migratory tendency, and the antigenicity of parasitic residues. Surgical complications that have resulted from ascarid infestations include brain abscess, larval granulomatosis of the retina, eustachian tube obstruction with otitis, pulmonary abscess, cholangiohepatitis, liver abscess, common bile duct obstruction, acute cholecystitis, cholelithiasis, pancreatitis, intestinal obstruction, small-bowel volvulus, intestinal perforation, acute appendicitis, and cystitis (Fig. 24-16).

Quiescent infestation has been discovered on plain films of the abdomen, on barium studies of the gut, and incidentally at laparotomy. Eosinophilia is present in 5% to 25% of patients infested, but in these patients other parasitic infestations are so common that this is rarely helpful in establishing the diagnosis. A history of passing worms in the stool or of coughing up worms may be obtained.

Biliary and pancreatic involvement with ascarid infestation is common in the Far East and in Africa. In children, biliary involvement is most common between the ages of 4 and 8; intestinal obstruction usually occurs at a younger age.

Mild symptoms of abdominal pain, with shifting soft abdominal masses, are often seen in patients with this disease. The most common of the abdominal manifestations of massive ascarid infestation is mechanical intestinal obstruction. The lumen may be blocked by a bolus of worms.

Fig. 24-16. Ascaris in the small bowel, causing obstruction.

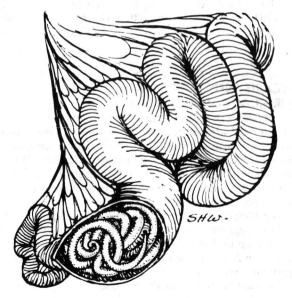

Crane reported the case of a child from Korea, who weighed 25 kg, with a gangrenous segment of ileum from a volvulus. In the resected bowel there were 1063 roundworms, and the bowel segment weighed 4 kg. The child died after resection.

The ascarids can cause spasm of smooth muscle, and spasm with contraction, producing obstruction at the ileocecal valve, has been reported. Loops of bowel may be matted together at sites occupied by the worms. Volvulus, intussusception, and band obstruction related to the infestation may cause intestinal obstruction. The vomiting of worms may be a grave sign in obstruction.

If small-bowel obstruction due to ascarids is suspected and the patient does not respond to intravenous fluids and tube suction, surgery is indicated. Signs pointing to an urgent need for laparotomy are multiple fluid levels on x-ray films, the passage of blood by rectum, or a distended abdomen and rebound tenderness (usually seen in a child).

Louw reported from Cape Town on 731 acute abdominal emergencies in children, 70% of whom harbored the parasite; 100 emergencies, or 12.8%, were due to ascaris infestation. Only appendicitis was a more common cause of acute abdominal emergencies. There were eight deaths in the 731 children; three were due to ascarids, accounting for 37.5% of all deaths. Intestinal obstruction was due to ascaris infestation in 68 instances and to other causes in 185 cases. Biliary disease was due to ascaris in 17 cases and to other causes in five instances.

The ascaris may migrate through the suture line and may live in the peritoneal cavity for as long as 2 weeks. The anthelmintic of choice is piperazine citrate, which causes muscular paralysis of the ascaris. In cases requiring laparotomy, the piperazine should not be started before the seventh to tenth postoperative day because dead and dying worms may impact in the terminal ileum.

INFECTIVE ENTERITIS

As a rule, bacterial conditions of the small intestine are not considered surgical problems, but in many parts of the world, tuberculosis (*Mycobacterium tuberculosis*) and typhoid (*Salmonella typhosa*) still constitute important causes of small-bowel pathology that can produce complications of surgical significance. Of course, these potential causes of diarrhea and gut stenosis, hemorrhage, or perforation must be distinguished from the host of other potential causes of diarrhea, infectious and otherwise.

In general, enteric tuberculosis is a granulomatous process that produces fibrosis, stricture, shortening, and changes in the mucosa visible on barium study. Effective drug therapy is usually successful, and operation is reserved for the rare complications of hemorrhage, perforation, or obstruction.

With typhoid fever, drug therapy (chloramphenicol, ampicillin) is usually successful, but surgery is occasionally required for hemorrhage that has not responded to conservative measures or for perforation, usually through ulcerated Peyer's patches.

BIBLIOGRAPHY

ABOURJAILY GS, MIKAL S, CHRISTIAN JH: Multifocal trichobezoars of the gastrointestinal tract. Am J Gastroenterol 47:287, 1967

ALLEN AC, BOLEY SJ, SCHULTZ L et al: Potassium induced lesions of the small bowel: II. Pathology and pathogenesis. JAMA 193:1001, 1965

AUSTAD WI, CORNES JS, GOUGH KR et al: Steatorrhea and malignant lymphoma. Am J Dig Dis 12:475, 1967

BERG EH, SCHUSTER F, SEGAL GA: Thiazides with potassium producing intestinal stenosis. Arch Surg 91:998, 1965

BOLEY SJ, ALLEN AC, SCHULTZ J et al: Potassium induced lesions of the small bowel: I. Clinical aspects. JAMA 193:997, 1965

BUCHHOLZ RR, HAISTEN AS: Phytobezoars following gastric surgery for duodenal ulcer. Surg Clin North Am 52:341, 1972

CIVETTA JM, DAGGETT WM: Gastrointestinal bleeding from jejunal diverticula. Am Surg 166:976, 1967

CRANE PS, PAK YH, LEE HK: Surgical complications of massive infestations with *Ascaris lumbricoides*. Ann Surg 162:34, 1965

DUNCAN W, LEONARD JD: The malabsorption syndrome following radiotherapy. Q J Med 34:319, 1965

FIDLER M: Foreign body perforation of a jejunal diverticulum. Br J Surg 59:744, 1972

GUEST JT: Collective review: Non-specific ulceration of the intestine. Int Abstr Surg 117:509, 1967

GUNN A: Intestinal perforation due to swallowed fish or meat bone. Lancet 1:125, 1966

KUSHLAN SD: Pneumatosis cystoides intestinalis. JAMA 179:699, 1962

LOUW JH: Abdominal complications of *Ascaris lumbricoides* infestation in children. Br J Surg 53:510, 1966

McMANUS JE: Perforations of the intestine by ingested foreign bodies: Report of two cases and review of the literature. Am J Surg 53:393, 1941

MAYO CW, BASKIN RH, HAGEDORN AB: Hemorrhagic jejunal diverticulitis. Am Surg 136:691, 1952

MIR AM, MIR MA: Phytobezoar after vagotomy with drainage or resection. Br J Surg 60:846, 1973

RAVITCH MM: Bezoars, old or new. Med Times 98:158, 1970

SCHANG HA, McHENRY LE: Obstruction of the small bowel by orange in the postgastrectomy patient. Ann Surg 159:611, 1964

SHACKELFORD RT, MARCUS WY: Jejunal diverticula: A cause of gastrointestinal hemorrhage. Am Surg 151:930, 1960

SHANDS WC, GATLING RR: Circumferential small bowel ulcers. Ann Surg 165:894, 1967

THOMAS C, CORNWELL EE: Perforation of the terminal ileum by foreign bodies: Report of two cases and review of the literature. J Nat Med Assoc 57:494, 1965

WELCH JW, HELLWIG CA, PAKORNY C: Intestinal pneumatosis. Am Surg 26:494, 1960

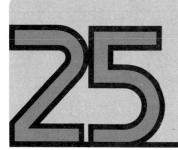

Harvey I. Pass/James D. Hardy

The Appendix

The appendix is a true diverticulum of the cecum, averaging about 10 cm in length. Its base is located at the site of convergence of the teniae of the colon, a fact that can be useful in locating it at operation. It is approximately 2.5 cm below the ileocecal valve. The appendix usually lies in the peritoneal cavity, although in many different positions, but is located retrocecally in 19% of adults.

The appendix has a microscopic appearance similar to that of the colon. Its mucosa of columnar epithelium is originally rich in lymphoid follicles, but these atrophy with adulthood. A circular and an outer longitudinal muscle layer surrounds the mucosa. The appendiceal artery is a branch of the ileocolic artery, and occlusion of the arterial supply can lead to distal gangrene in the appendix.

The function of the appendix may well be related to the role of the lymphoid follicles in developing and maintaining the immune capability of the host.

INFLAMMATION OF THE APPENDIX

ACUTE APPENDICITIS

The first clear description of appendicitis is generally attributed to Reginald Fitz of Boston. Although there had been numerous previous reports of suppuration in the region of the appendix termed perityphlitis, it was Fitz who in 1886 accurately summarized the pathology and recommended early diagnosis and treatment. McBurney extended clinical

ACUTE APPENDICITIS	
Etiology	Luminal obstruction causing bacterial stasis, distention, ischemia, focal necrosis and perforation

Dx	Symptoms:
	   Periumbilical pain, moving to right lower quadrant
	   Anorexia, nausea, at times vomiting; many variations
	 Signs:
	   Right lower quadrant tenderness, at times rigidity
	     Diffuse findings if perforated with spreading peritonitis
	 Laboratory:
	   Leukocytosis with shift to left, in typical case
	 Roentgenograms:
	   May demonstrate a fecalith and may exclude significant small bowel obstruction

Rx	Appropriate preparation and then appendectomy

knowledge of this condition and championed diagnosis and operation prior to rupture. McBurney's point was the name given to the site of maximal tenderness in the right lower quadrant of the abdomen, and the McBurney muscle splitting or gridiron incision became the usual surgical approach to appendectomy.

INCIDENCE

Acute appendicitis is the most common acute surgical condition in the abdomen. It should always be at least considered in the differential diagnosis of abdominal pain in any age group unless the appendix has previously been removed. It is estimated that about 6% of the population will have appendicitis at some time in their lives. Appendicitis is rare in the very young, occurring most often in the second and third decades of life. The incidence in the two sexes is approximately equal except for a definitely greater incidence in males in the 20- to 30-year-old age group. The overall incidence in the United States and abroad appears to be slowly declining for reasons that are not clear.

ETIOLOGY AND PATHOGENESIS

Acute appendicitis is almost always due to obstruction of the lumen. In the young this obstruction is often caused by lymphoid tissue, but in older persons it is commonly caused by a fecalith. The luminal obstruction leads to distention and stasis, bacterial overgrowth and suppuration, arterial ischemia and venous thrombosis, and ultimately perforation at the site of or distal to the fecalith. Rarely, the obstruction may be caused by parasites, foreign body, or tumor.

COMPLICATIONS

As the secretion of mucus with sepsis continues, the appendix becomes progressively distended, occluding the blood supply as previously noted and producing gangrene. Thus perforation may occur, with release of bacteria-laden pus and feculent appendiceal contents into the surrounding tissues (Fig. 25-1). Frequently, the appendix does not rupture but produces surrounding inflammation and cellulitis, which may be palpated as a tender mass on physical examination; a localized abscess after rupture of the appendix produces the same tenderness. However, if the escape of pus is not contained by the omentum and surrounding tissues in the form of a localized abscess, a much more widespread peritonitis will ensue if the appendix lies free in the peritoneal cavity or a large phlegmon will occur in the retroperitoneal space if the perforation is so situated. Widespread peritonitis can result in scattered intra-abdominal abscesses, including infection in the portal vein radicles (pylephlebitis) and multiple liver abscesses—all of which represent serious complications and grave threats to the life of the patient. Clearly, it is extremely desirable to diagnose and treat appendicitis before rupture.

DIAGNOSIS

The diagnosis of appendicitis is usually relatively simple but can be extremely difficult, and even after every precaution it will at times be found to be in error at operation. The diagnosis rests on the history and physical examination, laboratory studies, and roentgenograms. Many other acute intra-abdominal or even systemic conditions may mimic appendicitis, and the differential diagnosis must therefore consider other disorders that may require different treatment or no operation at all. Thus the basic decision often boils down to whether or not to operate (for appendicitis or some other condition requiring surgery).

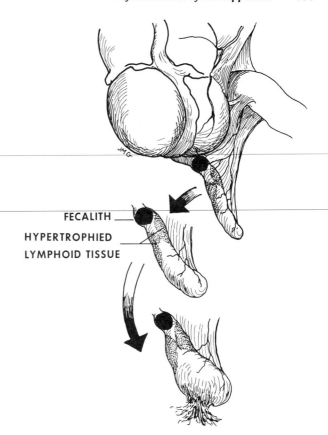

FECALITH

HYPERTROPHIED
LYMPHOID TISSUE

Fig. 25-1. Perforation of the appendix. Appendiceal perforation is almost always due to obstruction of its lumen, either by a fecalith or by lymphoid deposits in its wall. (Condon RE, Gleysteen JJ: Appendicitis, peritonitis, and intra-abdominal abscess. In Hardy JD [ed]: Rhoads Textbook of Surgery, 5th ed. Philadelphia, J B Lippincott, 1977)

Clinical Manifestations

The first symptom of acute appendicitis is usually abdominal pain, especially in the periumbilical region but at times in the epigastrium. Later, the pain shifts to the right lower quadrant and becomes localized. Meanwhile, the patient commonly feels nausea and anorexia; in fact, if the patient remains really hungry, the diagnosis of appendicitis should be questioned. If vomiting occurs it does not usually persist, and it follows the onset of abdominal pain in most instances.

Atypical pain patterns are common, especially in older patients. The pain may originate in the right lower quadrant and remain there, or there may be relatively little pain but deep tenderness associated with nausea, anorexia, and at times vomiting. Otherwise unexplained small bowel obstruction, especially in the elderly, may be due to appendicitis. In part, the variations in symptom complexes are due to the many different possible locations of the appendix, although the base of course remains attached to the cecum. The retrocecal appendix may present pain mainly in the flank, perhaps with walking or coughing or perhaps with urinary symptoms due to the contiguous ureter or bladder. The appendix situated in the pelvis may produce urinary frequency, diarrhea, tenesmus, and pain on rectal or pelvic examination. Abdominal signs may be minimal. A high cecum may place the appendix in the right upper quadrant, where appendicitis can be confused with acute cholecystitis, perforated ulcer, or pancreatitis.

On auscultation the abdomen is either quiet or normal.

The local findings are usually right lower quadrant tenderness and perhaps a mass, with or without rigidity and rebound tenderness (Fig. 25-2). Pressure and release in the left lower quadrant may produce pain on the right (Rovsing's sign). On rectal examination there may be tenderness on the right side that can be quite sharp if a pelvic appendix is palpated. Of course, the pelvic examination should be employed in women to exclude uterine or ectopic inflammatory disease, torsion of the ovary, or ectopic pregnancy.

Aside from pain, the patient usually exhibits a mild elevation of body temperature and some increase in pulse rate.

Laboratory Values

The hematocrit may be mildly elevated owing to dehydration. The white blood cell count is usually elevated but is rarely above 18,000 cells/mm³. There is usually a shift to the left, that is, an increased percentage of immature cells. The urinalysis may contain a few white blood cells, and albuminuria is present in about 20% of cases. Red blood cells may also be present but should not in themselves dissuade one from the diagnosis of appendicitis. In young black patients, a sickle cell preparation should be obtained.

Roentgenograms

Films of the abdomen are frequently nonrevealing, but at times a fecalith is disclosed. Otherwise, one of the principal dividends of films is evidence of other conditions such as calculous cholecystitis, intestinal obstruction, perforated ulcer, ureterolithiasis, or pancreatitis. Should the appendix fill normally on (rarely performed) barium enema, appendicitis is virtually excluded.

DIFFERENTIAL DIAGNOSIS

A remarkable number of disorders may be confused with appendicitis. They include the following:

Gastroenteritis. Diarrhea, uncommon in appendicitis. Nausea, vomiting *before* onset of pain, "flu-like." Abdomen

Fig. 25-2. Some physical signs of appendicitis prior to rupture. (Gelin LE, Nyhus LM, Condon RE: Abdominal Pain: A Guide to Rapid Diagnosis. Philadelphia, J B Lippincott, 1969)

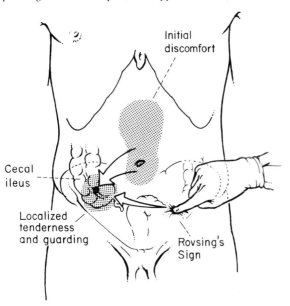

diffusely tender with hyperperistalsis. Laboratory tests essentially normal. X-ray film may show gas in the small bowel, an abnormal finding in most adults.

Mesenteric Lymphadenitis. Not usually diagnosed preoperatively. Recent upper respiratory infection, normal appendix, and large mesenteric lymph nodes.

Urinary Tract Infection. High fever, dysuria and frequency, often chills. Costovertebral angle tenderness. White blood cells and bacteria in urine.

Regional Enteritis. No anorexia. Minimal nausea, perhaps diarrhea. Often past history. Leukocytosis. Usually diagnosed at laparotomy if symptoms simulate appendicitis. Gastrointestinal series may be useful.

Ureteral or Renal Calculi. Colic, with radiation to groin. Often vomiting. Costovertebral angle tenderness. No focal peritoneal signs, hematuria. Plain film or intravenous pyelogram shows stones.

Pelvic Inflammatory Disease. Recent intercourse. Vaginal discharge. Treatment in past. High fever. Diffuse tenderness, bilateral. Tender cervix on pelvic examination. Gram-negative intracellular diplococci on cervical smear.

Ectopic Pregnancy. Cessation of menses. "Sudden" pain. Hypovolemia, perhaps shock. Anemia. Pelvic tenderness, perhaps a mass. Culdocentesis positive for blood.

Torsion Ovarian Cyst. Acute onset of pain. Afebrile. Mass and pain on pelvic examination, laboratory tests normal.

Ruptured Ovarian Follicle (Mittelschmerz). Midmenstrual cycle pain. Diffuse pain, not severe. Laboratory tests normal.

Others. Cholecystitis; perforated ulcer; pancreatitis; diverticulitis, especially of cecum or sigmoid colon; intestinal obstruction; Meckel's diverticulitis; perforated colon; carcinoma; intussusception in children; mesenteric vascular occlusion; infarcted epiploic appendages; primary peritonitis; pneumonitis; torsion of testis; acute epididymitis; other gynecologic disorders; hematoma of the abdominal wall; various systemic diseases such as Henoch-Schoenlein's purpura, sickle cell disease, diabetic acidosis, black widow spider bite, porphyria, and many others.

SPECIAL PROBLEMS IN THE VERY YOUNG AND THE ELDERLY

The diagnosis of appendicitis in the very young can be difficult, in part because children react sharply to most stimuli and of course are hard to question and to examine. Also the omentum is small and is less able to wall off a perforation. A period of observation in quiet surroundings in the hospital with subsequent reexamination can be very helpful.

Conversely, the elderly person often does not react with normal vigor to appendicitis. Symptoms and signs may be minimal, and the white cell count may show only a mild elevation, if any. At times an ileal obstruction suspected of being caused by a cecal carcinoma is in fact caused by entrapment of the small bowel in an appendiceal inflammatory mass. The substantial morbidity in the elderly is due to their diminished physiological reserve.

TREATMENT

Appendicitis can usually be diagnosed from the history and the physical examination of the patient. The operative diagnosis should be correct in 65% to 75% of the cases. If a surgeon's percentage is higher than this, it is possible that he is too conservative in recommending operation.

There will be some patients in whom the surgeon is not certain of the diagnosis either because the patient presents early in the course of the disease or because part of the symptom complex is absent. In these patients, many of whom have been unable to eat, it is reasonable to establish intravenous therapy and to monitor the patient either in an emergency room observation area or in the hospital for 8 hr to 12 hr. This is particularly valuable in children. During this period the patient should be examined at least two or three times, with palpation of the abdomen for increased or localizing tenderness. Repeat determinations of the leukocyte count and the vital signs can also be made. Antibiotics are often given in this situation, although there is no firm evidence that their administration will alter the course of an already suppurative appendicitis. No analgesia is given during this period of observation in most clinics until it is certain that the diagnosis is not appendicitis.

Appendectomy

Preoperative Considerations. Patients with presumed appendicitis can be prepared for surgery quickly and efficiently using the following techniques: (1) Intravenous fluid therapy should be instituted, with lactated Ringer's or other physiological substitute at a rate sufficient to establish adequate diuresis, usually 125 to 200 ml/hr; (2) nasogastric intubation, usually with a sump type tube, should be performed to prevent vomiting with aspiration or acute gastric dilation; (3) intravenous antibiotics should be administered prior to surgery. Since the organisms found in the appendix are predominantly of the gram-negative and anaerobic variety, a broad-spectrum antibiotic or combination of antibiotics can be used. Keflin, cefamandole, Mefoxin, or aqueous penicillin with tetracycline are satisfactory choices. For greater anaerobic coverage, clindamycin may be given. The purpose of these preoperative or prophylactic antibiotics is to reduce the incidence of postoperative intraperitoneal and wound complications,

For hyperpyrexia in cases of appendiceal rupture with peritonitis, the cooling blanket, Tylenol if feasible, alcohol sponging, or aspirin suppositories may be used.

Choice of Incision. The incisions used are the McBurney incision, an oblique muscle-splitting incision one third the distance from the iliac crest on a line with the umbilicus (Fig. 25-3), and the Rockey-Davis incision, a 5-cm to 7-cm transverse skin incision in the direction of Langer's lines at about the level of the anterior superior iliac spine. Both these incisions are similar after the skin incision is completed. The external oblique, internal oblique, and transversus abdominis muscles are split in the direction of their fibers and bluntly separated. The transversalis fascia and the peritoneum are divided transversely. With both incisions, the surgeon tries to preserve the iliohypogastric nerve lying under the internal oblique muscle (Fig. 25-3).

Midline and paramedian incisions are generally discouraged when one is confident of the diagnosis of appendicitis preoperatively because they are associated with a higher morbidity if a postoperative wound complication should occur. They are often used, however, when the diagnosis is in doubt and wide abdominal exploration may be required.

Exposure and Initial Evaluation of Peritoneal Fluid. After the peritoneum is entered, the cecum may be identified by its longitudinal muscle bands, the teniae, which should lead the surgeon to the base of the appendix. By grasping the cecum near the ileocecal valve with a wet sponge, the cecum may be drawn up into the wound, facilitating

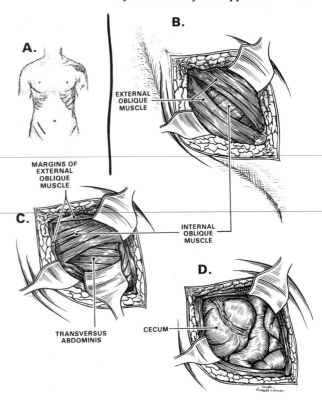

Fig. 25-3. Gridiron (McBurney, muscle-splitting) incision for appendectomy. (*A*) Placement of oblique skin incision. (*B*) The external oblique is split in direction of its fibers. (*C*) The internal oblique and transversus abdominis are similarly split in direction of their fibers. (*D*) Incision through peritoneum and retraction exposes cecum and appendix. (Condon RE, Gleysteen JJ: Appendicitis, peritonitis and intra-abdominal abscess. In Hardy JD [ed]: Rhoads Textbook of Surgery, 5th ed. Philadelphia, J B Lippincott, 1977)

exposure of the appendix. Palpation will also disclose the general direction of the appendix.

The quality of the peritoneal fluid (clear or turbid) should be noted; if it is turbid, a sample for culture of aerobic and anaerobic organisms may be taken. Once the appendix is visualized, its gross appearance is noted. Before the appendix is even visualized, the probing finger may break into an unsuspected loculation of pus, usually an indication of rupture.

Removal of the Appendix. Once the appendix is out of the abdomen and into the wound, the mesoappendix can be serially divided between hemostats, commencing at the tip. The mesoappendix is ligated, and a pursestring suture of 2–0 silk is placed in the seromuscular layer of the cecum. A clamp is placed near the base of the appendix, and the base is then tied securely with 2–0 chromic catgut. The appendix is then divided and, depending upon the surgeon, the divided stump is "treated" with the Bovie unit, phenol, Betadine, or alcohol. If there is a great deal of inflammation and edema at the base of the appendix, making inversion by way of a pursestring suture hazardous, simple ligation of the stump will suffice. In most cases, however, the appendiceal stump may be inverted with a hemostat, after which the pursestring suture is tied. A "Z stitch" or Lembert suture may be used as an alternative means of inversion or as a supplement to the pursestring.

What If the Appendix Is Normal at Operation? If the appendix is normal, a thorough exploration of the abdomen should be performed. In the female one must rule out pelvic inflammatory disease, corpus luteum cysts, ectopic pregnancy, and torsion of the ovary. The small bowel should be visualized by sequential examination to rule out regional enteritis or Meckel's diverticulitis. If regional enteritis is found, the appendix should be removed unless its base is involved in the disease process, to avoid diagnostic confusion should abdominal pain recur in the future. Mesenteric lymph nodes should be examined to exclude mesenteric adenitis. If upper abdominal pathology such as cholecystitis, perforated peptic ulcer, or pancreatitis is suspected, one may elect to perform a separate upper abdominal midline incision and close the right lower quadrant incision. Colon pathology such as diverticulitis should also be excluded; this may necessitate a new lower midline incision in order to perform proximal colostomy and resection if indicated. If no other abdominal pathology is found and exploration is indeed "negative," appendectomy should be performed and the family so informed.

Irrigation and Drainage. If pus is found in the abdomen, most of the fluid should be removed from the pelvis and lateral gutter with suction. Irrigation of the abdomen with saline solution may be performed until the effluent solution is clear. There is controversy about the efficacy of placing antibiotics intraperitoneally to decrease the incidence of wound and abscess complications, and this decision is up to the individual surgeon. When an appendiceal abscess is found, soft Penrose drains may be brought out through a separate stab wound, but in general uncomplicated appendicitis does not merit peritoneal irrigation or drainage.

Closure of the Incision. When there is obvious contamination, it is preferable to close the peritoneum, muscle, and fascia with absorbable sutures such as chromic catgut or Dexon or with a monofilament nonabsorbable suture such as prolene or steel wire. The skin and subcutaneous tissue are often left open if there is purulent abdominal drainage, to be closed secondarily after 48 hr to 72 hr.

Postoperative Care. Antibiotic therapy is indicated postoperatively for appendiceal abscess, gangrenous appendicitis, localized peritonitis, and spreading peritonitis. Therapy is based on the assumption that gram-negative and anaerobic organisms predominate and also on the culture reports at the time of surgery. Three to five days of antibiotic therapy are indicated, or until the patient has been afebrile for 24 hr. Early ambulation is important, and pulmonary physiotherapy with deep breathing is started.

In patients with uncomplicated appendicitis the nasogastric tube may be removed on the first postoperative day. Otherwise, it is removed when peristalsis has resumed. As soon as the patient passes flatus or has a bowel movement, a soft diet is given. Liquids may be started even earlier when peristalsis resumes, taking care not to produce more ileus with distention, nausea, and vomiting. When liquids are taken without difficulty and antibiotic therapy is completed, intravenous fluid therapy may be discontinued.

CLINICAL SITUATIONS OTHER THAN UNCOMPLICATED APPENDICITIS

Perforated Appendicitis

Patients with a perforated appendix are usually more toxic than patients with simple appendicitis. Generalized abdominal pain may be present with dehydration, hyperpyrexia, and even hypotension and tachycardia, either from sepsis, hypovolemia, or both. Diffuse rebound tenderness is often present if the process is not localized to the right lower quadrant and the pelvis, and no mass may be felt. Bowel sounds are usually decreased, and rectus spasm, either unilateral or bilateral, is present. Marked leukocytosis, more than 15,000 cells/mm^3 and even up to 25,000 cells/mm^3, may be present with a significant shift to the left. Treatment for these patients consists of the following measures: (1) rapid intravenous hydration, bladder catheterization, and establishment of a positive central venous pressure or adequate diuresis; (2) high dose antibiotics with established combination therapy of Keflin and tobramycin with clindamycin, or the newer antibiotics for anaerobes such as Mefoxin; (3) surgical therapy with appendectomy, aspiration of pus, irrigation, and peritoneal drainage if localized abscess is found.

The Appendiceal Mass

In addition to patients with uncomplicated appendicitis or rapidly progressive appendicitis with peritonitis, there is a group of patients who present with a symptom complex consistent with appendicitis but on physical examination are found to have a mobile or fixed mass in the right lower quadrant. Mobility of the mass in the patient with recent onset of symptoms leads the examiner to a diagnosis of appendiceal phlegmon, the mass being a gangrenous appendix surrounded by omentum and possibly small bowel. Treatment for this patient should consist of appendectomy with or without stump inversion, depending upon the extent of edema in the cecal wall. There is usually no gross pus with an appendiceal phlegmon, thus obviating the necessity for peritoneal drainage.

Patients who present with a fixed mass in the right lower quadrant usually have had sympoms for a longer period, and the mass is most likely a localized appendiceal abscess. These patients present with varying symptoms, including diarrhea or ileus, small bowel obstruction, or pelvic pain with tenesmus due to extrinsic pressure on the sigmoid colon. Intravenous pyelography may even depict a hydroureteronephrosis on the right side. On the other hand, the laboratory findings reveal only a mild leukocytosis. It is permissible to observe the patient for 24 hr; if he improves, elective appendectomy may be performed at 6 weeks. Deterioration in the clinical condition with spiking fever, leukocytosis, and continued paralytic ileus is an indication for drainage of the abscess through a muscle-splitting incision made directly over or slightly lateral to the mass. Once the pus is drained, a search for the partially autolyzed appendix should be made, and appendectomy with stump ligation should be accomplished if feasible. The incision should be kept extraperitoneal. After gentle irrigation of the abscess with antibiotic solution and breaking up of loculations, Penrose drains should be placed in the abscess cavity through the wound along with a small, flexible Foley catheter. This Foley catheter can serve as a type of sump drain and is also useful for performing sequential sinograms to document healing of the abscess. The wound is partially closed to allow drainage, and the drains are advanced after 72 hr. Interval appendectomy can be performed electively at 6 weeks if the appendix could not be removed safely at the first exploration.

Appendicitis and Pregnancy

Appendicitis is the most common extrauterine surgical emergency during pregnancy, occurring in most patients in the second trimester. Early diagnosis may be difficult owing to the upward displacement of the cecum by the uterus, which causes confusion in the physical examination, and nausea and vomiting may simply be attributed to the pregnancy. When there is perforation with peritonitis, the chance of fetal loss is greater than it is in uncomplicated appendicitis, in which 90% to 95% of pregnancies go on to maturity. Treatment of appendicitis in pregnancy consists of appendectomy, and progesterone given before and after the operation may aid in the prevention of abortion or premature labor.

COMPLICATIONS OF APPENDECTOMY

Wound infection is fairly common. If postoperative fever and leukocytosis occur after 5 days, intra-abdominal abscess must be considered and may be detected by rectal examination. A bulging on rectal examination, usually felt posterolaterally, may be a pelvic abscess, which may be drained through the rectum. Subphrenic and subhepatic abscess must also be considered and ruled out by sonography or CT scan. Acute paralytic ileus or late intestinal obstruction may occur.

Fecal fistula from appendicular stump blowout is usually self-limiting, and if there is no distal colonic obstruction it will usually heal spontaneously. Some fistulas require the use of intravenous alimentation or even late operation for closure. Hemorrhage can occur.

Pylephlebitis (portal vein phlebitis) due to appendiceal bacteremia may lead to hepatic abscesses with fever, right upper quadrant pain, jaundice, and leukocytosis. High-dose antibiotics to cover gram-negative and anaerobic organisms usually control this complication. Occasionally, open drainage of a large solitary hepatic abscess, usually in the right lobe, is required.

PROGNOSIS AND CONCLUSIONS

The mortality from appendicitis has decreased dramatically in the last 50 years as a result of better surgical intensive care, newer antibiotics, better anesthetic techniques, and better noninvasive diagnostic methods. Mortality ultimately depends on the age of the patient and the progression of the disease at the time of surgical intervention. Uncomplicated appendicitis is associated with a mortality of well under 0.5% in most large series. Gangrenous or perforative appendicitis is associated with a 2.4% mortality at this time, and perforation in the elderly has a mortality of 10% to 15%.

RECURRENT APPENDICITIS AND CHRONIC APPENDICITIS

In the past, there has been considerable debate about whether or not there is such an entity as "chronic appendicitis" or "recurrent acute appendicitis." In a sense, a matter of semantics is involved here. We have operated upon patients whose recurrent symptoms led to a confirmed diagnosis of suppurative or even ruptured appendicitis. There is no doubt that the patient may have had more than one attack of acute appendicitis, just as an intermittently obstructed cystic duct may produce recurrent attacks of acute cholecystitis in a gallbladder, which is thus the site of progressive scarring as repeated bouts of acute inflammation produce "chronic cholecystitis." The same thing occurs with the appendix—any type of prolonged recurrent inflammation, anywhere in the body, is likely to subside with some degree of surrounding fibrosis. Hence the diagnosis of chronic appendicitis, which need not imply a continuous, constantly smoldering inflammatory process.

TUMORS

Tumors of the appendix are not common but when encountered important decisions must be made.

CARCINOID

The most common tumor of the appendix is the carcinoid, which is variously reported to have an incidence of approximately 0.5%, compared with 0.08% for primary adenocarcinomas and 0.2% for mucocele, which may have a malignant element in some instances.

Almost one half of all carcinoid tumors of the alimentary tract arise in the appendix. Curiously, the appendiceal carcinoid very rarely gives rise to the carcinoid syndrome, which is associated with carcinoids of the jejunum and ileum. This circumstance is partly explained by the fact that only about 3% of appendiceal carcinoids show evidence of biologic malignancy with metastases, although a considerably higher percentage may exhibit some cytologic evidence of malignancy.

Treatment is the usual management of benign or malignant tumors of the alimentary tract, namely, excision when possible. Actually, most appendiceal carcinoids are discovered at appendectomy or at laparotomy for some other purpose. Appendectomy is all that is necessary for benign appendiceal carcinoids (*i.e.*, generally those less than 1 cm in diameter), but wide *en bloc* excision of the appendix, cecum, and regional lymphatics and lymph nodes is recommended whenever the carcinoid is larger or exhibits malignant histologic changes or invasion. Radiation is of little value, and chemotherapy is still experimental.

ADENOCARCINOMA

Adenocarcinoma is usually discovered at appendectomy or at laparotomy for other indications. Preoperatively, it may have perforated to simulate appendicitis, or it may have caused intestinal obstruction or be visible on barium enema.

Treatment consists of wide *en bloc* excision of the appendix and cecum, which is usually accomplished by a formal right radical colectomy as for any other type of colonic cancer.

MUCOCELE

The mucocele of the appendix arises when the mucus-secreting cells of its mucosa continue to secrete mucus in the presence of proximal appendiceal obstruction. The organ may enlarge to a surprising degree without rupture, since the process proceeds slowly, allowing time for the appendiceal wall to expand without rupture. However, some mucoceles do rupture, and we have seen an instance of widespread pseudomyxoma peritonei secondary to rupture of an appendiceal mucocele.

Most mucoceles of the appendix are benign, but some have malignant elements. Therefore, care should be exercised at operation to avoid spilling the mucoid material into the peritoneal cavity.

OTHER TUMORS

Very rarely, the appendix may be involved with other tumors arising from other cellular elements in its wall.

Leiomyoma, villous adenoma, neurofibroma, and other lesions such as adenomatous polyps have also been reported.

BIBLIOGRAPHY

Appendix

ALTEMEIER WA, CULBERTSON WR, FULLEN WD et al: Intra-abdominal abscesses. Am J Surg 125:70, 1973

ANDERSON M, LILYA T, LUNDELL L et al: Clinical and laboratory findings in patients subjected to laparotomy for suspected acute appendicitis. Acta Chir Scand 146:55, 1980

FITZ RH: Perforating inflammation of the vermiform appendix: With special reference to its early diagnosis and treatment. Trans Assoc Am Physicians 1:107, 1886

GRAHAM JM, POKORNY WJ, HARBERG FJ: Acute appendicitis in preschool age children. Am J Surg 139:247, 1980

GROSFELD JL, SOLIT RW: Prevention of wound infection in perforated appendicitis: Experiences with delayed primary wound closure. Ann Surg 168:891, 1968

GROSSMAN EB JR: Chronic appendicitis. Surg Gynecol Obstet 146:596, 1978

HALLER JA JR, SHAKER IJ, DONAHOO JS et al: Peritoneal drainage versus non-drainage for generalized peritonitis from ruptured appendicitis in children. Ann Surg 177:595, 1973

HAUSWALD KR, BIVINS BA, MEEKER WR JR et al: Analysis of the causes of mortality from appendicitis. Am Surg 42:761, 1976

HOMER MJ, BRAVER JM: Recurrent appendicitis: Reevaluation of a controversial disease. Gastrointest Radiol 4:295, 1979

LEAPE LL, RAMENOFSKY ML: Laparoscopy for questionable appendicitis: Can it reduce the negative appendectomy rate? Ann Surg 191:410, 1980

MCBURNEY C: Experience with early operative interference in cases of disease of the vermiform appendix. NY State Med J 50:676, 1889

OWENS BJ, HAMIT HF: Appendicitis in the elderly. Ann Surg 187:392, 1978

SAVRIN RA, CLATWORTHY HW JR: Appendiceal rupture: A continuing diagnostic problem. Pediatrics 63:36, 1979

SCHER KS, COIL JA: The continuing challenge of perforating appendicitis. Surg Gynecol Obstet 150:535, 1980

SIMONOWITZ DA, WHITE TT: The colon: III. Postoperative complications of appendectomy (including adhesions). Clin Gastroenterol 8:429, 1979

SMITH DE, KIRCHMER NA, STEWART DR: Use of the barium enema in the diagnosis of acute appendicitis and its complications. Am J Surg 138:829, 1979

SYRACUSE DC, PERZIN KH, PRICE JB et al: Carcinoid tumors of the appendix. Meso appendiceal extension and nodal metastases. Ann Surg 190:58, 1979

VAN ZWALENBURG C: Strangulation resulting from strangulation of hollow viscera, its bearing upon appendicitis, strangulated hernia and gallbladder disease. Ann Surg 46:780, 1907

WAKELEY CPG: Position of vermiform appendix as ascertained by analysis of 10,000 cases. J Anat 67:277, 1933

WANGENSTEEN O, DENNIS C: Experimental proof of the obstructive origin of appendicitis in man. Ann Surg 110:629, 1939

Tumors

AHO AJ, HEINONEN R, LAUREN P: Benign and malignant mucocele of the appendix. Histological types and prognosis. Acta Chir Scand 139:392, 1973

ANDERSSON A, BERGDAHL L: Carcinoid tumors of the appendix in children. A report of 25 cases. Acta Chir Scand 143:173, 1977

ARANHA GV, REYES CV: Primary epithelial tumors of the appendix and reappraisal of the appendiceal "mucocele." Dis Colon Rectum 22:472, 1979

GLASSER CM, BHAGAVAN BS: Carcinoid tumors of the appendix. Arch Pathol Lab Med 104:272, 1980

HERCZEG E, WINTER S, WEISSBERG D: Primary carcinoma of the appendix. JAMA 238:51, 1977

JAFARI N: Villous adenoma of appendix—report of a case and review of the literature. Am J Proctol Gastroenterol Colon Rectal Surg 30:30, 1970

PAI AM, VINZE HL, ATTAR-AZIZ et al: Leiomyoma of the appendix (a case report). J Postgrad Med 23:39, 1977

WOLFF M, AHMED N: Epithelial neoplasms of the vermiform appendix (exclusive of carcinoid): I. Adeno-carcinoma of the appendix. Cancer 37:2493, 1976

James D. Hardy

The Colon, Rectum, and Anus

2b

565

ANATOMIC CONSIDERATIONS

The colon is approximately 1.5 meters long and extends from the terminal ileum to the anus. The diameter is greatest (8.5 cm) in the cecum, diminishing to about 2.5 cm in the sigmoid. It becomes slightly more dilated in the rectum. The ascending and the descending portions are mostly retroperitoneal, whereas the sigmoid and the transverse portions are on mesenteries and thus are intraperitoneal. There are two sharp bends: the hepatic and the splenic flexures.

Several features distinguish the colon from the small intestine (Fig. 26-1): The large bowel has teniae coli, three separate longitudinal muscular bands that converge at the base of the appendix. The teniae represent the longitudinal

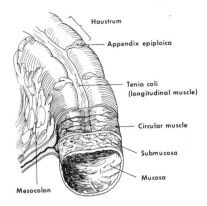

Fig. 26-1.   Gross anatomy of the colon wall.

muscle layer that completely covers the small bowel. The colon has sacculations, called haustra. Separating the haustra are incomplete, internal folds, called plicae semilunares, which are transient structures that depend on the segmenting actions of the colon for their existence. On plain abdominal films, when the small bowel is distended by air, valvulae conniventes traverse its entire diameter while the folds of the colon do not extend beyond the midline. The serosa of the large bowel has appendices epiploicae, which are fatty appendages. Most of these are attached to the medial wall of the colon, predominantly in its distal parts. In the sigmoid area, they appear in two rows, one on either side of the anterior tenia. In contrast to the mobile small bowel, the position of the colon is relatively fixed because of its retroperitoneal attachments. The omentum is attached to the transverse colon.

The wall of the colon has the standard four layers: serosa, muscularis, submucosa, and mucosa. The outer longitudinal muscle layer is incomplete and also forms three separate teniae; however, in the rectum these teniae no longer appear as separate bands. The peritoneum usually does not cover the posterior areas of the ascending and the descending colon or the posterior and part of the lateral walls of the rectum. The distal third of the rectum has no serosal covering. The mucosa is flat and has no villi. There are numerous tubular crypts, which in their lower half have mucus-secreting goblet cells. The mucosa is composed of simple columnar epithelium. The ganglion cells of the myenteric plexus of Auerbach are located mainly along the external surface of the circular muscle coat.

Vascular Supply

The colon is supplied by the superior and inferior mesenteric arteries (Fig. 26-2). The superior mesenteric artery gives off the ileocolic, right colic, and middle colic arteries. The inferior mesenteric artery divides into the left colic, the superior hemorrhoidal (rectal), and the sigmoid arteries. Each of the above-named arteries anastomoses with the adjacent artery to form a continuous vessel around the whole colon, called the marginal "artery" of Drummond. This is situated about 1 cm from the margin of the large bowel, the closest points being along the descending and the sigmoid colon. It is this rich collateral that permits the colon to be used for esophageal bypass surgery. The rectum is supplied in its upper half by the superior hemorrhoidal artery, the final branch of the inferior mesenteric. The middle hemorrhoidal arteries arise from the internal iliacs and are often a minor part of the rectal blood supply. The

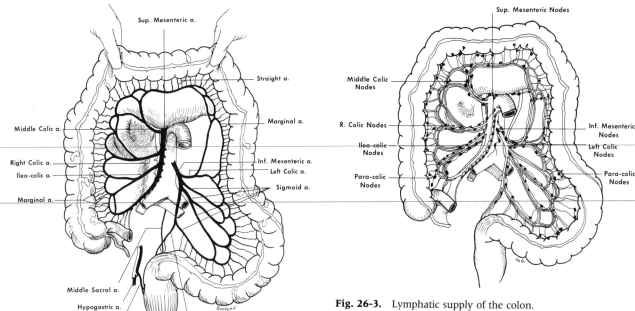

Fig. 26-2. Blood supply of the colon.

Fig. 26-3. Lymphatic supply of the colon.

inferior hemorrhoidal arteries arise from the internal pudendal arteries and supply the anus and the lower part of the rectum. All three of these hemorrhoidal arteries anastomose freely in the rectum. The venous drainage of the colon parallels the arteries except that it does not enter the caval system. The superior and inferior mesenteric veins join the splenic vein to form the portal vein and enter the liver. The rectum has an extensive plexus of venous anastomoses. Most of the rectal blood drains to the portal system, but, in the event of increased portal pressure, the flow is easily reversed to drain into the internal iliac veins.

Lymphatics

The colon is drained by a rich lymphatic network (Fig. 26-3). These lymphatics follow the regional arteries to the preaortic nodes at the roots of the superior and inferior mesenteric arteries. From there, they drain into the cisterna chyli, part of the thoracic duct, which, in turn, empties into the venous system at the left jugulosubclavian angle. Because of this relationship, metastatic carcinoma may appear in the neck as a Virchow's node. The rectum is drained upward along the superior hemorrhoidal vessels. The lymphatics of the anal canal can spread either upward or to the internal iliac nodes; the lymphatics of the anus at the perineal skin drain into the superficial inguinal nodes.

Innervation

The nerve supply of the colon is autonomic. *Sympathetic fibers* pass from the thoracic and lumbar portions of the spinal cord, through the sympthetic chains, to the preaortic sympathetic ganglia, where they synapse with the postganglionic fibers, which follow the major arteries to terminate in the submucosal (Meissner's) and myenteric (Auerbach's) plexuses. The rectum is supplied by the presacral or hypogastric nerves, which are extensions of the preaortic plexuses and the lumbar splanchnic nerves. The presacral nerve

originates just below the bifurcation of the aorta and divides to descend on either side of the pelvis, where it joins fibers of the sacral parasympathetic nerves (nervi erigentes) to form two pelvic plexuses, from which fibers go directly to all the viscera of the pelvis. The *parasympathetic innervation* is from fibers of the vagus and the nervi erigentes. The vagus fibers join the sympathetic fibers at the celiac axis and pass with them to the bowel but do not synapse until reaching the plexuses in the bowel itself. This vagus innervation passes as far down as the transverse colon. The distal part of the colon is innervated by the second through the fourth sacral segments of the cord by way of the nervi erigentes, which pass into the pelvic plexuses. Fibers going to the distal transverse colon, descending colon, and sigmoid pass upward through the presacral nerves to join the sympathetics at the inferior mesenteric ganglion, from which point they follow the arteries to the colon.

Sympathetic activity is mainly inhibitory to the colon and motor to the internal sphincter, and parasympathetic activity has the opposite action; however, the more important control of the bowel is the local reflex activity mediated by the intramural nerve plexuses of Meissner and Auerbach and their interconnections. Thus, despite cord transection or vagotomy, bowel function can continue essentially normally. Conversely, patients lacking these plexuses, as in Hirschsprung's disease, have very abnormal motor activity. It is important that the pelvic autonomics not be damaged during rectal surgery, since impotence or poor bladder function may follow. The sensory afferent fibers are sympathetic and react to distention, stretching, or spasm. The voluntary muscles, (*i.e.,* the levator ani, coccygeus, and external sphincter) are supplied by fibers from the fourth sacral segment.

Segmental Characteristics

The ileocecal valve is composed of two transverse folds that functionally can act as a valve to prevent reflux into the ileum. The appendix is attached to the medial aspect of the cecum. The cecum is fully covered by serosa and thus has some mobility. The ascending colon is usually fixed in position, having peritoneum on only three sides. The transverse colon is the most mobile segment of the colon. The splenic flexure is usually higher than the hepatic flexure and forms the most acute angle of the colon. The distal descending colon has the smallest diameter of any part of the colon. The sigmoid colon extends from the pelvic brim to the rectum. It is on a mesentery and can be very redundant, which accounts for its being the most common site of volvulus. The rectum follows the curve of the sacrum. The upper valve of Houston (10 cm from the anus) is generally considered to represent the abdominal portion of the rectum that is almost fully covered by peritoneum. The anal canal is the terminal 3 cm of the colon.

PHYSIOLOGICAL CONSIDERATIONS

The main functions of the colon are storage and expulsion of waste material and absorption of water and electrolytes. Most of the absorptive functions are in the right colon; the storage and expulsion functions are in the left.

Absorption and Secretion

Sodium is actively absorbed by the colon, which has a marked ability to conserve sodium, especially under conditions of sodium restriction. Water is absorbed mainly in the ascending colon and also in all other parts of the large intestine, the least amount being absorbed in the rectum. Water is passively absorbed in association with sodium. The terminal ileum presents 500 ml to 600 ml of water per day to the colon and the water content of stool is 100 ml to 150 ml per day; thus on the average, 350 ml to 500 ml is absorbed daily. The maximum capacity for water absorption is approximately 2.5 liters per day. Potassium is passively diffused from blood to bowel lumen in association with the electrochemical gradient created by the active sodium transport. Adrenal hormones can affect the transport of both sodium and potassium.

Bile acids are absorbed by passive diffusion. This becomes important mainly if the ileum is absent or nonfunctioning, since most (95%) of the bile is absorbed in the terminal ileum. Bacteria in the colon deconjugate bile acids. In increasing concentrations, this can block sodium and water absorption, leading to diarrhea.

Diseased states can alter colon physiology. Chronic inflammation, such as in ulcerative colitis and Crohn's disease, significantly decreases water and sodium absorption, leading to diarrhea. Potassium is affected to a much lesser degree. If an increased load is presented to the colon or if there is abnormal motility, contact time between mucosa and luminal contents is shortened and, thus, electrolytes and water are lost. The composition of diarrheal fluid can approach that of plasma. After subtotal colectomy, the rectum can accommodate and assume much of the role of the colon; thus many such patients have only two to three formed stools per day.

Motility

The motor activity of the colon falls into three categories: (1) local segmental activity, (2) mass movements, and (3) short propulsive movements. Local segmental contractions are present primarily in the right colon and serve to delay transit, to allow maximum time for surface absorption, and to mix the intestinal contents with a to-and-fro action. With mass movements, there is rapid transit of material from the right colon to the left. The gastroileal reflex is a form of such activity: food entering the upper small bowel initiates a reflex that leads to movement of material from the distal small bowel to the cecum. This is not dependent on an intact vagus or on gastrin, although the latter may play a role. The left colon initially has a decrease in its phasic activity but then resumes segmental contractions to slow down and mix the contents. Mass movements of material across the entire colon are rarely observed except in diseased states. Shorter propulsive activity is the more common mechanism of movement of material, but these are not the segmental contractions that mainly mix contents by a back-and-forth motion. This propulsive activity cannot be considered true peristalsis, because it is not proceeded by a decrease in pressure. It is not clear whether the short propulsive movements that account for most of the transport of fecal material represent a localized mass movement or a multisegmental contraction; however, this activity is more prominent in the left colon and is responsible for most of the evacuation of the colon.

The autonomic nervous system mainly has an inhibitory effect on the colon. Emotions have some effect on bowel motility. Physical activity increases motor activity of the colon. Several drugs affect the colon. Methacholine and acetylcholine increase the pressure in the right colon and decrease phasic activity on the left. Morphine sulfate causes increased pressure in the colon, especially if the colon is abnormal. Pressures of 40 torr have been recorded, and this can last 20 to 30 minutes. Codeine has the same effect but to a lesser degree. Pressures greater than 50 torr can be caused by morphine. Meperidine (Demerol) does not cause an increase in pressure and should probably be used in diverticular disease rather than morphine. Diphenoxylate (Lomotil), a meperidine analogue, has an inhibitory effect on colon activity. Anticholinergics such as propantheline (Pro-Banthine) have an atropinelike effect that decreases activity. Serotonin (5-hydroxytryptamine) increases segmenting activity. Distention of the colon stimulates motility, and this is the basis of action for many laxatives.

Rectal Continence and Defecation

The internal anorectal sphincter is an involuntary, circular, smooth muscle. The voluntary muscles are the external sphincter and the anorectal ring, consisting primarily of the levatores ani and the puborectalis. Both the internal and external sphincters remain in a state of tonus. This tone increases in response to an increase in intra-abdominal pressure, thus preserving continence. When fecal matter enters the rectum and causes distention, the internal sphincter relaxes and the external sphincter contracts. By this means defecation can be delayed until an appropriate time. When conditions are right for defecation, the external sphincter is voluntarily relaxed and defecation proceeds. Also involved in the voluntary mechanism are an increase in intra-abdominal pressure and relaxation of the pelvic floor. At the same time, the rectum and sigmoid contract and shorten, propelling the material outward. In patients with spinal cord injury, there is still much reflex control in both the internal and the external sphincters. In these patients, incontinence can often be controlled, but defecation is inefficient. In these situations, enemas will usually cause sufficient distention to initiate the reflexes for adequate evacuation.

Intestinal Gas

Swallowed air accounts for up to 70% of the intestinal gas, mainly in the form of nitrogen and oxygen. Hydrogen, carbon dioxide, and methane occur from bacterial metabolism of carbohydrates and account for up to 50% of flatus. Both high altitude and a decreased bowel transit time (e.g., from a high bulk diet) increase the amount of flatus, whereas constipation, with its increased transit time, leads to a decrease in flatus.

Dysmotility and Irritable Colon

Inadequate motility, sometimes found in the elderly and especially in those in nursing homes and in patients with neurologic disorders, can prove to be a very difficult problem to manage. It leads to pseudo-obstruction of the colon (Ogilvie's syndrome), with or without the presence of fecal impaction. It is important not to confuse this functional condition with organic colon obstruction. Although tedious, nonoperative management with stool softeners, optimal diet, more physical activity, mild laxatives, and enemas when necessary is preferable to colostomy or even to the resection of redundant colon. It is important to differentiate chronic pseudo-obstruction from acute pseudo-obstruction, which is more of a surgical emergency and represents true Ogilvie's syndrome. At times it can be very difficult to distinguish acute pseudo-obstruction, which usually responds to nonoperative treatments, from organic obstruction, which requires operation.

Irritable colon syndrome is one of the most common gastrointestinal disorders. It does not represent a precise set of symptoms, which may range from abdominal pain to constipation to diarrhea. The pain is usually associated with a spastic colon with small, constipated bowel movements. A painless diarrhea, often consisting of mucus, commonly represents the other end of the spectrum. In a given patient, symptoms may alternate. It has been shown that symptoms are worse during times of emotional stress. Motility studies of the bowel show that these disturbances of colonic function are reflections of the emotional state of the patient and are probably normal manifestations of emotional tension, just as are sweating, facial flushing, and weeping. Other factors such as diet and laxatives also play a role.

The diagnosis of irritable colon is based both on exclusion and on recognition of the multiple patterns in which it may present. To be excluded are other colonic disorders such as Crohn's disease, ulcerative colitis, carcinoma, and diverticular disease. Bacterial and parasitic infections and lactase deficiency, as well as other abdominal disorders not related to the colon, should also be excluded, as should systemic diseases such as hypothyroidism, scleroderma, Addison's disease, Graves' disease, and the carcinoid syndrome. A search for associations between stressful periods of life, emotional tension, and the manifestation of colonic symptoms must be made.

The management of the irritable colon syndrome consists first of assuring the patient that, on the basis of sigmoidoscopy, colonoscopy, barium enema, stool examination for parasites, and upper gastrointestinal series, none of the disorders mentioned above exists. Next is the education of the patient in regard to the relationship between his bowel problems and his emotions and stressful situations and helping him find ways to alter either his environment or his attitude about it. Last but very important is a continued concern for the patient. Occasionally the placebo effect of low dose phenobarbital or belladonna may help exacerbations. Some diet changes, such as omission of onions, cabbage, beans, and strong seasonings, may help. Severe pain may be controlled temporarily with codeine or propantheline but opiates should not be abused. Diphenoxylate will help diarrhea. Emphasis should be placed on helping the patient cope with his life situations rather than relying heavily on medications, although the latter do have a role.

INFLAMMATORY DISEASES

GRANULOMATOUS COLITIS AND ULCERATIVE COLITIS

Granulomatous colitis and ulcerative colitis have in common many clinical symptoms and pathologic and roentgenologic findings. Differentiation between the two is important for both prognostic and therapeutic purposes.

Granulomatous colitis is a disease, acute or chronic, involving all layers of the colon and is commonly called Crohn's disease of the colon. Crohn's disease may involve any part of the gastrointestinal tract and is characterized by segmental areas of involvement with normal intervening skip areas. Crohn's disease of the colon frequently extends into the terminal ileum and characteristically spares the rectum. No specific infectious agent has been found in granulomatous colitis.

Ulcerative colitis is an inflammatory disease of the colon. It is acute or chronic and involves primarily the mucosa and submucosa. The rectal mucosa and varying portions of the more proximal colon are usually involved without skip areas. No infectious agent has been identified.

Differentiation of granulomatous colitis from ulcerative colitis depends primarily on the gross and microscopic findings. Typically, ulcerative colitis begins in the rectum and extends proximally throughout the large intestine. The serosa of the colon is intact in ulcerative colitis, except in the acute fulminating form (toxic megacolon). The inflammation is confined to the mucosa and submucosa, and ulceration is patchy. Areas of intact mucosa within a denuded area may give rise to pseudopolyps. The colon is shortened, with loss of the haustral markings as a result of contraction of the musculature. The ileum may be involved secondarily by "backwash ileitis." Microscopic examination reveals increased vascularity, with loss of goblet cells and a relative lack of fibrosis. Crypt abscesses are common.

The gross pathology of granulomatous colitis is characterized by segmental involvement, with intervening segments of normal intestine. The bowel wall is thickened, owing to the transmural inflammation. The serosa is involved and may be studded with tiny tubercles, which represent noncaseating granulomas. The mesentery is usually thick, and regional lymph nodes are enlarged. The mucosa may have a cobblestone appearance where intercommunicating fissures surround islands of mucosa elevated by underlying inflammation and edema. Noncaseating granulomas represent a typical microscopic feature of granulomatous colitis. These lesions resemble the reaction seen in sarcoidosis. Granulomas may be found in 50% to 70% of patients. Crypt abscesses are less frequent than in ulcerative colitis but may be present. Fissuring (knifelike clefts into the wall of the intestine) may occur, with development of fistulas into the small intestine, bladder, vagina, or abdominal wall. The typical pathologic findings are shown in Table 26-1.

TABLE 26-1   COMPARATIVE FEATURES OF ULCERATIVE AND GRANULOMATOUS COLITIS

	ULCERATIVE COLITIS	GRANULOMATOUS COLITIS
Clinical		
Usual location	Rectum, left colon	Ileum and right colon
Diarrhea	Severe	Present, moderate
Rectal bleeding	Common (almost 100%)	Intermittent (about 50%)
Rectal involvement	Almost 100%	About 20%
Perianal disease	Fistulas rare	Fistulas and abscesses common
Abdominal wall and internal fistulas	Rare	Frequent
Sigmoidoscopy	Uniform, diffuse friability with shaggy irregular ulcers	Patchy involvement Linear ulcers (cobblestone mucosa)
Colon radiographic findings	Diffuse, tiny serrations (crypt abscess), uniform loss of haustration, shortening of colon	Segmental, skip areas, internal fistulas No shortening
Carcinoma	10% in 10 years	Rare
Toxic megacolon	Common	Rare
Associated systemic disease (arthritis, uveitis, pyoderma)	Common	Infrequent
Recurrent ileitis after colectomy	Rare	Frequent
Pathologic		
Gross appearance of colon	Confluent involvement, mesentery normal, pseudopolyps common, bowel wall thin or normal	Segmental involvement, mesentery thickened, lymph nodes enlarged, cobblestone mucosa, bowel wall thickened
Microscopic appearance of colon	Inflammation limited to mucosa and submucosa No granulomas No serositis Crypt abscesses	Transmural inflammation Frequent granulomas Serositis always present Rare crypt abscesses
Surgical Treatment	Proctocolectomy with ileostomy	Subtotal or total colectomy; rectum frequently preserved

GRANULOMATOUS COLITIS (CROHN'S DISEASE)

Granulomatous disease of the bowel was first recognized in 1932, when Crohn, Ginzburg, and Oppenheimer published their description of regional ileitis. According to that report, Crohn thought that the disease was confined to the distal small bowel. It is now known that "Crohn's disease" may involve any portion of the gastrointestinal tract. British writers prefer the term *Crohn's disease* for this condition wherever it occurs, but American authors vary the name with the area involved by the disease: *granulomatous gastritis* for disease in the stomach, *regional enteritis* for disease in the small bowel, *granulomatous ileocolitis* for disease in small bowel and colon, and *granulomatous colitis* for disease in the large intestine. It was not until 1959 that granulomatous colitis was clearly defined as an entity separate from ulcerative colitis by Morson and Lockhart-Mummery. Regardless of location in the gastrointestinal tract, the pathologic findings are the same.

Etiology (Unknown)

The cause of granulomatous colitis is not known. The search for an infectious agent continues. Immunologic factors are being studied.

The same basic causal factor may be present in both granulomatous and ulcerative colitis.

The disease may occur in any age-group and is more serious in children and geriatric patients. There is an increased incidence in families—between parent and child as well as between siblings. Although not recognized as a specific entity until 1959, the disease has been reported in most countries throughout the world. In the United States, about 30% of patients with inflammatory bowel disease have granulomatous colitis; ulcerative colitis accounts for approximately 60%. In about 10% of patients inflammatory bowel disease cannot be classified as either granulomatous or ulcerative colitis but has some characteristics of both.

Clinical Manifestations

The onset of symptoms from granulomatous colitis is usually insidious. Abdominal pain and diarrhea are the most prominent symptoms and may be accompanied by weight loss, anorexia, fever, and malaise. Abdominal pain unrelieved by defecation has been described as characteristic of granulomatous colitis. The pain may be generalized or localized to the lower abdomen and is usually constant. Diarrhea is usually less severe than in patients with ulcerative colitis and consists of frequent watery stools without blood. Patients with rectal involvement may complain of tenesmus, but patients seldom have proctitis. Rectal sphincter control is usually not impaired. However, the presence of perianal fistulas or granulomas should suggest the presence of granulomatous colitis.

Symptoms may occur from complications of obstruction in the distal segments of the colon, usually the descending or the sigmoid colon. In patients with ileocolitis, obstruction is commonly seen in the terminal ileum from fibrosis and lymphedema. Internal fistulas are common in patients with chronic disease and may occur to adjacent loops of bowel or to ureter, vagina, or bladder. External fistulas may develop through the abdominal wall. Abdominal masses consisting of dilated loops of small bowel or of abscesses may be palpated, usually in the right lower quadrant or deep in the left pelvis. Extra-intestinal manifestations are common and are very similar to those listed for ulcerative colitis.

Endoscopic examination may show a normal mucosa, friability, patchy areas of redness, or linear lesions that intersect, leaving the mucosa raised and nodular, like a cobblestone road.

The roentgenographic appearance has been well described by Marshak. The disease occurs predominantly in the right colon. Skip areas of normal colon are frequent. The ileum is commonly involved; the rectum usually appears normal.

Treatment

The treatment of granulomatous colitis consists of both nonoperative and operative measures. Since the etiology remains unknown, medical therapy is empirical and consists of antidiarrheal drugs and antibiotics when indicated. Corticosteroids and azathioprine (Imuran) have been rather ineffective. Azulfidine has been employed.

Surgery is used as conservatively as possible. Unlike ulcerative colitis in which colectomy with proctectomy and permanent ileostomy are curative, no operation cures granulomatous colitis with certainty. Recurrence following segmental colon resection will occur in about half the patients. The small bowel may be or may become involved. Fistula formation is common. Therefore, operation is reserved for demanding complications such as intestinal obstruction,

IDIOPATHIC CHRONIC ULCERATIVE COLITIS	
Etiology and Pathology	Unknown, but various theories. Mucosal lesions. Rectum almost always involved; spread in continuity to rest of colon. Substantial malignant potential. Extensive small bowel involvement rare. Fistulas to adjacent gut or abdominal wall almost never
Dx	Symptoms of diarrhea, often bloody. Extensive mucosal involvement on proctoscopic exam. Typical "hose-pipe" appearance on barium enema (loss of haustral markings). Exclude other causes of diarrhea, including granulomatous colitis
Rx	Nonoperative measures including diet, antimicrobials, antidiarrheal drugs, and steroids. Surgery for remote or even systemic complications where necessary, for toxic megacolon or malignancy. Excision of colon and rectum with permanent ileostomy curative

protracted bloody diarrhea, perforation with peritonitis, or fistula formation that cannot be ignored. However, even here the amount of colon resected should be the minimum consistent with achieving the necessary objectives.

The long-term prognosis in the patient with granulomatous colitis is fairly good.

ULCERATIVE COLITIS

Although ulcerative colitis has been recognized for more than a century, the cause remains unknown. Psychosomatic mechanisms were postulated 20 years ago but have not been substantiated. No causal relationship between ulcerative colitis and depression has been established. Emotional improvement following psychiatric care is not associated with reversal of the disease process in the colon. Controlled studies have failed to distinguish between patients with ulcerative colitis and patients with irritable colons. It is of course important to exclude amebiasis and other causes of colitis.

Genetic defects have also been studied as a cause for ulcerative colitis. Singer reported a threefold increase in the incidence of ulcerative colitis in relatives of patients. Jews have been reported to have an incidence significantly higher than that of other groups, whereas in our experience, blacks have a low incidence.

Clinical Manifestations

Ulcerative colitis may occur as an acute or a chronic inflammatory disease. Chronic disease is associated with mild to severe acute exacerbations.

Diarrhea, rectal bleeding, and abdominal pain are the principal symptoms of ulcerative colitis. Fever, weight loss, tenesmus, and vomiting are common additional symptoms.

The diarrhea consists of frequent loose bowel movements (10 to 20 per day) and occurs during the day and at night after the patient has gone to bed. Normal absorption of the

GRANULOMATOUS COLITIS (CROHN'S DISEASE)	
Etiology and Pathology	Unknown, but various theories: a granulomatous disease, may involve any part of alimentary tract but principally ileum and/or right colon. Fistulas and abscesses common. Involves full-thickness bowel wall
Dx	Diarrhea, fever, malaise, weight loss. Exclude infectious agents such as bacterial dysentery, bacteria, or amebiasis. Rectum often disease-free on endoscopic exam; sigmoid colon may exhibit inflammation, friability, granularity. Barium enema—predominantly right colon; loss of normal haustral markings; skip areas. Distinguish from ulcerative colitis, where rectum almost always involved. Perianal involvement more common in Crohn's disease
Rx	Steroids, azathioprine relatively ineffective. Antibiotics for cellulitis and abscess formation. Minimal excisional surgery, resorted to only when necessary for complications such as hemorrhage, perforation and abscess, cicatrization and obstruction, the rare malignant change—and very infrequently intractable diarrhea. No operation curative; prognosis fairly good long-term

colon is impaired, with loose, watery, or mushy stools. Mucus and pus may be abundant. Blood per rectum may be bright red or mixed with the stool and results from the increased vascularity and ulceration of the mucosa. At times, brisk massive rectal hemorrhage may occur.

Lower abdominal cramping is frequently present with urgency. Tenesmus may be a prominent feature if the rectal capacity is reduced by fibrosis. In the later stages of the disease, defecation may occur without warning, leading to the increased anxiety and insecurity so often exhibited by ulcerative colitis patients.

Systemic complications of ulcerative colitis are numerous and may be related to hypersensitivity. These symptoms include iritis, uveitis, arthritis, spondylitis, hepatitis, pyoderma gangrenosum, and erythema nodosum. Dramatic clearing of the symptoms may occur after proctocolectomy.

Absolute Indications for Operation

Absolute indications for surgical treatment include perforation, hemorrhage, obstruction, cancer, and acute fulminating disease with or without toxic megacolon. Free perforation of the colon usually occurs in association with toxic megacolon, which is much more common in patients with ulcerative colitis but can occur in patients with granulomatous colitis. Perforations may be single or multiple. Omentum may be adherent to the colon at the site of an impending perforation and should not be dissected from the bowel wall, but the adherent omentum should be resected along with the colon. In some patients, the signs and symptoms of colonic perforation are present, but no free perforation can be found. The purulent exudate in the peritoneal cavity is probably secondary to the acute, diffuse serosal inflammation developing in patients with granulomatous colitis. Perforating lesions resulting in abscess or fistula formation are characteristic of granulomatous disease of the colon because of the transmural extension of the inflammatory process. Fistulas in Crohn's disease are usually an indication for surgical intervention.

Repeated and massive hemorrhage may occur in patients with ulcerative colitis but seldom in patients with granulomatous colitis. Hemorrhage may occur in association with an acute attack of colitis and not necessarily in disease of long duration. In most patients, bleeding may be managed by multiple blood transfusions, but when life-threatening uncontrolled hemorrhage develops, urgent surgical intervention to perform proctocolectomy and ileostomy is necessary. This is a difficult decision, but both internists and surgeons should be aware that procrastination while giving multiple blood transfusions will cause the patient to become more debilitated and thus will increase the operative risk.

Obstruction secondary to inflammatory disease of the colon is seldom acute. Chronic obstructive symptoms may develop from stricture formation and occur in patients with granulomatous colitis. Tight stricture formation causing colonic obstruction in patients with ulcerative colitis arouses suspicion of cancer.

The diagnosis of cancer is an indication for surgical intervention to eradicate not only the malignant tumor but also the basic disease in the colon. Goligher's studies indicate that the risk of cancer is very low during the first 10 years after the onset of ulcerative colitis but rises thereafter at an increasing rate, reaching 41.8% after 25 years. MacDougall's studies indicate that this very high risk of colon cancer in patients with ulcerative colitis is found only in patients with diffuse disease involving the entire colon. When ulcerative colitis is limited to the distal end of the colon, the risk of cancer is the same as the general population.

It has been thought that the incidence of colon cancer in patients with granulomatous colitis is no greater than in the general population, but Weedon and associates reported from the Mayo Clinic that the incidence of colorectal cancer was 20 times greater in patients with Crohn's enteritis than in a control population. All the patients with cancer of the colon in this report had histologically confirmed, coexistent granulomatous colitis, and care was taken by the investigators to exclude any patients with chronic ulcerative colitis.

The onset of ulcerative colitis in childhood is associated with a high risk of colonic cancer. Not only do these younger patients have an opportunity to live long enough to enter the high cancer-risk category of patients who have had disease for longer than 10 years, but their disease is more likely to involve the entire colon, which puts them at greater risk. In a study by Michener, 46 of 401 children with ulcerative colitis developed colon cancer.

Colon cancer occurring in association with ulcerative colitis is difficult to recognize. The tumors are often multicentric and small and invade rapidly into the bowel wall. They tend to produce infiltrating lesions that mimic fibrous strictures in the colon. Aggressive surgical management (proctocolectomy with ileostomy) can lead to long-term survival. Hinton reported a 40% 5-year survival rate in patients with ulcerative colitis developing colon cancer. Menguy states that prophylactic colectomy for patients with active "universal" ulcerative colitis of long duration (more than 10 years) should receive "thoughtful consideration."

Relative Indications for Operation: Further Comment

Relative indications for surgical treatment include failure to respond to medical management, growth retardation in children, and recurring disease in the elderly. The frequency with which operation is required as an elective procedure varies with the philosophy of the medical-surgical team. Increasing acceptance of a permanent ileostomy because of improved patient education and availability of trained enterostomal therapists may liberalize the indications for elective surgery in patients with inflammatory bowel disease.

The most frequent indication for elective operation is failure of the patient's symptoms to respond to medical management with sulfasalazine (Azulfidine) or corticosteroids. Azathioprine has also been tried to ameliorate the symptoms of most patients with inflammatory colitis prior to surgical intervention. Intractable diarrhea with its restrictions on the patient's occupation and social life plus the side-effects of anemia, malnutrition, water and electrolyte depletion, and repeated hospitalizations for treatment of exacerbations of their disease finally force patient and internist to seek relief by surgical management even though this necessitates a permanent ileostomy. Children with intractable colitis have the additional problem of possible retardation of their growth. Elderly patients (over 60 years of age) with ulcerative colitis have an average annual mortality rate of almost 5% when managed by medical treatment with operation reserved for life-threatening complications. Elective operation in the elderly should be considered to reduce the high mortality risk associated with emergency operation and to prevent the complications of inflammatory colitis that are so difficult and hazardous for the elderly patient.

Choice of Operative Procedure

Choice of the correct operative procedure requires that the surgeon differentiate between ulcerative and granulomatous colitis. Patients with ulcerative colitis can be cured of inflammatory bowel disease by proctocolectomy. Except for possible complications related to their ileostomy, these patients have an excellent prognosis. In patients with granulomatous colitis, however, there is always the possibility of subsequent development of small bowel disease, and the choice of operation varies with the extent of the individual patient's disease. For example, ileostomy alone, which has been used to defunctionalize the colon, no longer has a role in the modern treatment of ulcerative colitis but may be worthwhile for patients with granulomatous colitis. Oberhelman has reported 10 patients with granulomatous colitis who had complete remission of their colonic symptoms following ileostomy alone. Menguy lists three indications for simple ileostomy in patients with granulomatous colitis: (1) patients with regional enteritis needing operation who have early, poorly delineated colon involvement, (2) patients with severe exacerbation of diffuse colon disease when colostomy cannot be performed for reasons of associated disorders or patient refusal, and (3) patients with severe systemic manifestations of disease with relatively benign pathologic changes in the colon. In patients with ulcerative colitis, the entire diseased colon and rectal mucosa must be excised, with permanent ileostomy. Because granulomatous colitis tends to segmental involvement, the surgeon may be able to do a segmental resection of localized disease, with end-to-end anastomosis. It is imperative, however, that both proximal and distal ends of the bowel are free of gross disease to reduce complications from disruption of the anastomosis. Granulomatous colitis limited to the distal colon and rectum may be successfully managed by abdominoperineal resection, with a permanent colostomy. The operative procedure varies with the extent and location of disease in patients with granulomatous colitis, but proctocolectomy with ileostomy is the indicated operative procedure for patients with ulcerative colitis. There is risk of producing impotence in males, but this risk is reduced by keeping the dissection close to the bowel wall.

Preoperative Preparation

Mechanical cleansing with or without oral antibiotics is routine preoperative preparation for elective colon operations. In patients with active inflammatory bowel disease, vigorous efforts at mechanical cleansing should be avoided, not only to prevent local damage to the colon but also to prevent serious water and electrolyte depletion. Laxatives and enemas are omitted in patients with active colitis who are having severe diarrhea. Patients are maintained on a clear liquid diet for 2 to 3 days prior to operation. Many different antibiotic regimens are employed, but we prefer neomycin sulfate 1 g PO q6h for 48 hours before operation and may add erythromycin base or kanamycin over the last 24 hours. Antibiotics may also be given intravenously.

Patients with anemia and hypoproteinemia should have these conditions improved prior to operation by blood transfusions and intravenous albumin solutions. Severe diarrhea may deplete potassium, magnesium, and calcium stores. Serum levels for these elements should be checked, and deficiencies corrected prior to operation.

Most patients requiring operative therapy for inflammatory bowel disease have been on corticosteroid therapy. Supplemental corticosteroid medication should be given during operation and gradually discontinued in the late postoperative period. If patients have been off corticosteroid therapy for more than a year, supplemental corticosteroid therapy is unnecessary; otherwise, supplemental corticosteroid medication is given prior to the initiation of anesthesia and is continued during operation and throughout the early postoperative period.

Preoperative emotional preparation of the patient for a permanent ileostomy is made easier by having a member of the local ileostomy club visit the patient. Patients can better accept their ileostomy when they realize that others lead a happy, useful life with a similar disability. The enterostomal therapist is an important member of the medical-surgical team caring for these patients. Preoperative visits should be made by the stomal therapist who will be caring for the patient after operation. The patient must be reassured that continuing assistance will be provided him in regard to the care of his ileostomy. It is also essential that the site of the ileostomy be selected prior to the operation. The patient should be examined in the sitting, standing, and lying positions. Men often prefer the stoma to be situated at the belt line while women prefer a site located halfway between the umbilicus and anterior-superior iliac spine. The flange of the ileostomy device should lie on a smooth, slightly convex skin surface away from the incision, the anterior-superior iliac spine, and the umbilicus. The Kock continent ileostomy may improve patient acceptance; this type of ileostomy, with a reservoir function, is electively emptied every few hours by temporary introduction of a catheter. The endorectal pull-through operation has been used in highly selected patients.

Operative Technique

There are two commonly used positions for the patient on the operating table. In both the abdominal part of the operation is done first, and then the patient either remains supine and the legs are put up in leg rests and abducted or is turned onto his side (Sims position) to permit completion of the perineal part of the operation. We prefer the supine position (see Fig. 26-6).

An indwelling bladder catheter is inserted, and a nasogastric tube is introduced after the induction of general anesthesia with the use of an endotracheal tube. The abdomen is opened through a midline incision carried up to the xiphoid process and curved to the left of the umbilicus. After identification of the ureters, the sigmoid colon and rectum are mobilized down to the levator ani muscles. Care must be taken to keep the dissection close to the rectal wall to avoid injury to the presacral nerves during the dissection of the rectum from the sacral concavity and to the nervi erigentes, which are contained in the lateral rectal stalks. This is important to prevent postoperative impotence in the male undergoing proctocolectomy. The cecum, hepatic flexure, and transverse colon are then freed. The omentum may be dissected from the transverse colon and saved, although some surgeons prefer to remove the greater omentum with the colon. The descending colon is then mobilized as is, finally, the splenic flexure, which is usually the most difficult because of its high location under the left costal margin. The colonic mesentery is then divided. The ileum is transected between clamps, the rectum is divided between clamps, and the colon is removed (Fig. 26-4).

The ileum is usually divided 10 cm to 12 cm proximal to the ileocecal valve. Diseased ileum is avoided. The site

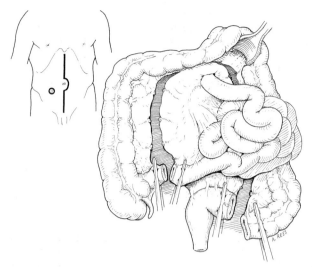

Fig. 26-4. In single-stage proctocolectomy, the colon is excised through a midline abdominal incision. The ileum and rectum are divided between clamps, and the entire colon is removed. (Sawyers JL: Granulomatous colitis and ulcerative colitis including toxic megacolon. In Hardy JD [ed]: Rhoads Textbook of Surgery, 5th ed. Philadelphia, J B Lippincott, 1977)

for ileostomy is marked prior to operation. After applying traction on Kocher clamps placed on the peritoneal, fascial, and subcutaneous layers of the right side of the abdominal incision to prevent distortion of the tissue planes, a circular incision is made through skin, subcutaneous tissue, and abdominal muscles down to the peritoneum, which is opened through a cruciate incision. The stoma should admit two fingers snugly. The ileum is brought through the opening and everted by the Brooke technique to obtain a mucosal covered stoma projecting 2 cm to 2.5 cm above the abdominal wall (Fig. 26-5). A plastic disposable ileostomy appliance is placed over the stoma before the patient leaves the operating room. Beahrs has reported the use of an ileal reservoir in 37 patients and believes that this procedure offers patients a better quality of life than ileostomy alone, since an appliance need not be worn constantly.

Fig. 26-5. Permanent ileostomy is performed by the Brooke technique. The ileum is brought through a separate opening and everted to obtain a mucosa-covered stoma. (Sawyers JL: Granulomatous colitis and ulcerative colitis including toxic megacolon. In Hardy JD [ed]: Rhoads Textbook of Surgery, 5th ed. Philadelphia, J B Lippincott, 1977)

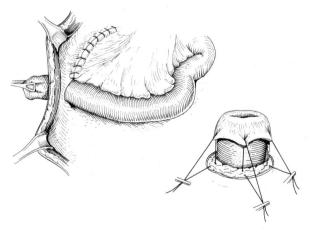

After completing the abdominal phase of the operation, the patient is turned on his side for the perineal procedure. The anal canal is separated from the skin and subcutaneous tissue by a circumferential incision. The dissection continues through the ischiorectal fat to the levator ani muscles, which are divided, allowing the rectal stump to be removed (Fig. 26-6). The perineal wound is either left open or closed in layers. Suction catheters are left in the pelvis for drainage and exteriorized lateral to the suture line. Alternatively, Penrose drains may be brought out through a small central drainage tract.

Postoperative Care

The pertinent problems in the early postoperative care of patients undergoing proctocolectomy with ileostomy are maintenance of fluid and electrolyte balance, supervision of corticosteroid medication, perineal wound care, and supervision of ileostomy function.

The clear plastic ileostomy bag applied in the operating room should be cut to fit exactly over the ileostomy stoma and not permit ileal contents to irritate the peristomal skin. The stoma can be examined through the bag at frequent intervals without having to remove the bag for 2 to 3 days. A temporary appliance with a small plastic faceplate and underlying karaya gum ring may then be applied. A permanent ileostomy appliance is usually fitted to the patient before discharge from the hospital. Commercial permanent ileostomy appliances may be two piece, consisting of a faceplate and bag, or one piece in which the faceplate is made to order for each patient. Because the stoma shrinks during the first 6 months, only the two-piece appliance should be used during this interval, because only the

Fig. 26-6. After the abdominal colectomy is completed, the perineum is exposed and the rectal stump and anus are excised from below. (Sawyers JL: Granulomatous colitis and ulcerative colitis including toxic megacolon. In Hardy JD [ed]: Rhoads Textbook of Surgery, 5th ed. Philadelphia, J B Lippincott, 1977)

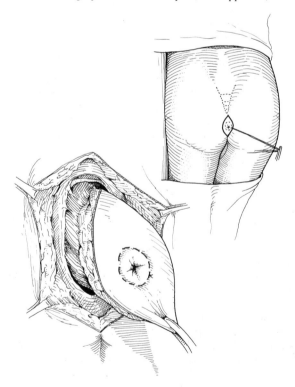

faceplate will need to be changed to fit around the stoma and prevent leakage of effluent between the faceplate and skin. Patients are advised to change their appliance twice a week.

A matured ileostomy of the Brooke type has reduced the frequency of late complications related to the ileostomy. Patients with an ileostomy can enjoy a reasonably healthy life and almost normal activity.

Toxic Megacolon

The dread complication of ulcerative colitis is toxic megacolon. Acute, fulminating, deeply penetrating ulcerative changes develop in the colonic wall and can result in severe hemorrhage, perforation, peritonitis, sepsis, and death. Fortunately, toxic megacolon occurs in only 2% to 5% of patients with inflammatory bowel disease; when these changes occur, the patient usually presents with acutely rising fever, tachycardia, abdominal pain and distention, bloody diarrhea, and the general manifestations of severe toxicity. Roentgenograms of the abdomen show gaseous dilatation of the colon.

The etiology and pathogenesis of toxic dilatation of the colon are obscure, and optimal management remains controversial. In addition to antibiotics and vigorous supportive measures, most physicians initiate treatment with high doses of corticosteroids, while in recent years most surgeons have advocated emergency resection of the colon with ileostomy. Turnbull and his associates, concerned with the high mortality of colectomy in toxic megacolon, have recommended initial surgical treatment by emergency loop ileostomy and so-called blowhole transverse or sigmoid colostomy.

Again, the proper course of treatment of toxic dilatation remains controversial. Spiro summarized collective experience by stating that about 25% of such patients treated medically will die and 25% to 40% of those who do not respond to medical therapy and must undergo emergency colectomy will also die. Medical therapy is usually initiated, but, if the patient fails to improve within a few hours, early emergency operation should be considered to avoid later operation when the patient is then almost moribund.

The results of prolonged medical therapy indicate an increased incidence of perforation of the colon when operation was delayed. Furthermore, serious deterioration in the patient's condition had occurred when operation was finally resorted to in every instance of prolonged delay. Scott and co-workers advocated that resuscitative treatment be given on a life-threatening emergency basis and should include parenteral fluids, electrolytes, blood, broad-spectrum antibiotics, vitamins, corticosteroids, and nasogastric suction. Operation should be performed urgently after 12 to 24 hours of resuscitative treatment. They preferred one-stage proctocolectomy with ileostomy. The operative mortality rate with this plan of management had been under 6%.

Results of Surgical Therapy

Satisfactory rehabilitation may be anticipated in all survivors after single-stage total proctocolectomy for ulcerative colitis. However, the long-term results after operation for granulomatous colitis are difficult to ascertain. This disease entity has been recognized only since 1959. Many patients with granulomatous colitis were undoubtedly operated on with an erroneous diagnosis of ulcerative colitis, and this has confused the evaluation of long-term surgical results. Because granulomatous colitis occurs much less frequently than ulcerative colitis, data are difficult to obtain. Evaluation of surgical therapy is also confused by the variety of operative procedures used in the treatment of granulomatous colitis. Unlike ulcerative colitis, which is cured by proctocolectomy, Crohn's disease may occur in other parts of the gastrointestinal tract after operation for granulomatous colitis. Nevertheless, the prognosis in patients with Crohn's disease limited to the colon (granulomatous colitis) is better than in patients with regional enteritis. Goligher reported a recurrence rate of 20% after partial colectomy and anastomosis for granulomatous colitis. Most surgeons tend to adopt a selective and conservative approach to the operative treatment of granulomatous colitis and accept the risk of ileal and colonic recurrences.

Yersinia enterocolitis can confuse the diagnostic picture and has not infrequently resulted in appendectomy.

DIVERTICULAR DISEASE OF THE COLON

Diverticular disease is described as a malady of Western civilization related to low residue diet and emotional stress. Diverticula of the colon are of two types: (1) *true,* the rare solitary congenital diverticulum of the cecum or right colon, consisting of all layers of the bowel, and (2) *false,* the common acquired diverticula presenting as mucosal outpouchings covered with serosa. Acquired diverticular disease is rarely encountered before age 35 but is seen with increasing frequency thereafter, so that, as noted by Rodkey and Welch, by the ninth decade it is found in two thirds of the population. The sigmoid colon is the usual site of involvement, and the lesion occurs with decreasing frequency with ascent into the more proximal colon. The potential for life-threatening complications increases with increase in the number and duration of diverticula present.

Fig. 26-7. Classic location of diverticula as pulsion mucosal outpouchings at point of entry of penetrating arterial branches. (Johnston JH Jr: Diverticular disease of the colon. In Hardy JD [ed]: Rhoads Textbook of Surgery, 5th ed. Philadelphia, J B Lippincott, 1977)

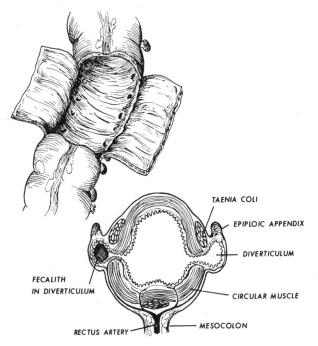

TAENIA COLI

EPIPLOIC APPENDIX

DIVERTICULUM

FECALITH IN DIVERTICULUM

CIRCULAR MUSCLE

MESOCOLON

RECTUS ARTERY

Acquired diverticula are pulsion outpouchings developing in a rather classic pattern in two rows between the tenia through defects in the circular musculature at the point of entry of blood vessels (Fig. 26-7). Their development is related to localized areas of high intraluminal pressure between haustral contraction rings. Painter and Arfwidsson independently used open-ended water-filled polyethylene tubes inserted into the colon to simultaneously coordinate intraluminal pressures with cineradiographic findings. High intrasigmoidal pressures were demonstrated in patients with the prediverticular state and overt diverticulosis and were considered to be an important factor in the genesis of diverticula. In the sigmoid with diverticulosis, the intraluminal pressure could be dramatically raised to 90 torr with morphine. The sigmoid had the potential for segmenting itself into a series of closed chambers with localized areas of high intraluminal pressure, initiating and perpetuating herniation of colonic mucosa through weak spots in the circular musculature. These localized areas of high intraluminal pressure are abolished with propantheline and, surprisingly, were not produced with meperidine, indicating that the latter would be the analgesic of choice in a patient with diverticular disease.

There is increasing agreement that the irritable colon syndrome may be a precursor to diverticulosis. In a follow-up study of 88 patients with irritable colon syndrome, it was noted that diverticula developed in 24%, which was twice the expected incidence, suggesting that tension-elevated intraluminal pressures are important in the development of diverticulosis.

Fleischner described two forms of diverticulosis of the left colon: (1) *simple massed diverticulosis*, in which the descending and the sigmoid colon are studded with diverticula decreasing the diameter and length of the colon, may be related to the diarrheal, painless variety of the irritable colon syndrome; and (2) the more frequently occurring *spastic colon diverticulosis* is limited to the sigmoid or the lower descending colon, with the circular muscle heaped into thick spastic rolls, creating the classic sawtoothed deformity (Fig. 26-8), erroneously ascribed in the past to the inflammatory changes of diverticulitis.

TREATMENT

Concepts of therapy for diverticular disease of the colon have undergone revision in recent years. Diverticula were first described in the 19th century and regarded only as pathologic curiosities. Beer has described the clinical and pathologic aspects of diverticulitis, including stenosis, perforation, and fistulization. Diverting colostomy and resection for the complications of sigmoid diverticulitis was first suggested by Mayo.

The increasing safety of colon surgery and appreciation of the potential complications of diverticulitis have made it a surgical disease (Fig. 26-9). Our aging population abounds with diverticula with the potential for bleeding and infection with localized abscess, fistulization, and spreading peritonitis. The ingenuity and resourcefulness of the surgeon are taxed to the fullest in dealing with this unpredictable disease. The conventional three-stage resection in diverticulitis is gradually being replaced by primary resection. The timing of such resection is of great importance. The use of exteriorization procedures permitting resection of the offending septic focus in perforated diverticulitis with abscess and spreading peritonitis is lowering the mortality and morbidity of perforation. Surgeons are still confronted with patients in extremis from ruptured diverticulitis with fecal peritonitis who cannot be salvaged even with the most vigorous therapeutic endeavors. This places real responsibility on all physicians to attempt to ferret out of the large group of patients with diverticula those more prone to develop serious complications.

Conventionally, diverticular disease is categorized into

DIVERTICULAR DISEASE (OF COLON)	
Etiology	Diverticula of the colon are usually acquired defects, most common in western countries
	Incidence increases with age and progression from right to left colon, rare before age 35; rectum usually spared
	Complications include inflammation with perforation—peritonitis—abscess-fistula, colon obstruction, and hemorrhage
Dx	Principally barium enema showing diverticula and/or mucosal changes
	Exclude other causes of inflammation, obstruction, or hemorrhage
Rx	*Diverticulitis:* For acute episode, antibiotics, IV maintenance, bed rest
	Surgery reserved for commanding complications—transverse loop colostomy with drainage, resection with immediate end-to-end anastomosis, resection of mass with both ends of colon brought out as proximal colostomy and distal mucous fistula, or Hartmann's procedure (resect mass, perform proximal end colostomy, and invert distal stump and drop back)
	Diverticular hemorrhage: Identify site by arteriographic or isotopic procedures and exclude other causes
	If operation mandatory, appropriate colon resection

Fig. 26-8. Roentgenographic appearance typical of sawtooth deformity. This was formerly considered pathognomonic of diverticulitis, but it may be due to smooth muscle abnormality of diverticulosis. (Johnston JH Jr: Diverticular disease of the colon. In Hardy JD [ed]: Rhoads Textbook of Surgery, 5th ed. Philadelphia, J B Lippincott, 1977)

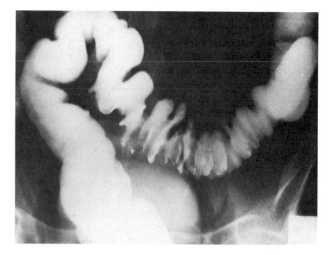

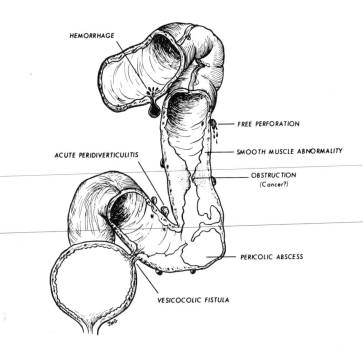

HEMORRHAGE

FREE PERFORATION

ACUTE PERIDIVERTICULITIS

SMOOTH MUSCLE ABNORMALITY

OBSTRUCTION (Cancer?)

PERICOLIC ABSCESS

VESICOCOLIC FISTULA

Fig. 26-9. Commonly occurring complications of diverticular disease. (Johnston JH Jr: Diverticular disease of the colon. In Hardy JD [ed]: Rhoads Textbook of Surgery, 5th ed. Philadelphia, J B Lippincott, 1977)

diverticulosis or *diverticulitis*. The former implies absence of infection with minimal symptoms, the latter, varying degrees of overt infection. However, studies have shown this classification to be too arbitrary, since there is considerable overlap. Indeed, diverticulosis and diverticulitis may be indistinguishable clinically and radiologically, because diverticulosis may be associated with pain, change in bowel habit, and rarely even palpable mass and obstruction.

Treatment in the past featured a low residue diet, but this has been well discounted by studies demonstrating that a high fiber diet, perhaps with bran, is helpful in diverticular disease, increasing the transit time and decreasing intraluminal pressures. The minimizing of emotional stress factors will decrease the intensity of spastic colon sequelae with potentiation of diverticulosis.

Diverticulitis denotes microperforation or macroperforation of a diverticulum. The management of varying stages of diverticulitis is discussed below:

Acute Peridiverticulitis (Pericolitis, Diverticulitis)

Acute peridiverticulitis arises from a microperforation in a single diverticulum in the sigmoid colon; other sites are relatively infrequent. Entrapped fecaliths erode the mucosa and allow infection to spread into the adjacent bowel wall, often occluding the necks of other diverticula, or through the apex of the diverticulum into the pericolic fat. The commonly used term *diverticulitis* really indicates peridiverticulitis from perforation of a diverticulum.

Peridiverticulitis is characterized by left lower quadrant or suprapubic pain and tenderness associated with constipation, mild distention, low grade fever, and leukocytosis. A mass is usually palpable per abdomen, rectum, or vagina, which emphasizes the importance of these examinations. In 15% to 20% of patients, the mass is palpable with rectal or vaginal examination only. Sigmoidoscopic examination is helpful in ruling out colitis and malignancy and gives

indirect evidence of diverticulitis if one encounters mucosal edema at 15 cm to 18 cm and minimal manipulation of the scope reproduces the pain of the disease. Differential diagnosis includes appendicitis, inflammatory adnexal diseases and carcinoma of the ovary in females and prostatitis in males, carcinoma of the sigmoid, and various forms of colitis (amebic, granulomatous, ulcerative, or ischemic).

If the sigmoid is redundant, peridiverticulitis can mimic appendicitis quite closely. Careful assessment may fail to rule out acute appendicitis, and exploration becomes necessary. If acute sigmoid diverticulitis is found even to the point of having free turbid fluid in the peritoneal cavity, appendectomy only should be done, because the acute peridiverticulitis will respond to conservative therapy. Primary bowel resection, exteriorization, or diverting colostomy is not necessary unless there is evidence of spreading fecal peritonitis.

Treatment of acute peridiverticulitis should be conservative, with bowel rest and antibiotics. Often a liquid diet will suffice; nasogastric suction is used only when there is adynamic ileus. Combinations of broad-spectrum antibiotics are indicated, employing either ampicillin or cephalothin or cefamandole with gentamicin or kanamycin. A good regimen is cefamandole 500 mg intramuscularly every 8 hours, alternating with gentamicin, 60 mg to 80 mg every 8 hours. However, gentamicin carries a risk of nephrotoxicity and appropriate precautions must be taken. After the acute symptoms have subsided, oral tetracycline may be used for minor recrudescences.

Barium enema is an essential diagnostic study but is usually deferred during the acute stage. After the acute episode subsides, preparation of the bowel with gentle cleansing enemas rather than catharsis is carried out. Criteria for diagnosis of acute diverticulitis have changed in recent years. Serrated, sawtooth patterns with spiked diverticula and luminal narrowing are no longer valid evidence of inflammation (see Fig. 26-8). Diagnostic criteria for acute diverticulitis are based on perforation of one or more diverticula with small pericolic extravasations. Only a tiny fleck of barium outside the diverticulum means that perforation exists. Small abscess formation around the perforation produces an eccentric mass indenting the lumen of the bowel and is the most common radiographic manifestation of infection. Marshak and colleagues emphasized that a longitudinal, intramural fistulous tract extending parallel to the lumen, 10 cm or more in length, is indicative of granulomatous colitis even when associated diverticula are demonstrated.

It should be strongly emphasized that *radiographic findings can often be subtle and minimal in patients with acute and chronic diverticulitis*. One study by Nicholas and associates of 51 patients with resected diverticulitis failed to demonstrate radiographic evidence of diverticulitis in 14% with demanding retrospective study. In the usual hospital, the incidence of missed diverticulitis is perhaps in the range of 25% to 30%, since the radiologist reports only diverticulosis, missing the subtle extravasations and extraluminal indentations diagnostic of diverticulitis. The clinician responsible should review the films with the radiologist in order to reduce the chances of overlooking radiographic evidence of microperforation.

Perforation with Localized Abscess (Small, Large)

The inflammatory process in acute diverticulitis may be walled off by surrounding abdominal parietes, omentum, pelvic viscera, and intestine into a localized abscess that is readily palpable by abdominal or rectal examination. If the process seems well walled off with no evidence of spreading peritonitis, intensive conservative therapy is indicated. Nasogastric suction to combat distention, along with intravenously administered fluids to maintain fluid and electrolyte balance, are often necessary because of associated adynamic or mechanical ileus. The probability of *Bacteroides* infection in such cases must be strongly considered and appropriate antibacteroidal therapy given. Clindamycin in a dosage of 300 mg every 6 hours, recognizing the possibility of a complicating coloproctitis, is the drug of choice and is often used in combination with ampicillin and gentamicin. Chloramphenicol is effective against *Bacteroides* but should be reserved for life-threatening complications because of its rare, but potentially fatal, bone marrow depressive effect. Often the abscess will resolve with such intensive therapy, allowing interval colon resection in 3 to 4 months.

Persistence or enlargement of the inflammatory mass, with associated fever, increasing pain, tenderness, and leukocytosis, demands operative intervention. This may be of three types:

Extraperitoneal Drainage. A fluctuant mass may present low in the pelvis and can be drained (after needle aspiration has shown the presence of pus) through the vagina or through the anterior wall of the rectum. More often it is possible to drain the abscess through a muscle-splitting extraperitoneal approach without violating the peritoneal cavity. Should fecal fistula develop with extraperitoneal drainage, it will often regress or heal, permitting subsequent one-stage resection. If regression does not occur, proximal diversionary colostomy is indicated.

Drainage with Diverting Transverse Colostomy. When operative intervention is necessary and extraperitoneal drainage is not feasible, drainage with defunctionalizing colostomy should be strongly considered unless there is an obvious defect in the bowel wall, allowing the escape of feces. In such cases, an exteriorization or Hartmann procedure is decidedly preferable. After colostomy with drainage, definitive bowel resection is possible in 3 to 4 months, with closure of the colostomy either at the time of resection or 2 to 4 weeks later. If closure of the colostomy is to be done as a third-stage procedure, one should have a barium enema evaluation of the anastomotic line before closure. Occasionally, there will be anastomotic extravasation, indicating abscess that is not discernible clinically. Deferring of colostomy closure permits spontaneous healing of the anastomotic leak.

Exteriorization or Hartmann Procedure; Immediate Resection with Anastomosis (?). In the past decade there has been increasing use of Mikulicz exteriorization or the Hartmann modification of this (Laimon). Both remove the source of the major pathologic process and the point of perforation, preventing further fecal soilage of the peritoneal cavity. Exteriorization may not be feasible because of inflammatory shortening of bowel mesentery or perforation low in the sigmoid. One may then resect the diseased, perforated segment, close the rectosigmoidal stump, and create a proximal sigmoid skin level colostomy (Hartmann procedure). Resection with anastomosis has also been used.

Perforation with Spreading Peritonitis

The pathology varies from minimal leakage of an abscess to frank feculent peritonitis. It is often caused by rupture of a previously walled off abscess. These patients may be gravely ill, presenting evidence of shock with hypotension, tachycardia, and oliguria. The abdomen is distended and diffusely tender, with varying degrees of rigidity. Roentgenograms of the abdomen show free gas in 25% to 30%, with evidence of ileus in most.

If there is a long-standing history of diverticulitis, the diagnosis is obvious. Differential diagnosis may be trying, for the picture of peritonitis with shock may be caused by ruptured appendicitis, perforated peptic ulcer, gangrenous bowel, and pancreatitis. Lavage with Gram stain of the aspirated fluid can be helpful in diagnosis. This can be done while the patient is being resuscitated with intravenous fluids; central venous pressure and 30-minute urine excretions are monitored, and massive doses of antibiotics are given intravenously. A foul smelling aspirate with a mixed flora and gram-negative rods points to peritonitis from a leak in the lower intestinal tract (*i.e.*, ruptured appendicitis or ruptured diverticulitis). A low midline incision will allow the surgeon to quickly assess and correct the underlying pathologic process.

In the past, traditional treatment for perforated diverticulitis with diffusing peritonitis was diversion of the fecal stream by proximal transverse colostomy, attempted suture of the perforation, and insertion of drains. Despite improvement in antibiotic and resuscitative therapy, the mortality rate remained at 35% to 50% with this approach. In spite of diverting colostomy, there continued to be discharge into the peritoneal cavity from the feces-filled left colon. Recently, the traditional three-stage operation for perforated diverticulitis has been challenged, with increasing emphasis being placed on removing the site of continuing contamination. Ryan, Large, Madden, and others have favored resection with primary anastomosis, claiming lessened mortality and morbidity. Large reported 18 patients with peritonitis due either to free perforation or to rupture of a pericolic abscess into the peritoneal cavity treated by primary resection with anastomosis, with only two deaths. Madden reported a series of 25 patients who had primary resections for perforated diverticulitis or malignancy of the left colon, who, he claimed, were "too ill to withstand other than a primary resection," with two deaths due to peritonitis, a mortality of 8%. Despite the relatively low mortality, 8 of the 25 patients with primary anastomosis developed an anastomotic leak, with one death and seven fecal fistulas.

Most surgeons agree that excision of the site of continuing spillage is essential, but they prefer *delayed* to primary anastomosis in the face of such obvious infection. In thin patients with redundant mesocolons, this may be accomplished by exteriorization. More often the Hartmann procedure (*i.e.*, sigmoid resection with closure of the rectosigmoidal stump and skin level sigmoid colostomy) is the procedure of choice. Copious lavage of the peritoneal cavity with 5 to 10 liters of warm saline is useful to cleanse the many potential spaces for subsequent abscess formation. Intraperitoneal instillation of antibiotics (penicillin, kanamycin, cephalothin, cephamandole) is advocated by some but apparently has no advantage over parenteral administration.

A distinct advantage of primary resection is that unsuspected adenocarcinomas misdiagnosed as diverticulitis are removed earlier, rather than being discovered weeks or months later, as often happened with the conventional three-stage procedure. Large reports that of 18 patients with peritonitis believed to be due to perforated diverticulitis and treated by primary resection, 5 proved to have unsuspected carcinoma.

PERFORATION ASSOCIATED WITH CORTICOSTEROID THERAPY

Perforation of colonic diverticula is being increasingly recognized as a complication of long-term adrenocorticosteroid therapy, which apparently predisposes to free perforation. Often there is no antecedent history of diverticulitis. Diffuse spreading peritonitis without localization is typical and related to the anti-inflammatory properties of corticosteroids. Exteriorization or the Hartmann procedure is mandatory to avoid continued contamination of the peritoneal cavity. Discontinuation of corticosteroid therapy 3 to 4 months prior to primary anastomosis is indicated. If the severity of the underlying disease contraindicates corticosteroid withdrawal, three-stage resection is preferable.

OBSTRUCTION

Colon obstruction from long-standing diverticulitis results from narrowing and distortion of the lumen from muscle hypertrophy and spasm, inflammatory edema, encroachment from intramural or pericolic abscesses, and fibrosis from repeated attacks. Usually colon obstruction is partial and responds to conservative therapy with bowel rest and antibiotics. Endoscopic viewing of the strictured area and biopsy should be performed soon after the obstruction has resolved, to exclude a malignant tumor. Infrequently the obstruction is complete, closely simulating neoplastic obstruction. Should obstruction persist despite conservative therapy, transverse colostomy as an initial decompressive procedure is indicated. In these patients with complete obstruction there is always the worry of an underlying malignancy, and therefore definitive resection is usually carried out within 2 to 3 weeks, with subsequent closure of the colostomy. Some surgeons would operate immediately and perform primary resection with colostomy–Hartmann pouch, to remove a possible cancer.

Occasionally, typical mechanical small bowel obstruction occurs secondary to the small intestine being plastered to an abscess arising from perforated sigmoid diverticulitis. An attempt at decompression with a long tube (Miller-Abbott) with intensive antibiotic therapy should be carried out. If there is not improvement with such a regimen in 7 to 10 days, laparotomy, with lysis of small bowel adhesions and resection of the sigmoid and offending abscess by Hartmann procedure, should be performed.

INDICATIONS FOR ELECTIVE SURGERY

Persistent or Recurrent Peridiverticulitis

The most common indication for surgery in diverticulitis is for persistent or recurrent peridiverticulitis; it is well recognized that repeated attacks significantly increase the chance for serious perforative complications. Early surgery in younger patients (particularly those under age 55) is strongly indicated. Elective resection can be done with a mortality and recurrence rate of less than 2%. In the majority of cases, sigmoidectomy alone is sufficient. In good-risk patients with a significant number of diverticula in the descending colon, left hemicolectomy is the procedure of choice. It is mandatory that all diverticula in the rectosigmoidal and upper rectal area be resected to avoid faulty anastomotic healing and persistence of symptoms. Diverticula remaining in other parts of the colon can be left without particular concern, since they rarely cause difficulty. Reilly advocated sigmoid colomyotomy with division of the thickened circular muscle in the distal colon as being logical and effective treatment. This operation has few advocates in the United States.

Cancer and Diverticulitis

Diverticula and cancer often coexist. Approximately 20% of resections for sigmoid malignancy present with associated diverticula. Bacon and associates in a review of 351 patients undergoing resection for diverticulitis found 27 (7.7%) to have coexisting carcinoma in the same segment of bowel. Distressingly, half of these were not suspected until operation and a few were not recognized until the resected specimen was opened for pathologic examination.

The differential diagnosis depends on barium enema examination, which gives an accurate appraisal in 85% to 90% of cases. In diverticulitis there is a long, narrow, conical deformity with a normal mucosal pattern thrown into folds. Cancer presents as a shorter defect with absent mucosa and more sharply defined margins ("apple core deformity"). The sigmoid flexure is difficult to examine radiologically, owing to redundancy and difficulty in palpation; clear distinction between malignancy and diverticulitis is impossible in 5% to 10% of patients.

The history is helpful in that the patient with diverticulitis is more likely to have had recurrent episodes of pain and fever and the patient with malignancy is likely to have had intermittent bleeding per rectum, but it is not diagnostic. Colonoscopy can be helpful in excluding malignancy, but is not successful in all cases. Dean and Newell noted that colonoscopy is particularly difficult in such patients: In 17 of 36 patients in whom colonoscopy was attempted because barium enema suggested the possibility of carcinoma there was failure to examine the diseased segment. The colonoscope could not be passed into the diseased segment, owing to sharp angulation of the bowel or to stenosis. We have had good success in these patients with use of a small diameter pediatric gastrointestinal fiberscope to traverse a narrowed angulated sigmoid lumen. Colonoscopy seems to have its greatest application in elderly poor-risk patients who are not suitable candidates for surgery without compelling indications. In the usual patient with diverticulitis severe enough to produce a radiologically confusing mass defect, resection is indicated.

Radioimmunoassay of carcinoembryonic antigen (CEA) may be helpful but rarely diagnostic in that high titers are often obtained in patients with colon carcinoma. However, CEA assay is not an absolute test for cancer. Elevated CEA levels may occur in certain benign disorders, including alcoholic cirrhosis, ulcerative colitis, and pulmonary emphysema. The CT scan may be helpful.

Emphasis should be given to the fact that *repetitious bleeding from the rectum in a patient with diverticular disease often indicates associated neoplastic disease (polyp or cancer) and is a compelling indication for surgical intervention.* It is tragic to find patients who have lost their chance for cure from malignancy because of procrastination when rectal bleeding has been ascribed to diverticular disease after a single proctoscopic and barium enema examination. The accuracy of these examinations is not greater than 90%, and continued bleeding demands repeat examinations to exclude malignancy. Surgical intervention may be necessary to decide the issue.

FISTULAS

Fistulization to adjacent hollow viscera, especially the bladder, vagina, or small bowel and, less frequently, the uterus, salpinx, adjacent colon or ureter, occurs when the pericolic abscess adheres to a hollow viscus and erodes into it. Sigmoidocutaneous fistulas may follow surgical incision and drainage of diverticular abscesses.

The most frequent internal fistula is sigmoidovesical which is more prone to occur in men or in women who have had a hysterectomy, because the uterus seems to act as a protective barrier. Proximity of the inflammatory process to the dome of the bladder causes genitourinary symptoms such as urgency, frequency, and dysuria. A common complaint is of pain induced by the act of micturition. The onset of urinary tract symptoms in a patient with diverticulitis should alert one to the possibility of impending fistulization and is an indication for elective resection when the acute episode subsides. The most dramatic symptom is pneumaturia with interruption of the urinary stream by the passage of gas. This is virtually pathognomonic of an enterovesical fistula but has been reported in cystitis associated with gas-producing organisms, as well as oral–genital sexual contact.

Sigmoidovesical fistulas may be difficult to demonstrate. One is usually unable to reach the level of fistulization with a proctoscope. A barium enema demonstrates the fistula in only 20% to 30% of patients. Cystoscopy is valuable in diagnosis and may demonstrate the fistulous opening. Should this not be evident, florid cystitis in the dome of the bladder heralds the possibility of fistulization.

Vaginal fistulas are characterized by the passage of purulent vaginal discharge with occasional passage of flatus and feces from the vagina. Fistulous communications between the colon and small bowel are often associated with diarrhea and can usually be demonstrated by barium enema or small bowel series.

In the past, the presence of a fistula was immediate indication for a colostomy as the first step in the usual three-stage procedure. More and more, good results are being reported following one-stage resection for sigmoidovesical, sigmoidovaginal, and sigmoidoenteric fistulas. The timing of one-stage operations is of utmost importance. The danger of an overwhelming ascending urinary tract infection in a patient with sigmoidovesical fistula has been overemphasized in the past. With conservative therapy, despite fistulization, much of the inflammatory reaction will subside, allowing a one-stage procedure to be performed with safety. All inflamed colon should be resected.

Should fistulization to the adjacent small bowel exist, it should be resected and end-to-end anastomosis effected. Hysterectomy is indicated if there is fistulization into the uterus. With fistulization into the bladder or vagina, resection of a portion of the bladder or vagina is usually not necessary, for prompt healing occurs when the offending sigmoid colon is resected.

DIVERTICULITIS OF THE CECUM AND RIGHT COLON

Diverticulitis of the cecum and right colon is an infrequent disease, with problems in diagnosis and therapy. Acquired diverticula of the right colon occur in approximately 5% of patients with colonic diverticulosis. Diverticulosis confined to the cecum and ascending colon without involvement of the sigmoid is rare in whites but may be the type of diverticulosis seen most commonly in certain Oriental races, as noted by Perry and Morson.

A true diverticulum of the cecum occasionally occurs and is usually located within 2 cm of the ileocecal valve. It may be the source of major hemorrhage or diverticulitis. Diverticulitis of the right colon usually mimics appendicitis and is rarely diagnosed preoperatively. A palpable right lower quadrant mass is present in one third of patients, raising the possibility of neoplasm.

The diagnosis is established at the time of exploration in over half of the cases when one finds a normal appendix and an obviously inflamed diverticulum. Resection of the diverticulum and adjacent inflamed bowel wall, with closure without tension, avoiding encroachment on the ileocecal valve, is preferred treatment. The inflammatory mass may be so dense that malignancy or inflammatory bowel disease such as granulomatous colitis, actinomycosis, or tuberculosis cannot be excluded. In such cases, resection of the cecum or right hemicolectomy can usually be done with safety and with good result. At times one may establish the diagnosis at operation by palpating the ostium of the diverticulum through the opposite wall of the cecum.

DIVERTICULITIS OF THE RECTUM (RARE)

Only 1% or 2% of diverticula occur in the rectum. Infection may occur, mimicking rectal malignancy in symptomatology and in gross and radiographic appearance. Unnecessary abdominoperineal resections have been done, emphasizing the need for histologic diagnosis in all cases before resorting to this ablative procedure.

HEMORRHAGE IN DIVERTICULITIS

One of the most serious complications of a colonic diverticulum is massive hemorrhage. Often this severe hemorrhage has been preceded by minor hemorrhage in the past. Some authors prefer to refer to *diverticulosis* when the presenting problem is hemorrhage, reserving the term *diverticulitis* for those instances when the major problem is inflammation and infection. However, this seems a rather arbitrary distinction, since it is likely that at least some degree of infection existed to cause erosion of the artery and bleeding in the first place.

Right colon diverticula, while far less numerous than left colon diverticula, appear to have a much greater propensity for bleeding. This *apparent* difference may be due in part to confusion with arteriovenous (AV) malformations in the right colon. These AV malformations may be missed if a very careful search is not made and, in some cases, this requires actual injection of the arterial supply with radiopaque medium and the use of roentgenography.

The precise diagnosis of colon hemorrhage can be a very difficult matter. The first thing to do is to inspect the anal area for hemorrhoids; then digital examination and anoscopy or sigmoidoscopy are performed prior to a barium enema. Indeed, if these measures fail to disclose the source or at least the approximate site or area of the bleeding, it may be desirable to proceed to radioisotope scanning with intravenously injected tagged erythrocytes or to arteriography. Certainly, it is important to perform arteriography at a time when the colon does not contain barium from a barium enema. However, usually the bleeding is not massive or life threatening, and under these circumstances a barium enema is appropriately performed after the sigmoidoscopy because it is less expensive and trying to the patient. Colonoscopy may follow barium enema, but it is not often helpful in acute colonic hemorrhage.

Colon malignancies do not often bleed massively. If such

massive bleeding does occur, it will most likely be associated with diverticulosis or AV malformation. Patients with ulcerative colitis or Crohn's disease may bleed substantially, but usually the history and physical examination will have suggested a chronic inflammatory condition, often with diarrhea. It is always to be remembered that this "colonic hemorrhage" may be derived from the small bowel or even the stomach and duodenum (ulcer). For example, an ulcerated leiomyoma can bleed massively. Some causes of bleeding from the rectum are shown in Fig. 26-10.

MISCELLANEOUS INFLAMMATORY CONDITIONS OF THE COLON AND RECTUM

RADIATION COLITIS

Radiation colitis is also discussed under radiation injury to the small intestine, but it should be considered here. Radiation colitis is a cicatrizing obliterative colitis. It is most often found in the rectum after radiation treatment of carcinoma of the prostate or uterus. It is usually transient and subsides in a month or so after cessation of radiation therapy, but at times it persists for a long while and may produce intractable tenesmus, pain and diarrhea, stricture, perforation with fistula formation, or bleeding. Of course, recurrence of the malignancy must always be excluded. Again, in most patients the condition is self-limited, but in others distressing symptoms and complications may require proximal colostomy or even resection. Early treatment is symptomatic, and encouragement is provided.

PSEUDOMEMBRANOUS ENTEROCOLITIS AND DRUG-INDUCED COLITIS

Pseudomembranous colitis is an uncommon disorder but may be lethal. For a time it was believed that it most commonly followed antibiotic therapy to which staphylococci were resistant and which therefore overgrew in vast numbers, in the absence of competing other normal intestinal flora. However, this theory failed to account for the fact that the condition had been reported long before

Fig. 26-10. Sites of origin of rectal bleeding. (Welch CE: Colon hemorrhage. In Hardy JD [ed]: Rhoads Textbook of Surgery, 5th ed. Philadelphia, J B Lippincott, 1977)

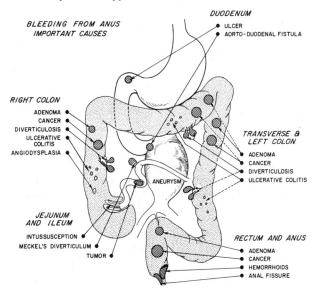

antibiotics were available (*e.g.,* in patients who had been in severe shock). Also, the overgrowth of staphylococci could not be demonstrated in some patients with the condition. Thus the condition is now perceived to be much more complex than once supposed. Severe ischemia can certainly cause sloughing of the mucosa almost in a cast, and some broad-spectrum antibiotics (*e.g.,* clindamycin) may have a direct toxic effect on the colorectal mucosa. In addition, nutritional deficits may play a role. The etiologic agent in some patients is an overgrowth of *Clostridium difficile,* which elaborates a toxin. Here vancomycin is the treatment of choice.

Whatever the etiology in the given case, the onset of pseudomembranous enterocolitis is an extremely serious development, with a substantial mortality rate, in part because the condition often occurs in patients who are severely ill. Basically, the integrity of the gut mucosa is impaired, and thus its protective effect against bacterial invasion may be lost. The clinical picture consists of fever, abdominal pain and distention, diarrhea and shock due to fluid loss, and bacterial invasion in some patients. The mucosa of the colon is covered with a pseudomembrane of fibrin, mucus, necrotic cells, and leukocytes. Proctoscopy and Gram stain of the membrane may provide a diagnosis of staphylococcal overgrowth, but bacterial cultures should also be made. Treatment consists of appropriate antibiotics (often methicillin), fluid, plasma, and blood replacement and of nasogastric suction to diminish gaseous distention of the intestine. The mortality remains high but has declined somewhat in recent years.

AMEBIASIS

The infestation with *Entamoeba histolytica* is not usually a "surgical" disease, but it may become so for several reasons:

The minor bleeding from the colorectum may camouflage the presence of a colon malignancy.

Amebiasis of the colon, often the cecum, may cause perforation of the colon, at times with the presence of a tumefaction, termed an *ameboma.*

Amebic infection around the anorectal canal can result in severe excoriation and even necrosis of surrounding tissues.

Amebiasis of the colon may produce liver abscess, which is usually single rather than multiple as might be met in ascending cholangitis.

The clinical picture of colonic amebiasis may range from no symptoms, to bloody diarrhea, to full-blown ulcerating colitis. Amebiasis must be differentiated especially from ulcerative colitis, dysentery, diverticulitis, carcinoma, and even appendicitis. The diagnosis is established by finding the parasites in fresh stool immediately examined, and then excluding the other possible causes of the symptomatology. If no amebas are found but the patient exhibits a liver abscess, serologic tests may be helpful.

Treatment consists of infectious precautions for stools, plus the drug therapy. The intraluminal form of the disease is usually treated with diiodohydroxyquin (Diodoquin) and tetracycline; for the extraluminal form metronidazole (Flagyl) is used. Perforation of the colon requires operation, but otherwise conservative therapy is usually successful.

ISCHEMIC COLITIS

In essence, ischemic colitis is a response of the colon to vascular insufficiency. The severity of the condition will be correlated with the degree of ischemia imposed, plus other as yet obscure factors. It may be transient, and relatively mild; it may be associated with mucosal slough but not with colonic perforation; or it may entail frank gangrene of the colon, most often the left colon but at any level on occasion. Late stricture may develop. It is now known that arterial ischemic insults to the colon are fairly common in older people, and we have observed this problem in younger people with some type of inflammatory arteritis, such as thromboarteritis obliterans (Buerger's disease).

The diagnosis is made on the basis of findings of abdominal examination and a carefully performed barium enema, which discloses the characteristic "thumbprint" sign. Treatment consists of bowel rest, administration of broad-spectrum antibiotics and intravenous fluids, and operative intervention when indicated for evidence of perforation or gangrene. In general, the clinical results are fairly good for isolated colon ischemia.

PROCTITIS

Inflammatory irritation of the rectum can be an annoying or even distressing condition when caused by agents other than those previously discussed. Various drugs (*e.g.,* quinidine sulfate) may be irritating in some patients. Rectal manipulation in sexual perversion or various medication instillations may also be a factor. Treatment consists primarily in detection and removal of the etiologic factor. Meanwhile, zinc oxide ointment, a local anesthetic ointment, or even corticosteroid ointment may be helpful. The condition is usually self-limited if etiologic agents are discontinued.

ACUTE TRAUMATIC PERFORATIONS OF THE COLON AND RECTUM

Traumatic perforations of the colon are very serious injuries, and the general management of knife, gunshot, and similar external traumatic injuries is surveyed in Chapter 10. Here brief consideration will be directed toward traumatic injuries caused by the introduction of objects into the rectum or colostomy, often for diagnostic purposes.

Acute traumatic perforations of the colon and rectum may result from the willful introduction of mechanical devices into the rectum or colostomy or may be part of a planned procedure conducted by medical or paramedical personnel. Most of these have one thing in common, namely, that the force producing the perforation acts from within the lumen of the bowel outward. These perforations may be caused by diagnostic and therapeutic medical procedures, such as cleansing enemas, endoscopy, or radiographic examinations using contrast material; introduction of mechanical objects into the rectum as acts of sexual perversion; and pranks such as the discharging of compressed air hoses aimed at the perineum of the victim.

Scattered reports of these injuries have appeared in the literature for many years. Abrasion injury to the rectal wall from enema tips is one of the most common lesions seen in proctoscopic examinations, but serious injury or perforation is not common. The paucity of reports does not give a true incidence, since there is probably reluctance on the part of physicians to report these cases. Nearly every surgeon will be called on to care for patients suffering from this type of accident.

As the surgeon has extended the scope of his field and has required more accurate diagnoses, the risk of injury to the colon and rectum has increased. One must ensure that the value of the examination justifies the risk involved. Hard data are not available, but it seems reasonable that proctoscopic and barium enema examinations are worthwhile for examining symptomatic patients, for screening asymptomatic patients past 45 years of age at intervals of 2 or 3 years, and for following certain conditions such as familial multiple polyposis and chronic idiopathic ulcerative colitis. Colonoscopy, which carries more risk of perforation, should be reserved for more specific purposes than routine screening of asymptomatic patients.

Two factors influence the incidence and site of perforation. One is the condition of the bowel—its involvement with a disease process such as ulcerative colitis or fixation by adhesions and inflammatory reaction. It has long been recognized that perforation is more likely to occur in such a segment of bowel. The skill of the examiner is an obvious factor. Undue and inept force on the instrument may result in injury.

The clinical picture and plan of management are related to the location of the injury in reference to the site of reflection of the peritoneum on the upper rectum. Those above that level communicate with the peritoneal cavity and those below open into the perirectal structures.

PERFORATION ABOVE THE PERITONEAL REFLECTION

A perforation above the peritoneal reflection enters into the peritoneal cavity. The injury may be caused by endoscopy, cleansing enema, barium enema radiographic examination, or air pressure insufflation. The junction of the rectum and sigmoid colon where the bowel is sharply angulated is a common site of perforation. Although the exact cause is not clear, perforation of a colostomy may well be due to the balloon or similar device intended to prevent extrusion of barium from the stoma.

Hydrostatic pressure *per se* is rarely the cause of perforation of the colon and is also rarely the cause of injury in barium enema examination but it can be. In accord with LaPlace's law, the likelihood of rupture of the intestinal wall is proportional to the product of the pressure times the radius of the lumen of the intestine. Thus, the greater diameter of the lumen of the cecum partly accounts for its increased vulnerability. Even in perforations resulting from air pressure hose injections, the velocity of the airstream striking the bowel wall rather than intraluminal pressure is the important factor.

Any foreign material introduced into the peritoneal cavity causes some inflammatory response, and it is likely that the composition influences the degree only. Some of the controversy in regard to tissue response to barium may stem from differences in the suspension used in animal experiments. There is no question that barium contaminated with feces produces a violent inflammatory reaction.

A clinical picture of perforation of the intestine following colon examination readily suggests the diagnosis. The patient complains of pain associated with inadequate return of the barium enema fluid. With extravasation of barium onto the peritoneal surface, there is outpouring of a large quantity of extracellular fluid. Shortly, there follows some degree of hypovolemic shock, owing to loss of extracellular fluid into the peritoneal cavity. Signs of peritoneal irritation may occur immediately, or these symptoms may be delayed until peritonitis has developed 12 to 24 hours later. In paraplegic patients, the injury may not be recognized immediately because of the loss of sensory perception. Radiographic examination discloses free air in the peritoneal cavity (Fig. 26-11). If the perforation resulted from a barium enema, the barium is seen outside the lumen of the bowel.

On recognition of the injury, treatment consisting of analgesics for pain, intravenous balanced salt solution to combat hypovolemia, and broad-spectrum antibiotics is instituted. Immediate abdominal laparotomy is mandatory. The operation is concerned with two things: (1) the perforation in the bowel and (2) the peritoneal contamination. The laceration is identified and, depending on the findings, the injured bowel may be treated by simple suture, revision of an existing colostomy, exteriorization, repair with a proximal diverting colostomy, resection of a segment of injured bowel with a colostomy, and drainage. A most important consideration is do not procrastinate—operate at once.

Since many of these patients have a mechanically clean bowel and are operated on soon after injury, simple suture closure of the perforation will suffice. If the perforation is located just proximal to a colostomy, resection of the injured segment and creation of a new colostomy proximally is the simplest procedure. The bowel adjacent to the laceration may show so much reaction that simple closure is not considered wise or the closure may not be secure, in which case the segment of bowel may be exteriorized. If the suture line in the exteriorized bowel breaks down, it becomes a colostomy; if it remains intact and heals satisfactorily, the bowel may be replaced into the peritoneal cavity in 5 to 7 days. (However, it may have had to be opened to relieve obstruction at the level of the abdominal wall.) Should the injury be in a segment of colon that cannot be exteriorized, the laceration may be repaired and a proximal diverting colostomy performed. If the perforation is on the mesenteric border and there is dissection into the leaf of the mesentery, that segment of bowel with its mesentery may be resected and the first stage of a definitive procedure accomplished. A proximal diverting colostomy should be performed.

The second aim of surgical intervention is to perform a satisfactory peritoneal toilet. All of the foreign material (enema water, barium, and feces) should be removed by suction and the region irrigated with copious amounts of normal saline. Adherent barium should be disregarded, because it is impossible to remove all these clumps of barium that are covered by a thin film of fibrin. Attempts at mechanical wiping only increase the local inflammatory response and increase chances for the formation of adhesions. The greater omentum to which barium has become adherent should be removed in an effort to decrease the magnitude of the inflammatory response. Resulting fibrosis and adhesions are responsible for the recurrent bouts of intestinal obstruction that occur in as many as 30% of these patients in later years.

PERFORATION BELOW THE PERITONEAL REFLECTION

In addition to frank perforations through all layers of the bowel wall, a laceration of the mucosa may occur and the enema water or barium suspension may dissect in the submucosal plane. This can be just as serious a problem as a frank perforation of the entire thickness of the bowel.

Often the patient complains of pain at the time of injury, and bright red bleeding per rectum may follow. Some degree of shock may be apparent. Although massive hemorrhage is not usually a problem unless a major vessel is damaged, hematoma formation is common because it is difficult to obtain complete hemostasis. The nature of the material injected into tissue influences the reaction that follows. As one would expect, with the inoculation of foreign material containing feces and with the presence of hematoma, the substantial morbidity and mortality are due to infection. The inflammatory reaction is intense and proceeds from cellulitis to necrosis and suppuration with abscess formation.

From the history of intrarectal manipulation, the diagnosis is suspected. Therapy consisting of sufficient analgesics to relieve pain, fluids and blood to treat shock, and antibiotics is instituted before beginning anoscopic and proctoscopic examination to identify the site and extent of the injury. As soon as the diagnosis is confirmed, a proximal colostomy is fashioned to divert the fecal stream from passing through the injured bowel. Usually, the sigmoid colon is brought out as a colostomy. At the time the abdomen is open, the lower sigmoid and upper rectum can be examined to make certain that the injury to the bowel is below the peritoneal reflection.

The patient is then placed in the lithotomy position and adequate drainage of serum and blood from the presacral space through a separate dependent perineal incision is accomplished. Debridement of necrotic tissue must be performed. In patients seen late after injury, debridement may be extensive enough to include removal of segments of bowel wall. The drain may be brought out between the anus and coccyx or, if the injury is located in a lateral wall, the drain may be brought out lateral to the anus. This is preferable to bringing the drain out through the anterior abdominal wall. Specimens for culture and sensitivity studies are obtained. Until the specific antibiotic can be chosen from these studies, an antibiotic effective against gram-negative organisms, such as a cephalosporin, should be administered. The importance of thorough cleansing of the segment of bowel between the colostomy and the anus has been emphasized. In some patients who are operated on early after injury, it is feasible to repair the laceration in the

Fig. 26-11. Roentgenographic features of acute perforation of colon above peritoneal reflection include air under the diaphragm. The intraperitoneal colon may be perforated by instrumentation as illustrated, as well as by barium enema or forced air pressure. (Kurzweg FT: Acute traumatic perforations of the colon and rectum. In Hardy JD [ed]: Rhoads Textbook of Surgery, 5th ed. Philadelphia, J B Lippincott, 1977)

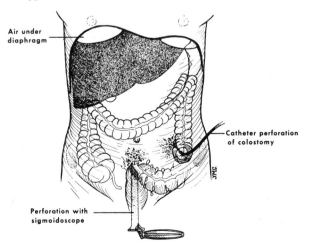

Air under diaphragm

Catheter perforation of colostomy

Perforation with sigmoidoscope

bowel. This is a decision requiring experienced judgment, and the procedure is only occasionally practicable.

On the other hand, there are reported instances of barium entering lacerations of the mucosa and dissecting submucosally that produced little disability and were managed expectantly. Small deposits of barium in the submucosa may not be recognized until years later when a granuloma results. Then it may be mistaken for a tumor.

Complications are related to sepsis. So much tissue may be destroyed that resection of the rectum and anus is necessary, leaving the patient with a permanent colostomy.

There is not a sufficient number of recent cases managed by modern techniques to indicate accurately the mortality following these injuries. The 40% to 50% mortality rates reported several decades ago are unreasonably high.

OTHER CAUSES OF TRAUMATIC PERFORATION

As yet, few cases of perforation have been reported following the removal of polyps with the flexible fiberoptic colonoscope, but probably few of these cases are reported. Certainly more of these cases will be seen as this instrument gains still wider use. The perforation may occur immediately if the snare cuts through the bowel wall, or it may be delayed until the fulgurated base of the polyp sloughs. Usually the colon has been mechanically cleansed and occasionally prepared with antibiotics so that contamination of the peritoneal cavity is not extensive. The bowel may be closed by direct suture and peritoneal toilet may be accomplished. A proximal colostomy will usually not be necessary.

Perforation of the colon following catheterization of the umbilical vein or artery for exchange transfusion or administration of intravenous fluids has been reported. The pathologic findings may resemble those found in acute necrotizing enterocolitis in adults. The etiology is not understood but may be related to a vascular accident occurring as a mechanical result of the exchange transfusion or may be related to hypoxia and superimposed infection. The treatment includes antibiotics and laparotomy (Table 26-2).

TUMORS OF THE COLON AND RECTUM

Carcinoma of the colon represents perhaps the most major consideration among diseases of this organ. Whereas breast carcinoma is the most common malignancy in women and

TABLE 26-2 PLAN OF MANAGEMENT OF PERFORATION OF THE COLON AND RECTUM: POSSIBLE CONSIDERATIONS

BELOW PERITONEAL REFLECTION	ABOVE PERITONEAL REFLECTION
Intravenous fluids, blood	Intravenous fluids, blood
Antibiotics	Antibiotics
Colostomy	Simple suture
Débridement	Revision of colostomy if colostomy was perforated
Drain posteriorly	(Exteriorization?)
Wash-out of distal segment	(Repair with proximal colostomy?)
	(Resection with colostomy?)
	Peritoneal toilet

CARCINOMA OF THE COLON AND RECTUM

Etiology	Most common major cancer (both sexes combined). Genetic aspects in some patients, especially as related to polyps. Cause of most cancers unknown, but environmental factors, especially diet, suspected because of varied geographical incidence. Most common in rectum and sigmoid colon; multiple in 5% to 10% of cases
Dx	Symptoms of bleeding, change in bowel habits with or without obstruction; pain late; mass often palpable late. Digital rectal examination, proctosigmoidoscopy, barium enema, and, if indicated, air-contrast colonoscopy; CEA for liver metastases (?)
Rx	Surgical resection or palliation where feasible Radiation and chemotherapy relatively ineffective

carcinoma of the lung is the most common malignancy in men, carcinoma of the colon is the most important major malignancy in both sexes combined. Moreover, regardless of what disease is under consideration in adults nearing or beyond middle age, the possibility of carcinoma of the colon lies always in the background and must be excluded in the course of reaching a definitive diagnosis. According to Cohn and Nelson, in the United States in 1975 an estimated 100,000 people developed carcinoma of the colorectum. An estimated 50,000 deaths resulted, exceeded only by the number of deaths from lung cancer. Thus the importance of this problem is apparent.

POLYPS

MALIGNANT POTENTIAL OF COLORECTAL POLYPS

Polyps constitute a very important consideration in the genesis, diagnosis, and management of carcinoma of the colon and rectum. Some observers believe that many or even most colon cancers arise from polyps or in association with polyps. However, there are several varieties of polyps, and some of these lesions have little or no malignant potential. In contrast to these almost invariably benign polyps, the villous adenoma, the large adenomatous polyps, and polyps occurring in the genetically determined multiple familial polyposis do have a very significant malignant potential. Therefore, it is important to examine the given polyp microscopically and to determine its classification.

CLASSIFICATION OF COLORECTAL POLYPS

A classification of colorectal polyps is presented in Table 26-3. It will be seen that a number of these conditions are benign and that others are so uncommon that they rarely present a clinical problem. Nonetheless, even nonmalignant polyps may have various complications, including bleeding or intestinal obstruction as the leading edge of an intussusception, for example.

ADENOMATOUS POLYPS

Adenomatous polyps are the most common neoplasms of the colorectum and occur eight times more frequently than

TABLE 26-3 CLASSIFICATION OF COLORECTAL POLYPS

Neoplastic
Adenomatous (polypoid adenoma)
Villous (papillary adenoma)
Villoglandular (mixed adenoma)
Adenomatous familial polyposis syndromes
Multiple familial polyposis
Gardner's syndrome
Other hereditary syndromes
Turcot syndrome
Oldfield syndrome
Cronkhite-Canada syndrome
Leiomyoma; lipoma; carcinoid; neurofibroma;
hemangioma

Inflammatory
Pseudopolyps
Ulcerative colitis
Granulomatous colitis (Crohn's disease)
Inflammatory (nonspecific)
Lymphoid polyp
Colitis cystica profunda

Hamartomatous
Juvenile (retention)
Juvenile polyposis coli (familial)
Peutz-Jeghers syndrome

Unclassified
Hyperplastic (metaplastic) polyp
Pneumatosis cystoides intestinalis

been variously estimated at from 15% to 30%. However, large adenomatous polyps must be distinguished from malignancy. Most clinicians view adenomatous polyps at a size of from 1 cm to 2 cm as either premalignant or potentially malignant lesions, because of foci of adenocarcinoma in 15% to 20%, and manage them accordingly.

VILLOUS ADENOMAS

Villous polyps are called papillary adenomas because of their frondlike projections (Fig. 26-13). They occur primarily in the rectum, sigmoid colon, and cecum and are rarely

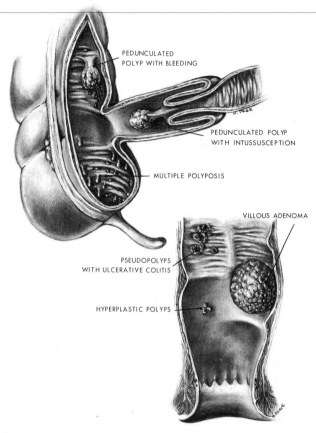

Fig. 26-13. Representative colorectal polyps. (Leffall LD Jr: Polyps of the colon and rectum. In Hardy JD [ed]: Rhoads Textbook of Surgery, 5th ed. Philadelphia, J B Lippincott, 1977)

villous adenomas. Recent studies indicate a fairly uniform distribution, but greater in the rectum and sigmoid. These polyps are usually pedunculated, firm tumors, but small lesions (3 mm to 5 mm) are often sessile (Fig. 26-12). They are often asymptomatic and are found on routine examinations. They usually manifest themselves with rectal bleeding, although prolapse through the anus and, rarely, intussusception may occur. Most polypoid cancers are sessile, but some are pedunculated and grossly resemble adenomatous polyps. The incidence of cancer in polyps less than 1.5 cm is low, 1% to 2%. This is in marked contrast to the malignancy rate ascribed to villous adenomas, which has

Fig. 26-12. Contrast between invasion as noted in a pedunculated adenomatous polyp and that in a sessile villous polyp. (Fenoglio CM, Lane N: The anatomic precursor of colorectal carcinoma. JAMA, 231:640, 1975. Copyright 1975, American Medical Association)

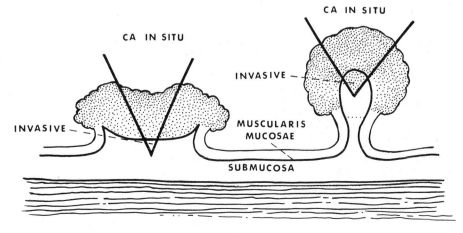

seen in patients under 45 years of age. They are characteristically soft, smooth, and velvety and are notoriously difficult to recognize by palpation. Large size (over 2.5 cm) and induration are the best clinical criteria for malignancy (Fig. 26-14). The incidence of invasive cancer in villous adenomas is, as mentioned previously, between 15% and 30%, depending on the source of the investigation. If induration is present, invasive cancer is likely. Furthermore, regardless of the biopsy report from the surface of a large villous adenoma, the surgeon must always remain concerned that there may be cancer much deeper in the villous adenoma and it should be managed accordingly. Symptoms are usually rectal bleeding, passage of bloody mucus, and a feeling of incomplete evacuation (for rectal lesions). A syndrome of rectal mucorrhea and hypoelectrolytemia has been described.

The diagnosis of a villous adenoma is usually made by sigmoidoscopy because these tumors are commonly located in the rectum or rectosigmoid. The results of digital rectal examination are unreliable at times because the tumors are soft and easily overlooked. Villous adenomas below the peritoneal reflection should be completely excised by transanal approach and examined for invasive adenocarcinoma; if present, abdominoperineal resection is preferably performed. Those above the peritoneal reflection should be completely removed by colonoscopy or, if this is not possible, by a laparotomy and appropriate colon resection.

VILLOGLANDULAR POLYPS (MIXED ADENOMA)

A mixed type of polyp has been recognized with increasing frequency over the past few years. This lesion is termed a *villoglandular polyp* and presents features of both adenomatous and villous tumors grossly and microscopically. These lesions have a malignant potential that lies somewhere between that of the adenomatous polyp and the villous adenoma; according to Leffall, cancer is present is about 7% of such lesions.

JUVENILE POLYPS

Juvenile polyps (hamartomatous mucous or retention polyps) occur principally in children under 12 years of age and are nearly always pedunculated; they are rare in adults. Grossly these lesions are smooth, round, shiny, cherry-red

Fig. 26-14. A large villous adenoma is shown in a resected colon specimen. Invasive cancer was present on histological examination. (Leffall LD Jr: Polyps of the colon and rectum. In Hardy JD [ed]: Rhoads Textbook of Surgery, 5th ed. Philadelphia, J B Lippincott, 1977)

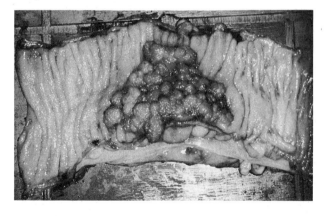

masses. As with most colorectal polyps the usual symptom is rectal bleeding, but intussusception and prolapse through the anus may occur. (Should the physician see the polyp protruding through the anus, it should be grasped at once, since it may be on a long stalk and once retracted may be difficult to retrieve.) These polyps are not premalignant. Histologically they consist of large, dilated mucus-filled glands with an abundance of supporting stroma. Those polyps within the range of the sigmoidoscope (about 60%) should be removed. Those at a higher level should be removed by colonoscopy or colotomy with polypectomy, if warranted by symptoms such as hemorrhage. If the polyps are asymptomatic, however, it should be remembered that about 10% or more undergo autoamputation or spontaneous disappearance, and indeed most disappear before puberty. When polypectomy is contemplated, a recent barium enema with air contrast is essential to verify the presence of the presumed symptomatic polyp. For the rare hereditary disorder, juvenile polyposis coli, colectomy may be indicated. Carcinoma of the colon almost never occurs before the age of puberty.

MULTIPLE FAMILIAL POLYPOSIS

Familial polyposis is an inherited autosomal-dominant disorder characterized by the appearance early in life of large numbers of adenomatous polyps of the colon and rectum. It is present in about one half of the children of an affected parent. If the disease is left untreated, practically all patients will have developed carcinoma of the colorectum by the time they are between 40 and 50 years of age. Males and females are equally affected and either may transmit the disease. Children of polyposis families who themselves do not have polyps do not transmit the disease in the colon because only those with polyps are carriers. Symptoms usually begin in the third or fourth decade, although polyposis occurs earlier. Cancer usually develops 10 to 15 years after the onset of symptoms. Cancer in patients with familial polyposis appears much earlier and the incidence of multicancer is 12 times greater than in nonpolyposis patients. The colonic polyps, usually not present at birth, start appearing somewhat before the age of puberty until, at about age 20, the entire colon and rectum may be covered by hundreds to thousands of polyps of varying sizes (Fig. 26-15). The small intestine is not involved; the distal portions of the colon and rectum are usually involved initially. The polyps are mostly sessile in younger patients, often becoming pedunculated later. The usual symptoms are abdominal pain, rectal bleeding with mucus, diarrhea, weight loss, and anemia. The diagnosis is made by sigmoidoscopy and barium enema with air contrast. Suspicious lesions noted at sigmoidoscopy should be biopsied. The treatment is surgical. Total colectomy with ileoproctostomy and fulguration of remaining polyps in the rectal segment may be preferred in children. However, in the adult the writer favors total colectomy with total excision of the rectal segment and permanent ileostomy, since leaving even the rectal segment incurs considerable risk of carcinoma in this segment eventually. If total colectomy with ileoproctostomy and fulguration of the remaining polyps in the rectal segment is to be employed, the following criteria must be met: cancer of the rectum must not be present; there must not be so many polyps in the terminal rectum that all cannot be fulgurated; the patient must be reliable and amenable to follow-up and fulguration of new polyps; and the retained rectal segment must be short enough (15 cm or less) to permit ready

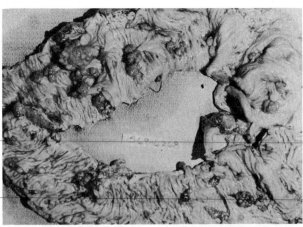

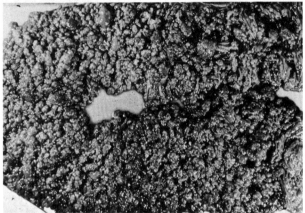

Fig. 26-15. These are gross specimens of patients with multiple familial polyposis. Note that polyps are much more numerous in the colon shown at *bottom*, with virtually the entire colorectal mucosa being replaced by polyps. (Courtesy of Dr EE Cornwell and Dr W Lawrence Jr; Leffall LD Jr: Polyps of the colon and rectum. In Hardy JD [ed]: Rhoads Textbook of Surgery, 5th ed. Philadelphia, J B Lippincott, 1977)

examination by sigmoidoscopy. If these criteria cannot be met, total colectomy with abdominoperineal resection and permanent ileostomy must always be performed. Periodic proctoscopic examinations (every 3 months) are mandatory, to ensure inspection and fulguration of any new lesions in the rectal stump. All members of the family must be investigated for familial polyposis.

Again, the decision to perform ileoproctoscopy, leaving the rectal segment, is flawed with the risk that the patient may not continue adequately in follow-up and that a carcinoma of the rectum may develop and be incurable before recognized. Having had some such experiences with total colectomy with ileoproctostomy and the subsequent development of cancer in the rectum, we prefer total ablation of the colon and rectum with permanent ileostomy in any patient over 20 years of age. It cannot be overemphasized that virtually all of these patients will eventually die of colorectal carcinoma unless this structure is completely excised or managed as outlined above.

GARDNER'S SYNDROME

Gardner's syndrome, a variant of familial polyposis coli, is characterized by multiple colorectal polyps; hard tissue tumors (*e.g.*, osteomas and exostoses of the mandible, skull, or sinuses); soft tissue tumors (*e.g.*, epidermal inclusion or sebaceous cysts); desmoid tumors; postoperative mesenteric

fibromatosis; and dental anomalies. This disorder is inherited as an autosomal dominant non-sex-linked gene of varying penetrance. In contrast to familial polyposis, in Gardner's syndrome the colonic polyps are less numerous and more scattered, and some polyps may also appear in the small intestine. Further, in Gardner's syndrome the polyps may not develop until after age 30 or 40, with the onset of colorectal cancer being later in life. The treatment of this type of intestinal polyposis is essentially the same as outlined for familial polyposis.

Multiple colonic polyps of other varieties may still be derived from genetically determined origins. For example, at times the siblings of a family will not have the hundreds or thousands of polyps characteristic of the usual multiple familial polyposis, but they may have multiple adenomatous polyps, some of which may eventually become malignant. Thus, genetically determined polyposis covers a wide range of possible lesions, and there are doubtless many incomplete manifestations of the syndromes described above or similar pathologic entities.

PEUTZ-JEGHERS SYNDROME

Peutz-Jeghers syndrome is a hereditary autosomal-dominant disorder characterized by melanin spots on the buccal mucosa, lips, digits, palms, and soles. It is associated with polyps, which may be scattered throughout the entire gastrointestinal tract. The small intestine is most frequently involved, but colorectal polyps also occur. These polyps are hamartomas and are not prone to malignant change. Approximately 5% of female patients with this syndrome have been noted to develop ovarian tumors. These polyps are not present at birth, but most patients become symptomatic before age 25. Presenting symptoms are usually those of intermittent colicky abdominal pain due to intussusception. Rectal bleeding may also occur. Treatment is designed to remove large polyps with minimal sacrifice of intestine. In adult female patients, the ovaries should be examined carefully because of the association with ovarian malignancy.

OTHER HEREDITARY SYNDROMES

Other hereditary diseases include colonic polyposis and a neurogenic tumor (Turcot syndrome); stomach and small and large intestinal polyposis associated with diarrhea, alopecia, hyperpigmentation, and nail atrophy (Cronkhite-Canada syndrome); and colonic polyposis and multiple epidermoid cysts (Oldfield syndrome).

HYPERPLASTIC POLYPS AND PSEUDOPOLYPS

Hyperplastic polyps are the polyps most commonly occurring in the colorectum and generally appear as small, sessile, smooth-surfaced mucosal excrescenses or dewdrop elevations in the 1- to 3-mm range. These polyps are not associated with the development of adenomas or carcinoma. Lane and associates found, in a detailed histologic examination of polypoid lesions of the colon and rectum measuring less than 3 mm in diameter, that well over 90% of the polyps were hyperplastic in type. When larger polyps were studied, the incidence of hyperplastic polyps decreased and the incidence of adenomatous polyps increased. Hyperplastic polyps may be transient and undergo spontaneous regression.

The pseudopolyps noted in ulcerative colitis and granulomatous colitis are not premalignant. However, there is an increased incidence of cancer in both diseases, which is noted to a considerably greater degree in ulcerative colitis. Apparently some neoplastic alteration occurs in the colorectal epithelium leading to the development of such cancer.

COMPLICATIONS

The complications of polyps are several, depending on whether they are sessile or pedunculated or eroded or premalignant. Perhaps the most common symptom is rectal bleeding. A pedunculated polyp or even some sessile polyps may become the leading edge of an intussusception and cause intermittent abdominal cramps or even frank colon obstruction, although this is more common in the small intestine. Different types of polyps have a different potential for predisposing to malignancy, if they are not frankly malignant at the outset.

The bleeding from a polyp is usually not severe, but often it is intermittent and is due to erosion of the surface of the polyp with exposure and erosion of its vasculature.

DIAGNOSIS

The diagnosis of polyps, many if not most of which are asymptomatic, is achieved by noting clinical features that lead to digital and proctoscopic examination or colonoscopy, in combination with barium enema and air-contrast barium enema. The importance of air-contrast barium enema in delineating polyps as an etiology of lower gastrointestinal bleeding renders it superior to conventional barium enema in the evaluation of hematochezia or occult GI bleeding.

TREATMENT

The treatment of polyps depends on the symptomatology and the potential for malignant change that the biopsy findings disclose. The advent and routine use of the colonoscope, in addition to the long-employed sigmoidoscope, has radically changed the management of most polyps (Fig. 26-16). The polyp can frequently be snared, particularly if it is pedunculated, and thus delivered for examination having in many or most instances been completely excised. The base may be fulgurated to diminish the possibility for postextraction bleeding. The management of the polyp that cannot be excised and appropriately examined will depend on the biopsy findings and whether the polyp is causing symptoms. Whether the polyp is causing intussusception or hemorrhage, exhibits premalignant change, or is a frank carcinoma will determine the type and extent of ablative surgery required.

CARCINOMA OF THE COLON AND RECTUM

CARCINOMA OF THE COLON

Incidence

Adenocarcinoma of the colon, the most common abdominal visceral malignancy, is more prevalent in the United States than in many other areas of the world. In this country, in 1975, an estimated 100,000 persons developed carcinoma of the colon. The estimated 50,000 deaths that resulted are exceeded only by the numbers of deaths from lung cancer. The frequency with which cancer of the colon occurs makes some knowledge of its development and therapy mandatory for all physicians.

The large bowel is divided descriptively into the "right colon" and the "left colon." The right colon is defined embryologically as that portion of the colon derived from the foregut and nourished by the tributaries of the superior mesenteric artery. Included are the colonic segments prox-

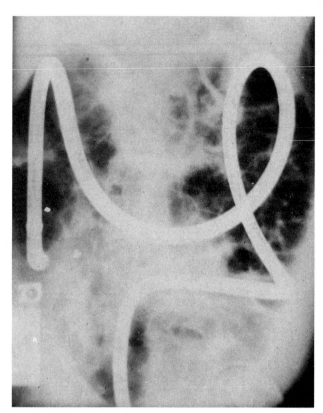

Fig. 26-16. X-ray film of the abdomen, revealing the colonoscope extending from the anus to the cecum.

imal to the splenic flexure: cecum, ascending colon, hepatic flexure, and most of the transverse colon. Its function is primarily one of absorption. The left colon, derived from the hindgut, has its blood supply from the inferior mesenteric artery by way of the left colic, the sigmoid, and the superior hemorrhoidal arteries. The major functions are storage and excretion.

Adenocarcinoma developing in the left colon is distinctive from similar disease in the right colon. Right-sided and left-sided lesions differ in occurrence rate, pathologic appearance, signs and symptoms, and ease of diagnosis.

The colon has three primary functions: absorption, storage, and excretion. The storage function and its relationship to diet may be a contributing factor in the etiology of carcinoma of the colon. Hill and colleagues suggest that the higher incidence of cancer of the colon in North America, Great Britain, and Northwest Europe is related to the higher fat content and lower residue of the Western diet. Burkitt hypothesizes that the "fecal arrest" that occurs in the colon as a result of fiber-depleted diet enhances whatever carcinogenic process may be operating in the bowel. Although the etiology of colon carcinoma remains unknown, the incidence in the United States and the predominance of left-sided colon cancer lend credence to the "fecal arrest" concept.

In Figure 26-17 is shown that the largest incidence of colon carcinoma is in the rectum and that about half of these tumors occur in either the rectum or the sigmoid colon. Cancer of the colon is usually a disease of older persons. The peak incidence occurs in the seventh decade of life and over 90% of patients are over 40 years of age. There appears to be no clear dominance of either sex in incidence.

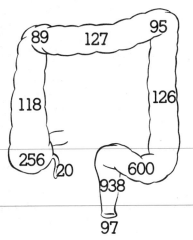

Fig. 26-17. Anatomic location of 2466 colorectal cancers in 2313 patients at Charity Hospital in New Orleans. (Falterman KW, Hill CB, Markey JC et al: Cancer of the colon, rectum, and anus: A review of 2313 cases. Cancer 34:951, 1974)

Clinical Manifestations

The malignant lesion in the right colon is typically a bulky, fungating, ulcerating carcinoma that projects into the lumen of the bowel. This type of lesion is in contrast to the annular, stenosing carcinoma of the left colon. The difference in pathologic characteristics accounts in part for the difference in the clinical syndrome produced by right- or left-sided lesions. Although the cauliflower type of malignancy predominates in the right colon and the scirrhous, obstructing carcinoma is more common in the left, one may find either pathologic type in any segment of the colon.

The napkin ring tumor of the left colon often produces obstruction. Crampy pain, constipation, diarrhea, or alternating periods of constipation and diarrhea may be the first features noted by the patient. Obstructive symptoms (pain), blood in the stool, weight loss, and a change in bowel habit are seen commonly (Table 26-4). Obstructive symptoms are related to the circumferential growth of the tumor and the solid nature of the feces. Obstruction may be minor, progressive, or total and acute when the patient first becomes aware of the lesion. Unfortunately, the presence of obstruction alters the prognosis. The cecum may perforate even

though the obstruction is in the sigmoid colon, owing to the greater distensibility of the right colon.

Among the various signs and symptoms of left colon carcinoma, the importance of change in bowel habit, blood in the stool, pain, and weight loss cannot be overemphasized. A cardinal rule for all physicians should be that *any change in bowel habit or the presence of blood (gross or occult) in the stool in an individual over age 40 demands investigation.*

Right colon cancer in its early stage of development is more difficult to detect than is carcinoma of the left colon. The delay in diagnosis occurs because early change in bowel habit and overt bleeding are not so common as in lesions of the left colon. Abdominal pain is the symptom most common in patients with right colon cancer (Table 26-5). Initially the pain may be one of dyspepsia, only later may it become localized to the right lower quadrant (for example, in the case of carcinoma of the cecum), arousing one's suspicions. Initially, because of its vagueness and lack of severity, the pain may be dismissed as an insignificant complaint. Weight loss and anemia are two systemic findings common to patients with right colon cancer. Any degree of weight loss in an older person suggests malignancy. If this weight loss is associated with a blood loss anemia (microcytic, hypochromic), right colon malignancy is suggested. The insidious onset of carcinoma of the right colon (cecum, in particular) is implied by the fact that many patients have a palpable mass at the time of diagnosis.

A presumptive diagnosis of carcinoma of the right colon can be made in the middle-aged or older patient with vague or crampy abdominal pains, anemia, and weight loss and in whom a mass (sometimes tender) can be palpated in the right side or upper midabdomen. Routine hemoccult testing in persons over 40 has been suggested.

Diagnosis

In the patient suspected of having carcinoma of the colon, sigmoidoscopy should be routine. This procedure can be accomplished during the patient's initial visit to the physician's office. Cancer below the distal sigmoid colon can be visualized and the diagnosis established.

Barium enema follows sigmoidoscopy in the patient suspected of having carcinoma of the colon. The cardinal radiographic sign of colon carcinoma is a filling defect in the barium shadow. This finding usually confirms the diagnosis. However, roentgenographic examination of the colon is not always easily accomplished. The cecum is the most common site of error (as high as 15%) in roentgenographic diagnosis of lesions of the large bowel. The colon (particularly the right colon) may be difficult to fill with barium because of the discomfort to the patient. Conse-

TABLE 26-4 SYMPTOMS AND SIGNS IN 725 PATIENTS WITH CARCINOMA OF THE LEFT COLON

	% PRESENT	% UNKNOWN
Abdominal pain	73	8
Blood (gross or occult) in stools	64	18
Weight loss	51	13
Change in bowel habit	43	18
Obstruction (partial or complete)	42	10
Anemia (less than 12 g Hgb)	32	10
Palpable mass	28	10

(Cohn IJ, Nelson JL: Carcinoma of the colon [excluding the rectum]. In Hardy JD [ed]: Rhoads Textbook of Surgery, 5th ed. Philadelphia, J B Lippincott, 1977)

TABLE 26-5 SYMPTOMS AND SIGNS IN PATIENTS WITH CARCINOMA OF THE RIGHT COLON

	% PRESENT	% UNKNOWN
Abdominal pain	76	6
Weight loss	60	13
Anemia	51	10
Palpable mass	49	8
Obstruction	20	9

(Cohn IJ, Nelson JL: Carcinoma of the colon [excluding the rectum]. In Hardy JD [ed]: Rhoads Textbook of Surgery, 5th ed. Philadelphia, J B Lippincott, 1977)

quently, the interpretation of filling defects or mucosal detail may be subject to question. Contributing to the problem of barium studies is that preparatory cleansing may not be effective and that fecal material may obscure abnormal findings. The films should always be reviewed by the clinician with the radiologist. The radiographic examination is repeated if there is any doubt in interpretation. Small or polypoid lesions are best visualized by air-contrast barium studies.

Direct visualization of the entire colon is now possible with the fiberoptic colonoscope. Colonoscopy has become a routine diagnostic procedure. It is particularly useful when routine studies are inconclusive or when a patient with suspected colon cancer has a negative barium enema. Direct visualization of the left colon can be done with ease; visualization of the right colon can be accomplished in the majority of the cases attempted. The procedure can be performed usually on outpatients who have been prepared with a liquid diet, castor oil, and cleansing enemas. Although not required for routine examinations of the left colon, fluoroscopic guidance is helpful in passing the scope into the right colon. Fluoroscopy correlates the viewing tip with the colonic area in question. Contrast material may be introduced through the instrument to outline the abnormal area. Biopsy should be performed.

The description of the carcinoembryonic antigen (CEA) by Gold and Freedman, in 1965, gave rise to the hope of a simple, dependable blood test for the diagnosis of carcinoma of the colon. However, the results of a collaborative study (sponsored by the National Cancer Institute of Canada and the American Cancer Society) suggest that the test's lack of sensitivity and specificity precludes its use for screening. However, if previously normal and then later elevated, cancer recurrence perhaps in the form of liver metastases must be suspected.

Benign polyps, diverticulitis, ulcerative colitis, and appendicitis are the most important differential diagnoses. A thorough history is helpful; radiographic examination is often diagnostic. Biopsy is the only way absolute differentiation can be made. Fiberoptic colonoscopy may facilitate visualization of the suspicious area. Whenever the diagnosis of cancer cannot be excluded, surgical exploration is required.

Treatment

Surgical removal is the only acceptable curative therapy for most cancers of the colon. Fulguration, with or without radiation therapy, has been advocated by some for certain carcinomas of the rectum in high-risk patients. A rational operative technique designed to give optimal control of the disease involves a consideration of six factors in the spread of the tumor:

Intramural Spread. Any curative resection should be performed with sufficient margin on each side of the lesion to provide a cut edge of the specimen free of tumor. Marginal growth is more rapid in the transverse than in the longitudinal axis of the bowel. Carcinoma of the left colon characteristically assumes an annular form. Right colon lesions protrude in a polypoid fashion into the lumen of the bowel. A 5-cm segment of grossly normal wall beyond the tumor usually provides the minimal margin free of microscopic extension. At the time of surgical excision, frozen section examination of the margins of resection is helpful.

Lymphatic Spread. The importance of spread of carcinoma

of the colon by means of extramural lymphatic channels, with the production of metastases in the related lymph glands, will become apparent when prognosis is discussed. The direction and extent of such spread primarily determines the scope of operation. First metastases usually occur in the paracolic glands nearest to the primary growth. With progression, the process extends to the chain of glands on the blood vessels. The lymphatic spread follows closely the course of the blood vessels feeding the site of the carcinoma. Therefore the field of excision of colon malignancies is based on the distribution of the arterial blood supply.

Venous Spread. Bloodborne metastases may occur to the liver, lung, adrenal glands, kidneys or bones. Fisher and Turnbull found tumor cells in the blood of the major mesenteric venous channels in patients being operated on for colorectal cancer. As an outgrowth of the conceptual relationship between distant metastases and tumor cells in the venous effluent of a colon cancer, Turnbull emphasized the advantages of early ligation of the venous supply from the tumor-bearing segment of the colon. His "no touch" technique, in which "the cancer-bearing segment was not manipulated or handled in any manner until after the lymphovascular pedicles were divided at the elected sites for resection," appeared to result in a better survival rate.

The relationship of the demonstration of tumor cells in venous blood to the development of metastatic implants is not clear. Griffiths and his colleagues found that the presence

Fig. 26-18. Dilated colon characteristic of obstruction. (Barnett WO: Large bowel obstruction: Approach to management. In Hardy JD [ed]: Rhoads Textbook of Surgery, 5th ed. Philadelphia, J B Lippincott, 1977)

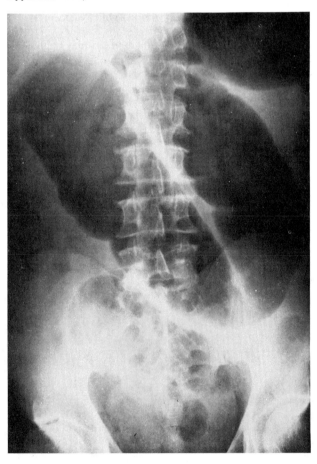

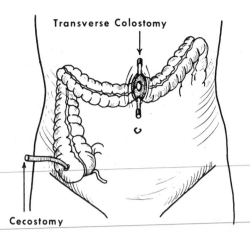

Fig. 26-19. Transverse colostomy and cecostomy are most often used at the sites indicated, for proximal colon decompression. (Barnett WO: Large bowel obstruction: Approach to management. In Hardy JD [ed]: Rhoads Textbook of Surgery, 5th ed. Philadelphia, J B Lippincott, 1977)

of tumor cells in venous blood had little influence on the 5-year survival rate. Cure appears related more to the extent of the colonic and mesocolic resection than to preliminary ligation of the lymphovascular pedicles.

Implantation of Tumor Cells in the Anastomosis. A suture line recurrence (10%-15% incidence) is apparently dependent on the cancer cells being implanted in the anastomotic area by the suture material, rather than by direct growth on the mucosal surface. Cole's suggestion of isolating the segment of bowel containing the cancer to prevent any spillage of tumor cells has been used widely.

Direct Extension. Tumors of the colon may break through the serosa and invade any organ in contact with the colon. Adjacent structures sometimes invaded by colon lesions include small bowel, bladder, abdominal wall, and stomach. These involved organs (or portions of organs) can be removed with the primary lesion. Extension to another organ is not necessarily a reason to abandon resection. Moreover, at times the adherence is due to inflammation rather than to actual tumor invasion.

Transperitoneal Spread. Spread by this route usually means widespread involvement and, in general, indicates an incurable lesion.

Preparation for Surgery. Since excision of some or all of the large bowel is a major operation, it is important that the patient be in optimal preoperative condition for the surgical procedure. The following should be considered a minimum for any prospective colon operation:

Complete blood cell count, to detect any anemia

Chest radiography, as part of any preoperative workup and to detect the presence of metastases

Electrocardiography

Sigmoidoscopy, as part of routine for any patient with colon disease

Barium enema, even when a lesion has been seen sigmoidoscopically, to detect the presence of other lesions in the large bowel (omit if perforation of the colon has occurred and do not force barium through a severely stenotic site, which may thus be caused to obstruct completely). Colon cancers are multiple in 5% to 10% of patients.

Intravenous pyelography, to determine number, location,

and function of the kidneys and to detect any displacement or obstruction of the ureters

Electrolyte studies, in patients with any evidence of volume or electrolyte abnormalities

Preoperative CEA to monitor changes after resection as a guide to nonsurgical therapy plans

Ancillary preoperative studies may include:

Liver function studies, such as evaluation of alkaline phosphatase, bilirubin, serum albumin, and prothrombin time

Liver scan or computed tomographic scan, when liver function studies suggest abnormality

Colonoscopy, to extend the range of endoscopic study of the colon

Air contrast barium enema, when coexisting polyps are suspected

Specific preparation of the patient for the elective operation procedure should include cleansing of the bowel. The routine is as follows:
1. Preparation in the hospital for 72 hours
2. Low residue diet for this period, preferably one of the commercially available nonresidue diets or clear liquids
3. A cathartic the first day. Cathartic administration: We prefer repeated 30-cc doses of 15% $MgSO_4$ solution given 5 to 10 times daily, until clear, watery stool results by 48 to 72 hours.
4. Isotonic saline enemas each day during the period. The last one should be administered the night before operation, not the morning of operation, to be sure the operative field is not flooded with liquid bowel contents. Enema returns should be seen by a responsible person to be sure the colon is clean.
5. Intestinal antisepsis for 72 hours as an adjunct for controlling infectious complications of colon surgery. One may use kanamycin as follows: 1 g every hour for 4 hours, then every 6 hours for the total 72 hours. The antibiotic is given orally; systemic effects are neither required nor expected. Neomycin is also satisfactory.

Parenteral hyperalimentation may be indicated in the anorectic patient who has lost weight and whose surgical therapy is being delayed.

Individuals who are cachectic because of the presence of malignancy usually possess total erythrocyte volumes that are smaller than those of normal persons of similar size, while their total blood volumes relative to body weight are the same as those of lean normal persons. A cachectic patient with colon cancer should have a preoperative determination of erythrocyte and plasma volumes. Abnormalities are corrected with the transfusion of packed red blood cells or whole blood, depending on the type of deficit (erythrocyte mass and/or plasma volume).

A central venous (subclavian) catheter is inserted in poor-risk patients or in those in whom considerable blood loss is anticipated. This is accomplished the day or evening prior to operation so that a chest film may be obtained confirming the accurate placement of the catheter. The immediate preoperative preparation is completed on the morning of the operation. In the surgical suite a Foley catheter and a nasogastric tube are inserted.

Management of colon obstruction. The presence of colon obstruction creates special problems. First, the fact that the obstruction is due to carcinoma may not be certain. Additional causes of colon obstruction in adults in order of frequency include volvulus; diverticulitis; adhesions; intussusception; external hernia; pseudo-obstruction due to dysmotility (Ogilvie's Syndrome) with or without fecal impaction; extrinsic compression by noncolonic carcinoma; endometriosis or stricture due to lymphogranuloma venereum, especially in females; pelvic abscess; and still other causes. Moreover, the colon proximal to the obstruction will often be filled with feces and a single-stage resection of a carcinoma may not be feasible. Furthermore, the patient may have been vomiting for several days, with water and salt depletion, and the proximal colon may be greatly dilated (Fig. 26-18). In this case it will be wise to prepare the patient for a few hours and then perform either a right transverse colostomy or, less optimally, a cecostomy (Fig. 26-19).

Operations. As suggested by the description of the six factors involved with the spread of cancer, an adequate cancer operation should remove all the appropriate vascular and lymphatic pathways. Of primary importance is the wide removal of bowel mesentery down to its base along the superior or inferior mesenteric arteries so as to include the lymphatic drainage routes.

Lesions of the splenic flexure or descending colon are ideally treated by left hemicolectomy with inclusion of the middle colic vessels for the more proximally located lesions or the inferior mesenteric vessels for the more distally located tumors (Fig. 26-20). Tumors of the sigmoid are treated by resection of the sigmoid colon with the mesentery to the origin of the inferior mesenteric artery. A proximally located tumor of the sigmoid is treated by a left hemicolectomy.

Cecal tumors are treated usually by right hemicolectomy, but an extended right colectomy is suggested for lesions of the right colon distal to the cecum (ascending colon, hepatic flexure, or transverse colon). This resection may include the ileocolic, right colic, and middle colic arteries and veins, 15 cm to 20 cm of terminal ileum and ascending and transverse colon (Fig. 26-21). An ileodescending colostomy restores bowel continuity.

Many surgeons employ a vertical incision for all colon resections, but a right transverse incision is especially convenient for right hemicolectomy. A careful exploration of the abdominal cavity for evidence of metastatic disease is performed prior to approaching the region of the tumor. The tumor is palpated to reassure the surgeon of the diagnosis, to determine operability, and to identify any problem that might influence treatment. Dissection of the root of the mesentery exposes the origin of the appropriate mesenteric vessels, which are ligated. Tape ligatures are placed about the colon proximal and distal to the tumor (Figs. 26-20 and 26-21). After thus "surrounding" the cancer, the right or the left colon is mobilized to the midsagittal plane. Mobilization requires division of the lateral peritoneal reflection, the splenic or hepatic flexure attachments, and the gastrocolic ligament (preserving usu-

Fig. 26-20. The steps in resecting the left colon include (1) ligation of the inferior mesenteric artery and vein at the root of the mesentery, (2) placement of tape ligatures proximal and distal to the tumor, (3) mobilization of the left colon, and (4) resection of the left colon with its lymph-bearing mesocolon. *Inset* shows anastomosis between the transverse colon and the distal sigmoid or proximal rectum. (Cohn I Jr, and Nelson, JL: Carcinoma of the colon (excluding the rectum). In JD Hardy [ed]: Rhoads Textbook of Surgery, 5th ed. Philadelphia, J B Lippincott, 1977)

Fig. 26-21. The steps in an extended right colectomy include (1) ligation of the ileocolic, right, and middle colic arteries and veins at the root of the mesentery, (2) placement of tape ligatures proximal and distal to the tumor, (3) mobilization of the right colon and splenic fixtures, and (4) resection of the colon and its lymph-bearing mesocolon. *Inset* shows anastomosis between the ileum and descending colon. (Cohn I Jr, and Nelson JL: Carcinoma of the colon (excluding the rectum). In Hardy JD [ed]: Rhoads Textbook of Surgery, 5th ed. Philadelphia, J B Lippincott, 1977)

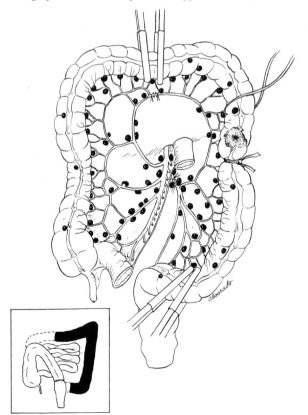

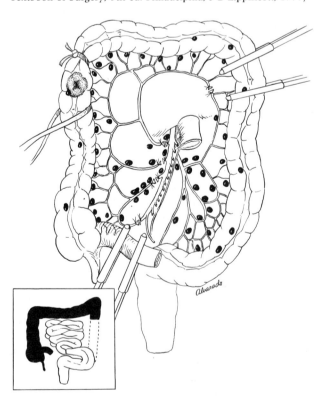

ally the gastroepiploic artery). The ureter and ovarian or spermatic vessels are identified and left behind on the retroperitoneal muscles. While performing an extended right colectomy, the surgeon is careful not to disturb the underlying duodenum. The tumor-bearing segment, mesentery, and attached omentum are resected. The two ends of bowel to be used for the anastomosis should have normal color and arterial bleeding from the cut edges. A colocolostomy is usually an end-to-end anastomosis. An ileocolostomy is an end-to-end anastomosis, although some surgeons prefer the side-to-end variety, particularly if there is a marked discrepancy in the diameter of the two ends of bowel.

In addition to the formal resection of colon, mesocolon, and lymphatic tissues as indicated, it is sometimes necessary to excise part or all of an involved adjacent viscus, such as the stomach, a loop of small intestine, or a portion of the abdominal wall. Cure has been accomplished by such radical resections. Fixation of a colon carcinoma to surrounding structures should not necessarily deter the surgeon from resecting the tumor.

The presence of metastases in the liver alters the prognosis but is not a contraindication to excision of the primary carcinoma. Removal of the colon lesion eliminates or diminishes the possibility of obstruction, bleeding, perforation, fistulization, and infection, which so often accompany colon carcinoma. Patients with hepatic metastases may live 18 months to 2 years. Rarely, a solitary hepatic metastasis can be removed with cure. Since widespread peritoneal deposits mean a short survival, palliative resection here is often contraindicated.

Management of the Obstructed Colon: Further Comment.
Carcinoma of the left colon frequently becomes apparent only after obstruction occurs. There are special problems related to surgical care of the obstructing lesion. The proximal colon is filled with fecal material; the bowel is dilated, edematous, and, often, friable. Staged operations remain the procedures of choice. The first stage is decompression via a transverse loop colostomy. A colostomy placed in this location accomplishes relief of obstruction and will not compromise the extent of resection during the second stage. After a suitable period of recovery and preparation (usually 7 to 10 days), the definitive resection is performed. The transverse colostomy is closed at the second operation as the third stage.

Although considered to be an uncommon complication, obstruction may result from carcinoma of the right colon. The obstruction may be caused by adhesions of the small bowel secondary to the inflammatory reaction generated by some tumors. The ileocecal valve may become directly involved, setting the stage for intussusception, or the obstruction may be due to the less commonly found annular growth of a right colon carcinoma. Contrary to the case of an obstructing lesion on the left side, the patient with an obstructing right-sided lesion usually should have a one-stage resection and primary anastomosis even when this must be done as an emergency procedure. The ileocolostomy, rather than colocolostomy associated with a left colon resection, following resection of an obstructed right colon appears to be the important factor in making this an acceptable procedure. The nutrient blood supply to the ileocolostomy is better. Liquid feces channeled through a healing ileocolostomy are perhaps less disruptive than the more solid feces of the left colon.

Management of the Perforated Colon.
Perforation of the colon in association with cancer is a calamity presenting a difficult surgical problem. Surgical care of the perforation and its resultant peritonitis or abscess must take precedence over that of the cancer. The risk of death from peritonitis exceeds that of the malignancy. Management of free perforation of the left colon should include resection of the involved colon with the required mesentery. In the presence of generalized peritonitis, the proximal end of the colon is managed as a colostomy, the distal end oversewn or exteriorized as a fistula. Bowel continuity is reestablished at a later date. Perforation of the left colon, with local abscess formation, may be managed by resection and primary anastomosis.

Management of free perforation of the right colon should include resection of the involved colon with the required mesentery. Generally, bowel continuity is reestablished during the primary procedure, or a temporary ileostomy can be constructed.

In any case, prior to closing the abdomen, the cavity is irrigated with a copious volume of saline. Following the irrigation, an antibiotic solution is poured into the peritoneal cavity.

Perforation into an adjacent viscus, with formation of a fistula, is treated as a nonemergency colon resection, with appropriate preoperative evaluation and preparation.

Postoperative Care.
Proximal decompression of postoperative ileus is maintained by either a Levin (nasogastric) tube, a Miller-Abbott (long) tube, or a gastrostomy catheter. Oral feedings begin following a return of peristalsis (usually in 3 to 5 days) and a bowel movement. Ambulation is not delayed. Systemic antibiotics are not always used unless there has been gross contamination at the time of operation or the presence of infection becomes evident, but many surgeons give antibiotics routinely. Multiple loose stools may follow right colectomy but usually decline to normal in a few weeks.

Complications.
The septic complications of anastomotic leakage or wound infection may occur to some degree in up to 20% of patients following resection of the left colon. However, most anastomotic leaks are minimal and self-limited. Those that cause abdominal pain and tenderness, a clinical picture of sepsis, or an external fistula with copious discharge require a diverting proximal colostomy.

A smooth postoperative course is common to the patient who has had a right colectomy. Although septic complications such as anastomotic leak and wound infection may occur, the incidence is less than that seen in patients following resection of the left colon.

Wound infection can be managed in most instances by removal of skin sutures and evacuation of purulent material.

Follow-up Care.
Those patients who have had less than curative resections may receive chemotherapy (usually 5-fluorouracil). Those who have had curative resections should preferably have a barium enema 6 to 8 weeks after operation. This will provide a visual index of the normal anastomotic deformity to which future radiographic studies may be compared. CEA may be a useful prognostic indicator, since an increase in the serum CEA level may indicate an otherwise occult recurrence or progression of the malignancy.

Annual reevaluation should include pertinent history, abdominal and rectal examination, chest films, barium enema, and liver function studies. Those patients who have had a left hemicolectomy should have, in addition, a sigmoidoscopic examination. Follow-up evaluation and care should be continued indefinitely. Colonoscopy may be performed periodically to exclude new polyps.

Prognosis and Results. Cohn and co-workers reported an overall 5-year survival rate of 29% for carcinoma of the splenic flexure, descending colon, and sigmoid (Fig. 26-22). The 5-year survival rate for the cecum and right colon was 21% (Fig. 26-23). These survival rates were somewhat lower than often reported, perhaps reflecting the patient population studied by Cohn and co-workers. For those patients who had had a "curative" resection (all gross evidence of tumor being removed) of either right- or left-sided malignancies, the 5-year survival was approximately 50%. Improved survival rates were noted in those patients whose malignancy was limited not only grossly but also microscopically. Using Dukes' classification as a method of staging carcinoma microscopically, they noted a correlation between the microscopic extent of the disease and prognosis. One expects at least 60% of patients with carcinoma of either the right or the left colon confined microscopically to the bowel to survive 5 years. Cancer in the lymph nodes (Dukes' C) reduces the 5-year survival rate to 20% to 30%.

Fig. 26-22. Five-year survival for all patients with left colon cancers, for those presenting with obstruction, for those with perforation, and for 725 members of the general population of similar ages. (Cohn I Jr, Nelson JL: Carcinoma of the colon (excluding the rectum). In Hardy JD [ed]: Rhoads Textbook of Surgery, 5th ed. Philadelphia, J B Lippincott, 1977)

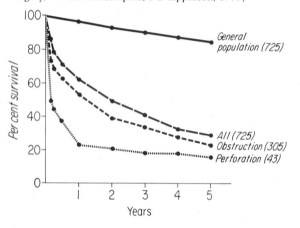

Fig. 26-23. Five-year survival for all patients with right colon cancers, for those presenting with obstruction, for those with perforation, and for 501 members of the general population of similar ages. (Cohn I Jr, Nelson JL: Carcinoma of the colon (excluding the rectum). In Hardy JD [ed]: Rhoads Textbook of Surgery, 5th ed. Philadelphia, J B Lippincott, 1977)

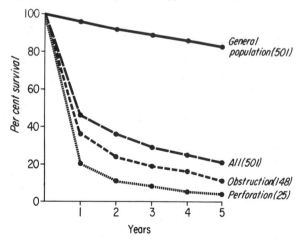

Obstruction or perforation associated with left colon malignancies lowers the 5-year survival rate to 23% and 16%, respectively (Fig. 26-22). Right colon carcinoma associated with obstruction or perforation lowers the 5-year survival rate to a dismal 11% and 4%, respectively (Fig. 26-23).

Clearly the key to improved survival rates for carcinoma of the colon is early diagnosis and appropriate surgical treatment. Early diagnosis is facilitated by education of both patients and physicians so that the relatively simple diagnostic tests will be done. Appropriate surgical treatment is accomplished by proper preoperative preparation of the patient and by practicing good surgical techniques based on a knowledge of routes of tumor spread. Identification of the etiologic agent(s) remains the ultimate objective.

CARCINOMA OF THE RECTUM

Diagnosis

The parameters of the clinical features, diagnosis, and management of rectal carcinoma are similar to those for the rest of the colon, but certain special considerations deserve emphasis.

Bleeding is the most prominent sign of rectal cancer, and 40% to 50% of all colorectal cancers are within reach of the sigmoidoscope. The bleeding is usually bright red, as opposed to bleeding from the right colon or the intestine more proximally. Moreover, it is usually on the stool rather than admixed with the stool. Change in bowel habits is the next common feature, followed by pain. Clearly, these signs and symptoms may also occur with hemorrhoids, which often is a cause for delay in diagnosis.

One third of all rectal cancers are readily palpable on digital examination. The digital examination gives vital information that may determine the choice of operative procedure and often indicates to the examiner the likelihood of cure after the proposed operation.

The level of the tumor above the anal verge can be assessed at the time of digital examination. During assessment of the level of the tumor, the examiner must be certain that he is feeling the tumor itself and not indirectly feeling it through a fold in the rectal wall. This would incorrectly locate the tumor at a level lower than its actual site.

The shape of the lesion may be determined at the time of rectal examination. Is the tumor ulcerating? Is the tumor polypoid and exophytic? These assessments may be of prognostic importance. The consistency of the tumor is also important. Soft, velvetlike tumors may have large areas of benign villous adenoma mixed with the cancer; thus, the actual cancerous lesion may be smaller than the grossly palpable tumor. Hard lesions that infiltrate into the bowel on the periphery of the major tumor tend to have a poor prognosis. The degree of tumor spread along the bowel wall and beyond the rectal wall into adjacent structures should be evaluated. Such spread may occur laterally along the lateral ligaments of the rectum into the walls of the pelvis or posteriorly to the sacrum and anteriorly to involve the vagina, prostate, urethra, or bladder. The degree of fixation of the tumor to these other structures should be assessed. The size of the lesion may be estimated at the time of rectal examination. Not all large tumors are associated with a poor outlook, but large growths often have had an opportunity to spread beyond the rectum.

The position of the tumor on the bowel wall must be

determined. Anterior tumors in women may spread into and through the rectovaginal septum and may require removal of the posterior vaginal wall and uterus as part of the surgical extirpation of the tumor. Circumferential tumors may produce obstruction and require special preparation of the patient for operation to avoid further obstruction from the introduction of barium into the colon and to avoid distress to the patient at the time of mechanical cleansing of the bowel. Posteriorly located tumors may be amenable to local excision through a posterior approach in poor-risk patients.

Pelvic lymph nodes are often palpable in the presence of inflammatory and neoplastic disease of the anorectal region. A search for nodes along the lateral ligaments and lateral pelvic walls should be instituted. Nodes may be felt in the presacral region in many patients with cancer of the rectum. An assessment of the size and degree of firmness of these nodes may give a useful preoperative clue in regard to the likelihood of involvement of these nodes by tumor.

As the examining finger is removed from the rectum, it should be inspected for the presence of blood or mucus.

Proctosigmoidoscopy permits direct visualization of the tumor and supplies information additional to that already obtained from the digital rectal examination. Multiple biopsies should be taken from several areas of the tumor. Barium enema is performed to exclude other lesions of the colon. However, barium should not be forced through a stricture, since absorption of its water content may result in complete obstruction. The CT scan is increasingly useful in detecting lymph nodal enlargement and local invasion of pelvic neoplasm such as rectal cancer.

Fig. 26-24. Vascular and lymphatic anatomy of the rectum. The lymphatic drainage follows the venous return. (Veidenheimer MC: Carcinoma of the rectum. In Hardy JD [ed]: Rhoads Textbook of Surgery, 5th ed. Philadelphia, J B Lippincott, 1977)

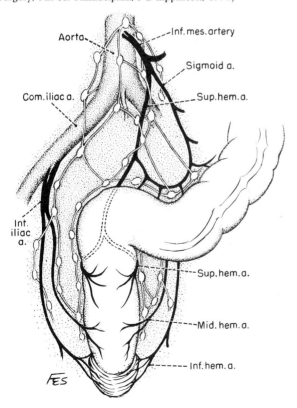

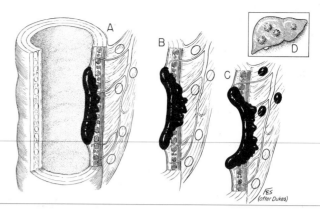

Fig. 26-25. Dukes' classification of cancer of the colon and rectum. Dukes' *A* cancer: tumor confined to bowel wall; Dukes' *B* cancer: tumor infiltrates through the full thickness of the bowel into surrounding tissues; Dukes' *C* cancer: tumor involves lymph nodes; Dukes' *D* cancer: tumor involves other organs that cannot be removed with the removal of the primary tumor. (Veidenheimer MC: Carcinoma of the rectum. In Hardy JD [ed]: Rhoads Textbook of Surgery, 5th ed. Philadelphia, J B Lippincott, 1977)

Treatment

The management of rectal carcinoma entails special anatomical considerations (Fig. 26-24). The confluence of the portal venous drainage with systemic venous drainage may lead to pulmonary metastases in addition to the far more common liver metastases.

The prognosis for the patient harboring a specific tumor prior to operation will be decided primarily by the extent of local invasion or metastasis (Fig. 26-25).

Preoperative radiotherapy was first proposed in 1959 by the Memorial Hospital group, with apparent improvement in survival rates in patients with Dukes' C cancer. However, subsequent experience there and elsewhere has failed to demonstrate improved survival rates. Even so, large tumors may be reduced in size and rendered more operable.

Choice of Operation

Anterior resection of the rectum is of course desirable when the lesion is situated appropriately. Tumors that lie in the lower third of the rectum require abdominoperineal resection with colostomy in order to achieve satisfactory surgical excision of the tumor mass. Lesions in the upper rectum and rectosigmoid region permit excision of tumor and 2 inches of normal bowel distal to the tumor, with ample distal rectum remaining for good function after anastomosis (Fig. 26-26). Lesions at this site may usually be removed without ligation of the middle hemorrhoidal vessels. Because the operation is performed through the anterior abdominal wall, the rectal resection is known as an anterior resection of the rectum. In the above instance, the operation is referred to as a high anterior resection.

Lesions of the midrectum require careful judgment in the choice of operation. A rectal stump less than 4 cm in length will result in incontinence of flatus and stool. Excision of lesions that have a lower border 10 cm from the anal verge results in a rectal stump measuring 5 cm in length. Theoretically any lesion 10 cm or higher can be removed, with a functional anastomosis. Obese patients or patients with a very narrow pelvis may make such a low anastomosis technically impossible.

The stapling instruments can be especially useful for the low anterior anastomosis (Fig. 26-27).

Complications of End Colostomy (Fig. 26-28)

Necrosis is due to an inadequate blood supply that may be caused by misjudgment of the adequacy of the circulation at the time of operation or by encroachment on the mesocolon by too tight an orifice in the abdominal wall. The necrosis may be mucosal only or may involve only that portion of the bowel that lies exterior to the peritoneal cavity; in these instances, no treatment other than observation may be required. If the bowel is seen to be necrotic through the abdominal wall and into the abdominal cavity, reresection is indicated, often with establishment of a transverse colostomy.

Retraction of the stoma may occur as a result of necrosis of the stoma or as a consequence of inadequate mobilization of the bowel with implantation of the stoma under tension on its mesocolon. Often a retracted stoma will function adequately, but in some instances the abdomen may have to be reopened and the bowel may have to be mobilized further.

Stricture formation was common at the skin level in colostomies fashioned by the technique of natural sloughing within a clamp. Modern techniques of primary suture maturation have largely eliminated this problem. Skin level strictures may be treated adequately by simple excision of the mucocutaneous junction, including the strictured area. Resuture of the bowel to the healthy skin is then performed with interrupted, absorbable sutures. Deeper strictures may occur as a sequel to bleeding into the colostomy incision, with subsequent fibrosis of the subcutaneous tissues. Deeper dissection is required to excise this type of stricture, and healthier, more pliable proximal bowel may have to be mobilized from within the abdominal cavity in order to fashion a satisfactory new colostomy.

Prolapse of an end colostomy is unusual. When prolapse occurs, it may be associated with the use of a large-ringed appliance tightly applied to the abdominal wall that permits the stoma to protrude into the ring at times of increased intra-abdominal pressure. Loop colostomy, however, has a greater tendency to prolapse, and, for reasons not understood, the distal or efferent limb is that portion of the bowel with the greater tendency to undergo prolapse.

Fig. 26-26. Rectal anatomy: Division of the rectum into upper, middle, and lower thirds. Tumors that lie in the lower third of the rectum require abdominoperineal resection for cure. Tumors in the upper third of the rectum may be treated satisfactorily by anterior resection of the rectum. Tumors in the middle third of the rectum require individual consideration in the operating room to determine whether they can safely be removed with an anastomotic procedure rather than abdominoperineal resection. (Veidenheimer MC: Carcinoma of the rectum. In Hardy JD [ed]: Rhoads Textbook of Surgery, 5th ed. Philadelphia, J B Lippincott, 1977)

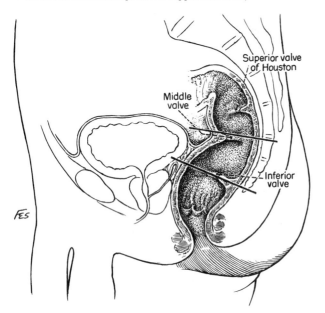

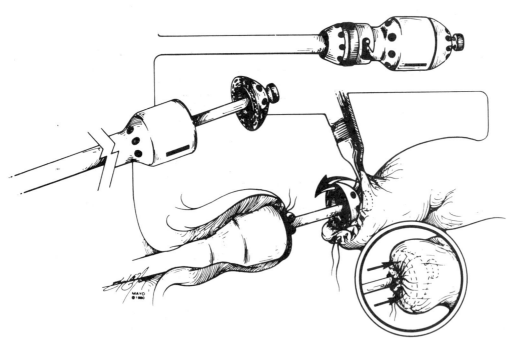

Fig. 26-27. The judicious use of stapling devices has added an important new dimension in intestinal surgery. (Beart RW Jr, Wolff BG: The use of staplers for interior anastomoses. World J Surg 6:525, 1982.)

Herniation may occur with the passage of time. Thus, paracolostomy hernia is a common sequel to colostomy operations. Herniation may also occur internally lateral to the limb of the colostomy. If the space lateral to the bowel is large, then such herniation does not usually cause symptoms. However, herniation may cause obstruction or may result in adhesions that lead to twisting and thus require surgical intervention to relieve the obstructive symptoms. In such instances, the gutter should then be closed to prevent a recurrence of this problem.

Bleeding from the stoma may indicate a problem higher in the gastrointestinal tract, but it commonly occurs as a result of trauma to the exposed bowel by dressings, appliances, clothing, or irrigating catheter. Care must be taken to prevent such trauma. If no logical cause for the bleeding is evident, the patient must be studied for a lesion higher in the gastrointestinal tract.

Infection at the site of a primarily matured colostomy is rare unless there is retraction of the stoma or separation of a portion of the mucocutaneous suture line. Usually, simple drainage of the area will allow resolution of the infection, and the granulation tissue at the site of separation will then heal readily.

Perforation of the colon during irrigation has occurred even in the patient experienced in handling his colostomy. Often a paracolostomy hernia causes some tortuosity of the colon as it passes through the abdominal wall, and forceful insertion of the irrigating catheter causes perforation of the bowel by the catheter. Extraperitoneal perforation results in cellulitis of the abdominal wall and occasionally in a colocutaneous fistula. Perforation of the intra-abdominal colon causes peritonitis. Treatment of this mishap requires resection of the colon to include the perforation, and reestablishment of a new colostomy at a higher level of the colon, usually at an alternative site on the abdominal wall.

Postoperative complications of abdominoperineal resection include urinary tract retention or injury, disorders of sexual function in males, and perineal wound problems such as bleeding, infection, persistent perineal sinus, perineal pain, or perineal hernia. Late perineal pain is usually due to recurrent cancer but occasionally is due to abscess formation.

Alternative Methods of Therapy

Pull-through operations have been used in the management of rectal cancer. Many believe that this operation offers no advantage over low anterior resection as a sphincter-saving procedure. Lesions too low to permit anterior resection with anastomosis should have the levators excised by the abdominoperineal technique in order to ensure wide removal of all areas of potential spread of cancer. We prefer to reserve the use of pull-through and other sphincter-saving procedures for nonmalignant rectal conditions.

Electrocoagulation was used for the destruction of rectal tumors early in this century. Interest in this technique has been renewed, largely owing to the experience of Madden in New York. There is a definite role for electrocoagulation in small lesions less than 10 cm from the anal verge. This technique may be especially useful if the lesion is exophytic or if the patient is a poor risk for major resective surgery. Electrocoagulation obviously will not cure those 20 per cent of patients with cancer of the rectum who have Dukes' C lesions, but only about 20% of these patients achieve a 5-year survival after conventional abdominoperineal resection.

Cryosurgical destruction of rectal tumors has been effec-

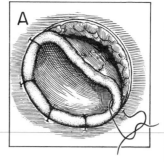
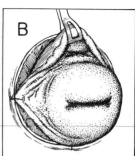
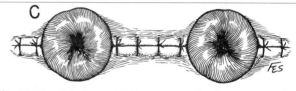

Fig. 26-28. Colostomy. (*A*) Permanent end colostomy. Bowel is being sutured to the skin with several interrupted absorbable sutures. (*B*) Loop colostomy. The proximal afferent functional limb is placed inferior to the nonfunctioning distal limb, the orifice of which is in relation to the Babcock clamp. (*C*) Divided colostomy with a bridge of skin between the afferent and efferent limbs. (Veidenheimer MC: Carcinoma of the rectum. In Hardy JD [ed]: Rhoads Textbook of Surgery, 5th ed. Philadelphia, J B Lippincott, 1977)

tive in a limited experience for indications similar to those used in electrocoagulation therapy.

Radiotherapy has been used by Papillon and others for primary treatment of rectal cancer. A special intraluminal tube has been designed for direct application of radiation onto the surface of the tumor after insertion of the tube into the rectum. This technique may be used on an outpatient basis and often is supplemented by insertion of radon seeds. Papillon has obtained a 5-year survival rate of 72% with radiotherapy in a highly selected series of patients who had largely Dukes' A and B lesions.

Results of Treatment

The 5-year survival rate for cancer of the rectum across the United States is about 45%. The operative mortality rate for abdominoperineal resection is in the range of 10%. A combination of radiotherapy and chemotherapy with 5-fluorouracil may be helpful in controlling symptoms from tumor regrowth.

OTHER TUMORS OF THE COLON AND RECTUM

CARCINOID

About 2% of gastrointestinal carcinoids occur in the colon and 17% occur in the rectum. Carcinoids of the colon and rectum rarely cause the malignant carcinoid syndrome, which is usually associated with carcinoids of the ileum with hepatic metastases. Colonic carcinoids smaller than 1 cm are rarely malignant and are usually asymptomatic. However, the larger the carcinoid, the greater is the malignant potential. The malignant carcinoid exhibits much the same clinical picture as carcinoma, and the principles of management are similar. These carcinoid tumors are often seen as submucosal masses with a yellow-orange configuration at sigmoidoscopy or colonoscopy.

LIPOMA

Most colon lipomas are asymptomatic, but rarely they may cause intussusception. The lipoma is the second most common benign tumor of the colon; only benign polyps occur more frequently. These lesions are submucosal and most often are found on the right side of the colon.

LYMPHOMA AND LYMPHOSARCOMA

Benign "lymphomas" occur in the rectum and rectosigmoid as a sessile or polypoid increase in the lymphoid tissue of the mucosa. They are removed locally only if symptomatic.

Lymphosarcoma may involve any part of the alimentary tract, with the colon and rectum being no exception. However, the colonic lesion may be predominant in this usually systemic disease. If systemic disease exists, radiation or chemotherapy will suffice for the local lesion. If the colorectal tumor is an isolated lesion, the usual operative measures used for colorectal carcinoma should be employed.

ENDOMETRIOSIS

Endometriosis may involve the colon externally and simulate cancer. It of course derives from the uterus, and hormonal suppression of menstruation will usually afford eventual relief. Rarely, the compression or constriction of the distal colon may require operative intervention, pending regression of the lesion under hormonal suppression.

EXTRINSIC CARCINOMA (BLUMER'S SHELF)

Intra-abdominal malignancies such as carcinoma of the stomach or of the ovary may result in metastatic deposits in the pelvis that can be palpated through the wall of the rectum on digital examination.

LEIOMYOMA AND LEIOMYOSARCOMA

Leiomyoma and leiomyosarcoma are smooth muscle tumors that may affect any portion of the alimentary tract.

CHORDOMA

A chordoma is a rare malignant tumor that arises from elements of the primitive notochord. When arising near the coccyx, it may be palpated through the rectal wall.

VOLVULUS OF THE COLON

Volvulus of the colon is defined as a twisting or rotation of a mobile segment of the colon about its mesentery. The degree of rotation may vary from 180° to as many as four or five complete revolutions. Depending on the degree of twist, either partial or complete obstruction is produced, which may advance to circulatory embarrassment and gangrene. The sigmoid colon is the most common site, accounting for about 80% of the cases, and the cecum is the next most common site, accounting for about 15% of the cases. Volvulus may also occur in the transverse colon and splenic flexure, but these cases are quite rare. Even though volvulus of the colon is the second most common cause of colonic obstruction, ranking behind cancer but slightly more frequent than diverticulitis, it accounts for only 3% to 5% of the total number of large bowel obstructions. It is, however, probably the most common cause of strangulated colon obstruction.

SIGMOID VOLVULUS

There is a variable geographic distribution of sigmoid volvulus. It has a low incidence in North America, Western Europe and Great Britain, but in Eastern Europe, Russia, Scandinavia, India, Africa, and South America it is common, accounting for perhaps 30% to 50% of all colon obstructions. There is a slight predominance in males, with a ratio of 2.5:1, and approximately two-thirds of the patients are over 50 years of age.

PATHOGENESIS

Sigmoid volvulus consists of the twisting of the sigmoid colon on its mesenteric base. This is associated with torsion along the longitudinal axis of the bowel. The combination of these two twisting forces results in obstruction (Fig. 26-29). The anatomical prerequisites for sigmoid volvulus include a redundant, elongated sigmoid colon and a narrow mesenteric base holding the two limbs of the sigmoid in close approximation, allowing easy rotation of the loop. Narrowing of the sigmoid mesenteric base may be secondary to previous intraperitoneal inflammatory disease or scarring from multiple episodes of twisting. The direction of the twist may be either clockwise or counterclockwise, and the degree of rotation varies from 180° to several complete rotations. A sigmoid volvulus produces a closed loop obstruction in the twisted segment, and if the ileocecal valve is competent, preventing reflux decompression of the proximal colon into the small bowel, a double loop obstruction occurs with distention of the proximal colon. Peristaltic forces tend to add additional amounts of liquid stool and gas into the closed loop, increasing the intraluminal pressure and producing massive distention. When the intraluminal pressure exceeds initially the venous pressure and later the arterial pressure, circulatory embarrassment and bowel necrosis occur if the obstruction is not relieved. The wall of the sigmoid colon is usually thickened in elderly patients who have experienced multiple episodes of volvulus with incomplete obstruction. This probably accounts for the ability of the bowel to withstand the massive distention and high intraluminal pressure without perforation, frequently allowing viability for several days.

Factors thought to be contributory in the pathogenesis of sigmoid volvulus include a high residue diet producing bulky stools, neglected bowel habits with chronic constipation, chronic laxative abuse, and pregnancy. As many as 40% of the cases of sigmoid volvulus are associated with various diseases of the nervous system, approximately equally divided between psychiatric illness and organic neurologic diseases such as chronic brain syndrome, parkinsonism, cerebrovascular accidents, and muscular dystrophy. Commonly a sigmoid volvulus occurs in association with acquired megacolon, which is also known to be increased in frequency in mental institutions and thought to result from chronic constipation and recurrent fecal impactions. Megacolon due to Chagas' disease and Hirschsprung's disease likewise predisposes the sigmoid to volvulus but accounts for only a small percentage of cases.

DIAGNOSIS

The patient usually presents with progressive abdominal distention, anorexia, and constipation that has been present for several days. Cramping lower abdominal pain may or may not accompany the illness. Frequently there is a history of chronic constipation and laxative abuse. Many patients will relate previous episodes of abdominal distention, which have been relieved by enemas or the knee-chest position and followed by the passage of large amounts of flatus and stool.

Massive abdominal distention and tympany are charac-

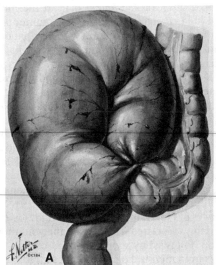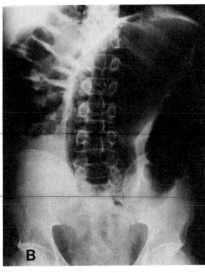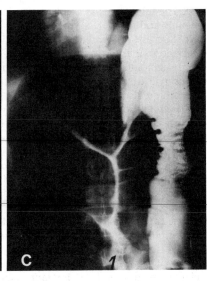

Fig. 26-29. Features of sigmoid volvulus. (*A*) Gross appearance. (*B*) Plain film of abdomen: note "bent inner tube" sign. (*C*) Barium colon exam: note obstruction of colon, gas filled loop, and "beak" deformity at end of barium column. (Fig. 26-29 *A*, copyright © 1962 CIBA Pharmaceutical Company, Division of CIBA-GEIGY Corporation. Reproduced with permission from The CIBA Collection of Medical Illustrations by Frank H Netter MD. All rights reserved)

teristic of sigmoid volvulus, with tenderness being remarkably mild or absent. Bowel sounds vary from hypoactive to hyperactive. Occasionally loops of distended bowel are visible through the abdominal wall. Rectal examination usually reveals the vault to be empty or filled with liquid stool. Varying degrees of dehydration may be present and respiratory distress secondary to massive abdominal distention may be an accompaniment. The temperature is usually normal, the pulse rate is only moderately elevated, and the blood pressure is unremarkable except when septic shock accompanies gangrenous bowel. When the volvulus is gangrenous, the findings on physical examination are not strikingly altered, as might be expected. Tachycardia is much more prominent, but the degree of direct and rebound tenderness may not be striking.

The leukocyte count may be normal or moderately elevated in cases without strangulation. When strangulation is present, the white count is markedly elevated, often above 25,000 cu mm with a marked left shift. Occasionally with advanced gangrene in elderly patients, the leukocyte count may be normal or low but have a marked left shift. This is a grave prognostic sign. Serum electrolytes often reveal hypokalemia and decreased bicarbonate. The blood urea nitrogen is often elevated, as is the urine specific gravity, indicating dehydration.

Although the diagnosis may be suspected from the history and physical examination, sigmoidoscopy or radiographic examination is required for confirmation. Plain abdominal films in the supine and upright positions are diagnostic in 60% of the patients, showing the characteristic bent innertube or omega sign (see Fig. 26-29) created by the markedly distended loop of sigmoid colon arising from the pelvis and frequently filling most of the abdominal cavity.

Sigmoidoscopy is helpful in establishing the diagnosis in the majority of patients. Either a characteristic point of twist is observed or an obstruction is encountered that releases large volumes of liquid stool and flatus on advancement of the sigmoidoscope or insertion of a colon tube. Barium enema is required as an emergency procedure only if

sigmoidoscopy fails to substantiate the diagnosis. Barium enema will demonstrate a characteristic "bird's beak" or "ace of spades" deformity (see Fig. 26-29) and, depending on the degree of obstruction, barium may or may not enter the loop of volvulus. Barium enema obtained after relief of the volvulus will demonstrate the predisposing redundant sigmoid colon with narrow base, and if obtained within a few days after an episode of volvulus, may demonstrate the point of twist as an area of narrowing and edema in the wall of the bowel.

TREATMENT

The foremost question in management is whether or not the sigmoid volvulus is strangulated. Strangulation may be suspected on the basis of physical examination and laboratory findings and may be confirmed at the time of sigmoidoscopy if the area of twist is visible. Findings include bluish-purple discoloration or hemorrhagic mucosa, bloody fluid in the rectum, or frank ulceration and necrosis of the bowel at the point of twist. If strangulation is present, no attempt should be made at sigmoidoscopic reduction of the volvulus because of the extreme risk of perforation. The patient should be prepared immediately for surgery with appropriate intravenous fluids and antibiotics. The surgical procedure consists of resection of the gangrenous sigmoid loop, accompanied by a double barrel colostomy or an end colostomy with closure of the rectal stump, if the length is inadequate to reach the abdominal wall. The mortality rate for strangulated volvulus with gangrene is high, approximately 50%. Without operation, death is inevitable.

If strangulation is not present, sigmoidoscopic reduction of the volvulus should be attempted. As the sigmoidoscope is advanced to the point of obstruction, usually encountered between 15 cm and 25 cm, the scope is gently and carefully negotiated into the obstructed loop. This frequently results in forceful release of massive amounts of flatus and liquid fecal material. (The wise sigmoidoscopist will be prepared for this.) A lubricated colon tube is then inserted through the sigmoidoscope and passed well up into the sigmoid loop. The tube serves as a stent to prevent recurrence of the volvulus and is firmly secured and left in place for several days. Successful sigmoidoscopic reduction of the volvulus can be accomplished in about 80% of the cases. Occasionally when sigmoidoscopic reduction is unsuccessful, barium enema will untwist the colon. When this occurs, a colon tube should also be inserted to prevent recurrence.

If sigmoidoscopic or barium enema reduction fails, laparotomy and operative detorsion should be performed. After the loop is untwisted, a colon tube should be passed up through the rectum from below by an assistant and advanced into the sigmoid loop to prevent postoperative recurrence. Mortality from operative reduction of volvulus without gangrene is low. Resection at this time has been advocated by some; however, this procedure is not recommended because the mortality rate is significantly higher, since the colon is obstructed and has not been properly prepared.

After decompression of the volvulus by either operative or nonoperative means, the patient should be prepared for elective resection of the redundant sigmoid, usually during the same hospitalization. Elective resection in the average patient carries a low mortality. If resection is not done, many patients will have a recurrence of the volvulus. Only in patients who have a high operative risk because of complicating medical conditions should one consider not resecting the sigmoid. Sigmoid resection is usually curative; however, a few cases of recurrent sigmoid volvulus have occurred following resection. In these cases, acquired megacolon has usually been present and a more extensive procedure such as total abdominal colectomy with ileoproctostomy may be required.

CECAL VOLVULUS

Even though *volvulus of the cecum* is a term in common usage, it is somewhat of a misnomer because the volvulus actually involves a significant portion of the ascending colon or terminal ileum. Cecal volvulus is much less common than sigmoid volvulus and accounts for only 10% to 15% of the cases of volvulus of the colon.

PATHOGENESIS

In the etiology of cecal volvulus two factors are necessary: (1) a congenital predisposition and (2) an acquired, precipitating event. The congenital predisposition is "hypofixation" or excessive mobility of the cecum resulting from failure of descent during the eighth month in utero or failure of fixation during the first 4 months of life.

The acquired precipitating factors are varied and include trauma, pregnancy, parturition, high residue diet, constipation, or hyperperistalsis due to a distal colon lesion, ascites, immediate postoperative status, and previous abdominal surgery. The association with previous surgery is particularly strong, occurring in 50% of Wilson's cases, with the adhesions from the previous operation providing the fixed point about which the cecum twists. The volvulus usually occurs in a clockwise fashion, and a 360° rotation is characteristic. Acute severe upward angulation of the cecum may produce the same findings without an actual twist (cecal bascule).

DIAGNOSIS

The symptom complex typical of cecal volvulus falls into two patterns: acute and chronic recurrent. In the acute variety there is rapid onset of abdominal pain in the mid abdomen or right side. It may be colicky or continuous. Nausea and vomiting follow, and distention with obstipation complete the syndrome. The majority of patients may have a history of antecedent similar episodes. Physical findings include abdominal distention, hyperperistalsis, and mild to moderate tenderness, especially with pressure on the distended loop. Sometimes the cecum may be palpated as a mass and it may be found in any quadrant. In a certain number of the acute cases, the volvulus will progress rapidly to strangulation and gangrene. In this group the duration of symptoms may be quite short, and distention will be minimal; the history of bowel function is of no significance. Signs of peritonitis will be present on abdominal examination and septic shock may occur. In the chronic recurrent variety, the history is one of multiple attacks of right lower quadrant pain, variably associated with nausea and vomiting and mild distention, followed by spontaneous resolution.

Radiographic examination is diagnostic in about 90% of the cases. Plain films of the abdomen reveal a characteristically dilated cecum, usually with a single large air fluid level on upright examination. The cecum may be found in any quadrant, with the mid abdomen and left upper quadrant being frequent locations. Additional contributory findings include associated small bowel gas, indicating obstruction of the terminal ileum, especially if the small bowel gas is to the *right* of the cecum; indentation of the ileocecal valve on the *right* of the cecum; and empty distal colon. Barium examination of the colon is usually pathognomonic. The barium passes up to the right transverse or hepatic flexure, excluding sigmoid volvulus, and stops by outlining the point of obstruction in a "spiraling" mucosal pattern, terminating in a "beak" deformity. In the chronic intermittent variety, only a large mobile cecum will be demonstrated unless fortuitously fluoroscopy reveals twisting and spontaneous untwisting of the cecum.

TREATMENT

If the cecal volvulus cannot be reduced by colonoscopy, operation is required. The patient should be expeditiously prepared for surgery and emergency operation performed. The status of the bowel and the condition of the patient determine what procedure is to be chosen. If the cecum is viable and is not tensely distended, detorsion and fixation of the cecum in the right lower quadrant may be carried out. If the cecum is tense and rupture appears imminent as indicated by serosal tears, decompression by needle or trochar should be performed before detorsion is attempted. There are various methods of anchoring the cecum in the right lower quadrant, including lateral cecopexy, cecostomy, and retroperitoneal tunneling. If trochar decompression is used, cecostomy through the same site is particularly advantageous. Since some cases of subsequent small bowel volvulus have occurred around an anterior cecostomy site, it is good practice to place the cecostomy as far lateral as possible and obliterate the "gutter." If the cecum is gangrenous, right hemicolectomy will be necessary unless the patient is an especially poor risk, in which case a Mikulicz type resection with double stoma might be chosen. In some cases where only a small patch of gangrene is present, cecostomy can be performed through this area, provided that the pursestring suture is placed well back into healthy tissue. The mortality rate varies from 10% to 40%, depending on the frequency of gangrene.

RARE TYPES OF COLON VOLVULUS

Volvulus of the splenic flexure or transverse colon occurs very infrequently. Also, a volvulus may occur in two different areas of the colon at the same time. The majority of all examples of colon volvulus occur in adults beyond middle age. The entity is also occasionally encountered in children. Volvulus of the splenic flexure and transverse colon in adults and almost all cases of volvulus seen in children are due to congenital abnormalities associated with a lack of proper fixation of the colon to the posterior abdominal wall. The principles of diagnosis and management previously outlined apply to these more rare forms of colon obstruction also.

Megacolon due to the variety of possible causes must be distinguished from true volvulus, although of course the presence of megacolon may predispose to volvulus.

RECTAL PROLAPSE

Rectal prolapse or procidentia is a condition in which part or all of the layers of the rectum are extruded through the anal sphincter (Fig. 26-30). There has been considerable confusion in regard to this lesion because of the many variations encountered to which the generic term *prolapse* has been assigned and because of some attempts to differentiate between prolapse and procidentia which, by definition, are synonymous.

Anatomical and pathophysiological factors in rectal prolapse are listed below:

Complete rectal prolapse is essentially a *sliding hernia.*

There is an associated large defect in the pelvic diaphragm.

There is elongation and redundancy of rectosigmoid and sigmoid colon with thickened, heavy, and distorted mesentery.

The prolapsed bowel is edematous, hyperemic, and often superficially ulcerated.

Continuation of the prolapse produces stretching and paralysis of the external sphincter muscle and a wide patulous anus.

Patients with this condition are often elderly, debilitated, and poor surgical risks, with multiple associated diseases.

TYPES

Altemeier recognizes three types of rectal prolapse:

Type I, the most common form, is a protrusion of the mucosal layer of the rectum for a distance of 1 cm to 3 cm, the mucous membrane being redundant, hypertrophied, and abnormally loose. It represents a *false prolapse* and it is usually associated with internal and external hemorrhoids.

Type II consists of the protrusion of all layers of the rectum through the anus, being essentially an intussusception. It begins at a level above the anus and is considered to be an *incomplete prolapse.* It does not have the associated sliding hernia of cul-de-sac characteristic of type III.

Type III is considered to be a *true* or *complete prolapse* of the rectum (Fig. 26-31). It is in reality a perineal sliding hernia of the peritoneum of the cul-de-sac. Through a defect in the pelvic diaphragm (levator ani muscle), the cul-de-sac hernia invaginates the anterior rectal wall to produce an intussusception through the rectal and anal canals, with its further protrusion through the anal sphincter. The posterior wall of the cul-de-sac peritoneum is carried along as the serosa adherent to the anterior wall of the rectosigmoid, in characteristic sliding hernia fashion (see Fig. 26-31). With repeated and prolonged protrusion, the anal sphincter becomes relaxed, progressively stretched, and ultimately paralyzed.

CLINICAL PICTURE

Rectal prolapse occurs most frequently in the extremes of life—in children below the age of 3 and in the elderly—with a reported predilection for females. Altemeier found the incidence of prolapse to be about 60% for females and 40% for males. His youngest patient in 159 cases was 2½ months of age and the oldest, 97 years, the average being 72 years. Of particular interest was the fact that approximately 50% of the patients were between 70 and 97 years of age, and the mean was 78 years.

Fig. 26-30. A large type III rectal prolapse with anterior bulge indicative of position of cul-de-sac hernia. Note thickening, ulceration, and changes in rectal mucosa.

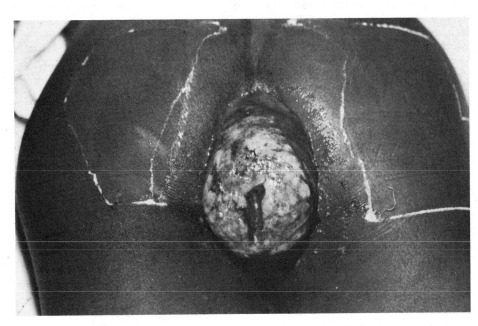

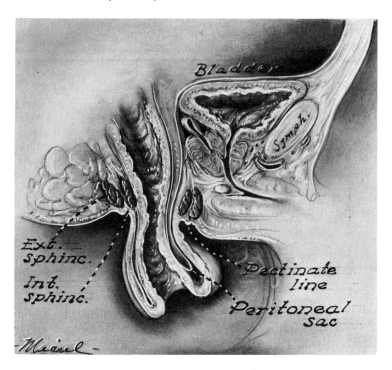

Fig. 26-31. Diagrammatic illustration of a true rectal prolapse indicating the presence of herniation of the cul-de-sac through the anterior rectal wall. (Altemeier WA: Rectal prolapse. In Hardy JD [ed]: Rhoads Textbook of Surgery, 5th ed. Philadelphia, J B Lippincott, 1977)

In the usual case, the rectal wall, including the muscular layers, turns inside out as it protrudes through the dilated anal sphincter in the presence of increased intra-abdominal pressure. The rectum may prolapse for 3 to 6 or more inches. Its outer surface of mucous membrane becomes hyperemic and at times cyanotic. It secretes increased amounts of mucus, which causes soilage, perineal excoriation, discomfort, embarrassment, and, ultimately, social rejection or voluntary seclusion. As the process progresses, the prolapse occurs more easily with activities such as coughing, lifting, walking, and micturition. Ulcerations may appear on the mucosal surface, and these may become the source of active bleeding. At times the prolapse may be due to a tumor.

Inspection and digital examination demonstrate the laxity or paralysis of the anal sphincteric muscles. It is a recognized fact that approximately 65% of patients with rectal prolapse are incontinent of feces preoperatively. In this regard, it has been generally believed that there were no significant associated neurologic defects. This has not been the case in Altemeier's experience, however. Fifty-three percent of his 159 patients had a diagnosis of established psychiatric disease and 30% had obvious neurological disease or injury. The neurologic disorders included cerebral thrombosis and hemorrhage, chronic brain syndrome, muscular dystrophy, poliomyelitis, mental retardation, birth injuries, fractured vertebrae, and other spinal injuries. Thus 83% had psychiatric or central nervous system lesions. In my experience, in some instances the patient has been in prison and involved in homosexual activity.

TREATMENT

There has been considerable confusion and discussion as to the essential factors characterizing true rectal prolapse and the most effective surgical operation. More than 54 different operative procedures have been devised to cure rectal prolapse since the report of Moschcowitz in 1912. These operations have been based on six general principles: (1) resection of the prolapsing and redundant bowel, (2) reduction of the size of the anus, (3) plastic reconstruction or reinforcement of the perineal floor, (4) transabdominal suspension or fixation of the prolapsed bowel, (5) obliteration of the cul-de-sac, or (6) repair of the perineal sliding hernia.

It has been generally believed that the cure of a type III prolapse is difficult under any circumstance, and there has been no consensus as to the most effective operation or agreement as to the results obtainable with each.

Altemeier and associates prefer a one-stage perineal procedure with resection of the rectal prolapse and involved rectosigmoid, ablation of the sliding perineal cul-de-sac hernia, repair of the defect in the pelvic diaphragm, and anorectosigmoidal end-to-end anastomosis. This procedure as used for types II and III is described below. Type I cases are treated by a radical hemorrhoidectomy. In a much less extensive experience, I have had considerable success with a combined abdominal and perineal approach. At laparotomy the rectosigmoid is retracted upward and excessive redundancy is actually resected when appropriate. The lower sigmoid and rectum are then fixed with silk sutures to the pelvic fascia at many points. Finally, after the abdomen has been closed, a heavy subcutaneous circular suture is placed to narrow the anus to the size of the index finger, since repeated prolapse of the large tissue bolus through the anus will usually have led to anal incontinence and sphincter tone must be restored.

Postoperative measures are similar to those for colon resection. There should be careful avoidance of straining at stool by using a low residue diet and stool softeners.

RESULTS

Permanent success including restoration of anal sphincter control can be expected in the majority of patients. However, recurrence will occur in a substantial number of patients, especially those in psychiatric institutions, ones with neurologic defects who are unable to defecate normally, and some in prison with abnormal sex practices.

ANORECTUM

The anorectum is 4 cm in length and includes all of the anal canal and the lower 2 cm of the rectum and their juncture within the sphincter mechanism (Fig. 26-32). The anal canal is of ectodermal origin and the rectum is of entodermal origin. The junction of the entoderm of the rectum and the ectoderm of the anal canal is an irregular, serrated line known as the dentate or mucocutaneous line. At the dentate line there may be as many as eight minute teatlike structures known as anal papillae, which are vestiges of the ectodermal anal plate. The anal crypts represent ectodermal folds from the proctodeal membrane bridging between the columns of Morgagni.

The anal canal is lined with true skin at the anal verge; however, as the skin enters the anal canal, it loses its skin glandular elements, changing gradually to a more modified stratified squamous epithelium, which terminates at the dentate line; the modified squamous epithelium may be overridden to some extent by the columnar epithelium of the rectum.

ANORECTAL EXAMINATION

First, the patient should be made to feel at ease with the maximum privacy and the least possible embarrassment. Next, careful inspection of the anus in a good light with the patient in a prone, semi-jackknifed position may afford much information. One may see excoriation, inflammation, excessive mucous drainage, perhaps traces of blood, hemorrhoids, rectal prolapse, sinuses or fistulas, condylomata, ulcerations, sentinel pile suggesting anal fissure, frank malignancy, and still other lesions. A good visual examination should always precede digital examination and endoscopy.

Digital examination should be performed gently and slowly, with adequate verbal preparation of the patient, using a well-lubricated gloved digit. Most patients are somewhat ill at ease and tense when undergoing rectal examination, and a better examination will be achieved if the external sphincter can be gradually dilated. Of course, some lesions cause the patient so much pain and spasm that adequate digital and endoscopic examination can only be accomplished with the use of anesthesia. This is especially true in the presence of perirectal abscess, for example. The character of lesions both within the rectum and without (including the prostate in males) should be noted, as well as the presence of blood on the withdrawn finger.

The lubricated anoscope is placed at the anus, and with gentle intermittent pressure the sphincters will relax, permitting the anoscope to enter the rectum with minimal discomfort. Anoscopy permits evaluation of the pecten and lower rectum simultaneously for anal fissures, anal squamous epitheliomas, internal hemorrhoids, hypertrophied anal papillae, low rectal polyps, carcinoma, cryptitis, acute papillitis, and the primary opening of a fistula-in-ano. Better evaluation of internal hemorrhoids is obtained if the patient is requested to strain and engorge the hemorrhoid during anoscopy.

Proctoscopy should be included as routine in patients over 40 years of age.

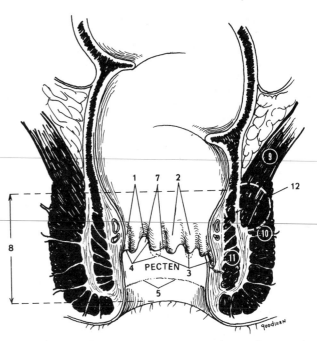

Fig. 26-32. Anatomy of the anorectum: (1) columns of Morgagni; (2) sinuses of Morgagni; (3) anal valves with crypts; (4) dentate line and upper limits of pecten; (5) intersphincteric line and lower limits of pecten (Hilton's line); (7) anal papillae (cephalic dentation of pecten); (8) anorectum (anal canal of Milligan and Morgan); (9) levator ani muscle; (10) deep portion external sphincter muscle; (11) internal sphincter muscle; (12) conjoined longitudinal muscle. (After Schutte AG, Tolentino MG: A second study of anal papillae. Dis Colon Rectum 14:435, 1971. Ted Conde, Medical Illustrator)

HEMORRHOIDS

Numerous etiologic factors are mentioned in the literature. Heredity is an important factor, and the majority of patients with symptomatic hemorrhoids have a familial history of the disorder.

In 2000 consecutive proctologic examinations reported by Hanley and Hines, the incidence of internal hemorrhoids was 72%. Internal hemorrhoids result from enlargement of the terminal veins of the three primary and secondary hemorrhoidal plexuses in the lower rectum. When the hemorrhoidal varicosities become large, the stool during defecation gradually pushes the hemorrhoid downward into the anal canal, stretching its submucosal attachment and further dilating the veins. This process eventually results in overstretching of its support and in chronic prolapse of the hemorrhoid.

The internal hemorrhoidal plexus is separated from the external hemorrhoidal plexus at the intersphincteric line, but there is a capillary anastomosis of the two plexuses in the subepithelial tissue of the pecten. The left primary internal hemorrhoid is located in the midlateral position. On the right side there are two primary groups in the posterior lateral and anterior positions, respectively. Frequently, secondary internal hemorrhoids of smaller size are adjacent to the primary internal hemorrhoids.

INTERNAL HEMORRHOIDS

Classification

The anatomical relationship of the hemorrhoidal plexus to the dentate line and not the size of the hemorrhoidal plexus determines the degree of hemorrhoids.

First-Degree Internal Hemorrhoids. The hemorrhoidal plexuses may be small or of moderate size. However, the patient gives no history of protrusion of the internal hemorrhoid and, on anoscopic examination, the hemorrhoids will not descend below the dentate line when the patient is instructed to strain as if he were attempting to evacuate his bowel.

Second-Degree Internal Hemorrhoids. The hemorrhoidal plexuses may be as large as first-degree hemorrhoids or larger; however, the submucosal support is not adequate to hold the hemorrhoid in its normal position, and it will protrude into the lower anal canal on straining. However, after defecation or cessation of straining, the protruding hemorrhoidal mass will spontaneously and immediately retract to its normal position in the rectum above the dentate line.

Third-Degree Internal Hemorrhoids. The submucosal support, because of repeated stretching by the passage of stool and straining, has become weakened and, after prolapsing, the hemorrhoidal mass is unable to retract spontaneously into the rectum. Manual manipulation is needed to push the hemorrhoids back into the rectum, where they will remain until the next bowel movement.

Fourth-Degree Internal Hemorrhoids. At this stage the rectal mucosa is redundant and submucosal attachments have been overstretched over a long period of time and are unable to retain the internal hemorrhoids in their normal location above the dentate line after manual replacement, thus resulting in chronic prolapse of the internal hemorrhoids.

Clinical Manifestations

Many signs and symptoms, such as anorectal pain, backache, thigh pain, bleeding, lassitude, blockage of evacuation, and pain with evacuation, are attributed to hemorrhoids by the patient, but actually are due to other anorectal problems, the most common of which are anal fissure and systemic disease. Internal hemorrhoids are asymptomatic except when they prolapse or become strangulated.

The only significant sign due to internal hemorrhoids is painless bleeding of bright red blood per rectum during or after defecation, noticed as blood streaking on the toilet tissue or dripping into the commode. This is a very common complaint for patients with first- to third-degree internal hemorrhoids. Over a period of months, painless blood loss may be of such quantity that the patient's hemoglobin may decrease to an alarming 3 g to 6 g. It is not uncommon for some patients with third- and fourth-degree internal hemorrhoids not to bleed; however, if the prolapsed hemorrhoids are not reduced by manual manipulation, the mucus secretion from the mucosa will cause a "wet bottom," resulting in soiling of the underclothing. This may also give rise to pruritic symptoms and maceration of the perianal skin that may lead to soreness. Metaplasia of the mucosa over the base of chronic prolapsing hemorrhoids is common. Some patients with large internal hemorrhoids complain of blockage of the rectal passage during defecation and pressure in the rectum. The most frequent complaint is difficulty in cleaning the anus after bowel movement.

Treatment

Patients with asymptomatic first- or second-degree internal hemorrhoids should be instructed in good bowel habits and anal hygiene that may postpone development of symptoms.

If bleeding is the only symptom in a patient with first-degree internal hemorrhoids, the physician must exclude carcinoma, polyps, inflammatory disease, or other etiologic factors that may cause bleeding from the colon before treating the hemorrhoids. Bleeding hemorrhoids frequently respond to conservative medical management: hydrophilic bulk laxative, rectal suppositories, and good anal hygiene. If bleeding persists, sclerotherapy (injection of a sclerosing solution) may stop the bleeding and provide complete relief.

In second-degree internal hemorrhoids, the same treatment as that given patients with first-degree hemorrhoids is recommended. Rubber band ligation (strangulation) of the larger internal hemorrhoid may be appropriate and dramatic in controlling the bleeding and preventing further prolapse of the hemorrhoidal mass.

In symptomatic patients with third- and fourth-degree internal hemorrhoids, surgical excision offers the highest percentage of cure. Surgical excision is not recommended for patients with severe systemic disease (ulcerative colitis, portal hypertension, Crohn's disease, leukemia, renal or cardiac disease) or in aged patients who may obtain adequate palliation by either the rubber band ligation or the injection treatment.

The type of surgical procedure depends on the degree of anatomical alteration. The surgical principle is to excise by sharp dissection the external and internal hemorrhoidal plexus en masse and to restore the anorectum to as near normal as possible. More than one technical approach in the same patient may be required to accomplish this result.

Hemorrhoidectomy. Under satisfactory caudal, spinal, or general anesthesia the patient is placed in a modified semi-jackknife prone position and 3-inch adhesive tape is placed over each side of the buttocks to partially evert the anal canal. If the anorectum is soft and pliable, and not restricted on a two-finger digital examination, dilatation of the anorectum is not done. The perianal area is prepared and draped with sterile sheets. If desired, approximately 3 ml 1% lidocaine (Xylocaine) with 1:200,000 epinephrine may be injected subcutaneously to each external hemorrhoid and into the submucosa deep to the internal hemorrhoids (Fig. 26-33). The solution separates the tissue planes, facilitates dissection, and minimizes bleeding during the dissection.

The base of the hemorrhoidal mass just above the dentate line is grasped with a hemostat and pulled out of the rectum. A catgut transfixion suture is then placed around the pedicle vessels proximal to the hemorrhoidal plexus. This is accomplished by placing the first suture superficially and the second suture deeper to ligate the hemorrhoidal vessels in the submucosa. The deeper suture is carefully placed so as not to include the internal sphincter muscle (Fig. 26-34). A second hemostat is placed just distal to the external hemorrhoids. An elliptical incision is made through the skin and mucosa about the external and the internal hemorrhoidal plexuses, which are dissected free from the underlying tissue. During a routine hemorrhoidectomy the subcutaneous dark red external sphincter muscle is completely relaxed lateral to the corrugator cutis ani and it is seldom seen. The hemorrhoids are excised en masse. When the dissection reaches the catgut transfixion suture, the external hemorrhoids under the skin are excised. After securing hemostasis, the mucosa and anal skin are closed longitudinally with a simple running stitch. The mucosa and the skin are not anchored to the underlying muscle or the subcutaneous tissue. Some surgeons prefer to leave the wound open to heal by secondary intention. Other modifications and variations in the details of the above basic procedure are in widespread use.

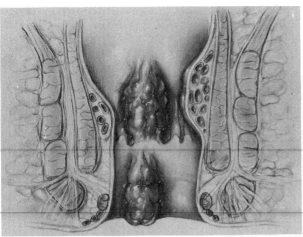

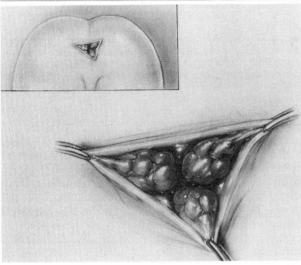

Fig. 26-33. *(Top)* The anatomical location of the internal and external hemorrhoids and their relation to the sphincters of the anorectum. *(Bottom)* Location of the three primary internal hemorrhoids in the anorectum. (Hanley PH: Anorectum. In Hardy JD [ed]: Rhoads Textbook of Surgery, 5th ed. Philadelphia, J B Lippincott, 1977)

Fig. 26-34. The internal hemorrhoid is pulled out of the rectum and a transfixion suture is placed about the vessels proximal to the hemorrhoidal plexus. (Hanley PH: Anorectum. In Hardy JD [ed]: Rhoads Textbook of Surgery, 5th ed. Philadelphia, J B Lippincott, 1977)

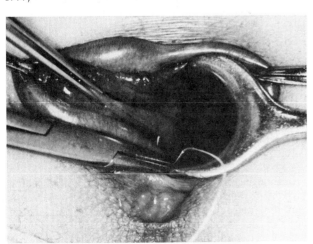

On completion of the operation, two small strips of Gelfoam soaked in lidocaine-epinephrine solution may be placed in the anorectum. A light dressing is applied without pressure.

One ounce of mineral oil is given twice a day until the patient has his first bowel movement; then the mineral oil is discontinued and a teaspoon of bulk laxative is given twice a day. Adequate and complete analgesia is provided. The patients are usually discharged on the third to fifth day after operation. Three to 4 weeks postoperatively a gentle digital examination should be done to assess the anorectum.

Bleeding immediately after hemorrhoidectomy is usually the result of a technical error in obtaining hemostasis. On the other hand, bleeding 7 to 9 days after hemorrhoidectomy results from sloughing of the wound. The bleeding site is usually from a hemorrhoidal artery at the level of the anorectal ring. In either instance, the bleeding should be controlled by fulguration or transfixion sutures with the patient under appropriate anesthesia. In early postoperative bleeding, heavy sedation may provide adequate analgesia. In late bleeding, the tissues are friable, and the ligature is gently tightened to stop the bleeding so as not to cut through the healing granulation tissue.

Urinary retention is caused by a combination of factors: overhydration prior to, during, and after anorectal surgery when the anesthesia is still interfering with bladder and urethral sphincter function; anxiety; excessive sedation; prostatic obstruction; and spasm of the anal sphincter postoperatively.

Urinary retention may resolve with relatively simple measures such as a hot sitz bath or administration of urecholine or hot compresses to abdomen. If these measures fail, catheterization may be necessary. If urinary retention is due to prostatic hypertrophy, consultation with the urologist is necessary.

Post-hemorrhoidectomy *stricture* of the anorectum may result from technical lapses at the time of surgery, such as circumferential removal of mucosa or anoderm, as well as from poor postoperative care of patients.

Frequent loose bowel movements in the postoperative period, owing to an irritable colon or excessive administration of laxatives, prevent anal dilation by formed feces during the critical healing period. Frequent manual dilation (twice daily) will be necessary until healing is complete to prevent stricture formation in these patients. Cicatricial stenosis of the anorectum may be cured only by a surgical procedure.

Fecal impaction may occasionally occur either before the patient leaves the hospital or up to 14 days after surgery, usually in a patient who is reluctant to defecate because of fear of pain. The impaction is usually soft and can be broken with the index finger and easily evacuated following enema. On rare occasions, it may be necessary to remove the impaction manually, and, in this case, light anesthesia may be necessary.

Ectropion of the rectal mucosa can occur if the mucosa was sutured to the lower anal canal of the dentate line. In these patients the anus is covered with rectal mucosa, resulting in a "wet bottom" and perianal irritation. Excision of the mucosa in the anal canal and covering the raw surface with an anal skin flap is curative for most patients.

Injection. Sclerotherapy of hemorrhoids was originally described by Mitchell in 1871. Injection therapy can be a good method of treatment in well-selected cases, especially in bleeding first- and second-degree hemorrhoids. It may also be used to render temporary palliative benefit to an elderly patient who is not a candidate for surgical procedure or to relieve a patient who must postpone a surgical procedure because of personal reasons.

In patients with third- and fourth-degree internal hemorrhoids, surgical excision is preferred to sclerotherapy, because the latter yields inferior results. Injection is contraindicated in the presence of symptomatic anal fissure, abscess, or fistula-in-ano.

Two to 3 ml of a sclerosing solution (5% phenol in clear vegetable oil or 5% quinine urea hydrochloride) are injected around the pedicle of each hemorrhoid through a lighted anoscope. Serious complications are rare after injection therapy. Occasionally, complications such as rectal stricture, postinjection bleeding, mesenteric thrombosis, abscess of the liver, vasomotor collapse, and pulmonary infarct have been reported. One of the more common complications of injection therapy when using a mineral oil and phenol solution is rectal oleo-granuloma.

In 1939, Milligan reported the results of 200 cases of hemorrhoids treated by sclerosing injection. First-degree internal hemorrhoids were cured in 90% of cases. In second-degree hemorrhoids the cure was uncertain in 25%, and in third-degree internal hemorrhoids, the injections were ineffectual for cure.

Office Ligation. Because the tissues in the upper anorectum receive visceral innervation, ligation treatment can be done as an office procedure without anesthesia. The internal hemorrhoids are visualized with a proximal lighted anoscope. The grasping forceps is passed through the double cylinder ligator loaded with two rubber bands over the edge of the inner cylinder. The most prominent proximal portion of the internal hemorrhoidal plexus is grasped and pulled into the double-sleeve cylinder. The ligator is triggered, forcing the outer cylinder over the inner cylinder and pushing the rubber bands off so that they encircle and strangulate the internal hemorrhoidal plexus mass and redundant mucosa. If the rubber band is too close to the dentate line, pain will result and immediate removal and reapplication 2 mm to 3 mm higher will be necessary. In 3 to 5 days, the strangulated internal hemorrhoid will become gangrenous. Eight to 10 days after ligation the gangrenous hemorrhoid and rubber bands will slough off, leaving a small raw area that heals in a few days.

It is desirable to treat a single group of internal hemorrhoids at one time, repeating the treatment at intervals of 2 to 3 weeks until all hemorrhoids are destroyed. Large hemorrhoids may require more than one application of rubber bands. The ligation treatment is used in small to medium-sized second-degree hemorrhoids and secondary hemorrhoids and in patients who are poor surgical and anesthetic risks. Salvati reported a statistical review of 490 consecutive patients who received 1625 ligation treatments by the Barron rubber band technique. His incidence of postoperative ligation bleeding was 1.8% and of pain, 7%.

EXTERNAL THROMBOTIC HEMORRHOIDS

A vein or veins in the anal canal may rupture and blood will extravasate under the anoderm, forming a clot varying from a few millimeters to as large as 2.5 cm. Rupture of the blood vessel may occur spontaneously or from straining, passage of stool, diarrhea, sneezing, coughing, or sudden movement of buttocks while seated.

The acute onset of pain is caused by separating of the anoderm from the underlying tissue by the extravasating

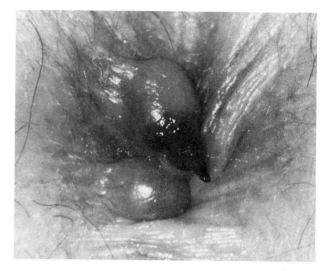

Fig. 26-35. Multiple thrombotic external hemorrhoids may occur. The skin over the clot may become ischemic, and the clot may be expelled spontaneously. (Hanley PH: Anorectum. In Hardy JD [ed]: Rhoads Textbook of Surgery, 5th ed. Philadelphia, J B Lippincott, 1977)

blood. The pain is severe during the first 48 hours and gradually diminishes, leaving a painless clot in the lower anal canal. In some patients pain may be minimal. On frequent occasions the skin and subcutaneous tissue adjacent to the thrombotic hemorrhoid become edematous. After several hours the bleeding ceases and the clot will not increase in size. At times the size of the clot may exert such a pressure on the anoderm that ischemic necrosis of the anoderm occurs on the third or fourth day. The clot will then ooze blood, soiling the underclothes or, at times, be expelled spontaneously (Fig. 26-35).

If the patient is seen when the thrombotic external hemorrhoid is very painful, the clot may be excised as an office procedure, using a local anesthetic. After a lapse of 48 hours, thrombotic external hemorrhoid is no longer painful and surgery is not necessary. The clot will be absorbed in about 3 weeks. Rubber band ligation is not suitable for treatment of external hemorrhoids due to the pain fibers below the dentate line.

STRANGULATED INTERNAL HEMORRHOIDS

If large second- and third-degree internal hemorrhoids prolapse, sphincter spasm may make it impossible for the internal hemorrhoids to retract into the rectum spontaneously. The prolapse usually follows a bowel movement or physical exertion. The pain increases in severity and edema of the hemorrhoids and perianal tissue rapidly occurs. The patient is unable to sit. After a few hours, the edematous internal hemorrhoids exude a serosanguineous transudate. In 24 to 38 hours, ischemic necrosis of the internal hemorrhoid develops. When all of the hemorrhoidal groups are strangulated, the edema is circumferential. If one primary hemorrhoidal group is strangulated, the swelling is limited to that area. The swollen hemorrhoids are tense and painful on palpation.

During the first several hours, the edematous swelling and pain are due to mechanical obstruction of venous return from the internal hemorrhoidal plexuses. Strangulation causes thrombosis of the internal and external hemorrhoids after 12 to 24 hours. After several days the base of the internal hemorrhoid near the dentate line becomes gangrenous and necrotic and sloughs (autohemorrhoidectomy).

For patients seen before ischemic gangrene and infection occur, emergency closed hemorrhoidectomy is recommended. Unfortunately, most patients are seen after the strangulation has caused thrombosis, gangrene, and infection of the base of the internal hemorrhoid. At this stage, nonoperative treatment is necessary. Bed rest, warm compresses to the anus, hot sitz bath, mineral oil, sedatives, and analgesic medication will make the patient comfortable. In a few days the devitalized tissue separates, leaving an ulcerated area that heals in approximately 3 weeks. On examination several weeks later, the residual hemorrhoids may be small and asymptomatic. However, the great majority of patients will require further elective surgical excision.

FISSURE-IN-ANO

Fissure-in-ano is an elongated tear of the anoderm of the proximal anal canal over the pecten. The tear usually begins about 2 mm below the dentate line and extends distally to the lower anal canal. Most acute fissures heal spontaneously; however, a large percentage require surgical treatment.

The most common cause of a tear of the anoderm in the posterior midline is overstretching during the passage of a large hard stool. Infection of the anal glands causes the anoderm to lose its normal elasticity and predisposes to formation of fissure-in-ano. Inflammatory conditions such as cryptitis, proctitis, and acute infectious diarrhea leading to inflammation of the anal gland may result in fissure formation. Crohn's disease and ulcerative colitis are associated with a high incidence of anal fissure. Not infrequently the presence of an anal fissure is the first clinical evidence of inflammatory bowel disease.

PATHOLOGY

At the onset, a fissure is a simple linear tear of the epithelium over the pecten, usually in the posterior midline, less frequently in the anterior midline, and rarely in the lateral position of the anal canal. Two or 3 mm of normal-appearing anoderm usually separate the dentate line from the fissure. The fissure extends downward toward the anal verge. When traction is applied on each side of the anus, the fissure appears to be triangular in shape, with the apex near the dentate line and the base over the lower anal canal. The submucosa muscularis forms the floor of the superficial acute fissure. The skin edges are not edematous and are well defined. The base is extremely tender and there is associated spasm of the sphincters. As the ulcer penetrates through the submucosa muscularis, circular fibers of the lower edge of the internal sphincter become visible in the ulcer base. In the past, the ulcer was frequently erroneously referred to in the literature as lying over the subcutaneous external sphincter muscle.

As a result of long-standing recurrent infection, the papilla proximal to the chronic anal ulcer becomes hypertrophied, varying in size from a few millimeters to a large anal fibroma. On digital examination a hypertrophied anal papilla is frequently mistaken for a rectal polyp. The hypertrophied anal papillae are readily diagnosed by anoscopy because they are of ectodermal origin. The subcutaneous external sphincter, being distal to the fissure, impairs the drainage from the fissure. The skin edge at the base of the fissure becomes undermined and edematous (Fig. 26-36).

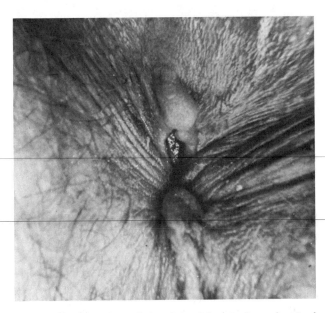

Fig. 26-36. Subacute and chronic anal fissure; the undermined skin is edematous. "Sentinel pile" or subcutaneous abscess could develop. The fissure is posterior in the vast majority of cases. (Hanley PH: Anorectum. In Hardy JD [ed]: Rhoads Textbook of Surgery, 5th ed. Philadelphia, J B Lippincott, 1977)

Occasionally a subcutaneous abscess develops from a fissure in the superficial postanal space. They usually rupture spontaneously 1 cm or 2 cm posterior to the fissure in the midline, forming a subcutaneous fistula-in-ano. Recurrent infection and chronic lymphedema result in formation of a prominent skin tag at the distal edge of the fissure, which has been called a sentinel pile by Brodie. The presence of a sentinel pile and a hypertrophied anal papilla is pathognomonic of a chronic anal ulcer.

An acute fissure causes excruciating pain and spasm of the sphincters, especially the internal sphincter. The base of the fissure is on the lowest part of the internal sphincter muscle, and persistent or recurrent exacerbation of infection will result in inflammatory fibrosis and contracture of this portion of internal sphincter. Patients suffering with pain during the passage of a hard stool often take mineral oil or laxatives to keep the stool soft. This results in a minimal physiological dilatation, and the contracture becomes worse.

Anal fissures complicate Crohn's disease in over 60% of the patients. The fissures are large and frequently multiple, and the base is usually covered with purulent exudate. Fissures that involve the lateral aspect of the anal canal in adults are considered to be complications of inflammatory disease of the intestine such as Crohn's disease and ulcerative colitis until proved otherwise. Anal fissures complicating ulcerative colitis and Crohn's disease usually respond to medical treatment, and surgery is contraindicated.

INCIDENCE

In 2000 consecutive proctologic examinations, anal fissure was present in 216 patients (12.55%). Of these, 86% were located posteriorly, 10.75% anteriorly, 1.59% in the lateral position, and 1.59% were multiple.

CLINICAL MANIFESTATIONS

At the onset, pain can be excruciating during and after defecation and may persist for several hours. The extreme distress associated with pain from a fissure is frequently disabling. With medical treatment the pain may gradually become less severe. The fissure may become asymptomatic and quiescent for weeks or months, followed by repeated acute exacerbations when overstretching of the pecten area of the anal canal occurs. In addition to forming an abscess in the superficial postanal space or a collar button abscess between the lower edge of the internal and subcutaneous external sphincter, fissures may cause intermuscular abscess with cephalad extension into the supralevator spaces or transsphincteric extension to involve the infralevator spaces. Bleeding after bowel movement is noticed as streaks of blood on the toilet tissue or stool or as a few drops in the commode.

Constipation is frequently associated with fissure. Because of fear of pain, patients postpone defecation.

DIAGNOSIS

The characteristic history invariably suggests the diagnosis. The fissure can usually be seen on gentle traction on each side of the anus. A medium-sized anoscope can be inserted without too much discomfort after application of topical anesthetic, in order to confirm the diagnosis. Proctosigmoidoscopy is deferred. In some apprehensive patients suffering with great pain, anoscopy may be deferred if the diagnosis can be made by inspection. On rare occasions, the pain and the degree of stenosis require examination under anesthesia.

TREATMENT

Over 50% of patients with acute superficial fissure respond to conservative treatment. The patient is placed on a restricted fiber diet and a bulk laxative to minimize straining at defecation and to maintain regular bowel movements. Topical application of anesthetic ointments gives temporary relief of pain. If the conservative treatment fails to give adequate relief from pain, posterior injection of 2 ml to 4 ml of long-lasting anesthetic solution in oil will give immediate relief by relaxation of the anal sphincter. The needle is inserted in the skin ½ inch below the fissure and is placed deeply into the sphincters on each side of the posterior midline and deep to the fissure itself. The satisfactory permanent healing that may result is attributed to relaxation of the sphincters.

Lateral Internal Anal Sphincterotomy

Eisenhammer was the first to recommend internal sphincterotomy in the treatment of anal fissures. The procedure yields good functional results, with relief of pain and a negligible recurrence. The procedure is recommended as a primary operation for anal fissures by many authors. Lateral internal sphincterotomy is contraindicated in patients with abscess of fistula.

If large sentinel piles or hypertrophied anal papillae are associated with the fissure, they are excised. The patient remains in the hospital until the first bowel action and then goes home with a prescription for oral bulk stool laxative. He is seen in the office 1 week after surgery. No special anal care is necessary. The fissure heals in about 2 to 4 weeks, with only occasionally a minor defect of anal control.

Chronic anal ulcer persists because of inadequate drainage caused by spasm of the internal sphincter. The pain is also attributed to the spasm. The lateral internal sphincterotomy removes the spasm of the sphincter muscles, allowing adequate drainage and permitting normal healing to take place. Some authors believe that widening of the anal canal in the pecten portion plays an important part in healing.

Surgical Excision

After satisfactory caudal anesthesia, the anal canal is gradually dilated to three fingers breadths. A hemostat is placed on the base of the secondary hemorrhoid in the posterior midline and it is pulled out of the rectum. A transfixion suture is placed proximal to the hemorrhoid in the manner described under closed hemorrhoidectomy. Beginning at the anal verge, an elliptical incision is made about the fissure to include the sentinel pile, anal fissure, papilla, crypts, and internal hemorrhoid. The sentinel pile, fissure, papilla, crypt, and internal hemorrhoids are excised en masse (Fig. 26-37). An internal sphincterotomy in the posterior midline to the level of the conjoined longitudinal muscle is carried out, with the cephalad extension of the incision terminating at the level of the dentate line. The mucosa is dissected from the internal sphincter for a short distance before closing the wound transversely up to the lower edge of the internal sphincter at the level of the

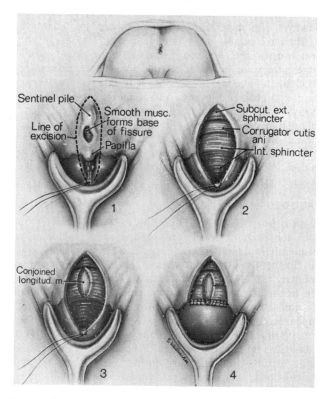

Fig. 26-37. Excision of anal fissure. (1) A submucosal transfixion suture is placed proximal to the posterior secondary hemorrhoid. The elliptical incision is illustrated to include "sentinel pile," fissure, papilla, crypts, posterior secondary internal hemorrhoids, and subepithelial tissue of the pecten. (2) The relationship of the subcutaneous external anal sphincter to the corrugator cutis ani and internal sphincter muscles after *en masse* excision of sentinel pile, fissure, papilla, crypts, and subepithelial tissue of the pecten. (3) The corrugator cutis ani and lower portion of the internal sphincter are severed to the anterior surface of the conjoined longitudinal muscle. The internal sphincterotomy extends cephalad to the level of the dentate line. (4) The rectal mucosa is sutured to the internal sphincter transversely. This increases the diameter of the pecten area of the anal canal. The sutures do not include the skin. The wound distal to the dentate line heals by secondary intention. (Hanley PH: Anorectum. In Hardy JD [ed]: Rhoads Textbook of Surgery, 5th ed. Philadelphia, J B Lippincott, 1977)

dentate line with a running lockstitch of plain No. 0 catgut. The suture is tied at the mucocutaneous junction, leaving the external part of the wound open. Suturing the elliptical incision transversely increases the diameter of the lower anorectum.

The wound may take 4 to 5 weeks to heal completely; however, the patient is relieved of pain and the amount of anal discharge from the healing wound seldom requires an anal dressing after 4 or 5 days. The results after complete healing have been excellent in regard to relief of pain, recurrence, continence, control of flatus, and soiling and are comparable to the present popular lateral internal sphincterotomy. Hanley has used this technique successfully over a period of 25 years.

Anal fissure is by far the most common anorectal disease in infancy and early childhood, with the majority of cases occurring from age 4 months through the second year. Although adults frequently require surgical treatment, infants usually respond to conservative medical management. Of 117 cases of pediatric anal fissure reported by Ellison, only one had to be treated surgically. Usually, 6 to 8 weeks of treatment are required to cure an anal fissure.

ABSCESS AND FISTULA-IN-ANO

With few exceptions, anorectal abscess fistula-in-ano is due to infection of anal glands in the space between the internal sphincter and the longitudinal muscle. From January 1950 to December 1974, 763 anorectal abscesses and 1432 anorectal fistulas-in-ano were treated at the Ochsner Clinic.

In most cases of acute abscess a curative operative procedure can be accomplished by a simpler procedure than that necessary to treat the complicated chronic fistulas-in-ano that may follow some anorectal abscesses.

Cultures from anorectal abscess fistulas usually are mixed infection, with *Escherichia coli* predominating; however, several organisms may be present, among which are *Pseudomonas aeruginosa*, *Staphylococcus aureus*, hemolytic streptococci, *Streptococcus faecalis*, *Enterobacter*, *Bacteroides*, and *Clostridium welchii*.

The consensus among anorectal surgeons is that there is no place for conservative medical treatment of anorectal abscess. Anorectal abscess should be considered a surgical emergency. Delay in surgical treatment only results in further destruction of tissue. Excision of the skin over the abscess cavity or skin grafting of the defect is not recommended. Usually, healing by secondary intention results in less scarring and deformity. The seton may be used as an adjunct in the surgical management of certain types of abscess fistula-in-ano with satisfactory results.

PERIANAL ABSCESS AND FISTULA-IN-ANO

The origin is from infected anal glands located in the lower intermuscular space (Fig. 26-38). Most frequently, the anal gland abscess ruptures into the perianal space, where it may remain confined. Less frequently, the abscess may form medially to the subcutaneous external sphincter. On rare occasions the pus ruptures transsphincterically into the ischiorectal space.

Most perianal abscesses are adjacent to the anus. Cellulitis, swelling, redness of the anal skin, and pain occur early. The cellulitis may be extensive and extend toward the buttocks and may be mistaken for an ischiorectal abscess. The cavity of a perianal abscess usually varies in size but seldom reaches 20 ml in capacity. The abscess will rupture

spontaneously through the skin, forming a secondary drainage site 3 cm to 6 cm from the anus, if not incised and drained. The pus is thick and creamy and has a foul odor.

Perianal abscess includes 50% to 75% anorectal abscesses and 35% to 40% will not recur as a fistula. Hughes stated that 75% of patients who have incision and drainage for perianal abscess have further problems: of 4000 cases taken consecutively and without selection at St. Marks Hospital, there were 196 abscesses, of which 151 recurred subsequently as fistulas. Infants rarely develop a fistula-in-ano after incision and drainage. If they do, the fistula may heal spontaneously. In selected cases in adults, fistulotomy at the time of incision and drainage may be appropriate. When a perianal abscess does not recur as a fistula, it is probably because of the inflammatory destruction of the anal duct or crypt. This prevents the infectious organisms from perpetuating the suppurative process, and resolution occurs without fistula formation. If fistula follows incision and drainage, the tract usually extends radially from the anus in a straight line for a short distance (3 cm to 5 cm). A fistulotomy to lay open the tract in its entirety is necessary to cure these. Some perianal abscesses in adults may be incised with the use of local anesthesia as an office procedure, making an incision over the abscess radially from the anus. Fluctuation of complicated abscesses should be evaluated using regional or general anesthesia because definitive treatment may be feasible to avoid the formation of complicated fistula-in-ano.

POSSIBLE SITES OF FISTULA AND ABSCESS

While the internal opening of the fistula will usually be at the dentate line in a crypt of Morgagni, the infection may force its way in a variety of directions as the abscess expands, finally to rupture at one site or another of the perineum. Goodsall's rule holds that if the external opening is anterior to an imaginary line drawn transversely across the midpoint of the anus, the fistula usually runs directly into the anal canal. If the external opening is posterior to the transverse line, the tract will usually curve to the posterior midline of the anal canal.

The locations of abscesses resulting from invasion of bacteria through the colon wall at the dentate line include most of the tissues and spaces surrounding the rectum. Moreover, there may be many branches of the fistulous process associated with a single internal opening. All ramifications must be identified and unroofed at the time of fistulotomy or fistulectomy. Injection of the external opening often assists in locating the internal opening and in identifying branches. There may of course be multiple external openings.

CHRONIC HORSESHOE FISTULA-IN-ANO

If a postanal abscess ruptures spontaneously or is incised over the ischiorectal fossa, the suppurative process will continue to recur, with periods of exacerbation and formation of new abscesses. Branching of the tracts with multiple secondary openings develops on one or both buttocks. The fistulous tracts from secondary skin openings converge, one with the other, to enter the deep postanal space as a common tract (Fig. 26-39).

A satisfactory method of treating chronic horseshoe fistula (Fig. 26-39) is similar to that used for the acute abscess. An incision in the posterior midline is made to sever in the coronal plane the subcutaneous external sphincter, the lower edge of the internal sphincter, and the superficial external

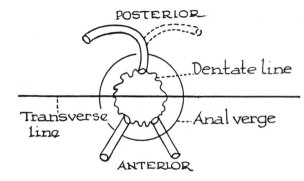

Fig. 26-38. *(Top)* Goodsall's rule—a transverse line divides fistula-in-ano into two groups: (1) When the secondary opening is anterior to a transverse line bisecting the anal canal into anterior and posterior halves, it is usually connected to the primary opening by a straight fistulous tract. (2) Secondary opening posterior to the transverse line is connected to a primary opening in the midline by a curved fistulous tract that may be horseshoe or semihorseshoe in pattern. *(Bottom)* Left side of illustration demonstrates the usual location of the anal gland and its duct. *(A)* Abscess in low intermuscular space may rupture through the medial termination of the longitudinal muscle superior to the subcutaneous external sphincter into the perianal space *(C)*. *(B)* Rupture between subcutaneous external sphincter and lower internal sphincter forms a subcutaneous abscess in the lower anal canal. *(C)* Perianal space referred to in *(A)*. *(D)* Rarely the low intermuscular abscess ruptures transsphincterically into the ischiorectal fossa. *(E)* Ischioanal abscess with fistulous tract passing between deep and superficial external anal sphincter. *(F)* Submucous abscess with resulting fistulous tract. (Hanley P, Hines MO: Anus, perianal and rectal regions. In Ochsner A, DeBakey ME [eds]: Christopher's Minor Surgery. Philadelphia, W B Saunders, 1955)

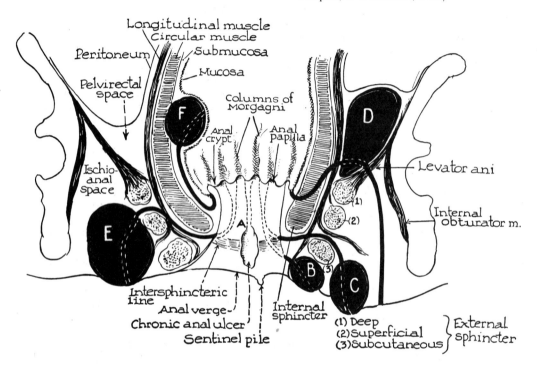

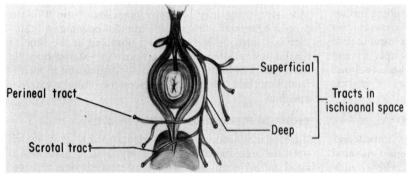

Fig. 26-39. In chronic horseshoe abscess fistula-in-ano with multiple secondary skin openings, the tracts join one with the other to enter the deep postanal space as a common tract. (Hanley PH: Anorectum. In Hardy JD [ed]: Rhoads Textbook of Surgery, 5th ed. Philadelphia, J B Lippincott, 1977)

sphincter muscles into halves. The incision opens the deep postanal space and exposes the chronic fistulous tract. The tract is easily identified by inspection and palpation. It is directly posterior to the deep external sphincter muscle. The tract at its point of bifurcation into left and right branches is grasped with a forceps and is excised by sharp dissection, including 1 cm of the tract that extends under the superficial external sphincter.

In some cases, it is feasible to core the tract out with sharp dissection without severing the superficial external sphincter muscle. In subacute horseshoe abscess fistulas, fistulotomy of the T-portion of the tract followed by curettage with a sharp bone forceps of the entire tract is all that is necessary. The secondary openings of the fistulous tracts are enlarged by incision to permit curettage of the granulation tissue. The wounds heal in 5 to 12 weeks with minimal posterior defect of the anus and with no complaint of incontinence.

SUPERFICIAL ANTERIOR PERIANAL SPACE ABSCESS FISTULA-IN-ANO

Superficial anterior anal space abscess fistula without sphincter involvement is treated by simple fistulotomy incision. However, if the tract passes superior to the subcutaneous external sphincter, in a female patient, it is advisable to place an elastic seton around the subcutaneous external sphincter after incision and drainage if a primary opening is present (Fig. 26-40).

ISCHIORECTAL ABSCESS FISTULA-IN-ANO

The most frequent cause of suppuration in the ischiorectal fossae is extension of pus from a deep postanal abscess and, rarely, from the deep anterior anal space. Very rarely,

Fig. 26-40. Fistulotomy. *Top,* for superficial subcutaneous fistula-in-ano: *(A)* skin incised over probe, *(B)* skin edges excised with scissors, *(C)* granulating wounds heal from within outward. *Bottom:* Under local anesthesia a fistulotomy incision is made to the subcutaneous external sphincter muscle. Rubber-band seton is used in female patients. (Hanley PH: Anorectum. In Hardy JD [ed]: Rhoads Textbook of Surgery, 5th ed. Philadelphia, J B Lippincott, 1977)

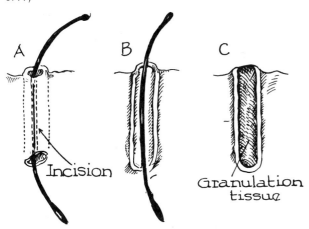

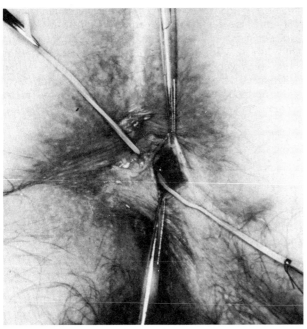

intermuscular suppuration may rupture directly in a lateral direction into the ischiorectal fossa without first involving the deep anal spaces. Rarely, suppuration from supralevator abscess may dissect downward through the levator or between the puborectalis and the rectal wall to involve the ischiorectal space. Although pus in the ischiorectal fossa from a deep posterior or a deep anterior anal space abscess can extend anterior to the scrotum, groin, or thighs, a primary ischiorectal abscess usually extends into the perianal space. It is more likely to rupture and surface to the skin over the ischiorectal fossa.

Deep ischiorectal abscess should be treated under anesthesia to detect primary posterior and anterior anal space suppuration. When found, as is commonly the case, treatment is as described under deep anal space abscess. If the abscess is diagnosed as a very rare primary ischiorectal abscess without evidence of a primary fistulous opening in a lateral crypt, simple drainage should suffice. If there is a primary fistulous opening in a lateral crypt, with the tract entering the ischiorectal fossa in a straight line between the superficial and deep components of the external sphincters or, more rarely, between the deep and puborectalis muscle, a staged procedure with the use of an elastic seton is recommended.

SUPRALEVATOR ABSCESS

Over 90% of intermuscular abscesses rupture into the infralevator spaces. On rare occasions an intermuscular abscess enlarges cephalad above the anorectal ring and ruptures through the longitudinal muscle, which is poorly supported at this level, into the supralevator space. Infrequently, the intermuscular abscess may rupture through the thin circular muscle layer of the rectum above the thick internal sphincter, into the rectum.

SUBCUTANEOUS ANAL CANAL ABSCESS

Subcutaneous abscess originates from infected anal glands located in the subepithelial space of the pecten. The abscess involves the lower anal canal presenting at the anal verge, medial to the subcutaneous external sphincter, but the tract subcutaneously connects to a crypt and does not penetrate the internal sphincter muscle and is not of intermuscular origin. These abscesses usually rupture spontaneously through the anal skin if they are not incised and drained. Abscess of this type is usually treated in the office under local anesthesia. If a subcutaneous fistula subsequently occurs, simple fistulotomy of the tract is all that is necessary.

ANAL INCONTINENCE

Anal incontinence may be due to a wide variety of causes, including old age, neurologic defects, hemorrhoids or hemorrhoid surgery, rectal prolapse, chronic inflammation with suppuration and fibrosis (as in granulomatous colitis), as well as many other factors. Neoplasm must be ruled out. Specific treatment directed to the underlying cause may permit recovery of bowel control. If the external sphincter was divided at a previous operation, it may be exposed beneath the mucosa and repaired. However, in extreme instances a permanent sigmoid colostomy may be required.

ANAL STRICTURE

Anal stricture may follow many of the conditions that cause anal incontinence. Here again, neoplasm must be excluded, by biopsy if necessary. If the stricture is "soft" and the disease process has been arrested, progressive dilatations aided by oral intake of stool softeners, may provide and maintain a lumen of adequate size. A "hard" fibrous stricture usually is not improved by efforts at dilatation. Operations on the stricture itself are usually unsuccessful. Occasionally, permanent sigmoid colostomy is required.

VENEREAL DISEASES

CONDYLOMATA ACUMINATA

Condylomata acuminata, or anal venereal warts, are apparently caused by a papillomavirus. They occur principally on the perineum and around the anus, often involving the squamous epithelium of the anal canal. They may be small or large and extensive.

This condition can be most difficult to cure. Small warts are usually treated with application of podophyllin solution, while large ones that obstruct the anal canal may be cauterized or excised. Unfortunately, they are very likely to recur and rarely may be associated with carcinoma. At times an abdominoperineal resection with permanent sigmoid colostomy will be required.

LYMPHOGRANULOMA VENEREUM

Lymphogranuloma venereum is caused by *Chlamydia trachomatis*. It is sexually transmitted and primarily involves the genitals and regional lymph nodes, although in one fourth of the patients the rectum is involved. Diagnosis of the rectal disease is made by proctoscopy with biopsy of the mucosa, as well as the Frei test and complement fixation. Treatment is usually with tetracycline. Late complications may include rectal stricture, rectovaginal or anal fistulas, and destruction of the anal canal. The rectal stricture usually occurs 3 cm to 5 cm from the anus, but the entire rectum may be involved. Occasionally, rectal dilatation is sufficient treatment for the stricture; advanced cases of any of the complications mentioned above may require colostomy and abdominoperineal resection.

PRURITUS ANI

Pruritus ani is a chronic itching in the anal area that can be very distressing in its intensity and, at times, even painful. The symptoms reflect inflammation, which may be secondary to poor hygiene, hemorrhoids, fungus infections, parasites (including pinworms), and many other conditions. After infectious conditions and lesions such as hemorrhoids have been excluded, symptomatic relief may be obtained with locally applied zinc oxide ointment, anesthetic ointment or corticosteroid cream. Hot sitz baths twice daily, followed by careful drying and application of an absorbent nonirritating powder, may be helpful. In some patients there is a considerable emotional element to the symptoms, and, if present, this must be handled appropriately.

NEOPLASMS OF THE ANUS

EPIDERMOID CARCINOMA

Anal carcinoma represents about 2% of cancers of the large bowel (Fig. 26-41). In 204 patients reported from the Mayo

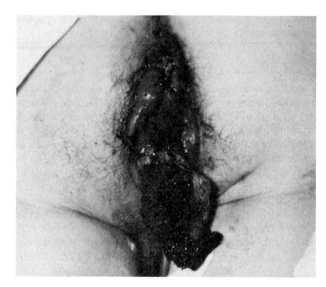

Fig. 26-41. Anal carcinoma.

Clinic, 113 had squamous carcinoma (31 perianal), 64 had basaloid squamous carcinoma, 8 had Paget's disease of the anus, 7 had melanoma, 6 had basal cell carcinoma, and 6 had adenocarcinoma. Combined abdominoperineal resection was the treatment of choice except for perianal lesions, for which local excision was used most frequently. Inguinal node excision was used infrequently. The 5-year survival rate varied with the presence of lymph node involvement and, in certain circumstances, with the histologic type. The 5-year survival rate reported by Beahrs and Wilson for squamous cell carcinoma was 58% following abdominoperineal resection. At present, local excision, rather than abdominoperineal resection, is used more often.

MALIGNANT MELANOMA

Malignant melanoma of the anal canal is a rare condition and represents something less than 1% of anal tumors. These melanomas are less common only than those of the skin or eye and arise mainly from the epidermoid layer, adjacent to the dentate line. Features such as pain, itching, or bleeding can result in a diagnosis of hemorrhoids, and biopsy is essential, especially with the amelanotic type. As a rule, however, the tumor is pigmented. Spread of the malignancy is by lymphatics (perhaps one third of cases) or by the bloodstream. Widespread hematogenous spread is common and usually is the cause of death. Radical resection with abdominoperineal technique is usually employed, but early metastasis prevents cure in most patients.

MELANOSIS COLI AND FECAL IMPACTION

Melanosis coli is a benign black or brown pigmentation of the colon, occurring in patients ingesting anthracene cathartics (cascara, senna) for long periods. It is also occasionally seen in patients with carcinoma of the colon, possibly as a result of stasis. It usually resolves in a few months to a year, if the predisposing conditions are eliminated.

Fecal impaction is most often seen in patients that are inactive or at bed rest, in those that are older, and in those with mental illness. Although these patients may present with obstruction, the clinical pattern most often consists of watery diarrhea or constipation. The diagnosis is made by rectal and abdominal examination. Treatment is by digital manipulation and extraction, followed by oil and saline enemas. Occasionally, general anesthesia and rectal dilatation may be necessary and, very rarely, laparotomy. Prevention is by bulk laxatives as well as cathartics, stool softeners, and occasionally enemas.

In the preparation of this chapter the author has drawn on material presented in *Rhoads Textbook of Surgery, 5th edition* (JD Hardy, editor), Philadelphia, JB Lippincott, 1977, by the following authors: Hardy JD, Bailey RV: Anatomy and Physiology of the Colon and Rectum; Sawyers JL: Granulomatous Colitis and Ulcerative Colitis Including Toxic Megacolon; Welch CE: Colon Hemorrhage; Kurzweg FT: Acute Traumatic Perforations of the Colon and Rectum; Barnett WO: Large Bowel Obstruction: Approach to Management; Johnston JH, Jr: Diverticular Disease of the Colon; Wilson H, Cheek RC: Volvulus of the Colon; Leffall LD Jr: Polyps of the Colon and Rectum; Cohn I, Jr, Nelson JL: Carcinoma of the Colon (Excluding the Rectum); Hunt TK, Schrock TR: Colonic Anastomosis: Healing and Problems; Veidenheimer MC: Carcinoma of the Rectum; Altemeier WA: Rectal Prolapse; Hanley PH: Anorectum; and Hardy JD, Bailey RV: Other Disorders of the Colon, Rectum, and Anus.

BIBLIOGRAPHY

Inflammatory Diseases: Granulomatous Colitis and Ulcerative Colitis

BEAHRS OH: Use of ileal reservoir following proctocolectomy. Surg Gynecol Obstet 141:363, 1975

BERCOVITZ ZT, KIRSNER JB, LINDNER AE et al: Ulcerative and Granulomatous Colitis. Springfield, IL, Charles C Thomas, 1973

BROOKE BN: Management of ileostomy. Lancet II:102, 1952

CROHN BB, GINZBURG L, OPPENHEIMER GD: Regional ileitis: A pathologic and clinical entity. JAMA 99:1323, 1932

GOLIGHER JC: Treatment of chronic ulcerative colitis. Curr Prob Surg 2:1, 1965

HINTON JM: Risk of malignant change in ulcerative colitis. Gut 7:427, 1966

MacDOUGALL IPM: The cancer risk in ulcerative colitis. Lancet II:655, 1964

MARSHAK RH, LESTER LJ, FRIEDMAN AI: Megacolon: A complication of ulcerative colitis. Gastroenterology 16:768, 1950

MENGUY RB: Indications for surgery. In Bercovitz ZT, Kirsner JB, Lindner AE et al: Ulcerative and Granulomatous Colitis. Springfield, IL, Charles C Thomas, 1973

MORSON BC, LOCKHART-MUMMERY HE: Crohn's disease of the colon. Gastroenterologia 92:168, 1959

OBERHELMAN HA, KOHATSU S, TAYLOR KB et al: Diverting ileostomy in the surgical management of Crohn's disease of the colon. Am J Surg 115:231, 1968

RITCHIE JK, HAWLEY PR, LENNARD-JONES JE: Prognosis of carcinoma in ulcerative colitis. Gut 22:752, 1981

SCOTT HW JR, SAWYERS JL, GOBBEL WG Jr et al: Surgical management of toxic dilatation of the colon in ulcerative colitis. Ann Surg 179:647, 1974

SERRANO A, MICHEL L, WARSAW, AL et al: Colonic obstruction as a complication of ulcerative colitis. Dis Colon Rectum 24:487, 1981

SINGER HC, ANDERSON JGD, FRISCHER H et al: Familial aspects of inflammatory bowel disease. Gastroenterology 61:423, 1971

SPIRO HM: Complications of colitis. In Clinical Gastroenterology. London, Collier-Macmillan, 1979

TELANDER RL, SMITH SL, MARCINEK HM et al: Surgical treatment of ulcerative colitis in children. Surgery 90:787, 1981

TURNBULL RB, HAWK WA, WEAKLEY FL: Surgical treatment of toxic megacolon: Ileostomy and colostomy to prepare patients for colectomy. Am J Surg 122:325, 1971

WEEDON DD, SHORTER RG, ILSTRUP DM et al: Crohn's disease and cancer. N Engl J Med 289:1099, 1973

Diverticular Disease of the Colon

BACON HE, TSE GN, HERABAT T: Coexisting carcinoma with diverticulitis of the colon. Dis Colon Rectum 16:500, 1973

BEER E: Some pathological and clinical aspects of acquired (false) diverticula of the intestine. Am J Med Sci 128:135, 1904

COLCOCK BP, STAHMANN FD: Fistulas complicating diverticular disease of the sigmoid colon. Ann Surg 175:838, 1972

LABOW SB, SALVATI EP, RUBIN RJ: The Hartmann procedure in the treatment of diverticular disease. Dis Colon Rectum 16:392, 1973

Limitations of radiology in differentiation of diverticulitis and diverticulosis of the colon. Br Med J 2:136, 1970

MADDEN JL: Primary resection in the treatment of perforated lesions of the colon. Am Surg 31:781, 1965

MAYO CW, BLUNT CP: Vesicosigmoidal fistulas complicating diverticulitis. Surg Gynecol Obstet 61:612, 1950

MAYO WJ, WILSON LB, GRIFFIN HZ: Acquired diverticulitis of the large intestine. Surg Gynecol Obstet 5:8, 1907

MORSON BC: The muscle abnormality in diverticular disease of the sigmoid colon. Br J Radiol 36:385, 1963

PERRY PM, MORSON BC: Right-sided diverticulosis of colon. Br J Surg 38:902, 1971

REILLY M: Sigmoid myotomy for acute diverticulitis. Dis Colon Rectum 8:42, 1965

RYAN P: Emergency resection and anastomosis for perforated sigmoid diverticulitis. Br J Surg 45:611, 1958

Acute Traumatic Perforations of the Colon and Rectum

ANDRESEN AFR: Perforations from proctoscopy. Gastroenterology 9:32, 1947

CORKERY JJ, DUBOWITZ V, LISTER J et al: Colonic perforation after exchange transfusion. Br Med J 4:345, 1968

GANCHROW MI, LAVENSON GS JR, McNAMARA JJ: Surgical management of traumatic injuries of the colon and rectum. Arch Surg 100:515, 1970

NOVEROSKE RJ: Perforation of a normal colon by too much pressure. J Indiana State Med Assoc 65:23, 1972

WESTFALL RH, NELSON RH, MUSSELMAN MM: Barium peritonitis. Am J Surg 112:760, 1966

Tumors of the Colon and Rectum
Polyps

CASTLEMAN B, KRICKSTEIN HD: Do adenomatous polyps of the colon become malignant? N Engl J Med 26:469, 1962

COLACCHIO TA, FORDE KA, SCANTLEBURY VP: Endoscopic polypectomy: Inadequate treatment for invasive colorectal carcinoma. Ann Surg 194:704, 1981

CRONKHITE LW JR, CANADA WJ: Generalized gastrointestinal polyposis. N Engl J Med 252:1014, 1955

FENOGLIO CM, LANE N: The anatomic precursor of colorectal carcinoma. JAMA 231:640, 1975

MORSON BC, BUSSEY HR: Predisposing causes of intestinal cancer. Curr Probl Surg 7:3, February 1970

SACHATELLO CR, GRIFFEN WO: Hereditary polypoid diseases of the gastrointestinal tract. Am J Surg 128:198, 1975

SHERLOCK P, LIPKIN M, WINAWER SJ: Predisposing factors in colon carcinoma. Adv Intern Med 20:121, 1975

WOLFF WE, SHINYA H: A new approach to colonic polyps. Ann Surg 178:367, 1973

Carcinoma of the Colon

BOEY J, CHOI TK, WONG J et al: Carcinoma of the colon and rectum with liver involvement. Surg Gynecol Obstet 153:864, 1981

BURKITT DP: An epidemiologic approach to cancer of the large intestine: The significance of disease relationships. Dis Colon Rectum 17:456, 1974

FISHER ER, TURNBULL RB JR: The cytologic demonstration and significance of tumor cells in the mesenteric venous blood in patients with colorectal carcinoma. Surg Gynecol Obstet 100:102, 1955

GOLD P, FREEDMAN SO: Demonstration of tumor-specific antigens in human colonic carcinomata by immunological tolerance and absorption techniques. J Exp Med 121:439, 1965

GOLD P, FREEDMAN SO: Specific carcinoembryonic antigens of the human digestive system. J Exp Med 122:467, 1965

GOLIGHER JC: Surgery of the Anus, Rectum and Colon. Springfield, IL, Charles C Thomas, 1967

GOLIGHER JC, GRAHAM NG, DEDOMBAL FT: Anastomotic dehiscence after anterior resection of rectum and sigmoid. Br J Surg 57:109, 1970

GRIFFITHS JD, MCKINNA JA, ROWBOTHAM HD et al: Carcinoma of the colon and rectum: Circulating malignant cells and five-year survival. Cancer 31:226, 1973

HILL MJ, ARIES VC: Faecal steroid composition and its relationship to cancer of the large bowel. J Pathol 104:129, 1971

IRVIN TT, HUNT TK: Pathogenesis and prevention of disruption of colonic anastomoses in traumatized rats. Br J Surg 61:437, 1974

KIRWAN WO: Integrity of low colorectal EEA-stapled anastomosis. Br J Surg 68:539, 1981

KLEIN PJ, OSMERS R, VIERBUCHEN M et al: The importance of lectin-binding sites and carcinoembryonic antigen with regard to normal, hyperplastic, adenomatous and carcinomatous mucosa. Recent Results Cancer Res 79:1, 1981

SCHROCK TR, DEVENEY CW, DUNPHY JE: Factors contributing to leakage of colonic anastomoses. Ann Surg 177:513, 1973

TURNBULL RB, JR, KYLE K, WATSON FR et al: Cancer of the colon: The influence of the no-touch isolation technic on survival rates. Ann Surg 166:420, 1967

WOLFF WI, SHINYA H, GEFFEN A et al: Colonofiberoscopy: A new and valuable diagnostic modality. Am J Surg 123:180, 1972

Carcinoma of the Rectum

BLACK BM, WALLS JT: Combined abdominoendorectal resection: Reappraisal of a pull-through procedure. Surg Clin North Am 47:977, 1967

BURKITT DP: Epidemiology of cancer of the colon and rectum. Cancer 28:3, 1971

CADY B, PERSSON AV, MONSON DO et al: Changing patterns of colorectal cancer. Cancer 33:422, 1974

DUKES CE: Cancer of rectum: Analysis of 1000 cases. J Pathol 50:527, 1940

GOLD P, FREEDMAN SO: Demonstration of tumor-specific antigens in human colonic carcinoma by immunological tolerance and absorption techniques. J Exp Med 121:439, 1965

GOLIGHER JC, GRAHAM NG, DEDOMBAL FT: Anastomotic dehiscence after anterior resection of rectum and sigmoid. Br J Surg 57:109, 1970

GRINNELL RS: Distal intramural spread of carcinoma of rectum and rectosigmoid. Surg Gynecol Obstet 99:421, 1954

HIGGINS GA, JR, DWIGHT RW, WALSH WS et al: Preoperative radiation therapy as an adjuvant to surgery for carcinoma of the colon and rectum. Am J Surg 115:241, 1968

MADDEN JL, KANDALAFT S: Electrocoagulation in the treatment of cancer of the rectum: A continuing study. Ann Surg 174:530, 1971

PAPILLON J: Radiation therapy in the management of epidermoid carcinoma of the anal region. Dis Colon Rectum 17:181, 1974

SPRATT JS, JR, ACKERMAN LB: Pathologic significance of polyps of the rectum and colon. Dis Colon Rectum 3:330, 1960

STRAUSS AA, STRAUSS SF, CRAWFORD RA et al: Surgical diathermy of carcinoma of rectum: Its clinical end results. JAMA 104:1480, 1935

VEIDENHEIMER MC: Alternatives to surgery in the treatment of carcinoma of the rectum. Surg Clin North Am 41:815, 1971

Volvulus of the Colon

Sigmoid Volvulus

ARNOLD GJ, NANCE FC: Volvulus of the sigmoid colon. Ann Surg 177:427, 1973

BALLANTYNE GH: Sigmoid volvulus: High mortality in county hospital patients. Dis Colon Rectum 24:515, 1981

SHEPHERD JJ: The epidemiology and clinical presentation of sigmoid volvulus. Br J Surg 46:353, 1969

WILSON H, DUNAVANT WD: Volvulus of the sigmoid colon. Surg Clin North Am 45:1245, 1965

Cecal Volvulus

WOLFE RY, WILSON H: Emergency operation for volvulus of the cecum: Review of twenty-two cases. Am Surg 32:96, 1966

Rare Types

CUDERMAN BS, ROBACH SA, WEINTRAUB WH et al: Volvulus of transverse colon. Surgery 69:797, 1971

MCGARITY WC, BOBO WE, HAYNES CD: Volvulus of splenic flexure of the colon: Report of two cases and literature review. Am Surg 32:425, 1966

Rectal Prolapse

ALTEMEIER WA, CULBERTSON WR, SCHOWENGERDT C et al: Nineteen years' experience with the one-stage perineal repair of rectal prolapse. Ann Surg 173:993, 1971

ALTEMEIER WA, GIUSEFFI J, HOXWORTH P: Treatment of extensive prolapse of rectum in aged and debilitated patients. Arch Surg 65:72, 1952

BADEN H, MIKKELSEN O: Results of rectopexy in complete prolapse of rectum in adults. Acta Chir Scand 116:230, 1959

GRAHAM RR: The operative repair of massive rectal prolapse. Ann Surg 115:1007, 1942

MILES WE: Rectosigmoidectomy as method of treatment for procidentia recti. Proc R Soc Lond 26:1445, 1933

MORGAN CN: Prolapse of rectum: Use of Ivalon sponge. Proc R Soc Lond 55:1084, 1962

MOSCHCOWITZ AV: Pathogenesis, anatomy, and cure of prolapse of rectum. Surg Gynecol Obstet 15:7, 1912

RIPSTEIN CB, LANTER B: Etiology and surgical therapy of massive prolapse of rectum. Ann Surg 157:259, 1963

TODD TW: Anatomical considerations in rectal prolapse of infants. Ann Surg 71:163, 1920

WELLS C: New operation for prolapse of rectum. Proc R Soc Lond 52:602, 1959

Anorectum

BEAHRS OH, WILSON SM: Carcinoma of the anus. Ann Surg 184:422, 1976

BARRON J: Office ligation of internal hemorrhoids. Am J Surg 105:563, 1963

BARRON J: Office ligation and treatment of hemorrhoids. Dis Colon Rectum 6:109, 1963

BERKOW SG, TOLK NR: Ischiorectal abscess followed by gas gangrene: Gas gangrene following trauma. JAMA 80:1689, 1923

BRODIE BC: Clinical Lectures on Surgery, Vol 36, p. 322. Philadelphia, Lea & Febiger, 1846

CALDAROLA VT, JACKMAN RJ, MOERTEL CG et al: Carcinoid tumors of the rectum. Am J Surg 107:844, 1964

CAMMERER RC, ANDERSON DL, BOYCE HW JR et al: Clinical spectrum of pseudomembraneous colitis. JAMA 235:2502, 1976

CAMPBELL ED: Prevention of urinary retention after anorectal operations. Dis Colon Rectum 15:69, 1972

CATTERALL RD: Sexually transmitted diseases of the anus and rectum. Clin Gastroenterol 4:659, 1975

EISENHAMMER S: The surgical correction of chronic anal (sphincteric) contracture. S Afr Med J 25:486, 1951

ELLISON FS: Anal fissure occurring in infants and children. Dis Colon Rectum 3:161, 1960

FERGUSON JA, HEATON JR: Closed hemorrhoidectomy. Dis Colon Rectum 2:176, 1959

GRACE R: Problems of minor anal surgery: A review. J R Soc Med 73:576, 1980

HANLEY PH, HINES MO: Analysis of two thousand consecutive proctologic examinations. South Med J 49:475, 1956

HUGHES ESR: Inflammation and infection of the anus. In Turrell R (ed): Disease of the Colon and Anorectum, Chap 44. Philadelphia, WB Saunders, 1959

JEFFERY PJ, MILLER W, RITCHIE SM, et al: The treatment of hemorrhoids by rubber band ligation at St. Mark's Hospital. Postgrad Med J 56:847, 1980

LEWIS MI: Cryosurgical hemorrhoidectomy: A follow-up report. Dis Colon Rectum 15:128, 1972

MADDEN MV, ELLIOTT MS, BOTHA JBC et al: The management of anal carcinoma. Br J Surg 68:287, 1981

McGIVNEY J: Ligation treatment of internal hemorrhoids. Tex Med 63:56, 1967

MENTZER CG: Symposium on pediatric proctology. Anorectal disease. Pediatr Clin North Am 3:113, 1956

MILLIGAN ETC: Summary of Proceedings of 107th Annual Meeting British Medical Association—Section of Surgery. Br Med J 2:412, 1939

PARKS AG: Hemorrhoidectomy. Adv Surg 51:1, 1971

PESSEL JF: Intestinal endometriosis. In Bockus HL (ed): Gastroenterology, 2nd ed, Vol 11, Chap 74. Philadelphia, WB Saunders, 1964

QUAN SHQ: Factitial proctitis due to irradiation for cancer of the cervix uteri. Surg Gynecol Obstet 126:70, 1968

ROSSER C: Chemical rectal stricture. JAMA 96:1762, 1931

SALVATI EP: Evaluation of ligation of hemorrhoids as an office procedure. Dis Colon Rectum 10:53, 1967

WANEBO HJ, WOODRUFF JM, QUAN SH: Anorectal melanoma. Cancer 47:1891, 1981

27

The Liver, Gallbladder, and Biliary Tract

George Johnson, Jr./C. Thomas Nuzum

Anatomy, Physiology, Pathophysiology, and Portal Hypertension

The liver has a tremendous influence on essentially every biochemical and physiological function in the body. Unlike other organs, it has been impossible to substitute for the liver in any meaningful fashion. It has enormous influence on glucose, protein, and fat metabolism, as well as on some of the many humoral agents. The diseases are mainly those related to destruction of the hepatic parenchyma with the resulting scarring. As the liver parenchyma repairs itself, abnormal distortions of the portal hemodynamics may develop. Where the portal system attempts to correct these hemodynamics, other pathological entities develop, and thus the patient may die of the secondary pathology of cirrhosis of the liver rather than of liver failure *per se*.

The therapy of portal hypertension and its associated complications has vacillated frequently throughout the years. Current thoughts on controlling the portal hypertension or at least the esophageal varices that result include total shunts, selective shunts, and procedures that attempt to ablate the esophageal collateral circulation.

ANATOMY

A thorough understanding of the blood supply to and of the liver is necessary if one is to appreciate the gross and microscopic anatomy. Grisham (1976) says "form and function of the liver are stringently dependent on the characteristics of blood supply to this organ." This was true even in the developing embryo (Fig. 27-1). The celiac and mesenteric arteries are developed in the dorsal mesentery of the foregut and enter into the septum transversum. The vitelline veins from the yolk sac enter the septum transversum to form a mass of anastomosing veins.

A hollow endothelial bud from the foregut enters the septum transversum, bifurcates, and produces epithelial trabeculae, which enter the area of the anastomosing veins in the septum transversum. The endodermal bud becomes the liver cells, and the spaces between them become the sinusoids. The vitelline vein becomes the portal and hepatic veins and the terminal segment of the inferior vena cava.

The gallbladder develops as a separate bud from the main hollow endothelial bud that arose from the foregut.

Although there were two umbilical veins, only the one on the left persists; it enters into the left branch of the portal vein. The ductus venosus allows the liver to be bypassed by connecting the left portal vein to the inferior vena cava. The umbilical vein closes after birth and becomes the ligamentum teres; the ductus venosus closes and becomes the ligamentum venosum.

The ability to dilate and cannulate the remnant of the umbilical vein that enters the left portal vein has been used as a method to gain access to the portal venous circulation for physiological, biochemical, and radiologic studies.

BLOOD SUPPLY

Approximately 25% of the cardiac output goes through the liver. The liver weighs 1200 g to 1400 g. Thus, it receives 1 ml/minute/g of blood. Only 30% of this is supplied by the hepatic artery at arterial pressure, whereas 70% comes from the splanchnic vascular bed through the portal vein at a pressure of 7 torr to 10 torr.

The extrahepatic portion of the hepatic artery (Fig. 27-2) arises from the celiac axis and gives origin to the cystic and gastroduodenal branches, as well as to the vasa vasorum, which supply the hepatic vessels in the hepatic hilus and then go to a diffuse plexus over the hepatic capsule. This capsular plexus, which anastomoses with branches of the inferior phrenic artery, may become very important in supplying arterial blood to the liver when the hepatic arterial flow is deficient. The hepatic artery terminates by dividing into right and left branches just before entering the liver.

The portal vein is formed by the confluence of the splenic and superior mesenteric veins. It also receives blood from small pancreatic veins and the right and left pyloric veins. The right pyloric vein (coronary vein) may become a major collateral channel connecting the splanchnic circulation to the systemic circulation by the azygos system. The submucosal veins in the esophagus are a part of this collateral channel. They are poorly supported by connective tissue and thus are prone to rupture and bleed. The portal vein, as it enters the liver, divides into right and left branches. The right branch receives the cystic vein, and the left branch, at which the ligamentum teres ends, receives a number of small paraumbilical veins. In portal hypertension, the umbilical vein at times becomes widely patent and a caput medusae surrounding the umbilicus develops.

The extrahepatic portal venous drainage is composed of the greater and lesser splanchnic systems (Fig. 27-3). The greater splanchnic system drains the large and small intestine and consists of the superior and inferior mesenteric veins and the portal vein. The lesser splanchnic system drains the stomach, pancreas, and spleen and consists of the splenic vein, the pancreatic veins that drain into the splenic and portal veins, the right (coronary) and left pyloric veins, and the right and left gastroepiploic veins. When normal portal venous hemodynamics are present, most of the blood flows into the liver. There are several actual and potential anastomoses between the portal and the systemic venous circulation; these include the coronary–esophageal–azygos, hemorrhoidals–internal iliac, umbilical–epigastrics, splenic–adrenal, capsular–diaphragmatic–inferior vena cava, and duodenal–inferior vena cava, to name a few. In portal hypertension, these collateral channels may carry consid-

Fig. 27-1. Development of the liver and its vascular supply.

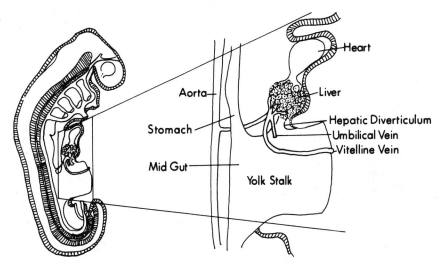

Aorta

Stomach

Mid Gut

Heart

Liver

Hepatic Diverticulum

Umbilical Vein

Vitelline Vein

Yolk Stalk

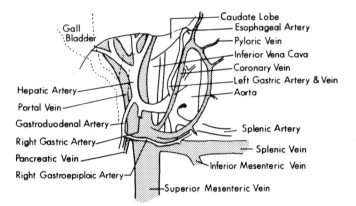

Fig. 27-2. Arteries and veins to the liver.

erable blood in an attempt to decompress the portal venous system. In ablative or selective shunt operations, to be discussed, it is important to know of their existence.

The intrahepatic vessels form a skeleton of the liver, which is strengthened by the investment of afferent vessels with areolar connective tissues continuous with the surface capsule. After entering the liver, the right and left portal veins divide into rami that supply the various segments of the liver (Fig. 27-4). Conducting and distributing portal veins give origin to the inlet or terminal portal veins, which pierce the limiting plate of the portal tract. The branches of the hepatic artery and portal vein and the ductules and ducts of the biliary system, with accompanying nerves, lymphatics, and supporting areolar connective tissue, make up the portal tract.

The inlet venules empty into the plexus of anastomosing sinusoids, which are lined by nonphagocytic endothelial cells interspersed with phagocytes (Kupffer's cells). Thus, the hepatocytes have easy access to the blood in the sinusoids. The sinusoids then empty into the hepatic (central) vein, which weaves throughout the course of the hepatic parenchyma without ever connecting directly to the portal tract. There are three major groups of hepatic veins located between parenchymal segments.

Fig. 27-3. Schema of the extrahepatic venous system (*IVC,* inferior vena cava).

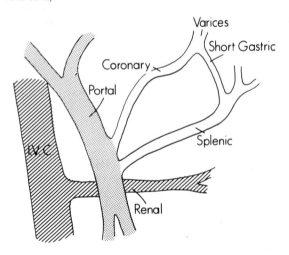

Ⓖ Greater Splanchnic Circulation

Ⓞ Lesser Splanchnic Circulation

Ⓢ Systemic Venous Circulation

The course of the hepatic artery is similar to that of the portal vein. Within the portal tract, the artery supplies a diffuse system of capillaries within the connective tissue and a more distinct peribiliary plexus. Portal vein branches connect with the peribiliary plexus, creating a presinusoidal arteriovenous fistula. The physiological importance of these arteriovenous communications is not determined. They may be especially prominent in cirrhosis and thus contribute to the portal vein hypertension.

MICROSTRUCTURE

The parenchyma of the normal liver is continuous throughout, with no structural subunit that can be dissected along connective tissue planes. The hepatocytes are rhomboidal in shape and are stacked to form continuous plates. Sinusoids fill the spaces between parenchymal plates. Disse's spaces in the subendothelium of the sinusoids develop from numerous enfoldings of the plasma membrane and give an increased surface area between the hepatocyte and the sinusoid for exchange of substrate, electrolytes, fluid, and other substances. Fluid from these spaces drains into the lymphatics of the portal tracts.

BILIARY DRAINAGE

The hepatocyte has 8 to 12 sharply faceted surfaces every one of which not in contact with a sinusoid is occupied by a canaliculus. After passing through the limiting plate, these canaliculi merge to form the smallest radicle of the biliary system, the ductule. The ductules empty into the bile duct of the portal tract, which in turn closely follows the branches of the portal vein to drain eventually into the common bile duct.

INNERVATION

The nerves to the liver derive from both the vagus and the right phrenic nerves, and from the celiac axis. These form a plexus around the vessels and ducts in the hepatoduodenal ligament and enter the liver at the hilus. There is little evidence that hepatic parenchyma is directly innervated. Hepatic vessels receive only adrenergic fibers, stimulation of which causes action on vascular smooth muscle that produces active vasomotion in both portal venous and hepatic arterial beds. Although these may have to do with intrahepatic distribution of blood, it is doubtful if they have any influence on the total volume of hepatic blood flow; this is primarily determined by conditions in the splanchnic bed.

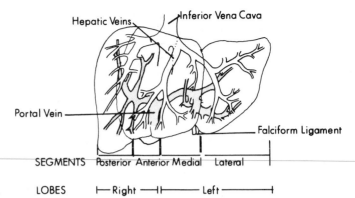

Fig. 27-4. Venous inflow and outflow.

Pain is created only by distention of the liver. It is dull and localized deeply in the right upper quadrant, although it may be referred to the neck, right shoulder, and back. Cutaneous hyperesthesia, or muscle rigidity, occurs only if there is irritation of the parietal peritoneum.

LYMPHATICS

There are two groups of lymphatic vessels that drain the liver: superficial and deep. The superficial vessels from the surface capsule penetrate the diaphragm and end in nodes near the terminal inferior vena cava; those from the concave or undersurface of the liver converge to the porta hepatis and accompany the deep lymphatics. The deep lymphatics originate in the hepatic substance, follow the portal and hepatic veins, and emerge from the hilus as several large trunks, which end in nodes along the hepatic artery or accompany the hepatic veins and terminate in nodes adjacent to the inferior vena cava. The lymphatic drainage from the liver accounts for 25% to 50% of total thoracic lymph flow. Blockage of the lymphatics, such as may occur in cirrhosis of the liver with scarring in the areolar connective tissues of the portal triad, may block the deep lymphatics and be a major contribution to the development of ascites.

LIGAMENTS

The liver is the largest solid organ in the body. It is in the right hypochondrium and epigastrium of the abdomen. The superior surface conforms to the undersurface of the diaphragm, and the inferior surface rests on the viscera of the upper abdomen. It extends from the right nipple down to the costal margin. The undersurface of the liver is in contact with the duodenum, colon, kidney, and adrenal gland on the right and with the esophagus and stomach on the left. It is covered by peritoneum except for the bare area in the posterior superior surface adjacent to the inferior vena cava, which is in direct contact with the diaphragm. Although there are many peritoneal attachments and ligaments, the liver is held in place primarily by intra-abdominal pressure. The falciform ligament stretches from the anterior abdominal wall to the liver and extends from the umbilicus to the diaphragm as far back as the opening for the inferior vena cava. The ligamentum teres contains the obliterated umbilical vein and lies in the posterior portion of the falciform ligament. The left triangular ligament suspends the lateral part of the left lobe of the liver to the undersurface of the diaphragm. The left phrenic vessels run close to the diaphragmatic attachment of this ligament. Division of the left triangular ligament allows the lateral part of the left lobe of

the liver to be free and mobile, giving better exposure to the lower esophagus and upper stomach. The right triangular ligament, which forms at the lateral portion of the bare area, attaches the lateral portion of the right lobe to the undersurface of the diaphragm. Division of the right triangular ligament and the two diverging peritoneal reflections that surround the bare area of the liver mobilizes the right lobe of the liver and allows access to its posterior surface.

LOBES AND SEGMENTS

On the surface, the ligamentum teres divides the liver into two lobes. However, the functional or anatomical separation of the two lobes lies 4 cm to 5 cm to the right of the falciform ligament (Fig. 27-5). Successful operations upon the liver have demonstrated the importance of the functional anatomy that follows the blood supply and biliary drainage of the liver. Knowledge of this allows resection of the liver along segmental planes. Thus, the true functional left lobe consists of a medial segment that lies to the right of the falciform ligament and the topographical left lobe (see Fig. 27-4). The quadrate lobe is part of the functional left lobe, whereas the caudate lobe is divided between the functional right and left lobes. The right lobe consists of an anterior

Fig. 27-5. Surface anatomy vs. functional anatomy.

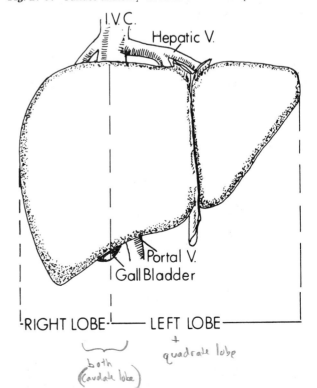

and posterior segment. The line of division between the functional right and left lobe is a line from the gallbladder fossa below to the inferior vena cava above. The hepatic veins have an interlobar distribution between the liver segments.

PHYSIOLOGY

In ancient and medieval history, the liver had an eminence it has never again achieved. As the organ of greatest mass and blood content, it was central to humoral theories of medicine. The story of Prometheus* is an unending myth that prefigures current interest in hepatic regeneration. Yet as discovery of circulation dramatized the heart, vessels, and blood itself, the liver went into an eclipse from which it has not emerged. Modern medicine began in the measurement of motions: blood moves, the heart pushes it, vessels carry it; air moves, urine moves, chyme moves, hormones act at distant sites; the liver sits still and percolates its contents. Simpler glands are supplanted by exogenous supplies of their products, and even the kidney can be replaced by mechanical imitations, but the liver seems too complex and refractory to control. Only its plumbing is subject to major interventions. Once the seat of the soul, the liver became the seat of biochemistry. When a liver function can be influenced or supplanted, a complication of liver disease may be ameliorated, but there is no tonic for the general well-being of the liver, nor for the body when it fails.

Liver physiology may be viewed in vascular, biliary, or parenchymal terms, although hepatic microanatomy, a suspension of parenchyma amid countercurrents of blood and bile, renders such fine distinctions difficult. Is hyperammonemia due to shunts or to the failure of hepatocytes to transform the ammonia that reaches them? The answer seems clear in the Eck fistula dog and in the child with a genetic defect of urea synthesis; however, on the middle ground of common diseases, it is hard to tell whether the circulatory or the metabolic derangement is primary. Cirrhosis lies toward the vascular end of this spectrum; fulminant hepatitis is more parenchymal. The biliary–parenchymal distinction, so obvious when stone or tumor blocks the common bile duct, blurs in many instances of intrahepatic cholestasis. These questions are writ large in the differential diagnosis.

The liver is the most versatile organ for chemical processing. Its functions include uptake, storage, transformation, release, and regulation of exogenous and endogenous substrates. Perfused by the gut's entire venous effluent, it is exposed to all absorbed nutrients, drugs, toxins, and organisms before they reach systemic circulation. In addition to protective detoxification and excretion, the liver's manifold capacities for transformation and synthesis provide vital substances both for export to other tissues and for its own maintenance. Although not classified in the endocrine system the liver activates hormones such as aldosterone and vitamin D and produces their sterol nucleus. It is a site of "lethal synthesis" in the biotransformation of prototoxic compounds such as carbon tetrachloride and acetamino-

---

* Prometheus stole fire from the gods and brought it to man. Zeus had him chained to a mountainside, where a vulture came daily to devour his liver, which grew back overnight. This myth represents man's bold quest for enlightenment and the endless suffering it causes.

phen. As a reticuloendothelial filter astride the portal circulation, stopover for myriads of wandering lymphocytes, and prime suspect in endotoxic shock, the liver may be as important in immunochemistry as in intermediary metabolism. The following discussion emphasizes those aspects of physiology that can be identified in clinical syndromes, either as isolated defects or in the composite picture of liver failure.

STORAGE

The liver is a reservoir or a potential reservoir of fat, amino acids, glycogen, vitamin B_{12}, the fat-soluble vitamins, and certain metals. Excessive stores are implicated in the cirrhosis of Wilson's disease (copper), hemochromatosis (iron), vitamin A toxicity, and several glycogenoses. The acute fatty change of Reye's syndrome or tetracycline poisoning is considered an effect rather than a cause of injury. Whether chronic fat accumulation evokes cirrhosis in alcoholics and jejunal–ileal bypass patients is still debated.

GLUCOSE HOMEOSTASIS

The liver has a central role in glucose metabolism. Hypoglycemia is a complication of liver failure and the earliest cause of death after total hepatectomy. Under the influence of insulin, the liver stores absorbed glucose as glycogen. As insulin falls in fasting, glycogenolysis ensues and glucose is released. The liver converts the milk sugar galactose to glucose; genetic defects of enzymes catalyzing this process result in cirrhosis, retardation, and cataracts.

Normal hepatic glycogen stores comprise only 80 g to 100 g of glucose. Brain, kidney, and red blood cells must draw on hepatic gluconeogenesis for energy substrate to survive a fast over 12 to 24 hours. New glucose formation from amino acids, lactate, and glycerol is promoted by glucagon and glucocorticoid hormones. The process reduces nicotinamide–adenine dinucleotide (NAD) to NADH. When alcohol metabolism preempts the reduction of NAD, failure of gluconeogenesis causes hypoglycemia, particularly in ill-fed persons lacking glucose input and glycogen stores.

AMINONITROGEN TRANSFORMATIONS

Whereas carbon chains of amino acids, particularly alanine, are the components of new glucose, amino groups are the potentially toxic by-product of gluconeogenesis. Deamination yields ammonia directly, but much of the waste nitrogen is first affixed to α-ketoglutarate, yielding glutamic acid. Glutamic–pyruvic transaminase (GPT) catalyzes the reversible amino transfer from alanine. Glutamic–oxaloacetic transaminase (GOT) serves aspartate similarly. Additional waste nitrogen enters the synthesis of glutamine from glutamic acid. Formation of glutamate and glutamine is a transient, reversible mode of nitrogen storage. If hormones and energy balance do not favor anabolism, these amino acids yield ammonia through the actions of glutamic dehydrogenase and glutaminase. The latter enzyme in liver, kidney, brain, and intestinal mucosa is activated by an acid pH and seems central in the regulation of ammoniagenesis.

Replenished with exogenous glucose, the hepatectomized animal lives long enough to die in hyperammonemic coma. The glutamate system has a limited capacity to detoxify ammonia; if exogenous and endogenous aminonitrogen exceeds anabolic requirements, the excess is normally converted to urea in the liver, the only site of the cycle of urea synthesis. Genetic defects of each of the five urea cycle enzymes cause protein intolerance, manifested by encephalopathy, seizures, and retardation without the other evidence of liver disease. Approximately 20% of urea nitrogen is conserved by bacterial ureolysis in the colon, contributing ammonia to the portal circulation. Small bowel glutaminase yields approximately as much ammonia from arterial glutamine as colonic bacteria produce from urea. In gut mucosa as in renal epithelium glutamine-dependent ammoniagenesis increases with acidosis.

Hepatic amino acid interconversion has functions other than gluconeogenesis. The amino acid composition of systemic circulation differs from portal venous blood. In liver failure, aminoaciduria and hyperaminoacidemia may represent excess catabolism, deficient protein synthesis, or a "backup" due to limited urea synthesis. The molar ratio of branched-chain amino acids to aromatic amino acids (normally 3.5:1) correlates with histology and prognosis in chronic active liver disease. A ratio under 2:1 marks severe liver dysfunction, often with encephalopathy. Specific toxicity of excess aromatic amino acids or deficient branched-chain amino acids is not yet proved.

PROTEIN SYNTHESIS

The liver synthesizes the protein required for its own maintenance and regeneration, plus many circulating proteins. Albumin, quantitatively the predominant plasma protein, is made by a hepatic process that can increase up to threefold in response to albumin loss or decreased oncotic pressure. In addition to supporting osmotic equilibrium, albumin binds and carries fatty acids, bilirubin, and certain hormones, metals, and drugs. The half-life of albumin is 2 to 3 weeks. If prior nutrition is adequate and losses through the gut and kidneys are not excessive, serum albumin levels are normal in acute liver diseases. Hypoalbuminemia accompanies severe chronic liver disease. The α-globulins and β-globulins are made by the liver, but most γ-globulins are made by plasma cells.

The liver makes most of the blood clotting factors, including factors I (fibrinogen), II (prothrombin), V, VII, IX, and X. As the vitamin K–dependent factors (II, VII, IX, and X) have short half-lives (hours to days), prolongation of the prothrombin time is an early sign of severe liver damage. In cholestasis, the bile salt–dependent absorption of fat and fat-soluble vitamins (A, D, E, and K) is impaired. Vitamin K deficiency may be compounded by deficient intake and by use of antibiotics that deplete vitamin K–synthesizing bacteria. The resulting coagulation defect is an operative hazard readily corrected by parenteral administration of vitamin K, provided that hepatocellular function is adequate. Fibrinogen deficiency in liver failure is due to diminished synthesis or excess plasma proteolytic activity. The liver synthesizes antithrombin III, the deficiency of which is seldom recognized in liver failure because of the deficiencies of procoagulants. Lack of this inhibitor may contribute to portal vein thrombosis in some cirrhotics. The liver assists in clearance or inactivation of procoagulants and inhibitors.

The liver produces the transport proteins haptoglobin, ceruloplasmin, and transferrin. The latter two are implicated in Wilson's disease and hemochromatosis. The liver makes α₁-antitrypsin. When genetic variants render this protein less exportable, the high levels in hepatocytes may be associated with cholestasis in infants or chronic hepatitis and cirrhosis in children and young adults. A transplanted normal liver produces its own protein phenotype, which enters the circulation and may prevent the emphysema of antitrypsin deficiency. Transplantation has corrected the abnormal copper metabolism of Wilson's disease. As a nonspecific acute-phase reaction to tissue injury, the liver increases synthesis of α₁-antitrypsin, haptoglobin, ceruloplasmin, transferrin, fibrinogen, orosomucoid, and C-reactive protein.

Protein synthesis is necessary for the liver to release otherwise insoluble cholesterol, phospholipid, and triglyceride into plasma. Apoproteins wrap lipid aggregates that are secreted by the liver as triglyceride-rich VLDL (very low density lipoprotein) and cholesterol-rich HDL (high-density lipoprotein). In addition to solubilizing lipids for transport, hepatic apoproteins activate lecithin/cholesterol acyltransferase (LCAT) and tissue lipoprotein lipase, enzymes of peripheral lipid metabolism. The liver synthesizes and secretes LCAT, which acts peripherally to form most of the cholesterol esters found in the circulation. Genetic deficiency of LCAT results in excess unesterified cholesterol, producing hemolysis and premature atherosclerosis. Catabolism of lipoprotein remnants and esterified HDL cholesterol seems to be initiated by hepatic triglyceride lipase (H-TGL).

LIPID METABOLISM

Fatty acids from diet and adipose tissue enter the liver and follow two major pathways. (1) In the fed state, fatty acids are esterified to form triglycerides, phospholipids, and cholesterol esters. Normally, most of the products are secreted as lipoprotein, but agents interfering with apoprotein synthesis (carbon tetrachloride, phosphorus, excess tetracycline) cause acute fat retention. (2) In diabetes and fasting (with low insulin and high glucagon levels), fatty acids are oxidized to ketones and CO_2. Mitochondrial fatty acid oxidation is the major source of energy for gluconeogenesis. In Reye's syndrome, impaired mitochondrial function appears responsible for both hypoglycemia and fat retention. Acute interference with energy generation and protein synthesis—a process requiring much adenosine triphosphate (ATP)—is often fatal. The more common chronic fatty livers of alcoholism, diabetes, corticosteroid excess, starvation, total parenteral nutrition, and obesity are not so dysfunctional. Other possible mechanisms of fat accumulation include excess fatty acid influx, excess fatty acid synthesis in hepatocytes, impaired union of apoprotein with lipid, and impaired excretion of lipoprotein.

Acute hepatitis increases plasma triglycerides and decreases the esterified fraction of cholesterol. LCAT and H-TGL activity levels fall. On lipoprotein electrophoresis, the alpha (HDL) and prebeta (VLDL) bands disappear, while the beta (low-density lipoprotein, LDL) band becomes broader and denser with abnormal lipoproteins, perhaps due to failure to clear remnants. Plasma is not grossly lipemic because the excess triglycerides are in the LDL fraction. Patients with hepatitis have increased plasma lecithin and unesterified cholesterol and decreased lysolecithin and esterified cholesterol, findings similar to familial LCAT deficiency. Lesser abnormalities occur in cirrhosis and chronic hepatitis. In cholestasis, total cholesterol levels are high. Cholestasis has an additional marker, lipoprotein-X, an amalgam of phospholipid, cholesterol, bile acids, albumin, and group-C apoproteins. Its appearance is attributed to bile regurgitation or diminished LCAT activity. Levels rise higher in extrahepatic obstruction than in intrahepatic cholestasis.

The liver is the major site of cholesterol and bile acid synthesis. The biliary tract is the subject of another chapter, but it should be noted here that enterohepatic circulation of bile acids is essential to normal fat digestion (serving as cofactor to lipase) and absorption (emulsifying fat in mixed micelles). The serum bile acid level reflects the fraction of bile acids reabsorbed from the ileum and not extracted on first pass through the liver. It increases in any form of liver disease. Cholestasis is broadly construed to include impaired bile secretion from liver cells into canaliculi, as well as mechanical obstruction of the ductal system. It usually entails decreased bile flow to the intestines, increased serum bile acids, and the abnormal lipid patterns noted above. Elevated serum levels of hepatic alkaline phosphatase, an enzyme of unknown physiological significance concentrated in lipid membranes near bile canaliculi, usually accompany cholestasis. Alkaline phosphatase is excreted in bile, and its synthesis increases in response to increasing intracanalicular pressure. Focal intrahepatic cholestasis can raise serum alkaline phosphatase with little other abnormality of serum or enteric bile. Itching, due to an unidentified "pruritogenic factor," is a major but inconstant symptom of cholestasis. Jaundice is not an essential feature.

In summary, the liver is the nexus of carbohydrate, protein, and fat metabolism. Its functions comprise a host of cyclic interactions with the gut and with peripheral tissue, as though situated in the center of a figure eight:

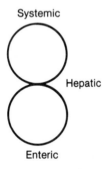

Systemic

Hepatic

Enteric

Cyclic pathways promote conservation of nutrients and reuse of certain products synthesized by the liver.

OTHER BIOTRANSFORMATIONS

The varieties of intervening biochemical steps and of enterohepatic or systemic–hepatic metabolite recycling make hepatic clearance more complex than renal clearance. The liver removes galactose, ammonia, and many other metabolites from plasma by unique substrate-specific pathways, but two broader excretory functions, each shared by several substrates, dominate the concept of hepatic clearance: (1) secretion into bile of cholesterol derivatives (bile acids, steroid hormones) coordinated to some extent with bilirubin excretion (see below) and (2) the mixed-function enzyme system shared by many drugs. The concept of clearance is implicit in the use of the postprandial serum bile acid level as a screening test for liver dysfunction. The microsomal mixed-function oxidase system is assessed by breath analysis of $^{14}CO_2$ following administration of (^{14}C) aminopyrine, a test under investigation for possible prognostic value in liver disease. Pharmacologic clearance is also illustrated by the

potentiating effect of portacaval shunting on an orally administered agent with a high hepatic extraction ratio, such as propranolol. Cimetidine, which decreases liver blood flow and inhibits the microsomal oxidase system, reduces both uptake and oxidation of propranolol.

Processes considered excretory for some substrates may activate others (*i.e.*, the mixed-function oxidase system, which degrades barbiturates, coumarin, digitoxin, and quinidine, produces potentially toxic intermediates from acetaminophen). Induction of these enzymes by alcohol explains in part the alcoholic's resistance to sedatives and susceptibility to acetaminophen poisoning. Even when two substrates are inactivated by this mechanism, their acute and chronic interactions may be opposite. Barbiturates acutely potentiate alcohol, by competing with its degradation, but chronically induce the enzyme system, which in turn raises the alcohol dose requirement for intoxication. Mixing liquor and barbiturate produces, for the naive subject, the notorious Mickey Finn, but it takes a lot of liquor to make a barbiturate addict drunk. Partly due to the heme requirements of cytochrome P-450 and associated microsomal oxidases, the liver is a major site of porphyrin synthesis.

The liver makes no hormones but has a central role in endocrine metabolism. Peptide hormones such as insulin and glucagon are inactivated by hepatic proteolysis. Thyroid hormones are degraded in the liver. The liver isomerizes testosterone, hydroxylates dietary vitamin D (an activating step), and converts cortisol to cortisone and estradiol to estriol and estrone. The final common path of hepatic steroid metabolism is inactivation by reduction and solubilization by conjugation with sulfates or glucuronic acid. Making the fat-soluble, protein-bound steroids water soluble permits their excretion in urine. It was once assumed that inhibition of hepatic degradation of aldosterone and sex steroids explained respectively sodium retention and feminization in cirrhosis. Altered aldosterone production and peripheral androgen–estrogen conversion now seem more important. By unknown means, liver disease reduces effective renal plasma flow, releasing aldosterone by renin–angiotensin activation. The effects of liver disease on plasma-binding proteins and on pituitary gonadotropins probably outweigh any changes in hepatic excretory metabolism of sex steroids.

BILIRUBIN

Bilirubin excretion is the most extensively studied liver function, not so much for its importance to life (bilirubin retention *per se* is relatively harmless after infancy) as for its diagnostic significance. Jaundice is the cardinal sign of liver disease, although absent in a majority of episodes of hepatitis, in many cases of cirrhosis, and in a few deaths from liver failure. Bilirubin excretion, a model for many organic anions, involves seven steps: (1) delivery by the circulation, (2) uptake across the sinusoidal membrane of the liver cell, (3) storage (binding) in the liver cell, (4) biotransformation (conjugation) in the liver cell, (5) secretion into the bile canaliculus, (6) delivery to the gut through the biliary tract, and (7) recycling of a portion of the product from the gut.

Over 80% of bilirubin normally comes from the degradation of senescent red blood cells in the reticuloendothelial system. The remainder is derived from the turnover of hepatic heme proteins such as cytochrome P-450, with a small fraction from the heme wasted in marrow during red blood cell maturation. Hemolysis is the most common cause of increased bilirubin production, but the mild jaundice of pernicious anemia or thalassemia is due to ineffective erythropoiesis. Color changes in a bruise reflect the oxidation of blue deoxyhemoglobin to green biliverdin, which is reduced to yellow bilirubin. The capacity of microsomal heme oxygenase and biliverdin reductase exceeds the liver's capacity to conjugate and excrete bilirubin. Thus, unconjugated hyperbilirubinemia is common in hemolysis, but hemoglobinuria and methemalbuminemia are minimal except in massive hemolysis.

Unconjugated bilirubin, insoluble in water and firmly protein bound, does not enter bile or urine. It diffuses across lipid membranes and is toxic to the neonatal brain. The more polar conjugated form is weakly bound and subject to biliary excretion. If regurgitated into serum, conjugated bilirubin readily traverses the glomerular membrane. Albumin is the plasma binding protein for both unconjugated and conjugated bilirubin. Cysts, cerebrospinal fluid, and effusions contain bilirubin in proportion to their albumin content, exudates being more icteric than transudates.

UPTAKE

A hepatocyte surface membrane receptor facilitates detachment of bilirubin from albumin. Transport is a carrier-mediated, saturable process that is competitively inhibited by organic anions such as Bromsulphalein (BSP). Binding by ligandin or other cytoplasmic proteins prevents reflux into plasma.

CONJUGATION

Bilirubin IX-α, the predominant isomer in humans, is not water soluble. In conjugation, propionate groups are esterified with glucuronate, which increases polarity and prevents intramolecular hydrogen bonds from holding the molecule in a hydrophobic configuration. The reaction is catalyzed by bilirubin glucuronyl transferase in the endoplasmic reticulum. Unconjugated hyperbilirubinemia is due to either overproduction or impaired clearance of bilirubin. Genetic defects of uptake (Gilbert's syndrome) and conjugation (Gilbert's, Crigler-Najjar syndromes I and II) have been identified in patients with no other impairment of liver function.

Little conjugated bilirubin is found in normal serum, whereas little unconjugated bilirubin is found in normal bile. In both hepatocellular and cholestatic jaundice, the serum monoglucuronide conjugates exceed the diglucuronide and free fractions. Normal bile contains diglucuronide in excess of monoglucuronide. Unconjugated bilirubin in bile, the substance of pigment gallstones, arises from bacterial hydrolysis of conjugated bilirubin and from the excretion of soluble photoisomers of unconjugated bilirubin.

EXCRETION

Conjugated bilirubin enters bile against a concentration gradient through a saturable transport mechanism subject to competitive inhibition. This transport system is separable from bile acid transport insofar as patients with a genetic defect in conjugated bilirubin excretion (Dubin-Johnson syndrome) excrete bile acids normally. In common liver diseases, jaundice may be deep while cholestasis is minimal, or mild while cholestasis is severe. Nevertheless, the maximal rate of bilirubin secretion seems linked to bile acid–dependent bile flow, as though a "micellar sink" holds bilirubin at concentrations that might otherwise reverse its transport equilibrium.

FATE IN THE GUT

Conjugated bilirubin, being water soluble, is not reabsorbed. Because little deconjugation occurs in the small bowel, bilirubin enterohepatic circulation is minimal in adults. In the colon and terminal ileum, bacterial β-glucuronidase starts a sequence of anaerobic reactions yielding colorless tetrapyrroles called urobilinogens. A small fraction of urobilinogen is reabsorbed and excreted by the liver and kidney. The amount of urinary urobilinogen depends on production, fraction absorbed (clostridia population may influence this), and hepatic clearance, as well as renal function, urinary volume, and pH. Urinary urobilinogen, high in hemolytic jaundice, is low in obstructive jaundice unless the biliary tract is heavily infected. Oxidized colored derivatives of urobilinogen (urobilins) have long been blamed for the brown color of stool, but, because a pigment-free diet yields clay-colored stool in normal persons, it is hypothesized that dietary pigment undergoes enterohepatic circulation and contributes to the color of stool.

PHYSIOLOGY VS. FUNCTION TESTS

Physiology and liver function tests are treated separately. Many tests have diagnostic use out of proportion to their functional significance. The most vital functions are discerned through remote end points: malnutrition, debility, coagulopathy, sepsis, hypotension, and death. Serum bilirubin is a cardinal sign and chemical measure, but bilirubin excretion is less important to health than is the liver's roles in glucose homeostasis or amino acid metabolism. Measures of the latter may be properly regarded as function tests but are used infrequently because of poor sensitivity, specificity, and quantitative correlation. Serum enzymes that signify hepatitis or bile stasis reflect neither their own function in the liver nor the extent of liver insufficiency; transaminases and alkaline phosphatase should be called diagnostic markers rather than function tests. The antimitochondrial antibody is a hallmark of primary biliary cirrhosis, a disease with no known mitochondrial injury, but is not found in the putative mitochondrial disorder, Reye's syndrome.

DIAGNOSIS OF LIVER DISEASES

As implied by the complexity of liver physiology, no liver test is a shortcut to diagnosis. History and physical examination, plus routine blood, urine, stool, and radiographic examinations, are as important as biochemical tests. The findings on general workup are combined with several liver function tests to classify jaundice as hemolytic, hepatocellular, or cholestatic (obstructive). This initial triage determines the need for supplementary procedures. Hyperbilirubinemia is subclassified extensively, but all liver diseases, with and without jaundice, may be categorized as hepatocellular or cholestatic. If cholestatic, the physician is obliged to rule out extrahepatic biliary obstruction.

HISTORY

The history should note the course regarding anorexia, nausea, pruritus, fever, and pain, as well as the background of operations, drugs, toxins, and exposures to infection. Patients with hepatocellular disease usually seem more ill than patients with cholestasis, unless the latter develop biliary sepsis. Although fever and pain are common in alcoholic hepatitis, rigors and sudden severe pain are more consistent with cholangitis. Relentless progression of jaundice, weight loss, pruritus, and pale stool suggests malignant extrahepatic obstruction. Prior biliary surgery also directs attention to the common duct. Transfusion, injections, polypharmacy, promiscuity, or contacts with drug abusers, dialysis patients, or jaundiced persons raise the question of hepatitis. Patients with viral hepatitis are generally younger than patients with common duct stones or cancers of the pancreas and bile ducts. A cancer history brings to mind both metastases and the hepatitis exposure of oncology patients. Jaundice in pregnancy may denote choledocholithiasis or "physiologic" cholestasis induced by sex-steroid hormones but is usually due to viral hepatitis. Jaundice in the postoperative setting is reviewed later in this chapter. The patient's occupation may entail exposure to hepatitis virus (blood products, closed institutions), alcohol, or toxins such as vinyl choloride. Family history may suggest hemolytic jaundice, congenital hyperbilirubinemia, or gallstones.

The importance of an exhaustive drug history cannot be overemphasized. Alcohol leads the list. Methyldopa isoniazid, (INH), and nitrofurantoin cause acute and chronic hepatitis. Manifestations of hepatocellular and cholestatic injury mingle in varying proportions in the jaundice induced by benzodiazepine, thiazide, and antithyroid drugs and in the hypersensitivity reactions to phenytoin, phenylbutazone, sulfonamides, quinidine, allopurinol, and para-aminosalicylic acid (PAS). Phenothiazines, tricyclic antidepressants, erythromycin estolate, oral contraceptive steroids, and C_{17} substituted androgens cause cholestasis. The liver is susceptible to so many other drugs that the clinician cannot rely on memory. Detective work often obviates the need for invasive procedures. Most forms of drug hepatitis, which may be fatal or may progress to cirrhosis, abate upon timely withdrawal of the agent.

EXAMINATION

Jaundice, ecchymoses, ascites, gastrointestinal tract bleeding, and encephalopathy often occur together in severe acute hepatitis (massive or submassive necrosis) and deteriorating of chronic liver disease. Jaundice is hard to detect when the total serum bilirubin is under 3 mg/dl. Hemolysis presents mild scleral icterus, whereas patients with prolonged cholestatic jaundice develop a green-tinged bronze color. Excoriations and xanthomas mark prolonged cholestasis. The combination of anemia and malnutrition suggests cancer or cirrhosis. Lymphadenopathy and signs of primary gastrointestinal, pulmonary, breast, genital, endocrine, or hematologic neoplasm should be sought. Patients with pancreatic cancer may bend forward to reduce pain. They occasionally suffer multiple venous thromboses (Trousseau's syndrome). Although not specific, spider angiomas are the most useful skin signs of cirrhosis, particularly when accompanied by palmar erythema and nutritional findings, such as muscle wasting, white nails, and diminished secondary sexual hair. Testicular atrophy, gynecomastia, parotid enlargement, and Dupuytren's contracture suggest an alcoholic etiology. Bruising reflects the clotting defects characteristic of vitamin K deficiency or severe liver disease. Intellectual deterioration, asterixis (flapping tremor), and "mousy" fetor indicate impending hepatic coma.

Liver size, consistency, and tenderness are estimated by percussion and palpation. The normal span (10 ± 2 cm in adults) extends from the right fifth intercostal space to the costal margin in the midclavicular line, descending 1 cm to 4 cm on deep inspiration. The left lobe extends 4 cm to 7 cm in the midsternal line. In acute hepatitis or intrahepatic cholestasis, the liver is moderately enlarged, but it is abnormally small in fulminant hepatitis. Greater enlargement occurs with fat infiltration, extrahepatic biliary obstruction, pericardial constriction, or right ventricular failure. A cirrhotic liver may be large, medium-sized, or small. Its edges are blunt and firm, perhaps irregular. Primary or metastatic cancer can make the liver very large, hard, and nodular. The liver may be tender in viral or drug hepatitis and more painful in alcoholic hepatitis, acute heart failure, cholangitis, abscess, or cancer. Gallbladder inflammation can mimic hepatic enlargement and tenderness. A palpable gallbladder is associated with periampullary cancer (especially pancreatic). A systolic bruit over the liver suggests hepatocellular cancer or alcoholic hepatitis. A rub implies abscess, necrotic tumor, infarction, or gonoccocal perihepatitis.

Dilated abdominal wall veins draining centrifugally from the umbilicus signify portal hypertension. The same process engorges hemorrhoids. Common causes of splenomegaly related to jaundice or liver disease are portal hypertension, hemolysis, hematologic cancer, sarcoidosis, and certain infections. Cirrhosis with portal hypertension is most prevalent of the many causes of ascites.

The patient's report on urine and stool color should be checked by direct examination (see bilirubin metabolism). Bilirubinuria accompanies a rise in conjugated bilirubin level before jaundice appears, so a positive "dipstick" occasionally calls attention to occult hepatitis or cirrhosis. The urinary urobilinogen value falls initially in hepatitis and rises before recovery. Prolonged absence of urinary urobilinogen implies total (malignant) bile duct obstruction. Dark brown stools and high urinary urobilinogen values (without bilirubinuria) accompany hemolysis. Pale stools result from cholestasis, which can occur in many liver diseases, including hepatitis and cirrhosis, but clay-colored stools devoid of urobilin denote complete biliary obstruction. Stool color varies widely in the course of choledocholithiasis. Among the hepatobiliary causes of blood in stool are varices, periampullary cancers, and hematobilia (usually from stones or cancer), but cirrhotics as often bleed from gastritis and ulcers as from varices.

Hematology also figures in preliminary diagnoses. Marked leukocytosis suggests biliary sepsis, although neutrophil counts are also high in alcoholic hepatitis and fulminant liver failure. Neutropenia and atypical lymphocytes accompany viral hepatitis as well as infectious mononucleosis. Some drug allergies produce eosinophilia, but many drug-induced liver disorders have no hematologic signs. Pancytopenia suggests hypersplenism and cirrhosis.

Plain films of the abdomen aid assessment of liver and spleen size and reveal biliary, hepatic, and vascular calcifications. On chest film the position of the right hemidiaphragm, changes at the right base, pleural fluid, tumor, granulomas, pneumonia, and signs of heart failure may pertain to liver disorders.

LIVER TESTS

Classification of jaundice based on alterations of bilirubin excretion serves as a prologue to conventional liver function tests and serologic tests, which often must be parlayed with procedures (sonography, radioisotope scans, computed tomography—CT scan, cholangiography, and liver biopsy) to identify hepatic lesions or to distinguish between extrahepatic and intrahepatic cholestasis. A later chapter describes their roles defining extrahepatic biliary pathology.

CAUSES OF JAUNDICE

The ranges of bilirubin are typical but not all-inclusive. Many forms of hepatitis and chronic active liver disease are anicteric.

I. Unconjugated hyperbilirubinemia
  A. Increased bilirubin formation
    1. Hemolysis, which may be intravascular (hemolytic anemia) or extravascular (infarction or hematoma), 2 mg to 5 mg/dl
    2. Ineffective erythropoiesis (as in pernicious anemia and thalassemia), 1 mg to 3 mg/dl
  B. Impaired hepatic uptake
    1. Drug competition (cholecystographic dyes), 1 mg to 2 mg/dl
    2. Gilbert's syndrome (some patients have both decreased uptake and a mild conjugation defect), 1 mg to 5 mg/dl
    3. Fasting (also unmasks Gilbert's syndrome), 0.7 mg to 1.5 mg/dl
  C. Impaired conjugation due to glucuronyl transferase deficiency
    1. Neonatal jaundice (transferase low relative to pigment load, subject to inhibition by pregnanediol and chloramphenicol), normally 1 mg to 5 mg/dl, little danger up to 10 mg/dl
    2. Crigler-Najjar syndrome I (transferase absent), 20 mg to 50 mg/dl
    3. Crigler-Najjar syndrome II (transferase markedly reduced), 5 mg to 15 mg/dl
    4. Gilbert's syndrome (transferase mildly reduced), 1 mg to 5 mg/dl

II. Conjugated hyperbilirubinemia (direct fraction >15% of total and usually >50%)
  A. Impaired hepatocanalicular excretion
    1. Dubin-Johnson and Rotor's syndromes, 1 mg to 7 mg/dl
    2. Hormone-induced cholestasis (contraceptives, androgens, pregnancy), 1 mg to 7 mg/dl
    3. Drug-induced cholestasis (chlorpromazine), 2 mg to 15 mg/dl
    4. Postoperative intrahepatic cholestasis, 5 mg to 30 mg/dl
    5. Hypoxemia and vascular congestion, 5 mg to 20 mg/dl
    6. Viral or drug-induced hepatitis, 5 mg to 30 mg/dl
    7. Systemic sepsis, 1 mg to 7 mg/dl
       Disorders 4, 5, 6, and 7 also affect uptake and conjugation, but excretion, the rate-limiting step, is most sensitive and the elevated bilirubin is mainly conjugated.
  B. Distortion of intrahepatic bile ducts
    1. Hepatitis
    2. Cirrhosis, 1 mg to 10 mg/dl
    3. Sclerosing cholangitis and primary biliary cirrhosis, bilirubin slowly rises to 20 mg to 30 mg/dl
    4. Tumors and granulomas affect bilirubin variably, depending on extent and site.
  C. Extrahepatic mechanical obstruction
    1. Stones or stricture, 5 mg to 15 mg/dl
    2. Pancreatic, bile duct, or other periampullary cancer, progressive jaundice to 20 mg to 30 mg/dl

BILIRUBIN

Serum bilirubin concentration is usually determined by allowing the pigment to combine with diazotized sulfanilic acid and measuring the colored product. In aqueous solution, conjugated bilirubin reacts faster than unconjugated bilirubin. This early color is measured in a time-limited assay to obtain the "direct"-reacting bilirubin fraction, normally less than 0.2 mg/dl. The "indirect" reaction of unconjugated bilirubin is accelerated by caffeine or alcohol solvents. Total bilirubin is measured by an accelerated assay (normal value <1.2 mg/dl). The amount of unconjugated bilirubin is estimated as total bilirubin − direct bilirubin = indirect bilirubin.

Direct and total bilirubin, properly assayed, provide a sensitive sign of the presence or absence of diffuse liver damage. Direct bilirubin levels greater than 0.3 mg/dl with a normal total bilirubin implies latent disease. If the direct fraction comprises less than 10% of an elevated total bilirubin, the disease is probably hemolysis or a benign defect of bilirubin metabolism rather than hepatitis, cirrhosis, or biliary obstruction. On the other hand, a direct fraction greater than 15% implies hepatobiliary disease even when hemolysis accounts for most of the total.

The serum bilirubin concentration relates directly to bilirubin turnover and inversely to bilirubin clearance. Concurrent changes in production and clearance may exaggerate or obscure each other's effect. The rate of rise or fall in bilirubin level has more prognostic significance than the absolute level. It has been estimated that total interruption of bile flow with no alteration in bilirubin production or renal excretion would result in equilibrium at a serum bilirubin around 25 mg/dl. Coincidental hemolysis or renal insufficiency is usually found when the total bilirubin level exceeds 30 mg/dl.

Jaundice is attributed to unconjugated bilirubin if the urine contains no bilirubin. Overproduction of bilirubin may be distinguished from defects of uptake and conjugation by high urinary urobilinogen, but urobilinogen is seldom measured because the reticulocyte count is a simpler screening test for hemolysis. In adults, unconjugated hyperbilirubinemia has a benign prognosis regarding liver function. It may indicate a serious hematologic problem or a specific liver defect that does not influence more vital functions. Lipid-soluble unconjugated bilirubin damages the neonate's brain (kernicterus) but seems harmless in the older child and adult. Patients with the rare Crigler-Najjar syndrome II develop kernicterus in infancy. Crigler-Najjar syndrome I may be the homozygous form of Gilbert's disease. Perhaps 5% of the population has the impaired bilirubin clearance of Gilbert's syndrome, but most cases are not recognized unless bilirubin is measured during such stresses as fasting, hemolysis, surgery, and sepsis.

Conjugated hyperbilirubinemia is accompanied by bilirubinuria. Familial defects in the excretion of conjugated bilirubin are benign except for the cosmetic problem of intermittent jaundice and the hazards of excessive diagnostic intervention. Dubin-Johnson and Rotor's syndromes are rare. Patients susceptible to sex-steroid cholestasis have no extraordinary susceptibility to the hepatic vascular tumors caused by the same hormones. Upon withdrawal, their jaundice and pruritus abate without residual liver damage. Women who develop benign cholestasis in the third trimester of pregnancy are prone to the same problem when given oral contraceptives. It occurs in men on oral (C_{17}-substituted) androgens. Phenothiazines have occasionally induced biliary cirrhosis. Prolonged large obstruction of the bile duct causes secondary biliary cirrhosis. In the absence of cholangitis, however, the liver changes of a month's obstruction are reversible. Hepatocellular injury affects uptake, conjugation, and excretion of bilirubin: The predominance of conjugated bilirubin in serum reflects the sensitivity of the final step. Jaundice in cirrhosis probably stems from diminished vascular access to hepatocytes (intrahepatic shunting), as well as from biliary distortion and liver cell necrosis.

SERUM BILE ACIDS

BSP and indocyanine green excretion tests are seldom used clinically, but serum bile acid determination serves similar purposes of detecting minimal liver disease and shunts. Although elevated in anicteric cholestasis, bile acid levels are normal in discrete defects of bilirubin metabolism, such as Gilbert's or Dubin-Johnson syndrome. Postprandial serum is most useful, as the normal rise due to enterohepatic circulation of bile acids is exaggerated by defective hepatic clearance. Total bile acid elevation, like conjugated bilirubin elevation, merely indicates liver damage without clue as to type. Although the ratio of trihydroxy to dihydroxy bile acids (cholic/chenodeoxycholic) is high in cholestasis and low in hepatocellular dysfunction, these difficult assays do not make the crucial distinction between intrahepatic cholestasis and extrahepatic obstruction.

SERUM ENZYMES

Assays of alkaline phosphatase and aminotransferases (usually called transaminases), together with bilirubin, constitute the simplest and most popular panel of liver function tests. The enzymes are sensitive markers of injury, crudely proportional to severity (Table 27-1). Their levels often indicate the predominance of cholestasis or necrosis in a given case. They are empirical rather than physiological tests insofar as serum levels do not reflect their functions in the liver. They are of little use in distinguishing extrahepatic from intrahepatic cholestasis. They are not liver specific because other tissues contribute to the enzymes measured in serum.

Although hepatic alkaline phosphatase is excreted into bile, its serum elevation owes as much to increased synthesis as to mechanical diversion. Diseases of canaliculi (drug or hormone cholestasis) and infiltrative partial obstruction (metastases or granulomas impinging unevenly on the intrahepatic ductal system, cancer of one hepatic duct) can raise serum levels as high as in common bile duct obstruction. Total bilirubin often remains normal in such cases. Great elevations of alkaline phosphatase (tenfold or more) in severe chronic cholestatic disorders, such as primary biliary cirrhosis and sclerosing cholangitis, may precede jaundice by years. A threefold or greater elevation in alkaline phosphatase level suggests cholestasis. Lesser increases are common in hepatitis or cirrhosis. High levels accompany transient cholestatic phases of any liver disease, particularly alcoholic hepatitis and postoperative jaundice. Serum alkaline phosphatase activity may fall dramatically upon relief of bile duct obstruction.

Bone, gut, and placenta also contribute to the total serum alkaline phosphatase. Elevations occur in growing children, osteomalacia, Paget's disease, bone metastases, and the third trimester of pregnancy. Hepatic, placental, and bone isoenzymes are imprecisely separated by differences in heat

stability. In determining whether liver or bone disease is the cause of an elevated alkaline phosphatase level, gammaglutamyl transpeptidase (GGT) elevation indicates liver injury. GGT is also used to detect early alcohol damage.

Serum glutamic–oxaloacetic transaminase (SGOT) and serum glutamic–pyruvic transaminase (SGPT) are the most practical measures of hepatocellular necrosis. In acute viral hepatitis, levels usually increase over tenfold. Extensive necrosis causes elevations up to 100-fold, but enzyme activity is not always proportional to severity. Chronic active hepatitis typically shows transaminases 5 to 20 times their upper normal limits. Persistent hepatitis, cirrhosis, granulomas, and tumors usually result in less than fivefold elevations. Levels in alcoholic hepatitis are lower than in viral hepatitis of like severity. In alcoholic hepatitis, the SGOT usually exceeds the SGPT (the OT/PT "split"); the reverse is common in viral hepatitis. Serial transaminase changes roughly mark the course of acute or chronic hepatitis.

Many tissues contain transaminases. This nonspecificity is a diagnostic hindrance, as serum levels rise with necrosis of gut, limb, lung, myocardium, kidney, and brain. Measurement of SGOT is a routine test for myocardial infarction and rhabdomyolysis as well as hepatitis. Creatine phosphokinase isoenzymes distinguish myocardial, skeletal muscle, and brain necrosis. Ornithine transcarbamylase, an enzyme of the urea cycle, rises in serum as a virtually liver-specific response, but its assay is more difficult than are transaminase assays. Lactate dehydrogenase (LDH) is even less specific than the transaminases and is seldom useful. Separation of the five isoenzymes helps distinguish the LDH contributions of liver disease, hemolysis, and myocardial infarction. High levels are common in metastatic cancer.

No other enzymes serve as well as alkaline phosphatase and transaminases in most questions of liver and biliary tract disease. An alkaline phosphatase elevation at least three times the normal limit, with less than fivefold elevation of transaminase, indicates intrahepatic or extrahepatic cholestasis without much parenchymal necrosis. Conversely, a tenfold elevation of transaminase, with less than a twofold excess of alkaline phosphatase, strongly favors hepatocellular injury. Occasionally, the expected findings are reversed, as in choledocholithiasis presenting with the sudden onset of cholangitis and high transaminase levels, or alcoholic hepatitis presenting as cholestatic jaundice. Often a "mixed" picture combining hepatocellular and cholestatic components calls for ancillary tests.

CLOTTING FACTORS

Blood tests of procoagulants made by the liver are diagnostically and prognostically useful. The prothrombin time reflects activities of factors II (prothrombin), VII, IX, and X, which depend on both hepatic synthesis and the availability of vitamin K, as well as factors I (fibrinogen) and V, which are made by the liver and are not vitamin K dependent. The prothrombin time is prolonged in severe hepatitis or cirrhosis, when hepatic synthesis fails despite parenteral administration of vitamin K (see Table 27-1). Prolongation of the prothrombin time is an ominous sign in acute hepatitis, but in cirrhosis the prothrombin time may stabilize a few seconds beyond control values. Bile duct obstruction and prolonged intrahepatic cholestasis reduce vitamin K absorption, because low enteric bile acid levels impair lipid absorption. If hepatocellular function remains adequate, one

TABLE 27-1   TYPICAL CHEMICAL FINDINGS IN LIVER DISORDERS

	NORMAL	EXTRAHEPATIC BILIARY OBSTRUCTION (PROLONGED)	CIRRHOSIS LATENT	CIRRHOSIS ACTIVE / CHRONIC ACTIVE HEPATITIS	*ORDINARY HEPATITIS	*FULMINANT HEPATITIS	*INTRA-HEPATIC CHOLESTASIS
Bilirubin (mg/dl)	<1.2 (total)	15	2	8	5	12	5
Alkaline Phosphatase (units/liter)	20 to 90	350	130	200	100	100	300
Transaminase (units/liter)	10 to 30	80	40	150	600	1500	60
Prothrombin Time	11 to 12 sec (control)	Prolonged but corrected by vitamin K injection	Slightly prolonged	Prolonged	Normal	Markedly prolonged	Normal or prolonged/correctable
Albumin (g/dl)	3.5 to 5.0	4.0	3.0	2.0		3.5	4.0

* Although most cases of viral hepatitis show a hepatocellular necrosis pattern and certain drugs and hormones are invariably cholestatic, most forms of drug hepatitis are biochemically indistinguishable from viral hepatitis.

or two injections of 10 mg vitamin K correct the prothrombin time and the clotting defect. Fibrinogen depletion usually reflects consumption coagulopathy as well as decreased synthesis. When clotting factors are assayed individually in severe liver disease, all are reduced except factor VIII, which is not made by liver and is often increased. This "compensatory" rise in factor VIII may explain the disparity between prolonged prothrombin time and nearly normal partial thromboplastin time in stable cirrhosis. The partial thromboplastin time lengthens progressively in impending liver failure. Some patients with chronic liver disease have relatively normal prothrombin and partial thromboplastin times, while their prolonged thrombin clotting times imply inadequate polymerization of fibrinogen.

Prothrombin time, partial thromboplastin time, and platelet count should precede invasive procedures in patients with liver disease. Bleeding time and thrombin-activated clotting time may also be indicated. Abnormal values refractory to parenteral administration of vitamin K can be corrected by blood products such as fresh frozen plasma. It is desirable to keep the prothrombin time within 3 seconds and the partial thromboplastin time within 10 seconds of control values, while maintaining at least 50,000 functioning platelets. Thrombocytopenia due to hypersplenism, intravascular consumption, or marrow suppression frequently compounds the coagulopathy of liver disease, particularly in alcoholics.

OTHER PROTEINS

Serum albumin has a longer half-life than the clotting factors. Its depression (below the normal 3.5-g–5-g/dl range) implies liver disease of several weeks' duration, unless the patient is already malnourished or losing protein through the kidney or gastrointestinal tract. Low levels are found in cirrhosis and chronic active hepatitis and in those who survive more than a few days with massive or submassive necrosis (see Table 27-1). Patients with cholestatic disease often maintain a normal albumin level. It is a valuable test of protein nutrition as well as of liver function.

Hyperglobulinemia suggests chronic inflammation (*i.e.*, the IgG elevation of chronic active hepatitis and the broad IgA, IgG peaks of cirrhosis). β-globulin levels rise in cholestatic jaundice. A high IgM accompanies primary biliary cirrhosis. None of these changes is diagnostically specific.

Several other protein assays are useful. Young persons with unexplained liver disease should be checked for α_1-antitrypsin deficiency and for Wilson's disease (marked by decreased ceruloplasmin). Although uncommon, the latter is an important diagnosis because its progression to cirrhosis and neurologic disability can be arrested by penicillamine therapy. Transferrin saturation with iron is normally around 30%, but in hemochromatosis, which also raises serum ferritin, it is over 80%. In the United States, α-fetoprotein is elevated in about half the patients with primary liver cancer, a majority of patients with embryonal cell gonadal cancers, and a few patients with gastrointestinal cancers metastatic to the liver.

IMMUNOLOGIC TESTS

IgM antibodies to hepatitis virus A appear in the acute phase and are replaced by IgG antibodies in convalescence. Hepatitis A has no late sequelae. Predominance of IgG antibodies to hepatitis A rules out hepatitis A as the cause of current illness.

The current serology of hepatitis B involves two antigens and three antibodies. Hepatitis B surface antigen (HB$_s$Ag)

is the first sign of infection. Typically, it appears 1 to 2 months after exposure and 2 weeks before transaminase elevation and symptoms; HB$_s$Ag usually disappears with resolution of symptoms, but 5% to 10% of patients remain positive over 3 months. Some of these carriers are infectious, and some have chronic liver disease. Antibody to HB$_s$Ag (anti-HB$_s$Ag) appears 2 weeks to several months after HB$_s$Ag disappears. About 5% of adults in the United States have anti-HB$_s$Ag, a persistent marker of immunity. Antibody to the viral core antigen (anti-HB$_c$Ag) arises near the onset of symptoms (after transaminase elevation and before HB$_s$Ag disappears) and persists indefinitely. Its elevation is useful diagnostically during the gap between the fall in HB$_s$Ag and the rise of anti-HB$_s$Ag. The hepatitis B "e" antigen appears soon after HB$_s$Ag. In uncomplicated cases, it disappears in about a month, marking the start of recovery. Persistent HB$_e$Ag signifies infectivity and an increased risk of chronic liver disease.

Some forms of chronic active hepatitis have several nonspecific immunologic abnormalities such as LE cells and antinuclear antibodies. Antimitochondrial antibodies are found in 80% to 90% of patients with primary biliary cirrhosis and are uncommon in other liver diseases.

AMMONIA

Serum ammonia increases in severe hepatic necrosis, portosystemic shunts, and specific defects of urea synthesis. The test sometimes aids the diagnosis of hepatic encephalopathy. Because ammonia rises spontaneously in shed blood and its venous levels vary widely, a specimen should be drawn from an artery, placed on ice, and assayed without delay. The true normal serum ammonia may be zero, but in most assays the upper limit of normal is 50μg to 70μg/dl. Even under optimal methods, the correlation with encephalopathy is imprecise. Serum and cerebrospinal fluid glutamine levels likewise reflect the disposition of waste nitrogen but are equally variable. Other measures of abnormal amino acid metabolism, such as methionine, tryptophan, or the ratio of aromatic to branched-chain amino acids, are not widely available.

LIPIDS

Total serum cholesterol (normally 130 mg–230 mg/dl) increases in cholestasis and remains normal or falls in hepatocellular disease. The fraction of cholesterol esterified (normally 50% to 70%) decreases in either type of disorder. Cholestasis raises serum triglycerides and produces lipoprotein-X. Differential diagnoses seldom depend on these phenomena.

PATTERNS OF FINDINGS

Conventional "liver chemistries" provide valuable clues to type, severity, and duration of disease. Hemolytic jaundice is usually identified by unconjugated hyperbilirubinemia and reticulocytosis. Inborn errors of metabolism manifest unconjugated hyperbilirubinemia without hemolysis, or conjugated hyperbilirubinemia with other liver functions normal. Cholestasis is characterized by alkaline phosphatase elevated out of proportion to the transaminases; hepatocellular necrosis reverses this pattern. Cholestasis is a common cause of vitamin K malabsorption. Refractory prolongation of the prothrombin time develops early in severe liver disease. A low albumin level implies chronic severe parenchymal injury or poor protein intake. Hypercholesterolemia suggests chronic cholestasis. Hyperglobulinemia suggests chronic hepatocellular damage. Additional clotting tests and the ammonia level delineate aspects of the pathophysiology of liver failure and portal–systemic shunting.

Other methods reveal etiology. Serologic tests identify hepatitis A and B, as well as infectious mononucleosis. Cytomegalovirus is isolated from secretions. Intranuclear herpesvirus inclusions may be found on liver biopsy. The correlation of granulomas on biopsy with a positive skin test or serology identifies diseases such as tuberculosis, syphilis, brucellosis, and Q fever. The diagnosis of drug injury is usually inferential, although biopsy can confirm the history of alcoholic liver disease.

Certain forms of cirrhosis or chronic hepatitis may be diagnosed specifically. Hemochromatosis, Wilson's disease, and α_1-antitrypsin deficiency have fairly specific serum screening tests and biopsy findings. Patients with persistent HB$_s$Ag are usually suffering the sequelae of that viral infection. Young women with immunoserologic abnormalities and no other apparent cause seem to have a different type of chronic active liver disease. Classification is important because hemochromatosis can be reversed by phlebotomy; Wilson's disease, by penicillamine; and lupoid hepatitis, by steroids. The most common reversible chronic liver diseases are those induced by alcohol and other drugs. Withdrawal lengthens survival in cirrhosis but may not prevent portal hypertension or the development of hepatoma.

Few blood tests pertain to cause or level of biliary obstruction. Extrahepatic lesions have no marker as specific as antimitochondrial antibodies in primary biliary cirrhosis. Clinical impressions are fairly reliable regarding extrahepatic or intrahepatic cholestasis if the history strongly favors one cause that acts at a predictable level of the biliary tree (drugs, hormones, infectious or infiltrative disorders, stones, and tumor) and tends to exclude other possibilities. Unfortunately, in many cases, no cause is apparent, several possibilities seem equally plausible, or a known disease such as pancreatic cancer affects more than one level of biliary function. The need to locate lesions and assess feasibility of mechanical decompression justifies many of the diagnostic procedures noted below.

SUPPLEMENTARY DIAGNOSTIC PROCEDURES

The procedures available to test primary diagnoses are expensive and may entail discomfort and hazard. Costs vary, but a rough 1983 approximation would price ultrasound, liver biopsy, and scintiscans at $125 to $200, with percutaneous transhepatic cholangiography (PTC), abdominal CT scan, and endoscopic retrograde cholangiopancreatography (ERCP) two to three times higher and angiography five times higher.

BILIARY TRACT RADIOGRAPHY

ORAL CHOLECYSTOGRAPHY

Oral cholecystography is valuable when liver function is normal but is useless in the jaundiced patient. The dye must be excreted by the liver, a function that does not return immediately after recovery from hepatitis or common duct obstruction. Intravenous cholangiography serves to localize lesions of the larger bile ducts but allergic reactions, dependence on hepatic function (bilirubin <4), and the availability of alternative procedures have reduced the use of this test.

PERCUTANEOUS TRANSHEPATIC CHOLANGIOGRAPHY

PTC is performed to demonstrate mechanical obstruction of the biliary tract, particularly when liver dysfunction precludes intravenous cholangiography and ultrasound or CT scan shows the ductal system to be dilated. Under fluoroscopic guidance, a thin (20 to 25-gauge), flexible needle is inserted into the liver through an intercostal space, and dye is injected as it is slowly withdrawn. Normal ducts may be seen with a 50% to 70% success rate if up to ten attempts are made. Coagulopathy, ascites, perihepatic or intrahepatic sepsis, and disease of the right lower lung or pleura are contraindications. Antibiotic prophylaxis is required. The technique is an adjunct to passage of a catheter through an obstruction for internal drainage.

ENDOSCOPIC RETROGRADE CHOLANGIOPANCREATOGRAPHY

ERCP is performed for similar indications but is less constrained by coagulopathy, pleurisy, or ascites and is more apt to be successful when ducts are not dilated. It is particularly useful when stones, stricture, or tumor affect the extrahepatic biliary tree and in pancreatic diseases causing jaundice. The endoscopist often obtains cytologic diagnosis of periampullary tumors. Intrahepatic ductal lesions and the upper border of a complete obstruction are shown best by PTC, but diffuse disorders, such as sclerosing cholangitis, are usually diagnosed by ERCP. As liver capsule and ducts are not punctured, the risks of bleeding and peritonitis are avoided. Pancreatitis is a complication for 1% to 2% of patients; hyperamylasemia occurs in more. Active pancreatitis or cholangitis is a contraindication. Endoscopic sphincterotomy, stone extraction, and insertion of drainage stents are based on this technique.

ULTRASOUND

High-frequency sound waves are beamed at tissues whose characteristics influence the reflected waves. The signal is processed to yield a composite picture in varying shades of gray and may be adapted to sequential scans of moving organs (real-time imaging). Ultrasound distinguishes hollow structures from parenchyma and identifies dense objects such as stones. Harmless and relatively inexpensive, this test is the usual procedure after the general workup reveals cholestasis. It can show stones in the gallbladder, dilated intrahepatic or extrahepatic bile ducts, and swelling or cysts in the pancreas. Diagnostic sensitivity is limited by the failure of ducts to dilate in early or partial obstruction. If serum bilirubin is over 10 mg/dl, a nondilated duct system is firm evidence against extrahepatic obstruction. Ascites and the relations of other organs to the liver are displayed. Although resolution is as low as a few millimeters, it depends on sharp contrasts of density. Fat and gas distort echoes more than radiation. Ultrasound distinguishes cystic from solid defects in the liver, but many solid lesions blend with the parenchyma, and the consistency differences between cirrhotic, fatty, and normal livers are subtle.

COMPUTED TOMOGRAPHY

The CT scan provides images of viscera more familiar than echoes for size, shape, and relations, and more reliable for tissue fat consistency. The images may be enhanced by vascular or gut contrast material. It is an expensive alternative to ultrasound for assessing the biliary tree and detecting hepatic, pancreatic, or other abdominal masses. The radiation exposure is roughly equivalent to a barium enema. CT-guided skinny-needle aspirations are used in the cytologic diagnosis of cancer and in obtaining microbiological culture material. Risks of bleeding and peritonitis are less than for conventional biopsy, but the specimen yields cells without the architecture of a tissue block.

RADIOISOTOPE SCANS

Two types of scan involve gamma-emitting isotopes extracted by the liver. The reticuloendothelial system takes up ^{99m}Tc sulfur colloid to display both spleen and liver. Although physical examination supplemented by plain abdominal films usually defines liver size, shape, and position, as well as spleen size, a scan occasionally serves this purpose when ascites or obesity interferes with simpler, less expensive methods. As normal liver is homogeneous, lesions such as tumor or abscess appear as focal defects. Irregular uptake of colloid due to shunting in cirrhotic liver may produce pseudotumors. Scintillation density is a semi-quantitative reflection of liver function: Colloid escaping the liver increases the density of spleen and vertebrae, a common picture in chronic liver disease. Because colloid is extracted by the reticuloendothelial system rather than by parenchyma, the scan may be misleadingly normal in diffuse hepatitis. Technetium scanning is usually limited to the search for focal lesions. Resolution is approximately 2 cm. The cost-effectiveness of scan screening for metastases is doubtful in view of the fact that true positive scans *without* alkaline phosphatase elevation are scarcer than false-negative scans *with* alkaline phosphatase elevation.

The second type of scanning agent is taken up by liver cells and excreted into the biliary tract. A family of radiopharmaceuticals, whose common iminodiacetic acid derivatives are abbreviated IDA, has replaced rose bengal for this purpose. Such scans are particularly reliable in assessing patency of the cystic duct when acute cholecystitis is suspected. Nonvisualization of the gallbladder for 2 hours is diagnostic, provided the common bile duct is well seen. A dilated common duct and poor excretion into the gut suggest common duct obstruction. IDA scans are occasionally used to determine the completeness of extrahepatic obstruction, but hepatic secretion of the agent decreases as serum bilirubin exceeds 5 mg/dl. Prolonged scans are sometimes attempted for differential diagnosis of neonatal hepatitis/biliary atresia.

Because the radionuclide ^{67}Ga is better concentrated in cancer cells and inflammatory cells than in hepatocytes, a "hole" on technetium scan may appear as a "hot spot" on gallium scan. Gallium scan is seldom used as a liver test, but liver lesions may be found when it is used in search of abdominal sepsis or neoplasia. In cirrhotic liver, a lesion cold on technetium scan and hot on gallium scan is likely to be hepatocellular carcinoma.

BIOPSY

Percutaneous needle biopsy by the Menghini technique is a simple, safe diagnostic procedure (0.02% mortality rate in experienced hands). Metabolic defects may be diagnosed specifically, and cultures occasionally are positive, but more common diseases are usually characterized by type of abnormality rather than etiology. Biopsy readings identify diffuse parenchymal abnormalities (fatty change, hepatitis, cirrhosis) and disseminated focal lesions (granulomas, metastases). Specific diagnoses are usually reached by combining biopsy findings with other data.

Indications for biopsy include hepatomegaly or splenomegaly; persistent liver function abnormalities, particularly in prolonged cholestasis without evidence of extrahepatic obstruction; suspicion of infectious or infiltrative disorders; suspicion of relatively specific primary liver pathology (such as the acute fatty change of Reye's syndrome), or the constellation of findings in alcoholic hepatitis (mimicked by the hepatitis of jejunoileal bypass); biochemical assay diagnosis of genetic disorders, including storage diseases and defects of intermediary metabolism; and prognostic assessment of liver disease, particularly chronic hepatitis. The procedure is most frequently performed to confirm a clinical diagnosis of liver disease, to seek metastases or granulomas, to stage chronic hepatitis and evaluate its therapy, and to investigate fever of unknown origin. Histologic appearance seldom distinguishes among causes of hepatitis but often reveals the severity of cholestatic versus hepatocellular injury and occasionally signifies extrahepatic obstruction (bile infarcts) and cholangitis.

The most frequent severe complication is massive hemorrhage. Pleurisy and perihepatitis cause pain after the procedure, but pneumothorax or local sepsis is rare. Septicemia may complicate biopsy during untreated cholangitis. Punctures of the gallbladder or dilated ducts can cause biliary peritonitis. Other complications, such as hemobilia, intrahepatic arteriovenous fistula, and needle fracture, are rare. Accidental puncture of kidney or bowel seldom requires further intervention. The contraindications to biopsy are coagulation disorders, gross ascites (which increases the risk of bleeding and peritoneal sepsis), high-pressure extrahepatic obstruction, vascular lesions or severe passive congestion, disease of the right lower lobe of the lung or its pleura, and an uncooperative patient.

LAPAROTOMY

Laparotomy is the ultimate liver investigation, but its use for purely diagnostic purposes has been largely supplanted by the newer methods of cholangiography and imaging. The hazard of postoperative liver failure makes acute hepatitis a relative contraindication to surgery. Exploration is still an important recourse in fever of unknown origin. Liver biopsy is also indicated as a secondary feature of many abdominal operations. Abnormalities of gross appearance call for biopsy: A report of cirrhosis is not as persuasive as tissue, particularly if the diagnosis was not suspected previously. Optimal operative biopsies comprise both wedge and needle specimens. If only one sample can be taken, the needle specimen is preferable, unless a discrete superficial lesion is found. The capsule and its septa distort the architecture of a wedge. Incising the capsule, boring a 1-cm trocar cannula to a depth of 2 cm, removing the cannula, and extracting the specimen with blunt forceps have been recommended as optimal surgical biopsy technique.

LAPAROSCOPY

Laparoscopy offers some of the advantages of operative biopsy. These are a view of gross anatomy (peritoneal surface, liver, gallbladder, and spleen), direct guidance of the needle, and early knowledge of bleeding. It is particularly valuable in finding focal lesions, including hepatocellular cancer, and in recognizing macronodular cirrhosis when blind biopsies are nondiagnostic. Pelvic and upper abdominal examinations may be diagnostic in ascites of unknown cause. Prior surgery is a relative contraindication, because adhesions may impede maneuverability or bleed as they tear.

SYSTEMATIC USE OF SECONDARY OR TERTIARY PROCEDURES

Many algorithms have been devised for distinguishing between medical and surgical causes of cholestasis. Ultrasound is the best screening test after initial assessment. If the duct system is not dilated, liver biopsy is considered next. If, despite normal ultrasound, an extrahepatic lesion is strongly suspected or if biopsy is contraindicated, ERCP usually follows. If the ultrasound appearance is equivocal, the choice between PTC and ERCP may depend on local talent, assuming neither procedure is contraindicated. ERCP is often preferable when obstruction is incomplete and evidence about the pancreas seems pertinent. If ultrasound shows dilated ducts, either procedure is indicated. PTC is often chosen in complete obstruction because the proximal anatomy determines possibilities of drainage. In general, PTC seems preferable for lesions suspected at or above the cystic duct and ERCP seems preferable for periampullary lesions that may yield positive cytology. ERCP is safer in the presence of ascites or coagulopathy.

Is such extensive preoperative investigation necessary in patients with obvious "surgical jaundice"? Unless a downhill course calls for immediate relief, the answer is usually yes: (1) The nature and extent of obstruction can be evaluated better with the manipulation feasible on the fluoroscopy table than by intraoperative cholangiography. (High biliary tumors are particularly hard to find.) (2) Coincidental intrahepatic lesions, as in sclerosing cholangitis, will be observed and misoperations on patients with medical jaundice will be avoided. (3) Both ERCP and PTC are opening new avenues for stone removal and palliative drainage of malignant obstruction. In some cases, preoperative drainage reduces the hazards of subsequent surgery. In practice, however, these theoretical advantages may be obviated by the morbidity and delay of the procedures, particularly in inexperienced hands. Some of the greatest errors occur when a careless primary assessment incurs an expensive invasive approach to unrecognized medical illness, such as Laennec's cirrhosis, a reversible drug- or steroid-induced disorder, or the cholestatic variant of viral hepatitis.

PATHOPHYSIOLOGY

PORTAL HYPERTENSION

MEASUREMENT

Portal hypertension is usually considered to be present when the pressure in the portal vein is greater than 20 cm of saline (15 torr). Measurement of the portal pressure may be accomplished by wedged hepatic vein pressure (WHVP), by intrasplenic pressure (ISP), or by a needle or catheter in the portal vein. The WHVP is measured by threading a catheter percutaneously from a peripheral vein to the vena cava into a hepatic vein and "wedging" it (advancing it

ESOPHAGEAL VARICES AND PORTAL HYPERTENSION	
Etiology	Cirrhosis, hepatitis, parasite infection, portal venous obstruction and collateral veins, alcoholism
Dx	Signs of liver disease: ascites, encephalopathy, jaundice, cutaneous stigmata, hematemesis/melena; esophagogastroduodenoscopy, visceral angiography; ↑ hepatic venous pressure
Rx	Transfusion, balloon tamponade, vasopressin infusion, variceal sclerotherapy, portosystemic decompression

into a small hepatic vein so it is tightly surrounded by vein wall). If there is no prehepatic occlusion such as portal vein thrombosis, this will accurately reflect the pressure in the portal vein. The ISP is determined by percutaneously inserting a needle into the spleen and measuring the pulp pressure with a manometer. This again correlates closely with portal venous pressure. The insertion of a needle or catheter into the portal vein can be performed at operation, by disobliterating the umbilical vein through a small incision in the epigastrium and passing a catheter through the umbilical vein remnant into the left branch of the portal vein and subsequently into the main portal vein, or transhepatically, by inserting a catheter percutaneously into the intrahepatic portal venous system and threading it retrograde into the portal vein. Although there is a significant variation in portal pressure with alterations in systemic hemodynamics, measurement is extremely helpful in appraising the hemodynamic pathophysiology of the portal system.

ETIOLOGY

Although numerous valid classifications have been presented for the etiology of portal hypertension, the most practical seems to be the division into intrahepatic obstructive disease and extrahepatic obstructive disease of the venous inflow or outflow system. In over 95% of the patients, portal hypertension results from intrahepatic obstruction; of these, a great majority will be due to alcoholic cirrhosis or posthepatic cirrhosis, the relative proportion of each depending on the type of patients seen. The remaining causes of intrahepatic obstructive disease are varied and include biliary cirrhosis, cirrhosis secondary to chemicals and drugs, schistosomiasis, congenital hepatic fibrosis, and hemochromatosis, to name a few.

Extrahepatic causes of portal hypertension are most often associated with thrombosis of the portal vein. This may occur as a result of neonatal omphalitis, but often the etiology is unknown. Although operation is infrequently required, when it is, the anatomical distortions of the portal venous system can sometimes make selection of the procedure difficult. Obstruction of the outflow system can be due to constrictive pericarditis, congestive heart failure, or obstruction of the hepatic vein (Budd-Chiari syndrome). Outflow obstruction is often associated with hepatomegaly and ascites.

Portal hypertension is a result of inadequate outflow channels relative to the portal venous flow. Thus, portal hypertension can develop from an increased resistance to outflow or an increased inflow, or both. An increase in the precapillary flow of blood from the arterial to the venous system may contribute to portal hypertension. It has been shown as an example that there are presinusoidal arteriovenous communications between small branches of the hepatic artery and the inlet venules of the portal vein. These arteriovenous communications may increase in the presence of sinusoidal obstruction, allowing the hepatic arterial inflow to contribute to the portal hypertension. An increase in flow in microscopic arteriovenous shunts in the spleen, stomach, and esophagus, as well as in the mesenteric system, would increase the volume of blood in the portal venous system and exaggerate portal hypertension. Although gross arteriovenous communications between the hepatic and portal systems such as result from trauma or congenital abnormalities have been well documented as a cause of portal hypertension and bleeding esophageal varices, it has not been determined how much the microscopic shunts contribute to portal hypertension.

CIRRHOSIS

Cirrhosis is widespread hepatic fibrosis with nodule formation. It follows necrosis of liver cells. It is not simply fibrosis, nor is it nodule formation without fibrosis.

Liver cells become necrotic and degenerate secondary to a number of causes. Fibrosis develops, causing approximation of the portal and central zones (bridging). Some of the liver cells attempt to regenerate, developing nodules of liver tissue in between the acellular permanent septa that have developed in the portal zones of hepatic parenchyma. Sinusoids at the periphery of the regenerating nodule may shunt blood directly from the portal zone to the hepatic vein without significant distribution to the functioning hepatic cells. The thick fibrous-tissue septa that develop compress the hepatic vein branches, interfering with the drainage of blood from the liver, one of the main causes of portal hypertension. The number and size of the regenerative nodules have been found to have some relationship to the degree of portal hypertension and cirrhosis. The smaller and more numerous the nodules, the greater is their compression effect.

PATHOLOGIC ANATOMY

In an attempt to decompress the portal system, the blood seeks detour routes such as have been described. The most vulnerable of these as far as the function of the human body is concerned are the veins that traverse through the esophageal submucosa. These thin-walled veins just under the mucosa have no valves and very little supporting connective tissue and thus are prone to break down, causing bleeding into the esophagus and into the stomach. Hemorrhoids, caput medusae around the umbilicus, and duodenal varices are other manifestations of attempts to create portosystemic shunting but are infrequently pathologic.

PATHOPHYSIOLOGY

The consequences of portal hypertension are compounded and sometimes inseparable from the pathology associated with cirrhosis of the liver.

Ascites

Ascites is frequently associated with lymphatic outflow obstruction of the postsinusoidal area, such as in the Budd-Chiari syndrome or with constrictive pericarditis. It rarely occurs with portal hypertension *per se* without associated cirrhosis. When portal hypertension and cirrhosis coexist, if ascites is present, it can usually be controlled with intense medical management. Several factors other than portal hypertension contribute to the development of ascites. Portal hypertension, especially if the block is at the postpresinusoidal area, causes an increase in hilar and perihepatic lymph flow. Portal venous hypertension leads to an increased hydrostatic pressure and a low albumin causes an increased oncotic pressure at the capillaries, both of which by Starling's law would result in forces causing fluid to leave the vascular system. There is an increase in aldosterone secretion either from a hepatic humoral event related to an elevated portal pressure or secondary to a decreased nonsplanchnic blood volume. The complicated interrelationships of these factors will be discussed.

Gastrointestinal Hemorrhage

Gastrointestinal hemorrhage in association with cirrhosis of the liver usually occurs from the esophageal veins but can occur from gastric, duodenal, or hemorrhoidal varices. Although esophagogastritis from various causes and the coagulopathy frequently associated with cirrhosis may contribute to the tendency to bleed, the primary etiology seems to be related to the portal hypertension. There is no demonstrable relation between the amount of portal venous pressure and the tendency to bleed from varices; however, it is rare for a patient to have varices without portal hypertension.

Hypersplenism

Hypersplenism with anemia, leukopenia, or thrombocytopenia develops in about 10% of the patients with portal hypertension. Whether it is due to sequestration and destruction or to a decrease in the production of the various blood elements has not been determined. It is usually associated with splenomegaly and is usually not associated with severe hematologic problems.

Encephalopathy

Hepatic metabolic encephalopathy results from toxic substances from the mesenteric venous circulation entering the systemic circulation before being broken down by the hepatic cells. It is unusual to find it in patients with extrahepatic portal vein occlusion. Recent evidence suggests encephalopathy is primarily a result of aromatic amino acids and can be alleviated by branched-chain amino acids. It may occur with the development of portosystemic collaterals or surgically created portosystemic shunts. It seems to be worse in patients with poor liver function. Serum ammonia is used as an indication of encephalopathy, but although it can cause encephalopathy, it is not always elevated when the patient has this disorder.

NATURAL HISTORY

With improved medical management, the course of the patient with cirrhosis of the liver is rapidly changing, and current data on this subject are not available. Roughly 35% of the patients with cirrhosis develop esophageal varices, and 25% of these will bleed from the varices. Thirty to 40 years ago, three fourths of the patients who bled from esophageal varices died in the hospital; today, the prognosis has markedly improved. Although it has been stated that once a patient bleeds from varices, 50% will bleed again within 2 years if not operated upon, this is probably incorrect with current nonoperative modes of therapy. The prognosis for 5-year survival for the patient with alcoholic cirrhosis who has bled from esophageal varices is currently reported to be about 25%. Although this is a selected group, the 5-year survival for those operated upon is 50%. Prospective randomization of patients having therapeutic portacaval shunts has not demonstrated prolonged survival when compared with those not operated on. Most series suggest that patients with nonalcoholic cirrhosis fare better than those with alcohol-induced cirrhosis. These data do not reflect current medical management and better rehabilitation, including cessation of drinking.

ASCITES

Ascites is accumulation of fluid in the peritoneal cavity, eventually evident as abdominal distention with full flanks. "Shifting dullness" is the best physical sign but is often misleading. Gross ascites promotes umbilical and other hernias and scrotal edema. In ascites related to portal hypertension, abdominal wall veins are dilated and the spleen is often palpable. Indeed, the combination of ascites, dilated veins, and splenomegaly with a soft liver suggests presinusoidal block. A large firm liver with ascites, splenomegaly, and abdominal veins draining from the groin toward the chest suggests inferior vena cava obstruction. Ballottement may be necessary to feel the liver and spleen beneath ascites. Ascites may be mimicked by pancreatic pseudocyst, pregnancy, ovarian cyst, and pseudomyxoma. Minimal ascites or ascites obscured by obesity can be detected by ultrasound or CT scan.

PATHOGENESIS AND DIFFERENTIAL DIAGNOSIS

Cirrhotic portal hypertension is the most common cause, but ascites may result from other types of portal hypertension and from diseases that do not affect portal pressure. As prehepatic portal hypertension in the absence of liver disease produces less ascites than cirrhotic portal hypertension, factors other than portal pressure must contribute to ascites in cirrhosis. Examples of noncirrhotic ascites indicate these factors.

Ascites occurs with the fluid retention and transudation from vessels that accompany severe hypoalbuminemia in nephrotic syndrome, protein-losing enteropathy, and kwashiorkor. These disorders and the inverse relation between serum albumin and fluid accumulation in cirrhosis place ascites within the framework of the Starling equilibrium. Portal pressure pushing fluid through capillary walls exceeds the osmotic pressure, which depends on albumin, a molecule large enough not to escape the vascular bed except into hepatic lymph.

Ascites also forms when obstruction or trauma causes lymphatic vessels to leak. In such cases, the fluid usually contains fat and is called chylous ascites. It looks milky. Fat may be distinguished from other turbidity by Sudan stain or ether extraction. Cirrhotic ascites is seldom chylous, but increased hepatic production and "weeping" of lymph may explain higher protein content in cirrhotic ascites than in ascites of prehepatic portal hypertension or the nephrotic syndrome. Lymphatic drainage plays a larger part in the ascites that occasionally accompanies liver metastases or granulomas and in the ascites of hepatic vein or vena cava obstruction.

Ascites occurs in severe heart failure (particularly right-sided failure) and with impaired return of blood from the inferior vena cava to the right heart chambers (constrictive pericarditis, obstruction by clot or tumor). In addition to increased portal pressure secondary to passive congestion of the liver, ascites in heart failure owes much to the general fluid overload resulting from low cardiac output and renal sodium retention. Renal function in cirrhosis is like renal function in heart failure insofar as the kidney responds to poor perfusion by increasing sodium and water retention. Both the renin–aldosterone system and less-defined abnormalities of intrarenal circulation are involved.

It is easy to imagine local factors increasing hepatic lymphatic pressure and portal pressure in the Budd-Chiari syndrome. The most common cause is thrombosis of the hepatic vein and inferior vena cava, whether spontaneous, as in polycythemia or oral contraceptive use, or induced by mechanical obstruction, as in extensive liver, kidney, and adrenal cancers. Obstruction site (hepatic veins versus vena cava) may be inferred from the severity of leg edema, superficial vein dilation, and proteinuria, but venography and pressure studies are necessary for accurate definition. Veno-occlusive disease of the small hepatic veins, the most proximal postsinusoidal cause of portal hypertension and ascites, results from pyrrolizidine alkaloids (in bush teas), irradiation, chemotherapy, and graft vs. host reaction. Transient ascites in alcoholic hepatitis may have a similar mechanism (central hyaline sclerosis).

In the instances noted above, as in uncomplicated cirrhotic ascites, the fluid is a transudate; inflammation of the peritoneum produces exudative ascites, which is generally richer in protein and cells. Causes include infarction or perforation of any viscus, bacterial peritonitis, pancreatitis, tuberculous peritonitis, and cancer involving the peritoneum. Spontaneous bacterial peritonitis is a dangerous complication of chronic ascites, particularly in the cirrhotic patient. The distinction between transudate and exudate is important because conditions associated with exudates usually require more urgent treatment than do conditions associated with transudates. Unfortunately, the criteria of specific gravity and protein content become difficult to interpret in long-standing ascitic fluid. The ratio of LDH to serum LDH (>0.6 suggesting exudate) seems less reliable for abdominal than pleural fluid.

A diagnostic abdominal tap is almost always indicated upon first recognition of ascites, whatever the presumed cause. If possible, 50 ml to 100 ml should be taken to have sufficient volume for cytology as well as other tests. If abdominal distention is symptomatic, removal of 500 ml to 1000 ml may bring temporary relief, but tapping more than a liter risks hypotension and oliguria. The laboratory findings in various kinds of ascites are listed in Table 27-2. Protein content is somewhat more reliable than specific gravity in distinguishing exudates from transudates, but both are listed because specific gravity can be measured at the bedside.

Each case of ascites should be considered in terms of local and systemic factors. The paucity of ascites in extrahepatic portal vein obstruction suggests that portal hypertension may not be a primary and sufficient cause in the ascites of liver disease, but it is certainly an important localizing factor. Cirrhotics have ascites out of proportion to edema elsewhere. Increased formation and extrusion of hepatic lymph is the second local factor and probably accounts for the protein-rich ascites of the Budd-Chiari syndrome, constrictive pericarditis, and congestive failure. Systemic factors include decreased plasma oncotic pressure (hypoalbuminemia from inadequate synthesis, dilution by excess retained fluid, and loss into the peritoneal cavity);

TABLE 27-2 **LABORATORY FINDINGS IN ASCITES OF VARYING ETIOLOGY**

DISEASE	APPEARANCE	SPECIFIC GRAVITY	PROTEIN (g/dl)	CELLS	OTHER
Cirrhosis	Pale—deep yellow or green	<1.016	<2.5	<300 with 100 white cells/cu mm	
Comment: Chronicity raises specific gravity, protein, and mesothelial cell content. Other causes of portal hypertension produce similar fluid, with higher specific gravity and protein in postsinusoidal block.					
Nephrosis	Pale yellow, occasionally chylous	<1.016	<2.0	<200 (mesothelial)	
Comment: The purest transudate					
Peritoneal Cancer	Pale, hemorrhagic, chylous, or mucinous	>1.016 —variable—	>2.5	>500 (malignant and other types)	± red cells ↑ LDH
Comment: Tuberculosis peritonitis has a similar range of findings, but the predominant cells are lymphocytes; as in cancer, peritoneal biopsy increases the diagnostic yield.					
Bacterial Peritonitis	Turbid or purulent	>1.016	>2.5	>300 polymorphonuclear leukocytes per cu mm + Gram stain	pH <7.3
Comment: Spontaneous peritonitis need not have a high specific gravity and protein content; polymorphonuclear content and a low pH seem to be the most sensitive signs. The combination of bile and elevated amylase in abdominal fluid of the nonjaundiced patient suggests biliary or upper gut perforation or infarction, but long-standing jaundice imparts bilirubin to any fluid with albumin to bind it.					
Pancreatic Ascites	Turbid, hemorrhagic, or chylous	>1.016 —variable—	>2.5	Variable	↑ amylase

secondary hyperaldosteronism, due to increased secretion secondary to ineffective renal perfusion activating the renin–angiotension system and to impaired hepatic metabolism of aldosterone; and diminished water clearance related to abnormal intrarenal circulation and perhaps to increased antidiuretic hormone effect. Little-known effects of liver disease on renal function initiate salt and water retention.

MANAGEMENT

After assessment and diagnostic tap, the treatment depends on the underlying disease and the degree of disability ascites causes for the patient. The following guidelines apply to ascites in cirrhosis. Ascites should be reduced slowly because dangerous changes in plasma volume, blood pressure, and renal perfusion follow large diuresis or paracentesis. Generally, paracentesis volume should be less than a liter and net daily fluid loss measured by body weight should be less than a kilogram. As the maximal rate of ascites reabsorption is less than a liter per day, a larger diuresis represents fluid from other sites or depletion of vascular volume. Other forms of edema can be mobilized faster. Therapeutic paracentesis is seldom necessary, but for the patient with tense ascites and ulcerated umbilical eversion portending dehiscence, tapping 1 or 2 liters may be lifesaving. Respiratory embarrassment is another indication for removing several liters. Such large taps are usually prolonged over several hours by intermittently clamping an abdominal cannula. The hemodynamic hazards may be reduced by simultaneous infusion of colloid.

Graded treatment starts with bed rest and salt restriction. Ascites often abates spontaneously when the underlying liver disease improves. Because urinary sodium loss may be less than 10 mEq/liter, a sodium intake of less than 25mEq/day is desirable. Although serum sodium concentration may be low, total body sodium is excessive in patients with edema

or ascites. Sodium supplementation is occasionally necessary for symptomatic patients with serum concentrations well below 120 mEq/liter. If the patient is hyponatremic, fluid restriction to 1000 ml to 1500 ml/day is indicated. A low-sodium diet is distasteful and often requires low-sodium, high-calorie snacks. Weight should be recorded daily. If no diuresis begins after several days, spironolactone, an aldosterone antagonist, is added in doses of 75 mg to 150 mg a day. The dose may be doubled if there is no effect in another week, but increasing the total daily dose beyond 400 mg is unavailing. Urinary sodium should rise to exceed the potassium concentration; spot checks of urine are used to guide dosage. An additional diuretic, if necessary, will be more effective after the urinary sodium/potassium ratio exceeds 1. If ascites remains refractory, furosemide, 40 mg to 80 mg, may be added, preferably in intermittent rather than daily doses. Spironolactone induces gynecomastia and hyperkalemia. Cirrhotics presenting with ascites are usually potassium depleted, but hyperkalemia is a dangerous effect of combining spironolactone with potassium supplements. Furosemide induces volume depletion, which may precipitate hepatorenal syndrome (HRS), and hypokalemic alkalosis, which may precipitate encephalopathy. Periodic electrolyte and creatinine determinations are indicated in patients on diuretic therapy.

Symptomatic ascites refractory to conservative management usually must await spontaneous improvement of the liver. Occasionally, a 750-ml to 1000-ml paracentesis, combined with infusion of 25 g salt-poor albumin and 120 mg furosemide, will precipitate a diuresis. Removal and reinfusion of ascitic fluid has been attempted by many techniques over many years without consistent success. The LeVeen shunt, a subcutaneous tube connecting the abdominal cavity with the internal jugular vein through a pressure-sensitive one-way valve, has a few dramatic successes in reducing ascites and improving renal function. Complicating peritonitis, septicemia, and disseminated intravascular coagulation limit its use. A side-to-side portacaval shunt can reduce otherwise intractable ascites, but such patients are poor operative risks.

Patients with cirrhosis and ascites, particularly alcoholics, are susceptible to spontaneous bacterial peritonitis, involving enteric gram-negative organisms usually and pneumococci occasionally. Pain is common. Fever and signs of peritoneal irritation are variable, but the fluid is usually cloudy, with over 300 polymorphonuclear leukocytes per cubic millimeter and a *p*H more than 0.1 unit below plasma *p*H. Gram's stain and culture of centrifuged fluid are essential. Treatment is started on the basis of the stain. Coverage for anaerobes is unnecessary. The febrile alcoholic with lymphocyte–monocyte predominance in a peritoneal exudate may have tuberculous peritonitis.

HEPATORENAL SYNDROME

HRS is reversible renal failure due to liver failure, without histologic signs of kidney damage. The pathophysiology is unknown but seems to combine two sets of findings. First, it seems to be an ultimate expression of ordinary adaptation to liver insufficiency: sodium retention, impaired free water excretion, reduced "effective" central plasma volume despite normal or increased total plasma and extracellular fluid volumes, and the pressure effects of ascites. Second, distinct peculiarities of renal circulation are recorded by angiography, xenon washout, and radiohippuran clearance: intense afferent vasoconstriction, reduced cortical perfusion sparing juxtamedullary glomeruli, and vasolability. The perfusion pattern is ever changing, as though intrarenal shunts continually open and close. Endotoxemia and a host of steroid, polypeptide, and prostaglandin abnormalities have been adduced in explanation of the above finding. The firmest generalizations are that HRS is a circulatory disorder precipitated by events known to affect blood volume or distribution and characterized by intrarenal circulatory changes and avid sodium and water retention.

The clinical picture consists of oliguria (200 ml–500 ml/day) and uremia (creatinine 2 mg–3 mg/dl, blood urea nitrogen 50 mg–70 mg/dl) in a patient with severe hepatitis or deteriorating cirrhosis. The syndrome is often precipitated by bleeding, sepsis, paracentesis, or diuresis, but one third of episodes seem spontaneous. The onset may be sudden or gradual. Declining blood pressure is a common warning. Except in patients with superimposed acute tubular necrosis (ATN), the renal failure usually does not progress to severe acidosis and hyperkalemia. (Cirrhotics have a propensity to renal tubular acidosis unassociated with HRS.) Although renal failure *per se* has a minor role in the outcome, 80% of patients with HRS die of their liver disease. The course depends upon the liver. Transplants of liver and kidney have demonstrated rapid complete reversal of the syndrome when the dysfunctional kidney is in a normal hepatic milieu.

The "functional" nature of the lesion contrasts with ATN, which is associated with anatomical changes and risk of uremic death. Patients with severe liver disease are subject to many of the hypotensive calamities known to precipitate ATN. A few cases document spontaneous transition from HRS to ATN. Differential diagnosis is important in determining how to treat the renal failure (*i.e.*, whether or not to dialyze). The patient with HRS is likely to be at a terminal stage of liver disease. The renal failure *per se* is not severe enough to require dialysis, and the prognosis is poor regardless of intervention. The patient with ATN *may* have less severe liver disease, which could improve if he is successfully tided through renal failure.

The abnormalities in HRS are of the type found in severe prerenal azotemia, but they do not respond to volume expansion. Urinary sediment is relatively normal. The urine/plasma creatinine ratio is over 20, the serum urea/creatinine ratio is often over 20, but a low urea due to poor protein nutrition or impaired urea synthesis may obscure this sign. In distinguishing HRS from ATN a urinary sodium concentration under 12 mEq/liter is the best discriminant and a urine/plasma osmolality ratio greater than 1.1 is second best. In typical ATN, urinary sediment is abnormal, sodium concentration is over 40 mEq/liter, urine osmolality is less than 350 mOsm/kg, and the ratios of urine/plasma creatinine and serum urea/serum creatinine are both under 20. Jaundiced patients undergoing biliary surgery seem particularly prone to develop ATN. Distinction between ATN and HRS is most difficult during pharmacologic diuresis.

It is important to exclude other common forms of renal failure. Prerenal azotemia can be recognized by fluid loss history, low central venous pressure, and response to hydration. Obstruction may also present as a low urinary sodium but should be readily identified by catheterization for residual volume and ultrasonic exam for a dilated collecting system. Nephritis, especially drug-induced interstitial disease, is common in the same population but should be distinguished by history, abnormal sediment, and higher urinary sodium. Infection differs from HRS in presentation, sediment, culture, and response to treatment. Like obstruction, this possibility should be tested early, because its reversal removes a factor that might otherwise exacerbate liver failure.

The term *hepatorenal* also suggests a number of uncommon afflictions shared by liver and kidney: infections (leptospirosis, tuberculosis, and yellow fever), toxins (carbon tetrachloride and amanita mushroom poison), immunologic disorders (polyarteritis and the nephritis of acute or chronic hepatitis), macrocirculatory syndromes (severe congestive failure, toxemia of pregnancy, endotoxemia, and ischemic shock), and a miscellany including polycystic disease, amyloidosis, and renal cell carcinoma.

Current treatment of HRS is that of other forms of oliguric renal failure, except that dialysis is rarely appropriate. The clinician should look for pseudohepatorenal situations and treat their causes (obstruction, hypovolemia, urinary tract infection, aminoglycoside toxicity). Paracentesis and volume expansion may correct the prerenal element in HRS, but variceal bleeding is a hazard. The LeVeen shunt dramatically improves renal function but has its own complications and cannot improve the underlying liver disease. Chronic HRS is occasionally relieved by portacaval shunt. The failures of dopa and dopamine infusions and of adrenergic blockers discredit the false neurotransmitter theory of the genesis of HRS. Agents inhibiting angiotensin formation may benefit intrarenal circulation at the cost of systemic hypotension.

HEPATIC ENCEPHALOPATHY

The neuropsychiatric syndrome of hepatic encephalopathy in acute liver failure is fully reversible if the patient survives. In chronic active hepatitis and cirrhosis, it usually reverses with treatment but may accumulate subtle irreversible effects. After portosystemic shunt, its severity varies with the size of the shunt and in many cases cannot be fully controlled. Increased size and numbers of astrocytes (Alzheimer type 2) in the cerebrum, cerebellum, and basal ganglia are the characteristic pathologic changes. Acute histologic changes are probably reversible, but some of the chronic syndromes are associated with cortical thinning, basal ganglia degeneration, and (rarely) pyramidal tract demyelination.

The clinical picture is variable. Disturbances of consciousness reduce alertness, slur speech, impair sleep rhythm, and generally promote somnolence. Some patients with fulminant liver failure, particularly children, enter coma through delirium, and a few present with choreoathetosis. Intellectual defects usually involve the ability to organize objects in space: Serial handwriting, matchstick stars, or the Reitan trail test are often more sensitive than ordinary examinations. In chronic syndromes, personality changes of apathy, irritability, or inappropriate euphoria may persist when other psychological and neurologic signs have reverted.

Asterixis is the most characteristic sign. Consisting of sudden lapses in posture, it is absent at rest. It is elicited by having the patient hyperextend his wrist while his forearm is flexed. A flap can seldom be shown in the lightest or deepest stages of encephalopathy. Muscle tone and deep tendon reflexes tend to increase until, deep in coma, limbs become limp and the Babinski sign emerges. Pyramidal tract signs occasionally dominate the course. Transverse myelitis with paraplegia has followed shunt surgery. Cirrhotics with large shunts may develop irreversible parkinsonian features.

Sherlock employs a five-step clinical grading scale: (1) confused, with altered mood and psychometric testing, (2) drowsy, with inappropriate behavior, (3) stuporous, with impaired speech and responsive only to simple command, (4) coma, and (5) deep coma unresponsive to painful stimuli.

None of the manifestations of hepatic coma is pathognomonic. Many signs including flap are common to other metabolic encephalopathies, such as uremia, CO_2 narcosis, and severe heart failure. Slowing of electroencephalographic waves from the alpha to the delta range precedes clinical signs but is not specific for liver disease. Hyperammonemia is a useful marker of liver insufficiency but is not present in every patient with liver coma (see section on laboratory tests). Simple screening tests exclude other metabolic encephalopathies, but the possibilities of delirium tremens and Wernicke-Korsakoff syndrome may obscure the differential diagnosis in the alcoholic. Fine tremor, insomnia, hyperactivity, and extreme anxiety usually distinguishes the alcohol withdrawal syndrome. Sometimes the issue is only resolved by cautious attempts at sedation with an agent such as diazepam or chlordiazepoxide. Thiamine is a harmless cure for acute Wernicke-Korsakoff syndrome, but the chronic disorder sometimes merges with chronic hepatic encephalopathy and alcohol's direct brain toxicity.

The encephalopathic toxin (or toxins?) is unknown, but it seems to arise in the portal circulation and escape metabolism by the failing or bypassed liver. No alternative agent has displaced ammonia from its putative role, but biochemical synergism with mercaptans, free tryptophan, and short-chain fatty acids may be analogous to the clinical synergism between protein intolerance and sensitivity to sedatives. The supposed importance of false neurotransmitters has been diminished by direct measurement and application of octopamine.

Whatever the final neurotoxic pathway, it must account for a wide variety of coma precipitants. The two most common causes are uremia and sedative and analgesic drugs. Spontaneous HRS and obvious dehydrating events (diuresis, paracentesis, vomiting) account for most episodes of uremia. Gastrointestinal bleeding produces coma more often than does dietary protein. Hyperaldosteronism promotes hypokalemic alkalosis, a tendency exaggerated by many diuretics. Hypokalemic alkalosis increases both formation and reabsorption of renal ammonia. Ammonia has a pKa of 9. The equilibrium $NH_4^+ \rightleftarrows NH_3 + H^+$ favors diffusible NH_3 in an alkaline environment. Thus, alkaline urine favors ammonia reabsorption and systemic alkalosis favors ammonia diffusion across the blood–brain barrier. Constipation and infection are less commonly recognized factors. (The role of infection, particularly endotoxemia, in deterioration of liver disease is probably underestimated.)

Chronic relapsing encephalopathy in an otherwise stable shunt patient differs from coma as one aspect of fulminant hepatitis (along with coagulopathy, hypoglycemia, respiratory distress syndrome and so forth), but the following discussion emphasizes common features in management:

The patient must be protected by measures related to the severity of the syndrome regardless of etiology or pathogenesis. This entails social and occupational precautions in grade 1; special nursing or household support in grade 2; parenteral nutrition in grade 3; nasogastric suction, turning, and bowel and bladder hygiene in grade 4; and mechanical ventilation in grade 5.

Precipitating or contributing factors must be found and corrected. Drugs must be reviewed compulsively to exclude sedatives, opiates, and most diuretics and to reevaluate the need for any agent known to affect blood pressure, metabolism, coagulation, or fluid–electrolyte and acid–base balance. Dehydration should be repaired and renal insufficiency corrected insofar as possible. A single measure, such as correction of hypokalemic alkalosis with administration of potassium chloride, sometimes reverses encephalopathy. Enemas and cathartics are necessary to remove blood and stool from the gastrointestinal tract. Infection should be sought and treated.

Two classes of therapeutic agents are employed to reduce toxic influx from the gut to the portal circulation: (1) Poorly absorbed antibiotics such as neomycin reduce the ureolytic and proteolytic bacterial flora of the colon. (2) Unabsorbed sugars such as lactulose interfere with bacterial amino acid metabolism, decreasing ammonia production and perhaps fostering ammonia incorporation in the flora. Carbohydrate fermentation products acidify colonic contents, which tends to keep free ammonia in the unabsorbable NH_4^+ form. Finally, these agents serve as cathartics. Enemas using the carbohydrate lactose may prove an effective alternative to oral neomycin therapy combined with cleansing enemas. Neomycin therapy has the enteric complications of small-intestinal malabsorption and staphylococcal enterocolitis. Ototoxicity and nephrotoxicity result from the fraction absorbed in long-term use. Treatment may be started at 4 g/day, but the dose should be reduced to 2 g/day for long-term use. Diarrhea is the main side-effect of lactulose. Doses of 10 ml to 30 ml three times a day are used. It is uncertain whether neomycin and lactulose effects are additive. The choice of one or both agents must be individualized. In nonemergency and chronic situations, lactulose is preferable because of its lesser toxicity.

Nutritional support must be carefully selected. Calorie

and nitrogen input must be sufficient to keep catabolism from increasing the waste nitrogen load. Dietary protein is usually restricted to less than 0.75 g/kg and more than 0.4 g/kg. Because vegetable proteins are less ammoniagenic than meat proteins, patients with chronic encephalopathy may benefit from a modified vegetarian diet. Caloric input is best estimated from basal energy expenditure multiplied by appropriate activity and stress factors. Most patients need at least 1500 calories a day.

The extent to which the abnormal plasma aminogram (increases in methionine and the aromatic amino acids phenylalanine, tyrosine, and tryptophan and decreases in the branched-chain amino acids valine, leucine, and isoleucine) should influence therapy is unknown. Conventional therapy can reduce plasma ammonia and restore normal mental status without changing the aminogram. Trials of amino acid infusion designed to normalize the aminogram have had conflicting results. Preparations enriched in branched-chain amino acids and low in aromatic amino acids have not yet proved worth their high cost. Use of the ornithine salts of ketoanalogues of essential amino acid is a more promising approach. Trials of levodopa and bromocriptine as agents influencing adrenergic central nervous system function have had equivocal results.

SURGERY AND THE LIVER

Operations on the liver, bile ducts, and vessels are described elsewhere; the role of the liver in the outcome of other operations is considered here. Data on operative risks imposed by liver diseases are sparse. Surgery appears to delay recovery from any form of acute hepatitis and is said to induce hepatic coma in up to 10% of patients with viral hepatitis. Alcoholic hepatitis is associated with a high perioperative mortality, as well as prolonged postoperative jaundice. In general, operative complications appear related to the acuteness and severity of hepatitis. Patients with latent cirrhosis are at less risk. They too may suffer transient encephalopathy and jaundice, but they usually do well with a forewarned anesthetist and vigilant postoperative prevention of hypotension and hypoxia. If any rule is applicable, it is to defer elective procedures on patients with acute hepatitis or deteriorating chronic liver disease but not to procrastinate unduly for stable cirrhosis. Intraoperative liver biopsy should be obtained whenever feasible on any patient with suspected liver disease.

Postoperative liver dysfunction is also common in patients without recognized liver disease. Brief transaminase elevation without jaundice occurs 1 to 3 days after major procedures in many patients with normal livers. Hemolysis in the postoperative patient may result in elevated conjugated as well as unconjugated bilirubin levels due to nonspecific (ischemic?) impairment of excretion. The problem may be anticipated in patients receiving much stored blood before and during surgery. Trauma and vascular procedures produce pigment overload from both hematomas and transfusions. Fifty milliliters, the amount hemolyzed per unit of stored blood in the first day after transfusion, equals normal daily bilirubin production of 250 mg. Immunotransfusion reactions may go undetected amid other problems, and the patient may be given drugs that induce hemolysis. Hemoglobinopathies, such as S-C disease, and enzyme defects, such as glucose-6-phosphate dehydrogenase deficiency, may be unmasked. Cardiac valve suture leaks induce microangiopathic hemolysis, as does disseminated intravascular coagulation.

Benign postoperative cholestasis results from multiple problems such as hypotension, congestive failure, septicemia, and pneumonia, usually combined with some degree of pigment overload. Jaundice (predominantly conjugated) is evident in a few days. Bilirubin and alkaline phosphatase levels usually peak in a week and remain elevated or fall depending on the patient's general course. Bilirubin levels may exceed 30 mg/dl, being magnified by hemolysis and renal insufficiency. Transaminase levels rise early but seldom persist over 250 IU. The syndrome is particularly prominent in circumstances combining hypotension with a heavy blood pigment load (*e.g.*, surgery for ruptured aneurysm). It should be recognized as intrahepatic cholestasis (confirmed by ultrasound if necessary) to prevent unnecessary biliary exploration. Such patients have high mortality, although their jaundice seldom signifies liver failure. It is a result rather than a major cofactor of their dire illnesses. Liver ischemia after cardiopulmonary bypass causes jaundice and occasional liver failure due to centrilobular necrosis. Transaminase levels are high relative to alkaline phosphatase.

Acute postoperative cholecystitis presents as jaundice and high alkaline phosphatase in a third of patients. This syndrome, often acalculous and affecting men more frequently than women, has a high mortality. Pain may not be prominent, but fever, leukocytosis, and right upper quadrant tenderness help make the diagnosis. Erythromycin estolate cholestasis occasionally mimics acute cholecystitis.

Liver dysfunction is sometimes an important sign of sepsis from peritonitis, abscess, renal infection, or pneumonia. Any severe septicemia may produce jaundice (conjugated) with nonspecific intrahepatic cholestasis and focal necrosis. Transaminase and alkaline phosphatase levels are slightly elevated. Hepatitis within 2 weeks of an operation cannot be attributed to intraoperative transfusions. The usual incubation period for hepatitis B or non-A, non-B hepatitis is at least 1 month. Cytomegalovirus postperfusion syndrome is usually anicteric.

Drug toxicity should be carefully sought in the patient with perioperative liver dysfunction. The fluorinated anesthetics halothane and methoxyflurane (Penthrane) are of special interest because of their characteristic allergic syndrome with its high mortality. A majority of the jaundiced and 90% of those who die had prior exposure to the agent. Recent repeated exposures seem most hazardous. About a week after initial exposure, the susceptible patient may have fever, nausea, and eosinophilia accompanied by a threefold to fivefold elevation in transaminase and occasionally followed by a rise in bilirubin level. After subsequent exposure, latency may be as short as 1 to 5 days, but jaundice usually is not evident for a week, which tends to exclude the pigment overload–cholestasis–ischemia syndromes. Transaminases rise to levels found in viral hepatitis. Full-fledged icteric halothane hepatitis has a 20% to 40% mortality rate. Patients with unexplained fever after halothane or Penthrane should not be tried on either agent again.

Transplantation surgery has several associated liver disorders. Multiple transfusions increase the probability of contracting hepatitis B and non-A, non-B hepatitis. Immunosuppression may promote chronic viral hepatitis. These patients are subject to cytomegalovirus and herpes simplex hepatitis. They are also at risk of septicemia with associated liver dysfunction, and they often take drugs such as α-methyldopa and isoniazid, which can induce acute or chronic liver disease. Severe postoperative pancreatitis with jaundice is an occasional complication of renal transplantation. Azathioprine hepatitis is ill characterized but often proposed as a diagnosis of exclusion. Graft-versus-host disease, common after marrow transplantation, starts with skin signs a few days before gastrointestinal symptoms and jaundice (usually in the third week of the transplant). Transaminase levels rise fivefold to 20-fold, and alkaline phosphatase rises later. Veno-occlusive disease is attributed to the graft-versus-host reaction and to the chemotherapy these patients undergo.

The long-debated relations of nutrition and the liver have been elucidated somewhat by two recent trends in surgery: the continuing advances in parenteral nutrition and the ill-fated venture of jejunoileal bypass. Early amino acid and peptide mixtures contained enough ammonia to induce encephalopathy in infants. Cholestasis is still a predictable problem in premature infants on parenteral nutrition for 6 weeks or longer. The most common hepatic complication of parenteral nutrition in adults could be termed the pâté de foie gras effect, the fatty infiltration resulting from caloric input in excess of maintenance and anabolic requirements. It appears analogous to the European custom of force-feeding geese to fatten their livers for pâté. Mild transaminase elevations are common early in total parenteral nutrition. Persistent overfeeding results in hyperbilirubinemia and a moderate rise in alkaline phosphatase after about 2 weeks. Biopsies show excess periportal fat but none of the inflammation and necrosis that precede lasting liver damage in jejunoileal bypass or alcoholic hepatitis. The same effect has been attributed to essential fatty acid deficiency but not to the usual doses of lipid in total parenteral nutrition. Caloric deprivation also can cause hyperbilirubinemia, unmasking generic defects such as Gilbert's and Dubin-Johnson syndromes. Other liver tests are normal, and jaundice abates with refeeding.

Hepatic complications led to abandonment of jejunoileal bypass in the treatment of morbid obesity. Moderately fat livers are common in obesity, but fat increases greatly in the first year after bypass. In 20% to 30% of patients, periportal fibrosis becomes prominent, and in half of these, inflammation, necrosis, and cholestasis imply hepatitis. In a few patients, the combination of Mallory hyaline, polys, and fat is indistinguishable from alcoholic hepatitis. The disease has progressed in so many patients that liver failure is the operation's foremost cause of death. Recognition of

the hepatic syndrome and timely reanastomosis often reverses the hepatitis, but some cases have gone on to cirrhosis.

BLEEDING ESOPHAGEAL VARICES

DIAGNOSIS

The patient who presents with a history and physical examination leading to the suspicion of bleeding from esophageal varices must be thoroughly evaluated. It must be established that the patient has bled and has done so from the upper gastrointestinal tract. Examination of the stools for blood, a hemogram profile, a history compatible with gastrointestinal bleeding, and aspiration of the stomach all contribute to the appropriate diagnosis. A history of alcoholism or hepatitis and a physical examination revealing the stigmas of cirrhosis contribute to the diagnosis. Splenomegaly and abnormal hepatic function tests are helpful but not diagnostic.

The venous phase of a celiac or superior mesenteric artery angiogram may demonstrate esophageal varices, as may a percutaneously performed splenoportogram (Fig. 27-6). Currently, the most definitive diagnosis of esophageal varices is made with the endoscope. This can be performed with the flexible esophagoscope under local anesthesia with a minimum risk of major complications. Since varices frequently stop bleeding spontaneously, the actual bleeding site may not be demonstrated. Another advantage of endoscopy is that other pathology of the upper gastrointestinal tract may be identified. The barium swallow at times is very diagnostic of esophageal varices, but its lack of sensitivity has led to its being replaced by other procedures (Fig. 27-7).

MANAGEMENT

The management of the patient with bleeding esophageal varices is rapidly evolving. Operative therapy, which has been the only effective form of therapy since the early part of the century, is being reexamined and replaced by nonoperative management in many instances. It will require several decades to adequately evaluate some of the newer methods presented in this chapter.

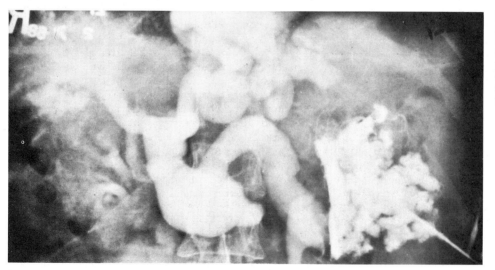

Fig. 27-6. This splenoportogram demonstrates an unusually large splenic vein and coronary vein arising from the portal vein. The gastric and esophageal varices are easily seen at the top midportion of the figure.

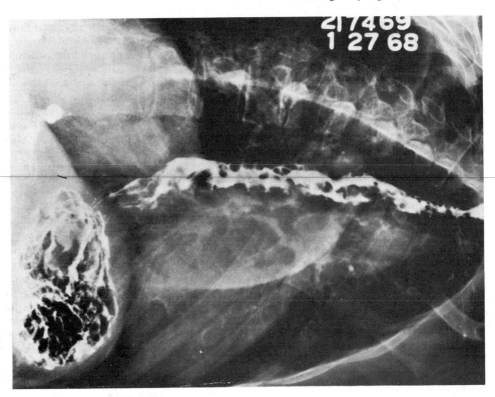

Fig. 27-7. Extensive esophageal and gastric varices demonstrated by a barium esophagogram.

A current method of management of the patient who presents with upper gastrointestinal tract hemorrhage due to esophageal varices is outlined in the algorithm presented in Figure 27-8. Patients cannot be managed by algorithm or checklists, since each patient must be treated as an individual and the resources of the institution and the expertise of the physician will vary.

RESUSCITATION

Immediate measures should be aimed at resuscitation of the patient should this be indicated. Blood pressure should be closely followed. Central venous lines for therapy and hemodynamics should be inserted. Urine output should be monitored by an indwelling Foley catheter. The patient should be immediately typed and cross matched for blood; blood incompatibility is frequently found in these patients, especially those who have had multiple blood transfusions. Electrolytes, liver function studies, coagulation studies, and arterial blood gases should be obtained in all patients with altered hemodynamics and in others as indicated.

It is very important not to make these patients hypervolemic, since this may inappropriately raise the portal

Fig. 27-8. Algorithm for management of the patient with bleeding esophageal varices.

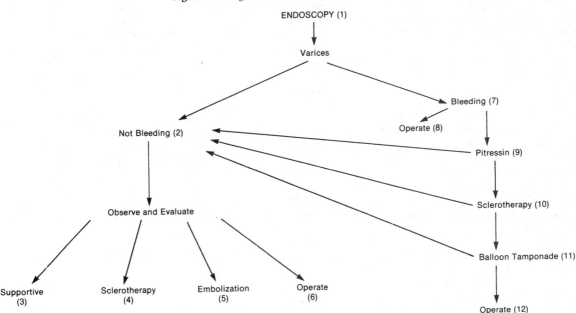

pressure, causing continued bleeding from the varices. The hematocrit should not be used as a criterion for the blood transfusions because the plasma volume is frequently expanded, causing a low hematocrit but an adequate blood volume. Fluid therapy also needs to be carefully monitored and restricted as much as possible; these patients frequently have an excess of fluid and salt as a result of an increased aldosterone mechanism.

Coagulation problems should be corrected. Prothrombin time, partial thromboplastin time, thrombin clotting time, and platelet count should be monitored carefully, and appropriate therapy should be instituted. Fresh blood should be given if readily available.

Prophylaxis against hepatic coma should be instituted as soon as possible. Hepatic encephalopathy seems to result from the absorption of certain amino acids from the intestine. This can be altered by measures such as iced gastric lavage to remove blood from the stomach, catharsis (magnesium sulfate), and a nonabsorbable antibiotic in the gastrointestinal tube to neutralize the bacteria of the intestinal tract which act on the protein substrate.

Metabolic alkalosis is usually due to hypokalemia and should be corrected with potassium chloride as rapidly as is safe. This condition not only potentiates encephalopathy, but the hypokalemia can lead to cardiac arrhythmias. Refractory alkalosis at times responds to carefully administered intravenous hydrochloric acid.

NONOPERATIVE

Patients should be admitted and carefully observed. Most of the patients will stop bleeding before or soon after admission to the emergency room.

Esophagoscopy (No. 1, Fig. 27-8) should be performed as soon as possible in an attempt to make a definitive diagnosis and outline a plan of therapy for the specific problem. The flexible endoscope can be used for this, and the procedure is performed under local anesthesia with a minimum of danger to the patient.

Should varices not bleeding (No. 2, Fig. 27-8) be seen on endoscopy, therapy is directed at preventing further bleeding. One must, of course, consider that the varices were not the source of bleeding. Once the varices bleed, they will usually rebleed; therefore, supportive therapy (No. 3, Fig. 27-8) is usually reserved for those patients in whom the diagnosis is in doubt. This consists of careful follow-up aimed toward the avoidance of alcohol. Should rebleeding occur, immediate endoscopy should be performed.

If bleeding varices (No. 7, Fig. 27-8) are found on endoscopy, intravenous pitressin (No. 9, Fig. 27-8) is begun. A bolus of 20 units of pitressin in 200 ml 5% dextrose in water is given over a 20-minute period. Following this, 0.2 unit/ml/minute is started. The dosage is increased to 0.4 unit/ml/minute if bleeding persists. Selective mesenteric intra-arterial injection seems to have no benefit over the intravenous route. Should intravenous pitressin fail to control slow but continuous bleeding, sclerotherapy (No. 10, Fig. 27-8), to be described, should be considered. It is difficult to perform this procedure if there is rapid bleeding from the varices.

Balloon tamponade (No. 11, Fig. 27-8) is a very effective yet dangerous method of controlling bleeding from gastric and esophageal varices. The method consists of a long gastric tube with two attached balloons, one for compressing the gastric varices and another for compressing the esophageal varices. The bleeding can usually be controlled by the gastric balloon (prevents blood flow into the esophageal varices). Aspiration of blood into the lungs from the esophagus is a real danger, and the patient needs to be monitored continually. It is not a definitive form of therapy for bleeding esophageal varices.

Sclerotherapy (No. 4, Fig. 27-8) as primary treatment of bleeding esophageal varices is currently being evaluated by numerous centers throughout the world. It may be performed by rigid esophagoscope or flexible endoscope. Five percent sodium morrhuate is injected directly into the varix or into the perivascular tissue. Recurrent hemorrhage develops in 30% to 40% of these patients; therefore, repeated injections are required. Stricture formation and other complications have been infrequently reported. The advantages of this therapy include simplicity, rapidity, no alterations in portal hemodynamics, no effect on the potential of performing a shunt in the future, and minimal hospitalization. The disadvantages primarily relate to its effectiveness and lack of long-term follow-up data.

Percutaneous embolization (No. 5, Fig. 27-8) of the coronary vein and short gastric vein by threading a catheter into the portal vein has been effective in some institutions in selected patients. The incidence of rebleeding and bleeding from the liver has hindered its widespread application. In addition, it has not proved effective in control of bleeding from esophageal varices by many who have used it.

SPECIAL STUDIES

Some of the special studies for evaluating the patient with portal hypertension have previously been described. The activity of the cirrhosis should be evaluated by liver function studies, level of hepatitis B antigen, and needle biopsy of the liver, as indicated. The portal system anatomy and hemodynamics can be evaluated by several methods. Hepatic vein catheterization, in which a catheter is inserted and then wedged into the hepatic vein, is of benefit in diagnosing cirrhosis by hepatic venography, but, more important, the pressure measurement accurately reflects the pressure in the portal veins. Percutaneous splenoportography gives an opportunity to accurately measure portal pressure (splenic pulp pressure) and obtain an angiogram demonstrating the complete portal venous system. Although it has amazingly few complications, the potential of necessitating an immediate operation always exists. Celiac and superior mesenteric arteriography demonstrates anatomical variations that are of help in diagnosis and outlining therapy. This also excludes arteriovenous fistula of the portal system. The venous phase of this is most helpful in demonstrating a patent portal and splenic vein, perhaps even demonstrating the coronary and short gastric veins along with the esophageal varices and, frequently, hepatopetal flow through the portal vein. Barium contrast studies of the upper gastrointestinal tract are useful in demonstrating the varices and excluding other pathology. Visualization of the upper gastrointestinal tract using the flexible endoscope has superseded the usefulness of the barium study. Transhepatic or transumbilical vein catheterization of the portal veins is used in a few centers for anatomical and hemodynamic appraisal of the portal venous system.

OPERATIVE (NOS. 6, 8, 12, FIG. 27-8; Figs. 27-9 and 27-10)

Types of Operations

Therapeutic measures to control the bleeding from esophagogastric varices are best understood by a thorough understanding of the pathologic anatomy, physiology, and biochemistry associated with portal hypertension with and without cirrhosis of the liver. A number of these procedures depend on the ability to separate the portal venous system into the greater and lesser systems (see Fig. 27-3). Thus, the end-to-side portacaval, side-to-side portacaval, side-to-side splenorenal, and mesocaval shunts direct the blood flow from the liver to a systemic vein (total shunt) and by this means decompress the hypertension in the esophageal varices.

The ablative operations attempt to separate the greater and lesser splanchnic systems by obliterating part or all of the lesser splanchnic circulation. These procedures range from complete devascularization of the intraesophageal and paraesophageal collateral circulations to embolization of the coronary and short gastric veins. The Womack ablative operation includes splenectomy, resection of the greater curvature of the stomach, oversewing the varices, and extensive ligation of vessels around the stomach. The Sugiura blocking procedure in addition transects and reanastomoses the esophagus, thus obliterating the esophageal veins. Cur-

rent reports of the use of a stapling device to simplify this part of the operation may make it very attractive for the control of bleeding esophageal varices.

The distal splenorenal and coronary vein–inferior vena caval shunts are designed to decompress the varices without diverting the portal venous blood from the liver directly into the systemic circulation (selective shunt). The remainder of the communications between the lesser splanchnic circulation and the greater splanchnic circulation must be obliterated. If this is not done, the operation in effect becomes a total shunt and is no longer selective for the lesser splanchnic system.

An estimate of the current results of these various procedures appears at the top of the next page.

Indications
The indications for an elective operation (No. 6, Fig. 27-8) are not well defined at present, since other forms of therapy are being extensively evaluated. Repetitive small hemorrhages or one life-threatening hemorrhage in a good-risk

Fig. 27-9. Total shunt operations used in the treatment of portal hypertension.

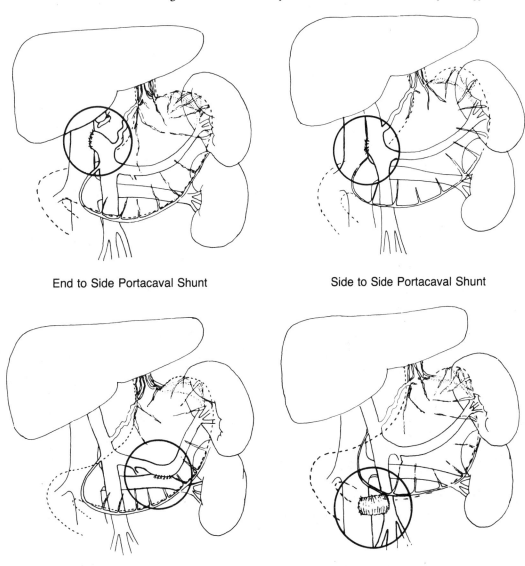

End to Side Portacaval Shunt

Side to Side Portacaval Shunt

Splenorenal Shunt

Mesocaval Shunt

	TOTAL SHUNTS	ABLA-TIVE OPERA-TIONS	SELEC-TIVE SHUNTS
Mortality	5%	25%	5%
Rebleed	5%	25%	10%
Encephalopathy	15%	0%	0%
Decreased liver flow	yes	no	no
Follow-up	25 years	20 years	5 years
(All figures are estimates)			

patient would lend strong support to operative intervention. Some authors believe that sclerotherapy or coronary–short gastric vein embolization should be used as measures to allow better preparation for the patient for elective operations.

Choice of Operation

A choice of an operation depends on the experience of the surgeon, the condition of the patient, and the support facilities available. The total shunt operation should be done on high-risk patients or when an emergency operation is

Fig. 27-10. Ablative and selective operations used in treatment of portal hypertension.

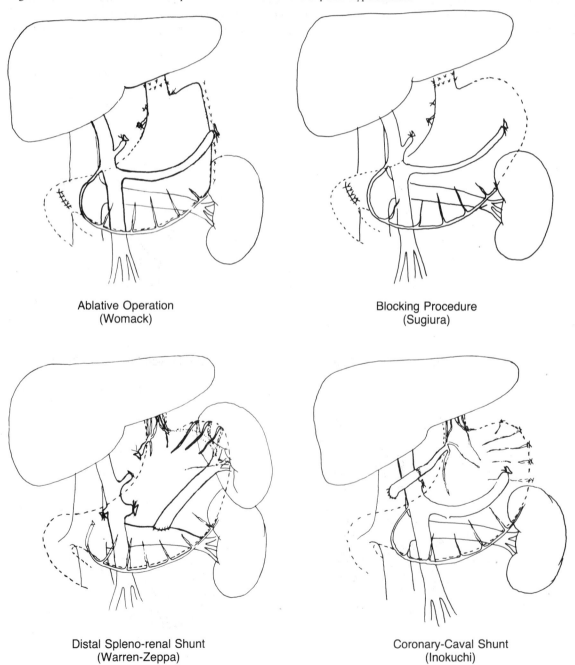

Ablative Operation
(Womack)

Blocking Procedure
(Sugiura)

Distal Spleno-renal Shunt
(Warren-Zeppa)

Coronary-Caval Shunt
(Inokuchi)

being performed. They are technically easier, and the primary requirement in these instances is that they control bleeding. Some reserve these operations for patients with hepatofugal flow (away from the liver); in this instance, there is no need to attempt to preserve flow into the liver. The total shunts direct portal blood into the systemic circulation, with a potential to cause serious encephalopathy. Longevity has not been shown to be improved by the procedure, although if it is successful, bleeding from the varices stops. The procedure does decompress the intrahepatic portal pressure and thus may be helpful in controlling ascites.

Selective shunts are usually reserved for good-risk patients and surgeons who are thoroughly familiar with the operative techniques. The selective shunt will not benefit ascites and may make it more difficult to control. It should not lead to encephalopathy, since no portal blood is shunted into the systemic circulation. If a complete separation of the greater and lesser splanchnic circulations is not performed, or if recommunications later develop, it becomes a physiologically "total" shunt.

Ablative or devascularization procedures have had repeated resurgences of popularity over the past 100 years. The main problems have been associated with a high operative mortality and recurrent bleeding from esophageal varices. Sugiura, Hassab, and Johnson have each reported a number of patients having extensive devascularization procedures. The reported results from Japan and Egypt are much better than those reported from the United States. The difference may be in patient selection or in operative techniques. The Womack operation has been discarded as a primary operation because of the high mortality and high incidence of rebleeding following its use. The Sugiura blocking procedure is widely and effectively used in Japan for patients with nonalcoholic cirrhosis. This procedure calls for transection of the esophagus, which may prevent the high incidence of rebleeding found with the Womack operation.

If the variceal bleeding cannot be controlled in spite of appropriate attempts at nonoperative methods, an emergency portacaval shunt should be considered (No. 12, Fig. 27-8). The precise time when this is indicated is a judgment decision. The patient is an unacceptable risk when he arrives in the operating room in shock with deep encephalopathy and has abnormal coagulation parameters.

Immediate operations (No. 8, Fig. 27-8) have been recommended by Orloff. Although he had a 50% mortality rate, this is compensated by data demonstrating that only 30% of those who bleed from esophageal varices will survive the hospitalization without an operation. Most centers seem to feel that they are able to improve the overall mortality by attempting to perform an elective operation.

Postoperative Care

Postoperative management of the patient requires extensive hemodynamic fluid and electrolyte monitoring. Coagulation parameters and liver function studies must be closely followed. The tendency to develop metabolic alkalosis and hypokalemia must be recognized, and if they develop, treatment must be appropriate. Special care must be taken not to give these patients too much fluid, since ascites may become difficult to control. These patients are frequently malnourished, and appropriate attention to nutrition must be given. Delirium tremens, hepatic failure, and renal failure are not infrequent complications and, if not prevented, should be treated appropriately.

BIBLIOGRAPHY

CONN HO: Portal hypertension and its consequences. In Gitnick GL (ed): Current Gastroenterology and Hepatology. Boston, Houghton Mifflin, 1979

COOPERMAN M, FABRI PJ, MARTIN EW, JR et al: EEA esophageal stapling for control of bleeding esophageal varices. Am J Surg 140:821, 1980

FUTAGAWA S, SUGIURA M, HIDAI K et al: Emergency esophageal transection with paraesophagogastric devascularization for variceal bleeding. World J Surg 3:229, 1979

GRISHAM JW: Liver and biliary tract. In Dietschy, JM (ed): The Science and Practice of Clinical Medicine, Vol 1, Disorders of Gastrointestinal Tract, Disorders of Liver, Nutritional Disorders. New York, Grune & Stratton, 1976

HANNA SS, WARREN WD, GALAMBOS JT et al: Bleeding varices: I. Emergency management; II. Elective management. Can Med Assoc J 124:29, 1981

JOHNSON G JR: Surgery for bleeding esophageal varices. In Jordan G (ed): Advances in Surgery. Chicago, Year Book Medical Publishers, 1980

ORLOFF MJ, DUGUAY LR, KOSTA LD: Criteria for selection of patients for emergency portacaval shunt. Am J Surg 134:146, 1977

RIKKERS LF, RUDMAN D, GALAMBOS JT et al: A randomized, controlled trial of the distal splenorenal shunt. Ann Surg 188:271, 1978

SHERLOCK S: Diseases of the Liver and Biliary System, 6th ed. Oxford, Blackwell Scientific Publications, 1981

TERBLANCHE J, YAKOOB HI, BORNMAN PC et al: Acute bleeding varices: A five-year prospective evaluation of tamponade and sclerotherapy. Ann Surg 194:521, 1981

Lewis M. Flint, Jr./Hiram C. Polk, Jr.

Liver Injury, Abscess, Cysts, and Tumors

LIVER TRAUMA	
Etiology	Blunt or penetrating injury such as occurs in deceleration vehicle accidents or with knife or gunshot wounds
	Numerous other types of trauma, such as too vigorous retraction at laparotomy
Dx	Evidence of internal bleeding in blunt injury or probable penetration in bullet or knife wounds
	Definitive diagnosis is usually made at laparotomy but is suggested by sonography, CT scan, or arteriogram
Rx	Celiotomy with surgical control of hemorrhage
	Repair of liver or resection of devitalized portion; major resection usually not necessary
	Vena caval and hepatic vein injury must be repaired
	Prognosis directly correlated with severity of liver and associated injuries

HEPATIC INJURY

Despite the location of the liver in a relatively protected area of the upper abdominal region, injury to this organ is frequent. Studies analyzing the relative risk of injury to individual abdominal organs indicate that the liver is the fourth most commonly injured structure in patients subjected to motor vehicle trauma. Because of the structural characteristics of the liver, and possibly the force-absorbing capacity of the overlying ribs and soft tissues, the vast majority of liver injuries are not life-threatening. However, when large amounts of hepatic parenchyma are damaged, massive hemorrhage may ensue, with consequent exsanguination and death. Indeed, uncontrolled parenchymal hemorrhage is the most common cause of early death following hepatic injury. Later, if adequate debridement and hemostasis have not been carried out, sepsis with hepatic failure is the greatest threat to life. Penetrating injuries, usually the result of crimes of violence or passion, also frequently involve the liver. Similarly, the amount of hepatic parenchymal damage is directly related to the threat to life. Gunshot wounds and stab wounds of the upper abdomen and lower chest frequently involve the liver. Injuries that are transthoracic may present diagnostic problems. The liver lies under the dome of the diaphragm on both sides, and diaphragmatic excursion from the 5th intercostal space to the 12th intercostal space with each respiratory cycle places the liver in a wide range of exposed locations, subjecting it to possible injury whenever the entry wound lies within the excursion area.

CLASSIFICATION

Because of the observed relationship between the extent of hepatic parenchymal damage and the threat of death from hemorrhage, classification schemes have been useful in establishing indications for therapeutic modalities and for determining, at least in part, prognosis for hepatic injury. A system that has been useful to us is demonstrated in Table 27-3. The immediate threat to life is hemorrhage. Disruptions

TABLE 27-3 GRADES OF INJURY

I	Capsular tears
II	Non-bleeding (<5 cm)
	Through and through missile tracts (non-bleeding)
III	Small actively bleeding lacerations
	Bleeding missile tracts
	Subsegmental tissue destruction (non-bleeding)
IV	Large fractures
	Lobar tissue destruction
V	Extensive parenchymal disruption with hepatic arterial or venous injury

(Flint LM, Mays ET, Aaron WS et al: Selectivity in the management of hepatic trauma. Ann Surg 185:613, 1977)

of the hepatic parenchyma from blunt trauma result in transections of branches of the hepatic artery and portal vein as the force transfer causes irregular tears in liver tissue. Most such transected arteries and veins are subject to the spontaneous hemostatic mechanisms of the liver, resulting in cessation of hemorrhage. However, when the injury crosses or extends along the long axis of subsegmental or segmental planes, longitudinal tears may occur in the hepatic arteries, portal veins, and particularly the hepatic veins draining directly into the vena cava, resulting in failure of the spontaneous hemostatic mechanisms. Indeed, hepatic venous lacerations either within the liver substance or at the retrohepatic vena cava itself comprise the most dangerous liver injuries and those leading to the highest mortality. Table 27-4 shows the relationship between the type of hepatic parenchymal wound and the subsequent mortality and indicates the lethality of major hepatic vascular injuries. Similarly, the presence of associated injuries contributes to the risk of mortality and morbidity. Madding and Kennedy first observed this "multiplicity phenomenon." Table 27-5 shows the contributions made by other injured organs to the risk incurred by the patient with hepatic injury. For each additional organ system injured there is a definite increment in risk.

DIAGNOSIS

In the setting of penetrating injuries to the abdomen, hepatic injury should be suspected whenever the projected trajectory of the injuring agent crosses the anatomic plane in which the liver is located. Figure 27-11 illustrates the external landmarks that define the usual location of the adult human liver. Prediction of the trajectory of a single-missile gunshot is hazardous. Therefore, patients who have sustained gunshot wounds in the vicinity of the peritoneal cavity should be subjected to exploratory laparotomy. Stab wounds of the abdominal wall, flank, or back in the area of the liver present difficult diagnostic problems. Anterior stab wounds are explored under local anesthesia, and if penetration past the deep fascia is noted, exploratory laparotomy may be indicated. In deep anterior stab wounds, we have used diagnostic peritoneal lavage, employing exploratory laparotomy according to the presence of significant blood, bile, or leukocytosis in the peritoneal fluid. Flank and back wounds are selectively subjected to exploratory laparotomy on the basis of position of the injury, depth of penetration, and clinical signs. In the patient who has sustained blunt trauma, the physical signs are useful when physical examination is reliable. Alcohol, drugs, and associated head injury may make patient cooperation impossible, and thus another diagnostic test for intraperitoneal injury is required.

TABLE 27-4 HEPATIC TRAUMA IN 178 PATIENTS

GRADE	TOTAL DEATHS	SEPTIC DEATHS	
I	8	0	
II	10	2/8	(25%)
III	36	10/16	(63%)
IV	41	11/13	(86%)
V	10	1/1	(100%)

(Flint LM, Mays ET, Aaron WS et al: Selectivity in the management of hepatic trauma. Ann Surg 185:613, 1977)

TABLE 27-5 EFFECT OF MULTIPLE ORGAN INVOLVEMENT ON MORTALITY RATE (829 CASES)

INVOLVEMENT	MORTALITY RATE (%)
Liver, uncomplicated	9.7
Liver plus one other organ	26.5
Liver plus two other organs	39.7
Liver plus three other organs	54.8
Liver plus four or more other organs	84.6

(Madding GF, Lawrence KB, Kennedy PA: Forward surgery of the severely wounded. Second Aux. Surgical Group 1:307, 1942–1945)

Peritoneal lavage has been very effective in detecting blood in the peritoneal cavity of patients with suspected abdominal trauma and represents the main adjunct to physical diagnosis in such patients. Radiologic studies are of limited usefulness in adults with suspected liver injury. Routine anteroposterior and lateral chest films and flat abdominal films may provide indirect evidence of injury by showing signs of lower rib fracture, pulmonary contusion, or the presence of intra-abdominal fluid. Imaging of the liver with radioisotopes or computed tomography (CT scan) has not been sufficiently studied to recommend the routine use of these modalities in the management of adult trauma patients. Children's liver and spleen injuries have been documented on the basis of nuclear imaging, and this information may be useful in the management of this highly select group. Similarly, visceral angiography is not usually employed in the early management of the patient with abdominal trauma. When exploratory laparotomy is delayed and significant hepatic injury is suspected, the surgeon may be guided by angiography in managing the very infrequent patient who must undergo definitive laparotomy and operative therapy on the third or fourth day following injury.

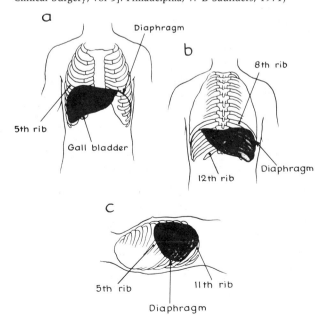

Fig. 27-11. Cutaneous projection of the liver in three views: (*a*) anteroposterior. (*b*) posteroanterior. (*c*) right lateral. (Madding GF, Kennedy PA: Trauma to the Liver, 2nd ed [Major Problems in Clinical Surgery, vol 3]. Philadelphia, W B Saunders, 1971)

The usual biochemical studies of liver function are of no diagnostic or therapeutic value in early evaluation. They supply baseline data, however, that may aid the clinician in establishing the presence of preexisting liver disease. We obtain baseline hepatic function studies, including coagulation values, in the early evaluation of trauma patients to facilitate trend analysis of hepatic function and to determine the course of post-traumatic liver failure, which is encountered frequently in patients sustaining severe injury, those requiring anatomic hepatic lobectomy for trauma, and those developing postinjury sepsis with the multiple organ failure syndrome.

MANAGEMENT

The initial effort in patients with hepatic injury is directed toward maintenance of oxygenation and restoration of intravascular volume and circulatory stability.

In the patient sustaining abdominal trauma who has a significant degree of hypovolemic shock, a major vascular injury within the peritoneal cavity should be assumed until it can be excluded by direct observation. Large volumes of blood and blood components should be available for the management of such patients. We routinely prepare 10 units of blood or packed red cells, alerting the blood bank to the fact that blood components, particularly platelet infusions, may be necessary. A broad-spectrum antibiotic (usually cefazolin 1.0 g intravenously) is administered as soon as the decision to operate is made.

In the operating room the patient is positioned to allow full preparation of the entire ventral surface of the body from the sternal notch to the knees. Median sternotomy is frequently required in addition to the midline laparotomy incision to gain vascular control of the liver when severe liver injury is present. In addition, left thoracotomy is occasionally needed prior to laparotomy, as mentioned previously. Adequate preparation for such an eventuality will save time if extension of the incision is required. A warming blanket is utilized routinely to prevent intraoper-

ative hypothermia. In addition, it may be beneficial to administer warmed intravenous fluids to such patients. In the hectic period of initial control when hemorrhage may be proceeding rapidly, we have not been able to warm blood effectively by passing it rapidly through commercially available warming devices. Therefore, hypothermia with its attendant cardiac and coagulation effects is a significant hazard in the patient with severe liver injury.

A long midline incision (xiphoid to pubis) is used to expose the intra-abdominal injury. Inspection of the liver and palpation of its dorsal aspects will allow delineation of the extent of laceration. Minor nonbleeding parenchymal wounds are treated by drainage alone. The contribution of drainage to reduced mortality in minor hepatic wounds remains somewhat controversial. Several patients have been reported who sustained minor liver injury and received no drainage treatment, and no increased septic morbidity was observed. We prefer to place suction drains; if no bile drainage is observed on the second postoperative day, the drains are removed. The nature of the hemorrhage originating in the liver is noted, and the injury is packed and other clots evacuated. Initial packing of the injury with compression of the hepatic parenchyma will control most actively bleeding lesions. If effective control of hemorrhage is not achieved by packing, inflow to the liver may be controlled by cross-clamping the vascular and ductal structures at the hepatic hilus (the Pringle maneuver). Figure 27-12 indicates the method of manual compression of stellate liver lacerations; this maneuver is effective in controlling hemorrhage in most instances. If hemorrhage persists following compression and control of hepatic inflow, hepatic venous injury is present, and further vascular control of the liver is indicated. It is extremely important to control the bleeding from the liver substance with intermittent pressure, allowing the anesthetist to maintain normal intravascular volume. Persistence of exploration in the face of continued bleeding and hypovolemia is an invitation to cardiac arrest, which is extremely difficult to reverse in such patients. Rapid infusion of banked blood results in a sig-

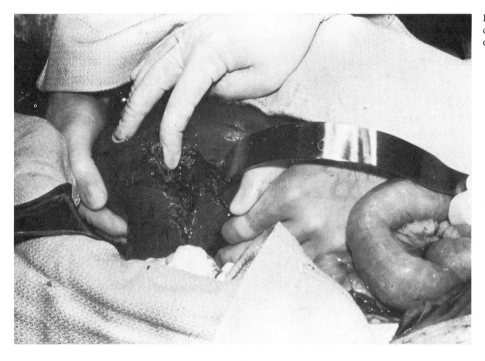

Fig. 27-12. Method of manual compression of stellate liver laceration to control hemorrhage.

nificant reduction of circulating ionized calcium. We supplement the patient at risk for hypocalcemia with intermittent doses of calcium chloride (1 ampule given by slow intravenous infusion for each 4 units of blood transfused rapidly).

When further vascular control of the liver is necessary, the incision is extended to encompass a full median sternotomy. When the sternal edges are retracted, the pericardium can be opened, and intrapericardial control of the inferior vena cava can be obtained by encircling this vessel below the right atrium. Subsequent control of the infradiaphragmatic inferior vena cava is obtained by encircling the area with Latex tape after mobilizing the suspensory ligaments of the liver. The infrahepatic suprarenal inferior vena cava is then controlled in a similar fashion. These maneuvers, when combined with occlusion of hepatic inflow and occlusion of the lower thoracic or upper abdominal aorta, provide total, though temporary, control of inflow to the liver and will reduce hemorrhage, allowing further evaluation of the injury. Warm ischemic injury to the liver is not incurred until approximately 30 min after full vascular occlusion. This period, according to Longmire and associates, may be extended to approximately 1 hour if hypothermia is induced. The protective effect of systemic hypothermia in the hypovolemic patient is unclear. However, the use of regional hypothermia, obtained by enclosing the liver in packs saturated with Ringer's lactate at 4°C, may provide some additional protection of the liver parenchyma while vascular occlusion is undertaken. Extensive vascular injuries to the hepatic veins may require the insertion of an intracaval shunt to preclude lower body ischemia and sequestration of venous blood in the lower extremities during the course of vascular isolation of the liver. The use of such a shunt is depicted in Figure 27-13. A No. 34 or No. 36 thoracostomy catheter is placed through the right atrial appendage and threaded down into the inferior vena cava. A hole is cut in the chest tube corresponding to the location of the tube in the right atrium. This tube may also be utilized for infusion of fluid and blood into the atrium. When the previously placed suprarenal, infradiaphragmatic, and intrapericardial tapes are tightened, the presence of the inlying tube allows continuation of flow through the catheter into the right atrium from the lower extremities while providing effective vascular isolation for the retrohepatic vena cava.

Definitive control of hemorrhage within the hepatic parenchyma is achieved by several methods. The underlying principle is that direct suture or ligation of the lacerated vascular channel is preferable. Specific permanent control of bleeding cannot be obtained as long as devitalized tissue is present, and therefore débridement of obviously devitalized liver tissue is necessary. Lobar hepatic resection is rarely indicated in trauma patients. Most observers agree that anatomic lobectomy is a major undertaking in trauma patients that may easily be avoided by judicious débridement and direct control of lacerated vascular structures. We prefer to retract the edges or even extend the limits of a hepatic laceration to approach the bleeding vessels within the parenchyma, controlling these with suture ligature or hemostatic clips. Obviously devitalized tissue is resected, usually along segmental planes, and control of the bleeding vessels in the liver surface is obtained with direct suture ligature. In certain complex bilobar injuries resulting from blunt or penetrating trauma (approximately 5%–10% of severe injuries), persistent arterial or venous bleeding may be controlled by anatomic lobar devascularization. Either

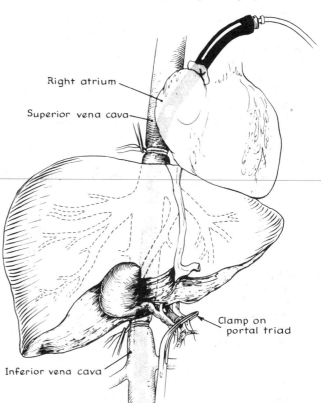

Fig. 27-13. Intracaval shunt inserted by way of the right atrium. (Madding GF, Kennedy PA: Trauma to the Liver, 2nd ed [Major Problems in Clinical Surgery, vol 3].Philadelphia, W B Saunders, 1971)

the hepatic artery to the bleeding area or the portal vein may be ligated. When such bleeding persists and when there is no hepatic venous injury, we selectively occlude the artery to the bleeding area. If this measure controls the bleeding, ligation of the appropriate feeding arteries is then performed. If bleeding persists despite occlusion of the artery, then the portal venous branch to the bleeding area is occluded. If this maneuver results in cessation of hemorrhage, the venous branch is ligated. It is important to remember that ligation of the lobar arterial or venous branch should be performed as distally as possible to maximize control of hemorrhage. In addition, the decision to use lobar dearterialization should be considered prior to mobilization of the suspensory ligaments of the liver, since these areas supply most of the collaterals that will supply nutrients to the dearterialized portion of the liver subsequent to operation. Portal venous anatomy is relatively constant. Hepatic arterial anatomy, in contrast, is variable. Ligation of the proper hepatic artery or the common hepatic artery is rarely indicated. Use of the collateral vessels in the dearterialized structure proceeds rapidly, and angiographic evidence of collateralization is usually present within a matter of hours following initial dearterialization.

Laceration of hepatic veins close to the vena cava or laceration of the retrohepatic vena cava itself is the most difficult liver injury to manage. Exposure of the entire retrohepatic vena cava with the three large and numerous small veins draining the liver directly into the vena cava is possible only after anatomic right lobectomy. Thus, if severe injury to the retrohepatic vena cava or to the hepatic veins is suspected and if , with complete mobilization of the liver, the site of this injury cannot be exposed, rapid anatomic right lobectomy will be necessary. The decision to perform hepatic lobectomy either as a definitive treatment of liver injury or as a method of exposure of complex hepatic venous injuries must be made early in the course of the patient's care. Resort to hepatic lobectomy as a late decision is almost uniformly fatal.

Wide drainage of the potential areas of fluid collection and bile leakage is recommended for most liver injuries. Dependent drainage is possible using a combination of active suction and passive rubber drains through the bed of the 12th rib for the right lobe and through the right flank for the left lobe of the liver. Passive drainage devices are removed early in the course of the patient's convalescence, leaving the suction drains to be removed later. If bile leakage is not apparent on the second postoperative day, sequential removal of the drainage devices is feasible. The wound is closed with interrupted heavy polypropylene sutures in a single layer. If extensive injury, contamination, or prolonged shock has been encountered, the skin and subcutaneous tissue are left open to be closed in delayed primary fashion.

Because of the wide variety of bleeding hepatic wounds, it is important for the surgeon to be aware of the surgical techniques outlined above and, in addition, to use selectively maneuvers such as temporary gauze packing and vascularized tissue packs (omentum). It is obvious from several reported series that some patients will require temporary or permanent packing of the laceration for effective control of hemorrhage. We have used gauze packing on several occasions to control hemorrhage that was unresponsive to other methods. Gauze packs are removed 48 hr following the initial operation, and definitive therapies are then planned, based upon the appearance of the liver and the persistence of hemorrhage at that time.

Most hepatic wounds produce significant intra-abdominal bleeding, necessitating operation. Subcapsular hematoma of the liver, however, may present diagnostic and therapeutic difficulties. Patients seen late after the injury with nonspecific complaints and a lesion on radionuclide liver scan have been treated by nonoperative means with a presumptive diagnosis of subcapsular hematoma. Observation and serial scans are utilized.

Although there is controversy about the management of subcapsular hematoma, our approach has been nonoperative in patients who present late with minimal symptoms. Small hematomas (less than 3 cm) discovered at operation that are not expanding may be treated similarly. Large or expanding hematomas are opened and drained, and specific hemostasis is obtained.

Injuries of extrahepatic segments of the portal vein and hepatic artery are usually encountered in patients sustaining penetrating injuries. Portal venous injuries are managed by repair, although ligation of the splenic or superior mesenteric vein may be accomplished successfully with splenectomy. In the case of superior mesenteric vein ligation, fluid volume lost owing to mesenteric venous congestion may be replaced. Hepatic arterial injuries usually respond to ligation of the injured segment.

POSTOPERATIVE MANAGEMENT

All methods of dealing with liver injury are associated with a risk of early postoperative rebleeding. Particularly in the patient with a severe injury, wound closure is necessary before hemodynamic stability has been obtained. Rebleeding as blood volume returns to normal in the early postoperative period is a continuing hazard. Table 27-6, reproduced from Lucas' prospective study of hemostatic methods in liver trauma, shows the relative risk of rebleeding following commonly employed methods of hepatic hemostasis.

Coagulopathy is also frequently encountered following severe liver injury. The basis of this disorder is usually not a deficiency in liver synthesis of clotting factors but consumptive and dilutional effects of massive transfusion. Thrombocytopenia, either absolute or functional, is the disorder most commonly encountered. Through use of platelet transfusions, we attempt to maintain platelet counts of $100,000/mm^3$ or greater in the early postoperative period. Correction of hypothermia and the selective use of other blood components such as fresh frozen plasma are also necessary.

Other post-traumatic complications, such as renal failure or upper gastrointestinal bleeding due to stress, are encountered in association with sepsis, which is a persistent threat in the patient sustaining severe liver injury. Hepatic failure, shown by abnormalities of biochemical tests of hepatic function, regularly accompanies significant liver injury, and such abnormalities indicate the extent of injury and the therapy utilized. Almost all of the biochemical abnormalities are transient; if they persist, the clinician should be alert to the potential development of a septic complication. Strawn studied the postoperative course of hepatic biochemical abnormalities in patients with liver injuries. Changes in enzymes were regularly observed fol-

TABLE 27-6   RESULTS OF VARIOUS HEMOSTATIC TECHNIQUES FOR LIVER BLEEDING

	NUMBER OF PATIENTS	REBLEEDING*	HEPATIC ISCHEMIA	ABSCESS*	DEATH
Liver sutures	244	14 (7)	2	22 (7)	53
Nonanatomic resection	30	1	0	8 (1)	2
Anatomic resection	21	4 (4)	0	7 (1)	10
Hepatic artery ligation	9	3 (3)	0	2	4
Hepatotomy-vascular control	5	0	0	0	0
Temporary internal pack	3	0	0	1	0
Totals	312	22 (14)	2	40 (9)	69

* Numbers of patients who died shown in parentheses
(Lucas CE, Ledgerwood AM: Prospective evaluation of hemostatic techniques for liver injuries. J Trauma 16:442, 1976)

lowing mild liver injury. Hyperbilirubinemia was a sign of significant liver injury, and if jaundice appeared and persisted (bilirubin level greater than 3mg/dl for more than 72 hr) perihepatic sepsis was a likely possibility. In fact, 75% of patients with persistent jaundice subsequently proved to have a septic focus at operation. Although the area of liver injury is routinely drained widely, perihepatic abscess or subphrenic abscess is the most common long-term postoperative complication. Detection and management of sepsis in injured patients is a difficult diagnostic problem. Most often exploratory laparotomy is required to exclude the presence of drainable abscesses in the patient with manifestations of hepatic failure, pulmonary failure, stress gastrointestinal bleeding, or renal failure following operation for liver trauma. This complex multiple system organ failure syndrome is a late manifestation of the septic response and represents the combined effects of acquired immunodeficiency, nutritional depletion, and invasive infection.

Hemobilia is a rare complication of liver injury. Intrahepatic hematoma may rupture into the biliary tract, giving rise to symptoms of bile duct obstruction and gastrointestinal hemorrhage. Sandblom has provided a definitive description of the syndrome. Diagnosis is confirmed in suspected cases by angiography. Treatment is based upon the initial presentation of intrahepatic hematoma and consists of provision of good drainage for all liver lacerations. The liver capsule should not be closed over intrahepatic cavities. Once symptoms occur, definitive treatment should include evacuation of the intrahepatic cavity and closure of the arterial–biliary fistula. Liver resection or hepatic artery ligation may occasionally be necessary.

CYSTIC DISEASE

PARASITIC LIVER CYSTS

Echinococcosis is distributed worldwide but is particularly prevalent where liver tache occurs frequently; Alaska and the southern United States are examples of such areas in North America. As a portion of its life cycle, *Echinococcus granulosis* has a transient residence attached to the villi of the small intestine of certain meat-eating hosts, commonly dogs, wolves, and foxes. After the parasite is excreted in the host's feces, it is swallowed by an intermediate host such as sheep, cattle, or humans. It then penetrates the intestinal wall directly and enters the portal venous system. The liver is the most common site of echinoccocal cysts, but the lung and other tissues may be involved. The cysts grow progressively and slowly and may reach enormous size; one cyst reportedly contained 16 liters of fluid! Cyst fluid is highly antigenic, and contact with the peritoneal or pleural

membranes may result in a total anaphylactic reaction. In addition, this fluid contains infective daughter cysts and scolices that can further infect the organism. Although the cystic form of the disease is the most common hepatic manifestation of echinococcosis, there are other, less commonly encountered forms, including the alveolar form, which involves a diffuse hepatic tissue infiltration by the parasite, resulting in liver failure. Leakage of daughter cysts or scolices into the biliary tract may give rise to symptoms of biliary colic or obstructive jaundice.

CLINICAL MANIFESTATIONS

Most of the clinical symptoms of echinococcal cysts result from the increasing size of the cyst, which compresses adjacent organs. Abdominal mass, pain, and jaundice may be present. Most often, attention is attracted to the cyst by the development of complications. It has been reported that 40% of patients with echinococcosis developed a complication of the hydatid disease prior to diagnosis of the cyst. Examples of such complications are rupture into the biliary tract and through the diaphragm into the pleural space and rupture into the free peritoneal cavity with acute circulatory collapse.

When there are no acute emergency clinical complications, physical examination, serologic tests, and x-ray examinations are important diagnostic adjuncts. The immunologic response to the antigenic material in the cyst is the basis of diagnostic serologic studies. The classic Casoni skin test is done by injecting hydatid fluid intradermally. More recently, complement fixation and immunoelectrophoretic tests with improved diagnostic accuracy have been developed. Systemic eosinophilia is a common finding. Radionuclide imaging, CT scans, and ultrasound reveal the presence of the fluid-filled cyst. Other radiologic studies may disclose extension of hydatid disease into the lung or primary pulmonary cyst. In addition, abdominal calcifications may be noted. Arteriography is an important adjunct prior to operation.

MANAGEMENT

Most parasitic cysts require excision. If the patient is asymptomatic, however, and if calcification of the cyst is present and serologic studies are negative, operation may not be required. If operation is chosen or if a suspected echinococcal cyst is encountered at operation, evacuation of the cyst should be preceded in all cases by aspiration of the fluid, taking great care not to spill the highly antigenic material into the peritoneal cavity. Following aspiration, an equal volume of a scolicidal agent, usually hypertonic glucose or hypertonic saline, is injected into the cyst cavity. The scolicidal agent should be left in the cyst for 10 min; the cyst is then opened, and all fluid and daughter cysts are removed.

Although many operative procedures, including marsupialization and external drainage, have been suggested, the most appealing surgical procedure is evacuation of the cyst including as much of the cyst wall as possible and closure of the cyst cavity using a viable omental pedicle pack.

NONPARASITIC LIVER CYSTS

Nonparasitic cystic disease of the liver may be congenital, polycystic, inflammatory, or traumatic. Most of these cysts are congenital and usually require no operative therapy. Longmire estimated that 15% or less of congenital cysts

LIVER CYSTS	
Etiology	Congenital, inflammatory, traumatic, or parasitic (*e.g.*, echinococcal)
Dx	Sonography, radioisotope scan, CT scan, arteriography
Rx	Depends on etiology; echinococcal cysts are usually excised

would require operation; those patients who did require surgery would need it because of space-occupying symptomatology. Congenital cysts, whether single or multiple, are the result of failure of involution of embryonic biliary ductal structures. Thus, parenchymal liver cysts are related to other forms of cystic disease of the hepatobiliary apparatus. Longmire and associates have provided a useful classification of such conditions (Table 27-7).

Because liver function is usually well preserved in parenchymal and polycystic liver disease, operative intervention is based on the presence of symptoms of expansion of the mass, not on the need to preserve liver tissue.

Polycystic disease of the liver and kidney usually requires no treatment directed toward the liver. Progressive renal disease is the principal manifestation of this condition.

CLINICAL MANIFESTATIONS

Abdominal fullness, pain, and mass comprise the presenting symptom complex. Physical examination discloses a mass, sometimes cystic in nature, and adjunctive radiologic studies such as ultrasound and CT scan disclose the fluid-filled cyst. Arteriography is usually required prior to elective surgery for suspected hepatic cyst.

MANAGEMENT

Decisions about management of the cyst are best made in a series of steps. If a large hepatic cyst is encountered at operation for another disease process, the fluid should be aspirated. If echinococcal cystic disease is suspected, a scolicidal agent should be used prior to aspiration. If there is a nonparasitic cyst with a clear fluid, the cyst may be unroofed and placed in free communication with the peritoneal cavity. If bilious material is encountered, decompression into a defunctionalized loop of jejunum is necessary. Traumatic and inflammatory cysts are frequently associated with infectious biliary tract disease, particularly cholangitis. Gallstone disease should be dealt with definitively, and adequate cholangiograms should be obtained before or during operation to allow appropriate decompression, thus ensuring adequate resolution of the cholangitis process. Adjunctive antibiotics are indicated when there are septic complications such as cholangitis. Occasionally, anatomic lobectomy or segmentectomy is necessary for the management of hepatic cysts. If complete excision is contemplated, anatomic liver resection is the procedure of choice.

HEPATIC ABSCESS

Because liver abscesses occur very infrequently in North America they are diagnosed relatively slowly. Amebic abscess classically follows exposure to *Entamoeba histolytica*, which is indigenous to the warmer parts of the world; however, with increasing worldwide travel and immigration, amebic abscess is occurring steadily and more frequently in North America. Gram-negative or mixed bacterial abscesses often form after biliary operation or disease or after appendiceal or colonic diverticulitis. These abscesses are often clinically more occult than one would suspect. Intra-abdominal injury is another important cause of abscess (Fig. 27-14).

PATHOGENESIS

Pyogenic hepatic abscesses depend on systemic or portal liver nutrient flow for their derivation and distribution.

Fig. 27-14. Frequent sources of pyogenic liver abscess.

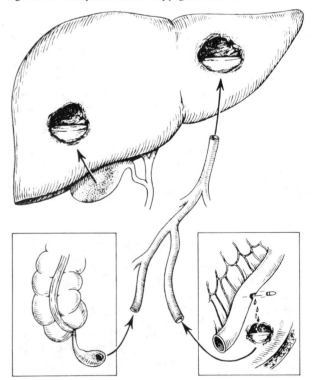

TABLE 27-7

CLASSIFICATION CYSTIC CONDITION	NO. LESIONS
I. Intrahepatic	
A. Primarily parenchymal	
1. Solitary with or without communication with biliary system	9
2. Polycystic disease	23
B. Primarily ductal	
1. Localized dilatation of a major intrahepatic duct	
a. Congenital	3
b. Acquired	2
2. Multiple cystic dilatations of intrahepatic ducts	
a. Congenital	2
b. Acquired	4
II. Extrahepatic	
A. Alonso-Lej Type A. Choledochal cyst	
1. Typical	9
2. Localized	1
3. Fusiform	1
B. Alonso-Lej Type B. Congenital diverticulum	
1. Arising from common bile duct, hepatic ducts, or gallbladder	2
C. Alonso-Lej Type C. Choledochocele	0
D. Multiple cystic dilatations	2
E. Unexplained diffuse ductal dilatation	
1. Congenital	3
2. Acquired	1

(Longmire WP, Mandiola SA, Gordon HE: Congenital cystic disease of the liver and biliary system. Ann Surg 171:712, 1971)

LIVER ABSCESS	
Etiology	Bacterial—from hematogenic dissemination
	Amebic—*Entamoeba histolytica* from colon to portal vein
	Risk factors, bacterial—abdominal infection, sepsis, drug abuse, biliary tract disease; amebic—travel to endemic areas of amebiasis
Dx	Upper abdominal pain, palpable mass (variable), fever, leukocytosis, variable jaundice, abnormal liver function tests
	Blood culture
	Serology for amebic infection
	Chest roentgenogram—pleural effusion or elevated diaphragm on right
	CT scan, ultrasound
Rx	Bacterial—antibiotics, surgical drainage for macroabscesses
	Amebic—metronidazole (systemic), surgical drainage for rare metronidazole failure

Hepatic abscesses are primarily derived from systemic bacteremias, typically caused by gram-positive bacteria, or from portal bacteremias, which are classically associated with gram-negative or mixed infections of alimentary origin.

Gram-positive bacterial, fungal, or mycobacterial abscesses are seen more often in persons with histories of drug abuse or prolonged hospitalization associated with defined or occult septicemias. Pyelonephritis, a more common occurrence in preantibiotic days, represents septic thrombosis of the portal vein and typically is derived from advanced or neglected appendiceal disease. Tables 27-8 through 27-11 show the prevalence of etiologic factors, signs and symptoms, microbiology, and pertinent radiographic and laboratory findings.

Amebic liver abscesses, by contrast, most typically occur in middle-aged men. The route of access is through the portal venous system from a focus of ulceration in the intestine. However, neither microbiologic nor clinical examination of the gastrointestinal tract, including endoscopy, often discloses signs of active intestinal disease in patients who develop amebic liver abscess.

CLINICAL MANIFESTATIONS

Patients with hepatic abscesses characteristically manifest malaise, fever, loss of appetite, and upper abdominal signs ranging from vague discomfort to an overly tender mass. The illicit drug abuser is usually the easiest to spot because he has telltale venous lesions on the extremities as well as other sociologic traits including a personal or hospital history positive for drug abuse. These patients tend to have multiple abscesses, and specific culture data are very important because vigorous and prolonged systemic antibody therapy is needed, even if most large abscesses are surgically drained. The patient whose liver abscesses are due to socially acceptable bacteremia may present a diagnostic dilemma; the diagnosis is clear enough if there are recognized septic episodes, no matter how remote or how slightly defined. If, however, the inciting illness was very mild, misdiagnosed, or clinically overlooked, the diagnosis can represent an especially obscure clinical problem.

The diagnosis of amebic liver abscess is obvious when the history and geographic exposure are compatible; with continuing immigration and worldwide travel the typical cases are less clear than they were two decades ago. The signs and symptoms of an intrahepatic collection are more definitive with amebic infection than with pyogenic liver abscess.

TABLE 27-8 ETIOLOGY OF PYOGENIC HEPATIC ABSCESSES

	PERCENT
Biliary	33
Portal	22
Unknown	21
Hematogenous	13
Contiguous spread	5
Trauma	3
Metastases	3
	100

(After McDonald AP, Howard RJ: Pyogenic liver abscess. World J. Surg 4:369, 1980)

TABLE 27-9 MICROBIOLOGY IN PATIENTS WITH PYOGENIC HEPATIC ABSCESSES

	PERCENT
Proteus	13
Klebsiella-Enterobacter	12
Enterococcus	10
No growth	7

(After McDonald AP, Howard RJ: Pyogenic liver abscess. World J. Surg 4:369, 1980)

TABLE 27-10 PRESENTING SIGNS AND SYMPTOMS AS PERCENT OF ALL PATIENTS WITH PYOGENIC HEPATIC ABSCESSES

	PERCENT
Symptoms	
Fever	81
Pain	51
Rigors	36
Nausea and vomiting	33
Weight loss	31
Anorexia	27
Malaise	20
Signs	
Hepatomegaly	50
Tenderness	50
Jaundice	27
Abnormal chest roentgenogram	18

(After McDonald AP, Howard RJ: Pyogenic liver abscess. World J. Surg 4:369, 1980)

TABLE 27-11 **LABORATORY AND RADIOGRAPHIC FINDINGS IN PATIENTS WITH PYOGENIC HEPATIC ABSCESSES**

	PERCENT
Leukocytosis (WBC > 10^4mm³)	71
Anemia (Hgb < 12 g/dl)	47
Elevated serum bilirubin (>2 mg/dl)	39
Hypoalbuminemia (<2 g/dl)	55
Elevated serum alkaline phosphatase	46
Abnormal chest roentgenogram	53
Abnormal liver–spleen scintiscan	80

(After McDonald AP, Howard RJ: Pyogenic liver abscess. World J Surg 4:369, 1980)

DIAGNOSIS

Depending upon the acuteness of the process, the patient may be acutely ill; more often one sees an acute exacerbation superimposed upon a relatively chronic process. Aside from historical signs, such as a history of septic phlebitis in the extremities of the drug abuser or the presence of an abdominal incision for a remote or recent alimentary inflammatory disease, the physical examination focuses on the right upper quadrant for signs of acute or chronic inflammation with or without a mass. Biliary tract disease with complications is a frequent misdiagnosis. In pyogenic liver abscess, abnormal laboratory values may include leukocytosis and elevated levels in several hepatic function tests. Appropriate blood cultures must be obtained, both to affirm the diagnosis and to assist with very specific microbial chemotherapy. When the diagnosis of amebic abscess is considered, the abnormalities of liver function are more clearly defined. As opposed to the limited value of laboratory studies with pyogenic liver abscess, serologic tests, particularly the hemagglutination test as well as precipitant and latex agglutination tests, are positive in nearly all patients with amebic liver abscess.

The radiologist is an especially helpful consultant in patients with suspected liver abscess. Pleural effusion may be present on the chest x-ray, and calcifications are frequently observed in cases of amebic abscess. Depending on the specific case, both ultrasound and CT scanning can play very important roles in locating the lesion and assessing its multiplicity. Previously, in patients likely to have multiple lesions, hepatic arteriography was found to be essential; to what extent it can be replaced by the new scanning devices remains to be seen.

THERAPY

Treatment is determined by the location, multiplicity, and microbial origin of the abscess. When dealing with a single pyogenic collection, the requisite therapy includes perioperative antibiotics selected as specifically as possible according to preoperative cultures. If no cultures are positive, we believe a safe broad-spectrum antibiotic directed toward aerobic alimentary organisms is in order, with further adjunctive therapy as needed depending upon the clinical response and further careful cultures taken at operation. The arguments for and against extraserous (*i.e.*, extraperitoneal) drainage of septic collections continue without

resolution. When the presence of a single lesion is virtually certain and is amenable to extraserous drainage, so much the better; otherwise, the transperitoneal approach allows much practical safety and better definition of disease, especially if a primary infection of biliary or intestinal origin has never been established or treated. In general, we prefer both active (suction) and passive drains, and we determine by sinus tract injection when drain removal is safe. If there is operative or other evidence that the pyogenic infective process involves multiple abscesses, drainage of all identifiable and accessible macroabscesses should be followed by 4 to 6 weeks of vigorous antimicrobial therapy to sterilize those small collections remaining. The utility of direct intraportal infusion of antibiotics for multiple liver abscesses is unclear but may be an appealing method as a last resort. If liver abscesses as well as untreated or incompletely treated intraperitoneal disease are encountered at operation, careful clinical judgment is needed about which of the processes is clinically dominant and whether the patient can safely tolerate an operative attack on both. The results of this regimen for fewer than four abscesses derived from intraperitoneal sepsis are generally good, although patient disparity precludes specific figures. Multiple lesions in the drug abuser who is likely to continue his habit obviously carry the worst prognosis.

Amebic lesions warrant a trifocal attack, with chemotherapy for the parasitic state and the abscess itself and surgical drainage employed selectively as well. Systemic treatment with a combination of drugs may be warranted. Metronidazole (Flagyl) has recently become the mainstay of therapy. This compound is safe and effective against both hepatic and intestinal amebae. Rare failures are reported, however, indicating that follow-up scanning and ultrasound examinations are necessary to select patients in whom combined drug treatment would be beneficial. The most feared complication of amebic liver abscess is secondary pyogenic infection. Deterioration of the patient being treated for amebic abscess may represent the emergence of this complication and warrants consideration of direct operative evacuation by the extraserous route with careful cultures. Aggressive systemic treatment of amebic liver abscess, reserving surgical intervention for abscesses that persist or enlarge, yields a survival rate of more than 95% at present, a sharp improvement over the rate seen in recent years.

It remains to be seen whether ultrasound-guided percutaneous drainage of hepatic abscesses will become a major therapeutic adjunct, although Druzthoff and associates have found this method promising.

HEPATIC TUMORS

Benign hepatic tumors are infrequently diagnosed during life and when so identified become clinical puzzles. Autopsy studies invariably show that benign tumors are more frequent than they appear to be in life, but these observations are not relevant to the clinician.

CLASSIFICATION

Hepatic adenomas have lately assumed much greater clinical significance because of their association with acute intraperitoneal hemorrhage and, in some cases, the necessity of differentiating adenomas from focal nodular hyperplasia. Also, the growth or shrinkage of these liver tumors is apparently correlated with the institution or cessation of

LIVER TUMORS	
Etiology	Benign: hepatic adenoma—birth control pills, focal nodular hyperplasia in women; hemangioma, hamartoma
	Malignant: hepatocellular carcinoma, associated with cirrhosis; cholangiocarcinoma, associated with parasites; metastatic tumors—colorectal, breast, pancreatobiliary
Dx	Pain, weight loss
	Palpable mass, occasional intraperitoneal hemorrhage
	Variable jaundice, abnormal liver function tests, especially alkaline phosphatase
	CEA, α-fetoprotein
	Radionuclide liver scan
	CT scan
	Hepatic angiography
	Percutaneous hepatic biopsy
Rx	Surgical resection if possible technically
	Chemotherapy

birth control medications. Adenomas, which will be combined with focal nodular hyperplasia for much of this discussion, make up the majority of all liver tumors. Their classic clinical presentation causes much consternation when it occurs as an unsuspected mass in the course of a careful physical examination or laparotomy. Documentation by biopsy or angiography is essential in view of the ominous significance of other masses to be discussed subsequently. The innate clinical significance of an otherwise asymptomatic adenoma is apparently very small. If biopsy is unequivocal, one may either ignore the lesion, since malignant change is very uncommon, or excise it if it is sufficiently accessible to render resection safe.

When an adenoma is associated with exsanguinating intraperitoneal hemorrhage, as it often is in a young woman taking birth control medication, immediate laparotomy for hemostasis is essential. The etiology of focal nodular hyperplasia, particularly in relation to hormone medication, is disputed. Clearly, the majority of recognized cases have occurred in young women taking hormone medication, and some impressive regressions of measurable abnormalities have occurred after termination of birth control agents. Still, these correlations show impressive expectations that have not yet yielded results from the microscope or the experimental laboratory.

Hepatic angiomas are common but are of limited clinical concern. On the other hand, hamartomas are common and are important because palpation, especially at laparotomy, suggests a metastatic origin. When they occur, these developmentally derived lesions warrant biopsy definition but no specific therapy.

Malignant hepatic tumors are absolute threats to life and are a primary clinical concern when they are suspected or known to be present. Expanding neoplasms cause pain and disability, and their replacement of viable hepatic parenchyma eventually causes death. As with lung and brain tumors, both primary and metastatic neoplasms are so important that they warrant immediate definitive therapy, if possible; the prognosis varies only slightly with classification or tumor cell type. Primary hepatocellular carcinoma is associated in western society with cirrhosis, usually of alcoholic or nutritional origin. In North America, hepatocellular carcinoma constitutes about 1% of all primary malignant tumors. Etiologically, hepatic cell injury by alcohol is predominant, although there have been important studies of industrially caused carcinomas, notably hepatic angiosarcoma induced by polyvinylchloride, as described from our institution. As attention to occupational safety becomes more necessary, industrial hepatic carcinogens may assume even greater clinical and societal importance.

Cholangiocarcinoma is the predominant form of primary malignant liver neoplasm in oriental societies and in others where the liver fluke (*Clonorchis sinensis*) is endemic. Its clinical presentation is less frequently associated with cirrhosis and often masquerades as obstructive jaundice. Treatment consists of resectional therapy, a technique pioneered by Ong.

Tumors developing in childhood warrant special attention and must, of course, be clinically differentiated from the more common Wilms' tumor of the kidney and from neuroblastoma. Malignant liver tumors are the third most common intra-abdominal cancer in children; most often they are hepatocellular carcinomas.

Metastatic malignant hepatic tumors outnumber primary neoplasms in North America and are especially important in relation to the state of the primary. If the primary is newly diagnosed, documentation of the state of the liver is indispensable to proper treatment of the primary; if hepatic disease is suspected before the primary is discovered, its importance is assessed in relation to whether the primary is otherwise, especially locally, controlled. Common primary sites include the colorectum, breast, and pancreaticobiliary system, although any cancer, notably malignant melanoma, can and does metastasize to the liver. When a particularly favorable clinical situation exists, treatment of metastatic disease, particularly if limited, by resection will bring about a satisfactory result. Hepatic metastatic disease may have a much worse or a much better prognosis than is commonly thought (Table 27-12). For example, a single metastasis from a primary tumor of the colon that has been controlled for 2 years locally has an extremely good prognosis after resection, with more than one third of patients being cured. Although visceral disease responds less well than disease from local or skeletal dissemination, a young woman with hepatic metastasis due to estrogen receptor–positive breast cancer has an excellent chance of significant remission when treated with hormones.

DIAGNOSIS

The clinical appearance is dominated by the presence of a palpable mass in the upper abdomen. The mass is hard, nontender, and moves freely with inspiration. Other features include liver function abnormalities, positive results on liver scan or other imaging tests, and discovery of metastasis at the time of laparotomy for another illness (laparotomy is most commonly undertaken for attention to the putative primary). As noted previously, liver neoplasms are a rare cause of an acute condition of the abdomen; examples include hemoperitoneum, often with hemodynamic instability due to rupture of a hepatic primary or metastasis, and sudden subcapsular expansion of the tumor masquerading as acute cholecystitis.

As an initial laboratory test, the alkaline phosphatase

TABLE 27-12   **RELATIONSHIP OF LIFE EXPECTANCY TO CERTAIN EVIDENCE OF HEPATIC METASTASES**

CHARACTERISTIC	ESTIMATED MEDIAN SURVIVAL AFTER DIAGNOSIS OF HEPATIC METASTASES (DAYS)
Metastases	
Multiple in one lobe	95
Multiple in both lobes	70
Solitary	140
Ascites	
Present	30
Absent	100
Jaundice	
Present	30
Absent	80
BSP retention	
<10%	140
>11%	30
Alkaline phosphatase	
<5.0	140
5.1–15.0	70
>15.1	20

(Polk HC Jr: Principles of preoperative preparation of the surgical patient. In Sabiston DC Jr (ed): Textbook of Surgery. Philadelphia, W B Saunders, 1977, pp 119–130)

determination (especially when fractionated) continues to be both reliable and specific. False negatives and false positives abound, but this test often shows the first routine abnormality that suggests hepatic neoplasm. Bilirubin elevation often occurs but seldom in the absence of overt metastatic disease, and it implies a poor outlook. Carcinoembryonic antigen studies may be elevated when recurrent disease of colorectal origin is present; however, this test is more specific for the diagnosis of liver involvement than it is for detection of primary or recurrent local disease. A relatively specific laboratory test for liver tumor is the α-fetoprotein determination; it is elevated in about one third of patients with primary liver tumors, but it is also often positive in tumors metastatic to the liver. Levels above 500 ng/ml in the adult male strongly suggest primary liver cancer.

Radiologic diagnostic techniques are used to attempt to determine resectability of the tumor prior to exploration. Only 15% to 20% of malignant liver tumors are resectable for cure. Preoperative staging is then of great potential benefit.

Although the traditional liver scan has earned the enmity of most clinicians because it is more often wrong than right, the new generation of imaging techniques have much to offer when clinically needed. When cystic disease of the liver is a realistic possibility, ultrasonography can be helpful while at the same time establishing the presence or absence of biliary lithiasis, an occasionally important differential feature. CT scans have replaced angiography as the next best method; the continuingly improved resolution offers extraordinarily detailed data. Hepatic arteriography is es-

sential when resection is contemplated, both to define arterial and portal venous anatomy and to provide evidence of the extent of disease. With the need for accuracy and specificity clinical decisions referable to life and death in these matters should seldom be made without biopsy and exploration. Needle biopsy is a convenient method for establishing a preoperative diagnosis. Laparoscopy, utilizing flexible fiberoptic devices, may be helpful in localizing and taking biopsies of the liver mass preoperatively.

MANAGEMENT

The management of hepatic tumors is determined by the severity of the clinical process and by whether the lesion is deemed likely to be malignant or benign. The surgeon caring for such a patient must appreciate both the acute nature of the tumor and the long-term biologic process of chronic neoplastic disease. A tumor that produces intraperitoneal bleeding is best treated by (1) suture hemostasis, immediate workup, and definitive treatment; (2) lobar dearterialization, workup, and consideration of further treatment; or (3) resection if the tumor is very peripherally located to facilitate safe excision.

A necrotic tumor that ruptures is usually best treated by evacuation of necrotic tissue, specific hemostasis, and drainage. Such rupture seldom occurs without overt evidence of dissemination and warrants palliative supportive care. An occasional favorably located lesion justifies excision. Therapy for other tumors that typically present with less acute clinical findings is, however, determined ultimately by the responsiveness of the systemic disease; we have already described a hormonally sensitive breast cancer. Similar considerations obtain for hepatic disease associated with unequivocal dissemination; a careful program of supportive measures plus chemotherapy that is as specific as possible is the principal plan of treatment.

When a favorable primary or a very favorable metastatic neoplasm is known to exist, resection may be justified. Such a decision must be tempered by the probable failure of the treatment to control the total disease and by the substantial risk of major hepatic resection, even in the hands of particularly skilled surgeons. Table 27-13 outlines the risk

TABLE 27-13   **OPERATIVE RISK AND OUTCOME**

	HOSPITAL DEATHS (%)	5-YEAR SURVIVAL (%)
Metastatic colorectal cancer		
Hepatic lobectomy	11	13
Segmental resection	0	21
Wedge resection	3	24
Metastases from other primaries		
All types of resections	13	14
Primary adult liver cancer		
All types of resections		
Asian patients	24	6
Non-Asian patients	22	36

(After Foster JH: Survival after liver resection for secondary tumors. Am J Surg 135:389, 1978; and Jones CE, Polk HC Jr: Abdominal mass. In Gardner B, Polk HC Jr, Stone HH et al (eds): Basic Surgery. New York, Appleton-Century-Crofts, 1978, pp 363–389)

involved. When such an undertaking is warranted, special anesthetic and blood-bank support is in order. The basic anatomy and technical procedures are examined in a subsequent section. The collective results of hepatic resection for various tumors are shown in Table 27-14.

Because much of the specific tumor blood flow is derived from the nutrient hepatic artery, hepatic dearterialization as a palliative measure or as a preoperative maneuver for very large tumors has been the subject of numerous, perhaps overly optimistic, reports. The studies of Mays and associates of patients subjected to hepatic artery ligation for trauma are helpful in assessing this process; although specific hepatic ischemia is produced, revascularization occurs rather promptly in the period of relative hepatic and tumor ischemias measured in terms of days. Complete dearterialization of the liver has, however, been reported to produce relief of tumor-related syndromes, particularly when carcinoid metastases are involved. Whether systemic or intra-arterial chemotherapy is helpful remains to be determined, as does the impact of local hepatic hypothermia. Studies of multiple drug chemotherapy for hepatic cancer have occasionally been encouraging (Table 27-14). Irradiation of the liver is, in general, poorly tolerated and has not been popular for liver neoplasms except for rapidly expanding tumors.

ELECTIVE HEPATIC RESECTION

Although removal of small portions of the liver has been reported frequently since the late 17th century, it was not until 1910 that Wendell first completed a successful anatomic right hepatic lobectomy. Subsequently, surgeons have utilized knowledge of various studies, particularly those elucidating the segmental distribution of hepatic blood vessels and biliary ductal system, to perform elective and emergency excision of hepatic tissue amounting to as much as 80% to 85% of the organ. Elective hepatic resection for tumor has been standardized through the contributions of Longmire, Adson, and Starzl. Table 27-15 shows the strategic approach to the patient who is a candidate for elective hepatic resection for tumor. Most authors prefer initially a right subcostal incision to determine the resectability of the tumor. Should hepatic resection then be contemplated, the incision is extended either as a thoracoabdominal incision or as a large bilateral subcostal approach. Liver resection can also be accomplished through a long midline incision with possible extension as a median sternotomy, as described by Miller and associates. Central to the strategy for elective hepatic resection is the assurance of adequate vascular control. The studies of Haney have provided definitive techniques for vascular isolation of the liver. Although hypothermic total vascular isolation has been suggested for elective excision of extensive hepatic tumors, current data indicate that mortality and morbidity are not improved with this adjunct.

Successful hepatic resection requires an understanding of hepatic segmental anatomy. The fissure between the right and left lobes of the liver (see Fig. 27-4) lies just to the left of the gallbladder fossa and extends to the midpoint of the retrohepatic vena cava. The portion of the liver intervening between this lobar fissure and the ligamentum teres is the medial segment of the left lobe. The right lobe as well as both segments of the left lobe are further subdivided into superior and inferior segments. Anatomic lobectomy proceeds by totally mobilizing the liver by dividing its attachments to the dorsal retroperitoneum and the diaphragm.

TABLE 27-14   RELATIVE SURVIVAL RATES

TREATMENT (1955–1964)[a]	NO. CASES	TIME (% SURVIVAL)		
		1 YR	3 YR	5 YR
All cases	913	8	3	3
Surgery only	64	34[a]	24[a]	20[a]
Radiation only	43	22[a]	3[a]	3[a]
Chemotherapy only[b]	101	12	3	4
No therapy[c]	680	4	1	1

[a]Rates have a standard error between 5% and 10%
[b]Route of administration not stated
[c]No tumor-directed therapy initiated within 4 months of diagnosis
(After Longmire WP: Liver tumors and cysts. In Hardy JD (ed): Rhoads Textbook of Surgery, 5th ed. Philadelphia, J B Lippincott, 1977, pp 938–947)

TABLE 27-15   STEPS IN ELECTIVE HEPATIC RESECTION

1. Abdominal incision
2. Exploration and biopsy
3. Extension of incision into thorax (for right hepatic lobectomy)
4. Mobilization of lobe
5. Division and individual ligation of lobar branch of hepatic artery, portal vein, and hepatic duct. Cholecystectomy
6. Division of segmental hepatic veins on dorsal surface of liver
7. Division of right or left hepatic vein
8. Division of parenchyma with ligation of biliary–vascular branches
9. Drainage
10. Closure of incision

(Longmire WP, Trout HH, Greenfield J et al: Elective hepatic surgery. Ann Surg 179:712, 1974)

The liver is delivered into the operative incision, taking care to avoid torsion on the vena cava and reduction of venous return. The hilar structures to the lobe being resected are isolated and encircled. After ligation of the hepatic artery, portal venous branch, and biliary duct, a line of demarcation is delineated indicating the line of incision for removal of the selected lobe. Storm and Longmire, as well as Lin, have suggested the use of hemostatic clamps encircling the liver. Although these instruments are of value in selected cases, most surgeons employ a modification of the "finger fracture" technique reported by Lin. The principles underlying successful hepatic resection include positive identification of ducts and vessels within the hepatic parenchyma and control of these prior to division. Individual suture ligatures or hemostatic clips are satisfactory approaches to vascular control within the hepatic parenchyma. A particular strategy is necessary for removal of the medial segment of the left lobe during the course of extended right hepatic lobectomy or trisegmentectomy. In contrast to right hepatic lobectomy, in which dissection is begun on the diaphragmatic surface of the liver, dissection for trisegmentectomy is begun in the umbilical fissure on the inferior surface of the liver so that the vessels that course from the left hepatic artery and the left branch of the portal vein back to the median segment of the left lobe will be encountered early and controlled. Starzl and associates pointed out that these "feedback" vessels are extremely important if the medial segment of the left lobe requires preservation. These vessels are also important in the course of trisegmentectomy because beginning the dissection on the dorsal surface of the liver would entail a risk of major hemorrhage from these vessels while the surgeon was trying to identify them. Control of the major hepatic veins running within the lobar segmental fissures is achieved before these veins enter the vena cava. Three large veins and up to 12 small veins within the hepatic parenchyma are identified so that a sufficient length of vein is obtained for positive control.

Extensive preparations for appropriate anesthetic support, oxygenation, and maintenance of blood volume are necessary. Intravascular monitoring devices are helpful in such patients, as is preparation for the use of temperature control devices. Blood and blood components are prepared in appropriate volumes and used as necessary.

Following hepatic lobectomy, a transient period of hepatic insufficiency that is directly related to the amount of liver removed may occur. Should signs of liver failure be prolonged, however, perihepatic sepsis is highly likely. Active and passive drains are used in the perihepatic space, and these are brought out in dependent portions of the abdominal wall, particularly the bed of the 12th rib. There seems to be no specific need for the administration of hypertonic glucose to patients following anatomic hepatic lobectomy or trisegmentectomy. Five percent dextrose solutions provide an adequate glucose supply to prevent hypoglycemia. Nutritional deficits may be incurred by patients with massive hepatic resection because of either the operation itself or the underlying disease process. Total parenteral nutrition is indicated as an early postoperative adjunct. Despite the fact that the liver is the main site for albumin synthesis, large volumes of intravenous albumin are infrequently required following liver resection. Pharmacologic attempts to improve hepatic blood supply are of potential benefit in patients who have had extensive liver resections, particularly after trauma. Glucagon given at 4- to 6-hr intervals in 1 mg intravenous doses may increase portal flow as well as hepatic arterial flow and thus improve hepatic oxygenation.

Perihepatic sepsis is a life-threatening complication of elective and emergency liver resection. The diagnosis of such infection may be difficult, however, because fever is frequently observed in patients who do not have sepsis. Quattlebaum was the first to identify this fever of unknown origin in the postoperative hepatic resection patient. He hypothesized that resorption of necrotic liver tissue at the line of resection was the cause of the fever.

General support of the patient should include appropriate infusions of blood and blood products and maintenance of oxygenation including selective use of adjuvant ventilator support. The use of adjunctive broad-spectrum antibiotics in the perioperative period completes the usual features of postoperative care.

Elective hepatic lobectomy or extended resection such as trisegmentectomy can be carried out for appropriately staged liver tumors with a mortality of under 10% for the operation itself. Standard operation can thus be recommended for patients with appropriately staged tumors when an experienced surgeon and the necessary supportive services are available.

BIBLIOGRAPHY

ADAM YG, ANDREW GH, FORTNER JC: Giant hemangiomas of the liver. Ann Surg 172:239, 1970

ADSON MA, BEART RW: Elective hepatic resections. Surg Clin North Am 57:339, 1977

ADSON MA, VAN HEERDEN JA: Major hepatic resections for metastatic colorectal cancer. Ann Surg 191:576, 1980

CHEATHAM JE JR, SMITH EI, TUNELL WP et al: Nonoperative management of subcapsular hematomas of the liver. Am J Surg 140:852, 1980

CRANE PS, LEE YT, SEEL DJ: Experience in the treatment of two hundred patients with amebic abscess of the liver in Korea. Am J Surg 123:332, 1972

EGGLESTON FC, VERGHESE M, HANDA AK et al: The results of surgery in amebic liver abscess: Experience in eighty-three patients. Surgery 83:536, 1978

FLINT LM JR, POLK HC JR: Selective hepatic artery ligation: Limitations and failures. J Trauma 19:319, 1979

FORTNER JG, KIM DK, MACLEAN BJ et al: Major hepatic resection for neoplasia: Personal experience in 108 patients. Ann Surg 188:363, 1978

GERZHOF SG, ROBBINS AH, BIRKETT DH et al: Percutaneous catheter drainage of abdominal abscesses guided by ultrasound and computed tomography. Am J Roentgenol Radium Ther Nucl Med 133:1, 1979

HADAD AR, WESTBROOK KC, GRAHAM GG et al: Symptomatic nonparasitic liver cysts. Am J Surg 134:739, 1977

LEDGERWOOD AM, KAZMERS M, LUCAS CE: The role of thoracic aortic occlusion for massive hemoperitoneum. J Trauma 16:610, 1976

LEWIS JW, KOSS N, KERSTEIN MD: A review of echinococcal disease. Ann Surg 181:390, 1976

MATTOX KL, ESPADA R, BEALL AC JR: Traumatic injury to the portal vein. Ann Surg 181:519, 1975

McDONALD AP, HOWARD RJ: Pyogenic liver abscess. World J Surg 4:369, 1980

McGEHEE RN, TOWNSEND CM JR, THOMPSON JC et al: Traumatic hemobilia. Ann Surg 179:311, 1974

NORTON L, MOORE G, EISEMAN B: Liver failure in the postoperative patient: The role of sepsis and immunologic deficiency. Surgery 78:6, 1975

POLK HC JR, JONES CE: Abdominal mass. In Gardner B, Polk HC Jr, Stone HH (eds): Basic Surgery, pp 362–389. New York, Appleton-Century-Crofts, 1978.

RANSON JHC, MADAYAG MA, LACABO SA et al: New diagnostic and therapeutic techniques in the management of pyogenic liver abscesses. Am J Surg 181:508, 1975

REYNOLDS TB: Amoebic abscess of the liver. Gastroenterology 60:952, 1971

ROMERO-TORRES R, CAMPBELL JR: An interpretive review of the surgical treatment of hydatid disease. Surg Gynecol Obstet 121:851, 1965

SCHROCK T, BLAISDELL FW, MATHEWSON C JR: Management of blunt trauma to the liver and hepatic veins. Arch Surg 96:698, 1968

STONE HH, LAMB JM: Use of pedicled omentum as an autogenous pack for control of hemorrhage in major injuries of the liver. Surg Gynecol Obstet 141:92, 1975

THAL ER: Evaluation of peritoneal lavage and local exploration in lower chest and abdominal stab wounds. J Trauma 17:642, 1977

VANA J, MURPHY GP, ARONOFF BL et al: Primary liver tumors and oral contraceptives. JAMA 238:2154, 1977

VIAMONTE M JR, SCHIFF E: Diagnostic approach to hepatic malignant neoplasms. JAMA 238:2191, 1977

John M. Beal

Gallbladder and Biliary Tract

ANATOMY

The extrahepatic biliary system includes the gallbladder, cystic duct, and common duct. The gallbladder is normally thin-walled and pear-shaped and has a normal capacity of 35 ml to 50 ml. It lies in the gallbladder fossa on the inferior surface of the liver and is covered by the peritoneum. The peritoneal reflection over the gallbladder may provide a short mesenteric attachment to the liver, or the gallbladder may be partially or nearly completely covered by adjacent folds of liver substance. The gallbladder is connected to the common duct by the cystic duct. The cystic duct varies considerably in length. Although normally it joins the common bile duct at about the junction of the upper and middle third of the common duct, the cystic duct may enter the common duct at any point more distally, including the ampulla of Vater. The lining of the cystic duct is arranged in a series of folds, the spiral valves of Heister, which may interfere with the passage of probes or catheters.

The common hepatic duct is formed by the union of the left and right hepatic ducts and becomes the common bile duct when joined by the cystic duct. The common duct is a passive conduit, 10 cm to 12 cm in length, and terminates in the papilla of Vater, which is 8 cm to 10 cm distal to the pylorus on the lesser curvature of the second portion of the duodenum. The common duct passes through the hepatoduodenal ligament adjacent to the portal vein and hepatic artery. The common duct passes behind the duodenum, becomes partially surrounded by pancreas, and enters the ampulla of Vater obliquely. Thus, the common duct can be described as having supraduodenal, retroduodenal, and pancreatic segments.

The common duct is joined by the pancreatic duct (duct of Wirsung) in its intraduodenal portion to form the ampulla of Vater, which enters the duodenum as the duodenal papilla or duodenal papilloma. There is variation in the manner in which the bile and pancreatic ducts enter the ampullary area. They may form a common channel in the ampulla, terminate in the papilla as separate ducts, or open into the duodenum separately.

The vessels that are related to the extrahepatic biliary tract are the portal vein and the hepatic artery. The portal vein lies posterior and superior to the common duct. The hepatic artery is one of three major branches of the celiac axis. The gastroduodenal artery arises as a branch of the hepatic artery posterior and superior to the pylorus. The hepatic artery then courses through the hepatoduodenal ligament superior to the common duct and divides into right and left hepatic branches to supply the liver. One or more cystic arteries are present, usually arising from the right branch of the hepatic artery. The cystic artery may cross posterior to the common hepatic duct or right hepatic duct or may arise to the right of the hepatic duct.

The gallbladder and extrahepatic biliary tract receive vagal fibers from the hepatic branch of the anterior vagal trunk. Stimuli from the vagus cause contraction of the gallbladder and relaxation of the sphincter of Oddi. Vagal innervation does not seem to be as important as humoral factors for gallbladder function. Cholecystokinin (CCK) is formed in the duodenal mucosa. CCK is a polypeptide with the same terminal pentapeptide as gastrin. Its secretion is stimulated by the entry of the products of gastric digestion into the duodenum. CCK causes contraction of the gallbladder, relaxation of the sphincter of Oddi, and secretion of enzymes by the pancreas. (See the section Gastrointestinal Hormones in Chapter 20.)

The common bile duct is a passive conduit in humans. The sphincter of Oddi has an intrinsic contractile rhythm that releases bile intermittently into the duodenum. The resting pressure of bile in the common duct is between 10 mm and 15 mm of water. The flow rate of bile in the common duct is difficult to measure accurately but appears to be 10 ml to 25 ml per hour in the fasting state. The administration of morphine causes profound contraction of the sphincter of Oddi that may persist for 12 hours or longer. In the presence of obstruction of the common bile duct, secretion of bile by the liver ceases when the intraductal pressure reaches 35 mm of water.

"White bile" is an uncommon complication of biliary tract disease and may occur in the presence of complete obstruction of either the gallbladder or the common bile duct. "White bile" is a colorless, viscid, bilirubin-free fluid. With complete obstruction of the cystic duct, the gallbladder becomes distended with fluid produced by its mucosal glands. When long-standing, this may lead to hydrops of the gallbladder.

ABNORMALITIES OF THE BILIARY TRACT

The majority of anatomic anomalies are variations in arterial relations rather than in the ducts. More ductal abnormalities are related to variations in length, number, and mode of junction.

ARTERIAL ANOMALIES

The textbook description of the arterial blood supply of the liver and biliary tract is present in approximately 55% of autopsy dissections, which stresses the frequency of variation in arterial relationships. The left hepatic artery originates from the left gastric artery in approximately 25% and in about 50% is the only artery to the left lobe of the liver. Occasionally the celiac artery does not have a hepatic artery branch, and the blood supply of the liver is provided by a hepatic trunk from the superior mesenteric artery. More frequently, the right hepatic artery arises from the superior mesenteric artery, and the celiac artery provides a hepatic branch that divides into a gastroduodenal artery and a left hepatic artery.

The cystic artery is single in 75% of cases and arises from the right hepatic artery. Dual cystic arteries are frequent and may originate from different hepatic arteries or from the gastroduodenal artery. When the right hepatic artery is furnished by the superior mesenteric artery, it frequently supplies the cystic artery.

ABNORMALITIES OF THE GALLBLADDER

The gallbladder, which is normally absent in the elephant, horse, deer, rat, and rhinoceros, may also be absent in the human. Among more than 150 recorded cases of agenesis of the gallbladder, a high incidence of other pathology, including common duct stones, has been reported.

Bilobed gallbladders may occur with either a longitudinal or a transverse septum. At least one patient had a central transverse septum with stones in the portion adjacent to the cystic duct.

Double gallbladder, vesica fellea duplex, is a rare anomaly. Double gallbladders may have union of their cystic ducts with one duct joining the common duct, or there may be two separate cystic ducts. There is a report of an instance in which removal of a stone-filled gallbladder failed to relieve a patient's symptoms, and exploration revealed another gallbladder, also containing calculi.

True diverticula of the gallbladder are rare and are usually asymptomatic. Diverticula may contain stones and thus must be distinguished from pseudodiverticula, which are intramural ulcerations caused by calculi.

Gallbladders may be partially or totally surrounded by hepatic parenchyma, the latter being called intrahepatic gallbladder. Intrahepatic gallbladders are difficult to detect. Calculi have been reported to be present in more than half the cases of intrahepatic calculi, which suggests an increased incidence of cholelithiasis in this abnormality.

"Left-sided" gallbladder is rare in patients without situs inversus. Such gallbladders have cystic ducts that terminate either in the right or left hepatic ducts. The gallbladder fossa is empty, and the gallbladder is found beneath the falciform ligament.

A frequent variation in the contour of the gallbladder is responsible for the descriptive term "Phrygian cap." In nearly one fifth of gallbladders, a fold in the fundus produces a characteristic radiologic appearance reminiscent of the conical cap with the top turned forward that was used in Phrygia and became a symbol of liberty in the French Revolution.

Variations in the cystic duct are encountered with sufficient frequency to have clinical significance. The cystic duct may be absent or short or have abnormal sites of entrance into the bile ducts. It may enter the left or right hepatic duct or at their junction. The right hepatic duct may open into the gallbladder, usually in the region of the gallbladder ampulla (Hartmann's pouch). The cystic duct may enter the common duct at any point, including the ampulla of Vater. The entrance into the common duct varies from direct to spiral insertion, and at times the cystic and common ducts may share a common wall (Fig. 27-15).

CLINICAL IMPLICATIONS OF VASCULAR AND BILIARY DUCT ANOMALIES

Recognition of anomalous arterial and biliary ductal anatomy during operation is essential for safe patient management. For example, ligation of a right hepatic artery that originates from the superior mesenteric artery may lead to ischemia and necrosis of a major segment of the right lobe in the liver.

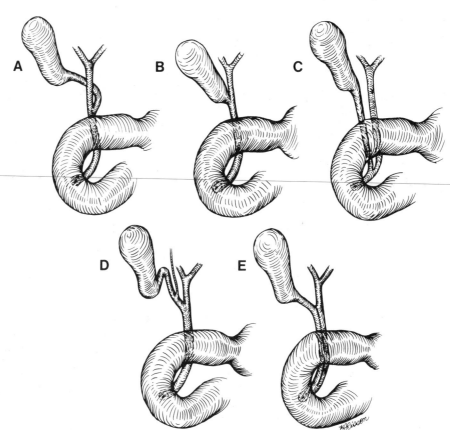

Fig. 27-15. Diagrammatic representation of variations of insertion of cystic duct into the common bile duct; (*A*) spiral insertion, (*B*) short or absent cystic duct, (*C*) insertion of cystic duct proximal to ampulla of Vater, (*D*) accessory bile duct entering cystic duct, and (*E*) long segment of cystic duct sharing wall with common bile duct.

Abnormalities of the major bile ducts may contribute to injury of the common bile duct during cholecystectomy. The variations in the entry of the cystic duct are numerous and must be anticipated. Careful identification of the junction of the cystic duct and common duct is essential in the prevention of injury to the common duct. Anomalies of the ductal system are of more frequent clinical significance than are vascular anomalies. Unusual relationships between the cystic duct and the common duct may be responsible for long cystic duct remnants after cholecystectomy. Patients who have cystic duct remnants that are longer than 1.5 cm after removal of the gallbladder may develop symptoms of biliary tract disease. Pain is the commonest symptom associated with cystic duct remnants and may resemble that experienced by the patient before cholecystectomy. Jaundice has been reported in 25% to 35% of these patients, with approximately 40% of reported cases having calculi in the retained segment of cystic duct. The stones may have been present in the duct at the time of cholecystectomy or may have developed later as a result of stasis within the ductal remnant.

It is uncertain how often cystic duct remnants cause symptoms. Many years may elapse between the removal of the gallbladder and development of symptoms attributed to the residual cystic duct. It should be recalled, however, that residual or recurrent symptoms after cholecystectomy may be caused by a cystic duct remnant.

Intravenous cholangiography and endoscopic retrograde cholangiopancreatography (ERCP) are useful in detection of a cystic duct remnant. However, if the cystic duct is occluded by stone or inflammation, the remnant will not be visualized. The majority of cholangiograms show other abnormalities, such as common duct calculi or abnormal ductal dilatation, which may lead to operation and detection of the cystic duct remnant.

COMPOSITION OF BILE

CHARACTERISTICS OF BILE

Bile, as secreted by the liver, is an isosmotic aqueous solution that contains a variety of soluble and insoluble substances. Bile is approximately 97% water and contains bilirubin, lipids, cholesterol, and organic and inorganic ions, as well as small amounts of protein. The normal adult secretes 750 ml to 1000 ml of bile daily (Table 27-16).

Bilirubin is responsible for the characteristic color of bile and is the product of the breakdown of hemoglobin into a protein fraction and heme. Heme is converted to bilirubin in the cells of the reticuloendothelial system. The normal daily destruction of erythrocytes yields 7.5 g of hemoglobin a day, which in turn forms approximately 250 mg of bilirubin daily. Bilirubin is a highly insoluble tetrapyrrole that is bound to the plasma proteins during transport to the liver. Bilirubin is conjugated in the liver for secretion. Conjugation is necessary for the secretion of bilirubin in bile. Normal bilirubin is esterified and secreted into the bile as a water-soluble glucuronide.

Bile contains three lipids: cholesterol, phospholipid, and bile acid. Phospholipid is chiefly lecithin, which constitutes more than 90% of phospholipid in the bile. Cholesterol and

TABLE 27-16   COMPOSITION OF HUMAN HEPATIC BILE

Specific gravity	$1.012 \pm .004$
Water	97%
Bilirubin	17–70 mg/dl
Bile acids	$1.48 \text{ g} \pm 0.24 \text{ g/dl}$
Cholesterol	$130 \text{ mg} \pm 45 \text{ mg/dl}$
Fatty acids	100–440 mg/dl
Phospholipid	220–6050 mg/dl
Chloride	90–120 mEq/liter
Bicarbonate	20–25 mEq/liter
Calcium	10 mg/dl
pH	7.3–7.45
K^+	4.8 mEq/liter
Na^+	146 mEq/liter

lecithin are highly insoluble in aqueous solution, and it is the interaction of bile acids with lecithin that results in the micellar solubilization of cholesterol in bile.

Cholesterol in bile originates from endogenous synthesis and from dietary sources. Synthesis of cholesterol occurs primarily in the liver and intestine. The intestine contains a mixture of free and esterified cholesterol from dietary and endogenous sources. The esterified cholesterol is hydrolyzed to free cholesterol by pancreatic esterase and is either excreted in the stool or solubilized for return to the liver. About 40% of dietary cholesterol is normally absorbed.

Bile acids are synthesized from cholesterol in the liver and are important in maintaining solubility of cholesterol in bile. The two primary bile acids are conjugated in the liver with the amino acids taurine and glycine. Conjugated bile acids are secreted into canalicular bile at high concentrations by active transport.

ENTEROHEPATIC CIRCULATION

When the bile acids reach the intestine, approximately 80% are resorbed in the distal ileum and transported in the portal blood back to the liver in a conjugated form, to be reexcreted in the bile. This excretion and reabsorption cycle is termed the enterohepatic circulation (EHC) of bile acids. Most of the remaining conjugated bile acid is deconjugated by bacterial action in the distal ileum and in the colon. The major portion of these deconjugated bile acids is hydroxylated and forms secondary bile acids, lithocholic acid, and deoxycholic acid. The secondary bile acids are resorbed in the colon. They are then conjugated in the liver with glycine and taurine and excreted in the bile. Between 2% and 5% of the total circulating bile salts escape reabsorption and appear in the feces, giving a fecal bile salt excretion of 200 mg to 600 mg per day.

The gallbladder is important in the EHC. The gallbladder stores and concentrates hepatic bile during fasting. With feeding, the gallbladder empties and, in addition, hepatic bile enters the intestine directly.

Of the bile acids that are produced by the liver and excreted into the intestine, more than 95% are returned to the liver by the EHC. The bile acid pool contains 3 g to 5 g of bile acid, which recirculates 6 to 10 times daily. The hepatic synthesis of bile acids is regulated by the size of the bile acid pool in the EHC. Thus, loss of bile acids from the intestinal tract results in increased synthesis of bile acids by the liver.

In addition to their function of solubilizing cholesterol

by micellar formation with lecithin, bile acids play an important role in the absorption of lipids from the intestine.

Phospholipids (more than 90% lecithin) are synthesized in the liver from choline. The secretion of phospholipids by the liver is increased sixfold during digestion when compared to the fasting state. Lecithin does not participate significantly in the EHC.

GALLSTONE FORMATION

The incidence of gallstones in the general population in the United States has been estimated to be between 8% and 10%. Gallstones are rare before the age of 10 years. The incidence of cholelithiasis, however, increases with age, and by 80 years of age approximately 30% are found to have stones at autopsy.

In general, gallstones may be classified as cholesterol stones, those composed primarily of cholesterol; and pigment stones, those containing less than 25% cholesterol. Cholesterol stones are present in more than 75% of patients with cholelithiasis in the United States. In some parts of the world, however—for example, Japan—two thirds of gallstones are of the pigment type.

The formation of *cholesterol gallstones* seems to be initiated by the liver's production of bile that is supersaturated with cholesterol. There are probably both genetic and metabolic factors that predispose patients to the production of supersaturated bile. Partial evidence that such supersaturated bile is lithogenic has been the appearance of cholesterol monohydrate crystals in fresh bile from patients without stones. These microscopic crystals may then agglomerate into macroscopic particles. As bile is concentrated in the gallbladder, the micellar particles increase to macromolecular size, which favors the precipitation of cholesterol into macroaggregates and, later, cholesterol stones.

Thus most patients with cholesterol gallstones have an abnormal or lithogenic bile because a portion of biliary cholesterol is not in micellar solution. Conversion of normal bile, in which all the biliary cholesterol is in solution, to an abnormal bile saturated or supersaturated with cholesterol, may result from a decrease in the biliary content of either phospholipids or bile salts. Individuals with cholesterol gallstones secrete bile with increased amount of cholesterol relative to bile acid and phospholipid content. The size of their bile acid pools is decreased to approximately 50% of normal. The amount of bile acid excreted in the stool each day, however, is the same as normal subjects.

Evidence has been presented to support the concept that normal bile, with cholesterol in stable micellar solution, may be converted to an abnormal bile, saturated with cholesterol, by a decrease in bile acid content. Decreased bile acid synthesis and increased cholesterol synthesis could produce increased biliary cholesterol secretion and fail to provide adequate amounts of bile acid to solubilize the cholesterol.

When normal intestinal absorption of bile acids is interrupted (short bowel syndrome, inflammatory bowel disease, and so on), the feedback inhibition of bile acid synthesis from bile acids returning to the liver is decreased. Although this leads to increased bile acid synthesis, the bile acid pool may become depleted and result in decreased micellar solubilization of cholesterol. A higher incidence of cholesterol gallstones has been reported in patients when normal bile acid absorption has been disturbed and fecal loss increased. Thus, the pathogenesis of cholesterol gallstone disease is complex, involving genetic and metabolic alterations of hepatic, gallbladder, and intestinal function.

Pigment stones are usually dark brown or black in color, either irregular or smooth, 5 mm or less in diameter, and multiple. Although pigment stones represent 25% or less among gallstones in the general population, the incidence increases with age. Intrahepatic gallstones and stones caused by stasis or cirrhosis are usually pigment stones. An increased incidence of pigment stones occurs in hemolytic disease such as hereditary spherocytosis and sickle cell anemia. The reported incidence of gallstones in hereditary spherocytosis varies from 43% to 85%. One of the side-effects after insertion of prosthetic cardiac valves is increased destruction of erythrocytes. Approximately one third of patients with prosthetic valves have been found to have pigment stones, in contrast to less than 15% of those with valvular disease. Men and women are affected with equal frequency in this country and in the Orient.

Dietary factors have been implicated in the pathogenesis of pigment stones. The incidence of pigment stones decreases among Japanese when a Western diet has been adopted. Other factors may be present, however. For example, a high incidence of parasites, especially *Ascaris lumbricoides,* has been detected in the pigment stones of Japanese patients.

In contrast to cholesterol stones, the mechanisms for the formation of pigment stones remain largely unproven. When compared to the bile from patients with cholesterol stones, the bile of patients with pigment stones generally contains less cholesterol but similar amounts of bile acid, phospholipid, and total bilirubin. Evidence for the hepatic secretion of an abnormal pigment that precipitates readily or for excessive secretion of bilirubin that exceeds its solubility in bile is lacking. In the Orient, gallbladder bile is often infected, usually with *Escherichia coli.* Bilirubin is normally secreted by the liver as a water-soluble glucuronide. Coliform infection produces β-glucuronidase, which deconjugates bilirubin glucuronide. Unconjugated bilirubin may combine with calcium to produce insoluble calcium bilirubinate stones. In contrast to patients in the Orient, the majority of patients in the United States with chronic cholecystitis and cholelithiasis have gallbladders that contain sterile bile. Stasis appears to be a factor in the formation of the pigment stones, which suggests that incomplete emptying might lead to increased concentration of bilirubin and calcium within the gallbladder, favoring the precipitation of sparingly soluble compounds. In addition, bilirubin secretion appears to be increased significantly in the bile of patients with hemolytic conditions and cirrhosis when studied by using duodenal perfusion techniques. Further studies are needed to elucidate the mechanism of the formation of pigment stones.

DISSOLUTION OF GALLSTONES

The dissolution of gallstones is based on the premise that cholesterol gallstone formation in humans is the result of supersaturation of bile by cholesterol. Chenodeoxycholic acid (3α, 7α-dihydroxy-5β cholanoic acid; CDCA) and ursodeoxycholic acid (3α, 7β-dihydroxy-5 β cholanoic acid; UDCA) have been demonstrated to be capable of dissolving cholesterol gallstones in humans. These bile acids decrease hepatic synthesis and secretion of bile.

CDCA has been investigated in a National Cooperative Gallstone Study. When oral doses of 750 mg daily were used, partial or complete dissolution of gallstones occurred in nearly half the patients. One problem is to determine when cholesterol stones are present in the gallbladder, because not all radiolucent stones are composed chiefly of cholesterol, and CDCA and UDCA are not effective against pigment stones.

Side-effects of CDCA include diarrhea and abdominal cramping pain. A more serious potential complication has been hepatotoxicity, which might result from the conversion of CDCA to lithocholic acid. Alteration of liver function, however, has been infrequent and has returned to normal when CDCA has been discontinued. An increase in the serum cholesterol level in some patients receiving CDCA therapy is apparently related to inhibition of biliary secretion of cholesterol. Theoretically, this alteration of cholesterol metabolism may increase the frequency of atherosclerosis when CDCA is administered over a long period.

UDCA has been investigated more extensively in Japan than in the United States and appears to compare favorably with CDCA in regard to therapeutic effectiveness. Significant elevation of lithocholic acid is less frequent; thus, liver function abnormalities are not encountered as often. Similarly, diarrhea is uncommon when UDCA is administered.

Symptoms continue during therapy until gallstones have been dissolved. Treatment must be continued indefinitely after gallstone dissolution has occurred. At the present time, the therapeutic role of secondary bile acids for the dissolution of gallstones has not been established and remains experimental.

BILIARY BACTERIA

Bile, as secreted by the liver and transported through the extrahepatic biliary tract, is sterile in humans. Cultures of the gallbladder and gallbladder bile in patients with gallstone disease, however, yield organisms in 20% to 25% of patients. Positive cultures are obtained with greater frequency in patients with acute cholecystitis, ranging from 50% to 70%. Cultures of common duct bile are usually sterile unless stones or stricture are present. The incidence increases in such cases to 80% to 95%. The frequency of positive cultures also increases with age and is significantly greater in patients over 70. The types of organisms cultured from the biliary tract are listed in Table 27-17. These bacteria are characteristically found in the intestinal tract. There remains, however, considerable controversy concerning the route by which the biliary tract becomes infected.

The incidence of positive bile cultures is reflected in the incidence of wound infections after biliary tract surgery. Wound infection is infrequent after cholecystectomy for chronic cholecystitis and cholelithiasis, usually 2% or less. The most frequent organism cultured is *Staphylococcus aureus.* The incidence of wound infection increases after cholecystectomy for acute cholecystitis and following common duct exploration for stone, where wound infection occurs in 4% to 8% of patients.

TABLE 27-17 BILIARY BACTERIA IN GALLSTONE DISEASE

AEROBES (60%)	ANAEROBES (40%)
Escherichia coli	Propionobacterium
Klebsiella, enterobacter	Peptostreptococcus
Streptococcus faecalis	Clostridium species
nonhemolytic streptococcus	*Bacteroides fragilis*
α-hemolytic streptococcus	Microaerophilic streptococcus

Bile is seldom infected in patients with obstruction of the common duct caused by neoplasms of the pancreas or bile ducts. Thus, partial obstruction and the presence of calculi are important factors in the development of biliary tract infections.

CHRONIC CHOLECYSTITIS AND CHOLELITHIASIS

Chronic inflammation of the gallbladder is associated with gallstones in more than 90% of instances. Gallstones occur in 8% to 10% of the adult population in the United States. Cholecystectomy for cholelithiasis is one of the most common abdominal operations, and more than 600,000 cholecystectomies are performed annually in this country. Women have chronic cholecystitis and cholelithiasis more often than men, and the incidence is increased among women who have been pregnant. It has been estimated that 50% of women over the age of 60 years have gallstones.

The pathogenesis of chronic cholecystitis has not been completely elucidated. The gallbladder seems to be an important site for the precipitation of macromolecular aggregates of cholesterol and for the development of pigment stones. This finding, as well as the frequent impaction of stones in the cystic duct or in the ampulla of the gallbladder, supports the contention that many of the changes in the gallbladder wall in the presence of cholelithiasis are the result of irritation from the stones or of chemical damage by the bile in combination with damage by the gallstones. Bacteria do not seem to play an important role in the development of chronic cholecystitis in the majority of patients. Cultures of the gallbladder wall or bile are usually sterile. In our experience, approximately 20% of cultures of the gallbladder were positive. In addition, the route by which bacteria reach the biliary tract remains uncertain. The majority of organisms are of enteric origin and may gain entry through either the portal vein or the common bile duct.

CLINICAL FINDINGS

The symptoms which are associated with gallstone disease are variable. Some patients have intermittent flatulence and vague abdominal distress in the upper abdomen, while others suffer from severe episodes of colicky right upper quadrant pain, nausea, and vomiting. Biliary colic may last from a few minutes to several hours. The patient with gallbladder colic is usually restless and is unable to find a comfortable position. Pain of gallbladder origin may radiate along the costal margin to the tip of the scapula or to the right shoulder region. Occasionally, patients with choleli-

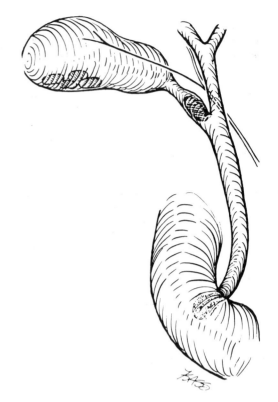

Fig. 27-16.   Biliary colic is caused by impaction of stone in cystic duct.

thiasis have radiation of pain substernally that may be confused with pain of cardiac origin. Pain in patients with cholelithiasis often occurs at night and frequently after a large meal, dietary indiscretion, or the ingestion of fatty food. The pain may be followed by nausea and vomiting. The patient may observe some lessening of pain after vomiting; during subsequent attacks, vomiting may be self-induced.

Biliary colic is caused by distention of the gallbladder or common bile duct, which results from obstruction of the cystic duct or common bile duct (Fig. 27-16). Obstruction of the gallbladder may cause the gallbladder mucosa to secrete calcium, which may be precipitated on the surface of the calculi or gallbladder wall (Fig. 27-17). The concentric rings on gallstones are evidence of intermittent obstruction of the gallbladder.

In the majority of patients with chronic cholecystitis, physical examination is not remarkable unless there is associated inflammation. During the attacks of biliary colic, the patient may have transient tenderness in the upper abdomen. When stones pass from the gallbladder through the common duct into the duodenum, mild icterus may be detected.

RADIOLOGIC DIAGNOSIS

The detection of gallstones depends on radiologic imaging techniques in the majority of patients. In a few individuals, cholelithiasis may be found when an operation is performed for an unrelated problem and the gallbladder is palpated by the surgeon.

For many years, oral cholecystography has been the standard radiologic study for detection of gallstones. Radio-

CHRONIC CHOLECYSTITIS	
Etiology	Precipitation of cholesterol in the gallbladder; obstruction of cystic duct; irritation of gallbladder wall
Dx	Episodic right upper quadrant pain, nausea, vomiting, flatulence. Stones detected by ultrasonography or oral cholecystography
Rx	Appropriate evaluation and cholecystectomy for symptomatic gallstones

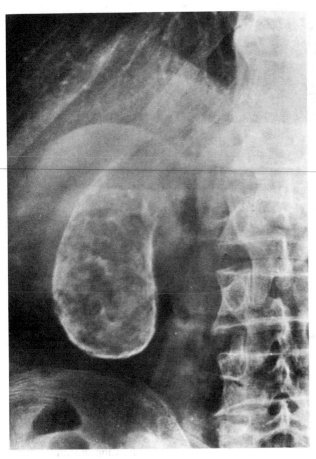

Fig. 27-17. Obstruction of the cystic duct has resulted in deposition of calcium in the gallbladder wall, which produces a "porcelain" gallbladder. (This patient had not received contrast material for cholecystography.)

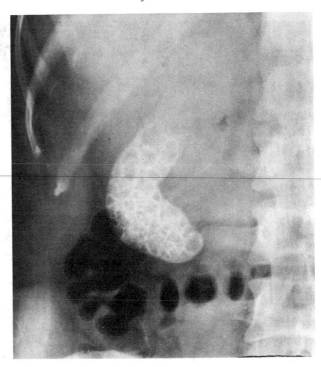

Fig. 27-18. Oral cholecystogram reveals multiple radiolucent gallstones within the gallbladder.

paque stones are seen in less than 10% of patients with cholelithiasis when plain abdominal films are obtained. Oral cholecystography is accurate and is associated with few side-effects. Usually 3 g of an iodinated compound, iopanoic acid, is given orally the evening before the radiologic study is to be performed. Iopanoic acid is absorbed from the small intestine and transported in the portal vein blood to the liver, where it is excreted in the bile. In the fasting state, the contrast agent enters the gallbladder, where it is concentrated 8 to 10 times. Thus, the gallbladder is visible when roentgenograms are obtained and, when present, stones appear as defects within the opacified gallbladder (Fig. 27-18).

Failure to visualize the gallbladder when oral cholecystography is performed on two successive days indicates that the gallbladder is diseased. The gallbladder mucosa may be sufficiently damaged so that the contrast agent cannot be concentrated or, usually, the contrast material is prevented from gaining entry into the gallbladder by a stone lodged in the cystic duct. Other causes of failure to visualize the gallbladder (aside from the patient's failure to take the tablets of iopanoic acid) are gastric outlet obstruction, malabsorption syndromes, diarrhea, or liver disease. In the presence of obstructive jaundice, the gallbladder will not be seen if the bilirubin level exceeds 3 mg/dl.

Ultrasonography is replacing oral cholecystography as the preferred method for initial screening of patients with suspected biliary tract disease (Fig. 27-19). The introduction of improvements in ultrasonography, such as gray scale and "real time" techniques, has provided better images and rapid study. The gallbladder is one of the abdominal organs that is particularly appropriate for ultrasound scanning because of its location and its anatomical configuration as a fluid-filled viscus.

Ultrasonography is a noninvasive method with accuracy similar to that of oral cholecystography. The study does not require the ingestion of contrast material and thus may be applied to patients who suffer from nausea and vomiting or who cannot take oral medication. The study is not influenced by problems that interfere with the absorption of contrast agents from the intestinal tract or excretion by the liver. Thus, ultrasonography may be applied in patients with acute or chronic cholecystitis, pancreatitis, hepatitis, or jaundice. It is applicable in pregnant patients and in those who are allergic to iodinated compounds. Gallstones appear as echo-dense structures in the gallbladder on sonograms (Fig. 27-20). If stones are not seen, oral cholecystography or radionuclide study using iminodiacetic derivatives (*e.g.*, HIDA, PIPIDA) may be helpful.

The radionuclide study uses a radioisotope scanning agent which is injected intravenously. Images of the liver and biliary tract are obtained with a scintillation camera that is placed over the abdomen. Normally the isotope is detected in the liver within five minutes and outlines the common bile duct, gallbladder, and duodenum in 10 to 20 minutes. If the cystic duct is obstructed, the isotope cannot enter the gallbladder, and thus an image of the gallbladder will not be seen. If the common bile duct is completely obstructed, the isotope will not enter the duodenum. When partial obstruction of the common duct is present, the duct will appear dilated and there will be a delay in the appearance of the radioisotope in the duodenum.

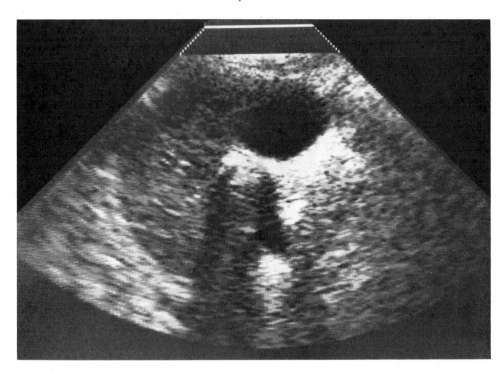

Fig. 27-19. "Real-time" ultrasonography shows a gallbladder without intraluminal echo or other defects: a normal gallbladder.

DIFFERENTIAL DIAGNOSIS

Gallstone disease is probably the most common cause of recurring right upper quadrant abdominal pain in adults. When the symptoms are vague or atypical, however, even though gallstones are present, consideration should be given to the possibility of peptic ulceration, hiatal hernia, pancreatitis, or hepatitis. The differentiation between gallstone disease and coronary artery disease may be difficult in some patients. Frequently, cholelithiasis and coronary artery disease are present in the same patient.

It has been reported that gallbladder disease occurs more often with coronary artery disease than in patients with normal coronary arteries. This may merely reflect increasing incidence of both diseases with age. Differentiating between symptoms due to myocardial ischemia and those resulting from biliary tract disease is necessary and important and, at times, difficult. There is increased incidence of gallstones in hemolytic disease, such as hereditary spherocytosis and sickle cell anemia. Hemolysis associated with red cell destruction is followed by increased bilirubin production, and these patients are found to have bile pigment stones. Approximately 33% of patients over the age of 10 years with homozygous sickle cell anemia and more than 50% of patients with hereditary spherocytosis have gallstones. An increased incidence of gallstones attributed to increased hemolysis has been reported in patients after the insertion of prosthetic cardiac valves.

Pancreatitis may be a manifestation of underlying gallstone disease and in some patients may be the initial presentation of chronic cholecystitis and cholelithiasis. The incidence of biliary tract disease in patients with pancreatitis has been reported to be as high as 60%. Cholelithiasis is the most common cause of pancreatitis in adult women. Pancreatitis that is associated with gallstone disease tends to recur until the biliary tract disease is treated, but it usually does not recur after the underlying gallstone disease has been corrected.

TREATMENT

The most satisfactory treatment of symptomatic gallstones is cholecystectomy. As an elective operation, this procedure is accomplished with a low operative mortality and provides relief of symptoms in more than 90% of these patients. Removal of the gallbladder prevents the major complications of gallstone disease, acute cholecystitis and choledocholithiasis.

TECHNIQUE OF CHOLECYSTECTOMY

Cholecystectomy may be performed through an upper midline incision or an incision placed obliquely or transversely beneath the right costal margin. After the peritoneal cavity is opened, a careful manual exploration of the abdominal cavity is performed, to make certain that other pathologic problems are not present.

The gallbladder is explored by depressing the hepatic flexure of the colon inferiorly and by retracting the omentum and duodenum medially. The peritoneum overlying the cystic duct is carefully incised, and the gallbladder is grasped by a clamp so that it can be retracted upward. The next step in the operation is most important: identification of the junction of the cystic duct and the common bile duct. This is achieved optimally by identifying the triangle of Calot, bounded by the common duct inferiorly, the cystic duct medially, and the cystic artery laterally.

When the cystic duct is isolated, a single tie is placed around it with a single loop that is designed to prevent migration of calculi through the cystic duct during manipulation of the gallbladder. The peritoneum is then incised about the gallbladder 10 mm to 12 mm from the liver. Beginning at the fundus of the gallbladder, the organ is dissected free from its bed until the only remaining attachment is the cystic duct. The cystic artery is ligated when encountered arborizing on the wall of the gallbladder.

At this point, an operative cholangiogram is usually performed. It is a matter of individual preference and

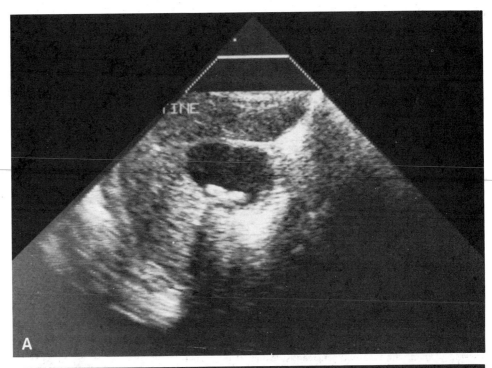

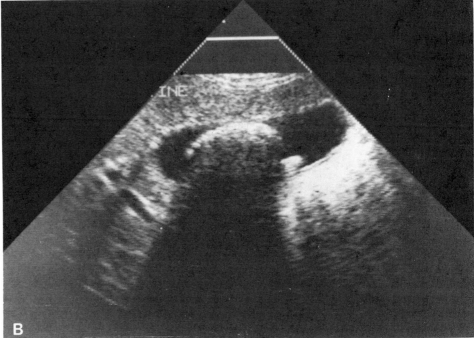

Fig. 27-20. (*A*) Demonstrations of cholelithiasis. This longitudinal section, using "realtime" ultrasonography, shows multiple stones in the central portion of the gallbladder with acoustic shadows extending beneath the stones. (*B*) Transverse section of the gallbladder demonstrating cholelithiasis.

experience whether the operative cholangiogram is performed before the gallbladder is removed or through the cystic duct stump after the gallbladder has been excised. In either case, a small plastic catheter is inserted through the cystic duct and 10 ml to 20 ml of an iodinated contrast agent (20%–25% concentration) is injected (Fig. 27-21). If stones are not present in the common bile duct, the catheter is removed and the cystic duct is tied carefully so that injury to the wall of the common duct is avoided.

If the gallbladder bed is "dry," without bleeding or bile leakage, and if there has not been spilling of gallbladder or common duct contents into the infrahepatic fossa (Morison's pouch), then the abdomen may be closed without drainage. Many surgeons prefer to insert a single Penrose (cigarette) drain routinely into the infrahepatic fossa, citing the occasional small bile duct that may be transected in the gallbladder fossa.

INDICATIONS FOR COMMON DUCT EXPLORATION

The indications for common duct exploration are changing somewhat because of the more frequent use of intraoperative cholangiography. Operative cholangiography is valuable in the assessment of the common duct at the time of cholecystectomy, as well as in patients with a history of jaundice

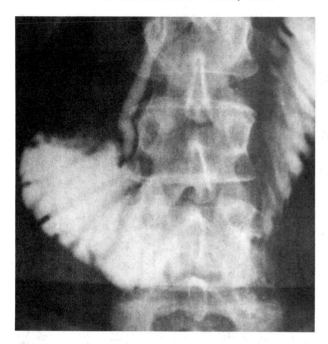

Fig. 27-21. This normal intraoperative cholangiogram in a 40-year-old woman with gallstone pancreatitis demonstrates normal common duct without defects or obstruction and with free flow into the duodenum.

and in those with multiple small stones within the gallbladder. The presence of jaundice, palpable common duct calculi, and a dilated common duct are findings that indicate the need for choledochotomy. Relative indications for exploration of the common duct are recent cholangitis or acute pancreatitis because of the associated frequency of choledocholithiasis.

ASYMPTOMATIC GALLSTONES

The incidence of asymptomatic ("silent") gallstones is uncertain. Some patients are found to have gallstones during study for unrelated diseases, and others are discovered to have cholelithiasis during abdominal operations for problems which do not involve the biliary tract. With increased use of noninvasive techniques such as ultrasonography, an increasing number of asymptomatic gallstones are being detected.

Studies of the natural course of gallstone disease indicate that approximately 50% of these patients with "silent" cholelithiasis will develop symptomatic gallbladder disease. With increasing age, the incidence of complications of gallstone disease increases, as does the risk of operation. Patients who are found to have gallstones should be advised of their presence. Elective cholecystectomy is usually recommended, unless the patient has some associated disease that presents an unwarranted risk to operation. Although common duct calculi are uncommon in this group of patients, incidence of choledocholithiasis increases in asymptomatic patients with gallstones.

ACALCULOUS CHOLECYSTITIS

Patients who have symptoms suggestive of biliary tract disease, in whom cholecystograms or ultrasonograms visualize the gallbladder without evidence of cholelithiasis, present difficult therapeutic problems. Removal of gallblad-

ders that do not contain stones results in relief of symptoms less often than does cholecystectomy for symptomatic cholelithiasis. In some patients, operation is undertaken with the impression that cholelithiasis is present but is not found when laparotomy is performed. It is possible that the gallstones may have passed spontaneously in some of these patients. In other patients, symptoms are attributed to the biliary tract when other gastrointestinal conditions are responsible for the patient's complaints. Cholesterosis of the gallbladder is a pathological process caused by the deposition of cholesterol in the gallbladder mucosa. These punctate yellow spots have resulted in the gross description of "strawberry" gallbladder. Although attempts have been made to correlate cholesterosis with clinical gallbladder disease (hyperplastic cholecystosis), these gallbladders probably reflect metabolic alterations and are not clinically significant unless cholelithiasis is present.

When patients have complaints, thought to be of biliary tract origin, but with normal cholecystograms, careful evaluation of the gastrointestinal tract should be undertaken, including repeated imaging of the gallbladder either by cholecystogram or ultrasound. It has been suggested that persistent visualization of the gallbladder after 36 hours is evidence of obstruction to the gallbladder and supports the diagnosis of acalculous cholecystitis. CCK has been administered to patients with symptoms of gallbladder disease who have normal cholecystograms as a diagnostic method. The patient is considered to have evidence of obstruction of the gallbladder if right upper quadrant pain occurs following injection of the CCK or if the gallbladder fails to empty following the injection. These conclusions have not been adequately supported. In most patients who do not have demonstrable cholelithiasis, therapy should be conservative, with dietary management and symptomatic medication. Operation is not recommended, and cholecystectomy should be performed only for patients whose symptoms are severe and persistent, closely resembling those of gallbladder disease. Relief of symptoms after cholecystectomy has been obtained in 50% to 65% of carefully selected patients with acalculous cholecystitis.

POSTCHOLECYSTECTOMY SYNDROME

More than 90% of patients who have cholecystectomy for symptomatic gallstone disease are relieved of their symptoms. The term *postcholecystectomy syndrome* has been applied to patients who have continued or recurrent symptoms of biliary tract disease for which the cholecystectomy was performed. Perhaps the term is inappropriate because, in the majority of patients, an organic lesion can be found explaining persistent symptoms of biliary tract disease after cholecystectomy. The most common of these may be placed in one of the following categories: residual gallstones, cystic duct remnant, neoplasm of the biliary tract, common duct stricture, or papillitis or stenosis of the sphincter of Oddi. If patients develop recurrent symptoms of gallstone disease after cholecystectomy, a careful evaluation of the biliary tree should be undertaken. Residual stones in the common bile duct, cystic duct remnant, or in the intrahepatic bile ducts occasionally will be found. The association of intermittent jaundice with biliary tract symptoms is suggestive of residual calculi. Ultrasound and radionuclide studies and retrograde cholangiography are useful techniques in the detection of residual stones. An occasional cause of symptoms is the retention of a long cystic duct which may behave as a "mini-gallbladder," with or without stones. When symptomatic, such cystic duct stumps will present with evidence of inflammatory disease and occasionally may be associated with jaundice.

Persistent symptoms after cholecystectomy should lead to the consideration that a malignant process might be present in either the bile ducts or the head of the pancreas. Approximately 30% of patients with periampullary carcinomas have had cholecystectomies within six months of the time that the neoplasm was detected.

Ultrasound, CT scans, and ERCP are useful techniques in the detection of malignant disease of the biliary tract. Papillitis or stenosis involving the ampulla of Vater is uncommon but occasionally causes persistent pain after cholecystectomy. Endoscopic visualization of the papilla is useful. Occasionally the problem may be corrected by endoscopic sphincteroplasty; in other patients, an operative procedure is required. If a common duct stricture is present from injury to the bile duct at the time of operation, this may be detected by percutaneous transhepatic cholangiography (PTC) or ERCP.

When intrinsic lesions of the biliary tract have been excluded by appropriate studies, a search should be conducted for disease processes that are extrinsic to the biliary tract. These extrinsic problems include peptic ulcer, neoplastic disease of the stomach or colon, coronary artery disease, and diseases of the pancreas, including pancreatitis. If a specific cause of the pain cannot be demonstrated, one should question whether the original symptoms were due to gallbladder disease. In some patients, dietary management, weight reduction, and symptomatic treatment will result in relief of symptoms.

ACUTE CHOLECYSTITIS

Acute cholecystitis is the most common complication of chronic gallbladder disease and is said to develop in approximately 25% of patients with chronic symptomatic cholecystitis. Gallstones are present in 90% to 95% of patients with acute cholecystitis. The relative frequency of acute cholecystitis increases with age among patients with cholelithiasis. In general, acute cholecystitis develops in less than 20% of patients under the age of 50 years who have chronic cholecystitis and cholelithiasis, but occurs in 30% or more of patients with chronic gallbladder disease who are 65 years or older.

At least three etiologic factors contribute to the development of acute cholecystitis. These are infection, obstruction, and ischemia (Fig. 27-22). Although any one of these may be the initiating cause, obstruction of the cystic duct by stone appears to be most frequent and is present in at least 90% of cases. Acute cholecystitis occurs without cholelithiasis and has been reported in association with anomalies of the cystic duct, tumors of the bile ducts, blood clots, and vascular lesions such as arteritis and thrombosis of the cystic artery. Acute cholecystitis may develop after operations remote to the biliary tract or following trauma. Factors other than simple obstruction are involved in the development of acute inflammation of the gallbladder. Ligation of the cystic duct does not produce acute cholecystitis but results only in distention or hydrops of the gallbladder. Increasing intraluminal pressure in the gallbladder may interfere with venous or lymphatic drainage with resultant edema of the gallbladder wall, followed by interference with the arterial supply, which may lead to ischemia and necrosis of a portion of the gallbladder wall. Pressure from calculi results in necrosis of the mucosa, ulceration, secondary imflammatory changes, and edema. Bacteria of enteric origin may be cultured from the gallbladder in approximately two thirds of patients with acute cholecystitis, but the frequency of positive cultures is highest 4 to 8 days after the onset of illness, suggesting a secondary, rather than an initiating, factor in the development of acute cholecystitis.

CLINICAL FINDINGS

Although acute cholecystitis may be the initial manifestation of biliary tract disease, the majority of patients develop acute inflammation of the gallbladder following previous episodes of upper abdominal pain compatible with chronic gallbladder disease. Typically, the patient has a knowledge of previous demonstrable gallstones or episodic, colicky, right upper quadrant pain. The development of acute cholecystitis usually begins with an episode of abdominal pain similar to previous experiences. The pain, however, becomes constant and is frequently exacerbated by deep inspiration. Anorexia, nausea and occasionally vomiting are present. Moderate elevation of the temperature may be detected. Examination of the abdomen discloses moderate to marked tenderness in the right hypochondrium, and in approximately 20% of patients a tender enlarged gallbladder may be felt. Laboratory studies may indicate an increase in

ACUTE CHOLECYSTITIS	
Etiology	Obstruction of cystic duct, usually by stone, distention of gallbladder, ischemia, secondary infection
Dx	Previous history of chronic cholecystitis or gallstones; severe right upper quadrant pain, right upper abdominal tenderness Tender palpable gallbladder in 20 percent Ultrasonography and radionuclide scan of common duct helpful
Rx	Nasogastric suction and parenteral fluid Careful evaluation for systemic disease Cholecystectomy unless contraindicated

Fig. 27-22. The mechanism for development of acute cholecystitis includes impaction of stone in cystic duct or ampulla of gallbladder, distention of gallbladder, and ischemia. Associated edema may partially occlude the common duct.

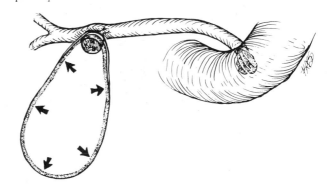

peripheral leukocyte count, and in some patients an elevation of the serum amylase and bilirubin are found. The initial management of patients with acute cholecystitis is directed toward the establishment of the diagnosis, relief of symptoms, and assessment of potentially serious associated diseases.

DIFFERENTIAL DIAGNOSIS

The differential diagnosis includes hepatitis, acute pancreatitis, perforated ulcer, and acute appendicitis. Occasionally, carcinoma of the gallbladder and hemorrhage into metastatic hepatic lesions may mimic acute cholecystitis. Acute pancreatitis may be present in association with acute cholecystitis.

INITIAL TREATMENT

The initial treatment of the patient usually includes nasogastric intubation and parenteral fluids. In the older individual an electrocardiogram is essential as an aid in cardiac evaluation. An attempt to visualize the gallbladder or to detect cholelithiasis by means of ultrasound is indicated. This noninvasive technique provides information concerning the caliber of the extrahepatic biliary system as well. If acute cholecystitis is suspected and the ultrasonographic study is inconclusive, radionuclide scans (HIDA or PIPIDA, for example) are useful. Characteristically, in acute cholecystitis, the cystic duct is occluded. The radionuclide scan will demonstrate the common duct but will not visualize the gallbladder (Fig. 27-23). This study has replaced intravenous cholangiography in many institutions. Successful intravenous cholangiography depends upon satisfactory hepatic function and does not provide satisfactory visualization of the biliary tree in the presence of elevation of the serum bilirubin level or severe parenchymal liver disease. Satisfac-

Fig. 27-23. Radionuclide study (IDA) demonstrates patent common duct with prompt excretion of the isotope by the liver and entry into the duodenum. The gallbladder was not visualized, which supports the diagnosis of acute cholecystitis.

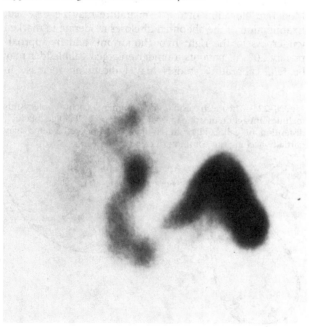

tory intravenous cholangiography demonstrates the common duct, but the contrast agent does not enter the gallbladder because of cystic duct obstruction.

CLINICAL COURSE

The clinical course of acute cholecystitis is unpredictable. In younger patients, the complications of perforation and peritonitis are infrequent. When acute cholecystitis occurs in young women who are pregnant, the acute process will often resolve and the patients can be operated upon at an interval after delivery. In patients over the age of 65 years, however, acute cholecystitis is often a progressive disease, and it is in this group of patients that coronary artery disease, congestive heart failure, chronic obstructive pulmonary disease, and diabetes mellitus present serious complications in the management of acute biliary tract disease.

The objective of the management of the patient with acute cholecystitis is to prepare the patient for cholecystectomy. If there is prompt abatement of the signs and symptoms of the acute phase of the disease, operation may be postponed and evaluation of the patient may be accomplished in a deliberate manner. Cholecystectomy can then be performed as an elective procedure. Prompt cholecystectomy for acute cholecystitis is the procedure of choice if contraindications to operation are not present.

TIMING OF OPERATION

There has been considerable controversy in regard to the timing of operation in patients with acute cholecystitis. If the signs of peritoneal irritation increase and other signs of inflammation become more marked, operation should be undertaken promptly. Cholecystectomy can be accomplished in a majority of patients. Cholecystostomy is reserved for patients who have serious complicating disease or when the inflammatory reaction at the time of operation is so marked that identification of the structures in the region of the gallbladder is seriously impaired. Cholecystostomy is indicated in less than 15% of patients with acute cholecystitis.

The presence of jaundice presents a significant problem in patients with acute cholecystitis. Jaundice is associated with acute cholecystitis in 20% to 30% of cases, and the serum bilirubin is greater than 1.5 mg in approximately one third of these patients. Icterus in acute gallbladder disease may be caused by pressure on the common duct by an edematous, acutely inflamed gallbladder, or by obstruction by common duct stone, ascending cholangitis, pancreatitis, and, rarely, tumor. The incidence of common duct stones has been reported to range from 10% to 25% in patients with acute cholecystitis (in our experience, 13% of patients with histologically proven acute cholecystitis had choledocholithiasis). If the serum bilirubin is greater than 3 mg/dl, the incidence of choledocholithiasis increases, but an increased serum bilirubin or serum alkaline phosphatase level is an unreliable indicator of common duct calculi.

Patients with acute cholecystitis who have evidence of cholangitis or acute pancreatitis also have an increased incidence of common duct calculi. More than 15% of patients with acute cholecystitis have evidence of acute pancreatitis as demonstrated by elevation of serum amylase levels. Because of the frequency of common duct stones, operative cholangiography is recommended at the time of cholecystectomy for acute cholecystitis.

Cholecystectomy for acute cholecystitis is associated with a mortality rate of 2% to 4%, whereas cholecystostomy carries a mortality of 10% to 15%. The latter figure indicates the serious nature of the associated disease problems that result in the performance of the technically less complicated operation. The mortality rate for cholecystectomy in patients 65 years and older approaches 10%, in contrast to an operative mortality of less than 2% for patients under the age of 65 years. This higher mortality in the older age group represents the limited capacity of the elderly to withstand surgical procedures and the influence of associated disease processes on the surgical mortality.

ACUTE CHOLECYSTITIS FOLLOWING OPERATION OR TRAUMA

Acute cholecystitis may occur following the surgical treatment of unrelated disease, trauma, and burns. This is a serious complication in such patients, differing in a number of respects from acute cholecystitis which presents as a primary problem. The mortality has been reported to range from 30% to 75%, which reflects the advanced stage of the pathologic process found in such patients. Men outnumber women, and the average age range is higher than in primary acute cholecystitis. Gallstones are frequently absent in patients who develop acute cholecystitis after trauma, injury, or operation. In two reported series of acute cholecystitis in Vietnam casualties, all patients were found to have acalculous cholecystitis. The pathogenesis of postoperative or post-traumatic cholecystitis is obscure. There is evidence of stasis and inspissation of gallbladder bile in the postoperative period. Other factors that seem to contribute are dehydration, the use of narcotics, and hemolysis from blood transfusion.

The diagnosis of acute cholecystitis is often obscured in traumatized patients because of the symptoms associated with trauma. Similarly, delay in diagnosis has been observed in the postoperative period. Pain is difficult to interpret in many of these patients. The most reliable physical finding is tenderness in the right hypochondrium, with signs of local peritoneal irritation. Delay in diagnosis is perhaps responsible for the high incidence of gangrene, perforation, empyema, and cholangitis that occurs in these patients. Ultrasonography and radionuclide scans may be of assistance in diagnosis.

When acute cholecystitis is suspected in the postoperative period or following trauma, operation should be performed. Cholecystectomy is the operation of choice, particularly in patients who have gangrene of the wall of the gallbladder. Cholecystostomy, which can be performed with local anesthesia, should be reserved for patients whose complicating disease processes will not permit cholecystectomy.

EMPYEMA OF THE GALLBLADDER

Empyema of the gallbladder is one of the serious complications of acute cholecystitis and is characterized by the presence of a suppurative exudate within the gallbladder. Extrahepatic abscesses are common in association with empyema of the gallbladder and include abdominal abscesses in the region of the gallbladder. Enteric organisms are usually found on culture, *E. coli* and Klebsiella species being most common. Empyema of the gallbladder is usually found in patients who have been treated for several days and in whom the correct diagnosis has been obscure or operation delayed. The findings of empyema of the gallbladder are indistinguishable from those of acute cholecystitis unless the patient has symptoms of clinical sepsis, peritonitis and jaundice.

The appropriate treatment is cholecystectomy. Whenever

Fig. 27-24. Gas within the lumen of and in the wall of the gallbladder is typical of emphysematous cholecystitis and was noted in this patient when an upper gastrointestinal barium study was performed.

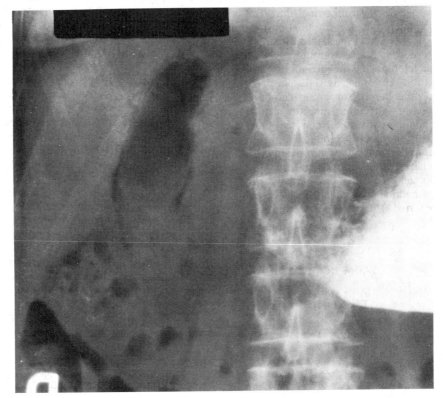

possible, an operative cholangiogram should be performed because of the high incidence of associated common duct calculi. Postoperative morbidity and mortality are usually higher in this group of patients because of the septic nature of the disease and the associated extrabiliary abscesses.

EMPHYSEMATOUS CHOLECYSTITIS

Emphysematous cholecystitis is a type of cholecystitis that is characterized by gas in the lumen or wall of the gallbladder. The clinical picture is that of acute cholecystitis, and the diagnosis is made by the recognition of gas in the gallbladder or gallbladder wall when abdominal films are obtained (Fig. 27-24). Gas has also been detected in the biliary radicles. An important feature of this problem is that gangrene and perforation occur with great frequency. Emphysematous cholecystitis is more common in men, and gallstones are found in only 75% of these patients.

Cultures of the gallbladder usually yield clostridial organisms. Diabetes mellitus has been reported to be present in more than one third of patients with this variety of acute cholecystitis. A higher mortality rate has been recorded in patients with emphysematous cholecystitis. Although emphysematous cholecystitis is uncommon, it has been recommended that plain abdominal films should be done prior to the diagnostic evaluation of all patients suspected of having acute cholecystitis because of the significant prognostic and therapeutic implications that go with the recognition of the presence of emphysematous cholecystitis as manifested by air in the gallbladder or bile ducts. Cholecystectomy is required because of the frequent presence of gangrene and perforation.

GALLSTONE ILEUS

Gallstone ileus is the term applied to mechanical intestinal obstruction caused by impaction of one or more gallstones within the gastrointestinal tract. Gallstone ileus is an uncommon cause of intestinal obstruction and accounts for less than 2% of mechanical small bowel obstruction. Gallstone ileus is a complication in less than 5% of all cases of cholelithiasis. Women outnumber men approximately 10 to 1 in gallstone ileus. Gallstone ileus is usually encountered in either the sixth or seventh decade of life. Serious associated diseases, including diabetes, cardiovascular disease, and pulmonary disease, are present in the majority of patients. Gallstone ileus is produced by the passage of a gallstone from the gallbladder into the intestinal tract by means of a biliary enteric fistula. The fistula is usually a cholecystoduodenal fistula, although occasional reports of fistula formation between the gallbladder and the colon have been reported. The site of obstruction is in the terminal ileum in

approximately 70% of cases, because this is the most narrow portion of the small intestine. Reported sites of obstruction also include the sigmoid colon and the duodenum. Stones producing obstruction are usually larger than 2.5 cm in diameter. Fewer than half the stones entering the gastrointestinal tract will cause obstruction, because stones smaller than 2.5 cm usually pass in the stool.

CLINICAL PICTURE

The clinical picture of gallstone ileus is that of mechanical small bowel obstruction. Approximately 50% of patients give a prior history of gallbladder disease, and 25% have symptoms of recent acute biliary tract problems. The symptoms may be intermittent and have been described as "tumbling obstruction." The intermittent nature of the symptomatology often delays diagnosis. Jaundice is uncommon. The patients have cramping abdominal pain, nausea, vomiting, abdominal distention, and obstipation—findings typical of mechanical small bowel obstruction.

Physical examination is characterized by abdominal distention, dehydration, and hyperactive bowel sounds. Laboratory findings are compatible with fluid losses, reflecting the fluid and electrolyte imbalance of intestinal obstruction. Plain films of the abdomen may be helpful. The triad of Rigler has been used to describe the characteristic findings: (1) air in the biliary tree, (2) radiologic evidence of small bowel obstruction, and (3) visualization of the gallstone in the right lower quadrant. In occasional patients who have radiopaque gallstones, a change in position of previously observed stones from the right upper quadrant to a different position in the abdomen has been detected.

SURGICAL TREATMENT

When the stone is found impacted in the distal ileum, surgeons prefer to gently displace and remove it through an incision in healthy proximal bowel. If the stone cannot be displaced, resection of the bowel, which contains the impacted stone and is frequently necrotic, may be necessary. At the time of operation, it is important to examine the entire gastrointestinal tract to detect other calculi. There is controversy concerning the advisability of simultaneous cholecystectomy and repair of the cholecystoenteric fistula. Because of the presence of intestinal obstruction and associated serious illnesses, many patients are not candidates for such an extensive operation. As long as the fistula remains patent, however, additional stones may pass into the gastrointestinal tract. The patient is also a candidate for the development of cholangitis. Recurrent gallstone ileus has been reported. With suitable preparation and careful patient selection, one-stage cholecystectomy, fistula repair, and enteral lithotomy for gallstone ileus can be performed without increasing the mortality and morbidity. Postoperative wound infections are high in this group of patients and have been attributed to the unavoidable contamination from enterotomy in an obstructed intestine.

BILIARY TRACT DISEASE

PRIMARY SCLEROSING CHOLANGITIS

Primary sclerosing cholangitis (stenosing cholangitis, obliterative cholangitis) is a progressive, nonspecific inflam-

---

COMPLICATIONS OF GALLSTONES

Acute and chronic cholecystitis
Obstructive jaundice
Pancreatitis
Cholangitis
Biliary-enteric fistula
Gallstone ileus (intestinal obstruction)
Gallbladder carcinoma

matory process of unknown etiology that produces fibrosis and obliteration of the biliary ducts. Three general types have been described. There may be dense fibrosis of the extrahepatic biliary tree, presenting with diffuse fibrosis which makes identification of the biliary system difficult; there may be segmental disease that is seen to involve portions of the biliary tract on cholangiogram; or there may be fibrosis of the entire biliary ductal system. Fortunately, the disease is uncommon.

DIAGNOSIS

In establishing the diagnosis, primary sclerosing cholangitis must be differentiated from secondary sclerosing cholangitis, choledocholithiasis, cholangiocarcinoma, and congenital biliary abnormalities. There must be an absence of the cholestatic jaundice from drug or viral hepatitis, and the jaundice must be progressive and obstructive. Common duct stones must be absent, and there must not have been previous bile duct surgery. Malignancy may be difficult to exclude except by long-term follow-up or autopsy. The presence of thickening and fibrosis of the extrahepatic biliary system is typical. Symptoms are nonspecific and may resemble those of chronic gallstone disease. The patient's complaint of pain is often intermittent and located in the right upper abdomen. Jaundice and pruritus are common. Fever, weight loss, anorexia, and malaise are present in many patients.

CLINICAL FINDINGS

Jaundice is usually present. Hepatomegaly and splenomegaly are often found. In the presence of cirrhosis, spider angiomas and ascites may be present. The disease is more frequent in the third to fifth decades of life and affects men predominantly. The serum alkaline phosphatase is usually elevated, and hyperbilirubinemia occurs in approximately two thirds of the patients.

The diagnosis is usually established at the time of operation, when an indurated thick-walled common duct is found. The appearance of the cholangiogram is typical and shows narrowing, beading, and irregularity of the bile ducts. Both the extrahepatic and intrahepatic portions of the biliary system are involved in approximately two thirds of the patients; in those remaining, only the extrahepatic portion of the biliary tract is fibrotic.

Other methods of diagnosis include ERCP, which has been reported to be accurate when used, and PTC, which is helpful in approximately 50% of the patients in which it has been employed.

Liver biopsies present evidence of cholestasis with portal edema, bile duct proliferation, centrilobular bile stasis, and evidence of secondary biliary cirrhosis. Primary sclerosing cholangitis resembles primary biliary cirrhosis in that there is hepatic copper overload. The role of copper in the pathogenesis of liver or bile duct injury in this disease remains unknown.

TREATMENT

The medical treatment of primary sclerosing cholangitis has included corticosteroids, immunosuppressants, and cholecystagogues, alone or in combination, but the results have been discouraging.

Surgical treatment has consisted primarily of drainage of the biliary tract by means of choledochoenterostomy or T-tube drainage. Surgical treatment may relieve pruritus or jaundice, but it does not affect the underlying process.

Primary sclerosing cholangitis has been associated with several other diseases, including chronic ulcerative colitis, granulomas, ileocolitis, ulcerative proctitis, thyroiditis, and chronic active hepatitis. It has been suggested that, in the presence of chronic ulcerative colitis, colectomy may result in improvement of the cholangitis.

ACUTE CHOLANGITIS

Cholangitis is defined as inflammation of the bile ducts and results from biliary tract infection and obstruction. The commonest causes of cholangitis are common duct stone and stricture. Occasionally, patients with neoplastic obstruction may develop cholangitis. Cholangitis may also occur following biliary enteric anastomoses. Another cause is sclerosing cholangitis. Cholangitis recurs frequently if not treated, and repeated attacks of cholangitis result in secondary biliary cirrhosis, hepatic abscess, liver failure, and portal hypertension.

CLINICAL FEATURES

Cholangitis is somewhat more frequent in women than in men and occurs more often after the age of 50. In 1877, Charcot described a triad of symptoms associated with cholangitis from common duct calculi that included chills and fever, abdominal pain, and jaundice. Of these symptoms, chills and fever are most commonly present and may be the presenting findings, particularly in elderly patients. Next in frequency is abdominal pain, and approximately 75% of the patients with cholangitis have clinical icterus.

As might be expected from review of the common causes of cholangitis, the majority of patients with cholangitis have had previous operations upon the biliary tract, most commonly cholecystectomy. Other operations include the previous removal of common duct stones or biliary enteric anastomoses.

PHYSICAL FINDINGS

The majority of patients with cholangitis have abdominal tenderness that is usually maximal in the right upper quadrant of the abdomen. Signs of peritoneal irritation may be present, and an occasional patient will be found to have a tender, palpable, enlarged gallbladder. Hepatomegaly may be detected, reflecting the chronic nature of the problem. Patients with severe cholangitis may be hypotensive and present with varying degrees of mental confusion. The symptom complex of chills and fever, abdominal pain, jaundice, hypotension, and alteration of mental state has been referred to as Reynolds' pentad.

ACUTE CHOLANGITIS	
Etiology	Common duct stone and/or stricture
Dx	Chills, fever, right upper quadrant pain, jaundice; history of previous biliary operation frequent Ultrasonography, PTC, and ERCP most important diagnostic methods
Rx	Antibiotics, adequate fluid therapy; common duct exploration and cholecystectomy, if gallbladder is present

LABORATORY FINDINGS

Leukocytosis is usually present, often ranging above 20,000. In those patients without leukocytosis, a marked left shift in the white cell count is common. More than three fourths of patients with cholangitis have serum bilirubin levels greater than 2 mg/dl, and the majority have significant elevation of the serum alkaline phosphatase. Transaminase levels usually are not of diagnostic significance but may become markedly elevated in patients with long-standing recurrent cholangitis and biliary cirrhosis. Elevations in serum amylase have been detected in patients with associated pancreatitis.

Blood cultures should be obtained in patients who have chills and fever and are suspected of having cholangitis. Positive blood cultures are frequent in these patients and usually yield a single organism. *E. coli* is the most common organism detected. Other organisms are usually gram negative and include Klebsiella, pseudomonas, and enterococcus.

DIFFERENTIAL DIAGNOSIS

The problems most commonly confused with acute cholangitis are acute cholecystitis, acute pancreatitis, and perforating peptic ulcer. These can usually be differentiated by careful history, physical examination, and radiologic studies. It must be remembered, however, that patients with acute cholecystitis may have common duct stones *and* associated cholangitis and that pancreatitis may be the result of common duct calculi, thus secondary to the cause of cholangitis.

DIAGNOSTIC STUDIES

Ultrasonography may provide assistance and is the preferred initial diagnostic method. In patients with an intact biliary tree, gallstones may be demonstrated in the gallbladder. In addition, distention of the biliary tract is readily demonstrated by ultrasonography. This method has been of limited value in the detection of common duct stones. Oral cholecystography is of little value and should not be ordered in icteric patients. Intravenous cholangiography has been useful in some patients but is limited by elevation of the serum bilirubin in more than 50% of patients with cholangitis. Radionuclide scans—for example, HIDA scans—provide more information when dilatation of the extrahepatic biliary tree is suspected or demonstrated by ultrasonography. PTC is useful in demonstrating the cause and location of the obstructing lesion of the biliary tract. ERCP is also effective in demonstrating benign stricture and sclerosing cholangitis. Computed tomography (CT) is of assistance if neoplastic obstruction is suspected and may be used to supplement the findings on ultrasonography.

MANAGEMENT

Patients who have diagnosis of acute cholangitis based on clinical findings and initial laboratory studies should be treated promptly with antibiotics and fluid therapy. Antibiotics that are most effective against gram-negative organisms should be used, such as cephalothin, cefazolin, or chloramphenicol. Intravenous fluid therapy is particularly important in stabilizing these individuals. Adequacy of fluid replacement requires monitoring serum electrolytes and urinary output. The majority of patients with cholangitis respond promptly to antibiotics and fluid therapy, which will permit careful investigation of the underlying cause of the problem.

ACUTE SUPPURATIVE CHOLANGITIS

Acute suppurative cholangitis is a particularly virulent form of cholangitis associated with ductal obstruction. Suppurative cholangitis may develop rapidly and may develop in patients without previous known biliary tract disease. It should be suspected in those patients who have evidence of biliary tract disease with increasing abdominal pain, rising fever, and hypotension. Acute suppurative cholangitis is a life-threatening disease associated with a high mortality rate primarily related to delay in diagnosis and treatment.

Surgical treatment is directed at relieving the biliary tract obstruction and requires decompression of the common duct. If the patient's condition permits, common duct stones may be removed, a cholecystectomy or cholecystostomy performed, and a T-tube placed in the common duct. Cholecystostomy alone is inadequate. T-tube drainage of the common duct is essential even though the gallbladder cannot be removed. Cultures of the common duct should be obtained at the time of operation. A gram stain of the common duct bile may provide immediate information concerning the organisms that are producing the infection.

BILE PERITONITIS AND BILE ASCITES

Bile in the peritoneal cavity is sufficiently toxic and irritating to produce signs and symptoms of acute peritonitis in the majority of patients and usually results in prompt surgical intervention. Some patients, however, may accumulate large quantities of bile in the peritoneal cavity and tolerate bile ascites for prolonged periods.

BILE ASCITES IN INFANCY

In infants, spontaneous infantile bile peritonitis is encountered during the first month of life and is associated with slight jaundice, acholic stools, and abdominal swelling with clinical ascites. Scrotal swelling may be present in male infants. Because this is an uncommon condition, diagnosis is often delayed. The babies do not appear to be ill but are apathetic and fail to gain. The presence of jaundice should suggest biliary tract disease in these infants. The diagnosis may be established by paracentesis, which will reveal bile-stained ascitic fluid. Biliary tract abnormalities, including stenosis, perforation of the common duct, and cholelithiasis, have all been implicated in the pathogenesis. Surgical correction is required.

BILE PERITONITIS IN ADULTHOOD

Bile peritonitis in adults is usually the result of gallbladder perforation in cholecystitis or injury to the bile ducts. Acute cholecystitis is followed by perforation in approximately 10% of cases. Many of these produce walled-off pericholecystic abscesses, but approximately one fourth of the perforations lead to bile peritonitis. Perforation of the gallbladder is a late complication of the obstruction of the distal common duct from carcinoma of the head of the pancreas and is usually a terminal event. Penetration of the gallbladder or the common duct by an instrument during operation in the vicinity of the common duct or gallbladder may be followed by bile peritonitis.

Wounds of the liver produce severe abdominal pain because of extravasation of bile, as well as blood, into the peritoneal cavity. In a few patients a choledochal cyst has ruptured and produced bile peritonitis. Bile peritonitis also may follow percutaneous cholangiography if the common bile duct is obstructed. The adverse effects of bile in the peritoneal cavity have been attributed to the chemical toxicity of the bile, the fluid and electrolyte imbalance which follows, and the associated bacterial infection. Bile salts produce bradycardia, hypotension and muscular hyperactivity, spasm, and twitching when absorbed. Bacterial infection occurs when perforations develop after acute inflammatory biliary tract lesions. In general, bile that is not infected or contaminated with other fluids is well tolerated by the peritoneal cavity. When bile is infected, however, or mixed with blood or radiologic contrast agents, significant peritoneal signs result. Treatment includes adequate parenteral fluid therapy, systemic antibiotics, and surgical correction of the defect in the biliary tract.

CHOLEDOCHOLITHIASIS

Common duct stones (choledocholithiasis) are usually a complication of long-standing gallstone disease and are the commonest cause of extrahepatic biliary obstruction. The majority of stones in the common bile duct originate in the gallbladder and are present in 10% to 15% of patients with cholecystitis. The frequency of choledocholithiasis increases with age and is more common in patient 50 years or older. In many instances the stones in the common bile duct are faceted and match those present in the gallbladder. In other instances it is likely that fragments of stones pass through the cystic duct into the common duct and become enlarged, possibly due to associated infection. Common duct calculi may become symptomatic months or years after cholecystectomy. There has been debate as to whether these represent primary common duct stones or whether they are residual fragments of calculi present at the time of cholecystectomy.

SYMPTOMATOLOGY

The usual pattern of symptoms associated with common duct stones includes pain, jaundice, and fever. The pain is usually colicky in nature and is present in the midepigastrium or right hypochondrium. Radiation to the back along the costal margins and to the right subscapular area is frequent. Pain from choledocholithiasis is attributed to distention of the common bile duct, and the colicky nature resembles that associated with gallbladder disease. It is often accompanied by nausea and vomiting. If the pain persists for a few hours, bile is often detected in the urine.

Also typical of common duct stones is the development of jaundice following 1 to 3 days of pain. Chills and fever

occur in approximately 33% of patients with common duct stones and are typically a spiking, intermittent, febrile response. Pain is present in approximately 90% of patients with common duct stones, and 75% of patients with choledocholithiasis become icteric. It should be remembered that the most frequent cause of obstructive jaundice is calculous biliary tract disease. Jaundice in patients with stones is usually fluctuating in nature (Fig. 27-25), in contrast to the persistent progressive jaundice associated with neoplastic obstruction of the bile duct. In a few patients, common duct calculi are discovered without having produced any symptoms.

PHYSICAL EXAMINATION

Physical examination should include careful examination of the sclerae and skin for evidence of jaundice. This requires good lighting. In addition, scratch marks may be found on the abdomen as a result of pruritus, which is often associated with obstructive jaundice. Epigastric and right upper quadrant tenderness and guarding may be present during periods of pain and fever. Hepatomegaly may be present, and the liver may be tender during episodes of cholangitis. The gallbladder usually is not palpable, although a tender, enlarged gallbladder is sometimes detected in patients with common bile duct obstruction from stone.

LABORATORY FINDINGS

Laboratory findings in the patient who is not jaundiced may be unremarkable. A persistently elevated serum alkaline phosphatase level may be present and suggests common duct calculi. The customary biochemical tests of liver function, however, often are unremarkable. In a study of 150 patients with acute cholecystitis, 17 were found to have common duct stones at the time of operation. Preoperative

Fig. 27-25. Intermittent jaundice in choledocholithiasis results from movement of a stone that sporadically occludes the distal end of the common duct.

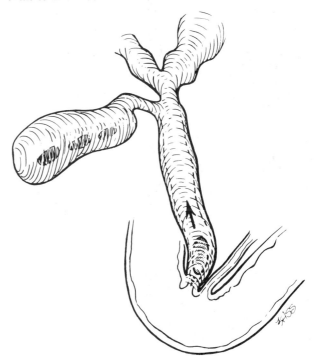

CHOLEDOCHOLITHIASIS	
Etiology	Majority originate in gallbladder Infection and stasis are also factors in pathogenesis
Dx	History of gallstone disease or cholecystectomy for cholelithiasis Pain in right hypochondrium, intermittent fever, jaundice Ultrasound, ERCP, and PTC are useful studies
Rx	Surgical: removal of gallbladder, when present, and common duct stones; operative cholangiogram and choledochoscopy are intraoperative aids

evaluation by means of serum bilirubin and alkaline phosphatase levels failed to be reliable in predicting the presence of choledocholithiasis in these patients.

Gallstone disease should be suspected in the patient who presents with acute pancreatitis without a history of alcohol abuse. The initial diagnostic step in both groups of patients should be ultrasonography. This may lead to the detection of gallstones in the gallbladder and, in some cases, a dilatation of the biliary tree despite the absence of jaundice. Stones within the common duct are not detected by ultrasound with regularity but may be demonstrated by intravenous cholangiography. Radionuclide studies (HIDA scan) may demonstrate delayed emptying of the isotope into the duodenum, suggesting partial obstruction. When the patient is icteric, differential diagnosis of obstructive jaundice arises. The most helpful initial study, again, is ultrasonography to determine the presence or absence of calculi in the gallbladder and dilatation of the ductal system. CT is useful in determining the presence or absence of masses in the region of the head of the pancreas and may be employed in the place of ultrasonography.

If dilated ducts are found, the extrahepatic biliary tree may be visualized by either PTC or ERCP (Fig. 27-26). It is important in those patients who have had evidence of infection, as manifested by chills and fever, to administer antibiotics for at least 24 hours prior to instrumentation of

Fig. 27-26. Common duct stones were demonstrated by percutaneous cholangiography in a 76-year-old man who developed chills, fever, and icterus 20 years after cholecystectomy.

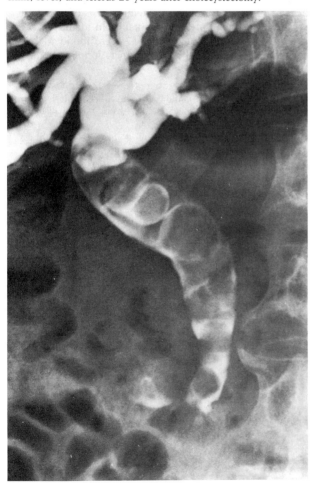

the biliary tract. An adequate prothrombin time should be obtained prior to PTC.

TREATMENT

Surgical treatment is indicated in patients with an intact biliary tree who are suspected of having common duct calculi. The operation involves cholecystectomy to remove the primary source of the calculous disease. At the time of operation, findings that confirm or suggest the presence of choledocholithiasis include palpable stones in the common bile duct, dilatation of the extrahepatic biliary tree, and evidence of pancreatitis. If common duct stones are palpable, or have been demonstrated by preoperative cholangiography, an incision is made in the common duct (choledochotomy) and the common bile duct is carefully explored. The opening in the common bile duct is made in a longitudinal direction to prevent later stricture, as well as to facilitate exploration. A variety of instruments and catheters are employed in common duct exploration, and in addition the interior of the extrahepatic biliary tree can be visualized by means of a choledochoscope.

After removal of common duct stones and careful thorough exploration and irrigation, an operative cholangiogram is obtained by means of the placement of a T-tube in the common bile duct. The operative cholangiogram is useful in searching for residual stones and other defects in the bile ducts and to determine if the contrast agent passes readily into the duodenum. The common duct exploration must be thorough, because common duct calculi are multiple in more than 70% of patients. Thorough irrigation is utilized to remove fragments, stones, and calcareous debris. Usually the T-tube utilized for postoperative cholangiography remains in place for 8 to 12 days after completion of the operation in order that a cholangiogram may be obtained during the postoperative period.

RETAINED BILIARY TRACT CALCULI

Despite careful common duct exploration and intraoperative cholangiography, retained or overlooked calculi are detected occasionally in postoperative cholangiograms. It is estimated that retained or recurrent choledocholithiasis occurs in 5% to 10% of patients who have had a common duct exploration for the removal of common duct stones. Following common duct exploration, drainage of the common duct is usually instituted by means of a T-tube. During the first 24 hours after operation, the volume of T-tube drainage normally ranges between 300 ml and 500 ml. During the next 3 to 4 days, the volume of drainage generally decreases to approximately 200 ml/24 hr. Biliary drainage that exceeds 500 ml/24 hr is suggestive of some type of occlusion of the distal common duct, most commonly a retained stone, although pancreatitis and inflammation of the ampulla of Vater may produce the same type of obstruction. Continued loss of this quantity of bile, if not replaced, results in lassitude and loss of appetite. Prolonged unreplaced biliary drainage can produce significant extracellular fluid deficits, with the consequent symptomatology associated with hypovolemia and hyponatremia.

The postoperative cholangiogram for detection of residual calculi is usually obtained 8 to 12 days following common duct exploration. Defects found within the biliary system at the time of postoperative cholangiography include not only calculi but air bubbles or clots as well. Differentiation of clots, air bubbles, and stone may be difficult at times. If there is uncertainty as to the nature of the defect that has been demonstrated by postoperative cholangiography, the study should be repeated in 5 to 7 days. If the postoperative cholangiogram demonstrated retained common duct calculi, the T-tube should be left in place in order that nonoperative removal of the retained calculi may be attempted. Small stones have been found to disappear with irrigation of the common duct using normal saline solution. A variety of solvents have been recommended, and varying degrees of success have been reported. Solutions containing heparin, sodium cholate, bile acids, clofibrate, and mono-octanoin (a medium chain monoglyceride) have been recommended. Cholesterol stones have been reported to dissolve in 30% to 70% of instances, and side-effects are infrequent. The symptoms associated with these solutions include pain, fever, elevation of liver enzymes, cholangitis, and pancreatitis in less than 10% of patients. The precise efficacy of these solvents remains to be demonstrated, but attempts at dissolution of pigment stones generally are not successful. The use of low flow rates and low pressure under adequate antiseptic control is a reasonable initial approach, however, when residual cholesterol calculi are demonstrated by T-tube cholangiogram.

If the retained calculi are still present in the common duct after a period of six to eight weeks, mechanical extraction of the stones can be attempted through the T-tube tract. When special forceps and Dormia baskets are used, the success rate of retrieval of residual calculi through the fibrous tract formed by the placement of the T-tube has been reported as high as 95%.

Another means of approach to residual choledocholithiasis is by transduodenal endoscopy. This is applicable to retained or recurrent calculi detected after the removal of T-tubes. The common duct is cannulated by means of a duodenoscope, and endoscopic sphincterotomy is accomplished. The procedure is associated with a morbidity rate of between 5% and 10%, the most frequent complications being hemorrhage, cholangitis, pancreatitis, and perforation. Experienced endoscopists, however, are able to retrieve approximately 90% of recurrent calculi with a low mortality rate.

Despite attempts at stone dissolution, mechanical extraction, and endoscopic sphincterotomy, operation may be required. Untreated recurrent or residual common duct stones lead to common duct obstruction, cholangitis, secondary biliary cirrhosis, and pancreatitis. The mortality rate of reoperation for common duct stones has been reported to be approximately 2%. The incidence of recurrent or residual stones, however, increases following reoperation. For patients who have had recurrence of calculi after two or three choledocholithotomies, or who develop multiple recurrent stones, choledochojejunostomy or choledochoduodenostomy has been suggested. The approach to residual or recurrent common duct stones requires careful individual assessment. Both mechanical extraction through the T-tube tract and endoscopic sphincterotomy and transduodenal removal require experience and special skills. At the present time, mortality rates associated with endoscopic sphincterotomy and operative choledocholithotomy are comparable.

BILE DUCT STENOSIS AND TRAUMATIC INJURIES OF THE GALLBLADDER AND BILE DUCTS

The commonest cause of benign stenosis or stricture of the common bile duct is operative trauma. Penetrating or blunt abdominal trauma accounts for less than 5% of injuries of the gallbladder and bile ducts. Other causes include choledocholithiasis, pancreatitis, inflammation secondary to peptic ulceration, pericholedochal abscess, and upper abdominal radiation therapy. More than 95% of injuries to the common duct are the result of damage at the time of operation, usually in association with cholecystectomy. Injury may also occur during operations for gastroduodenal ulcer, portacaval shunting, and pancreatic disease. Because most strictures of the bile duct occur after surgery for gallstone disease, this problem is encountered more often in women than in men. The common hepatic duct is the site of injury in most patients, and 10% to 15% of strictures involve the bifurcation or right or left main hepatic duct.

CLINICAL FINDINGS

Injury of the gallbladder is usually noted by signs of bile peritonitis or by bile staining at celiotomy performed for trauma or other reasons. Cholecystectomy is the recommended treatment, with cholangiography if the integrity of the bile ducts is uncertain.

The clinical manifestations of bile duct injuries depend upon the type of injury. The bile duct may be ligated. In some instances there is division of the common duct, with or without ligation, and a portion of the bile duct may actually be removed. In other patients, there may be injury to a portion of the wall of the common duct without complete transection or ligation of the duct. Patients in this last group may not manifest evidence of common duct injury or obstruction for many months or years. Patients who develop chills and fever and upper abdominal distress months or years after cholecystectomy should be suspected of having a biliary tract stricture or common duct stone. If the bile duct has been ligated, bile may be detected in the urine within 24 hours and jaundice becomes evident within 48 hours. If the bile duct has been divided without ligation, excessive drainage of bile from the drain site or wound becomes evident in the immediate postoperative period and a biliary fistula develops. When the bile duct has been ligated and divided, the appearance of a biliary fistula may be delayed for a period of 5 to 7 days. In the immediate postoperative period, bile duct injury must be differentiated from biliary obstruction from a retained common duct stone.

In the presence of long-standing biliary tract obstruction, the cause of persistent jaundice can be studied by means of ultrasound and PTC. If prolonged biliary drainage occurs, the biliary tract can be visualized by means of a catheter placed in the draining fistula and by injection of a contrast agent through the catheter. If injury to the common bile duct is suspected, operation should be undertaken as soon as possible. The presence of obstructive jaundice within 48 hours following cholecystectomy is sufficient evidence for immediate reexploration.

TREATMENT

The treatment of biliary strictures is primarily surgical. Plastic repair of common duct strictures is seldom possible or advisable. There is debate as to the preferred method of repair of common duct injuries that are detected in the immediate postoperative period after cholecystectomy. The method of repair depends on the status of the ductal system, the extent of loss of the common duct, and the level of injury (Fig. 27-27). End-to-end repair of the common duct is possible in some of these patients if the injured segment

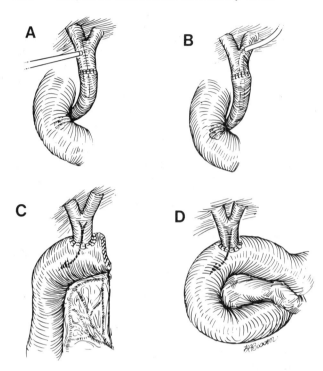

Fig. 27-27. Various methods of reconstruction of common bile duct: (*A*) end-to-end anastomosis over T-tube, (*B*) end-to-end anastomosis with catheter that exits through left hepatic duct, (*C*) end-to-side choledochojejunostomy, and (*D*) choledochoduodenostomy.

is short and the surrounding inflammatory reaction is minimal. It is recommended by many surgeons that the end-to-end anastomosis should be splinted by means of a T-tube or catheter, but it is imperative that the anastomosis be accomplished without tension on the suture line. If a splinting T-tube or catheter is used, it must be brought out through a separate incision and not through the anastomosis.

Objections to the end-to-end anastomosis have been based on long-term results that suggest a high rate of recurrent stricture. For that reason choledochojejunostomy has been recommended with an end-to-side anastomosis between the divided common duct and a Roux-en-Y segment of jejunum. In patients where there has been delay in recognition of the biliary stricture, reconstruction of the biliary tract is accomplished satisfactorily by either choledochojejunostomy or choledochoduodenostomy. Choledochoduodenostomy is effective if the diameter of the proximal common duct exceeds 2 cm and if the duodenum can be attached to the common duct remnant without tension. The debate concerning the advisability of stenting the anastomosis after common duct repair has not been resolved. Most surgeons appear to advocate stenting of the anastomosis, but the length of time before removal of these tubes has varied widely. In occasional patients, the proximal portion of the bile duct cannot be found at the time of exploration. In such patients, intrahepatic cholangiojejunostomy can be performed by anastomosing one of the major intrahepatic bile ducts, usually the left hepatic duct, to the defunctionalized Roux-en-Y segment of jejunum. The dilated bile duct can be found within the liver substance and attached to the segment of the jejunum after resection of a portion of the intervening liver substance. This procedure is helpful in patients where exposure of the bile ducts at the hilum in the porta hepatis is not feasible and in occasional patients who have developed evidence of portal hypertension.

The complications of reconstruction of the bile ducts are related to the degree of hepatic damage that the patient has suffered and the problems associated with cholangitis. In patients with biliary strictures who have a high incidence of infected bile, wound infection, septicemia, and intra-abdominal abscess are serious complications.

Recurrent stricture has been reported to occur in 25% to 45% of patients. The prognosis is influenced by the quality of the bile duct used for repair and whether it is possible to attain a satisfactory anastomosis between the bile duct and the mucosa of the bowel. Recurrent stricture after reconstruction usually presents as cholangitis and frequently occurs within 2 years of the repair. If patients do not have evidence of recurrent stricture within 2 years of reconstruction, there is a 90% chance of permanent relief from biliary obstruction.

INTRAHEPATIC GALLSTONES

Intrahepatic gallstones—that is, gallstones within the intrahepatic ducts above the junction of the right and left hepatic ducts—are uncommon in the United States. In the Orient, however, the incidence ranges as high as 10% of all patients with cholelithiasis. The reasons for the higher incidence in the Orient is uncertain but may be related to the greater frequency of infestation of the bile ducts with parasites and subsequent infection.

Intrahepatic gallstones are associated with serious problems in management. Liver damage and cholangitis are frequent, and long-standing presence of stones leads to stricture formation. Hepatic insufficiency and suppurative cholangitis are among the most serious complications associated with this problem.

Removal of intrahepatic stones presents a number of therapeutic problems. Successful removal of stones from within the liver can be accomplished by lithotomy in less than 60%. In the majority of patients, choledochoduodenostomy or choledochojejunostomy is required to eliminate obstruction and to permit the passage of stones retained within the hepatic radicles. Because intrahepatic calculi are usually pigment stones, attempts at dissolution are unsuccessful.

CARCINOMA OF THE GALLBLADDER

Carcinoma of the gallbladder is the fifth commonest gastrointestinal malignancy and is responsible for approximately 6,500 deaths a year in the United States. It accounts for 3% to 4% of all malignant lesions. Analysis of collective reviews indicates that carcinoma of the gallbladder is encountered in approximately 2% of operations upon the biliary tract. The peak incidence of carcinoma of the gallbladder is in the seventh decade of life, and 75% of the patients are over the age of 65 years. The majority are women. The cause of carcinoma of the gallbladder remains unknown. Cholelithiasis has been suggested as a causative agent because, in most series, 70% to 90% of patients have associated gallstone disease. In some series, however, the incidence of gallstones has been as low as 26%, and thus a causative relation has not been established for cholelithiasis.

SIGNS AND SYMPTOMS

The symptoms of carcinoma of the gallbladder resemble those of benign biliary tract disease. Pain in the right hypochondrium is the most frequent symptom. Other frequent clinical features include abdominal mass, jaundice, weight loss, nausea, and vomiting. Symptoms are usually present from 4 to 6 months before diagnosis. Jaundice is present in approximately 50% of the patients and is obstructive in nature. The gallbladder may be palpated in approximately 25% of the patients.

DIAGNOSIS

The diagnosis is usually not made before operation. Most frequently, patients are thought to have benign biliary tract disease or carcinoma of the pancreas or bile ducts. Oral cholecystography demonstrates nonvisualization of the gallbladder in approximately two thirds of the patients and is usually not diagnostic. Ultrasonography has not been helpful. PTC usually demonstrates extrahepatic biliary obstruction and, in some instances, has been diagnostic. Hepatic and celiac angiography may demonstrate tumor vascularity, and radioisotope liver scans may demonstrate hepatic metastasis. The correct diagnosis, however, is usually not made until the extrahepatic biliary tract is explored.

TREATMENT

The surgical treatment of carcinoma of the gallbladder has yielded poor results. At the time of operation, the gallbladder appears to be profusely thickened or occupied by a polypoid nodular lesion. The majority of the tumors are adenocarcinoma, and early metastasis is frequent. Long-term survival is unusual if there is extension of the tumor beyond the gallbladder. When cholecystectomy is performed as a curative procedure, the survival rate is less than 10%. The overall 5-year survival rate is 2% or less, although radical resection of the gallbladder, including all or part of the right lobe of the liver, has been suggested. This approach has been associated with a high postoperative mortality rate and few survivals.

CARCINOMA OF THE EXTRAHEPATIC BILE DUCTS

Carcinoma of the common bile duct is uncommon and has an autopsy incidence of 0.2% to 0.5%. Although this neoplasm occurs in a wide age range, the peak incidence is in the seventh and eighth decades of life. Carcinoma of the extrahepatic biliary system is encountered more frequently in Israelis, American Indians, and Japanese than it is in Americans. It is more common in men than in women.

PATHOGENESIS

As with other gastrointestinal neoplasms, the cause of biliary tract carcinoma remains obscure. Certain chemical agents (*e.g.,* methylcholanthrene) have been found to produce biliary tract cancer in animals either by direct contact or after ingestion. In addition, there is an increased incidence of bile duct carcinoma with ulcerative colitis and, perhaps, in patients with granulomatous colitis. In the Orient where there is a higher incidence of bile duct carcinoma, a causal relationship has been postulated with biliary parasites (*Ascaris lumbricoides* and *Clonorchis sinensis*) and with intrahepatic stones, which are more frequent than in the United States.

CLINICAL FINDINGS

The most common symptoms are those associated with obstructive jaundice. The patients usually have mild to moderate upper abdominal pain associated with jaundice. Weight loss and fatigue are common. Diarrhea is a frequent symptom, and the stools are usually clay colored. Some patients notice dark "tea colored" urine. The most striking findings on physical examination are scleral icterus and jaundice. Hepatomegaly is common. If the distal portion of the common duct is involved, an enlarged, nontender gallbladder may be felt.

The customary laboratory studies do not yield specific information other than that found in obstructive jaundice. Anemia is often present. The patients are found to have an elevated bilirubin level and an increase in serum alkaline phosphatase and transaminase values.

DIAGNOSIS

The diagnosis of bile duct carcinoma may be difficult and is often not made until the time of operation. Ultrasonography will commonly demonstrate dilated intrahepatic radicles of the biliary tract, and the diagnosis may be suspected by percutaneous transhepatic angiography or ERCP. Angiography and percutaneous transhepatic portography (PTP) have been suggested as methods to detect invasion of the hepatic artery or portal vein. Diagnosis may be difficult to establish at the time of operation. The differentiation between infiltrating ductal carcinoma and benign sclerosing cholangitis may arise. Choledochoscopy and study of cell cytology from specimens obtained by intraluminal scraping may be helpful. Biopsies of the common duct wall are often difficult to interpret.

The extrahepatic biliary system is often divided into thirds: the upper third is that portion which lies above the cystic duct, the middle third is between the cystic duct and the pancreas, and the distal third is the intrapancreatic portion. Unfortunately, bile duct carcinoma is more common in the upper two thirds of the extrahepatic biliary system, with only approximately 20% of these neoplasms occurring in the distal third.

TREATMENT

Bile duct carcinoma is usually associated with poor survival. The 5-year survival rate is less than 10%. The treatment is surgical. Resectability rates, however, are low because of local invasion with involvement of the hepatic artery and portal vein. Prolonged palliation may be obtained by insertion of tubes through the tumor into the intrahepatic portion of the bile duct. Prolonged relief of jaundice and associated symptoms may be obtained by this means because of the slow growth of the tumor. The use of U-tubes has found an important role in the palliative therapy of carcinoma of the bile ducts, particularly when the neoplasms arise at the junction of the right and left hepatic ducts. These tubes are inserted through the common bile duct into the liver and are brought to the surface of the skin at either end. This permits irrigation and replacement of the tubes should the tubes become occluded.

Neoplasms which arise in the lower third of the common bile duct may be treated with pancreatoduodenectomy and offer the most likely opportunity for cure. Carcinoma of the bile duct arising in this area is associated with approximately 20% 5-year survival rates when pancreatoduodenectomy is performed, providing a better outlook than pancreatic carcinoma.

BIBLIOGRAPHY

GIRAR RM, LEGROS G: Retained and recurrent bile duct stones. Ann Surg 193:150, 1981

GLENN F: Silent gallstones. Ann Surg 193:251, 1981

KOO J, WONG J, CHENG FCY et al: Carcinoma of the gallbladder. Br J Surg 68:161, 1981

LEOPOLD GR: The use of ultrasonography in the diagnosis of liver, biliary tract, and pancreas. Viewpoints on Digestive Diseases 12:17, 1980

LILLY JR: Surgical jaundice in infancy. Ann Surg 186:549, 1977

MICHELS NA: New anatomy of liver-variant blood supply and collateral circulation. JAMA 172:125, 1960

SOLOWAY RD, TROTMAN BW, OSTROW JD: Pigment gallstones. Gastroenterology 72:167, 1977

WEISNER RH, LA RUSSO NF: Clinicopathologic features of the syndrome of primary sclerosing cholangitis. Gastroenterology 79:200, 1980

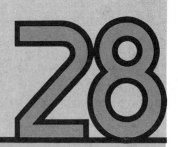

The Pancreas

George L. Nardi

Surgical Anatomy, Physiology, and Pancreatitis

EMBRYOLOGY

EMBRYOGENESIS

The pancreas is formed by fusion of dorsal and ventral segments (Fig. 28-1). During the fourth week of embryonic development, the endodermal hepatic bud grows into the ventral mesentery and the ventral and dorsal endodermal outgrowths, which will form the pancreas, take origin from the abdominal foregut. The smaller ventral bud arises from the lateral aspect of the hepatic duct, and the larger dorsal bud arises from the dorsal aspect of the gut (Fig. 28-1, *A*). By the sixth week of gestation, both buds have ductal communication with the gut (Fig. 28-1, *B*). At this time, rotation of the stomach and growth of the liver displace the duodenum to the right and posteriorly (Fig. 28-1, *C*). In this rotation, the duodenum loses its dorsal mesentery and becomes retroperitoneal, and the ventral pancreas fuses with the dorsal segment during the seventh week and becomes the lower part of the head and uncinate process of the fused gland (Fig. 28-1, *D*). The two ductal systems also fuse, and either or both may provide drainage for the gland's exocrine secretions.

The duct of the dorsal pancreas opens directly into the gut lumen as the duct of Santorini. The duct of the ventral pancreas opens into the termination of the common bile duct as the duct of Wirsung.

ANOMALIES

Congenital malformations of the pancreas may produce clinical symptoms in humans. Clinically recognized malformations are agenesis, ectopia, annular pancreas, and pancreas divisum.

AGENESIS

Complete agenesis of the pancreas has been reported. This has usually been associated with multiple anomalies in infancy. Agenesis of either the dorsal or the ventral pancreas may occur, the former being more common.

ECTOPIC PANCREAS

Ectopic pancreas is pancreatic tissue in an aberrant location not contiguous with the main pancreas. It may be found in up to 5% of autopsies and is most frequently seen clinically in the fourth and fifth decades. The most common sites for ectopia are the stomach and duodenum. The aberrant tissue,

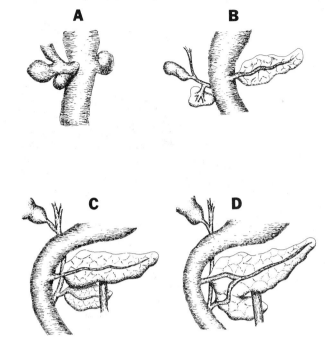

Fig. 28-1. Embryology of the pancreas. (Organ CH Jr: The pancreas: Surgical anatomy, physiology, and pathology. In Hardy JD [ed]: Rhoads Textbook of Surgery, 5th ed. Philadelphia, J B Lippincott, 1977)

usually 1 cm to 2 cm, is most commonly located in the submucosa. Microscopically, normal pancreatic acini and ducts are found. Islet cells and Brunnerlike glands are also frequently present.

The small intestine is the most common site for ectopic pancreatic tissue. The aberrant tissue may undergo the same pathology occurring in the pancreas itself. The most common symptoms are those of peptic ulcer disease or pyloric obstruction. Symptoms may be due to obstruction with secondary inflammatory changes. Because of the alkaline secretions, sustained gastrin release with hyperacidity may result. Hemorrhage may occur from ulceration or gastritis in the mucosa overlying the ectopic tissue.

Treatment is local excision. Although malignancy rarely occurs, frozen section should be performed at the time of operation.

ANNULAR PANCREAS

Annular pancreas is another rare anatomical anomaly that may not become apparent until adult life. It is thought to result from fixation of the free end of the ventral pancreas, which then results in encirclement of the duodenum by this tissue as it rotates around to the right posteriorly to fuse with the dorsal anlage.

This condition may be asymptomatic or may present as complete obstruction associated with other anomalies in the newborn. It may become symptomatic in adults, most commonly in the fourth decade. The most common symptom in the adult is colicky abdominal pain. The most common complication is duodenal ulcer.

Treatment consists in performance of bypass procedures such as gastroenterostomy rather than division of the encircling pancreas. When duodenal ulcer is present, it should also be corrected by appropriate treatment.

PANCREAS DIVISUM

With the advent of fiberoptic endoscopy and retrograde duct cannulation, another anomaly, pancreas divisum, to which we have previously alluded, has been defined. In this condition, there is failure of fusion of the ductal systems of the dorsal and ventral pancreatic anlage. It is believed that the duct of Santorini draining through the minor papilla is inadequate for the normal volume of pancreatic secretion, therefore causing a relative obstruction. Symptoms are those of epigastric pain as seen in recurrent pancreatitis. Surgical efforts to provide relief have consisted in resection to lower the exocrine load and sphincteroplasty to the minor papilla to reduce the resistance to flow.

ANATOMY

The human pancreas is a solid retroperitoneal organ extending transversely between the duodenum and hilus of the spleen behind the stomach. Its length varies between 15 and 20 cm, and its weight is between 80 and 90 g.

The pancreas is roughly divided into four parts: head, neck, body, and tail. The head is in intimate contact with the C loop of the pancreas, with which it shares its blood supply. Posteriorly, it lies on the vena cava, renal vein, and renal artery. The inferior extension, known as the uncinate process, lies between the portal vein and the vena cava. The common bile duct runs through the head of the pancreas. The neck is that part of the gland overlying the superior mesenteric vessels anterior to the uncinate process. The body continues into the tail, which may be of varying length. The relationships of anatomical features to certain surgical lesions are shown in Figure 28-2.

The pancreas has a very rich blood supply. The head of the pancreas and the duodenum are supplied by two arterial arcades, the anterior and posterior pancreaticoduodenal arteries, which are derived from the celiac trunk and superior mesenteric artery. The transverse pancreatic artery courses along the inferior border of the pancreas and has multiple anastomoses with the splenic artery, which runs along the superoposterior margin of the gland (Fig. 28-3).

Venous drainage is through the splenic and inferior pancreatic veins. The head of the pancreas is drained by branches that pass directly into the portal vein.

Tumors of the head may involve the portal vein, causing portal hypertension and ascites. Pancreatitis may involve the splenic vein and produce local venous hypertension with gastric hemorrhage.

The lymphatic drainage of the pancreas is diffuse and complex. Surface lymphatics follow the blood vessels. From the upper part of the head, the neck, and the body, drainage is into the celiac nodes; from the lower portion of the head, the lymphatics drain into the superior mesenteric nodes.

The pancreas is supplied by the autonomic nervous system, both sympathetic and parasympathetic. The sympathetics arise from the fifth to tenth thoracic ganglia as the greater and lesser splanchnic nerve and terminate in the celiac ganglion. From this ganglion, postganglionic sympathetics as well as parasympathetic fibers from the vagus travel with arteries to the pancreas. It is believed that the sympathetic fibers, particularly the splanchnic nerves, are the principal pathways for pancreatic pain (Fig. 28-4). Splanchnicectomy has therefore become an accepted surgical procedure for the relief of pancreatic pain. Clinical results have not been uniformly satisfactory, however.

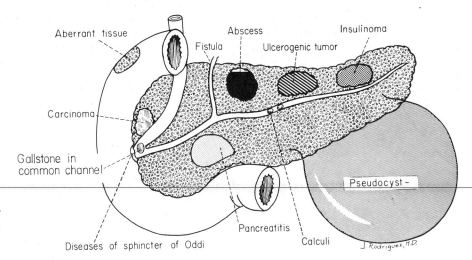

Fig. 28-2. Some surgical lesions of the pancreas. (Hardy JD: Pathophysiology in Surgery, p 258. Baltimore, Williams & Wilkins, 1958)

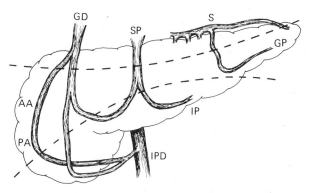

Fig. 28-3. Arterial supply to the pancreas. The dashed lines represent peritoneal reflections. *GD*, gastroduodenal; *SP*, superior pancreatic; *AA*, anterior arcade; *PA*, posterior arcade; *IPD*, inferior pancreaticoduodenal; *IP*, inferior pancreatic; *S*, splenic; *GP*, great pancreatic. (Organ CH Jr: The pancreas: Surgical anatomy, physiology, and pathology. In Hardy JD [ed]: Rhoads Textbook of Surgery, 5th ed. Philadelphia, J B Lippincott, 1977)

PHYSIOLOGY

The pancreas consists of two independent physiological units, exocrine and endocrine. The exocrine acinar cells make up most of the pancreas. They synthesize digestive enzymes that enter the duodenum through the pancreatic ducts. The endocrine secretions are produced by the islets of Langerhans, which represent less than 2% of the total mass of the pancreas and number from 1 million to 2 million. Each islet measures about 200 μ in diameter, is highly vascularized, and secretes its hormones into these vessels and eventually into the portal system. This section limits discussion to the exocrine functions of the pancreas, normal and abnormal, as a basis for diagnosis and therapy.

The functional unit of the exocrine pancreas is the acinus. The acinus, spherical in shape, is composed of a single layer of pyramidal cells with narrow apical ends bordering the duct lumen. The lumen draining the acinus is termed an intercalated duct; it drains in turn through intralobular and interlobular ducts into the main pancreatic duct.

The acinar cells produce a mixture of 20 or more enzymes that are involved in digestion. In the pioneering studies of Jamieson and Palade, radioautography was used to elucidate the intracellular transport and discharge of pancreatic en-

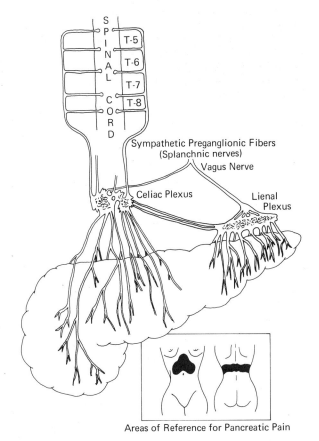

Areas of Reference for Pancreatic Pain

Fig. 28-4. Innervation of the pancreas. (Organ CH Jr: The pancreas: Surgical anatomy, physiology, and pathology. In Hardy JD [ed]: Rhoads Textbook of Surgery, 5th ed. Philadelphia, J B Lippincott, 1977)

zymes. They found that ribonucleoprotein particles on the endoplasmic reticulum of the acinar cell are the sites of protein–enzyme synthesis. The Golgi apparatus packages the protein by providing a limiting membrane and forming a zymogen granule. A single granule may contain all the different enzymes. These enzymes are discharged from the apical portion of the cell into the ductal system by a process of membrane fusion, rupture, and discharge into the centroacinar lumen. Under normal conditions of stimulation, it has been estimated that this process of synthesis to discharge requires approximately 30 minutes.

The presence of enzyme inhibitors and the secretion of proteolytic enzymes in inactive form provide a protective mechanism to autodigestion of the gland.

It was originally believed that pancreatic enzymes were synthesized and secreted in fixed ratios to one another. Recent observations, however, suggest that the pancreas can modify its enzyme output in response to diet and stimuli. Herein may lie a possible explanation of the varying degrees of severity of pancreatitis seen in persons of varying dietary habits.

Under normal conditions, the enzymes discharged into the ductal system are transported through the ductal system in pancreatic juice. Most of the 1 or 2 liters of pancreatic juice secreted daily is formed by the intercalated duct cells. This juice is clear and contains water, electrolytes, and protein. Its pH ranges from 7.6 to 8.3. The principal cations present are sodium and potassium in the same concentration as in plasma. This juice has a high bicarbonate content, which increases with increasing rates of secretion.

Pancreatic secretion is not constant but responds to a variety of digestive stimuli to maintain the duodenal pH and provide a properly timed supply of enzymes to the gut. With maximal stimulation, enough bicarbonate can be delivered to neutralize all gastric acid production. Clinical studies in which duodenal intubation has been used have demonstrated a rise in bicarbonate and a fall in chloride concentration, with the increased flow resulting from secretin stimulation. These studies have also demonstrated that there is loss of ability to secrete bicarbonate in pancreatitis but that bicarbonate concentration is normal in cancer with ductal obstruction, but the volume of juice is diminished.

Pancreatic juice is discharged into the duodenum through the ducts of Wirsung and Santorini. In most cases, the duct of Wirsung, draining through the major papilla (Vater), is the main drainage system and the duct of Santorini, opening in the more proximally situated minor papilla, plays a lesser role. The point of fusion of the ducts may be incomplete, resulting in stenosis at this point with obstruction to outflow from the caudal pancreas.

The so-called minor papilla draining the duct of Santorini is almost always present but is patent in only 60% of persons. A high incidence of obliteration of this orifice is found in patients with duodenal ulcer. The duct of Santorini communicates with the duct of Wirsung 75% of the time, and there is a 10% incidence of the duct of Santorini serving as the main drainage route for the pancreas. Since the advent of retrograde cholangiopancreatography, this latter situation has been noted with increasing frequency in patients suffering from abdominal pain typical of recurrent pancreatitis. This finding has been termed pancreas divisum. It is thought to be a congenital defect, a complete failure of fusion of the ducts of the pancreatic buds with persistence of two independent ductal systems.

The major duodenal papilla, containing the ampulla of Vater, represents the common termination of the duct of Wirsung and the bile duct. Boyden's classic study of this area showed that the musculature surrounding the terminal portions of these ducts within the papilla was not merely a prolongation of the intestinal musculature that they pierced in their course through the duodenal wall. Rather, they demonstrated an upper and lower choledochal sphincter, a pancreatic duct sphincter about 25 mm proximal to the tip of the papilla, and an ampullary sphincter.

This complex musculature ensheathed within the duodenal wall responds to a variety of neurohumoral stimuli to permit timely passage of bile and pancreatic juice into the intestine. The major papilla and the ampulla of Vater have been of interest to surgeons for many years, since there is evidence that dysfunction and inflammatory changes in this area may be a cause of pancreatitis, and are discussed in further detail in the discussion of recurrent pancreatitis.

In the duodenum, the pancreatic enzymes break down the larger molecules of food. Amylase digests large starch molecules into sugar, and lipases, in conjunction with bile salts, hydrolyze neutral fats to monoglycerides, glycerol, and free fatty acids. The proteolytic enzymes break down peptide bonds and liberate amino acids. Pancreatic juice itself, with its high pH, neutralizes the acid contents of the stomach to produce the neutral pH necessary for enzymatic action.

Obstruction of the pancreatic duct and pancreatic secretion, whether by stone, inflammation, or cancer, results in pancreatic insufficiency, malabsorption, and steatorrhea. In humans, it has been shown that a decrease in exocrine secretion cannot be detected until more than 60% of the total length of the main pancreatic duct has been obstructed.

Under basal conditions, the pancreas secretes at a slow, steady rate. Stimulation of secretion results from the sight, smell, and ingestion of food and occurs in three phases of stimulation identical to the phases of stimulation of gastric secretion: (1) cephalic, by way of the vagus nerves, (2) gastric, involving humoral and nervous stimuli, and (3) intestinal, by secretin and cholecystokinin. The cephalic phase is dependent entirely on the vagus nerves. Release of acetylcholine at vagal cholinergic nerve endings, release of gastrin from the gastric antrum, and acid stimulation of secretin from the duodenum result in a generous flow of enzyme-rich secretion. The same mechanism plus release of gastrin by antral distention play a role in the gastric phase of stimulation. The intestinal phase of pancreatic stimulation is dependent on two hormones: secretin, secreted by the crypt cells in the duodenum and proximal small intestine in response to the H^+ of gastric acid, and cholecystokinin (pancreozymin), secreted by the proximal jejunum in response to fatty and amino acids in the bowel lumen. Secretin appears primarily responsible for stimulating the flow of water and bicarbonate. Cholecystokinin stimulates the discharge of pancreatic enzymes from the zymogen granules.

Data for normal pancreatic secretory pressure in humans are understandably fragmentary. In one patient with an apparently normal pancreas, resting pressures of 7 cm to 12 cm of water with a rise to 22 cm during secretion were observed. In patients with pancreatitis, higher pressures have been recorded, with resting pressures from 15 cm to 22 cm. Pressure was elevated by giving morphine, and pain was noted when the intraductal pressure rose to about 25 cm. In dogs with outlet obstruction, secretory pressures as high as 80 cm of water have been achieved. It would thus seem that even in the presence of a common biliary–pancreatic channel, sphincter spasm or obstruction would result in pancreatic juice entering the biliary tree rather than the reverse.

Because of ease of measurement, amylase determinations have been widely used as an index of pancreatic disease. Serum amylase is not only of pancreatic origin but is also produced by the liver, salivary glands, fallopian tubes, and intestines. Nevertheless, serum amylase determinations have proved a pragmatically useful index of pancreatic disease, particularly in acute pancreatitis, in which abnormal elevations may persist for several days after the onset of the acute episode. A major portion of the serum amylase is excreted in the urine with no tubular reabsorption. The renal excretion rate is quite constant, and measurement of 24-hour urinary amylase excretion has been considered to be an even more reliable index of pancreatitis than is serum amylase.

Some patients suffering with abdominal pain have been found to have a high serum amylase but low urinary amylase excretion. The reason for this impaired excretion is that the amylase is bound to an abnormally large serum globulin molecule, the condition thus being termed macroamylasemia.

Renal disease may hamper amylase clearance and result in false elevations. Amylase is excreted, however, in direct proportion to creatinine, and the amylase/creatinine clearance ratio may provide a useful test for pancreatitis. Amylase clearance/creatinine clearance has a normal ratio of 1%: 4%. Similar values are found in patients with renal failure. In macroamylasemia, the ratio is below normal, suggesting that the elevated serum amylase is due to a different amylase and is not the result of pancreatic hypersecretion.

Another modification of the serum amylase determination is its fractionation into isoamylases on the basis of their isoelectric points. Amylase with an isoelectric point of 7 is the only isoamylase of pancreatic origin. It disappears from the serum after pancreatectomy. By this technique, it has been shown that about 35% of normal serum amylase is of pancreatic origin and the rest is of salivary origin. The diagnostic value of this technique is limited, however, and it has not found much use in clinical practice.

Elevation of the serum lipase may provide a more specific index of pancreatic dysfunction, but the time required to perform the assay has discouraged its routine use. Nevertheless, it has some possible advantages in diagnosis; it not only may remain elevated for longer periods of time than the serum amylase but also, coupled with a low serum calcium, may be a predictor of a more severe form of pancreatitis with fat necrosis. Recent development of a quicker assay may result in more frequent use of lipase levels.

Since the pancreas is the only organ that synthesizes proteolytic enzymes, such an assay might provide the most specific diagnostic test for pancreatitis. These assays are indeed feasible but because of their complexity have not achieved general use.

Because of difficulties in establishing a diagnosis of acute or chronic pancreatitis, evocative enzyme tests have been used in an attempt to improve on the accuracy of serum tests. These tests are basically an attempt to stimulate pancreatic secretion by a pharmacologic agent to see if the patient's symptoms can be reproduced and if a rise in serum pancreatic enzymes can be detected. Injection of secretin and cholecystokinin intravenously and analysis of duodenal drainage for enzymes, water, and bicarbonate have permitted identification of patients with pancreatic dysfunction. Cytologic study of the aspirated secretions may also be of value in the diagnosis of pancreatic cancer by identification of malignant cells. This type of examination, however, has not gained wide acceptance and is rarely used.

A combination of morphine and neostigmine (Prostigmin) administered intramuscularly has been used as an evocative test. Blood is sampled for amylase and lipase after administration of the drugs. Reproduction of the patient's pain and elevation of serum enzymes constitute a positive test result. This test has been of value in selecting patients with recurrent abdominal pain of presumed pancreatic origin who might respond to section of the pancreatic duct sphincter.

PANCREATITIS

Pancreatitis was first described at the Massachusetts General Hospital in 1889 by Fitz, who distinguished suppurative, hemorrhagic, and gangrenous forms. Subsequent refinements in diagnostic techniques have shown that pancreatitis may exist in many different forms, and a confusing plethora of clinicopathologic terms evolved. In an attempt to clarify this situation, Sarles, in 1963, proposed a clinical classification of pancreatitis that has gained wide acceptance and will serve as the basis of this presentation:

I. Acute reversible forms
   1. Acute pancreatitis
   2. Recurrent acute pancreatitis
II. Chronic progressive forms
   3. Recurrent chronic pancreatitis
   4. Chronic pancreatitis

In groups 1 and 2, the pancreas returns to normal after each attack. It is unusual for acute pancreatitis to develop into chronic pancreatitis, but it may occur. In groups 3 and 4, the disease is progressive and the distinction is clinical and not morphologic. Chronic pancreatitis may result from chronic recurrent pancreatitis or from acute pancreatitis or may manifest itself initially as the chronic form.

ACUTE

Acute pancreatitis is a clinical syndrome of epigastric pain, often radiating to the back, associated in varying degree with fever, tachycardia, ileus, hemorrhage, and shock. These pathologic manifestations are presumably the result of obstruction, complete or partial, to the secreting, stimulated gland. Such obstruction may be of any kind, from a tumor at the ductal orifice to a metabolic block at the cell membrane. The combination of obstruction and secretion results in extravasation and activation of pancreatic enzymes and in the production of vasoactive polypeptides. The presence of these agents in the tissues and circulation accounts for the local and systemic manifestations of the disease.

ETIOLOGY

In most patients, acute pancreatitis is associated with biliary tract disease or alcoholism. Gallstones are thought to be in some way responsible for about one third of the cases of pancreatitis in men and for about one half of the cases in women. The exact mechanism by which they induce this disease remains obscure. The common-channel theory of biliary reflux secondary to a calculus lodged in the ampulla is rarely found. Edema and ductal obstruction secondary to cholecystitis, alcoholic duodenitis, or peptic ulcer seem a more likely precipitating cause. Alcoholism is commonly associated with pancreatitis, particularly in men under 40 years of age. Again, the exact mechanism is unknown. A direct toxic effect, nutritional changes, duodenitis, and gastric hypersecretion may all play a role.

ACUTE PANCREATITIS

Etiology	Autodigestion of pancreas from extravasated pancreatic enzymes in gland
	Alcohol, biliary stones, post-traumatic, hyperlipidemia, hypercalcemia, and other associated factors
Dx	Midepigastric pain, back pain, vomiting
	Tachycardia, fever, shock
	Abdominal tenderness, $\pm$ rebound tenderness
	Abdominal x-ray film: ileus, pancreatic calcification
	Hyperamylasemia, hyperlipasemia
	Other surgical emergencies excluded
Rx	Relieve pain
	Intravenous hydration, Na^+, K^+, Ca^{2+}, blood replacement
	NPO, nasogastric decompression
	Monitor for multisystem failure (cardiac–pulmonary–renal)
	Celiotomy if surgical emergency cannot be excluded
	Treatment of alcoholism, gallstones, hypercalcemia, and other etiologic factors to prevent recurrence
	Surgery for complicating pseudocyst, abscess, ascites

After their convalescence, these patients should be carefully evaluated to ascertain whether they may be suffering from mumps, collagen disease, hyperlipidemia, or hyperparathyroidism. It must be emphasized that when no causal factor can be identified, the presence of a primary cancer obstructing or infiltrating the pancreas must be considered.

DIAGNOSIS

There is no characteristic clinical picture in acute pancreatitis. The symptomatic manifestations may vary from a bout of vague dyspepsia and slight abdominal pain to irreversible fulminating collapse, with shock and death. More often than not, the outstanding symptom is steady, severe epigastric pain, frequently radiating to the back. Nausea and vomiting are often present. A careful history will often reveal that the patient has had many prior episodes of "indigestion" and perhaps milder episodes of his current symptoms.

Clinical or chemical jaundice is not uncommon. This may be due to associated biliary tract disease or to obstruction of the common duct in its intrapancreatic portion secondary to edema in the head of the pancreas. The serum alkaline phosphatase is often an earlier and more sensitive index of such obstruction than is the serum bilirubin. Occasionally, jaundice is nonobstructive and is a manifestation of a toxic hepatitis secondary to portal absorption of toxic products.

Depending on the severity of the attack, the patient may be cold, clammy, and dehydrated, with tachycardia and hypotension. Spasm and rigidity may be absent, and the edematous, swollen pancreas may be palpated in the upper abdomen. Bluish discoloration in the flanks (Grey Turner's sign) or around the umbilicus (Cullen's sign) indicates the bloody retroperitoneal dissection of hemorrhagic pancreatitis and augurs a fatal prognosis.

The clinical diagnosis is confirmed by finding a significant elevation of the serum amylase. The more elevated the serum amylase, the more certain is the diagnosis. There is no relation, however, between the severity of the illness or its prognosis and the degree of elevation of serum amylase. Urinary amylase determinations are also of value in diagnosis but generally are more tedious and take longer.

Serum lipase determinations should be performed at the same time that the initial serum amylase is done. Newer substrates permit more rapid and accurate determination of lipase values. Elevations are a more specific index of pancreatic disease and may be present when amylase levels have returned to normal.

When the lipase values are elevated, serum calcium levels may be lowered. The exact mechanism of such a hypocalcemia is not clear. Some have believed it to be secondary to sequestration of calcium in the saponification (fat necrosis) activity of the lipolytic enzymes and to impaired resorption from bone secondary to calcitonin liberated by glucagon. A serum calcium level below 7.0 mg/dl has been considered to indicate a poor prognosis, not because of the hypocalcemia *per se* but rather as a reflection of the severity and extent of the primary disease. However, patients with much lower serum calcium levels have survived. Such patients may develop severe and bizarre leg pains easily misinterpreted as manifestations of thrombophlebitis. Usually these pains are the result of fat necrosis in the marrow of the long bones. Tetany as a result of this hypocalcemia is very unusual, presumably because, with the associated hypoproteinemia, the ionized calcium remains at a relatively normal level.

In hyperparathyroidism, a normal calcium level may exist in the presence of a severe attack of pancreatitis. The explanation for this apparent paradox is that the acute attack has indeed lowered the serum calcium from a hypercalcemic level to a normal value.

X-ray examination of the abdomen has been advocated as a diagnostic measure. Visualization of a distended, gas-filled segment of small bowel in the upper abdomen, the "sentinel loop," has been considered pathognomonic. This finding has, in my opinion, been much overrated. It is not uniformly seen, and, when present, it is usually a part of a generalized configuration of small-bowel distention and ileus. Roentgenography has much more diagnostic value in uncovering gallstones and in contributing to the differential diagnosis of perforated peptic ulcer or other acute conditions. Accordingly, films should be taken in the upright or lateral decubitus position. Chest films may demonstrate a pleural effusion on the left.

Abdominal paracentesis has been advocated as a safe and valuable diagnostic maneuver. Taps in all four quadrants, with examination, smear, culture, and enzyme analysis, may provide very useful information. I have not often used this technique and have little experience with it.

The serum amylase concentration remains the single most valuable diagnostic agent in this disease. Amylase is secreted by the parotid gland, small bowel, liver, and fallopian tubes, in addition to the pancreas, and it must be recognized that elevations of this enzyme may occur in pathologic states of these tissues (*e.g.*, parotitis). In addition, cholecystitis, alcoholism, peptic ulcer, and excessive opiate administration result in elevations of the serum amylase.

These are not false-positives but are indications of "neighborhood pancreatitis" secondary to low-grade obstruction caused by the primary condition. It is the surgeon who must interpret the test accordingly and evaluate the patient properly on the basis of all the evidence available to him.

TREATMENT

The immediate treatment of acute pancreatitis is nonoperative. However, in the differential diagnosis of pancreatitis, one must consider acute cholecystitis, perforated ulcer, intestinal obstruction, and mesenteric infarction; all of these conditions require immediate surgery. If there is any uncertainty about the diagnosis, laparotomy should be performed. There is little evidence that the effects of laparotomy undertaken for diagnosis or in error are catastrophic, and the outcome is more likely to be dictated by the course of the patient's disease than by the incidental laparotomy. In this situation, it is probably wiser to do whatever might be helpful and technically feasible than to hurriedly back out. If gallstones are present, a cholecystostomy or cholecystectomy might be indicated. If stones are present in the common duct, biliary drainage might be appropriate. A gastrostomy might prove an effective and comfortable substitute for a nasogastric tube.

The objectives of therapy include relief of pain, treatment of shock, replacement of fluid and electrolytes, suppression of pancreatic stimuli and reduction or neutralization of pancreatic secretions, and prevention of infection.

Relief of Pain

Pain medication should be used adequately but judiciously. Both morphine and meperidine (Demerol) produce spasm of the ampulla of Vater, but meperidine has a lesser effect. In alcoholics, death may result from delirium tremens, and sedatives such as chlorpromazine (Thorazine) may be of value.

Sympathetic or splanchnic nerve block, intravenous procaine, and epidural anesthesia have also been advocated for the relief of pain, but I have rarely found them necessary.

Treatment of Shock

A shocklike picture may appear early in the course of acute pancreatitis. The deficits in the circulating blood volume are akin to those seen in thermal trauma, and, from this point of view, the condition may indeed be considered an internal "burn." Intravenous administration of plasma and blood, together with water and electrolyte solutions, should be expeditiously performed. The amount and quality of replacement are dictated by central venous pressure, hematocrit, serum electrolytes, and urinary output. Urinary output is best evaluated by monitoring the hourly intake and output sheet.

A blood sugar value should be obtained before beginning intravenous glucose infusion. Pancreatitis has a relatively high incidence in diabetics, and awareness of this disease as a preexisting condition may be critical in the patient's management. Should the patient indeed be diabetic, insulin "by test" is given, the dosage tempered by the presence of an intravenous glucose infusion. Insulin overdose should be assiduously avoided, since hypoglycemia, with its vagotonic action on gastric secretion, could prove deleterious.

Intravenously or intramuscularly administered calcium is indicated for any clinical manifestations of tetany. However, I have found this to be an exceedingly rare complication. Whether or not calcium should be given for chemical hypocalcemia *per se* is a moot point. Its administration seems to have little effect on the serum calcium level. Theoretically, a contraindication to its use is that it may play a role in the activation of pancreatic proteolytic enzymes.

Dextran is an agent that is too rarely used in therapy. It not only serves as an effective plasma substitute but also has been shown to inhibit pancreatic secretion.

Inhibition of Pancreatic Secretion

Whether there is any great value in "splinting" the pancreas is not certain; if the basic pathogenesis of the disease is enzymatic, it would seem a logical measure. Continuous gastric suction by nasogastric tube reduces the acid stimulation to the duodenum and minimizes the production of secretin and pancreozymin, the intrinsic pancreatic secretagogues. In addition, it is an effective measure for the gastric distention or ileus that frequently accompanies the disease. Instantly, this measure alone often brings a degree of welcome relief to the patient. Subcutaneous atropine 0.3 mg to 0.6 mg administered every 4 to 6 hours, or propantheline bromide (Pro-banthine), 15 mg administered every 6 hours, may reduce pancreatic secretion.

Antienzyme preparations capable of inhibiting trypsin and chymotrypsin are widely used abroad. The best known of these is aprotinin (Trasylol), a polypeptide extracted from the lungs of cattle and used intravenously. This agent has been shown to be a potent inhibitor of kallikrein *in vitro*. Kallikrein is a pancreatic enzyme that, by its action on a circulating serum globulin, produces kallidin, a biologically active polypeptide with a marked vasodilating effect. The latter mechanism is believed to be important in producing the shock phase of acute pancreatitis. Originally, numerous clinical reports from other countries attested to the therapeutic effectiveness of such antienzymes in acute pancreatitis and shock. Recent clinical trials, however, have been much less impressive and have not justified making the agent available for general use. Quinine is another antienzymatic agent that has been shown to be effective in neutralizing pancreatic lipase *in vitro*. Limited reports have suggested that intravenous administration of somatostatin produces a beneficial clinical and chemical response in acute pancreatitis.

Antibiotics

Although infection is probably not a primary factor, its eventual appearance in the form of pancreatic abscess is a common complication (see Fig. 28-5). For this reason, as well as for their prophylactic value against concomitant pneumonitis, cystitis, and septicemia, antibiotics may have value. Peritoneal taps in the early phases of acute pancreatitis have revealed a mixed enteric flora. Accordingly, therapy with a broad-spectrum antibiotic seems to be a reasonable precaution.

Other Agents

Acetazolamide (Diamox), because it inhibits water and bicarbonate secretion by the pancreatic ductule cells, has been administered to reduce pancreatic flow. Because of its ability to reduce cellular metabolism, propylthiouracil has been administered. In a similar fashion, hypothermia has been used in an attempt to halt or retard the progressive pathologic changes of pancreatitis. Intravenous glucagon has been alleged to be of benefit. This is difficult to understand, since glucagon levels have been found elevated in pancreatitis. The clinical usefulness of these agents, like that of the antienzymes, remains to be established.

Convalescence

When the patient has recovered from his acute attack, a careful retrospective study of his clinical history should be undertaken. Cholecystography is done 4 to 8 weeks after discharge from the hospital. If biliary tract disease is discovered, appropriate surgical measures should be undertaken, with a high probability of protection against future attacks. There is no indication for removal of a normal gallbladder in the treatment of acute pancreatitis.

If the biliary tree is normal, the possibility of peptic ulcer must be investigated. At a time when the calcium values may have returned to a high level, serum calcium levels are determined to diagnose hyperparathyroidism. A low-fat diet should be advocated and antialcoholic therapy undertaken whenever necessary.

The possibility that the acute episode was due to a carcinoma of the pancreas must always be kept in mind. This occurs in approximately 3% to 5% of such patients. Occasionally, it will be discovered that the acute episode was only the most recent of other similar attacks, thus establishing a diagnosis of recurrent acute pancreatitis.

COMPLICATIONS

The complications of acute pancreatitis may pose a greater challenge in diagnosis and management than the primary attack. In all the complications, ultrasound examination and CT scanning may provide valuable information in regard to localization, evolution, and timing of operative procedures.

Phlegmon

The large epigastric mass paplable early in the course of the disease has been termed a phlegmon, and the usual clinical course is one of slow resolution. Persistence for more than 3 weeks may require surgical exploration.

Pseudocyst

Pancreatic pseudocysts are encapsulated collections of necrotic tissue, old blood, and secretions from the pancreas. The prefix *pseudo* is used to emphasize the fact that these collections frequently have no true capsules and that the cyst wall is made up of the adjacent viscera, such as stomach and colon (see Fig. 28-5).

Unlike a phlegmon, a pseudocyst usually forms late in the course of the acute disease and manifests itself as a palpable mass associated with a persistently elevated amylase and white blood cell count. Depending on their size and location, pseudocysts may cause gastroduodenal obstruction, splenic rupture, hemorrhage, or perforation into an adjacent viscus. Surgical drainage is required for the management of these pseudocysts. External drainage is indicated for the critically ill. In general, it is much safer to wait 3 to 4 weeks, allowing the cyst to ''mature,'' before performing internal drainage, that is, cystogastrostomy or cystojejunostomy (Fig. 28-5, *D*).

When operating for a presumed pseudocyst, the surgeon must be certain that the lesion does not represent a true cyst. True cysts, which have an epithelial lining, may be congenital or acquired. The acquired true cyst may harbor neoplastic elements, such as a *benign cystadenoma* or *malig-*

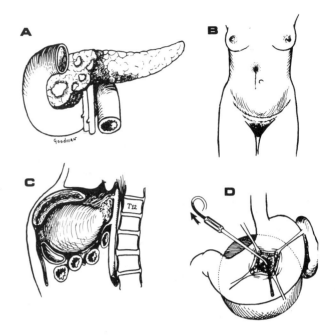

Fig. 28-5. *(A)* Multiple abscesses in the head of the pancreas secondary to acute necrotizing pancreatitis. *(B)* Pancreatic fistula draining onto the abdominal wall. *(C)* Large pancreatic pseudocyst behind the stomach in the lesser peritoneal sac. *(D)* Drainage of pancreatic pseudocyst into the stomach (cystogastrostomy).

nant cystadenocarcinoma or teratoma. Such neoplasms should be excised whenever possible.

Abscess

Pancreatic abscess is the result of infection of a necrotic pancreas and retroperitoneal tissue or infection of a pseudocyst. It is alleged to occur in 4% of patients with pancreatitis. Diagnosis is not difficult in the toxic febrile patient and should be suspected even when there is no palpable mass. Despite timely and adequate drainage, the mortality rate may be as high as 30%.

PANCREATIC ASCITES

During the past 10 years, the diagnosis of nonmalignant pancreatic disease as the source of ascites has been made more frequently. In the majority of patients, this form of ascites can be managed best by surgical intervention. Difficulty arises in the differential diagnosis. Major points of diagnostic value in pancreatic ascites are increased protein content (3.0 g/dl or greater) and high amylase levels in the ascitic fluid. The ascitic fluid in cirrhosis usually has a protein content of less than 1.5 g/dl and normal levels of amylase. The absence of cirrhosis in the presence of ascites is a strong supportive factor. However, since both cirrhosis and pancreatic disease are frequent in the alcoholic patient, analysis of ascitic fluid is imperative. The patient with pancreatic ascites is often refractory to therapy with salt restriction and diuretics because of the high protein content of the ascitic fluid. The incidence is twice as high in males as in females, and 78% of all cases are in chronic alcoholics. Age is not an important factor, and the pediatric patients with ascites must be investigated, especially if there is a history of blunt abdominal trauma. Associated complaints may include weight loss, weakness, anorexia, and diarrhea.

All recent investigators have found that disruption of the

pancreatic duct, with or without pseudocyst formation, is the most common cause of pancreatic ascites. The free leakage of pancreatic fluid into the peritoneal cavity may be demonstrated preoperatively by endoscopic cannulation of the pancreatic duct with pancreatography or by pancreatogram at operation. Identification of a specific site of leakage also aids the surgeon in the selection of the appropriate operation. Treatment is internal drainage of a pseudocyst if it cannot be excised or Roux-en-Y internal drainage of any specific site of leakage. If the tail only is involved, distal pancreatectomy may be appropriate.

NECROTIZING PANCREATITIS

The overall mortality rate of acute pancreatitis varies greatly, but most figures lie between 10% and 25%. Death is usually quite early or late. The rapid, irreversible, shocklike picture ending in death over a few hours or days is difficult to explain and may in part be the result of vasoactive substances previously discussed. The late deaths usually occur after several weeks of a progressive downhill course and result from toxemia, hemorrhage, or sepsis secondary to autodigested, necrotic pancreatic and retroperitoneal tissue. It becomes rapidly apparent that conservative measures have little effect on the course of the disease. Energetic measures to provide proper pulmonary ventilation with intubation, tracheostomy, and ventilatory support are indicated. Peritoneal dialysis may remove toxic pancreatic exudates. Should these measures prove ineffective, consideration should be given to operation that includes cholecystostomy, gastrostomy, feeding jejunostomy, and sump drainage of the lesser sac (Fig. 28-6).

Total pancreatectomy has been suggested as a lifesaving measure in patients with necrotizing pancreatitis; however, the procedure must be done early, and it is difficult to select the patient whose disease process will progress in this fashion. The overall results and mortality with radical resection have been no better than with more conservative surgical measures.

TRAUMATIC PANCREATITIS

Traumatic pancreatitis is most commonly seen in patients involved in automobile accidents and usually is part of multiple abdominal trauma. When there is extensive injury to the pancreas, duodenum, and bile ducts, pancreaticoduodenal resection is probably the procedure of choice.

Fig. 28-6. The multiple procedures performed for necrotizing pancreatitis.

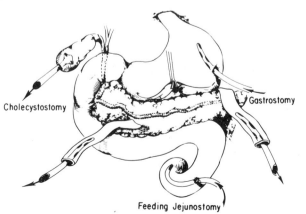

POSTOPERATIVE PANCREATITIS

A form of traumatic pancreatitis, postoperative pancreatitis is usually seen after cholecystectomy, gastrectomy, splenectomy, and aortic aneurysmectomy.

HEREDITARY PANCREATITIS

The hereditary form of the disease is inherited through an autosomal dominant gene, not sex linked. In this form, the disease begins in childhood and is rapidly progressive, and the incidence of cancer is high. The only effective treatment is excisional surgery.

RECURRENT ACUTE

Patients with recurrent bouts of epigastric pain, sometimes radiating to the back, may be considered as having recurrent bouts of acute pancreatitis. Obviously, some patients who initially are considered to be in Sarles' category 1 eventually are reclassified into this group. It must also be admitted that we are unable to differentiate category 2 from category 3, the recurrent chronic form of disease, on clinical grounds alone; yet this is a distinction that is of utmost importance, since in the latter, the patient may not respond to decompressive or drainage procedures. Attempts may be made to exclude the recurrent chronic pancreatitis on the basis of various diagnostic tests, but all too often such patients are identified only by their failure to respond to conservative surgical measures such as sphincteroplasty or internal drainage procedures. These patients have often had prior cholecystectomy, hiatal hernia repair, and other operations that have been ineffective in providing relief. Physical examination and routine x-ray studies are of little help, and laboratory values are usually normal. Over a period of months and years, these symptoms continue unabated despite antacids, antispasmodics, tranquilizers, sedatives, and analgesics.

In my experience, most of these patients are suffering from odditis or fibrosis of the sphincter of Oddi. It must be realized that partial or intermittent obstruction to the outflow of biliary and pancreatic secretions by the sphincter of Oddi may cause episodes of recurrent abdominal pain. Occasionally, both the biliary and the pancreatic ductal systems may be affected. In some patients, the chief manifestation is that of biliary obstruction with cholangitis, but most frequently the presenting symptoms are those of pancreatitis. In general, this symptom complex has been referred to as recurrent pancreatitis, although papillitis, odditis, and obstructive pancreatopathy might be more appropriate terms.

DIAGNOSIS

To make the diagnosis, the single most important item is an awareness that functional and organic obstruction at the ampulla of Vater or duct of Wirsung can occur. Peptic ulcer disease, gallstones, hiatal hernia, renal calculi, and cancer must all be eliminated as a possible cause of trouble.

An elevated serum alkaline phosphatase may be the first clue to obstruction. Serum amylase and lipase elevations provide additional diagnostic support, but these elevations are rare except in an acute bout of pain. Determinations of serum calcium, cholesterol, and triglycerides should be performed to rule out hyperparathyroidism and lipoprotein disturbances.

Ultrasound examination permits a safe and simple method of evaluating the size of the pancreas, determining whether or not there is dilatation of the biliary and pancreatic ducts, and ruling out the presence of residual common duct stones in the postcholecystectomy patient.

The next diagnostic maneuver to be considered is performance of an evocative test. Although secretin and pancreozymin are the natural pancreatic stimulants and would be the ideal pharmacologic agents to use, they must be administered intravenously, they are expensive, and they are difficult to obtain. As a practical substitute, I have used a combination of morphine, 10 mg, and neostigmine methylsulfate, 1 mg. These may be injected parenterally, and fasting blood samples are obtained before and after injection. The patient is not told what type of reaction he may expect. Four blood samples are drawn at hourly intervals after the injection, and each sample is analyzed for amylase and lipase, since only one enzyme may show a rise. The interpretation of the test depends on the extent of the enzyme elevations, regardless of whether or not the patient's symptoms were reproduced. In my opinion, the evocation of symptoms alone may constitute a positive test result. Elevation of the amylase above normal values by a factor of 2 or less without subjective response should be considered a normal reaction ascribable to the spastic effect of the morphine on the papillary and duodenal musculature.

Patients with a positive test result have an 80% chance of relief of symptoms by a drainage procedure such as sphincteroplasty, perhaps an indication that they represent Sarles' type 2 rather than type 3 disease.

The final diagnostic procedure is endoscopic retrograde cholangiopancreatography (ERCP). The endoscopist is able to evaluate reliably the presence of gastritis, ulcer, and residual biliary calculi; to estimate the size of the biliary and pancreatic ducts; and, to a reasonable degree, to rule out the presence of cancer.

SPHINCTEROPLASTY

The operation to be performed in patients with recurrent acute pancreatitis is one to provide relief of outflow obstruction due to spasm or narrowing. This can usually be accomplished by transduodenal sphincteroplasty. Pancreatography must always be performed to define the type of pathology and to ensure adequate drainage of the pancreatic ductal system.

If the patient has a reliable history and a positive evocative test result and ERCP reveals no other abnormalities, surgery should be performed. A careful exploration is first performed to rule out undiagnosed disease. If the gallbladder is present, it should be removed even if there are no stones. The common duct is then carefully examined. Cholangiography may substitute for choledochotomy. If common duct calculi are found, these are removed. Whether or not to proceed with sphincterotomy after removal of stones is a matter of judgment. I have usually been satisfied to dilate the ampulla gently with Bakes dilators and then terminate the operation.

If the gallbladder has been previously removed and if the common duct is normal, I have usually omitted choledochotomy and proceeded directly to transduodenal exposure of the ampulla.

After the major papilla is identified, a catheter is inserted into the ampulla and a pancreatogram is obtained by slowly injecting 2 ml to 3 ml of 50% Hypaque solution. The pancreatogram obtained indicates the type of surgery to be performed (Fig. 28-7). This may be omitted if the information is available from a previous ERCP examination.

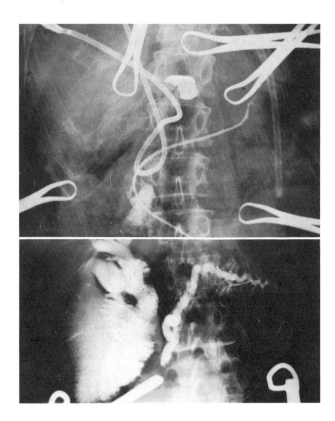

Fig. 28-7. *(Top)* A normal pancreatogram, demonstrating a smooth tapering duct that fills throughout. *(Bottom)* Dilatation and tortuosity of the pancreatic duct and filling of secondary branches. (Nardi GL, Acosta JM: Papillitis as a cause of pancreatitis and abdominal pain. Ann Surg 164:611, 1966)

A patent pancreatic duct should be drained adequately by transduodenal sphincteroplasty (Fig. 28-8). An obstructed duct requires caudal resection with or without pancreaticojejunostomy (see Fig. 28-8). The finding of intraductal obstruction is almost always associated with intrinsic pancreatic pathology and is therefore more properly categorized in group 3 or, perhaps, group 4. A fibrosed, sclerotic gland with ductal ectasia requires resection. This represents chronic pancreatitis and should be classified in Sarles' group 4.

In the performance of sphincteroplasty, it is important to unroof the common duct and expose the pancreatic duct orifice. A sphincteroplasty is then performed on the orifice of the duct of Wirsung (Fig. 28-9). It is the omission of this step, the decompression of the duct of Wirsung, that frequently results in operative failure.

CHRONIC

Patients suffering with chronic pancreatitis may have recurrent or continuous pain. In either case, there is a progressive, destructive process in the pancreas, with cellular infiltration, fibrosis, necrosis, and calcification with loss of functioning exocrine and endocrine tissue. In a few patients, pancreatic insufficiency may result from progressive painless pancreatitis. Again, cancer may be the basis of the patient's symptoms. Weight loss, steatorrhea, diabetes, and pancreatic calcification are frequently present, and alcoholism and drug addiction are not uncommon findings. Primary biliary tract disease is not a consideration.

In my experience, the majority of these patients are men

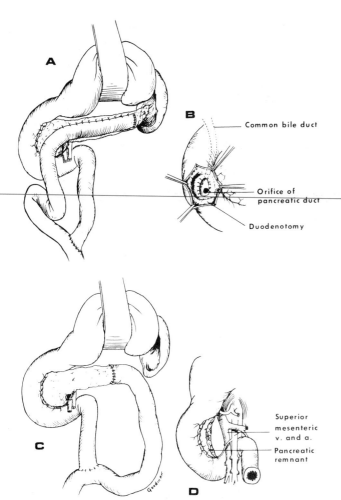

CHRONIC PANCREATITIS	
Etiology	Pancreatic fibrosis and scarring with ductal obstruction from multiple recurrent episodes of acute pancreatitis
Dx	Chronic abdominal pain Alcohol, narcotic use Diabetes mellitus, exocrine insufficiency Abdominal x-ray film: calcification in pancreas CT scan, ultrasonogram Endoscopic retrograde cholangiopancreatography Evocative testing
Rx	Avoidance and treatment of etiologic factors (especially alcohol) Surgery for recalcitrant pain: sphincteroplasty, pancreaticojejunostomy, distal pancreatic resection, pancreaticoduodenectomy, splanchnicectomy

Fig. 28-8. Operative management of chronic relapsing pancreatitis. *(A)* Onlay of defunctionalized jejunal loop for drainage of the unroofed pancreatic duct for proximal duct obstruction. *(B)* Overview of sphincteroplasty (see Fig. 28-9 for detail). *(C)* Similar use of defunctionalized jejunal loop for drainage of the tail of the transected pancreas in the presence of proximal pancreatic duct obstruction. *(D)* A 95% resection of the pancreas. The common bile duct is carefully preserved as it courses through the remaining small portion of the head of the pancreas adjacent to the duodenum.

and alcoholics. In most cases, the primary pathologic process is not remediable. Surgical efforts in this group of patients are directed chiefly toward relief of pain. Alcoholism and dependence on narcotics make evaluation of any procedure in the group most difficult. In patients with ductal dilatation and calcification, consideration should be given to the longitudinal pancreaticojejunostomy of Gillesby and Puestow. This parenchyma-sparing procedure may sometimes provide dramatic relief of pain, as well as preserving any residual exocrine and endocrine tissue and providing the best chance for long-term survival.

Distal resection of the pancreas should be considered when the pathologic changes are limited to the left side of the gland. A complementary pancreaticojejunostomy should be performed when pancreatography of the remaining ductal system reveals residual obstruction or when the duct is abnormally dilated (see Fig. 28-8).

All too often, a diffusely sclerotic pancreas is found, and the only effective procedure is total pancreatectomy. Oc-

Fig. 28-9. Removal of the septum between the common duct and the duct of Wirsung achieves satisfactory decompression of the pancreatic duct.

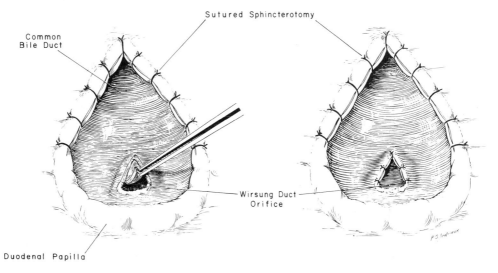

casionally, splanchnicectomy may provide relief of pain, but success with this procedure has been infrequent and short-lived.

One should be cautious, however, in performing resective procedures in confirmed alcoholics, since they will not be able to properly manage their exocrine and endocrine deficiencies. Leger and associates have demonstrated, in a personal series of 148 patients followed from 5 to 20 years, that although the immediate results of pancreaticoduodenectomy were superior functionally, compared with those of lesser resections and drainage, the advantage was eventually counterbalanced by a high late mortality. Pancreatic insufficiency after extensive resection was frequently complicated by malnutrition, sepsis, diabetes, and cirrhosis.

In the nonalcoholic who has no evidence of endocrine insufficiency, it may be possible to prevent development of diabetes by reimplanting pancreatic islets after total pancreatectomy. This has been accomplished by two techniques. The body and tail of the pancreas may be implanted into the pelvis or groin by vascular anastomosis of the splenic vessels, the duct being ligated or injected with plastic. The alternative method is to digest the excised gland with collagenase and inject a suspension of the islets into the portal system. These procedures are still in an investigational phase, but they do offer some hope of making total pancreatectomy a more acceptable therapeutic procedure.

BIBLIOGRAPHY

ACOSTA JM, CIVANTOS F, NARDI GL et al: Fibrosis of the papilla of Vater. Surg Gynecol Obstet 124:787, 1967

ACOSTA JM, NARDI GL, CIVANTOS F: Distal pancreatic duct inflammation. Ann Surg 172:256, 1970

BECKER V: Pathological anatomy and pathogenesis of acute pancreatitis. World J Surg 5:303, 1981

CAREY LC: The Pancreas. St. Louis, C V Mosby, 1973

COPE O, CULVER PJ, MIXTER C, JR et al: Pancreatitis: A diagnostic clue to hyperparathyroidism. Ann Surg 145:857, 1957

CRENTZFELDT W: Intensive medical treatment of severe acute pancreatitis. World J Surg 5:341, 1981

FITZ H: Acute pancreatitis. Boston Med Surg J 120:181, 1889

GIRARD RM, ARCHAMBAUKT A: Hereditary chronic pancreatitis. N Engl J Med 303:286, 1980

GREGG JA, GEOFFREY C, BARR C et al: Postcholecystectomy syndrome and its association with ampullary stenosis. Am J Surg 139:374, 1980

HOWAT HT, SARLES H: The Exocrine Pancreas. Philadelphia, W B Saunders, 1979

KÜMMERLE F, NEHER M: Management of complications after operations for acute pancreatitis. World J Surg 5:387, 1981

LEGER L, LENRIOT JP, LEMAIGRE G: Five to twenty year follow-up after surgery for chronic pancreatitis. Ann Surg 180:185, 1974

LIMBERG B, KOMMERELL B: Treatment of acute pancreatitis with somatostatin. N Engl J Med 303:284, 1980

MADURA JA, McCAMMON RL, PARIS JM et al: The Nardi test and biliary manometry in the diagnosis of pancreatico-biliary sphincter dysfunction. Surgery 90:588, 1981

MERCADIER M: Surgical treatment of acute pancreatitis: Tactics, techniques, and results. World J Surg 5:393, 1981

NARDI GL: Technique of sphincteroplasty in recurrent pancreatitis. Surg Gynecol Obstet 110:639, 1960

NARDI GL: Remediable chronic pancreatitis. Surg Clin North Am 54:613, 1974

RANSON JH: Conservative surgical treatment of acute pancreatitis. World J Surg 5:351, 1981

SARLES H (ed): Pancreatitis. Symposium, Marseilles, April 25 and 26, pp VII–VIII. New York, S. Karger, AG, 1965

SAXON A, REYNOLDS JT, DOOLAS A: Management of pancreatic abscess. Ann Surg 194:545, 1981

SHANAHAN F, CROWE J: Cimetidine and the control of pain in chronic relapsing pancreatitis. N Engl J Med 305:644, 1981

SKINNER DB, CORSON JG, NARDI GL: Aprotinin therapy as prophylaxis against postoperative pancreatitis in humans: A controlled evaluation. JAMA 204:945, 1968

SMITH RB, WARREN WD, RIVARD AA, JR et al: Pancreatic ascites: Diagnosis and management with particular reference to surgical technics. Ann Surg 177:538, 1973

WARSHAW AL: Inflammatory masses following acute pancreatitis. Surg Clin North Am 54:621, 1974

WARSHAW AL, IMBEMBO AL, CIVETTA JM et al: Surgical intervention in acute necrotizing pancreatitis. Am J Surg 127:484, 1974

John M. Howard

Cancer of the Pancreas

Recorded deaths from cancer of the pancreas have been progressively increasing in the United States since 1920, and at present cancer of the pancreas is the fourth or fifth most common cause of cancer death in this country. Among

TABLE 28-1 SELECTED FACTORS AND THEIR ETIOLOGICAL SIGNIFICANCE IN CANCER OF THE PANCREAS

FACTOR	CAUSATIVE RELATIONSHIP?
Cigarette smoking	Probable; 250% increase in smokers over nonsmokers reported
Cigar smoking	Possible
Diabetes	Probably not a factor
Pancreatic calcification	Probably not a factor
Chronic pancreatitis without calcification	No
Chronic alcoholism	No
Sex	Slight preponderance among males
Race	More frequent in Jews and blacks
Industrial chemicals	Several suggestive findings with exposure to nitrosourethane; acetaminofluorene; paradimethylamino azobenzene; methylcholanthrene; betanaphthylamine; benzidine
Atomic bomb exposure	No increased incidence found in Japan
Infectious agents	No evidence as causative agents in humans
Gallstones	No
Coffee drinking	Suggested in preliminary report

cancers of the digestive tract, cancer of the pancreas is second only to colo-rectal cancer in frequency. It was estimated (Cancer Facts and Figures, 1980) that there were 24,000 new cases of cancer of the pancreas per year among Americans (12,500 men and 11,500 women) and that 20,900 persons die of it annually. The incidence continues to increase.

Although cancer of the pancreas has been reported in childhood, it is extremely rare under the age of 40 years. The incidence increases steadily with age after the age of 45 and is higher in the black than in the white population.

Several reports indicate a higher incidence of cancer of the pancreas among cigarette smokers than among nonsmokers (Table 28-1) and a median age of its diagnosis among smokers that is at least 10 years younger than among nonsmokers.

The problems with cancer of the pancreas are that its incidence is apparently progressively increasing in the United States, its diagnosis is usually delayed and is usually dependent on its extension to adjacent tissues, its operative removal is hazardous, and the results of all forms of treatment are disappointing. On the encouraging side are the progressive improvement in operative techniques and the promising diagnostic advances with transoral pancreatography, cytological studies of pancreatic juice, computed tomography, percutaneous transhepatic cholangiography, and possibly percutaneous biopsy.

CLASSIFICATION

Pancreatic cancer, or cancer often indistinguishable preoperatively from pancreatic cancer, is usually an adenocarcinoma and is usually classified as follows:

Adenocarcinoma
    Cancer of the head of the pancreas
    Cancer of the body and tail of the pancreas
    Cancer of the ampulla of Vater
    Cancer of the distal end of the common bile duct
    Cancer of the duodenum
    Cystadenocarcinoma of the pancreas
    Malignant carcinoid of pancreas or duodenum
    Islet cell carcinoma (see Chapter 20)
Adenosquamous or squamous carcinoma
Sarcoma (an exceedingly rare tumor)

Except for the islet cell tumors, pathologists consider most pancreatic cancers to arise from the pancreatic ducts rather than from the pancreatic acini. The basis for this deduction may not be entirely justified. In general, histologic variations and staging of these cancers have not been classified as precisely as those of cancers arising in other parts of the body.

Cubilla and Fitzgerald, in an excellent study of 508 patients with cancer of the nonendocrine pancreas, proposed the following classification:

	PATIENTS	
	Number	Percent
Duct cell origin		
Duct cell adenocarcinoma	380	75
Giant cell carcinoma	22	4
Giant cell Ca (epulis with osteoid)	1	—
Adenosquamous carcinoma	18	4
Microadenocarcinoma	15	3
Mucinous ("colloid") carcinoma	9	2
Cystadenocarcinoma (mucinous)	3	1
Acinar cell origin		
Acinar cell adenocarcinoma	6	1
Uncertain histogenesis		
Pancreaticoblastoma	1	—
Papillary cystic tumor	1	—
Mixed type—acinar, duct, and islet cell carcinoma	1	—
Unclassified	51	10
Large cell (43)		
Small cell (7)		
Clear cell (1)		
Totals	508	100

CANCER IN AND AROUND THE HEAD OF THE PANCREAS

DIAGNOSIS

Cancer of the head of the pancreas is fundamentally a clinical diagnosis, usually without radiologic or histologic confirmation prior to laparotomy.

Cancer in and around the head of the pancreas is seldom diagnosed until it produces obstruction of the common bile duct, with resulting obstructive jaundice. The jaundice resulting from cancer of the head of the pancreas is usually (but not always) progressive, with obstruction usually becoming complete and unremitting. The stools become clay colored, pruritus is often severe, and the gallbladder (but seldom the tumor) becomes palpable. Most such patients are past the age of 50 years.

The basis of the clinical diagnosis includes confirmation or negation of a history of (or exposure to) hepatitis; exposure to any drugs that predispose to severe jaundice; and gallstones and biliary colic, peptic ulcer, chronic pancreatitis, or recent operation on the biliary tract that might have led to a stricture of the common bile duct. Since exclusion of these diagnoses is quite important in permitting the establishment of a diagnosis of cancer of the head of the pancreas, they should be explored carefully, at the bedside and by appropriate laboratory and radiologic studies.

CLINICAL MANIFESTATIONS

Clinically, cancer of the pancreas often causes pain. The concept that painless jaundice is typical of cancer of the pancreas is no longer justified. It is true that the cancer may be painless in its early course; however, obstruction of the pancreatic ducts leads to their distension, to pancreatic juice under pressure, and mild pain in the epigastrium or across the back. As the cancer spreads to invade pancreatic and peripancreatic nerves, backache and abdominal pain increase. Painless jaundice from cancer of the pancreas therefore results in a better prognosis than does painful jaundice from the same disease.

Except in the very slender patient, the tumor is usually not palpable and is seldom tender.

Stool habits may be normal. The absence of pancreatic lipase in the stool tends to increase the fat content and, thereby, the volume and number of the stools. On the other hand, the absence of bile salts in the stool promotes constipation. As a result, the frequency of stools is not predictable.

No clinical examination is complete without the physician's personally looking at the stool to verify its acholic color. This responsibility cannot be delegated to the patient, the house officer, the nurse, or the laboratory. Several specimens, however, should be sent to the laboratory to be tested for occult blood—a finding more suggestive of ampullary or other intestinal tumors or ulcers than of cancer of the pancreas.

LABORATORY STUDIES

Initial laboratory studies should document the increased serum bilirubin level and provide an initial baseline of prothrombin activity. Hepatic enzyme studies and serum hepatitis antigen assays should be obtained in order to exclude hepatitis. Serum amylase and lipase levels are usually normal in patients with cancer of the head of the pancreas, but elevated levels may occur, especially during the early phases of obstruction of the pancreatic ducts. Blood glucose levels may be normal or elevated; diabetes becomes more frequent as the pancreas is destroyed by the disease.

RADIOLOGIC STUDIES

Radiologic studies are essential. The abdominal roentgenogram is helpful in looking for pancreatic calculi. Pancreatic calculi are strongly suggestive of chronic pancreatitis, often alcoholic in origin. Although the presence of pancreatic calculi tends to provide assurance of a benign disease process, this assurance is not complete; in 1% to 4% of patients with radiologically demonstrable pancreatic calcification, the calcification will be located within the carcinoma of the pancreas. The flat plate should also be inspected for evidence of radiopaque gallstones in the gallbladder and in the lower end of the common bile duct.

Because of the effects of obstruction of the common bile duct, oral or intravenous cholecystography or cholangiography is seldom justified. Gastrointestinal (barium) studies of the stomach and duodenum, while usually negative, are invaluable. A large duodenal loop is *not* characteristic of pancreatic cancer. Its most frequent cause is a variation of normal anatomy, and its next most frequent cause is a pseudocyst in the head of the pancreas. An "inverted-3 sign" at the duodenal ampulla is suggestive of malignancy.

Several radiologic techniques deserve special attention.

Pancreatic Arteriography

Pancreatic arteriography has made a limited yet significant contribution to the diagnosis of pancreatic tumors (Fig. 28-10). Actually, it is of more value in localizing a tumor than in diagnosing its presence. Its usefulness is based on four factors. First, tumors, especially benign tumors, may result in displacement of arteries, so that indirectly the tumor may be outlined. Second, depending on the vascularity of the tumor, a rich capillary vascularity may result in a radiographic "blush" that actually localizes the tumor. In general, adenocarcinomas of the pancreas are relatively

PANCREATIC CANCER	
Etiology	Ductal adenocarcinoma most common, predominantly in pancreatic head, frequent nodal or hepatic metastases
	Cigarette smoking—risk factor among others
Dx	Obstructive jaundice ± pain, weight loss, ± palpable mass or gallbladder
	Ultrasonogram, CT scan
	Upper gastrointestinal radiography and endoscopy
	Percutaneous transhepatic cholangiography
	Endoscopic retrograde pancreatogram
	Pancreatic arteriography
Rx	Correct coagulopathy (vitamin K) and nutrition
	Consider percutaneous biliary drainage
	Surgery: Pancreaticoduodenectomy or distal resection if resectable (unlikely)
	Palliative cholecystojejunostomy and gastrojejunostomy

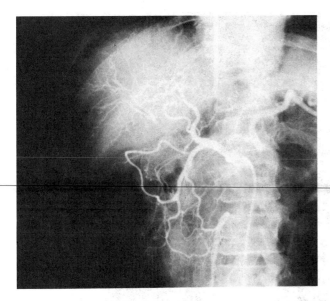

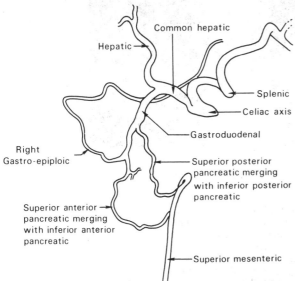

Common hepatic

Hepatic

Splenic

Celiac axis

Gastroduodenal

Right
Gastro-epiploic

Superior posterior
pancreatic merging
with inferior posterior
pancreatic

Superior anterior
pancreatic merging
with inferior anterior
pancreatic

Superior mesenteric

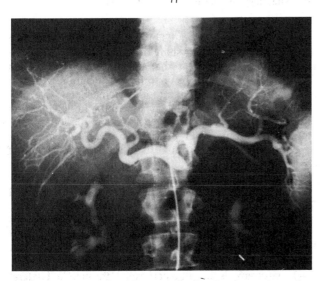

Fig. 28-10. *(Top* and *middle)* Normal celiac arteriogram, revealing retrograde filling of the superior mesenteric artery from the branches of the hepatic artery. (The catheter is seen in the celiac axis.) *(Bottom)* Celiac arteriogram, revealing obstruction of the gastroduodenal artery by carcinoma of the pancreas.

avascular and therefore fail to give a blush, whereas islet cell tumors, cystadenocarcinomas, and malignant carcinoids of the pancreas tend to have a rich capillary vascularity and do provide such a blush. Third, as carcinoma of the pancreas extends, it may invade arteries or veins, with resultant obstruction of the vessels, which may be delineated radiographically. Fourth, the demonstration of normal vascular anomalies, such as the origin of the hepatic artery from the superior mesenteric artery, may be of significant assistance to the surgeon at the time of operation, especially in cancers arising in the uncinate process. Nevertheless, the use of arteriography in patients with pancreatic cancer is probably diminishing.

Endoscopic Retrograde Cholangiopancreatography (ERCP)

Japanese surgeons and endoscopists, using the fiberscope, have made preoperative pancreatography and cholangiography useful (Fig. 28-11). The technique is widely available across the United States. It involves the transoral introduction of the fiberscope and the direct visualization of the stomach and duodenum. It can usually be carried out under analgesics or sedation, often including a drug such as glucagon to diminish peristalsis in the duodenum. An ulcer or tumor that originates in the stomach or the duodenum can usually be visualized, making feasible the preoperative biopsy of ampullary or duodenal carcinomas but seldom permitting preoperative biopsies of carcinomas of the head of the pancreas. Through the fiberscope the ampulla of Vater can be visualized and, with experience, the operator can cannulate the pancreatic and the common bile duct. The injection of a radiopaque medium then permits radiographic delineation of the duct. Cancer of the head of the pancreas tends to obstruct completely the pancreatic duct, whereas chronic pancreatitis results in strictures but seldom results in complete obstruction. Pancreatography by this method has led to a low complication rate. Cholangiography has a somewhat higher complication rate, owing to the exacerbation of any smoldering cholangitis. Collection of juice from the pancreatic duct for cytological study is being evaluated.

Computed Tomography (CT Scan)

CT scanning of the pancreas is making a definite contribution to the preoperative evaluation of patients with pancreatic cancer, but it does not yet provide a basis for the detection of the small, early lesion. CT scans may show large metastases in the liver, pseudocysts, early calcification of the pancreas, dilated bile ducts, and pancreatic tumors—all useful findings.

Under CT guidance, percutaneous "skinny needle" biopsy of pancreatic tumors is being evaluated.

Percutaneous Transhepatic Cholangiography with Catheter Drainage of Biliary Ducts

This study permits preoperative definition of the presence and location of obstruction of the bile ducts and often provides information on which an intelligent, although presumptive, etiological diagnosis can be made (e.g., stone, cancer, pancreatitis). The catheter can be left indwelling in the bile duct and connected to continuous gravity drainage, permitting preoperative improvement in hepatic function. This may prove to be a significant adjunct to therapy, although problems of dislodgement of the catheter, intraperitoneal bleeding, and cholangitis require continued evaluation and improvement.

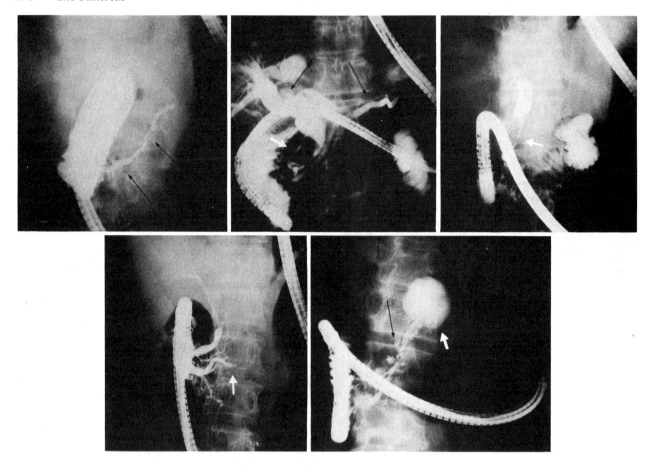

Fig. 28-11. *(Top, left)* The pancreatic duct *(arrows)* in chronic pancreatitis reveals irregularities and "stiffness," but the duct is patent. The fiberoptiscope is seen in this and the succeeding figures. *(Top, middle)* Combined cholangiogram and pancreatogram reveal an obstructing stone in the common bile duct *(white arrow)* with dilatation of both the common bile duct and pancreatic ducts *(black arrows.)* *(Top, right)* Cholangiogram reveals dilatation of common bile duct behind an obstructing carcinoma *(arrow)* of the terminal common duct. *(Bottom, left)* Obstruction of the pancreatic duct *(arrow)* by carcinoma of the pancreas. The common bile duct is not obstructed. *(Bottom, right)* Carcinoma of the pancreas with cyst. White arrow identifies the pancreatic cyst, which communicates with an irregular, deformed pancreatic duct *(black arrow).* Transoral Pancreatocholangiography via Fibro-Optiscope (Reproduced by permission of Satake, Howard and Associates, and Surgery, Gynecology and Obstetrics)

PREOPERATIVE MANAGEMENT

Once the decision has been made to operate on the patient, a normal prothrombin activity should be demonstrated, following the continued parenteral administration of vitamin K. A low-residue diet, intestinal cleaning agents (laxatives and enemas), and nonabsorbable oral antibiotics should be employed in preparing the bowel for operation. Baseline studies of hepatic function, arterial blood gases, renal function (blood urea nitrogen and creatinine levels), electrocardiogram, chest film, and serum albumin and electrolyte levels should be obtained. It is usually helpful to position a central venous catheter before operation. If the patient has had an external biliary fistula established at a prior exploration, every effort should be made to replace sodium and potassium reserves before surgery. The serum albumin level, if low, should be restored to normal by the administration of human serum albumin.

OPERATION

An experienced anesthetic team is an essential part of the operative team. It is their responsibility to be certain that

two or more portals for rapid blood and crystalloid infusion are available, and they share the responsibility with the surgeon of making certain that adequate amounts of blood are available for transfusion prior to operation. A Levin tube should be inserted into the stomach and a Foley catheter into the urinary bladder, with the urine collection bag *at the head of the table* so that the anesthesiologist can measure the urinary output *hourly as a vital sign during the operative procedure.* He should share in the responsibility of seeing that adequate fluid is administered during the operation so that oliguria does not result. The author's preference is for general anesthesia, achieved by endotracheal techniques.

The radiologist should verify that the technique for obtaining abdominal films in the operating room is correct *prior to operation,* so that, if operative pancreatography or cholangiography is employed, the studies will be satisfactory.

Laparotomy is usually performed through a bilateral subcostal incision, with the right subcostal portion of the incision made first. If hepatic metastases are demonstrated, the complete incision may not be necessary.

The aims of the operation are (1) to determine whether

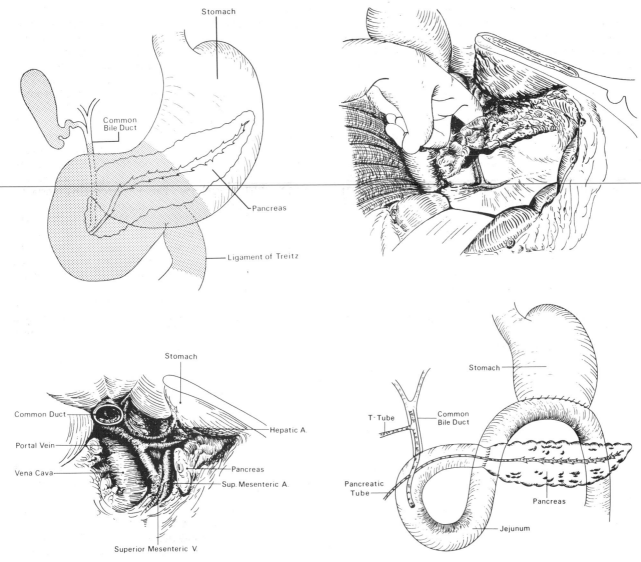

Fig. 28-12. Pancreaticoduodenectomy (Whipple resection). *(Top, left)* The shaded areas represent the areas to be resected, including lower portion of the stomach, head of the pancreas, entire duodenum, gallbladder, and terminal end of the common bile duct. *(Top, right)* The neck of the pancreas overlies the superior mesenteric vessels. Mobilization of the pancreas from these vessels is a crucial step, usually performed by finger dissection, as indicated. *(Bottom, left)* By the conclusion of the resection, the mesenteric vessels and the vessels of portal triad have been completely exposed and the common bile duct, the pancreas, and the stomach have been transected. *(Bottom, right)* Reconstruction after resection allows alkaline pancreatic juice and bile to enter the "isolated" limb of jejunum proximal to the acid gastric juice. Both the bile duct and the pancreatic duct are temporarily cannulated, with the catheters being exteriorized.

or not a malignancy is present and, if not, to identify another cause for the obstructive jaundice; (2) to determine whether or not the malignancy has spread to the liver or to other areas of the abdomen beyond the lines of potential resection; (3) to resect the tumor in toto; and (4) to restore continuity to the biliary, pancreatic, and gastrointestinal tracts (Fig. 28-12).

Resectability of the tumor varies tremendously, depending on its site of origin. In the Mayo Clinic experience, resectability has been as follows: cancer of the head of the pancreas 10%, cancer of the ampulla of Vater 72%, and carcinoma of duodenum and bile ducts intermediate to these two.

Demonstration of the presence of a tumor in the head

of the pancreas is achieved by the Kocher maneuver, which includes mobilization of the duodenum and head of the pancreas by division of the peritoneum from the right side of the duodenum through a relatively avascular area. This allows the operator to place his fingers behind the pancreas and palpate the head of the pancreas between thumb and fingers. A hard mass, limited to the head of the pancreas, can be almost diagnostic to the experienced pancreatic surgeon. A common duct gallstone may also be palpated by this maneuver. The surgeon examines the liver for evidence of spread and abandons resection of the pancreas if hepatic metastases are demonstrable. Biopsy of the tumor, with a prompt confirmation of malignancy by frozen section, is desirable in the management of pancreatic cancer, as it is in the operative management of other malignant tumors. A negative frozen section, however, does not exclude the presence of a malignant tumor, and the surgeon should not accept a negative report if the characteristics of the gross tumor, as determined by palpation, are those of carcinoma. Under such circumstances, it is best after careful deliberation to proceed with resection of the tumor in the absence of histologic verification of malignancy.

Because the arterial blood supply to the head of the pancreas and to the duodenum are essentially identical, one cannot resect the "periduodenal" pancreas without resecting the duodenum. The resection of the head of the pancreas, as described by Whipple, includes resection of the gastric antrum and pylorus, the entire duodenum, the terminal end of the common bile duct, and the head of the pancreas over to the left of the superior mesenteric vein.

Reconstruction following resection of the head of the pancreas includes approximation of the end of the jejunum, distal to a total duodenectomy, to the divided end of the pancreas for a pancreaticojejunostomy, using nonabsorbable sutures. Many variations of technique are used, including the insertion of a small polyethylene catheter into the pancreatic duct through the pancreaticojejunostomy, which is then brought through the wall of the jejunum and anterior abdominal wall to permit suction in the postoperative period. Distal to the pancreaticojejunostomy, the end of the divided common bile duct is sutured to the side of the jejunum, often over a long-arm T-tube. Finally, the limb of the jejunum is approximated to the divided end of the stomach for a gastrojejunostomy. This sequence in reconstruction permits alkaline bile and pancreatic secretions to flow across the gastrojejunostomy and thus minimizes the possibility of marginal ulceration of the jejunum. Some surgeons perform a vagotomy to further reduce gastric acidity. Drains are placed near the choledochojejunostomy and the pancreaticojejunostomy and beneath each hemidiaphragm to minimize potential problems of technical errors, most frequent of which is a delayed leak in the pancreaticojejunostomy.

POSTOPERATIVE CARE

Postoperatively, the patients are treated—as is any patient with major injuries—in an intensive care setting, with serial monitoring of vital signs, including hourly urinary output and possibly central venous blood pressure, and repetitive monitoring of hemoglobin, hematocrit, arterial blood gases, and *p*H. The problems of postoperative acute renal failure have largely disappeared as experience has emphasized the operative and postoperative maintenance of adequate capillary perfusion in the lungs and kidneys. Efforts are directed toward minimizing the secretin stimulation of the pancreas during the early postoperative period by the use of gastric suction, to remove gastric acid, and by the avoidance of oral feedings. In addition, patients are usually maintained on prophylactic antibiotics and vitamin K. The author uses large quantities of intravenous fluid and human serum albumin during the first two or three days after operation, because patients appear to lose tremendous volumes of water and albumin into the peritoneal cavity and the intestinal tract. Without such treatment, hemoconcentration develops during the early hours after operation.

Through the development of a team of professionals who are interested in diseases of the pancreas and are careful and meticulous in their operative techniques, and with intensive support of the patient in the postoperative period

by the nurses and surgical residents, as well as by the surgeons, it has been possible to steadily reduce the operative mortality from the Whipple resection. Across the country it has been demonstrated in a number of surgical centers that the concentration of experience in the hands of one or more senior surgeons has sharply reduced the risk of operative mortality. In almost every reported series, the operative mortality rate has been approximately twice as high in patients with carcinoma of the head of the pancreas (10% to 20%) as in those with carcinoma of the ampulla of Vater (5% to 10%). The author, after the earlier loss of several patients, has successfully performed the resection in the last 65 consecutive patients (a series which includes several patients with benign disease) without an operative mortality.

Owing to the possibility of intrapancreatic spread of malignancy, interest has developed in regard to the advisability of total pancreatectomy in the treatment of carcinoma of the head of the pancreas, rather than resection of the head only. The operative mortality rate following total pancreatectomy is also diminishing in experienced hands. Disadvantages of such a procedure include total loss of endogenous insulin and of the pancreatic enzymes that promote digestion in the intestine, as well as the fact that total pancreatectomy usually requires splenectomy also. Experience does not yet permit definition of the 5-year survival rate, but it suggests a rate approximating that of the Whipple resection.

PALLIATIVE TREATMENT

SURGICAL

If, at the time of laparotomy, the surgeon finds metastatic spread of the cancer to the liver or for other reasons finds the cancer inoperable, a cholecystojejunostomy and a gastrojejunostomy are usually performed. The cholecystojejunostomy is performed to relieve the obstructive jaundice, and the gastrojejunostomy is performed to relieve the existing or potential duodenal obstruction. If the lesion is locally invasive but there is no evidence of distant metastases, the surgeon should also ring the tumor with silver clips as a subsequent aid to the radiotherapist in the exact localization of the malignancy.

NONSURGICAL

Radiotherapists have demonstrated prolongation of survival following intensive radiotherapy in patients in whom the tumor was found to be unresectable because of local invasion but distant metastases had not been demonstrated. The value of chemotherapy in the treatment of cancer of the head of the pancreas has not been clearly defined.

FOLLOW-UP RESULTS

A series of 239 patients at the Mayo Clinic with cancer in or around the head of the pancreas were treated by a pancreatic resection. The results are shown in Table 28-2.

These results, while not as impressive as those seen following the treatment of several nonintestinal malignancies, represent a striking improvement over earlier years and indicate resection to be the treatment of choice until a better method of therapy has been demonstrated. Although the 5-year survival rates in the Mayo Clinic series are encouraging, the postoperative life span of non-5-year survivors averaged only 8 to 9 months. The life expectancy

TABLE 28-2   **RESULTS OF THE WHIPPLE RESECTION**

LOCATION OF THE MALIGNANCY	NUMBER OF PATIENTS	OPERATIVE MORTALITY RATE (PERCENT)	5-YEAR SURVIVAL RATE (PERCENT)
Head of the pancreas	119	21	14*
Ampulla of Vater	77	15	39
Adjacent duodenum	25	24	39
Terminal common bile duct	18	17	11
Total	239	Average 19	Average 26

* Including 4 survivors with islet cell carcinoma, the 5-year survival rate was 18 among 66 patients.

of those patients whose lesions are not resectable is even less.

Adenosquamous carcinoma and squamous carcinoma have not been adequately described as to prognosis, but the former would appear to parallel that of the adenocarcinomas.

OTHER CANCERS OF THE PANCREAS

CARCINOMA OF THE BODY AND TAIL OF THE PANCREAS

Carcinoma of the body and tail of the pancreas apparently has the same growth characteristics as does cancer of the head of the pancreas; however, limitations of specific radiographic techniques and failure of the tumor to obstruct the common bile duct early in its course have, in the past, resulted in delayed diagnosis of the cancer, permitting an almost hopeless state of invasion and metastasis to develop. Up until the present, diagnosis has been based on unremitting pain in the back and deep in the upper abdomen, in association with negative gastrointestinal and renal films. Under these circumstances, laparotomy has almost always demonstrated advanced malignancy. It is hoped that transoral pancreatography may permit a more successful approach to an earlier diagnosis.

CYSTADENOCARCINOMA

Cystadenocarcinoma constitutes approximately 1% to 2% of malignant pancreatic tumors. There is no clear-cut proof that a *benign cystadenoma* is a premalignant lesion leading secondarily to the cystadenocarcinoma. Histologically, several forms of cystadenocarcinoma have been described with a common feature: The cystic spaces in the tumor are lined by malignant epithelial cells. This is to be distinguished from a pseudocyst, which may develop behind an obstructing carcinoma of the pancreas. The cystadenocarcinoma has no distinguishing clinical features that help to differentiate it from other malignancies of the pancreas. It occurs somewhat more frequently in women and more commonly in the body and tail of the pancreas.

The diagnosis of cystadenocarcinoma of the pancreas is aided somewhat by arteriography that demonstrates an increased vascularity of the tumor, in contrast to other ductal adenocarcinomas of the pancreas, which tend to be relatively avascular by arteriographic criteria. The operative finding of a mucus-filled pancreatic cyst is suggestive of cystadenoma or cystadenocarcinoma.

The treatment of cystadenocarcinoma of the pancreas is resection; but, because this tumor most often occurs in the body and tail of the pancreas, diagnosis is usually delayed and the opportunity for resection before the lesion becomes inoperable is infrequent.

MALIGNANT CARCINOID

Malignant carcinoid of the pancreas or duodenum has occasionally been reported and has often metastasized to the liver prior to diagnosis. The systemic manifestations parallel those of carcinoid tumors found in the other parts of the body: growth is usually slow, permitting a life expectancy of several years in spite of the presence of distant metastases at the time of diagnosis.

SARCOMAS

Sarcomas constitute approximately 0.5% of malignant tumors of the pancreas. Fibrosarcoma, leiomyosarcoma, malignant neurilemmoma, neuroblastoma, extra-medullary plasmacytoma, and lymphomas, as well as unclassified sarcomas, have been reported. Although surgical excision is accepted as the treatment of choice, experience has been too limited to permit generalization.

POSTOPERATIVE LONG-TERM TREATMENT

Humans and other animals with a normal pancreas can maintain a normal state of nutrition so long as 20% to 25% or more of the pancreas is functioning. With varying degrees of damage to the pancreas, before or as a result of operation, and with varying degrees of diabetes having preceded an operative resection, one cannot predict with accuracy that a given patient's nutrition will be adequately maintained by any postresection pancreatic remnant.

Total pancreatectomy, of course, results in diabetes. Postpancreatectomy diabetes requires insulin and is often difficult to regulate. Approximately 20 to 25 units of insulin usually suffice, but small variations in dosage may evoke changes ranging between diabetic coma and hypoglycemic shock. As compared to the normal, *insulin after total pancreatectomy results in a more pronounced and a more prolonged drop in the blood sugar level.* This increased sensitivity to insulin after total pancreatectomy appears to result from the simultaneous loss of pancreatic glucagon and its normal feedback mechanism for the regulation of the blood glucose level.

The patient with a total pancreatectomy will have a significant steatorrhea, manifesting itself as frequent bulky stools—3 to 10 (or more) daily. The orally administered

TABLE 28-3   ENZYME ANALYSES OF PANCREATIC SUPPLEMENT ACTIVITY PER TABLET OR CAPSULE

DRUG (TRADE NAME)	TRYPSIN (BAPA SUBSTRATE)	AMYLASE (SOMOGYI UNITS)	LIPASE (CHERRY CRANDALL UNITS)
Accelerase	10,300	19,850	2,600
Cotazym	63,800	60,470	4,630
Lipan	7,400	27,510	2,380
Pancreatin	2,460	17,190	1,620
Viokase	2,440	25,590	2,230

pancreatic supplements that are commercially available do not, by any means, quantitatively replace the enzymes normally secreted into the intestine by the pancreas. However, the better supplements will reduce the number and volume of stools and fecal fat to levels commensurate with a reasonably normal state of nutrition. The amount of pancreatic extract necessary for control cannot be completely predicted but must be evaluated by trials of therapy. Although a number of the commercially available extracts are acceptable (Table 28-3), pancreatin, in 300-mg tablets, is the standard on which many physicians base therapy. An initial program of therapy for evaluation would be 3 or 4 such tablets of pancreatin or other extract by mouth at each meal and again at bedtime. Minor modifications of such a program should result in the patient having one to three formed stools per day and permit him to maintain his body weight at a stationary level.

BIBLIOGRAPHY

American Cancer Society: Cancer Facts and Figures, 1980

Brooks JR, Culebras, JM: Cancer of the pancreas, palliative operation, Whipple procedure or total pancreatectomy. Am J Surg 131:516, 1976

Cubilla AL, Fitzgerald PJ: Cancer of the pancreas (nonendocrine): A suggested morphologic classification. Semin Oncol 6:285, 1979

Howard JM: Pancreatico-duodenectomy: Forty-one consecutive Whipple resections without an operative mortality. Ann Surg 168:629, 1968

Maniz D, Webster PD III: Pancreatic carcinoma. A review of etiologic considerations. Dig Dis Sci 19:459, 1974

Monge JJ, Judd ES, Gage RP: Radical pancreatoduodenectomy. A 22-year experience with the complications, mortality rate and survival rate. Ann Surg 160:711, 1964

Pairent FW, Howard JM: The treatment of pancreatic insufficiency. IV. The enzyme content of commercial pancreatic supplements. Arch Surg 110:739, 1975

Satake K, Umeyama K, Kobayashi K et al: An evaluation of endoscopic pancreatocholangiography in surgical patients. Surg Gynecol Obstet 140:349, 1975

Whipple AO Parsons WB, Mullins CR: Treatment of carcinoma of the ampulla of Vater. Ann Surg 102:763, 1935

Wynder WL, Mabuchi K, Maruchi N et al: Epidemiology and carcinoma of the pancreas. JNCI 50:645, 1973

James W. Maher

Pancreatic Trauma

MECHANISM OF INJURY
DIAGNOSIS
  Signs and Symptoms
  Serum Amylase Determination
  Radiologic Studies
  Peritoneal Lavage
TREATMENT
  Exposure
  Management
    Contusions Without Capsular Injury
    Capsular Laceration Without Ductal Disruption
    Severe Injury with Ductal Disruption
    Combined Pancreaticoduodenal Injury
COMPLICATIONS
  Fistula
  Pseudocyst
  Abscess

Pancreatic trauma requires of the surgeon a wide repertoire of procedures suited to the individual circumstance and condition of the patient. Strict adherence to the principles of débridement of devitalized tissue and good drainage, whether internal or external, will result in a high percentage of excellent results.

Recognition of the significance of pancreatic injuries has markedly increased since the original report of Travers in 1827, who described a classic pancreatic transection sustained by an intoxicated woman knocked down by the wheel of a stagecoach. Only occasional patients with injuries of this type were reported for the next 100 years. Even in wartime, few of these injuries were noted (World War II, 62 patients; Korean War, 9 patients). This relative rarity may be explained in part by the close association of the pancreas with major vascular structures that, when injured by the typical high-velocity military missile, resulted in the patient's dying before reaching medical care. It is only within the past 25 years that enough experience has been accumulated to allow formulation of certain basic principles for the optimum care of these patients.

MECHANISM OF INJURY

Pancreatic injuries account for only 1% or 2% of all abdominal trauma. Penetrating trauma accounts for two thirds of these injuries. The mortality rate for penetrating injuries is approximately 19%; however, almost half these deaths are related to shotgun wounds, which carry a 61% mortality rate. This high death rate primarily reflects injuries to the major vascular structures intimately associated with the pancreas. Blunt trauma accounts for the remaining one third of pancreatic injuries. The anatomic derangements associated with blunt trauma correlate well with the mechanism of injury. Forces concentrated to the right of the vertebral column produce crushing injuries to the head of the pancreas that may be associated with hepatic lacerations, avulsion of the common bile duct from the duodenum, or rupture of the duodenum. Forces concentrated on the vertebrae result in classic pancreatic transections over the superior mesenteric vessels, while forces localized to the left usually result in trauma to the distal pancreas and spleen. Again it is injury of associated vascular structures that accounts for the higher mortality rate associated with injuries to the pancreatic head and body (head 22%, body 18%, tail 12%).

DIAGNOSIS

SIGNS AND SYMPTOMS

The diagnosis of pancreatic trauma is based upon a complete history and physical examination of the patient. The history of blunt trauma to the abdomen may be the only clue to pancreatic injury, because definitive symptoms are characteristically slow to appear. There is usually at least some mild midepigastric tenderness, although, at the other extreme, some patients present with severe pain, guarding, and rigidity, which suggest the need for immediate laparotomy. The delayed appearance of signs and symptoms in isolated pancreatic injuries is probably secondary to failure of pancreatic enzymes to be activated in the absence of duodenal enterokinase. In fact, some patients may be asymptomatic for years following an episode of blunt trauma before a pseudocyst suddenly appears. The decision for laparotomy in penetrating trauma poses no such dilemmas, since all penetrating injuries of the peritoneal cavity require surgical exploration.

SERUM AMYLASE DETERMINATION

In 1943, Naffziger and McCorkle were the first to suggest serum amylase determination as a useful indicator for pancreatic injury. Subsequent studies have demonstrated elevated serum amylase values in from 60% to 90% of patients with blunt pancreatic trauma. An elevated amylase value is not diagnostic of pancreatic injury, however, since it is elevated in many other visceral injuries, as well as in up to 50% of patients shown at laparotomy to have no injury whatsoever. An elevated serum amylase value cannot be considered sufficient justification for laparotomy unless accompanied by other confirmatory evidence.

PANCREATIC TRAUMA	
Etiology	Penetrating trauma accounts for two thirds of injuries; blunt trauma, which crushes the pancreas against vertebrae, one third
Dx	Symptoms: Mild midepigastric tenderness with slow progression; extremely variable Amylase: Usually elevated in blunt trauma; however, it is nondiagnostic since it may be elevated in patients with no intra-abdominal injury Radiologic: Usually normal; may show retroperitoneal air Peritoneal lavage: Unreliable
Rx	Wide exposure of pancreas and control of hemorrhage Lesions without ductal injury may be treated with external drainage. Ductal disruption may be treated with either resection and external drainage or internal drainage into a Roux-en-Y jejunal limb. Pancreaticoduodenal injury, carrying highest mortality, is best treated with duodenal diverticulization or, in particularly severe cases, pancreaticoduodenectomy
Complications	Fistulas: Overwhelming majority close spontaneously Pseudocyst: Internal drainage to stomach or jejunum Pancreatic abscess: Result of inadequate drainage and débridement, treated by external drainage

RADIOLOGIC STUDIES

Plain films of the abdomen are typically normal; however, they may demonstrate obliteration of the psoas margin, displacement of the stomach, or, in the case of duodenal rupture, retroperitoneal air around the right kidney or psoas muscle. Gastrografin upper gastrointestinal tract series may demonstrate leakage from retroperitoneal duodenal injuries, while sonograms may demonstrate an evolving mass in the lesser sac. Any of the above findings make the decision for laparotomy easier.

PERITONEAL LAVAGE

The retroperitoneal position of the pancreas makes peritoneal lavage an unreliable indicator of pancreatic injury unless associated trauma to other organs contributes to a positive lavage. The presence, however, of an elevated amylase value or bile in the peritoneal effluent is an indication for exploration.

TREATMENT

EXPOSURE

When preoperative studies indicate the need for laparotomy, it is important to visualize the pancreas thoroughly in all cases. The body and tail may be adequately visualized by dividing the omentum just below the greater curvature of the stomach, entering the lesser sac, and reflecting the stomach cephalad. The tail of the gland may be mobilized by freeing the spleen and retracting it medially with the tail of the pancreas, allowing direct visualization and bimanual palpation. The head of the gland and the duodenum should be mobilized from their retroperitoneal position (the Kocher maneuver). This allows inspection not only of the head of the pancreas and the duodenum but also of the inferior vena cava, the aorta, and the renal vessels for associated injuries. It is important to note that all hematomas in this areas *must* be explored to rule out occult injuries to major vascular and ductal structures.

MANAGEMENT

The goals of operative treatment of pancreatic injuries are to control hemorrhage, conserve pancreatic function, and drain pancreatic exocrine secretion. Hemorrhage can best be controlled initially by antero-posterior compression of the mobilized gland. Devitalized tissues are then carefully débrided, allowing precise placement of hemostatic sutures. Clamps should be avoided because they may avulse these flimsy vessels and further damage pancreatic tissue. Sutures should be of nonabsorbable material (absorbable sutures are rapidly digested by the pancreatic enzymes). Deep sutures or mass ligatures are also contraindicated because they may obstruct major pancreaticobiliary ducts or injure the superior mesenteric vessels. The secure control of hemorrhage allows time for a more adequate assessment of the degree of injury. Pancreatic injuries may be classified in order of increasing severity as (1) contusion of the pancreas without rupture of the capsule, (2) capsular and parenchymal disruption without injury of the major pancreatic duct, (3) severe injury with rupture of the major duct, and (4) combined pancreatic and duodenal injuries.

CONTUSIONS WITHOUT CAPSULAR INJURY

Contusions without capsular injury require neither débridement nor sutures. This class of injury should, however, be drained because of the risk of unrecognized breaches in the capsule that could result in collection of pancreatic secretions with subsequent abscess or pseudocyst formation. A soft Silastic sump drain, as well as several Penrose drains, should be left in the area of injury and brought out through a generous stab wound in the flank. They should be left in place for 10 days, since there may not be significant drainage until after the patient resumes oral intake.

CAPSULAR LACERATION WITHOUT DUCTAL DISRUPTION

Laceration of the capsule without ductal disruption may be treated with simple suture with nonabsorbable sutures, followed by wide drainage as described above. One should always remember that in these situations a pancreatic fistula is not necessarily a complication, since it is infinitely preferable to the sequelae of inadequate drainage, namely, pseudocyst or abscess formation.

SEVERE INJURY WITH DUCTAL DISRUPTION

Severe injury with ductal disruption requires careful individualization of management. Inadequate drainage invariably leads to pseudocyst or abscess formation, and external drainage alone usually results in a pancreatic fistula that may be particularly persistent either because of discontinuity of the duct, or because of obstruction of the proximal duct.

The best way to treat ductal injuries in the body or tail is with a distal pancreatectomy. In this procedure, the pancreas is usually transected at the area of ductal injury and resected in continuity with the spleen and its vessels. Alternately, the tail of the pancreas may be resected without sacrificing the spleen by dissecting the pancreas free from its intimate association with the splenic vein and dividing the short venous tributaries encountered. This is a particularly useful maneuver in children when preservation of the spleen is a desirable goal. The proximal pancreas may be treated with ligation of the duct of Wirsung and closure of the pancreas with sutures or with application of a double line of stainless steel staples with one of the many available stapling intruments. Complementary external drainage is mandatory. Jones and Shires have advocated a different method of treating total transection of the pancreas. They describe a technique that sutures both ends of the transected pancreas to a Roux-en-Y limb of jejunum (Fig. 28-13). This procedure, combined with wide external drainage, has the theoretical advantages of leaving all functioning pancreatic tissue, thereby avoiding the possibility of pancreatic exocrine insufficiency or diabetes. In fact, these difficulties rarely arise following major pancreatic resection for trauma. Yellin and associates reported only one case of diabetes in over 60 patients undergoing distal pancreatectomy. Nevertheless, Roux-en-Y pancreaticojejunostomy remains a useful alternative to resection in isolated pancreatic injuries, when the increased time required to perform this procedure is not a liability. Patients with severe injury to the tail and body of the pancreas combined with contusions and edema of the head of the pancreas may develop a persistent pancreatic fistula due to ductal obstruction if treated with distal pancreatectomy and external drainage. Therefore, it may be wise to manage this situation with distal pancreatectomy combined with drainage of the proximal pancreas into a defunctionalized Roux-en-Y. Again, it must be emphasized that all forms of internal drainage procedures must be supplemented by external sump drainage.

Severe ductal injuries in which the posterior capsule is intact may be treated by suturing a Roux-en-Y limb to the defect anteriorly. Shattering injuries to the head of the pancreas without duodenal involvement can be treated by either 95% pancreatectomy or the Jones-Shires maneuver (see Fig. 28-13).

COMBINED PANCREATICODUODENAL INJURY

The mortality rate in combined pancreaticoduodenal injury is 44%, much of which is due to injuries to the major vascular structures in the area. Nevertheless, nearly 30% of mortalities in this group of patients are related to septic complications from duodenal and pancreatic fistulas.

In the past, the favored treatment of this injury has been simple closure of the duodenal defect and wide external pancreatic drainage. Berne and associates have reported that this approach may result in a high incidence of duodenal fistula and have therefore designed an approach that diverts gastric chyme from the duodenum. They have called this procedure duodenal diverticulization. The salient features of this approach are closure of the duodenal defect, tube duodenostomy, antrectomy and gastrojejunostomy to divert the gastric contents, vagotomy to prevent marginal ulceration, and wide external drainage (Fig. 28-14). In Berne's

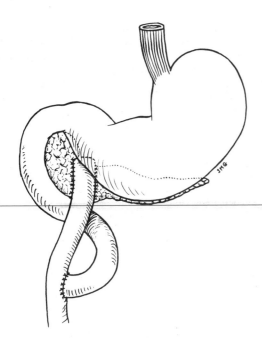

Fig. 28-13. This double pancreaticojejunostomy anastomoses both ends of the transected pancreas to the defunctionalized Roux-en-Y limb of jejunum. It should be combined with external drainage.

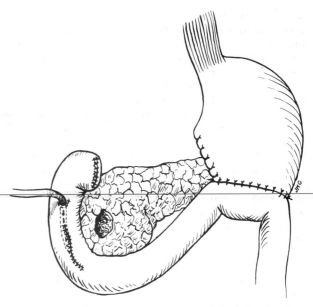

Fig. 28-14. Duodenal diverticulization partially defunctionalizes the duodenum by diverting the gastric contents, making duodenal fistula less likely.

experience, this procedure is associated with a 16% mortality rate, a commendable result in these difficult patients.

Other options to duodenal diverticulization include the Thal serosal patch or a Roux-en-Y jejunoduodenostomy as described by Jones and Joergenson to patch the duodenal wall with well-vascularized bowel (Fig. 28-15). These procedures have never been tested in large groups of patients but have the advantage of being more rapid to perform than duodenal diverticulization.

Pancreaticoduodenectomy (the Whipple procedure) should be reserved for shattering devitalizing injuries of the pancreas and duodenum, especially those in which the common duct

is avulsed from the duodenum. The mortality rate for this procedure averages 30%; however, small series have been reported without mortality.

COMPLICATIONS

The complications of pancreatic injuries, as noted before, are fistula, pancreatic abscess, necrosis of vessels with hemorrhage from drain sites, pseudocyst formation, and duodenal fistula.

FISTULA

Pancreatic fistulas occur in 35% of cases of pancreatic trauma (most commonly blunt). Most of these fistulas are mild and

Fig. 28-15. The Thal serosal patch patches the duodenal wall with pliable well-vascularized jejunum.

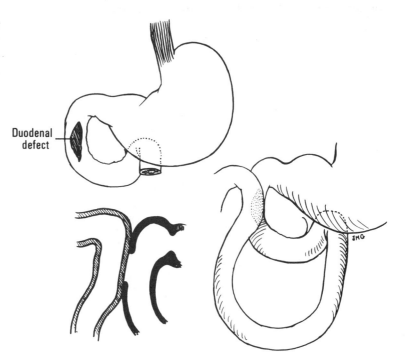

Duodenal defect

will close spontaneously in less than 1 month. Fistulas that persist for longer than 1 month are arbitrarily considered to be major; 95% of major pancreatic fistulas will also close spontaneously. However, there are several goals that are useful to keep in mind when caring for these patients.

The skin must be meticulously protected from autodigestion. This is best accomplished using Stomahesive. An opening is cut in the sheet of Stomahesive just large enough to permit passage of drains from the fistula. This remarkable material adheres well to the skin for several days, protecting it from the excoriating fistula output. A special drainable ostomy appliance is applied to the Stomahesive, allowing measurement of fluid losses.

Pancreatic fluid should be replaced either by refeeding or by using a balanced salt solution with extra bicarbonate.

Parenteral nutrition is unnecessary unless the fistula drains more than 500 ml/day. Nevertheless, if feeding causes a large increase in drainage, parenteral nutrition is the preferred course, since it will maintain an anabolic state while reducing pancreatic exocrine secretion by at least 50%.

The 5% of patients with persistent drainage may be adequately treated by implantation of the fistula into a Roux-en-Y limb of jejunum.

PSEUDOCYST

A pseudocyst is a cystic structure without epithelial lining that results from a collection of pancreatic fluid within the lesser sac. Its walls are usually made up of the structures bordering on the lesser sac. The most common symptoms and signs are pain, nausea and vomiting, and an abdominal mass. Serum amylase is usually elevated. These cysts rarely resolve spontaneously and are best treated with internal drainage with a Roux-en-Y–cystojejunostomy or a cysto-gastrostomy.

ABSCESS

Lesser sac abscesses are the usual result of poor drainage of pancreatic injuries. These abscesses routinely erode into adjacent major vascular structures, as well as hollow viscera. Cultures usually reveal mixed aerobic and anaerobic gram-negative flora, although staphylococci and enterococci are not rare. The only treatment for a pancreatic abscess is external drainage and parenteral administration of antibiotics. Mortality is high. The best treatment is, of course, prevention by adequate débridement and wide external drainage initially.

BIBLIOGRAPHY

Baker RJ, Bass RT, Zajtchuk R et al: External pancreatic fistula following abdominal injury. Arch Surg 95:556, 1967

Berne CJ, Donovan AJ, White EJ et al: Duodenal "diverticulization" for duodenal and pancreatic injury. Am J Surg 127:503, 1974

Howell JF, Burrus GB, Jordan GL: Surgical management of pancreatic injuries. J Trauma 1:32, 1961

Jones RC, Shires GT: The management of pancreatic injuries. Arch Surg 90:502, 1965

Jones RC, Shires GT: Pancreatic trauma. Arch Surg 102:424, 1971

Jones SA, Joergenson EJ: Closure of duodenal wall defects. Surgery 53:438, 1963

Kobold EE, Thal AP: A simple method for the management of experimental wounds of the duodenum. Surg Gynecol Obstet 116:340, 1963

Letton AH, Wilson JP: Traumatic severance of pancreas treated by Roux-Y anastomosis. Surg Gynecol Obstet 109:473, 1959

Moretz JA, Campbell DP, Parker DE et al: Significance of serum amylase level in evaluating pancreatic trauma. Am J Surg 130:739, 1975

Naffziger HC, McCorkle HJ: The recognition and management of acute trauma to the pancreas: With particular reference to the use of the serum amylase test. Ann Surg 118:594, 1943

Travers B: Rupture of the pancreas. Lancet xii:384, 1827

White RH, Benfield JR: Amylase in the management of pancreatic trauma. Arch Surg 105:152, 1972

Yellin AE, Rosoff L: Pancreatoduodenectomy for combined pancreatoduodenal injuries. Arch Surg 110:1177, 1975

Yellin AE, Vecchione TR, Donovan AJ: Distal pancreatectomy for pancreatic trauma. Am Surg 124:135, 1972

Joaquin S. Aldrete/Henry L. Laws

The Spleen

29

References to the spleen and speculation about its functions have appeared since 250 BC. Galen found a place for the spleen in his humoral theory of health and disease. Interesting functions were attributed to the spleen; it was believed to control anger, laughter, and even a runner's speed. During the flourishing periods of the Greek and later the Roman cultures, splenomegaly was recognized. Arataeus of Cappadocia (c. AD 150) believed, still within the humoral theory of medicine, that the spleen strained black blood or black bile; thus for the first time, the "filtering" function of the spleen was recognized. In 1659, Malpighi first described some of the microscopic anatomy of the spleen, including the corpuscles that bear his name.

Only scant references can be found during the Middle Ages to operations involving the spleen; most of them were performed to treat traumatic ruptures of this organ. The first nontraumatic splenectomy recorded in modern times was done in 1826 by Quittenbaum of Rostock, but it was not until 1881 that Spencer Wells reported for the first time the survival of a patient after splenectomy for spherocytosis. The pioneering formal chapter on surgery of the spleen was written in 1908 by Moynihan, who dealt primarily with traumatic and neoplastic lesions. Thirteen years later, the same author wrote a monograph on splenectomy, this time detailing the indications for this operation for the treatment of some hematologic diseases. As splenectomy was done with increasing frequency, its indications became more specific. In recent years, perhaps the most important development in surgery of the spleen has been the recognition that children subjected to splenectomy have a higher incidence of overwhelming and often fatal sepsis than the population with intact spleens.

EMBRYOLOGY AND GROSS ANATOMY

The spleen develops from several mesenchymal swellings in the dorsal mesogastrium. With growth, these masses coalesce and project to the left side. The point where the future spleen joins the dorsal mesogastrium, or greater omentum, gradually narrows and becomes the gastrosplenic ligament. By the end of the third gestational month, the spleen has almost reached its mature form.

The normal adult spleen is a purplish, rounded, flat, highly vascular organ situated deep in the left upper abdomen at the level of the 8th to the 11th ribs, tucked between the diaphragm, the gastric fundus, the splenic flexure of the colon, and the anterior surface of the left kidney (Fig. 29-1). The adult spleen weighs 100 g to 150 g, measures about 12 cm × 7 cm × 4 cm and can be palpated in only 5% of the normal population. It is attached to adjacent viscera and to the abdominal wall by numerous peritoneal folds or ligaments (Fig. 29-2) that are avascular normally but under pathologic circumstances, specifically portal hypertension, can carry large collateral veins. The spleen is encased in a capsule of peritoneum overlying a 1 mm to 2 mm fibroelastic layer that sends into the splenic parenchyma numerous fibrous bands (trabeculae) that form the framework of the spleen.

The splenic artery and vein run along the upper border of the body and tail of the pancreas. The artery enters the spleen at its hilum and branches along the trabeculae (trabecular arteries), which terminate in branches that enter the white and red pulps that extend peripherally to communicate through capillaries and sinuses with the more peripheral venous channels. The white pulp is composed of lymphatic tissue and lymphoid follicles containing mainly lymphocytes, plasma cells, and macrophages distributed throughout a reticular network. The marginal zone between the white and red pulps is a poorly defined vascular space of variable size. Sometimes it contains only plasma and at other times a variety of cellular elements or foreign materials. Abnormal cellular elements are often found sequestered in this zone.

The red pulp is made up of cords of reticular cells and sinuses forming a honeycombed vascular space. The sinuses lie between the cords of cells and provide an extensive net of channels from the arterial to the venous circulations (Fig. 29-3).

PHYSIOLOGY AND PATHOPHYSIOLOGY

Although the physiology and pathophysiology of the spleen is incompletely understood, recent research and clinical observations indicate that the spleen has unique and vital functions. Approximately 350 liters of blood flow through the spleen in a 24-hr period. Normal blood cellular elements usually pass rapidly through the spleen, but aged and abnormal blood cells, as well as foreign materials, are impeded or removed, strongly suggesting a remarkable ability to discriminate by the spleen. Chromium (^{51}Cr)-tagging experiments have shown that under normal circumstances few blood cells are filtered in one passage through the spleen. The bone marrow, however, does produce a number of cells with abnormal inclusion particles that usually appear in the circulation after the spleen has been removed. These include Howell-Jolly, Pappenheimer, and Heinz bodies. The spleen is capable of removing some of these nuclear remnants, leaving the parent erythrocyte intact.

The alterations in the erythrocyte that make it susceptible to removal or destruction by the spleen after 105 days in the circulation remain to be fully understood. Similarly, the enzyme activity, and therefore the metabolic capacity, of the red cell diminishes with aging of the cell. A variety of erythrocytes altered by intrinsic factors (membrane, hemoglobin, or enzymatic abnormalities) or extrinsic factors (antibody and nonantibody injury) may be prematurely removed by the spleen. On the other hand, the presence of a normal erythrocyte lifespan in asplenic subjects suggests that red cell aging occurs independently of splenic function. Normal leukocytes are removed from the circulation by the reticuloendothelial system, including the spleen. Neutrophils

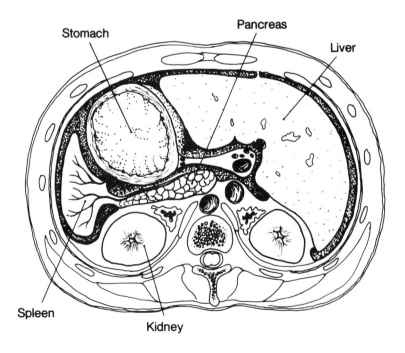

Fig. 29-1.   The spleen lies behind the stomach and beneath the diaphragm. The pancreas almost touches the splenic hilum. The spleen is also in close contact with the anterior portion of the upper pole of the left kidney.

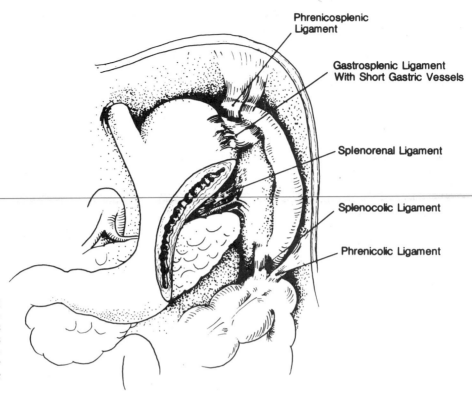

Fig. 29-2. The spleen is suspended by a number of ligamentous attachments to several of the nearby organs and structures. Since these ligaments attach to the splenic capsule, excessive traction during operation easily results in avulsion of the capsule with bleeding.

Fig. 29-3. Diagram of the spleen's circulation. The spleen is divided into multiple compartments by thin fibrous walls or trabeculae that are extensions of the fibrous capsule. The trabecular arteries and veins that are branches of the splenic artery and vein penetrate the spleen along the trabeculae, becoming the central artery, which is enclosed in a lymphatic sheath or white pulp. Further branching arterioles extend into the red pulp. Blood flows from them into the venous system through the sinuses. The sinuses then empty into pulp veins, which in turn empty into the trabecular veins.

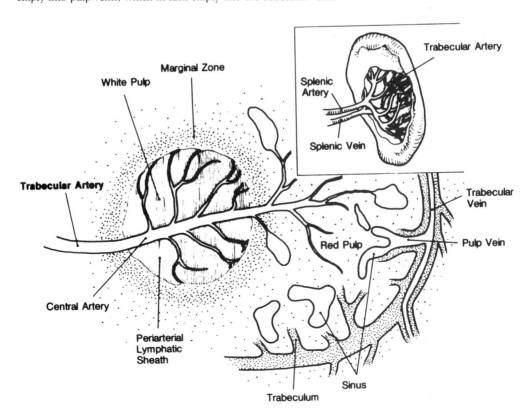

are removed from the circulation with a half-life of about 6 hr; thus, 85% of the neutrophils either emigrate into tissues or are destroyed within 24 hr. Platelets (thrombocytes) are also filtered out of the circulation by the spleen. Under normal circumstances, thrombocytes have a finite survival period in the circulation of about 10 days. One third of the total platelet pool is normally sequestered in the spleen. In the presence of splenomegaly and when platelets are coated by antibodies, a larger proportion or a faster rate of sequestration of these cells by the spleen takes place, leading to thrombocytopenia. The reticuloendothelial cells in the adult spleen are involved in the normal production of monocytes, lymphocytes, and plasma cells.

The spleen is also an important and even an essential line of defense when the host is invaded by blood-borne bacteria to which it has few or no preexisting antibodies. The unique splenic circulation makes it the main site of clearance of microorganisms and the initial site of synthesis of specific immunoglobulin M (IgM) antibody. The liver clears most of the well-opsonized bacteria from the blood, but the spleen, a more efficient filter than the liver, removes poorly opsonized bacteria more effectively. When no specific antibody is present to allow efficient liver uptake, clearance of blood-borne bacteria is delayed and depends on effective splenic function. The unique microcirculation of the spleen also facilitates the immune response to intravenously administered particulate antigens. When blood enters the spleen, the soluble antigens are skimmed off with much of the plasma to enter the arterioles of the white pulp. When the splenic microcirculation is impaired, as in sickle cell anemia, or when the spleen has been removed, the antibody response to blood-borne antigen is blunted, and serum IgM levels fall.

The spleen is also a major site of synthesis of tuftsin and properdin, two proteins that serve as opsonins. Serum levels of tuftsin, a basic tetrapeptide that coats blood polymorphonuclear leukocytes to promote phagocytosis, are subnormal after splenectomy. Serum levels of properdin, a vital component of the alternate pathway of complement activation, are also subnormal after splenectomy. The spleen can also remove parasites, such as the malarial organism, from the red blood cells.

DIAGNOSIS OF SPLENIC DISEASE

PHYSICAL EXAMINATION

The normal-sized spleen is almost always nonpalpable. An enlarged spleen, before it becomes palpable, may cause dullness to percussion above the left ninth intercostal space. Bimanual examination, with the left side of the patient tilted upward, will often help to differentiate an enlarged spleen with its typical notch from other palpable masses in the left upper abdomen, such as the left lobe of the liver, a pancreatic pseudocyst, an enlarged left kidney, or a colonic tumor.

RADIOGRAPHY

A normal spleen usually can be outlined on a supine x-ray film of the abdomen. In the same films, splenomegaly can be detected by the medial displacement of the stomach and the downward displacement of the transverse segment and splenic flexure of the colon. Selective splenic arteriography is useful when necessary to differentiate the spleen from nearby anatomic structures and to detect subcapsular hematomas.

IMAGING TECHNIQUES

Radioisotope scanning, sonography, and computed tomography (CT scanning) are of great assistance in clearly establishing the exact location and size of the spleen. Radioisotope scanning of the spleen provides an accurate method of outlining the organ, differentiating it from other masses in the left upper abdomen, and even detecting rapid changes in size. The most commonly used method is the technetium (^{99m}Tc–sulfur colloid) scan. It depends on the capacity of the spleen to take up and retain the radiocolloid. CT scan is an accurate and noninvasive method of assessing splenic size. Sonography is of comparable accuracy.

CELL SURVIVAL–TAGGING TECHNIQUES

Reduced red cell or platelet survival can be measured by labeling the patient's cells with ^{51}Cr and measuring its disappearance rate from the circulation. The role of the spleen in removing erythrocytes or thrombocytes can be assessed by measuring the ratio of radioactivity that accumulates in the liver, spleen, and heart during removal of the tagged cells. As a general rule, if the concentration of radioactivity appears to be greater in the spleen than in the liver, splenectomy may alleviate the hemolytic process under investigation.

CONSEQUENCES OF SPLENECTOMY

A relatively small number of cases of congenital absence of the spleen have been reported. The great majority of asplenic patients have had their spleens removed deliberately, for trauma, hematologic diseases, or, less commonly, as an incidental procedure during the course of a surgical intervention. Currently, it is well recognized that removal of the spleen is not innocuous. The peripheral blood smear of patients who have undergone splenectomy is recognizable because of the presence of numerous abnormal red cells, including those that contain Howell-Jolly bodies, siderocytes, target cells, and others with abnormal shapes. The reticulocyte count is only mildly elevated, but asplenic patients show a permanent abnormal reticulocyte response. The hemoglobin level is normal, and except in rare circumstances, the total red blood cell count as well as the estimated lifespan of erythrocytes in the circulation are within normal limits. Target cells temporarily appear shortly after splenectomy, suggesting a disproportionate shrinkage in erythrocyte volume until other tissue in the body takes over the function of the spleen. After splenectomy in patients without hematologic disease, anemia and polycythemia do not occur, and red cell survival remains unchanged. These facts suggest that the filtering function of the spleen is quickly assumed by remaining reticuloendothelial tissue.

After splenectomy a temporary leukocytosis, predominantly lymphocytosis, occurs, and the circulating levels of platelets rise, sometimes to more than one million per cubic millimeter. The cause of this thrombocytosis has never been adequately determined. One hypothesis is that it is simply a matter of decreasing sequestration and destruction of platelets. Another hypothesis is that splenectomy also removes a suppressor of bone marrow platelet production or release. Still another theory is that the bone marrow is geared to regulate the overall platelet mass at a certain size, and when a compartment normally containing a significant proportion of the platelet pool is removed, the overall platelet concentration rises. In most normal adult patients, the hematologic changes described above usually return to near normal after a few months following splenectomy. Some patients maintain an abnormal leukocyte response to stimuli, suggesting decreased defenses for infection. Because antibodies are normally produced by cells within the spleen, splenectomy can lead to a slight temporary reduction in antibody formation. In acquired hemolytic anemia, splenic leukopenia, and idiopathic thrombocytopenic purpura, antibodies to specific cellular elements are produced. Splenectomy then not only will remove an organ designed to sequester antibody-coated cells but will also reduce antibody production, at least temporarily.

It is now well established that the loss of the spleen renders some patients more susceptible to infections, and, although this complication afflicts only a small proportion of the asplenic population, nevertheless it appears to be a direct consequence of splenectomy.

HYPERSPLENISM

In an oversimplified manner, hypersplenism has been defined as sequestration and destruction of blood elements with reduction of circulating erythrocytes, leukocytes, or thrombocytes. Traditionally, hypersplenism has been categorized as primary and secondary. *Primary hypersplenism* includes a group of diseases in which there is splenic hyperfunction in response to a sustained and heavy work load. Under these conditions, the abnormal blood cells are removed so efficiently that the resulting cytopenia becomes of greater concern than the presence of the abnormal cells. *Secondary hypersplenism* is most often due to congestive splenomegaly caused by portal hypertension secondary to cirrhosis, or to thrombosis of the portal or splenic veins. Sometimes inflammatory diseases or neoplastic diseases involving the spleen (*e.g.,* Hodgkin's disease, lymphomas, leukemias) produce secondary hypersplenism.

Currently, it is clear that hypersplenism is a relatively imprecise term. Classically, it refers to splenomegaly; any combination of anemia, leukopenia, and thrombocytopenia; compensatory bone marrow hyperplasia; and improvement after splenectomy. Within this framework, however, different diseases may cause different forms of hypersplenism.

CAUSES OF PRIMARY HYPERSPLENISM

Congenital hemolytic anemias
    Hereditary spherocytosis
    Hereditary elliptocytosis
    Pyruvate kinase deficiency
    Hemoglobinopathies (*e.g.,* sickle cell anemia)
    Thalassemia
    Porphyria hematopoietica
Acquired hemolytic anemia ("autoimmune")
Idiopathic thrombocytopenic purpura
Thrombotic thrombocytopenic purpura
Primary splenic neutropenia
Primary splenic pancytopenia

An enlarged spleen can cause problems for the patient without meeting the aforementioned definition of hypersplenism. Furthermore, the spleen is usually not enlarged in thrombocytopenic purpura. Thus, hypersplenism can be redefined to mean that the spleen in question has become more harmful than beneficial. Examples of diseases in which massive splenomegaly causes symptoms without fulfilling the strict definition of hypersplenism include chronic myelocytic leukemia and agnogenic myeloid metaplasia.

The most commonly encountered form of secondary hypersplenism is that associated with portal hypertension, which is usually produced by hepatic cirrhosis and occasionally by splenic vein thrombosis. These cause pancytopenia because the normal splenic pool of blood cells is enlarged. Normally, about 30% of the blood platelets in the body are pooled in the spleen. In addition, the spleen contains approximately 20 ml of erythrocytes and an unknown but probably marginal fraction of granulocytes. When the spleen is greatly enlarged, however, there is considerably more pooling of these blood cells, and pancytopenia may result. When hypersplenism is caused by simple pooling, as in congestive splenomegaly, the leukopenia is often characterized by a "balanced" diminution, so that the ratio of polymorphonuclear leukocytes to lymphocytes and monocytes stays normal. Also, because the leukocytes may be available when needed, the risk of infection is not so great.

DIAGNOSTIC EVALUATION OF HYPERSPLENISM

SYMPTOMS AND SIGNS

The clinical findings of hypersplenism depend largely on the underlying disorder. They usually develop gradually, and the diagnosis is often made at a routine physical or laboratory examination. Some patients experience left upper quadrant fullness or discomfort; others have hematemesis due to bleeding gastroesophageal varices. Purpura, bruising, and diffuse mucous membrane bleeding are unusual symptoms unless thrombocytopenia is severe. Recurring infections and chronic leg ulcers are sometimes seen in patients with Felty's syndrome and severe leukopenia.

LABORATORY FINDINGS

The normocytic normochromic anemia is usually only moderately severe. Hemoglobin values below 10 g suggest one of the following complications: (1) chronic blood loss, possibly from esophageal varices secondary to portal hypertension; (2) simultaneous hemolysis in the liver; (3) autoimmune hemolytic anemia; or (4) marrow failure (as in cirrhosis). Secondary folic acid deficiency and megaloblastic anemia may develop. If the patient has a primary condition such as myelofibrosis or thalassemia, the red cells have the characteristic morphologic abnormalities of these disorders. Despite the anemia, the total red cell mass may be normal or even increased because so much blood is pooled in the enlarged spleen. In some cases, expansion of plasma volume aggravates the anemia. The reticulocyte count is usually slightly elevated. The white blood cell count is usually 2000 to 4000/mm³ but may be lower. The leukopenia is confined to the granulocytes, especially the polymorphonuclear cells. Platelet counts are usually about 100,000/mm³ but may fall much lower. The bone marrow shows various degrees of generalized hyperplasia.

HYPOSPLENISM

The concept of hyposplenism is not as time-honored as that of hypersplenism, but severe hyposplenism is a potentially lethal condition. The findings in the peripheral blood smear and hemograms of asplenic patients have been described in the earlier section on consequences of splenectomy. These hematologic clues should alert the physician to suspect hyposplenism. Confirmatory tests include splenic scan, quantification by interference-phase microscopy of red blood cells, surface pits or craters that are increased after splenectomy, and determination of splenic uptake of heat-damaged radio-labeled blood cells. Clinically, complete lack of uptake in the splenic area confirms the diagnosis of hyposplenism.

Another clinical prototype of hyposplenism is the child with sickle cell anemia who is vulnerable to overwhelming, often fatal, pneumococcemia. Ironically, the child is at greatest risk when the spleen is enlarged, not when it is later atrophic (autosplenectomy). Children with sickle cell anemia and enlarged spleens have functional asplenia. Transfusion can temporarily reverse this phenomenon, presumably by restoring the splenic and phagocytic activity to normal by reducing the load of irreversible sickle cells. As the child grows older, the spleen shrinks because of repeated infarcts. However, the child gains immunity to the different serotypes of pneumococcus, and more reliance can be placed on the liver for clearance of blood-borne pneumococci.

A wide variety of conditions is associated with hyposplenism. The classic association has been splenic atrophy with celiac sprue or idiopathic steatorrhea; more than 50 such cases have been reported. Although the mechanism of hyposplenism and these disorders remains unknown, it has been linked with the generalized lymphoreticular atrophy noted in celiac sprue.

Next to sickle cell anemia, perhaps the most convincing link between a disease and hyposplenism is ulcerative colitis. Although patients with ulcerative colitis do not have hyposplenism at the time of diagnosis, it develops in about 40% during the course of the disease, and the magnitude of the hyposplenism fluctuates with the activity of the colitis. Hyposplenism becomes more severe when the active colon becomes severely and totally involved with the colitis. This helps to explain the link between thrombocytosis and active severe ulcerative colitis. Patients with pancolitis and hyposplenism who require colectomy have a high risk of postoperative sepsis.

FULMINANT BACTEREMIA AND HYPOSPLENISM

The hyposplenic state is potentially lethal because of the risk of fulminant bacteremia. The risk is greatest in young children who have had splenectomy, especially for the first 2 years after surgery (80% of the cases) and when the disorder for which the splenectomy was required is a disease of the reticuloendothelial system. Fulminant septicemia seems rare after splenectomy for hereditary spherocytosis. In recent years, up to 50 cases of serious and often fatal postsplenectomy septicemia have been reported in adults, many of whom underwent splenectomy for trauma. Although the actual risk of fulminant bacteremia in these normal subjects remains unknown, some investigators have estimated it to be as high as 0.5% to 1% per year after splenectomy. The longest reported interval between incidental splenectomy and overwhelming bacteremia has been

25 years. In the typical instance, a previously healthy, normal adult has a high fever, usually after a brief mild upper respiratory tract infection, and within hours experiences shock and disseminated intravascular coagulation that often proves fatal. These patients may have no obvious site of pneumococcal infection. However, it is speculated that the nasopharynx may be the site of infection and that a synergistic viral infection is sufficient to convert an asymptomatic carrier state into a fulminant pneumococcemia. In this fulminant syndrome, blood levels of pneumococci reach extraordinary proportions, which are seen only in patients with hyposplenism, and the capsular polysaccharides of these organisms trigger bacterial shock and disseminated intravascular coagulation. The peripheral blood smear shows vacuolated polymorphonuclear leukocytes, thrombocytopenia, and even pneumococci, both free and within polymorphonuclear leukocytes. Although the pneumococcus has accounted for most cases, there have been reports, especially in children, of fatal septicemia caused by meningococcus, *Hemophilus influenzae*, and *Escherichia coli.*

A hypothesis to explain the infrequency of fatal pneumococcemia after splenectomy for trauma has suggested that certain patients preserve some splenic function originating in the splenic tissue implants (splenosis) that often occur at the time of traumatic splenic rupture. Although this novel suggestion merits study, there are reports in children and adults of lethal postsplenectomy septicemia despite the presence of at least 25 g of residual splenic tissue at autopsy. Furthermore, animal work has shown that splenic autotransplants, although they restore the normal immunoglobulin response to intravenously administered particulate antigen, do not protect the organism from death from intravenous pneumococci. The doses of antigen in these studies, however, were high.

SPLENOMEGALY

Palpable spleens are not always abnormal, and hyperfunctioning spleens are not always palpable. Patients with emphysema and low hemidiaphragms commonly have palpable spleens. One study showed that 63 (3%) of 2200 healthy college freshmen had palpable spleens, and a more recent study showed that almost 5% of hospital patients with normal spleens by scan were thought to have palpable spleens by their physicians. In contrast, clinical splenomegaly is rarely noted in idiopathic (autoimmune) thrombocytopenia purpura, despite avid destruction of antibody-coated platelets by the spleen.

Mild splenomegaly occurs with many diseases. Rather than making a list, it is more productive to consider the mechanisms of splenomegaly and then the relatively few diseases that cause either massive splenomegaly (10 times or more its usual weight of about 200 g) or hypersplenism. Table 29-1 presents some postulated mechanisms of splenomegaly and gives examples of common diseases in each category. The most common cause of splenomegaly is liver disease. "Work hypertrophy," if it exists, is due to increased removal of diseased cellular elements. Cirrhosis and splenic vein thrombosis produce splenomegaly by venous congestion. In the myeloproliferative disorders, such as myeloid metaplasia and polycythemia vera, splenomegaly is caused by extramedullary hematopoiesis. In chronic myelocytic leukemia, splenomegaly occurs mainly because of leukemic infiltration. Splenomegaly sometimes results when the spleen

TABLE 29-1 **CLASSIFICATION OF SPLENOMEGALY ACCORDING TO ETIOLOGIC MECHANISM**

MECHANISM	COMMON EXAMPLES
Increased erythrocyte destruction	Spherocytosis, thalassemia major, pyruvate kinase deficiency
Possible immune reaction	Felty's syndrome, infectious mononucleosis
Congestion	Cirrhosis, splenic vein thrombosis
Myeloproliferation	Chronic myelocytic leukemia, myeloid metaplasia
Infiltration	Sarcoidosis, amyloid, Gaucher's disease
Neoplastic involvement	Lymphoma, chronic lymphocytic leukemia, metastatic cancer

TABLE 29-2 **INDICATIONS FOR SPLENECTOMY 1966–1975 AT THE HOSPITALS OF THE UNIVERSITY OF ALABAMA IN BIRMINGHAM**

	NO. OF CASES	PERCENT
Trauma	223	47
Iatrogenic or incidental procedures	102	21
Diagnosis and staging for Hodgkin's disease	68	14
Hematologic disease	88	18
TOTAL	481	100

is infiltrated by granulomatous tissue or by amyloidosis, or when the reticuloendothelial cells contain an indigestible lipid, such as glucocerebroside in Gaucher's disease. Also, neoplastic disorders such as lymphoma, chronic leukemias, and, very rarely, metastatic cancer can cause splenomegaly. Because the spleen apparently lacks afferent lymphatics, lymphatic spread of cancer to the spleen is rare. Even carcinomas that spread to the spleen by way of the splenic artery rarely grow large, suggesting that the rich lymphoid tissue of the human spleen may suppress growth of carcinoma. Lastly, splenomegaly may arise from cysts, hemangiomas, or other malformations.

MASSIVE SPLENOMEGALY

In the United States, relatively few diseases now cause massive splenomegaly as a presenting or early feature. The largest spleens, weighing up to 5000 g, are usually found in the myeloproliferative disorders, agnogenic myeloid metaplasia, and chronic myeloid leukemia. Hairy cell leukemia is a newly recognized cause of massive splenomegaly and hypersplenism. Isolated splenic lymphoma causes splenomegaly, and prior reports of this disorder probably include some patients with hairy cell leukemia. Hypersplenism is occasionally the presenting feature of Gaucher's disease. In the tropics, splenomegaly (tropical splenomegaly) results from a hyperimmune response to malaria, in which serum IgM levels are elevated. The very advanced stages of chronic lymphocytic leukemia and polycythemia vera often cause considerable splenomegaly, as does long-standing thalassemia major. Finally, rare causes of massive splenomegaly include sarcoidosis, in which hypersplenism may be a presenting or major feature, and chronic congestive splenomegaly.

INDICATIONS FOR SPLENECTOMY

Removal of the spleen can be an effective therapeutic measure under the right circumstances, as in a variety of congenital, acquired, traumatic, inflammatory, degenerative, and neoplastic disease processes involving the spleen and its blood vessels. Until the present, the most common reason for splenectomy has been trauma (Table 29-2).

During the last 30 years, the indications for splenectomy have changed. Splenectomy has become almost routine for the staging of Hodgkin's disease. Although splenectomy is often effective in controlling hypersplenism, the total number of patients undergoing splenectomy for this reason has declined in many medical centers. In the last 10 years, the increasing frequency of splenectomy as part of a staging celiotomy for Hodgkin's disease has also influenced the statistics of indications for splenectomy. The mortality and morbidity attributable to or coexisting with incidental splenectomy cannot be ignored, particularly when splenectomy is performed for this reason in as many as 20% of cases.

In systemic diseases involving the spleen, the indications for splenectomy raise some controversy. Some of the so-called medical indications for splenectomy are listed in Table 29-3. In many instances, splenectomy controls but does not cure the disease; a good example is hereditary spherocytosis. However, the patient lives a normal life despite the spherocytes present in the blood. Similarly, the spleen is the dominant organ of cell destruction and a source of antibody production in autoimmune thrombocytopenia and in autoimmune hemolytic anemia of the warm antibody type. In these disorders splenectomy offers good control of the disease in up to 70% of patients, although low-grade destruction of the blood cells continues in other reticuloendothelial organs such as the liver. When the spleen is removed as part of a staging celiotomy for Hodgkin's disease

TABLE 29-3 **MEDICAL INDICATIONS FOR SPLENECTOMY**

To control basic disease
Hereditary spherocytosis
Autoimmune thrombocytopenia or hemolysis
Hairy cell leukemia

If hypersplenic symptoms are chronic or severe
Felty's syndrome
Agnogenic myeloid metaplasia
Thalassemia major
Gaucher's disease
Splenomegaly with hemodialysis
Splenic vein thrombosis

To stage the basic disease and select most appropriate treatment
Hodgkin's disease

in children, it involves a risk of lethal septicemia as high as 10%. Splenic vein thrombosis, usually caused by pancreatitis, is a cause of hypersplenism and variceal bleeding, which can be cured by splenectomy.

Other reasons have been advocated for splenectomy, including discomfort from massive splenomegaly; facilitation of treatment, using splenectomy as an adjunctive measure; splenomegaly, using splenectomy as a diagnostic maneuver; and fever of undetermined origin. These remain disputable as established indications for splenectomy because factual data proving their beneficial effect are not available. Table 29-4 shows the indications for splenectomy according to the expected degree of benefit obtained from splenectomy. To select objectively the indications for splenectomy under different circumstances, it is essential to know the alternatives available.

TABLE 29-4 CURRENT INDICATIONS FOR SPLENECTOMY ACCORDING TO EXPECTED DEGREE OF BENEFIT

Splenectomy almost always indicated
Primary splenic tumor (rare)
Splenic abscess (rare)
Hereditary spherocytosis (congenital hemolytic anemia)

Splenectomy usually indicated
Severe splenic injury (common)
Primary hypersplenism
Chronic idiopathic thrombocytopenic purpura
Ovalocytosis or spherocytosis with hemolysis
Splenic vein thrombosis causing bleeding esophageal varices

Splenectomy sometimes indicated
Autoimmune hemolytic disease
Thrombotic thrombocytopenic purpura
Nonspherocytic congenital hemolytic anemias (*e.g.,* pyruvate kinase deficiency)
Hemoglobin H disease
Hodgkin's disease (for staging)
Hairy cell leukemia
Felty's syndrome
Certain patients with unstable hemoglobin

Splenectomy rarely indicated
Chronic lymphatic leukemia
Lymphosarcoma
Hodgkin's disease (except for staging)
Myelofibrosis
Thalassemia major and intermedia
Splenic artery aneurysm
Sickle cell anemia
Congestive splenomegaly and hypersplenism due to portal hypertension
Sarcoidosis
Splenomegaly with hemodialysis
Gaucher's disease

Splenectomy not indicated
Asymptomatic hypersplenism
Splenomegaly with infection
Splenomegaly associated with elevated IgM
Acute leukemia
Agranulocytosis

HEMATOLOGIC DISEASES TREATABLE BY SPLENECTOMY

HEMOLYTIC ANEMIAS

The category of hemolytic anemia includes a spectrum of diseases characterized by accelerated destruction of mature erythrocytes. Hemolytic anemias can be divided into two groups—congenital and acquired. Congenital anemias are due to an intrinsic abnormality of the erythrocytes, and acquired anemias are usually related to an extracorpuscular factor acting on an intrinsically normal cell. In both types, there is a decreased survival period of the erythrocytes, which can be documented by measuring their rate of disappearance from the patient's circulation.

HEREDITARY SPHEROCYTOSIS

Also known as congenital hemolytic jaundice or familial hemolytic anemia, hereditary spherocytosis is transmitted as an autosomal dominant trait and is the most common of the symptomatic familial hemolytic anemias. Occasionally, the diagnosis is not made until late in adult life, but it is usually discovered in the first three decades. The basic defect is a defective erythrocyte membrane, which results in a smaller, very thick cell with increased osmotic fragility and a rigid spherical, nondeformable shape. The membrane abnormality causes premature destruction of the erythrocyte.

The prominent clinical features are splenomegaly, anemia, and frequently jaundice. Periodic and sudden increases in the intensity of the anemia and jaundice may occur, and rare, fatal crises have been described. Cholelithiasis of the biliary pigment type occurs in 30% to 60% of patients but is rare in children below 10 years of age.

The usual complaints are easy fatigability and fullness and discomfort in the left upper abdomen due to the enlarged spleen. However, the diagnosis is usually made during a family survey when the patient is asymptomatic.

Diagnosis can usually be established by the peripheral blood smear, which shows the spherocytic-shaped erythrocytes that are thicker and smaller in diameter than normal. The red cell count (3–4 million/mm³) and hemoglobin (9–12 g/dl) may be moderately reduced. The reticulocyte count is often increased from 5% to 20%. The indirect serum

---

CONGENITAL HEMOLYTIC ANEMIA	
Etiology	Red cell membrane defect with excessive splenic red cell destruction
	Spherocytosis, elliptocytosis, other genetic red cell disorders
Dx	Anemia, reticulocytosis, jaundice, splenomegaly
	Seek associated gallstone
	Peripheral blood smear (altered RBC shapes)
	Osmotic fragility tests
	Red cell survival
Rx	Age 4 or less: supportive transfusion
	Over age 4: Splenectomy, cholecystectomy if gallstones are present

bilirubin and stool urobilinogen values are usually elevated, and the serum haptoglobin value is usually decreased or absent. The Coombs' test is negative. Osmotic fragility is increased; hemolysis of 5% to 10% of cells may be observed at saline concentrations of 0.6%. Infusion of the patient's own red blood cells labeled with ^{51}Cr shows a greatly shortened red cell lifespan and sequestration in the spleen. Normal erythrocytes labeled with ^{51}Cr have a normal lifespan when transfused into a spherocytotic patient, indicating that splenic function is normal.

Splenectomy is the only treatment for hereditary spherocytosis, even when the anemia is fully controlled and the patient is asymptomatic. In the presence of cholelithiasis, cholecystectomy should be done after the spleen has been removed. A search should be made for accessory spleens, and those found should be removed. Splenectomy corrects the anemia and jaundice in all patients. The increased osmotic fragility, the spherocytosis, and the membrane abnormalities persist, but the erythrocyte lifespan becomes nearly normal.

HEREDITARY NONSPHEROCYTIC HEMOLYTIC ANEMIA

Hemolytic anemia of the hereditary nonspherocytic type is a heterogeneous group of hemolytic anemias caused by inherited intrinsic red cell defects. Included in this group are (1) enzyme deficiencies in anaerobic glycolytic pathways, the prototype of which is pyruvate-kinase (PK) deficiency, and (2) enzyme deficiencies in the hexosemonophosphate shunt, the prototype of which is glucose-6-phosphate dehydrogenase (G6PD) deficiency. These deficiencies render the cells susceptible to increased hemolysis. PK deficiency is usually manifest in early childhood with anemia, jaundice, reticulocytosis, erythroid hyperplasia of the marrow, and normal osmotic fragility. Cholelithiasis is also frequently encountered.

Most patients maintain hemoglobin levels of over 8 g/dl, are free of symptoms, and require no treatment. In the presence of severe anemia, multiple blood transfusions are required. Splenectomy, while not curative, may ameliorate some of these conditions, especially PK deficiency. Splenectomy is not beneficial for G6PD deficiency.

HEREDITARY ELLIPTOCYTOSIS

Also known as ovalocytosis, elliptocytosis is a familial disorder that usually exists as a harmless trait. Normally, up to 15% of the cells in a peripheral blood smear are oval or elliptic; however, if 50% to 90% of the erythrocytes have these deformities, clinical manifestations indistinguishable from those noted with hereditary spherocytosis may occur. Faulty permeability of the erythrocyte membrane is responsible for the abnormal shape and increased destruction by the spleen. Symptomatic patients will benefit from splenectomy and cholecystectomy if gallstones are found. The erythrocyte defect persists after splenectomy, but the hemolysis and anemia return to normal.

THALASSEMIA MAJOR

Also known as Cooley's or Mediterranean anemia, thalassemia major is transmitted as a dominant trait and involves primarily a defective hemoglobin synthesis caused by a structural defect in one of the globin chains of the hemoglobin molecule that produces abnormal erythrocytes (e.g., target cells). Heterozygotes usually have minor anemia (thalassemia minor); however, starting early in infancy, homozygotes have severe chronic anemia associated with jaundice, hepatosplenomegaly (often massive), retarded growth, and enlargement of the head.

In the United States, most patients are of southern European origin. Clinical manifestations of thalassemia major usually occur in the first year of life. The manifestations of thalassemia minor vary. Most of these patients live a normal life, but some have a more severe expression of their disease (thalassemia intermedia) and generally have signs and symptoms attributable to mild anemia, chronic mild jaundice, and moderate splenomegaly. The peripheral blood smear reveals hypochromic, microcytic anemia with target cells, nucleated red cells, reticulocytosis, and leukocytosis. Gallstones are present in about 25% of patients. Features that are helpful in establishing the diagnosis are the presence of increased quantities of A_2 and fetal hemoglobin. Importantly, both parents should have evidence of thalassemia minor.

Splenectomy is indicated only in symptomatic patients requiring frequent blood transfusions. Although splenectomy does not modify the basic hematologic disorder, it may decrease the hemolytic process significantly, reducing the frequency of needed transfusion.

SICKLE CELL DISEASE

This hereditary hemolytic anemia, which is seen predominantly but not exclusively in blacks, is characterized by the presence of sickle and crescent-shaped erythrocytes. It is a hemoglobinopathy in which the normal Hb A is replaced by an abnormal form of hemoglobin called sickle hemoglobin (Hb S). Hb F is also mildly elevated in some cases. Combinations of Hb S with other hemoglobin variants also occur owing to an abnormal trait inherited from each parent (*e.g.*, Hb S/Hb C or Hb S/thalassemia with high percentages of Hb S). Circulatory stasis occurs, leading ultimately to thrombosis in small vessels and then to ischemia, necrosis, and organ fibrosis. The role of the spleen in sickle cell anemia is not clear. Early in the course of the disease, the spleen becomes enlarged, but often after some time it undergoes infarction and contraction, resulting in obliteration of splenic function (autosplenectomy).

The diagnosis is established by the presence of anemia, the characteristic sickle cells in blood smears, high levels of Hb S in hemoglobin electrophoresis, positive sickle cell preparation, and the presence of the trait in both parents. Cholelithiasis is often found as well. For most patients, only palliative and supportive treatment is possible. Splenectomy may offer benefit only in a few selected patients in whom excessive splenic sequestration of red cells is demonstrated. Certain groups of patients with unstable hemoglobin values benefit from splenectomy.

IDIOPATHIC AUTOIMMUNE HEMOLYTIC ANEMIA

In idiopathic autoimmune hemolytic anemia, the lifespan of a presumably normal erythrocyte is shortened when exposed to an endogenous hemolytic mechanism. The presence of antibodies reacting with the patient's normal red cells has been suggested as the autoimmune reaction that produces this disease. Autoimmune hemolytic anemia may be encountered at any age but occurs more frequently after the age of 50 and twice as often in women. Mild jaundice is often present. Splenomegaly is found in half and gallstones in a quarter of all cases. The detection of hemolysis is made by demonstrating the presence of anemia and sustained reticulocytosis accompanied by the products of red cell destruction in the blood, urine, and stool. The bone marrow is hypercellular with an increase in erythroid precursors. The direct Coombs' test documents the presence of autoantibodies in the erythrocytes. Excessive splenic sequestration of ^{51}Cr-tagged red cells, which occurs in about 80% of patients, offers a guide for the selection of patients who may respond favorably to splenectomy.

Occasionally, the disease runs an acute, self-limiting course, and no treatment is necessary. If anemia becomes severe, corticosteroids and blood transfusions may be required. Immunosuppressive drugs such as azathioprine have also been used for treatment of these patients. Splenectomy should be considered when treatment with steroids or immunosuppressives has been ineffective or is not feasible.

IDIOPATHIC THROMBOCYTOPENIC PURPURA

Idiopathic thrombocytopenic purpura (ITP) is a hemorrhagic syndrome characterized by a decreased number of circulating platelets, abundant megakaryocytes in the bone marrow, and a shortened platelet lifespan; it has an immunologic pathogenesis. The term ITP includes a number of disorders involving purpura secondary to drug or toxic reactions, resulting in much confusion. Furthermore, purpura and thrombocytopenic states resulting from viral and bacterial infections, lymphoproliferative disorders, and disseminated lupus erythematosus have also been included under the term ITP. However, as the name implies, the etiology is unknown, and currently the term ITP should be reserved exclusively for disease in which the well-known causes of secondary thrombocytopenia cannot be identified.

Most patients with the chronic form of the disease have platelet-agglutinating antibodies. A circulating antiplatelet factor, probably an antibody, can often be demonstrated. Normal platelets are rapidly destroyed when they are transfused into patients with ITP. The onset may be acute, with extensive petechiae and ecchymosis often associated with bleeding from the gums, gastrointestinal tract, and genitourinary tract. The acute form is most common in children under 8 years of age. The chronic form, which is more common, may start at any age and is three times more common in women. It begins insidiously with a history of easy bruisability and menorrhagia. Cyclic remissions and exacerbations may continue for several years, but the thrombocytopenia is frequently persistent. Owing to the thrombocytopenia, the bleeding time is prolonged, capillary fragility (Rumpel-Leede test) is increased, and clot retraction capability is poor. Usually, other aspects of coagulation function are normal.

Corticosteroids are indicated in patients with moderate to severe purpura of short duration. Steroids increase the platelet count in 75% of patients which will avert the danger of severe hemorrhage. Corticosteroids produce sustained remission in about 20% of adults. Because in patients with ITP the spleen not only sequestrates and removes coated platelets but may also contribute to the production of antiplatelet antibodies and may even have some suppressive effect on the maturation or release of thrombocytes by the bone marrow, splenectomy is the most effective form of therapy and is indicated for patients who do not respond to corticosteroids. Intracranial bleeding indicates a need for emergency splenectomy. Splenectomy produces a sustained remission in about 70% of patients.

THROMBOTIC THROMBOCYTOPENIC PURPURA

Thrombotic thrombocytopenic purpura (TTP) is an acute, often fatal disease involving primarily the arterioles or capillaries. However, there are associated hematologic abnormalities that may respond favorably to splenectomy. Classically, five clinical features have been described for TTP: (1) fever, (2) thrombocytopenic purpura, (3) hemolytic anemia, (4) neurologic abnormalities, and (5) renal dysfunction. The cause is unknown, but autoimmunity is the most probable hypothesis. Anemia is often severe, and hepatomegaly and splenomegaly occur in 35% of cases.

The clinical diagnosis can be confirmed only by biopsy, which shows a characteristic vascular lesion located at the arteriocapillary junctions. Neurologic manifestations due to involvement of small cerebral vessels are frequent and tend to fluctuate rapidly. Intracerebral hemorrhage is a common cause of death.

In most untreated cases, the disease has a fulminating course and a fatal outcome. There have been reports of remissions following treatment with heparin, corticosteroids, dextran, fibrinolytic agents, antimetabolites, plasmapheresis, or splenectomy, but the long-term survival rate is unpredictable with any form of treatment. Higher survival rates have been obtained with treatment combining high doses of corticosteroids with prompt splenectomy. The efficacy of plasmapheresis is currently being investigated.

SPLENIC NEUTROPENIA AND SPLENIC PANCYTOPENIA

Splenic neutropenia and splenic pancytopenia are two rare conditions of unknown etiology that usually are grouped under the term primary hypersplenism. These diseases are characterized by splenomegaly, leukopenia, or varying degrees of pancytopenia; the bone marrow is normal or hyperplastic. The clinical manifestations include fever, recurrent infections, purpura, and pallor. Corticosteroids are of questionable therapeutic value. The diagnosis is difficult to establish firmly, and lymphoma or lymphoproliferative disorders are hard to exclude. Splenectomy is usually effective in controlling these diseases.

IDIOPATHIC THROMBOCYTOPENIC PURPURA	
Etiology	Autoimmune platelet destruction by antiplatelets
	Antibody and reticuloendothelial (splenic) clearance
	Postviral, drug-induced, collagen-vascular associations
Dx	Bleeding diathesis: mucous membrane hemorrhage, petechiae, hemarthrosis, etc.
	Normal prothrombin, partial thromboplastin, activated thrombin times
	Decreased platelet counts (<100,000/mm³)
	Bone marrow has increased megakaryocytes
	Decreased platelet survival
Rx	Await spontaneous remission in mild cases
	Corticosteroid treatment in severe cases
	Splenectomy for corticosteroid failures
	Immunosuppression

MYELOID METAPLASIA

A proliferative disorder of unknown etiology, myeloid metaplasia is often referred to as agnogenic myeloid metaplasia. It is closely related to myelofibrosis, polycythemia vera, and myeloid leukemia. The bone marrow is progressively replaced by fibrous tissue, although early in the disease it can be hyperplastic with less fibrosis. There is a leukoerythroblastic blood reaction, and the spleen is usually very large, hard, and irregular. Extramedullary hematopoiesis develops, mainly in the spleen and liver. Symptoms are usually those of anemia and splenomegaly. Late in the course of the disease, spontaneous bleeding, secondary infections, spleen infarcts, and bone pain are frequently encountered.

Hepatomegaly is present in 75% of cases, and overt portal hypertension sometimes develops. Secondary hypersplenism is common and may lead to thrombocytopenia and hemolytic anemia. About 30% of the patients are asymptomatic and require no treatment at the time of diagnosis. When anemia and splenomegaly produce symptoms, transfusions are necessary and splenectomy should be considered. Splenectomy is also indicated when massive splenomegaly produces severe discomfort; however, it should not be undertaken until the patient develops thrombocytopenia (platelets <100,000/mm³). Otherwise, rebound thrombocytosis may occur, which can result in thrombosis or hemorrhage.

FELTY'S SYNDROME

The triad of chronic, deforming rheumatoid arthritis, splenomegaly, and granulocytopenia, which occurs in up to 1% of patients with rheumatoid arthritis, may represent a unique variant of hypersplenism in which the spleen appears to be acting as if it were a giant lymph node. Mild anemia or thrombocytopenia (or both) have been noted in most cases. Gastric achlorhydria is common, as are extreme susceptibility to infections and sometimes leg ulcers.

Possible explanations for the granulocytopenia of Felty's syndrome include (1) decreased marrow granulopoiesis, (2) increased margination of granulocytes from the peripheral blood, (3) increased splenic sequestration of granulocytes, and (4) antigranulocyte antibodies. Granulocytes in Felty's syndrome may be coated with immunoglobulin, which is either an antigranulocyte antibody or part of an immune complex adsorbed to granulocytes.

Corticosteroids and splenectomy have been used to reverse the neutropenia in order to reduce the susceptibility to infection. The response to steroids is usually not long-lasting, and splenectomy for Felty's syndrome has long been debatable. A number of studies show good long-term results after splenectomy. Although it is not unanimous, common opinion holds that splenectomy is the treatment of choice for patients with this syndrome. Splenectomy at least remains the standard against which to test proposed newer therapies such as testosterone, lithium, and gold.

SARCOIDOSIS

Sarcoidosis affects mainly young adults. Among the vague symptoms are nocturnal diaphoresis, low-grade fever, dyspnea, or a combination of these. Skin lesions appear in about 50% of the patients, and generalized lymphadenopathy is frequent. Hepatomegaly and splenomegaly are present in about 25% of patients, suggesting involvement of these organs. About 20% of patients with splenomegaly develop the manifestations of hypersplenism, particularly thrombocytopenic purpura, but hemolytic anemia, neutropenia, pancytopenia, and spontaneous splenic rupture have also been observed. Splenectomy should be considered for such patients to correct the hematologic abnormality.

CHRONIC LEUKEMIA

The spleen can be involved in various stages of the different kinds of leukemia, particularly in the chronic myeloid and lymphoid types. In these circumstances, manifestations of secondary hypersplenism may be apparent, and splenectomy may be suggested, either as a palliative measure or to facilitate or enhance the effectiveness of more direct treatment such as chemotherapy. Current data show that splenectomy for palliation of advanced chronic myeloid and lymphoid leukemias has produced only marginal gains in survival with considerable operative morbidity. Although it may be helpful in selected individual cases, at this time there is no evidence that early splenectomy prolongs overall survival in chronic leukemia.

HAIRY CELL LEUKEMIA

Hairy cell leukemia is an uncommon form of chronic leukemia (leukemic reticuloendotheliosis). Serious infections develop in approximately 40% of the patients. Bacterial infections are linked with granulocytopenia and opportunistic fungal and tuberculosis infections. Splenic histology in this disease shows massive congestion of the red pulp; the characteristic pancytopenia may occur because this large mass of rigid cells cannot easily traverse the red pulp. Chemotherapy has not yet been shown to prolong the survival of patients with this disease, so splenectomy is still the treatment of choice.

CIRRHOSIS AND PORTAL HYPERTENSION

Approximately 60% of patients with cirrhosis develop splenomegaly, and 15% develop hypersplenism. Splenomegaly is due partly to elevated portal pressures and passive congestion, but other factors must be involved because splenic size does not correlate well with the severity of the cirrhosis or with the magnitude of elevation of the portal vein pressure. The hypersplenism of cirrhosis is seldom of clinical significance; anemia and thrombocytopenia are usually mild and cannot be considered as indications for splenectomy.

When portal decompression becomes necessary because of massive bleeding from esophageal varices that complicate the cirrhotic state, the selection of the type of shunt should be made without considering the presence of hypersplenism. Any procedure that lowers the portal pressure tends to improve the thrombocytopenia and anemia and reduces the size of the spleen. It is very rare for hypersplenism to develop after a portal systemic shunt. Bleeding esophageal varices resulting from thrombosis of the splenic vein, usually in association with pancreatitis, can be successfully treated with splenectomy and devascularization of the gastric fundus and lower esophagus. In some other cases of extrahepatic portal occlusion—specifically, thrombosis of the extrahepatic portal vein—surgical decompression of the portal system is usually not feasible. When recurrent and severe variceal bleeding becomes a problem, devascularization of the gastroesophageal region is indicated. Whether splenectomy should be performed also remains controversial owing to lack of factual information.

PORPHYRIA ERYTHROPOIETICA

Porphyria erythropoietica is a congenital disorder of the erythrocyte pyrrole metabolism. This disease, which is transmitted as a recessive trait, is characterized by excessive deposition of porphyrins in tissues, resulting in pronounced sensitivity to light and severe bullous dermatitis. Premature erythrocyte destruction within the spleen contributes to severe anemia. When the disease is complicated by hemolysis or splenomegaly, splenectomy is usually followed not only by improvement of the anemia but also by a decrease in the concentration of porphyrins in the red cells, bone marrow, and urine.

SPLENOMEGALY WITH HEMODIALYSIS

Recent information suggests that hypersplenism develops in 5% to 10% of patients with end-stage renal disease who are being treated with long-term hemodialysis. Hypersplenism in these patients apparently results from "combined work" hypertrophy. The reticuloendothelial system of the spleen is hypertrophied because of accelerated red blood cell destruction, perhaps partly attributable to the defect in uremia and the red cell hexose monophosphate shunt, and the immune system of the spleen is hypertrophied apparently because of repeated viral infections including hepatitis or antigenic challenge from blood transfusions or dialysis. In patients with extreme hypersplenism, splenectomy should be considered.

GAUCHER'S DISEASE

A familial disorder, Gaucher's disease is characterized by abnormal storage or retention of β-glucocerebrosidase in reticuloendothelial cells. Proliferation and enlargement of these cells produces enlargement of the spleen, liver, and lymph nodes. The disease is generally discovered in childhood but may become evident either early in infancy or late in adult life. Usually the earlier the symptoms appear, the more severe the disease. The adult form of the disease is often undetected.

The main clinical manifestation may be an awareness of a progressively enlarging abdominal mass, which is primarily caused by splenomegaly and, to a lesser extent, by hepatomegaly. A yellowish brown pigmentation of the head and extremities occurs in 45% to 75% of cases. Bone pain and pathologic fractures may develop in long-standing cases. Sequestration by the spleen of formed blood elements may occur in a number of patients. Moderate to severe thrombocytopenia and normocytic anemia are almost always present, and often there is mild leukopenia. Pancytopenia is thought to be caused by increased pooling due to the increased reticuloendothelial cell function with fibrocytosis of platelets and by a dilution anemia in which a flow-induced portal hypertension expands the portal vascular space, decreases the effective intravascular volume, and causes an acceleration of albumin synthesis and expansion of the plasma volume. This dilution anemia is also thought to occur in certain other varieties of giant splenomegaly. The age-dependent adult type is often manifested by mild splenomegaly and hemolysis. In patients with hypersplenism

and massive splenomegaly, splenectomy is almost uniformly beneficial in correcting the hematologic disorder, but there is no evidence that the operation influences the course of the basic disease.

SPLENECTOMY AS PART OF STAGING CELIOTOMY FOR HODGKIN'S DISEASE

Advances in the therapy of Hodgkin's disease, utilizing radiation, multidrug chemotherapy, or both, have greatly improved the outlook of victims of this disease. Whereas in the 1950s only 15% of patients could anticipate a 5-year survival, now 85% can expect to live this long. A major step in improving therapy was the development of a rational classification of the disease based on the stage of involvement. Table 29-5 depicts the classification currently used. It was established by Carbone and associates at the University of Michigan and called the Ann Arbor Classification.

In most patients, Hodgkin's disease initially affects the mediastinal or cervical lymph nodes. The disease almost always spreads from a single nodal site in a stepwise fashion to contiguous lymph nodes. Below the mediastinum and diaphragm the disease spreads contiguously to the lymph nodes in the upper abdomen, specifically those around the celiac trunk. At present, clinical methods of assessment short of celiotomy cannot accurately estimate the presence or extent of abdominal involvement. Lymphangiography for this purpose has not proved to be sufficiently reliable. Ultrasonography and CT scanning may in the future prove to be useful in this regard.

Staging celiotomy is usually performed on most patients over the age of 15 who have clinical Stage I or II disease and in patients with Stage III-A disease. At celiotomy, about 25% of patients who have clinical Stage I or II disease are found to have unsuspected disease in the abdomen. Patients with unequivocal evidence of Stage III-B or Stage IV disease as manifested by hepatic or bone marrow involvement usually do not benefit from staging celiotomy. The presence of splenic involvement changes the clinical stage from I or II to at least III. Celiotomy for staging is indicated only when its results may influence therapy. When Hodgkin's disease involves the bone marrow or viscera other than the

TABLE 29-5   ANN ARBOR STAGING CLASSIFICATION FOR HODGKIN'S DISEASE

STAGE*	DEFINITION
0	No detectable disease due to prior excisional biopsy
I	Involvement of a single lymph node region
II	Involvement of two or more lymph node regions; limited to one side of diaphragm
III	Involvement on both sides of diaphragm but limited to the lymph nodes, spleen, or Waldeyer's ring
IV	Involvement of bone, bone marrow, lung parenchyma, pleura, liver, skin, gastrointestinal tract, CNS, kidney, or sites other than lymph nodes, spleen, or Waldeyer's ring

* All stages are subclassified to describe the absence (A) or presence (B) of systemic symptoms, (*e.g.*, fever, more than 10% weight loss, night sweats).

spleen (Stage IV) it is considered diffuse disease that cannot be cured by radiation and requires chemotherapy. Staging celiotomy can be avoided by demonstration of intrapulmonary disease, bone marrow involvement, liver disease (by needle liver biopsy), or involvement of the lymph nodes on both sides of the diaphragm (*i.e.*, cervical and inguinal lymph nodes).

For the staging celiotomy, a long midline incision provides adequate exposure for a careful general exploration of the abdomen. After the initial exploration, the liver is examined, and wedge and needle biopsies of both lobes are performed. The abdominal exploration is terminated if the pathologist confirms hepatic involvement because this is considered Stage IV disease. Splenectomy is performed next. It not only will allow careful pathologic assessment of the spleen but will also provide a more limited central radiation portal to the abdomen, thus preventing radiation nephritis and pneumonitis. When removing the spleen, all hilar lymph nodes should be removed as well, and accessory splenic tissue must be sought in the usual locations. The splenic pedicle is then marked for the radiotherapist by metal clips. Any obviously abnormal intra-abdominal lymph nodes are excised and sent for histologic evaluation. If regional lymph node involvement is documented, it is no longer necessary to continue the dissection. At this point, the lateral extent of any grossly abnormal lymph nodes is marked with metal clips to aid the radiotherapist in adequately treating all abdominal disease. Biopsies of representative celiac, para-aortic, and mesenteric lymph nodes should be obtained. In women of childbearing age, the ovaries should be transposed behind the uterus to prevent ovarian injury secondary to radiotherapy. A final optional portion of the staging laparotomy is open iliac crest bone marrow biopsy. If staging laparotomy does not demonstrate subdiaphragmatic spread of Hodgkin's disease, radiotherapy is usually given.

RUPTURE OF THE SPLEEN

In spite of the fact that the spleen seems well protected by the ribs and the muscles of the thoracic and abdominal walls, splenic rupture, defined as disruption of the parenchyma, capsule, or blood supply to the spleen, is the most common indication for splenectomy and the most common major injury resulting from blunt abdominal trauma. The spleen may also be ruptured by penetrating trauma (transabdominal or transthoracic), by nonpenetrating trauma (which can produce an immediate rupture or a delayed rupture), or by operative iatrogenic trauma; in some instances, the spleen appears to rupture spontaneously. Mortality with splenic rupture is usually associated with other concomitant injuries or other associated systemic diseases.

PENETRATING TRAUMA

Most penetrating abdominal injuries are obvious; however, the spleen can be injured when the site of penetration appears to be in the mid or lower chest, and a thoracic penetrating injury can injure the lung, pleura, and diaphragm before finally reaching the spleen. The spleen is a highly vascular organ and bleeds profusely when injured even minimally. With penetrating injuries to the spleen, the most commonly associated injured organs include the stomach, the left kidney, the pancreas, and the vascular structures at the root of the mesentery.

SPLENIC TRAUMA	
Etiology	Penetrating or blunt trauma Iatrogenic injury Spontaneous with splenomegaly
Dx	Abdominal pain, tenderness Hypotension, shock External signs of abdominal trauma Abdominal x-ray—gastric displacement, fluid Chest x-ray film—elevated diaphragm, left rib fractures Peritoneal lavage—hemoperitoneum CT scan
Rx	Treatment of hypovolemic shock Celiotomy, splenorrhaphy, splenectomy

NONPENETRATING TRAUMA

Automobile accidents are the most common cause of blunt trauma to the spleen. With blunt injury, the spleen may be fractured through the parenchyma and capsule, avulsed from its pedicle, or disrupted beneath an intact capsule, producing a subcapsular or contained hematoma. Even trivial blunt trauma has been reported to cause splenic injury. Although bleeding is usually profuse, approximately 5% of blunt injuries to the spleen appear to result in delayed rupture, which begins as a subcapsular hematoma that grows and becomes clinically manifest days to weeks later. Although the incidence of delayed rupture to the spleen has been exaggerated in the past, this entity is nevertheless real and should be considered in all cases of blunt thoracoabdominal trauma.

OPERATIVE TRAUMA

Iatrogenic injuries to the spleen occurring during surgical intervention account for an estimated 20% of all splenectomies. The usual mechanism of injury is avulsion of the splenic capsule by traction on the peritoneal attachments and sometimes direct injury by a misplaced retractor. The mortality after this type of splenectomy remains above 10%. With the new interest in preservation of the spleen and the advent of new techniques using hemostatic substances to cover the area of avulsion of the splenic capsule, the so-called incidental splenectomy can and should be avoided.

SPONTANEOUS RUPTURE

The spleen may also rupture spontaneously (no history of trauma). Although spontaneous rupture of the normal spleen has been reported, it more commonly occurs when the spleen is involved with a hematologic disorder. It is logical to think that most so-called spontaneous ruptures followed some minor trauma that went unnoticed. Spontaneous rupture of the spleen is a complication to be looked for particularly in patients with infectious mononucleosis, but the entity has also been described in patients with spleens enlarged because of malaria, lymphoma, leukemia, typhoid fever, and other conditions in which splenomegaly occurs. Spontaneous rupture of the spleen is a rare complication of oral anticoagulant therapy.

CLINICAL FINDINGS

Clinical signs vary from severe hypovolemic shock to minimal or no symptoms. There is usually a history of a blow to the upper abdomen, specifically to the left flank, and some evidence of injury to the skin in this area can sometimes be detected; however, all these signs and symptoms can be lacking, and no early clues may be present in delayed splenic rupture or spontaneous splenic rupture. Most patients with ruptured spleens complain of generalized abdominal pain; about one third of them have pain confined to the left upper quadrant, and they frequently describe pain in the left shoulder and cervical region.

The abdominal findings are those of low-grade peritoneal irritation, mostly tenderness, mild muscular spasm, and abdominal distention. With rapid bleeding, the abdomen may distend quickly, and the characteristic signs of acute blood loss (*i.e.,* tachycardia, hypotension, and shock) will appear. Delay in the diagnosis may result in a fatal outcome. Plain films of the abdomen may show fractured ribs in the left lower chest; often the gastric air bubble may be displaced medially. Peritoneal lavage should be done when serious doubt exists about the possibility of major intra-abdominal bleeding from rupture of the spleen or other viscera, or when accurate evaluation of the injured patient is precluded because of unconsciousness, intoxication, or paraplegia. The presence of a suspected subcapsular hematoma of the spleen can be confirmed by sonography or a technetium-sulfur colloid scan of the spleen, thereby alerting the surgeon to the possibility of sudden delayed rupture. Selective splenic arteriograms can also be helpful in selected situations.

TREATMENT

Traditional surgical teaching notwithstanding, the injured spleen is capable of adequate healing, either spontaneously or after operative repair. That is, splenic injury does not inevitably lead to delayed rupture, enlarging splenic hematomas, or cyst formation, and nonoperative management and operative repair of the injured spleen under properly selected circumstances are realistic alternatives to the traditional but now obsolete concept of ''splenectomy for injured spleens.''

Nonoperative management can be successfully applied to patients with suspected splenic injuries when the hemodynamics of the injured patient are stable and can be observed in an intensive care setting. Because of the difficulty in assessing the magnitude of the splenic injury and in excluding the possibility of other intra-abdominal injuries, nonoperative management is applicable only to a very carefully selected group of patients.

Celiotomy should be performed in all patients suspected of having a splenic injury who have signs and symptoms of intra-abdominal injury, obvious peritoneal irritation, or positive findings on peritoneal lavage. In severe injuries of the spleen, splenectomy is required, but it is now well established that repair of many splenic injuries is feasible, safe, and effective in controlling hemorrhage. Small capsular tears can be successfully treated by application of hemostatic agents; larger injuries that do not involve the hilar vessels can be repaired by débridement, ligation of individual vessels, and approximation of the remaining cut surfaces by sutures (splenorrhaphy). Another method, reported by the pediatric surgeons of our department to be successful for treating children with shattering or deep lacerations of the spleen, consists in snug approximation of the tissue fractures and restoration of the normal contour of the spleen without needle sutures. This tight but gentle compression is exerted by a ladderlike net constructed of absorbable suture material that is carefully tied around the mobilized spleen. Partial removal of the spleen (hemisplenectomy) has also been successful in treating splenic ruptures localized to either the upper or the lower pole of the spleen (Fig. 29-4). It must be noted that in order to perform any kind of major splenic repair it is essential to mobilize the spleen extensively and deliver it almost completely into the abdominal incision.

Because of the possibility of fatal postsplenectomy sepsis, every effort should be made to preserve the injured spleen not only in children but also in adults. However, splenic repair should be attempted only in patients who are he-

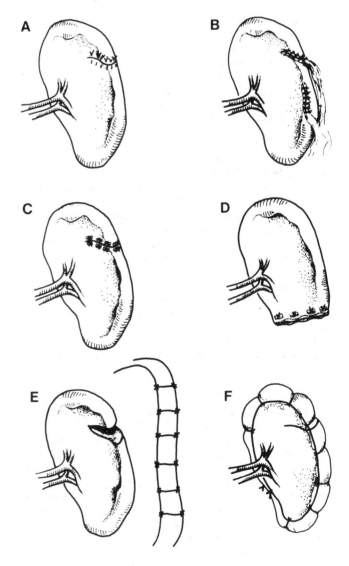

Fig. 29-4. Various methods of repairing splenic lacerations. *(A)* Simple multiple sutures. *(B)* Sutures placed after packing the laceration with a segment of omentum to better achieve hemostasis. *(C)* U sutures placed using Teflon pledgets to prevent the sutures from cutting through the splenic capsule. *(D)* Partial splenectomy; notice the same U sutures with pledgets used to approximate the edges of the cut splenic surface. *(E)* Ladderlike device constructed from absorbable suture material to approximate the edges of the splenic laceration. *(F)* The ladder is tied around the entire spleen and the bleeding is arrested.

modynamically stable or in whom, because of the severe associated intra-abdominal injuries, the inevitable increase in operating time and intraoperative blood loss will not jeopardize their chances for survival. Massive fecal contamination resulting from severe colonic injuries is also a contraindication for splenic repair. It appears inevitable that in a small proportion of cases splenic repair will fail to control the hemorrhage; therefore, splenic repair should not be used in patients in whom a second operation would seriously reduce their chance for survival. The possibility that repaired spleens may be more susceptible to future trauma must be considered, but there is no evidence of this at present.

Criteria for the absolute need and justification for splenic repair are not yet final. Only further experience will allow a definitive determination of the exact risks, early and late, of splenic salvage procedures. At present, splenorrhaphy appears to be both safe and effective in most patients. The deliberate induction of splenosis at the time of splenectomy is probably not effective in preventing postsplenectomy sepsis. When removal of the spleen is unavoidable, the surgeon should document his reasons for electing such a course of action. The patient should be informed of his potentially vulnerable state and should be protected as far as possible by currently available vaccines and early aggressive treatment of all infections.

MISCELLANEOUS LESIONS OF THE SPLEEN

SPLENOSIS

Splenosis results from the dissemination and autotransplantation of fragments of splenic parenchyma that are scattered throughout the peritoneal surfaces in the abdomen after traumatic rupture of the spleen. It has been postulated that these splenic tissue implants can carry on, at least partially, the functions of the normal intact spleen, including preservation of immunocompetence, but to date this remains unproved. Occasionally, loops of small intestine become firmly attached to the segments of spleen, resulting in partial or complete small bowel obstruction. Splenosis is usually an incidental finding at an operation performed for other purposes. Because of the low possibility of complications and the extent of the dissemination of the splenic fragments throughout the abdomen, aggressive surgical attempts to excise all of them are not warranted. They differ histologically from accessory spleens by the absence of elastic or smooth muscle fibers that characterize the capsule of intact and accessory spleens.

ECTOPIC SPLEENS

Occasionally during the course of splenectomy or any other operation near the splenic hilum, one or several small spleens are found. These accessory spleens are sometimes attached to a long pedicle, producing what has been called "wandering accessory spleens," which may present as a mobile mass; in some instances, even acute torsion of the pedicle can occur, requiring surgical removal. Accessory spleens are clinically important if, when the spleen is removed to ameliorate or correct a hematologic condition, one or more accessory spleens are overlooked at the time of splenectomy. Subsequently, some functions of the spleen proper are taken up by the accessory spleens, resulting in

perpetuation of the hematologic condition despite splenectomy. For this reason it is advisable to make a reasonable search for accessory spleens during the course of splenectomy performed for hematologic disease. The presence of functionally important accessory spleens can be excluded if Howell-Jolly bodies are present in the blood smear.

ANEURYSMS OF THE SPLENIC ARTERY

The splenic artery is the most common site for intra-abdominal aneurysms outside the infrarenal abdominal aorta (see also Chapter 36). This lesion occurs more frequently in females. Patients with aneurysms of the splenic artery can be classified in two groups: (1) elderly people in whom the aneurysm is a manifestation of atherosclerotic generalized disease, and (2) young women with apparently congenital aneurysms that may rupture during the last stages of pregnancy. Splenic artery aneurysms are usually discovered incidentally in abdominal radiographs, where they appear as round calcified masses in the splenic hilum. The frequency of rupture ranges from less than 10% to 46%; about 20% of ruptures occur during the last trimester of pregnancy. Ligation of the splenic artery proximal and distal to the aneurysm with or without splenectomy is recommended for enlarging or symptomatic splenic artery aneurysms, particularly in women of childbearing age. Many asymptomatic small aneurysms in males and in women past the childbearing age justify close observation.

SPLENIC ARTERIOVENOUS FISTULA

Abnormal communications between the main splenic artery and vein have been described. Most splenic arteriovenous fistulas are associated with aneurysms of the splenic artery. These patients often have clinical signs and symptoms of portal hypertension including esophageal varices, hematemesis, melena, ascites, and splenomegaly. Most splenic arteriovenous fistulas are manifested by the presence of a loud bruit in the left upper abdomen that eventually leads to selective celiac arteriography, which demonstrates the splenic arteriovenous communication. Splenic arteriovenous fistula should be suspected in patients who have a loud bruit in the left upper abdomen, particularly if they have portal hypertension, a history of previous abdominal trauma, splenic artery aneurysm, or an unusually large number of pregnancies. Because it appears that most of these arteriovenous splenic communications eventually lead to portal hypertension and its complications, splenectomy has been advocated. Recently, successful and permanent control of these fistulas has been obtained by catheter occlusion of the fistula in patients in whom surgical intervention was estimated to carry a very high risk.

NEOPLASMS

The spleen is an uncommon site for primary tumors; however, primary lymphomas, sarcomas, hemangiomas, and hamartomas of the splenic parenchyma have been reported. They are difficult to differentiate from splenic involvement by Hodgkin's disease or systemic lymphomas. Primary neoplastic lesions of the spleen are usually asymptomatic until splenomegaly causes abdominal discomfort or a palpable mass. Benign vascular tumors of the spleen such as angiomas have also been reported. Primary splenic tumors may be divided as follows: (1) capsular and trabecular framework tumors, (2) lymphoid element tumors, (3) vascular or sinus endothelium tumors, and (4) embryonic inclusion tumors. Neoplasms arising from the lymphoid elements of the spleen occur more commonly.

Splenectomy is recommended in patients suspected of having a primary neoplasm of the spleen. Although the number of tumors studied by any given group is very small, the 5-year survival rate quoted for patients with primary malignant neoplasms of the spleen has been around 30%.

The spleen is a relatively common site for metastases and advanced malignancies, especially when the primary tumor is located in the lung or breast. Splenic metastases are usually found at autopsy but rarely are clinically significant. They are usually considered a manifestation of extensive spread of the primary tumor.

CYSTS OF THE SPLEEN

Cysts of the spleen occur rarely. For the sake of simplicity, they can be classified as parasitic and nonparasitic. *Echinococcus* is the only parasitic infection reported to cause splenic cysts. Cysts may be asymptomatic and are usually detected on routine physical examination owing to the presence of splenomegaly, or the calcification of the cyst wall may be noted underneath the left diaphragm on routine chest or abdominal films. CT scan is particularly useful in determining the size and location of splenic cysts (Fig. 29-5). Serologic tests may confirm the diagnosis of *Echinococcus* infestation. Because of the possibility of rupture, the treatment of choice of parasitic cysts of the spleen is splenectomy. Nonparasitic cysts can be classified either as true cysts, lined by epithelium and of dermoid, epidermoid, or endothelial type, or as pseudocysts, which probably arise from old hematomas or splenic infarcts. Because of the uncertain course of splenic cysts and the real possibility of rupture, splenectomy rather than aspiration has been advocated for all splenic cysts.

SPLENIC ABSCESS

Abscesses within the spleen can be simple or multiple. They are uncommon but are important when present because of

their high mortality rate. The possible causes of splenic abscess include (1) an overwhelming bacteremia from a source such as endocarditis, pyelonephritis, or the generalized sepsis that often occurs in debilitated patients, (2) an intrinsic splenic lesion such as a hematoma or an infected infarct that forms an abscess, and (3) an extrinsic lesion such as gastric or colonic perforations or pancreatic or perinephric abscesses that extend and penetrate into the splenic parenchyma. They can also be caused by hematogenous seeding of bacteria from a remote site of sepsis. In most cases, one or more abscesses already exist in organs other than the spleen and develop in the spleen as a terminal manifestation of uncontrolled systemic sepsis. The presenting signs and symptoms are tenderness in the left upper abdomen, referred pain to the left shoulder, weight loss, and other indications of long-standing infection. Splenomegaly or a left upper quadrant mass exists in approximately half of the patients, and leukocytosis is present in approximately 70%. The chest film reveals such abnormalities as left lower lobe atelectasis, left pleural effusion, and elevated left hemidiaphragm; extraluminal gas can be found in the left upper abdomen in 70% of these patients. Sonograms and scans are the most important diagnostic tests.

When a splenic abscess is diagnosed, treatment should include intravenous broad-spectrum antibiotics followed by splenectomy. Initial control of the splenic vein and artery prior to mobilization of the spleen and wide drainage of the splenic fossa appear to be very important.

TECHNICAL ASPECTS AND COMPLICATIONS OF SPLENECTOMY

PREOPERATIVE PREPARATION

Because emergency splenectomy is seldom necessary except in cases of splenic rupture, careful preparation prior to operation is usually possible. In these circumstances, anemia, coagulation abnormalities, and metabolic disturbances can be corrected or improved. Systemic infections should be treated. Coagulation disorders should be improved by giving transfusions of the specific depleted factors. Patients with

Fig. 29-5. CT scan on the left and left lateral ^{99}Tc scan on the right show a large splenic cyst. Note that the size of the cyst and the thickness of its wall can easily be assessed from both studies.

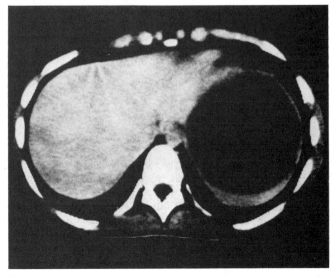
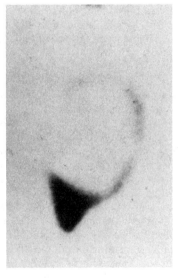

severe immune thrombocytopenia usually benefit from platelet concentrates that should be given only after the splenic artery has been ligated. Antibodies in the patient's serum may complicate the cross-matching of blood. Many patients require corticosteroid coverage in the preoperative period. In emergency splenectomy, hypovolemia should be corrected as much as possible by transfusion of whole blood after initial resuscitation with crystalloid solutions.

TECHNIQUES OF SPLENECTOMY

The spleen can be reached through a variety of incisions, but the upper midline or left oblique are most commonly used. The choice of incision is dictated by the indications for operation and by the individual preference of the surgeon. A midline incision is preferable for ruptured spleens, staging celiotomies, and massive splenomegaly and when the patient has a severe coagulation disorder. For splenectomy alone, a left oblique incision below the costal cartilages also gives excellent exposure. Thoracoabdominal incisions are seldom necessary and should be avoided.

There are two operative techniques for splenectomy. In one approach, which is of value chiefly for traumatic rupture of the spleen or when the spleen is readily movable and absolute hemostasis is not essential, the organ is first mobilized by dividing the peritoneal attachments to the colon, left kidney, and diaphragm. These ligaments are usually avascular or contain only a few small blood vessels except when the patient has portal hypertension. Adhesions to the diaphragm are often present and must be divided with care because they sometimes can cause troublesome hemorrhage. The short gastric vessels must be ligated accurately, avoiding injury to the gastric fundus. After all the attachments have been transected, the spleen is retracted medially by gentle traction, and a large gauze pad is inserted and placed in the splenic fossa. The spleen is carefully mobilized toward the incision (Fig. 29-6), and clamps are placed across the splenic artery and vein close to their entrance to the spleen, making sure that the tail of the pancreas is not injured or included in the clamps. It is best to ligate the vein and artery separately by accurately placed suture ligatures.

The other operative technique for splenectomy is the method of choice for removing massively enlarged spleens or in patients with portal hypertension. In this technique, the splenic vessels are ligated before the spleen is mobilized by ligating and partially transecting the gastrocolic ligament to gain access to the lesser sac. The usually avascular adhesions between the anterior surface of the pancreas and the posterior wall of the stomach are transected, and the stomach is retracted anteriorly, clearly exposing the distal body and tail of the pancreas (Fig. 29-7). The splenic artery and vein, which run along the superior border of the pancreas, are located and isolated. The artery is usually ligated first with a double proximal ligature, and then the splenic vein is carefully dissected, avoiding tearing the small branches entering the pancreas; the splenic vein is then ligated and transected. Initial ligation of the splenic artery allows most of the blood contained in the spleen to empty through the splenic vein, thus minimizing the loss of blood.

After the spleen has been removed, meticulous hemostasis of the splenic fossa should be accomplished. The pancreas and the stomach are carefully examined for any injury. Drainage is not necessary unless there is a question of damage to the pancreas or unless sutures had to be placed in the distal portion of this organ to control hemorrhage.

MANAGEMENT OF POSTOPERATIVE COMPLICATIONS

Persistent bleeding can occur in the immediate postoperative period owing to thrombocytopenia or incomplete surgical hemostasis. If continued transfusions are required and the abdominal girth is increasing, reexploration of the abdomen is mandatory. Often in such situations, intraperitoneal blood and clots are found, but a specific bleeding site is not found. Evacuation of the clots, irrigation with saline solution, and

Fig. 29-6. Method of quick splenectomy. The spleen is first mobilized from its fossa and lifted to near the incision; the splenic vessels are then ligated.

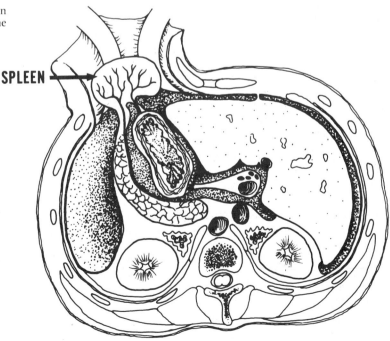

SPLEEN →

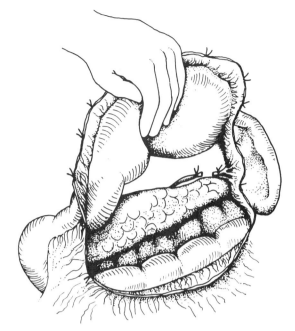

Fig. 29-7. Method for splenectomy with minimal blood loss. The lesser sac is entered first, and the splenic vessels are located and ligated on the superior border of the pancreas near the splenic hilum. The splenic artery should be ligated first.

packing the splenic fossa for several minutes with a gauze pad will usually control the oozing while the coagulopathy is actively treated.

The most common complication after splenectomy is atelectasis of the left lower lung. Blunting of the left costophrenic angle and a small pleural effusion are not uncommon findings in chest films of patients recovering from splenectomy. A large pleural effusion a few days after splenectomy is always suspicious of the development of a left subphrenic abscess. Injury to the pancreas or stomach is not common but does occur. Gastric injury usually results in a subphrenic abscess with a gastrocutaneous fistula. Pancreatic injury can result in a pancreatic fistula with or without concomitant pancreatitis, and even a pseudocyst may form.

Another frequent occurrence after splenectomy that can become a serious complication is thrombocytosis. Although most patients do not have thrombotic complications, when the platelet count rises over one million per cubic millimeter, thrombosis of the peripheral and splanchnic veins can occur. Thrombocytosis in myeloproliferative diseases is particularly subject to thrombotic and bleeding complications. Anticoagulants, antiplatelet drugs, and sometimes antimetabolites have been successfully used to prevent venous thrombosis after splenectomy when the platelet count rises over one million. In the majority of cases, however, thrombocytosis is of no consequence. At present, most surgeons would agree that some type of anticoagulant prophylactic therapy is indicated in well-hydrated patients without anemia when the platelet count exceeds 1.5 million in the immediate postsplenectomy period.

Overwhelming postsplenectomy infection occurs most frequently in asplenic patients with serious systemic disease affecting the lymphoid or reticuloendothelial system. It can, however, occur in a healthy person who has lost the spleen because of trauma or because of complications incidental to operations in the upper abdomen. The incidence of overwhelming postsplenectomy sepsis in such patients is very low (0.5%–0.8%) but is still much higher than that in the normal population (0.01%). Overwhelming postsplenectomy sepsis most commonly affects patients who undergo splenectomy within the first 4 years of life, but it can afflict persons at any age. Approximately 80% of septic episodes occur within 2 years of operation, but the syndrome has been described as late as 25 years after operation. The clinical manifestations of overwhelming postsplenectomy sepsis are the same, whether splenectomy has been a recent or distant event. Patients who have undergone splenectomy should be informed of the potential for developing overwhelming sepsis.

The current consensus suggests that asplenic children and adults should receive the polyvalent pneumococcal vaccine and should be advised to seek prompt medical attention when they develop even the minor symptoms of a cold or "flu." In the same population, when fever of 38.8°C or more develops and there is no obvious site of infection, it should be managed as a medical emergency, and treatment with penicillin should be started immediately. Infants and children who cannot communicate the symptoms of early infection adequately should be protected by continued prophylactic penicillin. Similar protection should be given to asplenic patients of any age who have systemic diseases that affect the lymphoid or reticuloendothelial system.

BIBLIOGRAPHY

Pathophysiology
CHEN L-T: Microcirculation of the spleen: An open or closed circulation. Science 201:157, 1978
EICHNER ER: Splenic function: Normal, too much and too little. Am J Med 66:311, 1979
SULLIVAN HL, OCHS HD, SCHIFFMAN G et al: Immune response after splenectomy. Lancet 1:178, 1978

Diagnostic Studies
MITTELSTAEDT CA, PARTAIN CL: Ultrasonic-pathologic classification of splenic abnormalities: Gray-scale patterns. Radiology 134:697, 1980
SOLHEIM K, NERDRUM HJ: Radionuclide imaging of splenic laceration and trauma. Clin Nucl Med 4:528, 1979

Hypersplenism
CHRISTENSEN BE: Pathophysiology of "hypersplenism syndrome." Scand J Haematol 11:5, 1973
JACOB HS: Hypersplenism: Mechanisms and management. Br J Haematol 27:1, 1974

Hyposplenism
DAMESHEK W: Hyposplenism (letter). JAMA 157:613, 1955
WALDROP CAJ, LEE FD, DYET JF et al: Immunological abnormalities in splenic atrophy. Lancet II:4, 1975

Sepsis in Hyposplenism
DICKERMAN JD: Bacterial infection and the asplenic host: A review. J Trauma 16:662, 1976
GOPAL V, BISNO AL: Fulminant pneumococcal infections in "normal" asplenic hosts. Arch Int Med 173:1526, 1977
LEONARD AS, GIEBINK GS, BAESL TJ et al: The overwhelming postsplenectomy sepsis problem. World J Surg 4:423, 1980

Splenomegaly
SULLIVAN S, WILLIAMS R: Reliability of clinical techniques for detecting splenic enlargement. Br Med J 4:1043, 1976

General Indications for Splenectomy
DAMESHEK HL, ELLIS LD: Hematologic indications for splenectomy. Surg Clin North Am 55:253, 1975

LAWS HL, BURLINGAME MW, CARPENTER JT et al: Splenectomy for hematologic disease. Surg Gynecol Obstet 149:509, 1979

TRAETOW WD, FABRI PJ, CAREY LC: Changing indications for splenectomy. 30 years' experience. Arch Surg 115:447, 1980

Hemolytic Anemias

FRANK MM: Pathophysiology of immune hemolytic anemia. Ann Int Med 87:210, 1977

LAWRIE GM, HAM JM: The surgical treatment of hereditary spherocytosis. Surg Gynecol Obstet 139:208, 1974

ZAIL SS: The erythrocytic membrane abnormality of hereditary spherocytosis. Br J Haematol 37:305, 1977

Idiopathic Thrombocytopenic Purpura

DIFINO SM, LACHANT NA, KIRSHNER JJ et al: Adult idiopathic thrombocytopenic purpura. Clinical findings and response to therapy. Am J Med 69:430, 1980

PICOZZI VJ, ROESKE WP, CREGER WP: Fate of therapy failures in adult idiopathic thrombocytopenic purpura. Am J Med 69:690, 1980

RUTKOW IM: Thrombotic thrombocytopenic purpura (TTP) and splenectomy: A current appraisal. Ann Surg 188:701, 1978

Agnogenic Myeloid Metaplasia

SCHWARTZ SI: Myeloproliferative disorders. Ann Surg 182:464, 1975

Felty's Syndrome

LASZLO J, JONES R, SILBERMAN HR et al: Splenectomy for Felty's syndrome. Clinicopathological study of 27 patients. Arch Int Med 138:597, 1978

RILEY SM, ALDRETE JS: Role of splenectomy in Felty's syndrome. Am J Surg 130:51, 1975

Sarcoidosis and Gaucher's Disease

SALKY B, KREEL I, GELERNT I et al: Splenectomy for Gaucher's disease. Ann Surg 190:592, 1979

WEBB AK, MITCHELL DN, BRADSTREET CM et al: Splenomegaly and splenectomy in sarcoidosis. J Clin Pathol 32:1050, 1979

Leukemia

CHRISTENSEN BE, HANSEN MM, VIDEBAEK A: Splenectomy in chronic lymphocytic leukemia. Scand J Haematol 18:279, 1977

GOLOMB HM, CATOVSKY D, GOLDE DW: Hairy cell leukemia. A clinical review based on 71 cases. Ann Int Med 89:677, 1978

GOMEZ GA, SOKAL JE, MITTELMAN A et al: Splenectomy for palliation of chronic myelocytic leukemia. Am J Med 61:14, 1976

Portal Hypertension

FELIX WR, MYERSON RM, SIGEL B et al: The effect of portacaval shunt on hypersplenism. Surg Gynecol Obstet 139:899, 1974

Hypersplenism in Dialysis Patients

YAWATA Y, JACOB HS: Abnormal red cell metabolism in patients with chronic uremia. Nature of the defect and its persistence despite adequate hemodialysis. Blood 45:231, 1975

Hodgkin's Staging

CHABNER BA, FISHER RI, YOUNG RC et al: Staging of non-Hodgkin's lymphoma. Semin Oncol 7:285, 1980

JONES SE: Importance of staging in Hodgkin's disease. Semin Oncol 7:126, 1980

Ruptured Spleen

DANFORTH DN JR, THORBJARNARSON B: Incidental splenectomy: A review of the literature and the New York Hospital experience. Ann Surg 183:124, 1976

OAKS DD: Splenic trauma. Curr Probl Surg 18:6, 1981

SHERMAN R: Perspectives in management of trauma to the spleen. J Trauma 20:1, 1980

Delayed and Spontaneous Rupture

BENJAMIN CI, ENGRAV LH, PERRY JF JR: Delayed diagnosis of rupture of the spleen. Surg Gynecol Obstet 142:171, 1976

BIRD D, KELLY MJ, BAIRD RN: Spontaneous rupture of the normal spleen: Diagnosis by computerized tomography. Br J Surg 66:598, 1979

SOYER MT, MERCK DE, ALDRETE JS: Spontaneous rupture of the spleen: An unusual complication of anticoagulant therapy. Arch Surg 111:610, 1976

Repair of the Injured Spleen

BUNTAIN WL, LYNN HB: Splenorrhaphy: Changing concepts for the traumatized spleen. Surgery 86:748, 1979

HOWMAN-GILES R, GILDAY DL, VENAGOPAL S et al: Splenic trauma: Nonoperative management and long-term follow-up by scintiscan. J Pediatr Surg 13:121, 1978

MORGENSTERN L, SHAPIRO SJ: Techniques of splenic conservation. Arch Surg 114:449, 1979

STRAUCH GO: Preservation of splenic function in adults and children with injured spleen. Am J Surg 137:478, 1979

Splenosis

FLEMING CR, DICKSON ER, HARRISON EG JR: Splenosis: Autotransplantation of splenic tissue. Am J Med 61:414, 1976

RICHEY K, PEARSON HA, JOHNSON D: Splenosis following splenectomy for trauma in adults. Blood 52 (Suppl 1):88, 1978

Ectopic Spleens

APPEL MF, BART JB: The surgical and hematologic significance of accessory spleens. Surg Gynecol Obstet 143:191, 1976

Aneurysms and Arteriovenous Fistulas of the Splenic Artery

WESTCOTT JL, ZITER FM JR: Aneurysms of the splenic artery. Surg Gynecol Obstet 136:541, 1973

ZELCH JV, HERMANN RE: Control of arteriovenous fistula of splenic vessels by Fogarty catheter. Arch Surg 110:329, 1975

Abscess

CHUN CH, RAFF MJ, CONTRERAS L et al: Splenic abscess. Medicine 59:50, 1980

Complications After Splenectomy

BALFANZ JR, NEWBIT MD JR, JARVIS C et al: Overwhelming sepsis following splenectomy for trauma. J Pediatr 88:458, 1976

HARRISON BF, GLANGES E, SPARKMAN RS: Gastric fistula following splenectomy: Its cause and prevention. Ann Surg 185:210, 1977

30

Henry Buchwald/Richard B. Moore/Richard D. Rucker, Jr./Richard L. Varco

Management of Morbid Obesity and Hyperlipidemia (Metabolic Surgery)

Morbid obesity is a metabolic disease with a neurohumoral basis and a strong hereditary predisposition. There are no nonoperative diet or drug approaches to morbid obesity that offer even a modicum of success or promise. Surgery is the only reasonable therapy for this disease that is available. A thorough review of the literature, as well as the personal experience of the authors, leads us to conclude that the procedure of choice for treatment of morbid obesity today is a gastric bypass. This operation involves total cross-stapling of the stomach, leaving a very small upper reservoir, and anastomosis with approximately a 1-cm orifice of this reservoir, Roux-en-Y, to a loop of jejunum.

Partial ileal bypass is a time-proven therapeutic modality for treatment of the hyperlipidemias; indeed, it may be the treatment of choice for certain patients with hypercholesterolemia. Data clearly demonstrate that diet and drug therapy do not achieve the lipid reductions reached by partial ileal bypass, that their effects are not lasting, and that patient adherence to these therapies is poor. On the other hand, the effects of partial ileal bypass are lasting, its therapeutic effects are obligatory, and the lipid reductions are marked: 35% to 40% lowering of the total cholesterol, 45% reduction in the low density lipoprotein (LDL)–cholesterol level, no reduction in the high density lipoprotein (HDL)–cholesterol level, and an approximately 90% increase in the HDL-cholesterol to LDL-cholesterol ratio.

Metabolic surgery can be defined as the operative manipulation of a normal organ or organ system to achieve a biologic result for a potential health gain. In this chapter we will discuss metabolic operations that have been devised to intervene therapeutically in the disease processes of morbid obesity and hyperlipidemia.

OPERATIONS FOR MORBID OBESITY

DEFINITION AND ETIOLOGY OF MORBID OBESITY

In 1970 Scott and associates defined the morbidly obese individual as "one who has reached two to three or more times his ideal weight and who has maintained this level for five years or more despite efforts by himself, his family and his physician to bring about effective and sustained reduction of weight to acceptable medical standards." Numerous formulas have been used in an attempt to improve precision in the measurement of the excess adipose mass; yet, we, as well as the majority of practitioners in this area, simply define the weight limit for morbid obesity as greater than 100 pounds over insurance-table "ideal weight."

Obesity results when caloric intake exceeds expenditure. This excess is stored as fat. Thus, obesity is the result of overeating and massive obesity is the product of food "addiction."

Why does the obese individual overeat? We do not know the specific answer to that question. Several possible mechanisms may be operative in the etiology of obesity. It has been demonstrated that obesity occurs in families. In addition to the obvious familial environmental factor, a significant positive correlation between the weight of natural children and their parents has been demonstrated; no correlation between the weights of adopted children and their parents seems to exist. If one parent is obese, the likelihood of the child's being obese is about 40%; if both mother and father are obese, the likelihood of obesity in the child is about 75%. It is generally accepted that obesity in early childhood results in the formation of an excess number of fat cells and that, although these lipocytes vary their fat content during life, they do not diminish in number. Obese individuals may carry a "humoral" factor that triggers overeating and filling of lipocytes. The theory has also been advocated that, without chemical evidence of hypothyroidism, the morbidly obese have impaired thyroid utilization at the cellular level.

Physical activity is decreased in the obese, and this lack of physical activity results in decreased muscle insulin sensitivity, increased insulin release, secondary hypoglycemia, and stimulation of the central nervous system center for eating. An obvious area for metabolic research has been the intestinal absorption mechanisms; however, no absorptive capacity abnormality has been found in the obese.

Psychological or emotional factors must be included in a discussion of morbid obesity. Yet there has been no demonstration of a particular obese personality or psychopathic behavior disorder uniquely associated with obesity. Nisbett reported in 1972 that there are distinct differences in the types of cues that govern the eating behavior of obese and nonobese humans and that the peculiarities observed in the eating behavior of the obese human are displayed by several animal obesity preparations. Human obesity seems to involve abnormalities in satiety mechanisms, rather than differences in the hunger sensation. Furthermore, obese subjects demonstrate emotional attachment to the consumption of large amounts of food but not to the product of this activity; indeed, the personal body image of the obese individual is anything but complimentary.

Socioeconomic status is an influential factor for obesity, especially in the female. The higher the educational level of women and the greater their economic independence, the thinner they tend to become, with a role model akin to the high fashion model with amenorrhea.

COMPLICATIONS OF MORBID OBESITY

Obesity is not only a disease but it is also a harbinger of other diseases. The complications of obesity affect nearly every organ system and are both structural (bulk related) and functional. Obesity is correlated with the complications of atherosclerotic cardiovascular disease (*e.g.*, myocardial infarctions and strokes). Owing to the requirement for a greater cardiac output, at a cost of an increased heart rate or stroke volume, the obese patient with atherosclerotic or hypertensive heart disease has a greater risk of developing congestive heart failure. In addition, obesity *per se* results in cardiac hypertrophy, predominantly of the left ventricle, and can be responsible for heart failure without evidence of other heart disease. The incidence of hypertension is higher in an obese than in a nonobese population. Venous insufficiency and thrombophlebitis are more prevalent in the obese. The obese individual has, as a rule, impairment of ventilation parameters with a diminished pO_2. Chest wall bulk can be responsible for alveolar hypoventilation, resulting in drowsiness and episodic involuntary sleep (Pickwickian syndrome).

Chronic cholelithiasis and cholecystitis have been observed in 30% to 40% of morbidly obese persons. It has been suggested that obesity may be correlated with carcinoma of the stomach. Altered liver function has been described in the presence of morbid obesity, and most morbidly obese patients have some degree of fatty metamorphosis of the liver. The incidence of cirrhosis of the liver has been reported to be two and one-half times greater in the obese male and one and one-half times greater in the obese female than in the general population. Diabetes mellitus of adult onset is three to four times more prevalent in obese subjects. Orthopaedic problems are more frequent in the markedly obese and include osteoarthritis of the lumbar spine, herniated intervertebral disks, and osteoarthritic changes in the knees. The obese female is often subject to infertility problems, and birth complications are higher. There is a demonstrated increased incidence of carcinoma of the endometrium in association with excess body weight, possibly secondary to increased estrogen storage in and prolonged release from lipocytes. Intertriginous dermatitis and stasis dermatitis are two of the cutaneous problems encountered in obese subjects.

Insurance company statistics have clearly demonstrated the end-result of the summation of these obesity-induced problems. The mortality of obesity rises geometrically as a function of the percentage of increase in weight over the "ideal." In a Veterans Administration study in 1980 of 200 morbidly obese men, 23 to 70 years of age, with an average weight of 143.5 kg, Drenick and co-workers found a 12-fold increase in the expected mortality in the group 25 to 34 years of age and a 6-fold increase at ages 35 to 44. Significantly, there are also excellent data documenting that the increased risk of death for the obese individual diminishes with weight reduction.

It is important for the physician to appreciate that in addition to being a medical problem obesity is also a social, psychological, and economic problem. The obese can experience great difficulties in interpersonal relationships, courtship, marriage, and community acceptance. They often cannot find employment and tend to rely on welfare programs. Employers may believe that the obese are unable to cope with a job, unsightly to customers, and, most important, too expensive to insure.

DIET AND DRUG THERAPY

The treatment of choice for obesity is dietary management. Unfortunately, for those individuals who are 100 pounds or more overweight, dietary therapy has afforded little lasting success. Those obese individuals who can sustain a diet for even a short period of time, almost universally rapidly regain lost weight. Physician reinforcement of dietary measures, psychotherapy, hypnosis, group therapy, incarceration (voluntary hospitalization for about 1 year on acaloric liquids and vitamins), mobile incarceration (wiring of the jaws), and the lay counseling groups (*e.g.*, TOPS, Weight Watchers, Counter Weight) all have a near-zero record of lasting success in the management of the morbidly obese. Indeed, Stunkard and colleagues showed that somewhat less than 5% of morbidly obese individuals ever lose 40 pounds or more for even a transient time span.

Drug therapy has employed appetite suppressants (thyroid preparations and amphetamines), hormones, and commercial products with a dubious value. In addition to the toxicity, potential addiction, and side-effects of certain of these preparations, their success in providing a sustained weight loss has been as poor as dietary therapy alone. Obviously, the impetus for a surgical approach for the treatment of morbid obesity evolved from the general failure of available methods of nonsurgical therapy.

HISTORY OF SURGICAL MANAGEMENT

Varco performed the first intestinal bypass specifically to induce weight reduction in 1953; he never published this case report. In 1954, Kremen, in the discussion of his animal research paper on certain nutritional aspects of the small intestine, described a patient on whom he had performed an end-to-end jejunoileostomy for the reduction of body weight. In 1956, Payne initiated the first clinical program of massive small intestinal bypass for the management of morbid obesity. He sought rapid and marked weight reduction through bypass of nearly the entire small intestine, the right colon, and half of the transverse colon. Bowel continuity in his initial series of 11 patients was restored by end-to-side anastomosis of the proximal 15 inches of jejunum to the midtransverse colon. Weight loss following the jejuno-transverse colostomy was dramatic; however, the morbidity (from uncontrolled diarrhea, electrolyte imbalance, and liver failure) was prohibitive and, in at least one instance, fatal. Payne originally envisioned that his procedure would cause a relentless weight loss, with the patient never achieving a state in which calories absorbed balanced energy expenditure. Thus, a second operation would be needed to restore additional bowel length and weight equilibrium when ideal body weight was obtained. This operation was condemned by many; Payne concurred with this assessment and soon abandoned transverse colonic bypass.

Sherman and his associates, essentially simultaneously with Payne, proposed abandonment of primary anastomosis to any segment of the colon and restoration of bowel continuity proximal to the ileocecal valve by an end-to-side jejunoileostomy. The aim of this less radical bypass operation was to achieve an eventual balance between caloric intake and body caloric needs, with elimination of consideration of a second operation and minimization of postoperative side-effects and complications. Several refinements of the end-to-side jejunoileal bypass to provide an antireflux mechanism were proposed by others.

A return to end-to-end jejunoileal bypass was advocated independently by Scott and ourselves. Although different proportions of jejunum and ileum were employed, these procedures preserved the ileocecal valve as a means of diminishing postoperative diarrhea and electrolyte losses. Such procedures required the performance of a second anastomosis of the distal end of the bypassed segment to some segment of the colon.

Before turning from intestinal bypass procedures, certain imaginative derivations, as yet early in their history, should be mentioned, although they will not be discussed in detail in this chapter. Scopinaro and associates devised a procedure in 1976 that they call a "bypass bilio-pancreatico." This operation actually involves two procedures: (1) hemigastrectomy with Polya gastrojejunostomy to a Roux-en-Y loop deprived of the biliary-pancreatic secretions and (2) a jejunodistal ileostomy for drainage into the intestinal tract of the biliary-pancreatic secretions. Lavorato and associates described ileocholecystectomy, in which the gallbladder is bypassed into the terminal ileum, with anastomosis of the stomach, jejunum, and the remainder of the ileum end-to-side into the terminal ileal conduit. This procedure, as well as the bypass bilio-pancreatico, is designed to minimize diarrhea and electrolyte imbalance; to allow no segment of the intestinal tract to lie dormant and, thereby, to provide a site for unfavorable bacterial overgrowth and its possible sequelae; and yet to provide for a substantial weight reduction. These operative modifications have not been systematically used in the United States to date.

The history of gastric procedures for weight reduction began with Mason, who performed the first gastric bypass and the first gastroplasty. Gastric bypass refers to a complete functional separation of a small upper gastric pouch from the remainder of the stomach and drainage of that pouch into a segment of the jejunum. Gastroplasty refers to an incomplete division of the stomach, with a small upper pouch separated from the remainder of the stomach by a narrow orifice.

The report of the first 100 gastric bypass patients by Alden in 1977 served as a landmark in this field. The procedure was eloquently simplified. Alden, for the first time, did not transect the stomach. Instead, he anastomosed, with 1.2-cm stoma, the greater curvature of the stomach close to the esophagogastric junction to an antecolic loop of jejunum and then placed a complete staple line across the stomach. A major innovation that completely prevents bile reflux was introduced by Griffen: a retrocolic Roux-en-Y gastrojejunostomy reconstruction. At the University of Minnesota Medical School we have performed gastric bypasses in more than 350 patients, employing the Alden technique, the addition of an enteroenterostomy to the jejunal loop procedure, and, currently, a Roux-en-Y antecolic restoration of bowel continuity.

Gastroplasty was actually given prominence in the surgical arena by Gomez, who has attempted to perfect a method of maintaining the small luminal size of the connecting gastric stoma. The Gomez operation has had wide acceptance and immediate modification. Egan proposed to make the communicating stoma on the lesser curvature, and LaFave introduced total gastric cross-stapling and subsequent construction of a small gastrogastrostomy anterior to the staple line. Carey changed the name of gastroplasty to gastric partitioning, moved the orifice to the middle of the stomach, and performed his operation by the simple removal of the central staples prior to applying the stapling instrument to the stomach.

A myriad of gastric procedure modifications, limited only by the imagination of surgeons, have been proposed and include various plications, wrapping the stomach tightly with various nonreactive materials, and so on. Space does not permit their discussion. Indeed, truncal vagotomy alone, without a drainage procedure, has been proposed by Kral, who postulates that a lasting weight reduction can ensue by a central effect on the gastric hunger stimulus.

PATIENT SELECTION CRITERIA

Our criteria for patient selection for obesity surgery are as follows: weight greater than 100 pounds over insurance-table "ideal weight" for age and sex; a minimum 5-year effort at weight reduction by dietary means; no known causative correctable endocrine dysfunction; willingness to undergo the procedure after having the postoperative side-effects, potential complications, and chances of success fully explained; mental capacity and emotional stability to tolerate the operation and postoperative sequelae; and commitment to use the suggested postoperative dietary modifications and restrictions.

JEJUNOILEAL BYPASS

This segment of this chapter is written neither to praise nor to bury jejunoileal bypass. It is presented to tell the story of this operation in order that today's students of surgery understand the past and the management of patients who have had this operation, as well as to prepare students of the future for a possible resurgence of this procedure.

Bypass of a sufficient length of small intestine creates an absorptive caloric deficit and forced conversion of body depot fat (although some lean tissue mass is also lost) to energy, with a concomitant weight loss. This process continues until caloric absorption reaches equilibrium with the energy requirements of the smaller body mass. As a rule, absorptive compensation with weight adjustment occurs 1 to 3 years after jejunoileal bypass.

TECHNIQUE

The technique used at the University of Minnesota is shown in Figure 30-1.

IN-HOSPITAL STATISTICS AND MORTALITY

When surgeons began to perform the jejunoileal bypass the prevailing murmur of discontent was that this operation was dangerous *per se*; when surgeons took up the gastric bypass the statement was made that the jejunoileal bypass was a safe procedure but that gastric bypass posed great technical difficulties. We, as well as most other surgeons experienced in obesity surgery, have found neither procedure extraordinarily hazardous and both to be relatively safe.

After nearly 1,000 jejunoileal bypass operations in the past 10 years or so, our 30-day postoperative mortality from any cause has been under 0.5%. The morbidity rate for pneumonia, thrombophlebitis, pulmonary embolism, prolonged wound lipid drainage, and gastrointestinal hemorrhage have all been under 3%. The wound infection rate has been 4.5%. The presence of positive findings on urine culture postoperatively has been 12%, although overt urinary tract infection has been present less than 2% of the time. Only one patient in our entire series has ever experienced a wound dehiscence.

LONG-TERM SIDE-EFFECTS

The long-term side-effects of jejunoileal bypass are predictable and can, for the most part, be prevented. To avoid the inevitable hypokalemia and hypocalcemia, all patients at discharge were taking potassium and calcium supplements, as well as intramuscular vitamin B_{12} (1,000 μg) every 6 weeks. Diarrhea was the problem most universally annoying to the patient. We attempted to control this diarrhea with a constipating diet, diphenoxylate HCl and atropine sulfate (Lomotil), calcium carbonate to bind free fatty acids and bile acids, and a bulk-forming resin (*e.g.*, Effersyllium). Over the years, less than 5% of our patients have had uncontrollable diarrhea or electrolyte problems requiring take-down of the bypass. The incisional hernia rate following

Fig. 30-1. The jejunoileal bypass operation. *(1)* The entire bowel is measured along the mesenteric border, and division is planned at a point 40 cm distal to the ligament of Treitz; *(2)* the bowel is divided between marking sutures; *(3)* the distal end of this division is closed; *(4)* the bowel is also divided 4 cm proximal to the ileocecal valve; *(5)* the proximal 40 cm of jejunum is anastomosed, end to end, to the terminal 4 cm of ileum; *(6)* the distal end of the bypassed loop is anastomosed, end to side, to the cecum, the proximal end of the bypassed loop is tacked to prevent intussusception, and all mesenteric defects are carefully closed.

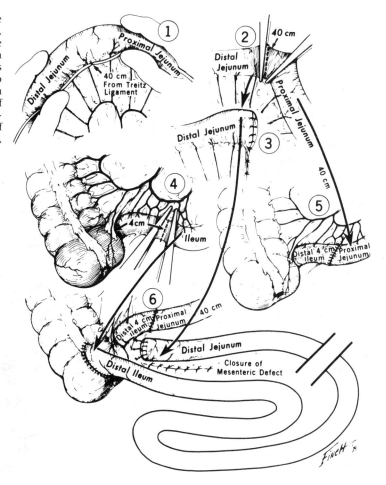

jejunoileal bypass, and in general after most obesity operations, has been approximately 5%.

UNIQUE COMPLICATIONS

The unique complications of jejunoileal bypass are well known. They include polyarthralgia or polyarthritis, urinary calculi, and hepatic decompensation.

Post-bypass *arthralgia* and arthritis is a diagnosis made by exclusion of rheumatoid, lupus, and other known forms of arthritis. Management has consisted of symptomatic treatment and, most effectively, of low-dose antibiotic therapy (tetracycline, 250 mg, or metronidazole 250 mg, two to three times daily) to combat microorganisms in the bypassed bowel ostensibly responsible for these symptoms.

Oxalate *nephrolithiasis* postjejunoileal bypass is the result of an excess of gut oxalate, due to a relative decrease in gut calcium ions secondary to binding of these ions to free fatty acids and bile acids to form soaps; hyperabsorption of oxalate; hyperoxalemia; hyperoxaluria; and, finally, calcium oxalate stone formation with a coefficient of formation of 40:1, making the serum calcium concentration quite irrelevant in this process. We have, therefore, prophylactically treated this problem with increasing the calcium in the diet. Our nephrolithiasis rate was thus reduced from about 11% to less than 5%.

Alterations in liver function and morphology in the morbidly obese not subjected to any operative intervention are well known. The primary pathologic alteration is fatty metamorphosis; but fibrosis, inflammatory changes, bile duct duplication, and hyaline body formation are not infrequent. As a rule, most of these changes progress after the jejunoileal bypass, as demonstrated in our hundreds of sequential postoperative percutaneous biopsy studies, then eventually regress and often leave the liver in a more normal state of histology than present before the operation. There are certain patients in whom the degenerative changes are progressive; however, frank liver failure has been seen in less than 5% of these patients, and half of these can be managed without the necessity for bypass take-down. It stands to reason that the hepatotoxicity associated with chronic alcoholism is a complicating factor well avoided in the patient with an intestinal shunt.

Hair loss following any massive weight reduction has been reported and has been attributed to diffuse protein deficiency. This alopecia has never been more than a thinning of hair, and full recovery has taken place.

It was predicted that intestinal bypass would cause cholelithiasis, but this prediction has not been borne out by actual experience. We also feared that jejunoileal bypass would be causative in the development of colon carcinoma, due to the effect of the bile acid irritation on the large bowel mucosa. This too has not been confirmed by any of the studies to date in the rather large number of jejunoileal bypass patients in this country, in Canada, and in Europe. Certain peripheral neuropathies, skin problems (*e.g.,* erythema nodosum), and other disease states may have some causative association with jejunoileal bypass, although they are rare and the mechanism for this association has not been defined.

At this time, it is impossible to state what percentage of jejunoileal bypass patients will eventually request, or be recommended to have, a take-down of the procedure because of unremitting complications. As gastric surgery meets the test of time, conversions are becoming more popular. It should not be forgotten that the greater majority

of jejunoileal bypass patients have had an excellent weight reduction and have mastered or avoided the side-effects and unique complications of this intervention.

POSITIVE RESULTS

The basic positive result of obesity surgery is, of course, weight reduction. Twelve months following jejunoileal bypass, our patients lost a mean of 40 kg, and at 36 months, a mean of 51 kg. Thus, weight loss occurs primarily in the first year but continues up to 3 years. In many of our patients, however, there has been a slight regaining of weight at the end of their weight-losing period. Looking at the weight loss as a percent of excess weight, the jejunoileal bypass patients lost 65% of their excess weight at 12 months and 76% at 36 months. An easily remembered fact is that the mean weight loss at 1 year is approximately 100 pounds (Fig. 30-2).

There is a marked and lasting plasma cholesterol concentration reduction after jejunoileal bypass, with a mean cholesterol value at 1 year postoperatively 42% lower than the average preoperative value; this effect has been maintained 36 months and longer. The serum triglyceride level is reduced 35% by the jejunoileal bypass procedure.

Nearly all of our hypertensive patients had significant blood pressure reduction after bypass, and many became normotensive. This correlation has been reported by others. With progressive weight loss, we have seen insulin-dependent diabetics convert to only dietary control or exhibit a marked reduction in their insulin requirement. There has been a definite symptomatic improvement of lower extremity varicosities, osteoarthritic spine and hip pathology, and respiratory distress states. Many of our female patients have given birth to normal children.

The statistics in regard to the long-term beneficial effect on longevity of obesity surgery have yet to be reported, although a positive influence can be expected. The deter-

Fig. 30-2. *(Left)* A morbidly obese patient weighed 343 pounds immediately preceding his jejunoileal bypass. *(Right)* The same patient 1 year later weighed 193 pounds. (Buchwald H, Varco RL, Moore RB et al: Intestinal bypass procedures. Curr Probl Surg 12:1, 1975)

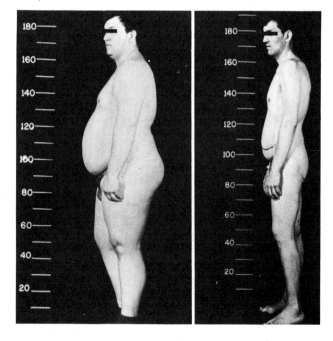

mination of cardiovascular disease risk is based on the presence of certain risk factors, including obesity, hyperlipidemia, hypertension, and diabetes. Since the massive weight loss following obesity surgery has been shown to reverse or mitigate these risk factors, it seems appropriate to assume that these procedures will eventually be demonstrated to prolong life.

The quality of life after marked weight reduction in morbidly obese individuals has improved significantly. Patients tend to make improved social adjustments, return to school, and plan a more productive future. The rate of gainful employment has increased after weight reduction. There has been marked improvement in self-image and interpersonal relationships.

GASTRIC BYPASSES

As previously stated, the gastric bypass procedures consist of construction of a small upper functioning gastric reservoir joined by an anastomosis with a small stoma to a loop of jejunum. On minimal food intake, ideally less than 50 ml, the patient should feel a sense of satiety (possibly, for the first time in his life) and stop eating. Persistence of food intake results in vomiting.

TECHNIQUE

The operative technique employed at the University of Minnesota is shown in Figure 30-3.

IN-HOSPITAL STATISTICS AND MORTALITY

Our 30-day perioperative mortality with gastric bypass is again less than 0.5%. Also, the incidence of pneumonia, thrombophlebitis, pulmonary embolism, excessive lipid wound drainage, and gastrointestinal hemorrhage has been under 3%. Positive results of postoperative urine cultures have been found in 4.9% of our gastric bypass patients. There has been no episode of wound dehiscence. Wound infections have been fewer than after jejunoileal bypass, with a 0.8% incidence.

After more than 350 gastric bypass procedures, we have had only two anastomotic leaks. In one patient, who had an incidental splenectomy for intraoperative splenic trauma, an anastomotic leak of the gastrojejunostomy was demonstrated after a prolonged course of pancreatitis and subphrenic abscess. Another patient developed an afferent loop obstruction and, at the time of exploration, methylene blue dye demonstrated a leak along the TA-90 staple line, which could no longer be seen after decompression of the distal gastric pouch. We had four additional episodes of functional afferent loop obstruction, prior to conversion of our operative technique from a simple loop gastrojejunostomy to a loop with an additional entero-enterostomy and, finally, a Roux-en-Y antecolic reconstruction.

LONG-TERM SIDE-EFFECTS

The long-term side-effects of gastric bypass are limited essentially to a 10% incidence of prolonged nausea and vomiting, sometimes requiring rehospitalization and rehydration. The diet education to a small meal program, given in the preoperative and postoperative periods, must often be reinforced.

UNIQUE COMPLICATIONS

The dumping syndrome has, surprisingly, been rarely seen. To this time, the arthralgias and arthritis, and nephrolithiasis,

which is sometimes seen after jejunoileal bypass, have not been experienced after the gastric procedures. Also, we have not witnessed liver failure; however, we were the first to report that after gastric bypass all individuals do not have an improvement in biopsy-determined liver histology; 12% of patients after gastric bypass actually show a progression in hepatic pathology 1 year after the operation.

POSITIVE RESULTS

Weight loss after gastric bypass in our series, as well as in those of others, has been comparable to that achieved after jejunoileal bypass. The mean weight reduction at 1 year has been 37 kg. This can be translated to an average loss of 62% of excess weight, or approximately 100 pounds.

The positive effects of weight reduction after gastric bypass with respect to reduction of blood pressure, improved diabetes, less osteoarthritis, and so on should be the same as those seen after jejunoileal bypass. This is not true for the lipid effects. Although the plasma triglyceride concentration is reduced an equivalent 35% after gastric bypass, the plasma cholesterol level is only lowered 14% by this operation.

On the other hand, the socioeconomic advantages after gastric bypass may exceed those following jejunoileal bypass; after gastric bypass, patients have fewer, if any, long-term side-effects or complications and often a greater sense of strength and well-being.

GASTROPLASTY AND GASTRIC PARTITIONING

The rationale for gastroplasty and gastric partitioning is the same as that for gastric bypass: the construction of a small upper gastric reservoir connected by a small orifice with the remainder of the gastrointestinal tract. With these procedures, the connection is to the residual distal stomach rather than to the jejunum.

TECHNIQUE

For these procedures, the reader is referred to the papers by Carey and Gomez.

IN-HOSPITAL STATISTICS AND MORTALITY

The operative mortality following gastroplasty and gastric partitioning has been low: 0.5% in over 200 patients reported by Gomez and 1.4% in approximately 400 patients reported by Carey. However, these percentages are not lower than those achieved with gastric bypass and the requisite one to two bowel anastomoses; in the case of Carey, with what appears to be the simplest of the gastric procedures, the perioperative mortality rate has been the highest.

The reported postoperative morbidity after gastroplasty and gastric partitioning has been comparable to that found after gastric bypass.

LONG-TERM SIDE-EFFECTS

The primary long-term side-effect of these operations has been technical failure. Gomez has a 12% revision rate in 200 patients, including 15 staple line disruptions, three enlarged channels, four channel stenoses, and two enlarged pouches. Carey reports an 85% technique failure rate in the 89 patients with the TA-55 stapling, with lower, but very substantial, technical failure and severe complication rates after each of his other operative innovations.

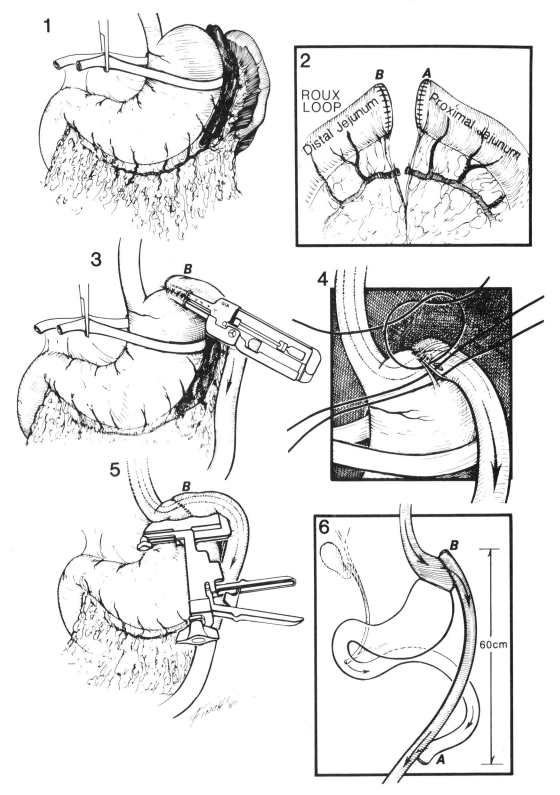

Fig. 30-3. The gastric bypass operation. *(1)* The upper one third of the short gastric vessels has been divided, the entire upper fundus of the stomach is mobilized, and the stomach is encircled with a Penrose drain below the first feeding vessels on the lesser curvature; *(2)* a Roux loop is created; *(3)* gastrojejunostomy is performed at the esophagogastric junction on the greater curvature with the GIA stapler approximately 1.0 cm in diameter; *(4)* both the anterior and the posterior aspect of this anastomosis are oversewn with 5-0 nonabsorbable sutures; *(5)* the stomach is totally cross stapled with the TA-90 stapler, leaving a small (~50 ml) upper reservoir; and *(6)* the operation is completed with a side-to-side anastomosis of the proximal jejunal limb to the Roux loop.

The groups performing these operations have come to recommend elaborate postoperative diets to minimize technical failures and enhance weight reduction. These diets consist of liquids or purees for several months, a situation untenable for most individuals and probably more so for the morbidly obese.

UNIQUE COMPLICATIONS

The long-term complications for the operation will, if the initial weight loss is successful, be comparable, we believe, to those experienced with gastric bypass.

POSITIVE RESULTS

The positive results, if comparable weight loss is achieved, should be the same as those seen after gastric bypass. Significantly, weight loss, even after technically successful gastric partitioning, may not equal that achieved by gastric bypass. A prospective randomized clinical trial by Laws in 1981 comparing gastric bypass to gastric partitioning clearly showed earlier, greater, and more sustained weight loss with the gastric bypass ($p < 0.01$).

Although thought and trial must be encouraged, the data currently available make us conclude that it is more difficult to achieve good weight loss with gastroplasty and gastric partitioning than with gastric bypass and that these operations, performed without an intestinal anastomosis or even opening the gastrointestinal tract, are no safer than the gastric bypass procedure.

SURGICAL OPERATIONS FOR FAILED BYPASSES

Certain advantages and disadvantages are associated with each of the two common classes of procedures, and both jejunoileal and gastric operations will require revision procedures or take-down under some circumstances.

When medical management of the unique side-effects and complications of jejunoileal bypass fails, take-down is recommended. Generally, individuals undergoing take-down or revision of a jejunoileal bypass have had an excellent weight response from the operation. This fact should be stressed; it is exceedingly rare that a patient will request a remedial operation for failure of weight loss after jejunoileal bypass.

Remedial surgery should not be done in haste, and reoperation is preferably undertaken as a strictly elective procedure. Quite often reoperation requires adequate preparation of the patient in-hospital with hyperalimentation, supplemental oral protein, restoration of body electrolyte balance, and replenishing of body vitamin stores. Early in the common experience with jejunoileal bypass, patients with life-threatening complications or with significant disturbances in the quality of life underwent bypass take-down only. Inevitably, after recovery, all of these patients regained their original weight. Also, operations that added or subtracted from the length of the bypassed segment failed in their intent better than 50% of the time. Therefore, unless the patient is extremely ill, when a jejunoileal bypass take-down is performed, a concurrent gastric operation to maintain the patient's weight response is done. We have published a description of the operative technique for jejunoileal bypass take-down and a concurrent construction of a gastric bypass.

Contrary to jejunoileal bypass, a failed gastric procedure is usually synonymous with a failure to achieve an adequate weight loss response. In distinction to a failed jejunoileal bypass, under certain circumstances remedial procedures on the stomach for failed gastric bypass, gastroplasty, or gastric partitioning can be recommended. These include appropriate operations for disruptions of the staple line, widening of the upper pouch or poorly constructed upper pouch, and enlargement of the connecting stoma. However, failure of weight loss is often not due to a technical problem, as determined by barium swallow under fluoroscopy. By eating small meals at frequent intervals (hourly or less), any person can outeat a gastric operation for weight reduction. Under these circumstances, we prefer not to attempt any gastric revison operation, since this more than likely would be a futile gesture. Instead, after thorough discussion with the patient, we proceed with a jejunoileal bypass in addition to, or after take-down of, the gastric operation. We have also published a description of a method for take-down of the gastric bypass and for concurrent construction of a jejunoileal bypass.

CONCLUSIONS

All surgical approaches to the management of morbid obesity are an approximation to rational therapy. Surgeons do not, at this time, deal with the primary etiology of this disease. Our own conviction, based on currently available genetic, experimental, and psychological-psychiatric data, is that morbid obesity is a metabolic disease with a neurohumoral basis and a strong hereditary predisposition. Obviously, opportunities for research on the cause or causes of morbid obesity are protean and future therapy will have to be based on a knowledge of mechanisms. There are today no recommendable operations on the endocrine or neurologic systems to modify morbid obesity. More strikingly, there are currently no nonoperative (diet [with or without support analysis and counseling] or drug) approaches to morbid obesity that offer even a modicum of success or promise. Operative therapy in this area has been designated by some as radical. Surgery, however, is the only reasonable and available therapy for this disease.

OPERATIONS FOR HYPERLIPIDEMIA

DEFINITION AND ETIOLOGY OF HYPERLIPIDEMIA

Hyperlipidemia is an excess of circulating lipids. Primarily, we are concerned with hypercholesterolemia, which can be arbitrarily defined as a circulating cholesterol concentration over 220 mg/dl, or possibly even over 200 mg/dl. If we examine the mean cholesterol concentration in middle-aged men in the United States, it is about 240 mg/dl; therefore, is it proper to call 200 mg/dl, or 220 mg/dl, the upper limit of a "normal" cholesterol? We believe it is. Children all over the world are born with essentially the same electrolytes and blood chemistries they will maintain for a lifetime. This is not the case for cholesterol. The average plasma cholesterol level in the neonate, except for familial hypercholesterolemic infants, is 65 mg/dl. The rise to an adult level is disproportionate in the world and even within a given population, with some well-nourished groups and individuals retaining a cholesterol level between 100 mg/dl and 150 mg/dl. More significantly, as the cholesterol concentration climbs over 200 mg/dl, there is a rapid and exponential increase in the incidence of atherosclerotic cardiovascular disease.

In the past, the designations of familial hypercholesterolemia, familial hypertriglyceridemia, and familial xanthomatosis were used to describe severe and hereditary forms of hyperlipidemias. Acquired cholesterolemia and hypertriglyceridemia indicated less florid manifestation of this spectrum of conditions. Fredrickson and his associates, more effectively, categorized such lipid elevations as functions of lipoprotein abnormalities. Their schema was subsequently revised by others as well as by themselves. The current format of dividing the hyperlipoproteinemias into five types provides a standard nomenclature and is widely accepted today for discussions of the hyperlipidemias. An alternative classification system has been proposed by Goldstein and co-workers based on the plasma lipid levels in the patient and his near relatives. The proportion of relatives having elevated plasma cholesterol or triglyceride levels and the proximity of their relationship to the patient with hyperlipidemia serve as the bases for classification into one of five categories, distinct from the Frederickson system.

LIPID-ATHEROSCLEROSIS HYPOTHESIS

Atherosclerosis is not equivalent to aging; it is a disease. Today, atherosclerosis is endemic in the United States. Diseases of the heart, strokes, and generalized arteriosclerosis account for approximately half of the total deaths in this country; 650,000 coronary deaths alone occur yearly in the United States. Over 10 million Americans alive today have a history of a heart attack or angina pectoris and over 1 million Americans will have a myocardial infarction this year. Since many myocardial infarction victims survive the insult, and only end-stage peripheral vascular disease results in death, clearly the pain, incapacitation, emotional impact, economic hardship, and career deprivation resulting from atherosclerotic cardiovascular disease create problems of substantial magnitude for those who treat these afflictions.

The primary instigating cause, or agent, responsible for atheroslerosis remains unknown. The disease epidemiology and incidence is described in terms of risk factors: family history, hypertension, cigarette smoking, and, of course, hyperlipidemia. The conclusion for a causative relationship of the plasma lipids, primarily the plasma cholesterol, in the development of atherosclerosis is derived from certain experiments of nature (*e.g.*, advanced atherosclerosis in children with hypercholesterolemia; premature development of atherosclerosis in diabetics); animal preparations; retrospective epidemiologic research; and prospective population studies, the most famous of which has been that conducted at Framingham, Massachusetts.

More recently, the role of cholesterol in atherogenesis has been further defined. Plasma total cholesterol is the sum of the cholesterol in the three major plasma lipoprotein classes: very low density lipoprotein (VLDL), low density lipoprotein (LDL), and high density lipoprotein (HDL). LDL-cholesterol is directly related to coronary heart disease risk and HDL-cholesterol seems to be inversely related to this risk; multivariant analysis has shown that these two lipoprotein fractions exert an independent effect on coronary heart disease risk. Davignon considers the LDL-cholesterol a chemical agent capable, as a function of its concentration in the plasma or in combination with injurious elements (*e.g.*, hemodynamic stress, carbon monoxide, catecholamines), of injuring the endothelium and infiltrating the intima to induce proliferation of smooth muscle cells and the initiation of the plaque lesion. The work of Brown and Goldstein has further broadened our understanding of the

role of LDL-cholesterol. They showed in human fibroblast and surface cells of the human aorta the existence of a cell surface receptor that binds and degrades plasma LDL. Individuals with heterozygous familial hypercholesterolemia have a reduced number of these receptors, and subjects with the homozygous form of this disease have none.

If an elevated plasma cholesterol is causally related to atherosclerosis, does a reduction in plasma cholesterol result in a decrease in the incidence of atherosclerosis and its clinical manifestations? This is an eminently logical conclusion but has yet to be definitively documented in humans. Since the mid 1950s there have been more than 20 major clinical lipid modification trials initiated. The "first generation" trials were all negative or inconclusive. The current six "second generation" clinical trials have either demonstrated no significant benefit with respect to atherosclerosis risk from cholesterol reduction or they are still in progress. Unfortunately, none of the completed trials provided a significant cholesterol reduction.

The Coronary Drug Project was the first "second generation" trial and was initiated in 1966 and completed in 1974. This was a secondary (*i.e.*, following myocardial infarction) intervention trial that showed no beneficial effect on the progression of coronary heart disease with the use of either clofibrate or nicotinic acid therapy. The degree of plasma total cholesterol reduction was, however, only 6.5% with clofibrate and 9.9% with nicotinic acid.

The Minnesota Coronary Survey, a primary (*i.e.*, in asymptomatic patients) intervention trial completed in 1973, also failed to show definitive beneficial effects (morbidity or mortality), with an average 14% cholesterol reduction with dietary modification therapy.

The European World Health Organization cooperative clofibrate trial, a primary intervention trial conducted from 1965 to 1976, showed no reduction in coronary heart disease mortality, with an average 9% plasma cholesterol lowering. However, this trial did report a lower incidence of nonfatal myocardial infarction in the clofibrate-treated group in comparison to the control group. On the other hand, there was a 25% increase in mortality in the clofibrate-treated group, primarily from noncardiovascular diseases, when compared with the controls. This study, obviously, raised the question of a long-term toxic effect of clofibrate and has, essentially, led to the discontinued use of this agent.

The Multiple Risk Factor Intervention Trial (MRFIT), recently completed, showed no noticeable reductions in atherosclerotic deaths by three concurrent intervention modalities: cholesterol reduction by diet (modest—about 5%—lowering effect), blood pressure control by drugs, and cessation of cigarette smoking by encouragement.

At the present time, there are basically two intervention trials, one primary and one secondary, using a unifactorial approach. The Coronary Primary Prevention Trial (CPPT) of the Lipid Research Clinics (LRC) Program is using the bile acid sequestrant cholestyramine for cholesterol reduction. This trial was designed for an average 24% reduction in the plasma total cholesterol level, but it is estimated that only about half of this degree of cholesterol reduction will actually be achieved, primarily because of the problems of long-term adherence to drug therapy.

The Program on the Surgical Control of the Hyperlipidemias (POSCH) is a secondary intervention trial using partial ileal bypass surgery to effect plasma cholesterol reduction. In this study, 1,000 subjects, 30 to 64 years of age and not hypertensive, obese, or diabetic, who have had only one documented myocardial infarction, are randomly assigned to a surgical or a control group. The follow-up will be a minimum of 5 years after entry into the trial. In addition to the determination of cardiovascular mortality and morbidity, the study will document the anatomical extent of atherosclerotic disease using peripheral and coronary arteriography prior to randomization and at two subsequent intervals. This trial is designed for an average 30% to 40% cholesterol reduction in the surgery group; the current lipid results in the POSCH trial are reviewed later in this chapter. A major advantage of using partial ileal bypass surgery as the treatment modality in a clinical trial is that the effects on body lipids and cholesterol metabolism are obligatory. This benefit minimizes or eliminates the problem of subject compliance. Thus, POSCH is providing maximum reduction of the major atherogenic risk factor with a negligible subject noncompliance rate, and it is the only lipid hypothesis clinical intervention trial employing serial arteriographic assessment. The trial is scheduled for completion between 1988 and 1990.

What can be recommended with respect to lipid modification therapy in the light of today's knowledge? The majority of clinicians have adopted the concept, and we would recommend that it is prudent to attempt atherosclerosis modification by plasma lipid reduction while awaiting the results of the current clinical trials, as long as the means used for lipid reduction are effective and safe.

DIET AND DRUG THERAPY

Based on retrospective and prospective studies of the influence of various diets on the circulating cholesterol concentration, the most effective diet regimen for lowering the cholesterol level includes a diet low in saturated fats, with a relative increase in the proportion of polyunsaturated fatty acids, and with a low daily dietary cholesterol intake. The following general rules seem sound: the total amount of fats is less than 30% of the total caloric intake; the polyunsaturated-saturated fatty acid ratio is at least 1.5; and the daily intake of cholesterol is less than 300 mg. An extensive literature review of dietary cholesterol modification offers two rather discouraging conclusions: (1) it is difficult to influence the cholesterol concentration significantly in an adult population by dietary means, mainly due to noncompliance over time and (2) the best long-term dietary results in at-risk adult populations range between 12% and 14%.

Turning to drugs, cholestyramine and similar sequestrants are relatively safe and moderately effective. The best cholesterol-lowering results reported for cholestyramine range between 20% and 25%; although as stated above, the results in the LRC trial are expected to be half of that amount. Clofibrate, initially an agent of promise, has been disappointing in all major trials and may, indeed (as indicated in the WHO trial) be dangerous. Numerous side-effects and toxic manifestations have been described for clofibrate, and even more have been documented for nicotinic acid. Flushing of the skin occurs initially in nearly all patients started on nicotinic acid therapy and persists in 10% to 15%. Other side-effects of nicotinic acid include erythematous rash, pruritus, hyperpigmentation, gastrointestinal disturbances, hyperglycemia, postural hypotension, hyperuricemia, and impairment of liver function. This agent, as well, has been disappointing in the cholesterol lowering achieved in a large randomized trial.

Probucol (a substituted dithioacetal) has been introduced as a lipid-lowering agent in adults. Approximately 10% of the patients receiving the recommended dose of 500 mg twice a day report mild side-effects consisting of diarrhea, flatulence, abdominal pain, and nausea; however, patient acceptance and adherence to the drug have been reported to be good. Initial results have shown a 10% to 20% reduction in plasma cholesterol levels. Unfortunately, both the LDL- and HDL-cholesterol were reduced, making the use of this drug, an agent that reduces the "protective" HDL-lipoprotein, questionable.

New drugs are continually being proposed for the management of the hyperlipidemias. Clinicians should be wary of recourse to such agents before their actions are well studied and their reactions characterized. Estrogen therapy has now been abandoned; it caused feminization in men and intravascular clotting, and its use was associated with an increased frequency of sudden deaths. Although the early reports on the use of dextrothyroxine were promising, other effects of this agent argued against its greater use. Dextrothyroxine can potentiate angina pectoris and arrhythmias, induce hypermetabolism, and lead to functional hyperthyroidism. Indeed, because these consequences were so deleterious, the code in the Coronary Drug Project was broken for dextrothyroxine and it was removed from the protocol.

HISTORY OF SURGICAL MANAGEMENT

From 1962 to 1964, the first experiments designed to develop the rationale for partial ileal bypass management of the hyperlipidemias were carried out by us at the University of Minnesota. Studies in white New Zealand rabbits, in pigs, and by retrospective analysis in patients who had undergone ileal resection for causes other than carcinoma showed that both the cholesterol absorption from the intestinal tract and the whole blood cholesterol concentration were markedly and significantly reduced, without concomitant weight loss, following diversion or loss of substantial lengths of distal bowel. We also demonstrated that bypass of the distal third of the small intestine interferes with the enterohepatic bile acid cycle and results in a loss of bile acids in the feces at a rate at least three times that of normal. Thus, the partial ileal bypass operation affects cholesterol homeostasis by a direct drain on the body cholesterol pool and by an indirect drain on the cholesterol pool through forced conversion of cholesterol to its metabolic end-product bile acids in order to maintain the stressed bile acid reservoir (Fig. 30-4).

An animal model of a reproducible 50% myocardial infarction attack rate has been developed by feeding rabbits a high cholesterol content diet for long periods of time. Using this model, we have demonstrated both for adult and infant rabbits that partial ileal bypass will prevent hypercholesterolemia and atherosclerosis despite consumption of a severely atherogenic (2% cholesterol) diet for 4 months. The operation in rabbits with established hypercholesterolemia and atherosclerosis returns the whole blood cholesterol values to below normal and reduces cholesterol xanthomatous accumulations, even though the animals remain on the 2% cholesterol diet. In addition, partial ileal bypass will arrest and reverse the atherosclerotic process in rabbits. Several other investigators have confirmed these findings in a variety of animal species.

The laboratory experience in the development of partial ileal bypass has been complemented by Moore and co-

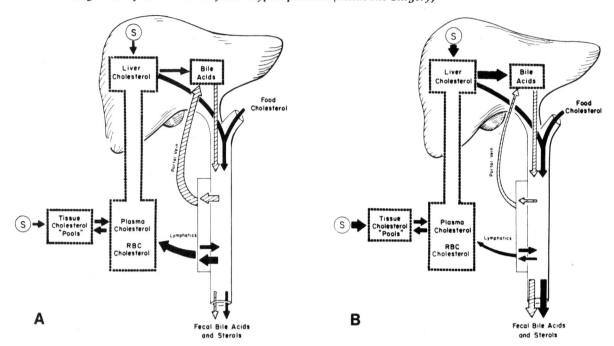

Fig. 30-4. Cholesterol enters the small intestine by way of food and bile and by direct secretion through the intestinal wall. *(A)* Preoperatively, the markedly efficient cholesterol and bile acid enterohepatic cycles account for maximum absorption. *(B)* Postoperatively, fecal cholesterol and bile acid excretion are increased, resulting in decreased absorption, a direct drain on the cholesterol pool, and an indirect drain on the cholesterol pool by the forced conversion of cholesterol to bile acids. In addition, there is an increase in cholesterol synthesis *(S)* mechanisms to attempt to offset these effects. (Buchwald H, Varco RL: Partial ileal bypass operation for control of hyperlipidemia and atherosclerosis. In Sabiston DC, Spencer FC (eds): Gibbon's Surgery of the Chest, 3rd ed. Philadelphia, W B Saunders, 1976)

workers in 1969 by human cholesterol dynamics studies using radioisotope methods. Cholesterol absorption is reduced 60% following partial ileal bypass. This state of reduced absorption capacity has been maintained for at least 10 years. Complementary data in humans show a 3.8-fold increase in total fecal steroid excretion, with a much greater increase in bile acids (4.9-fold) than in neutral steroids (2.7-fold). This state of increased steroid excretion has also been maintained for 10 years of follow-up. Compensatory cholesterol and bile acid absorptive adaptation by the functioning small intestine apparently does not occur. Thus, the effect of partial ileal bypass on the cholesterol and bile acid enterohepatic cycles appears to endure.

Other homeostatic mechanisms in humans do respond to the increased loss of cholesterol and bile acids by increasing cholesterol synthesis. Indeed, a 5.7-fold increase in cholesterol synthesis rate has been shown to occur following partial ileal bypass, and this effect, too, has been maintained. Concomitantly, the cholesterol turnover rate has been demonstrated to increase markedly. The total exchangeable cholesterol pool, on the other hand, is reduced by about one-third at 1 year after partial ileal bypass. This lowering is reflected in both the freely miscible cholesterol pool (*i.e.*, plasma, red blood cells, liver, intestinal mucosa) and the less freely miscible cholesterol pool (*i.e.*, depot fat, muscle, other organs). The less freely miscible cholesterol pool probably includes cholesterol in the arterial walls; therefore, loss of cholesterol from this pool can reflect a loss of cholesterol from atherosclerotic plaques. Cholesterol dynamics are graphically summarized in Figure 30-5.

We performed the first human partial ileal bypass op-

eration specifically for cholesterol reduction on May 29, 1963. Since that time, we have performed more than 350 partial ileal bypass procedures. Currently other institutions in the United States and Europe have programs employing this method of cholesterol lowering. Since this approach to lowering lipids is a surgical procedure, it has encountered resistance from the nonsurgical medical community. Nevertheless, in recent years, this reluctance is slowly giving way and we are beginning to see partial ileal bypass candidates at a rate of about one per week.

In 1973, Starzl clinically introduced end-to-side portacaval shunting for the management of type IIA homozygous hyperlipoproteinemic patients. A brief discussion of this innovative operation is included in this chapter.

PARTIAL ILEAL BYPASS

The flexible criteria for patient selection as candidates for partial ileal bypass are as follows:
1. Any adult under 60 years of age with a posthypocholesterolemic diet plasma cholesterol level greater than 200 mg/dl and who has manifest atherosclerotic cardiovascular disease.
2. Any adult under 60 years of age with a posthypocholesterolemic diet plasma cholesterol concentration greater than 2 SD above the mean level for the patient's age, if the individual has a family history for but no manifest features of atherosclerotic cardiovascular disease.
3. Any child over 6 years of age with documented familial hypercholesterolemia and with a cholesterol concentration 2 SD above the mean for the individual's age.

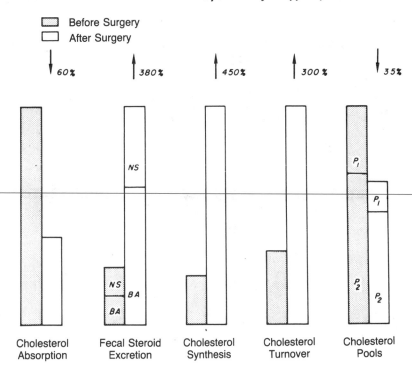

Fig. 30-5. Metabolic studies in partial ileal bypass patients (*NS*, neutral sterols; *BA*, bile acids; P_1, freely miscible pool; P_2, slowly miscible pool). (Buchwald H, Moore RM, Varco RL: Surgical treatment of hyperlipidemia. Circulation 49(suppl 1):1, 1974. By permission of the American Heart Association, Inc.)

TECHNIQUE

The operative technique for partial ileal bypass is shown in Figure 30-6.

IN-HOSPITAL STATISTICS AND MORTALITY

We believe, and our data confirm, that the partial ileal bypass procedure can be performed with an in-hospital mortality of less than 0.5%, with the presence of coexisting coronary artery disease in many of these patients notwithstanding. Wound infection, pulmonary emboli, or other serious postoperative complications that resulted in prolonging hospitalization beyond a week, have occurred in only 2% of these patients. To date, in the Minnesota series, no instance of intussusception of the proximal end of the bypassed bowel segment or obstruction secondary to internal hernia created by inadequate closure of the rotational mesenteric defect has occurred. These complications seem to be avoidable.

LONG-TERM SIDE-EFFECTS

Diarrhea is the one annoying side-effect experienced by the majority of individuals after partial ileal bypass. Commonly, it is not persistent. Within a year or so, approximately 90% of patients have fewer than five bowel movements daily and are taking no bowel controlling medications. Patients generally also report an increase in the firmness and consistency of stools with time. Only two patients (of 350) in our experience have requested operative restoration of bowel continuity because of intractable diarrhea.

Following partial ileal bypass, vitamin B_{12} absorption is either severely impaired or totally lost. After several years, however, absorptive adaptation for vitamin B_{12} occurs in about one half of these patients. Nevertheless, we believe it prudent to prescribe a parenteral vitamin B_{12} supplementation, 1,000 µg intramuscularly every 2 months, for all partial ileal bypass patients. We continue this regimen indefinitely.

Contrary to the often encountered experience with jejunoileal bypass for obesity, no change in the serum electrolyte values follows partial ileal bypass. Nutrient malabsorption has not been described following partial ileal bypass; no essential long-term weight loss occurs.

UNIQUE COMPLICATIONS

Neither arthritis phenomena nor an increased rate of nephrolithiasis as described following jejunoileal bypass has been reported after partial ileal bypass. Lithogenic bile and the formation of gallstones have not been causatively related to partial ileal bypass in our experience. It is of considerable importance in distinguishing partial ileal bypass from jejunoileal bypass that hepatic fatty infiltration or fibrosis has not occurred following clinical or experimental partial ileal bypass. Thus, for practical purposes, there are no unique complications related to the limited partial ileal bypass procedure.

EFFECT ON PLASMA LIPIDS AND LIPOPROTEINS

Total Cholesterol

In our experience prior to the POSCH trial, the circulating cholesterol concentration was reduced an average of 41% from the preoperative and postdietary baseline after partial ileal bypass. In combination with type-specific dietary management, a 53% cholesterol level lowering, on the average, has been achieved in type IIA individuals (Fig. 30-7). Parenthetically, certain type IIA patients are likely to be refractory to just dietary therapy or to drugs, singly or in combination. Partial ileal bypass, in addition to its effectiveness in the type IIA individual, lowers the cholesterol concentration in all of the hyperlipidemia types. These results have not been compromised by effect escape in our experience, which now extends for more than 18 years.

The cholesterol-lowering effect of the operation is neither uniform nor precisely predictable for each person. The lowering of cholesterol from the preoperative postdietary

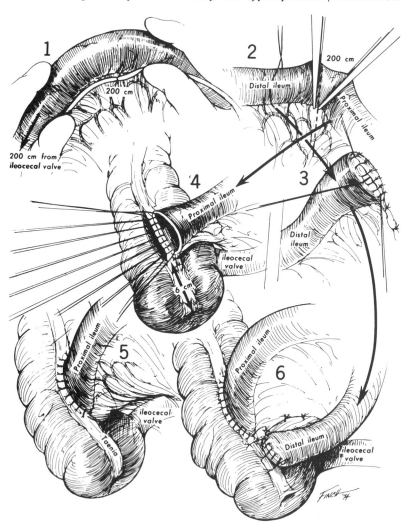

Fig. 30-6. The partial ileal bypass operation: *(1)* The entire bowel is measured along the mesenteric border, and division is planned at a point 200 cm proximal to the ileocecal valve (or at 250 cm if the total length exceeds 600 cm); *(2)* the bowel is divided between marking sutures; *(3)* the distal end of the division is closed; *(4)* the proximal end is anastomosed end-to-side into the cecum, about 6 cm above the appendiceal stump; *(5)* the anterior row of the two-layer open anastomosis is completed; *(6)* the proximal end of the bypassed loop is tacked to prevent intussusception, and all mesenteric defects are carefully closed. (Buchwald H, Varco RL: Partial ileal bypass operation for control of hyperlipidemia and atherosclerosis. In Sabiston DC, Spencer FC (eds): Gibbon's Surgery of the Chest, 3rd ed. Philadelphia, W B Saunders, 1976)

baseline has varied from 5% to 79%. However, in the series reported by investigative groups elsewhere in the United States and in Europe, the mean cholesterol concentration reduction after dietary therapy of 40% has been virtually identical to our findings. To date, the least impressive responders have been type IIA homozygous young people. Yet, Balfour and Kim reported two homozygous children observed for 3 years who had sustained cholesterol reductions of 42% and 33%.

The average preoperative cholesterol concentration reported for individuals who have undergone partial ileal bypass has been over 330 mg/dl. Following partial ileal bypass, better than 80% of these subjects have circulating cholesterol levels below 250 mg/dl and better than 50% have levels below 200 mg/dl.

The preliminary lipid findings in the POSCH trial have been reported. A recent analysis of the plasma lipids and lipoproteins in 165 operated individuals followed for up to 3 years in the POSCH trial reveals a significant and sustained reduction in the plasma total cholesterol, ranging from 35% at 3 months to 31% at 3 years.

Triglycerides

The best data with respect to postoperative triglyceride concentration following partial ileal bypass are those from the POSCH study. In this trial, there has been no significant average effect on plasma triglycerides in the overall group

of subjects, which includes both normotriglyceridemic and hypertriglyceridemic patients. In the 140 normotriglyceridemic subjects there was a slight, but not statistically significant, increase in plasma triglycerides, and in the 40 hypertriglyceridemic subjects there were variable individual responses with an overall average reduction (again, not statistically significant).

Lipoprotein Fractions

The best current data available with respect to the lipoprotein fraction effect of partial ileal bypass come from the POSCH trial. The LDL-cholesterol concentration has been reduced in a significant and sustained manner, ranging from 47% at 3 months to 43.5% at 3 years. There was no significant average effect on the VLDL-cholesterol level. HDL-cholesterol levels, interestingly, tended to increase after partial ileal bypass surgery; when the surgical group was compared with the control group, in which there was an average decrease in HDL-cholesterol over time, there was a significant ($p < 0.05$) difference between the two groups (10.4% at 1 year, 9.3% at 3 years). Following partial ileal bypass surgery, there was a marked increase in the ratio of HDL-cholesterol to LDL-cholesterol, ranging from 94% at 3 months to 79% at 3 years.

These results definitively show that partial ileal bypass results in a marked reduction in the total plasma cholesterol and in the major atherogenic plasma lipoprotein (LDL),

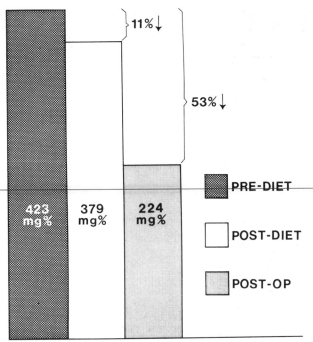

11% ↓

53% ↓

423 mg% | 379 mg% | 224 mg%

■ PRE-DIET

□ POST-DIET

▨ POST-OP

Fig. 30-7. Effect of cholesterol-lowering diet and partial ileal bypass on serum cholesterol levels in 24 type IIA patients. (Buchwald H, Moore RB, Varco RL: Surgical treatment of hyperlipidemia. Circulation 49(suppl 1):1, 1974. By permission of the American Heart Association, Inc.)

with an increase in the presumably protective plasma lipoprotein (HDL) and the HDL/LDL ratio.

CLINICAL OBSERVATIONS

Xanthomas, Xanthelasma

Investigators have reported a postoperative decrease in size, or even disappearance, of peripheral xanthelasma, subcutaneous xanthomas, and tendon xanthomas, especially of the plantor extensor tendons. By analogy, a reduction in size of xanthomatous lesions should indicate that other tissue stores of lipid have been mobilized and excreted from the body. During a period of rapid mobilization, lipid transport may occur at the expense of a reduction in circulating lipid concentration.

Angina Pectoris

Many individuals afflicted with angina pectoris have testified to a reduction in the frequency of these attacks or to the complete disappearance of these symptoms during comparable effort after partial ileal bypass. A survey of 104 patients, by personal interview, showed that of the 41 individuals who were angina pectoris negative prior to the partial ileal bypass, none developed these symptoms subsequently. Of the 63 preoperative angina positive patients, 7% stated that they were worse, 27% had no change, 23% reported moderate improvement as determined by a reduction in their use of nitroglycerin, 18% stated that they had marked improvement as determined by their reduced use of nitroglycerin and their increased exercise capacity, and 25% stated that they had complete remission of angina. Thus, 66% of the patients with angina pectoris prior to operation experienced improvement postoperatively. In certain of these patients, although not in all, there has been a concomitant improvement in exercise tolerance, free of the

development of ischemic ST-T changes, on the time- and grade-controlled treadmill exercise electrocardiogram. Although difficult to quantify, these findings may indicate an improvement in circulating hemodynamics or tissue oxygen availability. This concept is supported by demonstration that the red blood cell membrane thickens when the blood cholesterol content is elevated and that this increase in membrane diameter can serve as a barrier to oxygen diffusion.

Sequential Arteriography

Serial evaluation of coronary atherosclerotic plaque changes by arteriography yields data that must be viewed with caution, since a randomized control population for objective statistical comparison has not been available. Nevertheless, one of our preliminary studies indicated an apparent nonprogression rate of coronary artery disease in 55% of patients observed for up to 3 years by sequential assessments; comparable arteriographic studies of atherosclerotic individuals not on lipid reduction management have shown 50% to 60% progression rates over similar time spans. Apparent coronary arteriographic evidence of actual plaque regression was noted in three partial ileal bypass patients after 1 to 2 years (Fig. 30-8).

PORTACAVAL SHUNT FOR HYPERLIPIDEMIA

The portacaval shunt operation has essentially been limited to type IIA homozygous individuals, primarily children. However, Mieny has operated on at least one heterozygote.

TECHNIQUE

The technique is that of a standard end-to-side portacaval shunt.

IN-HOSPITAL STATISTICS AND MORTALITY

Only 43 patients have been reported in the literature, with an operative (30-day) mortality of 2.4%. There is little available in the way of statistics regarding the in-hospital course of these individuals.

LONG-TERM SIDE-EFFECTS

Little data are available or published concerning the long-term side-effects of portacaval shunting for hypercholesterolemia; however, increased platelet aggregation and female infertility have been reported.

UNIQUE COMPLICATIONS

The feared complication of portacaval shunting has always been encephalopathy. None has been reported in these patients, who are generally young and have a well-functioning liver free of cirrhosis. Nevertheless, the average time of follow-up has been short and subtle encephalopathy may go undetected (*e.g.*, a slight decrease in IQ).

EFFECT ON PLASMA LIPIDS AND LIPOPROTEINS

Total Cholesterol

The mean cholesterol reduction after portacaval shunting for hypercholesterolemia has been approximately 40%. This is interesting since it is essentially equivalent to the cholesterol lowering engendered by the enterohepatic mechanism of partial ileal bypass in heterozygous patients. We await with interest pending reports on the combined utilization of partial ileal bypass with the portacaval shunt.

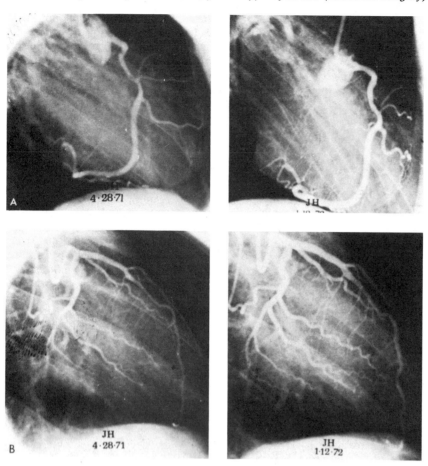

Fig. 30-8. *(A)* Preoperative and postoperative right coronary arteriograms show apparent regression of an atherosclerotic plaque. *(B)* Left coronary arteriograms of the same patient. (Buchwald H, Varco RL, Moore RB, et al: Intestinal bypass procedures. Partial ileal bypass for hyperlipidemia and jejunoileal bypass for obesity. In Ravitch MM et al [eds]: Current Problems in Surgery. Copyright © 1975 by Year Book Medical Publishers, Inc, Chicago)

Triglycerides

Little data have been published concerning the effect of portacaval shunting on plasma triglycerides; however, a reduction of triglycerides in patients who had elevated triglyceride levels preoperatively has been reported after portal diversion.

Lipoprotein Fractions

Again, little data are available regarding the lipoprotein effects of portacaval shunting. The reduction in total cholesterol seems to be due almost entirely to a decrease in the LDL-cholesterol fraction, with essentially no change in the HDL-cholesterol concentration.

CLINICAL OBSERVATIONS

No systematic prospective study is available on the long-term clinical effects of the portacaval shunt operation for hypercholesterolemia. It has been stated that, overall, approximately one third of patients following this operation experience clinical benefits; however, objective documentation has been scanty. The hardest data have been supplied by Starzl, who reported a decrease in the aortic valve gradient from 56 to 10 torr in one patient.

CONCLUSIONS

Surgical management of the hyperlipidemias deserves increased clinical attention since it offers a safe and effective approach to cholesterol lowering. The portacaval shunt for management of hypercholesterolemia should undergo fur-

ther careful appraisal. Partial ileal bypass is, currently, a time-proven therapeutic modality in the armamentarium of lipid management. The procedure is not proposed, at this time, as the treatment of choice for that segment of the population with hyperlipidemic, primarily hypercholesterolemic, disease; it may, however, be the treatment of choice for certain patients with hypercholesterolemia. The available data clearly show that diet and drug therapy, singly or in combination, rarely achieve the lipid reductions reached by partial ileal bypass. Contrary to the results of drug therapy, the cholesterol-lowering effect of partial ileal bypass is universally lasting. Patients may or may not adhere to diet or may or may not take pills, but once the operation is performed its therapeutic effects are obligatory.

BIBLIOGRAPHY

Operations for Morbid Obesity

ALDEN JF: Gastric and jejunoileal bypass: A comparison in the treatment of morbid obesity. Arch Surg 112:799, 1977

BUCHWALD H: Surgical approaches for failed jejunoileal bypass and failed gastric bypass. Surg Clin North Am 59:1121, 1979

CAREY LC, MARTIN EW JR: Treatment of morbid obesity by gastric partitioning. World J Surg 5:829, 1982

DRENICK EJ, BALE GS, SELTZER F, et al: Excessive mortality and causes of death in morbidly obese men. JAMA 243:443, 1980

EAGAN J: Personal communication, May 1981

GOMEZ CA: Gastroplasty in morbid obesity: A progress report. World J Surg 5:823, 1982

GRIFFEN WO, JR: Gastric bypass for morbid obesity. Surg Clin North Am 59:1103, 1979

Kral JG: Vagotomy as a treatment for morbid obesity. Surg Clin North Am 59:1131, 1979

Kremen AJ, Linner JH, Nelson C: An experimental evaluation of the nutritional importance of proximal and distal small intestine. Ann Surg 140:439, 1954

LaFave JW, Alden JF: Gastric bypass in the operative revision of the failed jejunoileal bypass. Arch Surg 114:438, 1979

Lavorato F, Doldi SB, Scaramella R et al: Evoluzione storica della terapia chirurgica della grade obesita. Min Med 69:3847, 1978

Laws HL, Piantadosi S: Superior gastric reduction procedure for morbid obesity: A prospective, randomized trial. Ann Surg 193:334, 1981

Mason EE, Ito C: Gastric bypass in obesity. Surg Clin North Am 47:1345, 1967

Mienyk: Personal communication, June 1980

Nisbett RE: Eating behavior and obesity in men and animals. Adv Psychosom Med 7:173, 1972

Payne JH: Metabolic observations in patients with jejuno-colic shunts. Am J Surg 106:273, 1963

Scopinaro N, Gianetta E, Pandolfo N, et al: Il bypass biliopancreatico. Minerva Chir 31:560, 1976

Scott HW Jr, Law DH IV, Sandstead HH, et al: Jejunoileal shunt in surgical treatment of morbid obesity. Ann Surg 171:770, 1970

Sherman CD Jr, May AG, Nye W, Waterhouse C: Clinical and metabolic studies following bowel bypassing for obesity. Ann NY Acad Sci 131:614, 1965

Stunkard A, McLaren-Hume M: The results of treatment for obesity: A review of the literature and report of a series. Arch Intern Med 103:79, 1959

Operations for Hyperlipidemia

Balfour JF, Kim R: Homozygous type II hyperlipoproteinemia treatment, partial ileal bypass in two children. JAMA 227:1145, 1974

Brown MS, Goldstein JL: Receptor-mediated control of cholesterol metabolism. Science 191:150, 1976

Buchwald H: Myocardial infarction in rabbits induced solely by a hypercholesterolemic diet. J Atheroscler Res 5:407, 1965

Buchwald H, Moore RB, Lee GB et al: Treatment of hypercholesterolemia: Combined dietary, surgical, and bile salt binding resin therapy. Arch Surg 97:275, 1968

Buchwald H, Moore RB, Varco RL: Surgical treatment of hyperlipidemia. Circulation 49(suppl 1):1, 1974

Buchwald H, Moore RB, Varco RL: Ten years' clinical experience with partial ileal bypass in management of the hyperlipidemias. Ann Surg 180:384, 1974

Davignon J: The lipid hypothesis: Pathophysiological basis. Arch Surg 113:28, 1978

Fredrickson DS, Levy RI, Lees RS: Fat transport in lipoproteins: An integrated approach to mechanisms and disorders. N Engl J Med 276:32, 94, 148, 215, 273, 1967

Goldstein JL, Brown MS: Lipoprotein receptors, cholesterol metabolism and atherosclerosis. Arch Pathol 99:181, 1975

Goldstein JL, Schrott HG, Hazzard WR et al: Genetic analysis of lipid levels in 176 families and delineation of a new inherited disorder, combined hyperlipidemia. J Clin Invest 52:1544, 1973

Moore RB, Buchwald H, Varco RL, POSCH Group: The effect of partial ileal bypass on plasma lipoproteins. Circulation 62:469, 1980

Moore RB, Frantz ID Jr, Buchwald H: Changes in cholesterol pool size, turnover rate, and fecal bile acid and sterol excretion after partial ileal bypass in hypercholesterolemic patients. Surgery 65:98, 1969

Starzl TE, Chase HP, Putnam CW et al: Portacaval shunt in hyperlipoproteinaemia. Lancet II:940, 1973

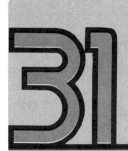

Lesions of the Umbilicus and Abdominal Wall, Abdominal Enlargement, the Peritoneum and Mesentery, Retroperitoneal Tumors and Other Conditions, and the Groin Mass

James A. Majeski/Charles T. Fitts

Umbilicus and Abdominal Wall

THE UMBILICUS

The umbilicus is at the level of the highest point of the iliac crest—that is, L3-L4. This point is almost equidistant along a line joining the tip of the xiphoid process and the top of the symphysis pubis. The position is, however, variable and unreliable as a landmark. The umbilicus is normally above the midpoint between the top of the head and the soles of the feet. When the abdomen is distended as a result of a pregnant uterus, the umbilicus is displaced cephalad; ascites will cause a downward displacement (Tanyol's sign). The skin in the umbilical area drains to the lymph nodes in both axilla and to both inguinal regions.

The prominence of the umbilicus and the depth of the umbilical pit are variable. A bluish discoloration of the umbilicus and surrounding skin (Cullen's sign) occurs in cases of ruptured ectopic pregnancy, hemorrhagic pancreatitis, and massive intraperitoneal bleeding. A yellow discoloration of the umbilicus is sometimes observed in acute pancreatitis, while an intraperitoneal rupture of a hydatid cyst may result in a dirty greenish stain of the umbilicus. Visible veins are occasionally seen, arranged radially from the umbilicus. The normal venous flow of blood is downward below the umbilicus; above it is upward. In portal vein obstruction, the direction of flow is unchanged. In obstruction of the inferior vena cava, the flow in veins below the umbilicus is reversed to an upward direction in order to shunt blood through superficial veins to the superior vena cava.

ABNORMALITIES

Abnormalities of the umbilicus may be divided into embryonic developmental defects and acquired lesions of the umbilicus that are similar to those in other areas of the body.

CONGENITAL DEFECTS

Embryonic development is characterized by an orderly formation or obliteration of various structures. Disruption of this sequence results in abnormalities primarily due to defects of the obliterative phase. The fetal umbilical cord contains (1) two umbilical arteries and a single vein, (2) the omphalomesenteric vessels, (3) the omphalomesenteric duct; (4) the allantois, and (5) the allantoic vessels.

Vascular abnormalities secondary to persistence of vascular structures are rare. The primary importance of these remnants is their ability to serve as conduits for invasive infection. Occasionally persistent fibrous bands remain intra-abdominally without external manifestations at the umbilicus.

Classification

The following classification of congenital umbilical abnormalities is useful:

Alimentary
    Complete patency of omphalomesenteric duct
    Partial patency of omphalomesenteric duct
        Distal (umbilical sinus)
        Middle (omphalomesenteric cyst)
        Proximal (Meckel's diverticulum)
    Band (obliterated omphalomesenteric duct)
    Umbilical polyp
Urinary
    Patent urachus (umbilical urinary fistula)
    Partial patency
        Distal (sinus)
        Middle (cyst)
        Proximal (diverticulum, bladder)
Vascular
    Umbilical vessels
    Omphalomesenteric vessels
    Urachal vessels

Anomalies of the Vitello-Intestinal Duct

The omphalomesenteric (vitelline) duct, formed from the narrowed yolk sac, connects the center of the yolk sac and the lumen of the midgut during intrauterine life. This duct becomes obliterated about the fifth week *in utero*. When this fails to occur, the degree of anomaly ranges from complete patency to a persistent fibrous band, thus allowing a variable symptom complex (Fig. 31-1). There is a 9:1 male predominance.

A patent vitello-intestinal duct, open in its whole length, usually is associated with a fecal discharge at the umbilicus. Occasionally, a patent duct is associated with atresia of the bowel at a lower level. The mucosa of a patent duct may prolapse at the umbilical fistula. Prolapse or intussusception of the ileum may also occur (rarely) through the patent mesenteric duct. An *enteroteratoma* (raspberry tumor) results when the umbilical extremity of the duct only remains patent and becomes everted through the navel. When

heterotopic gastric mucosa are present in a patent vitello-intestinal duct, redness and swelling may occur with every meal. When the proximal and distal ends of a vitello-intestinal duct close, a mucocele may form in the central section. This cyst is termed an *enterocytoma* and usually hangs from the antimesenteric border of the ileum, free in the peritoneal cavity.

Meckel's Diverticulum. The congenital antimesenteric diverticulum (**Meckel**) is a persistence of the duct to some degree in 10 males and 1 to 2 females per 1,000 population. It occurs on the antimesenteric border of the ileum, some 50 cm to 100 cm above the ileocecal valve, is 5 cm in length and of the same caliber as the ileum, and represents persistent patency of the intestinal portion of the vitello-intestinal duct. The mucous membrane of Meckel's diverticulum usually resembles that of the small intestine. Occasionally, patches of gastric mucosa or even small islets of pancreatic tissue may occur in a Meckel's diverticulum. Stagnation in Meckel's diverticulum may lead to inflammation, distention, perforation, and peritonitis. Symptoms are frequently identical with those of acute appendicitis.

Other Anomalies. Heterotopic gastric epithelium is present in 16% of diverticula, and pancreatic tissue is present in 5% of diverticula. Heterotopic gastric mucosa concentrates ^{99m}Tc sodium pertechnetate, and diverticula containing such tissue may be demonstrated by abdominal scan. The acid secretion in gastric mucosa-containing diverticula can lead to the development of a typical peptic ulcer in the bowel. The ulcer can be either acute or chronic, and is eight times more common in males than in females. The onset of symptoms occurs at an average age of 10 years, although adult cases occur occasionally. Melena is the most common symptom in children, and postprandial pain most common in adults.

The diverticulum may terminate as a whiplike process of fibrous tissue (vitello-intestinal cord), free at its outer end. This free extremity may adhere to another loop of bowel and obstruct it, or it may ensnare a loop, strangulating it. A diverticulum is more liable to perforation by sharp foreign bodies than any other part of the small intestine. Carcinoid is the most common tumor of the diverticulum, while adenoma, carcinoma, and sarcoma may also occur. All are extremely rare. The diverticulum may form part of the content of a hernia (Littre's hernia).

A vitello-intestinal band, as a fibrous remnant of an obliterated vitello-intestinal duct or an obliterated vitelline artery or vein, may entangle and strangulate a loop of small intestine, or it may serve as an axis around which a volvulus of the ileal loop to which it is attached may occur.

The umbilical area is one of several sites of communication between the portal and systemic circulations. The ligamentum teres carries small veins to the liver (portal) that communicate at the umbilicus with the veins of the anterior abdominal wall (systemic). The latter are radially arranged at the umbilicus and, when dilated, are called the *caput medusae*. Repair of an umbilical hernia in the presence of portal hypertension may interrupt important portosystemic connections.

Treatment. The most serious complication, intestinal obstruction, results from small bowel volvulus around a band or prolapse of intestine through a completely patent duct, and for this reason surgical intervention is indicated when the diagnosis is made. Excision of the umbilicus and intra-abdominal duct or band, with inversion of the intestinal portion of the tract, has been the usual treatment. However,

Fig. 31-1. Remnants of omphalomesenteric duct. (Britt LG, Sellers KD: Lesions of the umbilicus and the abdominal wall. In Hardy JD [ed]: Rhoads Textbook of Surgery, 5th ed. Philadelphia, J B Lippincott, 1977)

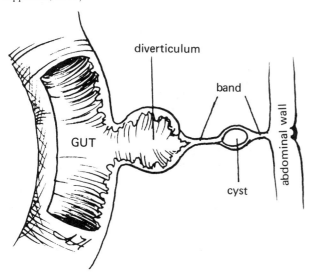

for cosmetic reasons, the umbilicus should be preserved when feasible.

Urinary Tract Abnormalities

Urinary abnormalities associated with the umbilicus are due to embryological abnormalities of the urachus (Fig. 31-2). The urachus, thought to be derived from the superior aspect of the allantois, connects the umbilicus and urinary bladder. It is normally present as a fibrous cord located between the peritoneum and the transversalis fascia. The inferior portion remains patent approximately one third of the time. Like intestinal abnormalities related to the umbilicus, urachal problems are much more common in males.

Umbilical-Urinary Fistula. Complete patency of the urachus results in an umbilical-urinary fistula, manifested by the

Fig. 31-2. Remnants of urachus. *(Center and bottom)* Patent urachus, showing catheter entering urethra and emerging from umbilicus, with a cystogram. (Benton BF, Langford HG, Hardy JD: Patent urachus. Am J Surg 88:513, 1954)

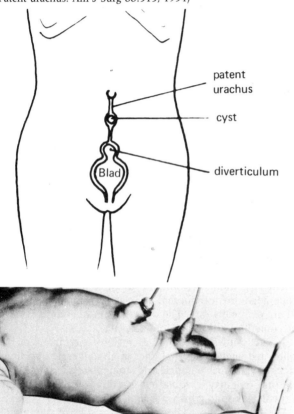

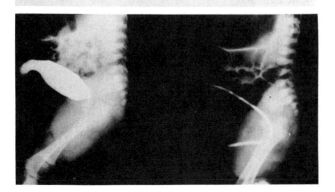

discharge of urine from the umbilicus. Skin excoriation is less severe than with the discharge of intestinal contents. The character of the discharge helps differentiate this lesion from umbilical intestinal fistula and the more common umbilical granuloma. Associated urinary tract abnormalities, particularly those producing outflow obstruction, should be sought, since they often play a significant role in the establishment of umbilical urinary fistulas.

Urachal Cyst. The most common abnormality is a urachal cyst, which results from partial obliteration of the urachus during embryologic development. Communications may exist to the urinary bladder or umbilicus. Clinically, urachal cysts may occur in the lower midline and are usually asymptomatic until they attain considerable size or become infected. Symptoms usually occur during childhood but may be seen later. Pain, the most frequent primary complaint, may be associated with fever, malaise, gastrointestinal upset, and urinary symptoms. Peritoneal irritation may give rise to findings that mimic an acute abdomen. Rupture of the cyst into the peritoneal cavity, bladder, or umbilicus may occur. Investigation of a lower midline mass should include radiologic evaluation of the lower urinary tract, since occasionally urachal cysts may be demonstrated. The most common tumors of the urachus are an adenocarcinoma and transitional cell carcinoma.

Treatment. Excision is indicated when the diagnosis is established, because of the risk of infection. Indefinitely delayed treatment may occasionally result in carcinoma of the urachal epithelial tissue.

Excision of the umbilicus, tract, and bladder apex is accomplished through a low midline approach. Dissection may be facilitated by catheterization or methylene blue injection of the fistulous tract. If associated urinary tract abnormalities have been found, particularly obstruction, they should be given priority. The umbilicus should be preserved when feasible.

Uncomplicated urachal cysts should be primarily resected, in addition to any communicating tracts. Infected cysts should be staged, with initial incision and drainage. Later excision of the remnants is recommended to prevent recurrence and the small but recognized risk of carcinoma in the urachal epithelium.

ACQUIRED UMBILICAL LESIONS

Omphalitis

Omphalitis has become infrequent in newborn nurseries since the advent of aseptic management of the umbilical stump. The majority of these infections are due to *Staphylococcus aureus.* It presents as erythema around the umbilical cord remnant and can spread quite rapidly. The vascular connections between the umbilicus and systemic circulation through the umbilical vein can introduce serious infection, including liver abscess, meningitis, pneumonia, arthritis, and peritonitis. Extrahepatic portal venous thrombosis may be related to neonatal omphalitis. For these reasons, a febrile illness in the neonate necessitates careful examination of the umbilicus and recognition that obscure infections may originate from this often overlooked site.

Obesity and diabetes are found frequently in association with adult omphalitis. Secondary infection with *Candida albicans* can be found by KOH prep. Persistent moisture and poor hygiene account for the majority of these infections. A pilonidal abscess may develop around hair buried in the navel.

Therapy is directed at improving hygiene and ensuring dryness and includes use of antifungal agents when appropriate. Systemic antibiotics are generally unnecessary in adults. Neonatal omphalitis requires aggressive therapy with systemic antibiotics and intensive local measures. Drainage or débridement of localized collections of purulent material should not be delayed. Active infection may produce abscesses in the ligamentum teres or iliac fossa (along the obliterated umbilical arteries), or a metastatic abscess in bones or joints.

Granulomas and Foreign Bodies

Two common problems of the umbilicus are umbilical granulomas and foreign bodies. The former occur in the first weeks of life; concretions may occur at any time.

Granulomas result from exuberant granulation tissue, secondary to umbilical stump infection, and are characterized by serosanguineous discharge. The base has the characteristic fiery-red appearance of granulation tissue. Foreign bodies of the umbilicus may produce inflammation as well as chronic discharge. Most concretions are debris from clothing or collections of desquamated epithelium.

Umbilical granuloma is easily managed by application of silver nitrate. Removal of the foreign body is a simple matter, and instructions in personal hygiene help prevent recurrence.

Endometriosis occasionally appears at the umbilicus, producing a confusing picture of intermittent bleeding, with asymptomatic intervals. Association with menstruation is the important clue.

Tumors

Primary tumors of the umbilicus are usually of an epidermoid type. Teratomas and desmoids occur but are extremely rare. Adenocarcinomas of urachal remnants have been reported, which emphasizes the need for early surgery in these congenital abnormalities.

In contrast to the rarity of primary umbilical tumors, the umbilicus is a common site for metastasis (Fig. 31-3). A malignancy of the umbilicus has been termed the *Sister Mary Joseph node*. It frequently is metastatic and points to a diagnosis of disseminated malignancy. Common sites of origin are pancreas, ovary, stomach, breast, and colon. These lesions signify a dismal prognosis.

THE ABDOMINAL WALL

Abdominal wall abnormalities are separated into congenital defects, inflammatory conditions, primary and metastatic tumors, painful syndromes, and rectus sheath hematomas.

CONGENITAL DEFECTS

Congenital defects of the abdominal wall are rare and occur almost exclusively in males. Complete absence (prune-belly syndrome) is extremely rare, a deficiency of one or more muscle groups being more common. The transverse abdominis muscle is most often affected, followed by the rectus abdominis below the umbilicus, internal oblique, external oblique, and rectus muscle above the umbilicus. Diastasis of the upper rectus abdominis muscles is common in newborns and does not require treatment unless there is an associated epigastric hernia. *Gastroschisis* is a defect in the abdominal wall lateral to the umbilical cord and is caused by a failure of closure of the body wall. The intestines

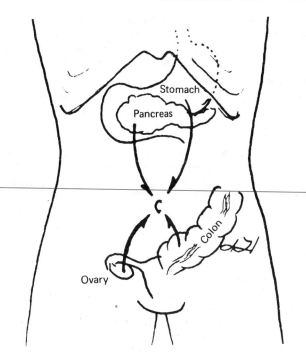

Fig. 31-3. Common sources of umbilical metastasis. (Britt LG, Sellers KD: Lesions of the umbilicus and the abdominal wall. In Hardy JD [ed]: Rhoads Textbook of Surgery, 5th ed. Philadelphia, J B Lippincott, 1977)

protrude through the defect, and no sac is present. Gastroschisis, omphalocele, umbilical hernia, and exstrophy of the bladder are discussed elsewhere.

ACQUIRED LESIONS

INFLAMMATORY CONDITIONS

Abdominal wall infections are generally seen in the postoperative state in association with abdominal incision. These vary in severity from localized cellulitis to necrotizing fasciitis. *Necrotizing fasciitis* is a mixed infection caused by aerobic and anaerobic bacteria. The infection is rapidly progressive, with necrosis of subcutaneous tissue and fascia. Immediate débridement of all involved tissue, antibiotics, and aggressive nutritional support is the only treatment.

Other inflammatory conditions of the abdominal wall include Weber-Christian panniculitis and insulin lipodystrophy. Relapsing nonsuppurative panniculitis, *Weber-Christian disease*, is a peculiar entity characterized by recurrent painful nodules of the abdominal wall as well as other areas of the body. Systemic manifestations include fever, malaise, and leukocytosis. Involvement of the small bowel mesentery gives rise to an intra-abdominal mass. These findings can present a confusing picture. The disease tends to subside spontaneously after days or weeks, only to recur. No satisfactory therapy is available; the importance of this entity lies in recognizing it, so that unnecessary laparotomy is avoided.

Another condition of interest is insulin lipodystrophy. Subcutaneous nodules or depressions may be found over the lower abdomen at sites of insulin injection. These areas represent hypertrophy or atrophy of subcutaneous adipose tissue. Pain may be a prominent finding in these areas, and secondary infection with abscess formation occurs when unsterile techniques are employed for insulin injection.

Elderly diabetics with poor vision are usually the victims of this complication. The enigma of multiple lower abdominal abscesses may not be resolved until the patient is questioned about the sites and methods of insulin injection.

TUMORS

The majority of abdominal wall tumors are benign, and their character and frequency parallel soft tissue tumors in other regions of the body. The most common tumor is the lipoma, followed by papilloma, fibroma, nevi, and keratoses. Therapy is simple excision. Neurofibroma may be single or multiple if in association with von Recklinghausen's disease. The malignant potential of the latter has been well documented.

Malignant tumors of the abdominal wall occur with equal frequency as primary malignancies or blood-borne metastases. Sarcomas are among the most common of the primary tumors. Epidermoid carcinoma and melanoma are the next most frequent abdominal-wall malignant tumors. Epidermoid carcinoma occurs often in areas of previous trauma, burns, or scar formation. Melanomas around the umbilicus are associated with an unfavorable prognosis, owing to the large network of lymphatics and surrounding blood vessels. Secondary malignancies of the abdominal wall may arise from the ovary, prostate, stomach, uterus, lung, kidney, breast, and colon. Resection of primary and metastatic tumors is the primary treatment; only minimal effectiveness has been obtained from radiation therapy and chemotherapy. Hyperthermia has been mildly successful in controlling these tumors.

Desmoid Tumor

The desmoid tumor seems to have a peculiar affinity for the abdominal wall. These tumors represent a curious proliferation of fibrous tissue with a pathologic appearance on the spectrum between fibroma and fibrosarcoma. They are histologically benign but are capable of local invasiveness. Distant metastasis probably does not occur. They are usually gray-white unencapsulated masses located in the myoaponeurotic layers of the abdominal wall. The tumor is more common in females, and its association with recent pregnancy suggests an endocrine dependency. Desmoids may be seen at any age, but the third and fourth decades represent the peak incidence. The lower abdomen near the midline in association with the rectus abdominis muscle is the most frequent site of occurrence.

No characteristic signs exist, and a clinical diagnosis can be made only with a high index of suspicion. Occasionally, these masses are confused with intra-abdominal tumors, but this dilemma should be resolved by physical examination. Intra-abdominal tumors cannot be felt with the abdominal wall tensed, whereas tumors arising in the wall become fixed and remain palpable. This sign, attributed to Fothergill, is of benefit in localizing these tumors to the abdominal wall.

Wide local excision is strongly recommended as treatment because of a high incidence (20%) of local recurrence. The abdominal wall musculature and fascia should be excised in a three-dimensional fashion with the tumor, and restoration of the abdominal wall accomplished with either prosthetic material or primary repair. Primary repair is usually possible because of the wall's elasticity.

Rectus Sheath Hematoma

Although not a tumor in the traditional sense, hematomas of the rectus sheath often simulate abdominal tumors (Fig.

31-4). Since its description in 1857, this condition has been recognized with increasing frequency.

The anatomic arrangement of the rectus abdominis muscles contributes to the formation of this condition. These are paired longitudinal muscles with the capability of stretching and contracting over a distance of 17 cm. The course of the muscle is interrupted by four or five tendinous inscriptions, which prevent bulging of the muscle with contraction and relaxation. The rectus muscle is surrounded by a strong sheath, except below the semilunar line of Douglas. From this line inferiorly, only a layer of transversalis fascia and preperitoneal fat separates the muscle from the peritoneum. In the lower abdomen, the inferior epigastric artery and veins course posterior to the rectus muscle and are joined in the upper abdomen by the inferior portion of the internal mammary artery. Shearing forces caused by muscle contraction or direct trauma result in disruption of these vessels and hematoma formation. In the upper abdomen, dissection of the hematoma is limited by the tendinous inscriptions and rectus sheath, whereas in the lower abdomen dissection of the hematoma is unimpeded.

Trauma plays the most significant role in the formation of hematomas of the rectus sheath. Other predisposing factors include pregnancy, anticoagulant therapy, degenerative states of the muscle or blood vessels, and the postoperative state.

The chief clinical finding is a painful abdominal mass. The onset may be sudden or gradual, and associated fever and leukocytosis are commonly seen. Skin discoloration is a late finding and not usually helpful in the early stages. Blood loss may be sufficient to cause anemia. Fothergill's sign may be present and helps localize the mass to the abdominal wall. Ultrasound has proved a reliable means of diagnosing and localizing a hematoma in the rectus sheath.

If the diagnosis can be established, conservative therapy is indicated. Bed rest, sedation, warm or cold packs, and

Fig. 31-4. Rectus sheath hematoma. (Britt LG, Sellers KD: Lesions of the umbilicus and the abdominal wall. In Hardy JD [ed]: Rhoads Textbook of Surgery, 5th ed. Philadelphia, J B Lippincott, 1977)

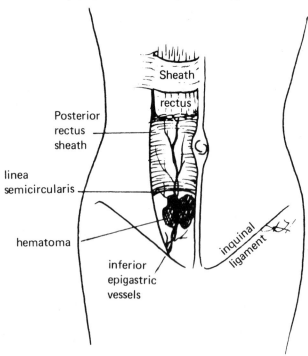

control of coagulation defects are indicated. In most cases the diagnosis is not made and operation is performed. A hematoma is encountered on entering the rectus sheath or posterior to the rectus muscle. The hematoma should be evacuated and the bleeding vessels ligated. Closure without drainage is preferred. If doubt exists in regard to the diagnosis, the peritoneal cavity should be entered.

PAINFUL SYNDROMES

Patients with localized pain and tenderness of the abdominal wall are often seen. If no organic cause can be found, the complaints are attributed to psychoneurotic factors. Local factors, as well as distant causes, should be sought. These include entrapment of cutaneous nerves, hernia, herpes zoster, and intercostal neuralgia.

Entrapment of cutaneous nerves can occur at several sites but, because of the arrangement of the muscular foramina there, the rectus margin is a common site of involvement. The neurovascular bundle emerges through this foramen, and any condition that produces narrowing may cause compression of the nerve, with resultant pain. These patients typically complain of dull, aching pain at the margin of the rectus muscle. The most important differential is the precise localization of the pain and, in particular, reproducible local tenderness.

Referred pain to the abdominal wall may occur from abdominal visceral disease or distension. This type of abdominal wall pain can be understood on an anatomic basis. The afferent sympathetic fibers innervate the abdominal viscera. These fibers join the central nervous system in a segmental fashion, as do the somatic afferent fibers arising from the abdominal wall (which perceive cutaneous pain). When visceral impulses are transmitted to the central nervous system, they are perceived as somatic or cutaneous pain in those segments of the body innervated from the same segment that receives the afferent sympathetic impulses. A common example occurs when a distended appendix has referred pain to the skin and abdominal wall around the umbilicus.

Immediate relief can be obtained by the injection of a local anesthetic directly into the area of localized tenderness. As well as affording immediate, albeit short-term, relief, this establishes the diagnosis and helps allay the patient's anxiety. Other symptomatic therapy may be used, consisting of heat or cold and abdominal binders. Operation is rarely necessary.

Before attributing complaints of abdominal wall pain to hysterical symptoms, consider that this might be referred pain of spinal origin, intercostal neuralgia, or a neurological condition such as tabes dorsalis or herpes zoster infection.

This section is a revision of the first section of Chapter 49, written by Louis G. Britt and Kenneth D. Sellers, in the fifth edition of *Rhoads Textbook of Surgery*.

BIBLIOGRAPHY

APPLEGATE WV: Abdominal cutaneous nerve entrapment syndrome. Surgery 71:118, 1972
BICHER HI: The physiological effects of hyperthermia. Radiology 137:511, 1981
BOURNE IH: Treatment of painful conditions of the abdominal wall with local injections. Practitioner 224:921, 1980
BRASFIELD RD, DASGUPTA TK: Desmoid tumors of the anterior abdominal wall. Surgery 65:241, 1969
COETZEE T: Clinical anatomy of the umbilicus. S Afr Med J 57:463, 1980
CRESSON SL, PILLING GP: Lesions about the umbilicus in infants and children. Pediatr Clin North Am 6:1085, 1959
CULLEN TS: Embryology, Anatomy and Disease of the Umbilicus Together with Disease of the Urachus. Philadelphia, W B Saunders, 1916
FOTHERGILL WE: Haematoma in the abdominal wall simulating pelvic new growth. Br Med J 1:941, 1926
HILDRETH D: Anticoagulant therapy and rectus sheath hematoma. Am J Surg 124:80, 1972
HITCHENS E, PLATT D: Fibrosarcoma. Cancer 29:1369, 1972
KLEIN MD, KOSLOSKE AM, HERTZLER JH: Congenital defects of the abdominal wall. JAMA 245:1643, 1981
SASMAZ O, PETRIDIS I, ALICAN F: Hematoma of the rectus abdominis muscle. Arch Surg 100:8, 1970
SCHRECK W, CAMPBELL W: The relation of bladder obstruction to urinary-umbilical fistula. J Urol 108:641, 1972
SHIU MH, FLANCBAUM L, HAJDU SI et al: Malignant soft tissue tumor of the anterior abdominal wall. Arch Surg 115:152, 1980
SILVERMAN F, HUANG N: Congenital absence of the abdominal muscles associated with malformation of genitourinary and alimentary tracts: Report of case and review of literature. Am J Dis Child 80:91, 1950
SOUTAR SF, DOUGLAS DM, DENNISON WM: Patent vitellointestinal duct—The risk of obstruction due to prolapse. Br J Surg 45:617, 1958
TITONE C, LIPSIUS M, KRAKAUER J: Spontaneous hematoma of the rectus abdominis muscle: Critical review of 50 cases with emphasis on early diagnosis and treatment. Surgery 72:568, 1972
WYATT GM, SPITZ HB: Ultrasound in the diagnosis of rectus sheath hematoma. JAMA 241:1499, 1979

Charles T. Fitts

Abdominal Enlargement and Diseases of the Mesentery, Omentum, and Peritoneum

EMBRYOLOGY AND PHYSIOLOGY
ABDOMINAL ENLARGEMENT
MESENTERY
  Mesenteric Cysts
  Tumors of the Mesentery
  Retractile Mesenteritis
OMENTUM

PERITONEUM
  Adhesions
  Primary Malignant Disease
  Metastatic Malignant Disease
  Pseudomyxoma Peritonei
  Starch Granulomas
  Peritoneal Dialysis and Lavage

EMBRYOLOGY AND PHYSIOLOGY

The peritoneum, mesentery, and omentum are intimately associated from the standpoints of embryology, physiology, pathology, and the disease processes that may involve them. Thus, it is appropriate that they be considered in one chapter. This chapter discusses evaluation of abdominal enlargement and the disease processes of the mesentery, diseases of the peritoneum other than peritonitis, and diseases of the omentum.

Embryologically, the primitive coelom initially is a single cavity, but by the seventh week of fetal life it is divided into pleural and peritoneal cavities by the pleuroperitoneal membrane, the future diaphragm. Initially, the peritoneal cavity is separated into right and left halves by the primitive gut and its mesentery. The mesentery is both dorsal and ventral to the gut, but the ventral mesentery eventually disappears, leaving the gut suspended on the dorsal mesentery. The gut then undergoes a series of herniations and rotations (which are well described in textbooks of embryology). During the process of herniation and rotation, the dorsal mesogastrium, which is actually the mesentery of the stomach, overlaps the transverse mesocolon and fuses with it so that the mesogastrium actually appears to take origin from the transverse colon itself. Considerable further overgrowth of the dorsal mesogastrium between the greater curvature of the stomach and the transverse colon produces an apron of redundant tissue that descends into the lower abdomen to form the greater omentum.

Consideration of the physiology of the peritoneum will be limited to absorption and transduction of fluid. We take advantage of this physiological process in the application of peritoneal dialysis for renal failure and in the use of ventriculoperitoneal shunts for hydrocephalus. It has been demonstrated in animals that the peritoneum can absorb fluid at a rate of up to 8% of the total body weight in 1 hour. Thus, in 12 to 30 hours, the peritoneum absorbs a quantity of fluid equal to the body weight. Toxins introduced into the peritoneal cavity are absorbed as rapidly as if injected into the circulation. This is also true for various bacteria and medications. Again, as surgeons, we take advantage of this physiological process by administering antibiotics intraperitoneally.

Normally, the peritoneal cavity contains only several milliliters of serous fluid to serve as lubricant for the viscera that slide over one another. Very few cells are in normal peritoneal fluid; the normal cell count is between 2000 and 2500/ml. Most of these cells are lymphocytes, basophils, and monocytes, with few neutrophils.

The physiological role of the mesentery is to support the viscera to which it is attached, that is, the small bowel, transverse colon, and sigmoid colon. Any disease process that involves the mesentery usually affects the adjacent viscera secondarily. The omentum has the same absorptive capability as the peritoneum but also serves an additional function in localization of inflammatory processes. The omentum has been called by many the abdominal leukocyte; others call it the great "policeman" of the abdomen. Inflammatory processes are walled off very quckly by the normal omentum unless it has previously become adherent to another structure by adhesions.

The total surface area of all of the peritoneum, mesentery, and omentum is approximately the same as the total surface area of the skin. Again, comparing the peritoneum with the skin, one can think of peritonitis as being an internal burn

that represents an insult to the body equal in magnitude to that from a third-degree burn of the skin.

ABDOMINAL ENLARGEMENT

Abdominal enlargement occasionally presents as the chief complaint in a patient. This may be due to any specific pathologic process that develops a space-occupying mass within the abdominal cavity that is of sufficient size. The diagnosis and management of these individual lesions is the subject of many of the chapters in this text and is beyond the scope of this particular chapter.

Abdominal enlargement not due to a specific space-occupying mass is almost always due to the accumulation of gas or fluid within the peritoneal cavity or the intestinal lumen. Accumulation within the intestinal lumen is almost invariably associated with intestinal obstruction and is probably the most common cause of diffuse abdominal enlargement. Chronic severe constipation and congenital megacolon also fit into this broad category of intestinal obstruction as a cause of abdominal enlargement. The diagnosis of these problems is usually obtained accurately by history, physical examination, and standard radiographic techniques without the necessity for newer sophisticated technology. Accumulation of gas within the peritoneal cavity may cause abdominal enlargement and is almost always due to a ruptured hollow viscus. The presence of free air in the peritoneal cavity is usually detectable by a plain upright or lateral decubitus film of the abdomen. It should be remembered that small amounts of free air may be found for several days after laparotomy. The accumulation of fluid within the free peritoneal cavity is probably the second most common cause of diffuse abdominal enlargement and is generally covered under the term *ascites*. Ascites is most frequently due to hepatic circulatory dysfunction or cardiac insufficiency. Less frequent causes are malignant ascites, chylous ascites, pancreatic ascites, biliary ascites, and inflammatory ascites (*e.g.*, bacterial, nephrogenic, or collagen disease–associated serositis).

The diagnosis is suspected from information in the history and physical examination together with standard radiographic techniques. Once it has been established that fluid accumulation within the peritoneal cavity is present, paracentesis and appropriate examination of the fluid itself is usually the key for planning further diagnostic steps.

Lastly, two extremely common causes of diffuse abdominal enlargement that are basically physiologic rather than pathologic entities should be mentioned: obesity and pregnancy.

MESENTERY

There are very few primary diseases of the intestinal mesentery. Diseases involving the blood vessels passing through the mesentery and diseases of adjacent viscera involving the mesentery only secondarily are discussed elsewhere. This leaves for consideration mesenteric cysts, tumors of the mesentery, and retractile mesenteritis.

MESENTERIC CYSTS

Mesenteric cysts are generally thought to arise from congenital abnormalities in the lymphatics of the mesentery that slowly result in the accumulation of lymph and cyst formation. The cysts are usually multiloculated and may vary in size from quite small to filling the entire abdominal cavity. Somewhat puzzling, considering the presumed congenital origin, is the fact that most cysts present after 10 years of age. Most commonly, patients present with a palpable mass unassociated with other symptomatology or with only vague visceral pain. As the cyst enlarges, however, a variety of symptoms may develop related most often to compression of adjacent viscera. Compression with obstruction of the intestine or ureters are examples. Classically, the palpable cyst is smooth, rounded, nontender, and more mobile from side to side than up and down.

Definitive preoperative diagnosis is not easily obtained. Both plain abdominal roentgenography and ultrasound may suggest a fluid-filled mass but cannot specify the origin. Arteriography may show an avascular mass within the mesentery with a thin, uniformly staining rim. These findings, together with the clinical picture, may give a high degree of suspicion, but absolutely definitive diagnosis basically requires laparotomy. The treatment of choice is complete enucleation of the cyst, which is usually technically feasible without damaging adjacent viscera or the blood supply to the intestine. On those rare occasions when dense adherence to adjacent vasculature or intestine precludes this approach, resection of a wedge of mesentery containing the cyst, together with the bowel served by that mesentery, should be carried out. If this is deemed technically too hazardous, internal drainage into the peritoneal cavity has been successful. Simple aspiration of the cyst is usually unacceptable because recurrence is the rule rather than the exception.

Very rarely, cysts have ruptured or have sustained hemorrhage into the cyst, or have contained sarcomatous changes in the wall. The basic therapy should be the same under these conditions, with the possible exception of a somewhat wider resection if a diagnosis of sarcoma has been fortuitously obtained. There is no evidence to support return to the abdomen and wide resection in the event of a pathologic report of sarcoma after the fact. On the other hand, if the surgeon feels certain he left gross tumor behind, this approach could be reasonably entertained.

TUMORS OF THE MESENTERY

The mesentery may rarely be the origin of a benign or, even more rarely, malignant tumor. Solitary neurofibroma or multiple neurofibromas associated with von Recklinghausen's disease or Gardner's syndrome are probably among the most common benign tumors, together with lipoma. Other benign tumors include neurilemoma, leiomyoma, fibromyoma, dermoid, and hemangioma. Each of these tumors has a malignant counterpart. Lymphomas may cause a solid tumor mass when the disease involves mesenteric lymph nodes.

The tumors usually present as a nontender abdominal mass that may be quite large. A great variety of symptoms may be present, all related to the position of the tumor and the effects of pressure on adjacent structures. Accurate preoperative diagnosis is usually not obtainable. The abdominal CT scan recently has facilitated the diagnosis of solid and cystic intra-abdominal masses.

The treatment of choice for benign or malignant lesions is surgical excision. The outlook for patients with malignant tumors is poor; however, very occasionally, patients survive for a long time even after partial resections.

RETRACTILE MESENTERITIS

Retractile mesenteritis (mesenteric lipodystrophy, mesenteric panniculitis) is a rare and poorly understood disorder of the intestinal mesentery. The pathology and clinical course are somewhat variable, so it is difficult to be certain that one basic process is responsible. At the present time, however, it seems most helpful to consider the problem as one pathologic process that starts as lipodystrophy in the fat of the mesentery with resultant masses or thickening of areas composed of foamy lipophages and only rarely collagen deposits or inflammatory cells. This may apparently progress to include an inflammatory response with lymphocyte and giant-cell accumulation and then progress even further to marked fibrosis, scarring, and retraction. The gross pathology is similarly variable. There are isolated firm grayish nodules or placques in some patients; in other patients, there is a diffuse, thickened, rubbery mesentery, especially at the root. In some instances, there is extensive scarring, retraction, and foreshortening of the mesentery with dense adhesions between adjacent mesenteric surfaces. The clinical picture may be mild, with low-grade fever, vague abdominal pain, and malaise, or severe, with the symptoms and signs of partial or complete intestinal obstruction. It should also be noted that diarrhea or rectal bleeding may occur.

The diagnosis is difficult to establish preoperatively. In the milder forms found at surgery, biopsy is probably all that is indicated. In the case of intestinal obstruction, however, corrective surgery of a conservative nature should be carried out. The overall prognosis is generally very good, but there are exceptions, and at least one reported patient has died from obstruction of mesenteric veins.

OMENTUM

The greater omentum may occasionally be involved with cysts similar to those described in the mesentery and is also rarely involved with all of the solid tumors described in the mesentery. In the case of the omentum, however, malignant lesions are more common than are benign; of these malignant lesions, leiomyosarcoma is the most common. The treatment is surgical excision.

Idiopathic segmental infarction and primary torsion of the omentum both result in the findings of localized peritonitis, most often on the right side. The etiology of idiopathic segmental infarction is not determined. Torsion is thought to occasionally result from excessive accumulation of fat, with the weight twisting a portion of the omentum on a pedicle with or without the aid of adhesions.

Torsion has been reported approximately twice as often as idiopathic infarction. Overall, there appears to be no significant age or sex preference. The clinical picture is essentially the same in both problems and is generally right-sided abdominal tenderness with signs of peritoneal irritation, fever, and leukocytosis. A mass is occasionally palpable. Most often, the patient is believed to have appendicitis. Retrospectively, most cases have been found to lack the prodromal periumbilical crampy pain typical of appendicitis, and nausea is practically never present. In addition, the course is relatively indolent; there is slow progression over a matter of days, with increasing pain, fever, and leukocytosis but without the development of nausea, vomiting, and systemic illness to be expected from neglected appendicitis. The treatment is excision of the infarcted mass, and the results are excellent.

Finally, it should be noted that the omentum has been used in many reconstructive procedures. The omentum may be used on a pedicle to cover wounds from the knee to the chest. In addition, with the advent of successful microsurgery, free omental flaps can be used almost anywhere in the body.

PERITONEUM

ADHESIONS

When abdominal surgical procedures were not as commonly performed as they are now, intra-abdominal adhesions were of little importance. In a review of cases of intestinal obstruction at hospitals throughout England in the 1920s, adhesions accounted for only 7% of the obstructions as compared to 49% due to incarcerated hernia. A review from the Massachusetts General Hospital in 1932 revealed that 30% of the cases of intestinal obstruction were related to adhesions. A review from New Orleans at about the same time showed that 27% of cases of intestinal obstruction were secondary to adhesions. This relatively low incidence of obstruction secondary to adhesions is still found in primitive areas of the world where little abdominal surgery is done.

In developed countries, adhesions are more common because more abdominal operations are being performed. Previous abdominal surgery accounted for 79% of adhesions in one large review, whereas 10% of the adhesions were related to previous inflammatory disease and 11% were congenital. Most inflammatory adhesions are secondary to appendicitis, but occasionally they occur after inflammation of the gallbladder or pelvic organs or even after inflammatory bowel disease. Postoperative adhesions are most common after appendectomy and pelvic surgery.

At one time it was believed that damage to the endothelium, as a result of rough handling, retraction, swabbing, or surgical denudation, necessarily was followed by persistent adhesions. On the basis of this concept, surgeons went to great lengths to completely cover all raw serosal surfaces within the abdominal cavity. Recently, however, this concept of adhesion formation has been opened to question. It has been demonstrated many times, experimentally and clinically, that the presence of raw surfaces of the peritoneum does not necessarily lead to the formation of adhesions.

After radical pelvic operations that completely denude the pelvis of its peritoneum, healing is frequently smooth, with no adhesions whatsoever. In contrast, several studies have shown that heroic attempts to patch or repair peritoneal defects actually increase the incidence of adhesions. Thomas and co-workers noted that excision of an area of peritoneum from the small intestine of guinea pigs resulted in adhesion formation in 31% of the instances. When the raw area was carefully oversewn, the incidence increased to 79%. Conolly and Stephens found in rats that laparotomy incisions closed without suturing of the peritoneum healed with a decreased incidence of adhesions to the wound. Gross and microscopic examination of adhesions produced in this manner revealed that tiny blood vessels accompany the adhesions, suggesting that the operative area was attempting to obtain a new blood supply from another source. This observation suggested that the stimulus for adhesion formation was not the peritoneal defect itself but rather the presence of ischemic

tissue resulting from pulling the edges of the tissue together by sutures in an attempt at repair. It is not totally understood how serosal defects heal, but the consensus among investigators is that cells deep to the injury differentiate into mesothelium rather than the mesothelium at the periphery of the injury extending laterally across the site of the injury.

Ischemic tissue is not the only stimulus of an inflammatory vascular response in neighboring structures. A study by Ryan and colleagues showed that drying, wiping, or wetting with saline causes the same degree of injury to the mesothelium of the peritoneum. All of these insults destroy the mesothelium and induce adhesions. Other irritating agents that enter the peritoneal cavity at the time of laparotomy may be responsible for the development of fibrous intra-abdominal adhesions. Granulomatous reactions to talcum and starch powder are examples of this.

Prevention of adhesions is a goal of all surgeons. This has been attempted by a number of different approaches. To prevent deposition of fibrin in the peritoneal exudate, sodium citrate, heparin, and other anticoagulants have been used. Enzymes such as trypsin, pepsin, hyaluronidase, streptokinase, and streptodornase have been used to remove fibrin; lavage has been used for mechanical removal. In an attempt to prevent fibrin-coated walls of the intestine from touching each other, the abdomen has been distended with oxygen, saline, olive oil, lanolin, dextrose solution, amniotic fluid, silicone, and various other solutions. Prevention of fibroblastic proliferation has been attempted with corticosteroids and cytotoxic agents. Attempts have been made to control the distribution and nature of forming adhesions by plication of the intestine. Recently, low-frequency sound has been used prophylactically in experimental animals with some success. At the present time, however, none of these procedures has accumulated enough evidence to be considered of proved routine clinical value.

Good surgical technique will decrease the incidence of unnecessary adhesion formation. This involves careful avoidance of foreign materials that induce granuloma formation, such as talcum powder, starch powder, and long redundant ends of suture material. Whenever possible, serosal defects are left open rather than pulled together under tension. Because adhesions represent neovascularity, an ischemic area should be covered with vascular omentum instead of allowing intestine to become adherent to the ischemic area, which would cause adhesions to arise from the intestine.

PRIMARY MALIGNANT DISEASE

The only primary cancer of the peritoneum is mesothelioma. It has been recognized with increased frequency recently, and there is no question that it is related to environment and occupation. A study in Canada showed an incidence of 0.1 case per 100,000 population in rural occupations. In contrast, in Holland the incidence was found to be 1 case per 100,000 population among workers in heavy industry and 100 cases per 100,000 population among shipyard workers. With the exception of lung cancer, there is no other neoplasm for which the relationship of environment to carcinogenesis has been so clearly established as it has for mesothelioma.

Asbestos exposure is definitely the responsible factor. Asbestos miners, shipyard workers, asbestos textile manufacturers, and insulation workers have an increased incidence of mesothelioma, and pleural mesothelioma occurs more often than peritoneal mesothelioma. Duration of exposure to asbestos has varied from less than 1 year to more than 50 years. However, not all cases of mesothelioma have had an association with exposure to asbestos. Mesothelioma in children has been reported and bears no relationship to asbestos exposure. At the present time, the overall incidence of mesothelioma in the United States is approximately 2.2 per million per year, and only 20% of these originate in the peritoneum.

Grossly, peritoneal mesothelioma occurs as two types. One is a large tumor in the upper abdomen with scattered small nodules, and the other consists of scattered small nodules and plaques over all peritoneal surfaces. The neoplasm is mostly local, and death usually occurs from local abdominal involvement rather than from visceral involvement. Metastasis to lungs and other distant organs is uncommon.

Patients have abdominal pain, cramping, weight loss, and abdominal distention, and 90% have ascites. Few have a palpable mass. An occasional patient has hypoglycemia (the cause of hypoglycemia with mesothelioma has not been determined; circulating insulin levels are normal). Preoperative diagnosis is rare, and even at operation it usually is thought that peritoneal carcinomatosis is present until biopsy proves mesothelioma.

If the disease is local, resection may be possible. In the usual case, in which there is involvement of all of the peritoneum, no form of surgical excision is feasible, and death usually ensues within a matter of months. Chemotherapy, either intra-abdominal or systemic, is rarely beneficial. Generalized abdominal irradiation usually does not control the symptoms. Frequently, palliation with narcotics and medical treatment of the ascites are all that can be provided. Peritoneal mesothelioma has a worse prognosis than does pleural mesothelioma because of the severe obstructive problems of the bowel that occur.

METASTATIC MALIGNANT DISEASE

Peritoneal carcinomatosis is distressingly frequent and is most often from visceral cancer. The stomach and pancreas are the most likely sources of carcinomatosis. Virtually any malignant tumor, including lesions of the lung and breast, can spread to the peritoneum and cause carcinomatosis. The symptoms are not only those of the primary tumor but also those of bowel obstruction and ascites. Peritoneal carcinomatosis is the third most common cause of small-bowel obstruction.

Chemotherapy may offer minimal palliation; surgical treatment relieves only the bowel obstruction. Strangulative obstruction is exceedingly rare; therefore, small-bowel obstruction from carcinomatosis is hardly ever a surgical emergency. Conservative management usually fails, but only 50% of patients operated on for obstruction from carcinomatosis have their symptoms relieved. The mean survival after palliative surgical treatment is only 4 months. When intestinal anastomosis is necessary because of bowel resection for carcinomatosis, it should be performed only in a segment of intestine that is free of peritoneal implants; otherwise, an intestinal fistula is likely to develop.

PSEUDOMYXOMA PERITONEI

Pseudomyxoma peritonei is a rare condition resulting from a ruptured mucin-producing lesion, usually of the appendix or ovary, although the uterus, bowel, and common bile duct are occasional sources. A mucocele of the appendix may rupture, seeding the entire peritoneum with mucous cells. A similar condition develops when an ovarian mucinous cystadenoma ruptures. The peritoneal lesions consist of edematous granulation tissue with abundant mucin and focal hemorrhage. Mucin-producing epithelium is found in the implants. Massive mucin production results, and mucinous ascites follows. Symptoms relate to the primary disease plus massive abdominal enlargement and intestinal obstruction.

Treatment is laparotomy with evacuation of as much of the mucus as possible plus treatment of the primary condition, usually by appendectomy or oophorectomy. Repeated laparotomy for recurrences is justified. Long disease-free intervals frequently occur between multiple laparotomies. Chemotherapy and radiation therapy contribute little to the management of pseudomyxoma peritonei. Very few cases have been reported to metastasize, and viscera are not invaded. Death may be secondary to intestinal obstruction or fistula formation.

STARCH GRANULOMAS

From the advent of use of rubber gloves during operations, various lubricants have been used to aid in donning the gloves. Talcum powder was used initially, but talcum granulomas, resulting in talcum peritonitis, adhesions, and bowel obstructions, were reported in the early 1930s. Corn starch was substituted in 1948. Shortly thereafter, starch granulomas began to be reported. Starch granules cause a foreign-body reaction that results in multiple peritoneal granulomas and the development of an abdominal mass, pain, fever, nausea, and symptoms of small-bowel obstruction. Sluggish recovery after an abdominal operation sometimes may be due to this.

When symptoms do justify abdominal reexploration, metastatic carcinoma or tuberculous peritonitis may be suspected at first. Biopsy reveals classic starch granulomas. Fortunately, the disease is self-limited, and the symptoms resolve as the starch is absorbed. Once the problem has been identified, symptomatic treatment is all that is indicated. Steroids have occasionally relieved the symptoms, but their use does not alter the overall course of the disease. Bloody ascites occasionally develops, making one suspect malignancy.

Rice powder was tried for a short time in place of starch powder as a glove lubricant, but the foreign-body reactions were even worse than with starch. The only prophylaxis is diligent removal of the powder from the gloves before the peritoneal cavity is entered.

PERITONEAL DIALYSIS AND LAVAGE

The peritoneum can be used as an absorptive and excretory organ in treating renal failure. Intermittent short-term peritoneal dialysis has been in use for years in treatment of acute renal failure but was often associated with complications such as peritonitis, fluid overload, intestinal perforation, and catheter obstruction. Development of the Tenckhoff catheter has permitted highly successful short-term and long-term dialysis even in renal failure requiring dialysis over a period of years. The Tenckhoff catheter is made of Silastic and has a Dacron bacteriostatic button that is placed in the subcutaneous tissues. When the catheter is inserted with appropriate aseptic techniques and precautions, the incidence of peritonitis is less than 1%. Heparin (1000 U) is added to each bottle of dialysis fluid to prevent catheter obstruction. Fever, turbidity of the returning fluid, and abdominal tenderness are indications for the use of antibiotics. At the present time, there is considerable interest in chronic ambulatory peritoneal dialysis, and it is to be expected that surgeons will be asked to contribute frequently to the management of chronic access to the peritoneal cavity for this purpose.

Enthusiasm varies regarding the use of peritoneal lavage as treatment for peritonitis unrelated to a perforated viscus. McKenna and associates stated that mechnical cleansing by continuous peritoneal lavage is of benefit to the inflamed peritoneal surface just as débridement is of benefit to surface wounds and skin burns. They suggested continuous lavage of the peritoneum with large volumes of crystalloid solution, with two catheters in the upper abdomen for instillation of fluid and two suction catheters in the lower abdomen.

The beneficial effect is from mechanical cleansing, and intravenous rather than intraperitoneal administration of antibiotics has been suggested. Experimental and clinical studies have proved that intraperitoneal antibiotic therapy is as efficient as intravenous therapy for obtaining therapeutic serum levels. Whether or not the topical effect of intraperitoneal therapy is beneficial is controversial. Artz and co-workers found that irrigation of the peritoneal cavity with a solution of penicillin and kanamycin decreased the mortality of patients with early peritonitis. Few surgeons rely completely on intraperitoneal antibiotic therapy for treating peritonitis, but many use this technique in addition to intravenous administration of antibiotics.

Peritonitis from a perforated viscus remains an absolute indication for formal laparotomy and systemic antibiotic therapy.

This section is a revision of the second section of Chapter 49, written by William J. Hardin, in the fifth edition of *Rhoads Textbook of Surgery.*

BIBLIOGRAPHY

ADAMS GT: Primary torsion of the omentum. Am J Surg 126:102, 1973

ARTZ CP, BARNETT WO, GROGAN JB: Further studies concerning the pathogenesis and treatment of peritonitis. Ann Surg 155:756, 1962

BURNETT WE, ROSEMOND GP, BUCHER RM: Mesenteric cysts: Report of 3 cases, in one of which calcified cyst was present. Arch Surg 60:699, 1950

COLASANTE DA, AU FC, SELL HW et al: Prophylaxis of adhesions with low frequency sound. Surg Gynecol Obstet 153:357, 1981

CONOLLY WB, STEPHENS FO: Factors influencing the incidence of intraperitoneal adhesions: An experimental study. Surgery 63:976, 1968

COX KR: Starch granuloma (pseudo-malignant seeding). Br J Surg 57:650, 1970

CROFOOT DD: Spontaneous segmental infarction of the greater omentum. Am J Surg 139:262, 1980

CURRIE DJ: Continuous peritoneal lavage. Surg Gynecol Obstet 135:951, 1972

DURST AL, FREUND H, ROSENMANN E et al: Mesenteric panniculitis: Review of the literature and presentation of cases. Surgery 81:203, 1977

ELLIS H: The cause and prevention of postoperative intraperitoneal adhesions. Surg Gynecol Obstet 133:497, 1971

GLASS RL, LEDUC RJ: Small intestinal obstruction from peritoneal carcinomatosis. Am J Surg 125:316, 1973

GRUNDY GW, MILLER RW: Malignant mesothelioma in childhood: Report of 13 cases. Cancer 30:1216, 1972

HUBBARD TB JR, KHAN MZ, CARAG VR JR et al: The pathology of peritoneal repair: Its relation to the formation of adhesions. Ann Surg 165:908, 1967

LANKISCH PG, TONNIS HJ, FERNANDEZ-REDO E et al: Use of Tenckhoff catheter for peritoneal dialysis in terminal renal failure. Br Med J 4:712, 1973

LEGHA SS, MUGGIA FM: Pleural mesothelioma: Clinical features and therapeutic implications. Ann Intern Med 87:613, 1977

LIMBER GK, KING RE, SILVERBURG SG: Pseudomyxoma peritonei: A report of ten cases. Ann Surg 178:587, 1973

MCDONALD AD, MAGNER D, EYSSEN G: Primary malignant mesothelial tumors in Canada, 1960–1968: A pathologic review by the mesothelioma panel of the Canadian Tumor Reference Centre. Cancer 31:869, 1973

MCIVER MA: Acute intestinal obstruction: General considerations. Arch Surg 25:1098, 1932

MCKENNA JP, CURRIE DJ, MACDONALD JA et al: The use of continuous postoperative peritoneal lavage in the management of diffuse peritonitis. Surg Gynecol Obstet 130:254, 1970

MOERTEL CG: Peritoneal mesothelioma. Gastroenterology 63:346, 1972

MOSS W, MCFETRIDGE EM: Acute intestinal obstruction: Comparative study of 511 cases, with special reference to lowered mortality achieved by modern methods of therapy. Ann Surg 100:158, 1934

NEELY J, DAVIES JD: Starch granulomatosis of the peritoneum. Br Med J 3:625, 1971

NOBEL TB JR: Plication of small intestine as prophylaxis against adhesions. Am J Surg 35:41, 1937

PARSONS J, GRAY GF, THORBJARNARSON B: Pseudomyxoma peritonei. Arch Surg 101:545, 1970

PERRY JF JR, SMITH GA, YONEHIRO EG: Intestinal obstruction caused by adhesions: Review of 388 cases. Ann Surg 142:810, 1955

ROBERTS GH, IRVINE RW: Peritoneal mesothelioma: A report of 4 cases. Br J Surg 57:645, 1970

RYAN GB, GROBETZ J, MAJNO G: Postoperative peritoneal adhesions: A study of the mechanisms. Am J Pathol 65:117, 1971

SAMSON R, PASTERNAK BM: Current status of surgery of the omentum. Surg Gynecol Obstet 149:437, 1979

SHARBAUGH RJ, RAMBO WM: Cephalothin and peritoneal lavage in the treatment of experimental peritonitis. Surg Gynecol Obstet 139:211, 1974

SOERGEL KH, HENSLEY GT: Fatal mesenteric panniculitis. Gastroenterology 51:529, 1966

STOUT AP, HENDRY J, PURDIE FJ: Primary solid tumours of the great omentum. Cancer 16:231, 1963

TAFT DA, LASERSOHN JT, HILL LD: Glove starch granulomatous peritonitis. Am J Surg 120:231, 1970

TENCKHOFF H, SCHECHTER H: A bacteriologically safe peritoneal access device. Trans Am Soc Artif Intern Organs 14:181, 1968

Charles T. Fitts

The Retroperitoneum: Tumors, Cysts, Abscesses, and Other Conditions

The retroperitoneum is a potential space lying between the peritoneum and the posterior wall of the abdominal cavity. It is bounded by the diaphragm superiorly and the pelvic brim inferiorly. The lateral margins of the area extend to the lateral borders of the quadratus lumborum muscles, which, in association with the medially placed psoas muscles, form the floor of the retroperitoneum.

Lying within the retroperitoneal space are structures that are either wholly located in the area or traverse it. These structures include the kidneys, ascending and descending colon, adrenals, ureters, abdominal aorta, inferior vena cava, pancreas, second and third portions of the duodenum, and the spermatic or ovarian vessels (Fig. 31-5).

PRIMARY RETROPERITONEAL TUMORS

The vast majority of masses that develop in the retroperitoneal space originate in the major organs that are located in this area—namely, the kidney, pancreas, adrenal, and retroperitoneal portions of the gastrointestinal tract (Table 31-1). Numerous diagnostic examinations can be performed to determine the organ responsible for development of a mass in the retroperitoneum, but these various studies are beyond the scope of this chapter and are adequately discussed in appropriate sections of this book.

After selective examinations have eliminated the major retroperitoneal organs as the cause of a retroperitoneal mass, and when no malignant focus has been discovered that could be the source of direct invasion or metastatic spread to the retroperitoneum or to one of its lymph nodes, there remains the probability that the unknown mass in the retroperitoneum is a primary retroperitoneal tumor. These tumors are uncommon but not rare. They develop from fat, areolar, fascial, muscle, nerve, vascular, urogenital ridge, or lymphatic tissue with no apparent connection to any organ or major blood vessel. They can be benign or malignant; the malignant varieties are four times more common.

Cystic development within a primary retroperitoneal tumor suggests that the lesion is benign, whereas a malignant retroperitoneal tumor has a greater tendency to be solid. Occasionally there is a combination of both cystic and solid elements.

The variety of tissues within the retroperitoneum creates the potential for a wide range of tumor types. The most frequent malignant retroperitoneal tumors are the lymphomas. Liposarcoma, fibrosarcoma, rhabdomyosarcoma, leiomyosarcoma, and sarcomas of undetermined origin are other major primary tumors of the retroperitoneum and are given in order of decreasing frequency. Histologic determination of a retroperitoneal tumor must be made eventually, since the exact pathologic diagnosis may influence subsequent treatment.

Fig. 31-5. Structures and organs beneath posterior peritoneum lie within retroperitoneum. (Goldsmith HS: The retroperitoneum: Diagnosis and management of tumors and other conditions. In Hardy JD [ed]: Rhoads Textbook of Surgery, 5th ed. Philadelphia, J B Lippincott, 1977)

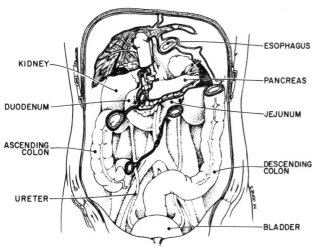

RETROPERITONEAL MASSES	
Trauma	Retroperitoneal hematoma
	Anticoagulants
	Pelvic fracture
	Vena caval injury
	Renal injury
Vascular	Abdominal aortic aneurysm
Infections	Tuberculosis
	Pyelonephritis
	Viscus perforation
	Psoas abscess
Tumor	Lymphoma
	Lymphosarcoma
	Fibrosarcoma
	Rhabdomyosarcoma
	Leiomyosarcoma
	Sarcoma, origin unknown
	Renal neoplasm or cyst
	Adrenal neoplasm or cyst

TABLE 31-1   HISTOGENESIS OF RETROPERITONEAL TUMORS*

	TUMORS	
TYPE OF TISSUE	**Benign**	**Malignant**
Mesoderm		
Adipose	Lipoma	Liposarcoma
Smooth muscle	Leiomyoma	Leiomyosarcoma
Connective	Fibroma	Fibrosarcoma
Striated	Rhabdomyoma	Rhabdomyosarcoma
Lymph vessel	Lymphangioma	Lymphangiosarcoma
Lymph node		Hodgkin's
		Lymphosarcoma
		Reticulum cell sarcoma
Blood vessel	Hemangioma	Hemangiosarcoma
		Hemangiopericytoma
Undetermined	Xanthogranuloma	Dysgerminoma
		Synovioma
		Undifferentiated malignant tumor
Nerve		
Nerve sheath	Nonencapsulated fibroma	Malignant schwannoma
Sympathetic nervous system	Encapsulated neurilemoma	Sympathicoblastoma
	Ganglioneuroma	
Heterotopic adrenocortical and chromaffin	Pheochromocytoma (benign)	Pheochromocytoma (malignant)
		Malignant nonchromaffin paraganglioma
Urogenital Ridge		
Embryonic Remnants	Teratoma (benign)	Teratoma (malignant)
	Nephrogenic cysts	
	Chordoma	

* In addition to the above conditions, a retroperitoneal mass may derive from any organ or structure normally present in the retroperitoneal space such as kidney, pancreas, adrenal, aorta, or bone.

CLINICAL FINDINGS

Retroperitoneal tumors most frequently develop in adults over 40 years of age, with approximately 10% to 15% occurring in children. Early symptoms caused by these tumors are frequently vague or lacking because they develop in the loose connective tissue that characterizes the retroperitoneal space. This space allows the retroperitoneal tumor to grow unrestricted except in a posterior direction, so that the tumor can expand to a large size before a patient becomes aware of symptoms and prior to objective evidence of an enlarging mass.

Symptomatic complaints of a patient with a retroperitoneal tumor depend on the structures that the mass is compressing, obstructing, or invading. Nausea, vomiting, and signs of intestinal obstruction may be the major problem if the gastrointestinal tract is compromised by the tumor. When the genitourinary system is involved, hematuria, dysuria, urgency, and frequency may result. Pressure or invasion of major retroperitoneal veins by an expanding mass can cause ascites, edema of one or both lower extremities, dilated superficial abdominal veins, and occasionally development of a varicocele.

A nontender abdominal mass is experienced by at least half of the patients with a primary retroperitoneal tumor. The mass may be considered to be either movable or fixed, and approximately 15% of the patients complain of tumor tenderness upon palpation. As the retroperitoneal mass continues to enlarge, it may invaginate into the peritoneal cavity, extend into one or both flanks, or progress into the pelvis, where it may be palpable through the rectum. The mass may continue to enlarge so that it appears to fill the entire abdominal cavity. Fixity of the tumor suggests malignancy, whereas if it is soft, movable, and ballottable there is a greater likelihood that it is cystic and benign. Even though the physical characteristics may suggest preoperatively whether a tumor is benign or malignant, the histologic origin of the mass can be established only by obtaining a suitable biopsy specimen for tissue diagnosis.

A primary retroperitoneal tumor is diagnosed principally through radiographic examinations of the urologic and gastrointestinal systems and by abdominal aortography. Ultrasound diagnostic techniques and computed tomography are also useful. The presence of an expanding retroperitoneal mass characteristically shows distortion and displacement of the kidney or ureters on intravenous and retrograde pyelograms. This urologic information is important in that it shows the extent of the retroperitoneal tumor and the functioning ability of each kidney. The latter information can be of vital significance because a kidney is the organ most frequently sacrificed when an *en bloc* retroperitoneal resection is performed. It is obvious that performance of a nephrectomy cannot be considered without complete assurance that the remaining kidney is functioning normally.

Retroperitoneal tumors have the potential for displacing and distorting practically the entire gastrointestinal tract, including the stomach. An upper gastrointestinal series or a barium enema will show whether an abdominal mass is intrinsic to the gastrointestinal tract. Abdominal aortography may be useful in delineating the size of the tumor and the blood vessels within the retroperitoneum that are supplying the mass. Selective radiographic views of the inferior vena cava can show whether this structure is inherently involved with a retroperitoneal mass and whether it must be sacrificed in the attempt to perform what would be considered ideally complete *en bloc* retroperitoneal resection.

SURGICAL APPROACH

Operation to remove a retroperitoneal mass is performed after the patient has been carefully evaluated and prepared for the operative procedure. Such preparation includes an adequate preoperative bowel preparation in case a portion of intestine must be resected while attempting to perform a complete tumor resection.

The most important step in the operation is to establish as early as possible the feasibility of total resection of the retroperitoneal mass. The major problem is deciding whether the retroperitoneal tumor is truly fixed and therefore nonresectable. This determination can be difficult because what appears initially to be a fixed retroperitoneal mass may, with appropriate surgical dissection, subsequently become mobile and can be completely excised. It is estimated that in a cancer hospital approximately 10% of the patients who have been operated on at another institution for what was described as a nonresectable tumor will subsequently be found to have a tumor that can be completely resected *en bloc;* this situation is especially true with retroperitoneal tumors. This suggests that there is a direct relationship between experience in retroperitoneal surgery and appreciation of tumor fixity and resectability.

During the performance of retroperitoneal surgery, certain structures must be carefully guarded. The second portion of the duodenum should be visualized and protected against injury when dissecting close to the right renal pedicle. The ureter in particular requires constant visualization during the operation. This structure or its ipsilateral kidney should be sacrificed only if it is involved in the retroperitoneal mass, and then only when the surgeon is convinced that a complete *en bloc* retroperitoneal resection is possible.

Certain aspects of the technical removal of a retroperitoneal mass merit emphasis, especially because there is an overall operative mortality of 10% to 25% associated with this type of surgery. A large incision is always necessary to give adequate exposure of the retroperitoneal space, and a thoracoabdominal incision should be performed whenever increased exposure of the upper retroperitoneum is needed.

Various points of fixity can be encountered while freeing a retroperitoneal mass from its surrounding environment. Whenever fixation at a particular place around the tumor develops into a technical problem, either alone or in association with bleeding, it is always a safe surgical maneuver to go to a distant location along the circumference of the tumor and begin dissection in this new area. Upon returning to the location of previous technical difficulty, there will often be increased tumor mobility and ease in dissection.

A surgical maneuver that is mentioned only to be condemned is blunt and, especially, sharp dissection performed directly beneath a retroperitoneal tumor. The reason this is so dangerous is that if bleeding in this area occurs before adequate exposure and mobility of the mass has been accomplished, it may be difficult and at times impossible to gain control of hemorrhaging vessels beneath the mass.

If early in an operation for a retroperitoneal tumor it is felt that a complete *en bloc* resection is not possible, or when there is incomplete excision of the tumor, metallic clips should be placed around the circumference of the tumor tissue so that postoperative radiation therapy can be accurately applied. Another technique is the insertion of low-energy radiation seeds (^{125}I) directly into the unresected malignant tissue. These permanently implanted seeds exert a very high radiation dose over an extended period and have been found effective for both palliation and cure. If this form of interstitial radiation is not available, metallic clips for outlining the field of external radiation should never be forgotten because only one third of patients with a retroperitoneal tumor have a lesion suitable for complete *en bloc* excision; the remaining patients are found at laparotomy to have either involvement or invasion of structures within the retroperitoneum that precludes the possibility of total tumor removal.

Occasionally, an operation may begin with the expectation that complete removal of a retroperitoneal tumor is possible, only to find during the course of the procedure that this is not technically possible. Being forced to abort an attempt at complete removal of a retroperitoneal mass is always unfortunate, but it is consoling for the surgeon to know that, according to current immunologic knowledge, removal of large amounts of tumor antigen may be helpful to the patient in mounting some form of immunologic response during his postoperative treatment.

RADIATION THERAPY

Radiation therapy plays a major role in the treatment and palliation of patients with a primary retroperitoneal tumor because it is employed when a tumor is nonresectable and when distant metastases are present. In addition, approximately half of the patients who have a retroperitoneal tumor that is believed to be totally removed at surgery subsequently develop local tumor recurrence. These patients also become candidates for radiation therapy.

Radiation therapy is the primary form of treatment for any tumor histologically proven to be a lymphoma. However, when the lymphoma is found to be small and easily resectable, it seems reasonable to remove it, following the resection by appropriate postoperative radiation therapy to the tumor base and surrounding area. In addition to lymphomas, liposarcomas tend to be radiosensitive, and survival statistics do improve when postoperative radiation therapy is given following their complete, or even incomplete, surgical excision.

Many retroperitoneal tumors are slow growing and have some degree of response to radiation therapy, although clinical experience has not unequivocally shown whether radiation therapy plays a significant role in the postoperative management of primary retroperitoneal tumors other than lymphomas and liposarcomas. Long-term palliation after radiation therapy occurs in approximately 10% of patients who have a nonresectable or incompletely removed retroperitoneal tumor. Although the results of chemotherapy have generally been disappointing, it plays a secondary role in the treatment of retroperitoneal tumors, and some authors are advocating adjuvant chemotherapy and irradiation for particular tumor types at the present time.

STATISTICS

Only one third of patients with a retroperitoneal tumor have what may be considered complete surgical excision of the mass, and of this number only 25% live 5 years. This means that the overall survival rate for all patients with a primary retroperitoneal tumor is less than 10%; most patients die within the first several years following surgery or radiation therapy from widespread metastases, intestinal or urinary tract obstruction, or hemorrhage due to invasion of a major blood vessel.

IDIOPATHIC RETROPERITONEAL FIBROSIS

Ormond described idiopathic retroperitoneal fibrosis in 1948. The cause has never been determined, although at least one drug, methysergide, has been definitely associated with some cases and several other drugs are currently suspected of a possible association. These include amphetamines, lysergic acid diethylamide, phenacetin, methyldopa, and propranolol.

Grossly, the retroperitoneum is found to be involved with a mat of dense fibrous tissue with a silvery-appearing surface; it is centrally located over the aorta and vertebral column and extends laterally. It characteristically extends from about the fourth lumbar vertebra to the sacrum. Microscopically, it is characterized by dense collagen with varying amounts of fibroblastic proliferation and round cell infiltration.

The clinical hallmark of this disease is obstruction of the ureters, usually bilaterally, but occasionally unilaterally. The intravenous pyelogram shows that the obstruction is most often distal but progresses upward so that long segments of the ureter are encased. Characteristically, the ureters deviate medially. The patient is most likely to complain of pain in the lower abdomen, flank, or back. There are no specific laboratory studies that will confirm or deny the diagnosis, although the sedimentation rate is often elevated. Both ultrasound and computed tomography have been used to help confirm the diagnosis.

The treatment is almost certainly surgical if obstruction is present. The ureters should be freed from the retroperitoneal fibrosis and transplanted to an intraperitoneal position if possible for their entire course. If severe obstruction and renal compromise are present, nephrostomy may be necessary. If there is no obstruction, a trial of steroid therapy may be utilized, and there are reports that postoperative steroids may be helpful in some cases. In patients with a definite history of methysergide ingestion and no obstruction, the problem will frequently be resolved by simple discontinuance of the drug. The methysergide patient who already has mild obstruction but no renal impairment may also be given a trial of conservative therapy, but it seems wisest to operate on patients who show severe obstruction and impairment of renal function. The overall prognosis of these patients is excellent, with the exception of a small number (8%) in whom the problem is found to coexist with a malignant tumor.

RETROPERITONEAL ABSCESS

An abscess in the retroperitoneum is relatively uncommon, difficult to diagnose, and associated with high morbidity and mortality. Any infection in this area is hazardous because of the looseness of tissue and lack of anatomic barriers that are necessary to impede the initial development of infection, progressive cellulitis, and eventual pus formation.

A retroperitoneal abscess secondary to tuberculosis of the spine (Pott's disease) formerly was a relatively common phenomenon, but this disease has become a rarity in the United States. Presently, the most common cause of a retroperitoneal infection results from pyelonephritis that progresses to a perinephric abscess. The second most common cause of pus in the retroperitoneum is perforation of a gastrointestinal structure such as the colon, appendix, or duodenum, which contaminates and infects the retroperitoneal area.

CLINICAL FINDINGS

Patients with a retroperitoneal abscess usually have generalized symptoms of infection such as chills, anorexia, weight loss, and malaise but few physical signs pointing to the diagnosis. Patients may appear ill far out of proportion to their symptoms, with the most persistent complaint being an elevated temperature that is often spiking in character.

Physical examination of a patient with a retroperitoneal abscess may demonstrate a tender mass in the abdomen, swelling or a sense of fullness in the flank, or tenderness in the costovertebral angles. If the infection involves the psoas muscle, the patient makes voluntary attempts to decrease the pain in this area by minimizing the activity of the muscle, positioning the hip in a flexed and somewhat externally rotated position. Suspicion that a retroperitoneal abscess is present should always be heightened if a patient complains of pain on hip extension in association with systemic signs of infection.

The only positive laboratory finding in a patient with a retroperitoneal abscess may be an elevated leukocyte count. When an infection in the retroperitoneum is secondary to a perinephric abscess, routine urinalysis may show pyuria, albuminuria, and bacteria even though urologic symptoms may be absent.

The loss of psoas muscle shadow detail and the appearance of an ill-defined mass in the retroperitoneal space are characteristic findings on abdominal films in a patient with a retroperitoneal abscess. This finding may generally be confirmed by ultrasonography or computed tomography. Radiographic examination is considered diagnostic if gas or fluid is visualized in the retroperitoneal space; however, this finding is rarely observed. When a retroperitoneal abscess is secondary to infection and destruction of a vertebral body, x-ray studies will confirm which segment is involved.

TREATMENT

It is important to understand the various routes by which infection spreads within the retroperitoneal area to treat an abscess in this location adequately. The retroperitoneum is divided anatomically by the kidney into anterior and posterior spaces, which cross the midline and descend toward the pelvis (Fig. 31-6). Infection in these spaces travels along the paths of least resistance. When pus accumulates within or above the psoas muscle, it tends to gravitate toward the inguinal ligament, where it may form a sinus tract to the skin; otherwise, it may continue along the lateral margin of the femoral vessels, eventually exiting through the skin in the thigh (Fig. 31-7). The last mentioned clinical presentation of a retroperitoneal abscess used to be seen during

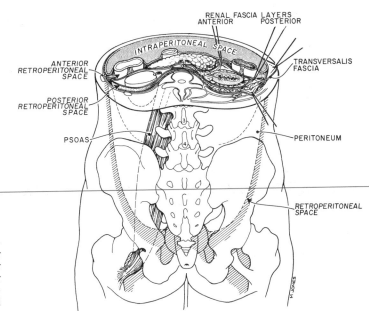

Fig. 31-6. Drawing shows how renal fascia compartmentalizes retroperitoneum into anterior and posterior spaces. The anterior space lies between the posterior peritoneum and the anterior renal fascia. The posterior space is between the posterior renal fascia and transversalis fascia. The spaces extend across the midline and toward the pelvis.

the era of Pott's disease when spinal tuberculosis was prevalent.

Knowledge of the retroperitoneal space is surgically essential in dealing with such lesions as a horseshoe type of infection originating from an appendiceal abscess. In this situation, the suppurative process can develop in the right lower quadrant, ascend, cross, and then descend retroperitoneally prior to exiting by way of a cutaneous opening in the left lower quadrant. Obviously, surgical drainage of the left lower quadrant would prove to be an inadequate operative treatment.

The surgical approach to a retroperitoneal abscess should be made through a muscle-splitting flank incision, taking

Fig. 31-7. Common routes of retroperitoneal infection. Pus tends to follow the psoas muscle inferiorly into the basin of the pelvis and may eventually reach adductor area of thigh. (Goldsmith HS: The retroperitoneum: Diagnosis and management of tumors and other conditions. In Hardy JD [ed]: Rhoads Textbook of Surgery, 5th ed. Philadelphia, J B Lippincott, 1977)

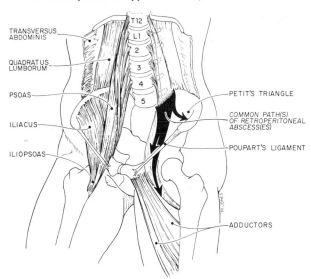

great care to keep from entering the peritoneal cavity. As pus is encountered in the surgical exploration, it should be removed and sent for culture and sensitivity evaluation so that appropriate antibiotic therapy can be initiated. No antibiotic is a substitute for adequate drainage of the retroperitoneal spaces. Failure to recognize and adequately drain an abscess in the retroperitoneum usually results in the death of the patient.

RETROPERITONEAL HEMATOMA

There are many blood vessels within the retroperitoneum that can bleed at the time of traumatic injury, resulting in a retroperitoneal hematoma. Collection of blood in the retroperitoneum most frequently results from pelvic fractures. However, retroperitoneal bleeding from this cause is usually not an isolated clinical finding because approximately half of these patients have associated injury to intraperitoneal organs such as the liver and spleen. Retroperitoneal bleeding may also occur in patients on anticoagulants.

Although blunt trauma continues to cause the majority of retroperitoneal hematomas, an ever-increasing number of persons experience retroperitoneal injury to the aorta or inferior vena cava owing to gun or knife wounds of the abdomen. There is every reason to believe that the incidence of wounds of this type will continue to increase. Rupture of an aortic aneurysm is another common cause of retroperitoneal hematoma (see Chapter 36).

CLINICAL FINDINGS

Patients with retroperitoneal bleeding frequently present in a state of shock owing to severe blood loss into the retroperitoneal space. Even though associated traumatic injuries may be the major cause of the hypovolemia, retroperitoneal bleeding alone can cause hypotension; it has been shown experimentally that the retroperitoneum has the ability to accommodate up to 4 liters of blood injected under arterial pressure. Retroperitoneal hemorrhage may produce bluish discoloration in the flanks (Grey Turner sign).

MANAGEMENT

Management of retroperitoneal hematoma is directed at correction of the causative pathology.

BIBLIOGRAPHY

ABERCROMBIE GF, VINNICOMBE J: Retroperitoneal fibrosis: Practical problems in management. Br J Urol 52:443, 1980

ACKERMAN LV: Tumors of the retroperitoneum, mesentery, and peritoneum. Atlas of Tumor Pathology, Section 6, Armed Forces Institute of Pathology, Washington DC, 1954

AHMAD S: Sclerosing peritonitis and propranolol. Chest 79:361, 1981

ALTEMEIER WA, ALEXANDER JW: Retroperitoneal abscess. Arch Surg 83:512, 1961

ARMSTRONG JR, COHN I JR: Primary malignant retroperitoneal tumors. Am J Surg 110:937, 1965

BRAASCH JW, MON AB: Primary retroperitoneal tumors. Surg Clin North Am 47:663, 1967

DONNELLY BA: Primary retroperitoneal tumors. Surg Gynecol Obstet 83:705, 1946

FELIX EL, WOOD DK, DAS GUPTA TK: Tumors of the retroperitoneum. Curr Probl Cancer 6:1, 1981

GOLDSMITH HS: The retroperitoneum: Diagnosis and management of tumors and other conditions. In Hardy JD (ed): Rhoads Textbook of Surgery, 5th ed. Philadelphia, J B Lippincott, 1977

GOMZYAKOR GA: Closed fractures of the pelvis complicated by retroperitoneal hematomas. Vestnik Khir 75:67, 1955

HENRIKSSON LE: Retroperitoneal abscess with gas after perforation. Acta Radiol 11:220, 1971

HILARIS BS: Techniques of interstitial and intracavitary radiation. Cancer 22:745, 1968

JONES JH, ROSS EJ, MATZ LR et al: Retroperitoneal fibrosis. Am J Med 48:203, 1970

KOEP L, ZUIDEMA GD: The clinical significance of retroperitoneal fibrosis. Surgery 81:250, 1977

LARRIEU AJ, WEINER I, ABSTON S et al: Retroperitoneal fibrosis. Surg Gynecol Obstet 150:699, 1980

LEPOR H, WALSH PC: Idiopathic retroperitoneal fibrosis. J Urol 122:1, 1979

LEVIN DC, WATSON RC, BALTAXE HA: Arteriography of retroperitoneal masses. Radiology 108:543, 1973

ORMOND JK: Bilateral ureteral obstructions due to envelopment and compression by an inflammatory retroperitoneal process. J Urol 59:1072, 1948

PACK GT, TABAH EJ: Primary retroperitoneal tumors. Surg Gynecol Obstet (Int Abstr) 99:209, 1954

PIERCE JR, JR, TROSTLE DC, WARNER JJ: Propranolol and retroperitoneal fibrosis. Ann Int Med 95:244, 1981

STEICHEN FM, DARGAN EL, PERLMAN DM et al: The management of retroperitoneal hematoma secondary to penetrating injuries. Surg Gynecol Obstet 123:581, 1966

STEVENSON EOS, OZERAN RS: Retroperitoneal space abscesses. Surg Gynecol Obstet 128:202, 1969

Charles T. Fitts/Albert Kreutner, Jr.

The Groin Mass: Differential Diagnosis

ANATOMY OF THE GROIN
HISTORY
PHYSICAL EXAMINATION
DIFFERENTIAL DIAGNOSIS BY PATHOLOGICAL ENTITY
THE ROLE OF SURGERY IN DIFFERENTIAL DIAGNOSIS

A mass in the groin is a moderately common presenting complaint frequently referred to the surgeon. Although in the great majority of cases the mass is either a lymph node (infectious or neoplastic in origin) or a hernia, the large number and variety of less common lesions of importance necessitate caution on the part of the diagnostician. In addition, the groin nodes drain such a large anatomic area that the primary infection or neoplasm resulting in the enlarged node may be relatively obscure, remote, or both, thus escaping detection. For these reasons it is appropriate to discuss the mass in the groin as a particular surgical diagnostic problem.

ANATOMY OF THE GROIN

There are numerous lymph glands located in the region of the groin. The inguinal glands, which number from 12 to 20, are divided into two groups. Those above the fossa ovalis—superficial inguinal nodes—drain the skin of the penis, scrotum or labia, perineum, buttocks, abdominal wall below the umbilicus, and the anus (but not the anal canal). Those below the fossa ovalis—subinguinal nodes—drain mostly the entire lower extremity but with some connections

THE GROIN MASS	
Etiology	Enlarged lymph nodes (inflammation, lymphoma, or metastatic cancer?), hernia (inguinal or femoral), vascular (arterial aneurysm or venous varix), "psoas" abscess, undescended testicle, cyst of the canal of Nuck, primary tumors or still more rare lesions, and vaginal disease
Dx	History of systemic disease, foot-leg infection or malignant neoplasm, trauma or hernial bulging Useful x-ray films such as lymphangiogram or arteriogram or CT scan when a retroperitoneal source is suspected Physical exam usually informative Needle aspiration or surgical exploration on occasion
Rx	Appropriate to diagnosis established

to the lower vagina or penis, scrotum or labia, perineum, and buttocks. These glands are primarily located on either side of the upper part of the greater saphenous vein superficial to the fascia lata. A small subgroup located medial to the femoral vein and under the fascia lata—deep subinguinal nodes—drains the glans penis and clitoris. The highest of these, situated in the femoral canal, is known as Cloquet's node. The external iliac nodes, which usually number 8 to 10, lie along the external iliac vessels and generally are considered part of the groin region. These glands drain the deep lymphatics of the abdominal wall below the umbilicus, the adductor region of the thigh, the glans penis and clitoris, the membranous urethra, the prostate, the fundus of the bladder, the cervix, the upper vagina, the seminal vesicles, and the ductus deferens. The lymphatic drainage of the testes and the ovaries is to the lumbar glands and thus generally not to any nodes in the groin region. The uterus above the cervix also drains primarily to lumbar glands, although some accessory connections may exist that would allow the drainage to reach the external iliac glands or even, occasionally, the subinguinal. It is worth noting that anastomotic connections do exist between the lymphatics in the right groin and those of the left groin.

HISTORY

When a patient presents with a groin lump, obtaining a standard complete history is mandatory because of the number and variety of illnesses that may be responsible. In addition, one should keep in mind specific aspects of the history that give clues to the more common causes of a lump in the groin, as well as those aspects that may point to less common causes that can be overlooked unless specifically sought. An inguinal or femoral hernia is one of the most common conditions presenting as a groin mass. The history as pertains to hernia is covered in Chapter 32.

A mass in the groin equally as frequent as hernia is an enlarged lymph node. An infection anywhere in the extensive area of the body drained by the groin nodes may result in an enlarged hyperplastic or inflammatory node. It is of great importance to recall those areas (listed earlier) and to question the patient concerning symptoms that could be related to infections there. Thus a history of a fungal infection of the feet, painful external hemorrhoids, urethral discharge, vaginal discharge, dysuria, frequency, and a host of other symptoms may point to the basic primary infection resulting in the enlarged lymph node in the groin. Relatively minor infections may result in very large nodes. Enlargement of a lymph node draining an infection is generally not as sudden as the development of a hernia, but it is usually faster than enlargement due to a malignant neoplasm. A lymph node draining an infection may double in size in a few days and double again in the next several days if the infection is not controlled; rarely does a tumor grow that fast. Enlarged lymph nodes secondary to infection may be mildly to moderately painful and call attention to themselves by this discomfort. Once enlargement has occurred, resolution may take place very slowly over a matter of weeks, so that a history of recent infection that has now cleared may be the only clue to the etiology. A history that the lump was larger and more painful at an earlier date is corroborative.

Any malignant tumor in the area of lymphatic drainage to the groin nodes may metastasize to these nodes and result in a mass. The same aspects of the history that draw attention to specific areas of primary infection may be equally indicative of a primary tumor. Thus a history of burning urination, blood in the urine, or some combination of urinary tract symptoms may lead the physician to diagnose either prostatitis or carcinoma of the prostate as a cause of the groin mass. In a woman, vaginal bleeding might lead to the discovery of either a chronic cervical infection or carcinoma of the cervix as the primary cause of a groin lump. Malignant melanoma, squamous cell carcinoma of the skin (including the anus), and other less common malignant growths may metastasize to the groin nodes.

Although the physical examination is of primary importance, the history may occasionally play a critical role. The patient should be questioned closely concerning previous removal, fulguration, or cauterization of any "lump, bump, mole, or spot," from the toes to the umbilicus. There have been instances of removal of such lesions, initially thought to be benign, in which subsequent analysis of the slides revealed malignancy. The patient should not necessarily be expected to volunteer such information. Following removal of a localized malignant lesion with clear margins, it is certainly considered good medical practice to reassure the patient by emphasizing that he should not spend the rest of his life dreading its return. However, the patient may present a year or two later with a groin lump that is a metastasis from a small malignant tumor removed completely in a 15-minute session in a physician's office under local anesthesia. The entire episode may have left a mark on the patient's memory as tiny as the scar.

There are many systemic diseases, malignant and non-malignant, that characteristically cause lymph node enlargement in the groin and elsewhere and that should be kept in mind during the taking of the history. Among the more common malignant diseases are the lymphomas and chronic lymphatic leukemia. Venereal disease such as syphilis, chancroid, and lymphogranuloma venereum probably rank high among the nonmalignant systemic diseases that result in a groin mass. A detailed sexual and genital tract history may clarify such a problem. A precise menstrual history may not only help in these areas but may lead to diagnosis of the very occasional case of endometriosis of the inguinal canal by uncovering the fact that the mass becomes tender, painful, and enlarged primarily during menstruation. Other systemic nonmalignant diseases that may result in a surprising degree of lymphadenopathy and thus possibly present with a groin mass are sarcoidosis, tuberculosis, and toxoplasmosis. Thyrotoxicosis, Addison's disease, and hypopituitarism can also be associated with adenopathy on occasion.

A history of trauma should be sought, especially in the area draining to the groin nodes. Cat-scratch fever is noted for marked enlargement of the nodes draining the area of the injury, as is tularemia. Sharp injuries to the groin area may result in immediate collections of blood or lymph, leading to formation of a mass. Relatively trivial sharp injuries of minor nature may heal without apparent incident, but subsequently the patient may present a mass due to a false aneurysm, an arteriovenous fistula, or a foreign body granuloma. Rotary power lawn mowers have been known to hurl tiny sharp objects hundreds of feet to strike and penetrate an unwary bystander, who notices only a tiny sting or sharp pain that quickly subsides. Later the victim may develop symptoms referred to the area injured. Such an event may lead to the development of a granuloma, arteriovenous fistula, false aneurysm, or other late manifestations of such an injury (Fig. 31-8). A direct blow to the groin area may result in a hemorrhagic mass that defies diagnosis unless the history of trauma is obtained. The hemophiliac or bleeder from other causes is especially subjected to this problem with even the most minor trauma.

The historian should ask about drug exposure. The serum sickness type of allergic reaction may cause adenopathy. Cases of spontaneous hemorrhage into the spermatic cord and testicle, misdiagnosed as incarcerated hernias, have been reported in patients undergoing anticoagulant therapy. The administration of phenytoin (Dilantin) may be associated with a striking degree of lymphadenopathy and should be considered as a possible etiologic agent.

Pseudocysts of the pancreas may rupture retroperito-

neally and track down the surface of the psoas muscle or through the internal inguinal ring to present as a groin mass. A previous history of pancreatitis and an abdominal mass can be indicative of this problem. Aortic aneurysms may rupture retroperitoneally and take the same route; a history of a pulsatile mass, severe back pain, or both could suggest this. Intraperitoneal hemorrhage from a ruptured spleen has been known to fill a previously present, but undiagnosed, hernial sac and present as an incarcerated hernia. Tubercular abscess of the spine may characteristically travel along the psoas muscle and present as a cold abscess in the groin (see Fig. 31-8). Other retroperitoneal infections may do likewise. We have had a patient who underwent proximal diverting colostomy and drainage of an intra-abdominal abscess from a perforated diverticulum of the sigmoid colon. Postoperatively he developed a tender crepitant subinguinal mass that was revealed to be a retroperitoneal extension of the abscess, containing gas-forming bacteria, that had taken the familiar route down the surface of the psoas muscle in the groin.

Fig. 31-8. *(Top)* On the left side are the three predominant groups of groin nodes; on the right side, a topographic representation of an inguinal hernia presenting above the inguinal ligament and a femoral hernia presenting below this structure. *(Bottom)* On the left side, the path of retroperitoneal fluid tracking down the surface of the psoas muscle, passing beneath the inguinal ligament, and presenting as a groin mass is illustrated. On the right, the relationship between the major blood vessels and the bony and ligamentous structures of this groin region is shown. (Fitts CT, Kreutner A Jr: The groin mass: Differential diagnosis. In Hardy JD [ed]: Rhoads Textbook of Surgery, 5th ed. Philadelphia, J B Lippincott, 1977)

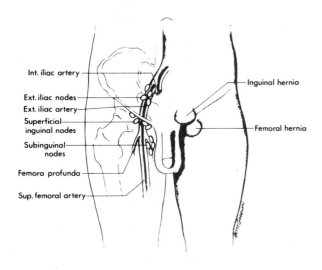

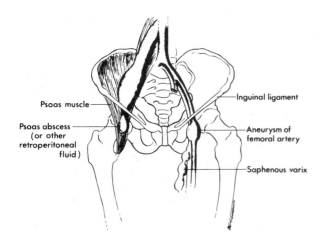

PHYSICAL EXAMINATION

When the patient presents with a lump in the groin, the physical examination is of considerable importance. Again, as in the taking of the history, a purely regional examination (as opposed to a complete and thorough one) may result in a missed diagnosis.

The examination should begin with the area under suspicion. Either the physician or the patient may be concerned over slight bilaterally symmetrical bulges in the groin area just above the inguinal ligament visible in some thin patients on coughing or straining. They are just what they appear to be—a slight give in the lowermost abdominal wall in response to the increased intra-abdominal pressure—known as Malgaigne's bulgings and of no pathologic significance. Patients may also be concerned over the discovery of an inguinal lymph node; these nodes are often palpable in thin, normal individuals. If the swellings under question are thought to be lymph nodes 1 cm or more in diameter, they probably should be considered enlarged. If the mass is located in the skin, subcutaneous tissue, intramuscularly, or deep to muscle and fascia, a different set of diagnoses is likely.

The consistency of the lump should be determined. Malignant lesions are likely to be stony hard. Benign solid tumors and hyperplastic lymph nodes are usually of a rubbery consistency, while those tumors with a high liquid content, such as hemangiomas, lymphangiomas, or lipomas, are generally quite soft. A saphenous varix is a soft lesion that may present as a groin mass in the area of the fossa ovalis. A visible varicose saphenous vein leading to the area or a slightly bluish color strongly suggests this. Lesions that contain fluid confined within a sac, with more or less pressure, generally are cystic to palpation: that is, there is a feeling of compressibility but with a definite elastic rebound.

Lesions that contain a clear or relatively clear fluid will almost always transilluminate brilliantly. Probably the most common cystic lesion in the groin is a hydrocele of the spermatic cord or of the canal of Nuck.

An abscess (other than tubercular) is usually associated with tenderness, heat, and reddening of the overlying skin. Fixation to adjacent structures should be determined. Fix-

TABLE 31-2 DIFFERENTIAL DIAGNOSIS BY PATHOLOGICAL ENTITY

SOLID MASSES

1. Neoplastic or proliferative solid masses other than lymph nodes

Fibrohistocytic tissue. Benign: congenital generalized fibromatosis, fibrous hamartoma of infancy, nodular fasciitis, fibromatoses,* musculoaponeurotic fibromatosis* (desmoid fibromatosis), pleomorphic fibrous histiocytoma, fibroepithelial polyp of skin.* Malignant: fibrosarcoma,* dermatofibrosarcoma protuberans, fibroxanthosarcoma.

Peripheral nerve tissue. Benign: traumatic neuroma, schwannoma, neurofibroma* or neurofibromatosis. Malignant: malignant schwannoma (neurofibrosarcoma).

Adipose tissue. Benign: lipoma.* Malignant: liposarcoma.*

Smooth muscle. Benign: leiomyoma. Malignant: leiomyosarcoma.

Vascular. Benign: hemangioma, hemangiopericytoma.

Striated muscle. Malignant: alveolar rhabdomyosarcoma, undifferentiated adult pleomorphic rhabodomyosarcoma.

Lymph vessels. Benign: lymphangioma. Malignant: lymphangiosarcoma.

Synovial tissue. Malignant: synovial sarcoma.

Uncertain origin. Granular cell tumor, alveolar soft-part sarcoma, clear cell sarcoma, epithelioid sarcoma.

Bone and cartilage. Benign: osteochondroma. Malignant: chondrosarcoma, osteosarcoma, Ewing's sarcoma.

Undescended testis (cryptorchidism). Malignant: seminoma, embryonal carcinoma, choriocarcinoma, teratoma, teratocarcinoma, mixed forms.

Skin and skin adnexae. Epidermis: epidermoid (squamous) carcinoma, basal cell carcinoma, seborrheic keratosis.

Adnexae. Eccrine spiradenoma, papillary hidradenoma, sweat gland adenocarcinoma.

Dermis. Nodular subepidermal fibrosis.

Metastatic carcinoma. Breast, gastrointestinal tract (stomach, colon, pancreas), lung, melanoma, kidney.

Malignant lymphoma. Malignant melanoma. Superficial spreading melanoma, nodular melanoma.

2. Non-neoplastic solid masses other than lymph nodes

Mechanical. Hernias.* Direct inguinal, indirect inguinal, femoral, obturator. Trauma. Hematoma,* foreign body granuloma.

Congenital. Undescended testicle.*

Developmental. Endometriosis.

Inflammatory. Abscess of skin or subcutaneous tissue, psoas abscess: Tuberculous, non-tuberculous, sparganosis.

Complex. Retroperitoneal fluid via psoas or internal inguinal ring: ruptured aortic or arterial aneurysm, ruptured pancreatic pseudocyst.

3. Lymph nodes, neoplastic, primary

Non-Hodgkin's lymphoma, Hodgkin's lymphoma, acute lymphatic leukemia, chronic lymphocytic leukemia.*

4. Lymph nodes, neoplastic, metastatic

Primary sites—Female: Vulva, clitoris, vagina, cervix uteri, corpus uteri, Fallopian tubes.

Primary sites—Male: Penis,* scrotum, testes.

Primary sites—Both: Anus, perianal region, distant sites.

5. Lymph nodes, non-neoplastic (lymphadenitis, lymphadenopathy). Probably most common cause of inguinal lymph node enlargement

Venereal disease. Gonorrhea,* syphilis, chancroid, lymphopathia venereum, granuloma inguinale, herpes (Type II) progenitalis.*

Inflammatory (infectious), local. Anal and perianal. * Hemorrhoids, inflamed or infected, and fissure, fissure in ano, perirectal abscess.

Vulva and vagina. * Herpes (Type II) progenitalis,* nonspecific bacterial vulvo vaginitis, senile vaginitis with secondary infection, trichomonal vulvo vaginitis, all causes of pruritus vulvae.*

Penis. Balanitis and posthitis, nonspecific bacterial,* herpes (Type II) progenitalis, monilial or trichomonal infection.

Scrotum. Cutaneous infections.

Infections of skin or subcutaneous tissues. Buttocks, extremities, perineum, lower abdomen, i.e., pediculosis pubis, scabies, pinworms.

Inflammatory (infectious), specific or systemic.

Granulomatous-suppurative. Cat-scratch disease, tularemia, tuberculosis.

Hyperplastic. Toxoplasmosis.

Reactive hyperplasia. Postvaccinial, infectious mononucleosis.

Granulomatous. Sarcoidosis, sarcoidlike granulomas in lymph nodes draining areas bearing malignant neoplasms.

Systemic. Rheumatoid arthritis, lupus erythematosus, thyrotoxicosis, Addison's disease, hypopituitarism, sinus histiocytosis (massive), chronic granulomatous disease of children, lymphangiogram effect.

CYSTIC MASSES

Hydrocele of spermatic cord or canal of Nuck, arterial aneurysm, saphenous varix, arteriovenous fistula, psoas bursitis, lymphocele, epidermal inclusion cyst, hematoma (liquefied), cystic metastatic epidermoid (squamous) carcinoma in a lymph node, dermoid cyst

* One of the more common lesions

ation in the absence of inflammation is very suggestive of a malignant lesion. Tenderness to palpation has some variants that are quite diagnostic. The characteristic severe pain associated with squeezing or striking the testicle may betray an undescended testicle as the source of a groin mass. Absence of the testicle in the scrotum on that side is confirmatory. Stimulation of an ovary descended into the hernial sac causes a similar type of pain. Neuroma and other tumors may involve the femoral nerve and, when briskly tapped, give a characteristic tingling or "pins and needles" feeling in the sensory distribution of the nerve.

Examination of a mass in the groin should always include an attempt to determine if it is pulsatile, in which case it may represent an aneurysm (true or false) of the femoral or iliac artery. A pulsatile mass associated with signs of inflammation is likely to be a mycotic aneurysm.

The mass should be auscultated with a stethoscope. Aneurysms are often associated with a systolic bruit and arteriovenous fistulas with a continuous bruit as well as a distinctly palpable thrill. Those features of a groin mass that are suggestive of hernia are included in Chapter 32.

Once this examination of the local mass has been concluded, the physician should examine the remainder of the body. Search the extremities carefully for any possible source of infection. Infections on the feet, including the common fungal infection, athlete's foot, are easily the most frequent cause of an enlarged inguinal node. This same search should be made for any pigmented lesion that might represent a malignant melanoma. These can occur in such easily overlooked locations as between the toes and on the soles of the feet. Attention can next be turned to the perineum and the external genitalia, pigmented lesions and foci of infection again being searched for.

Anal inspection and rectal examination are very important. Carcinoma of the anus may metastasize to groin nodes; carcinoma of the rectum and anal canal does not. A complete and organized pelvic examination is extremely important in women; vaginal, uterine, and cervical disease that may be contributing to a groin mass may be discovered.

Especially important in the remainder of the physical examination are signs of systemic disease. Since it is difficult to consider each of these possibilities in detail, we shall point out some of the more common ones as examples. Generalized adenopathy is a very important finding, immediately suggesting chronic lymphatic leukemia or lymphoma. General cachexia, fever, or both, together with generalized adenopathy, are even more suggestive of some such systemic disorder that is neoplastic, infectious, or metabolic in nature. Examination of the chest and lungs may provide the clue that tuberculosis or sarcoidosis is responsible for the adenopathy. Surprisingly, thyrotoxicosis is frequently associated with generalized adenopathy. A rapid pulse, enlarged thyroid gland, fine moist skin, tremor, or exophthalmos may lead to the discovery of this problem.

DIFFERENTIAL DIAGNOSIS BY PATHOLOGICAL ENTITY

Table 31-2 is a classification of possible lesions that might present as a groin mass. The great majority of groin masses will be either a hernia or neoplastic or proliferative involvement of the groin nodes. This extensive list should not serve to obscure this fact but rather help the astute physician in consideration of those masses that present unusual or puzzling features.

THE ROLE OF SURGERY IN DIFFERENTIAL DIAGNOSIS

Surgical exposure with the possibility of biopsy is practically always indicated in the presence of a groin mass in which a diagnosis has not been reached despite a thorough and complete evaluation. Needle biopsy may occasionally be employed in special circumstances, but it should be remembered that this technique suffers several drawbacks: It may not be representative of the lesion; the pathologist may not get enough tissue to interpret the lesion; and without exposure of the lesion, one may biopsy something one did not intend to biopsy, such as bowel or aneurysm.

Prior consultation with a pathologist is useful. The likely diagnoses are considered and the amount of specimen to be removed and the precise manner in which it is to be handled after removal are decided. Routine removal of a piece of tissue and "dumping it in formalin" may make it impossible to utilize many diagnostic techniques.

In those areas where a pathologist or laboratory is not immediately available to receive large pieces of tissue, it is suggested that these tissues be sectioned prior to immersion in fixative. Formalin penetrates tissues for a distance of only 3 mm to 5 mm in 12 to 24 hours. The interior of large masses may autolyze during that time. Cultures should be obtained in the operating room under sterile conditions. Aerobic and anaerobic cultures and acid fast and fungal stains should all be considered.

In addition to these general principles, the following guidelines are of value in the technique of lymph node excision:

1. A representative lymph node should be selected. If a lymph node is less than 1 cm, it is unlikely to be diseased. It may be necessary to bypass a more superficial small node and extend the dissection to a more suspicious example.
2. The node should be totally excised when possible. If one is not certain that one is dealing with a lymph node and there is a possibility that the mass is actually a soft-tissue neoplasm, an incisional biopsy is best, since wide *en bloc* excision may prove to be advisable immediately or in the very near future.
3. Frozen section should be avoided for diagnostic purposes in suspected lymphoma. Frozen section may be used to make certain that representative tissue is being biopsied.
4. In those cases in which a lump in the groin is the presenting symptom but generalized lymphadenopathy is subsequently detected, biopsy of the groin node is not the procedure of choice. An enlarged node from another site should be biopsied.

In developing this section, the author has drawn upon his own and the following material presented in Chapter 49 of the fifth edition of *Rhoads Textbook of Surgery:* William J. Hardin, Abdominal enlargement and certain lesions of the mesentery, omentum, and peritoneum; and Harry S. Goldsmith, The retroperitoneum: Diagnosis and management of tumors and other conditions.

BIBLIOGRAPHY

Barker K, Smiddy FG: Mass reduction of inguinal hernia: Description of a new physical sign of diagnostic value and aetiological significance. Br J Surg 57:264, 1970

Blum L, Kark A: Ruptured aneurysm of the abdominal aorta simulating incarcerated inguinal hernia, Am J Med Sci 252:97, 1966

Brightmore T: Dermoid cyst of the inguinal canal simulating a strangulated inguinal hernia. Br J Clin Pract 25:191, 1971

CLAIN A: Hamilton Bailey's Demonstrations of Physical Signs in Clinical Surgery. Baltimore, Williams & Wilkins, 1973

COBB O: Abdominal hematocele: Case report. J Urol 92:300, 1964

COLE AT, STRAUS FH, GILL WB: Malignant fibrous histiocytoma: An unusual inguinal tumor. J Urol 107:1005, 1971

COLODNY AH, HOLDER TM: Rectal examination: A useful maneuver to aid in differentiating an incarcerated inguinal hernia from a hydrocele in infancy. Surgery 53:544, 1963

GARGOUR G, WHITELAW GP: An extraordinary case of a right inguinal mass or serendipidity in the operating room. Boston Med J 16:87, 1965

HANDMAKER H, MEHN WH: Hemorrhage into spermatic cord and testicle simulating incarcerated inguinal hernia. Ill Med J 135:697, 1969

HIRA NR: Rare presentation of testicular neoplasm. Br J Clin Pract 19:533, 1965

HOFFMAN E: Multicystic retroperitoneal lymphangiomata presenting as an indirect inguinal hernia in a newborn. Am Surg 31:525, 1965

JIMENEZ J, MILES RM: Inguinal endometriosis. Ann Surg 151:903, 1960

JOHNSTONE JMS, RINTOUL RF: Unusual cause of inguinal mass. Br Med J 2:179, 1970

JU DM: Fibrosarcoma arising in surgical scars. Plast Reconstr Surg 38:429, 1966

KARNAUCHOW PN: Enterobius vermicularis granuloma in the inguinal canal. Can Med Assoc J 84:388, 1961

MARKS RM: Surprises in operations on the inguinal area in young children. Calif Med 97:76, 1962

MENDELSON E: Abdominal wall masses: The usefulness of the incomplete border sign. Radiol Clin North Am 2:61, 1964

PERKOFF M, SERLIN O, SKERRETT P: Retroperitoneal hemorrhage presenting as an inguinal mass. Arch Surg 80:660, 1960

RADMAN HM, GABY S: Inguinal endometriosis: Case report. Am Surg 32:69, 1966

SALAH MW: Retroperitoneal hemorrhage simulating a strangulated inguinal hernia. Br Med J 4:403, 1972

SALVO AF, NEMATOLAHI H: Distant dissection of a pancreatic pseudocyst into the right groin, Am J Surg 126:430, 1973

SPEED T: Inguinal liposarcoma. Surg Clin North Am 52:439, 1972

WAPNICK S, MACKINTOSH M, MAUCHAZA B: Shoelessness, enlarged femoral lymph nodes and femoral hernia. Am J Surg 126:108, 1963

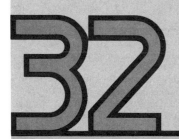

Abdominal Wall Hernias

Fred W. Rushton

Groin Hernias: Inguinal and Femoral

The term *hernia* applies to protrusion of tissue through an abnormal opening in a body cavity. Hernias of the groin are almost as old as the human race, having long been a source of disability, morbidity, and mortality. Although descriptions of hernias have been noted in cave drawings from primitive times, significant advances in hernia management have been made only within the past century. This discussion considers anatomy, epidemiology, morbidity, diagnosis, management, and problems of groin hernias.

ANATOMY

DEVELOPMENTAL

The genesis of the gonadal structure—testis in the male, ovary in the female—begins in the first month of intrauterine life at the caudal end of the genital ridge. By the eighth week, folds of peritoneum develop at both the upper and lower ends of the mesonephros. The lower fold, the processus vaginalis, is forced by increasing intra-abdominal pressure in a crowded abdomen around the sides of the gubernaculum, a fibromuscular band that anchors the testicle to the ventral wall of the fetus. As the gubernaculum invades the abdominal wall, forming the inguinal canal, the surrounding layers of transversus abdominis, internal oblique, and external oblique muscles are pushed aside by the processus vaginalis to form the internal spermatic fascia, cremaster muscle, and external spermatic fascia. As the weakened tissues of the ventral abdominal wall are forced outward, the scrotum is formed (Fig. 32-1). The round ligament of the ovary, the female counterpart of the gubernaculum, is far less bulky and "weakens" the lower abdominal fascia to a much lesser extent. Thus, although a processus vaginalis is formed, there is no scrotal pouch.

There is diverging theory as to whether the gubernaculum actually contracts, drawing the testis into the scrotum and the processus along with it, or simply anchors the testicle to the ventral fetal wall as the fetus elongates. The theory of "descent" of the testicle fails to explain the development of indirect inguinal hernia in females, since a processus vaginalis must be present in the absence of a testis.

Indirect inguinal hernia is the result of failure of the processus vaginalis to obliterate to a greater or lesser degree, complete failure leading to scrotal hernia, and partial obliteration resulting in indirect inguinal hernia. Narrowing of the processus with a persistent communication between the tunica vaginalis testis and the abdominal cavity constitutes a communicating hydrocele. An enlargement of the processus in the midportion of the scrotum is referred to as hydrocele of the spermatic cord.

NORMAL

Basically, the abdominal wall consists of three musculoaponeurotic layers, listed in Table 32-1.

The external oblique stratum consists of an anterior fascial plate, which was termed the innominate fascia by Gallaudet. This thick layer of collagenous fibers courses in a superolateral to inferomedial direction, that is, the direction of putting one's hands in one's pockets. All layers of the external oblique fuse at the free border of the inguinal ligament and are carried inferiorly below the inguinal ligament as the fascia lata of the thigh. The lowermost fibers of the external oblique fascia form the external spermatic

---

GROIN HERNIAS

Types
Inguinal
    Indirect: defect lateral to epigastric vessels; peritoneal sac protrudes through internal inguinal ring
    Direct: defect medial to epigastric vessels; sac protrudes through floor of inguinal canal
Femoral: enlargement of femoral ring with protrusion of sac medial to femoral sheath beneath inguinal ligament

Etiology
Inguinal
    Indirect: persistence of processus vaginalis from fetal life
    Direct: weakness in floor of inguinal canal
Femoral: enlarged femoral ring; increased intra-abdominal pressure forces sac into defect

Incidence and Associated Factors
Inguinal hernia seen in 10 of every 1000 births, 18 of every 1000 adult American men over age 25 (75% to 90% of all hernias are in males)
Increased incidence in cigarette smokers and patients with varicose veins, urinary obstruction, straining at stool, chronic obstructive pulmonary disease, and hemorrhoids

Dx
History of pain, groin mass
Physical examination most specific: finding of thickened spermatic cord, impulse in inguinal canal, palpable defect, palpable bulge

Rx
Inguinal
    Indirect: high ligation of peritoneal sac, with or without tightening of internal ring
    Direct: repair of defect in inguinal floor, preferably using transversalis fascia; types of repair: Bassini, Shouldice, Halsted, and McVay
Femoral: repair of defect with transversalis fascia (McVay repair)

---

fascia as this layer continues onto the spermatic cord passing into the scrotum. The origin of the external oblique stratum is from the iliopsoas fascia laterally, and in its medial portion it forms the anterior layer of the rectus sheath. A triangular cleft in the aponeurosis of the external oblique is the external

Fig. 32-1. *Descent of the testis.* (a) Protrusion of the testis and mesonephros into the coelomic cavity. (b) Formation of the processus vaginalis by folding of the peritoneum at the caudal end of the testis. (c) "Invasion" of the abdominal wall musculature by the swollen gubernaculum. (d) The intrascrotal testis. (Shrock P: The processus vaginalis and gubernaculum: Their raison d'être redefined. Surg Clin North Am 51:1263, 1971)

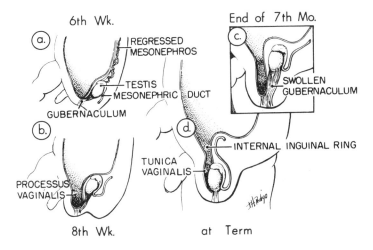

TABLE 32-1   LAYERS OF THE ABDOMINAL WALL

LAYER	DERIVED INGUINAL STRUCTURE
Skin	
Subcutaneous fat and Camper's fascia	
Scarpa's fascia	
External oblique	External spermatic fascia
Innominate fascia	
Muscle and aponeurosis	
Inner fascia	
Internal oblique	Cremaster muscle
External fascia	
Muscle and aponeurosis	
Inner fascia	
Transversus abdominis	Internal spermatic fascia
External fascia	
Muscle and aponeurosis	
Inner fascia	
Preperitoneal fat	
Peritoneum	Tunica vaginalis testis (or processus vaginalis)

inguinal ring, which allows exit of the spermatic cord into the scrotum.

The inguinal ligament (Poupart's ligament) is the slightly thickened inferior border of the external oblique aponeurosis, the lateral one fourth of which is densely bound to the iliopsoas fascia and the remainder of which is a free edge (Fig. 32-2). This ligament courses from the anterior superior iliac spine to the pubic tubercle.

The lacunar ligament (Gimbernat's ligament) is an extension of the external oblique aponeurosis that runs parallel to the inguinal ligament and inserts into the pecten of the pubis and the pectineal fascia. Contrary to several anatomical descriptions, the medial boundary of the femoral ring is formed not by the lacunar ligament but by the iliopubic tract.

The second stratum of the abdominal wall is that of the internal oblique muscle, fascia, and aponeurosis. As does the external oblique, the internal oblique exists as a layer of external fascia, a layer of muscle and aponeurotic fibers, and a layer of internal fascia. The inguinal portion of this stratum also arises from the iliopsoas fascia laterally and medially forms the second layer of the anterior rectus sheath. The fibers of the internal oblique follow an essentially perpendicular direction to those of the external oblique. The cremaster muscle is contiguous with the lowermost slips of the internal oblique muscle and arises from the iliopsoas fascia. The investing fascia of the internal oblique muscle and aponeurosis is very thin, and the aponeurosis may be deficient in its inferior portion. This stratum attaches inferiorly to the pubic pecten.

The transversus abdominis muscle, fascia, and aponeurosis is the investing layer that holds the abdominal contents in place and is thus the most important layer of the abdominal wall. As do the more superficial layers, it has an anterior fascial plate, a musculoaponeurotic middle layer, and a thin internal fascia. It also arises from the iliopsoas fascia and extends to and beyond the inguinal ligament inferiorly to form the anterior half of the femoral sheath. Medially, the transversus layer inserts into the pubis on a line beginning at the insertion of the pyramidalis muscle; this insertion continues laterally for the width of that muscle, then superiorly to the pubic tubercle, and finally along the pectinate line as far as the femoral ring. Beneath the semicircular line of Douglas, the transversalis fascia splits to surround the rectus muscle, forming portions of both the anterior and the posterior rectus sheath in this inferior location. The fibers of the transversus layer course in an almost horizontal direction. An opening in the transversalis layer, the internal inguinal ring, allows exit of the spermatic cord as it enters into the inguinal canal. The ligamentum interfoveolare is a thickening in the transversalis fascia at the medial side of the internal inguinal ring, the result of reduplication of this layer by the evaginated internal spermatic fascia.

Cooper's ligament (iliopectineal ligament) is a thickening in the transversalis fascia that fuses with the periosteum of the superior pubic ramus and extends from the pubic symphysis in a posterolateral direction until it thins and

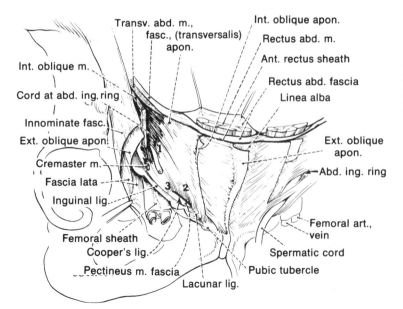

Fig. 32-2. Superficial and deep inguinal anatomy showing the inguinal ligament, the lacunar ligament, and Cooper's ligament, which courses along the superior pubic ramus from the pubic tubercle to the point where it blends into the periosteum of the pubic tubercle posterior to the iliac vessels. (McVay CB: Davis-Christopher's Textbook of Surgery. Philadelphia, W B Saunders, 1968)

Transv. abd. m., fasc., (transversalis) apon.
Int. oblique apon.
Rectus abd. m.
Ant. rectus sheath
Rectus abd. fascia
Linea alba
Int. oblique m.
Cord at abd. ing. ring
Innominate fasc.
Ext. oblique apon.
Cremaster m.
Fascia lata
Inguinal lig.
Ext. oblique apon.
Abd. ing. ring
Femoral sheath
Cooper's lig.
Pectineus m. fascia
Lacunar lig.
Femoral art., vein
Spermatic cord
Pubic tubercle

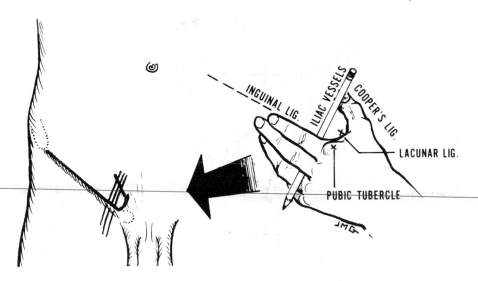

Fig. 32-3. Relationship of Cooper's ligament to the inguinal ligament and iliac vessels. Note that the two structures have a similar relationship to that of the thumb and the first finger when holding a pencil between the thumb and index finger, the index finger corresponding to the inguinal ligament and the thumb corresponding to Cooper's ligament. The first knuckle of the index finger would represent the pubic tubercle, and the web-space would correspond to the lacunar ligament. Cooper's ligament is thus noted to pass behind the iliac vessels in a posterolateral direction.

becomes indistinguishable from the periosteum (Fig. 32-2 and 32-3).

The iliopubic tract is an aponeurotic band, formed of transversalis fascia, that bridges across the iliac vessels from the iliopsoas fascia to the superior pubic ramus, immediately deep to the inguinal ligament. This transversalis analogue forms the medial border of the femoral ring.

The iliopsoas fascia gives attachment to the external oblique, internal oblique and cremaster, and transversus muscles. A slip of iliopsoas fascia forms the posterior aspect of the femoral sheath.

The funiculus spermaticus is the structure that covers the spermatic cord as it descends into the scrotum. It consists of four layers: the external spermatic fascia, derived from the external oblique aponeurosis; the cremaster muscular layer, derived from the internal oblique muscle; the internal spermatic fascia, which is a continuation of the transversalis fascia; and a preperitoneal fatty tissue layer surrounding and passing between the structures of the spermatic cord. The spermatic cord itself consists of the vas deferens, the external spermatic artery and vein, veins of the pampiniform plexus, and lymphatics.

As the femoral nerve and vessels course beneath the inguinal ligament, they are invested by a fascial sheath that is derived anteriorly from the transversalis fascia and posteriorly from a slip from the iliopsoas fascia. Between the medial portion of this femoral sheath and the lateral edge of the transversus abdominis aponeurosis that inserts into the pecten of the pubis, there is a funnel-shaped potential space, the femoral ring, usually occupied by lymphatic vessels and occasionally by lymph nodes, which may be the site of development of a hernia (Fig. 32-4). Within the femoral sheath proper, there is also a visceral sheath that is contiguous with the preperitoneal connective tissue.

The term *falx inguinalis* is given to an inconstant dense portion of the transversus abdominis aponeurosis that inserts into the pecten of the pubis rather than, as in the usual case, into the rectus sheath. The term *conjoined tendon* is considered to be synonymous with the term *falx inguinalis* when these transversus fibers are joined by fibers from the internal oblique aponeurosis.

The inguinal canal is defined as the potential space through which the spermatic cord courses between the internal inguinal ring and the external (superficial) inguinal ring. It is bounded posteriorly by the transversalis fascia and

internal oblique muscle and slips of the internal oblique aponeurosis. The posterior boundary or floor of the inguinal canal is the site of herniation in direct inguinal hernia. Hesselbach's triangle is the area within the inguinal canal classically bounded inferiorly by the inguinal ligament, superolaterally by the inferior epigastric vessels, and medially by the linea semilunaris, the line of fusion of the anterior and posterior rectus sheath (Fig. 32-5).

PATHOLOGIC

INDIRECT INGUINAL HERNIA

Protrusion of abdominal contents through a dilated internal inguinal ring into a patent processus vaginalis constitutes an indirect inguinal hernia (see Fig. 32-5). This hernia may range from a small bulge that is barely palpable within the inguinal canal to a large hernia that protrudes into the scrotum. The hernia sac, which consists of the processus vaginalis itself, is found in a position anteromedial to the spermatic cord structure. The protrusion is located lateral

Fig. 32-4. The femoral ring. The potential space between the medial side of the femoral sheath and the insertion of the transversalis fascia into the pecten of the pubis may be the site of herniation of a peritoneal sac. (McVay CB, Savage LE: Etiology of femoral hernia. Ann Surg 154:28, 1961)

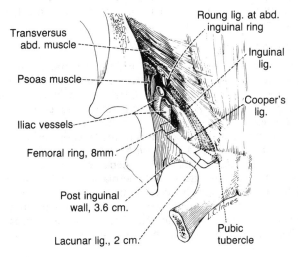

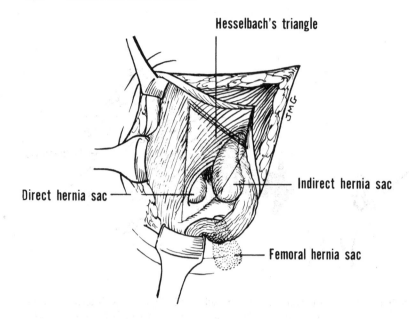

Hesselbach's triangle

Direct hernia sac

Indirect hernia sac

Femoral hernia sac

Fig. 32-5. Presentation of both direct and indirect inguinal and femoral hernia sacs with relation to Hesselbach's triangle. The indirect inguinal hernia presents through the internal inguinal ring lateral to the inferior epigastric vessels. The direct hernia presents through the floor of the inguinal canal medial to the inferior epigastric vessels in Hesselbach's triangle. The femoral hernia presents inferior to the inguinal ligament and medial to the femoral vessels.

to the inferior epigastric vessels and outside of Hesselbach's triangle. With continual pressure of abdominal contents through the defect, there is loss of the "shutter mechanism" by which the internal inguinal ring is normally closed during a Valsalva or coughing maneuver. With continued chronic pressure transmitted from the abdomen into a large indirect hernia sac, there is eventual destruction of the aponeuroticofascial plate that forms the floor of the inguinal canal, resulting in attenuation of the transversalis aponeurosis and fascia and leading to associated direct inguinal hernia.

DIRECT INGUINAL HERNIA

Attenuation of the transversalis aponeuroticofascial plate in the floor of the inguinal canal predisposes to development of hernia in that location. Direct inguinal hernia consists of a defect in the transversalis layer medial to the inferior epigastric vessels, with the protrusion of abdominal contents directly through the floor of Hesselbach's triangle (Fig. 32-5).

FEMORAL HERNIA

A funnel-shaped potential space exists within the femoral ring in a location medial to the insertion of the transversus abdominis muscle into Cooper's ligament and the femoral sheath (Fig. 32-5). Increased intra-abdominal pressure may cause protrusion of abdominal contents into this potential space, constituting a femoral hernia.

VARIANTS AND SPECIAL CASES

An inguinal hernia may have both direct and indirect components, that is, the hernia sac may protrude through the internal ring lateral to the inferior epigastric vessels, while a second component of the hernia protrudes medial to the epigastric vessels. The two hernia sacs give the appearance of a pantaloon astride the inferior epigastric vessels and are called a *pantaloon hernia.*

The term *sliding hernia* applies when an abdominal viscus makes up a portion of the wall of a hernia sac. The abdominal viscus involved may be cecum, sigmoid colon, urinary bladder, ovary or fallopian tube in the female, distal ileum, broad ligament, or appendix. The viscus is always at least a partially retroperitoneal structure. Sliding components

have been described in 2% to 5% of all inguinal hernias. It is important to note that a hernia sac that contains bowel is not necessarily a sliding hernia.

Protrusion of one wall of the intestine through a hernia defect without protrusion of the opposite wall constitutes a *Richter's hernia.* It is in this situation that a portion of the bowel may become incarcerated in a hernia defect without manifestations of intestinal obstruction, which may give the surgeon a false sense of security, allowing gangrene of the portion of the bowel with perforation and sepsis.

Lacunar ligament hernia is a defect in the lacunar ligament of Gimbernat. This may also be termed Velpeau's hernia or Laugier's hernia.

Cloquet's hernia is linked to an abnormal insertion of the pectineus muscle. The sac first enters the femoral canal and then perforates the aponeurosis of the pectineus muscle rather than protruding through the fossa ovalis as the common femoral hernia does. The sac remains between the pectineus muscle and its aponeurosis. It is also termed pectineal hernia.

The sac of *Hesselbach's hernia,* also called external femoral hernia, passes beneath the inguinal ligament but lateral to the femoral vessels and posterior to the iliopubic tract. It is usually associated with indirect inguinal hernia on the same side.

In *prevascular hernia,* the sac passes into the femoral sheath but in front of the femoral vessels rather than medial to them as in the usual femoral hernia.

Serafini's hernia is a rare defect in which the sac passes behind the femoral vessels inside the sheath of the femoral vein.

Rarely, a hernia defect develops in the transversalis fascia in the area of an aortofemoral arterial graft or beneath a femoral–femoral crossover graft in which the proximal limb of the graft has an origin from the common iliac artery; such a defect is called a *paragraft hernia.*

In *Cooper's hernia,* the main sac is within the femoral canal, but there are multilocular sacs that stretch toward the obturator foramen and may go preperitoneally into the labia majora or into the upper part of the scrotum.

Littre's hernia is one in which the sac contains a Meckel's diverticulum.

Maydl's hernia is a rare hernia that consists of two loops of bowel within the hernia sac with strangulation of the intra-abdominal portion of intestine between the loops. If one considers the bowel in the shape of the letter *W*, the lower loops of the *W* would correspond to the intestine within the hernia sac, while the upper midportion of the *W* would be held within the abdomen and strangulated.

Lipoma of the spermatic cord may be associated with, or mistaken for, inguinal hernias. When a "lipoma" is found in an operation, care must be taken to assure that there is not a peritoneal sac within the fatty structure.

EPIDEMIOLOGY

INCIDENCE

In the pediatric age-group, inguinal hernia is one of the most common surgical maladies, occurring in approximately 10 of every 1000 live births. Eighteen of every 1000 American men over the age of 25 years have inguinal hernia, and the incidence increases markedly after the fifth decade. Women over the age of 25 have fewer than ten hernias per 1000 population, and the incidence increases only slightly with advanced age. Sex distribution is heavily slanted toward the male population: Approximately 75% to 90% of hernias are reported in men. Groups at greatest risk for inguinal hernia include premature infants and adult males over 75 years of age.

ASSOCIATED FACTORS

Cigarette smoking has been shown to be associated with an increased incidence of inguinal hernia, as have varicose veins, urinary obstruction, straining at stool, chronic lung disease, and hemorrhoids. Obesity, once thought to be associated frequently with hernias, may in some instances be a protective factor associated with decreased incidence of inguinal hernia.

ETIOLOGY

Indirect hernia results from failure of the processus vaginalis to close completely with the subsequent protrusion of abdominal viscera into the processus or the remnant thereof. The question arises why an indirect hernia may remain undiagnosed for most of the patient's lifetime and then present as a hernial mass at an advanced age. Patent processus vaginalis may be found in patients who have no discernible hernia. Studies in rats have shown that although the processus vaginalis may be patent, herniation occurs only if the internal inguinal ring is dilated surgically and the rat is treated with a lathyrogenic agent such as β-aminoproprionitrile. Also, within the processus vaginalis in rats, fat pads have been discovered which when removed surgically lead to development of inguinal hernia. It is thus surmised that indirect inguinal hernia is manifest only when, in addition to persistence of the processus vaginalis, there is dilation of the internal inguinal ring through some mechanism.

The development of a direct inguinal hernia requires a combination of weakness in the transversalis fascia in the floor of the inguinal canal and increased intra-abdominal pressure leading to a defect in the fascia. Cigarette smokers have been found to have increased levels of circulating elastolytic activity and decreased α_1-antitrypsin inhibition. This may also be associated with pulmonary emphysema and the development of aortic aneurysm.

Femoral hernia occurs in the case of a congenitally narrow attachment of the transversalis fascia to Cooper's ligament, creating an enlarged femoral ring. With chronically increased intra-abdominal pressure, there is protrusion of abdominal contents through this ring. Pregnancy is felt to be a factor in the increased incidence of femoral hernia in women. An alternate theory of the development of femoral hernia involves infection in the lower extremity that leads to enlargement of femoral lymph nodes, which dilate the femoral ring. As these nodes shrink, the dilated ring may become the site of a hernia.

MORBIDITY

REDUCIBLE HERNIA

In most cases, the contents of a hernia sac may readily be returned to the abdominal cavity. The hernia may be virtually asymptomatic, with the first sign being swelling within the inguinal region. Only about one third of patients with reducible hernia complain of pain. In the case of the long-standing large hernia with a large amount of intestine within the sac, the hernial mass creates an inconvenience for the patient as well as a significant cosmetic defect.

According to insurance statistics, work disability due to symptomatic hernia occurs in 4.6 men and 0.9 women for every 1000 population.

INCARCERATION AND STRANGULATION

A hernia that is not reducible into the abdominal cavity is said to be *incarcerated*. If there is intestine within the incarcerated hernia sac, intestinal obstruction will result.

After a period of incarceration, *strangulation* may occur, with lymphatic obstruction leading to edema, further tightening the hernial ring. When the venous pressure is exceeded, capillary pressure may become increased, creating progression of edema and increased pressure within the hernia sac. This may eventually exceed the arterial pressure, leading to gangrene of the viscera incarcerated within the sac.

A simple analogy to differentiate between incarceration and strangulation relates to a penal system in which a criminal may be incarcerated in jail until he is strangulated by the hangman. Incarceration is seen most commonly in the age-groups under 2 years and over 60. Although inguinal hernias are much more common than femoral hernias, femoral hernias have a higher incidence of incarceration and strangulation. The mortality rate for a strangulated inguinal hernia is 12% to 13% as compared with up to 30% for a strangulated femoral hernia. When the bowel is frankly gangrenous, the mortality rate increases to approximately 50% to 75%.

RATIONALE FOR HERNIORRHAPHY

In the pediatric age-group, the mortality rate for both emergency and elective herniorrhaphy is very low, although the morbidity of incarcerated inguinal hernia is significant.

Since it is evident that a processus vaginalis that has not closed by the time of birth will in all likelihood not close spontaneously, this morbidity can be eliminated by elective herniorrhaphy. In the adult age-group, the mortality rate for elective herniorrhaphy is somewhat less than 1%, while that of an emergency operation increases to 10%. In patients over 60 years of age, the mortality rate for elective operation has been approximately 2%, with the emergency group having a 13% to 15% mortality rate. This would indicate that herniorrhaphy on an elective basis should decrease the overall mortality rate for inguinal and femoral hernia.

DIAGNOSIS

In the pediatric age-group, the most common presenting sign is swelling in the groin noted by the child's mother. The hernia may become incarcerated, and may present as such, or may have become spontaneously reduced prior to examination.

In adults, about one third of hernias are discovered at the time of a routine examination and the other two thirds are discovered when the patient presents with symptoms. Most commonly, there is swelling in the groin that may be associated with pain in one third of patients. A history of tenesmus, chronic obstructive pulmonary disease (COPD), urinary symptoms, or lifting a heavy object may be elicited.

PHYSICAL EXAMINATION

In children, a swelling may be present within the groin that may be visible on inspection. A hernia sac containing an abdominal viscus may be palpable, but it is difficult to feel a mass if the sac is empty. The "silk sign" consists of the sensation similar to two pieces of silk rubbing together as one passes a finger perpendicular to the spermatic cord with tension on the testicle. The most reliable physical finding in diagnosing inguinal hernia in a child is the presence of a thickened spermatic cord. Children with hydroceles or undescended testes frequently have inguinal hernia.

In adults, inspection of the groin may reveal a swelling with or without scrotal involvement. Palpation may elicit a mass within the inguinal canal, and there may be an impulse within the canal on cough or Valsalva's maneuver. A hernia sac palpable below the internal ring suggests direct hernia; if a finger placed over the internal ring after reduction of the hernia prevents presentation of the hernia sac, one may surmise that the hernia is indirect. *Reducibility* should be documented in the patient's record. Auscultation of the groin may elicit bowel sounds in a large hernia; when femoral aneurysm masquerades as femoral hernia, a bruit may be heard.

If the hernia cannot be reduced, a diagnosis of incarceration may be made, and tenderness or discoloration in the area of the hernia suggests strangulation.

DIAGNOSTIC TECHNIQUES

Sonography has recently been used to demonstrate inguinal and femoral hernias as well as other hernias of the abdominal wall. In my experience, it has not been extremely useful, although in the patient who complains of groin pain and in whom there is a question of femoral hernia, the technique can be particularly helpful in differentiating femoral hernia from femoral adenopathy or abscess.

Herniography involves the injection of radiopaque con- trast material into the abdominal cavity to identify a hernia sac. The patient is turned in different directions, allowing the contrast to gravitate into the pelvis and outline the peritoneal contour. This technique has been used most extensively in children, although its use in adults has recently been reported. Complications, although infrequent, are due to injury of either the intestine or the bladder. In my experience, there has been little need for herniography to diagnose inguinal or femoral hernia, since the clinical diagnosis is usually straightforward.

DIFFERENTIAL DIAGNOSIS

Inguinal hernia must often be differentiated from hydrocele or, more rarely, a retroperitoneal abscess presenting in the groin. Intra-abdominal hematomas from a number of sources, including ruptured aneurysm and hepatic fracture, may also present as groin "hernias."

Femoral hernia is often confused with femoral lymphadenopathy, saphenous varicosities, and femoral artery aneurysm.

MANAGEMENT

Taxis, the reduction of a hernia by external manipulation with truss support, dates back to the fifth century B.C. The first description of surgical treatment of incarcerated hernia is attributed to Celsus, a Roman who lived from 25 B.C. to A.D. 50. His technique, termed kelotomy, consisted of the cord being isolated and placed on stretch, the contents reduced, and the sac transected.

Delineation of the inguinal anatomy marked the beginning of a sequence of events that led to present-day methods of hernia management. In 1804, Sir Astley Cooper, in a study of femoral hernia, described the iliopectineal ligament that bears his name. In a classic book, Franz Kaspar Hasselbach, in 1814, described the triangle that bears his name, as well as the iliopubic tract. In 1837, Velpeau in France and Pancoast in the United States advocated the injection of sclerosing agents into hernia sacs. Complications of the technique included pain, hydrocele of the spermatic cord in the unobliterated part, bladder injury, allergy to the sclerosing agent, and strangulation. The recurrence rate proved to be higher than was originally thought by the proponents, and the technique fell into disfavor after a period of time, although it has been more recently used in the treatment of hydrocele.

Prior to 1881, all surgical attempts to repair inguinal hernia were associated with reluctance to incise fascial planes, the widespread belief being that to do so would invite infection and that the fasciae could not successfully be sutured together. In that year, Lucas-Championniére opened the inguinal canal for the first time, marking the transition from kelotomy to herniotomy.

Perhaps the first herniorrhaphy was described in 1884 by Edoardo Bassini of Padua, Italy. His technique, described in a later section, was associated with lower recurrence and mortality rates than any ever previously published. Almost simultaneously, in 1885, Henry O. Marcy of Boston innovated a method of closure of the internal ring. Also about 1885, William S. Halsted of Johns Hopkins University devised a procedure of *en masse* suturing of all the fascial layers with cord transposition. In 1889, this procedure was revised to close the layers separately and to leave the cord in its anatomical position.

In a series of papers from 1938 to 1942, McVay and Anson described their observations on the anatomy and physiology of the groin based on over 300 dissections using transillumination from within the abdominal cavity. They pointed out that the transversalis fascia does not insert at any time into Poupart's ligament but normally inserts into Cooper's ligament.

In 1953, E. E. Shouldice of Toronto devised a method with a 13-year recurrence rate of less than 0.2%. This technique is described in detail in a later section. Local anesthesia was used in 97% of his cases. In 1970, Usher described the technique in which the fascia is backed with polypropylene mesh with a repair using both Cooper's and Poupart's ligaments for recurrent hernias.

In 1964, Condon advocated the use of the iliopubic tract in the repair of inguinal hernias excluding femoral hernia or sliding hernia. The repair of indirect hernia was done much as a Bassini-type repair except that the iliopubic tract was used rather than Poupart's ligament. Direct hernia repair was similar to the McVay repair except that the iliopubic tract was used rather than Cooper's ligament. In 1978, Nyhus advocated the preperitoneal approach. This, he felt, was ideal for recurrent hernias because of the approach through previously unoperated tissue. Sliding hernias could easily be recognized and reduced, and femoral and indirect hernias could also be easily identified and repaired.

Today, surgical treatment of inguinal and femoral hernia has become a safe, common procedure and should be chosen over any nonoperative method. Primarily, the Marcy, Bassini, Halsted II, McVay, Shouldice, and preperitoneal repairs are used.

NONOPERATIVE

From the time of Paré, trusses have been used in patients who were felt not to be candidates for surgical management. Many variations have been devised, but all consist of external pressure applied constantly to the hernia defect. Since it is speculated that the use of a truss may predispose the patient to incarceration during the time that the truss is not in place, the truss should be worn at all times. Its use should be restricted to those patients who absolutely are not candidates for operation, such as those with advanced cancer or extremely severe cardiorespiratory disease. With today's excellent anesthesia and the greatly improved capacity for caring for ill patients in the postoperative period, the truss should seldom be used, giving way to surgical management in practically every case of groin hernia.

Prolonged periods of rest have been prescribed over the years for hernia patients. This method also gave way to routine surgical management.

Injection of the hernia sac using a sclerosing solution is at this point of historical note only. The late results have been almost uniformly poor.

OPERATIVE

PREOPERATIVE EVALUATION

The major factor of mortality in patients undergoing elective herniorrhaphy is related to the anesthetic, the most common postoperative complication of anesthesia being respiratory. Thirty percent of patients undergoing herniorrhaphy under general anesthesia and 13% of patients undergoing herni-orrhaphy under spinal anesthesia have respiratory complications. Since it is well known that the most common cause of death in elderly patients is pneumonia, people with chronic bronchopulmonary disease must be thoroughly evaluated as to their ability to withstand an operative procedure.

Cardiac disease is also a source of anesthetic-related mortality in patients who have had recent myocardial infarction.

In addition to its untoward effect on anesthetic risk, obstructive airway disease has been implicated as a major cause of chronically increased intra-abdominal pressure. Hernia recurrence is seen frequently in patients with chronic lung disease; therefore, every effort should be made to improve pulmonary function prior to any operative procedure.

Bladder outlet obstruction may also cause increased intra-abdominal pressure, leading to recurrence of inguinal hernia following repair. All patients undergoing herniorrhaphy should be questioned thoroughly for symptoms of bladder outlet obstruction, and a rectal examination should be done to determine the size of the prostate gland. If there is any question as to the severity of urinary obstruction, the postvoiding residual urine volume in the bladder, if significant, may indicate evaluation by a urologist prior to hernia repair. Urinary retention continues to be a common early postoperative complication following herniorrhaphy under spinal anesthesia.

Although the association of hernia with colon cancer is somewhat controversial, the incidence of inguinal hernia in patients with colon carcinoma has been reported as high as 22.5%. On the other hand, recent studies have shown that if a large group of patients with inguinal hernia are examined, the incidence of carcinoma of the colon will be no greater than in the general population. However, since patients who have partially obstructing lesions of the lower bowel have chronically increased intra-abdominal pressure, the incidence of recurrent hernia in these patients might be expected to be considerable; of course, if the obstructing lesion is malignant, it must be managed with priority. Patients undergoing herniorrhaphy should be carefully assessed for any history of change in bowel habits, diarrhea, or straining at stool. Those who have symptomatology should have proctoscopy and barium enema as a screening procedure and, if symptoms are felt to warrant it, endoscopic evaluation of the colon and rectum. Although young patients with inguinal hernia and without symptoms of gastrointestinal tract pathology should not be expected to have carcinoma of the colon, certainly those asymptomatic patients who are in the age-group at risk should undergo routine proctosigmoidoscopy prior to hernia repair.

Patients who have chronic ascites, whether due to portal hypertension, renal disease, or other causes, are at increased risk for development of hernia. In addition, their recurrence rate after repair will be considerably higher than in patients without chronic ascites. In patients with massive ascites, the risk of recurrence is so great as to be essentially prohibitive of any attempt at repair. However, those patients who have controlled ascites can undergo hernia repair with a considerable degree of safety.

Patients who are afflicted with systemic disease processes that impair wound healing must be identified prior to any operation because wound healing and long-term success in hernia repair may become impaired. Diabetes mellitus, collagen vascular disease, systemic malignancy, steroid hormones, and protein–calorie malnutrition have all been associated with poor wound healing. Patients undergoing radiotherapy probably should not have an elective surgical procedure until the course of radiation therapy is completed; elective operation is also contraindicated during therapy with many types of antineoplastic drugs.

CHOICE OF ANESTHETIC

The operative risk in elective inguinal or femoral herniorrhaphy is related primarily to the anesthetic. Three types of anesthesia are available, and considerations in making the choice should include cardiorespiratory status and patient acceptance.

The greatest risk of cardiorespiratory complications occurs with the general anesthetic; approximately 30% of patients have some respiratory complication, and a significant number have cardiac complications. In addition, some patients feel that in being anesthetized, they have no control over the situation and are completely dependent on the anesthetist. General anesthesia is, however, favored by some surgeons because the procedure may be done more rapidly. In addition, some surgeons feel a bit self-conscious in operating on an awake patient.

Spinal anesthesia may also have considerable effect on the heart due to the hypotension of vasodilatation following induction. There is also an increased incidence of urinary retention in patients undergoing spinal anesthesia for hernia repair, and approximately 13% of these patients also have respiratory complications. The operation may be done as rapidly as with general anesthesia, but because of unfounded fears of spinal cord injury and paralysis, spinal anesthesia may be poorly accepted by the patient.

The safest anesthesia for inguinal herniorrhaphy is local. Urinary retention, urinary sepsis, atelectasis, and phlebitis are virtually eliminated, and patients may be discharged on the day of operation. This type of anesthetic has been well accepted because the patient is conscious during the entire procedure and feels that by being aware of the surroundings he does not "lose control." Any type of conduction anesthetic may be used, and lidocaine and mepivacaine have been used in significant numbers of patients. Our preference is 0.25% bupivacaine, although 0.5% solution has also been reported to be efficacious. Anesthesia is obtained as follows: (1) Ten ml of the anesthetic is injected in a fanlike fashion approximately 1 cm medial to the anterior superior iliac spine. Resistance is felt as the needle passes beneath the external oblique aponeurosis, and the solution is injected to block the branches of the lumbar nerves that course through this potential space. (2) A cutaneous wheal of anesthetic is made along the line selected for skin incision, and the subcutaneous tissues are infiltrated. Short-acting agents such as lidocaine may be chosen for this injection because of rapidity of onset. (3) The cutaneous branch of the iliohypogastric nerve is then blocked by injection at the pubic tubercle. (4) The cutaneous incision is made, and more anesthetic is injected beneath the external oblique aponeurosis prior to its opening. (5) The floor of the inguinal canal, the pubic tubercle, and the medial portion of Cooper's ligament are injected. The lateral portion of Cooper's ligament is usually not innervated. (6) The ilioinguinal nerve is blocked by infiltration lateral to the internal ring. (7) The spermatic cord is mobilized, the base of the hernia sac is identified, and a wheal of anesthetic is made around the base of the sac.

The repair may then be completed as a Bassini operation,

Shouldice repair, McVay repair, or practically any type of repair desired. Hospital costs are cut essentially in half, so that with respect to both economy and decreased morbidity, local is the anesthetic of choice.

The disadvantages of local anesthesia include increased operating time, since the surgeon must be extremely gentle in handling tissues, and the fact that some surgeons feel somewhat ill at ease when the patient is awake and able to converse. If the operation becomes prolonged, the patient may complain of back pain from lying on the hard surface of the operating table for an extended period.

If the anesthetic becomes dissipated, additional amounts can be injected.

TECHNIQUES OF REPAIR

Although an almost unlimited number of different hernia operations have been described, a basic few have found widespread use in the modern repair of inguinal and femoral hernia.

Pediatric Hernia (see also Chapter 41)

In infants and young children, the hernia is practically always an indirect hernia or patent processus vaginalis. Direct hernias are infrequently seen in children and when present are usually associated with failure of repair of an indirect hernia. The technique of hernia repair in children is a simple one, consisting in identification of the indirect sac and high ligation of that sac. The sac may be transfixed to the undersurface of the internal oblique muscle to prevent protrusion of the stump of the sac into the internal ring. Although simple ligation is felt by many to be curative, some surgeons feel that some procedure to tighten the internal inguinal ring adds to the efficacy of the repair.

Bilateral hernia can be detected preoperatively in about 10% of infants and children undergoing inguinal herniorrhaphy. Controversy exists as to whether the contralateral side should be explored in patients who have clinically a unilateral hernia. When routine bilateral exploration has been done in these patients, a contralateral hernia has been found about half the time. However, the definition of a hernia may be somewhat liberal in that if one tugs on the spermatic cord sufficiently a small protrusion of peritoneum can almost always be found. A patent processus vaginalis may often be found without an associated hernial protrusion of abdominal contents; these patent processes may remain empty throughout life. After unilateral hernia repair, contralateral clinically detectable hernia develops in 15% to 20% of patients. It is our belief that because of the high incidence of bilaterality in children under 2 years of age and in female children, routine bilateral exploration may be warranted in these patients. In the older age-group, once the child has been anesthetized, a thickening of the spermatic cord should be evident with slight tension on the testicle in the presence of a hernia. Occasionally, the opposite internal ring can be palpated through the side being repaired, and a Bâkes dilator may be passed into the opposite internal ring to determine if a hernia sac is present.

The anesthetic of choice in infants and young children is general, although local anesthesia may be feasible in older adolescents.

Adult Hernia

Indirect Inguinal Hernia. Marcy Repair. The internal inguinal ring is a funnel-shaped structure with a lining of peritoneum, the most important fascial layer of the ring being the extension of transversalis fascia known as the

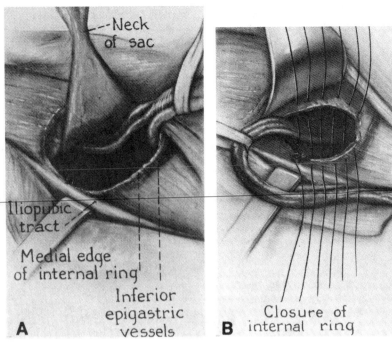

Fig. 32-6. Marcy repair of indirect inguinal hernia. *(A)* The vas deferens and vessels have been separated from the peritoneum, and the neck of the sac has been freed. The sac is ligated flush with the general peritoneal cavity. *(B)* After ligation and amputation of the hernia sac, sutures are placed through the transversalis fascia on either side of the defect in the internal ring so that the reconstructed ring admits only the tip of a hemostat. (Griffith CA: The Marcy repair of indirect inguinal hernia. Surg Clin North Am 39:531, 1959)

internal spermatic fascia. Since the defect involved in indirect hernia is that of the internal ring itself, it is desirable to close the ring snugly around the spermatic cord. This may be done from either an anterior or a preperitoneal approach. The hernia sac is identified and is ligated or oversewn flush with the peritoneal cavity. The defect in the transversalis fascia that constitutes the internal inguinal ring is identified, and the thickened bands of transversalis fascia that form the pillars of the ring (ligamentum interfoveolare) are sutured together until the ring is tightened around the spermatic cord, restoring the shutter mechanism (Fig. 32-6). In women, the round ligament of the uterus is divided and the internal ring is completely closed.

Indirect Inguinal Hernia. Bassini Repair. Although repair of the internal ring, if properly done, should ordinarily be curative of indirect hernia, the Bassini operation has been used extensively in adult patients. This technique does not adequately repair a direct hernia defect in the floor of the inguinal canal but can be used to tighten the internal inguinal ring as well as to reinforce the inguinal floor. After exposure of the external oblique aponeurosis, that aponeurosis is opened in the direction of its fibers into the external ring. The hernia sac is ligated flush with the abdominal cavity, and the conjoined tendon of internal oblique, transversus abdominis, and transversalis fascia is sutured to Poupart's ligament beginning with the pubic tubercle and continuing with interrupted sutures until the internal ring admits a fingertip alongside the spermatic cord (Fig. 32-7). The external oblique aponeurosis is then closed over the spermatic cord to the point that the external inguinal ring will admit a fingertip.

Direct Inguinal Hernia. Halsted Repair. The hernia repair originally described by William S. Halsted consisted of skeletonization of the spermatic cord with mass closure of the external oblique aponeurosis, internal oblique aponeurosis, and transversus muscles superiorly to the transversalis fascia and Poupart's ligament inferiorly, the spermatic cord

being transplanted into the subcutaneous tissue. This Halsted I operation gave way to the Halsted II procedure, which differed in that the spermatic cord was not transplanted but remained in the anatomical position within the inguinal canal and the closure was done in layers rather than as a mass closure. An incision was also made in the rectus sheath, with a flap of anterior rectus sheath folded over to reinforce the attenuated transversalis fascia in the floor of the inguinal canal.

Direct Inguinal Hernia. Preperitoneal Repair. The preperitoneal approach to hernia repair as popularized by Condon and Nyhus involves making a skin incision approximately 3 cm above the inguinal ligament and entering the preperitoneal space by transversely incising the external oblique, internal oblique, and transversus layers. Care is taken to avoid entering the peritoneal cavity. Retraction of the lower margin of the incision exposes the posterior inguinal wall and area of herniation. The peritoneum and preperitoneal fat are separated from the transversalis fascia by blunt dissection, and any hernia sac protruding through the transversalis becomes evident. The hernia sac may be oversewn flush with the general curvature of the peritoneum and the hernia defect closed. This is quite efficacious in dealing with indirect hernias.

In the case of a direct hernia, the upper border of the defect will be thickened transversalis fascia and the lower border will be the iliopubic tract. These two structures may be sutured together to obliterate the defect (Fig. 32-8). The first few sutures also commonly pass through Cooper's ligament; if the iliopubic tract is attenuated, the complete repair may be done using Cooper's ligament.

The distal hernia sac may protrude for such a distance into the inguinal canal that removal of the sac is not possible. The sac may be transected and left in place, the distal sac remaining open so that any fluid that accumulates may drain into the subcutaneous tissues and be absorbed.

Direct Inguinal Hernia. Shouldice Repair. The Shouldice

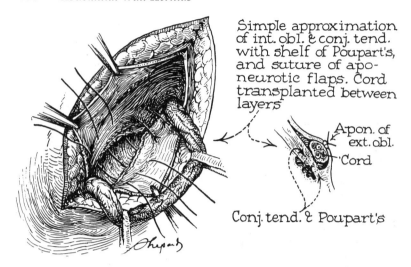

Simple approximation of int. obl. & conj. tend. with shelf of Poupart's, and suture of apo-neurotic flaps. Cord transplanted between layers

Apon. of ext. obl.

Cord

Conj. tend. & Poupart's

Fig. 32-7. Bassini repair of inguinal hernia. Sutures have been passed between the conjoined tendon of internal oblique and transversalis fascia and then approximated, on the inferior side of the defect, to the edge of Poupart's ligament. The external oblique aponeurosis is then approximated over the spermatic cord. (Bombeck CT, Nyhus LM: Hernia. In Nora PF [ed]: Operative Surgery: Principles and Techniques, chap 32, p 695. Philadelphia, Lea & Febiger, 1972)

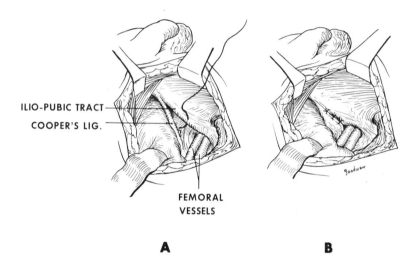

ILIO-PUBIC TRACT
COOPER'S LIG.

FEMORAL VESSELS

A   **B**

Fig. 32-8. Preperitoneal repair using the ilio-pubic tract. *(A)* The preperitoneal sac is removed from the fascial defect by traction and blunt dissection, and sutures are passed between the transversalis fascia superiorly and the iliopubic tract inferiorly. *(B)* Completed repair showing approximation of transversalis fascia to the ilio-pubic tract. If the iliopubic tract is attenuated, Cooper's ligament may be used. (Smith GV: Groin hernias in adults: Clinical management. In Hardy JD [ed]: Rhoads Textbook of Surgery, 5th ed. Philadelphia, J B Lippincott, 1977)

repair of inguinal hernia applies to direct as well as indirect hernias. A set routine is followed no matter what type of hernia so that no component of the repair will be omitted. After the skin and subcutaneous incision is made in a horizontal crease, the external oblique aponeurosis is opened in the direction of its fibers and the spermatic cord is exposed. It is felt important to remove the cremaster muscle from the cord, opening this muscle longitudinally for several centimeters up to the internal inguinal ring. Removal of the cremaster muscle facilitates exposure of any direct hernia defect; the stump of the cremaster muscle may be used to reinforce the repair at the level of the internal ring. Any indirect peritoneal sac is identified and is widely mobilized from the transversalis layer of the internal ring. This allows retraction of the peritoneal sac into the abdomen after its division and ligation. Transversalis fascia is then opened from the internal inguinal ring to the pubic tubercle. The leaves of the divided transversalis fascia are imbricated using a continuous suture, preferably of 34-gauge wire, the superomedial flap being brought over the inferolateral one (Fig. 32-9, *A*). The first suture line begins at the pubic tubercle and is brought in a continuous fashion up to the internal ring, suturing the free edge of the inferolateral flap to the undersurface of the superomedial flap. This suture line then is doubled back, bringing the leading edge of the superomedial flap to the shelving edge of Poupart's ligament.

The lacunar ligament is included in this suture line to obliterate the dead space medial to the femoral vessels. A second suture, beginning at the internal ring, brings the internal oblique and transversus muscles down to the deep surface of the inguinal ligament (Fig. 32-9, *B*). At the level of the pubic bone, this suture line doubles back, attaching the same structures in a more superficial plane, and the suture is tied to itself at the internal ring. No relaxing incision is made.

Since this repair does not include Cooper's ligament, it is not useful in repairing femoral hernias, and, in fact, most recurrences following Shouldice repair take the form of a femoral hernia.

Direct Inguinal Hernia. McVay (Cooper's Ligament) Repair.
The reconstruction of the posterior inguinal wall as described by McVay has been a great technical advance in modern surgery. It is primarily indicated in direct hernia but may be useful in repairing indirect hernias when a large sac has caused attenuation of the inguinal floor. The skin incision is made in a fashion similar to any other hernia repair and is carried down to the external oblique aponeurosis, which is opened in the direction of its fibers. Any indirect hernia sac is identified, and high ligation is done. Cooper's ligament is then exposed, and after a relaxing incision is made in the anterior rectus sheath, the transversalis fascia is sutured to Cooper's ligament beginning at the pubic tubercle. This line

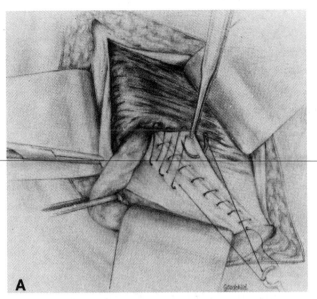

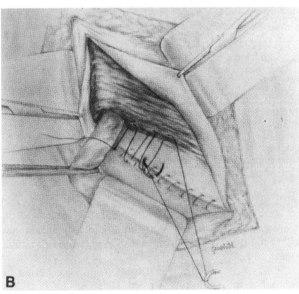

Fig. 32-9. Shouldice repair of inguinal hernia. *(A)* The transversalis fascia is imbricated using a continuous suture beginning at the pubic tubercle, continuing laterally to the internal ring, and then doubling back to the pubic tubercle. *(B)* A second suture reinforces the repair, beginning at the internal ring and approximating transversalis fascia and internal oblique aponeurosis to the inguinal ligament. This suture also doubles back to the internal ring, further reinforcing the repair. (Glassow F: The Shouldice repair for inguinal hernia. In Nyhus LM, Condon RE [eds]: Hernia, 2nd ed. Philadelphia, J B Lippincott, 1978)

of interrupted sutures is carried to within a few millimeters of the femoral vein. At this point, a transition suture is made encompassing Cooper's ligament as well as the anterior femoral sheath, which in reality consists of transversalis fascia. Some controversy exists as to whether the "shelving edge" of Poupart's ligament should be included in this transition suture. Some feel that failure to include Poupart's ligament weakens the repair, while others contend that suturing Poupart's ligament to Cooper's ligament prevents the functional closing of the internal inguinal ring. It

is our usual practice to include in the transition suture the iliopubic tract as it reflects on the undersurface of Poupart's ligament and to continue the repair laterally using the iliopubic tract to anchor the transversalis fascia. The suture line is continued until the internal inguinal ring admits a fingertip alongside the spermatic cord (Fig. 32-10). The cord is placed in the anatomical position within the inguinal canal, and the external oblique aponeurosis is closed. In the elderly patient in whom cord trauma is not an expected problem, the cord may be placed in the subcutaneous tissue and the external oblique aponeurosis imbricated beneath. The subcutaneous tissue is closed loosely, and the skin edges are closed, preferably with a subcuticular suture to avoid cutaneous sutures in a relatively contaminated area.

Femoral Hernia. Infrainguinal Approach. Although the infrainguinal approach for repair of femoral hernia is seldom used, it may be quite an acceptable alternative in the elderly woman. An oblique incision is made below the inguinal ligament, and the deep fascia of the thigh is incised transversely. The femoral hernia sac is usually surrounded by extraperitoneal fat; this is cleaned from the sac, and the sac is opened. Opening on the lateral side avoids injury to the bladder, which may be present within the sac. The contents of the sac are inspected and reduced, and the sac is transected and ligated. In men undergoing infrainguinal repair of a femoral hernia, it is advantageous also to open the fascia above the inguinal ligament. In addition to facilitating reduction of the hernia, an associated inguinal hernia may be thus demonstrated. In women, associated inguinal hernias are found less commonly. Reduction of the hernias may require incision of the transversalis fascia at the neck of the sac to loosen the hernial ring. The repair is done by approximating the inguinal ligament to Cooper's ligament. The femoral ring may be further closed by approximating Hey's ligament, the strip of fascia forming the superior border of the fossa ovalis, to the pectineal fascia. If the approximation of the inguinal ligament and Cooper's ligament is not feasible, synthetic mesh may also be used to obliterate the enlarged femoral ring.

Femoral Hernia. Suprainguinal Approach (McVay Repair). The preferred method of repairing femoral hernias is the Cooper's ligament repair described by McVay. The repair is done essentially as for inguinal hernia, the transversalis fascia being sutured to Cooper's ligament. The transition suture between Cooper's ligament and the anterior femoral sheath obliterates the femoral ring after reduction and ligation of the sac. The transversalis fascia in the case of femoral hernia is somewhat stronger than in direct inguinal hernia, and this repair is quite secure. Occasionally, in the man who has both inguinal and femoral hernia, Cooper's ligament repair is an excellent choice of operation. If no inguinal hernia is present, it is usually not necessary to make a relaxing incision.

Incarcerated or Strangulated Hernia. About 10% of hernias become incarcerated, leading to a mortality rate of 12% to 13% in inguinal hernia patients and 13% to 30% in femoral hernia patients. Gangrene of the associated bowel increases the mortality rate to 50% to 75%.

Nonoperative reduction may be either passive or active. It is more often possible to reduce an incarcerated hernia in a child than in an adult. This is accomplished by elevation of the feet and placing the patient at ease. Sedation and muscle relaxants may be used in adult patients. Since the incidence of bowel gangrene is low in infants and children,

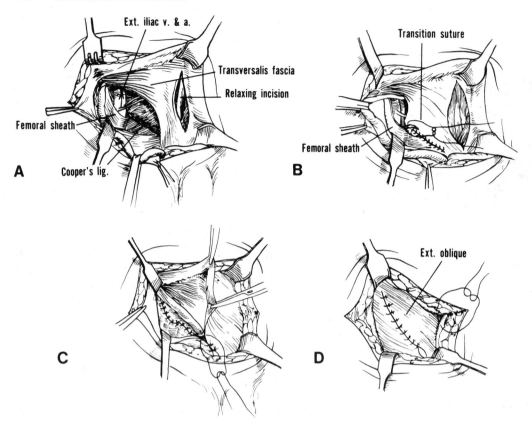

Fig. 32-10. McVay repair of inguinal or femoral hernia. After a generous relaxing incision is made in the anterior rectus sheath *(A),* the transversalis fascia is approximated to Cooper's ligament to the point that Cooper's ligament passes behind the iliac vessels. At this point, a transition suture is made *(B)* encompassing the transversalis fascia, Cooper's ligament, and the femoral sheath. The repair is then continued laterally *(C)* approximating the transversalis fascia to the femoral sheath until the internal ring admits a fingertip. The external oblique aponeurosis is then closed anterior to the spermatic cord *(D).* It is often beneficial to include the iliopubic tract in the transition suture and in the lateral continuation of the repair.

an attempt at passive reduction and even gentle manipulation is warranted in most cases.

In the adult, gangrenous bowel is found in 5% to 10% of incarcerated hernias. Bowel gangrene may be very difficult to diagnose preoperatively but can be suspected if the hernial mass is tender with associated induration and erythema of the surrounding tissues. Because of the high incidence of gangrene in adult patients, the safest method of treating incarcerated hernias is immediate operation. Although the mortality rate for emergency herniorrhaphy is significantly higher than that for elective operation, there are no definite criteria to determine if the bowel is gangrenous. Statistically, reduction attempts have not reduced the mortality in incarcerated hernia, since mortality occurs chiefly in patients in whom reduction attempts were unsuccessful.

In addition to the danger of reducing gangrenous bowel into the abdomen, there is also the consideration of reduction *en masse*. This is a rare occurrence, but it is associated with a very high mortality. There are three types of *en masse* reductions: Type I involves forcing the inguinal hernia sac contents into a preperitoneal location, the neck of the peritoneal sac remaining tightly about the hernial contents. Type II is a bilocular hernia in which the contents of the inguinal portion of the sac are forced into a preperitoneal extension of the sac. In Type III, the sac ruptures and the

incarcerated viscus with the remnant of the hernia sac bound tightly about it becomes displaced behind the pubic bone.

As has been mentioned, the reduction of a hernia by external manipulation is termed *taxis*. Although in the pediatric age-group taxis may be successful and allow an emergency situation to be transformed into an elective one, attempts at taxis should not persist in the adult patient.

The safest means of treating incarcerated hernia is immediate operation. Although in the young patient the operation may be quite straightforward, in the elderly patient there is no room for technical or anesthetic error. Great attention must be paid to detail. The sac is identified as usual, but great care must be taken that the contents of the sac are not allowed to retract into the abdomen before examination for nonviability. If the contents of the sac are lost into the abdomen, laparotomy is mandatory to examine the bowel for viability.

In the occasional patient in whom the hernia cannot be reduced by an anterior approach, the Laroque maneuver may be useful. An incision is made parallel to the inguinal incision at a point about 3 cm cephalad and is carried through the layers of the abdominal wall into the peritoneal cavity. This incision may be made through the same skin incision by retracting the skin. The hernia can be reduced from within the abdomen and the repair done as usual. The Laroque incision also affords an excellent opportunity to inspect the bowel.

Although there are more inguinal hernias than femoral hernias, more femoral hernias become strangulated. The femoral hernia sac and its contents may be resected *en bloc* by dividing the inguinal ligament. As the bowel is resected, an anastomosis is done and the bowel is reduced into the abdomen. This technique is felt to reduce the mortality for strangulated femoral hernia, since the strangulation fluid is not allowed to come into contact with the peritoneal cavity.

Sliding Hernia. The majority of sliding hernias are indirect, although direct and femoral hernias may have sliding components. The repair of a sliding hernia requires, first of all, identification of the presence of a sliding component. This should be suspected preoperatively if the hernia is difficult to reduce or if it does not remain so after initial reduction.

Operative repair of sliding hernias may be accomplished by dissecting the sac from the cord and transversalis fascia and placing the sac and the associated viscus beneath the transversalis fascia and securely tightening the internal ring. Peritonealization of the bowel surface probably serves no useful purpose and is thus omitted in this procedure.

A second type of repair of sliding hernia, more commonly used, is that of a purse-string closure of the sac with reduction of the viscus into the abdominal cavity. A Laroque-type counterincision may be beneficial in reduction of the viscus within the sac.

Pantaloon Hernia. Pantaloon hernia can be managed basically in two ways. The Hoguet maneuver involves conversion of the direct sac component to an indirect sac, by placing tension on the indirect sac as the direct sac is freed from beneath the inferior epigastric vessels. When the direct sac has been shifted beneath the epigastric vessels and the entire sac becomes indirect, simple high ligation is done.

This method, however, has given way to simple division of the inferior epigastric vessels to create one large hernia sac, which is repaired as a direct hernia.

POSTOPERATIVE CARE

EARLY POSTOPERATIVE PERIOD

In the very recent past, patients undergoing groin herniorrhaphy were kept at strict bed rest for 2 weeks following the procedure. Fortunately, this practice has given way to early ambulation, with a resultant decrease in the risk of deep venous thrombosis and pulmonary complications. Early ambulation may also actually decrease the risk of recurrence. Patients undergoing herniorrhaphy under local anesthesia may sometimes walk from the operating suite to their rooms, allowing the groin musculature to be stretched slightly and possibly decreasing the amount of postoperative incisional tenderness.

The postoperative diet should be a normal one, but the patient should be encouraged to eat high-bulk material to prevent constipation with resultant straining to defecate.

The wound should be covered for at least the first 48 hours. The patient may then shower, changing the dressing after the bath. The wound should be inspected on the seventh postoperative day for any evidence of infection.

DISCHARGE INSTRUCTIONS

The patient should be instructed to keep the wound dry except during showers and to dry the wound immediately as it becomes wet. Daily cleansing of the wound is desirable, removing any encrusted serum or exudate. After the first 48 hours, wound dressings are optional. The patient should be instructed to report in immediately if the wound becomes reddened, increasingly tender, or painful.

Herniorrhaphy patients should be instructed to refrain from driving an automobile for 10 days following the operation. It has long been felt by many that driving an automobile might require stressing an inguinal hernia repair if brakes were applied suddenly. This has not been shown to be the case, and recurrence is probably not fostered by early driving. However, reflex stopping time is increased in patients studied on the fifth and seventh days postoperatively and becomes normal at 10 days following the procedure.

Exercise is beneficial following any operation as long as the level of activity is kept reasonable. The patient who was in an exercise program prior to his operation may resume the exercise program at a decreased pace at 2 or 3 weeks following the operation. The patient should be instructed to begin slowly, to walk initially, and to refrain from any activity that is painful. The body will protect itself by eliciting a pain response.

COMPLICATIONS

SYSTEMIC

Exclusive of local complications, most morbidity associated with inguinal herniorrhaphy is associated with the anesthetic (Table 32-2). Respiratory complications occur in 13% of patients undergoing herniorrhaphy under spinal anesthesia and in 30% of those who have general anesthesia. The elderly patient may be prone to cardiac complications, and urinary retention may be seen in patients who have significant prostatic disease. Urinary retention occurs in patients who have bilateral simultaneous hernia repairs, particularly those who have spinal anesthesia.

LOCAL

A number of complications may occur due to technical errors during the performance of a herniorrhaphy. Nerve injury may lead to a significant source of pain in the postoperative period. Injury of the ilioinguinal nerve may lead to decreased sensation in the base of the penis, the upper scrotum, and the inner thigh. This injury usually occurs during opening of the external oblique aponeurosis. Injury to the iliohypogastric nerve denervates the suprapubic area and may occur with the relaxing incision of a McVay hernia repair. The genitofemoral nerve lies on the iliopsoas muscle and divides into its genital and femoral branches just internal and lateral to the internal inguinal ring. The genital branch perforates the internal oblique muscle at the origin of the cremaster muscle and gives motor innervation to the cremaster and sensory innervation to the skin of the penis and scrotum. The femoral branch provides sensation to the skin of the upper lateral thigh. Injury to this nerve may cause anesthesia in these areas and loss of the cremasteric reflex. The greatest morbidity involving the genitofemoral nerve is due to entrapment by suture in hernia repair, leading to chronic postoperative pain.

There is extensive cross connection between the nerves

TABLE 32-2 **COMPLICATIONS OF INGUINAL HERNIORRHAPHY**

EARLY POSTOPERATIVE PERIOD

Anesthetic complications
Nerve injury
Damage to testicular blood supply; testicular atrophy
Injury to vas deferens
Bladder injury
Vascular injury/hemorrhage
Bowel injury
Reduction of infarcted intestine
Scrotal swelling due to lymphatic obstruction
Hydrocele
Wound infection

LATE POSTOPERATIVE PERIOD

Pain
Recurrence

of the inguinal region, and transection of one does not necessarily cause great morbidity. Primary repair of these nerves is neither necessary nor often beneficial.

Damage to testicular blood supply may occur as internal spermatic artery injury. This vessel may be ligated with relative impunity if the testicle has not been delivered from the scrotum, since the testicle will not atrophy if scrotal collaterals are intact.

Injury to the vas deferens may take place during dissection of an indirect hernia sac. This injury should be repaired primarily at the time of injury, the vas deferens being anastomosed over a stainless steel wire stent using fine sutures with optical magnification.

Bladder injury may result from failure to identify the bladder on the medial side of the hernia sac. This injury should be closed in two layers and a Foley catheter left in place for 5 days following the operation.

The pubic branch of the obturator artery, the deep inferior epigastric vessels, the external iliac vessels, and the cremasteric artery are placed at risk for injury during an inguinal or femoral hernia repair. All of these, with the exception of the external iliac vessels, may be ligated with impunity when injured. Iliac artery or vein injury usually is controlled by direct pressure but may require vascular repair.

Bowel injury may occur if sutures are placed too deeply during ligation of the hernia sac. This may lead to fecal fistula if not recognized.

Loss of control of strangulated bowel is a difficult problem that may result from retraction of the bowel as the constricting band is divided. Laparotomy is mandatory in this situation.

Scrotal swelling may be due to lymphatic interruption, in which case external scrotal support is beneficial. Fluid collecting in the distal sac as a result of occlusion of the cut end of the sac results in hydrocele, often treatable by aspiration.

Wound infection is usually due to poor surgical technique in a clean wound such as a hernia repair. The infection must be drained by opening the surgical wound.

RECURRENT HERNIA

Recurrence takes place at some time following about 5% to 10% of all inguinal and femoral hernia repairs, although longer follow-up may prove the incidence to be somewhat higher. Right-sided hernias recur slightly more often than left-sided ones. The majority of hernias recur within 5 years after the operation; a significant number, however, may not recur until 10 to 20 years later.

CAUSES

Patient factors in hernia recurrence include presence of chronic pulmonary disease with associated chronic cough, bladder outlet obstruction, lower gastrointestinal tract pathology leading to chronically increased intra-abdominal pressure, ascites, and multiple pregnancies. Each of these conditions is associated with chronically increased intra-abdominal pressure, which places stress on the repair. In addition, most patients who have chronic pulmonary disease and continue smoking have been found to have increased levels of serum elastase.

Errors in operative technique may cause recurrence. In repair of indirect hernia, recurrence develops most commonly because of inadequate ligation of the hernia sac. In addition, improper closure of the internal inguinal ring, failure to recognize associated hernia, damage to the posterior inguinal wall, or failure to evaluate correctly the strength of the posterior inguinal wall may also lead to recurrence.

Use of an attenuated transversalis fascia for repair may lead to recurrence of a direct hernia. Tension at the suture line due to an inadequate relaxing incision, as well as failure to recognize a concomitant indirect or femoral hernia, may also doom the repair to failure.

Femoral hernia may recur because of injury to the transversalis fascia at the time of reduction of the hernia or because of undue tension on the closure of Cooper's ligament to the inguinal ligament.

Hernia recurrence may also be the result of wound hematomas, wound infection, or postoperative abdominal distention.

REPAIR

About half of hernia recurrences occur at the internal inguinal ring. In this case, simple repair of the defect is not a durable procedure. Elderly patients may benefit from resection of the spermatic cord and complete closure of the internal ring; orchiectomy then may or may not be necessary but must always be planned for. A Cooper's ligament (McVay) hernia repair is most efficacious.

Recurrence at the pubic tubercle constitutes approximately one fourth of hernia recurrences. In this case, simple closure will usually suffice.

In the case of recurrence through the floor of the inguinal canal, a Cooper's ligament repair is usually the procedure of choice. However, if the transversalis fascia is quite attenuated, if the previous repair was a Cooper's ligament repair, or if there have been multiple recurrences, prosthetic material is usually necessary. The prosthetic material can be stretched across the hernia defect, or, preferably, the fascia can be backed with the prosthetic material and a repair done.

The Usher repair of recurrent inguinal hernia involves backing of the transversalis fascia and internal oblique with polypropylene mesh and suturing the backed fascia to Cooper's ligament and to the iliopubic tract. The leading edge of this backed fascia is then sutured to Poupart's ligament. Tantalum mesh and polyglactin 910 mesh have also been used.

Recurrence as a femoral hernia may be due to tearing of the fascia at the transition suture of a Cooper's ligament (McVay) repair or where a femoral hernia was at the initial operation. This is usually repaired by McVay's technique of Cooper's ligament repair.

The preperitoneal approach has been advocated by many as the preferred approach to recurrent hernia. An iliopubic tract repair may be done, or prosthetic material may be inserted. This approach has the advantage of avoiding the scar tissue from the previous operation. Only surgeons experienced in the technique should use the preperitoneal approach.

SPECIAL PROBLEMS

BILATERAL HERNIA

The question often arises whether to repair bilateral hernias simultaneously or to delay the second operation. The recurrence rate is slightly but significantly increased when bilateral hernias are repaired less than 6 weeks apart. In addition, there is an increased incidence of scrotal swelling and urinary retention. However, if the patient is healthy and has good tissues and the economic impact of his second hospitalization is significant, bilateral repair is acceptable. Bilateral repair of indirect hernias is always appropriate.

INGUINAL HERNIA IN FEMALE PATIENTS

Although femoral hernias are relatively common in females, the most common hernia in the female is the indirect inguinal hernia; direct inguinal hernias are rare in female patients. The repair of an indirect hernia in a female is facilitated by the fact that the internal inguinal ring can be closed completely after the division of the round ligament. Bilaterality occurs in about 80% of female infants with inguinal hernia, and bilateral exploration is always justified. Some advocate palpation of the ovary or even biopsy to rule out testicular feminization in these patients.

APPENDECTOMY

The major objection to incidental appendectomy during herniorrhaphy is the added risk of wound infection. However, if the appendix presents within the hernia sac and there is no complicating disease that would contraindicate a 5- to 10-minute prolongation of operating time, and if the entire appendix can be delivered into the wound without extending the wound, many feel that incidental appendectomy is reasonable in right inguinal hernia repair.

ECONOMIC AND SOCIAL IMPACT OF GROIN HERNIA

A study in the British Isles of 261 men in the working age-group who had inguinal hernia repairs showed an average time off work of 51 days. This represents a significant economic impact on both the community and the persons involved. Most patients who had strenuous jobs, low sick pay, or family worries tended to remain off work longer, while those who had seen fit to estimate their time off work

prior to the operation and who had stopped smoking prior to the operation remained off work the least amount of time. A second British study indicated that the cost of inpatient stay and time off work combined to 2.5 million pounds per year, or $4.75 million.

Disability due to hernia occurs in 4.6 males and 0.9 females per 1000 population. Herniorrhaphy is felt to eliminate this disability.

Infertility following an inguinal hernia repair may, of course, be due to ligation of the vas deferans, but sperm antibodies have been reported following herniorrhaphy. The overall effect of herniorrhaphy on fertility requires further investigation.

In the year 1970, approximately 3000 people in the United States died as a result of the complications of inguinal or femoral hernia. In other years, the mortality has been reported as high as 8000 to 10,000. This represents a large number of preventable deaths.

THE CHALLENGE FOR IMPROVEMENT IN THE TREATMENT OF GROIN HERNIAS

Repair of hernias before they become incarcerated or before they reach such size that repair becomes of great risk to the patient is feasible only if the hernia is diagnosed before that time. Physicians must take the initiative with routine examination of the groin and must caution patients that procrastination in repair of what seems to be a simple malady may lead to dire consequences.

The risk of inguinal hernia should not be minimized in its portrayal to the public. The general public must be educated to the fact that hernias may be lethal, particularly as one becomes advanced in age, and that this great risk can easily be prevented by simple elective herniorrhaphy with very low operative risk.

BIBLIOGRAPHY

Developmental Anatomy
Davies J: Human Developmental Anatomy. New York, Ronald Press, 1963
Shrock. P: The processus vaginalis and gubernaculum: Raison d'être. Surg Clin North Am 51:1263, 1971

Normal Anatomy
McVay CB: The anatomic basis for inguinal and femoral hernioplasty. Surg Gynecol Obstet 139:1251, 1971
McVay CB: The normal and pathologic anatomy of the transversus abdominis muscle and inguinal and femoral hernia. Surg Clin North Am 51:931, 1974

Epidemiology
Abramson JH, Gofin J, Gopp C et al: The epidemiology of inguinal hernia. J Epidemiol Community Health 31:59, 1978

Etiology
McVay CB, Savage LE: Etiology of femoral hernia. Ann Surg 154:25, 1961
Peacock EE, Jr, Madden JW: Studies on the biology and treatment of recurrent inguinal hernia: II. Morphological changes. Ann Surg 179:567, 1974
Turner WT, Peacock EE Jr: Some studies on the etiology of inguinal hernia. Am J Surg 125:732, 1973

Morbidity
Nashville JW Jr, Davis WC, Jackson FC: Colon carcinoma and inguinal hernia. Surg Clin North Am 45:1165, 1965
Sanella N: Inguinal hernia and colon carcinoma: Presentation of a series and analysis. Surgery 73:434, 1973

SINGER RB, LIVENSON L: Medical Risks: Patterns of Mortality and Survival, 1st ed. Toronto, D C Heath and Co, 1976

Diagnosis
DIETCH EA, SONCHRANT MC: The value of ultrasound in the diagnosis of nonpalpable femoral hernias. Arch Surg 116:185, 1981

History
CARSON RI: The historical development of the surgical treatment of inguinal hernia. Surgery 39:1031, 1956
ZIMMERMAN LM, ZIMMERMAN JE: The history of hernia treatment. In Nyhus, LM, Condon RE (eds): Hernia, pp 3–13. Philadelphia, J B Lippincott, 1978

Operative Techniques
CONDON RE: Anterior iliopubic tract repair. In Nyhus LM, Condon RE (eds): Hernia, 2nd ed. Philadelphia, J B Lippincott, 1978
CONDON RE, NYHUS LM: Complications of groin hernia and of hernial repair. Surg Clin North Am 51:1325, 1971
GLASSOW F: Femoral hernia: Review of 1143 consecutive repairs. Ann Surg 163:227, 1966
GRIFFITH CA: The Marcy repair of indirect inguinal hernia. Surg Clin North Am 56:1309, 1971
HALVERSON K, MCVAY CB: Inguinal and femoral hernioplasty: A 22 year study of the authors' methods. Arch Surg 101:127, 1970
MADDEN JL, SAEED H, ATHANASIO B: The anatomy and repair of inguinal hernias. Surg Clin North Am 51:1269, 1971

NYHUS LM: The preperitoneal approach and iliopubic tract repair of inguinal hernia. In Nyhus LM, Condon RE (eds): Hernia. Philadelphia, J B Lippincott, 1978
SHEARBURN EW, MYERS RN: Shouldice repair for inguinal hernia. Surgery 66:450, 1969

Pediatric Hernia
DONOVAN EJ, STANLEY-BROWN EG: Inguinal hernia in female infants and children. Surg Gynecol Obstet 107:663, 1958
SPARKMAN RS: Bilateral exploration in inguinal hernia in juvenile patients: Review and appraisal. Surgery 51:393, 1962

Sliding Hernia
PIEDAD OH, STOESSER PN, WELS PB: Sliding inguinal hernia. Am J Surg 126:106, 1973
RYAN EA: An analysis of 313 consecutive cases of indirect sliding inguinal hernias. Surg Gynecol Obstet 102:45, 1956

Incarcerated and Strangulated Hernia
KAUFFMAN HM, JR, O'BRIEN DP: Selective reduction of incarcerated inguinal hernia. Am J Surg 119:660, 1970
ROGERS FA: Strangulated femoral hernia: Review of 170 Cases. Ann Surg 149:9, 1959
ROWE MI, CLATWORTHY HW: Incarcerated and strangulated hernias in children. Arch Surg 101:136, 1970

Ward O. Griffen, Jr.

Extrainguinal Abdominal Wall Hernias

UMBILICAL HERNIA
EPIGASTRIC HERNIA
SPIGELIAN HERNIA
LUMBAR HERNIA
OBTURATOR HERNIA
INCISIONAL HERNIA
**GENERAL MANAGEMENT OF EXTRAINGUINAL
    ABDOMINAL WALL HERNIAS**

Although inguinal and femoral hernias represent the great majority of protrusions of peritoneal contents beyond the confines of the coelomic cavity, a variety of other hernias have been described. As in inguinal hernias, the basic problem is a defect in the fascia immediately adjacent to the peritoneum. This defect can occur as a congenital mishap (umbilical hernia); as an attenuation of a fascial layer, perhaps beginning as a weakness in the layer caused by the presentation of a blood vessel (spigelian hernia); or as the result of a penetration of the fascial layer (incisional hernia). All of these hernias have the same potential for complications as do groin hernias, namely, incarceration or strangulation.

In this chapter, the variety of extrainguinal hernias, including umbilical hernia, epigastric hernia, spigelian hernia, lumbar hernia, obturator hernia, and incisional hernia, are presented. Although there are several different anatomical herniations, the basic principle of repair remains the same. To remove the hernia and its threat of incarceration or strangulation, it is necessary to reduce the hernial contents into the peritoneal cavity and to produce a firm closure of

the fascial defect either by approximating fascia or by using material, autologous or synthetic, to bridge the fascial defect.

UMBILICAL HERNIA

Prominence of the umbilicus was recorded by Benivieni in the 15th century. An early account of the surgical treatment of umbilical hernia appeared in 1740, when William Cheselden published his *Anatomy of the Human Body*. He recounted the case of a 50-year-old woman who presented with strangulated bowel protruding from the navel. The necrotic bowel was excised, and the patient lived for 23 years with an umbilical ileostomy. Elective repairs of umbilical hernias were rarely performed until William Mayo reported his imbrication technique, the so-called vest-over-pants maneuver, in 1907. It has now been shown that the important contribution by Mayo was not the technique as much as it was the concept of a transverse closure of the defect. Prior to that time, most surgeons had employed vertical closure after extensive dissection of the rectus muscles and sheaths. The results were disappointing.

ETIOLOGY AND ANATOMY

Umbilical hernia is a congenital defect that is estimated to occur in approximately 6% of all humans as a result of incomplete fusion of the fascial layers of the abdominal wall in the mid portion of the abdomen where the umbilical cord is found in the late stages of gestation. It is present in approximately 10% of all black infants and in 0.1% of white infants. It occurs in varying sizes, and many investigators point out that an omphalocele may be regarded simply as a large umbilical hernia.

SIGNS AND SYMPTOMS

An umbilical hernia usually presents as a protrusion of variable size at the umbilicus. Local pain or vague generalized abdominal pain may accompany the herniation. When the hernia is reducible, it is usually possible to feel the defect as a circular area bounded circumferentially by tough fascia. When it is irreducible, it may be difficult to feel the defect, and if the herniation has progressed superiorly, it may be impossible to distinguish from an epigastric hernia lying close to the umbilicus. Strangulation occurs only rarely.

MANAGEMENT

About 20 years ago, Kiesewetter outlined a succinct scheme of management for umbilical hernia:

Newborn to 6 months of age: If a defect is smaller than the tip of the index finger, observe only. If the defect admits the index finger or is slightly larger, use adhesive strapping. Surgical repair should be done only for specific indications, such as incarceration or strangulation.

Six to 12 months of age: Observe only, unless specific symptoms such as suspected strangulation dictate an operation.

One to 2 years of age: The indications for surgical repair should be individualized. Increasing defect size or marked symptoms are sufficient to warrant surgical correction.

Two years of age and older: Surgical correction will be necessary, since it is unlikely that the hernia will now close spontaneously.

The surgical technique is straightforward (Fig. 32-11). Excision of the umbilicus is rarely necessary. A transverse curvilinear incision is made 1 cm inferior to the umbilicus, and the skin flap is developed superiorly to expose the

Fig. 32-11. Repair of umbilical hernia. *(A)* Large umbilical hernia. *(B)* Transverse infraumbilical incision for umbilical hernia repair. *(C)* Imbrication of fascia, using "vest-over-pants" or Mayo repair. *(D)* Simple apposition of the fascia and peritoneum with permanent suture material.

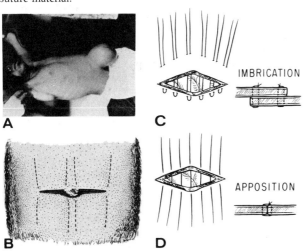

hernia. The hernia sac and protrusion usually contain preperitoneal fat and may be excised as the peritoneal cavity is entered. The umbilical defect is enlarged laterally on either side, and the fascia can then be closed directly with interrupted sutures. Experimentally, it has been shown that simple approximation of the fascia produces satisfactory results and a recurrence rate as low as that with the vest-over-pants technique. A single suture may be used to bring the umbilical dimple back down to the fascial layer, and the skin is closed as usual. Postoperative morbidity and mortality are low, and hospitalization rarely exceeds 36 hours. In fact, umbilical hernia repair is now being performed as outpatient surgery.

One specific pitfall is the repair of umbilical hernias in cirrhotic patients who have ascites. The mortality in this group of patients is high and often due to bleeding esophageal varices. It has been postulated that repair of the umbilical hernia interrupts portasystemic shunts; this leads to greater pressure in the varices, which disrupt and bleed. Moreover, the increased intra-abdominal pressue due to ascites may impair wound healing and increase the risk of recurrence of the hernia.

EPIGASTRIC HERNIA

The term *epigastric hernia,* used to describe small defects occurring in the linea alba between the xiphisternum and the umbilicus, was introduced in 1812. This was 70 years after the first clear-cut description of epigastric hernia had been made by H. F. LeDran and 10 years after the first report of a successful epigastric hernia repair. It was not until asepsis in surgical procedures became standard that the repair of epigastric hernias was undertaken as a routine matter. McCaughan has estimated the incidence of epigastric hernia at 5%.

ETIOLOGY AND ANATOMY

In 1914, Moschcowitz was of the opinion that epigastric hernias occurred in the linea alba between the xiphisternum and the umbilicus as the result of the enlargement of fascial defects where blood vessels came through that layer. More recently, however, blood vessels were not found in these defects, and most observers today feel that these also are congenital defects. The linea alba superior to the umbilicus is formed by fusion of the anterior and posterior layers of the rectus sheath. Failure of this fusion of the linea alba anywhere in its length will result in one or more lineal defects.

SIGNS AND SYMPTOMS

Many of these hernias do not cause symptoms and are found incidentally during physical examination (Fig. 32-12). Paradoxically, the large epigastric hernias with a fully developed peritoneal sac infrequently cause pain and rarely incarcerate. They present as a mass in the epigastrium, which is the most frequent manifestation associated with epigastric hernias. The small hernias, on the other hand, often contain a bit of incarcerated omentum and therefore are associated with pain, often brought on by exercise, and exquisite localized tenderness. Nausea and vomiting occurring after eating may be a presenting complaint, and sometimes the abdominal wall reaction to the pain is so severe that perforated ulcer may be suspected.

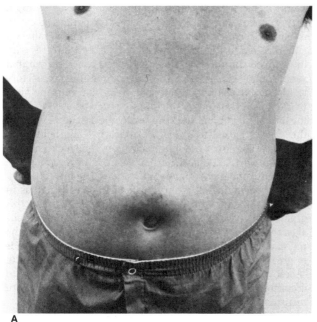
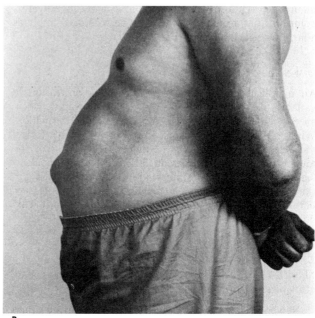

Fig. 32-12.   Supraumbilical epigastric hernia. *(A)* Front view. *(B)* Side view.

MANAGEMENT

The small epigastric hernia found in an infant, like the umbilical hernia, often requires no operation. Small asymptomatic hernias in the adult need not be treated surgically. It was recommended in the past that symptomatic hernias be treated in conjunction with an exploratory celiotomy to rule out intra-abdominal lesions; however, a careful history, along with modern diagnostic maneuvers, usually discloses any significant pathologic process that should be corrected in conjunction with the repair of the hernia. If no intra-abdominal lesions are found, simple repair of the hernia may be undertaken.

A variety of techniques have been described. These include reduction of the hernia and simple vertical closure of the defect; enlargement of the defect transversely with an imbricating or fascia-to-fascia closure; and a more extensive procedure, which involves opening the rectus sheath, approximating the posterior layer of the two sheaths in the midline, and bringing the rectus muscles together over the posterior fascial closure and completing the repair by approximating the anterior fascia.

The treatment of choice is to expose the linea alba from the xiphisternum to the umbilicus and to identify the hernia or hernias. The fascial defects are then joined vertically in the linea alba to form one large hernia. The falciform ligament and the peritoneum on the right side of the cut linea alba are dissected free, and the left edge of the linea alba is sutured to the posterior rectus sheath with vertical mattress sutures. The right edge of the linea alba is then brought over and approximated to the anterior left rectus sheath so that the fascia is closed in an imbricating vertical fashion, although simple closure without imbrication is often used. Since dissection in the subcutaneous tissue is limited, no drainage is necessary and the skin is closed primarily.

The most frequent complication is infection. Inadequate exposure or failure to identify all hernial defects in the linea alba also occurs. All of these factors have been cited as

reasons for the high reported recurrence rate of 10%. Another common factor in "recurrence" is that the epigastric hernia is frequently accompanied by an umbilical hernia, which, unless looked for during the repair process, is later interpreted as a recurrence. For this reason, total repair of the linea alba has been recommended.

SPIGELIAN HERNIA

Spigelian hernia is really a spontaneous lateral ventral hernia and thus is not to be confused with the midline hernias (umbilical and epigastric) or with hernias occurring after trauma or operations. It derives its name from Spieghel, who made the first accurate description of the semilunar line, a curved line of fascia just lateral to the outer border of the rectus abdominis muscle, extending from the tip of the ninth costal cartilage to the pubis. Anteriorly, this line is reinforced by fibers of the external oblique aponeurosis. However, posteriorly, the transversus abdominis fascia becomes attenuated in the lower one fourth of this semilunar line, and defects may appear at the level of the inferior epigastric vessels just at the lateral border of the rectus sheath.

In 1764, Klinkosch first described a hernia in this location, and only about 250 cases of spigelian hernia have been reported since, although, of course, a great many patients with this lesion go unreported.

ETIOLOGY AND ANATOMY

The structure of the rectus sheath and anterolateral abdominal muscles seems to be an obvious contributing factor to the formation of spigelian hernias. Above, the musculo-aponeurotic layers run at varying angles to each other, whereas below the umbilicus, the fibers run parallel to each other and slitlike defects appear in the various layers. Therefore, spigelian hernias are rare above the umbilicus. Although it was originally believed that the hernias occurred

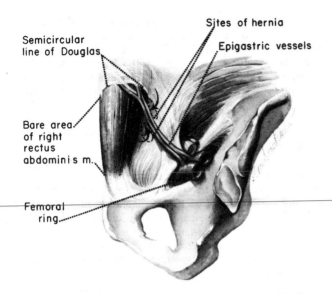

Semicircular line of Douglas

Sites of hernia

Epigastric vessels

Bare area of right rectus abdominis m.

Femoral ring

Fig. 32-13. Posterior view of the anterior abdominal wall indicates the sites of spigelian hernias in relationship to the deep epigastric vessels.

in sites where the vessels penetrated the fascial layers, this does not seem to be an important feature, and such factors as childbearing, obesity, muscle wasting, and chronic cough are important.

Anatomically, two types of spigelian hernias are described, depending on the location of the fascial defect in relation to the inferior epigastric vessels. A defect inferior to these vessels and lateral to the semilunar line is in Hesselbach's triangle and therefore is indistinguishable from a direct inguinal hernia. Thus, a true spigelian hernia is one that occurs superior to the inferior epigastric vessels (Fig. 32-13).

SIGNS AND SYMPTOMS

Small hernias often are responsible for vague symptoms over a long period. Localized pain or a "pulling" sensation at the site of the fascial defect may be constant or intermittent but usually is made worse by exertion and has no relationship to meals. If the external oblique fascia remains intact, the hernia sac contents, usually omentum and small bowel, may dissect intramuscularly and deeply, making it difficult to define the mass of herniated tissue and impossible to detect the fascial defect and make the diagnosis. Once the external oblique fascia is transgressed, the hernia sac and its contents become subcutaneous and usually present in front of the anterior superior iliac spine. The diagnosis is apparent. As more omentum occupies the hernia, the increasing traction on the omentum may lead to nausea and vomiting. These manifestations, in association with an irreducible abdominal wall mass, marked localized tenderness, and discoloration, signify incarceration or strangulation.

MANAGEMENT

The repair of spigelian hernias is usually not difficult. A transverse incision is made overlying the hernia, the sac is dissected from the subcutaneous tissue and opened, and the peritoneal contents are reduced into the abdomen. The sac is then isolated up to its neck and ligated high, and the

excess peritoneum is excised. The edges of the fascial defect are identified carefully and may be enlarged transversely to facilitate a linear or imbricating closure. The defects are rarely large enough to require foreign-body material to reinforce the repair. Again, infection is the biggest complication, but recurrence is an extremely infrequent event.

LUMBAR HERNIA

The lumbar region may be described as an area bounded inferiorly by the crest of the ilium, posteriorly by the paravertebral group of muscles, superiorly by the 12th rib, and anteriorly by the border of the external oblique aponeurosis. Hernias in this area have been variously described by eponyms such as Petit's, Lesshaft's, Larrey's, and Huguier's hernia. In 1672, Barbette first suggested that hernias could occur in this area, and in 1731, Garangeto described such a hernia that was reduced at autopsy. In 1750, Ravaton described the reduction of a strangulated hernia in this area in a pregnant woman. In 1783, Petit described a hernia through the lower lumbar region, and all lumbar hernias were known as Petit's hernia until 1866, when Grynfelt described a superior lumbar triangle bounded above by the 12th rib, medially by the quadratus lumborum, anterolaterally by the external oblique aponeurosis, and below by the internal oblique aponeurosis. This larger space is the site of more frequent herniation. Such hernias are referred to variously as Grynfelt's hernia and Lesshaft's hernia. In 1893, Macrady described 25 instances of lumbar hernia, and by 1925, Virgillo was able to report 109 cases, including several examples of lumbar hernia occurring following trauma or drainage of an abscess. The latter group now comprises about a third of those reported and often follows removal of the iliac crest.

ETIOLOGY AND ANATOMY

Lumbar hernia is considered to be both congenital and acquired; regardless of the etiology, it occurs at two areas of definite weakness in the lumbar musculature (Fig. 32-14). In the superior lumbar triangle of Grynfelt-Lesshaft, the most consistently weak point is situated immediately beneath the 12th rib, where the transversalis fascia is not covered by the external oblique fascia and muscle, at the point where the 12th intercostal neurovascular bundle penetrates the fascia right at the tip of the 12th rib. The inferior lumbar triangle of Petit has been described as being consistently present in the adult but not in the infant, thus raising speculation that this triangle develops as the infant grows. A small weak point at the apex of the triangle, where there may be some attenuation of the internal oblique, accounts for the majority of hernias in this triangle. Such hernias have been seen in infants and are thus felt to represent a congenital condition, perhaps because of lack of muscular growth or fusion. The great majority of these hernias, however, are seen in adults, suggesting an acquired nature. The spontaneous lumbar hernias probably represent true attenuation of fascial layers as a function of aging. Falls, motor vehicle accidents, and other mishaps have been associated with the subsequent development of lumbar hernias. Of course, these may occur in any part of the lumbar region. Of particular interest are lumbar hernias that are seen following removal of the iliac crest for bone grafts. A number of such iatrogenic hernias have been described in the literature.

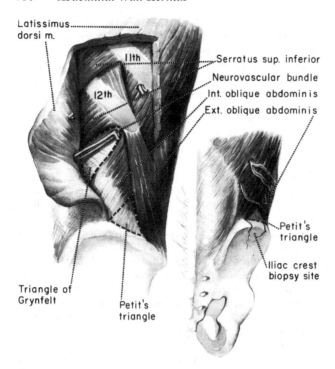

Latissimus dorsi m.

11th

12th

Serratus sup. inferior

Neurovascular bundle

Int. oblique abdominis

Ext. oblique abdominis

Petit's triangle

Iliac crest biopsy site

Triangle of Grynfelt

Petit's triangle

Fig. 32-14. Two triangular areas may be sites of lumbar hernias. Petit's triangle often overlies the area of iliac crest bone biopsy, a possible site of postoperative hernia.

SIGNS AND SYMPTOMS

A lumbar hernia invariably presents as a bulge in the lumbar area. It is usually soft and, in the case of the superior triangle hernia defect, is commonly reducible to some extent. A roentgenogram of the abdomen usually shows air-filled loops of bowel in the hernia sac. It must be distinguished from a mass lesion of some sort.

MANAGEMENT

Unfortunately, most lumbar hernias are not repaired until they have attained a large size. This means that there may be a considerable number of intra-abdominal organs in the subcutaneous space; therefore, a large incision with wide subcutaneous dissection is necessary. If a sac is present, it should be opened and the contents placed intra-abdominally again. The excess sac may be excised to expose the fascial edges. Since the fascial defect may be large, primary closure of the defect itself is often required, with reinforcement by other fascial tissues. The classic repair described by Dowd in 1907 or modifications thereof involve identification of the fascial defect and primary closure by approximating the external oblique and latissimus dorsi fascia. This closure is then reinforced by turning up a flap of fascia made up of the fascia lata and aponeurosis of the gluteus maximus muscle and suturing it to the lumbar fascia, external oblique, and latissimus dorsi. Three fascial flaps can then be used to reinforce any remaining tenuous area. All of these multiple flaps and suture lines must be placed accurately. It is now possible to reinforce the primary closure with a sheet of Marlex placed in the subcutaneous space and sutured to fascia. This has greatly simplified the repair of lumbar hernias and has shortened the operating time. Because of extensive subcutaneous dissection, it is usually necessary to use suction catheters to remove the serous drainage and decrease the

incidence of infection. In defects created by iliac bone biopsies, the mesh can be used very satisfactorily after reducing the hernia. The mesh may be used as a single subcutaneous layer or on either side of the bony defect. The recurrence rate should be low but is reported to be at 5%; this is increased, as in all hernia repairs, when postoperative infection develops.

OBTURATOR HERNIA

Herniation in the area of the obturator canal, even though it is uncommon, is important because of the frequency with which it causes strangulating obstruction of the bowel and the infrequency with which it is diagnosed prior to celiotomy. It was first noted in 1724 by deRonsil; in 1926, Kamper described the anatomical defect associated with obturator hernia. Hilton reported the first celiotomy for strangulated obturator hernia in 1848, but Obre is usually given credit for the first successful surgical procedure in 1851. In 1927, Horine reported on 258 cases from the literature, and by 1956, Harper and Holt had compiled 463 cases reported in the literature. Nevertheless, this figure is probably only a small percentage of the actual occurrence of this lesion.

ETIOLOGY AND ANATOMY

The obturator hernia is undoubtedly a combination of a generous obturator canal, where the obturator vessels pierce the pelvic fascia and musculature, and attenuation of the fascia in this area. The defect is usually situated anteromedially to the neurovascular bundle, which traverses the obturator canal. The preponderance of women to men in a ratio of 6:1 makes it likely that repeated pregnancies and pelvic relaxation contribute to the development of these hernias. The fact that the hernias often occur in the elderly suggests that continued attentuation of the fascia in this area contributes to the development of the hernia sac.

The obturator opening is approximately 1 cm in diameter. Through the opening goes the obturator neurovascular bundle. The defect invariably is anterior and medial to the neurovascular bundle and somewhat more triangular in women. Because of the pubic ramus superiorly and the tough ligamentous portion of the internal obturator muscle laterally and posteriorly, the fascial defect has little elasticity, thus accounting for the high incidence of gut strangulation.

SIGNS AND SYMPTOMS

The symptoms of obturator hernia are usually acute, with progressive increase in severity, and relief is obtained only by reduction of the hernia. Most frequently, the presenting complaints are of abdominal pain and vomiting. Abdominal distention and obstipation lead to a diagnosis of mechanical bowel obstruction. The next most common symptom is pain extending down the medial aspect of the thigh to the knee. Flexion of the thigh usually relieves the pain, whereas extension, abduction, or medial rotation of the thigh exacerbates it. This is known as the Howship–Romberg sign. On careful neurologic evaluation, both motor and sensory deficits can be demonstrated, affecting the skin of the medial aspect of the thigh and the abductor group of muscles. About a third of the patients give a history of having had a similar attack in the past. A mass palpable in the thigh is present in only about 20% of patients. Obstruction alone may be the only symptom.

MANAGEMENT

As suggested above, obturator hernia is associated with a very high incidence of bowel obstruction. Recurrent episodes of transitory intestinal obstruction indicate that a small-bowel loop may herniate into the obturator canal temporarily and reduce spontaneously. The loop may become incarcerated or, worse, strangulated, necessitating urgent surgical intervention. In 80% to 90% of reported cases of obturator hernia, the small intestine is present in the hernia. If the operation is performed early in the disease process, the intestinal loop is usually healthy and need only be reduced. If there is some delay in the surgical procedure, as there may be in the older patient who requires cardiopulmonary stabilization before undergoing the operation, the herniated loop may have a compromised blood supply, necessitating resection and primary anastomosis. If there has been significant delay, the strangulated loop may have perforated, leading to significant peritonitis. In this instance, it may be wiser to resect and fashion an ileostomy or jejunostomy and a mucous fistula.

Although there has been some controversy about the surgical approach, most surgeons prefer the direct abdominal approach. The other two surgical approaches are the perineal approach and the inguinal approach. The single advantage of the latter two approaches is the avoidance of entering the peritoneal cavity. They both give good results if the diagnosis of obturator hernia is firm and bowel resection is not required. However, if such an incision has been made and compromised bowel is found, an abdominal incision will be necessary. Thus, the abdominal approach as the primary incision is preferred because it permits intestinal resection when necessary. It has other advantages: It permits the management of bowel obstruction due to some other cause, and it provides the best exposure to the obturator canal and is most likely to avoid injury to the obturator neurovascular bundle.

As is the case in any other hernia, the contents of the sac should be reduced and gut resection done if necessary. The sac should be inverted and ligated at the level of the obturator foramen, and the excess peritoneum should be excised. Usually, the fascial defect can then be closed with two or three nonabsorbable sutures, incorporating the stump of the sac if desired. The closure may be reinforced with fascial flaps or a prosthetic material. With the use of this surgical approach, the recurrence rate of hernia is low. The mortality rate following repair of this hernia usually is reported to be about 10%, the highest reported for any abdominal hernia repair, and is due to the high incidence of strangulation.

INCISIONAL HERNIA

An incisional hernia usually occurs because of less-than-optimal surgical care; for this reason, the full history of incisional hernia may never be told. In 1916, Stanton reported the occurrence of three incisional hernias in 216 clean laparotomies, whereas 18 occurred in 186 infected laparotomy incisions. In the monograph by Zimmerman and Anson in 1967, the incidence of incisional hernia was 1.7% of all hernias operated on, but the range in various reported series was from 1.3% to 10.8%. The prevalence of incisional hernias is likely to increase for two reasons: More celiotomies are being performed, and the age of the population is increasing.

ABDOMINAL WALL HERNIAS (Excluding Groin Hernias)	
Etiology	Congenital, acquired, or traumatic causes Symptoms include mild to moderate pain, a dragging sensation that limits activity, intestinal obstruction, and marked pain and tenderness if incarcerated or strangulated Ventral incisional hernias commonly follow operation
Dx	Symptoms and physical examination; occasionally by x-ray film
Rx	Elective repair: hernia defects tend to enlarge, and early repair more successful Recurrence most common with incisional hernias

ETIOLOGY AND ANATOMY

Incisional hernia is obviously an iatrogenic disease. There are a number of factors in the etiology of incisional hernia, not the least of which is the choice of incision. While it is true that the operation should fit the patient rather than the patient fit the operation, in general, a transverse incision on the abdomen is followed by a lower incidence of evisceration and possibly by a lower incidence of wound infection. In an early randomized series from the University of Michigan, incisional hernia occurred three times more frequently with vertical incisions as compared to transverse incisions.

There are other factors that enter into the equation. The age bracket in which incisional hernia occurs most frequently is 30 to 59 years; however, this also represents the age at which most operations are performed. In most series, women have a higher incidence of ventral hernia than do men, but this may be related to the fact that incisional hernia is more frequently seen after hysterectomy, cesarean section, and appendectomy done through a right paramedian incision. Wound infection also plays a role in the development of postoperative incisional hernia, and, therefore, it is not surprising to find that incisions made for conditions in which sepsis is more likely (*e.g.*, appendectomy for acute appendicitis, closure of perforated duodenal ulcer, colectomy) are followed by a higher incidence of wound infection and late hernia formation.

Two other factors that seem to play a role in the development of postoperative incisional hernia are obesity and concomitant systemic diseases. Obesity not only increases operative time but also, because of retraction difficulties, predisposes to seromas and wound infections, which then lead to the hernia. Systemic diseases such as diabetes may be associated with a higher rate of wound infection, and chronic obstructive airway disease may lead to excessive coughing, which can weaken or disrupt a wound.

SIGNS AND SYMPTOMS

Invariably, this hernia presents as a defect in the posterior fascia that is palpable through the scarred area. The patient usually complains of a bulge at the incisional site, although occasionally, particularly in obese persons, the bulge is not apparent and the patient may complain only of pain in the incision, particularly with exercise or ambulation. Depending on the size of the fascial defect, incarceration or strangulation may occur.

MANAGEMENT

The point to be stressed in discussing incisional hernia is prevention. This means intelligent placement of abdominal incisions. Because of the somewhat lower incidence of ventral hernia in transverse incisions, many surgeons prefer this approach whenever possible. The use of retention sutures when delayed healing or excess stress is expected in the postoperative period may reduce the incidence of postoperative incisional hernia. Judicious use of nasogastric suction is important to minimize abdominal distention. Obviously, avoidance of wound infection will lead to a lower incidence of incisional hernia.

When a hernia has developed, however, certain basic principles apply in regard to its management. Closure of the fascial defect is best accomplished using the patient's own tissues. In fact, patients with very large fascial defects in the abdominal wall may at times best be treated nonoperatively. These patients are often asymptomatic except for the bulging of the peritoneal contents, and this can be handled by an appropriate corset. Because of the large size of the hernial defect, incarceration is infrequent and strangulation rare.

In contrast, small fascial defects are likely to be associated with incarceration and even strangulation. Moreover, the natural history of an incisional hernia is gradual enlargement of the defect with time. Therefore, it is important to urge the patient to undergo hernia repair as soon as feasible after the diagnosis is made. Pain at the hernia site, postprandial abdominal discomfort, and inability to reduce completely the contents of the hernia sac are indicative of incarceration. Obviously, patients with symptomatic hernias should undergo surgical repair.

The principles of the repair are standard. The hernia sac, if one is present, should be opened and the contents replaced into the peritoneal cavity. The excess peritoneum can then be trimmed back to the fascial edges, which should be clearly identified. If intra-abdominal contents are adherent to the fascial edges, they should be carefully dissected free for 3 cm to 4 cm to allow proper placement of sutures. Nonabsorbable sutures should be used in the fascial layer and placed in an interrupted fashion. Maximum relaxation is essential at the time of the tying down of the sutures. If the hernia sac has occupied a large subcutaneous space, subcutaneous suction catheters brought out through separate stab incisions are useful to evacuate blood and serous material to avoid postoperative wound infection. The nonabsorbable sutures are often "backed" with Marlex.

When large hernia defects are symptomatic, some sort of material must be used for repair. Autogenous tissue is still probably the best, and a large patch of fascia lata may be harvested to use in the defect. Tantalum mesh and nylon sheeting were once popular, but the material most used at present is a polyethylene sheet with wide interstices (Marlex) (Fig. 32-15). Marlex mesh has a number of advantages. It has great tensile strength and shows very little tendency to fragment. It is highly inert and is therefore well tolerated by tissues. It is the one prosthetic material that may be kept in place even in the face of infection; secondary healing takes place over the mesh. Some surgeons use Marlex

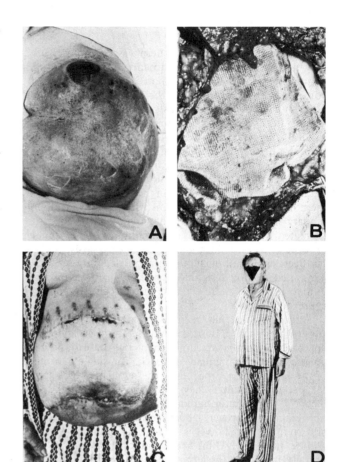

Fig. 32-15. Huge multiloculated, multirecurrent incisional hernia with resection of multiple segments of gangrenous small intestine. The repair of the large fascial defect was achieved using a double layer of Marlex. *(A)* Preoperative appearance. *(B)* Marlex sheets applied over abdominal viscera. *(C)* Postoperative appearance. *(D)* Patient on discharge from hospital. (University of Mississippi Hospital series)

almost routinely in the repair of many types of hernia simply as a reinforcing layer.

The recurrence rate for incisional hernia depends on a number of factors; it is generally reported to be about 5%. The reported mortality rate following repair of incisional hernia is less than 1%; usually, the risk is incurred when bowel resection, or other additional procedure, is necessary in the course of repair of the incisional hernia.

GENERAL MANAGEMENT OF EXTRAINGUINAL ABDOMINAL WALL HERNIAS

Some general elements in the surgical management of extrainguinal abdominal wall hernias are similar to those of any hernia. Irreducible incarceration or strangulation of a hernia dictates an urgent operative procedure. In either instance, but particularly when there may be compromised bowel, preoperative fluid and electrolyte administration is essential to replace third-space losses. Antibiotics should be given whenever necrotic bowel is suspected. The rate of recurrence is increased following repair for incarceration or strangulation. The mortality rate in repair of all extrainguinal hernias is less than 2%, whereas the fatality rate after repair of these strangulated hernias is approximately 8% to 10%.

Direct approximation of the fascial edges is the best surgical procedure for repair of these hernias. Large defects that require correction are a continual challenge to any surgeon's ingenuity and have led to many novel approaches. These techniques, some of which have withstood the test of time, include the use of relaxing incisions, usually at a distance from the hernia; movement of autologous tissues either as free grafts (*e.g.,* fascia lata) or as rotated pedicle grafts; preoperative instillation of progressively increasing amounts of intraperitoneal air every 2 or 3 days to "stretch" the remaining fascia; and use of foreign materials to complete or reinforce the repair. Many foreign materials have been used, including stainless steel mesh, tantalum mesh, nylon net, and, most recently and very successfully, Marlex mesh.

BIBLIOGRAPHY

FARRIS JM: Umbilical hernia. In Nyhus LM, Harkins HN (eds): Hernia. Philadelphia, J B Lippincott, 1964

GRAY SW, SHANDALAKIS JE, SORIA RE et al: Strangulated obturator hernia. Surgery 75:20, 1974

HARPER JR, HOLT JH: Obturator hernia. Am J Surg 92:562, 1956

ISAACSON HH: Spigelian hernia. In Nyhus LM, Harkins HN (eds): Hernia. Philadelphia, J B Lippincott, 1964

KIESEWETTER WB: Hernia: Inguinal and umbilical. Am J Surg 101:656, 1961

KOONTZ AR: An operation for large incisional epigastric hernias. Surg Gynecol Obstet 114:117, 1962

KOZOLL DD: Incisional hernia. In Nyhus LM, Harkins HN (eds): Hernia. Philadelphia, J B Lippincott, 1964

McCAUGHAN JJ JR: Epigastric hernia: Results obtained by surgery. Arch Surg 73:972, 1956

SWARTZ WT: Lumbar hernia. In Nyhus LM, Harkins HN (eds): Hernia. Philadelphia, J B Lippincott, 1964

THOMPSON JB, MacLEAN KF, COLLER FA: Role of the transverse abdominal incision and early ambulation in the reduction of postoperative complications. Arch Surg 59:1267, 1949

ZIMMERMAN LM, ANSON BJ: Anatomy and Surgery of Hernia, 2nd ed. Baltimore, Williams & Wilkins, 1967

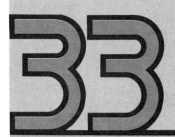

33

Trachea, Thoracic Wall, and Pleura

Hermes C. Grillo

The Trachea

The adult trachea averages 11 cm in length (10 cm–13 cm, depending on the person's size). There are approximately two cartilaginous rings in each centimeter. The subglottic intralaryngeal airway (to the inferior border of the cricoid cartilage) is about 1.5 cm in length. In the infant, the tracheal cross section is rounded; in the adult, it flattens anteroposteriorly to an ovoid shape. In chronic obstructive lung disease, the trachea may assume a "saber-sheath" shape in its lower two thirds, with marked narrowing from side to side, or it may splay out at the ends of the cartilage. In its short course, the trachea runs from the anterior neck to the posterior mediastinum, where it lies against the esophagus and vertebral bodies. It becomes much more transverse with aging and kyphosis. In youth, extension of the neck brings more than half of the trachea above the sternal notch. With advancing age, the trachea loses mobility and the larynx may lie at the sternal notch. These points are of critical importance in reconstructive tracheal surgery. The brachiocephalic artery crosses the trachea approximately below the midpoint.

With respiration and cough, the trachea narrows from side to side. The airway, however, does not close completely except with pathologic malacia. Calcification to a varying degree is common with age and also follows trauma. The trachea moves easily in the mediastinum with deglutition. The thyroid isthmus is fixed to the trachea at the level of the second or third ring.

The blood supply is shared with the esophagus laterally and with the main bronchi below. The vessels supplying the upper trachea originate principally from the inferior thyroid artery, and those supplying the lower trachea originate from the superior and middle bronchial arteries. Contributions may come from the subclavian, highest intercostal, internal thoracic, and brachiocephalic arteries. The supply is largely segmental, so great care must be taken to preserve vascularity during surgical dissection.

CONGENITAL DISORDERS

STENOSIS

Circumferential weblike stenosis is seen most frequently at the subcricoid level. More extensive stenoses have been grouped into three principal types: generalized stenosis of the trachea, usually with a normal larynx and main bronchi; funnellike narrowing at any level in the trachea; and segmental stenosis, most often in the lower trachea (Fig. 33-1). The right upper lobar bronchus may originate above such a segmental stenosis. Completely circular O rings of cartilage may be present in the stenotic segment. Degrees of cartilaginous disorganization are also seen with congenital stenosis. An aberrant left pulmonary artery originating from the right pulmonary artery and passing behind the trachea may be present in conjunction with a segmental stenosis of the lower trachea ("pulmonary artery sling"). About half of the patients with pulmonary artery sling have a concurrent segmental congenital stenosis with circular cartilages that cannot be relieved by transplantation of the artery. In the other cases, transplantation of the artery will relieve compression obstruction. In this case, the segment may remain malacic for a time following successful transposition. When true segmental stenosis exists, primary attack must be on the trachea.

MALACIA

Softening of the trachea is more often seen with compressive rings (double aortic arch, right aortic arch with patent ductus arteriosus or ligamentum arteriosum, aberrant subclavian artery, abnormal innominate artery) or with agenesis of the right lung and rotation of the heart and subsequent displacement of the aorta and left pulmonary artery. True congenital malacia as an isolated lesion is exceedingly rare, if it truly exists.

AGENESIS

Tracheal agenesis or atresia is usually fatal at birth.

Fig. 33-1. Congenital tracheal stenosis. *(Left)* Generalized hypoplasia of the trachea. The airway is of normal caliber at the level of the cricoid cartilage and also in the main bronchi. *(Center)* Funnellike narrowing. The trachea is of normal caliber immediately below the cricoid cartilage but funnels to a narrow point in the upper or lower trachea. *(Right)* Segmental stenosis. This may be accompanied by bronchial anomalies. The segmental stenosis may vary in length and be at varying levels. (Grillo HC: Congenital lesions, neoplasms, and injuries of the trachea. In Sabiston DC Jr, Spencer FC [eds]: Gibbon's Surgery of the Chest, 3rd ed. Philadelphia, W B Saunders, 1976; after Cantrell and Guild: Am J Surg 108:297, 1964)

CONGENITAL TRACHEOESOPHAGEAL FISTULA

There may be a communication to the esophagus. Congenital tracheoesophageal fistula is described in Chapter 41. The trachea is very rarely stenotic in these lesions.

Reconstruction of the infant and pediatric trachea may be accomplished. Risks are great because of the small diameter of the airway, its potential postoperative compromise by edema, and the susceptibility of the juvenile trachea to separation at lesser tensions than the adult trachea following reconstruction. If a conservative approach is possible, it is advisable to await growth of the child prior to undertaking repair.

TRAUMA

The trachea most often suffers external trauma from blunt cervical injury. The principal agents are the steering wheel or dashboard in a motor vehicle and the neck-high cable for the trail bike or skimobile operator. The trachea may be partially or completely torn from the larynx or separated below this level. Laryngeal injuries frequently occur from the same mechanism. One or both recurrent laryngeal nerves may be temporarily or permanently nonfunctional. The patient may have great respiratory distress to none at all, aphonia, hemoptysis, or cervical emphysema. Intubation with or without the aid of a bronchoscope may be impossible, and prompt tracheostomy is required. The severed trachea may have retracted into the mediastinum. Primary repair after adequate débridement is possible in skilled hands. A protective tracheostomy well below the repair is required, since the larynx may also be nonfunctional. If there is laryngeal injury, internal splinting by an otolaryngologist is required. There are often accompanying injuries to the esophagus and pharynx. Avulsion of the esophagus from the pharynx may occur. Cervical vertebral subluxation is also seen.

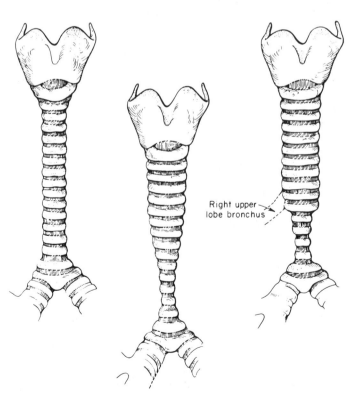

Right upper lobe bronchus

If a surgeon skilled in tracheal work is not available or if there are other injuries that take priority, a cervical tracheal separation may be handled with a tracheostomy tube placed in the severed end. Reconstruction may be done at a later date, after first stabilizing the glottic airway by appropriate procedures.

The intrathoracic trachea may be lacerated transversely concurrent with a sternal fracture or split vertically from the carina with blunt injuries to the thoracic cage. Mediastinal emphysema and unilateral or bilateral pneumothorax may be seen, responding promptly, slowly, or incompletely to tube thoracostomy and suction. Diagnosis is made by bronchoscopy, and repair is performed. Esophageal damage may also be present and may characteristically manifest itself a few days later as a tracheoesophageal fistula. Prompt repair is required through a thoracotomy to avoid the high mortality of such fistulas.

Penetrating wounds by knife or gunshot may occur in the neck. Appropriate débridement or resection with repair is indicated. Late injuries are handled by reconstruction. Penetrating injuries to the mediastinal trachea are rare because of its central position. The functional status of the larynx must always be clarified prior to surgical repair of the trachea.

TRACHEOSTOMY

INDICATIONS

Tracheostomy was formerly the principal method for relief of upper airway obstruction. Only in very rare circumstances is this now the case. Endotracheal intubation is usually used in an emergency. Even difficult intubations can usually be effected with the intubating flexible laryngoscope. Rigid bronchoscopy is another alternative for establishing an emergency airway. When acute obstruction has occurred in a nonmedical setting, for example by a bolus of food resting on the glottis, the Heimlich maneuver is usually successful. If not, emergency cricothyroidotomy may be performed. The cricothyroid membrane is the most superficial portion of the upper airway.

With contemporary chest physiotherapy, tracheostomy is rarely used simply as a means of controlling secretions. It does have such a role in some chronic situations. Tracheostomy is currently used most commonly as a route for the delivery of assisted mechanical ventilation. Ventilation is commenced in most patients through an endotracheal tube. Although there are widely differing opinions, if the ventilation is necessary for more than 1 or 2 weeks, tracheostomy is usually mechanically more satisfactory and more comfortable for the patient. In adults, the substitution of prolonged endotracheal tube intubation or cricothyroidostomy does not prevent airway complications but simply alters their location and type. This is discussed further in the section on postintubation injuries.

TECHNIQUE

Variations in the technique of tracheostomy are multiple. In almost every case, the tracheostomy is done electively after establishing an airway with an endotracheal tube. A short transverse incision is made 1 cm below the cricoid cartilage (Fig. 33-2, *A*). The sternal notch is *never* used as a reference point for the location of tracheostomy because

> **THE TRACHEA**
>
> **Congenital Disorders** Rare, may involve all or part of trachea; sometimes associated with pulmonary sling
>
> **Trauma** Cervical rupture most often due to blunt trauma; needs tracheostomy and repair
> Intrathoracic trauma may lead to tracheoesophageal fistula
>
> **Tracheostomy** Almost always elective; used principally as conduit for mechanical ventilation or for chronic upper airway obstruction
> Tube must be carefully selected and placed high enough to avoid late tracheoarterial fistula; most complications avoidable
>
> **Postintubation Injuries** Obstruction may develop at glottis from endotracheal tube; at subglottic level from endotracheal tube, cricothyroidostomy, or tracheostomy; at stomal level from tracheostomy tube; at cuff level from all tubes
> Airway obstruction following intubation indicates an organic lesion; most obstructive lesions of the trachea are surgically reparable when first seen
>
> **Tumors** Rare, most often malignant; squamous cell carcinoma and adenoid cystic carcinoma most common
> When extent of tumor permits, surgical resection, often followed by irradiation, is treatment of choice

movement of the neck changes the distance between the upper trachea and the sternum. After elevating the platysma, the strap muscles are separated in the midline and the thyroid isthmus is divided and sutured. The second tracheal ring is precisely identified and divided vertically in the midline, extending the incision through the third ring in most cases; the first ring is preserved (Fig. 32-2, *B*). Thyroid pole retractors gently spread the tracheal opening. The tracheostomy tube with obturator is introduced after withdrawing the endotracheal tube under direct vision to a point just above the stoma (Fig. 32-2, *C*). If more room is needed, the fourth ring may be partially divided. It is unnecessary to remove pieces of cartilage, although excision of a small bit will not lead to difficulties. Tracheal flaps contribute nothing. A transverse incision is to be avoided. The skin is closed loosely. The flange of the tracheostomy tube not only is tied with a tape around the neck but also is sutured to the skin. The endotracheal tube is removed only when the tracheostomy tube has been shown to provide a satisfactory airway. If there is any question about where the tip of the tube lies, a flexible bronchoscope may be used to check the distal position.

TUBES AND MANAGEMENT

The tracheostomy tube should be just large enough to provide an adequate airway for the patient. Larger tubes can only cause damage. It must be remembered that most women, even when obese, have tracheas smaller in diameter than those of men. There is almost never an indication for a tracheostomy tube larger than No. 7, even in a large man. Tubes should progress downward in size with smaller tracheas. A tube with an inner cannula is preferable, since it may be more easily cleaned; however, with modern

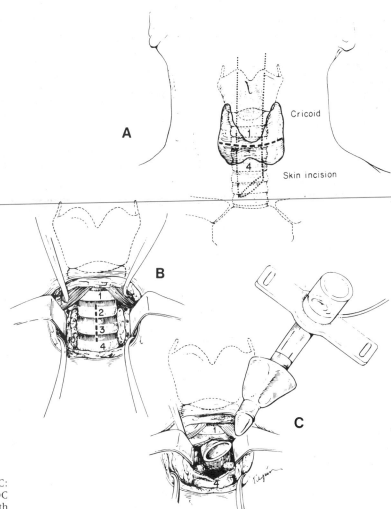

Fig. 33-2. Technique of tracheostomy. (Grillo HC: Tracheostomy and its complications. In Sabiston DC [ed]: Davis-Christopher Textbook of Surgery, 12th ed, p 2059. Philadelphia, W B Saunders, 1981)

humidification, this is not as critical in hospital patients. Standard tubes are useful for most patients, but in a few their anatomy makes a movable tracheostomy tube plate an advantage. As long as the material is not intrinsically irritating, there is little difference, since any tube rigid enough to stay open may potentially cause pressure injury. Thus, stainless steel and nonirritant plastics are equally acceptable.

If a cuff is necessary for ventilation or to seal the trachea to avoid aspiration, it should be a large-volume, low-pressure type. When the tracheal lumen is completely occluded, the cuff should not have been distended to greater than its "resting" full volume. This is the volume attained when the cuff is filled without placing any stretch on the material of which it is made. If a cuff is too small in resting size or if a large-volume cuff is inadvertently filled beyond its maximal resting volume, it converts into a high-pressure cuff at a rate that is dependent on the extensibility of the material of which it is made. Latex is much more extensible than are plastics thus far developed; unfortunately, its shelf-life characteristics and expenses of handling and fixing to tubes have led to its replacement by plastic materials. It is essential that those caring for the patient be aware of the characteristics and management of the cuffs being used, since almost every plastic cuff currently available has at one time or another been converted into a high-pressure cuff and caused severe tracheal damage. Accessory pressure-controlling balloons and systematic measurement of intra-cuff pressure may prevent injuries. Foam cuffs also avoid injuries but have other difficulties, including bulk, expense, and accumulation of secretions. It has also been impossible to manage most adult patients with severe failure by volume respirators alone.

Periodic deflation of cuffs is more useful for clearing secretions that may puddle above the cuff rather than for protecting the tracheal mucosa from injury at the cuff site. Care must be taken to deflate the cuff completely and actively each time, so that reinflation does not add to the volume of air in the cuff. Refilling should best be done with pressure control or filling until a seal is just achieved.

It is very important that the weight of the connecting tubing not be allowed to lever the tube against the tissues of the trachea and neck. This is the most frequent cause of erosion of the stoma, which may lead to later stenosis.

Tracheostomy should be done under sterile technique, and care should be taken to keep the stomas and tubes as clean as possible. All tracheostomies become contaminated after a period of time, usually with *Staphylococcus aureus* and *Pseudomonas aeruginosa,* but invasive infection can usually be avoided. If it occurs, it must be treated.

Adequate humidification and frequent cleaning of the inner cannula, as well as routine suctioning, will usually prevent obstruction of the tube.

TRACHEOSTOMY IN CHILDREN

In infants and small children, the use of the Aberdeen tube or tubes of similar construction with a size, curve, and plate designed for the young has eliminated many of the granulomas, depressed tracheal walls, and stenoses formerly seen. However, the softness and delicacy of the juvenile trachea is such that even with care a common result of a prolonged tracheostomy is depression of the tracheal wall just above the stoma, often with a little granuloma at its tip. The use of endotracheal tubes for prolonged ventilation in infants and children has been generally more successful. The size of the tube is very carefully selected, since a large tube may cause severe damage to the glottis and subglottic larynx.

COMPLICATIONS

IMMEDIATE

Many of the immediate complications of tracheostomy were the result of doing the procedure as an emergency for the establishment of an airway in a patient who was asphyxiating. With elective tracheostomy, these complications have largely vanished. Such complications included cardiac arrhythmias and cardiac arrest due to asphyxia during the procedure, hemorrhage from veins or even arteries injured during a hastily performed procedure done under poor conditions of lighting and equipment, injuries to adjacent structures (including recurrent laryngeal nerves and esophagus), and pneumothorax (especially in children).

EARLY

With better understanding and management, most of the early complications have also disappeared. Thus, obstruction of the tube due to dried blood and crusts has been avoided by adequate humidification. Slippage of the tube out of the trachea rarely occurs following deliberate placement and careful fixation of the tracheostomy flange to the skin. Some prefer to put sutures on either side of the trachea itself and lead these out through the incision so that a tube may be replaced if necessary. Early infection is less likely, since the tracheostomy is done in the operating room.

LATE

Infection of an erosive and invasive type occurs rarely. Treatment is meticulous local care and systemic antibiotics selected on the basis of sensitivities. Hemorrhage results from diffuse tracheitis in patients receiving prolonged ventilation. Most commonly, significant bleeding is from erosion of the brachiocephalic artery. This occurs from two sources. Less common in this era of improved equipment is direct erosion through the anterior wall of the trachea by either a high-pressure cuff or the tip of the tracheostomy tube into the artery. The more common occurrence is from a low-placed stoma, which allows the tube to rest essentially on the artery. Erosion then occurs directly into the artery just below the stoma. This is avoided by the proper placement of the stoma with relation to the cricoid cartilage rather than with relation to the sternal notch. As mentioned earlier, in a young person, the trachea and the brachiocephalic artery are pulled up into the neck in hyperextension. This is why most such fistulas are seen in children or young adults.

The emergency management of the two arterial fistulas is different. The rare fistula occurring due to cuff or tube tip can be controlled only by inserting an endotracheal tube and overdistending the cuff to achieve temporary tamponade. The second and more common type may be controlled by finger pressure against the fistula itself, while replacing the tracheostomy tube with an endotracheal tube with an inflated cuff.

In both cases, immediate surgery is required. Exposure is through a collar incision with an upper sternal or full sternal division. The artery is controlled and resected and the ends sutured and buried in appropriate local tissue. Neurologic sequelae are exceedingly rare with innominate division only. If time permits, electroencephalographic monitoring and back pressure readings are added safeguards. In the case of erosion by a cuff, the trachea must also be resected and reconstructed. In the case of the more common type of erosion at a stoma, nothing need be done to the trachea at this time.

A variety of other obstructive and erosive lesions may follow tracheostomy. These are discussed in the next section.

POSTINTUBATION INJURIES

ETIOLOGY

Most intubation injuries of the airways are seen in patients who have had mechanical assisted ventilation. Although tracheostomies done for other reasons may result in injury, it is extremely rare. Any mechanical airway can produce complications. The differences are in the location of the injuries, their frequency, and their potential correctability (Fig. 33-3). It is almost impossible to compare frequency because of the heterogeneous nature of the patient groups, the care systems, and the equipment used. The relative infrequency of any of these injuries would make enormous randomized series necessary to establish these facts. What is a fact is that any method that has been used—endotracheal tubes, cricoidothyroidostomy, or tracheostomy—has produced serious injuries. The injuries have one common factor: They are the result of pressure necrosis. Many factors have been studied and incriminated in the production of these injuries. Many of these factors do play a role, but none is critical unless there is also pressure on the tissue. Factors that have been studied include the irritant nature of specific materials from which the cuffs are constructed, the elution of acids from plastics by inadequate aeration following ethylene oxide sterilization, local infection, the prolonged use of cortisone, and hypotension with poor perfusion.

Postmortem and *in vivo* studies early demonstrated that high-pressure cuffs caused necrosis of the mucous membrane of the airway, followed by ulceration and necrosis of the cartilage. These lesions have also been reproduced experimentally. A study of surgically removed specimens also correlated with these findings. Conversely, the use of low-pressure cuffs (within a low-pressure range) has eliminated such injuries even when other factors are still present.

Endotracheal tubes can produce inflammation, erosion, and ulceration, particularly at the two narrow points of the airway, the glottis and the subglottic intracricoid level of the larynx. This is particularly true when an excessively large tube is used. While the majority of more superficial laryngeal injuries will regress with time, greater depths of erosion lead to cicatricial healing, with posterior commissural stenosis, subglottic narrowing, and circumferential stenosis at the cricoid level. In extreme cases, the stenosis will extend from the glottis to the upper trachea. Acute

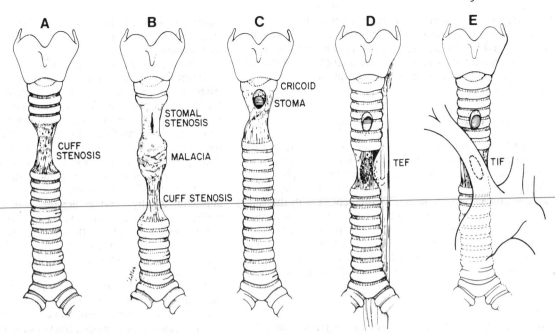

Fig. 33-3. Diagram of principal postintubation lesions. *(A)* Cuff lesion following endotracheal intubation alone. *(B)* Lesions that may follow tracheostomy. Malacia may also occur instead of stenosis at the level of the cuff. *(C)* Erosion of the cricoid by a high-placed stoma. *(D)* The tracheoesophageal fistula (TEF) is at the level of the cuff, where there has usually been pressure against an in-lying esophageal tube. *(E)* Tracheoinnominate fistula (TIF) caused by erosion due to a high-pressure cuff or an angulated tip of tracheostomy tube. The more common arterial fistula is where a low-placed stoma is immediately adjacent to the artery. (Grillo HC: Surgical treatment of postintubation tracheal injuries. J Thorac Cardiovasc Surg 78:860, 1979)

intubation injuries include laceration of the posterior pharyngeal wall, the esophagus, and the tracheal wall and tracheoesophageal fistula.

Cricoidothyroidostomy can and does produce severe subglottic intralaryngeal injury when there has been necrosis around the stoma and cicatricial healing. Tracheostomy tubes have the potential for causing injury at the stoma. Injury is caused most often by leverage of the weighty equipment on the tube; this erodes the stoma to a larger size, which in healing cicatrizes to cause anterolateral stenosis. This differs from the circumferential stenosis produced by a cuff. Careful attention to avoiding this leverage and the use of flexible swivel connectors have minimized such injuries. The creation of too large a stoma surgically can also contribute to the problem.

Varying degrees of malacia may also occur in the trachea at or above the level of a cuff. Segmental malacia may not be demonstrated on standard x-ray film, but the malacic segment may be seen on fluoroscopy to collapse on forced respiration or cough.

CLINICAL PRESENTATION

Shortness of breath on exertion, episodes of difficulty in raising secretions, and, later, stridorous breathing in any patient who has been intubated in the recent past should suggest the probability of organic obstruction until proved otherwise. Occasionally, patients will also present with unilateral or bilateral pneumonia. These symptoms will not appear in a totally sedentary patient until the airway is reduced to 5 mm or less in diameter. With activity, symptoms become manifest earlier. Since the airway may get to such critical levels in the sedentary patient, prompt diagnosis and treatment are necessary. Tracheoinnominate and tracheo-

esophageal fistulas usually appear in patients who are still on ventilators or intubated. In the case of arterial fistula, there may be a premonitory hemorrhage. Such bleeding should be investigated rapidly with endoscopy and sometimes angiography. The patient with an esophageal fistula will have a sudden increase in tracheal secretions. If he is eating, food or liquid will appear in the trachea. Ingested methylene blue will appear immediately in the tracheal secretions. X-ray film often demonstrates a dilated esophagus below the level of the stoma.

EVALUATION

Simple tracheal radiographs taken with soft-tissue technique will show the status of the entire airway, including the glottis, the subglottic region, the trachea, and the carina. Contrast medium is not necessary. Fluoroscopy can demonstrate the functional status of the glottis and the presence of malacic segments. Many patients with postintubation injuries of the trachea also have glottic dysfunction and sometimes glottic stenosis. Glottic problems must be thoroughly appreciated prior to any attempt at repair of the distal lesion. With increasing experience, tomograms are rarely necessary for full evaluation of the lesion. It is as important to establish the amount of unaffected airway as it is the level, extent, and severity of the lesion itself. A cautious swallow of nonirritant contrast material is indicated in cases of suspected tracheoesophageal fistula.

If a tracheostomy tube has been placed for management of these lesions, it should be removed at the time of the x-ray studies. A responsible surgeon should be on hand to replace the tube. He should have adequate equipment for rapid dilatation of a tightening stoma or stenosis and reestablishment of the airway.

Endoscopy is performed in many cases under the same anesthesia used for surgical correction if the case is straightforward and the lesion well defined. In complex lesions, it may be preferable to perform bronchoscopy as a separate procedure. This is done under general anesthesia without paralyzing agents.

ANESTHESIA FOR CORRECTIVE OPERATION

If a tracheostomy tube is in place, the tube is replaced with a similarly sized armored flexible endotracheal tube, and anesthesia is thus administered. Halothane is preferred. Paralyzing agents are avoided. If there is a high degree of airway obstruction, induction is commenced with the surgeon at hand with a range of pediatric and adult bronchoscopes and esophageal dilators. Airways smaller than 5 mm in diameter are electively dilated to avoid arrhythmias during the operation. In other cases, an endotracheal tube may be placed above the stenosis unless it is a high subglottic lesion.

OPERATION

Almost all postintubation stenoses of the trachea may be corrected by a single-stage resection of the lesion and end-to-end anastomosis (Fig. 33-4). In rare cases in which multiple tracheostomies have been done at different levels with multiple areas of injury and in cases in which unskilled surgery has been performed with failure of the initial procedure, sufficient trachea may be destroyed that reconstruction is not possible. In the latter case, it is preferable to dilate the stenotic areas and place an in-lying Montgomery silicone rubber tracheal T tube. This provides a mechanism for breathing and speaking by the normal route with the side-arm of the tube plugged. This is far better than performing a hazardous introduction of a prosthetic by open operation, with all the hazards of obstruction by granulations, distal sepsis, prosthetic migration, and major arterial hemorrhage.

Almost all of these lesions can be approached through a collar incision and sometimes through upper sternal division. After the anterior surface of the trachea is dissected, the lesion is isolated; division is made above or below the lesion, depending on its level; and intubation is carried out across the operative field. The lesion is dissected away from the esophagus and the mediastinal structures. With dissection against the trachea, the recurrent nerves will not be injured. Great attention is paid to avoiding devascularization of the trachea during this dissection. The majority can be approximated by cervical flexion alone. In other cases, additional maneuvers are required, including suprahyoid laryngeal release. The transthoracic approach is almost never required. Tracheostomies are avoided. The patients are extubated under spontaneous respiration at the conclusion of the procedure.

Lesions involving the lower part of the larynx present more difficulty. In some cases, the stenosis has been the result of endotracheal intubation or cricoidothyroidostomy; in other cases, a high-placed tracheostomy tube has eroded through the cricoid cartilage into the subglottic larynx. Partial antero inferior laryngeal removal and tailored excision of the stenosis, especially posteriorly, must be done, preserving the cricoid plate to protect recurrent laryngeal nerves. The trachea is appropriately beveled, and direct anastomosis is performed.

Results of treatment are summarized in Table 33-1.

POSTOPERATIVE CARE

The airway is kept clear postoperatively by physiotherapy. Bronchoscopy is sometimes required. A chin stitch is placed

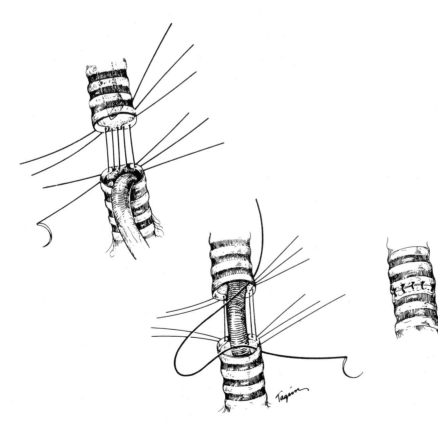

Fig. 33-4. Reconstruction of the upper trachea. (Grillo HC: Surgery of the trachea. In Ravitch MM et al [eds]: Current Problems In Surgery. Copyright © 1970 by Year Book Medical Publishers, Inc., Chicago)

TABLE 33-1 POSTINTUBATION TRACHEAL LESIONS: RESULTS OF SURGICAL RECONSTRUCTION

RESULT	NUMBER OF PATIENTS	PERCENT
Good	168	83
Satisfactory	21	10
Failure	9	5
Death	5	2
Total	203	

(After Grillo HC: Surgical treatment of postintubation tracheal injuries. J Thorac Cardiovasc Surg 78:860, 1979)

in the operating room to prevent forceful extension of the neck for 1 week. The result is checked early and late by appropriate radiologic studies.

POSTOPERATIVE COMPLICATIONS

Intraoperative complications include injury to the innominate artery in a secondary procedure for tracheal reconstruction, damage to a recurrent laryngeal nerve by carrying the dissection too far away from the trachea or larynx, and devascularization of the trachea by excessive mobilization of that portion of the trachea, especially distally, that is to remain within the patient. Injury to a single remaining functional nerve may lead to glottic inadequacy postoperatively. This in turn may necessitate the placement of a tracheostomy tube, which may be very difficult if a significant segment of trachea has been removed. It is important not to place a tracheostomy tube adjacent to an anastomosis, since it will destroy the anastomosis. In extreme cases, a small endotracheal tube may be required for a number of days; later, a tracheostomy tube is placed away from a previously walled-off anastomosis. Necrosis that follows excessive devascularization can lead to restenosis at a later date, which will then require further reoperative surgery or placement of a T tube as a permanent stent.

Granulations at the suture line used to be a serious complication of this type of reconstructive surgery, but this problem has essentially vanished with the use of polyglycolic acid polymeric sutures. The preferred sutures are 4-0 coated Vicril.

The most serious problem is that of separation due to excessive tension. This should be prevented by judging in advance whether a lesion is indeed resectable or not. If there is tension in a more extensive removal, it may be necessary to add procedures such as laryngeal release. If separation has occurred, the patient will require a repeat tracheostomy or later a Montgomery T tube. After 4 to 6 months have elapsed, it may be possible to consider re-resection in expert hands.

TUMORS

PRIMARY

Primary tracheal tumors are rare. Approximately one third of these tumors are squamous cell carcinoma (excluding secondary invasion by laryngeal, bronchogenic, or esophageal carcinoma). Another one third are adenoid cystic carcinoma (formerly called cylindroma). The remaining one third are a mixed group of malignant tumors and benign tumors. These include carcinoid tumors, adenocarcinoma, carcinosarcoma, mucoepidermoid tumor, fibrosarcoma, spindle cell sarcoma, plasmacytoma, fibroma, granular cell tumor, chondroma, chondroblastoma, chondrosarcoma, lymphangioma, hemangioma, and squamous papilloma (single and multiple).

SECONDARY

The trachea may be invaded by squamous carcinoma of the larynx and bronchogenic carcinomas of various types, principally squamous cell, oat cell, and large cell. Carcinoma of the esophagus may invade the trachea at any point, frequently at the carina at the junction with the left main bronchus. Postcricoidal carcinomas of the esophagus also invade the back of the upper trachea. Tumors metastatic to the mediastinum, such as breast carcinoma, may also invade the trachea. Patients with cancer of the thyroid may present initially with symptoms due to invasion of the trachea. This occurs at the level of the thyroid isthmus in papillary, follicular, and mixed papillary and follicular carcinoma. Hemoptysis is the usual initial sign. Obstruction of the trachea is seen also with tumors of this same histology and with the undifferentiated carcinomas of the thyroid. In many cases, a cancer of the thyroid is treated initially with thyroidectomy, and the surgeon describes tumor being "shaved off" the trachea. Sometimes radiotherapy is then given. In such cases, recurrence is the rule rather than the exception, and, ultimately, airway obstruction or bleeding develops. The cancer may involve the larynx as well as the upper trachea.

CLINICAL PRESENTATION

Because of their rarity and the fact that the chest film usually shows normal lung fields, tracheal tumors tend to be diagnosed late. Often, the patient presents with signs and symptoms of upper airway obstruction, and the diagnosis of adult-onset asthma is made. The patient is progressively treated to include high-dose steroids but does not improve. This is most commonly seen with benign tumors, which do not produce hemoptysis, and with adenoid cystic carcinoma, which may not produce hemoptysis until later in its course. Squamous cell carcinoma is more likely to cause hemoptysis, which leads to bronchoscopy and to earlier diagnosis. Another presentation is with unilateral or bilateral recurrent pneumonitis; initially, this responds to antibiotics. Although tumors are often seen retrospectively on standard chest films, special radiologic studies of the trachea will in almost every case demonstrate the tumor. If there is any question, early bronchoscopy is advisable.

TREATMENT

The full extent of the tumor must be evaluated radiologically, as previously described. A contrast study of the esophagus is indicated in the case of tumors. Studies for remote metastases are only indicated in selected cases. Squamous cell carcinoma metastasizes frequently to mediastinal and subcarinal lymph nodes and also invades mediastinal structures. Adenoid cystic carcinoma, on the other hand, will extend for long distances submucosally and perineurally and only later and in the more aggressive cases will present with numerous pulmonary metastases and remote metastases, especially to bone.

In the extensive cases, bronchoscopic evaluation with biopsies above and below the visible extent of the tumor may be indicated. Usually the patient can be intubated on the side of the trachea uninvolved by tumor. On occasions when the tumor is circumferential or when the patient's condition does not permit immediate operation, a highly obstructing tumor may be treated in a preliminary way by coring out tumor. The laser is useful for this maneuver. Except in the case of multiple papillomas, the laser is useless for definitive treatment of tracheal tumors, since the base of the tumor in the tracheal wall cannot be eliminated without destroying the trachea.

The preferred treatment for any primary tracheal tumor, whether benign or malignant, is primary excision with primary reconstruction of the trachea. Planning must be done very carefully, since only about one half of the adult trachea can generally be resected and primary reconstruction guaranteed. A variety of adjunctive maneuvers are available. Tumors of the upper trachea are usually approached anteriorly but with the patient positioned so that the options are open to include intrathoracic extension for anatomical mobilization to permit approximation. Laryngeal release has its place in upper tracheal tumors; it has a lesser place in tumors of the distal trachea and carina. Tumors of the middle and lower trachea are best approached through various combined incisions, but a right posterolateral thoracotomy is preferred for the distal third and carina (Fig. 33-5). All of these procedures are done under inhalation anesthesia. Cardiopulmonary bypass is of no value, since heparinization would not be tolerated in the extensive manipulations wherein bypass would even have to be considered. Radiotherapy is used adjunctively either preoperatively or postoperatively in lesions in which the margins are small or there is lymphatic or perineural invasion or lymph node involvement. In upper tracheal tumors, individually designed partial removal of the larynx with salvage of at least one functional side of the larynx may be accomplished to give a margin around the tumor and yet preserve vocal function. In the small number of cases in which the tumor appears potentially curable but the larynx is also widely involved, laryngotrachiectomy with cervical or mediastinal tracheostomy may be indicated. Partial excisions of the esophagus are also required in some cases.

The principal role of tracheal resection in secondary tumors is in the treatment of papillary and follicular carcinoma of the thyroid that involves trachea either initially or as a recurrence. While cure of secondary involvement has been rare, the periods of palliation have been extended and appear to justify the procedure. In most cases, laryngeal function may be preserved. Clearly, if a thyroid tumor involves the trachea at the time of initial resection, the tracheal resection should ideally be performed at that time. Otherwise, it should be planned for an early date following its discovery. In selected patients, carinal resection may be the optimal method of treatment of proximal cancer of the lung that otherwise fulfills criteria of resectability.

Results of treatment are noted in Table 33-2.

OTHER LESIONS

INFLAMMATION AND INFECTIONS

Tuberculous strictures may obstruct the bronchi, the lower trachea, and, less often, the entire trachea. A complex seen on several occasions includes stenosis of the lower trachea

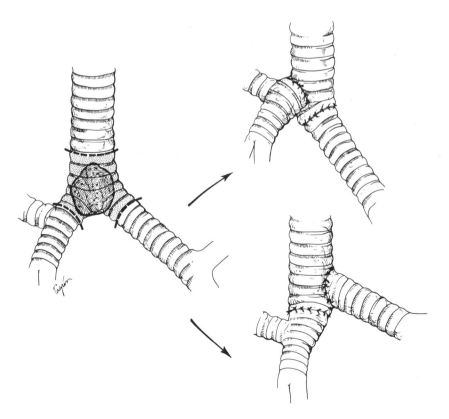

Fig. 33-5. Reconstruction of the carina. While a wide variety of modes have been used, two of the more commonly applied methods are illustrated. (Grillo HC: Tracheal tumors: Surgical management. Ann Thorac Surg 26:112, 1978)

TABLE 33-2 RESULTS FROM PRIMARY RESECTION AND ANASTOMOSIS OF TUMORS INVOLVING THE TRACHEA, 1962–1977

	SQUAMOUS CELL CARCINOMA	ADENOID CYSTIC CARCINOMA	OTHER TUMORS	SECONDARY TUMORS
Postoperative Deaths	2	1	1	1
Alive Without Disease	13 yr 7 mo	15 yr 1 mo	15 yr 1 mo	4 yr 4 mo
	7 yr 7 mo	7 yr 3 mo	8 yr	10 mo
	2 yr 5 mo	5 yr 8 mo	7 yr 3 mo	
	1 yr 11 mo	4 yr 3 mo	3 yr 6 mo	
	10 mo	1 yr 5 mo	2 yr 9 mo	
		1 yr 3 mo	1 yr 10 mo	
			1 yr 1 mo	
Alive with Disease	1 yr 6 mo	5 yr 8 mo		
		1 yr 6 mo		
Dead Without Disease	2 yr			
Dead with Disease	2 yr 8 mo			8 yr
				6 yr 6 mo
				3 yr 6 mo
				2 yr
				6 mo

(Grillo HC: Tracheal tumors: Surgical management. Ann Thorac Surg 26:112, 1978)

and right main bronchus and contraction of the right upper lobe. The process is often submucosal fibrosis of dense type. Externally, the cartilaginous rings appear to be of normal caliber. Tuberculosis is rare in the United States. Strictures due to diphtheria are usually residual cases that occurred in childhood. Syphilis, typhoid, scleroma, and blastomycosis may cause tracheal stenosis, but such cases are exceedingly rare in the United States.

Fibrosing mediastinitis, often identified as being caused by histoplasmosis, may severely involve the trachea and main bronchi. The extent of the fibrosis in many cases precludes reconstruction. There is no known effective treatment for this manifestation of the disease.

IDIOPATHIC OBSTRUCTION

Idiopathic strictures of the trachea may occur. These are seen most often in the upper trachea at the junction with the cricoid cartilage. There is no history of intubation, infection, or trauma. Resection, somewhat surprisingly, has been curative. Amyloidosis, Wegener's granuloma, and tracheopathia osteoplastica may all obstruct the trachea. Relapsing polychondritis also destroys cartilages in both the larynx and the trachea with obstructive results.

EXTRINSIC OBSTRUCTION

A variety of lesions may obstruct the trachea by extrinsic compression. These include massive goiter, parathyroid cyst, other mediastinal tumors of wide variety, and aneurysms. In most of these cases, correction of the obstructive lesion, if possible, leads to relief of the airway obstruction.

Long-term compression by goiter, although rarely seen today, can lead to a thinning of the cartilages so that when the goiter is finally removed there is a segmental obstruction due to malacia. If the trachea is splinted for a time, the cartilages will become firm in the splinted position and the airway will be restored. This has been accomplished in

varying ways in the past, including tracheostomy, intubation followed by tracheostomy or placement of a T tube, the use of traction sutures through the tracheal wall to buttons placed superficial to the sternocleidomastoid muscles, and the placement of inert plastic rings around the malacic segment.

BIBLIOGRAPHY

CANTRELL JR, GUILD HG: Congenital stenosis of the trachea. Am J Surg 108:297, 1964

ECKER RR, LIBERTINI RV, REA WJ et al: Injuries of the trachea and bronchi. Ann Thorac Surg 11:289, 1971

ESCHAPASSE H: Les tumeurs trachéales primitives: Traitement chirurgical. Rev Fr Malad Resp 2:425, 1974

GRILLO HC: Surgery of the trachea. In Keen G (ed): Operative Surgery and Management, pp 657–660. Bristol, England, John Wright & Sons, 1971

GRILLO HC: Tracheal tumors: Surgical management. Ann Thorac Surg 26:112, 1978

GRILLO HC: Complications of tracheal operation. In Cordell AR, Ellison R (eds): Complications in Thoracic Surgery, pp 278–288. Boston, Little, Brown & Co, 1979

GRILLO HC: Surgical treatment of postintubation tracheal injuries. J Thorac Cardiovasc Surg 78:860, 1979

GRILLO HC: Tracheostomy and its complications. In Sabiston DC (ed): Davis-Christopher Textbook of Surgery, 12th ed. Philadelphia, W B Saunders, 1981

GRILLO HC: Carinal reconstruction. Ann Thorac Surg 34:356, 1982

GRILLO HC: Primary reconstruction of airway after resection of subglottic laryngeal and upper tracheal stenosis. Ann Thorac Surg 33:3, 1982

GRILLO HC, MONCURE AC, MCENANY MT: Repair of inflammatory tracheo-esophageal fistula. Ann Thorac Surg 22:112, 1976

KIRSH MM: Blunt Chest Trauma: General Principles of Management. Boston, Little, Brown & Co, 1977

PEARSON FG, THOMPSON DW, WEISSBERG D et al: Adenoid cystic carcinoma of the trachea: Experience with 16 patients managed by tracheal resection. Ann Thorac Surg 18:16, 1974

SADE RM, ROSENTHAL A, FELLOWS K et al: Pulmonary artery sling. J Thorac Cardiovasc Surg 69:333, 1975

SALASSA JR, PEARSON BW, PAYNE WS: Gross and microscopical blood supply of the trachea. Ann Thorac Surg 24:100, 1977

Lyman A. Brewer III/G. Arnold Mulder

Thoracic Wall and Pleura

CHEST WALL

CONGENITAL DEFORMITIES

RIB DEFORMITIES

Chest films often demonstrate abnormalities of the ribs. These are rarely appreciated clinically and are usually asymptomatic. They include fork shape, fusion, or complete absence of one or multiple ribs. Fusion of multiple ribs may cause severe scoliosis as a child grows. There may also be extra ribs. These are very rare except in cervical ribs. In multiple absence of ribs, hernia of the lung may thrust through the defect. This can be closed in infancy, when the ribs are malleable.

CERVICAL RIBS

Cervical ribs may be single or bilateral and are usually not symptomatic at all. Patients with symptoms develop them after the third decade. The problem is that the lower portion of the brachial plexus and the subclavian artery are tented up over the ribs before going to the arm. The compression causes neurologic symptoms, such as pain and weakness, in the hands and arms. There may also be vascular obstructive symptoms. These may be continuous or related only to certain positions or to exercise. The standard treatment is to remove the cervical and first ribs. The problem as to who should be operated and by what approach is discussed under "Thoracic Outlet Syndromes" in Chapter 36.

STERNAL ABNORMALITIES

Incomplete fusion of the embryonic sternal bars may cause defects at the top or bottom of the sternum. These sternal clefts are uncommon and are rarely symptomatic. Complete failure of fusion is much more serious. It can vary from a slightly unstable defect to complete ectopia cordis. This requires emergency closure in infancy and is often fatal.

Other chest deformities include an association of midline defects of the sternum, diaphragm, and sometimes the heart, described by Cantrell. Similar abnormalities were reported by Ravitch. Poland's syndrome is part of a rare group of abnormalities involving the chest, hand, arms, and thighs. It particularly relates to absence of costal cartilages, ribs, breasts, and pectoralis muscles.

LUNG HERNIAS

A congenital weakness in the fascia at the dome of the pleural cavity can result in a supraclavicular hernia of the lung. Hernias can also occur through areas where ribs are absent or areas of weakness following chest surgery. A slight bulge on straining may be noted, usually anteriorly or posteriorly where the intercostal muscles are single thickness. Glassblowers and musicians apparently are affected most frequently. These hernias can be repaired by approximating the ribs with pericostal sutures and buttressing the repair with muscle.

SPINAL ABNORMALITIES

In severe kyphoscoliosis and also in Pott's disease of the spine, there can be impairment of respiratory function. Because of the chest deformity, the intercostal muscles may work poorly and the diaphragm may be almost flat. Spinal fusion procedures, particularly in children, may improve ventilation considerably.

TUMORS

In our experience, the most common tumors palpated in the chest wall are lipomas and metastatic malignancies. All chest tumors should be strongly suspected of being malignant.

BENIGN

Benign skeletal tumors have many forms. Fibrous dysplasia is considered the most common. It may present as a solitary rib lesion, as polyostotic fibrous dysplasia, and in Albright's syndrome. The monostotic form can be locally invasive. Eosinophilic granuloma (histiocytosis X) may present as an expanding rib lesion with a punched-out appearance on x-ray film. Usually, there are lesions in other bones. Rarely, osteoma, osteoid osteoma, osteofibroma, and hemangioma are seen in ribs. Desmoid tumors may progress to frank fibrosarcoma.

Lipomas are common and may have a dumbbell shape protruding through fascia. They may become very large. During palpation, fibromas and neuromas may feel the same. Chondromas are discussed below. Other "benign" chest masses include a prominent ensiform process, foreign body, fat necrosis, organized hematoma, ectopic breast tissue, aneurysms of the intercostal vessels, and fracture callus.

MALIGNANT

The most common malignant skeletal tumor in the chest wall is chondrosarcoma. These tumors can develop in any portion of rib, cartilage, or sternum and may become huge. Occasionally they metastasize. A cure rate of around 20% has been achieved by wide *en bloc* resection of the chest wall with margins around the tumor. The differentiation of chondrosarcoma from chondroma may be extremely difficult. The physical examination, x-ray findings, and history may be identical, although the malignant form usually occurs in people over 20 years of age. Histologically, areas of chondrosarcoma may appear benign, and, conversely, what appears to be a benign chondroma may prove subsequently to be malignant. Therefore, it is generally recommended that most skeletal masses of the chest be treated with wide resection.

Other malignant tumors often seen in the ribs are osteogenic sarcoma and Ewing's tumor, which are almost invariably lethal. Ewing's tumor is usually treated by radiation therapy if the diagnosis is made by a needle biopsy. Frequently, these are initially resected widely and subsequently irradiated. Metastatic tumor to the rib is common, and all rib tumors should include investigation of possible primary sites. Multiple myeloma is frequently first diagnosed through its appearance in the ribs. We have seen several cases of so-called poorly healing fractures that proved to be due to myeloma and metastatic cancer. Other tumors of the reticuloendothelial system and marrow are sometimes first diagnosed as rib tumors. Rhabdomyosarcoma may involve the adjacent ribs.

Treatment of chest tumors often involves extensive *en bloc* dissection and repair of these large defects. The surgery can be challenging. The resection may need to include portions of lung, pleura, sternum, and diaphragm, as well as chest wall. Many techniques of reconstruction are recommended in the literature. Woven stainless steel wire or fascia has worked well in the past. Rib struts can be fixed across the defect. Recently, Marlex mesh with acrylic plates has been sewn in place, although many reports have shown that the paradoxical respiration associated with only a superficial closure may be well tolerated physiologically. When large blocks of skin and muscle must be removed, repair using myocutaneous flaps or muscle pedicles rotated on their blood supply and then skin grafted have worked amazingly well.

PAIN SYNDROMES

Pain radiating in the distribution of an intercostal nerve is a common temporary annoyance following thoracotomy. The pain of intercostal neuralgia is usually burning and radiates in the distribution of the nerve; occasionally this pain is confused with that of angina or hiatal hernia. Chest wall tumors are frequently painless, but tumor and inflammation can cause nerve pain. Other causes of the neuralgia are arthritic osteophytes, nerve tumors, herpes zoster, and unsuspected rib fractures. The treatment is usually expectant, but on some occasions a neurectomy may be necessary.

Tietze's syndrome is a rare, tender, nonseptic swelling of the anterior costal cartilages. The cause is not clear and no specific treatment is successful, but it can last for months and be very annoying to the patient.

INFLAMMATORY CONDITIONS

Chest wall infections usually follow surgery or trauma. They can also be associated with abscesses, carbuncles, and cellulitis and may follow empyema necessitatis. They must be managed with the usual surgical principles, with adequate drainage and antibiotic therapy.

SUBPECTORAL AND SUBSCAPULAR ABSCESSES

Subpectoral and subscapular infections are under the chest wall muscle flap and may be difficult to recognize. They are seen occasionally following empyema, thoracic wounds and trauma, lymphadenitis, and even operations such as pacemaker insertion. They are best drained at the edge of the muscle flaps and may require immobilization of the arm.

Chronic chest wall sinuses may follow deep-space infections and other abscesses, particularly if a foreign body is present. Chronic sinuses may also follow radiation necrosis, osteomyelitis of a rib, or an infected deep suture. Often, tuberculosis or fungi, such as actinomycosis, are implicated. In the worst of these cases, sophisticated plastic techniques, such as myocutaneous flaps, must be used to cover the area after the underlying disease has been treated.

PRIMARY OSTEOMYELITIS OF THE RIBS

Prior to antibiotics, primary osteomyelitis was common and the ribs were often involved. Now rare, it can occur in persons more susceptible to infection and in drug addicts. Tuberculous osteomyelitis has a characteristic punched-out x-ray appearance.

Sternal infections, after sternal splitting operations, are usually mild and related to sutures or wax in the wounds. Rarely, these are serious and require extensive drainage procedures. Chronic sternal instability may result.

Costochondritis is an infection in the anterior costal cartilages. It is one of the most insidious and malignant inflammatory processes in the body and is frequently undertreated. Because the anterior costal cartilages communicate with each other over a large area of the anterior chest and are extremely avascular, it is possible for infection to persist in them for a long time. The initial symptom of fever is followed by anterior chest wall tenderness and then induration of subcutaneous tissues and skin. If an abscess points, it is followed by a chronic draining sinus. Treatment is to resect all of the contiguous cartilage. Sometimes this seems to be a much more radical procedure than a small sinus drainage would warrant, but the lesser procedures are usually followed by recurrent inflammation. Once all the contiguous cartilage tissue has been excised, the infection disappears. Many bacterial species can produce this syndrome, but the most common is *Pseudomonas* species.

PLEURA

The pleura completely invests the thoracic cavity, covering the lung as the visceral pleura and covering the chest wall, mediastinum, and diaphragm as the parietal pleura. Because of its intimate relationship with the heart, great vessels, and lungs, pathologic conditions of the pleura may profoundly alter the physiological action of these organs in the following ways. The acute pain of pleurisy may make respirations and cough weak and ineffectual. The accumulation of large amounts of fluids in the pleural space markedly collapses the lungs and displaces the heart and great vessels, so as to seriously impair their function. In empyema, the absorption of potent toxins and the depletion of protein in the subacute and chronic states adversely affect the general well-being of the patient. Pleural diseases become important mainly as they affect cardiopulmonary function or the general condition of the patient.

PLEURAL EFFUSION

Hydrostatic changes across the visceral and parietal pleural membranes and inflammation result in the formation of fluid in the pleural cavity. Thoracentesis will determine the presence and type of pleural fluids as suspected by physical and roentgenographic examination. The five main types of pleural fluid are transudates, exudates, bloody effusion or hemothorax, chylous effusion, and purulent effusion or empyema.

TRANSUDATES

Pleural transudates are formed as the result of noninflammatory and inflammatory conditions (Fig. 33-6). Noninflammatory types of pleural transudates may be a prominent part of the clinical picture in a variety of diseases in which the fluid persists as a transudate. However, in malignant disease of the pleura, the fluid is serous at the outset and then becomes grossly bloody.

The inflammatory pleural fluids all start as transudates; as the disease process progresses, an exudate or even a grossly purulent type of fluid (empyema) develops. Thus, in these diseases, the transudate state merely represents the early developmental phase of a purely exudative process. Effective antibiotic or antimicrobial therapy may abort the exudate phase or stop the formation of fluid. The diagnostic points of the most common types of disease causing transudates are shown in Table 33-3.

In the case of hepatic and congestive cardiac failure, the nephrotic syndrome and Meigs' syndrome, and early exudative disease, the fluid is not diagnostic in itself. The

Fig. 33-6.   Etiology of pleural transudates.

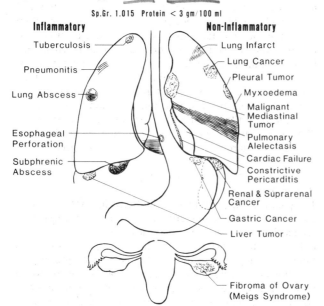

Sp.Gr. 1.015   Protein < 3 gm/100 ml

Inflammatory	Non-Inflammatory
Tuberculosis	Lung Infarct
Pneumonitis	Lung Cancer
Lung Abscess	Pleural Tumor
	Myxoedema
	Malignant Mediastinal Tumor
Esophageal Perforation	Pulmonary Alelectasis
Subphrenic Abscess	Cardiac Failure
	Constrictive Pericarditis
	Renal & Suprarenal Cancer
	Gastric Cancer
	Liver Tumor
	Fibroma of Ovary (Meigs Syndrome)

TABLE 33-3   PLEURAL TRANSUDATES*

ETIOLOGY	KEY DIAGNOSTIC FEATURES
Congestive heart failure	Enlarged, failing heart
Nephrotic syndrome	Kidney failure; high creatinine
Hepatic failure	High SGOT; ascites; jaundice; liver biopsy
Meigs' syndrome	Laparotomy; finding of fibroma of the ovary
Early infections	Early fever; pleurisy; later infectious organism in pleural fluid
Early malignancy of pleura	Early clear fluid, later bloody fluid, contains malignant cells; pleural biopsy

* Specific gravity, 1.015; protein, 3 g/dl; no Ca cells; sterile.

TABLE 33-4   PLEURAL EXUDATES*

ETIOLOGY	KEY DIAGNOSTIC FEATURES
Rheumatoid arthritis	Fluid not diagnostic; joint disease and subcutaneous nodules
Collagen disease	Fluid not diagnostic; joint disease and subcutaneous nodules; LE prep positive
Radiation pleuropneumonitis	Irradiation of chest—must rule out malignancy of pleura
Subphrenic abscess	Subphrenic abscess proved by liver/lung scan, ultrasound
Neoplastic disease	Malignancy in lungs or elsewhere; malignant cells in chest fluid
Bacterial pneumonia	Signs of pneumonia and effusion; infectious organisms found in sputum and pleural fluid
Chronic granuloma	Finding of TBC, coccidioidomycosis, and other fungi in fluid or sputum

* Specific gravity over 1.015; protein, more than 3 g/dl.

identification of the underlying disease process will indicate the cause of the fluid formations. In pleural transudates secondary to malignancy of the pleura, the finding of the malignant cells in the fluid or pleural biopsy confirms the diagnosis.

EXUDATES

In the noninflammatory pleural exudates secondary to rheumatoid arthritis, collagen disease, and radiation pleuropneumonitis, there is nothing diagnostic about the fluid itself, and diagnosis is based on identification of the basic disease (Table 33-4). Cancer cells and virulent organisms and fungi are absent in the fluid. In pleural exudates secondary to subphrenic abscess, the fluid is not diagnostic. The identification of the subphrenic abscess is made by clinical signs, liver and lung scans, ultrasound, and so forth.

In exudative pleural effusion secondary to various infections, the recovery of bacteria, fungi, or tubercle bacilli in the pleural fluid by smear and culture methods or in the sputum establishes the diagnosis. The diagnosis of chronic granulomas may depend on guinea pig inoculation, precipitins, or complement fixation, fluorescent antibody, and immunodiffusion tests.

BLOODY EFFUSION (HEMOTHORAX)

In hemothorax, there is grossly bloody pleural fluid (Table 33-5). Trauma and thoracotomies are the two most common forms of bloody pleural effusion. Spontaneous hemothorax or hemopneumothorax are rare conditions in which the rupture of a vascular intrapleural adhesion or a lung cyst during hard coughing is the source of the blood or air in the pleural cavity. Conservative treatment is usually effective, and thoracotomy is reserved for the life-threatening types of intrapleural hemorrhage.

A ruptured intrathoracic aneurysm may be suspected by demonstration of a wide mediastinum on x-ray film, with or without a massive hemothorax; it is definitively diagnosed by angiography, ultrasound, or CT scan. Immediate surgery may be lifesaving.

CHYLOTHORAX

The finding of an opalescent, creamy pleural fluid on aspiration at first suggests empyema. However, when the fluid remains sterile and is often formed in prodigious amounts, chylothorax may be suspected. The finding of fat droplets by osmic acid and scarlet R fat stains confirms the diagnosis (Table 33-6). Trauma or neoplasm commonly causes perforation of the thoracic duct and the resultant chylothorax. In our series, 7 of 24 cases were secondary to trauma. In the trauma group, ligation of the leaking lymphatic vessel is curative. However, the management of the malignant cases is more difficult. The diagnosis is made by biopsy of available cervical, mediastinal, or regional lymph nodes. Radiation therapy should be tried first and surgery attempted as a last resort.

Pseudochylous effusions are due to long-standing "burnt-out" pyogenic or granulomatous lesions. Cholesterol crystals rather than fat droplets are found in the sputum.

PURULENT EFFUSION (EMPYEMA)

Empyema is most often diagnosed by the aspiration of grossly recognizable pus from the pleural cavity (Table 33-7). The number of acute empyemas has been reduced by the administration of antibiotics, which cure the pneumonia that caused the pleural infection. Conversely, the use of antibiotics, which attenuate the organisms so that they do not grow on culture, often makes the diagnosis of pleural empyema difficult. Although pneumococcal and streptococcal empyemas were formerly the most common types, with the advent of antibiotics, these forms of pneumonia are controlled and a new spectrum of infecting organisms have taken their place. These include *Staphylococcus aureus, Bacteroides, Escherichia coli, Klebsiella, Aerobacter aerogenes, Bacillus pyocyaneus, Proteus,* and *Streptococcus pyogenes.* The pleural cavity becomes involved from direct extension of the infection in adjacent organs (lung, mediastinum, diaphragm, and chest wall) and the blood or lymph. Refractory pneumonitis or septicemia may be the result of a debilitating disease or immunosuppression. The diagnosis of empyema is made by the aspiration of pus from the pleural cavity, although the prior use of antibiotics may make the identification of the infective organism difficult.

TABLE 33-6 CHYLOTHORAX

ETIOLOGY	KEY DIAGNOSTIC FEATURES
Trauma	Fat cells in pleural fluid shown by fat stains
Malignant tumor	Fat cells in pleural fluid; biopsy of pleura, lung, mediastinum reveals malignant cells
Pseudochylous effusion	Cholesterol crystals not fat in pleural fluid formed from burnt-out chronic infection

TABLE 33-7 ACUTE EMPYEMA

ETIOLOGY	KEY DIAGNOSTIC FEATURES
Pneumonia	Gross pus; positive smear and culture
Lung abscess	Gross pus; positive smear and culture
Lung abscess, acute rupture	Pyopneumothorax (surgical emergency!); mandatory closed pleural drainage
Trauma/surgery	Infected hemothorax; positive smear or culture
Subphrenic abscess	Serous/purulent pleural fluid; subphrenic abscess diagnosed by liver/lung scan, CT scan, or ultrasound
Amebic	Brown red pus; hepatic abscess; recovery of amebae from pleural fluid, hepatic abscess pus, or stools
Granulomatous disease Tuberculosis	Usually active pulmonary TB; acid-fast bacillus in sputum or pleural fluid
Fungi	Usually active pulmonary infection; fungi in sputum or pleural fluid or positive precipitin and complement fixation tests

TABLE 33-5 BLOODY PLEURAL EFFUSION

ETIOLOGY	KEY DIAGNOSTIC FEATURES
Trauma/surgery	Blunt trauma, penetrating wound, or surgery
Ruptured aneurysm	Chest pain; wide mediastinum; angiogram
Spontaneous hemothorax	Chest pain; shock; ruptured adhesion or lung cyst
Neoplasm	Evidence of malignancy; malignant cells in fluid
Pulmonary infarction	Chest pain; positive lung scan or angiogram
Pulmonary TB	TBC in fluid, sputum, or pleural biopsy
Periarteritis nodosa	Systemic disease; pleural or cutaneous biopsy

Acute

Essentially, the treatment of acute empyema is the evacuation of pus from the pleural cavity so that the lung will expand completely. With the coaptation of the pleural surfaces, the infection will then be controlled. This may be effected in a number of ways: (1) early local and systemic administration of antibiotics as determined by culture and sensitivity tests, (2) closed dependent pleural drainage, (3) open dependent pleural drainage, and (4) decortication for multiloculated empyema. When the empyema fluid is thin and readily aspirated by thoracentesis, it may be possible to sterilize the empyemic pocket with aspiration and instillation of large doses of the proper antibiotic. This treatment may be successful if bactericidal doses of antibiotic have been determined by culture and sensitivity tests. However, the lung must be capable of expanding to fill the pleural space. A bronchopleural fistula contraindicates this treatment, and immediate closed pleural drainage is mandatory.

Dependent closed thoracostomy is used early in the development of the empyema when, owing to lack of intrapleural adhesions, the mediastinum is not fixed. An effective irrigating closed drainage catheter may be made from an intratracheal tube. It provides a means to instill higher concentrations of antibiotic in the pleural space than is achieved by parenteral administration. The irrigation also flushes out the pus from the pleural space. The use of this irrigating catheter has cut down on the number of rib resections for drainage of empyema. However, when the pus is thick and time has elapsed to permit the development of intrapleural adhesions and a fixed mediastinum, rib resection provides the classic and effective method of empyema drainage. Because it may be difficult to determine the bottom of the pleural pocket, a vertical incision is made over the rib that has been carefully selected by posteroanterior and lateral chest films or fluoroscopy and needle aspirations. If the cavity is lower than anticipated, a second or third rib segment is resected until the large-bore drainage tubes rest at the bottom of the empyemic pocket. When selecting the site for the drainage, it is well to leave the aspirating needle in place and remove the rib above the most dependent site where pus was obtained. In most instances, when the needle cannot find the pus, the knife will fail. The patient must be operated upon in the upright position when a bronchopleural fistula is present, to avoid flooding the opposite lung with the infected pus.

When the drainage track is less than 6 ml and the lung is completely expanded, the tube may be removed. However, it is most important that the patient realize what an important role this drainage tube plays in the recovery. If the drainage tube falls into or out of the pleural cavity, the surgeon must be consulted at once for the replacement or the retrieval of the tube, before the pleura seals over (often in 48 hours).

Postpneumonectomy

During the past decade, we have treated postpneumonectomy empyema by biweekly instillation of massive doses of the proper antibiotic, as determined by sensitivity tests. Doses of from 2 g to 4 g of methicillin sodium (Staphcillin), for example, can be injected intrapleurally because there is little systemic absorption. This method is an improvement over the classic open drainage followed by the painful, deforming multistaged thoracoplasty for the obliteration of the pleural space.

In a similar manner, open drainage and lavage with neomycin or the proper antibiotic as determined by sensitivity tests may successfully sterilize the pleural pocket, permitting closure of the drainage site and obviating thoracoplasty. In cases of bronchopleural fistulas, resection of the bronchial stump and resuture of the bronchus, with reinforcement by means of a pedicled pericardial fat or muscle graft, has been successful in our experience.

Empyema Necessitatis

When pleural infection burrows into the chest wall and forms an abscess, the bulge in the thoracic cage is called an *empyema necessitatis*. The empyema is usually subacute or chronic and often is associated with osteomyelitis of the ribs or osteochondritis of the cartilages. Adequate dependent drainage of the pleural cavity is the treatment of choice, with secondary incision and drainage of the chest wall infection. Frequently, the optimum drainage of the pleural abscess may be much lower than the level of the abscess in the chest wall.

Pyopneumothorax

The rupture of a pulmonary abscess into the pleural cavity without pleural adhesions results in a collapse of the lung and a violent pleuritis that often places the patient into septic shock. It is a true surgical emergency. The rapid outpouring of pleural fluid may be aspirated into the opposite lung, producing a fatal contralateral pneumonia or asphyxia in a debilitated patient. Dependent closed thoracostomy must be immediately performed to prevent the aspiration of the rapidly forming pleural fluid. The salient features of the various types of acute pyopneumothorax are shown on Table 33-8.

Following wounds of the major airways, fluid and air collect in the affected pleural space and the large volume of air that escapes may not be adequately handled with closed pleural drainage. Open operation and closure of the traumatic air leak is the procedure of choice. Following perforation of the thoracic esophagus, air and fluid accumulate in the mediastinum, which usually breaks rapidly into the pleural cavity. Most often there is the history of esophageal instrumentation. If the diagnosis is confirmed by Hypaque swallow within 12 to 18 hours after the perforation, the immediate repair of the esophageal rent or

TABLE 33-8 PYOPNEUMOTHORAX

ETIOLOGY	KEY DIAGNOSTIC FEATURES
Acute rupture of lung abscess	Shock; violent pleural effusion secondary to bronchopleural fistula
Rupture of TB cavity	Pyopneumothorax; mixed TB and pyogenic organisms in fluid, less virulent than above
Rupture of fungous cavity	Similar to TB cavity rupture; pyogenes and fungi in pleural fluid
Wound of major airway	Pus and air in pleural cavity; air escapes violently with large major airway tear
Perforation of esophagus	Air and pus in pleural cavity; Hypaque swallow confirms esophageal perforation

Hypaque: H_2O soluble contrast medium

perforation should be carried out. If more time has elapsed, then drainage of the pleura and the mediastinum should be performed. Frequently, it is necessary to isolate the esophagus by means of a cervical esophagostomy and ligation of the esophagus at the gastroesophageal junction. At a later date, if the esophageal wound has not healed, the esophagus may be resected and a colon esophageal substitution operation performed.

Chronic

Empyema becomes chronic secondary to a variety of pathologic conditions outlined in Figure 33-7. On the left-hand side of the diagram are seen primarily chronic infection of this lung: lung abscess, granulomas of the lung (tuberculosis, fungi), and infected cysts spread by direct extension or rupture into the pleura, as discussed in pyopneumothorax. If a small bronchopleural fistula is present, the patient may be able to cough up the pleural fluid without severely contaminating the opposite side.

On the right-hand side of the diagram is seen the thickened pleural membrane formed from layers of fibrin laid down parallel to the visceral pleura. Regardless of the etiology of the empyema, the ultimate pathologic state is the thick pleural membrane and permanent collapse of the lung held captive in this unyielding cuirass. Untreated hemothorax following trauma and retained foreign bodies (often chest tubes that have dropped into the pleural space without the knowledge of the patient or the physician) lead to chronic empyema. Similarly, drainage tubes inserted too high in the pleural cavity so that they act like smokestacks and fail to completely empty out the pus cause chronic pleural infection. Adequate drainage, removal of the source of the chronicity, and decortication of the inelastic visceral pleural membrane will liberate the lung so that it may fill the pleural space.

Tuberculous

When pulmonary tuberculosis was treated with artificial pneumothorax, tuberculosis of the pleura was common (21% of the cases). Now that the multiple powerful antituberculous drugs have proved so effective in controlling the pulmonary disease, the incidence of pleural tuberculous infection is low. There are five main types: (1) Pure tuberculous empyema without pulmonary disease is treated with antituberculous drugs administered systemically and by pleural aspiration and local instillation. (2) Tuberculous

empyema with pulmonary disease is usually treated the same as for the first type. (3) In mixed pyogenic and tuberculous empyema without pulmonary disease, pleural drainage is the treatment of choice; in addition, antibiotics and drugs to combat the pyogenic and tuberculous infections are administered. (4) In a mixed tuberculous and pyogenic empyema with tuberculous pulmonary disease, the treatment is similar to that for type 3; however, pulmonary resection with or without thoracoplasty or decortication of the remaining lobes may be necessary. (5) Mixed tuberculous and pyogenic empyema with a pulmonary tuberculous cavity that has ruptured into the pleura is treated by immediate pleural drainage to preserve function in the contralateral lung; later, any of the procedures outlined in type 4 may be employed. Low pulmonary function may contraindicate major surgery.

CALCIFICATION

In cases of chronic empyema secondary to prolonged pyogenic, tuberculous, or fungal infections, calcification of the pleura occurs when calcium carbonate is deposited in the pleural membrane. It is believed that the calcium salts are slowly deposited at sites of caseous necrosis in the infected pleural membrane, usually over a period of time. Fibrin from the purulent pleural exudate is deposited in layers parallel to the visceral and parietal pleura and forms a true pleural membrane, making decortication possible. We have, however, successfully decorticated calcified pleural membrane in both tuberculous and nontuberculous pleural disease. If there has been subpleural infection of the lung with necrosis, then the pleura and the pleural membrane are fused to the lung and decortication is impossible.

An exception to the chronic infectious etiology of pleural plaques is found in heroin addicts. It is common to cut the heroin "on the street" with talcum powder, since it looks like heroin. When injected intravenously, a talc granuloma of the lung and pleura is formed. Solitary or coalescent calcified granulomas of the lung and calcification of the diaphragmatic pleura are the hallmarks of this condition. No treatment is indicated.

TUMORS

Primary tumors of the pleura are rare. They generally arise from the visceral pleura. Only mesotheliomas are clearly of parietal pleura origin. Seventy percent of solitary pleural tumors are benign. Multiple pleural tumors are generally malignant. The diagnosis is confirmed by findings of malignant cells in a specimen obtained by aspiration with a large-bore Silverman or other suitable needle. In contrast to carcinoma of the lung with secondary pleural involvement and bloody pleural effusion, which occurs in 10% to 15% of the pleural tumor cases, the fluid early may not show evidence of malignancy. Pulmonary osteoarthropathy occurs in 60% to 70% of the primary pleural tumor cases, while in cancer of the lung it is seen in only 5% to 6%. Hypoglycemia leading to syncope, convulsion, or coma occurs in a small percentage of patients. Because of syncope, carcinomatous metastases to the brain are usually suspected but are not found on CT scan of the brain.

Localized pleural mesotheliomas, whether benign or malignant, most often can be completely excised. In multiple malignant pleural mesotheliomas, especially if bloody pleural

Fig. 33-7. Etiology of chronic empyema.

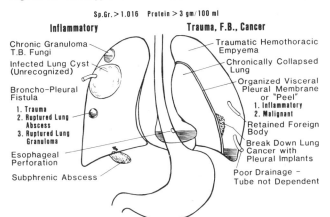

Sp.Gr. > 1.016   Protein > 3 gm/100 ml

Inflammatory

- Chronic Granuloma T.B. Fungi
- Infected Lung Cyst (Unrecognized)
- Broncho-Pleural Fistula
  1. Trauma
  2. Ruptured Lung Abscess
  3. Ruptured Lung Granuloma
- Esophageal Perforation
- Subphrenic Abscess

Trauma, F.B., Cancer

- Traumatic Hemothoracic Empyema
- Chronically Collapsed Lung
- Organized Visceral Pleural Membrane or "Peel"
  1. Inflammatory
  2. Malignant
- Retained Foreign Body
- Break Down Lung Cancer with Pleural Implants
- Poor Drainage – Tube not Dependent

fluid is present, complete resection is usually impossible. Palliation with irradiation and chemotherapy has been disappointing, although symptoms may be alleviated.

Secondary pleural tumors are quite common, especially in cancer of the lung. Invasion of the pleura may be direct extension from carcinomatous processes in the lung or mediastinum or the chest wall. Bloodstream or lymph stream metastases from a primary malignancy elsewhere in the body are fairly frequent. Diffuse seeding of the pleura makes the case inoperable. These cases may be refractory to chemotherapeutic and roentgen therapy, and the treatment is primarily symptomatic.

BIBLIOGRAPHY

AISNER J, WIERNIK PH: Malignant mesothelioma: Current status and future prospects. Chest 74:438, 1978

ANDREWS NC: The surgical treatment of chronic empyema. Dis Chest 47:533, 1965

BAILIERE JL, BISTRONG HW, SPENCE WF: Streptococcal pneumonia: Recent outbreaks in military populations. Am J Med 44:580, 1968

BARRETT NR: Primary tumors of rib. Br J Surg 43:113, 1955

BARRETT NR: The pleura. Thorax 25:515, 1970

BELL JW: Management of post-resection space in tuberculosis. J Thorac Surg 31:442, 1956

BESSONE LN, FERGUSON TB, BURFORD TH: Chylothorax: A collective review. Ann Thorac Surg 12:527, 1970

BLADES B, PAUL JS: Chest wall tumors. Ann Surg 131:976, 1950

BOYD JW: The intrathoracic complication of subphrenic abscess. J Thorac Cardiovasc Surg 38:771, 1959

BREWER LA III: Tuberculous empyema and bronchopleural fistula. In American College of Chest Physicians: Clinical Tuberculosis. Springfield, IL, Charles C Thomas, 1966

BROWN RB, TRENTON J: Chronic abscesses and sinuses of chest wall: Treatment of costal chondritis and sternal osteomyelitis. Ann Surg 135:44, 1952

CLAGETT OT, McDONALD JR, SCHMIDT HW: Localized fibrous mesothelioma of the pleura. J Thorac Surg 24:213, 1952

CONDON WB, HARPER FT: Tumors of the chest wall. Dis Chest 17:741, 1950

CROSBY IK, CROUCH J, REED WA: Chylopericardium and chylothorax. J Thorac Cardiovasc Surg 65:935, 1973

DOLLINGER MR: Management of recurrent malignant effusions. Cancer 22:138, 1972

DONOHOE RF, KATZ S, MATHEWS MJ: Pleural biopsy as an aid in etiologic diagnosis of pleural effusions. Ann Int Med 48:344, 1958

FLEISHMAN SJ, LICHTER AI, BUCHANAN G et al: Investigation of idiopathic pleural effusions by thoracoscopy. Thorax 11:324, 1956

GAERCHI EG, CLAGETT OT: Post-pneumonectomy empyema. J Thorac Cardiovasc Surg 63:771, 1972

GRAH J, USHER FC, PERRY JL et al: Marlex mesh as a prosthesis in repair of thoracic wall defects. Ann Surg 141:469, 1960

GRAHAM EA, BELL RD: Open pneumothorax: Its relation to treatment of acute empyema. Am J Med Sci 156:839, 1918

GROFF DB, ADKINS PC: Collective review: Chest wall tumors. Ann Thorac Surg 4:260, 1967

HEIMLICH HJ: Valve drainage of the pleural cavity. Dis Chest 53:282, 1968

JANES RM: Primary tumors of the ribs. J Thorac Surg 9:145, 1939

KAYSER HL: Tietze's syndrome: A review of the literature. Am J Med 21:982, 1956

MAHER GG, BERGER HW: Massive pleural effusion: Malignant and non-malignant causes in 46 patients. Am Rev Respir Dis 105:458, 1972

MEIGS JF, CASS JW: Fibroma of the ovary with ascites and hydrothorax. Am J Obstet Gynecol 33:249, 1937

OCHSNER A, LUCAS G, McFARLAND G: Tumors of the thoracic skeleton. J Thorac Cardiovasc Surg 52:311, 1966

OKIKE H, BERNATZ PE, WOOLNER LB: Localized mesothelioma of the pleura: Benign and malignant variants. J Thorac Cardiovasc Surg 75:363, 1978

PAYNE WS, CARDIOZA F, WEED LA: Chronic draining sinuses of the chest wall. Surg Clin North Am 53:927, 1973

RIPSTEIN JR, ROHMAN M, WALLACH JB: Endometriosis involving the pleura. J Thorac Surg 37:382, 1959

SAMSON PC, BURFORD TH: Total pulmonary decortication. J Thorac Surg 16:127, 1947

TILLETT WS, SHERRY S, READ CT: The use of streptoferrase and streptodornase in treatment of chronic empyema. J Thorac Surg 21:325, 1951

TRAPNELL DH, THURSTON JGB: Unilateral pulmonary edema after pleural aspiration. Lancet 1:1367, 1970

URSCHEL HC, PAULSON DL: Mesotheliomas of the pleura. Ann Thorac Surg 1:559, 1965

VIANNA NJ: Nontuberculous bacterial empyema in patients with and without underlying disease. JAMA 215:69, 1971

WAGNER JC, SLEGGS CA, MARCHAND P: Diffuse pleural mesotheliomas and asbestos exposure in North Western Cape Province. Br J Ind Med 17:260, 1960

YEH TJ, HALL DP, ELLISON RG: Empyema thoracis: A review of 110 cases. Am Rev Respir Dis 88:785, 1963

The Lung

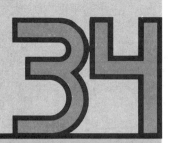

34

Mark A. Kelley/L. Henry Edmunds, Jr.

Overview: Pathophysiology, Manifestations of Disease, and Modern Diagnostic Techniques

A variety of pathologic conditions afflict the lung and chest wall and, by interfering with lung function, threaten life.

Often two or more diseases are present simultaneously, as when carcinoma develops in a patient with chronic obstructive lung disease. Not infrequently one pathologic process leads to another, as when empyema develops after pneumonia. The successful thoracic surgeon needs clear knowledge of pulmonary structure, function, and pathology. Because of space limitations, none of these important topics can be covered here. Instead, this chapter focuses on the pathologic physiology of common pulmonary diseases treated by surgeons, reviews diagnostic methods, and offers some guidelines for operability.

SYMPTOMS OF RESPIRATORY DISEASE

DYSPNEA

Dyspnea is the subjective sensation of breathlessness, which is normal after appropriate exercise but abnormal if it occurs after mild exercise or at rest. The symptom is a common manifestation of both pulmonary disease and heart failure. Unfortunately, the peripheral receptors and sensory pathways that initiate and transmit the signals interpreted as dyspnea are not known. Current knowledge supports a central role for J receptors located in the interstitium of some alveoli and irritant receptors located in airways. J receptors are thought to be stimulated by interstitial edema or inflammation, with impulses transmitted by vagal fibers. Signals from irritant receptors also travel along vagal afferent fibers. In some conditions bilateral vagal block alleviates or obliterates the sensation of dyspnea, but in others the symptom is not affected. Without a clear understanding of the pathologic physiology of dyspnea, we can only conclude that its presence signifies important pulmonary disease or heart failure.

<table>
<tr><td colspan="2">**PREOPERATIVE EVALUATION OF THE PATIENT WITH LUNG DISEASE**</td></tr>
<tr><td>**History**</td><td>Dyspnea, cough, hemoptysis, pain</td></tr>
<tr><td>**Physical Exam**</td><td>Barrel chest, tachypnea, restricted diaphragm movement, chest accessory muscles of respiration, cyanosis, clubbing, decreased exercise tolerance</td></tr>
<tr><td>**Dx**</td><td>Chest films, arterial blood gases, pulmonary function tests, bronchoscopy or bronchography, staging, ventilation-perfusion scanning, needle biopsy</td></tr>
<tr><td>**Operability**</td><td>FEV_1/FVC ratio, hypercarbia, pulmonary arterial pressure, MVV</td></tr>
</table>

COUGH

Cough is a normal reflex that is an important part of the mucociliary transport system for removing inhaled particles. Persistent, frequent, or productive cough is also a symptom of pulmonary disease. The cough reflex originates from stimulation of afferent vagal irritant receptors in the trachea and major (to second order) bronchi. Irritant receptors are stimulated by noxious gases, inhaled particles, accumulations of mucus, distortion of the trachea or bronchi, and local inflammation (*e.g.*, bronchitis). The act of coughing is a complex coordinated act that requires a deep inspiration, closure of the glottis, compression of the thoracic cavity by diaphragm and chest wall, and sudden opening of the glottis with release of the compressed air within the airways. After a deep inspiration with lung volume high, cough most effectively clears large airways. At lower lung volumes, as occurs with repetitive coughing, smaller airways are cleared. During compression of the chest, intrapleural pressures increase to 50 to 300 torr and airways are compressed and narrowed, thereby increasing air flow when the glottis opens.

Postoperatively, suppression of cough by drugs and pain increases the likelihood of postoperative atelectasis and pneumonia. A tracheostomy greatly reduces the effectiveness of cough. Without glottic closure, the rise in intrathoracic pressure and the degree of airway compression are greatly reduced. This slows the velocity of airflow within the airways as compared to that during a normal cough.

PAIN

The lung parenchyma and visceral pleura do not contain pain fibers, but pain fibers are present in the parietal pleura and chest wall. In addition, pain can originate from the trachea during episodes of acute inflammation. Pleuritic pain is well localized and most pronounced during inspiration, when the pleura and endothoracic fascia are stretched. Pleuritic pain is usually associated with infection but can be caused by pulmonary infarction or tumor. Pleuritic pain is easily distinguished from pain of cardiac, great vessel, or esophageal origin but is sometimes difficult to distinguish from pain originating in the pericardium or that due to inflammation of intercostal nerves (*e.g.*, herpes zoster). Diaphragmatic pleuritic pain sometimes is referred to the shoulder or abdomen.

Pain from a thoracotomy incision originates in the chest wall and not in the pleura. It is often associated with paresthesias and areas of numbness as severed intercostal nerves regenerate. Prolonged postoperative chest pain can be due to chronic inflammation of an intercostal nerve caused by an encircling or adjacent suture. Chest wall pain due to trauma (fractured rib) or direct invasion of tumor is similar to that which occurs in other bony and muscular structures.

HEMOPTYSIS

A variety of pulmonary lesions may cause bleeding into airways that is then coughed up and recognized as hemoptysis. Occasionally, tight mitral stenosis causes hemoptysis when one or more dilated submucosal bronchial veins ruptures into an airway. In most patients, sputum is merely blood-tinged and indicates the need for workup and diagnosis of the causative pulmonary lesion. Hemoptysis can be due to either benign or malignant tumors; infections, including bronchitis, lung abscess, bronchiectasis, tuberculosis, pneumonia, and fungal infections; pulmonary infarction; trauma; or various miscellaneous lesions such as pulmonary arteriovenous fistula.

Massive hemoptysis, defined as over 200 ml in 12 hours (300 ml in 24 hours), is potentially life-threatening and requires immediate steps to control the hemorrhage and to establish the cause. Most often, mild sedation (without suppressing cough) and correction of coagulation deficiencies result in gradual cessation of hemorrhage. If bleeding is so brisk that the patient cannot maintain a clear airway, immediate bronchoscopy (rigid scope) is required to localize the source of bleeding. This is followed by thoracotomy and preferably lobectomy, to excise the source of bleeding.

Aspirated blood is exceedingly harmful within the lung. Clots obstruct airways, and blood reaching alveoli inactivate surfactant and lead to atelectasis and often pneumonia.

DIAGNOSTIC INDICATIONS OF PULMONARY DISEASE

ATELECTASIS

The term *atelectasis* is used to describe collapse of lung units in the absence of infection. It differs from consolidation, wherein alveoli are filled with a transudate, exudate, or blood. In atelectasis, alveoli are empty. The condition usually develops from partial or complete obstruction of airways or from persistent hypoventilation of susceptible (*i.e.*, basilar or edematous) lung units.

At transalveolar gas pressures that normally occur during respiration, all alveoli would collapse during expiration in accordance with Laplace's law were it not for pulmonary surfactant and the interdependence of each lung unit on surrounding lung units. Within an alveolus, Laplace's law relates the distending pressure, P (normally between 2 and 20 torr) to surface tension, T, and radius, R (normally about 280 to 330 μ): $P = 2T/R$. Thus during expiration when P and R are lowest, high surface tension tends to collapse small alveoli but is less likely to collapse larger blebs or bullae because radii are larger. A phopholipid secreted by type II alveolar cells called *pulmonary surfactant* has the remarkable property of reducing alveolar surface tension from approximately 20 dynes/cm at end inspiration to 1 or

2 dynes/cm at end expiration. The reduced surface tension prevents alveolar collapse during expiration. Pulmonary surfactant also reduces the tendency of alveolar surface tension to draw fluid from alveolar insterstitial spaces to alveolar surfaces. This helps to keep alveoli dry.

The second mechanism preventing atelectasis is called *interdependence*. Except beneath the visceral pleura, each alveolus is surrounded by other alveoli. When one group of alveoli collapses, expanding forces due to radial traction from surrounding ventilated units increase and thus tend to reexpand collapsed lung units.

Complete obstruction of a bronchus causes collapse of distal lung units as alveolar gas is absorbed into pulmonary capillary blood that has lower partial pressures. Although nitrogen is poorly soluble in blood, absorption occurs if alveolar gas is not replenished. Collateral ventilation from surrounding lung units can sometimes replenish alveolar gas in small areas of collapsed lung within a lobe but does not occur between lobes. Localized hypoventilation due to partial obstruction or reduced tidal volume also leads to collapse as the delicate balance between surface tension and alveolar pressure and radius breaks down. A third mechanism causing atelectasis is due to inactivation of alveolar surfactant, when proteinaceous fluid leaks into alveoli. Aspiration causes atelectasis by a similar mechanism.

Perfusion of atelectatic lung units reduces arterial pO_2, since the perfusate cannot exchange oxygen or carbon dioxide. However, persistent atelectasis usually causes localized pulmonary arterial vasoconstriction, which reduces the amount of unventilated blood reaching the left atrium.

HYPOXIA

Hypoxia may be caused by one of four mechanisms: hypoventilation, a right-to-left shunt, a marked reduction in diffusing capacity, or an imbalance between alveolar ventilation and perfusion. By far the most common cause of hypoxia due to lung disease is mismatch of alveolar ventilation and perfusion. Although often more than one cause of hypoxia is present, it is possible to pinpoint the pathologic physiology by measuring arterial blood gases when the patient breathes room air and 100% oxygen.

Pure oxygen markedly raises arterial pO_2 to nearly that of alveolar gas in patients who are hypoventilating, who have an impairment in diffusion, or who have an imbalance between alveolar ventilation and perfusion. Oxygen breathing only slightly increases (owing to the increase in plasma pO_2) arterial pO_2 in patients with right-to-left shunts. Aside from certain congenital heart lesions, right-to-left shunts result from pulmonary arteriovenous fistulas or perfusion of unventilated lung units, as may occur in pneumonia.

In surgical patients, hypoventilation most commonly occurs as a result of pain or pharmacologic depression of respiration. Less commonly, multiple rib fractures or upper airway obstructive lesions cause hypoventilation. By definition, alveolar hypoventilation is present when arterial pCO_2 is elevated and is not present when arterial pCO_2 is normal or low.

Hypoxia due primarily or predominantly to an impairment in diffusing capacity is uncommon, since normally pulmonary capillary red cells are fully saturated with oxygen after traversing only the proximal third of the capillary. A variety of interstitial lung diseases that increase the thickness of the alveolar–capillary barrier (normally 0.5μ thick) may impair diffusion and cause hypoxia, particularly during exercise. Chemoreceptors maintain arterial pCO_2 at normal levels, and an increase in alveolar pO_2 with oxygen breathing increases the O_2 diffusion gradient and raises arterial pO_2. If interstitial disease and impairment of diffusion are suspected, diffusing capacity can be easily measured by the single-breath carbon monoxide technique.

For maximum efficiency, alveolar ventilation should precisely match alveolar perfusion throughout the lung. In normal lungs this does not occur for several anatomic and physiologic reasons. In an upright individual, both alveolar ventilation and alveolar perfusion are greater at lung bases than at the apexes; however, the difference in perfusion across the vertical axis of the lung is much greater than the difference in ventilation. At the apexes the ventilation–perfusion (V/Q) ratio is high, largely because pulmonary blood flow is low. Pulmonary capillary blood is fully saturated, but the pO_2 of alveolar gas is relatively high (compared to the rest of the lung), since diminished amounts of oxygen diffuse into poorly perfused capillaries. At lung bases V/Q ratio is low, resulting in lower oxygen tensions and higher CO_2 tensions in pulmonary capillary blood. Since proportionately more blood from lung bases than lung apexes reaches the left atrium, the net effect is that mean arterial pO_2 is 4 to 5 torr lower than the mean pO_2 of alveolar gas. Arterial CO_2 is slightly higher than mean alveolar CO_2, but this difference is insignificant.

In pathologic states, V/Q imbalances can greatly increase differences between alveolar and arterial pO_2 (A–a O_2 gradient) to 50 and 60 torr during air breathing. Although abnormal A–a O_2 gradients are due to lung units with both high and low V/Q ratios, most of the hypoxia is due to units with low V/Q ratios (Fig. 34-1). Consequently, it is often convenient to calculate the physiologic shunt ratio to obtain semiquantitative measurements of the severity of the V/Q imbalance. Physiologic shunt ratios are calculated from measurements of arterial and mixed venous blood O_2 content and a calculation of what alveolar pO_2 would be if all lung units were uniformly ventilated. The physiologic shunt ratio (Qps/Qt) equals $(C_1 - Ca)/(C_1 - C_v)$, where C_1 is the calculated oxygen content of capillary blood in equilibrium with the calculated "ideal" alveolar pO_2, and Ca and C_v are

Fig. 34-1. Ventilation and blood flow plotted against ventilation–perfusion ratios. Ventilation and perfusion are matched when the ratio is 1. In this patient, considerable blood flow to poorly ventilated lung units causes a "physiologic shunt" and hypoxemia.

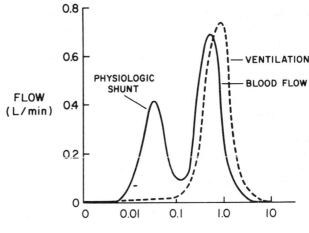

the oxygen contents of arterial and mixed venous bloods, respectively. Normally the physiologic shunt is less than 5%, but it may exceed 50% in patients with severe imbalance between ventilation and perfusion.

HYPERCARBIA

The respiratory center in the brain stem controls respiration and contains central chemoreceptors that are sensitive to small changes in arterial pCO_2. In contrast, peripheral chemoreceptors located in the carotid body are particularly sensitive to changes in arterial pO_2 and are less responsive than central chemoreceptors to changes in arterial pCO_2. Small increases in arterial pCO_2 stimulate the respiratory center to increase ventilation and reduce the CO_2 concentration of alveolar gas. *A priori*, hypercarbia indicates hypoventilation of alveoli. The feedback mechanism between arterial pCO_2 and central chemoreceptors of the respiratory center is so sensitive and strong that arterial pCO_2 remains within the normal range (35 to 40 torr) in most pulmonary disease states.

An exception is severe chronic obstructive pulmonary disease (COPD), in which the increase in airway resistance (and the work of breathing) is very marked. In these patients, who also have reduced arterial pO_2, arterial pCO_2 may be chronically increased. Because the resulting respiratory acidosis is chronic, kidneys conserve base and excrete acid (compensatory metabolic acidosis) to maintain a normal arterial pH. CO_2 retention is the hallmark of very severe COPD.

DISEASE SYNDROMES

CHRONIC OBSTRUCTIVE PULMONARY DISEASE (COPD)

COPD is a very common, insidious lung disease affecting primarily, but not exclusively, middle-aged and older individuals and characterized by an increase in airway resistance. Patients generally have a mixture of emphysema and chronic bronchitis, but one or the other of the two conditions may predominate. The emphysematous process results in destruction of alveolar walls and capillaries, narrowing of small bronchi and respiratory bronchioles, destruction of some large airways, and creation of an irregular honeycomb of large dilated airspaces, blebs, and sometimes bullae across which thin strands of tissue are stretched. The process may be present throughout the lung or near central portions of the lobule, or near the septal portions. In chronic bronchitis, airway mucous glands hypertrophy and increase mucus production. Small airways are narrowed by inflammatory cells and edema of their walls, which may progress to peribronchial fibrosis. The association of cigarette smoking and COPD is well known.

Emphysema causes loss of elastic recoil of the lung and an increase in total lung capacity (TLC), residual volume (RV), and functional residual capacity (FRC). Compliance is increased and vital capacity plus diffusing capacity are often reduced. Airway resistance is increased primarily as a result of the loss of elastic recoil and radial traction on airways. Consequently, forced expiratory volume in one second (FEV_1), peak expiratory flow rate (PEFR), and maximum mid-expiratory flow rates (MMEFR) are all decreased. Hypoxemia results from severe imbalances between alveolar ventilation and perfusion and may or may not be associated with CO_2 retention. Alveolar–arterial oxygen difference is increased, as are physiologic deadspace and physiologic shunt. Pulmonary vascular resistance increases in advanced cases.

When chronic bronchitis predominates, increases in lung volumes are less marked; but measurements of airway resistance all indicate significant airway obstruction, which may or may not improve with bronchodilators. Diffusion capacity is normal, as are elastic recoil and compliance. Severe V/Q imbalance leads to hypoxia and eventually an increase in pulmonary vascular resistance. CO_2 retention may occur if airway obstruction is severe.

RESTRICTIVE LUNG DISEASES

The hallmark of this group of lung diseases, many of which have an unknown etiology, is diffuse interstitial fibrosis with eventual destruction of alveoli and development of cysts and collagen strands throughout the lung. Plasma cells and lymphocytes first invade the interstitium of the alveolar–capillary barrier, after which fibrosis and thickening of the alveolar interstitium occur.

Restrictive lung diseases cause hypoxemia without hypercarbia. Cyanosis is increased with exercise, caused by an imbalance of ventilation and perfusion and impairment of diffusion. Diffusing capacity measurements are low and do not increase with exercise. The fibrotic interstitial process causes a proportionate reduction of all lung volumes and compliance but does not increase airway resistance. Therefore, although total FEV and FEV_1 may be low, the ratio FEV_1/FEV is normal or high. MMEFR is normal when related to the percentage of the reduced total lung volume. Hypoxia increases pulmonary vascular resistance.

AIRWAY OBSTRUCTION

Tumors, strictures, and foreign bodies are the most common causes of partial obstruction of the trachea and major airways. Occasionally the airways may be compressed externally by enlarged lymph nodes, tumor, or vascular ring. Tracheal obstructions are more serious than bronchial obstructions and cause dyspnea, inspiratory and expiratory stridor, wheezing, and often chronic cough as the patient tries to raise mucus beyond the lesions. Critical obstruction resulting in inadequate alveolar ventilation causes severe dyspnea, CO_2 retention, and hypoxia and may rapidly result in death. Partial obstructions of the trachea may become critical if bronchoscopy beyond the lesion causes bleeding or edema.

Tracheal obstructions increase airway resistance and the work of breathing. The flow-volume loop obtained by plotting velocity of inspiratory and expiratory airflow against changes in lung volume is always abnormal. The location and the flexibility of the tracheal lesion determine whether the obstruction is more severe in inspiration or expiration. FEV_1 may be nearly normal or only slightly reduced; however, depending on the type of lesion, maximum flow rates in inspiration and expiration are reduced (Fig. 34-2). Severe tracheal obstructions may reduce vital capacity and inspiratory reserve volume and increase residual volume. V/Q relationships and diffusing capacity are not altered. CO_2 retention will occur if fatigue leads to alveolar hypoventilation. Patients are more susceptible to lung infections because of difficulties in clearing mucus beyond the obstructing lesion.

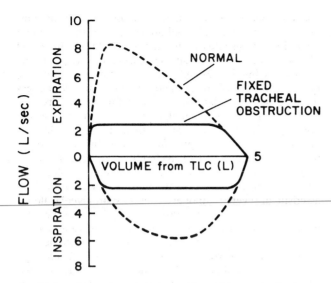

Fig. 34-2. Flow volume loop in a patient with a tracheal stricture before (solid line) and after (dotted line) resection. The postoperative flow volume is normal. (TLC = total lung capacity)

Partial obstructing lesions of the major bronchi affect the unilateral lung and are more insidious than tracheal lesions. Dyspnea, unilateral stridor and wheezing, and cough are prominent early symptoms. Of necessity, ventilation is shifted to unobstructed lobes or the opposite lung, but air trapping may occur in the obstructed lung if the lesion exerts a ball valve effect. This produces a hyperinflated lobe or lung that may be apparent by inspection or on chest x-ray film.

More often, a partial obstructing lesion of a major lobe or segmental bronchus leads to complete obstruction. Bronchial obstructions interfere with mucus transport and often become complete when mucus impacts the narrowed airway. Atelectasis and an increase in physiologic shunt occur. If infection does not develop, the obstructed lung may gradually fill with inspissated mucus and be impossible to reexpand at a later date. More often, infection develops and leads to pneumonia, destruction of the lung, or a lung abscess.

COMPRESSION

Lobes, segments, or an entire lung can be compressed by accumulation of air, blood, pus, tumor, or transudates or exudates within the pleural space. If an organized fibrotic peel develops over compressed parenchyma, the lung cannot be reexpanded until the peel is removed (decortication).

Intrapleural pressure is normally negative (approximately −5 torr) with respect to atmospheric pressure. Open pneumothorax—the occasional result of trauma, but more often the result of poor technique during tube thoracostomy—permits air to enter through a hole in the chest wall. The elastic recoil of the lung leads to partial or complete collapse of the unilateral lung. In spontaneous pneumothorax, air enters the pleural space from ruptured apical blebs or bullae. Spontaneous pneumothorax can also result from rupture of emphysematous cysts or bullae or as a complication of high airway pressures during assisted ventilation. Tension pneumothorax occurs if exaggerated respiratory efforts continue to draw air into the pleural space during inspiration and do not permit escape of air during expiration. If trapped pleural

air breaks through the parietal pleura, or if traumatic rupture of a bronchus occurs, mediastinal and subcutaneous emphysema may develop as air escapes the pleural cavity along tissue planes. Tension pneumothorax is a medical emergency, since high (above atmospheric) intrapleural pressure may compress the mediastinum, interfere with ventilation of the opposite lung, and reduce cardiac output.

Blood, transudate, exudate, pus, or tumor may also appear in the intrapleural space and compress the underlying lung. With the exception of hemothorax in association with trauma, pleural fluid accumulation is slower and more insidious than pneumothorax. Gas exchange in the compressed lung, which is easily recognized by chest radiograph, is compromised. This results in reduced lung volumes and vital capacity. Some degree of hypoxia occurs from the mismatch of ventilation and perfusion in the compressed lung units. Airway resistance is not affected. Diffusing capacity may be decreased slightly and pulmonary arterial pressure increased slightly if a large amount of lung parenchyma is compressed.

Usually the compressed lung does not develop infection unless infection was present before compression occurs, as when empyema complicates pneumonia or a tuberculous infection. In the absence of infection, the compressed lung parenchyma may be reexpanded even after weeks, months, or years, once the compressing force is relieved.

INFECTION

The lung is an external organ and therefore is constantly exposed to potentially pathogenic microorganisms. The mucociliary transport system and alveolar macrophages are the lungs' defense against infection.

Inhaled particles greater than 5μ are primarily trapped in the nose and pharynx. Small particles less than 1μ are exhaled. Particles between 1μ and 5μ are cleared by the mucociliary transport system. As velocity of airflow slows in the small peripheral airways (terminal bronchioles and respiratory ducts), these particles fall upon the mucous blanket, where they are trapped. The mucous blanket, which contains the immunoglobulin IgA, is produced by bronchial mucous glands and goblet cells and consists of a superficial viscous gel layer and a deeper serous layer. Noninnervated cilia beating up to 20 times/sec move in the serous layer and propel the viscous gel layer outward at rates ranging from mm/min in small airways up to 2 to 3 cm/min in the trachea. Ciliary activity is inhibited by heat, drying, and a variety of noxious gases.

In large bronchi and the trachea, the outward transport of mucus is aided by occasional coughs produced in response to stimulation of irritant receptors in the large airways. Eventually, particles trapped in the mucous gel reach the pharynx, where the mucus is expectorated or swallowed.

Particles that are deposited in alveoli are engulfed by alveolar macrophages that continuously travel over alveolar surfaces. Macrophages contain lysosomes and can engulf and kill organisms. Particle-laden macrophages may travel outward along alveolar ducts to reach the mucous blanket or deposit foreign particles outside the walls of respiratory bronchioles. These particles may be cleared by lymphatics or remain in deposits to produce the anthracotic, mottled appearance beneath the visceral pleura of many adult lungs.

Acute or chronic bronchitis produces acute or chronic inflammation of portions of the bronchi. The inflammation may destroy areas of the ciliated bronchial epithelium and interfere with mucus transport. The inflammation usually causes increased mucus production and, if chronic, hypertrophy of mucous glands. The inflammation and increased mucus production increase airway resistance and not infrequently result in airway obstruction, with subsequent atelectasis or pneumonia.

Once infection becomes established in alveoli and terminal airways, the resulting pathology and outcome are determined by the virulence and type of organism, the host defenses, and treatment. Pneumonia involves inflammation and often destruction of alveolar septae and formation of an exudate that completely fills alveolar spaces. Ventilation is impossible, but perfusion may continue, producing a right-to-left shunt and hypoxemia. If alveoli are destroyed, healing occurs by fibrosis and scarring; alveoli do not appear to regenerate. Abscesses or cavities (tuberculosis and certain fungal diseases) result if relatively large areas of lung are destroyed and the suppurative products of infection cannot be cleared by white cells.

Pneumonia may produce a pleural effusion, which can be a transudate that is low in protein or an exudate that is high in protein and may contain viable organisms: that is, an empyema. Pleural transudates are easily aspirated, since they are generally not loculated. Exudates and empyemas are frequently loculated and therefore are more difficult to remove. Reexpansion of the underlying compressed lung requires removal of pleural fluid or pus, resolution of the pneumonia process, and removal of any visceral peel that may have formed.

Pleural air above fluid in the chest radiograph, in the absence of trauma, indicates a bronchopleural fistula. Infection of the pleural fluid can be assumed. If the bronchial communication is large, as may occur postoperatively due to disruption of the bronchial staple line, drowning may occur if pleural fluid massively enters the bronchus. Immediate aspiration or preferably tube thoracostomy drainage of the fluid may be lifesaving. In all bronchopleural fistulas, surgical closure of the bronchus is required, in addition to drainage of the pleural fluid or pus.

PULMONARY CONGESTION

The term *pulmonary congestion* describes an increase in the fluid content of the lung, which most commonly occurs as a result of left heart failure. Other causes of pulmonary congestion include mitral stenosis; over transfusion, particularly with crystalloids; inhalation of toxins, including high oxygen concentrations; and obstruction of pulmonary lymphatics by fibrosis or tumor.

Starling's law for fluid exchange across capillaries describes the factors that determine whether or not excess fluid will enter alveolar interstitial spaces or the alveoli themselves. Fluid exchange is affected by capillary wall permeability, capillary hydrostatic pressure, capillary colloid osmotic pressure, interstitial hydrostatic pressure, and interstitial colloid osmotic pressure. Capillary hydrostatic pressure and interstitial colloid osmotic pressure tend to pull fluid out of capillaries, and capillary colloid osmotic pressure and interstitial hydrostatic pressure keep it in. Capillary endothelium is permeable to water, ions, and small molecules but resists transfer of proteins.

When the Starling equation becomes unbalanced in favor of fluid leakage out of the capillaries, excess fluid accumulates in alveolar interstitial spaces (interstitial edema) and widens alveolar–capillary barriers. Excess interstitial fluid spreads to the loose tissue around the small bronchi

and pulmonary vessels, where some of it enters the lymphatic system. Normally, pulmonary lymph flow is about 20 ml/hr, but this rate can increase manyfold. The increased interstitial and peribronchial–perivascular fluid reduces lung compliance but does not affect gas exchange, lung volumes, or airway resistance and does not cause measurable changes in pulmonary vascular resistance or diffusing capacity.

Further increases in capillary leakage result in alveolar flooding. Although alveolar epithelium is normally impermeable to solutes and proteins, severe pulmonary congestion causes fluid to progressively fill alveoli. This produces V/Q imbalance and hypoxemia, since flooded alveoli cannot be ventilated, and produces the pink, frothy sputum characteristic of severe pulmonary edema. With alveolar flooding, pulmonary vascular resistance may increase, perhaps in part due to vasoconstriction of vessels perfusing flooded lung units. Compliance is decreased, lung volumes are reduced, and airway resistance is increased. There is a propensity for unflooded lung units to collapse. Assisted ventilation with increased end expiratory airway pressures may be necessary to prevent atelectasis and more severe hypoxia. CO_2 retention is a late and often preterminal manifestation.

OXYGEN TOXICITY

Pure oxygen breathing causes direct injury to the alveolar–capillary barrier that can be recognized histologically within 36 to 48 hours. During the acute exudative phase of the injury, capillary endothelial cells swell and begin to leak, allowing edema fluid to enter the interstitial space and eventually the alveoli. Type I alveolar epithelial cells disappear and are replaced with type II cells. These changes cause a reduction in vital capacity, compliance, and diffusing capacity and an increase in alveolar arterial oxygen difference. If high oxygen exposure is continued, death ensues.

Oxygen toxicity is related to both the concentration and duration of inspired oxygen. Although not well documented, probably any concentration of inspired oxygen over 50% for several days causes injury to pulmonary capillary endothelial cells. As a rule of thumb, 100% oxygen should not be continued more than 24 hours, 80% more than 48 hours, and 60% more than 4 days. In all instances, the lowest concentration of inspired oxygen that will maintain arterial pO_2 between 60 and 70 torr (approximately 90% hemoglobin saturation) is recommended until the pathologic process causing the hypoxemia is reversed.

ACUTE RESPIRATORY DISTRESS SYNDROME (ARDS)

A diverse group of diseases or events may result in acute respiratory distress syndrome (ARDS), which has as a common manifestation the development of hemorrhagic consolidation of the lung (Fig. 34-3). The syndrome may develop after chest trauma, massive transfusions, fat embolism, septicemia, cardiopulmonary bypass, aspiration, inhalation of smoke or noxious gases, oxygen toxicity, viral pneumonia, toxemia of pregnancy, or acute pancreatitis. It is not clear how the multiple causes of ARDS produce the marked increase in capillary permeability that allows first fluid, then protein, and eventually red cells to reach the alveolar interstitial space and eventually the alveolar surface.

Early in ARDS, signs, symptoms, and findings of interstitial edema and later alveolar flooding develop. The chest film shows diffuse infiltrates throughout both lung fields that may progress to nearly total opacification. Severe

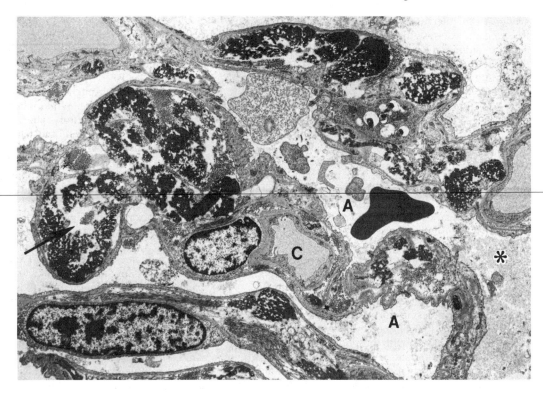

Fig. 34-3. Electron micrograph from the lung of a patient dying 5 days after severe trauma and hemorrhage. There is interstitial and alveolar edema and hemorrhage. At this stage, the capillary endothelium and the alveolar epithelium appear anatomically intact. The lung was fixed immediately after the patient was pronounced dead. Magnification ×9,000. A = alveoli; C = capillary; arrow = interstitial edema; * = alveolar edema. (Pietra GT, Rüttner JR, Wüst W et al: The lung after trauma and shock. . . . J Trauma 21:454, 1981. Copyright © 1981 by The Williams & Wilkins Co., Baltimore)

hypoxemia develops, lungs become noncompliant, the work of breathing increases, lung volumes decrease, and pulmonary vascular resistance increases. Patients require assisted ventilation with increased end expiratory pressures, markedly increased peak inspiratory airway pressures, and progressively increasing inspired oxygen concentrations to avoid life-threatening hypoxia. Catecholamine infusions may be necessary to maintain an adequate cardiac output. When arterial pO_2 remains below 50 torr at inspired oxygen concentrations of 60% or greater, mortality exceeds 90%.

If the patient survives the acute phase and does not develop an intervening bacterial pneumonia, the lung often heals by fibrosis. As red cells, macrophages, and polymorphonuclear cells are removed, alveolar interstitium may remain thickened by fibrous tissue. If interstitial fibrosis occurs, the pathologic and functional picture of restrictive lung disease develops.

DIAGNOSTIC METHODS

GENERAL HISTORY

A careful and complete history can provide important information in the diagnosis of pulmonary disease and often determines which additional diagnostic tests to order. The history should include not only documentation of the patient's present illness but also a careful review of systems and relevant family, occupational, and environmental history. For example, a nonsmoker is much less likely to have

lung disease than a smoker. A family history of chronic lung disease, particularly at an early age, suggests an inherited lung disorder such as alpha$_1$-antitrypsin deficiency. Patients with a history of asthma, seasonal rhinitis, or bronchitis may be prone to bronchospasm in the perioperative period. An occupational history may reveal previous exposure to coal, silica, or asbestos dusts. These substances are encountered in a variety of occupations and are associated with characteristic chest radiographic abnormalities. In addition, asbestos exposure is associated with an increased risk of lung cancer, interstitial and pleural disease, and pleural mesothelioma. Since tuberculosis enters the differential diagnosis of many pulmonary disorders, a history of tuberculosis and PPD skin testing should be elicited in every patient.

A careful review of systems may provide clues about extrathoracic malignancy or a systemic disorder with pulmonary manifestations. Symptoms of pulmonary disorders may not be confined to the thorax. Serious debilitating processes, such as tuberculosis or malignancy, produce constitutional complaints of fever, night sweats, anorexia, and weight loss. With malignancy, constitutional symptoms strongly suggest widely metastatic disease. Neurologic or muscular complaints may be from paraneoplastic syndromes, such as myopathy and peripheral neuropathy. Skeletal pain may represent metastases. Arthritis symptoms can be from hypertrophic osteoarthropathy associated with thoracic neoplasm or inflammatory disease.

Potential candidates for operation should also be questioned about exercise tolerance to assess cardiopulmonary performance. Patients who can easily perform everyday activities can tolerate most surgical procedures involving the lung. In contrast, those who complain of significant exercise limitation should undergo detailed physiologic testing to document pulmonary and cardiac performance. The results may influence decisions regarding surgical intervention.

PHYSICAL EXAMINATION

Physical findings provide not only important diagnostic clues but also important information regarding diseases of other organ systems and the patient's cardiopulmonary reserve. Some of the more common physical findings in patients with lung disease underscore the importance of a thorough physical examination. For instance, pulsus paradoxus may be seen with severe obstructive pulmonary disease and can be used to monitor efficacy of bronchodilator therapy. Respiratory rate can reflect the degree of respiratory insufficiency. Tachypnea with shallow, rapid respirations over 40/min signifies impending respiratory failure.

Cyanosis is a difficult sign to assess since 5 g of desaturated hemoglobin are necessary for its appearance. Nonetheless, obvious cyanosis is indicative of severe hypoxemia. Clubbing of the digits can be seen with intrathoracic neoplasms, both benign and malignant, and with chronic infections such as bronchiectasis. Clubbing may resolve when these conditions have been reversed. Erythema nodosum—painful erythematous nodules over the anterior tibia—is associated with sarcoidosis, fungal infections, and tuberculosis.

Lymphadenopathy may signify extrathoracic metastatic disease or the presence of infection. Lymph nodes in the cervical and supraclavicular areas are most often involved in pulmonary disorders. Palpation of the trachea will detect tracheal deviation suggestive of volume change of the lung. Thyroid enlargement can produce upper airway obstruction and may affect the technical approach to upper mediastinal surgery. Careful assessment of the nasal and oral passages may reveal processes, such as sinusitis or poor dentition, associated with chronic respiratory infections. Elevated jugular venous pressure can occur with cor pulmonale, superior vena cava obstruction, pericardial tamponade, or constrictive pericarditis, and occasionally in severe obstructive pulmonary disease.

The chest examination may reveal an increased anterior-posterior diameter consistent with chronic obstructive pulmonary disease. Asymmetrical expansion of either hemithorax occurs with a paralyzed hemidiaphragm, splinting from chest pain, or the compression of underlying lung by a pleural effusion or pneumothorax.

Increased tactile fremitus indicates pulmonary consolidation, while decreased tactile fremitus occurs in pleural effusions or pneumothorax. Percussion of the chest is helpful in detecting diaphragmatic movement and pleural effusion.

On auscultation, normal breath sounds are distant from the ear because air turbulence in the tracheobronchial tree is muffled by alveolar air. Tubular breath sounds, also termed bronchial sounds, occur when breath sounds seem close to the examiner's ear. Pulmonary consolidation, such as pneumonia, obliterates alveolar air and allows sound waves to be transmitted more clearly from large airways to the chest wall. Decreased breath sounds, which seem distant to the examiner's ear, occur with pleural effusion or pneumothorax.

Coarse sounds in mid inspiration and expiration, termed *rhonchi*, indicate fluid or mucus in larger airways. *Rales*,

fine crackling sounds late in inspiration, indicate interstitial disease, such as pulmonary edema or pulmonary fibrosis. Generally both these findings occur with diffuse disorders and are heard throughout the chest, particularly in the lower lung fields.

Wheezing, a high-pitched musical sound, indicates obstructive airway disease. While wheezing is usually heard during expiration, inspiratory wheezing can occur in severe obstructive disease. Generalized wheezing suggests diffuse obstructive disease, while an area of localized wheezing is more consistent with an anatomic obstruction, such as a mass lesion. Wheezing heard both on inspiration and expiration over the tracheal area suggests tracheal obstruction from scar or neoplasm.

Cardiac examination may suggest right or left ventricular failure, pulmonary hypertension, or intrinsic valvular disease of the heart. Hepatomegaly may suggest metastatic disease from a primary lung carcinoma. Examination of the genitourinary system and the rectum may detect occult malignancy. Examination of the musculoskeletal and neurologic systems may suggest metastatic disease in the skeleton or central nervous system.

ROUTINE LABORATORY TESTING

Certain routine and relatively inexpensive laboratory tests are helpful in evaluating pulmonary disorders. An elevated hemoglobin may be seen with long-standing tissue hypoxia. Elevated platelet count is often a subtle sign of either acute inflammatory disease or tumor. Hypercalcemia can be found with skeletal metastases from lung carcinoma or from the secretion of parathyroid hormonelike substance from carcinoma of the lung. Elevated liver enzymes may suggest metastatic disease.

Several other studies should be performed routinely. Microscopic examination of a specimen of sputum from deep within the tracheobronchial tree can provide information about infection or malignancy. The induced sputum specimen should contain alveolar macrophages, indicating that it came from the lower respiratory tract. Gram stain of the sputum is the most accurate way to diagnose bacterial infection. Fluorescent or acid-fast stains may identify tuberculosis bacilli. Sputum can also be cultured for bacteria, fungi, and mycobacteria. Cytologic examination of the sputum can be highly rewarding in carcinoma of the lung if the specimens are properly induced and processed.

Arterial blood gases accurately document arterial oxygenation and alveolar ventilation. Because of the shape of the hemoglobin dissociation curve, any arterial pO_2 greater than 60 mm saturates over 90% of the hemoglobin molecule and therefore is adequate for normal tissue oxygenation. Arterial blood gases are particularly important if the disease appears to compromise lung function: pneumothorax, empyema, or thoracic trauma, for example.

PULMONARY FUNCTION STUDIES

Pulmonary function studies are helpful in the diagnosis of many pulmonary pathologic processes and in assessing lung function. Function studies define the pathologic physiology of the disease in quantitative terms and therefore replace the qualitative bedside tests of yesteryear. Since age, size, and sex alter normal values, both raw numbers and the percentage of predicted values are reported. Essentially all patients scheduled for elective pulmonary surgery should have at least simple spirometry and analysis of blood gases prior to operation.

Simple spirometry measures vital capacity and expiratory flow rates. After a maximum inspiration, air is forcibly expired as volume and time are recorded. Air flow is commonly reported as a ratio of the FEV_1 to the FVC. An FEV_1/FVC less than 70% indicates significant obstructive disease. If abnormal flows are detected, it is important to retest the patient after bronchodilator therapy. Improvement of flows indicates reversible airways disease, as seen in asthma.

Lung volumes (Fig. 34-4) may be useful in accurately identifying either restrictive or obstructive pulmonary disease. Restrictive lung disease, as in interstitial fibrosis, is characterized by reductions in all lung volumes, particularly the FVC. Obstructive lung disease, as in asthma or emphysema, features a normal or moderately reduced vital capacity with increased total lung capacity, functional residual capacity, and residual volume. Measurement of lung volumes can be performed with the helium dilution method or the body plethysmograph. The helium dilution method may be influenced by poor air mixing within the airways and may provide somewhat inaccurate results in the presence of severe obstructive disease. The body plethysmograph method, which measures only pressure and volume changes, is not influenced by air mixing and is the more accurate and preferred method for measuring lung volumes.

Other pulmonary function tests, performed less commonly, may be indicated in special situations. The single-breath diffusing capacity measures the amount of carbon monoxide transferred from the lung to the blood in a single breath. This test, an index of lung capillary surface area, is reduced in diseases which destroy alveolar units, as seen in emphysema or interstitial fibrosis.

The maximum voluntary ventilation (MVV) is a maneu-ver where the patient breathes as fast and as deeply as possible over a 12-second period. The MVV depends on patient cooperation, motivation, neuromuscular function, and pulmonary function. All these elements may be important in deciding a patient's operative suitability. The MVV has a predictable relationship to the FEV_1. The FEV_1 × 35 should equal the MVV in liters per minute.

If the MVV is less than predicted, the problem may be abnormal inspiratory flow, a parameter often not measured in pulmonary function testing. The forced inspiratory flow between 25% and 75% of the forced inspiratory capacity (FIF 25–75) should be 50% greater than the similarly measured forced expiratory flow (FEF 25–75).

If the inspiratory flow is reduced, upper airway obstruction should be suspected and investigated by means of a flow-volume loop. This plot of lung volume vs. flow may be done manually from a simple spirogram; more commonly it is performed by computer. As mentioned, several characteristic flow-volume loop patterns have been described with obstructing lesions of the upper airway. These patterns can provide precise information about the location as well as the character of the obstructing lesion.

RADIOLOGIC TECHNIQUES

The chest radiograph is essential in the evaluation of the pulmonary patient. While a complete discussion is beyond the scope of this chapter, several elements of the conventional chest radiograph are worth emphasizing. First, chest radiographs are extremely helpful in judging the activity of any pulmonary process. Lung nodules or masses, unchanged over a 2-year period, are rarely malignant. Similarly, a pulmonary process which changes dramatically within 1 to 2 weeks is nearly always inflammatory. In practical terms, a lung nodule must be at least 1 cm in diameter to be seen prospectively in a chest radiograph. Lateral chest films, and sometimes oblique views, are required to locate abnormal pulmonary shadows or nodules accurately. A nodule not seen on the lateral film may not be in the lung at all but may lie in the chest wall or represent an artifact.

Tomography provides sequential views at different levels of the lung and may be helpful in demonstrating central calcification within a nodule, cavitation, or vascular shadows. Whole lung tomography may also detect multiple nodules when metastatic disease to the lung is suspected. Tomograms taken at 55° oblique position may demonstrate hilar and mediastinal adenopathy that is not apparent on the plain chest radiograph.

Radiographic imaging of many organs including the lung has been enhanced by the use of computed tomography (CT scan) (Fig. 34-5). Since conventional pulmonary radiographs already provide much information, the impact of lung CT scans has been less than that of CT scans of some other organs. The lung CT scan, particularly with the use of contrast agents, provides an excellent three-dimensional view of the mediastinum. Vascular and soft tissue structures can be easily distinguished. In patients with abnormal mediastinal radiographs, the CT scan may accurately define the structure and location of the abnormality. Unfortunately, the CT scan has not proven sensitive enough to detect small lymph nodes with metastatic disease. The CT scan is also an excellent method for studying the pleural–parenchymal interface and may be useful in designing diagnostic or therapeutic approaches when conventional radiographs do not distinguish between parenchymal and pleural lesions.

Fig. 34-4. The effect of lung disease on lung volume in a 40-year-old 180 cm man. In interstitial fibrosis, all lung volumes—especially VC—are reduced. With bronchitis and emphysema, air trapping from obstruction results in increased lung volumes but a reduced VC. (VC = vital capacity; RV = residual volume; TLC = total lung capacity; FRC = functional residual capacity)

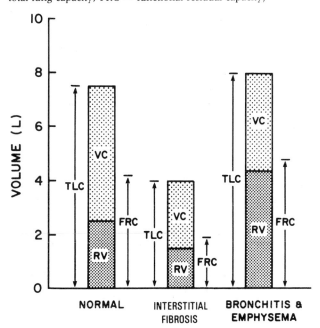

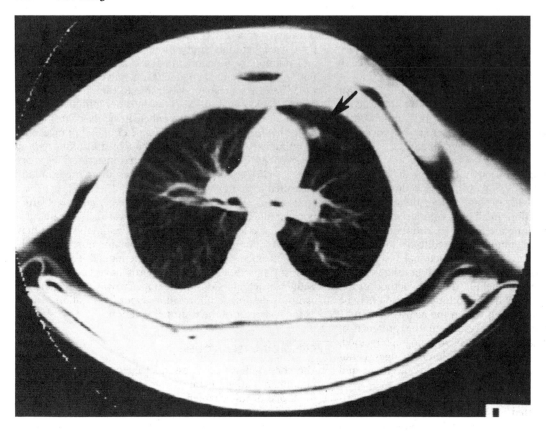

Fig. 34-5. CT scan in a woman with Wilms' tumor shows an 8-mm metastatic nodule along the left cardiac border *(arrow).* The chest roentgenogram was normal.

A third application of CT scanning is in the evaluation of the solitary pulmonary nodule. The CT scan can resolve lesions as small as a fraction of a millimeter and provide clues as to the benign or malignant nature of the lesion. Although this high-resolution technology is not generally available, the technique is promising for the noninvasive evaluation of solitary pulmonary nodules.

RADIONUCLIDE SCANNING

Radionuclide lung scans provide detailed information about ventilation and perfusion of the pulmonary parenchyma. Perfusion scanning is performed with macroaggregated albumin tagged with a radionuclide such as technetium. Injected intravenously, the material lodges in the pulmonary circulation and provides an image of blood flow through the pulmonary capillary bed. Destruction of this capillary network, as in emphysema, or obstruction of blood flow, as with pulmonary emboli, produces perfusion defects. Ventilation abnormalities are detected by the use of inert, nonabsorbable radioactive gases such as xenon. Inhaled xenon is distributed according to the ventilatory pattern of the lung. Areas of V/Q imbalance can then be documented with these complementary methods of lung scanning.

V/Q scanning is commonly employed in two situations: the diagnosis of pulmonary embolism and the preoperative evaluation for lung surgery. A normal perfusion scan rules out the diagnosis of pulmonary embolism. Scans with perfusion defects corresponding to segmental or lobar areas of the lung associated with normal ventilation are diagnostic of pulmonary embolism with at least 80% certainty. In contrast, multiple non-segmental defects (particularly when matched by ventilation defects) suggest diffuse parenchymal disease, such as chronic obstructive lung disease. Such a pattern is associated with a less than 15% likelihood of pulmonary embolism. In doubtful cases, the diagnosis should be clarified with a pulmonary angiogram.

The lung scan can be helpful in evaluating pulmonary function before pulmonary surgery. By quantifying the radioactivity over different areas of the lung, the perfusion scan can document the contribution of any anatomic area to the patient's overall pulmonary function. This permits an accurate assessment of the physiologic effect of any contemplated pulmonary resection.

A different radionuclide technique, gallium lung scanning, is useful for detecting inflammation. Radioactive gallium is actively taken up by inflammatory cells such as polymorphonuclear leukocytes. While the gallium scan is sensitive for detecting areas of active disease, it provides very little information about the specific disease process. In the lung, the gallium scan is useful in two situations: staging of lung carcinoma and assessment of inflammation in diffuse inflammatory parenchymal diseases such as idiopathic pulmonary fibrosis. Gallium is taken up by most primary carcinomas of the lung, except adenocarcinoma. When the tumor does concentrate gallium, metastatic disease within the thorax may also be detected. Several small studies have suggested that gallium scanning may be a useful screening technique to determine the need for mediastinal exploration prior to resection of lung carcinoma.

Liver and bone scans may be useful in staging patients with lung cancer. These studies are not recommended routinely because of frequent false positive results. However, in patients with constitutional symptoms, abnormal liver function tests, or bone pain, positive scans may confirm suspicions of metastatic disease. Brain scanning is indicated for lung cancer patients with neurologic signs and symptoms. However, this technique may be supplanted by computed tomography (CT) scans of the brain.

BRONCHOSCOPY

A specific tissue diagnosis is usually desirable before lung surgery is undertaken. Specimens of pulmonary tissue can be obtained in several different ways. With fiberoptic bronchoscopy, the tracheobronchial tree may be inspected, airway secretions obtained, and bronchial and alveolar tissue sampled. Under local or general anesthesia, the flexible fiberoptic bronchoscope is inserted through the nasal or oral passages. Lesions visualized through the bronchoscope can be easily brushed for cytology and biopsied.

If the lesion is beyond the visualization of the fiberoptic bronchoscope, fluoroscopy may be used to guide the placement of biopsy brush or forceps. For a transbronchial biopsy, the forceps are wedged into a distant bronchus during expiration. When the forceps ensnare the entrapped bronchial wall, areas of peribronchial alveolar tissue are included in the specimen. With this technique some diffuse parenchymal processes such as lymphangitic spread of carcinoma, sarcoidosis, or miliary tuberculosis can be accurately diagnosed.

In experienced hands, fiberoptic bronchoscopy and its biopsy techniques have very little morbidity and mortality. In patients with underlying bronchospasm, bronchoscopy may provoke airway obstruction easily reversible with bronchodilators. The rare patient develops a postbronchoscopy pneumonitis that is usually mild and self-limiting. With bronchoscopic biopsy two major complications have been observed. Pneumothorax can occur with transbronchial biopsy, but the use of fluoroscopy during the procedure has virtually eliminated this problem. Endobronchial bleeding from biopsies, while usually mild, can occasionally be life-threatening. Avoiding bronchoscopic biopsies in patients with bleeding disorders, pulmonary hypertension, or uremia has reduced this complication.

In malignancy, the diagnostic accuracy of fiberoptic bronchoscopy is dependent on the size and location of the lesion. Endoscopically visible tumors can be diagnosed with over 90% accuracy. For small lesions close to the mediastinum or in the far edges of the lung, accurate placement of biopsy forceps is difficult even with fluoroscopy. Consequently, diagnostic accuracy in these circumstances is under 40%. Moderate-sized malignant lesions in the mid-lung fields can be accurately diagnosed in about 60% to 70% of patients, by a combination of cytology and histologic examination of biopsied tissue.

NEEDLE ASPIRATION

For small nodules or infiltrates in areas of the lung inaccessible to the bronchoscope, needle aspiration is a useful diagnostic technique. With this method, a long needle (usually 18 to 25 gauge) is passed through the chest wall under fluoroscopy into the abnormal area of the lung. When the needle is in the correct position, gentle suction is applied to obtain a small sample of cells for cytology and culture. The technique is relatively easy to perform, with an acceptably low complication rate; hemoptysis occurs infre-

quently, and pneumothorax occurs in 20% of patients, with only a fifth of this group requiring chest tube drainage. In the presence of malignancy or infection, the "skinny needle" aspiration is about 90% sensitive, but inconclusive results do not rule out any diagnosis. This technique has replaced the use of large cutting biopsy needles and trephine core drills, which were associated with high incidences of hemothorax and pneumothorax.

THORACENTESIS AND PLEURAL BIOPSY

Disorders in the pleural space often produce pleural effusions that are easily aspirated. For nonloculated effusions, the pleural fluid may be located by percussion and auscultation. Thoracentesis is easily accomplished using local anesthesia. Loculated fluid with high fibrin content may be difficult to aspirate. The precise location of a pocket of free fluid can be identified with the use of ultrasound or with fluoroscopic examination of the chest.

Aspirated pleural fluid should be examined for protein content, cell count, cytology, pH, and culture. Exudative fluid, characterized by a protein concentration which is at least 50% that of serum, always indicates some inflammatory process in or near the pleural space. Frankly bloody effusion with red cell count in excess of 100,000 is seen in thoracic trauma, pulmonary infarct, malignancy, and (rarely) tuberculosis. Aspiration of frank pus on thoracentesis indicates empyema. Opalescent fluid with a high triglyceride content is seen in chylothorax. Culture of pleural fluid is often highly rewarding, particularly in tuberculosis effusions.

Biopsy of the parietal pleura with a Cope or Abrams needle is particularly useful for the diagnosis of pleural malignancy and tuberculosis. Multiple samples of the pleura can be obtained at the same time as thoracentesis. In addition to histologic examination, these samples can be cultured to improve diagnostic yield. In malignancy of the pleural space, the combination of pleural fluid and pleural biopsy yields a diagnosis in 90% of cases. In tuberculous pleurisy the figure is similar, with nearly 80% of patients diagnosed by culture of pleural fluid and pleural biopsy. With care to avoid intercostal arteries, pleural biopsy is a safe technique with a low incidence of pneumo- or hemothorax.

Thoracoscopy is another technique for obtaining fluid or tissue from the parietal or visceral pleura. A fiberoptic or rigid instrument is introduced into the pleural space through a small incision in the chest wall. Biopsies of suspicious areas can be obtained under direct visual control. Although infrequently used, this technique in selected patients can provide accurate diagnostic information.

SKIN TESTING

Cellular immunity is often assessed in patients with lung disease. Previous exposure to tuberculosis is documented by skin testing with tuberculin antigen. Intermediate-strength PPD of 5 tine units (TU) is injected intradermally and examined for induration 48 hours later. Induration 10 mm or greater is considered significant and indicative of previous tuberculin exposure. If the exposure was in the distant past, it may be necessary to repeat skin testing two weeks later to evoke a diagnostic response. Importantly, a falsely negative skin test can occur because cellular immunity is too low to produce any delayed hypersensitivity reaction to common antigens. This state, termed anergy, can be documented by the presence of negative skin tests to common antigens, such as mumps and candida. Anergy occurs with debilitating disorders such as malnutrition, systemic infection, and advanced malignancy, particularly lymphoma.

More specific information about immunologic reactions within the lung can be obtained with the technique of bronchoalveolar lavage. Immunologically active cells such as lymphocytes and alveolar macrophages can be harvested directly from the lung by segmental saline lavage through the fiberoptic bronchoscope. With special immunologic techniques, T-cell and B-cell lymphocytes can be identified and their numbers compared to other harvested cells, such as macrophages and neutrophils. Certain cellular patterns have been associated with various inflammatory diseases in the lung, including sarcoidosis and interstitial fibrosis.

BRONCHOGRAPHY

Bronchography, once widely used as a diagnostic procedure, has largely been replaced by studies such as fiberoptic bronchoscopy and noninvasive radiologic techniques such as CT scanning. For the bronchogram, a contrast agent, usually an iodinated liquid, is instilled into the tracheobronchial tree either through a tracheal catheter or a fiberoptic bronchoscope. The topography of the airways can then be defined. The risks of this procedure are dye reaction, bronchial obstruction, infection, and reduced pulmonary function.

Bronchography can be useful if precise anatomic definition of a bronchial abnormality is necessary. For example, a cinetracheogram may help distinguish malacia from stenosis. Bronchography may also define the extent of bronchiectasis if surgical resection is contemplated. Occasionally a bronchopleural fistula or congenital anomalies of the tracheobronchial tree may be visualized only in the bronchogram. However, these clinical situations occur infrequently, and for most purposes other safer diagnostic studies generally provide as much or more information.

ANGIOGRAPHY

The pulmonary angiogram is commonly used to establish the diagnosis of pulmonary embolism. In experienced hands the technique has minimal risk, particularly if patients with dye reactions and severe pulmonary hypertension are excluded. The accuracy of angiography for pulmonary embolism is nearly 100% if selective segmental injections and magnification views are employed. The pulmonary angiogram may also be used to diagnose other vascular problems, such as arteriovenous malformations, vasculitis, or compression of pulmonary vasculature by bulla or tumor.

Angiography of the systemic arterial circulation occasionally can be helpful in diagnosing and treating massive hemoptysis. Most brisk bleeding from the lung comes from the bronchial arterial circulation. Sometimes, the exact site of bleeding can be identified by bronchial angiography. This may facilitate surgery, but if surgery is not feasible, embolization of the bleeding bronchial vessel may stop the lung hemorrhage. Angiography can identify the vascular supply of a different condition, pulmonary sequestration, which originates from the systemic circulation.

ASSESSMENT OF OPERABILITY

The normal lung has an enormous functional reserve such that oxygen uptake can increase from 250 or 300 ml/min at rest to nearly 2000 ml/min during maximum exercise. Consequently, an individual can lose a large percentage of pulmonary functional capacity to an insidious disease process and still remain asymptomatic at rest and during ordinary activity. Since many operations involve resection of lung parenchyma, an assessment of functional reserve is an important criterion to determine operability.

In determining operability, clinical factors such as age, alertness, motivation to recover, nutritional status, and presence of disease in other organ systems must be considered. Sometimes these factors alone argue for nonoperative treatment, even though long-term results are clearly better from a successful operation.

Although many sophisticated pulmonary function tests are available to define specifically the pathologic physiology of lung disease, only a few relatively simple tests are helpful in determining operability. The most useful tests include vital capacity (VC), FEV, FEV_1, and MVV. These tests are easily obtained by spirometry before and after administration of a bronchodilator. In addition, arterial oxygen and carbon dioxide tensions and pH at rest are important. If pneumonectomy is contemplated, a single-breath CO measurement of diffusing capacity and measurement of mean pulmonary arterial pressure by a Swan-Ganz catheter may add important information in borderline cases.

After thoracotomy, inspiratory capacity, VC, and FRC are all reduced primarily because of pain. Reduced ventilation and reluctance to cough or sigh encourage atelectasis.

No constellation of criteria defines the borderline between safe and unsafe lung resections. It must be remembered that pulmonary function in patients with chronic bronchitis can be often improved by an intensive period of medical management that includes abstinence from smoking, antibiotic bronchodilators, and chest physiotherapy. Usually, if patients can tolerate thoracotomy, lobectomy is well tolerated, since only 15% to 25% of the lung mass is removed by an upper or lower lobectomy. Pneumonectomy, on the other hand, is a mutilating operation which removes approximately 50% of the lung mass. After pneumonectomy, VC, compliance, and diffusing capacity are reduced but airway resistance and arterial blood gases do not change. If the remaining lung is normal, pulmonary arterial pressure does not increase except during moderate exercise.

Some clinical and laboratory criteria argue against successful pneumonectomy. Severe dyspnea unimproved by good medical management, severe hypoxia ($paO_2 < 55$ torr) at rest, or CO_2 retention ($pCO_2 > 55$ torr) in patients with COPD indicate little pulmonary reserve. An FEV_1 less than 1.5, diffusing capacity or MVV less than 50% of normal, or pulmonary hypertension (mean pulmonary artery pressure >25 torr) do not favor successful pneumonectomy. The final decision often requires considerable judgment, weighing the natural history and time course of the disease and other therapeutic options against the estimated risk of resection.

BIBLIOGRAPHY

FISHMAN AP: Pulmonary Disease and Disorders. New York, McGraw-Hill, 1980

HOPEWELL PC, MURRAY JF: The adult respiratory distress syndrome. Ann Rev Med 27:343, 1976

LILLINGTON GA: The solitary nodule. Am Rev Resp Dis 110:699, 1977

MITTMAN C, BRUDERMAN I: Lung cancer: To operate or not? Am Rev Resp Dis 116:477, 1977

WEST JB: Pulmonary Pathophysiology: The Essentials. Baltimore, Williams & Wilkins, 1977

WEST JB: Respiratory Physiology: The Essentials, 2nd ed. Baltimore, Williams & Wilkins, 1979

Harvey I. Pass

Suppurative Conditions of the Lung, Tuberculosis, and Fungal Disease

PNEUMONITIS

Diffuse pulmonary disease, or pneumonitis, may have many causes and may be acute or chronic, symptomatic or asymptomatic, benign or malignant. The role of the surgeon in the diagnosis and treatment of pneumonitis has been expanded with the application of fiberoptic bronchoscopy, transthoracic needle biopsy, mediastinoscopy, and open lung biopsy. The diagnosis of a new pulmonary infiltrate in the patient who has an obvious history of postoperative aspiration of gastric contents is academic. The thoracic surgeon, on the other hand, is usually presented with a patient who does not have such an obvious history. The first portion of this chapter is concerned with the classification of diffuse lung disease and the diagnostic workup of patients with this disorder.

CLASSIFICATION OF DIFFUSE LUNG DISEASE

More than 100 diseases belong in the category of pneumonitis, and most are associated with a specific etiologic agent, either infectious, occupational, immunologic, or idiopathic. Pneumonitis may also be characterized by its radiographic appearance—hilar enlargement, diffuse nodular lesions, miliary or reticular pattern, or "honeycomb lung." Table 34-1 provides a partial classification of these disorders.

HISTORY AND SYMPTOMATOLOGY

The characteristic complaint in patients afflicted with symptomatic pneumonitis is *dyspnea* associated with a feeling of easy fatigability or nonproductive cough. An accurate history will make the diagnosis in 21% of the cases. Key points include the following:

Occupation: Present and past, types of material used, exposure to fumes, spray, or dust, tools used, and the relation of the onset of symptoms to the time and type of occupation

Environment: Exposure to pets, travel history (especially in regions endemic to certain lung infections), hobbies

Infection: Exposure to tuberculosis in the past, past documentation of TB skin test, family members with recent onset of pulmonary disease

Previous Illnesses: Diabetes, rheumatoid arthritis, leukemia, cystic fibrosis, seizure disorder, gammaglobulin deficiency, alcoholism, previous medications, associated abdominal symptoms

Habits: Smoking history, use of mineral oil for laxation, or oily nose drops

Fever, chest pain, and hemoptysis, as well as the quality and quantity of sputum should be carefully documented.

PHYSICAL EXAMINATION

The presence of peripheral adenopathy, clubbing, or extrathoracic manifestations of pulmonary malignancy should be ascertained. The *respiratory pattern,* labored or relaxed, with splinting or retraction, defines the severity of the illness. Tactile fremitus, bronchophony, and whispered pec-

TABLE 34-1 CLASSIFICATION OF DIFFUSE LUNG DISEASE

I. Infectious pneumonitis
Bacterial
Fungal
Viral
Parasitic
II. Occupational
Silicosis
Anthracosis
Asbestosis
III. Organic dust
Spores
Avian-related antigens
IV. Irritant gases
V. Aspiration pneumonia
VI. Oxygen toxicity
VII. Burn injury
VIII. Radiation
IX. Drug induced
X. Idiopathic
Sarcoid
Wegener's granulomatosis
XI. Idiopathic interstitial pneumonitis
Desquamative
"Usual"
Giant cell
Lymphocytic
XII. Collagen vascular disease

toriloquy, as well as rales, wheezes, or friction rubs, should be correlated with the radiographic location of the pneumonitis.

Pulmonary function testing in patients with pneumonitis should be performed before and after treatment. The changes seen with early diffuse lung disease include

Normal maximal breathing capacity with normal FEV_1

Increased dead space

Reduced oxygen tension with exercise

Increased alveolar–arterial oxygen gradient

Hypocapnia and respiratory alkalosis

With more severe disease vital capacity and total lung capacity are diminished. There is always a ventilation–perfusion imbalance with physiological right to left shunting. Pulmonary function testing in itself, however, cannot distinguish the cause of one pneumonitis from another.

DIAGNOSTIC EVALUATION

X-RAY FILMS

Despite many classifications of the x-ray appearance of diffuse lung disease, the spectrum is wide, and it is rarely possible to make a specific diagnosis from x-ray appearance alone (Fig. 34-6). X-ray films, therefore, in most cases simply confirm the presence of a pulmonary infiltrate and document improvement after treatment has started. Tomograms may delineate mediastinal adenopathy, calcification patterns, or cavitary disease.

SPUTUM EXAMINATION

Sputum examination for routine culture, along with acid-fast smears and fungal cultures, must be obtained. If the patient cannot produce sufficient quantities on his own, induction with an ultrasonic nebulizer may be useful. Sulfur granules of actinomycosis, asbestos bodies, lipid-containing macrophages of lipoid pneumonia, or *Pneumocystis carinii* parasites on methenamine silver staining may be seen on sputum cytologies.

SKIN TESTING

Tuberculin skin testing should be applied to rule out the presence of tuberculosis. The Kveim test for sarcoid and the Caroni skin test for hydatid cyst disease are of doubtful use.

LABORATORY BLOOD TESTS

Rheumatoid factor, antinuclear antibody, cold agglutinins, and complement fixation testing for fungal diseases are often useful in the workup of diffuse lung disease. Peripheral blood smears should also be examined, and the calcium level, which may correlate with malignancy, sarcoidosis, or myelomas, should be determined.

THORACENTESIS AND PLEURAL BIOPSY

When a pleural effusion is demonstrated on chest x-ray, thoracentesis and pleural biopsy should be performed. Gram stain, cultures, and cytologic examination should be recorded as well as rheumatoid factor, pH, specific gravity, protein, cell count, and differential cell count. Glucose determinations as well as LDH are also useful. A low pH (less than 7.2) usually indicates empyema, and neutrophils tend to predominate in inflammatory pleural effusion, whereas mononuclear cells are more commonly associated with malignancy, lymphoma, and tuberculosis. Before thoracentesis a pleural biopsy should be performed with a Cope or Abrams needle.

BRONCHOSCOPY

The fiberoptic bronchoscope permits examination of the segmental and subsegmental bronchi to the fourth and fifth order. Mucosal abnormalities consistent with inflammation or neoplasm should be identified by biopsy. Bronchial brushings should be performed but are mainly used in diseases with endobronchial manifestations. Bronchoscope placement in abnormal segments can be assured by using fluoroscopy, and transbronchial biopsy can then be performed to obtain specimens from the peripheral parenchyma for histologic evaluation, of which the overall accuracy is approximately 52%. This yield is even higher when transbronchial biopsy is combined with bronchial brushing and selective washings for culture and cytology.

TRANSTHORACIC NEEDLE ASPIRATION BIOPSY

Under fluoroscopic control, transthoracic needle biopsy of the area of pneumonitis may be performed if bronchial washings, brushings, and transbronchial biopsy are not diagnostic. Material is obtained for a bacteriologic smear and culture as well as cytologic study. Rates of accuracy of diagnosis reach 96%. Pneumothorax and mild hemoptysis may occur, and biopsy is contraindicated in patients with pulmonary hypertension, bleeding diathesis, or bullous emphysema.

OPEN LUNG BIOPSY

When all the above methods do not lead to a conclusive etiology for the pneumonitis and the patient's condition permits general anesthesia, open lung biopsy may be performed. *Progressive undiagnosed illness* and anticipated use of

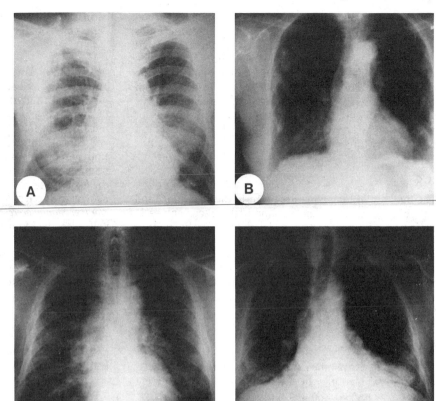

Fig. 34-6. Four examples of diffuse lung disease. *(A)* Anthracosis. *(B)* Asbestosis. *(C)* Idiopathic pulmonary fibrosis. *(D)* Desquamative interstitial pneumonitis.

corticosteroids are also indications for open lung biopsy. Biopsies are taken from the diseased segment with the lung fully expanded. One portion of the specimen is fixed immediately, and other portions of the specimen are dispatched for electron microscopy and assorted cultures.

TREATMENT

The treatment of diffuse lung disease will be influenced not only by the etiology of the disease but also by its severity. Antibiotic therapy, either singly or in combination with other drugs, must be used against specific organisms as determined by sensitivity testing. The use of supportive treatment with oxygen therapy as well as tracheal intubation will be determined by the patient's clinical appearance together with arterial blood gas parameters. *Stable preexisting fibrosis requires no specific treatment,* and specific indications for steroid use include collagen vascular disease, hypersensitivity pneumonitis, and selected cases of interstitial pneumonitis. Finally, elimination of offending environmental factors must be accomplished either by use of a protective mask for the patient on the job or by change of occupation.

LUNG ABSCESS

HISTORY

Hawthorne provided one of the earliest descriptions of the diagnosis and surgical management of lung abscess in 1819. Drainage of a lung abscess in an alcoholic patient resulted in the discharge of "twelve pounds of vitiated matter." Early medical treatment of this condition led to a mortality of 90%, and surgical drainage also had a prohibitive mortality of 40%. Improvement in the treatment of lung abscess resulted from control of infection by antibiotics, use of postural drainage based on knowledge of segmental anatomy, and earlier surgical treatment with either drainage or resection. Although the majority of lung abscesses can now be controlled without thoracotomy, surgical therapy remains important because of bacterial resistance, incomplete resolution with antibiotics (resulting in a continuing illness), and the need to rule out neoplasms.

DEFINITION AND ETIOLOGY

A lung abscess can be defined as a pus-containing cavity within the lung parenchyma that develops from a localized area of suppurative pneumonitis. Lung abscess may be *primary* (as with aspiration) or *secondary.* Etiologically, lung abscess may be grouped into five major categories as follows:

Bronchial occlusion by aspiration of septic material, bronchial carcinoma or benign bronchial tumors, or by interbronchial foreign body

Specific pneumonias such as *Staphylococcus,* actinomycosis, and anaerobic organisms

Nonspecific suppurative pneumonia such as occurs with aspiration pneumonitis or from vascular occlusion by emboli

Trauma that produces an infected hematoma or persistence of a foreign body within the parenchyma of the lung

Esophageal disorders due to cricopharyngeal or epiphrenic diverticuli, achalasia, or esophageal neoplasm.

Lung abscesses are usually associated with gingival or oral disease, aspiration due to alcoholism, anesthesia, diabetic coma, or drug addiction. After bronchial occlusion causes atelectasis, the aspirated material may infect this atelectatic area, producing a suppurative pneumonia that leads to the lung abscess. With opportunistic lung abscesses, normal host defenses are usually diminished, as in the elderly. In children, lung abscesses may be associated with congenital defects, prematurity, or bronchopneumonia. Patients who require immunosuppression with steroids or Imuran or who are undergoing radiation therapy are subject to secondary lung abscesses.

LOCATION

The majority of lung abscesses occur in the right lung, and 75% of lung abscesses can be found in three segments—(1) the superior segment of the right lower lobe, (2) the superior segment of the left lower lobe, and (3) the posterior segment of the right upper lobe.

When the patient is supine, aspirated contents gravitate to the dependent apical bronchi of the lower lobe, and when the patient is on his side the posterior segments of the upper lobes are affected.

SYMPTOMS AND SIGNS

With an *acute abscess,* the patient usually presents with fever, malaise, and pleuritic chest pain. Cough may be present but rarely hemoptysis. With rupture into the bronchial tree, copious amounts (50 to 500 ml per day) of foul-smelling sputum may be produced. If the patient presents with acute shortness of breath with hyperpnea and peripheral vascular collapse, an acute *pyopneumothorax* must be ruled out. Signs of a lung abscess include fetid breath, rapid and labored breathing, and localized chest wall tenderness. Broncho-vesicular breath sounds and moist rales will be heard in the area of the lung abscess. An inspection of the oropharynx may reveal poor dentition. The signs of a *chronic abscess* may

be masked by antibiotics, but the patient usually presents with pain, cough, and sputum production.

DIAGNOSIS

The key to the diagnosis of lung abscess involves sputum examination and roentgenography of the chest. The quantity of sputum produced must be measured daily, and samples must be sent for routine bacterial culture and tuberculous and fungal culture, as well as for cytologic examination. Both aerobic and anaerobic cultures must be performed. In primary lung abscesses, anaerobic causative bacteria include the fusiform bacilli, anaerobic streptococci, spirochetes, and *Bacteroides* species. Aerobic bacteria such as *Diplococcus pneumoniae, Staphylococcus aureus,* and β-hemolytic streptococci will also be found. *Staphylococcus aureus* as well as α-streptococci, *Neisseria, Klebsiella, Proteus,* and *Escherichia coli* are usually associated with opportunistic lung abscesses.

When ordering radiographs of the chest in patients with suspected lung abscess, four views of the chest are helpful for localization. Early in the course of disease only segmental atelectasis with pneumonitis may be seen. With communication to a bronchus an air–fluid level will be visualized. With successful treatment the cavity will decrease in size and disappear altogether. Occasionally, however, the cavity will form a more organized wall and remain as a chronic abscess, appearing as a thin- or thick-walled cyst. In cases of chronic abscess, bronchography may be useful in demonstrating early filling of the cavity and associated bronchiectasis (Fig. 34-7).

COMPLICATIONS

Insufficiently treated lung abscess can lead to life-threatening complications. There can be spread to the noninvolved pulmonary segments, leading to diffuse bronchopneumonia and multiple abscesses that are more difficult to treat.

Fig. 34-7. Chronic lung abscess. *(A)* Thick-walled cavity with air–fluid level. *(B)* Bronchography reveals splaying of bronchi to the anterior and posterior segments of the right upper lobe.

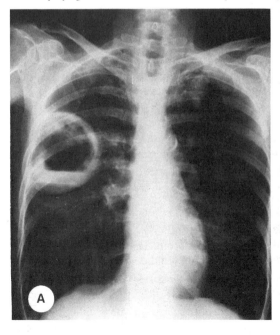 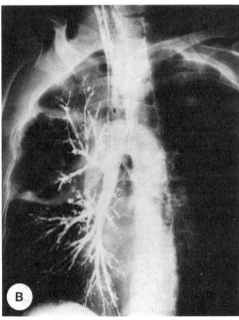

Rupture into the pleural cavity causing a tension pyopneumothorax as well as rupture into the bronchial artery with life-threatening hemoptysis are morbid complications. Generalized dissemination with overwhelming sepsis as well as a brain abscess that is difficult to diagnose may also occur. Finally, the development of a chronic lung abscess will only increase the difficulty of resolving the disease with antibiotic therapy.

TREATMENT

Antibiotic therapy remains the mainstay of management of lung abscess. Twenty million units per day of penicillin for a duration of 4 weeks should be started when the disease is diagnosed. It should be given parenterally for at least 2 weeks. Additional or substitution of other antibiotics are dictated by the results of sputum culture with sensitivity testing. If fever and toxicity persist, bronchoscopy must be performed, sometimes daily, to obtain anaerobic brushings and washings. Selective bronchial catheterization is also necessary for drainage by fluoroscopy. Coordination with a respiratory therapy team should be initiated early, with the use of chest physiotherapy and postural drainage. If fever and sputum production decrease and if the chest x-ray film shows improvement, the abscess will usually resolve with no sequelae.

Surgical therapy is indicated during the fulminating stage of lung abscess in which the patient appears toxic and when there is no resolution of fever despite antibiotic treatment. Closed tube thoracostomy should be performed only if there is associated empyema or if the physician is confident that there has been pleural symphysis. With chronic nonresolving lung abscess, location by aspiration, rib resection (Fig. 34-8), and opening of the cavity with insertion of a tube can be curative. Life-threatening hemoptysis calls for emergent lobectomy. If there is a large residual cavity (greater than 2 cm) despite clinical improvement after 4 to 6 weeks of antibiotic therapy, the diagnosis of malignancy must be entertained. Pyopneumothorax, due to bronchopleural fistula and empyema, should be treated initially with closed tube thoracostomy. Patients who have suffered destruction of a lobe with continuing symptomatology (sputum production, hemoptysis) require lobectomy.

Operative management of lung abscess by thoracotomy must be approached with extreme caution. Adequate preoperative antibiotics must be given to prevent possible dissemination with resulting cerebral abscess. Use of a double lumen tube (Carlen's) or selective ventilation (Fig. 34-9) is mandatory to prevent aspiration of contents in the dependent lung. Early clamping of the bronchus will also prevent interbronchial dissemination. The treatment of lung abscess by surgical techniques should encompass no less than a lobectomy to decrease the incidence of postoperative complications including bronchopleural fistula and empyema.

RESULTS OF TREATMENT

The treatment of primary lung abscess with antibiotics has resulted in a decrease in mortality from 25% to 5%. However, opportunistic lung abscess still has a mortality of approximately 75%, despite all treatment modalities.

BRONCHIECTASIS

Bronchiectasis is a suppurative pulmonary disease whose clinical course is characterized by infection of dilated bronchi with purulent sputum and recurrent respiratory infection. The incidence of new cases of bronchiectasis has markedly decreased since its discovery in 1819 by Laennec owing to the use of antibiotics for childhood respiratory disorders. Pulmonary resection, however, remains the best hope of cure for long-standing localized disease that is resistant to primary medical therapy.

ETIOLOGY

The development of bronchiectasis can be traced in most instances to one of four causes— (1) infection, (2) bronchial obstruction, (3) congenital causes, including immune deficiency, or (4) deficiency of bronchial cartilage.

Fig. 34-8. Steps in rib resection. *(A)* Incision carried down to musculature after localization with needle. *(B)* Subperiosteal rib removal. *(C)* Closure of muscle around a large bore tube, which now drains the abscess cavity.

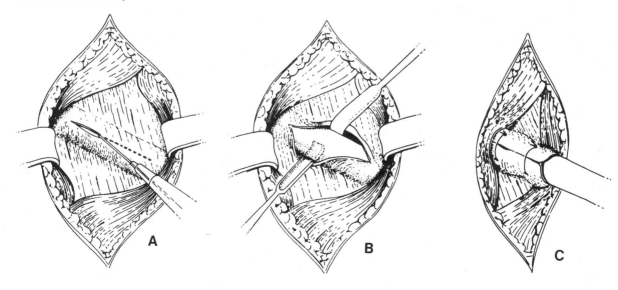

A   **B**   **C**

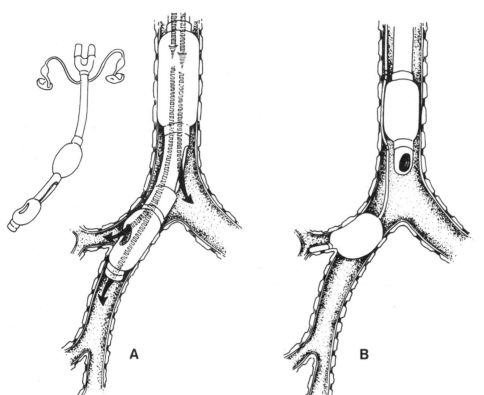

Fig. 34-9. Methods of selective ventilation. *(A)* Robert-Shaw tube. *(B)* Large intrabronchial Fogarty catheter (No. 6 or 7).

INFECTION

The childhood illnesses associated with bronchiectasis are well-managed medically and prophylactically at this time with vaccines and antibiotics. Tuberculosis and diffuse pneumonitis, however, remain a challenge, and in spite of vigorous treatment may cause bronchiectasis through residual scarring and contracture. This inflammatory process creates external traction of the cartilages with the least support, the second through the fourth order bronchi, causing dilation. This is the so-called traction theory.

BRONCHIAL OBSTRUCTION

Bronchial obstruction from any cause, including foreign body, tumor, or inflammatory stenosis, may cause bronchial dilation and infection. Extrinsic pressure by nodes involved with tuberculosis or fungal pneumonitis may give rise to middle lobe bronchiectasis by producing the middle lobe syndrome. It has been shown that completion of the fissure between the upper and middle lobe also plays a role, because an incomplete fissure will allow collateral ventilation and improve atelectasis, thus decreasing the chance of middle lobe bronchiectasis.

CONGENITAL DISORDERS

A number of congenital disorders are associated with bronchiectasis. In most cases, however, congenital cystic bronchiectasis is really an early acquired disease associated with unrecognized infection. *Kartagener's syndrome* of pansinusitis, situs inversus, and bronchiectasis is an associated genetic disorder of faulty respiratory cilia causing insufficient mucociliary transport. *Deficiency of α_1-antitrypsin*, a protease inhibitor, may subject the lung elastin and collagen to abnormally high levels of proteases released from leukocytes. This can lead to the production of bronchiectasis if the patient experiences recurrent respiratory infections. *Cystic fibrosis*, by affecting the properties of the tracheobronchial mucus and adequacy of ciliary clearance, causes retention of secretions, plugging of the airways, and overgrowth of bacteria with bronchial destruction.

PATHOLOGY

Bronchiectasis is a segmental disease that primarily involves the lower lobes and basal segments. The superior segments are usually spared, but the right middle lobe (40%) and lingula (70%) are often affected. The shape of the dilated bronchi may give a clue to the stage of development of the disease because early dilation is often cylindrical and more advanced disease tends to be saccular or fusiform. The classification of bronchiectasis by shape, however, indicates neither the prognosis nor the severity of the disease (Fig. 34-10).

Grossly, the lung may have a normal external appearance with areas of atelectasis. Bronchial structures are thickened when palpated, and there is extensive destruction of the bronchial wall with peribronchial pneumonitis. Microscopically, there is an intense cellular inflammatory response with destruction of the bronchial mucosa.

CLINICAL MANIFESTATIONS

Recurrent pneumonia, productive cough, and the presence of purulent fetid sputum are the usual clinical manifestations of bronchiectasis. Symptomatic patients may complain of seasonal exacerbations, especially in cold weather. With long-standing disease the patient may complain of dyspnea and typically is asthenic, pale, and chronically ill. Only long-standing disease will exhibit pulmonary osteoarthropathy. Hemoptysis occurs in 50% of the patients, especially those with diffuse disease and disease localized to the upper

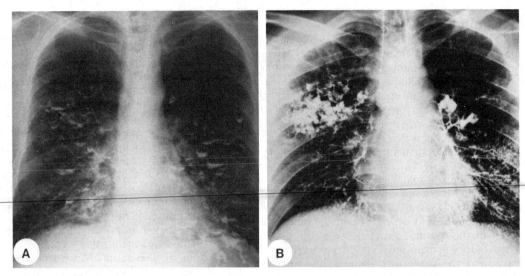

Fig. 34-10. Cystic bronchiectasis. *(A)* Diffuse disease. *(B)* Disease localized to the upper lobe, primarily the right. (This patient would have a significantly higher chance of a good result with pulmonary resection than the patient in *A*.) (The definitive diagnosis of bronchiectasis requires a bronchogram.)

lobes as a result of old tuberculosis. Physical examination reveals dullness to percussion with diminished breath sounds in the affected lobe and the presence of moist rales or expiratory rhonchi.

DIAGNOSIS

The diagnosis of bronchiectasis is rarely made with the conventional roentgenogram of the chest. Increased pulmonary vascularity, honeycombing, or prominent bronchial markings are nonspecific findings. Bronchoscopy will reveal bronchial erythema with copious mucopurulent sputum. The particular segment affected by the disease may appear inflamed and dilated, and bronchoscopy will help to rule out the possibility of endobronchial lesions, strictures, and foreign bodies. Sputa, uncontaminated by the nasopharynx, can be collected for microbiologic examination from the obviously affected segment.

Bronchography is the definitive diagnostic modality for demonstrating the extent and localization of bronchiectatic segments. Most secretions must be drained prior to the study by good postural drainage, and the patient must not have acute widespread infection. It is best to study one lung at a time because the chemical pneumonitis attending the procedure can significantly decrease vital capacity. The patient fasts after midnight and is given premedication with a barbiturate for sedation. Codeine may also be given as a premedication to depress the cough reflex. Topical anesthesia with Pontocaine, lidocaine, or cocaine is applied to the oropharynx, pyriform sinuses, and vocal cords. A well-lubricated rubber catheter is introduced transnasally into the trachea, and contrast material at room temperature is given slowly while the patient is positioned for appropriate segmental filling. Usually 10 to 20 ml of oily Dionosil is sufficient to study a whole lung. Films are taken in all projections, and the area of bronchiectasis will appear as segmental areas of blunted and dilated bronchial outlines.

TREATMENT

Medical treatment of bronchiectasis demands the identification of the offending organisms and proper antibiotic therapy. Postural drainage, endotracheal suction, bronchodilators, and pulmonary physiotherapy will aid in the clearing of purulent secretions. Repeated bronchoscopies may be necessary for adequate clearing of the airway. The antibiotics chosen should be of a broad spectrum (*e.g.,* tetracycline, oxytetracycline, or ampicillin). The most common organisms associated with the disease are *Haemophilus influenzae, Streptococcus,* and *Staphylococcus.* It goes without saying that cessation of smoking is crucial for proper therapy.

Indications for surgical therapy include recurrent exacerbations of pulmonary disease due to a bronchiectatic segment, and recurrent hemoptysis. All patients should have adequate cardiopulmonary reserve, and there should be no other concurrent disease. Chronic bronchitis as well as asthma must be ruled out. Ideally, the disease is unilateral, but if bronchograms reveal bilateral localized disease, at least a 3-month interval should be allowed before the other side is operated on. When bilateral disease is present, the most diseased side, as determined by bronchography, is operated on first. A double lumen tube is indispensable not only to protect the other lung but to aid in the dissection. Postoperative complications include atelectasis, empyema, and bronchopleural fistula.

RESULTS OF TREATMENT

In the preantibiotic era, 82% of patients afflicted with bronchiectasis died from the disease, whereas in the postantibiotic era 28% die at a later age as a result of bronchiectasis. A number of patients surviving with medical treatment alone present with cor pulmonale. Of patients who are operated upon for bronchiectasis, 80% are cured if disease is unilateral and another 10% are improved. With multisegmental disease, only 36% of the patients operated on are cured. A basic tenet of surgical therapy is the preservation of lung parenchyma, because the more lung removed the greater the chance of cor pulmonale. Nine percent of patients present with recurrent bronchiectasis after surgical intervention. The cause of these failures can usually be traced to inability to resect localized disease completely or failure to take care of the aforementioned postoperative complications.

TUBERCULOSIS

The surgical treatment of tuberculosis has been modified in the twentieth century by two major factors. First, beginning before the era of chemotherapy, the incidence of new cases of pulmonary tuberculosis has decreased 3% to 5% per year. Second, the advent of effective chemotherapeutic agents has resulted in an ability to control the infection and render the sputum negative in more than 95% of patients within a 3-month period. Twenty years ago as many as 33% of hospitalized patients may have undergone operation. Today only 2% to 3% of patients with tuberculosis need thoracotomy, a 20-fold decrease in some centers.

Tuberculosis is caused by *Mycobacterium tuberculosis*, the tubercle bacillus spread by airborne transmission of droplet nuclei. Transmission depends upon the number of viable bacilli in the sputum, susceptibility of the host, and the length of time of exposure. Rates vary markedly with ethnic origin and are higher in nonwhites. The initial portal of entry is almost always the lung, in which the tubercle bacilli produce a characteristic cellular reaction resulting in the so-called epithelioid cell tubercle. There is an inflammatory cell infiltrate that includes lymphocytes, plasma cells, and macrophages interspersed with Langhans type giant cells. Fibroblastic proliferation occurs, and a chronic, indolent, necrotizing, caseating cavitary pneumonitis and bronchitis result. Healing occurs by fibrosis and often by calcification. There is usually resolution of the initial infection with "healed" lesions appearing on chest x-ray films as calcified parenchymal nodules (Ghon lesion). The late residua include

1. Cavitation with or without bronchial communication
2. Bronchiectasis with lobar destruction
3. Hemoptysis
4. Localized bronchostenosis with stricture.

Pleural involvement can progress to empyema with ensuing lung entrapment. Healed lesions may be reactivated by numerous conditions including malnutrition, alcoholism, and immunosuppression.

DIAGNOSIS

The patient usually complains of cough, fever with nightsweats, and general debilitation with weight loss and anorexia. Hemoptysis can be mild to severe, or absent. Chest roentgenograms may reveal a fluffy alveolar infiltrate usually confined to the upper lobes, a diffuse process (miliary pattern), or the sequelae of an ongoing process including cavitation or pneumothorax. Diagnosis is made by culture of the organisms either by routine sputum collections or occasionally by bronchial washings. A major disadvantage is that 4 weeks to 8 weeks are required to obtain results. Skin testing, by intracutaneous injection of a standardized, stabilized dose of purified protein derivative (PPD) is invaluable in investigating tuberculous infections. The test, which is read at 48 hr to 72 hr, is positive if 10 mm of induration or greater is present. Pleural involvement with pleural effusion demands thoracentesis, the fluid being exudative and predominantly lymphocytic. Pleural biopsy, in combination with analysis of pleural fluid, documents a tuberculous cause in 80% of cases.

TREATMENT

MEDICAL TREATMENT

Medical therapy of tuberculosis with multidrug chemotherapy is the mainstay of treatment at this time. The use of three first-line drugs in continuity for 18 to 24 months has resulted in relapse rates of only 0% to 2%. First-line drugs include isoniazid, 5 mg/kg to 300 mg/day; ethambutol, 15 to 20 mg/kg/day orally; and rifampin, 600 mg daily. Complications attend each of these agents: isoniazid may produce hepatotoxicity and peripheral neuritis, which can be lessened by prophylactic pyridoxine, 100 mg/day; ethambutol can cause optic neuritis, and rifampin can lead to hepatotoxicity. Approximately 50% of patients will have a negative smear and culture after 2 months, and more than 95% will be negative after 6 months.

SURGICAL THERAPY

Early operations for tuberculosis involved collapse procedures. These included pneumothorax, in which repeated refills of air at regular intervals were instilled into the affected hemithorax in order to maintain the desired degree of collapse. Phrenic nerve paralysis, either temporary or permanent, elevated the diaphragm. Extraperiosteal thoracoplasty with plombage involved depression of the periosteum and intercostal muscles as well as both pleural layers of the lung with insertion of prosthetic devices to cause lobar collapse. Formal thoracoplasty with removal of ribs over the diseased area was refined to resection of ribs 1, 2, and 3, including the transverse processes of the corresponding vertebrae as a first stage. In ensuing stages lengths of other ribs through the seventh were removed. With time, thoracoplasty became the primary procedure for treatment of stable unilateral pulmonary tuberculosis. It was gratifyingly successful—75% to 90% effective even without chemotherapy.

Indications for Resection

The basic indication for resectional therapy in the treatment of tuberculosis is localized disease that does not respond to chemotherapy.

Primary indications include

SUPPURATIVE AND INFECTIVE DISEASES OF THE LUNG

Definition	Parenchymal lung inflammation that becomes clinically significant
Etiology	Occupational disease, tuberculosis, bacterial, fungal, viral infection
Symptoms	Cough, hemoptysis, fever, chills, dyspnea
Dx	Physical examination and history, skin tests, sputum culture, radiography of the chest, bronchoscopy or bronchography in selected cases
Rx	Medical—Antibiotics depending on the etiology; respiratory therapy depending on the severity Surgical—For complications of the disease including nonresolution, destroyed lung, abscess, hemoptysis, bronchopleural fistula

1. Persistently positive sputum culture after 6 months of continuous chemotherapy with two drugs in the presence of an open cavitary lesion or nonhealable anatomic residua of infection such as bronchiectasis, destroyed lobe, or significant bronchial stenosis
2. The presence of localized infection with a typical group 3 (Battey) organism
3. Suspected presence of a concomitant neoplasm with tuberculosis
4. Life-threatening hemoptysis
5. Nonresponding spontaneous bronchopleural fistula or any postoperative bronchopleural fistula

Secondary indications include

1. Negative sputum in a patient whose symptoms are referrable to permanently altered anatomy secondary to infection
2. Negative sputum in a patient whose disease is localized and in whom reactivation is likely
3. Entrapped lung following tuberculous or mixed pleural empyema

Preoperative Assessment

Patients should be in the best possible nutritional state even if it means continued hospitalization and nutritional supplementation by the alimentary or parenteral route with correction of blood volume and vitamin deficiencies. Pulmonary reserve must be investigated by room air and exercise blood gases, and by spirometry with the addition of bronchodilators as necessary. Adequate localization of the disease by bronchography is essential to define preoperatively the extent of the intended resection. Fiberoptic bronchoscopy should be done several days prior to operation to ensure the absence of active endobronchial disease and to rule out bronchostenosis. Streptomycin 500 mg intramuscularly should be given preoperatively and 10 to 14 days postoperatively, after which oral agents are continued for 18 to 24 months.

Conduct of the Operation and Choice of Resection

Pulmonary resection for the sequelae of tuberculosis can be a formidable undertaking. Selective ventilation using either a double lumen Carlen's tube or peroral intrabronchial placement of a No. 6 or No. 7 Fogarty will aid not only in the prevention of spillage and debris to the dependent lung but also in the dissection. The preferred approach is by way of the standard posterolateral thoracotomy, which will give adequate exposure for clearing of adhesions and mobilization of bronchovascular structures. (For the general approach to thoracotomy, see Fig. 34-11.) The dissection of the involved lobe begins in the plane between the fused visceral and parietal pleura, taking care not to enter any cavities demonstrated on preoperative bronchography. This precaution occasionally forces the surgeon to adapt an extrapleural approach using electrocautery, carefully avoiding the major vascular structures in the apex as well as the intercostal neurovascular bundle. Isolation of the pulmonary artery and veins may be tedious owing to the dense perivascular inflammatory reaction, and isolation of the main pulmonary artery using a Penrose drain is suggested. The bronchus is freed of investing nodes without devascularization; it is divided with a scalpel at a point that will not leave an excessive amount of bronchial stump. Bronchial

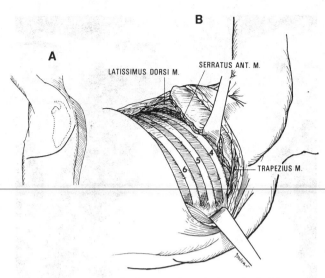

Fig. 34-11. *(A)* Standard posterolateral thoracic incision. *(B)* Division of muscles of the chest wall. (After Johnson J, McVaugh H III, Waldhausen JA: Surgery of the Chest, 4th ed, Chap 5. Chicago, Year Book Medical Publishers, 1970)

stapling devices have proved to be a useful technique without increased possibility of bronchopleural fistula compared with hand-sewn techniques. Although the basic goal is to conserve as much parenchyma as possible while eradicating the disease and to obliterate the remaining pleural space by compensatory expansion of other lobes, lobectomy is the most common procedure performed. Because of the high incidence of postoperative bronchopleural fistula, many surgeons no longer perform formal segmentectomy. All raw surfaces with bronchopleural fistulas should be controlled by suture or staple obliteration. Hemostasis must be diligent, and two chest tubes are placed for closed chest drainage. Bacteriologic and pathologic examinations of the specimen are performed, and, before discharge, thoracentesis is performed for routine tuberculous and fungal cultures. If a residual space problem persists after resection, a formal six-rib tailoring thoracoplasty can be performed at a second stage.

Complications

The two most common complications of resection for tuberculosis include bronchopleural fistula and postresection empyema. The incidence of bronchopleural fistula is 3% to 7% with a mortality of 25%. The diagnosis is usually heralded by uncontrollable coughing, and once established, adequate pleural drainage must be instituted immediately. Attempts at operative closure are usually doomed to failure unless the fistula becomes apparent within 3 to 4 days after the operation. Alternate treatment is limited to resection of diseased lung tissue, decortication, and six-rib thoracoplasty (Fig. 34-12). If this still does not control the fistula, closure with muscle periosteal flaps may be necessary.

Postresection empyema may be due to non–acid-fast organisms and is usually managed by pleural drainage or rib resection with the appropriate antibiotics. Postresection tuberculous empyema or mixed empyema may necessitate decortication and thoracoplasty with combined chemotherapy.

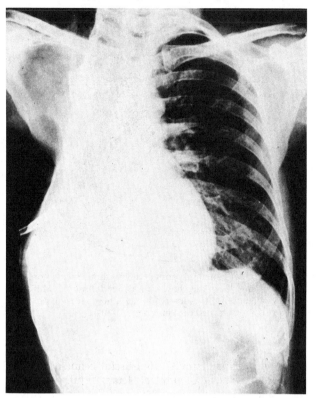

Fig. 34-12. Right thoracoplasty in a patient with persistent empyema following pulmonary resection for tuberculosis. (Stauss HK, Hardy JD: Tuberculosis and fungous diseases of the lungs. In Hardy JD [ed]: Rhoads Textbook of Surgery, 5th ed. Philadelphia, J B Lippincott, 1977)

SPECIAL SITUATIONS

PLEURAL DISEASE

Pleural tuberculosis may be manifest as a pure tuberculous empyema with or without bronchopleural fistula or as a mixed tuberculous, pyogenic empyema with or without bronchopleural fistula. Once the diagnosis is established by thoracentesis and pleural biopsy with the appropriate studies, chemotherapy must be started in all instances. If the empyema is purely tuberculous, multiple thoracenteses in combination with lengthy chemotherapy will usually control the situation. Mixed tuberculous pyogenic empyema, however, usually demands closed thoracotomy drainage in addition to chemotherapy for all organisms. Rib resection may eventually prove necessary. In both instances, if the lung becomes entrapped by a "thick peel," decortication with removal of the thickened parietal pleura and incision of portions of the visceral pleura should be performed. Resection of involved parenchymal disease should also be done if the empyema was originally accompanied by bronchopleural fistula.

ATYPICAL STRAINS

Atypical mycobacteria cause a clinically significant infection in 2% of patients with tuberculosis. The group 3, or Battey bacilli, located predominantly in the South Atlantic and Gulf Coast states, are notoriously resistant to chemotherapy in 60% to 70% of cases. All patients with group 3 infection or localized disease are candidates for resection. Chemotherapy, including four drugs for a period of 4 to 6 months, is attempted to eradicate the disease and remove the organ-

isms from the sputum. If this is unsuccessful, a fifth drug (usually streptomycin) is added preoperatively, and a lobar resection is performed with the realization that a higher incidence of recurrence and postoperative complications may ensue.

RESULTS OF TREATMENT

Surgical resection of tuberculosis remains a safe method of treatment. An expected operative mortality of 2.5% is fairly consistent at this time with most of the deaths resulting from coronary thrombosis. Morbidity in the form of bronchopleural fistula or empyema occurs in 1% to 5% of cases, the lowest incidence of complications occurring in patients treated by lobectomy.

FUNGAL DISEASE OF THE LUNG

As pulmonary tuberculosis has receded from the truly awesome threat it posed to the infected patient 30 years ago, the importance of fungal disease has increased. Pulmonary mycoses still do not represent major surgical problems very frequently, but their diagnosis and effective management can pose difficult challenges. As Buechener said, "There are few areas in the total sphere of medicine in which the average physician seems to have less confidence in his ability to judge the indications for therapy and to administer his therapy than in the field of systemic mycosis." The more prominent pulmonary fungal infections include histoplasmosis, coccidioidomycosis, aspergillosis, cryptococcosis, actinomycosis, nocardiosis, blastomycosis, mucormycosis, sporotrichosis, and candidiasis (Table 34-2 and Figs. 34-13 and 34-14).

HISTOPLASMOSIS

Histoplasmosis is caused by the organism *Histoplasma capsulatum*, which is endemic in the central United States and

TABLE 34-2   THERAPY IN PULMONARY MYCOSES

DISEASE	ANTIFUNGAL AGENT
Actinomycosis	Penicillin; erythromycin; broad spectrum antibiotics
Aspergillosis, invasive type	Amphotericin B
Candidiasis, systemic	Amphotericin B or amphotericin B and 5-fluorocytosine
Coccidioidomycosis	Amphotericin B
Cryptococcosis	Amphotericin B or amphotericin B and 5-fluorocytosine
Histoplasmosis	Amphotericin B; saramycetin
Mucormycosis (phycomycosis)	Amphotericin B; iodides
Nocardiosis	Sulfadiazine
North American blastomycosis	Amphotericin B; 2-hydroxystilbamidine
South American blastomycosis	Amphotericin B; sulfonamides
Sporotrichosis, pulmonary	Iodides; amphotericin B; saramycetin

(Busey J.: Modern concepts in the diagnosis and management of pulmonary mycoses. Clin Notes Resp Dis 14:1, 1976)

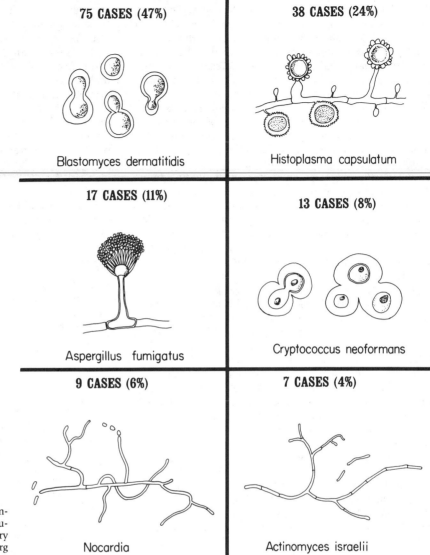

75 CASES (47%)

Blastomyces dermatitidis

38 CASES (24%)

Histoplasma capsulatum

17 CASES (11%)

Aspergillus fumigatus

13 CASES (8%)

Cryptococcus neoformans

9 CASES (6%)

Nocardia

7 CASES (4%)

Actinomyces israelii

Fig. 34-13. Morphology of fungi commonly producing pulmonary disease in humans. (Newsom BD, Hardy JD: Pulmonary fungal infections. J Thorac Cardiovasc Surg 83:218, 1982)

Fig. 34-14. Some complications of pulmonary fungal disease. (Newsom BD, Hardy JD: Pulmonary fungal infections. J Thorac Cardiovasc Surg 83:218, 1982)

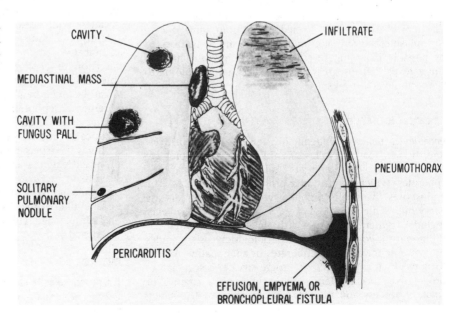

CAVITY

INFILTRATE

MEDIASTINAL MASS

CAVITY WITH FUNGUS FALL

PNEUMOTHORAX

SOLITARY PULMONARY NODULE

PERICARDITIS

EFFUSION, EMPYEMA, OR BRONCHOPLEURAL FISTULA

the Mississippi and Ohio river basins. Infection occurs by the inhalation of micronidia from bird droppings. The yeast proliferates in the lung, peaking in 1 and 2 weeks, and spreading to the pulmonary lymph nodes and through the blood. *Histoplasma* organisms are contained within granulomas that may calcify. The primary infection is usually asymptomatic; however, it can be an acute flulike illness with bronchopneumonia on chest roentgenograms. Diagnosis can be made by skin testing and complement fixation.

Surgical therapy depends on the stage of the disease—(1) acute, (2) healed asymptomatic chronic granulomas, (3) chronic cavitary disease, or (4) mediastinal disease. When the disease is acute and is limited to the lung, with confluence or cavitation in infiltrates, amphotericin should be administered. For disseminated disease, intravenous amphotericin (more than 2 g) should be given for 6 to 12 weeks, especially in immunosuppressed patients. Wedge resection of a healed granuloma is performed to rule out carcinoma when it appears as an unexplained solitary nodule. No postoperative amphotericin coverage is needed in this instance.

Patients with chronic pulmonary histoplasmosis usually are middle-aged white men with preexisting chronic obstructive pulmonary disease. These patients usually present with infected emphysematous areas in the apical and posterior segments of the upper lobe. In 20% the disease progresses to cavitary disease manifested by fever, malaise, weight loss, cough, and hemoptysis. Thick-walled cavities (3 to 4 mm in thickness or greater) may develop. The diagnosis of chronic pulmonary histoplasmosis is usually confirmed by culture of the organism combined with radiographic and cytologic studies. Surgical intervention is used (1) in diagnosis, (2) if there has been no change in the areas of cavitation with multiple courses of amphotericin, or (3) if there is progressive disease. Resection, which has a 6% to 9% mortality and a 13% to 20% morbidity, is performed to prevent dissemination and to control the disease. Amphotericin B (up to 2 g) should be administered either 1 month preoperatively or postoperatively if the diagnosis was not established before surgical intervention.

Mediastinal involvement with histoplasmosis may be manifest as mediastinal granuloma with broncholithiasis, hemoptysis, atelectasis, and mediastinal fibrosis with trapping of the superior vena cava, esophagus, trachea, or atria. If the patient presents with a noncalcified mediastinal mass, exploratory thoracotomy may be needed to diagnose mediastinal histoplasmosis. If mediastinal granuloma due to histoplasmosis is found, as much disease should be resected as possible including resection of bronchiectatic lung in order to prevent progression of mediastinal granuloma to sclerosing mediastinitis.

COCCIDIOIDOMYCOSIS

Coccidioides immitis is endemic in the soil of the southwest and the San Joaquin Valley of California. Arthrospores are inhaled in the lung and are transformed into parasitic spherules, which rupture and proliferate endospores. The endospores give rise to a flulike syndrome, but the disease is asymptomatic in 60% of cases. San Joaquin Valley Fever includes erythema nodosum, arthralgias, malaise, and fever. Pulmonary involvement with coccidioidomycosis includes bronchopneumonia with infiltrates or adenopathy. After 6 to 8 weeks it is classifed as progressive. The sequelae of progressive coccidioidomycosis include open cavities or cavitary abscess and nodules of various sizes. The cavity

may rupture, bleed, or close spontaneously. A *coccidioidoma* represents the residua of active pulmonary disease. Diagnosis is made by skin test (which will be positive for life), precipitin test, and complement fixation test.

The surgical approach is used for (1) diagnosis of persistent pneumonias, (2) diagnosis of the solitary pulmonary nodule, possibly a coccidioidoma, and (3) resection of destroyed lung. Cavitary lesions have been known to expand to cause bronchopleural fistula, empyema, or pyopneumothorax. Lesions more than 2 cm in diameter that persist for more than 6 months should be removed, especially when there are multiple fluid-filled cavities surrounded by infiltrates; diabetic and pregnant patients are at particularly high risk for dissemination. Established cavitary disease is not responsive to amphotericin B parenterally. Resection of the cavity should be done by lobectomy because of the possibility of satellite nodules of active disease around the cavity. Amphotericin B should be instituted postoperatively.

ASPERGILLOSIS

Aspergillus fumigatus, A. niger, and *A. flavus* are the causative fungi of aspergillosis. Pulmonary manifestations of aspergillus include
1. Bronchial involvement with or without allergic sensitization
2. Aspergilloma or intracavitary mycetoma
3. Pneumonic or invasive aspergillosis
4. Disseminated aspergillosis

Thoracic surgeons are most concerned with intercavitary mycetoma and invasive aspergillosis. An aspergilloma is a rounded necrotic mass of matted hyphae, fibrin, and inflammatory cells superimposed upon underlying chronic lung disease, such as tuberculosis, histoplasmosis, or obstructive pulmonary disease. Positive serum precipitins, positive culture, and plain radiographs will make the diagnosis. Mycetomas usually occur in the upper lobes, and an intracavitary *fungus ball* surrounded by gross disease in the lung parenchyma forms a Belcher's complex (Fig. 34-15). Hemoptysis will occur in 45% to 85% of cases of aspergilloma and can be massive. In patients with massive or recurrent hemoptysis with reasonable pulmonary function, the cavity containing the aspergilloma should be resected by lobectomy. Prophylactic resection is not indicated in asymptomatic patients. If the aspergilloma is associated with coexisting tuberculosis, hemoptysis is frequently fatal, and resection after lesser degrees of hemoptysis is indicated. Amphotericin B should be given at the time of resection to prevent dissemination. In poor-risk patients intercavitary treatment with sodium iodide or amphotericin B can be given by percutaneous or intrabronchial catheter. Parenteral amphotericin B has been found to be useless for cavitary disease associated with aspergillosis except as an adjunct to surgical resection.

Invasive aspergillosis is usually seen in immunocompromised patients and manifests itself as bilateral, patchy, necrotizing bronchopneumonia. Diagnosis is made by transbronchial biopsy or by open lung biopsy with demonstration of aspergillosis invading pulmonary vessels with infarction and hemorrhage. This condition is highly fatal except when diagnosed early.

CRYPTOCOCCOSIS

Cryptococcosis is caused by the single budding yeast *Cryptococcus neoformans,* which exists saprophytically in the soil.

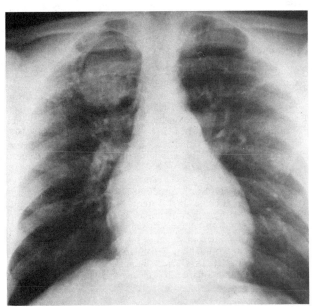

Fig. 34-15. Fungus ball (aspergilloma) in the right upper lobe of a patient with old tuberculous bronchiectasis.

The organism is inhaled into the lungs with air contaminated from soil containing pigeon dung. There is a high association with meningitis. Symptomatology includes cough, fever, and weight loss, and granulomas of up to 4 cm occur in the lower lobes. Surgery has a role in cryptococcosis in the diagnosis of these unexplained pulmonary nodules. If thoracotomy has been performed and *Cryptococcus* is found in the nodules, drug treatment with a half dose of amphotericin B or 5-fluorocytosine should be initiated if the disease is active. Because 10% of patients with cryptococcosis will develop meningitis after resection, a spinal tap should be performed to detect the characteristic organism with India ink preparation. Resection is curative in 90% of the cases.

ACTINOMYCETACEA AND NOCARDIOSIS

Actinomycetacea and Nocardia are classified as bacteria, not fungi, despite the fact that they form hyphae and are spore producers. They do not respond to amphotericin B. *Actinomyces israelii* are anaerobic or microaerophylic organisms that normally inhabit the oral cavity. Pulmonary manifestations of actinomycosis include fever, cough, and weight loss with cervicofacial, thoracic, or abdominal draining sinuses. On chest x-ray film an infiltrative process with or without cavitation is seen that is difficult to distinguish from malignancy. The infiltrative process is due to chronic suppuration with superinfection of material aspirated from the oropharynx. There is usually no lymph node involvement, and the diagnosis can be made when sulfur granules are detected in material obtained from an abscess, draining sinus, or pleural biopsy. Pulmonary resection is performed to rule out a neoplastic process or other disease. When the diagnosis is made, treatment is initiated with intravenous penicillin G for a period of 2 to 4 weeks followed by oral penicillin for 1 year.

Nocardiosis, caused by another actinomycete, can be an infectious process limited to the lungs or may be systemic involving the central nervous system. It occurs in patients who are immunosuppressed or immunodeficient. Recovery of organisms from the sputum or from the pleura should be regarded as pathogenic. Nocardiosis causes pathologic changes similar to those seen in actinomycosis. The diagnosis can be made by brush biopsy, needle biopsy, or culture of organisms from an empyema or abscess cavity. Treatment is with intravenous sulfa drugs or Septra.

BLASTOMYCOSIS

North American blastomycosis is caused by *Blastomyces dermatitidis,* which is endemic in the soil of the Mississippi and Ohio River Valleys in the south central states. Infectious spores are inhaled and produce a flulike syndrome, cutaneous disease, or disseminated disease. The simultaneous appearance of a chronic papulopustular skin lesion and a pulmonary infiltrate should lead to the suspicion of blastomycosis. Symptoms include weight loss, anorexia, fever, chills, and hemoptysis. The diagnosis can be made by sputum culture, which requires 3 weeks for growth, or by complement fixation analysis. Organisms may also be identified in the sputum or in gastric aspirates.

Chronic blastomycosis will lead to cavitary disease, with multiple or single nodules in the lung. When there is a residual cavity and positive sputa, cavitary disease should be resected by lobectomy, and antibiotic therapy should be instituted with amphotericin B or hydroxystilbamidine to prevent recurrence.

MUCORMYCOSIS

Mucormycosis causes a pulmonary infection by inhalation of spores and is seen in patients with impaired immunocompetence or diabetes mellitus. A characteristic pathologic feature of mucormycosis is the thrombosis of blood vessels in the pulmonary circuit resulting in infarcted lung. Because of poor penetration of antifungal agents due to blood vessel thrombosis, the only hope of cure is early recognition with removal of infected lung and supportive treatment of the immune system.

SPOROTRICHOSIS

Sporotrichosis rarely causes pulmonary infection but may cause hilar adenopathy accompanied by upper lobe infiltrates and multiple thin-walled cavities. Diagnosis is made by a sputum culture, washings, brushings, and serologic testing. Surgical intervention is necessary for undiagnosed pulmonary lesions or for cavitary disease, and resection of persistent cavitary disease is performed after adequate parenteral treatment. Conservative resection is the rule, and despite the fact that recurrence is rare, amphotericin B should be given preoperatively and postoperatively.

CANDIDIASIS

Candida albicans, a yeastlike budding fungus, causes a hemorrhagic bronchopneumonia in patients who are immunosuppressed or chronically ill. The role of surgery in pulmonary candidiasis is to confirm this diagnosis by lung biopsy and institute treatment with amphotericin B.

BIBLIOGRAPHY

Diffuse Lung Disease and Pneumonitis
BECKLAKE NR: Asbestos related disease of the lung and other organs. Am Rev Resp Dis 114:187, 1976

DEREMEE RA: The present status of treatment of pulmonary sarcoidosis. Chest 71:388, 1977

ELLIS JH, JR: Transbronchial lung biopsy via the fiberoptic bronchoscope. Chest 68:524, 1975

FINT JN: Hypersensitivity pneumonitis due to organic dust. Clin Notes Resp Dis 13:3, 1974

GAENSLER EA, MASTER VB, HAMM J: Open lung biopsy in diffuse pulmonary disease. N Engl J Med 270:1319, 1964

GAENSLER EA, CARRINGTON CB, COUTER RE et al: Chronic interstitial pneumonias. Clin Notes Resp Dis 10:1, 1972

HANSON RR: Transbronchial biopsy via the flexible fiberoptic bronchoscope: Results in 164 patients. Am Rev Resp Dis 114:67, 1976

MARKS A: Diffuse pulmonary fibrosis. Med Clin North Am 51:439, 1967

MEYER JE, GANDBHIR LH, MILNER LB et al: Percutaneous aspiration biopsy of nodular lung lesions. J Thorac Cardiovasc Surg 73:787, 1977

SAGEL SS, FERGUSON TB, FORREST JV et al: Percutaneous transthoracic aspiration needle biopsy. Ann Thorac Surg 26:399, 1978

ZISKIND A, JONES RN, WEIL H: Silicosis. Am Rev Resp Dis 113:643, 1976

Lung Abscess

ALEXANDER JC, WOLFE WG: Lung abscess and empyema of the thorax. Surg Clin North Am 60:835, 1980

BARNETT TB, HERRING CL: Lung abscess: Initial and late results of medical therapy. Arch Int Med 127:217, 1971

BORRIE J: Management of Thoracic Emergencies. New York, Appleton-Century-Crofts, 1980

GLENN WWL: Thoracic and Cardiovascular Surgery with Related Pathology, 3rd ed. New York, Appleton-Century-Crofts, 1975

TAKARO T, SETHI G, STEWART S: Suppurative diseases of the lungs, pleurae, and pericardium. Curr Prob Surg 14:6, 1977

Bronchiectasis

BOLMAN RM, WOLFE WG: Bronchiectasis and bronchopulmonary sequestration. Surg Clin North Am 60:867, 1980

GEORGE SA, LEONARDI HK, OVERHOLT RH: Bilateral pulmonary resection for bronchiectasis: A 40 year experience. Ann Thorac Surg 28:48, 1979

LINSKOG GE, HUBBELL DS: Analysis of 215 cases of bronchiectasis. Surg Gynecol Obstet 100:643, 1955

SANDERSON JN, KENNEDY MC, JOHNSON MF et al: Bronchiectasis: Results of surgical and conservative management. A review of 393 cases. Thorax 29:407, 1974

SEALY WC, YOUNG G: Surgical treatment of multisegmental and localized bronchiectasis. Surg Gynecol Obstet 123:80, 1966

TAKARO T, SETHI G, STEWART S: Suppurative diseases of the lungs, pleurae, and pericardium. Curr Prob Surg 14:6, 1977

Tuberculosis

BARKER WL, FABER LP, OSTERMILLER WE et al: Management of persistent bronchopleural fistulas. J Thorac Cardiovasc Surg 63:393, 1971

ELKADI A, SALAS R, ALMOND CH: Surgical treatment of atypical pulmonary tuberculosis. J Thorac Cardiovasc Surg 72:435, 1976

FLOYD RD, HOLLISTER WF, SEALY WC: Complications in 430 consecutive pulmonary resections for tuberculosis. Surg Gynecol Obstet 109:467, 1959

HARRISON LH: Current aspects of surgical management of tuberculosis. Surg Clin North Am 60:883, 1980

MCLAUGHLIN JS, HANKINS JR: Current aspects of surgery for pulmonary tuberculosis. Ann Thorac Surg 17:513, 1974

SHAH HH, HOLLAND RH, MEADOR RS et al: The surgical variations of pulmonary infections caused by different species of mycobacteria. Ann Thorac Surg 7:145, 1969

SHIELDS TW, FOX RT, LEES WM: Changing role of surgery in the treatment of pulmonary tuberculosis. Arch Surg 100:363, 1970

Fungal Disease

HAMMON JW JR, PRAGER RL: Surgical management of fungal diseases of the chest. Surg Clin North Am 60:897, 1980

HATCHER CR JR, SEHDEVA J, WATERS WC et al: Primary pulmonary cryptococcosis. J Thorac Surg 61:39, 1971

KARRAS A, HANKINS JR, ATTAR S et al: Pulmonary aspergillosis: An analysis of 41 patients. Ann Thorac Surg 22:1, 1976

LARSON RS, BERNATZ PE, GERACI JE: Results of surgical and nonoperative treatment for pulmonary North American blastomycosis. J Thorac Cardiovasc Surg 51:714, 1966

NELSON AR: The surgical treatment of pulmonary coccidioidomycosis. Curr Prob Surg 11:1, 1974

NEWSOM BD, HARDY JD: Pulmonary fungal infections: Survey of 159 cases with surgical implications. J Thorac Cardiovasc Surg 83:218, 1982

SAAB SB, UNGARO R, ALMOND C: The role of and results of surgery in the management of chronic pulmonary histoplasmosis. J Thorac Cardiovasc Surg 68:159, 1974

TAKARO T: Mycotic infections of interest to thoracic surgeons. Collective review. Ann Thorac Surg 3:71, 1967

TOMM KI, RALEIGH JW, GUINN GA: Thoracic actinomycosis. Am J Surg 124:46, 1972

Thomas W. Shields

Carcinoma and Other Lung Tumors

PRIMARY CARCINOMA OF THE LUNG
  Pathogenesis
    Cigarette Smoking
    Industrial Exposure
    Air Pollution
  Pathology
    Gross Characteristics
    Microscopic Characteristics
  Natural History
    Squamous Cell Carcinoma
    Adenocarcinoma (Including Alveolar Cell Type)
    Undifferentiated Large Cell Carcinoma
    Undifferentiated Small Cell Carcinoma
  Dissemination Pathways

  Clinical Manifestations
    Bronchopulmonary Symptoms
    Extrapulmonary Intrathoracic Symptoms
    Extrathoracic Metastatic Symptoms
    Extrathoracic Nonmetastatic Symptoms
  Roentgenographic Features
  Diagnostic Procedures
    Cytologic Studies
    Special Roentgenographic Examinations
    Radionuclide Scans
    Invasive Diagnostic Procedures
      Bronchoscopy and Biopsy
      Transthoracic Percutaneous Needle Biopsy
      Lymph Node Biopsy

PRIMARY CARCINOMA OF THE LUNG

During the past fifty years there has been an alarming increase in the incidence of bronchial carcinoma in all economically developed countries of the world, especially in the United Kingdom. In the United States at present over 110,000 new cases are diagnosed each year. The greater number of cases are observed in men, although the incidence in women is now increasing at a more rapid rate than is presently observed in men. The ratio formerly was 10:1, but in the 1970s it had decreased to 4:1.

In men, the number of deaths due to bronchial carcinoma exceeds the total of that from carcinoma in the next four common sites: colon and rectum, stomach, prostate, and pancreas. In women, only deaths due to breast tumor exceed those due to carcinoma of the lung.

PATHOGENESIS

The marked rise in the frequency of the disease during the twentieth century is believed to be related primarily to the presence of certain environmental factors: cigarette smoking, specific industrial exposure, and urban air pollution.

CIGARETTE SMOKING

The relationship between smoking and the development of bronchial carcinoma is supported by a vast amount of evidence: a dose-response relationship, demographic distribution correlating with long-term smoking habits, reduced rates among ex-smokers, and the successful production of cancer with tar or inhaled cigarette smoke in a number of animal species. The correlation of smoking is most evident in patients with squamous cell and undifferentiated small cell carcinomas, but a causal relationship is also believed to be present in those with adenocarcinoma as well.

INDUSTRIAL EXPOSURE

Many different industrial agents have been identified with the development of lung carcinoma. Cigarette smoking in association with exposure to such agents is believed to greatly increase the risk. This is especially true in individuals exposed to radioactive substances (*e.g.*, uranium miners) and to asbestos. Other specific agents are nickel, mustard gas, dichloromethyl ether, arsenic, chromium, and polycyclic hydrocarbons.

AIR POLLUTION

Coal tar and petroleum products are also present in varying quantities in the atmosphere, particularly in urban areas. However, the true role of such pollution is difficult to determine.

PATHOLOGY

GROSS CHARACTERISTICS

Bronchial carcinoma occurs more frequently in the right than in the left lung. The upper lobes (a predilection for the tumor to be located in the anterior segment) are involved more often than the lower lobes, and the middle lobe is involved least frequently of all. The tumor may be central or peripheral in origin. The central tumors are seen in the major bronchi and their subdivisions. These tumors present as firm irregular masses, and the endobronchial surface is almost always ulcerated. Obstruction of the bronchial lumen is frequent, and associated atelectasis or infection or both are commonly present. The peripheral tumors are firm, often spherical or ovoid, and frequently associated with umbilication or puckering of the overlying visceral pleura. The cut surface is homogeneous; the smaller lesions are usually solid, but larger ones may have central necrosis with cavitation. The blood supply of the primary bronchial carcinomas is from the bronchial arterial system.

MICROSCOPIC CHARACTERISTICS

Bronchial carcinomas are classified histologically into four main cell types: squamous cell carcinoma, adenocarcinoma, undifferentiated large cell carcinoma, and undifferentiated small cell carcinoma. Tumors of mixed cell types are also seen.

WORKUP OF THE PULMONARY MASS LESION	
Symptoms	Cough, hemoptysis, wheezing, pain, extrathoracic manifestation of malignancy
Dx	X-ray films: solitary nodule, mass lesion, hilar, peripheral Sputum cytologies Bronchoscopy: washings, brush, biopsy Mediastinoscopy, mediastinotomy Percutaneous needle biopsy
Staging	Liver enzymes, bone scan, brain scan when indicated
Physiologic Status	Pulmonary spirometry, arterial blood gases
Rx	Surgical resection and/or radiation and/or chemotherapy, if indicated

Squamous cell carcinomas are highly differentiated tumors in which there is abundant keratin with formation of epithelial pearls; moderately differentiated tumors with less keratinization but readily recognized intercellular bridges (Fig. 34-16); or less differentiated tumors composed of large cells having squamatoid appearance but without obvious keratinization and a few, or only questionable, intercellular bridges.

Adenocarcinomas may be well differentiated tumors composed of cubital to columnar epithelial cells with fairly

Fig. 34-16. Major cellular types of carcinoma of the lung. *(Top, left)* Squamous cell carcinoma. *(Top, right)* Undifferentiated small-cell carcinoma. *(Bottom, left)* Adenocarcinoma. *(Bottom, right)* Undifferentiated large-cell carcinoma. (Shields TW [ed]: Textbook of General Thoracic Surgery. Philadelphia, Lea & Febiger, 1972)

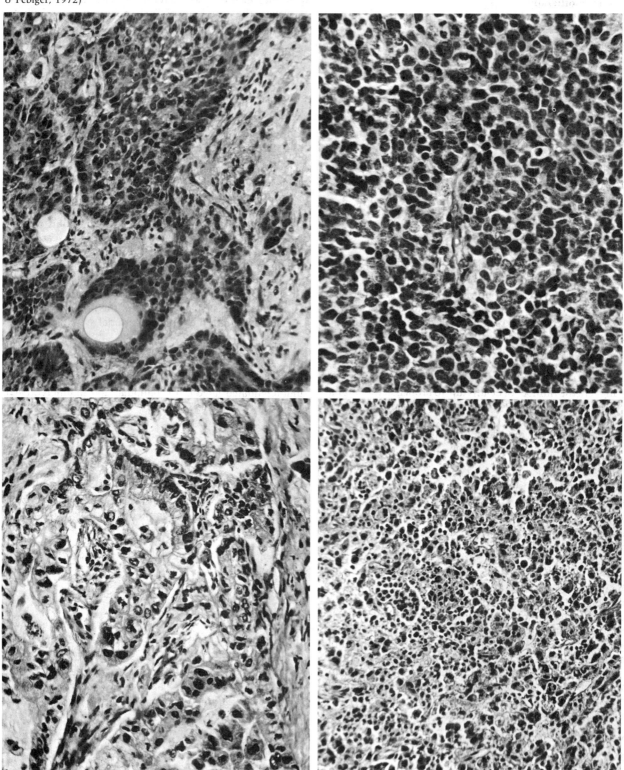

uniform round nuclei arranged in distinct acinar or glandular patterns (see Fig. 34-16). The moderately differentiated are composed of nests, cords, or isolated cells, occasionally arranged in acinar or glandular pattern. The poorly differentiated cells are composed predominantly of anaplastic cells but with distinct evidence of acinar formation. Bronchiolo-alveolar/papillary tumors are composed of tall columnar epithelial cells arranged in a dominant papillary pattern.

Comprising a number of heterogeneous tumors that cannot be classified readily as squamous cell carcinomas or as adenocarcinomas, *undifferentiated large cell carcinomas* of the lung are considered anaplastic tumors that show no apparent evidence of differentiation. Individual cells have enlarged irregular vesicular or hyperchromatic nuclei that may have prominent nucleoli. The cell may have abundant cytoplasm (Fig. 34-16).

Undifferentiated small cell carcinomas are composed of small round or oat-shaped cells which resemble lymphocytes (Fig. 34-16). An intermediate cell type and a combined oat cell type associated with foci of squamous or adenocarcinoma cells or both may be seen. Classically, in the small cell tumors there is a high nuclear cytoplasmic ratio, and several nucleoli may be present in the nuclei.

NATURAL HISTORY

SQUAMOUS CELL CARCINOMA

From 35% to 60% of all carcinomas of the lung are squamous cell carcinomas. They may occur in either the central or peripheral areas, although the former is more common, with two thirds of these tumors being found in this location. Squamous cell tumors tend to metastasize late. The centrally located lesions not only cause bronchial obstruction as a result of the intraluminal growth but also tend to extend peribronchially, so that not infrequently the lumen may be constricted by extrinsic pressure with a grossly normal-appearing mucosal pattern. The peripherally located squamous cell tumors have a tendency to undergo central necrosis with resultant cavitation.

ADENOCARCINOMA (INCLUDING ALVEOLAR CELL TYPE)

Approximately 15% to 20% of all carcinomas of the lung are adenocarcinomas. Most arise in the peripheral area of the lung, although one fourth may occur in the central area. These lesions tend to spread by way of the vascular system early in the course of the disease, but lymphatic spread is late. They also may attain a large size without undergoing central necrosis.

The *bronchiolo-alveolar/papillary tumor*, considered to represent a highly differentiated adenocarcinoma, comprises 1.5% to 6% of all bronchial carcinomas, with an average incidence of 2.5%. Grossly, it may occur in one of three forms: solitary nodule, multinodular, and diffuse or pneumonic type. The first is the most common and comprises two thirds of the tumors of this subclassification. The multinodular and diffuse forms, which comprise the remainder, do not often present surgical problems. However, the more common peripherally located solitary lesions of this cell type are encountered as asymptomatic peripheral lesions. Generally, the solitary type of this highly differentiated tumor has a much better prognosis than do the other types of adenocarcinoma arising in the lung. Hematogenous spread and nodal metastases are infrequent.

UNDIFFERENTIATED LARGE CELL CARCINOMA

As a result of the lack of uniformity in the criteria for the histologic diagnosis of undifferentiated large cell carcinomas, the actual incidence is unknown but probably is between 5% and 15%. These tumors may occur in either the central or the peripheral area, although the latter site is probably somewhat more common. They spread early in the course of the disease and have a relatively poor prognosis. The clinical course of giant cell tumors is rapidly fatal, but fortunately this is an uncommon lesion, representing less than 1% of all lung carcinomas.

UNDIFFERENTIATED SMALL CELL CARCINOMA

These anaplastic tumors comprise approximately 35% of all bronchial carcinomas. Approximately four fifths of them arise in the central area, and the remainder in the peripheral area of the lung. Tumors arising in either region involve the hilar and mediastinal lymph nodes early in the course of the disease. Hematogenous spread also occurs early and is frequently widespread. Twenty percent to 40% of patients with small cell carcinoma that appears limited to the hemithorax have bone marrow involvement. Central necrosis within the primary tumor or changes in the distal parenchyma of the lung are infrequent.

DISSEMINATION PATHWAYS

In all cell types, metastatic spread may be by direct extension to contiguous structures within the chest, by lymphatic pathways, and by hematogenous spread.

DIRECT EXTENSION

The tumor may extend directly into the adjacent pulmonary parenchyma, the adjacent visceral pleura, across the fissure, along the bronchus of origin, and also into adjacent structures in the thorax. The structures commonly involved are the parietal pleura, the pulmonary and other great vessels of the thorax, the chest wall, the superior sulcus area and its adjacent neurogenic and bony structures, the pericardium, and the diaphragm. Although direct extension of the tumor may involve the superior vena cava and contiguous nerves, the recurrent laryngeal and phrenic nerves, and the esophagus, these structures more frequently are invaded by secondary extension from metastatic disease within hilar and mediastinal lymph nodes.

LYMPHATIC METASTASIS

The lymphatic spread of the disease from the individual lobes is relatively constant. The important area in each lung is the lymphatic sump area. On the right this is the area about the bronchus intermedius and on the left the area between the upper lobe bronchus and the superior segmental bronchus of the lower lobe. Lymphatic spread on the right is most often ipsilateral to the broncho-pulmonary nodes and then to the tracheobronchial nodes (azygous nodes) and the high mediastinal nodes (Fig. 34-17). On the left, tumors of the upper lobe most often go to the ipsilateral bronchopulmonary nodes and tracheobronchial nodes (aortic window nodes) as well as to the anterior mediastinal nodes, although in 10% of the patients lymphatic metastasis may cross to the contralateral mediastinum. Lesions in the left lower lobe may metastasize to the same areas but also

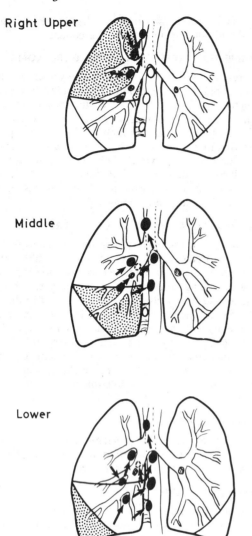

Right Upper

Middle

Lower

Fig. 34-17. Lymphatic drainage of the three lobes of the right lung. (After Nohl HC: An investigation into the lymphatic and vascular spread of carcinoma of the bronchus. Thorax 11:172, 1956)

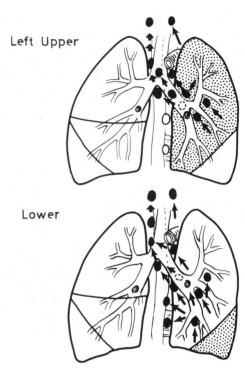

Left Upper

Lower

Fig. 34-18. Lymphatic drainage of the two lobes of the left lung. (After Nohl HC: An investigation of the lymphatic and vascular spread of carcinoma of the bronchus. Thorax, 11:179, 1956)

to the subcarinal nodes; in approximately 25% of the patients, spread may cross over from here to the right paratracheal nodes (Fig. 34-18). From the paratracheal node group of either side, as well as from the anterior mediastinal nodes, involvement of the respective supraclavicular nodes may occur. Lymphatic spread also occurs to nodes in the paraesophageal and para-aortic areas.

HEMATOGENOUS SPREAD

Blood-borne metastases are common in patients with bronchial carcinoma. The organs and structures most commonly involved are the liver, lungs, skeletal system, adrenal glands, kidneys, brain, and pancreas. Skeletal metastases are usually osteolytic. They occur most commonly in the ribs, spine, femur, humerus, and pelvis. Metastatic deposits distal to the knee or elbow are rare.

Metastatic deposits may occur in the skin and subcutaneous tissue, myocardium, thyroid gland, small intestine, spleen, and ovary. No distant site has been spared. Not infrequently, symptoms resulting from the metastatic spread of the tumor will be the first sign of the patient's disease.

CLINICAL MANIFESTATIONS

The clinical manifestations of bronchial carcinoma are protean. Approximately 5% of the patients are asymptomatic. In the others, symptoms are present in varying combinations and are related to the size and position of the tumor in the lung (bronchopulmonary manifestations) and its spread to extrapulmonary intrathoracic (extrapulmonary intrathoracic manifestations) and extrathoracic sites (extrathoracic metastatic manifestations), as well as to various substances with endocrine or toxic action or antigenic activity that the tumor may produce (extrathoracic nonmetastatic manifestations).

BRONCHOPULMONARY SYMPTOMS

Bronchopulmonary symptoms occur as a result of irritation, ulceration, or obstruction of a bronchus, with resulting collapse or occurrence of septic complications in the lung distal to the tumor, and include cough, hemoptysis, febrile respiratory symptoms, and, occasionally, dyspnea.

EXTRAPULMONARY INTRATHORACIC SYMPTOMS

Symptoms and signs may result from direct growth of the tumor onto the pleural surfaces or into the parietal pleura and chest wall or from direct involvement with other contiguous structures within the ipsilateral hemithorax. Extracapsular spread from lymph node metastases within the mediastinum also may involve the vena cava, the phrenic or recurrent nerves, and the esophagus. Hoarseness, superior vena caval syndrome, Horner's syndrome, dysphagia, dyspnea, and chest wall pain are some of the manifestations noted. In almost all instances, the occurrence of these symptoms supports nonresectability of the tumor.

EXTRATHORACIC METASTATIC SYMPTOMS

Symptoms resulting from metastatic spread of the tumor outside the thorax account for a small percentage of the presenting or major complaint of patients with carcinoma of the lung. Intracranial metastases may result in hemiplegia, epilepsy, personality changes, confusion, speech defects, or, at times, only headache. Bone pain and pathologic fracture from metastatic involvement may occur infrequently. Rarely, jaundice, ascites, or an abdominal mass may be the major complaint. Masses in the neck, muscle, or subcutaneous tissue are complained of only rarely.

EXTRATHORACIC NONMETASTATIC SYMPTOMS

Approximately 12% of patients with bronchial carcinoma will develop systemic symptoms and signs not related to metastatic spread of the tumor. None of these manifestations is specific, and all may occur in association with other malignant lesions.

Metabolic Manifestations

As a result of the secretion of endocrine or endocrinelike substances by the tumor, hormone-producing tumors may develop in any organ that contains cells originating in the primitive neural crest. Such cells have been demonstrated in organs derived from the foregut, including the bronchi. These cells can concentrate and decarboxylate precursors of the biogenic amines. These cells have been designated *APUD cells*, and they can produce a variety of polypeptide hormones. At times these symptoms may be produced by tumors that are still resectable, but unfortunately most are found in association with undifferentiated small cell carcinomas.

Cushing's syndrome is seen primarily in patients with undifferentiated small cell carcinoma. These patients comprise the majority of the reported individuals with this syndrome associated with nonadrenocortical, nonpituitary tumors. These patients differ from those with classic Cushing's syndrome, with reversal of the sex ratio, an older age incidence, the prominence of hypokalemia alkalosis, fewer physical stigmata of typical Cushing's syndrome, and a more rapid, fulminating clinical course.

Significant amounts of *adrenocorticotropic hormone* (ACTH) have been demonstrated in the tumor tissue and blood of many of these patients. By physiological, physiochemical, and immunochemical tests, the ectopic ACTH is indistinguishable from the normal hormone, although the tumors have physiologic autonomy since dexamethasone fails to suppress the levels of end products of ACTH in the urine. Excessive quantities of hydroxycorticosteroids, 17-OHCS, are readily demonstrable in the urine.

Excessive antidiuretic hormone production has been recognized in patients with undifferentiated small cell tumors. Positive immunoassay of an arginine-vasopressin-like material has been recorded. The symptoms are those of water intoxication with anorexia, nausea, and vomiting accompanied by increasingly severe neurologic complications. There is hypotonicity of the urine, absence of clinical evidence of fluid depletion, and normal renal and adrenal function.

Carcinoid syndrome is also seen in patients with undifferentiated small cell tumors. Neurosecretory granules similar to those seen in carcinoid tumor cells have been described in these tumor cells and are thought possibly to be the source of this and other materials.

The carcinoid syndrome is a well-defined clinical entity characterized by cutaneous, cardiovascular, gastrointestinal, and respiratory manifestations. Classically, the syndrome includes episodic signs and symptoms related to the release of various vasoactive amines. Flushing or edema, or both, of the face and upper body, hyperperistalsis and diarrhea, tachycardia, wheezing, pruritus, paresthesias, and vasomotor collapse may occur in varying combinations. Fibrosis of the right-sided heart valves due to superficial deposition of fibrous tissue with resultant cardiac decompensation may occur if the disease is long-standing, often not the case in association with carcinoma of the lung.

Many *vasoactive substances* in addition to serotonin (5-hydroxytryptamine), which was thought originally to be the cause of the clinical features, have been shown to be produced by these tumors; among these are 5-hydroxytryptophan, bradykinin and its precursor enzyme kallikrein, and various catecholamines.

Hypercalcemia is a frequent complication of malignant disease, and although it is often the result of the presence of bony metastases, it may be caused by excessive secretion of a polypeptide, similar to parathyroid hormone, by the tumor. An accompanying hypophosphatemia frequently is found. Most of these tumors are squamous cell in type. Clinically, the patient may have somnolence and mental changes as well as anorexia, nausea, vomiting, and weight loss. Frequently, the tumors are resectable, and this results in a reversal of the abnormal calcium levels in the blood.

Ectopic gonadotropin production is found rarely in association with carcinoma of the lung. There are a few male patients with tender gynecomastia, often associated with hypertrophic pulmonary osteoarthropathy, in whom production of gonadotropin may be documented.

Neuromuscular Manifestations

The neuromyopathies are the most frequent extrathoracic, nonmetastatic manifestations of carcinoma of the lung. If specifically looked for, one or more types of neuromyopathy may be found in approximately 15% of these patients. It may occur with any cell type. One half of the patients have no other symptoms of the lung tumor, and in one third the neuromyopathy may precede, by one year or more, the symptoms or the diagnosis of the carcinoma.

Carcinomatous myopathies consist mainly of two types: a myasthenialike syndrome and polymyositis. The former, probably a defect of neuromuscular conduction, is characterized by weakness and marked fatigability of the proximally located muscles of the extremities, particularly those of the pelvic girdle and thighs. The features of the latter are similar to those of the myasthenic syndrome, except that muscular wasting is more prominent and there is a primary degeneration of muscle fibers.

Peripheral neuropathy may be purely sensory, with pain and paresthesias followed by complete sensory loss in the extremities. Often, this is found in association with motor neuropathy, as evidenced by muscular weakness and wasting. Neuropathologic findings consist of loss of neurons in the dorsal root ganglia and selective degenerations of the posterior roots and columns of the spinal cord. The anterior roots are relatively unaffected.

Subacute cerebellar degeneration may result in a rapidly progressive loss of cerebellar function. Ataxic gait, lack of coordination, vertigo, nystagmus, and dysarthria are the characteristic features. Diffuse degeneration and depletion of Purkinje's cells, as well as other degenerative changes, occur in the cerebellum.

Encephalomyelopathy is manifested by a wide range of psychiatric disorders, such as dementia, deterioration of memory, and mood disorders. If the brain stem is involved, the symptoms depend upon the distribution of the lesions. Pyramidal tract signs and pseudobulbar palsy may occur.

The causes and pathogenesis of these neuropathies are unclear. The current hypothesis is that they arise as autoimmune or altered immune responses to substances produced by the tumor cells.

The recognition and differentiation of these neuromyopathies from metastatic lesions are important. Resection of the lung tumor, when possible, may result in remission of the symptoms.

Hypertrophic pulmonary osteoarthropathy consists of pain and swelling of the joints and periostitis, with elevation of the periosteum and new bone formation. Clubbing of the nails may be associated with this clinical syndrome. Clinically, the spectrum of symptomatology of hypertrophic pulmonary osteoarthropathy varies from minimal stiffness of the wrists to inability to walk. Edema of the joints may be marked, and joint and bone pain may be severe. The involvement is usually bilateral. The joints of the hand, ankle, knee, elbow, and shoulder are involved in that approximate order. Generalized malaise and even systemic toxicity with chills and spiking temperature and an elevated sedimentation rate may occur. The mechanism of development of the tissue changes is unknown. Hypertrophic pulmonary osteoarthropathy is not found in patients with undifferentiated small cell tumors, but it is distributed equally in patients with the other three major cell types.

Removal of the pulmonary lesion for the most part gives a dramatic remission of the arthralgia and peripheral edema. Osseous roentgenographic changes regress much more slowly.

Dermatologic Manifestations

Dermatologic manifestations consist of the acanthosis nigricans (usually associated with a bronchial adenocarcinoma), scleroderma, dermatomyositis, erythema gyratum, acquired ichthyosis, and nonspecific dermatoses.

Vascular Manifestations

Vascular manifestations such as thrombophlebitis, recurrent or migratory, may be the first indication of the presence of bronchial tumor. Nonbacterial verrucae—marantic endocarditis—characterized by deposition of sterile fibrin plaques on the heart valves and resultant arterial embolization, may occur. The mechanism by which either of these complications takes place is unknown.

Hematologic Manifestations

Hematologic findings are nonspecific. Normocytic normochromic anemia, fibrinolytic purpura, erythrocytosis, and nonspecific leukocytosis have been reported in patients with bronchial carcinoma.

Nonspecific Symptoms

Weight loss, weakness, anorexia, lassitude, and malaise occur in a large number of patients and may or may not be accompanied by other nonspecific symptoms. These symptoms may be the reason the patient seeks medical advice. Their causes are obscure but, when they are severe, suspicion of metastatic intra-abdominal spread of the tumor to liver, adrenal glands, pancreas, or para-aortic nodes should be considered.

ROENTGENOGRAPHIC FEATURES

The roentgenogram of the chest is abnormal in 98% of the patients and is strongly suggestive of tumor in approximately

80% percent of these. The early roentgenographic features are variable and are produced directly by the tumor itself. These may not be detectable until the tumor has completed three quarters of its normal existence.

USUAL ROENTGENOGRAPHIC FEATURES

The late and more usual manifestations are caused not only by the tumor itself but also by changes in the pulmonary parenchyma distal to the lesion and by changes resulting from extrapulmonary intrathoracic spread of the tumor. The usual roentgenographic abnormalities may be classified as hilar, parenchymal, and extrapulmonary. These abnormalities are best evaluated with posteroanterior (PA) and lateral roentgenograms of the chest.

The hilar abnormalities may be a unilateral hilar prominence, a distinct hilar mass, or a perihilar mass. Pulmonary parenchymal changes may consist of a peripheral mass of varying size (infrequently multiple masses), an apical opacification, regional hypertranslucency (rare), evidence of bronchial obstruction (regional atelectasis, consolidation, or pneumonitis), or abscess formation. Intrathoracic extrapulmonary changes may be represented by enlargement of the mediastinal shadow, erosion or disruption of the normal body structures of the chest wall, pleural effusion, and elevation of the hemidiaphragm.

INFLUENCE OF CELL TYPE

Commonly each cell type presents with relatively characteristic roentgenographic patterns.

Squamous Cell Carcinoma

Squamous cell tumors most often present the features of obstructive pneumonitis, parenchymal collapse, or consolidation (Fig. 34-19). One third may present as peripheral

Fig. 34-19. Roentgenogram of chest showing atelectasis of the right upper lobe due to obstructing tumor in the right upper lobe bronchial orifice.

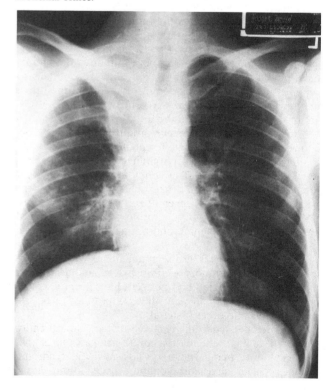

masses. Cavitation in these is relatively frequent, in contrast to the low incidence of cavitation in peripheral lesions caused by other cell types.

Adenocarcinoma

Adenocarcinomas are most often peripheral masses of varying size. Central lesions are relatively uncommon but are observed on occasion.

Undifferentiated Large Cell Carcinoma

Undifferentiated large cell carcinomas, likewise, are frequently peripheral. Hilar abnormalities with or without distal parenchymal changes may occur in one third of the patients with this type of tumor.

Undifferentiated Small Cell Carcinoma

Roentgenographically, undifferentiated small cell carcinomas most often present as hilar abnormalities, frequently with mediastinal widening. Distal parenchymal changes occur in only about two fifths of patients with these lesions; this is in contradistinction to the high incidence seen in patients with squamous cell tumors.

DIAGNOSTIC PROCEDURES

In addition to the history and physical, routine laboratory studies, and the PA and lateral roentgenograms of the chest, various diagnostic procedures including cytologic studies, special roentgenographic examinations, radionuclide scans, and invasive diagnostic procedures are required to establish the diagnosis and to stage the extent of the patient's disease process. It is certainly neither necessary nor appropriate to carry out all these various examinations in every patient. Each examination should be done only when it may resolve a diagnostic or therapeutic question.

CYTOLOGIC STUDIES

Cytologic examination of the sputum in patients with carcinoma of the lung may be positive in 45% to 90% of cases. Central lesions have a higher positive yield than do peripheral ones. Sputum from patients with small peripheral lesions are only infrequently positive. The cell type of the tumor may be determined reasonably well by the cytologic findings. Examination of smears obtained from bronchial brushing and from percutaneous needle aspiration of a suspicious pulmonary lesion is highly rewarding; cytologic examination of pleural fluid is less so.

SPECIAL ROENTGENOGRAPHIC EXAMINATIONS

Roentgenograms of the chest with the patient in various positions—oblique, lordotic, or kyphotic—may be helpful in various situations. Laminography of peripheral lesions and 55° oblique laminography of the ipsilateral hilus are useful. Laminographic examination of central lesions and of the mediastinum may be done but is not very rewarding. Contrast evaluation of the esophagus may be helpful in evaluating central lesions. Bronchography and venous angiographic studies are indicated only infrequently. The role of computed tomography of the chest in evaluating patients with carcinoma of the lung is yet to be determined.

RADIONUCLIDE SCANS

As a general principle, radionuclide scans of the liver, skeleton, or brain should only be performed when either signs or symptoms or laboratory findings of involvement of

the organ system are present. Exceptions to this may be a bone scan in those patients who are being considered for therapeutic irradiation or those few patients with undifferentiated small cell carcinoma who are being considered for possible resection. Gallium$_{67}$ scans with or without computed tomography appear to be indicated in the staging process of patients with undifferentiated small cell carcinoma. Their use in the evaluation of possible mediastinal lymph node metastases is under investigation.

Confirmation of a positive scan by an appropriate biopsy is indicated when the positive scan is the only contraindication to an otherwise indicated surgical resection.

INVASIVE DIAGNOSTIC PROCEDURES

It frequently is necessary to utilize one or more invasive diagnostic procedures to obtain tissues for diagnosis and to determine the appropriate therapeutic approach. These procedures include *bronchoscopy, percutaneous needle biopsy, mediastinal lymph node biopsy, and biopsy of suspected metastatic sites.*

Bronchoscopy and Biopsy

All patients with suspected bronchial carcinoma should undergo bronchoscopy, except those with readily documented distant metastasis. An additional exception may be the patient with a very small peripheral lesion in whom the examination most often is unrewarding. The flexible fiberoptic bronchoscope is utilized more frequently than the rigid scope, although the latter is very useful in patients with central lesions (Fig. 34-20).

Transthoracic Percutaneous Needle Biopsy

This procedure is highly accurate (90% to 97%) in obtaining tissue or cells for establishing the diagnosis of a peripheral carcinoma. Minimal complications are seen, the most common of which is a pneumothorax in approximately 20% of the procedures. Closed tube thoracotomy is required in approximately a third of these to control the complication. Despite its high diagnostic yield, this procedure is not

Fig. 34-20. Diagrammatic representation of the extent of visualization at bronchoscopy with the various bronchoscopic instruments. Fine diagonal lines: rigid bronchoscopic telescope; heavy diagonal lines: bronchoscopic telescope; horizontal lines: flexible fiberoptic bronchoscope. (Shields TW [ed]: Textbook of General Thoracic Surgery. Philadelphia, Lea & Febiger, 1972)

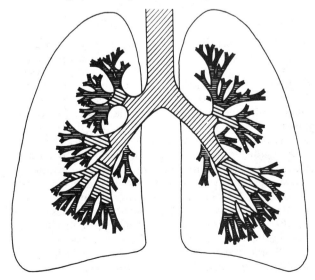

indicated routinely; it should be done only when it will influence the management of the patient.

Lymph Node Biopsy

The biopsy of the various lymph node groups which serve as reservoirs for the involved lung is indicated selectively.

Scalene Node Biopsy

Scalene node biopsy is indicated only when the nodes in the supraclavicular fossa are palpable. When nonpalpable, the diagnostic yield is too low (6% to 7%) to justify the procedure as supportive.

Mediastinal Node Biopsy

Mediastinal node biopsy, by mediastinoscopy or mediastinotomy, although recommended by some as routine for all surgical candidates, is indicated only under certain circumstances. These instances are when hilar enlargement is demonstrated on routine roentgenographic evaluation of the hilus; when hilar lymph node involvement has been suggested by 55° oblique tomograms of the hilar area; when the mediastinal shadow is abnormal, or suspiciously so, or when neither the hilus nor the mediastinum can be evaluated because parenchymal changes caused by the tumor obscure these structures. When computed tomography suggests enlarged mediastinal nodes, mediastinal exploration is also indicated.

Mediastinoscopy is carried out via a small cervical incision just above the sternal notch. It permits bilateral investigation of the mediastinum but does not afford accessibility to the lymph nodes in the aortic window area or to those in the anterior mediastinum.

Mediastinotomy is performed via a limited anterior thoracotomy. It provides access to the aforementioned areas and permits evaluation of the pulmonary artery and other hilar structures, but permits evaluation only of the ipsilateral mediastinum.

The findings which contraindicate surgical exploration for resection are gross extracapsular metastatic ipsilateral lymph node involvement, lymph node metastases above the midportion of the trachea or in the anterior mediastinum, contralateral lymph node involvement, or any direct invasion of other mediastinal structures or fixation or tumor involvement of the proximal portion of either pulmonary artery.

CLINICAL STAGING

Once the diagnosis has been established and the extent of the disease determined, the patient and the disease may be classified and staged by the TNM clinical staging system suggested by the American Joint Committee for Cancer Staging and End Results Reporting (see Table 14-3 in Chapter 14). In this classification, T designates the primary tumor, N the regional lymph nodes, and M distant metastasis. With the assignment of the TNM categories, the tumor may be grouped into Stage I, II, or III. Some modification in the stage grouping may be appropriate. The inclusion of $T_1N_1M_0$ lesions in Stage I disease is questioned, since metastases to hilar or lobar lymph nodes reduce the chance of long-term survival by at least half. Recent studies suggest that these $T_1N_1M_0$ lesions be placed in Stage II. An additional modification of the proposed stage grouping is to subdivide Stage III into that disease which is localized to the ipsilateral hemithorax and mediastinum—localized Stage II—and that

which is disseminated beyond these boundaries—disseminated Stage III. The stage grouping as suggested is primarily applicable to patients with tumors of a cell type other than undifferentiated small cell; however, tentative clinical classification of even patients with this cell type may be helpful in their management. Regardless of these suggested modifications, the TNM classification and staging system appears to be pertinent. However, before final decision as to therapy is made, the physiological and functional status of the patient should be determined.

PHYSIOLOGICAL EVALUATION

FUNCTIONAL CLASSIFICATION

The functional classification of Karnofsky (see Table 14-2 in Chapter 14) or one of its modifications is important in the overall evaluation of the patient as to the appropriateness of a proposed therapeutic course. This is particularly true for those patients with disseminated disease, since most surgical candidates are ambulatory and need little or no care preoperatively. However, in the latter group assessing the physiological status of the respiratory and cardiovascular systems is important in determining whether or not the patient will be able to tolerate the proposed surgical procedure.

EVALUATION OF PULMONARY FUNCTION

Pulmonary function is evaluated primarily to define which patients are at high risk for resection and which patients are unable to tolerate any resection. The estimation of extent of the maximum tolerated resection as well as prediction of the postresection ventilatory capacity may be accomplished.

In many instances, screening ventilatory tests are sufficient, but when significant impairment is detected, additional studies may be indicated. The most useful tests for initially assessing the status of the patient's pulmonary function are the forced vital capacity *(FVC)*, the forced expiratory volume in 1 second *(FEV_1)*, and the maximum voluntary ventilation *(MVV)*.

The measurements of FVC and FEV_1 may classify the nature of any existing ventilatory impairment as restrictive (FVC) or obstructive (FEV_1). When the FEV_1 is equal to 2.5 liters or more (85% of predicted normal), the patient can tolerate a pneumonectomy. When the FEV_1 is between 1 and 2.4 liters (40% to 80% of predicted normal), the patient has moderate to mild ventilatory impairment. In such instances the estimate of the extent and the risk of resection must be further evaluated. When the FEV_1 is less than 1 liter (40% of predicted normal) severe impairment is present and surgical resection is contraindicated (Fig. 34-21). When a MVV has been performed, a result of less than 45% to 50% of predicted normal contraindicates resection. Bronchoradiospirometry may be carried out to predict the postoperative FEV_1; when this is greater than 800 cc it is concluded that the patient can tolerate a pneumonectomy.

The final assessment of the ability of the patient to withstand the proposed pulmonary resection must be a clinical one. The pulmonary function studies must be viewed in the light of the age of the patient (although age *per se* is not a contraindication), the amount of loss of functioning lung tissue due to the tumor and its associated parenchymal changes as judged by the roentgenographic findings, the degree of cooperation of the patient, the presence or absence of toxicity and fatigue due to associated infection, and the status of the cardiovascular system.

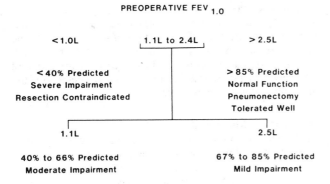

PREOPERATIVE FEV₁.₀

| <1.0L | 1.1L to 2.4L | >2.5L |

<40% Predicted
Severe Impairment
Resection Contraindicated

>85% Predicted
Normal Function
Pneumonectomy
Tolerated Well

1.1L

2.5L

40% to 66% Predicted
Moderate Impairment

67% to 85% Predicted
Mild Impairment

Maximum Tolerated Resection Judgemental

Greater Risk   Lesser Risk

Fig. 34-21. Preoperative FEV₁ relative to selection of operative procedure in patients with carcinoma of the lung. (Shields TW: Surgical therapy for carcinoma of the lung. In Matthay R [ed.]: Lung Cancer. Clinics in Chest Medicine 3:369, 1982)

CARDIAC CONTRAINDICATIONS TO OPERATION

The presence of uncontrolled cardiac failure or uncontrolled arrhythmia, or the history of a recent myocardial infarction, also contraindicates resection. Whether only a 3- or 6-month period should elapse after a myocardial infarction before resection is considered is questioned. Anesthesia and surgical intervention less than 3 months after an infarct are unwise.

A history of angina does not rule out pulmonary resection when the stress tests are negative. Electrocardiographic abnormalities are not unusual in the patient group under consideration for a pulmonary resection for carcinoma. A right bundle branch block does not increase the operative risk to any great extent. However, left posterior fascicular blocks have the highest risk.

IMMUNOLOGIC FEATURES

TUMOR ANTIGENS

As with other tumors of the body, it is believed there is an immunologic response to carcinoma of the lung. There is evidence that the tumor cells possess surface antigens that are capable of evoking an immune response in the host. Some of these antigens are specific for the cell type in question, while other antigens may evoke response to normal tissues. Fetal tissue antigens are encountered with particular frequency. Carcinoembryonic antigen may be identified in approximately 20% of patients with bronchial carcinoma but is identified infrequently in resectable patients.

TUMOR ANTIBODIES

There is only minimal demonstrated evidence of humoral immunity to lung tumors. This may be the result of only small amounts of antibody released into the circulation at irregular intervals or to the blocking of antibody in antigen–antibody complexes.

CELL-MEDIATED IMMUNITY

Although it appears that humoral immunity to carcinoma of the lung is weak, there appears to be a strong cell-mediated immunity. This has been observed to be associated with a better prognosis. Tests of cell-mediated immunity reveal that it is depressed in patients with advanced carcinoma of the lung. However, in patients with early (resectable) disease, the results are variable. In general, depression of DHS skin reactions to recall antigens has not been demonstrated. However, an impaired ability to become sensitized to DNCB frequently has been demonstrated. The degree of depression of lymphocyte function tests (Table 34-3) varies with different histologic cell types and with the extent of the disease process.

The significance of these studies in identifying resectable candidates is undetermined. However, most studies support the concept that impaired tests of lymphocyte function carry a poor prognosis.

TREATMENT

The treatment modalities available for patients with carcinoma of the lung are surgical resection, radiation therapy, chemotherapy, immunotherapy, and other nonspecific measures. The selection of the appropriate treatment regimen is dependent upon the stage and cell type of the patient's disease, functional status, and physiological capacity. As a general guide, most patients with undifferentiated small cell carcinoma, regardless of the stage of the disease, are managed by a regimen of combined chemotherapy and radiation therapy. Patients with the other three cell types are surgical candidates when the disease can be classified as Stage I or II (occasionally specific types of localized Stage III). Patients with localized Stage III disease are usually candidates for therapeutic irradiation. Patients with disseminated Stage III disease may receive palliative radiation therapy, chemotherapy, or other nonspecific palliative measures in varying combinations.

SURGICAL THERAPY

Approximately 20% to 25% of the patients with tumors of a cell type other than undifferentiated small cell carcinoma are surgical candidates. The extent of the disease process in the hemithorax at exploration and the pulmonary functional capacity of the patient determine the extent of the resectional procedure.

The operations employed are lobectomy, pneumonectomy, and segmental or wedge resection. Each procedure may be modified or extended to remove adjacent structures as indicated.

TABLE 34-3   TESTS OF LYMPHOCYTE FUNCTION

Delayed hypersensitivity skin tests	Recall antigens, *e.g.*, mumps, PPD, streptokinase/streptodornase
	New antigens, *e.g.*, DNCB
	Tumor extracts
Peripheral blood cell counts	Total lymphocytes
	T-cells
	B-cells
Lymphocyte transformation studies	Mitogens: PHA, pokeweed, concanavilin A
	Bacterial antigens: PPD, staphylococcal phage lysate
	Allogeneic lymphocytes
Leukocyte migration inhibition tests	

Operative Procedures

Lobectomy. Lobectomy is the most commonly done resection. It is indicated when the disease process is confined to a lobe and preferably when lymph node metastases are absent. The procedure permits conservation of lung tissue, it is better tolerated by the patient, and the morbidity and mortality are less than after a pneumonectomy. Modifications of the procedure are a bilobectomy on the right and a sleeve lobectomy when the tumor is in a lobar bronchus. The latter operation consists of resection of a lobe and a portion of the adjacent main stem bronchus, with bronchoplastic repair of the bronchus by an end-to-end anastomosis.

Pneumonectomy. Pneumonectomy is required when a lobectomy or one of its modifications is not sufficient to remove the local disease or its lobar or hilar lymph node metastases. The procedure may be modified to include an *en bloc* mediastinal lymph node dissection or by intrapericardial ligations of the pulmonary vessels or both. An infrequently used modification is a pneumonectomy with a tracheal sleeve resection.

Segmentectomy and Wedge Resections. Segmental and wedge resections may be used to remove small peripheral tumors (3 cm or less in size) without evidence of lymph node metastases.

Extended Resections. Extended resections to include local extension of the primary tumor into structures that may be removed *en bloc* without compromise of the patient's well-being may be added to any one of the aforementioned operative procedures. Such resections may include portions of the lateral chest wall, diaphragm, pericardium, superior vena cava, and apex of the chest cage.

Lung carcinoma at the apex that involves the apical parietal pleura and invades the soft tissue above this level is called *Pancoast's tumor*. Pain down the arm and, at times, Horner's syndrome are frequent symptoms of the lesion, because of invasion of the brachial plexus and sympathetic chain. These tumors are usually readily detected by chest roentgenogram or CT scan, but at times they may be very small and go undetected for some months. The prognosis is guarded, though a few have been cured by preoperative irradiation followed by extirpation of surrounding tissues.

Operative Technique

A posterolateral thoracotomy is used for most pulmonary resections. Individual dissection and ligation of the vascular structures and then isolation and division of the bronchus are carried out. Closure of the bronchial stump may be accomplished equally well by interrupted sutures or by a mechanical suturing device. All accessible lymph nodes should be removed and appropriately labeled as to their position relative to the tracheobronchial tree; no true *en bloc* removal of the lymph nodes can be performed.

Complications

After any procedure, the complications may be classified as those either unique to, or directly related to, the procedure—technical, pleural, pulmonary, cardiac, or septic—and as those related to the performance of any major operative procedure—cardiovascular, genitourinary, gastrointestinal, or peripheral-vascular.

The more commonly encountered complications related to the procedure are atelectasis, continued air leak, residual air space, disruption of the bronchial closure, empyema, cardiac arrhythmias, respiratory insufficiency, and postoperative hemorrhage.

Postoperative Mortality

Mortality rates vary with the magnitude of the procedure. After pneumonectomy for resection of a carcinoma of the lung, the incidence may vary from 5% to 10% to as high as 15%. After lobectomy this incidence is in the range of 2% to 8%. After segmentectomy or wedge resection, the mortality rates are approximately only 1%.

Adjunctive Measures

Additional treatment may include radiation therapy, chemotherapy, and immunotherapy. Each may be used alone or in combination with the others. The chosen modality may be used pre-, intra-, or postoperatively.

Radiation Therapy. Irradiation given preoperatively has been found to be of no benefit and is not recommended. Postoperative irradiation has been suggested to be of value in patients in whom mediastinal lymph nodes which have been resected are found to contain metastatic tumor. Randomized studies have not been done to confirm this reported benefit.

Chemotherapeutic Regimens. Regimens of one or more drugs given for varying periods of time postoperatively have not improved survival in the controlled studies reported to date. Except in a study situation, adjuvant chemotherapy is not recommended.

Immunotherapy. Specific and nonspecific immunotherapy as an adjuvant is under investigation. In patients with Stage I disease there is some evidence that nonspecific and specific immunotherapy may be of benefit, although more information is needed before it can be recommended as a routine. Immunorestorants have not been beneficial.

Results of Surgical Therapy

Long-term survival is dependent primarily upon the extent of the disease process, as determined by examination of the resected specimen, and to a lesser extent by the cell type. In patients without lymph node metastases, cell type (exclusive of undifferentiated small cell carcinoma) is of minimal importance. When lymph nodes are involved, patients with squamous cell carcinoma do better than those with either adenocarcinoma or undifferentiated large cell carcinoma; the more advanced the pathologic stage, the greater the difference.

Regardless of cell type, patients with $T_1N_0M_0$ lesions have a 5-year survival of between 55% and 70%. Patients with $T_2N_0M_0$ lesions have a 5-year survival of 40% to 45%. Patients with $T_1N_1M_0$ or $T_2N_1M_0$ lesions have a 5-year survival of 20% to 30%. Patients with Stage III disease (T_3 with any N, M_0, or N_2 with only T, M_0) have a 5-year survival well under 15%.

RADIATION THERAPY

Irradiation may be given in an attempt to cure (therapeutic irradiation) or only to ameliorate distressful symptomatology (palliative irradiation). The most radiosensitive cell type is undifferentiated small cell carcinoma. Squamous cell carcinoma is somewhat more sensitive than either adenocarcinoma or undifferentiated large cell carcinoma.

Therapeutic Irradiation

Radiation therapy in an attempt to cure is indicated in patients who have a tumor other than an undifferentiated small cell carcinoma and who have Stage III disease localized to the hemithorax which can be treated via relatively small ports (10 cm × 15 cm). The suggested total dose is between 5000 and 6000 rads in 6 weeks. Approximately 8% to 10% 5-year survival rate may be obtained. It also may be used for patients with Stage I or Stage II disease who either refuse operative removal of the lesion or are unable to undergo the indicated operation because of medical contraindications. Patients with undifferentiated small cell carcinoma may receive therapeutic irradiation to the primary lesion as part of a treatment regimen with chemotherapy.

Palliative Irradiation

Radiation therapy is useful in alleviating hemoptysis in 95% of instances; cough, dyspnea, and chest pain to some extent in 60% to 70% of patients; and bone pain and symptoms of intracranial metastases in most patients who present with these complaints. Patients with superior vena caval obstruction respond to radiation therapy, and this primary modality of treatment may be supplemented with diuretics, anticoagulants, and cortisone.

CHEMOTHERAPY

The management of patients with undifferentiated small cell carcinoma regardless of the extent of the disease process (with few exceptions) is chemotherapy. A multiple drug regimen using a combination of four or more drugs (cyclophosphamide, doxorubicin [Adriamycin], methotrexate, vincristine, VP-16, lomustine [CCNU], and others), along with therapeutic irradiation to the primary site plus prophylactic whole-brain irradiation, has resulted in complete remissions of the disease process and an increasing incidence of disease-free survival of 2 years or more. The incidence of complete response and the numbers of 2-year disease-free survivors are greater in those patients who have localized disease (10% to 15% 2-year survival) but improvement in median survival also has been noted in patients with extensive disease. The timing and dosage of irradiation to the local lesion continue under investigation. Prophylactic whole-brain irradiation (2000 to 3000 rads in 2 weeks) has been shown to reduce the incidence of cerebral manifestations of intracranial metastases from 25% to about 2%, although it has not increased the length of survival.

In patients with tumors other than undifferentiated small cell carcinoma, chemotherapy plays a minor role. Response rates vary from 10% to 30%. This is influenced by the performance status of the patient; the better the status, the better the chance of response. Patients who are confined to bed and require nursing care have minimal to no response to most drug regimens. Ideally, chemotherapy, as now available, should be employed only in symptomatic patients with disseminated disease who are ambulatory for at least half the day. Regimens of two or more drugs for each specific cell type have been recommended.

IMMUNOTHERAPY

At present immunotherapy, either specific (autologous or allogeneic tumor cells or extracts) or nonspecific (mycobacterial antigen-BCG or C Parvum or immunorestorants-levamisole), has been employed only as an adjuvant modality. Despite the intensive investigations that have been carried out, the results have not been very impressive. In only a few patients with localized disease treated by either resection or irradiation has some increase in survival and freedom from tumor recurrence been noted with the use of adjuvant immunotherapy.

PALLIATIVE MEDICAL MEASURES

Many patients with carcinoma of the lung eventually require palliative medical measures such as antibiotics, narcotics, and other supportive measures (orthopedic, neurosurgical) to relieve symptoms arising from the presence of the tumor within the chest or from its metastasis. Judicious use of all such modalities is indicated to keep the patient as comfortable as possible.

PROGNOSIS

The results obtained with a specific type of therapy depend upon the selection of patients in which it is employed. Only short-term prolongation of survival may be expected from the various chemotherapeutic regimens, since most patients who are candidates for this therapy have far-advanced disease. Radiation therapy may afford significant palliation, but long-term survival rarely follows. In the select group of patients with highly localized but unresectable Stage III disease and in the few with Stage I and II disease who undergo radiation therapy, the survival rate is better. As many as 50% may survive for 1 year, and 5% to 8% may survive for 5 years.

Patients with undifferentiated small cell tumors have a very poor prognosis, less than 1 year median survival with extensive disease. With limited disease, some 2-year survivals have been achieved with appropriate therapy.

After a definitive resection of tumors other than undifferentiated small cell in type, long-term survival depends upon the pathologic classification of the disease process. This reflects primarily the size, location, and extent of the primary tumor and the absence or presence of and site of intrathoracic lymph node metastasis. Patients with $T_1N_0M_0$ disease have the best prognosis, a 55% to 70% 5-year survival. Patients with $T_2N_0M_0$ disease may expect a 40% to 45% 5-year survival; those with $T_1N_1M_0$ or $T_2N_1M_0$ disease a 20% to 30%; those with Stage III disease, with few exceptions, a 5-year survival under 15% (Fig. 34-22). Most patients who die of recurrent disease will do so within the first or second postoperative year. The percentage is less in the third year and only a few in the fourth and fifth years. During the first 5 years after operation, 10% to 25% of the patients die of some disease other than their original tumor. After the fifth anniversary almost all patients will die of some cause other than the original tumor. Twenty percent will develop a second primary, half of which occur in the remaining lung tissue.

BRONCHIAL ADENOMA

Bronchial adenomas constitute 1% to 2% of all bronchial tumors. The name implies that the lesions are benign, but in fact these tumors are malignant, albeit generally low grade in nature, with long natural histories. Included in this category are carcinoid adenomas, cylindroma (adenoid cystic carcinoma), mucoepidermoid tumor, and other rare varieties: bronchial mucous gland adenoma and a mixed tumor of salivary gland type.

CARCINOID ADENOMA

INCIDENCE

Carcinoid adenoma is the most common of these tumors and comprises 85% to 90% of all bronchial adenomas. The

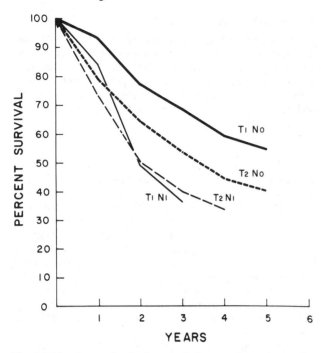

Fig. 34-22. Postrandomization survival curves for patients who have undergone successful resection of carcinoma of the lung with the various pathologic TNM classifications. (Shields TW: Pathological stage grouping of patients with resected carcinoma of the lung. J Thorac Cardiovasc Surg 80:400, 1980)

lesions occur with equal frequency in men and in women. They may occur in any age group but are most commonly discovered in young and middle-aged adults.

PATHOLOGY

Ninety percent of these lesions occur in the first to the third order bronchi; 10% occur as peripheral lesions. Grossly, the proximal lesions present as an endobronchial mass covered with an intact mucosa. The tumor may partially or completely block the bronchial lumen. Some of the lesions are polypoid, while others are infiltrating. In the latter the tumor extends extrabronchially into the surrounding peribronchial tissue and pulmonary parenchyma. This portion of the growth may be many times larger than the visualized endobronchial disease (an iceberg tumor). The peripheral lesion presents as a solitary firm nodule of varying size.

Microscopically, the typical carcinoid adenoma is made up of interlacing cords and masses of small uniform cells with oval nuclei containing granular chromatin (Fig. 34-23). The connective tissue is highly vascular; occasional osseous metaplasia may be seen. Atypical forms exist. Only few argentaffin-staining cells are seen, but electron microscopic studies reveal neurosecretory granules in varying numbers in the tumor cells. Bronchial carcinoids are thought to arise from the paraendocrine (APUD) system of cells. At times the tumor appears not unlike an undifferentiated small cell carcinoma.

CLINICAL FEATURES

Bronchial carcinoids may metastasize to the regional lymph nodes in 10% to 15% of instances. Distant dissemination is infrequent. Locally, the central tumors produce bronchial obstruction and its sequelae: cough, recurrent infection, and atelectasis. Hemoptysis is a not uncommon complaint. As a result of the slow growth of these lesions, these symptoms may be present for long periods of time before the diagnosis is established. Peripheral lesions are generally asymptomatic.

Fig. 34-23. Low- and high-power photomicrograph of a carcinoid adenoma with interlacing cords and masses of uniform cells. (Shields TW [ed]: Textbook of General Thoracic Surgery. Philadelphia, Lea & Febiger, 1972)

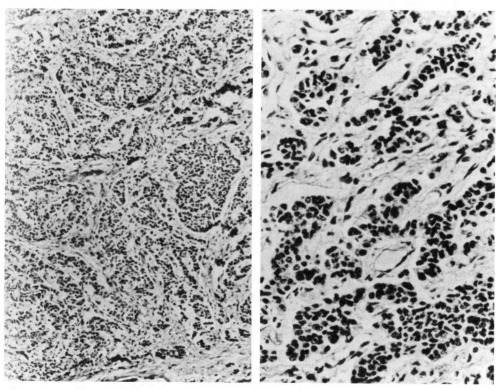

On occasion, significant amounts of biologically active substances are produced in these cells. The carcinoid syndrome and Cushing's syndrome are the more frequently recognized clinical entities. Rarely, gastrinlike substances, antidiureticlike hormone, and excessive insulin production have been identified in these patients.

DIAGNOSIS

Roentgenographic studies of the chest in patients with tracheal adenoma often will reveal the associated pulmonary parenchymal changes but only infrequently the tumor itself. In approximately 25% of the patients, roentgenograms of the chest will be normal.

Bronchoscopic examination is essential in making the diagnosis; at least 75% of the lesions may be identified by this examination. Despite the vascularity of the tumor, endobronchial biopsy is indicated to obtain tissue for diagnostic histologic examination.

Biochemical studies to screen patients with suspected bronchial adenomas for the presence of serotonin and its degradation products may be worthwhile. The blood levels and urinary levels may be elevated even in the absence of clinical symptomatology.

TREATMENT

Surgical resection is the treatment of choice. The most conservative resection necessary to remove the tumor is indicated. When irreversible parenchymal changes are not present, resection with bronchoplastic reconstruction of the bronchial tree is indicated. When irreversible changes, such as distal bronchiectasis or organized pneumonia, are present, the involved lung tissue also must be removed—again with as conservative resection as possible. A lobectomy is not uncommon, but fortunately pneumonectomy is infrequent.

When lymph nodes are involved by metastatic tumor, adequate lymph node dissection should be accomplished. Even if complete removal is not possible, as much of the involved tissue should be removed as feasible.

When the lesion is nonresectable, or medical contraindications to resection are present, endoscopic removal may be attempted. Postoperative hemorrhage is a serious complication after such procedures. Rarely, when the tumor is a polypoid lesion, endoscopic removal may be curative.

PROGNOSIS

In most series, 5- to 10-year survival rates are reportedly between 75% and 95%. Patients in whom the lesion has been removed completely and in whom no lymph node metastases were present may be considered cured. When metastatic lymph node involvement is demonstrated, only about 50% will develop recurrent disease.

CYLINDROMA (ADENOID CYSTIC CARCINOMA)

Cylindromas comprise 8% to 10% of all bronchial adenomas. These lesions tend to occur in the lower trachea near the level of the carina and the take-off of the stem bronchi; approximately one third occur near the origin of the major lobar bronchi. Rarely are they peripheral in location. These lesions are much more malignant than the carcinoid lesions, and one third of the patients have either local (regional lymph nodes) or distant metastases (liver, bone, and kidneys) or both at the time of diagnosis.

Microscopically there are two cellular patterns, pseudo-acinar (Fig. 34-24) or medullary. Distant submucosal spread and perineural lymphatic invasion are commonly demonstrated.

Treatment ideally is wide surgical excision with conser-

Fig. 34-24. Low- and high-power photomicrograph of an adenoid cystic carcinoma with pseudo-acinar pattern. (Shields TW [ed]: Textbook of General Thoracic Surgery. Philadelphia, Lea & Febiger, 1972)

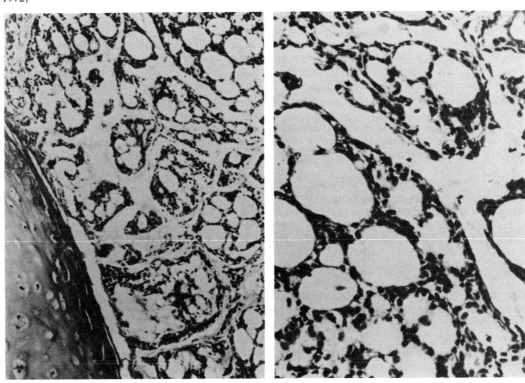

vation of distal lung tissue when possible by tracheal or bronchoplastic sleeve resection. Resection of distal lung is required when the lung has been destroyed by persistent infection. Extensive lymph node resection is indicated in all operations for the removal of this tumor. Endoscopic removal is ineffective for cure but may result in satisfactory palliation when the lesion cannot be removed surgically. Radiation therapy may result occasionally in long-term survival, but as a rule these lesions are radiation-resistant.

The prognosis for these patients for freedom from recurrent disease is poor (20% to 35%). Long-term survival with recurrent disease is not uncommon, but the majority of patients ultimately die of the disease process.

MUCOEPIDERMOID CARCINOMA

Mucoepidermoid carcinoma makes up about 2% of all bronchial adenomas. These may occur in either sex and at any age, although most commonly in the sixth decade of life. The anatomic distribution is similar to the carcinoid tumors. These tumors have characteristics similar to the mucoepidermoid tumors of the salivary glands. The principles of treatment and the prognosis of these lesions are similar to those described for the bronchial carcinoids.

LESS COMMON MALIGNANT TUMORS

Nonepithelial malignant tumors are exceedingly rare and constitute less than 1% of all lung cancers. Included are soft-tissue sarcomas and lymphomas.

SOFT TISSUE SARCOMA

Tumors of mesenchymal origin may arise from stromal elements of the bronchus, the vascular walls, or interstices of the lung parenchyma. They usually appear as well-circumscribed and encapsulated masses in the lung parenchyma. They spread by local invasion and metastasize by way of the bloodstream, rarely by lymphatic invasion. The tumor may originate from any one of the various mesenchymal cell types. Most are asymptomatic, although chest pain, cough, dyspnea, and hemoptysis may be present. Fever, fatigue, anorexia, and weight loss are late manifestations. The typical roentgenographic feature is a sharply demarcated mass within the lung substance, at the hilus or in the periphery.

Cytologic studies and bronchoscopy are usually unrewarding. Treatment is adequate resection of the lesion: sleeve resection, lobectomy, or pneumonectomy as necessary.

Most patients with soft tissue sarcoma succumb to their disease within 3 years. Patients with rhabdomyosarcoma have an extremely poor prognosis. In contrast to these and other soft tissue sarcomas, over 50% of patients with leiomyosarcoma of the lung survive 5 years or longer.

LYMPHOMA

All tumors originating in lymphoid tissue within the lung are lymphomas. Most types can be readily identified, but there is difficulty in differentiating benign lymphocytic and plasma cell tumors from their malignant counterparts.

The majority of primary pulmonary lymphomas are solid tumors. Cystic degeneration may be seen in reticulum cell sarcoma and in Hodgkin's disease. Most of these tumors remain localized. Regional node involvement is variable.

The symptomatology and roentgenographic features are indistinguishable from those due either to inflammatory or to other malignant processes. Few are correctly identified before operation. Both radiation therapy and resection are effective in the treatment of primary pulmonary lymphomas. The prognosis is better than for disseminated lymphomas or other lung cancers.

BENIGN LUNG TUMORS

Benign tumors of the lung are infrequently encountered. They may present as asymptomatic solitary peripheral nodules or may produce symptoms due to an endobronchial location with resultant hemoptysis, atelectasis, or distal infection.

BRONCHIAL HAMARTOMA

Hamartomas are the most common benign lung tumors. They are more common in the fifth and sixth decades of life, and are seen twice as often in men as in women. Ninety percent or more are peripheral in location; the remainder are located endobronchially. Infrequently the lesions may be multiple, and slow growth of the lesion may be observed.

Roentgenographically, a hamartoma presents a sharply demarcated peripheral mass, which may be lobulated (bosselated). Calcification within the mass is uncommon but may be seen in a popcorn distribution.

Surgical resection is the treatment of choice. Enucleation or wedge resection is done when possible; occasionally a more extensive resection will be required. In patients with an endobronchial hamartoma, as conservative a resection as possible to remove the tumor and the associated distal parenchymal changes is indicated. Recurrence after surgical excision is unknown.

OTHER BENIGN TUMORS

Benign tumors of epithelial, mesenchymal, and lymphoid origin may occur. Multiple papillary tumors and inflammatory polyps of the tracheobronchial tree may present troublesome clinical problems. Pulmonary hemangiomas are often associated with Rendu-Osler-Weber syndrome.

SECONDARY TUMORS IN THE LUNG

The lungs are common sites for the occurrence of metastatic disease. Approximately 20% to 30% of patients dying of cancer will have such disease. In one half of the patients, this is the only site of metastatic involvement. The lesions are most often multiple and bilateral. In 2% to 10% the lesion may be solitary.

PATHOLOGY

Metastatic spread to the lungs may occur by direct infiltration, may be lymphatic-borne and, most importantly, may be blood-borne. Lymphatic spread occurs less commonly and presents as lymphangitic carcinomatosis. Primary tumors of the stomach, breast, and lung occasionally spread to the lung in this manner. Most lesions, however, are solid, spherical masses.

RARE PULMONARY TUMORS

"Bronchial Adenoma"

Carcinoid tumor
Cylindroma
Mucoepidermoid tumor
Mucous gland adenoma

Other Tumors Derived from Bronchial Epithelium

Multiple papillomata
Inflammatory polyps
Solitary bronchial polyp

Tumors of Vascular Origin

Hemangioma
Lymphangioma
Lymphangioleiomyomatosis
Hemangioendothelioma
Pulmonary arteriovenous fistula
Hemangiopericytoma
Leiomyosarcoma of the pulmonary trunk

Tumors of Muscular Origin

Leiomyoma
Leiomyosarcoma
Rhabdomyosarcoma

Other Tumors of Mesenchymal Origin

Chondroma
Lipoma
Fibroma
Malignant mesenchymoma
Myxoma
Osteochondrosarcoma
Mesothelioma

Tumors of Lymphogenous Origin

Lymphosarcoma
Intrapulmonary Hodgkin's disease (primary)
Plasmacytoma
Lymphomatoid granulomatosis
Primary pulmonary histiocytosis X
Thymoma
Pulmonary pseudolymphoma

Tumors of Neural and Neural Crest Origin (Excluding Carcinoid)

Chemodectoma (nonchromaffin paraganglioma)
Benign clear cell tumor
Medullary carcinoma of the lung
Primary pulmonary melanoma
Oncocytoma
Granular cell myoblastoma
Neuroma
Neurofibromatosis
Neurilemmoma (Schwannoma)
Neurogenic sarcoma

Tumors of Mixed Cellular Origin

Hamartoma (chrondromatous hamartoma)
Congenital adenomatous malformation
Multiple nodular fibroleiomyomatous hamartoma
Blastoma (embryoma)
Carcinosarcoma
Teratoma

Pulmonary Pseudotumors

Tracheobronchopathia chondro-osteoplastica
Amyloidosis
Inflammatory pseudotumors (xanthomas, fibroxanthomas, fibrous histiocytoma)
Pulmonary infarction

Tumors of Uncertain Origin

Histiocytoma (plasma cell granuloma)
Sclerosing hemangioma

Aberrant Tissue

Endometriosis
Splenosis

Tumor doubling time may be calculated when several sequential films are available. Doubling time refers to increase in volume, not diameter. The method involves plotting diameter against time on semilogarithmic paper, since a doubling in diameter increases volume eight-fold. When a doubling time of less than 37 or more than 465 days is observed, the lesion is benign. Metastatic lesions and primary carcinomas of the lung will have doubling times somewhere in between these extremes. The more malignant, generally the more rapid the growth.

DIAGNOSIS

The diagnosis of metastatic tumor to the lungs is made readily by the history and roentgenographic findings. A tissue diagnosis may be established by bronchoscopy, cytologic examinations, percutaneous needle biopsy, and open lung biopsy.

In patients with a solitary lung lesion and a history of a previous primary malignancy in a different organ system, the new lesion may represent a benign lesion, a secondary lung primary, or a metastatic lesion. When the lesion is malignant, the new lung lesion most frequently is a new lung primary when the original tumor was a squamous cell carcinoma. When it was an adenocarcinoma, there is a 50–50 chance that the lung lesion is either a new primary or a metastatic lesion. When the original tumor was a sarcoma, the new lesion is almost always a metastasis.

TREATMENT

The management of a solitary metastasis is surgical resection if there are no signs or symptoms of recurrent or other metastatic disease. Five-year survival rates of 20% to 35% have been recorded.

When multiple metastatic disease is present, several courses of action are possible. When a satisfactory chemotherapeutic regimen is available, this should be initiated; residual lesions, if any, may be resected by multiple local excisions by a bilateral thoracotomy through a median sternotomy approach. When no satisfactory chemotherapeutic regimen is known, occasional bilateral resection may be attempted when the disease is relatively limited. However, in most instances, only palliative measures are available under these circumstances. Adjuvant radiation therapy may be used on occasion.

PROGNOSIS

Patients with multiple metastatic lesions have a poor prognosis unless a suitable, effective chemotherapeutic regimen for the specific tumor is available. This along with adjuvant irradiation and multiple local excisions may result in improved survival.

BIBLIOGRAPHY

American Joint Committee for Cancer Staging and End Results Reporting: Clinical Staging System for Carcinoma of the Lungs. Chicago, 1973

BEATTIE EJ JR (ed): Symposium on lung cancer. World J Surg 5:661, 1981

BOROW M: Mesothelioma following exposure to asbestos: A review of 72 cases. Chest 64:641, 1973

BURCHARTH F, AZELSON C: Bronchial adenomas. Thorax 27:442, 1972

BYRD RB, CARR DT, MILLER WE et al: Radiographic abnormalities in carcinoma of the lung as related to histological type. Thorax 24:573, 1969

DABEK FT: Bronchial carcinoid tumor with acromegaly in two patients. J Clin Endocrinol Metab 38:329, 1974

ERDMAN S: Lung pseudotumor caused by pulmonary infarction. Geriatrics 30:103, 1975

HAKIMI M: Endobronchial lipoma associated with squamous metaplasia of bronchial mucosa. Mich Med 74:129, 1975

HARDY JD, EWING HP, NEELY WA et al: Lung carcinoma: Survey of 2286 cases with emphasis on small cell type. Ann Surg 193:539, 1981

HORTON WA: Multiple endocrine adenomatosis presenting a Zollinger-Ellison syndrome, non β islet cell tumor, parathyroid adenoma, renal calculi, bronchial carcinoid, insulinoma, hepatic hamartoma. Birth Defects 7:275, 1971

JENSIK RJ, FABER LP, MILLOY FJ et al: Segmental resection for lung cancer: A 15-year experience. J Thorac Cardiovasc Surg 66:563, 1973

KIRSH MJ, KAHN DR, GAGO O et al: Treatment of bronchogenic carcinoma with mediastinal metastases. Ann Thorac Surg 12:11, 1971

KOIKKALAINEN E, KESKITALO E, LUOSTO R et al: Carcinoid tumors and cylindromas of the tracheobronchial tree. Ann Chir Gynaecol 63:332, 1974

LAUSTEDA E, KOSKINEN R, AHLQUIST J: Leiomyoma of the bronchus. Ann Chir Gynaecol 63:346, 1974

MALAISE EP: Relationship between the growth rate of human metastases, survival and pathologic type. Eur J Cancer 10:451, 1974

MARTINI N, BAINS MS, HUVOS AG et al: Surgical treatment of metastatic sarcoma to the lung. Surg Clin North Am 54:841, 1974

MATTHEWS MJ: Morphologic classification of bronchogenic carcinoma. Cancer Chemother Rep 4:299, 1973

MILLER DR: Benign tumors of lung and tracheobronchial tree. Ann Thorac Surg 8:542, 1969

NOHL-OSER HC: Lymphatics of the lung. In Shields TW (ed.): General Thoracic Surgery. Philadelphia, Lea & Febiger, 1972

PAULSON DL, URSCHEL HC JR, McNAMARA JJ et al: Bronchoplastic procedures for bronchogenic carcinoma. J Thorac Cardiovasc Surg 59:38, 1970

RICCI C, PATRASSI N, MASSA, R et al: Carcinoid syndrome in a bronchial adenoma. Am J Surg 126:671, 1973

SALTZSTEIN SL: Pulmonary malignant lymphomas and pseudolymphomas, classification, therapy and prognosis. Cancer 16:928, 1969

SCHWABER JR: Diagnostic approaches in metastatic lung disease. Med Clin North Am 59:277, 1975

SELAWRY OS: Monochemotherapy of bronchogenic carcinoma with special reference to cell type. Cancer Chemother Rep 4:177, 1973

SHERMATA DW, CARTER D, HALLER A: Chondroma of the bronchus in childhood: A case report illustrating problems in diagnosis and management. J Pediatr Surg 10:545, 1975

SHIELDS TW: Preoperative radiation therapy in the treatment of bronchial carcinoma. Cancer 30:1388, 1972

SHIELDS TW: Bronchial Carcinoma. Springfield, IL, Charles C Thomas, 1974

SHIELDS TW: The fate of patients after incomplete resection of bronchial carcinoma, Surg Gynecol Obstet 139:569, 1974

SHIELDS TW, ROBINETTE CD, KEEHN RJ: Bronchial carcinoma treated by adjuvant cancer chemotherapy. Arch Surg 109:329, 1974

SIBALA JC: Endobronchial hamartoma. Chest 62:631, 1972

STRUTYNSKY N: Inflammatory pseudotumors of the lung. Br J Radiol 47:94, 1974

THIIJ LG, KROON TAJ, VAN LEEUWEN TM: Leiomyosarcoma of the pulmonary trunk associated with pericardial effusion. Thorax 29:490, 1974

TURNBULL AD, HUVOS AG, GOODNER JT et al: The malignant potential of bronchial adenoma. Ann Thorac Surg 14:453, 1972

VOONTZ FK: Giant bronchial polyp treated by emergency thoracotomy. Chest 66:102, 1974

WADE A: Case report: Lymphangioma of the lung. Arch Pathol 98:211, 1974

WEINBERGER M: The adult form of pulmonary hamartoma, a reappraisal. Ann Thorac Surg 15:67, 1973

WYNDER EL: An appraisal of a smoking–lung-cancer issue. N Engl J Med 264:1235, 1961

H. Pat Ewing

Structural Lesions of the Lung: Cysts, Bullae, and Spontaneous Pneumothorax

LUNG BUD ANOMALIES
  Bronchogenic Cyst
  Cystic Adenomatoid Malformation
  Sequestration
  Congenital Lobar Emphysema
  Additional Anomalies of the Lung
BULLAE
  Etiology and Pathology
  Clinical Presentation
  Treatment

SPONTANEOUS PNEUMOTHORAX
  Incidence, Etiology, and Pathology
  Clinical Presentation
  Treatment

The first portion of this chapter deals with congenital anomalies of the lung. Embryologically, the complex and rapid development of the lower respiratory system begins as a longitudinal groove in the floor of the foregut during the fourth gestational week, with subsequent separation of the caudal portion to form the lung buds. By the fifth gestational week the secondary bronchi are developing, and by the seventh week, the tertiary bronchi appear. Meanwhile, the original vascular connections with the splanchnic plexus are lost, and connections with the sixth aortic arch and the primary pulmonary veins from the sinus venosus are established. Maldevelopment during this period may give rise to a number of pathologic entities of particular interest to the surgeon (Fig. 34-25). Among these are bronchogenic cysts, cystic adenomatoid malformation, sequestration, and congenital lobar emphysema. Although they may be asymptomatic, typically they present either in the newborn, causing problems of intrathoracic tension, airway obstruction, or heart failure, or in the older child, causing problems of recurrent and chronic pulmonary infection.

The second portion of this chapter deals with developmental anomalies of the lung and their complications. Specifically, these include bullous emphysema and spontaneous pneumothorax.

LUNG BUD ANOMALIES

BRONCHOGENIC CYST

Although not a common lesion, bronchogenic cysts comprise 10% of mediastinal masses in children and are an important diagnostic consideration. They develop from embryonic lung bud tissue before the development of bronchi and consequently seldom communicate initially with the bronchial tree. They are generally unilocular and are lined with respiratory epithelium, which is surrounded with varying amounts of mesenchymal elements including smooth muscle and cartilage. In keeping with their embryologic development, bronchogenic cysts are most commonly located near the root of the lungs or at the level of the carina in the posterior mediastinum. They may be found embedded in the wall of the trachea or bronchi. The right hemithorax

Fig. 34-25. Lung bud anomalies include cystic adenomatoid malformation, bronchogenic cyst, congenital lobar emphysema, and pulmonary sequestration. (Haller JA Jr, Galladay ES, Pickard LR et al: Surgical management of lung bud anomalies: Lobar emphysema, bronchogenic cyst, cystic adenomatoid malformation and intralobar pulmonary sequestration. Ann Thorac Surg 28:33, 1979)

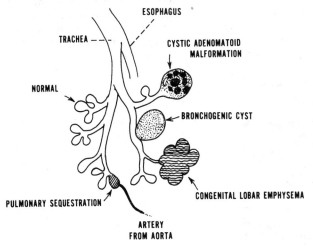

is reported to be involved slightly more frequently than the left, and males are affected more frequently than females. Size may vary from less than 1 cm to over 20 cm. Because of their close embryologic relationship, bronchogenic cysts are often difficult to differentiate from other foregut anomalies, including sequestration and duplication or esophageal cysts, which are lined with squamous or endodermal epithelium. Indeed, bronchogenic cysts may be found embedded in the esophageal wall itself, and the presence of respiratory epithelium may be the only indication of the true etiology.

If small, bronchogenic cysts may be asymptomatic. However, in the newborn, the characteristic presentation is airway obstruction. Dyspnea, stridor, cyanosis, and wheezing are often episodic and become worse with crying or feeding. In the older child or adult, recurrent pulmonary infection due to partial bronchial obstruction is the usual clinical presentation. Infection may occur in the cyst itself even with no apparent bronchial communication. Rarely, a pulmonary flow murmur secondary to pulmonary artery stenosis from extrinsic pressure may be present. When large, the cyst may be visible on chest radiographs as a mediastinal mass. However, less than 50% of bronchogenic cysts are visible radiographically. Barium swallow may demonstrate esophageal displacement, and computerized axial tomography may demonstrate an otherwise undetectable mass. The differential diagnosis usually includes a variety of mediastinal neoplasms, metastatic cancer, and duplication cysts. Bronchoscopy is generally not helpful, and mediastinoscopy is contraindicated when it may exclude later curative resection of neoplastic lesions. In some centers, diagnostic fine-needle aspiration biopsy of mediastinal and parahilar masses is being done with increasing frequency. In this circumstance, aspirate packed with characteristic respiratory epithelial cells is virtually diagnostic of a bronchogenic cyst.

Frequently, however, surgery is indicated for both diagnostic and therapeutic reasons. Symptomatic patients who have been treated nonsurgically because of normal chest radiographs and the lack of a definitive diagnosis have had a course characterized by continued complications and a high mortality. Surgical mortality, on the other hand, is low. Infection and injury to adjacent structures such as the phrenic or vagus nerves, esophagus, or aorta comprise the primary risks. The usual approach is through a posterolateral thoracotomy. The cyst may often be removed intact, but dense adhesions may make dissection difficult, especially if infection has been present. In such situations, a portion of the cyst wall may be left behind with little chance of compromising the expected curative results.

CYSTIC ADENOMATOID MALFORMATION

Cystic adenomatoid malformation is an uncommon lesion with less than 200 cases reported. It is nevertheless of great importance to the surgeon dealing with pediatric patients because it may present as a completely correctable surgical emergency. Pathologically, it is characterized by abnormal pulmonary tissue that is meaty, multicystic, and enlarged with malformed bronchial connections. Histologically, there is an absence of cartilage but an increase of terminal bronchiolar structures with varying-sized cysts lined with respiratory epithelium and containing foci of mucogenic cells. Reported cases have demonstrated no sexual predilection. The malformation may be seen in all of the pulmonary lobes and may involve more than one lobe. Associated congenital anomalies are rather common and include cardiac anomalies, diaphragmatic hernia, hypoplastic lungs, pectus excavatum, and gastrointestinal and renal anomalies.

In a recent review, 62% of cases of cystic adenomatoid malformation were found to be symptomatic in patients younger than 1 month of age, whereas 24% of patients presented after 1 month. Fourteen percent of cases are stillborn. Typically, the afflicted newborn demonstrates respiratory distress, tachypnea, subcostal retractions, cyanosis, and evidence of a mediastinal shift to the unaffected side. After 1 month of age, the characteristic pattern of presentation changes to one of chronic pulmonary infection with chronic cough, recurrent fever, and failure to thrive. Typically, there is a sharply defined intrapulmonary mass with scattered radiolucent areas representing air-filled cysts. The mediastinum is usually displaced to the unaffected side. However, the picture may be confused with lobar emphysema or, in the lower lobes, with sequestration or diaphragmatic hernia.

Treatment is surgical resection. Lobectomy is usually necessary, but segmentectomy may occasionally be possible. Complete removal of the affected region is necessary to avoid postoperative problems with persistent air leak or recurrent infection. Occasionally, with extensive involvement or hypoplastic lung, pneumonectomy may be necessary. Care must be taken to avoid mistaking atelectatic and compressed normal lung for diseased lung, but failure to remove all of the involved lung will frequently result in the need to reoperate. Survival rate after surgery is 95%.

SEQUESTRATION

The term *pulmonary sequestration* is applied to a portion of persistent embryonic accessory lung parenchyma that derives its blood supply from anomalous systemic vessels and generally does not communicate directly with the bronchial tree. Embryologically, pulmonary sequestration is felt to result from anomalous lung buds that probably develop before the completed separation of aortic and pulmonary circulations, thereby explaining the characteristic anomalous arterial connections. The anomalous lung tissue contains both bronchial and alveolar structures.

Sequestration may be either extralobar or intralobar, the former being completely separated from normal lung tissue and covered by its own pleural investment whereas the latter occurs within the pulmonary parenchyma proper and is seldom completely covered by its own pleura (Fig. 34-26). Various hybrid sequestrations with characteristics of both intralobar and extralobar varieties have been described. However, typically the two varieties differ in a number of respects (Table 34-4). Both varieties are more common in the left hemithorax, but the extralobar sequestration is most

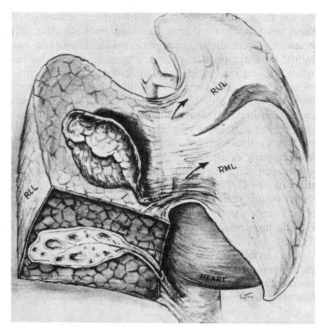

Fig. 34-26. An intralobar sequestration of the right lower lobe *(RLL)* and an extralobar sequestration in the major tissue that occurred in the same patient. *RUL,* right upper lobe; *RML,* right middle lobe. (Zumbro GL, Treasure RL, Seitter G et al: Pulmonary sequestration. Ann Thorac Surg 20:161, 1975)

frequently found in the left posterior hemithorax near the diaphragm, whereas the intralobar sequestration is most commonly seen in the left lower lobe. Other locations are possible. The arterial blood supply is quite variable. Most frequently it comes from the descending thoracic aortic, but it may come from the subclavian artery, abdominal aorta, superior mesenteric artery, intercostal arteries, or even the coronary arteries. The intralobar sequestration characteristically has a single large anomalous artery whereas the extralobar sequestration is more likely to have multiple smaller arterial connections. Venous drainage in the intralobar type is almost always by way of the pulmonary veins, but the extralobar veins generally drain into the azygos system. Although there are no direct bronchial communications, air reaches the intralobar sequestration by collateral ventilation from surrounding alveoli, and 90% of these are aerated on chest radiographs. On the other hand, extralobar sequestrations are rarely aerated, although persistent foregut communications are more frequent with these, and aeration by way of a patent connection with the esophagus is theoretically possible. Overall, intralobar sequestration is six times more frequent than extralobar, but additional associated anomalies are more frequent in the extralobar variety. Rarely, the two may coexist (Fig. 34-26).

TABLE 34-4	CHARACTERISTICS OF INTRALOBAR AND EXTRALOBAR SEQUESTRATION	
	INTRALOBAR	**EXTRALOBAR**
Pleural investment	None or partial	Always complete
Location	Left lower lobe (60%)	Left hemithorax (90%)
Arterial supply	Large, single aortic branch	Multiple small branches
Venous drainage	Pulmonary veins	Azygos veins
Aeration	Frequent	Rare
Associated anomalies	Rare	Frequent

Because they so rarely communicate with either the bronchial or the gastrointestinal systems, extralobar sequestrations rarely become infected and are frequently asymptomatic. Their discovery is often the result of a radiopaque density seen on a chest radiograph taken for an unrelated reason. Intralobar sequestrations may also be asymptomatic, but this is not characteristic. In the newborn, such lesions may produce a continuous murmur and congestive heart failure due to a large vascular shunt from the systemic to the pulmonary circulation. In the older child and adult, it is again chronic infection that brings the patient to the attention of a physician. Resultant cough, chest pain, hemoptysis, intrapleural hemorrhage, and eventual bronchiectasis are the presenting findings in such cases. Infection may be delayed if there is no bronchial communication. Arteriography demonstrates the arterial blood supply and is an important diagnostic tool.

Asymptomatic extralobar sequestration diagnosed on the basis of a characteristic radiographic density in the left lower hemithorax and an anomalous blood supply demonstrated arteriographically may be safely observed because of the low incidence of associated problems. However, these signs frequently cannot be differentiated from other lesions preoperatively and are found at diagnostic thoracotomy. Under these circumstances, simple excision is curative and recommended. Intralobar sequestrations generally require lobectomy, although segmentectomy is occasionally possible. The anomalous systemic blood supply must be carefully dissected, ligated, and divided. It is well known that careless division of the inferior pulmonary ligament, which frequently contains the anomalous arteries, may result in their premature division and retraction and subsequent serious or fatal hemorrhage.

CONGENITAL LOBAR EMPHYSEMA

Massive hyperinflation of one or more lobes of the lung in the newborn infant constitutes congenital lobar emphysema. It rarely presents in infants more than 1 year old, and a third of the affected infants present during the first month of life. In 97% of cases, it is the upper lobes or the right middle lobe that is involved. There is a high correlation with cardiac anomalies.

Although congenital lobar emphysema has been successfully managed with surgical resection since 1945 when Gross resected the first case, the etiology remains uncertain. It is possible that it is the common manifestation of multiple pathologic processes. Many investigators have felt that some form of bronchial obstruction is present. Associated congenital bronchial stenosis has been described but is rare. More frequently, the lesion has been attributed to a cartilaginous deficiency, mucous plugs, bronchiolar kinking, obstruction from aberrant pulmonary vessels or enlarged lymph nodes, or redundant bronchial mucosa. In one-half of the patients no cause is found. Of particular importance in discussing congenital lobar emphysema is the more recently described polyalveolar lung. Polyalveolar lung, first reported by Hislop and Reid in 1970, describes a congenital malformation in which there is a fivefold increase in alveoli in the involved lung with normal airways and arteries. Approximately 35% of infants with congenital lobar emphysema are found on examination to meet the criteria for polyalveolar lung, but it is unclear why patients with polyalveolar lung trap air and not all patients with areas of polyalveolar lung develop congenital lobar emphysema.

Nevertheless, these patients seem to form a distinct group, presenting at less than 1 month of age with severe dyspnea and requiring early surgery for survival.

Congenital lobar emphysema results in massive air trapping in the involved lung, compression of the normal lung, and mediastinal shift toward the uninvolved side. The infant develops hypoxia, cyanosis and hypercarbia, and respiratory distress that may become life-threatening. In severe cases venous return is decreased, further compromising cardiovascular instability. Breath sounds are decreased over the involved side, which is hyperresonant to percussion. Associated congenital heart disease such as ventricular septal defect, tetralogy of Fallot, or patent ductus arteriosus may further complicate the picture. Chest radiography is usually definitive, but care must be taken to rule out pneumothorax or, in some cases, diaphragmatic hernia. Bronchoscopy and bronchography are rarely helpful and are difficult to perform safely in the infant. Foreign body aspiration is generally not a consideration in the newborn infant.

In asymptomatic or mildly affected patients with radiographic features of congenital lobar emphysema, conservative and supportive treatment is indicated. Follow-up of these patients has demonstrated that the distended portions of the lung do not continue to enlarge. However, if the infant is symptomatic, conservative treatment is associated with a 50% mortality, whereas over 90% of infants treated surgically survive and are cured. Normally, lobectomy is the treatment of choice. Although initially vital capacity and total lung volume are decreased in proportion to the amount of lung resected, long-term follow-up at 15 to 30 years has shown normal lung volumes.

ADDITIONAL ANOMALIES OF THE LUNG

Wide variation in the degree of separation of the lobes and segments of the lung by their pleural investment is possible. Although these are of interest to the thoracic surgeon, they will not be discussed here. Azygos lobe is an anatomic variant created by malpositioning of the azygos vein and right upper lobe during development. The right upper lobe is crossed by the azygos vein, creating a deep cleft in the lobe that separates the medial and apical portion from the remainder. Radiographically, the variant azygos vein and its mesentery are seen as an inverted "comma" lateral to and paralleling the superior vena cava. Because of its anatomic separation, infection, atelectasis, and neoplastic disease may involve the azygos lobe without involving the remainder of the upper lobe. Developmental anomalies manifested by abnormalities of the spleen are well known indicators of congenital heart disease as well as congenital pulmonary anomalies. Asplenia is associated with mirror image development of lungs with both right and left lungs containing middle lobes. In polysplenia, both lungs lack middle lobes. Scimitar syndrome is named for the distinctive radiographic shadow produced in the right hemithorax by an anomalous pulmonary vein that passes through the diaphragm to the inferior vena cava. It is also associated with a hypoplastic right lung and an anomalous pulmonary artery coming from the descending aorta. Pulmonary vascular sling is created by an anomalous course of the left pulmonary artery, which passes posterior to the trachea, producing symptoms of bronchial, tracheal, or esophageal obstruction. Other variations in pulmonary vasculature are discussed in relation to associated anomalies.

BULLAE

ETIOLOGY AND PATHOLOGY

Pulmonary emphysema is characterized by an increase in size of the air spaces distal to the terminal bronchiole, with stretching, rupture, and destruction of alveolar wall secondary to loss of elasticity. It is a common disease whose precise etiology has remained obscure. However, it may be assumed to be related to abnormalities of proteolytic activity within the lung because it is seen in a panlobular form with α_1-antitrypsin deficiency and is associated with increased elastase production of pulmonary alveolar macrophages and polymorphonuclear leukocytes that are seen with cigarette smoking.

A major complication of emphysema is the progressive development of bullae, a term used to describe emphysematous spaces of more than 1 cm in diameter. Bullae may eventually become huge, occupying up to 90% of a hemithorax and severely compressing the remaining lung (Fig. 34-27). When they occupy more than 13% of the hemithorax, they are frequently referred to as giant bullae and become of particular importance to the surgeon.

Such lesions are thin-walled cystic structures with multiple small connections to the pulmonary bronchioles. They contain scattered trabeculae consisting of remnants of pulmonary parenchyma and blood vessels. In keeping with LaPlace's law, bullae tend to enlarge progressively because the pressure required to stretch the walls of the cyst decreases in inverse proportion to the diameter. Theoretically, giant bullae could result in a tremendous dead space ventilation, but in reality, they are usually poorly ventilated and do not contribute significantly to gas exchange. Rather, it is the compression of the relatively uninvolved lung and the subsequent ventilation–perfusion abnormalities that are the primary defects amenable to surgical correction. It should also be remembered that cigarette smoking is associated with both emphysema and bronchogenic carcinoma and that bronchogenic carcinoma has been reported to be especially common in young males with emphysematous bullae.

CLINICAL PRESENTATION

Patients with giant bullae are generally over 35 years old with a long history of smoking and varying degrees of

Fig. 34-27. Giant bullae of the left lung at operation. Much functional lung tissue was permitted to expand by resection of the bullae. (University of Mississippi Hospital series)

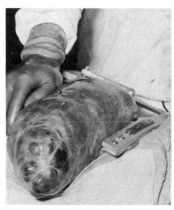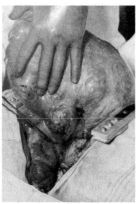

generalized emphysema. They may be asymptomatic, but if symptoms are present the primary one is dyspnea, which may be incapacitating. Complications include pneumothorax and infection of the bulla with subsequent lung abscess.

Diagnosis is usually readily apparent on chest radiographs, although giant bullae may sometimes be confused with pneumothorax. Careful examination will reveal the absence of the visceral pleural line seen with pneumothorax and the presence of trabeculae within the bulla. Tomograms may be helpful in ruling out pneumothorax in difficult cases.

However, it is generally not the diagnosis of bullous disease that is of first concern but rather the determination of the extent of generalized emphysematous changes and chronic obstructive disease in the remainder of the lung. In short, because the diagnosis of bullous emphysema is easily established, the most difficult problem is determining which patients will benefit from surgery. If bullous disease represents an exaggeration of diffusely involved emphysematous lungs, surgical interference will entail a significant mortality with little chance of symptomatic improvement. On the other hand, if there is a large percentage of compressed and atelectatic but potentially functional lung, resection of the bullae may result in dramatic symptomatic improvement and rehabilitation of the patient. Careful consideration of pulmonary function tests, forced vital capacity, residual volume, minute ventilation, diffusing capacity, and arterial P_{O_2} is useful in ruling out prohibitive underlying lung disease. A large difference between functional residual capacity (FRC) as measured by body plethysmography (which measures actual lung volume) and FRC as measured by closed circuit helium dilution (which measures the volume of ventilated parenchyma) indicates a large area of poorly ventilated lung and predicts a favorable response to surgery. A significant drop in arterial P_{O_2} with exercise may be an important preoperative indication to a gratifying response to surgery. Tomography and computerized axial tomography are of considerable importance in determining the presence of compressed, nonventilated lung. Pulmonary arteriography is also useful in this regard and allows the added benefit of determining pulmonary artery pressure and ruling out cor pulmonale. Ventilation–perfusion scans with ^{133}Xe have also proved useful in the hands of some. However, it is well recognized that the correlation between preoperative diagnostic assessment and symptomatic response to surgery is poor. Patients with severe generalized emphysema, hypoxia at rest, and cor pulmonale have prohibitive surgical mortalities and should be excluded from surgical resection. In the final analysis, given all the available facts, the surgeon must frequently rely upon his common sense because there are no absolute criteria to contraindicate surgery in these uniformly poor surgical candidates.

TREATMENT

A persistent pneumothorax or an infected bulla unresponsive to antibiotics is an indication for surgery, but the primary indication is disabling dyspnea that has been unresponsive to the best medical management. The combined experience of many surgeons has confirmed the premise that surgery for bullous disease of the lung should be characterized by conservation of lung tissue. Bullae are excised down to the lung parenchyma, the air leaks are oversewn with absorbable suture, and the base of the bulla is then closed in layers to obliterate dead space. Surgical stapling devices have been particularly useful in this circumstance, allowing resection of the diseased lung with minimal subsequent air leak. Segmental resection and lobectomy have occasionally been advocated in circumstances in which the entire area was thought to be involved in the emphysematous changes, but generally they are not necessary, and preservation of all functioning lung is mandatory. Approach through the fourth intercostal space from a standard posterolateral thoracotomy incision is usually indicated. However, with bilateral bullous disease adequate exposure for bilateral, simultaneous resection may be obtained through a median sternotomy incision. Complete re-expansion of the lungs postoperatively is of primary importance, and careful attention to detail in the placement and management of the chest tubes is necessary to prevent partial re-expansion and secondary infection, empyema, and respiratory insufficiency. Air leaks may persist for a prolonged period but usually stop after up to a week of drainage.

Mortality will depend upon patient selection but is reported to be 10% to 22%. Subjective improvement postoperatively has been shown to have little relationship to objective changes in pulmonary function. Objective improvement is demonstrated by a reduction in residual capacity, an increase in arterial Po_2, particularly after exercise, and a less prominent change in flow rates. In carefully selected patients with significant dyspnea, severe but localized bullous disease occupying more than 25% of the hemithorax, radiologic evidence of compressed lung, and minimal inflammatory disease, both symptomatic and objective evidence of improvement can be expected.

Finally, in very high risk patients with generalized emphysema and bullous disease, intracavitary tube drainage and suction (Monaldi drainage) has been used with some success and relatively low mortality. Overall, this treatment is seldom useful except in cases of infected bullae that are resistant to medical management.

SPONTANEOUS PNEUMOTHORAX

INCIDENCE, ETIOLOGY, AND PATHOLOGY

Spontaneous pneumothorax may be defined as an accumulation of air or gas within the pleural space occurring without external influence. It is usually distinguished from iatrogenic and traumatic pneumothorax, the two most common causes of pneumothorax. Nevertheless, it is a relatively common disease and is seen most frequently in men between the ages of 20 and 40 years. Consequently, it is a common problem around college campuses and in the military, but it may occur at any age and in women. Although it is slightly more frequent in the right hemithorax, it may occur on both sides, and in 5% of patients it will be bilateral.

A wide variety of pathologic problems have been associated with the occasional development of spontaneous pneumothorax. These have included most primary lung diseases, pneumonitis, pneumoconioses, bronchiolitis, endometriosis (catamenial pneumothorax), Marfan's syndrome, Wegener's granulomatosis, multiple sclerosis, sarcoidosis, metastatic lung disease, and bronchogenic carcinoma. Although these are important considerations in the evaluation of the individual patient, from a practical standpoint

SPONTANEOUS PNEUMOTHORAX	
Etiology	Diffuse lung disease (acquired or infectious), subpleural apical bleb disease
Presentation	Young persons, chest pain, possible tension pneumothorax
Dx	Hyperresonance of chest, diagnostic chest films
Rx	Closed chest drainage; if no resolution after 7 to 14 days or if multiple pneumothorax is present, then open thoracotomy with bleb resection and pleurodesis

it may be safely maintained that nearly all cases of spontaneous pneumothorax are caused by rupture of subpleural blebs, which are most commonly located in apical segments of the upper lobes. What causes the blebs to develop or to rupture is unknown. The onset of symptoms is often not associated with unusual exercise or position. Although some investigators have found no relationship to smoking, many of these patients do smoke. It has been suggested that subpleural blebs are developmental and secondary to chronic bronchiolitis with disturbances of collateral ventilation. Electron microscopic examination of pulmonary blebs demonstrates loss of mesothelial cells over the surface of the blebs with exposed naked collagen fibers forming the only barrier to bleb rupture. This sloughing of mesothelial cells may play an important role in the development of spontaneous pneumothorax. Disorganization of collagen and elastic fibers, along with chemical changes in the protein content of the lungs in patients with recurrent spontaneous pneumothoraces similar to those seen with emphysema, suggests a complex problem of tissue degeneration and loss rather than a problem purely of bronchiolar obstruction.

CLINICAL PRESENTATION

Typically, the onset of spontaneous pneumothorax is associated with sudden chest or shoulder pain, which abates after several hours and may be mild or severe. No doubt some patients with small pneumothoraces and minimal symptoms never see a physician, and their pneumothorax resolves as spontaneously as it occurred. However, with development of a significant pneumothorax, the onset of pain is followed by symptoms of dyspnea and nonproductive cough. In 15% to 30% of patients, the course is complicated by development of tension pneumothorax or hemopneumothorax due to tearing or adhesions. These patients may present with cardiovascular compromise or shock due to tamponade or hemorrhage.

Physical examination demonstrates hyperresonance to percussion and decreased breath sounds over the involved lung. The patient may be in respiratory distress, and, if tension pneumothorax is present, the trachea may be shifted toward the uninvolved side. The diagnosis is confirmed by the chest roentgenogram, which typically demonstrates the partially collapsed lung outlined by the faint line representing the visceral pleura with absence of lung markings peripherally. If the pneumothorax is not large and the roentgenogram is of poor quality and obtained with the patient in the supine position, these findings may not be apparent and the only indication of a pneumothorax may be hyperlucency of the lower thorax with visualization of the anterior costophrenic sulcus and a deep lateral costophrenic angle. Although it is common practice to estimate the percentage of hemithorax involved in a pneumothorax, such estimations are arbitrary, of questionable accuracy, and of no more clinical value than simply stating whether the pneumothorax is large, moderate, or small. Seventy-five percent of patients have a moderate to large pneumothorax. Care must be taken to avoid the mistaken diagnosis of pneumothorax in a patient with giant emphysematous bullae.

TREATMENT

A minimal pneumothorax may be safely treated with expectant observation, especially if it has been several hours since onset of symptoms and it may be assumed that the air leak has stopped. However, absorption of pleural air is slow, and moderate to large pneumothoraces are best treated with closed tube thoracostomy using a large-bore chest tube with multiple holes for drainage. Aspiration of air through a needle or catheter is frequently ineffective and seldom allows complete expansion of the lung. The chest tube is usually placed using sterile technique and local anesthesia. Placement through the second intercostal space in the midclavicular line or through the sixth or seventh intercostal space in the midaxillary line is acceptable (Fig. 34-28). The tube is sutured to the skin and connected to an underwater seal drainage system to which controlled negative pressure

Fig. 34-28. Diagram of two different sites of chest tube insertion for management of spontaneous pneumothorax. (Stauss HK, Hardy JD: Tuberculosis and fungous diseases of the lungs. In Hardy JD [ed]: Rhoads Textbook of Surgery, 5th ed. Philadelphia, J B Lippincott, 1977)

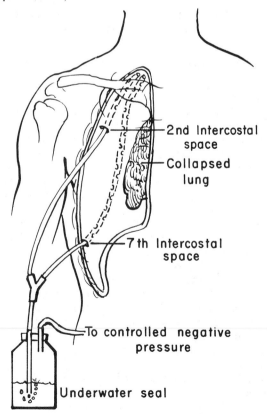

2nd Intercostal space

Collapsed lung

7th Intercostal space

To controlled negative pressure

Underwater seal

is applied. Usually, a minimal negative pressure of around 10 cm H_2O is all that is needed. But this should be increased as necessary up to 60 cm H_2O to maintain complete evacuation of a continued air leak and re-expansion of the lung. Usually, the tube is left in place for 1 to 2 days after the air leak has stopped and the lung remains expanded. Complications following closed tube thoracostomy are few in experienced hands. With inexperienced personnel, care must be taken to avoid malposition of the tube (inserting it below the diaphragm) and laceration of the lung. Poor positioning may result in incomplete lung expansion. An unusual complication that should be remembered nevertheless because of the potentially lethal results is ipsilateral pulmonary edema following lung re-expansion. It was first described following treatment of a pneumothorax by Carson et al. in 1959. The etiology is uncertain, but it is associated with prolonged atelectasis of the involved lung and the use of excessive negative pressure during re-expansion. However, neither of these two factors is a prerequisite. Some component of bronchial occlusion preventing adequate lung re-expansion is probably also a frequent factor. The syndrome is characterized by the onset of coughing and chest discomfort soon after tube placement. This is followed by progressive dyspnea, hypoxemia, cyanosis, and the production of the pink frothy sputum of fulminant pulmonary edema, which on chest roentgenograms is limited to the lung involved in the pneumothorax. Positive pressure ventilatory support may be necessary to prevent death from respiratory failure. Gradual clearing of the lung may be expected over 2 to 12 days.

Open thoracotomy is necessary in approximately 10% to 40% of patients with spontaneous pneumothorax. Indications for open thoracotomy are (1) persistent air leak after 7 to 14 days of chest drainage, (2) a large air leak that cannot be adequately handled by the chest tube, (3) recurrent ipsilateral pneumothorax, and (4) hemopneumothorax with evacuation of more than 1 liter of blood. Usually a standard posterolateral thoracotomy incision is used and the chest is entered through the fourth intercostal space. Approach through a median sternotomy with access to both lungs has been advocated. The apical blebs are ligated or plicated. The use of a surgical stapling device is particularly useful in this procedure because it allows resection of the lung with minimal problems with postoperative air leak. The superior segment of the lower lobe is also a frequent site of bleb formation and is readily amenable to resection. In addition to bleb resection, some means of vigorous pleural abrasion should be employed to promote pleural symphysis. Usually abrasion with dry gauze is adequate. Cauterization or resection of the parietal pleura is effective, but in our experience and that of others, it has not been necessary. Early and complete lung expansion is very important postoperatively. Chest tubes should be carefully placed and meticulously attended to postoperatively. Recurrence of spontaneous pneumothorax after open thoracotomy is very rare.

A variety of agents acting as pleural irritants, such as silver nitrate, nitrogen mustard, tetracycline, and talc, have been insufflated into the pleural space in efforts to obtain pleural symphysis in the treatment of recurrent spontaneous pneumothorax. In the occasional very elderly patient who is a poor surgical risk, such methods are still advocated by some. However, this method of management is very uncomfortable for the patient and is frequently ineffective. Surgery is the definitive method of management.

BIBLIOGRAPHY

Bolman RM III et al: Bronchiectasis and bronchopulmonary sequestration. Surg Clin North Am 60:867, 1980

Boushy SF, Billig DM, Kohen R: Changes in pulmonary function after bullectomy. Am J Med 47:916, 1969

Brennan NJ, Fitzgerald MX: Anatomically localised re-expansion pulmonary edema following pneumothorax drainage. Case report and literature review. Respiration 38:233, 1979

Brooks JW: Open thoracotomy in the management of spontaneous pneumothorax. Ann Surg 177:798, 1973

Buntain WL, Isaacs H Jr, Payne VC et al: Lobar emphysema, cystic adenomatoid malformation, pulmonary sequestration and bronchogenic cyst in infancy and childhood: A clinical group. J Pediatr Surg 9:85, 1974

Canty TG: Extralobar pulmonary sequestration. Unusual presentation and systemic vascular communication in association with a right-sided diaphragmatic hernia. J Thorac Cardiovasc Surg 81:96, 1981

Carlson RI, Claassen KL, Gallen F et al: Pulmonary edema following the rapid reexpansion of a totally collapsed lung due to pneumothorax: A clinical and experimental study. Surg Forum 9:37, 1959

Delarue NC, Pearson FG, Cooper JD et al: Developmental bronchopulmonary disease in adults: Practical clinical consideration. Can J Surg 24:23, 1981

Demos NJ, Trevesi A: Congenital lung malformations: A unified concept and a case report. J Thorac Cardiovasc Surg 70:260, 1975

DeVries WC, Wolfe WG: Spontaneous pneumothorax and bullous emphysema. Surg Clin North Am 60:851, 1980

Fain WR, Conn JJ, Campbell GD et al: Excision of giant pulmonary emphysematous cysts: Report of 20 cases without deaths. Surgery 62:552, 1967

Fitzgerald MX, Keelan PJ, Cugell DW et al: Long term results of surgery for bullous emphysema. J Thorac Cardiovasc Surgery 68:566, 1974

Flye MW, Carley M, Silver D: Spectrum of pulmonary sequestration. Ann Thorac Surg 22:478, 1976

Folger GM Jr, Lewis JW: Cardiovascular findings with bronchogenic cyst. Angiology 32:29, 1981

Haller JA, Jr, Galladay ES, Pickard LR et al: Surgical management of lung bud anomalies. Lobar emphysema, bronchogenic cyst, cystic adenomatoid malformation and intralobar pulmonary sequestration. Ann Thorac Surg 28:33, 1979

Harris J: Severe bullous emphysema: Successful surgical management despite poor preoperative blood gas levels and marked pulmonary hypertension. Chest 70:658, 1976

Hislop A, Reid L: New pathological findings in emphysema in childhood. Thorax 25:682, 1970

Hugh-Jones P: Surgery of emphysema in adults. Theoretical basis for surgery in emphysema and the means of pre-operative assessment. Bronchopneumologie 30:269, 1980

Kuwabana M, Taki T, Hatakenaka R et al: The surgical treatment of bullous emphysema. A new method for management of giant bullae. Bronchopneumologie 30:202, 1980

McBride JT et al: Lung growth and airway function after lobectomy in infancy for congenital lobar emphysema. J Clin Invest 66:962, 1980

Meng RL, Jensik RJ, Kittle F et al: Median sternotomy for synchronous bilateral pulmonary operations. J Thorac Cardiovasc Surg 80:1, 1980

Miller RK, Sieber WK, Ynis EJ: Congenital adenomatoid malformation of the lung. A report of 17 cases and review of the literature. Pathol Ann 15:387, 1980

Monaldi V: Endocavitary aspiration: Its practical applications. Tubercule 28:223, 1947

Murray GF: Congenital lobar emphysema (collective review). Surg Gynecol Obstet 124:611, 1967

Pride NB, Barter CE, Hugh-Jones P: The ventilation of bullae and the effect of their removal on thoracic gas volumes and tests of overall pulmonary function. Am Rev Resp Dis 107:83, 1973

Rivas AA et al: Intralobar pulmonary sequestration. Am Surg 45:754, 1979

Roe JP, Mack JW, Shirley JA: Bilateral pulmonary sequestration. J Thorac Cardiovasc Surg 80:8, 1980

Saha SP, Amants JE, Kosa A et al: Management of spontaneous pneumothorax. Ann Thorac Surg 19:561, 1975

Schmidt FE, Drapanas T: Congenital cystic lesions of the bronchi and lungs. Ann Thorac Surg 14:650, 1972

Tapper D, Schuster S, McBride J et al: Polyalveolar lobe: Anatomic and physiologic parameters and their relationship to congenital lobar emphysema. J Pediatr Surg 15:931, 1980

Wolf SA, Hertzler JH, Philippart AI: Cystic adenomatoid dysplasia of the lung. J Pediatr Surg 15:925, 1980

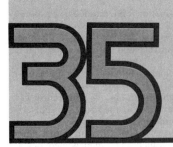

James D. Hardy

The Mediastinum

ANATOMY

It is important to have a clear concept of the anatomy of the mediastinum (Fig. 35-1) because the anatomic location of most masses gives a strong clue to the probable nature of the lesion; for example, because the nerves are mainly located posteriorly, a posterior mediastinal mass may represent a neurogenic tumor (or a pulmonary or esophageal mass or an aortic aneurysm). The curve of the aorta represents a major vascular landmark in the left hemithorax as does the azygous vein on the right. It is useful to divide the mediastinum into anterior, middle, superior (anterosuperior), and posterior compartments.

MEDIASTINAL MASSES—CYSTS, TUMORS, AND OTHER LESIONS

A mass in the mediastinum usually represents an important clinical problem. Many mediastinal masses are actually secondary, such as metastasis from a primary malignant tumor elsewhere. However, it is the primary mediastinal masses that are under consideration here. Such primary lesions, although not especially common, pose a wide range of clinical possibilities. Almost any histologic type that normally occurs in or around the mediastinum has on occasion given rise to a cyst, tumor, or other type of enlargement such as aneurysm, parasternal hernia, or abscess.

It is obvious that mediastinal masses can represent a wide range of pathologic entities. Because these conditions are divergent and often have virtually no clinical features in common except their anatomic location in and around the mediastinum, it is not surprising that, as in most clinical circumstances, therapy and prognosis cannot be determined until a specific diagnosis has been made. Indeed, the diagnosis itself can be difficult to achieve without thoracotomy, since many or most of the more common mediastinal masses do not communicate with a hollow viscus through which a radiopaque medium can be instilled, and endoscopic efforts at diagnosis may also be unrewarding. Nevertheless, preoperative studies can usually be depended upon either to identify the cytology of the lesion specifically or to limit the diagnostic possibilities in such a way that operative intervention can be planned accurately and successfully.

TYPES

Cytologic cell types of mediastinal masses cover a wide spectrum. Nevertheless, again more than in most other areas of the body, the *location* of the mass on chest roentgenograms commonly suggests specific diagnostic possibilities. The more important lesions shown in Table 35-1 and Figure 35-2 were derived from a consecutive series of 56 mediastinal masses treated by the author and his associates. When the mediastinal area is arbitrarily divided into anterior, middle, posterior, and superior compartments, it will be seen that specific pathologic types most commonly develop in specific compartments. For example, the mass most commonly found in the superior mediastinum is a goiter; in the anterior mediastinum, a thymoma or teratoma, including the dermoid cyst; in the middle mediastinum, lymphomatous tissue or bronchogenic cyst; in the posterior mediastinum, neurogenic tumor, aneurysm and, rarely, enteric cyst. Of course, in almost any series the most common mediastinal mass at the lung level is a bronchogenic carcinoma or, more rarely, a tumor of the esophagus. Aneurysm must always be considered, as must a solid lung or mediastinal abscess, granuloma, or idiopathic mediastinal fibrosis. Any of the

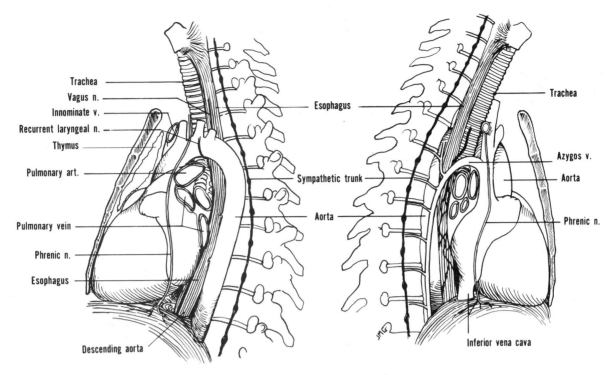

Fig. 35-1. The mediastinum. *(Left)* Left lateral view exhibiting prominence of the aortic arch. *(Right)* Right lateral view presenting the anatomical landmark represented by the azygos vein.

conditions shown in Table 35-1 as well as still other lesions may be found on occasion, and thus a wide range of diagnostic possibilities must be kept in mind. Finally, despite the generally specific location of the individual lesions cited above, there is some overlap in the anatomic sites at which a given entity may be found. For example, we have found a thymoma low in the posterior mediastinum. The pericardial cyst is usually found in the sulcus between the pericardium and the diaphragm.

DIAGNOSIS

The diagnosis of a mediastinal mass usually begins with its discovery, often the result of a roentgenogram made for any of a variety of symptoms, including venous distention, dysphagia, respiratory symptoms, pain, or other phenomena, but perhaps still more often because a mediastinal mass is noted on routine chest x-ray. The diagnostic value of its position in the mediastinum has been emphasized.

ROENTGENOGRAPHIC AND RADIOIODINE STUDIES

In addition to anterior–posterior, lateral, oblique and tomographic studies with which to localize the lesion and to search for cavitation or a fluid level therein, angiographic

TABLE 35-1   MEDIASTINAL MASSES*

LESION		NUMBER OF CASES
Substernal goiter		11
Thymoma		6
Teratoma		7
Lymphoma		7
Pericardial cyst		6
Parasternal (Morgagni) hernia		2
Parathyroid adenoma		1
Lipoma		1
Bronchogenic cyst		2
Angiomatous tumor		3
cystic hygroma	2	
hemangioma	1	
Neurogenic tumor		5
Esophageal leiomyoma		1
Undiagnosed masses (no operation)		4
		56

(Bronchogenic carcinoma)

(Lung abscess)

(Aneurysm)

(Lymphadenopathy of inflammation)

* The entities in parentheses frequently appeared as mediastinal masses, but they are not otherwise considered here.
(Hardy JD, Booth JE: Mediastinal masses. Survey of 56 cases. Am Surg 33:621, 1967)

Fig. 35-2. The location of a mass in the mediastinum suggests specific diagnostic possibilities. Some observers prefer to consider the anterior and superior compartments as one: "anterosuperior." (Hardy JD, Booth JE: Mediastinal masses. Am Surg 33:621, 1967)

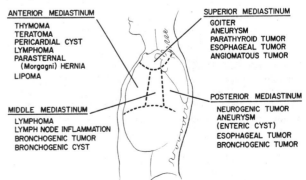

ANTERIOR MEDIASTINUM
THYMOMA
TERATOMA
PERICARDIAL CYST
LYMPHOMA
PARASTERNAL
   (Morgagni) HERNIA
LIPOMA

SUPERIOR MEDIASTINUM
GOITER
ANEURYSM
PARATHYROID TUMOR
ESOPHAGEAL TUMOR
ANGIOMATOUS TUMOR

MIDDLE MEDIASTINUM
LYMPHOMA
LYMPH NODE INFLAMMATION
BRONCHOGENIC TUMOR
BRONCHOGENIC CYST

POSTERIOR MEDIASTINUM
NEUROGENIC TUMOR
ANEURYSM
(ENTERIC CYST)
ESOPHAGEAL TUMOR
BRONCHOGENIC TUMOR

studies may exclude aneurysm and opacify bronchogenic carcinoma through the selective injection of the bronchial arteries that supply the lung tumor. Sonography is increasingly useful in distinguishing between solid and cystic lesions, and computed axial tomography (CT scan) is even more valuable. A calcified rim may suggest a teratoma (*e.g.*, a dermoid). Teeth are more likely to be found in an ovarian dermoid than in a mediastinal dermoid. Bone erosion in association with a posterior mediastinal mass may be due to a neurogenic tumor of one of the several cytologic varieties, malignant bronchial or esophageal tumor, or aneurysm. Of course, an infection may rarely cause bone erosion. Calcification in the center or rim of a mass suggests chronicity, often a degree of long-standing inflammation, and usually benignancy, although malignancy is not excluded by some degree of calcification.

An air–fluid level suggests communication with a bronchus (*e.g.*, bronchogenic cyst) or the esophagus (unusual with esophageal duplication). Thoracic duct opacification may occasionally be useful, as may azygous venography. A lipoma may appear less radiolucent in the chest in comparison with surrounding lung than it does in the thigh with surrounding muscle.

Radioiodine scan may indicate the nature of an intrathoracic thyroidal mass, but the goiter may fail to take up sufficient isotope to be identified. As a rule, intrathoracic or substernal goiter is associated with some thyroid enlargement in the neck (see Chapter 20). Isotopic study may identify a ventricular aneurysm or a pericardial defect or effusion.

Barium swallow may show esophageal distortion, and bronchograms may show bronchial encroachment or communication with the mass.

ENDOSCOPY AND BIOPSY

Bronchoscopy, esophagoscopy, or mediastinoscopy may prove useful, especially when mediastinoscopy provides diagnostic material as in the case of a goiter, thymoma, or lymphoma.

TRANSTHORACIC NEEDLE BIOPSY

Transthoracic needle biopsy of a mass for diagnosis may be justified, especially when there is evidence of unlikely cure, such as left vocal cord or phrenic nerve paralysis, bone erosion, or distant metastases.

EXPLORATORY THORACOTOMY

Despite the numerous diagnostic modalities available for the cytological identification of the mediastinal mass, exploratory thoracotomy is still commonly required to establish

a definitive diagnosis of the nature of the mediastinal lesion, and it is also usually necessary for therapeutic management.

MANAGEMENT

The majority of mediastinal masses require operative intervention, often for diagnosis if not also for therapy. The operative approach employed is usually a right or a left thoracotomy in an appropriate interspace, though lesions of the thyroid and occasionally of the thymus not accessible through a neck incision are approached with a splitting of the upper half of the sternum. Cystic hygroma also may require a combined approach.

SUPERIOR MEDIASTINAL MASSES (MOST OFTEN THYROID)

The mass most commonly encountered in the superior mediastinal compartment is the substernal goiter. As noted elsewhere, the substernal goiter demonstrated on roentgenogram is frequently associated with a palpable goiter in the neck, and a radioiodine uptake study may disclose that the substernal mass does in fact take up radioiodine. Occasionally selective arteriography may show perfusion of the mass in the superior mediastinum by the inferior thyroid artery. Characteristic displacement of the trachea and of the esophagus may occur. However, an aneurysm in the superior mediastinum may also displace surrounding structures, but would usually be identified with an aortogram. A pulsation in the suprasternal mediastinum may be due to an aneurysm itself, or to a transmitted pulsation through a substernal goiter. Rarely, a parathyroid cyst or a large parathyroid adenoma may be seen on roentgenogram. Cystic hygromas of the neck and the superior mediastinum are often associated with a similar type of mass in the neck itself. Lesions of the esophagus may also present as mass lesions. Superior mediastinal masses producing the superior vena caval syndrome are likely to be malignant but at times represent a chronic granulomatous process.

The management of substernal goiter is usually not difficult. In most instances the goiter can be removed through the usual collar or transverse cervical incision employed for a thyroidectomy, though it may be necessary to morcellate or break up the goiter into pieces to extract it. Since colloid goiters in the upper mediastinum have a relatively meager blood supply, serious hemorrhage is rarely encountered if one stays within the capsule of the goiter. Some goiters are too large to be delivered safely without splitting the sternum for about one half its length. It is virtually never necessary to split the entire sternum, and thus the possible complication of complete sternal separation is avoided. At times the goiter may have taken a position in the apex of the chest, situated posteriorly, and can be surprisingly difficult to deliver into the wound and to remove. In rare instances the goiter is situated well down in the thorax and has no connection with the inferior thyroid artery or elements of the thyroid in the neck.

Postoperatively, it is well to achieve the best possible hemostasis first and then not drain the superior mediastinum unless with closed underwater seal or suction drainage. The placing of unsealed drains through the neck wound into the superior mediastinum may result in air being sucked into the mediastinum with each inspiration; it then may not escape readily and may be forced into the subcutaneous tissues of the upper thorax, neck, and head, producing *massive subcutaneous emphysema*. This can present a very

---

MEDIASTINUM

The mediastinum is an extrapleural space, lying between the pleurae covering the lungs and bounded by the thoracic inlet above and the diaphragm below. Through this rather small space run many vital structures of cardiovascular, enteric, neural, and lymphatic importance. In addition to lesions of these tissues *per se*, other conditions such as developmental defects, represented by cysts or true tumors, may complicate diagnosis and therapy. Other disorders such as hemorrhage, emphysema, or infection occur occasionally.

disturbing appearance, at least to the patient and relatives, though it rarely occasions serious difficulty and is dissipated in several days.

THE ANTERIOR MEDIASTINUM

Lesions in the anterior mediastinum are primarily thymomas, teratomas including dermoid cysts, pericardial cysts, and lymphomas. Parathyroid tumor, lipoma, and Morgagni (parasternal) hernia were also represented in our series. Aneurysm should always be considered.

Thymoma

Thymoma may be either benign or malignant, the incidence of benign and malignant types being approximately equal in the series reported by Boyd and Midell. Thymomas may be lymphocytic (35%), spindle cell and epithelial (40%), and mixed lymphocytic and epithelial (25%). Thymomas, either benign or malignant, may or may not be associated with *myasthenia gravis,* and the myasthenia gravis may or may not be improved by removal of the thymoma (Fig. 35-3). Payne and Clagett found that about 10% of patients with myasthenia gravis had a thymoma, and one half of patients with thymoma had myasthenia gravis. The thymus has much to do with the development of immune capability and immunologic disorders and even anemia may be associated with diseases of this organ.

In general, we have preferred a posterolateral thoracotomy incision, largely anterior in extension, for the excision of a thymoma on either the right or the left side. A benign thymoma is usually removed with ease, but because a malignant thymoma may invade the surrounding structures it may be impossible to excise the lesion totally. In general, the tumor is sensitive to radiation, at least initially, and radiation was used in our series (six thymomas, three benign and three malignant) for the malignant thymomas that could not be excised. Three of the six were associated with myasthenia gravis and all tumors were of the lymphocyte (thymocyte) variety, with no squamous cell carcinoma derived from Hassall's epithelial corpuscles. However, mixed cytological types of thymic malignancy do occur. In the series reported by Boyd and Midell the patients with

Fig. 35-3.   Thymoma, associated with myasthenia gravis.

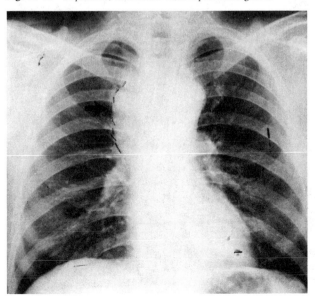

myasthenia typically had benign thymomas. These patients usually died from myasthenia, whereas those with malignant lesions usually died from the effects of the tumor itself.

Thymectomy for Myasthenia Gravis. On May 26, 1936, Blalock and his associates successfully resected a thymoma in a young woman with myasthenia gravis, with gradual but complete remission of symptoms thereafter. After this first and very encouraging experience, hundreds of thymectomies were performed as treatment for myasthenia gravis. Unfortunately, permanent cures were difficult to predict, whether the excised thymus contained a tumor or not; in fact, many patients showed no improvement, an important consideration when the risk of any major operation in a patient with myasthenia gravis is considered. One reason for the uncertain results of admittedly empirical thymectomy has been the lack of firm knowledge concerning the underlying cause of the disease. Over the years, myasthenia gravis has more and more been accepted as an autoimmune disease, and the slow beneficial response to operation, when achieved, has been believed to be due to the slow subsequent alteration in the immunological status of the patient with regard to depletion of activated lymphocytes over a period of months or even a year or so. Other explanations include the possibility that the autoimmune changes were irreversible at the time of operation or that not all of the thymus was removed.

At present, however, thymectomy for myasthenia gravis is giving much better results. If the operation is performed in a young woman early in the course of the disease and if the thymus exhibits hyperplasia, much improvement and even cure can often be achieved. With judicious use of prostigminelike drugs and steroids, plus optimal pulmonary toilet and support of respiration, most patients can be carried safely through the thymectomy. We prefer a short upper median sternotomy incision.

Teratoma (Including Dermoid Cyst)

Teratomas and thymomas occurred with almost equal incidence in our series, the teratoma most often taking the form of a dermoid cyst. The intramediastinal teratoma has various elements of skin, bronchus, blood vessel, and still other structures. It is frequently benign but may be malignant. A fairly common feature is the presence of calcium in the wall of the cyst, though the mediastinal dermoid is not as likely to contain tooth elements as is the ovarian dermoid cyst. All three germ layers are usually represented but in varying degrees. The ectodermal layer predominates in cystic lesions, the most common being the dermoid cyst, and the cyst may contain hair, hair follicles, sweat glands, and sebaceous material. These lesions are usually located anteriorly, and usually pose little difficulty in their excision through a lateral thoracotomy incision in the fourth or fifth intercostal space, on either the right or the left, depending on the major presentation of the mass. The postoperative problems presented by excision of benign tumors have been few, in our experience. Of seven teratomas in our series, five were benign and two were malignant. Other, less common germ cell tumors include embryonal carcinomas, choriocarcinomas, and endodermal sinus or yolk sac tumors.

Pericardial Cyst

The pericardial cyst usually consists of a very thin walled cyst containing clear fluid and usually attached to the pericardium, most often at the pericardiophrenic angle. In our experience these cysts have rarely if ever exhibited a functioning communication with the pericardial cavity. There has been no difficulty in excising the pericardial cyst, and there has been no recurrence in our experience.

Other mediastinal cysts include thymic cysts and nonspecific cysts, plus others discussed in this chapter.

Other Conditions

Additional lesions in the anterior mediastinum met in our series were Morgagni (parasternal) hernias containing omentum, and a very large parathyroid adenoma representing a fifth parathyroid gland. In one patient a huge parasternal hernia contained omentum, stomach, and colon, and had produced acute alimentary tract obstruction that required emergency operation. Mediastinal lipoma may be identifiable only by a thoracotomy, at least at the present time, though ultrasound and CT scan techniques may become more discriminating.

MIDDLE MEDIASTINAL MASSES

The surgical lesions of the middle mediastinum consist primarily of various types of lymphomas (Fig. 35-4), bronchogenic carcinoma, bronchogenic cysts, and in some instances lesions of the esophagus. In our series, only eight lymphomas presented as solitary or more or less unilateral masses in the mediastinum; in many patients, bilateral hilar masses represented intrathoracic manifestations of lymph node enlargement that were due to lymphosarcoma, Hodgkin's disease or various other neoplasms or infectious agents. If the cytologic diagnosis of lymphoma can be reached preoperatively, radiation or drug therapy is usually considered the management of choice.

Bronchogenic cysts may arise from accessory respiratory buds that originate from the primitive foregut, or they may be pinched from the tracheobronchial tree after it has arisen as a diverticulum from the foregut. They are lined by pseudostratified ciliated columnar epithelium, and the walls usually contain smooth muscle and occasionally cartilage. The cyst may be filled with a milky mucoid material and appear "solid" on chest roentgenogram (Fig. 35-4), or it may partially drain into a bronchus, contain air, and exhibit an air–fluid level. Nocturnal pulmonary aspiration of material from the cyst may produce pneumonitis and chronic lung damage. The bronchogenic cyst may be essentially asymptomatic, or it may be associated with a chronic or recurring productive cough and occasionally with hemoptysis. Characteristically, however, the cyst may fill up with secretions including pus, and it may then periodically be disgorged of this material, at which time the patient may exhibit copious sputum. If fever was a prominent feature prior to the spontaneous endobronchial drainage, it may then subside until the whole cycle repeats itself. When an air–fluid level is seen, the cyst may be still further delineated with a bronchogram, which may show the radiopaque medium entering the cyst.

Excision of the cyst at thoracotomy usually occasions no difficulty. One definite hazard of the operation is that the patient may aspirate infectious material from the cyst while under anesthesia, and this should be prevented by the use of a double-lumen endotracheal tube or other adequate precautions.

POSTERIOR MEDIASTINAL MASSES

The most commonly occurring lesions of the posterior mediastinum are bronchogenic carcinoma, carcinoma of the esophagus, aneurysms of the thoracic aorta, and neurogenic tumors. The first three are discussed elsewhere in this

Fig. 35-4. Large malignant lymphoma in right hemithorax. *(Left)* Roentgenogram. *(Right)* Lung retracted to expose lymphoma with extensive surface vasculature.

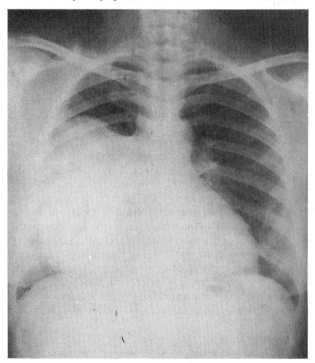
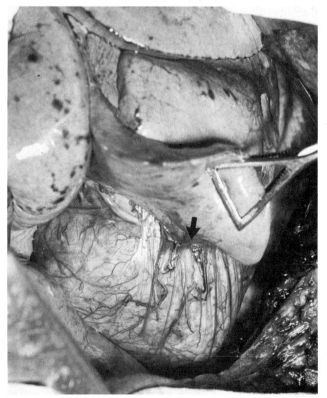

volume. Enteric cyst (duplication of the esophagus or stomach) is rare but will be met in most large series of mediastinal masses. These are excised.

The neurogenic tumor of the posterior mediastinum (Fig. 35-5) may arise either from a spinal nerve or from the sympathetic chain. Histologically, when the microscopic picture is largely of nervous and fibrous tissue, with relatively few ganglion cells, the lesion is commonly termed a *neurofibroma;* when many ganglion cells are present the lesion is termed a ganglioneuroma. In either instance, these tumors are usually benign, and the main symptom is pain due to bone erosion or neurologic deficits due to spinal cord damage. These tumors may become so large that they fill a significant part of the involved hemithorax, but as a rule they are discovered fairly early, either on routine chest x-ray or because of pain. The malignant variety is termed a neuroblastoma. A paraganglioma ("pheochromocytoma") may arise also from the sympathetic chain; it, and in varying degrees certain of the other intrathoracic neurogenic tumors, may elaborate catecholamine products that can be measured in the urine, affording an opportunity for surveillance for tumor recurrence.

These posterior mediastinal neurogenic tumors may assume a dumbbell shape with one portion of the tumor extending into the spinal canal. Both motor and sensory loss in the legs may occur, owing to spinal cord compression. The presence of café au lait spots of skin pigmentation, in the presence of a neurogenic tumor, may suggest von Recklinghausen's neurofibromatosis.

The neurogenic tumor is usually readily removed by

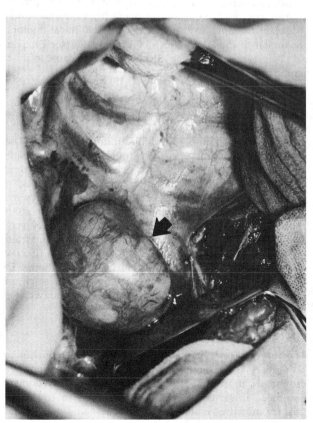

Fig. 35-5. Neurogenic tumor. These lesions are usually found in the posterior mediastinum, arising from spinal or sympathetic nerves.

thoracotomy, but occasionally a laminectomy is required to remove a portion of the tumor that lies within the spinal canal. At operation the tumor arising from sympathetic ganglia may be distinguished from the more common neurofibroma, in that it may have a fusiform shape and may run in a vertical direction, the sympathetic chain emerging at each end, at times from several fused enlargements of the tumor.

As noted, other "solid" lesions of the posterior mediastinum met in our series were aortic aneurysm, bronchogenic carcinoma, lung abscess without an air–fluid level, and lesions of the esophagus. Aortic aneurysms were identified with aortography, bronchogenic carcinomas with appropriate diagnostic studies, and esophageal lesions with barium swallow and esophagoscopy. However, despite all available diagnostic techniques, the definitive diagnosis of many mediastinal masses is achieved only by thoracotomy.

ENDOCRINE TUMORS

Various types of endocrine tumors may arise in the mediastinum. These include pheochromocytoma, parathyroid adenoma, and carcinoid tumor, which when malignant may secrete a variety of hormones including ACTH.

INFECTIONS

Mediastinal infections can range from acute to chronic and from those with effects that are mild to devastating. Certainly, the experienced surgeon approaches mediastinitis with care and much respect.

ACUTE MEDIASTINITIS

Apart from infected median sternotomy incisions for open heart surgery, acute mediastinitis is most often due to perforation of the esophagus by instrumentation, foreign body, or severe vomiting. However, it may also develop from contiguous infections of the neck, lung, or abdomen or from penetrating injuries. The predominant infecting bacteria are highly variable and will depend to a considerable extent on the source of the infection. Perforation of the esophagus admits gram-negative aerobic as well as anaerobic organisms, the most common being anaerobic *Streptococcus* and *Bacteroides.* Following median sternotomy an infection is likely to be due to *Staphylococcus.* Many other organisms have been reported on occasion.

DIAGNOSIS

The diagnosis of acute mediastinitis is not often a problem in patients whose infection is due to esophageal perforation. Pain, fever, dysphagia, leukocytosis, and roentgen findings of mediastinal widening and mediastinal air with or without air–fluid levels will prompt a study with water-soluble contrast medium or barium, and thus the disgnosis will usually be established promptly, provided that this possibility is suspected and acted upon. Unfortunately, the presence of a perforation may not be suspected early, and the patient's condition may deteriorate rapidly with shock if a major leak with massive mediastinal contamination has occurred. Also, the opaque contrast medium may occasionally fail to demonstrate the esophageal perforation, even when it is still open and leaking. We do not perform esophagoscopy for diagnosis except in rare instances.

TREATMENT

The management of acute mediastinitis will depend on the cause. In acute perforation of the esophagus, it is usually mandatory to perform a posterolateral thoracotomy, locate and close the esophageal defect, and institute tube underwater drainage. (However, minor perforations caused by dilatation of an esophageal stricture may occasionally be confined to the immediate periesophageal area by surrounding fibrosis and may not require thoracotomy; indeed, they may be so asymptomatic that they are discovered late on barium swallow, almost by accident.) Nasogastric tube suction may be employed if considered appropriate in the given case, and broad-spectrum antibiotics in heavy dosages and intravenous fluids and nutrients are provided. With such management, promptly initiated and vigorously pursued, most patients will survive. In perforations of the cervical esophagus, it is important to drain the neck so that infection will not build up and advance into the mediastinum. If the mediastinitis is secondary to a median sternotomy incision or spread from a primary infection elsewhere, the primary problem must also be handled appropriately.

CHRONIC MEDIASTINITIS

ETIOLOGY

Chronic mediastinitis has presented a confusing picture over the years. The remarkable and at times astonishing degrees of fibrosis have been attributed to a varied etiology including methysergide therapy, tuberculosis, syphilis, and histoplasmosis, among other agents. At present, most cases are thought to result from infection by the *Histoplasma capsulatum* fungus, but in many instances no specific etiology can be proved. Certainly, acute mediastinitis due to suppurative organisms rarely progresses to chronic fibrosis.

The degree of granulomatous reaction and fibrous proliferation can be extremely dense and thick. It can entrap the pulmonary arteries, producing right heart failure, or it can constrict the superior vena cava, causing the *superior vena caval syndrome*.

TREATMENT

In the absence of a specific etiologic diagnosis in many instances, exploratory thoracotomy has often been employed in the past for biopsy, at times with a surprise finding of bronchial malignancy, lymphoma, or other neoplasm. Some surgeons have advocated a more radical approach, with excision of granulomas, granulomatous lymph nodes, and fibrosis to the extent possible. However, we have generally adopted a conservative approach once the diagnosis of mediastinal fibrosis has been established. With neoplasia, symptomatic disease that is most amenable to surgical extirpation may respond somewhat to radiation therapy, and steroid therapy may be tried, though with limited expectations.

MEDIASTINAL COMPRESSION SYNDROMES

The structures in the mediastinum can be compressed by fluid (blood, effusion, pus), fibrosis, or neoplasm. Fibrous compression of the pulmonary arteries was mentioned above. Hemorrhage into the mediastinum, whatever the cause, can produce the symptoms and signs of pericardial tamponade.

SUPERIOR VENA CAVAL SYNDROME (due to Neoplasm, Thrombosis, Granuloma, Goiter, etc.)

The superior vena caval syndrome is fairly commonly encountered. Obstruction of the vena cava may be due to thrombosis from indwelling catheters or to extension from an arm vein. Compression may be due to mediastinal fibrosis, large intrathoracic goiter, benign or malignant neoplasm, or aneurysm, among other causes.

CLINICAL FINDINGS

The superior vena caval syndrome is discussed in Chapter 37, but, in brief, the result of increasingly elevated venous pressure is distention of the veins of the upper half of the body, edema of the face, arms and torso, and related symptomatology. Dyspnea may be prominent. Venography will demonstrate the site of obstruction or of external compression.

TREATMENT

The possible treatment will depend on the etiology. Malignant tumors causing superior vena caval obstruction are rarely completely resectable, but debulking may at times be helpful. However, in our experience radiation therapy is more likely to be helpful than surgery. Various types of vascular bypasses, for example, from the superior vena cava to the azygous vein or to the right atrium, have been tried, but success has been infrequent. Fortunately, most patients with benign conditions eventually develop sufficient collateral venous flow to the inferior vena cava to remain stable with symptomatic and supportive therapy.

HEMORRHAGE

Hemorrhage into the mediastinum can be due to penetrating injuries, ruptured aneurysm, bleeding from a tumor, anticoagulant therapy, and still other causes. Clinical findings are similar to those of pericardial tamponade (see Chapter 10). Management will be dictated by the cause of the hemorrhage.

MEDIASTINAL EMPHYSEMA

The escape of air into the mediastinum is not rare. The picture presented can be a very mild and asymptomatic emphysema, noted on a chest x-ray, or it can assume dramatic and at times even life-threatening proportions. In general, however, the remarkable subcutaneous emphysema that may involve the entire upper body down to the groin and at times further, with closing of the eyes, can be very distressing to the patient and the family. As pressure from the escape of air into the mediastinum increases, it may rupture through the pleura to produce a pneumothorax. In rare cases the great veins can be compressed to such an extent that venous return to the heart is compromised.

ETIOLOGY

The source of the air may be disruption of a bronchus or pulmonary tissue or blebs, penetrating injuries, ruptured esophagus, air from a perforation of a viscus in the abdomen, or other causes. Often it is "spontaneous" or caused by positive pressure ventilation.

MANAGEMENT

As startling as the patient's appearance may be from extensive subcutaneous emphysema due to extension of the mediastinal air into the neck, spontaneous mediastinal emphysema rarely requires more than supportive measures and reassurance. Operative intervention is rarely required. If pneumothorax should develop, however, closed thoracostomy tube (underwater) drainage should be instituted. If indicated, endotracheal intubation should be considered as a temporary measure.

If the emphysema is due to other causes such as perforation of the esophagus or the tracheobronchial tree, surgery should be directed toward management of the underlying condition.

BIBLIOGRAPHY

Boyd DP, Midell AT: Mediastinal cysts and tumors. An analysis of 96 cases. Surg Clin North Am 48:493, 1968

Fox MA, Vix VA: Endodermal sinus (yolk sac) tumors of the anterior mediastinum. Am J Roentgenol 135:291, 1980

Lichtenstein AK, Levine A, Taylor CR et al: Primary mediastinal lymphoma in adults. Am J Med 68:509, 1980

Pugatch RD, Faling LJ, Robbins AH et al: CT diagnosis of benign mediastinal abnormalities. Am J Roentgenol 134:685, 1980

Rastegar H, Arger P, Harken AH: Evaluation and therapy of mediastinal thymic cyst. Am Surg 46:236, 1980

Shields TW: The mediastinum: Primary tumors and cysts. In his General Thoracic Surgery, pp. 908–944. Philadelphia, Lea & Febiger, 1972

Silverman NA, Sabiston DC Jr: Mediastinal masses. Surg Clin North Am 60:757, 1980

Tsuchiya R, Sugiura Y, Oyata T et al: Thoracic duct cyst of the mediastinum. J Thorac Cardiovasc Surg 79:856, 1980

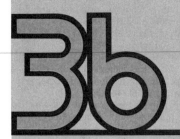

The Aorta and Its Branches

James D. Hardy

Overview

The major disorders that affect the cardiovascular system are either congenital or acquired. The major congenital lesions of the aorta and its branches are considered in Chapter 39. The acquired lesions of these vessels are represented largely by complications of atherosclerosis such as an aneurysm or occlusive disease, embolism, traumatic injuries, infection, and multiple diseases of small arteries.

The surgery of the aorta and its branches now comprises a wide range of specific clinical problems and objectives, most of which require a degree of expertise for optimal management and results. Most surgeons should be prepared at least to handle adequately such routine vascular emergencies as iatrogenic vascular injury in the course of some other operation or with injury from external trauma, when no vascular surgeon of special experience is available. In some circumstances or geographic areas the general surgeon will need to explore the peripheral artery for embolic occlusion or manage a ruptured abdominal aortic aneurysm. The transplant surgeon requires vascular experience, as does the urologist for renal vessels, the hepatobiliary surgeon for portosystemic venous shunts, the neurosurgeon for extracranial and intracranial arterial procedures, and so on. Clearly, so pervasive has the need for a reasonable degree of familiarity with vascular techniques become over the past 25 years that most residents progressing through training for almost any surgical specialty should achieve this capability.

The major advances in vascular surgery of the past two decades include constantly improving and more widely applied arteriographic techniques, better sutures and arterial substitution fabric materials, and the pervasive use of the Doppler flow principle in determining and imaging arterial and venous flow through specific vessels without the need for invasive arteriography in many instances. There is increasing experience to document when and what operations are most likely to be of benefit to the patient and which are not (cost/benefit ratios). Sonography and CT scan for diagnosis of aneurysm and the percutaneous catheter-balloon dilatation of arterial stenosis under fluoroscopic guidance have also made rapid strides in clinical usefulness.

Finally, especially when dealing with aneurysmal or atherosclerotic arterial occlusive disease—carotids, aortic arch, coronaries, renals, and femoral-popliteal systems—the physician should consider the body circulation as a whole (Fig. 36-1). Atherosclerosis is a generalized disease with segmental emphasis at bifurcations. The patient with coronary artery disease may well have a concomitant or future carotid or lower aortic disease. The entire system of accessible peripheral arteries should be assessed and the results recorded with the physical examination.

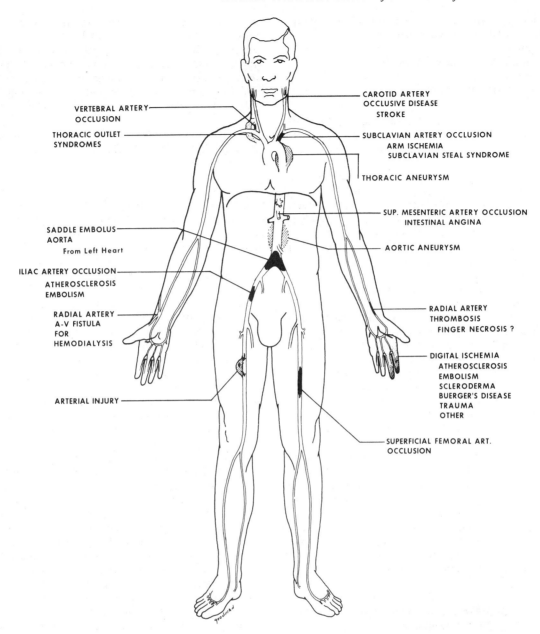

Fig. 36-1. Representative arterial lesions. Numerous additional arterial diseases may require surgical intervention, including renal artery stenosis causing hypertension. (For discussion see opposite page.)

Jesse E. Thompson

Thrombo-obliterative Disease of the Vessels of the Aortic Arch

Occlusive lesions of the great vessels arising from the aortic arch and in the extracranial branches of these vessels are responsible for symptoms of cerebral and upper extremity arterial insufficiency.

Until fairly recently, the prevailing notion held by most physicians was that strokes were caused by intracranial vascular disease, in spite of the fact that occlusive lesions in the extracranial segments of the main arteries supplying the brain had been described in the mid 1800s and their association with cerebral ischemia noted. With the development of cerebral arteriography by Moniz in 1927, a practical method for diagnosis became available. More widespread use of arteriography led to increasing awareness of the extracranial location and segmental nature of atherosclerotic occlusive lesions. This was followed by rapid development and employment of appropriate vascular surgical techniques for removing obstructive plaques and restoring cerebral blood flow. It is now estimated that 75% of patients with ischemic stroke syndromes have at least one obstructive lesion at a surgically accessible site and that upward of 50% have the principal occlusions confined to the extracranial vasculature.

Successful carotid reconstruction for stroke was first performed by Carrea and colleagues in Buenos Aires in 1951, and successful carotid endarterectomy was first done by DeBakey and associates in Houston in 1953. The operation that gave the greatest impetus to the development of surgery for cerebro-occlusive disease was that of Eastcott and co-workers, performed in 1954.

In 1954, Davis and associates performed the first innominate endarterectomy. DeBakey's group, in 1957, constructed a bypass graft from the innominate artery to the distal subclavian and carotid arteries and shortly thereafter

---

THROMBO-OBLITERATIVE DISEASES OF THE VESSELS OF THE AORTIC ARCH

Etiology	Usually atherosclerosis, resulting in emboli to the brain or arms, or reduction in cerebral or upper extremity blood flow
Dx	Symptoms of cerebral or arm ischemia, either transient or persistent. Noninvasive tests helpful Definitive diagnosis made by appropriate arteriography
Rx	Surgical therapy by endarterectomy or appropriate bypass graft, depending on the vessels involved
Results	Relief or improvement in symptoms in 90% of cases treated Sixfold reduction in stroke incidence in patients with transient ischemic attacks or asymptomatic carotid bruits when compared with untreated patients

---

successfully performed subclavian endarterectomy. In the same year, Cate and Scott carried out successful endarterectomy of the left subclavian and left vertebral arteries. In 1952, Crawford and co-workers described their management of basilar artery insufficiency by means of vertebral endarterectomy in one case and a bypass graft from the subclavian to the patent distal vertebral artery in another.

ANATOMY AND PATHOLOGY

MECHANISM OF SYMPTOM PRODUCTION

The main vessels supplying blood to the brain are the two carotid and two vertebral arteries and their branches. Many variations in the normal anatomy occur, and anomalies at all levels are not uncommon. In the absence of occlusive disease, each internal carotid carries 300 ml to 400 ml of blood per minute, whereas the two vertebrals together carry only 200 ml/minute. When major vessels are obstructed, the functional capacity of the brain is largely dependent on the integrity of the compensatory mechanisms responsible for collateral circulation, whose anatomical arrangement includes both extracranial and intracranial components.

Extracranial obstructive lesions responsible for cerebrovascular insufficiency are found in the aortic arch at the origins of the innominate, carotid, and subclavian arteries; in the vertebral arteries at their origins and beyond; in the common carotid bifurcations; and in the first portion of the internal and external carotid arteries (Fig. 36-2). Obstructions at the carotid bifurcation, which usually involve the first few centimeters of the internal carotid artery as well, are by far the most common. In many cases, the intracranial vessels are surprisingly free of demonstrable disease. The segmental nature of the cervical lesions makes possible restoration of blood flow by surgical means. Multiple-vessel involvement by stenotic plaques in the great vessels, the carotids, and the vertebrobasilar system is a frequent finding.

Most of the occlusions are caused by intimal atherosclerotic plaques that partially or completely obstruct the extracranial vessels. At times, the plaques become necrotic and ulcerated. This debris may become dislodged and embolize into the distal circulation to cause transient ischemic attacks (TIAs) or frank strokes. As a plaque enlarges and lumen size diminishes, blood flow decreases. The final episode is thrombosis, with complete occlusion of the artery. Other lesions that may be responsible for occlusions are aneurysms, arteritis, bony spurs, fibromuscular dysplasia, kinks and loops, thoracic outlet syndrome, Takayasu's disease, tumors, irradiation injuries, and trauma.

Thus, symptoms of cerebrovascular insufficiency result from two basic mechanisms: embolization into the brain of platelet aggregations or debris and reduction in cerebral blood flow, either total or regional.

SIGNIFICANCE OF STENOTIC LESIONS

The question arises as to the functional significance of occlusive lesions seen on the arteriograms of the extracranial vessels supplying the brain. A lesion that is significant on x-ray film may not be accompanied by clinical manifestations. Most of the significant carotid lesions show a reduction in diameter of the artery of 40% to 50% or more, as measured on the arteriogram. A 50% reduction in diameter results in a 75% reduction in cross-sectional area, at which

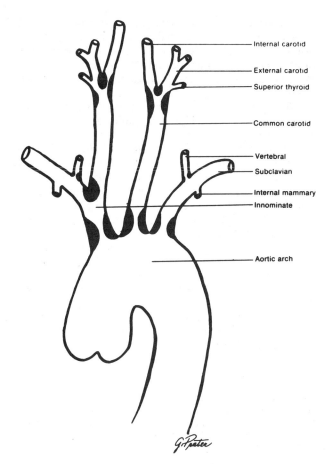

Fig. 36-2.   Usual extracranial locations of atherosclerotic plaques responsible for cerebrovascular insufficiency.

point significant pressure gradients begin to occur and blood flow begins to fall rather precipitously. A lumen of 1.0 mm diameter or less in the internal carotid artery always causes a significant pressure gradient and reduction in internal carotid artery flow. Stenoses of a lesser degree are of greater significance if the opposite carotid or the vertebral arteries are also compromised or if multiple stenotic lesions are present. A stenosis of any degree may be significant if its appearance suggests the deposition of platelet aggregations or the presence of an ulcerated plaque, which may be sources of cerebral emboli. Noninvasive studies, such as oculoplethysmography (OPG), are useful in evaluating the hemodynamic significance of stenotic lesions.

CLINICAL MANIFESTATIONS

The clinical syndromes of cerebrovascular insufficiency vary from a few minor symptoms to the catastrophic stroke with paralysis and coma. Manifestations may be related to the carotid system, to the vertebrobasilar system, or to a combination of the two systems. The most common extracranial occlusive lesions are found in the carotid system.

Dizziness, giddiness, light-headedness, and syncope or blackout spells may be seen in patients with cerebrovascular insufficiency but frequently accompany other disease states. True vertigo, implying an illusion of motion, occurs with vertebrobasilar disease but is a vestibular symptom that can arise from a variety of vestibular lesions other than vascular. Thus, the differential diagnosis of cerebrovascular insuffi-

ciency includes brain tumor, brain abscess, subdural hematoma, intracerebral hemorrhage, subarachnoid hemorrhage, carotid-sinus sensitivity, heart block, epilepsy, hypotension, hypoglycemia, vestibular disease (including Meniere's syndrome), migraine, hypertension with and without encephalopathy, temporal arteritis (transient blindness), hyperventilation, and psychosis.

Lesions of the great vessels of the aortic arch may give the clinical picture of either carotid or vertebrobasilar disease, depending upon the particular anatomical situation.

CAROTID SYSTEM

Patients with carotid occlusive disease have symptoms and signs that include headaches, dizziness, blackout spells, buzzing noises in the head and ear, and mental deterioration and loss of memory. There may be transient monocular blindness on the ipsilateral side of a carotid occlusion or homonymous visual-field defects. There may be numbness, weakness, or paralysis of an extremity or of one entire side of the body. Dysphasia or aphasia occurs if the dominant hemisphere is involved. Coma and convulsions also occur. In some patients, symptoms are minimal to absent and the only suggestion of occlusive disease is the finding of a bruit over the carotid artery in the neck.

VERTEBROBASILAR SYSTEM

The symptoms and signs of vertebrobasilar insufficiency include vertigo, headaches, bilateral visual disturbances, dysarthria, dysphagia, disorders of equilibrium, impairment of consciousness, and drop attacks. There may be monoparesis or paralysis shifting from side to side and involving any or all of the extremities. Sensory defects on both sides of the body, cranial nerve paralyses, and cerebellar signs with ataxia also occur.

CLASSIFICATION OF PATIENTS

It is important to classify patients with cerebrovascular insufficiency into specific clinical categories. Only in this way can proper selection of patients for operation be made and results of different methods of therapy within the same categories be compared. For purposes of surgical consideration, patients are classified into four clinical groups: frank stroke, transient cerebral ischemia, chronic cerebral ischemia, and asymptomatic bruit.

FRANK STROKE

Frank stroke includes all patients with a neurologic deficit at the time of operation, whether improving, progressively worsening, or stable. All degrees of severity may be present, ranging from mild residual deficits to profound strokes with hemiplegia, aphasia, and coma.

TRANSIENT CEREBRAL ISCHEMIA

Transient cerebral ischemia includes patients with focal attacks of neurologic dysfunction and transient symptoms of generalized cerebral ischemia, lasting minutes or hours, but without residual neurologic deficit at 24 hours. Focal attacks include ocular, speech, sensory, and motor disturbances. Features of generalized ischemia include dizziness, blackout spells, headaches, and other nonlocalizing symptoms.

CHRONIC CEREBRAL ISCHEMIA

Patients in the chronic cerebral ischemia category exhibit obvious cerebrovascular insufficiency, with loss of memory, impaired mentation, or overt motor or mental deterioration. These patients are not numerous and are difficult to classify but logically cannot be placed in any other group.

ASYMPTOMATIC BRUIT

Patients in the asymptomatic bruit group are without neurologic symptoms and are found to have cervical bruits during routine auscultation of the neck. These bruits may arise from the great vessels or the subclavian or cervical carotid arteries.

DIAGNOSTIC METHODS

HISTORY AND PHYSICAL EXAMINATION

In the workup of a patient with obvious or suspected cerebrovascular insufficiency, the complete history and physical examination should emphasize the salient features of the clinical syndromes outlined above. A history of diabetes, hypertension, or heart disease is particularly important.

The status of the carotid, superficial temporal, subclavian, and radial pulses should be carefully noted. An absent or diminished carotid pulsation in the neck aids in localizing lesions to the aortic arch area. Blood pressure readings in the two arms are helpful in the diagnosis of subclavian or innominate occlusions. It is especially important to listen for murmurs over the carotid artery in the neck, over the globe of the eye, in the supraclavicular region, and over the heart. A bell stethoscope is most useful for auscultation of these murmurs. Complete neurologic examination must be done.

LABORATORY FINDINGS

X-ray films of the chest are routinely obtained, as is an electrocardiogram. An electroencephalogram (EEG) is frequently done. Lumbar puncture may be performed to help substantiate the diagnosis and rule out hemorrhagic or expanding intracranial lesions.

Radionuclide scans and especially computed tomography (CT) scans have been used in the investigation of stroke syndromes, but their role is limited. There is little reason to perform these tests in patients with TIAs, the principal indication for carotid surgery. Scans have been employed in attempts to define the blood–brain barrier, as a guide in timing surgical revascularization, but most surgeons have applied clinical criteria to determine operability, using the brain scan as an adjunct. The CT scans are most useful in demonstrating infarcts, hemorrhage, cysts, and tumors.

ARTERIOGRAPHY

Following the studies outlined above, one should proceed directly to cerebral arteriography, since definitive evaluation is made only by this means. Four-vessel and arch studies should be considered in every case but may not be routinely carried out unless indicated. Retrograde catheter techniques through the femoral, brachial, or axillary arteries, using local anesthesia, are most commonly employed. By this means, one can not only visualize the aortic arch and upper extremity vessels but also study selectively the extracranial carotid and vertebral arteries and the intracranial vasculature. Serial biplane views are routinely obtained (Fig. 36-3).

When retrograde techniques are not possible, percutaneous carotid or brachial injections, antegrade or retrograde, may be used.

Complications of arteriography include cardiac problems, hematomas, peripheral embolization of debris, arterial thrombosis, false aneurysms, extravasation of contrast material, seizures, production or aggravation of neurologic deficits, and peripheral nerve paresis. Care in the technical performance of the procedure is of great importance in preventing these complications. The use of safe contrast material is most important. Hypotensive episodes may be avoided by the administration of lactated Ringer's solution during and after the procedure. Suction apparatus, oxygen, and cardiac drugs must be available in the x-ray department and recovery area.

Unless the diagnosis of ischemic stroke is in question, it is best to avoid cerebral arteriography during the acute phase of completed, progressing, fluctuating, or improving strokes. It is preferable to delay such procedures until a

Fig. 36-3. This left lateral carotid arteriogram of a 63-year-old man having recurrent attacks of amaurosis fugax in the left eye and a loud carotid bruit shows an ulcerated, stenotic atherosclerotic plaque involving the bifurcation and internal and external carotid arteries (*arrows*).

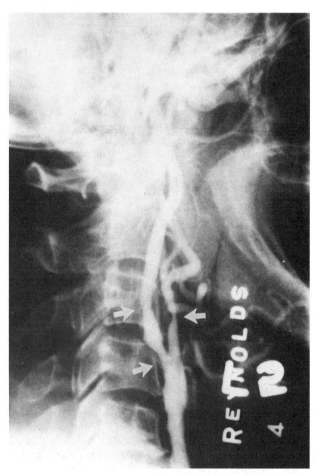

stable situation ensues, at which time arteriography can usually be performed safely. If there is some question as to the presence of subdural hematoma, intracerebral hemorrhage, or brain tumor, arteriography is justifiable in the acute situation, although the CT scan may make this unnecessary.

If total occlusion of a stenotic carotid artery results from the arteriographic procedure, emergency surgical intervention for restoration of cerebral blood flow becomes necessary.

Although the list of complications related to cerebral arteriography is an imposing one, their incidence is quite low and has continuously decreased with increasing experience of those performing the procedures and with increasing use of retrograde catheter techniques under local anesthesia. Cerebral angiography can be performed with a mortality rate of 0.2% or less and a procedure-related stroke rate of 0.5% or less. The occurrence of other less serious complications varies from 5% to 25% in reported series.

NONINVASIVE STUDIES

Since cerebral arteriography still poses certain hazards, although few in number, noninvasive methods of study have been sought in attempts to avoid unnecessary arteriograms in puzzling diagnostic situations and in the management of asymptomatic carotid bruits.

Bidirectional Doppler studies of supraorbital blood flow are in common use but have limited application because of poor correlation with arteriographic results. The phonoangiogram has been adapted for study of cervical bruits. It takes on added significance when used in conjunction with OPG. At present, the most helpful studies are the oculoplethysmograms and the various types of scans.

Oculopneumoplethysmography (OPG-Gee) measures ophthalmic artery pressure and when accompanied by carotid compression gives an estimate of internal carotid artery stump pressure. It thereby assesses collateral blood flow to the ipsilateral cerebral hemisphere. In Gee's hands, the results have been quite accurate.

Oculoplethysmography (OPG-Kartchner) compares the ocular pulse wave forms in the two eyes to assess the hemodynamic significance of internal carotid artery lesions. It has been combined with carotid phonoangiography (CPA) to increase its accuracy. Compared with arteriograms, this study gives about 85% correct interpretations.

Doppler imagery scans and ultrasonic scanning combined with Doppler studies and spectral analysis have given fairly accurate anatomical evaluations of the carotid bifurcation but leave much to be desired. A developing technique that appears very promising at this writing is computerized digital subtraction angiography (DSA), using only intravenous injections of contrast material. The technique may render the other noninvasive methods unnecessary or obsolete and indeed, with increasing refinements in technology, may eventually replace invasive arteriography in many areas.

SURGERY OF THE GREAT VESSELS

Occlusive lesions in the great vessels arising from the aortic arch and in the vertebral arteries may cause symptoms of cerebrovascular insufficiency. Such lesions are characteristically located at the origins of these vessels and are usually segmental in extent. Even with total occlusion of the innominate, subclavian, and common carotid arteries, the distal vasculature is nearly always patent. By virtue of this fact, most occlusions of the great vessels can be successfully reconstructed by surgical means. Numerically speaking, these lesions comprise only a small proportion of the total extracranial occlusions responsible for cerebrovascular insufficiency; those at the common carotid bifurcations are by far the ones most frequently encountered. Multiple stenoses may occur in the great vessels, the carotids, and the vertebral arteries.

Symptomatology varies depending upon the location of the lesions. Thus, one may find patterns of carotid insufficiency or vertebrobasilar insufficiency, or combinations. When the subclavian artery is involved, there may be symptoms of arterial insufficiency of the upper extremity, in addition to, or without, cerebral manifestations.

INNOMINATE AND COMMON CAROTID ARTERIES

When the innominate artery is stenotic or occluded, there may be symptoms arising from the distribution of the right carotid, the right subclavian, or the right vertebral artery systems. Diagnostic features include differences in blood pressure and arterial pulsations in the two arms and a murmur heard over the innominate artery. With occlusive lesions in the innominate artery, when the distal subclavian, carotid, and vertebral arteries are patent, one occasionally encounters the syndrome known as the innominate steal, with reversal of flow in both the right carotid and right vertebral arteries, giving symptoms of left hemiparesis and brain-stem ischemia.

SUBCLAVIAN ARTERIES AND SUBCLAVIAN STEAL SYNDROME

Subclavian occlusive lesions may cause vertebrobasilar insufficiency or arterial insufficiency of the corresponding arm or may give no symptoms whatsoever. Differences in blood pressure and arterial pulsations in the arms and bruits in the supraclavicular areas are diagnostic features of these lesions.

An interesting syndrome known as the subclavian steal syndrome has been described. In this situation, the proximal subclavian artery, usually the left, is occluded, while the ipsilateral vertebral artery is patent. There is reversal of flow in the vertebral artery, with blood flowing from the brain into the arm distal to the subclavian occlusion through the patent vertebral vessel. With loss of blood from the brain stem and cerebellum, one may have manifestations of vertebrobasilar insufficiency. Symptoms may be precipitated by exercise of the ipsilateral arm. Detailed serial arteriograms are necessary to establish the diagnosis of subclavian steal syndrome. Unless symptomatic, patients with subclavian steal syndromes need not be subjected to surgical reconstruction.

VERTEBRAL ARTERIES

Stenosis at the takeoff of the vertebral artery from the subclavian may cause symptoms of vertebrobasilar insufficiency. Anatomical variations in the origin of the vertebral artery are not uncommon. At times, the artery is vestigial or even completely absent on one side. Ordinarily, if one vertebral artery is widely patent, circulation in the vertebrobasilar system is adequate and symptoms are minimal or absent. The situation may vary, however, depending

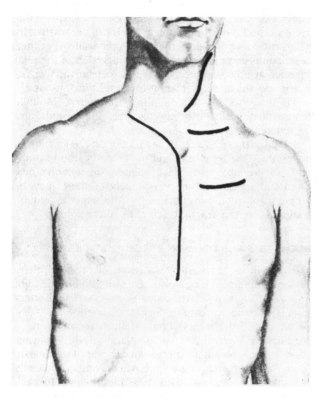

Fig. 36-4. Locations of sternal splitting, intercostal space, and cervical incisions used for operations on the aortic arch, and the common carotid, subclavian, vertebral, and internal carotid arteries.

upon the presence of occlusive lesions in the carotid system and in the basilar artery itself. Total occlusion of the vertebral artery at its origin is usually accompanied by thrombosis throughout the entire cervical extent of the vessel and precludes surgical restoration of patency.

Many patients with the clinical syndromes of vertebro-basilar insufficiency have occlusive lesions in the carotid system as well as the vertebral vessels. Endarterectomy of the carotid arteries may so favorably influence the vertebral symptoms that further surgery on the vertebral artery is not required. Surgical reconstruction of the vertebral artery is infrequently indicated. Patients with bilateral vertebral stenoses or with stenosis of a single remaining artery are the principal candidates for operation.

SURGICAL TECHNIQUES

Revascularization procedures for occlusions of the great vessels and vertebral arteries must be highly individualized because of the many possible sites of the lesions. Technical procedures include intrathoracic and extrathoracic cervical approaches. The former may be done through sternal splitting incisions, anterior thoracic incisions through the second or third intercostal space, or lateral thoracic incisions through the fifth intercostal space; the latter are approached through supraclavicular incisions (Fig. 36-4).

In the past, stenoses of the innominate, common carotid, and subclavian arteries were treated with direct endarterectomy or with bypass grafts taking origin from the arch of the aorta (Fig. 36-5). Although blood flow restoration was quite satisfactory, mortality and morbidity for these procedures were quite high. Consequently, new methods were devised, resulting in the use of extrathoracic cervical bypass

procedures almost exclusively. These operations are simple to perform, have low mortality and morbidity, and are quite satisfactory. Many variations in technique are possible.

In a good-risk patient, one may still elect to perform endarterectomy of the innominate artery using a cervical or an intrathoracic approach. A sternal splitting incision is usually employed. If the artery is totally occluded, there is little hazard in cross-clamping and performing a routine endarterectomy through a linear arteriotomy. In the presence of partially occlusive innominate lesions, however, one may wish to use a temporary inlying bypass shunt.

Stenoses of the common carotid and proximal subclavian arteries are best handled by means of the simpler cervical bypass maneuvers. Experience has shown that construction of these bypasses does not produce symptomatic steal syndromes. Compensatory increase in blood flow, sufficient to vascularize the various distal beds, occurs in the patent artery.

When there is a proximal common carotid artery stenosis, a bypass is constructed, employing either autologous vein or 6-mm Dacron, from the subclavian artery to the common carotid just distal to the stenosis through a supraclavicular incision in the neck (Fig. 36-6).

Occasionally, one may employ a long bypass graft from the subclavian artery to the bifurcation of the common

Fig. 36-5. This type of bypass graft may be used for reconstruction of occlusive lesions of the aortic arch vessels. Here, the occluded innominate artery has been bypassed with 8-mm Dacron from the aortic arch to the distal right subclavian and common carotid arteries. Many variations of this technique are possible. (Thompson JE: Cerebrovascular insufficiency. In Barker WF [ed]: Peripheral Arterial Disease. Philadelphia, W B Saunders, 1975)

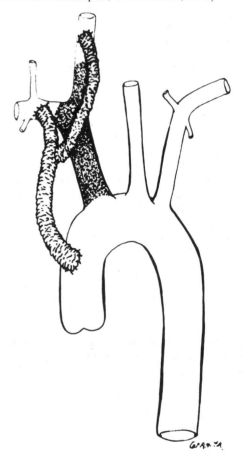

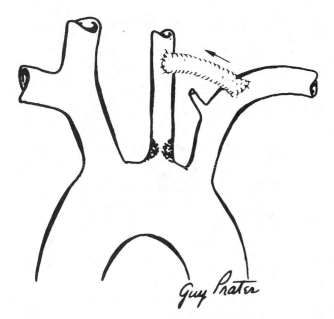

Fig. 36-6. An extrathoracic cervical bypass graft from the left subclavian artery to the left common carotid artery is used in the treatment of common carotid stenosis at its origin from the aortic arch. Either the saphenous vein or a 6-mm Dacron tube may be used. (Thompson JE: Cerebrovascular insufficiency. In Barker WF [ed]: Peripheral Arterial Disease. Philadelphia, W B Saunders, 1975)

carotid to avoid a long endarterectomy of a completely occluded common carotid.

For symptomatic subclavian steal syndromes or arm symptoms, a carotid-to-subclavian bypass graft is performed using the same approach as described for subclavian-to-carotid bypass. In this situation, however, since the carotid is the nonstenotic artery, it may be well to employ cerebral protection in the form of an inlying shunt in the carotid artery (Fig. 36-7).

One variation of this technique is ligation of the proximal subclavian artery, division, and anastomosis of the divided

Fig. 36-7. Extrathoracic cervical bypass from the left common carotid to the left subclavian artery restores blood flow into an occluded left subclavian artery. This same maneuver restores flow into the vertebral artery when it is patent and only the proximal portion of the subclavian is occluded, the subclavian steal syndrome. (Thompson JE: Cerebrovascular insufficiency. In Barker WF [ed]: Peripheral Arterial Disease. Philadelphia, W B Saunders, 1975)

distal end of the subclavian artery to the side of the proximal carotid. The use of a prosthesis is obviated.

To avoid the more serious intrathoracic operation for repair of an innominate artery stenosis, one may perform a cervical subclavian-to-subclavian bypass. Bilateral supraclavicular incisions are made. An 8-mm or 6-mm prosthetic graft or autologous vein is then sutured end to end to the left subclavian artery, and the graft is tunneled under the strap muscles across the anterior neck into the exposed right subclavian artery area. An end-to-side anastomosis is then performed between the graft and the right subclavian artery. Success of this operation depends upon the patency of the subclavian–carotid bifurcation in the innominate system.

A variation of the subclavian-to-subclavian bypass is the axillary-to-axillary bypass, with the prosthesis passing subcutaneously. It has been used to revascularize both subclavian arteries, as well as the innominate artery.

When vertebral artery reconstruction is required, a variety of techniques are available. An isolated vertebral stenosis is best approached through a standard supraclavicular incision. At times, this operation is difficult because of the depth of the operative field. Simple endarterectomy of the vertebral origin is usually inadvisable because of the small size of the artery and may be hazardous because of its friability. A vein patch graft is ordinarily used for reconstruction of the vertebral origin (Fig. 36-8, *A*).

When the vertebral artery is tortuous, arterioplasty may be performed by suturing the vertebral artery to the subclavian artery, employing a side-to-side anastomosis (Fig. 36-8, *B*). The artery may also be ligated and divided at its proximal takeoff and then reimplanted into the distal subclavian artery at a more convenient site, using an end-to-side anastomosis (Fig. 36-8, *C*).

In the presence of subclavian plaques, the orifice of the vertebral artery may be endarterectomized through the lumen of the subclavian artery to avoid direct incision into the small vertebral artery itself.

Bypass techniques are also useful for vertebral reconstruction. One such bypass is from the distal subclavian to the distal vertebral, employing a vein or a 6-mm Dacron

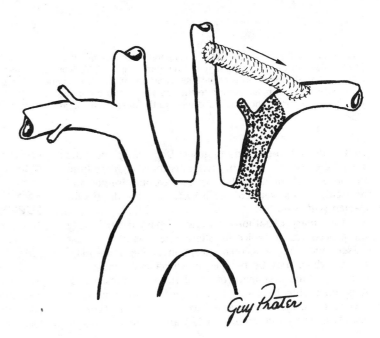

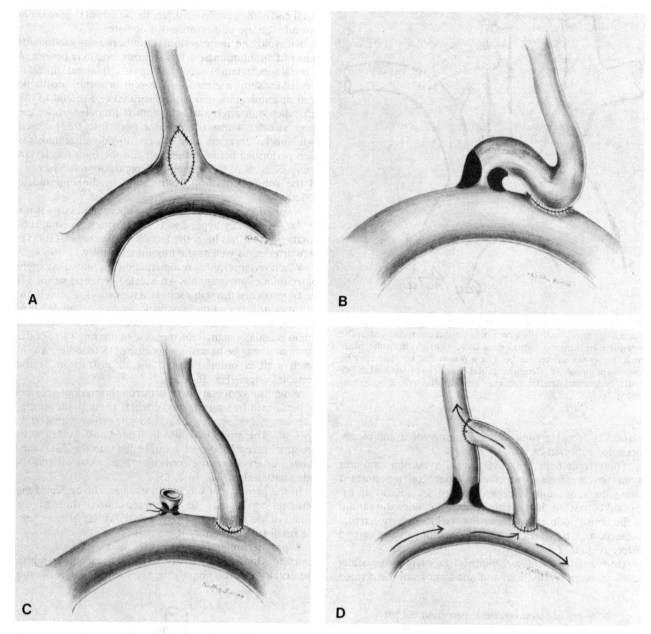

Fig. 36-8. Technical procedures for vertebral artery reconstruction. *(A)* Patch graft reconstruction (vein or Dacron) to enlarge the stenosed vertebral origin. *(B)* Vertebral arterioplasty of a tortuous artery with side-to-side anastomosis to the subclavian artery. *(C)* Ligation and division of the vertebral artery with end-to-end reimplantation into the subclavian at a more distal site. *(D)* Bypass graft, using the saphenous vein, from the distal subclavian to the distal vertebral artery beyond the stenosed orifice.

graft with end-to-side anastomoses. Depending upon the site of the lesions, other bypass grafts may originate from the aortic arch or from the common carotid arteries and revascularize the vertebrobasilar system by the distal subclavian (Fig. 36-8, *D*).

In summary, extrathoracic cervical bypass operations are the procedures of choice for stenotic lesions of the great vessels, with the occasional exception of the innominate artery, which may be handled by direct endarterectomy. Because of the excellence of distal runoff in most cases, these operations have very high immediate and long-term success rates. Patients subjected to operation for occlusive lesions in the aortic arch branches and vertebral arteries

become asymptomatic or improved in some 80% to 85% of the cases reported.

SURGERY OF THE CAROTID BIFURCATION

INDICATIONS FOR AND TIMING OF CAROTID ENDARTERECTOMY

By far the most common lesions amenable to surgical correction are found in the carotid system at the carotid bifurcation. The most frequently performed operation, therefore, is carotid endarterectomy. Clinical considerations in

TABLE 36-1   INDICATIONS FOR CAROTID ENDARTERECTOMY IN CEREBROVASCULAR INSUFFICIENCY

Indications
1. Transient cerebral ischemia
2. Stable strokes—selected
3. Asymptomatic bruits—selected
4. Chronic cerebral ischemia—selected

Contraindications
1. Acute profound strokes
2. Progressing strokes
3. Severe intracranial disease
4. Other severe generalized disorders (*e.g.*, cancer)

each of the four categories of patients determine the indications and contraindications for carotid endarterectomy. The indications for operation are listed in Table 36-1. The principal indication is transient cerebral ischemia, since strokes can be prevented and troublesome episodes of ischemia are largely abolished. Patients with recent mild stable strokes or those with old strokes who develop new symptoms may also be candidates. Operation is contraindicated for cervical occlusions in the presence of severe intracranial disease. Mild intracranial disease, however, is an indication rather than a contraindication for operation. Age itself is not necessarily a contraindication to operation when the patient's general condition otherwise does not pose undue hazard.

The chief contraindication to operation is acute stroke. Mortality rates up to 60% follow operations in the early phases of acute stroke because of the intracranial hemorrhage and cerebral edema that follow revascularization of an acute cerebral infarction. Patients with profound strokes, rapidly progressing strokes, and rapidly improving strokes should be allowed to stabilize for 3 to 6 weeks (or longer) before operation is considered.

Indication for operation is also based on a critical evaluation of operative risk, since a high proportion of these patients have hypertension and generalized atherosclerosis, especially coronary disease. Risk may be graded employing a combination of medical, neurologic, and angiographic factors.

Appropriate timing of operation for the various clinical categories is summarized in Table 36-2. Although delayed operation is an important principle in stroke surgery, emergency operation is not often indicated. There is considerable difference of opinion regarding operation for acute carotid thrombosis following arteriography or endarterectomy. If operation can be performed immediately (in 1 to 2 hours), then this is a justifiable and worthwhile procedure.

Likewise, controversy has arisen over the advisability of performing emergency endarterectomy on patients with unstable or fluctuating deficits and with crescendo TIAs. Management of these patients is fraught with difficulty. In the absence of reliable methods to distinguish between cerebral infarction and reversible ischemia without infarction, the results of therapy—whether surgical or medical—are unpredictable. In general, if the deficit is mild and the lesion severe, emergency operation may be justified. Best results are usually obtained, however, if the patient's situation can be stabilized before operation is performed.

Patients with significant bilateral lesions should have bilateral endarterectomies, but in separate stages, at least 1 to 2 weeks apart, or even longer. Bilateral operation in a single stage is inadvisable because of the complications that may ensue, including respiratory difficulties, postoperative hypertension, and aggravation of neurologic deficits.

Occasionally, one finds patients in whom occlusive lesions are located in the ipsilateral or paradoxical carotid artery, relative to the neurologic picture. Removal of these "inappropriate" lesions results in a clinical response to be expected had they been located on the appropriate side, because of collateral circulation.

TECHNIQUE OF CAROTID ENDARTERECTOMY

Technical considerations are of the utmost importance in carotid endarterectomy, since the limits of tolerance to temporary occlusion of the blood supply to the brain may be quite narrow. Safety factors that will eliminate in most instances the occurrence or aggravation of neurologic deficits must be employed. Carotid endarterectomy should be associated with low mortality, few complications, satisfactory immediate and long-term anatomical results, and good functional results relative to cerebrovascular insufficiency.

Operation is usually performed under light general anesthesia, although some surgeons prefer local or regional blocks. Successive steps in the operation are shown in Figure 36-9.

It is important that adequate levels of blood pressure be maintained during operation and in the immediate postoperative period to prevent thrombosis in the operative site or in the brain. This may be achieved by administration of 500 ml to 1000 ml lactated Ringer's solution or of vasopressor.

Rarely, one encounters patients with bilaterally occluded internal carotid arteries that cannot be opened. Under these circumstances, endarterectomy of the external carotid may be necessary to improve flow.

TABLE 36-2   TIMING OF CAROTID ENDARTERECTOMY FOR CEREBROVASCULAR INSUFFICIENCY

Elective operation
1. Stable stroke, recent or old
2. Transient cerebral ischemia
3. Asymptomatic bruit
4. Chronic cerebral ischemia (rare)

Delayed operation (days to weeks)
1. Mild stroke
2. Fluctuating stroke

Emergency operation (rarely necessary)
1. Frank stroke
   Disappearance of bruit
   Slowly worsening
   Fluctuating
2. Transient cerebral ischemia
   Severe stenosis, especially if bilateral
   Disappearance of bruit
3. Carotid thrombosis immediately following arteriography or endarterectomy

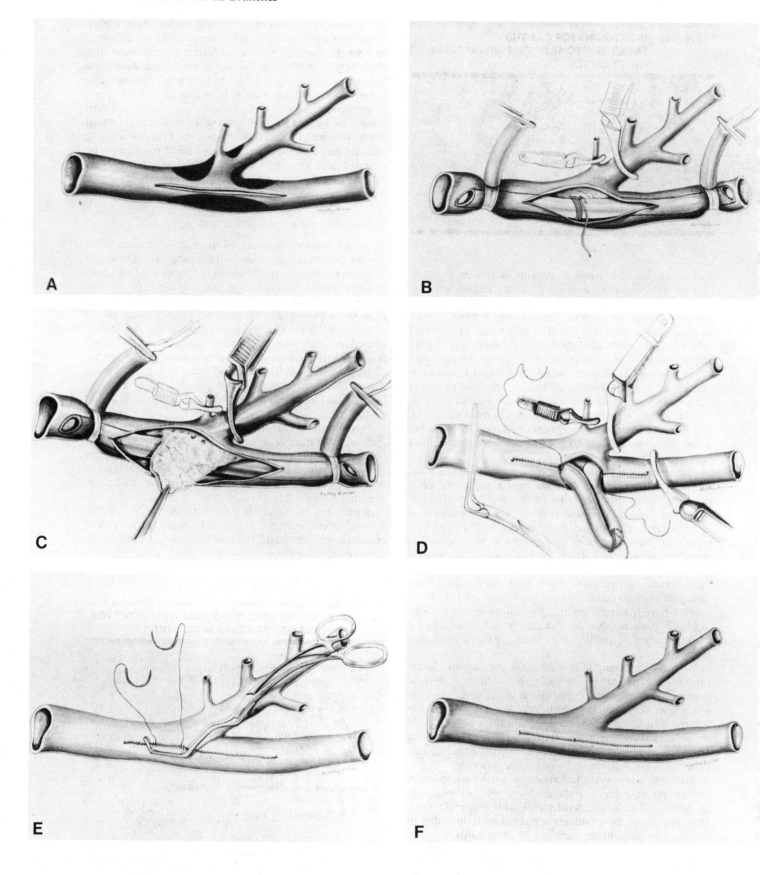

A

B

C

D

E

F

COMPLICATIONS

Complications associated with carotid endarterectomy are listed in Table 36-3. If one is meticulous with details of intraoperative and postoperative management, the actual incidence of complications is quite low. The occurrence of neurologic deficits should not exceed 2% to 3%, and the incidence of all remaining complications should be no more than 3% to 4%.

Excessively high levels of blood pressure postoperatively must be treated aggressively to prevent hematomas in the wound, disruption of the arterial reconstruction, and intracerebral hemorrhage and edema. If the blood pressure rises above 200 mm Hg, one should immediately employ an intravenous drip of nitroprusside or trimethaphan camsylate (Arfonad), which lower pressure within minutes.

The most serious complication of carotid endarterectomy is the occurrence or aggravation of neurologic deficits. Many of these episodes are transient, whereas others remain as permanent deficits, either mild or severe. A common cause of neurologic deficits is cerebral embolization of debris, owing to excessive manipulation of the artery or improper flushing of vessels following closure of the arteriotomy.

A second cause of operation-related deficits is cerebral ischemia, resulting from hypotension, intracerebral arterial thrombosis, or inadequate cerebral protection. Although many patients undergoing carotid endarterectomy can tolerate temporary clamping of the artery without deleterious effect, the rest require some form of cerebral protection if strokes are to be prevented. Patients with severe vascular disease and multiple large-vessel occlusions are least tolerant of carotid clamping.

Methods presently available to determine the adequacy of collateral blood flow during carotid clamping include temporary occlusion under local anesthesia while checking the neurologic status, determination of stump pressure in the occluded distal internal carotid artery, and EEG monitoring. Although actual determination of regional cerebral blood flow (rCBF) by the ^{133}Xe method would be ideal, the technique is rarely available. Clinical investigations indicate that carotid stump pressures of 50 to 55 torr or higher reflect adequate cerebral collateral.

TABLE 36-3 COMPLICATIONS OF CAROTID ENDARTERECTOMY

I. Related to anesthesia, general or local
  A. Cardiac problems
  B. Airway problems
  C. Hypotension

II. Related to cervical wound
  A. Infection
  B. Hematoma
  C. Nerve paresis
    1. Vagus
    2. Hypoglossal
    3. Marginal branch of facial
  D. Parotitis
  E. Tracheal obstruction

III. Related to carotid artery
  A. Disruption
  B. False aneurysms
  C. Carotid–cavernous arteriovenous fistula
  D. Infection of Dacron graft

IV. Production or aggravation of neurologic deficits
  A. Intraoperative causes
    1. Embolism
    2. Cerebral ischemia
  B. Postoperative causes
    1. Thrombosis of endarterectomized segment
    2. Hypotension
    3. Intracerebral hemorrhage or edema
    4. Hypertension

V. Miscellaneous
  A. Postoperative headache
  B. Cerebral edema

The use of a temporary inlying bypass shunt remains the most reliable method for cerebral support. Recent discussion has centered on the necessity for its routine use. Some surgeons employ it routinely in all partially occlusive lesions; others use it selectively, based on an assessment of cerebral

Fig. 36-9. Technique of carotid endarterectomy using a temporary inlying bypass shunt. An oblique incision is made in the neck along the anterior border of the sternocleidomastoid muscle and centered over the carotid bifurcation; it curves medialward at its lower end and slightly inferior to the lobe of the ear at its upper end. *(A)* Usual site of atherosclerotic plaque. Location of the linear arteriotomy is indicated from the common carotid into the internal carotid beyond the distal extent of the plaque so that its upper end is clearly visualized. *(B)* A 10 F plastic catheter 8 cm in length is first inserted into the distal internal carotid and allowed to backflow. The proximal end of the shunt is then placed into the common carotid lumen, and the umbilical tapes with rubber tourniquets are made snug. Cerebral blood flow is thus restored through the shunt, a step requiring approximately 60 seconds. *(C)* The appropriate plane is entered with a fine-pointed clamp, and endarterectomy of the common carotid bifurcation, the origin of the external carotid, and the internal carotid is accomplished under full visualization. The distal end of the plaque in the internal carotid usually feathers off quite smoothly. If not, the distal intima may be secured with a few interrupted sutures of 6-0 polyester to prevent dissection. *(D)* After flushing out the artery, the arteriotomy is closed with running sutures of 6-0 polyester beginning at each end. Immediately prior to placing the final three or four sutures, the common carotid and internal carotid are clamped and the shunt is removed. The vessels are flushed and the final sutures placed and tied. Flow is restored, first into the external carotid and finally into the internal carotid. *(E)* A variation on the technique of arteriotomy closure uses a thin-blade, partially occluding clamp to include the unfinished portion of the suture line after the shunt is removed. In this way, cerebral blood flow is more quickly reestablished. The suture line is then completed. *(F)* Appearance of the artery following final closure. A patch graft is rarely necessary unless the artery is unusually narrow. The wound in the neck is closed with two layers of fine cotton sutures about a small rubber drain, which is removed 24 hours postoperatively. (Thompson JE: Internal carotid and vertebral artery occlusive disease. In Hardy JD [ed]: Rhoads Textbook of Surgery, 5th ed. Philadelphia, J B Lippincott, 1977)

collateral circulation; and a few state that they rarely or never use it.

Those who advocate selective shunting base its use on the inadequacy of cerebral collateral circulation. Some test the patient under local anesthesia and use a shunt if temporary clamping cannot be tolerated. Others, using general anesthesia, insert a shunt if internal carotid artery stump pressure is below 50 torr to 55 torr or if EEG changes occur upon carotid clamping.

From the data in the literature on operative mortality and morbidity, it is clear that an assessment of collateral circulation is necessary in all patients and that provision for cerebral protection must be made for those with inadequate flow. Internal carotid artery stump pressure and EEGs appear to be fairly reliable indicators for the use of a shunt, although they are not infallible.

Since present methods of assessing adequacy of collateral circulation are not entirely infallible, the author recommends the use of a shunt routinely in all partially occlusive lesions, particularly for patients with TIAs and asymptomatic stenoses, who have no demonstrable neurologic deficit prior to operation and who should, therefore, have none postoperatively.

RESULTS OF CAROTID ENDARTERECTOMY

The purpose of carotid endarterectomy is to remove occlusive plaques. By so doing, one eliminates sources of cerebral emboli and increases cerebral blood flow.

Successful anatomical restoration of blood flow by operation may be accomplished in more than 98% of patients with partially occluded arteries. Carotid endarterectomy is a very durable operation. The total incidence of recurrent stenosis is between 3% and 5%. The incidence of symptomatic recurrence requiring reoperation is 1%. Early recurrence (*i.e.*, less than 1 year) takes the form of myointimal hyperplasia, while late stenosis is due to recurrent atherosclerosis. Reoperation requires patch-graft reconstruction.

OPERATIVE MORTALITY

Of primary concern is the operative mortality. The average age of patients undergoing operation is about 65 years. There is a high incidence of hypertension and diabetes, and atherosclerotic lesions are frequent in other areas of the peripheral vasculature, especially in the coronary arteries. At the outset, therefore, these patients constitute a high-risk group.

Operative mortality over a 23-year period is shown in Table 36-4 for 1298 private patients operated upon by the author and his associates. Mortality varies directly with the severity of the clinical category. Half of the deaths are from cerebral causes and half from cardiac complications.

In the past 17 years, with routine use of general anesthesia, together with use of a temporary inlying shunt and avoidance of operation on patients with acute and progressing strokes, the mortality rate in the frank stroke group has been reduced to 3.3% and that in the TIA group to 1.1%; the overall mortality rate is 1.4%.

In a follow-up study of patients subjected to carotid endarterectomy, it was found that 52.3% of the long-term deaths were from cardiac causes and only 13.4% of the deaths were due to strokes. These latter deaths represented 3.9% of the entire series of patients operated upon, a figure considerably lower than the expected mortality from stroke in patients with cerebrovascular insufficiency treated with nonsurgical methods.

OPERATIVE MORBIDITY

Complications related to carotid endarterectomy have been discussed above. The total incidence of all complications is about 5%. With provision for adequate cerebral protection during operation, permanent neurologic deficits should be no more than 2%.

FUNCTIONAL RESULTS

The goals of therapy should be kept in mind in every patient with cerebrovascular insufficiency. One is concerned almost as much with morbidity as with mortality; that is to say, the quality of survival is important. Thus, the principal goal is prevention of stroke.

Frank Stroke

The functional results of any method of treatment of frank stroke are difficult to assess because of the wide variation in severity of neurologic deficits at onset and the natural history of improvement without treatment. Long-term results after carotid endarterectomy in one series of 125 surviving patients followed up to 13 years showed 30.2% normal, 58.7% improved, 4.7% unchanged, and 6.4% worse. During follow-up, only 6.7% died of stroke. It appears that in selected patients with frank strokes, endarterectomy has lowered the incidence of recurrence of strokes and probably has been responsible for some improvement in neurologic status beyond that to be expected from the natural course of the disease.

Transient Cerebral Ischemia

Transient cerebral ischemia is the ideal stage for definitive therapy. No neurologic deficit is present, and if the causative lesion can be removed, strokes should be prevented in the majority of patients so treated. On the average, 35% of untreated patients with transient cerebral ischemia develop actual strokes if observed up to 5 years. In a series of 210 survivors observed up to 13 years, 18% had no further

---

TABLE 36-4   OPERATIVE MORTALITY FOLLOWING CAROTID ENDARTERECTOMY

CLINICAL CATEGORY	NO. PATIENTS	NO. OPERATIONS	NO. DEATHS	PATIENT MORTALITY	PROCEDURE MORTALITY
Frank stroke	352	427	21	6%	4.9%
Transient ischemia	733	936	11	1.5%	1.2%
Chronic ischemia	22	28	0	0	0
Asymptomatic bruit	191	236	0	0	0
Totals	1298	1627	32	2.5%	2%

attacks, while an additional 15.7% had fewer attacks of less severity. The incidence of both fatal and nonfatal strokes after endarterectomy is quite low and in reported series is between 5% and 7%, or about one sixth of that to be expected in untreated controls. Thus, endarterectomy is effective in relieving symptoms and in lowering the incidence of subsequent stroke.

Chronic Cerebral Ischemia

In patients with chronic cerebral ischemia, mental improvement has been limited. However, certain patients relate they can "think better" after carotid endarterectomy, although no gross changes in mentation were apparent preoperatively. Reports of neuropsychological tests before and after carotid endarterectomy show no postoperative deterioration following operation but actual improvement in function.

Total Carotid Occlusion

Most patients with total carotid occlusion are not candidates for operation. If the occlusion is chronic, operation is usually futile. If it is acute, operation is contraindicated in the presence of accompanying severe neurologic deficits. Occasionally, endarterectomy is justifiable and has a patency success rate of about 20%. Restoring flow in a tightly stenosed external carotid in the presence of a totally occluded internal carotid artery may be quite beneficial by increasing total cerebral blood flow.

Asymptomatic Carotid Bruits

The most controversial area concerns the advisability of performing arteriography and operation on patients with asymptomatic carotid bruits. Asymptomatic subclavian bruits, even with a demonstrated subclavian steal syndrome, do not require operative intervention. It has been observed that certain patients with asymptomatic carotid bruits are at definite risk for ischemic cerebral episodes, either transient attacks or frank strokes. In one study, among 132 patients undergoing prophylactic endarterectomy, the long-term incidence of TIAs was 4.5% and that of stroke was 4.6%. Among 138 patients observed but not operated upon primarily, the incidence of TIAs was 26.8% and that of stroke was 17.4%. Other studies have shown that among patients with asymptomatic carotid bruits not subjected to operation, those with positive OPG tests exhibit an incidence of TIAs up to 29% and of stroke to 12%, while those with negative OPG tests have TIA and stroke rates of 2%.

Based on the foregoing considerations, management of the patient with an asymptomatic carotid bruit follows three steps: (1) noninvasive screening, (2) cerebral arteriography, and (3) carotid endarterectomy. Noninvasive screening tests may be applied to all patients. A satisfactory combination is the OPG–CPA (Kartchner) and ultrasonic scanning. The ease and safety of such examinations make possible serial testing at regular intervals to determine if a bruit-producing lesion found initially to be insignificant is indeed progressing toward one of hemodynamic significance, in which arteriography may be required.

As cerebral arteriography has become increasingly safer with retrograde techniques and local anesthesia, it may be recommended more liberally than previously, *but not routinely,* in evaluating asymptomatic bruits. The overall general status of each patient should be considered very carefully. Arteriography should not be done if some contraindication to endarterectomy already exists. It is not to be recommended if the bruit is soft and unilateral, if other conditions take priority over study of the bruit, or if the noninvasive test results are negative. It may be recommended if bruits are bilateral and harsh, in patients with known progressive atherosclerosis elsewhere, prior to other major operations, when noninvasive test results are positive, and when one's best clinical judgment indicates that it is necessary.

If the arteriograms show a significant atherosclerotic stenosis in the common or internal carotid, endarterectomy may be recommended. Specific indications include bilateral stenoses; unilateral stenosis with contralateral occlusion; stenosis in the artery to the dominant hemisphere; known progressive atherosclerosis elsewhere in the peripheral vasculature, especially in younger patients; contemplated major operation of another sort, particularly open heart surgery; and a markedly ulcerated plaque.

If prophylactic carotid surgery is to be considered, multiple risk factors, such as a history of hypertension, myocardial infarction, and congestive heart failure in patients over 65, should not be present. This is pointed up by the distressingly high long-term mortality from heart disease during the early years of follow-up. Since no unnecessary technical risks should be taken, appropriate measures for cerebral protection must be used during endarterectomy to avoid producing neurologic deficits, such as the routine use of a temporary inlying shunt. Operative mortality rates should be below 1% and complication rates no more than 2%. Patients treated with operation appear to have a more favorable long-term outlook, from the standpoint of subsequent ischemic cerebral episodes, than their nonoperated counterparts.

MISCELLANEOUS LESIONS

The external carotid artery is an important source of intracranial collateral circulation in the presence of a stenosed or occluded internal carotid artery. During routine endarterectomy, any plaques in the origin or accessible portions of the external carotid artery should be removed.

Fibromuscular dysplasia of the internal carotid artery in most instances is an incidental finding on arteriograms, but in some patients it is a cause of cerebral symptoms. The lesions are frequently bilateral and are usually found in the distal portion of the cervical internal carotid artery extending to the base of the skull and beyond. The disorder may be associated with dysplasia of the renal, celiac, and superior mesenteric arteries and with multiple intracranial aneurysms.

Surgical treatment in symptomatic patients varies with the location of the lesion and any associated pathologic conditions, such as an atherosclerotic plaque, and includes resection with graft repair, patch-graft angioplasty, and, most often, graduated dilation of the stenotic areas with flexible coronary artery dilators. Results of operation are quite satisfactory.

The relationship of carotid coils and kinks to symptoms of cerebrovascular insufficiency remains a controversial subject. Many techniques of operation have been reported. Sometimes symptoms are clearly related to lesions, and operative repair is indicated. In the majority of cases, however, there are alternative explanations for the clinical picture and careful weighing of all factors must be made before surgical therapy is recommended.

UPPER EXTREMITY PROBLEMS

The arterial anatomy of the upper extremities is shown in Figure 36-10. Occlusive lesions in the major vessels to the arms are relatively uncommon. Etiology includes atherosclerosis at the origin of the subclavian artery, aneurysmal and fibrotic lesions resulting from cervical rib syndrome or thoracic outlet syndrome, embolism, and trauma, either violent or iatrogenic from catheters or needles. Symptoms may be absent or may include mild claudication, severe claudication, rest pain, and even gangrene. Arteriography is necessary in most cases to delineate the lesions and plan appropriate therapy.

Management of subclavian occlusion at the origin from the aortic arch has been discussed above. Lesions in the midportion of the subclavian artery and in the axillary artery are best handled by means of bypass grafts, either autologous vein or prosthetic. The same is true of the rare occlusive lesions found in the brachial, radial, and ulnar arteries, for which management must be individualized.

The treatment of thoracic outlet syndrome, arterial embolism, and vascular trauma is dealt with in other sections of this text.

BIBLIOGRAPHY

BAKER JD, GLUECKLICH B, WATSON CW et al: An evaluation of electroencephalographic monitoring for carotid study. Surgery 78:787, 1975

BOYSEN G: Cerebral hemodynamics in carotid surgery. Acta Neurol Scand 49 (Suppl 52), 1973

CALLOW AD: An overview of the stroke problem in the carotid territory. Am J Surg 140:181, 1980

CARLSON RE, EHRENFELD WK, STONEY RJ et al: Innominate endarterectomy: A 16-year experience. Arch Surg 112:1389, 1977

CONTORNI L: The vertebro-vertebral collateral circulation in obliteration of the subclavian artery at its origin. Minerva Chir 15:268, 1960

CRAWFORD ES, DEBAKEY ME, MORRIS GC, JR et al: Surgical treatment of occlusion of the innominate, common carotid, and subclavian arteries: A 10-year experience. Surgery 65:17, 1969

DEWEESE JA, ROB CG, SATRAN R et al: Results of carotid endarterectomies for transient ischemic attacks: Five years later. Ann Surg 178:258, 1973

EDWARDS WH, MULHERIN JL: The surgical approach to significant stenosis of vertebral and subclavian arteries. Surgery 87:20, 1980

EFFENEY DJ, EHRENFELD WK, STONEY RJ et al: Fibromuscular dysplasia of the internal carotid artery. World J Surg 3:179, 1979

GEE W, OLLER DW, AMUNDSEN DG et al: The asymptomatic bruit and the ocular pneumoplethysmography. Arch Surg 112:1381, 1977

Fig. 36-10. Upper extremity ischemia. *(A)* Representative causes of arm ischemia. *(B)* Arterial anatomy of the upper limb. (Hardy JD: Diseases involving arterial supply to the upper extremities. In Surgery of the Aorta and Its Branches. Philadelphia, J B Lippincott, 1960)

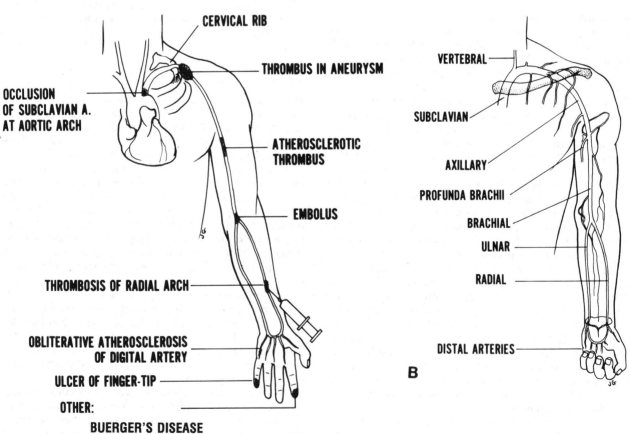

CERVICAL RIB

THROMBUS IN ANEURYSM

OCCLUSION OF SUBCLAVIAN A. AT AORTIC ARCH

ATHEROSCLEROTIC THROMBUS

EMBOLUS

THROMBOSIS OF RADIAL ARCH

OBLITERATIVE ATHEROSCLEROSIS OF DIGITAL ARTERY

ULCER OF FINGER-TIP

OTHER:
BUERGER'S DISEASE
RAYNAUD'S DISEASE
SCLERODERMA
VIBRATING TOOL SYNDROME

A

VERTEBRAL

SUBCLAVIAN

AXILLARY

PROFUNDA BRACHII

BRACHIAL

ULNAR

RADIAL

DISTAL ARTERIES

B

GOLDSTONE J, MOORE WS: Emergency carotid artery surgery in neurologically unstable patients. Arch Surg 111:1284, 1976

HAJJAR WM, SUMNER DS: Comparative study of carotid ultrasonic arteriography and oculoplethysmography and contrast angiography. Stroke 9:12, 1978

HOLLEMAN JH JR, HARDY JD, WILLIAMSON JW et al: Arterial surgery for arm ischemia: A survey of 136 patients. Ann Surg 191:727, 1980

HORNE DJL, ROYLE JP: Cognitive changes after carotid endarterectomy. Med J Aust 1:316, 1974

KARTCHNER MM, McRAE LP: Noninvasive evaluation and management of the "asymptomatic" carotid bruit. Surgery 82:840, 1977

MILLIKAN CH, McDOWELL FH: Treatment of transient ischemic attacks. Stroke 9:299, 1978

OLIVECRONA H: Complications of cerebral angiography. Neuroradiology 14:175, 1977

SUNDT TM, JR, HOUSER OW, SHARBROUGH FW et al: Carotid endarterectomy: Results, complications, and monitoring techniques. Adv Neurol 16:97, 1977

THOMPSON JE: Surgery for Cerebrovascular Insufficiency (Stroke). Springfield, IL, Charles C Thomas, 1968

THOMPSON JE: Complications of carotid endarterectomy and their prevention. World J Surg 3:155, 1979

THOMPSON JE, AUSTIN DJ, PATMAN RD: Carotid endarterectomy for cerebrovascular insufficiency: Long-term results in 592 patients followed up to thirteen years. Ann Surg 172:663, 1970

THOMPSON JE, PATMAN RD, TALKINGTON CM: Asymptomatic carotid bruit: Long-term outcome of patients having endarterectomy compared with unoperated controls. Ann Surg 188:308, 1978

THOMPSON JE, PATMAN RD, TALKINGTON CM: Carotid surgery for cerebrovascular insufficiency. In Ravitch MM (ed): Current Problems in Surgery, vol. 15. Chicago, Year Book Medical Publishers, 1978

Hilary H. Timmis

Thoracic Outlet Syndrome

INCIDENCE

ANATOMIC CONSIDERATIONS

ETIOLOGY AND PATHOGENESIS

COMPLICATIONS

DIAGNOSIS

DIFFERENTIAL DIAGNOSIS

THERAPY

Nonoperative

Operative

Morbidity

Recurrence

Results

Thoracic outlet syndrome (TOS) is a constellation of clinical entities that share a common symptomatology resulting from compression of the neurovascular bundle as it exits from the bony, ligamentous, and muscular relationships that exist at the thoracic apex. Although endowed with antiquity, cervicobrachial compression in the shoulder region is still an evolving clinical concept characterized by a multiplicity of attitudes regarding anatomic basis, etiology, diagnosis, and treatment. The problem has been addressed under many different titles, usually descriptive of pathogenesis. Chief among these are cervical rib syndrome, scalenus anticus syndrome, costoclavicular syndrome, and hyperabduction syndrome. Other synonyms are listed below.

First rib syndrome

Brachiocephalic syndrome

Cervicobrachial neuralgia

Scapulothoracic syndrome

Pectoralis minor syndrome

Cervicobrachial neurovascular compression

Steinbrocker's syndrome

Naffziger's syndrome

Rucksack paralysis

Paget-Schrötter syndrome

Shoulder-hand syndrome

Neurovascular entrapment by a cervical rib was first documented by Willshire in 1860. One decade later Gruber defined the various presentations of cervical rib in a treatise that is germane today. Murphy (1905) indicated the anterior scalene muscle as well as the cervical rib as a cause of vascular compression. In 1913, Todd broadened this concept by demonstrating the role of descent of the shoulder from infancy on, in the production of pressure on the brachial plexus. Brickner (1927) reported brachial plexus compression by a normal first rib. The results of surgical decompression of neurovascular structures at the thoracic outlet by Adson (1927), Ochsner, Gage, and DeBakey (1935), and Naffziger and Grant (1938) added validity to the concept of cervicobrachial compression syndromes. The mechanism of costoclavicular compression of the subclavian artery and brachial plexus was defined by Falconer and Weddell in

THORACIC OUTLET SYNDROME	
Etiology	Osseous, fibrous, and muscular neurovascular compression at the thoracic aperture
Dx	Symptoms: Pain in neck and upper extremity, arm weakness, hand paresthesias, especially over ulnar distribution Signs: Supraclavicular tenderness, reproduction of symptom with 90° abduction, flexion, and external rotation of arm Laboratory: Median and ulnar nerve conduction velocity, cervical spine and chest x-ray films; EMG to rule out cervical radiculopathy
Rx	Progressive shoulder strengthening exercises if acute or subacute without vascular compromise First rib resection if syndrome chronic, unrelieved by exercise program, or complicated by denervation or vascular compromise

1943, and two years later Wright reported on vascular obstruction of the arm induced by hyperabduction. In 1956, Peet coined the term "thoracic outlet syndrome," which Rob and Standeven popularized as a common designation for different mechanisms of neurovascular compression in the shoulder region that produce a similar clinical picture. Clagett (1962) introduced a unified approach to therapy by emphasizing the ubiquitous influence of the first rib in potentiating neurovascular compression and demonstrated effective decompression at all levels in the thoracic canal by first rib resection. The operative procedure was greatly expedited by the transaxillary technique described and popularized by Roos in 1966. A growing clinical experience by Roos, Urschel, and others since then continues to add to the body of knowledge surrounding TOS.

INCIDENCE

Thoracic outlet syndrome has been reported from infancy to advanced age, in both sexes, in all body builds, and at all levels of activity. However, it appears to be the purview of women with a prevalence as high as 80%. The majority of patients are in the 20- to 40-year age range, and the onset of TOS is greatly enhanced by chronic unsupported elevation of the upper extremities.

The chief sources of referral are twofold. About 40% come from the large group of women who have entered our country-wide work force where lifting, sorting, typing, and other sustained abductive activities are required. Another 40% present with a history of cervical hyperextention injuries produced by motor vehicle whiplash trauma or forceful jerking of the upper extremity. Despite the sexual prevalence of 4 in women, many of whom have an asthenic habitus, to 1 man, when TOS occurs in men it is likely to be seen in those with overdeveloped shoulder musculature (weight lifters, heavy laborers) or with an unusually S-shaped, posteriorly displaced clavicle. Other osseous anomalies are also pernicious in the production of TOS, especially accessory (cervical) ribs, which occur in 0.5% to 1% of the general population. Of this group about 10% develop symptomatic cervicobrachial compression.

We are all, to some extent, predisposed to neurovascular entrapment in the shoulder region by virtue of our upright posture, which drapes the weight of the shoulder girdles and upper extremities over the upper thorax. Symptoms are widespread following bouts of heavy exercise, especially with hyperabduction, but are short-lived in the absence of induced pathologic changes or a preexisting anatomic reason for sustained compression.

ANATOMIC CONSIDERATIONS

An understanding of the anatomy of the superior thoracic aperture is essential to appreciate the range of possibilities for neurovascular compression in this area. The structural relationships which permit passage of the neurovascular bundle have been likened to a canal, the entrance of which is bounded by the anterior scalene muscle in front, the medial scalene in back, and the first rib below—the interscalene triangle. Just medial to the first rib from front to back the subclavian vein, subclavian artery, and lower trunk of the brachial plexus line up in an almost horizontal plane. The first rib in turn descends anteriorly from its vertebral articulation at a 40° to 45° angle. The lower trunk of the

brachial plexus formed by a marriage of C8-T1 fibers crosses the sharp superior-medial edge of the rib or the overlying fibrous insertion of the medial scalene muscle in which it is frequently cradled. When the arm is abducted, the trunk is in a position to be bow-strung across this fulcrum point. The other two trunks of the brachial plexus cross at a higher level and are seldom compromised.

During passage across the first rib, the lower trunk and subclavian artery occupy a tract in the costoclavicular space. This region, which is also termed the proximal cervicoaxillary canal, is bounded by the clavicle and underlying subclavius muscle above, the outer surface of the first rib below and behind, and the clavipectoral fascia and costoclavicular ligament anteriorly.

The lower trunk continues as the medial cord of the brachial plexus in a similar posterior relationship along the first part of the axillary artery. Although the neurovascular bundle enjoys a more spacious position in the distal cervicoaxillary canal, the artery is again subject to compromise during passage under the coracoid process and behind the costocoracoid ligament and insertion of the pectoralis minor muscle.

ETIOLOGY AND PATHOGENESIS

Osseous anomalies of the first rib, partly or completely formed cervical ribs, fibrous bands from a long C7 transverse process, and other structures listed in Table 36-5 under A are all likely to exert a noxious influence on the unencumbered passage of the neurovascular bundle. The majority of patients, however, are symptomatic because of an upward impingement on the lower trunk of the brachial plexus by the knifelike superior border of the first rib or the sharp fibrous insertion of the medial scalene muscle overlying the rib posteriorly. Roos has demonstrated a variety of ligaments and fibrous bands enhancing truncal compression in this area by elevating the superior border of the thoracic outlet in a manner similar to that produced by the presence of an accessory rib (see Table 36-5B). The most common of these, the type 3 band, arises from the inner aspect of the neck of the rib and inserts at the scalene tubercle. Whatever the case, compression of the lower trunk of the brachial plexus or its major derivative, the medial cord, accounts for over 80% of the clinical experience.

The subclavian artery, because of its higher position relative to the inclined first rib, tends to be spared. Vascular entrapment may occur with an unusually narrow-based interscalene triangle but is most common in the presence of osseous anomalies such as a cervical rib. In this case the vessel is usually caught between the insertion of the cervical rib or its fibrous extension and the insertion of the anterior scalene muscle, producing a persistent arterial pinch. Poststenotic dilatation is common and may progress to a subclavian artery aneurysm. This, in turn, can either occlude or produce devastating peripheral arterial emboli.

In the costoclavicular area the neurovascular bundle can be caught by the scissorlike action of the clavicle and the first rib, especially with the shoulders thrust posteriorly and downward. The tendency for entrapment is increased by clavicular abnormalities or by any activity enhancing downward displacement of the shoulders, such as recumbency in the supine position, backpacking, and the counter support of pendulous breasts.

Although hyperabduction will tend to constrict the sub-

TABLE 36-5 MORPHOLOGIC PREDISPOSING FACTORS

A. OSSEOUS
Cervical rib
Long C7 transverse process
First rib abnormalities
  Fracture
  Exostoses
  Anomalous joint
Clavicular abnormalities
S-shaped clavicle
Exuberant callus
Malunion with angulation
Pseudoarthrosis

B. FIBROMUSCULAR
Scalene muscle hypertrophy
Scalene spasm or contracture
Narrow interscalene triangle
Scalenus minimus muscle
Congenital bands: pleural, clavipectoral, costocostal
  (type 3)
Fibrous extension of cervical rib
Continuity of scalene insertions

C. OTHER
Post-fixed brachial plexus with caudal displacement
Space-occupying lesions
  Subclavian aneurysm
  Lipoma and other benign tumors
  Lymphadenopathy
Pendulous breasts
Downward displacement of shoulders

clavian artery as it passes under the coracoid process, the vascular compression is rarely sustained and usually not symptomatic when the extremity is brought to the resting position. There has been no instance in our experience in which division of the pectoralis minor tendon appeared to be indicated.

In 1% to 2%, evidence of intermittent venous obstruction or frank subclavian vein thrombosis is the primary manifestation of thoracic outlet compression. With an unusually broad or forward-placed insertion of the anterior scalene muscle, the subclavian vein is subject to pressure from behind against the costoclavicular ligament and adjacent subclavius muscle. In a similar manner, hypertrophy of these structures may trap the vein against the anterior scalene muscle. Occasionally there is a history of unusual exertion or stretching just prior to the onset of venous occlusion, which was formerly termed effort thrombosis or the Paget-Schrötter syndrome.

COMPLICATIONS

The most dramatic and serious sequelae of thoracic outlet compression consist of peripheral gangrene, due to arterial occlusion or embolization, and denervation and severe muscle atrophy following prolonged entrapment of the lower trunk of the brachial plexus or the medial cord. Fortunately, the former is extremely rare and the latter uncommon. A far more frequent morbidity arises from the chronic, unrelenting pain and disability lending to catastrophic sociooccupational consequences. Dissolving mar-

riages, lost jobs, and broken lives are commonplace and are often associated with major emotional upheavals. These only serve to confuse the issue and render these people second-class patients to many physicians.

Sympathetic hyperactivity producing coldness and color change in the upper extremity is present in 10% and is probably an autonomic reflex reaction to somatic nerve trauma. Syncope is another dramatic manifestation of subclavian artery compression that can result in serious injury.

DIAGNOSIS

CLINICAL MANIFESTATIONS

The propensity for thoracic outlet syndrome in asthenic, anxious women in the third or fourth decade of life is due to the muscular weakness and poor posture native to this group, to the tendency toward intercostal breathing, and to the increased descent of the shoulders of women in general. When thoracic outlet syndrome occurs in the well-muscled man or woman, it appears to result from scalene muscle hypertrophy that crowds the neurovascular bundle, and from the wear and tear inherent in achieving this magnitude of muscle development. A rather characteristic constellation of complaints is commonly met consisting of neck, shoulder, and arm pain, weakness and postural discomfort of the arm, and dysesthesias of the forearm and hand.

Cervical pain may be aching, lancinating, or burning, is usually posterolateral in location, and is often associated with an adjacent suboccipital headache, especially when there is a history of cervical hyperextension injury. Radiation of pain is common, to the superior border of the trapezius muscle and down into the arm, to the interscapular area of the back, and to the pectoral area, where it may be confused with angina pectoris.

Pain in the upper extremity often has a toothachelike quality that may be confined to the arm and shoulder or may extend into the forearm and hand. Although it is sometimes intermittent and relieved by rest, arm pain is characteristically increased by activity, especially in the abducted position. Difficulty in driving, holding a book or newspaper, stacking dishes, brushing one's hair, and other abductive activities become progressively more difficult and eventually necessitate a change in life-style to accommodate the disability.

Weakness of the affected extremity is common and is almost certainly neurologic in origin. Early onset of fatigue, reduced lifting power, and declining strength of grip are all characteristic. The tendency to drop objects partly results from compromised innervation of the intrinsic hand muscles.

Sensory changes may be confined to the C8–T1 dermatomes or involve the entire hand. The former is caused by entrapment of the lower trunk of the brachial plexus, which produces dysesthesias over the peripheral distribution of the ulnar nerve and is manifested by numbness, hypesthesia or hypersensitivity over the ring and little finger and the medial aspect of the hand and forearm.

Numbness of the entire hand results from an associated compression of the median nerve at the wrist (carpal tunnel syndrome), which is seen in 15% of patients with thoracic outlet syndrome, or from compression of the subclavian-axillary artery and reduced blood supply to the hand. Generalized numbness of one or both hands is commonly

TABLE 36-6 FREQUENCY OF SYMPTOMS OF THORACIC OUTLET SYNDROME

SYMPTOMS	PERCENT
Posterolateral neck, shoulder, and arm pain	98
Upper extremity weakness	95
Chest pain, pectoral and scapular	80
Numbness and paresthesias	80
Suboccipital headache	60
Coolness and discoloration of hands	15
Tinnitis, dizziness, syncope	15
Pain over face and ear	10

reported during recumbency, even when the arms are not abducted to support the head. This results from critical narrowing of the costoclavicular space due to posterior and downward descent of the shoulders during complete relaxation.

Periodic duskiness or pallor of the hand is reported in about 15% to 20% of cases, often associated with a sense of coolness that may be striking and uncomfortable. These changes rarely occur in response to ambient temperature and are not a true Raynaud's phenomenon. They appear to be a reflex autonomic response to nerve trauma, or they may result from compression of sympathetic fibers that travel independently or within the lower trunk of the brachial plexus. If severe and persistent, the question of a therapeutic block or cervicodorsal sympathectomy is raised.

Suboccipital or occipital headache is a common complaint and is essentially an extension of posterolateral neck pain. In some instances, it is the major presenting symptom and is totally disabling in character. The association with syncope, tinnitis, and dizziness suggests vascular or intracranial pathology. Frontal headache is occasionally prominent and is probably related to the anxiety and tension that is almost palpable in some patients. Although it is difficult to determine if the distraught state is a precursor or sequel to chronic pain and disability, its presence tends to mitigate against a sustained good surgical result.

HISTORY

Because of the dearth of precise and accurate reliable objective tests, the diagnosis of TOS must be made basically from the history and physical examination. By and large, special roentgenographic, electrophysiologic, and other examinations are most useful to rule out other neuromuscular maladies. Knowledge of the symptomatic structure of TOS, its prevalence in women, and the high incidence of antecedent trauma is essential to get on the right track. Searching inquisition must be applied to elicit the characteristic triad of posterolateral neck, shoulder, and arm pain, early fatigue during abduction of the arm, and dysesthesias, numbness, and tingling of the forearm and hand. The absence of any one of these components reduces the likelihood of TOS. The onset of symptoms should be pinpointed as closely as possible along with its relationship to trauma, illness, or other notable events in the patient's life. The evolution of complaints up to the patient's present symptomatic status should also be charted; their relative frequency is shown in Table 36-6.

Usually these patients have been examined and treated by several other physicians, and oftentimes the results of previous tests must be documented as well as the nature and response to previous therapy. Cervical traction characteristically causes a sharp exacerbation of neck and arm discomfort and is a useful diagnostic sign. In many instances analgesics, muscle relaxants, antispasmodics, vasodilators, and other drugs have been prescribed and may be an index of the severity of complaints.

PHYSICAL EXAMINATION

The physical examination must be fastidiously performed and begins with inspection of body habitus, carriage of the shoulders, and gross abnormalities of the upper extremities. Deformities of the clavicle usually follow trauma and may impinge on the costoclavicular space and its contents. Healed scars with asymmetry and muscle atrophy may be the sequelae of former trauma or previous operation. Atrophy of the muscles of the shoulder, arm, and forearm (with the exception of the triceps, which are innervated by T7, points to spinal or nerve root pathology) may occur. Atrophy of the hypothenar and intrinsic hand muscles by virtue of their ulnar innervation, however, is more characteristic of TOS. Range of motion of the shoulder should be examined to rule out pathology in and around the joint. Signs of sustained vascular compromise occur in less than 25% of patients and may result from arterial or venous occlusion or more commonly from alterations of sympathetic tone in the arm and hand. Changes that occur in varying degree and combination include pallor, plethora, swelling, healed ulcerations, local ischemia, and gangrene. Raynaud's phenomenon is reported in 4%.

Tenderness in the supraclavicular fossa (Morley's sign), with or without swelling, is a cardinal if not pathognomonic sign of TOS. It apparently results from brachial plexus irritation or spasm of the scalene muscles or both. Tenderness is also common but less dramatic over the lateral neck and infraclavicular area. Roos has found that inciting symptoms of TOS by continuously applying pressure in the supraclavicular fossa for 30 seconds is an important diagnostic test. Tenderness over the volar aspect of the wrist (Tinel's sign) and the onset of pain with flexion of the wrist (Phalen's sign) suggest entrapment of the median nerve and are seen as associated findings in 10% to 15% of patients with TOS.

Demonstration of reduced grip is a significant sign and may be associated with hypesthesia over the ulnar distribution of the hand. Both findings and the characteristic symptoms of truncal compression can be accentuated by opening and closing the hands during 90% abduction of the arm, 90° flexion of the elbow, and 90° external rotation (*Roos test*). This same attitude (90° AER) may produce color changes of the affected hand, a bruit in the infraclavicular

---

SIGNS OF THORACIC OUTLET SYNDROME

Tenderness and swelling in supraclavicular fossa
Percussion tenderness of lateral neck
Arm fatigue during abduction
Infraclavicular bruit with 90° AER
Reduced grip
Hypesthesia of ring and little finger
Discoloration of hand with 90° AER

area, and a reduced radial pulse, indicating a tight axillary passage.

The three classic provocative maneuvers for TOS—the Adson test, the costoclavicular maneuver, and the hyperabduction maneuver—are now relegated to a secondary role in the diagnosis of most cases of TOS. They are used to amplify vascular compression, which is the primary pathologic finding in less than 15% of patients. At the same time, false positive findings are seen in 25% to 30% of normal people. Nevertheless, the subclavian artery and lower trunk of the brachial plexus literally cross the first rib side by side, and the inference is valid in some instances that detection of vascular compression increases the likelihood of nerve compression.

All tests for vascular compression should be performed during palpation of the radial pulse and auscultation of the subclavian artery in the infraclavicular area. The Adson test is performed with the arm extended and externally rotated and the neck extended and rotated to the side of examination during full inspiration. The costoclavicular maneuver (exaggerated military position) is carried out with the shoulders fully extended and externally rotated as if at crisp attention. The hyperabduction maneuver, which consists of full abduction of the arm and 90° external rotation, is the most likely of the three postures to induce symptoms. The anatomic basis for this observation is clear when the neurovascular structures are visualized through the opened axilla. Both the nerve trunk and, to a lesser extent, the artery are drawn taut over the superior border of the first rib. Thomas prefers the 90° AER test over the Adson maneuver because it closes the interscalene triangle more effectively; using this posture, Sanders reports reproduction of paresthesias in 95% and suppression of the radial pulse in 50%. McGough and associates were able to reproduce symptoms in 60% of their patients by downward traction on the externally rotated arm.

ADJUNCTS TO DIAGNOSIS

Accuracy in assessing reduction of subclavian flow during office examination can be enhanced by brachial oscillometry, finger plethysmography, and most effectively by ultrasonic bidirectional Doppler measurements during the hyperabduction, costoclavicular, and 90° AER maneuvers. All provide an objective record of circulatory dynamics to both the physician and patients in cases where subclavian-axillary compression is the dominant clinical feature.

Roentgenograms of the neck, shoulders, and chest should be performed routinely to pinpoint osseous abnormalities capable of producing TOS and to identify other lesions mimicking this syndrome. Included in the former are cervical rib, bifid first rib, elongated C7 transverse process, healed first rib fracture, and congenital and acquired clavicular abnormalities. In the latter group are degenerative disk disease, hypertrophic arthritic spurs, calcified residual of previous inflammatory disease, lytic lesions of the spine and bony thorax, and parenchymal lesions of the pulmonary apexes.

Contrast studies are reserved for further evaluation of documented morbid changes in the neck, shoulders, and upper extremities. Thus, cervical myelography is indicated with findings that suggest herniated disk, spinal cord tumor, or cervical root compression.

Subclavian arteriography and venography have well-defined indications that sharply limit their usefulness. In

---

INDICATIONS FOR ANGIOGRAPHY

Arterial
Subclavian bruit with arms at rest
Pulsatile mass
Recurrent embolization
Recurrent or sustained ischemia of hand
Severe dizziness or syncope with hyperabduction

Venous
Edema of hand and arm
Sustained cyanosis, plethora, or suffusion of hand

---

addition to defining thromboembolic events in the upper extremity, arteriograms are necessary to evaluate the impact of large cervical ribs and other osseous anomalies on the integrity of the subclavian-axillary system where static compression and post-stenotic dilatation are suspected. In addition, they are a critical part of the workup of patients with prominent vertebrobasilar symptoms.

Electrophysiologic studies are indicated to identify nerve compression and to rule out other neuromyopathic problems. The electromyogram (EMG) is used to diagnose cervical radiculopathy but is invariably negative in TOS (with the exception of polyphasic motor units in the intrinsic hand muscles) unless there is an associated cervical syndrome. Nerve conduction velocity studies will pinpoint ulnar nerve compression at the elbow and median nerve entrapment at the wrist; however, a range of opinion exists concerning the validity of ulnar nerve conduction velocity (UNCV) measurements across the thoracic outlet. Because the ulnar nerve is the peripheral representative of the lower trunk of the brachial plexus, determination of UNCV from Erb's point to the elbow was introduced by Caldwell in 1971 and used extensively by Urschel and others since then to evaluate TOS. Although false negative examinations do occur, thanks to the central location and intermittent character of compression and technical problems of proximal stimulation and standardization, an electrically confirmed diagnosis of TOS reassures the physician that the patient is relating organic symptoms. Average normal values across the shoulder, elbow, and wrist are 72, 55, and 59 meters/ second respectively but may vary somewhat between test facilities. To provide a more reliable method of appraising nerve function, analysis of F wave latency following stimulation of the ulnar nerve at the wrist has recently been used to evaluate TOS patients. This technique appears to offer considerable promise of ensuring that the conduction study crosses the compromised site at the thoracic apex.

The electronystagmogram (ENG), which examines the extraocular movements with the eyes closed, is used to detect the fine nystagmus that accompanies vertebrobasilar insufficiency and is ordinarily suppressed by extraneous stimuli. Vertebrobasilar symptoms such as dizziness, tinnitus, and syncope are produced by intermittent postural kinking of the vertebral artery, which arises just medial to the first rib, and may be the most distressing and dramatic presenting complaints. The examination should be performed at rest and during the provocative maneuvers.

Finally, an association exits between hypoglycemia and susceptibility to symptomatic nerve compression. A glucose tolerance test should be obtained and a high-protein hypoglycemia diet prescribed when indicated.

DIFFERENTIAL DIAGNOSIS

In most instances TOS is not difficult to diagnose in a youthful woman with asthenic habitus and a working history of antecedent cervical hyperextension injury. A greater challenge is met in the middle-aged patient or after complex head and neck injuries. Here ruptured intervertebral disk, degenerative disk disease, and hypertrophic arthritic spurs as well as trauma are likely to produce cervical radiculopathy.

The brachial plexus itself is vulnerable to local invasion by apical (superior sulcus) pulmonary tumors or to pressure by expanding subclavian aneurysm, benign tumor, or malignant lymphadenopathy.

Indistinguishable hand symptoms as well as proximally referred pain can be caused by ulnar entrapment at the medial epicondyle of the elbow or as the nerve passes through Guyon's loge at the wrist. Median nerve compression beneath the transverse carpal ligament may also pro-duce symptoms simulating TOS. Incapacitating chest pain, accompanied by discomfort and tingling of the hand, is often suggestive of coronary artery disease.

Signs of vascular insufficiency may be mistaken for intrinsic lesions of the subclavian artery and vein or their major derivatives. Pain, pallor or plethora, and reduced temperature of the hand and forearm must be distinguished from Raynaud's disease, thromboangiitis, reflex vasomotor dystrophy, causalgia, and collagen disease.

Arthritis, capsulitis, periarthrosis, subdeltoid bursitis, supraspinatus tendinitis, acromioclavicular separation, and other pathologic lesions in and around the shoulder joint may all be confused with TOS.

Intrathoracic pathology must also be ruled out when precordial, pectoral, and periscapular pain are a dominant feature.

DIFFERENTIAL DIAGNOSIS

1. CERVICAL RADICULOPATHY
  Cervical syndrome
  Ruptured disk
  Degenerative disk disease
  Cervical spondylosis
  Hypertrophic spurs, arthritic spurs

2. PERIPHERAL NERVE COMPRESSION
  Tardy ulnar palsy
  Ulnar neuritis
  Carpal tunnel syndrome

3. MYOFACIAL DISORDERS
  Tension neck syndrome
  Myofasciitis
  Humeral tendinitis (supraspinous and bicipital)
  Subdeltoid bursitis
  Capsulitis

4. VASCULAR DISEASE
  Arterial
  Arteriosclerosis (occlusion, aneurysm)
  Embolism
  Dysautonomias
    Raynaud's disease
    Reflex vasomotor dystrophy
  Causalgia
  Collagen disease

  Venous
  Thrombophlebitis
  Post-traumatic thrombosis
  Lymphedema

5. OTHER
  Metastatic neoplasms
  Coronary artery disease
  Noncardiac intrathoracic lesion
  Lesions of chest wall
  Lesions of spine and spinal cord
  Diaphragmatic irritation

THERAPY

NONOPERATIVE

When symptoms are of recent onset, follow a traumatic experience, and are significantly reduced or relieved by rest, 60% to 70% can be managed successfully by physiotherapy. On the other hand, conservative treatment tends to be ineffective in those with long-standing chronic pain, who are not improved with immobilization. Members of this group are more likely to have a fixed, congenital, anatomic cause for neurovascular compression. Often, thoracic outlet exercises increase disability, at least temporarily, and cervical traction so characteristically magnifies symptoms that it has come to be a valuable diagnostic sign. Nevertheless, if patients are symptomatic for less than 1 year and do not present with signs of vascular insufficiency or significant denervation of the hand, a physical therapy program extending over a period of months is indicated. This should begin with anti-inflammatory agents, analgesics, muscle relaxants, antispasmodics, hot packs, thermal energy, and ultrasound to relieve pain and muscle spasm, followed by muscle reeducation and strengthening of the suspensory muscles of the shoulders: that is, trapezius, levator scapulae, and rhomboid muscles. Nerve and scalene muscle blocks may be helpful in some cases. McGough advocates shoulder shrugging exercises 5 to 10 times daily, 7 to 15 times at each sitting. If these are well tolerated, progressive resistance exercises are added 1 or 2 times daily by having the patient hold weights during the shoulder elevation program. The affected shoulder should be elevated and abducted with pillows during repose and the upper extremity supported when upright to prevent drag on the arm and depression of the shoulder girdle. Weight reduction is essential for obese patients to reduce the drag of massive upper extremities and, in the case of women, pendulous breasts. At the same time, if operation becomes necessary, weight loss will substantially reduce operative risk and morbidity. Professional counseling may provide insight to meet this challenge and to integrate other emotional fall-out.

In practice, referrals for surgical evaluation are generally failures of nonoperative therapy. To demand arbitrarily an additional period of discomfort before offering surgical decompression of the thoracic outlet is ill advised, and simply to await consummation of litigation in trauma-associated cases as a prerequisite for operation is inexcusable.

We have now evaluated over 1500 patients with TOS symptomatology, most of whom were previously screened by neurological examination, roentgenograms, ENG, EMG, nerve conduction testing, and other studies. About 28% of this group have been operated upon for unilateral (396) or bilateral (32) neurovascular entrapment.

OPERATIVE

INDICATIONS

Indications for surgical treatment of TOS are:
1. Denervation of hand
2. Gangrene of hand
3. Sustained ischemia of hand
4. Recurrent severe ischemia of hand
5. Failure of conservative therapy to relieve pain
6. Presence of osseous anomaly
7. History of embolus to hand

Decompression of the thoracic outlet should be carried out promptly when osseous lesions, such as cervical rib, and deformities of the first rib or clavicle produce severe pain or cause local changes in the subclavian artery. Early operation is also recommended for recurrent peripheral ischemia accompanying incapacitating pain of the neck and upper extremity and a marked reduction of the UNCV.

Patients with TOS who have failed to respond to conservative measures over a period of months, those with persistent dysesthesias and atrophy of the intrinsic hand muscles, and those who have been severely symptomatic for more than 1 year are other bona fide surgical candidates.

TECHNIQUES

Effective decompression of the thoracic outlet was expedited enormously by the transaxillary technique of first rib resection described by Roos in 1966 (Fig. 36-11). In the ordinary case, it is superior to all other approaches from the standpoints of facility, overall exposure, operative trauma, recovery time, cosmetic appearance, and postoperative disability. The posterolateral incision is preferred by some for reoperation to remove a long residual posterior rib end, whereas the subclavian vessels are best exposed anteriorly. Whatever the approach, extraperiosteal resection of the rib is recommended to forestall recurrent entrapment by a regenerated rib.

Care must be taken to transect the rib posteriorly well beyond the crossing of the nerve trunk and to assiduously remove all bands, fibrous reflections, and filamentous shreds in the vicinity of the neurovascular structures. If a partially or completely formed cervical rib is present, both it and the first rib should be resected. Although the transected anterior scalene usually retracts upward, excision of 1 cm or 2 cm of muscle may forestall reattachment to the pleura. When venous compression is prominent, mobilization of the costoclavicular ligament and subclavius muscle are necessary

Fig. 36-11. Transaxillary technique of first rib resection. *(A)* Schematic view of the anatomy of the thoracic outlet showing relationship of the subclavian artery and vein, first rib, clavicle, and scalene muscles. *(B)* Elevation of the arm during surgery facilitates exposure of the thoracic outlet. *(C)* The transverse axillary incision used in first rib resection for thoracic outlet decompression. (Roos DB: Transaxillary approach for first rib resection to relieve thoracic outlet syndrome. Ann Surg 163:354, 1966)

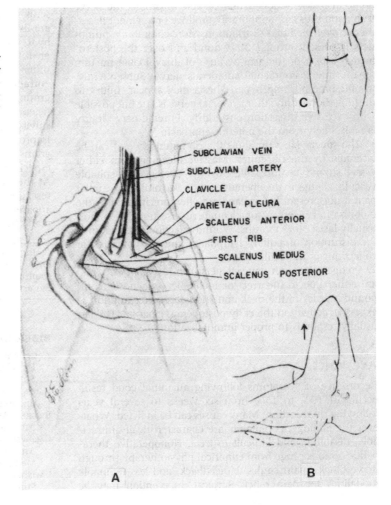

SUBCLAVIAN VEIN
SUBCLAVIAN ARTERY
CLAVICLE
PARIETAL PLEURA
SCALENUS ANTERIOR
FIRST RIB
SCALENUS MEDIUS
SCALENUS POSTERIOR

C

A

B

to permit resection of more rib anteriorly. Catheters are routinely positioned in the depths of the axilla for suction drainage for 24 to 48 hours. The pleura is also drained overnight if a pleural leak is present.

Lesions of the subclavian artery and vein should be identifiable before operation and intervention planned accordingly. Subclavian vein thrombosis is best managed conservatively with elevation and anticoagulation or, when acute, with streptokinase therapy. Associated arterial lesions, principally subclavian aneurysm and thrombosis, are managed by standard vascular techniques described elsewhere using an anterior supra or infraclavicular approach. Exposure can be supplemented by partial or complete resection of the clavicle. When subclavian artery compression is complicated by microembolism, cervicodorsal sympathectomy is recommended because of the prolonged nature of occlusive symptoms. In some instances, a combined transaxillary-supraclavicular technique will provide optimal access for rib resection, arterial repair, and extraction of clot.

In the postoperative period, motion of the shoulder is encouraged immediately and full range achieved at the time of discharge, usually within 5 days. The patient should avoid lifting and all but light activity for 4 to 6 weeks.

MORBIDITY

The lower trunk of the brachial plexus is vulnerable during rib resection by virtue of its depth in the operative field and its position, adjacent to the site of rib transection posteriorly. Some instrumentation is unavoidable to protect the nerve trunk and thus can temporarily produce or augment dysesthesias over the ulnar distribution. More commonly, numbness is present around the wound and over the posteromedial aspect of the arm because of unavoidable traction on the intercostobrachial cutaneous nerve. Subsequently, troublesome burning hyperesthesia may appear. Injury to the long thoracic and thoracodorsal nerve is rare but possible with excessive dissection posteriorly. Phrenic nerve injury is more likely from the anterior approach.

The subclavian vein abuts the rib anteriorly and can be lacerated by the rib cutter. Massive bleeding from either vessel should be forestalled by the presence of suitable vascular clamps in the operative setup. Pectoral and scapular pain if not present beforehand are often precipitated by the mobilization necessary for adequate rib resection. Discomfort usually lasts 1 to 2 months. Wound infection is rare despite the disruption of axillary lymphatics and the potential for collections in the axillary apex.

Preoperative pain patterns persist in less than 10% and are either due to incorrect or incomplete diagnosis, compound injuries of the neck and shoulder, or resumption of excessive activity in the early postoperative period. The last usually responds to proper immobilization.

RECURRENCE

Recurrence of symptoms following an initial good result occurs in 10% to 15% from six weeks to several years following rib resection. Many causes can be indicted. Whatever the etiology, complaints are characteristically intractable, disabling, and difficult to treat. Nonoperative therapeutic options range from empirical physiotherapy through nerve blocks, pain clinics, biofeedback, and less reputable modalities for pain relief. Surgical intervention may be

ETIOLOGY OF RECURRENT SYMPTOMS

Reattachment of anterior scalene
Unresected compressive bands
Reattachment of bands
Excessive posterior rib stump
Brachial neuritis
Adherence of medial cord to posterior scalene
Postoperative causalgia

directed to lysis of adhesions around the neurovascular bundle, excision of reattached scalene muscle fibers, reexcision of the posterior rib stump, resection of the second rib, and in some cases cervicodorsal sympathectomy.

RESULTS

With proper selection, expeditious operation, and confident aftercare, a striking uniformity of results continues to be reported which agrees with our own experience. Eighty percent achieve complete, or almost complete, lasting relief of symptoms; 10% are unimproved; and 10% develop recurrent complaints after an initial fair to good result. Restoration of neurologic function can be demonstrated in many patients by UNCV measurements, usually after several months.

Despite the steady stream of presentations and manuscripts dealing with current concepts of TOS, a few of which are listed in the Bibliography, this entity is still considered by too many to consist of subclavian artery compression by an impinging anterior scalene muscle or cervical rib. The other 90% of clinical material representing lower truncal entrapment is either overlooked or unaccepted. It is in this group, without the florid manifestations of vascular insufficiency, that an unusual degree of patience, insight, sensitivity, and credibility is required to give effective treatment. Improved and intelligently applied progressive exercise programs, coupled with appropriate periods of rest, are useful, especially in the relatively acute uncomplicated syndrome. At the same time, the recognition of the value of first rib resection to relieve unrelenting pain has become increasingly apparent, and the surgical treatment of TOS has produced many heart-warming clinical experiences.

In preparing this text, I am again indebted to Dr. Herbert Robb for his wealth of clinical experience, as well as for his sagacious counsel and the innovative concepts he has shared in managing thoracic outlet syndrome.

BIBLIOGRAPHY

ADSON AW, COFFEE JR: Cervical rib: A method of anterior approach for relief of symptoms by division of the scalenus anticus. Ann Surg 85:839, 1927

BANIS JC JR, RICH N, WHELAN TJ JR: Ischemia of the upper extremity due to noncardiac emboli. Am J Surg 134:131, 1977

BRICKNER WM: Brachial plexus pressure by the normal first ribs. Ann Surg 85:858, 1927

CALDWELL JW, CRANE CR, DRUSEN EM: Nerve conduction studies: An aid in the diagnosis of the thoracic outlet syndrome. South Med J 64:210, 1971

CAPISTRANT TD: Thoracic outlet syndrome in whiplash injury. Ann Surg 185:175, 1977

CLAGETT OT: Presidential address: Research and Prosearch. J Thorac Cardiovasc Surg 44:153, 1962

CRAWFORD FA JR: Thoracic outlet syndrome. Surg Clin North Am 60:947, 1980

FALCONER MA, WEDDELL G: Costoclavicular compression of the subclavian artery and veins: Relation to the scalenus anticus syndrome. Lancet 2:539, 1943

GRUBER W: Ueber die Halsrippen des Menschen mit vergleichend. Anatomischen Bemerkungen, Vol. XII. Mein Acad imp d.sc. St Petersberg 1869

KELLY TR: Thoracic outlet syndrome: Current concepts of treatment. Ann Surg 190:651, 1979

McGOUGH, EC, PEARCE MB, BYRNE JP: Management of thoracic outlet syndrome. J Thorac Cardiovasc Surg 77:169, 1979

MARTENS V, BUGDEN C: Thoracic outlet syndrome: A review of 67 cases. Can J Surg 23:357, 1980

MURPHY JB: A case of cervical rib with symptoms resembling subclavian aneurysm. Ann Surg 41:399, 1905

NAFFZIGER HC, GRANT WT: Neuritis of the brachial plexus mechanical in origin; the scalenus syndrome. Surg Gynecol Obstet 67:722, 1938

PEET BM, HENRIKSEN JD, ANDERSON TP et al: Thoracic outlet syndrome: Evaluation of a therapeutic exercise program. Mayo Clin Proc 31:265, 1956

POLCAK EW: Surgical anatomy of the thoracic outlet syndrome. Surg Gynecol Obstet 150:97, 1980

ROB CB, STANDEVEN A: Arterial occlusion complicating thoracic outlet compression syndrome. Brit Med J 2:709, 1958

ROOS DB: Transaxillary approach for first rib resection to relieve thoracic outlet syndrome. Ann Surg 163:354, 1966

ROOS DB: Congenital anomalies associated with thoracic outlet syndrome; anatomy symptoms diagnosis and treatment. Am J Surg 132:771, 1976

SANDERS RJ, MONSOUR JW, GERBER WF et al: Scalenectomy versus first rib resection for treatment of the thoracic outlet syndrome. Surgery 85:109, 1979

TODD TW: The arterial lesions in cases of cervical rib. J Anat 47:254, 1913

URSCHEL HC, ROZZUK MA, HYLAND JW et al: Thoracic outlet syndrome masquerading as coronary artery disease. Ann Thorac Surg 16:239, 1973

WEBER RJ, PIERO DL: F-wave evaluation of thoracic outlet syndrome. A multiple regression derived F wave latency predicting technique. Arch Phys Med Rehabil 59:464, 1978

WILLIAMS HT, CARPENTER NH: Surgical treatment of the thoracic outlet compression syndrome. Arch Surg 113:850, 1978

WILLSHIRE WH: Supernumerary first rib, clinical records. Lancet II:633, 1860

WRIGHT IS: The neurovascular syndrome produced by hyperabduction of the arms. Am Heart J 29:1, 1945

WULFF CH, GILLIATT RW: F-waves in patients with hand wasting caused by a cervical rib and band. Muscle Nerve 2:452, 1979

Scott J. Boley/Frank J. Veith

Mesenteric Ischemia

ANATOMY AND PHYSIOLOGY OF THE MESENTERIC CIRCULATION

ANATOMY AND PHYSIOLOGY OF THE MESENTERIC CIRCULATION

The mesenteric circulation can be defined as that portion of the splanchnic circulation supplying the small and large intestines. The major arteries contributing to this intestinal vascular bed are the superior and inferior mesenteric arteries, branches of the celiac axis, and the middle and inferior hemorrhoidal branches of the internal iliac artery.

The intestines are protected from ischemia to a great extent by their abundant collateral circulation. Communications between the celiac and the superior and inferior mesenteric beds are numerous, and a general rule that has proved valid over many years is that at least two of these vessels must be compromised to produce symptomatic intestinal ischemia. Moreover, occlusion of two of the vessels occurs frequently without evidence of ischemia, and total occlusion of all three vessels has been observed without symptoms.

The major collateral circulation from the celiac axis is through the superior pancreaticoduodenal artery into the inferior pancreaticoduodenal artery, which is the first branch of the superior mesenteric artery. Collateral blood flow from the inferior mesenteric artery comes primarily through the arch of Riolan ("meandering artery"), which connects the left colic and middle colic arteries (Fig. 36-12). The inferior mesenteric artery in turn may receive collateral circulation from the internal iliac artery through the inferior hemorrhoidal to superior hemorrhoidal arterial connections.

Collateral pathways around occlusions of smaller mesenteric arterial branches are provided by the primary, secondary, and tertiary arcades in the mesentery of the small bowel and by the marginal arterial complex of Drummond in the mesocolon. Within the bowel wall itself there is a network of communicating submucosal vessels that can maintain the viability of short segments of the intestine whose extramural arterial supply has been lost.

In the resting state the mesenteric circulation receives up to 25% of the cardiac output. This percentage may increase modestly after eating or decrease during exercise. Motor control of the mesenteric circulation is mediated primarily through the sympathetic nervous system; although beta adrenergic receptors are present, alpha adrenergic

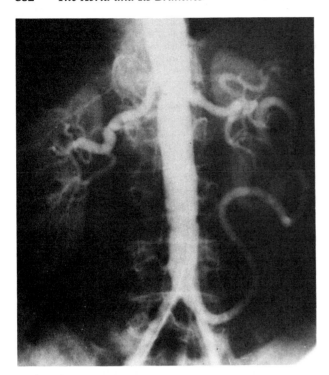

Fig. 36-12. Aortogram from patient with occlusion of the superior mesenteric artery (SMA). The large "meandering artery" is the dilated arch of Riolan, which provides collateral blood flow from the left colic artery to the middle colic artery. The presence of this large collateral indicates a chronic SMA occlusion.

receptors predominate. Thus increased sympathetic activity produces vasoconstriction, which increases resistance and decreases blood flow.

In response to the fall in arterial pressure distal to an obstruction, collateral pathways open immediately when a major vessel is occluded. Increased blood flow through this collateral circulation continues as long as the pressure in the vascular bed distal to the obstruction remains below the systemic pressure. If vasoconstriction develops in this distal bed, the arterial pressure there rises and causes diminution of collateral flow. Similarly, if normal blood flow is reconstituted, flow through collateral channels ceases.

The degree of reduction in blood flow that the bowel can tolerate without damage is remarkable. Reduction of mesenteric arterial flow of 75% or greater for up to 12 hours can be tolerated without morphologic changes in the bowel.

Intestinal ischemia may result from a reduction in blood flow, from redistribution of blood flow, or from a combination of both. A reduction in blood flow to the intestine may reflect generalized poor perfusion, as in shock or with a failing heart, or it may result from either local morphologic or functional changes. With hypertension there is both decreased splanchnic blood flow, as a result of vasoconstriction, and redistribution of flow away from the mucosa because of arteriovenous shunting within the bowel wall. Narrowings of the major mesenteric vessels, emboli, vasculitis as part of a systemic disease, or mesenteric vasoconstriction all can lead to inadequate circulation. However, whatever the cause, intestinal ischemia has the same end results: a spectrum ranging from completely reversible functional alterations to total hemorrhagic necrosis of por-

tions or all of the bowel. Two situations that can dramatically produce or sustain diminished intestinal blood flow in the absence of vascular occlusion are bowel distention and systemic conditions producing lowered cardiac output and transient falls in mesenteric arterial blood flow.

ACUTE MESENTERIC ISCHEMIA

The earliest report of a patient with acute mesenteric ischemia (AMI) was that of Tiedemann, who described the first clinical case of superior mesenteric artery occlusion in 1843. The first successful bowel resection for intestinal infarction was reported by Elliott in 1895. Further progress in the management of these catastrophes did not occur until the 1950s. Klass in 1950 attempted the first superior mesenteric artery embolectomy, and one year later Stewart performed the first successful operation of this type. Successful operative approaches to acute superior mesenteric artery thrombosis, as well as chronic mesenteric ischemia, were reported in that decade. Ende, in 1958, first described nonocclusive mesenteric ischemia, and during the 1960s various attempts to treat this latter condition using local and regional anesthetic blocks as well as systemic and intraarterial vasodilators were reported.

INCIDENCE

The exact incidence of AMI is difficult to ascertain. In one large metropolitan medical center, the incidence in the late 1970s was 1 per 1000 admissions. Recently, there appears to have been a real increase in the occurrence of AMI as well as in its recognition, and with this increased incidence there has been a change in the distribution of cases attributed to each of the different causes. Whereas, in the past, mesenteric venous and arterial thrombosis were most common, in recent series arterial emboli and nonocclusive mesenteric ischemia were responsible in 70% to 80% of patients.

MESENTERIC ARTERIAL ISCHEMIA	
Etiology	Atherosclerosis, embolus, vasculitis, drug-induced splanchnic vasoconstriction, low flow states
Symptoms	Abdominal pain, distention
History	Sudden pain, associated myocardial infarction, shock, past or present embolization
Dx	Abnormal bruit, leukocytosis, acute abdomen, GI bleeding
Angiography	Established collaterals vs. acute occlusion; presence or absence of flow restricting lesions
Rx	Intra-arterial papaverine Surgery: embolectomy, endarterectomy, bypass Resection: venous vs. arterial Embolus vs. atheroma: second-look operations

ETIOLOGY

SUPERIOR MESENTERIC ARTERY EMBOLUS (SMAE)

Today, emboli are responsible for 40% to 50% of episodes of AMI and usually originate from a mural or atrial thrombus. Formerly, such thrombi were most often due to rheumatic valvular disease, but arteriosclerotic heart disease is now the most common cause. Many patients have a previous history of peripheral arterial embolism, and approximately 20% have synchronous emboli in other arteries.

Arterial emboli tend to lodge at points of normal anatomic narrowings, usually just distal to the origin of a major branch, such as the inferior pancreaticoduodenal or middle colic artery (Fig. 36-13).

The artery may be completely occluded, but more often the embolus only partially obstructs blood flow. Mild to marked vasoconstriction is often present in arteries both proximal and distal to the embolus.

ACUTE SUPERIOR MESENTERIC ARTERY THROMBOSIS (SMAT)

Acute thrombosis of the SMA almost always is superimposed upon severe atherosclerotic narrowing, most commonly at its origin. Thirty to fifty percent of patients with SMAT give a history of abdominal pain during the preceding weeks or months. When total occlusion of the SMA is demonstrated by angiography in a patient with abdominal pain, but there are no abdominal findings, it is important to differentiate an acute occlusion from a long-standing one, as the latter may be coincidental to the present illness. The presence of prominent collaterals between the superior mesenteric and celiac or inferior mesenteric circulation in such a patient suggests a chronic occlusion, while the absence of collaterals indicates an acute occlusion.

NONOCCLUSIVE MESENTERIC ISCHEMIA (NOMI)

Since Ende's first description in 1958, the proportion of mesenteric vascular accidents resulting from NOMI has risen from 12% to over 50% in recently reported series. The pathogenesis of this entity is believed to be splanchnic vasoconstriction occurring in response to a decrease in cardiac output, hypovolemia, dehydration, vasopressor agents, or hypotension. This vasoconstriction may persist even after the initiating cause has been corrected. Predisposing conditions include myocardial infarction, congestive heart failure, aortic insufficiency, renal and hepatic disease, or major abdominal or cardiac operations. Digitalis and diuretic therapy have also been implicated. In addition, a more immediate precipitating cause such as pulmonary edema, cardiac arrhythmias, or shock is usually present, although the intestinal ischemic episode may not become manifest until hours or days later.

ACUTE MESENTERIC VENOUS THROMBOSIS (MVT)

Mesenteric venous thrombosis, cited as the most frequent cause of intestinal infarction 50 years ago, is uncommon today.

MVT can be primary ("agnogenic") or secondary to a variety of conditions, including hematologic disorders, hypercoagulable states, intra-abdominal sepsis, local venous stasis, and abdominal trauma. Recently there has been a spate of reports of minor and major mesenteric venous thromboses in patients taking oral contraceptives.

DIAGNOSIS

CLINICAL PRESENTATION

Early identification of AMI depends upon recognition of those patients who are at risk: patients over 50 years of age with heart disease and long-standing congestive heart failure, cardiac arrhythmias, or recent myocardial infarctions or patients with hypovolemia or hypotension, such as in burns, pancreatitis, or hemorrhage. The development of abdominal pain in a patient with one of those conditions should raise the suspicion of AMI. Previous or simultaneous arterial emboli increase the possibility of the ischemia being due to an SMA embolus.

Abdominal pain is present in 75% to 98% of patients with intestinal ischemia, but it varies in severity, nature, and location. A history of postprandial abdominal pain for several weeks or months preceding the acute episode is common in patients with SMA thrombosis. A characteristic early clinical feature is a disparity between the severity of the pain and the paucity of significant abdominal findings. Sudden severe pain accompanied by forceful intestinal emptying is strongly suggestive of an acute arterial occlusion, especially when there are minimal or no abdominal findings.

Unexplained abdominal distention or gastrointestinal bleeding may be the only indication of acute intestinal

Fig. 36-13. Sites where SMA emboli commonly lodge. Thromboses most commonly occur near the origin of the artery.

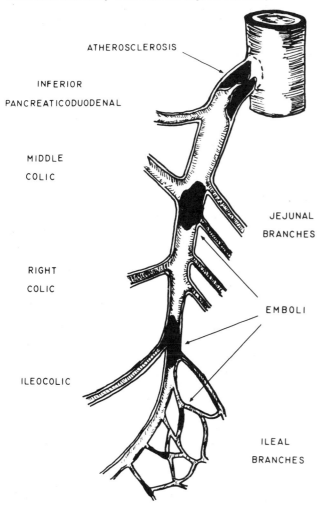

ATHEROSCLEROSIS

INFERIOR
PANCREATICODUODENAL

MIDDLE
COLIC

JEJUNAL
BRANCHES

RIGHT
COLIC

EMBOLI

ILEOCOLIC

ILEAL
BRANCHES

ischemia, since pain may be absent in up to 25% of patients. Distention, while usually absent early, may be the first sign of impending intestinal infarction. Gastrointestinal bleeding may precede any other symptom of mesenteric ischemia, and stools are positive for occult blood in up to 75% of patients.

Early in the course of an ischemic episode there are no abdominal findings; as infarction develops, increasing tenderness, rebound tenderness, and muscle guarding reflect the progressing intestinal changes. Significant abdominal findings are strong evidence for the presence of nonviable bowel. Nausea, vomiting, fever, rectal bleeding and even hematemesis, intestinal obstruction, back pain, shock, and increasing abdominal distention are other late signs.

LABORATORY VALUES

Leukocytosis above 15,000 cells/mm³ occurs in approximately 75% of patients with AMI, and a metabolic acidosis with increased base deficit is present in about 50%. Elevations in other serum and peritoneal fluid values have been reported, but the consistency and specificity of these findings have not been established.

ANCILLARY TECHNIQUES

Several diagnostic radioisotopic techniques have been developed in experimental animals but have not been evaluated clinically. Laparoscopy has been used to identify transmural infarction but is not reliable in the earlier stages of intestinal ischemia.

ROENTGENOLOGIC STUDIES

Signs of intestinal ischemia on plain film studies occur late and usually indicate bowel infarction. Ideally, all patients should be studied before the signs of ischemia develop. In series of cases in which a significant portion of the patients have had such signs, the mortality has been dismaying.

ANGIOGRAPHY

Angiography can establish AMI in most cases and will identify both the cause of the ischemia and the site of an SMA occlusion if one is present. Moreover, it provides the surgeon with a road map to accomplish adequate revascularization when it is indicated. Angiographic signs of mesenteric vasoconstriction in patients who clinically are suspected of having AMI, and who are not hypotensive or receiving vasopressors, are presumptive evidence of nonocclusive mesenteric ischemia. The angiographic catheter provides an access for the administration of vasodilators into the SMA as part of a management plan.

MANAGEMENT PLAN

Although the diagnosis of AMI has been made with increasing frequency during the past 20 years, until recently the mortality of this catastrophe remained at 70% to 90%. This poor outlook could be attributed mainly to three factors: inability to make the diagnosis before intestinal gangrene developed, progression of the bowel infarction after the primary initiating vascular or systemic cause had been corrected, and the increasing frequency of NOMI, with its reported mortality rate of over 90%. Improved survival of patients with AMI has been achieved with an aggressive approach directed at these factors. The new features in this approach are (1) the earlier and more extensive use of angiography to diagnose mesenteric ischemia and determine its cause before intestinal infarction occurs and (2) the intra-arterial infusion of papaverine to interrupt the splanchnic vasoconstriction that is the direct cause of NOMI and a major factor in occlusive forms of AMI, and that persists after successful management of the underlying local or systemic cardiovascular cause. These concepts are incorporated into a comprehensive roentgenologic and therapeutic plan.

GENERAL MANAGEMENT

When AMI is suspected, initial treatment is directed toward correction of predisposing or precipitating causes of the mesenteric ischemia. Relief of acute congestive heart failure, correction of cardiac arrhythmias, and replacement of blood volume precede any diagnostic studies. In general, efforts at increasing intestinal blood flow will be futile if low cardiac output, hypotension, or hypovolemia persist. Plain roentgenographic studies of the abdomen are then obtained, and subsequent abdominal angiography is routinely performed unless some other intra-abdominal condition is diagnosed on the plain film examination. Based on the angiographic findings and the presence or absence of signs of peritoneal irritation on physical examination, the individual patient is then treated according to the schema outlined in Figures 36-14, 36-15, and 36-16.

Even when a decision to operate has been made, an angiogram must be obtained to manage the patient properly at operation. Moreover, the relief of mesenteric vasoconstriction is an integral part of the therapy for emboli and thromboses, as well as the "low flow" states, and can best be achieved by intra-arterial infusion of papaverine through the angiography catheter in the SMA.

VASODILATOR THERAPY

When the therapeutic regimen includes the use of papaverine, the drug is infused at a constant rate of 30 mg/hr to 60 mg/hr using an infusion pump. Systemic arterial pressure and cardiac rate and rhythm are continuously monitored, as these amounts of papaverine theoretically could have systemic effects. The duration of the papaverine infusion varies with both the purpose for its use and the clinical and angiographic response of the patient.

SURGICAL PRINCIPLES

Laparotomy is indicated during the course of AMI either to restore intestinal arterial flow, such as after an embolus or thrombosis, or to resect irreparably damaged bowel. Revascularization should precede any evaluation of intestinal viability, since bowel that initially apears infarcted may show surprising recovery after restoration of blood flow.

After revascularization, if short segments of bowel are nonviable or questionably viable, these are resected. If extensive segments of bowel are involved, only the frankly necrotic bowel is resected and a planned reexploration or "second look" is performed within 12 to 24 hours.

A decision to perform a "second look" is made at the initial laparotomy if there is questionable viability of either a major portion or multiple segments of intestine. The purpose of the "second look," as proposed by Shaw, is "not just to allow a clear definition between dead and live bowel to take place, but also to allow time for the institution of supportive measures, which may render more of the bowel viable."

Embolectomy is indicated for all emboli impacting in the main SMA at or above the origin of the ileocolic artery

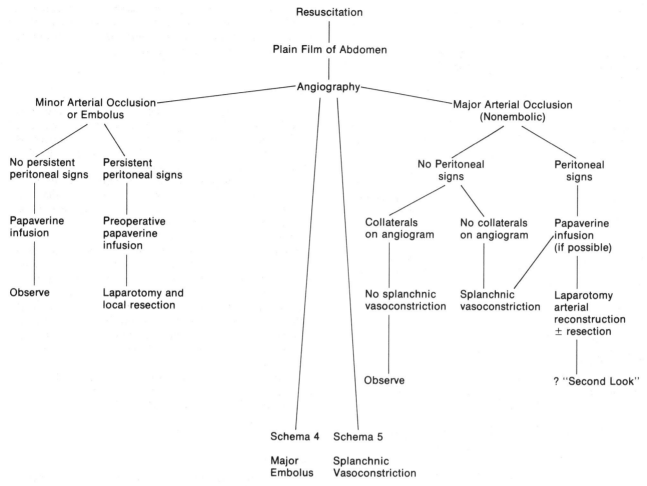

Fig. 36-14. Schema of plan of management for minor superior mesenteric artery occlusions (in branches of the SMA distal to the ileocolic artery) and acute thrombosis of the SMA at or proximal to the origin of the ileocolic artery.

unless the entire small bowel is obviously necrotic. A Fogarty balloon catheter is used to remove residual clots proximal and distal to the point of obstruction. For occlusions due to an acute thrombosis of the SMA, endarterectomy may be attempted, but an aorta-to-SMA bypass using a segment of saphenous vein is the preferred method of reestablishing flow to the distal SMA.

When mesenteric venous thrombosis is found at laparotomy, the nonviable bowel is resected and anticoagulant therapy begun. Isolated instances of venous thrombectomy have been reported, but this is usually not possible, as the thrombi are in the smaller mesenteric veins.

Extensive small intestinal resections of all but a foot of proximal jejunum, and often including the right colon, are frequently necessary when AMI is diagnosed late in the course of the disorder. In the past only a few patients survived with the "short bowel syndrome" resulting from such resections, but long-term home parenteral alimentation offers hope for better results.

PROGNOSIS

While mortality rates of 70% to 90% for AMI were consistently reported for almost 50 years, an aggressive approach to management has lowered the mortality to under 50%.

Although many patients with AMI are elderly and suffering from severe cardiovascular disease, they can survive the acute intestinal ischemic episode if diagnosed early and managed properly. A recent review of experience with 47 patients with SMA emboli showed that if the "doctor delay" was less than 12 hours, and the patient managed as described above, 2 out of 3 patients survived.

FOCAL INTESTINAL ISCHEMIA

Ischemic insults localized to short segments of the small bowel produce a broad spectrum of clinical features without the life-threatening systemic complications associated with ischemia of more extensive portions of the gut.

ETIOLOGY

The most frequent causes are atheromatous emboli, strangulated hernias, collagen diseases, blunt abdominal trauma, segmental venous thrombosis, and, especially during the 1960s, enteric-coated thiazide–potassium chloride preparations. Lesions associated with systemic diseases may occur late in the course of the illness or may be the heralding event of the generalized disorder.

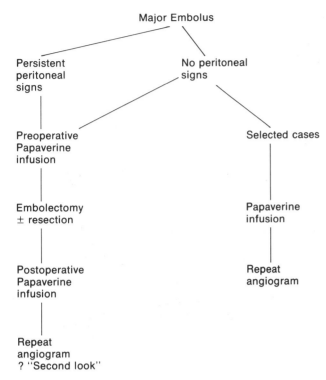

Fig. 36-15. Schema of plan of management for emboli in the SMA at or proximal to the origin of the ileocolic artery.

Fig. 36-16. Schema of plan of management for nonocclusive mesenteric ischemia (angiography revealing splanchnic vasoconstriction).

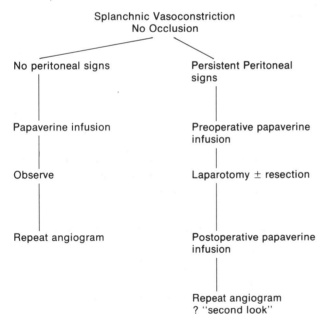

PATHOGENESIS

With focal ischemia there is usually adequate collateral circulation to prevent transmural hemorrhagic infarction. Hence, the commonest lesions are infected infarcts resulting from partial necrosis of the bowel wall and secondary invasion by the intestinal bacterial flora. Limited tissue necrosis may result in complete healing, a chronic enteritis

simulating Crohn's disease, or a stricture with partial or complete intestinal obstruction. When the local insult is severe enough to produce transmural necrosis, perforation or a localized peritonitis may ensue.

SYMPTOMS

Patients with short segment ischemia present in one of three clinical patterns, depending upon the severity of the infarct.

In the acute presentation, seen with transmural necrosis, there is a sudden onset of abdominal pain that often simulates an attack of acute appendicitis.

Another group of patients present with signs and symptoms of chronic enteritis, crampy abdominal pain, diarrhea, occasional fever, and weight loss. The clinical picture may be indistinguishable from that of Crohn's disease of the small bowel.

The most common presentation is that of chronic small bowel obstruction, with or without a history of some antecedent episode of trauma, pain, or hernia incarceration. Intermittent abdominal pain, distention, and vomiting are direct results of the obstruction, and bacterial overgrowth in the dilated loop proximal to the obstruction may lead to the metabolic and clinical derangements usually associated with the "blind loop syndrome": that is, anemia, diarrhea, and steatorrhea.

A preoperative diagnosis of focal ischemia is difficult to make. A previous episode of transient pain, trauma, incarcerated hernia, or a known systemic illness can suggest the correct diagnosis.

TREATMENT

The treatment of acute focal ischemia is usually surgical, but some patients without signs of peritonitis can be managed expectantly. In those instances the diagnosis is based on the roentgenographic findings of "thumbprints" indicative of acute ischemia; serial studies should reveal a changing pattern. Both clinical and roentgenographic findings must resolve or the nonsurgical approach is abandoned.

Patients who present with chronic enteritis or obstruction should be operated on immediately after proper preparation. Awareness of these lesions of segmental ischemia is essential, because a limited resection is the operation of choice both for obstructing lesions and for focal enteritis.

CHRONIC INTESTINAL ISCHEMIA

ETIOLOGY

In this entity, also known as abdominal angina, intestinal angina, or recurrent mesenteric ischemia, there is inadequate intestinal blood flow to satisfy the demands of the increased motility, secretion, and absorption that develop after meals. Thus patients with chronic intestinal ischemia are actually experiencing recurrent acute episodes of insufficient blood flow during periods of maximal intestinal work load. The ischemia is manifested either by ischemic visceral pain or abnormalities in gastrointestinal absorption (see Chapter 24, Malabsorption Syndromes) or motility. Therefore, the pain is similar to that arising in the myocardium with angina pectoris or in the calf muscles with intermittent claudication. Atherosclerotic involvement of the mesenteric vessels is almost always the cause of this form of intestinal ischemia. Although partial or complete occlusion of the SMA, CA, and IMA is fairly common, relatively few patients have documented chronic intestinal ischemia. Moreover, there are many patients with occlusion of two or even all three of these vessels who remain asymptomatic.

SYMPTOMS

The various small vessel diseases such as thromboangiitis obliterans (Buerger's disease) or periarteritis nodosa may also produce chronic intestinal ischemia and even lead to segmental intestinal gangrene.

The one consistent clinical feature of chronic mesenteric ischemia is abdominal discomfort or pain. Most commonly this occurs 10 to 15 minutes after eating, gradually increases in severity, reaches a plateau, and then slowly abates in 1 to 3 hours. The pain pattern is so intimately related to the ingestion of food that the patient will reduce the size of his meals, become reluctant to eat, and have massive weight loss. Bloating, flatulence, and derangements in motility with constipation or diarrhea are also seen.

DIAGNOSIS

There is no specific reliable diagnostic test for abdominal angina. The diagnosis must be based on the clinical symptoms, the arteriographic demonstration of an occlusive process of the splanchnic arteries, and, to a great measure, on the exclusion of other gastrointestinal disease. Angiographic evaluation includes flush aortography in frontal and lateral views and selective injections of the SMA, CA, and, if possible, the IMA. The degree of occlusive involvement of the three major arteries can be best assessed on the lateral projections, and the collateral circulation and pattern of flow are best seen on the frontal views. The presence of prominent collateral vessels indicates a significant stenosis of a major vessel but also connotes a chronic process. Angiographic demonstration of stenoses or occlusions of one, two, or all the major vessels does not by itself establish the diagnosis of arterial insufficiency.

In the past a major indication given for early operative intervention for chronic intestinal ischemia was the prevention of acute intestinal infarction. However, over 75% of cases of AMI are due to embolus or nonocclusive disease, and in neither condition are prodromal symptoms present. Neither has the incidence of intestinal infarction in patients with occlusive disease of the splanchnic vessels ever been established. Hence, the fear of impending intestinal infarction is not an indication for operation, if other criteria do not warrant it. There is one special situation in which reconstruction or bypass of obstructed splanchnic arteries is indicated in the absence of abdominal complaints. This indication arises in a patient who is undergoing an aortic operation for peripheral vascular disease and in whom aortography has demonstrated occlusive involvement of the SMA or CA and the presence of a large "meandering artery."

SURGICAL APPROACH

Although several procedures have been advocated for restoring normal flows and pressures distal to an occlusion in the CA or SMA, the present preferred operation is a bypass to the latter vessel. However, some surgeons believe that in the presence of CA and SMA occlusion, adequate surgical management must include restoration of normal pressure to both vessels and their branches. Autologous saphenous vein (reversed) is probably the graft material of choice if, after gentle distention, it is at least 5 mm in its smallest diameter. Knitted Dacron (6 mm to 8 mm) or polytetrafluoroethylene are acceptable substitutes.

Patency rates with such bypass grafts to the SMA or CA have generally been good, and symptomatic relief in properly selected patients has been excellent. However, Stoney and his associates have recently reported poor results with retrograde bypasses. They attribute this to an unusual and rapidly progressive form of atherosclerosis that involves the subdiaphragmatic aorta and that occurs more commonly in females and in relatively young subjects. On the basis of their series of 34 cases, they advocated either a thoracoabdominal retroperitoneal approach, with antegrade prosthetic grafts originating from the uninvolved distal thoracic aorta, or a "trapdoor" transaortic endarterectomy supplemented with venous patch grafts when indicated. How often this more complicated approach will prove to be necessary remains to be shown.

CELIAC AXIS COMPRESSION SYNDROME (CACS)

This controversial syndrome is included, although we and others do not consider it to be a manifestation of gastrointestinal ischemia. One of the major difficulties in assessing the validity of the CACS is that different criteria are used by various authors to define it. Postprandial abdominal pain, weight loss, diarrhea, an abdominal bruit and angiographic demonstration of extrinsic compression of the CA constitute the findings on which the diagnosis should be based. This compression is due to the crural fibers of the diaphragm, the celiac ganglion, or both, which produce a smooth asymmetric narrowing of the superior aspect of the CA. The surprisingly high frequency of CA narrowing among asymptomatic individuals and the lack of close correlation between the severity of symptoms and the degree of narrowing in symptomatic patients indicate the need for considerable caution in attributing a patient's symptoms to the arterial stenosis.

The most difficult aspect of the treatment of the CACS is the selection of patients for surgical relief of the compressed artery. Results of surgical procedures have varied from series to series, and no specific criteria can be well correlated with a successful outcome. In view of the continuing lack of objective evidence that stenosis of the CA produces any pathologic changes in the viscera supplied by that artery, we believe that only patients fulfilling strict criteria should be operated on. These criteria are abdominal pain, preferably related to eating; significant weight loss; an abdominal bruit; and angiographic demonstration of the typical narrowed celiac axis. In a large medical center with special interests in vascular surgery and vascular disorders of the gastrointestinal tract, we have not encountered a single patient with these findings during the past 10 years.

The surgical approach to CACS varies with the surgeon's beliefs concerning the cause of the pain. Those who believe it is ischemic emphasize the necessity for reestablishing CA blood flow. Those who believe that the pain is neurogenic emphasize the division or resection of the celiac ganglion. A practical approach includes incision of the median arcuate ligament and local resection of the periarterial portion of the celiac ganglion as an initial step. In a few cases where a significant aorta–celiac axis pressure gradient remains, dilatation or arterial reconstruction may be warranted.

BIBLIOGRAPHY

AAKHUS T, EVENSEN A: Angiography in acute mesenteric arterial insufficiency. Acta Radiol (Diagnosis) 19:945, 1978

BERGAN JJ, DEAN RH, CONN J JR, YAO JST: Revascularization in treatment of mesenteric infarction. Ann Surg 182:430, 1975

BOLEY SJ, BRANDT LJ, VEITH FJ: Ischemic disorders of the intestine. Curr Prob Surg 15:1, 1978

BOLEY SJ, FEINSTEIN FR, SAMMARTANO RJ, BRANDT LJ, SPRAYREGEN S: Superior mesenteric artery embolus: New concepts in management. Surg Gynecol Obstet 151:561, 1981

BOLEY SJ, REGAN JA, TUNICK PA et al: Persistent vasoconstriction a major factor in nonocclusive mesenteric ischemia. Curr Top Surg Res 3:425, 1971

BOLEY SJ, SPRAYREGEN S, SIEGELMAN SS et al: Initial results from an aggressive roentgenological and surgical approach to acute mesenteric ischemia. Surgery 82:848, 1977

BRANDT LJ, BOLEY SJ: Celiac axis compression syndrome: A critical review. Am J Dig Dis 23:633, 1978

CRAWFORD ES, MORRIS GC JR, MYHRE HO et al: Celiac axis, superior mesenteric artery and inferior mesenteric artery occlusion: Surgical considerations. Surgery 82:856, 1977

ENDE N: Infarction of the bowel in cardiac failure. N Engl J Med 258:879, 1958

HANSEN HJB: Abdominal angina. Acta Chir Scand 142:319, 1976

INAHARA T: Acute superior mesenteric venous thrombosis: Treatment by thrombectomy. Ann Surg 174:956, 1971

JACKSON BB: American Lectures in Surgery, Occlusion of the Superior Mesenteric Artery. Springfield, IL, Charles C Thomas, 1963

LINDHOLMER B, NYMAN E, RAF L: Nonspecific stenosing ulceration of the small bowel. Acta Chir Scand 128:310, 1964

MCCOLLUM CH, GRAHAM JM, DEBAKEY ME: Chronic mesenteric arterial insufficiency: Results of revascularization in 33 cases. South Med J 69:1266, 1976

OTTINGER LW, AUSTEN WG: A study of 136 patients with mesenteric infarction. Surg Gynecol Obstet 124:251, 1967

SHAW RS: The "second look" after superior mesenteric arterial embolectomy or reconstruction for mesenteric infarction. In Ellison EH, Friesen SR, Mulholland JH (eds): Current Surgical Management. Philadelphia, W B Saunders, 1965

SIEGELMAN SS, SPRAYREGEN S, BOLEY SJ: Angiographic diagnosis of mesenteric arterial vasoconstriction. Radiology 122:533, 1974

STONEY RJ, EHRENFELD WK, WYLIE EJ: Revascularization methods in chronic visceral ischemia caused by atherosclerosis. Ann Surg 186:468, 1979

SZILAGYI DE, RIAN RL, ELLIOT JP et al: The celiac artery compression syndrome: Does it exist? Surgery 72:849, 1972

TOMCHIK FS, WITTENBERG J, OTTINGER LW: The roentgenographic spectrum of bowel infarction. Radiology 96:249, 1970

WATSON WC, SADIKALI F: Celiac axis syndrome: Experience with 20 patients and a critical appraisal of the syndrome. Ann Intern Med 86:278, 1977

Charles G. Rob/Irwin N. Frank

Renal Artery Occlusive Disease with Hypertension

The problem of arterial hypertension has been the subject of wide current interest. Treatment or correction may alter the morbidity and mortality of this condition. Control of hypertension with drug therapy is an acceptable form of treatment, and in some instances surgical procedures may provide curative or palliative results.

Renal artery stenosis is only one of many surgically correctable causes of arterial hypertension. The importance of obstructive uropathy is often underestimated; it is probably the most common of the causes of high blood pressure that can be relieved by surgery. The incidence of high blood pressure in the general population of the United States is probably about 15%—approximately 23 million people. It is not known how many patients have sustained hypertension due to occlusive disease of the renal arteries.

Many causes of arterial hypertension are potentially correctable by surgery. In this chapter we shall discuss the management of hypertension due to occlusive disease of the renal arteries.

THE RENIN–ANGIOTENSIN SYSTEM

The first experiment of significance in this area was reported in 1898 by Tigerstedt and Bergman. They demonstrated that injection of a crude extract of kidney could produce hypertension in dogs. They called the active substance *renin* and opened the way for much further investigation of this enzyme and its relationship to hypertension in man. In 1934, Goldblatt and associates demonstrated that hypertension induced in the dog by partial constriction of the renal artery regressed after nephrectomy; these classic experiments suggested the release of a pressor substance from the kidney when its blood supply was decreased by constriction of the renal artery.

Further investigation has resulted in the identification of renin as a proteolytic enzyme found primarily in the granules of the juxtaglomerular cells of the kidney and secreted by that organ. Although some details of its location within the kidney, molecular weight, and function are known, it has not been obtained in a pure form; reninlike enzymes have been identified in extrarenal sites.

A variety of stimuli and factors are involved in the release of renin into the circulation. The substrate on which renin acts is an X^2 globulin synthesized in the liver, and the result is the formation of the decapeptide angiotensin I, which is relatively inactive. Enzymatic conversion of angiotensin I to the octapeptide angiotensin II occurs primarily in the pulmonary circulation. Angiotensin II is a potent pressor agent producing vasoconstriction by its action on arteries and arterioles. It is also the stimulus for aldosterone production and is therefore the key substance of this system in relationship to the problem of hypertension and the control of circulatory homeostasis. A simplified presentation of the renin–angiotensin system is:

Renin (kidney) + substrate (liver) → angiotensin I
Angiotensin I + converting enzyme (lung) → angiotensin II
Angiotensin II pressor arteries + arterioles → hypertension
Angiotensin II → ↑ aldosterone production

Since renin has not been isolated in the pure form, indirect methods of assay have evolved. Bioassays have proved difficult and often not reproducible. Radioimmunoassays for angiotensin II and angiotensin I have provided a degree of accuracy, sensitivity, and reproducibility that has correlated well with renin activity and clinical results. The final role of these determinations in the diagnosis of the etiology of hypertension and of the prognosis of therapy is yet to be determined. The area of angiotensin blockade for diagnosis and therapy will be further discussed and is the subject of considerable investigation.

PATIENT EVALUATION

Since there is no universally successful screening test to determine which patients with hypertension should be fully evaluated, the following procedure is recommended.

Screening
"Angiotensin antagonism"
(saralasin, captopril)

Evaluation
Excretory urogram
Renal arteriogram
Bilateral renal vein renin assay

Supplementary confirmatory tests
Isotopic renography, scans, and function tests
Differential renal function tests (ureteral catheters)

PHYSICAL EXAMINATION

First, a complete clinical examination is performed with special attention to whether there is an abdominal bruit. A bruit in the upper abdomen is usually due to atherosclerosis of the abdominal aorta, so this finding is often without true clinical significance. Wylie (1962) found that of 55 female hypertensive patients with an abdominal bruit, 73% had renal arterial lesions; of 37 patients without a bruit, only 32% had lesions. Abdominal auscultation may be a more useful diagnostic aid in the female hypertensive with fibromuscular hyperplasia as the cause than in the male with atherosclerosis.

EXCRETORY UROGRAPHY

Rapid-sequence intravenous pyelography with early films represents the first step in defining a possible renal etiology for hypertension. Disparity in renal length, calyceal appearance time, concentration on late films, and notching of the upper ureter and pelvis represent significant alterations. The involved kidney may be smaller and may show delay in calyceal appearance time, with hyperconcentration in late films, and the ureter may reveal notching secondary to collateralization. All these features are seldom present, but the existence of two or three is strongly suggestive of significant renal artery stenosis. Bilateral disease may be difficult to define, since comparison between kidneys is often required. The presence of hydronephrosis, calyceal deformity suggesting a mass, or lateral displacement of the upper pole by an adrenal lesion may offer information suggestive of conditions other than renal artery stenosis that could produce hypertension. The excretory urogram when performed properly can offer approximately 85% accuracy in suggesting the presence of a renal etiology for the blood pressure elevation, but it offers little prognostic information in regard to surgical correction.

RENAL ARTERIOGRAPHY

The transfemoral percutaneous renal arteriogram with selective angiography represents the most significant advance in the radiographic evaluation of the patient suspected of having renovascular hypertension. Definition of the nature of the vascular lesion and the potential for surgical correction should result from a satisfactory study. Approximately two out of three significant renal artery lesions prove to be atherosclerotic, with fibromuscular dysplasias and occasional aneurysms and other rare lesions of the renal artery making up the rest of the group. Angiography may also reveal a primary renal malignant tumor or benign reninsecreting lesion. The presence of bilateral disease can be defined, as well as the degree of collateralization. Flush films of the aorta demonstrate atherosclerotic lesions of the renal artery take-off junction, and selective studies may be useful for the demonstration of segmental occlusive vascular disease. This study should be performed on patients who have abnormalities on excretory urography as previously described, and also in high-risk patients with negative excretory urography. Complications secondary to the procedure include hemorrhage, thrombosis of femoral or iliac arteries, and renal injury. However, a review of 2089 transfemoral catheterizations revealed a fatality rate of 0.11% and a nonfatal major complication rate of 1.2%. Since renal arterial occlusive disease may be present without production of hypertension, one must supplement the patient evaluation with other studies to identify a relationship between this finding and the hypertension. The prognostic implication of surgical correction of an anatomical abnormality is most desirable.

BILATERAL RENAL VEIN RENIN ACTIVITY

Selective catheterization of both renal veins by the femoral vein route can provide blood samples for radioimmunoassay for renin (angiotensin). The technique is simple and usually is performed in conjunction with renal arteriography. Care should be taken to pass the catheter on the left side beyond the junction of the spermatic or ovarian vein so that an undiluted renal vein blood sample can be collected. Most investigators have agreed that a renal vein renin activity ratio of 1.5 to 1.0 or greater is suggestive of an increased renin secretion of significance and correlates well with anatomic abnormalities. The accuracy and value of the determinations are enhanced by renin stimulation prior to performance of the collections. The use of salt depletion, diuretics, and the upright position in preparation have been advocated and may result in an exaggeration of the differences in renin levels or change a test that is negative or equivocal to a positive one. Vena caval as well as both renal vein samples are collected and analyzed. Often the involved side is elevated significantly as compared to the contralateral side and vena caval samples. It is this determination that offers the best prognostic information in regard to the significance of the anatomic abnormality found on radiographic evaluation. Occasionally the unilateral elevation of renal vein renin levels on repeated studies may be the only significant finding in the presence of no diagnostic radiographic findings.

ISOTOPIC STUDIES

The ^{131}I renogram, renal scans, and isotopic evaluation of kidney function and renal blood flow represent relatively noninvasive means of demonstrating a circulatory reason for renal vein hypertension. They offer excellent means of differential evaluation and comparison of kidneys with little morbidity and can be performed without admission to the hospital. Blood flow and kidney function determinations may aid in the selection of patients for surgery and in the choice of surgical approach to be utilized. The renogram that shows dissimilar curves in the presence of a normal nonobstructive excretory urogram is suggestive of a vascular abnormality that may be significant. Scans may reveal kidney size and areas within a kidney with decreased vascularization secondary to segmental occlusive disease.

DIFFERENTIAL RENAL FUNCTION STUDIES

The collection of urine from both kidneys by ureteral catheterizations has proved to be a fairly reliable method of localizing the kidney that may be producing hypertension. The procedure is usually performed during diuresis, and the parameters include decreased urine volume, increased PAH concentration, decreased sodium concentration, and usually decreased PAH and inulin clearances on the involved side. Satisfactory collections of urine samples may offer information that suggests a segmental vascular lesion as well as a main renal artery stenosis and offer definitive differential renal function values. It is a physiological indication of degree of damage and is of prognostic significance. Prior to the development of satisfactory renin assay methods, this diagnostic technique was considered by many to be the only available means of determining the significance of arteriographic findings or localization of the kidney that may produce hypertension without positive radiographic evidence. With reliable renin assay, we seldom perform differential renal function tests, and utilize isotopic techniques for determining individual renal function. It appears that there is still a place for the method in selected cases when the level of suspicion is high and the renin assays do not confirm the clinical and radiographic findings.

ANGIOTENSIN BLOCKADE

The area that may prove to be the most valuable in providing a relatively simple means of screening hypertensive patients for a surgically correctable etiology is that of angiotensin "blockade," "inhibition," or "antagonism." It has been demonstrated that the infusion of certain substances intravenously in patients with "angiotensinogenic" hypertension results in a significant and measurable decrease in blood pressure. This does not seem to occur in those patients who have a normal or low plasma renin activity. Streeten has designated the first group as "responders" and the latter group as "nonresponders." He has used saralasin (1-sar-8-ala-angiotensin II) in his studies and appears to be able to separate the two groups. Identification of the angiotensinogenic hypertensives by this test for further evaluation and treatment would prove to be a great contribution to screening. The nonresponders with low plasma renin activity may be further evaluated for an adrenal etiology for hypertension.

The formation of angiotensin II can also be blocked by the use of captopril, which is a nonapeptide converting enzyme inhibitor. This agent does not have the pressor activity of saralasin and is available as an oral preparation. It may produce a more specific and complete blockade of angiotensin II generation and prevents the release of aldosterone from the adrenal glands. Captopril is an effective therapeutic drug in the management of hypertension and may play an increasing role in defining which patients to evaluate for possible renal artery occlusive disease.

SUMMARY OF PATIENT EVALUATION

The evaluation of patients for a possible renal etiology of hypertension requires more than one diagnostic test to establish that a lesion is present, that the lesion is causing the elevated blood pressure, and that surgical correction or extirpation will improve the patient's clinical situation. This must further be weighed against the benefits of a purely medical regimen before deciding which patients should be operated on. Evaluation can be commenced with angiotensin-inhibition screening to select the patients who might benefit from further diagnostic tests for adrenal or renal causes of hypertension. The techniques for this screening method and data are being evaluated.

The established diagnostic procedures include excretory urography, renal arteriography, and bilateral renal vein renin activity assays. These methods are most valuable in establishing a diagnosis and prognosis for correction. Isotopic renography, scans, and function tests, as well as differential renal function tests by ureteral catheterization, may be required to give supplementary, confirmatory, functional, and prognostic information in selected cases.

CAUSES OF HYPERTENSION POTENTIALLY CURABLE BY SURGERY

Obstructive uropathy
Renal artery occlusive disease
  Atherosclerosis
  Fibromuscular hyperplasia or dysplasia
  Aneurysm and arteriovenous fistula
  Arteritis and aortitis
  Embolism
  External compression
Coarctation of the aorta
Unilateral renal disease (e.g., tumor, infarction, inflammation, hydronephrosis)
Renal vein thrombosis
Pheochromocytoma
Cushing's syndrome
Primary aldosteronism
Cerebral tumor
Hyperthyroidism
Renin-secreting tumors of the kidney

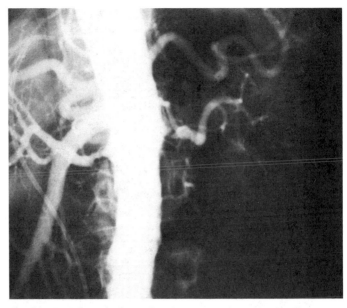

Fig. 36-17. Bilateral atherosclerotic stenosis of the renal arteries before transluminal balloon dilatation. (Courtesy of Dr Irwin S Johnsrude)

OPERATIVE TREATMENT

The operative treatment of hypertension secondary to occlusive disease of the renal arteries consists of three basic procedures: transluminal balloon dilatation under x-ray control, surgical restoration of full arterial blood flow, and nephrectomy or partial nephrectomy.

ABLATIVE THERAPY

The most radical procedures are nephrectomy or partial nephrectomy; they should be reserved for situations in which arterial repair is impossible or unusually hazardous and the disease is unilateral and likely to remain so. Partial nephrectomy is the best treatment for hypertension secondary to ischemia or infarction of a segment of one kidney.

BALLOON DILATATION

Since the modification by Gruntzig of Dotter and Judkins's method of transluminal dilatation of an artherosclerotic arterial stenosis, there has been increasing interest in the application of this method to the treatment of renovascular

hypertension. Today, this is a widely used procedure for the management of renovascular hypertension secondary to a localized stenosis of the renal arteries. The method works well over the short term, but the long-term results are not yet available. One of the first reports was by Gruntzig in 1978; in 1980 Schwarton and associates reported good results in more than 50 patients. Figures 36-17 and 36-18 show bilateral renal artery stenosis before and after transluminal balloon dilatation.

RENAL ARTERY BYPASS

If transluminal balloon dilatation fails or is technically not feasible, surgical reconstruction is indicated. The most widely used procedure is a bypass graft with a segment of the saphenous vein anastomosed to the side of the abdominal aorta and to the renal artery, distal to the stenosis (Figs. 36-19, 36-20, and 36-21). An alternative suggested by Wylie is to use a segment of autogenous artery, taken from the iliac or hypogastric artery and itself replaced when

Fig. 36-18. The patient shown in Figure 36-17 after transluminal balloon dilatation. Note the complete dilatation on the left and the partial dilatation on the right side. (Courtesy of Dr Irwin S Johnsrude)

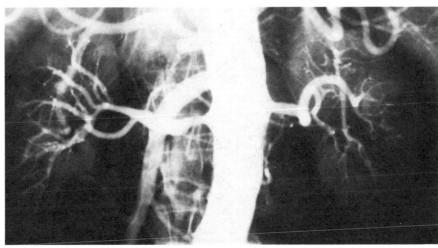

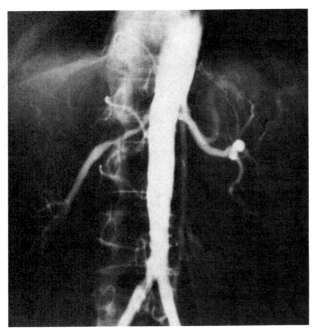

Fig. 36-19.   Stenosis of the right renal artery in a woman aged 41. The cause is probably fibromuscular hyperplasia.

necessary by a Dacron or similar prosthesis. This is of special value in children because the autogenous artery, if sutured in position with interrupted sutures, will grow in size as the child grows.

THROMBOENDARTERECTOMY

When the cause is atherosclerosis and the lesion is well localized, equally good results may be obtained by a throm-

Fig. 36-20.   An 8-mm Dacron prosthesis was placed as a bypass into the patient shown in Figure 36-19. Seventeen years later this patient has a normal blood pressure with an apparently open graft.

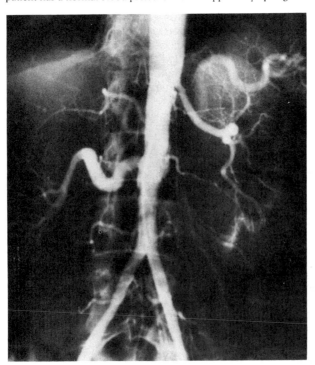

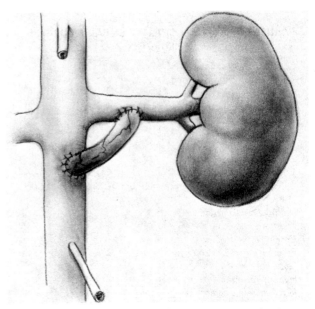

Fig. 36-21.   Aortorenal bypass graft, using a segment of saphenous vein.

boendarterectomy (Fig. 36-22). This operation may be performed through the abdominal aorta, a procedure that has special value when the origins of both renal arteries are stenosed, or through the renal artery, where closure with an autogenous venous patch graft ensures a wide lumen.

OTHER PROCEDURES

In the past the splenic artery has been used as a bypass to the left renal artery, and the renal artery has been implanted into the aorta, iliac, or superior mesenteric arteries. These operations are rarely performed today. Other procedures that have a limited use in special situations are resection of the diseased segment and reconstruction with an end-to-end anastomosis or, preferably, the insertion of an autogenous arterial graft taken from the iliac or hypogastric artery.

If the hypertension is caused by an aneurysm of the renal artery, then resection of the aneurysm is best followed by the insertion of a segment of autogenous vein or artery. Occasionally, when the aneurysm is small and saccular, it may be possible to repair the defect in the artery by direct end-to-end suture.

Fibromuscular hyperplasia may be treated by a venous bypass graft or an autogenous arterial graft taken from the hypogastric artery, if the disease does not extend too far into the smaller branches of the renal arteries. In some patients with fibromuscular hyperplasia, simple dilatation of the stenotic segments may be effective.

An exciting advance has been the extension of arterial reconstruction operations to patients with fibromuscular hyperplasia or aneurysm involving the secondary branches of the renal arteries. This is an *ex vivo* operation in which the main renal artery and vein are divided. The kidney is perfused with a continuous pulsatile flow using a Belzer pump or is preserved by cooling. The ureter is mobilized so that the kidney can be placed on a small table adjacent to the patient. The surgeon then uses magnification and 7-0 arterial sutures and reconstructs the secondary branches of the renal arteries and replaces them with saphenous vein or hypogastric artery autogenous grafts. At the conclusion

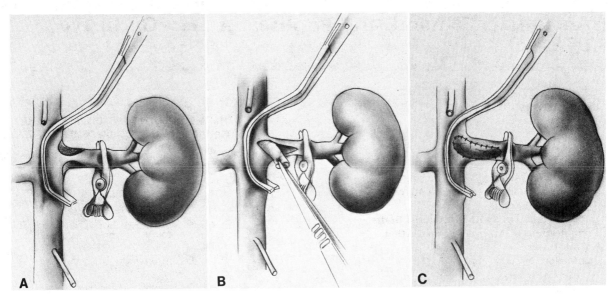

Fig. 36-22. Thromboendarterectomy of renal artery. *(A)* A localized plaque of atherosclerosis, suitable for the procedure of thromboendarterectomy. *(B)* The thromboendarterectomy is shown. *(C)* The arteriotomy incision is closed with a patch graft of saphenous vein.

of this phase of the operation, the kidney is returned to the patient, either at its original position or autotransplanted to another location, such as the side of the iliac artery and vein.

In some patients, renal artery stenosis and hypertension are associated with thrombosis or aneurysm formation in the aorta distal to the renal arteries. This combined problem is best treated by reconstruction of the renal arteries and of the abdominal aorta at one operation. The aorta is clamped above the renal arteries and transected below them. The atherosclerotic stenosis of the renal arteries is then removed by a thromboendarterectomy, performed through the divided end of the infrarenal abdominal aorta, after which the clamp is placed just below the renal arteries and the aorta anastomosed end-to-end to a Dacron prosthesis.

RESULTS

The results of surgery in patients with renovascular hypertension have been presented by the Cooperative Study of Renovascular Hypertension. Since these reports were published, the techniques of balloon dilatation and microsurgery of the secondary and tertiary branches of the renal arteries were developed. The Cooperative Study presented the results achieved by a group of top-quality surgeons treating patients before 1970. Their conclusion was that, in patients with unilateral lesions, corrective surgery is seldom indicated without evidence of disparity of renal function. In bilateral lesions, the side with the greater functional disparity should be repaired first. In general, patients with fibromuscular hyperplasia respond better than those with atherosclerosis. In patients with fibromuscular hyperplasia, 79.8% were benefited by operation, as compared to 63.4% with atherosclerosis.

BIBLIOGRAPHY

Belzer FO: Surgical correction of advanced fibromuscular hyperplasia of the renal arteries. Surgery 75:31, 1974

Case DB, Wallace JM, Keim HJ et al: Estimating renin participation in hypertension: Superiority of converting enzyme inhibitor over saralasin. Am J Med 61:790, 1976

Case DB, Wallace JM, Keim HJ et al: Possible role of renin in hypertension as suggested by renin-sodium profiling and inhibition of converting enzyme. N Engl J Med 296:641, 1977

Dotter CT, Judkins MD: Transluminal treatment of atherosclerotic stenosis. Circulation 30:654, 1964

Foster JH, Maxwell MH, Franklin SS et al: Renovascular occlusive disease: Results of operative treatment. JAMA 231:1043, 1975

Fry WJ, Brink BE, Thompson NW: New techniques in the treatment of extensive fibromuscular disease involving the renal arteries. Surgery 68:659, 1970

Goldblatt H, Lynch J, Hanzal RF et al: Studies on experimental hypertension: Production of persistent elevation of systolic blood pressure by means of renal ischemia. J Exp Med 59:347, 1934

Gruntzig A, Vetter W, Meier B: Treatment of renovascular hypertension with percutaneous transluminal dilatation of a renal artery stenosis. Lancet I: 801, 1978

Hirose M, Arakawa K, Kikuchi M, et al: Primary reninism with hamartomatous alteration. JAMA 230:1288, 1974

Lim RC, Eastman AB, Blaisdell FW: Renal autotransplantation, adjunct to repair of renal vascular lesions. Arch Surg 105:847, 1972

Marks LS, Maxwell MH, Kaufman JJ: Renin, sodium, and vasopressor response to saralasin in renovascular and essential hypertension. Ann Int Med 87:176, 1977

More IAR, Jackson AM, MacSween RNM: Renin-secreting tumor associated with hypertension. Cancer 34:2093, 1974

Reiss MD, Bookstein JJ, Bleifer KH: Radiologic aspects of renovascular hypertension. 4. Arteriographic complications. JAMA 221:374, 1972

Schwarton DE, Yune HY, Klatte EC et al: Clinical experience with percutaneous transluminal angioplasty of stenotic renal arteries. Radiology 135:601, 1980

Wylie EG, Perloff P, Wellington JS: Fibromuscular hyperplasia of the renal arteries. Ann Surg 156:592, 1962

Richard E. Fry/William J. Fry

Aortoiliac, Femoral, and Popliteal Artery Occlusive Disease

GENERAL CONSIDERATIONS

PATHOPHYSIOLOGY

Diseases of the aortoiliac, femoral, and popliteal arteries, along with coronary vascular and cerebrovascular disease, are among the most common manifestations of atherosclerosis obliterans (ASO). ASO is the most common cause of vascular occlusive disease. Other entities rarely produce disease in the aorta and lower extremities and will be discussed when relevant.

Theories of the causes of atherosclerosis involve the concept of intimal damage followed by activation and

THROMBO-OBLITERATIVE DISEASE OF THE AORTOILIAC, FEMORAL, AND POPLITEAL ARTERIES	
Etiology	Atherosclerosis, usually associated with smoking, diabetes, obesity, hyperlipidemia, and advanced age
Dx	Claudication, impotence, rest pain History, physical examination, Doppler ultrasound studies, arteriography
Rx	Reduce risk factors, undertake exercise regimen Transluminal balloon angioplasty (?), arterial bypass, thromboendarterectomy in selected patients

aggregation of platelets. This activity initiates further inflammation, which ultimately gives rise to deposition of lipoprotein and dystrophic calcification, leading to the development of an atheromatous plaque. Factors that may be related causally to the development of atherosclerosis include male sex and more than 45 years of age, hypertension, hyperlipidemia, hypercholesterolism, diabetes mellitus, tobacco ingestion, and obesity.

Traumatic thrombosis of the aorta or iliac arterial system is very rare and is associated with severe blunt abdominal trauma with multiple other injuries. On occasion, penetrating trauma will disrupt the distal aorta. Because of the nature of the injury, rapid attention is demanded to prevent exsanguination.

Rapid occlusion of the aorta or iliac system by embolus is a much more common problem than occlusion following trauma. Invariably, the source of the embolus is the heart, secondary to severe myocardial disease (the result of either valvular abnormalities or occlusive coronary artery disease). Sometimes, in the patient with ulcerated atheromata of the aorta and its bifurcation, chronic slow occlusion of the vessel may take place owing to repeated small emboli. Although this is well delineated in the literature, it has

CAUSES OF CHRONIC ARTERIAL OCCLUSION
1. Degenerative Atherosclerosis Cystic medial degeneration
2. Inflammatory Buerger's disease   (thromboangiitis obliterans) Livedo reticularis Arteritides
3. Other Fibromuscular hyperplasia Compression Atresia Dysplasia

become less common with advances in cardiac reconstructive procedures.

Because chronic occlusive disease of the distal aorta and iliac system is a local manifestation of a systemic disease, it is important to correlate these findings with involvement in other parts of the body, such as the coronary arteries and the vessels supplying the brain. Because atherosclerosis accounts for more deaths in the middle and elderly age groups than any other cause, symptoms of aortoiliac occlusive disease are common.

Atheromas tend to be more prevalent where vessels are fixed, either by branching or by fascial elements such as those in the adductor hiatus. Occluding atheromas tend to be more prevalent in the distal aorta toward the bifurcation. The aorta immediately distal to the renal artery is more commonly involved with the shaggy, ulcerating atherosclerotic plaques. Three types of aortic occlusive disease, which are simply a delineation of disease development and progression, have been described.

Type 1. In this process, the occlusion is limited to a short segment of the distal aorta or iliac system. This lesion accounts for approximately one third of all lesions.

Type 2. The occlusive process is found in the region of the aortic bifurcation, with either narrowing or complete occlusion of the common iliac arteries. This lesion produces the so-called Leriche syndrome, classically described as back or buttock pain, intermittent claudication, and impotence. It is the most common type of aortoiliac occlusive disease, accounting for approximately 60% of all lesions.

Type 3. High or complete distal aortic thrombosis is undoubtedly a progression of type 2, with occlusion of the distal aorta causing retrograde thrombosis of the aorta owing to lack of outflow from the lumbar segmental and inferior mesenteric arteries. This is a relatively rare manifestation of aortoiliac occlusive disease, accounting for no more than 10% of all lesions.

The age and sex distribution of this disease is the same as that for other manifestations of atherosclerosis—almost a 10:1 predominance of males over females. This ratio may be changing owing to the increased use of cigarettes by women.

COLLATERAL CIRCULATION

The collateral blood supply of the distal aorta and its branches is extensive and, in most cases, very efficient (Fig. 36-23). The multiple sources of collateral blood flow make it highly unlikely that necrosis will occur in the early progressive form of aortoiliac disease, particularly in types 1 and 2. Necrosis is most commonly associated with sudden occlusion of the aorta and is seen with embolus or hemorrhage under a partially occluding plaque that causes it suddenly to occlude the lumen of the vessel. As shown in Figure 36-23, the collateral blood supply is derived from several sources. The mesenteric system (by way of branches from the superior mesenteric, middle colic, left colic, and inferior mesenteric arteries) may supply the entire left colon, sigmoid, and rectum. Also, by communications with the internal iliac system, it may supply the pelvis and, in some cases, the lower extremities.

The lumbar segmental vessels with their extensive collateral network may supply the pelvis and the lower extremities through communications with not only the internal iliac artery system but also the femoral system by way of the iliac circumflex vessels.

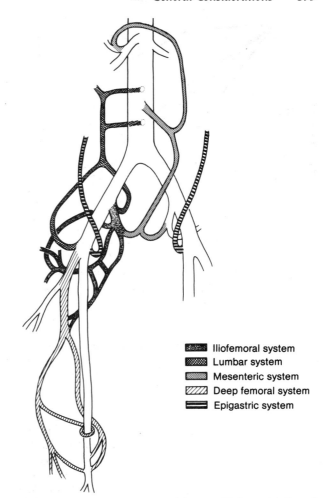

Fig. 36-23. Schematic diagram of the aortoiliofemoral collateral channels.

Legend:
- Iliofemoral system
- Lumbar system
- Mesenteric system
- Deep femoral system
- Epigastric system

The epigastric arteries, both superficial and deep, are important collaterals and may, by communications with the internal mammary and the intercostal and lumbar segmental branches, supply or add blood flow to the lower extremities and, in a retrograde fashion, to the pelvis.

The cruciate anastomosis within the iliofemoral system is an important network of communicating arteries between the internal iliac system, lumbar segmentals, iliac circumflex system, and the profunda femoris artery. When the primary disease is in one iliac artery, these vessels may supply the contralateral leg because of pelvic and buttock communications. The spermatic arteries may act as communications between the upper distal aorta and the pelvis. These vessels generally are small and rarely contribute significant amounts of collateral blood flow in the cases of aortic occlusion. On occasion, the renal artery, by way of branches to the pelvis with anastomoses along the ureteral arterial arcade, may supply significant blood flow to the region of the bladder and pelvis.

NATURAL HISTORY

Untreated symptomatic lower extremity atherosclerosis usually has a benign course, with only 10% to 15% of patients coming to amputation within 10 years after onset of symptoms. Related cardiac and cerebrovascular disease is responsible for an overall 5-year mortality of 40% to 50%

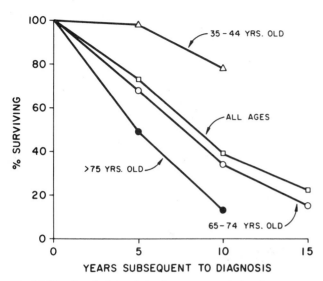

Fig. 36-24. Boyd's data relating long-term survival to the presence of intermittent claudication.

(Fig. 36-24, Table 36-7). The presence of lower extremity vascular disease in combination with other systemic manifestations of atherosclerosis carries a higher mortality.

SYMPTOMS

The most common symptom associated with peripheral vascular disease is *claudication.* Classically, this reproducible pain occurs with exercise in the calf as well as the thigh or buttock and is relieved by rest. The level of disease correlates well with the site of claudication—for example, a person with only calf pain has more distal disease than one with thigh or buttock claudication. The sural artery branches off the popliteal artery and feeds the gastrocnemius muscle. Impairment of blood flow through this artery will produce calf claudication, whereas disease in the common femoral artery and iliac vessels will cause thigh and buttock pain, respectively. *Pseudoclaudication* is pain similar to claudication but requires sitting or recumbency for relief. The pain may not disappear with rest and is also often associated with paresthesias and incoordination. This syndrome is thought to be related to spinal canal stenosis from bony or disc disease with secondary nerve compression and should not be confused with vascular insufficiency. *Rest pain* is constant discomfort that occurs without exercise in the area of the metatarsal heads, ankle, or forefoot. It is exacerbated by elevation and is relieved to some degree by dependency. Rest pain reflects severe atherosclerotic involvement of the

TABLE 36-7   INTERMITTENT CLAUDICATION AND COMPLICATIONS

	5 YEAR	10 YEAR
Nonfatal myocardial infarctions and cerebrovascular accidents	20%	39%
Progression of occlusions	21%	36%
Amputations	7%	12%

(Boyd AM: The natural course of atherosclerosis of the lower extremities. Angiology 11:10, 1960)

SYMPTOMS AND SIGNS OF EXTREMITY ISCHEMIA

Exercise tolerance
  Intermittent claudication
  Rest pain

Physical findings
  Loss of hair
  Atrophy of skin
  Dependent rubor
  Increased venous filling time
  Decreased capillary refill
  Muscle atrophy
  Impotence
  Tissue necrosis

extremity, and these patients are at high risk for tissue loss if they are not treated.

Impotence is a relatively rare phenomenon seen with occlusive disease of the distal aorta and iliac system and occurs in only about 20% of the patients seen. Great care must be taken in the interpretation of this symptom because it has many other causes, principally of psychogenic origin.

Most patients will have typical calf claudication as a presenting symptom. This and the above-described symptomatology are always associated with important physical findings that substantiate the diagnosis of occlusive arterial disease.

SIGNS

All signs of vascular disease are related to ischemia. The pulses will decrease as the arterial lumen becomes narrowed. Turbulent flow may result, producing a bruit or thrill. Atrophy of the skin with secondary hair loss and hypertrophied toenails are apparent. Decreased capillary refilling and increased venous filling time are seen after toe compression and leg elevation, respectively. *Dependent rubor* is an attempt at the arteriolar level to overcome the foot ischemia through maximum vasodilation. The foot becomes warm, dry, and erythematous, resembling the signs seen after sympathectomy.

The typical muscular atrophy seen in patients with occlusive vascular disease is readily apparent upon physical examination. In patients with aortoiliac occlusive disease, there will be atrophy of the calf, thigh, and buttock musculature. Buttock atrophy produces an appearance of flat buttocks that is particularly apparent when the patient is observed from the side. Careful observation and measurements may delineate segmental involvement if selective areas of muscular atrophy are found.

DIAGNOSIS

History and physical examination, with the above-described signs and symptoms as evidence, lead the clinician to further confirmation and localization of the vascular lesion. The location of the obstruction or stenosis can be approximated by palpating the pulse and by knowing the level at which claudication begins. Further localization can be obtained by using the Doppler blood flowmeter. This instrument uses ultrasonic signals that allow transcutaneous auscultation of blood flow. Its sensitivity is such that blood flow may be detected where no pulse is palpable. Evaluation of the signal

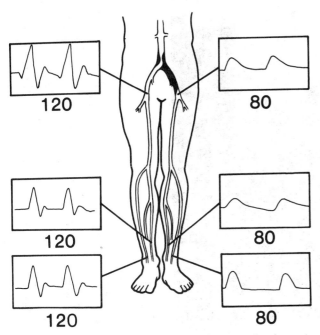

Fig. 36-25. Segmental Doppler examination. Note the change in waveform and pressure distal to the occlusion.

at various levels on the leg and thigh can aid in accurately locating a lesion (Fig. 36-25). Some idea of the degree of stenosis or obstruction may be obtained by taking segmental systolic blood pressures using the Doppler flowmeter. Bergan and Yao have developed the concept of the ankle pressure index (API), which compares a Doppler systolic blood pressure at the ankles with the blood pressure in the brachial arteries bilaterally. Normally, the ratio should be greater than or equal to 1.0 and, the pressure gradient should not be greater than 20 to 30 mmHg between levels. As vascular disease causes decreased blood flow, the ratio will decrease, and this can be correlated with symptoms. Claudication occurs in the 0.5 to 0.7 range. Rest pain occurs at values of less than 0.4 and gangrene at levels of less than 0.3. Calcified vessels may give falsely high readings because of the inability to compress them.

Exercise testing in conjunction with the Doppler flow-

meter can also be helpful. Ankle blood pressure does not vary significantly when a normal person exercises. If the blood pressure falls more than 20 mmHg and lasts for more than 2 minutes, blood is being shunted to muscle and away from the foot. This drop in the distal blood pressure reflects the lowering of blood flow distal to an obstruction. The time of onset of pain, the fall in blood pressure, and the response to treatment can be documented with serial measurements (Fig. 36-26). Digital pulses and pressures can be measured using plethysmography or infrared flow probes, thus giving a more sensitive indication of blood flow to the foot.

Arteriography remains the most accurate means of identifying vascular lesions. The transfemoral, translumbar, and transaxillary routes are the most commonly used. The femoral route is preferred because of its lower morbidity. Anatomy can be easily assessed in views encompassing the distal aorta, iliac, femoral, and infrapopliteal vessels. Oblique and lateral views may show lesions that cannot be demonstrated on standard posteroanterior (PA) and lateral views (Fig. 36-27). Arteriography is most useful in documenting the anatomic extent of the lesion, the presence of collateral flow, and synchronous lesions; in short, it is the road map that allows the surgeon to plan his operation.

TREATMENT

In peripheral vascular disease secondary to atherosclerosis, all treatment is palliative because no cure is available. Nonoperative or conservative treatment is used for patients in whom claudication is not severe. These patients show no evidence of tissue loss and have relatively normal noninvasive studies. Such patients are encouraged to stop smoking, lose weight, and exercise to the point of claudication every day. They should take good care of their feet and keep blood pressure and diabetes, if present, under control. Exercise and abstinence from smoking can bring significant improvement in exercise tolerance through an increase in collateral circulation.

Operative therapy is reserved for those patients with (1) disabling claudication that drastically alters life style and does not respond to conservative therapy, (2) rest pain, (3) tissue loss, such as a nonhealing ulcer, and (4) gangrene.

Fig. 36-26. Exercise tolerance test before and after femoral-popliteal reconstruction. Note the smaller drop in pressure after exercise and the quicker return to baseline in the upper curve.

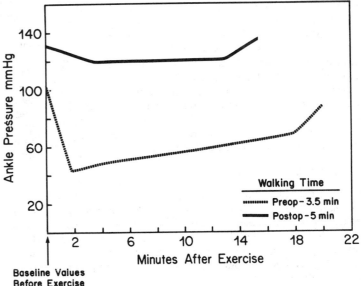

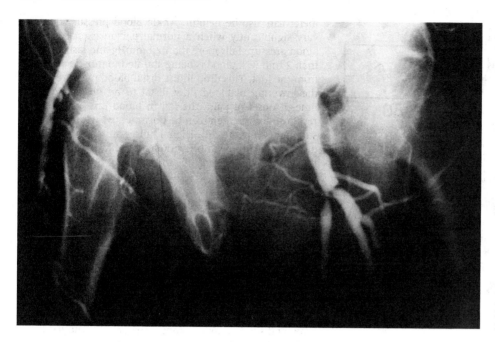

Fig. 36-27. Oblique iliofemoral arteriogram. The left profunda femoris stenosis was not visible in the standard AP views.

The most common approaches are bypass procedures and thromboendarterectomy (TEA). The TEA is used mainly for vessels such as the aorta, iliac, and common femoral arteries, although it has been used on smaller vessels such as the superficial femoral and popliteal arteries. It entails making an arteriotomy, stripping the diseased intima, and then closing the vessel (Fig. 36-28). It is indicated for segmental disease in vessels 7 mm to 8 mm in diameter. Vein patches of saphenous vein or Dacron may be used to prevent narrowing of the lumen after TEA.

The bypass procedure may be used on both large and small caliber vessels, using either a saphenous vein or plastic implant to go around the stenosis or obstruction. Autogenous tissue is used mainly for medium-sized arteries such as the superficial femoral and popliteal arteries, whereas Dacron prosthetic grafts are used for the larger vessels such as the aorta and iliac arteries. Because of the unsuitability of many patients' saphenous veins, substitutions with expanded polytetraflouroethylene (PTFE) and preserved human umbilical vein may be used, though they produce poorer results.

Transluminal angioplasty is a technique by which stenotic or occluded vessels may be dilated by use of a balloon catheter. The catheter is placed in the same manner as a standard angiographic catheter and is passed into the diseased vessel and expanded under fluoroscopic control. The balloon fractures the intima and media and dilates the diseased area. This technique holds promise, but long-term follow-up data are lacking, and more time is needed before its place in vascular reconstruction is decided.

GRAFT MATERIALS

Grafting materials should be durable, easy to work with, biologically inert, nonfibrogenic, able to withstand sterilization where applicable, and noncarcinogenic. Several materials that have most of these characteristics are in use. The major types of graft material are autologous, synthetic, heterologous, and homologous; the last two show poorer long-term results.

AUTOLOGOUS MATERIAL

Saphenous vein and iliac artery are the two most commonly employed autologous materials. They are useful because of their length, diameter, and wall strength. There is no problem with rejection and little with infection. They display long patency, even with low flow rates. They are used mainly for replacement of arteries less than 8 mm in diameter, such as the femoral, popliteal, splanchnic, renal, carotid, and coronary segments. The saphenous vein may also be used as a patch to increase luminal diameter after TEA. Because of its length, the saphenous vein is the most versatile and may be used in all procedures where its size is appropriate. Arterial autografts are shorter and are more useful for replacement of splanchnic branches, especially the renal arteries. Arteries already occluded by atherosclerosis may be salvaged and used as autogenous grafts by the technique of eversion endarterectomy. The vessel is inverted, the atheromas are stripped from it, and then it is reversed, producing a useful graft. Eversion TEA is especially useful in gaining long segments of autogenous tissue that can be used in reconstruction after aortic graft infection or if saphenous vein is not available.

Incorporation of autogenous material hinges upon the reestablishment of the vasa vasorum. Immediately after placement, the graft is nourished by diffusion from luminal blood. New vasa vasorum are established after 72 hours and are completely reformed in 2 months. The effectiveness of autogenous incorporation depends upon careful handling to minimize endothelial damage. Extensive damage to the intima will render the vein graft more thrombogenic and more susceptible to failure. Short ischemia time, avoiding overdistention, and use of cold isotonic fluids for preservation optimize vein graft patency and decrease endothelial damage. Long-term patency is excellent, with approximately 60% of autogenous grafts remaining open after 10 years. Causes of long-term graft failure are progression of atherosclerosis, intimal "hyperplasia," operative injury with secondary stricture, valvular fibrosis, and aneurysmal dilatation.

HOMOLOGOUS AND HETEROLOGOUS MATERIAL

Homologous materials are mainly of historical interest. Preserved cadaver aorta was the first grafting material used; however, it showed a tendency to degenerate early, often with fatal results. Recently, use of preserved human umbilical vein has been reported. Early results have been promising, but it is tedious to prepare and implant and must still be considered an experimental material. The major heterologous material in use is bovine carotid artery. It is prepared by tanning with glutaraldehyde to render it into an immunologically inert collagen tube. Although early results were encouraging, bovine grafts have shown an increasing tendency toward infection. They also degenerate early and have lower patency rates. This material is now used mainly for angioaccess in hemodialysis.

SYNTHETIC MATERIAL

Dacron and Teflon are the most popular synthetic grafting materials. They are used mainly in reconstruction of the aorta and its major branches (those greater than 8 mm in diameter). These grafts are either knitted or woven. The woven variety is less porous and does not need to be preclotted before implantation, a useful attribute in procedures in which blood loss should be kept to a minimum (e.g., ruptured aortic aneurysm). Because of the decreased porosity, woven grafts do not incorporate well nor does the neointima adhere well to the graft surface. This can result in fracture of the neointima and occlusion of the graft. The edges also have a tendency to fray with time, leading to suture line breakdown and pseudoaneurysmal formation. Certain early Dacron grafts developed seromas around them, which were felt to be due to the chemicals used in manufacture. Modifications in production have largely eliminated this problem.

Knitted grafts are more porous and must be preclotted with the patient's blood before implantation to seal the graft wall, or considerable blood loss will result. The greater porosity allows better ingrowth of the neointima and surrounding connective tissue with resultant better incorporation. There is little tendency to fraying.

INCORPORATION OF SYNTHETIC ARTERIAL GRAFTS

The graft acts as a framework for organization and eventual incorporation. There are four stages in this process:
1. *Sealing.* Sealing is the covering of the graft with fibrin and platelets immediately after placement.
2. *Connective tissue invasion.* Neovascularization and fibroblast proliferation smooth the surface of the graft and further seal the graft framework.
3. *Organization.* Eventual buildup of fibrous adventitia and neointima with further differentiation of the connective tissue elements give the graft a more "normal" appearance. No muscular or elastic layers form. This process occurs approximately 2 to 6 months after implantation.
4. *Degeneration.* In time, because of wear and tear from pulsatile flow, the graft may begin to exhibit signs of subintimal damage with secondary intimal hyperplasia, subintimal calcification, and hyalinization. This may cause intimal fracture with secondary thrombosis or stenosis of the graft. As the graft ages, it gains a thicker connective tissue covering and loses some of its flexibility, and these changes may result in intimal fracture if the graft crosses a joint surface. In patients more than 50 years old, graft endothelialization is poor, which may explain a slightly lower patency rate in this age group.

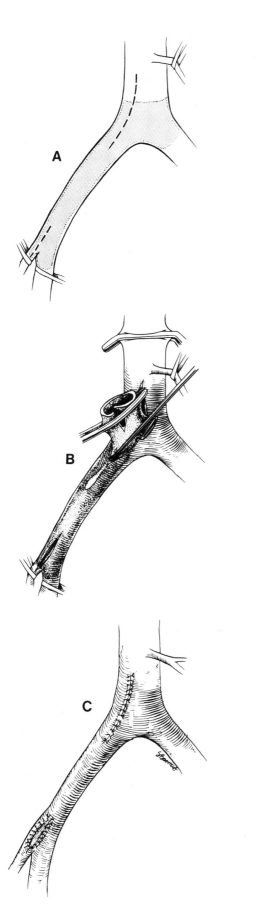

Fig. 36-28. Open iliac thromboendarterectomy (TEA). *(A)* Lines of arteriotomies and extent of lesion. *(B)* Removal of the intima. *(C)* Completed TEA with distal vein patch angioplasty.

To offset the problems of graft incorporation and degeneration, new materials and pharmacologic treatments have been developed. Expanded PTFE has the advantage of being watertight, obviating the necessity of preclotting. According to the manufacturer, it remains flexible for long periods. However, our experience has been that PTFE stiffens with age and tends to wrinkle. Its inner surface is negatively charged, which tends to repel the similarly charged platelets and other blood elements, thus reducing thrombogenicity. Double velour grafts have a large surface area of filaments projecting from both the inner and outer surfaces. These interspaces allow greater ingrowth of connective tissue elements and rapid and more complete incorporation. The use of salicylates and antimetabolites has been described to reduce the incidence of intimal hyperplasia and give a smoother neointima. Preseeding prosthetic plastic grafts with endothelial cells has been suggested as a way to speed organization and formation of a nonthrombogenic intima. These procedures must still be regarded as experimental and are not in general use at this time.

COMPLICATIONS OF ARTERIAL RECONSTRUCTION

Complications of vascular reconstruction can be categorized as early (first 30 days) and late (after 1 year). Early complications include thrombosis, infection, and edema, due mainly to technical factors. Late complications include infection, false aneurysm, and graft thrombosis. These are usually due to progression of primary atherosclerotic disease or degeneration of the graft material.

GRAFT FAILURE

Early graft failures are due entirely to technical factors. Poor anastomotic technique with kinking, twisting, or faulty suture placement are the most common causes of early thrombosis. Inadequate distal runoff, intimal flaps, and unrecognized clot in the graft are other causes. These pitfalls may be avoided by paying careful attention to technical details and obtaining a completion arteriogram at the end of the procedure. This radiographic study will reap dividends for the surgeon by helping to identify problems before they cause trouble (Fig. 36-29 *A, B*).

Early failures are best treated by thrombectomy or correction of technical errors. Expeditious treatment of early thrombosis can give good results in 70% to 80% of cases, including aortofemoral and femoropopliteal bypasses. Late failures usually need a re-bypass procedure because thrombectomy usually is not feasible. Success of revascularization after late failure depends entirely upon the state of the inflow and outflow vessels. Options may be limited by the progression of the atherosclerotic disease.

INFECTION

Of the possible complications of vascular reconstruction, graft infection is the most dreaded. Plastic grafts are the most commonly affected. The incidence of infected grafts ranges from 1.3% to 6%. Infection brings an attendant mortality of 30% to 37% and up to 75% for aortoenteric fistulas. As many as 40% of patients with infected grafts require a major amputation of the extremity.

Most graft infections are caused by wound infection (seeding from a remote infection, such as a foot ulcer or urinary tract infection) or concurrent or inadvertent opening of the gastrointestinal tract, especially the colon. Hematogenous seeding from remote sites and primary wound infections are by far the most common causes. Seventy-five percent of infections begin at the groin with breakdown of the skin incisions and secondary infection. This may be due to rough handling of the tissues with resultant devitalization, strangulating skin sutures with secondary wound dehiscence, or poor postoperative wound care. The more superficial the graft placement, the greater the chance of infection. If the graft lies at or below the inguinal ligament, the chance for infection is increased. Coliforms and *Staphylococcus aureus* are the most frequently cultured organisms from infected graft sites. Staphylococci are native skin flora and typically are found in graft infections with concurrent cutaneous lesions or wound infections. Coliforms may be found if a urinary tract infection is present, if the bowel was opened during surgery, or if an aortoenteric fistula is present.

Manifestations of graft infection are those of sepsis— fever, chills, leukocytosis, malaise, and erythema at the wound site. Late manifestations include false aneurysmal formation with secondary rupture or septic emboli. *All patients with a synthetic graft and fever should be considered to have an infected prosthesis until proved otherwise.* These patients should have serial urine and blood cultures, especially during times of elevated temperature. The sedimentation rate is frequently elevated and may help with the diagnosis. Patients with erosion of the aortic graft into the gastrointestinal tract may present with upper gastrointestinal bleeding as well as a history of sepsis. The combination of gastrointestinal bleeding and aortic prosthetic graft should alert the clinician to the presence of this highly lethal condition. Fiberoptic endoscopy and angiography may aid in the diagnosis of an aortoenteric fistula.

All patients who undergo aortoiliac-femoral-popliteal reconstruction should receive systemic preoperative antibiotics. Doses given 1 hr to 2 hr preoperatively, intraoperatively, and 24 hr to 48 hr postoperatively are sufficient. Most major reconstructions involve either a synthetic graft, a groin incision, or an ischemic ulcer, all of which are indications for prophylaxis. Double-blind randomized studies have documented that such treatment can significantly reduce the number of postoperative wound infections. Of course, if a patient has a grossly purulent ischemic ulcer, skin lesion, or other distant infection, it should be adequately treated before proceeding with elective reconstruction. Good operative technique with gentle handling of tissues can aid in avoiding wound infections. Covering the graft with extraperitoneal tissue or omentum can isolate the graft from the gastrointestinal tract and reduce the incidence of aortoenteric fistula. Fluid collections, such as seromas or hematomas, should be vigorously treated with initial aspiration or surgical drainage if necessary.

Treatment of infected grafts is constant. The prosthetic material should be removed, with closure of the aortic stump if an aortic graft is present. Circulation should be restored by placement of new grafts in uninfected tissue planes. All devitalized tissue should be debrided, and the

---

COMPLICATIONS OF ARTERIAL RECONSTRUCTION

1. Failure of reconstruction
   Early: Technical
   Late: Progression of disease
2. Pseudoaneurysm formation
3. Prosthetic graft infection
4. Edema

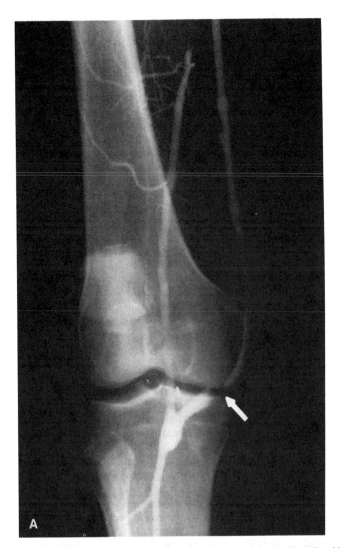
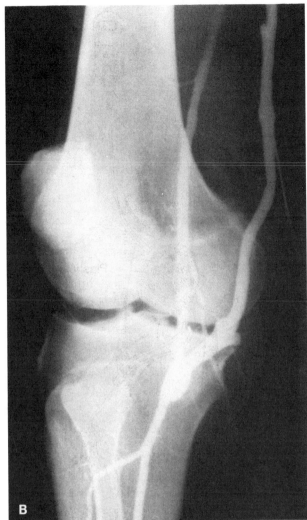

Fig. 36-29. Intraoperative arteriogram of the distal femoral-popliteal bypass. *(A)* Note the interruption of flow *(arrow)*. *(B)* Flow after correction of the error. In this case, the arteriogram and correction prevented early thrombosis.

patient should be treated with antibiotics. Axillofemoral and femorofemoral bypass grafts are the most commonly employed reconstructive procedures used in treating graft infections. These reestablish blood flow to the extremities without the risk of passing near the infected areas. Usually, a Dacron prosthesis is employed for the long subcuticular axillofemoral and femorofemoral bypasses. As an alternative, saphenous vein may be used for the femoral crossover. This procedure has the disadvantage of a subcutaneously placed synthetic graft, which may be seeded from an established infection or occluded from external pressure. For this reason, several investigators have employed retroperitoneal and obturator bypass to diminish the risks of subcutaneous graft placement.

There have been several reports of nonoperative treatment. This entails continous irrigation of the infected wound and graft area with povidone-iodine solution, followed by delayed wound closure when bacterial cultures are sterile (Fig. 36-30). Although the results of this approach have been promising, clinicians should assess the type, location, extent, and bacteriology of the infection accurately and meticulously before using irrigation as a primary treatment. Localized early infection in still patent peripherally located

grafts are best suited for such treatment. Sinograms with water-soluble contrast material may aid in identifying abscess cavities and showing the extent of infection. Later infections tend to involve the entire graft and cannot be treated in this conservative manner.

The most notable alternative to the classic extra-anatomic bypass has been the use of anatomic autogenous tissue reconstruction with endarterectomized arterial segments. Use of this method has significantly reduced mortality to 13% and amputation to 8% in the series reported by Ehrenfeld et al. The major vascular conduits are fashioned using the eversion thromboendarterectomy technique, which can salvage large segments of occluded iliac or femoral arteries for use in a unilateral aortofemoral bypass. Saphenous vein is then used for femorofemoral crossover graft to reestablish blood flow to the opposite leg (Fig. 36-31). Thromboendarterectomy, with or without vein patch and composite grafts, provides a viable alternative to the standard axillofemoral bypass. Besides obviating extra-anatomic bypass and lowering morbidity and mortality, there is no need for closure of the distal aorta with its risk of subsequent rupture or proximal propagation of thrombus to occlude the renal arteries.

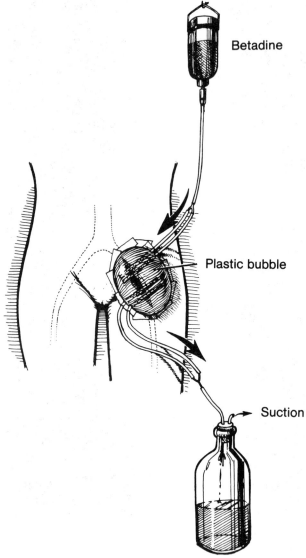

Betadine

Plastic bubble

Suction

Fig. 36-30. Continuous irrigation for isolated graft infection.

FALSE ANEURYSM

False aneurysms occur at anastomotic sites in approximately 2% to 5% of grafts, with 70% of these occurring in the groin. The aneurysm is formed by a partial disruption of a suture line with formation of a fibrin and platelet sac. The lack of true endothelium and vessel wall elements in the aneurysm gives the lesion its name. The incidence of false aneurysms is increased by the presence of graft infection, fraying of the prosthesis and suture line, and poor condition of the parent artery. The use of silk suture material that may degenerate, side-to-side anastomosis, arterial hypertension, and tension on the anastomosis can also contribute to the formation of false aneurysms.

Pseudoaneurysm presents as an expanding pulsatile mass in the area of weakness, usually the groin. This may be confirmed by the use of ultrasound or arteriography (Fig. 36-32). Ultrasound can show whether the mass is solid or cystic and may show confluence with the arterial lumen. Arteriography usually shows extravasation into the mass with free communication with the parent artery, thus confirming the diagnosis. Pseudoaneurysms may also cause distal thrombosis of the graft due to compression. Showers

of emboli from the laminated clot in the sac can cause acute distal ischemia to the foot and calf. Expansion may also compress the adjacent vein, causing secondary edema and venous insufficiency. Rupture, the most feared complication of pseudoaneurysm, is more commonly associated with plastic grafts than with those of autogenous tissue owing to the low anastomotic tensile strength of synthetic grafts, which allows larger aneurysmal formation.

Treatment consists of sac excision with primary repair of the anastomosis if the area is small, or regrafting with the anastomosis placed in an unaffected area of the vessel. Permanent sutures such as Dacron polypropylene should be used, taking care to take adequate "bites" of the parent vessel. Infection should be treated as previously described. One large series showed that 73% of patients with pseudoaneurysms can be treated electively; of these there was an attendant good result in 82%, an amputation rate of 4%, and a mortality rate of 4%. Twenty-seven percent were treated as emergency cases, mainly for rupture or acute ischemia of a limb. Of these emergency cases, good results occurred in 83%, 12% came to amputation, and 10% died. In contrast, a 30% mortality resulted from nonoperative treatment, thus emphasizing the need of operative treatment for these lesions.

EDEMA

Edema is the most common complication of lower extremity revascularization and is seen in up to 50% of all patients with this type of revascularization. The major cause is transection of the subcuticular and inguinal lymphatics. Fifty to 100% of inguinal incisions may cut across these bundles, predisposing them to lymphatic obstruction. Other causes are increased transcapillary pressure from an increased arterial inflow with exudation of fluid, and thrombophlebitis. Edema may also occur with secondary venous insufficiency that was asymptomatic because of low blood flow to the ischemic limb. Edema often resolves in the early postoperative period as the vascular tree accommodates the increased blood flow. If not treated adequately, however, the swelling may lead to wound dehiscence and secondary graft failure. Compressive stockings should be used with great care because of their potential for graft compression and secondary thrombosis. Longitudinal incisions that parallel the lines of lymphatic distribution or a lateral approach may lessen lymphatic damage and reduce the risk of edema.

AORTOILIAC OCCLUSIVE DISEASE

Partial and complete occlusion of the distal aorta and the iliac arterial system has been observed for centuries. As early as 1818, Goodison described not only atherosclerotic occlusions of the aortic bifurcation but included in his monograph a detailed description of the collateral blood supply to the pelvis and lower extremities. Although the clinical significance of these lesions was alluded to in early reports, it was not until the detailed report in 1923 by Leriche that anatomic findings were correlated with the clinical manifestations of occlusive disease. With the introduction of translumbar aortography by dos Santos 6 years later, accurate diagnosis of occlusive disease involving the distal aorta and iliac arteries became possible. Much credit must be given to dos Santos for demonstrating the radiographic findings of occlusive disease and correlating them not only with the earlier pathologic descriptions but also with the clinical manifestations exhibited by the patient.

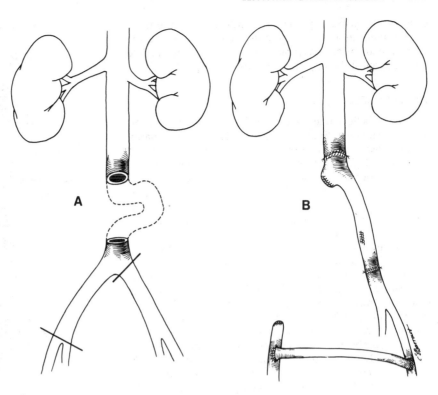

Fig. 36-31. Replacement of severely kinked and infected aortic tube graft with autogenous iliac segment and saphenous vein.

Fig. 36-32. Pseudoaneurysm formation *(arrows)* in the proximal *(left)* and distal *(right)* portions of an aortic bifurcation graft.

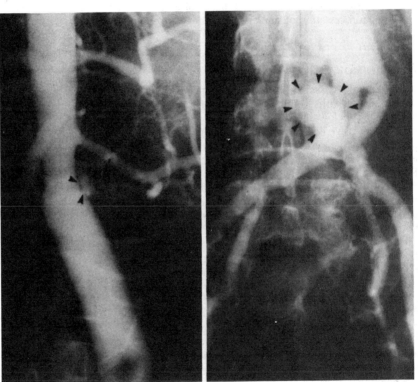

The first successful reconstructive procedure for aortic occlusive disease was done in 1951 by Oudot. He utilized resection of the involved segment and replacement with a homograft. As early as 1947 John Sid dos Santos demonstrated the feasibility of thromboendarterectomy of the distal external iliac artery and the femoral arteries. Soon after dos Santos' work was published, thromboendarterectomy quickly achieved popularity in the treatment of aortoiliac occlusive disease. In 1948 Kunlin introduced the bypass principle into operative therapy for femoropopliteal disease, and in 1954 it was extended to include the aortoiliac segment. Homografts were first used, and then in 1956 synthetic prostheses were introduced.

The pioneers in the treatment of this disease utilized accurate pathologic and anatomic descriptions as published a century before. These were combined with accurate assessment of the clinical manifestations of the disease. The techniques for arterial suture had been delineated in the early 1900s by Alexis Carrel, but it was not until the rapid advancement in anesthesia, the use of antibiotics, and the development of arterial replacements that it was possible for the surgical therapy of this disease to progress.

PATIENT SELECTION

We do not believe that intermittent claudication *per se* is an indication for operative therapy. This belief is based primarily on the classic work of Boyd, who demonstrated that (1) the prognosis for life after the onset of intermittent claudication is poor; (2) 50% of all persons with claudication improve, 30% reach a plateau, and only 20% progress to severe difficulty; and (3) amputation becomes necessary in only 5% to 7% of all patients within a 5-year period after the onset of claudication.

Patients with impending or true tissue loss, rest pain, and inability to move far enough to carry out ordinary activity, or those who are unable to perform their usual occupation because of claudication, are candidates for operative therapy. One additional group should be mentioned—those with rapidly progressive intermittent claudication that cannot be modified by conservative therapy.

Owing to the increasing safety of operative therapy, some surgeons advocate it for any patient with claudication. We do not believe this treatment to be indicated without at least a firm trial of conservative therapy composed of weight loss, control of hypertension and heart disease, graded exercise, and cessation of smoking.

TREATMENT

AORTOFEMORAL BYPASS

Aortofemoral bypass is the operative therapy of choice in most patients with aortoiliac occlusive disease. The aorta immediately below the renal artery is usually spared significant occlusive disease, providing adequate space for the insertion of the bypass graft. We prefer the end-to-end anastomosis of the graft to the aorta because we believe that the flow characteristics are better and that the graft lies in a position where it can more easily be covered with retroperitoneal tissue to protect it from the gastrointestinal tract. Many surgeons utilize the end-to-side anastomosis with a long suture line between the end of the graft and the side of the aorta. This is felt to be more expeditious; however, there is no difference in time between the two operative techniques and both seem to function well. The decision to use either the end-to-end or the end-to-side anastomosis is largely one of training and personal preference. Following the upper anastomosis the limbs of the graft are tunneled retroperitoneally beneath the ureters, through the pelvis, and into the groin, where anastomoses are carried out in an end-to-side fashion to the femoral or profunda femoris artery (Fig. 36-33), depending on the arteriographic distribution of the atheromatous disease.

THROMBOENDARTERECTOMY (TEA)

Thromboendarterectomy once was the most popular operative therapy for aortoiliac occlusive disease. Because of the extensive exposure required, the time needed for the operation, and the relatively high immediate occlusion rate, it is performed much less often now than in the past. It remains an excellent operation for limited disease in and about the bifurcation of the aorta. Indications for thromboendarterectomy in our practice are limited to the distal

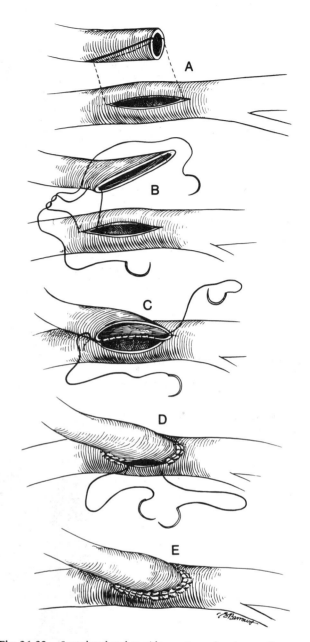

Fig. 36-33. Spatulated end-to-side anastomosis using continuous suture technique.

aorta and common iliac arteries only. If the disease process is extensive enough to require endarterectomy beyond the bifurcation of the iliac vessels, we feel that the bypass technique is preferable. Thromboendarterectomy has the advantage of eliminating the need for prosthetic material, thus reducing the risk of infection. In patients with small vessels this procedure may be complemented by the use of patch grafting to enlarge the ostia of the involved vessels.

There is a significant group of patients with localized disease involving one iliac artery predominantly. In such patients femorofemoral crossover bypass graft may be an appropriate therapy, particularly in patients who are poor operative risks because of severe cardiopulmonary disease. This operative therapy totally eliminates the need for an abdominal incision and can be done expeditiously without the use of general anesthesia.

Great care must be taken in the selection of patients for femorofemoral crossover bypass grafting. There must be adequate blood flow in the relatively nondiseased side to allow adequate perfusion of both legs. Determination of adequacy of flow is done by combining the findings of the physical examination with the noninvasive laboratory results and the arteriogram. Multiplane arteriographic views are required to ensure the adequacy of the donor femoral artery. This operation must be carefully planned, particularly for those patients with severe outflow disease, to ensure adequate runoff on the involved side. To achieve good blood flow it is often necessary to do a profundaplasty in conjunction with the crossover femorofemoral graft.

Occasionally, patients with severe aortoiliac disease and concomitant severe cardiopulmonary disease are encountered. These patients may not be candidates for aortofemoral bypass because of their precarious cardiac status. When there is rest pain or tissue loss indicating an imminent need for amputation, axillofemoral or femorofemoral bypass may be a safe alternative. Either procedure can generally be done with a much lower operative mortality and morbidity than an aortofemoral bypass. The choice is one of a lesser patency rate in a graft that is more vulnerable to occlusion than that of the aortofemoral bypass. It also demands an adequate subclavian-axillary system to accommodate the increased blood flow necessary to supply blood to both lower extremities. Under such circumstances it is useful for revascularization and salvage of markedly ischemic lower extremities.

PERIOPERATIVE THERAPY

Most patients with aortoiliac occlusive disease have concomitant cardiac disease and other manifestations of atherosclerosis, such as stroke syndrome and hypertension. Most have received some form of therapy, including digitalis, propranolol, diuretics, and insulin for diabetes.

Our experience has shown that most of these patients are hypovolemic. Careful assessment of fluid volume is mandatory prior to operation. Most patients should be monitored with the Swan–Ganz catheter before operative intervention, allowing the reestablishment of adequate fluid volume and correction of any electrolyte abnormalities that may be secondary to diuretic therapy. This careful fluid management provides a larger safety margin and virtually eliminates renal failure and intraoperative cardiac problems.

The routine use of antibiotics in the perioperative period, particularly when a foreign body is to be utilized, has been well documented. The source of contamination is primarily the skin, especially the skin of the groin. This area is particularly difficult to sterilize, and great care should be taken to reduce the bacterial flora to the minimum. It has been demonstrated that hematoma formation in the groin associated with recent arteriography has increased the incidence of groin infections following aortofemoral bypass. When large hematomas are present, it is wise to defer operation until these resolve.

Another source of bacterial contamination is the gastrointestinal tract, though this is relatively rare. Utilization of a broad-spectrum antibiotic or two specific antibiotics has been most helpful in reducing the incidence of graft infection from this source to 1%.

The choice of anesthesia must be mentioned, particularly in the patient with poor cardiac function. The overuse of some anesthetic agents (*e.g.,* Fluothane), can cause cardiac depression that may result in a disastrous chain of events such as multiple organ failure. Therefore, it is important for the surgeon to coordinate his management with that of the anesthesiologist prior to operation.

Patency of grafts for 5 years may be expected in 75% to over 90% of patients with adequate outflow. Attention to technical details has been responsible for improved patency rates. In most large series, decreased mortality rates of 3% to 5% have resulted from the use of cardiac monitoring.

PROFUNDAPLASTY

The profunda femoris artery is one of the most important collateral channels in the lower extremity. If this artery is patent, occlusion of the superficial femoral artery may be well tolerated. This artery has the potential to carry a large volume of blood and in fact will double the usual blood flow when the superficial femoral artery is occluded.

The anatomy of the profunda femoris artery is most significant in determining its effectiveness as a primary collateral conduit. The importance of the collateral conduits of the profunda femoris artery cannot be overemphasized. Vessels contributing to this collateral are the lateral circumflex femoral artery with its anastomoses to either the popliteal or the geniculate vessels. There are midthigh collaterals that also play an essential role in joining with the geniculates to supply the popliteal and tibial vessels. In selecting patients for profundaplasty, accurate assessment of the arteriogram is imperative in determining the success of the operation (Fig. 36-34). Great care must be taken to

Fig. 36-34. Major arteriographic points to be evaluated before performing a profundaplasty.

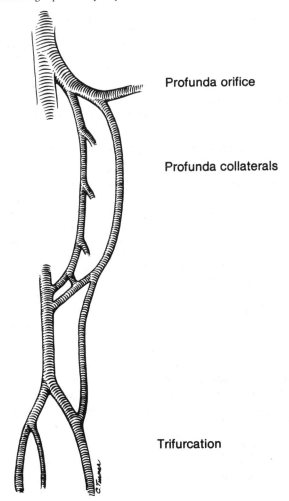

Profunda orifice

Profunda collaterals

Trifurcation

make sure that there are minimal distal profundal occlusive disease, disease-free profunda collaterals, and flow of collaterals into a patent superficial femoral or popliteal artery with subsequent good outflow of that vessel. In-depth knowledge of the anatomy of the profunda femoris artery is paramount in the decision-making process for selection of patients for isolated profundaplasty.

INDICATIONS FOR PROFUNDAPLASTY

Thirty-four percent of all patients with distal occlusive disease have stenosis of the profunda femoris vessel. It is important to consider some form of profundaplasty in aortofemoral bypass procedures. Generally, this will be necessary in approximately 80% of the cases encountered. It must be emphasized that the runoff for such operative procedures dictates long-term patency of the aortofemoral bypass. Without adequate attention to the profunda femoris artery in the selection of patients for this operative procedure, patency rates will be much below satisfactory levels.

Twenty percent of all patients operated upon for disabling claudication or limb salvage, done either alone or in conjunction with bypass procedures, have severe profunda femoris occlusive disease. Profundaplasty should be considered for these patients to increase blood flow to the extremity.

Isolated profundaplasty gives best results for disabling claudication, although this operative procedure can be considered in a small number of highly selected patients who face threatened tissue or limb loss.

Angiographic correlation with success cannot be over-emphasized. The criteria for success are as follows:
1. Severe profunda femoris orifice stenosis
2. A relatively disease-free segment of distal profunda femoris artery
3. Disease-free collaterals from the profunda femoris artery
4. Reconstitution of the distal superficial femoral artery or popliteal artery
5. Good outflow from the patent popliteal segment

TYPES OF PROFUNDAPLASTY—EXTENDED AND SIMPLE

The procedure of profundaplasty can be divided into two categories, extended and simple. Extended profundaplasty usually involves a thromboendarterectomy of a portion of the common femoral artery and the orifice of the profunda femoris artery down to a relatively disease-free segment. It is noteworthy that, in most instances, the distal intima does not feather as it usually does in the carotid artery. It may be necessary to tack the distal intima down carefully with fine arterial sutures. The ostium and the proximal portion of the profunda femoris artery can be widened by patch angioplasty using a patch of saphenous vein or the already occluded superficial femoral artery. Generally, we are hesitant to sacrifice the saphenous vein because it may be necessary for other reconstructive procedures. The superficial femoral artery may be dissected free to the proper length, transected and opened. After careful endarterectomy of this segment, it may be swung over the arteriotomy as a patch graft, thereby opening the proximal portion of the profunda femoris artery.

Simple profundaplasty is utilized either in conjunction with aortofemoral bypass or when the superficial femoral artery is free of disease. The latter is an infrequent finding in our experience. The operative techniques are much the same as those of the extended profundaplasty except that

a common femoral thromboendarterectomy is necessary. Because the profunda femoris artery is generally small in diameter even after endarterectomy, it is necessary to use the patch angioplasty technique.

RESULTS

The operative mortality of this procedure is low, ranging from 1% to 3%. With ideal radiologic criteria (*i.e.*, stenosis of the profunda femoris orifice, a disease-free distal profunda femoris, disease-free collaterals, and a patent popliteal with good runoff), our success with profundaplasty has been 100%. Our success rate drops to 27% when there is profunda orifice stenosis and either diseased collaterals, an occluded popliteal artery, or poor popliteal runoff.

Failure occurs when there is minimal profunda orifice stenosis and marked disease of the distal profunda femoris artery. In this setting our success with profundaplasty has been nil. Other authors have demonstrated a 77% patency rate over 5 years when this operative procedure is done for claudication alone. There is a patency rate of only 23% when the operation is done for limb salvage. This reflects extensive involvement of the profunda femoris artery and certainly governs the selection of patients for this operative procedure. There is a reported 20% to 40% amputation rate when this procedure is done alone for limb salvage, again emphasizing the need for careful assessment of the preoperative angiogram in determining the selection of patients for profundaplasty.

There is no question that in properly selected patients this is a durable procedure, particularly when it is done for claudication or in conjunction with an inflow procedure such as aortofemoral bypass. Careful attention must be paid to the radiographic anatomy as well as to the outflow tract to ensure optimal results.

FEMORAL, POPLITEAL, AND INFRAPOPLITEAL OCCLUSIVE DISEASE

Atherosclerosis again is the most common cause of femoropopliteal occlusive disease, affecting more than 95% of all patients with arterial disease. Theories of the pathophysiology and etiology of atherosclerosis are described in earlier sections.

Cystic adventitial degeneration is a condition affecting mainly men in the 30- to 50-year age group. Cysts form between the media and the adventitia or within the adventitia itself. These cysts are similar to those seen in synovial ganglion cysts. Clinical findings are the sudden onset of disabling claudication and the absence of pulses at the popliteal level and below. Arteriographic findings may reveal tapering of the arterial lumen to a tight stenosis or complete occlusion—the so-called "scimitar" sign. Vessel occlusion occurs as the cysts enlarge, causing a relatively short history of symptoms.

Entrapment of the popliteal vessel occurs when there is

CAUSES OF FEMORAL-POPLITEAL OCCLUSION
1. Atherosclerosis
2. Adventitial cystic disease of the popliteal artery
3. Popliteal artery entrapment
4. Chronic embolization

an anomalous medial course of the popliteal artery, causing it to bow around the medial head of the gastrocnemius muscle. Secondary occlusive symptoms occur in young people (30 to 40 years of age) upon exercise. Arteriographic findings show either aneurysmal dilatation, poststenotic dilatation, stenosis, or thrombosis (Fig. 36-35 *A, B, C*).

Embolic phenomena are more completely described elsewhere in this chapter. Although cardiac sources are the most common, emboli also originate from aneurysms or ulcerated atherosclerotic plaques. A laminated clot that partially fills an aneurysm of the aorta, iliac, femoral, or popliteal vessels may be a source of distal emboli. Throm-

bogenic ulcerations may form in atheromas, acting as a nidus for platelet and fibrin aggregation. The "blue toe" syndrome, an ischemic digit or forefoot, may be the presenting symptom of distal emboli. Acute ischemia with the loss of pulses, pain, pallor, paresthesia, and paralysis is also common in acute occlusion by a large embolus.

INCIDENCE

The femoropopliteal segment is involved in 50% of patients with peripheral vascular disease. Males outnumber females in a ratio of approximately 10:1, and most are in the 50-

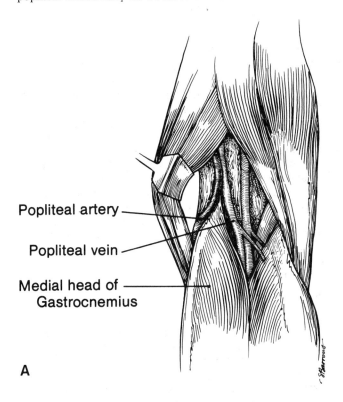

Popliteal artery

Popliteal vein

Medial head of Gastrocnemius

A

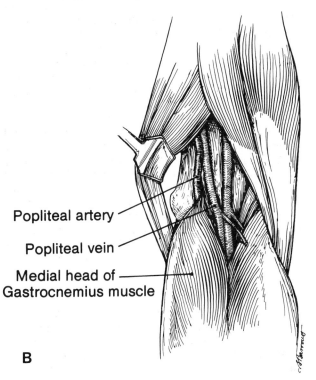

Popliteal artery

Popliteal vein

Medial head of Gastrocnemius muscle

B

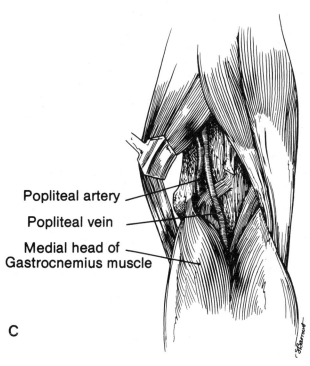

Popliteal artery

Popliteal vein

Medial head of Gastrocnemius muscle

C

Fig. 36-35. Popliteal artery entrapment. *(A)* Type I: pronounced looping of the popliteal artery around the medial head of the gastrocnemius muscle. *(B)* Type II: less pronounced medial course of popliteal artery. *(C)* Type III: compression of popliteal artery beneath an accessory gastrocnemius muscle.

to 69-year-old age group. There may be a slightly higher incidence of infrapopliteal disease in diabetics compared with the nondiabetic population.

ANATOMY

The femoropopliteal segment may be divided into three major sections—the superficial femoral artery segment, the popliteal segment, and the infrapopliteal branches. The superficial femoral artery is the section of the vessel that begins at the takeoff of the profunda femoris and ends at the adductor hiatus. The popliteal artery is a natural extension of the superficial femoral artery and begins below the adductor hiatus; it extends to the soleus arch, at which point the vessel branches. This artery may be further divided into three segments. The first segment extends from the adductor hiatus to the gastrocnemius tunnel and is fixed at both points. Most disease occurs at these fixed points. The high geniculate branches may originate here, but most will branch off higher with connections to the profunda femoris artery. The second segment extends from the gastrocnemius tunnel to the superior aspect of the tibia; and the third segment extends from the superior aspect of the tibia to the soleus arch. Collateral circulation to the popliteal artery segment is scanty. Major collaterals come from the geniculate vessels. The highest geniculate, the terminal branch of the profunda femoris, is the most important. Acute occlusion of the popliteal artery above the highest geniculate artery carries a 20% to 70% primary amputation rate, as seen from World War II experience. The infrapopliteal segments nourish the muscles of the calf as well as the foot. The major branches are the sural arteries, which come off the proximal popliteal artery and provide the major blood supply of the gastrocnemius muscle. One to three arteries may arise close together and may form one branch. They have sparse anastomoses with other muscular vessels of the lower leg and should not be considered a useful collateral pathway. Occlusion or stenosis of the sural artery will cause the classic symptom of intermittent claudication.

The anterior tibial artery crosses the upper edge of the interosseous membrane, enters the anterior compartment, and courses on the surface of the interosseous membrane. It becomes more superficial just above and at the ankle. At the point at which it crosses the ankle joint it becomes the dorsalis pedis artery. The branches of this artery may serve as major collateral pathways in the presence of trifurcation vessel disease. Major branches are the posterior and anterior tibial recurrent arteries, and the anterior medial and lateral malleolar arteries. The anterior tibial recurrent artery is a major collateral pathway between the geniculate arteries and the anterior muscle compartment. The posterior tibial recurrent vessel is of lesser importance and supplies blood mainly to the ligaments and articular structures. The malleolar branches are part of the anastomoses that circle the limb at the malleoli and anastomose with the other two major arteries in the lower leg, forming the major connection with other vessels supplying the plantar area.

The posterior tibial artery is usually considered the direct continuation of the popliteal. It courses from the midpopliteal fossa to a point around the medial malleolus, at which point it becomes superficial and palpable. The posterior tibial artery also forms the arterial arch of the foot and anastomoses with the anterior tibial and peroneal arteries at the malleolar level. The posterior tibial artery also supplies the major nutrient vessels to both the fibula and the tibia.

The peroneal artery is the third member of the popliteal trifurcation and usually branches directly off the posterior tibial artery. There is wide variation in the location of the takeoff of this vessel, and the variation in its location may be of importance in the formation of collateral pathways. At the ankle the peroneal may replace the anterior tibial and produce a dorsalis pedis artery by way of a large perforating branch in 5% of the population. It may also replace the lower posterior tibial artery by way of a communication branch in 2.5% of limbs. The peroneal artery also forms the nutrient artery to the fibula, as well as the calcaneal and numerous anastomotic branches to the posterior and anterior tibial vessels.

LOCATION OF DISEASE

Twenty percent of patients have disease involving a short segment of the superficial femoral or popliteal artery at or near the adductor hiatus. Sixty percent of patients with involvement of the femoropopliteal segment have extensive disease, defined as disease involving the superficial femoral artery from the profunda takeoff to the hiatus. Twenty percent of patients have disease intermediate between the two extremes. Approximately 4% of patients have a combination of disease in the proximal femoral segment and the trifurcation. There is some evidence that diabetics may have a slightly higher incidence of trifurcation involvement than nondiabetics. At least one trifurcation vessel is affected in 65% of diabetics, and two or three vessels are affected in 35%. Fifty percent of patients have severe bilateral extremity involvement.

SIGNS AND SYMPTOMS

The signs and symptoms of femoropopliteal occlusive disease are those of any vascular disease. Claudication involving the calf or thigh is the most common sign. Any involvement of the sural arteries will also produce the classic picture. As occlusive disease progresses, the patient may begin to experience symptoms of rest pain in the area of the metatarsal head or forefoot. Abnormal pulses will be evident upon physical examination, with diminution of pulse volume, evidence of bruits or thrills, or complete absence of pulses.

DIAGNOSIS

History and physical examination remain the cornerstone of the initial evaluation of patients with peripheral vascular disease. It is important always to evaluate inflow, the common femoral artery, and the iliac vessels as well as the more distal vessels. Noninvasive studies, such as the Doppler ultrasound examination with calculation of the API at rest and at exercise, will aid in identification of the severity and extent of the femoropopliteal lesion. Multiplane angiography will give a precise anatomic picture and help the surgeon plan surgical management.

PROGNOSIS

Approximately one third of patients with peripheral vascular disease involving the femoropopliteal segment will demonstrate rapid progression of this process; one third will show slow progress; and one third will remain stable. There is low risk of amputation in those with claudication only, with a 1.5% per year amputation rate for those treated nonsurgically. This rate may be further reduced if the patient stops smoking when the initial diagnosis is made. Patients with claudication alone have an average mortality of 4.5% per year, mostly from cardiac and cerebrovascular disease. The overall survival of those with femoropopliteal disease is approximately 10% higher over a 10-year period than that of those with aortoiliac disease (57% versus 47%), and this rate probably reflects the more severe systemic manifestations of aortoiliac disease.

INDICATIONS AND SELECTION FOR OPERATION

To ensure optimal operative results, patients considered for femoropopliteal reconstruction should have adequate inflow. The common femoral or superficial femoral artery should have a relatively disease-free proximal segment. The patient should also have good runoff, with two to three patent trifurcation vessels to ensure long-term patency of the graft. Approximately 20% of those who come to operation will be in this category. Relative contraindications to vascular reconstruction are combined proximal and distal occlusion with no patent distal vessels and patients who have severe respiratory or cardiac disease.

OPERATIVE CHOICES

Regardless of the operative procedure chosen, all patients undergoing vascular reconstructions involving the lower extremities should have a completion arteriogram before the operation is concluded. This study gives the surgeon a picture of his procedure and allows him to recognize and correct any technical errors before they become limb-threatening or life-threatening problems.

THROMBOENDARTERECTOMY

TEA entails making an arteriotomy over the site of disease and stripping out the diseased intima. The arteriotomy is closed primarily or with a vein or Dacron patch to widen the lumen. TEA is usually indicated for segmental disease of the superficial femoral or popliteal artery but not for smaller vessels because of the problem of luminal stenosis. The advantages of TEA are the short operative time required and the fact that no graft is needed, although a Dacron or vein patch may be used. *Extensive* TEAs usually require large patch grafts to prevent narrowing of the lumen and are technically difficult to perform because they can be tedious and time-consuming. The disadvantages of this procedure are frequent recurrence of the disease (30% over long-term follow-up) and the difficulty of revision. Revision may be so difficult that bypass is usually indicated following recurrence, especially when the lesion is extensive and the outflow poor. There is a risk of embolization if the diseased tissue is not completely stripped from the luminal surface. The success of TEA depends on "feathering" or "tapering" the diseased intima into normal intima. If this is not done, it is necessary to tack down the distal intima with several fine interrupted vascular sutures; otherwise, an intimal flap may result, causing obstruction and resultant thrombosis of the artery.

BYPASS PROCEDURES

Bypass procedures are usually indicated for extensive lesions or when TEA is not practical. Bypass entails taking an autogenous or artificial graft from a patent proximal vessel and placing it on a patent distal vessel, going around the area of obstruction or stenosis. The graft may be placed above or below the knee, either straight (*i.e.*, two points of anastomosis) or in a sequential fashion that entails an end-to-side anastomosis proximally, an intermediate side-to-side anastomosis, and a distal end-to-side anastomosis. These two different bypass techniques are illustrated in Figure 36-36.

The advantages of the bypass procedure are that it is easy to perform, and suitable autogenous vein is available in 85% to 90% of all patients. Recurrence of primary atherosclerosis is rare in the graft itself. The sequential graft has the advantage of two proximal anastomotic sites, both of which tend to increase total graft flow and may help with long-term graft patency. The disadvantages of bypass procedures are that they may be difficult to do and hard to revise if no autogenous vein is available. Other materials such as expanded PTFE, preserved human umbilical vein, and composite grafts made of both plastic and autogenous material have been used but have lower patency rates than those seen with autogenous tissue.

ALTERNATE TREATMENTS

LUMBAR SYMPATHECTOMY

Lumbar sympathectomy was the only operative procedure available before there were any vascular reconstructive techniques for peripheral vascular disease. The rationale for its use was based upon the vasodilation that occurred after the sympathetic constriction fibers were cut. In the presence of severe atherosclerotic or other obliterative vascular disease, there is no place for sympathectomy. There is no substitute for blood flow, and proximal and distal vasodilation will be of no avail if a high-grade stenosis or complete occlusion exists between the proximal and distal circulations. Blood will be shunted away from muscle and to the skin, further compromising an already ischemic extremity. At the present time, there is no real indication or benefit to be derived from the routine use of lumbar sympathectomy for peripheral vascular disease.

TRANSLUMINAL BALLOON ANGIOPLASTY

The transluminal angioplasty or balloon catheter dilatation was first developed by Dotter in the 1960s and further modified by Gruntzig in 1974. The instrument consists of a double-lumen catheter with a cylindrical plastic balloon for dilatation and an injection port for contrast material. This allows an even pressure of approximately 4 to 6 atmospheres to be generated within the balloon and thus within the lumen of the diseased vessel. The catheter is passed percutaneously according to standard angiographic procedure, or it may be used as an adjunct to operative therapy. After placing the catheter tip in the stenotic or occluded segment of the vessel, prestenotic and poststenotic pressures are taken. The balloon catheter is then placed in the stenotic area and inflated for approximately 4 to 6 seconds. The 4 to 6 atmospheres of pressure fracture the intimal plaque and separate it from the media in several places. The media is also stretched beyond its elastic limits, and the attached intima and atheromatous material adhere to it, although intimal fragments may project into the lumen. It is thought that once the media is freed from the constricting effects of the diseased intima, it remains expanded owing to the increased blood flow and that the arterial widening with patency of the vessel is due to this overstretching of the

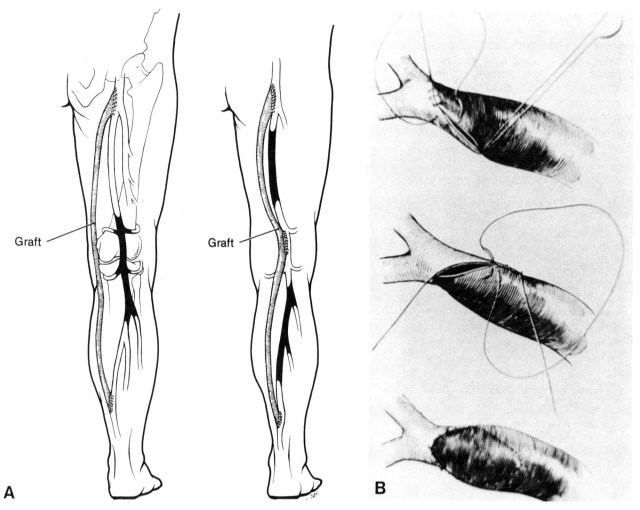

Fig. 36-36. *(A)* Standard *(left)* and sequential *(right)* femoropopliteal bypasses. Note the side-to-side anastomosis to the isolated popliteal segment. *(B)* Spatulated end-to-end anastomosis with continuous suture technique. Important for use in the distal bypass.

muscle fibers. It appears that the diseased intima itself is not expandable and that the success of balloon angioplasty is based upon the elastic properties of the media and adventitia. One study has shown that the increased caliber of arteries following angioplasty is believed to be caused by permanent overstretching of the media and that rupture of the intima and media results in longer-term widening of the arterial lumen.

The advantages of balloon angioplasty are (1) it has a less invasive nature with concurrent smaller risk of mortality and morbidity; (2) functional results should be similar to those seen in surgically treated atherosclerotic lesions; (3) the angioplasty can be repeated with no greater risk to the patient; and (4) if the dilatation fails, surgical options are still available. Enthusiasm for this procedure has led to its application in a wide variety of vascular conditions. Large vessels, such as the aortoiliac segment and common femoral artery, as well as smaller vessels such as those found at the ankle have been dilated in various trials. The balloon catheter has also been used in the coronary circulation as well as in the intracranial and extracranial vessels. At the present time, balloon angioplasty seems to be best suited for dilatation of the large caliber vessels. Patency rates after dilatation have been good, with 85% to 95% still open after 1-year follow-up. Longer-term follow-up is lacking due to the relatively

short time this procedure has been available. It appears that the larger vessels will probably have a 50% to 70% 2-year patency. Smaller vessels such as the superficial femoral, popliteal, and infrapopliteal segments, have decreasing success rates, with approximately 40% to 60% 2-year patency at the ankle, and the recurrence rates are high.

Transluminal angioplasty has also been used in conjunction with vascular reconstructive procedures (concurrent distal or proximal bypass) to augment either inflow or outflow. Initial results have been encouraging, more so with the combined procedure than with either procedure used alone. This holds promise in optimizing results of peripheral vascular construction, though again, long-term follow-up is lacking.

Due to the relatively recent employment of balloon angioplasty, complete guidelines for its use have yet to be established, but certain broad indications can be made. Isolated stenoses of large caliber vessels, such as the iliac and common femoral arteries and even the superficial femoral vessels, appear to be the best locations for use of the balloon. Stenotic lesions may also be dilated in conjunction with a bypass procedure, either proximally or distally, in the hope of augmenting the long-term patency of the graft. Use of the balloon may be indicated for patients who are prohibitive operative risks because of poor cardiopulmonary status. Whether balloon angioplasty should be used for limb salvage in the presence of gangrene is not clear, although it has resulted in effective palliation in some cases. At this time, however, it should not be thought of as a definitive procedure for this condition.

In summary, although percutaneous transluminal angioplasty appears to be an exciting development in vascular reconstruction, we must await the results of long-term studies before making firm comment on the place of this procedure in the vascular surgeon's armamentarium.

RESULTS

GRAFT PATENCY AND LIMB SALVAGE

The standard femoropopliteal (supragenicular) bypass graft using autogenous vein will show a 5-year patency rate of approximately 60% to 70%, with a 75% limb salvage rate. This success appears to be independent of the state of runoff, although an API of less than 20 carries a prohibitive risk of early thrombosis and failure. Infragenicular bypass carries a 5-year patency rate of approximately 40% to 60%, with limb salvage rates for nonsequential grafts of approximately 60%. The success of these grafts does depend upon the state of distal runoff vessels. Sequential grafts carry a 5-year patency rate of approximately 70% to 75%; however, this is based upon the patency of the two proximal anastomoses. The distal segment carries a 5-year patency rate that is identical to that of the nonsequential grafts.

Approximately 80% of patients with failed nonsequential distal grafts and approximately 50% of those with sequential bypass will come to amputation. The difference in amputation rates can be attributed to the increased flow through the middle side-to-side anastomosis, which is felt to increase distal blood flow enough to maintain limb viability despite distal graft thrombosis. If the entire sequential graft is thrombosed, it carries the same amputation risk as that of nonsequential grafts. There is some evidence that a failed distal bypass carries an increased risk for above-the-knee amputation (AKA) versus below-the-knee amputation (BKA) if the primary threat is to the segment below the knee.

The operative mortality for distal bypass ranges from 0.5% to 3%. Long-term analysis shows a 48% mortality at 5 years, which is almost completely due to the complications of systemic atherosclerosis. Only 14.1% of patients undergoing femoropopliteal bypass were alive after 10 years with limbs intact, while only 12% are alive with intact limbs after femorotibial bypass.

PRIMARY AMPUTATION VS. DISTAL RECONSTRUCTION FOR LIMB SALVAGE

More distal reconstructive procedures are done for limb salvage for impending gangrene or nonhealing trophic ulcers than for disabling claudication. For this reason, the failure rate is expected to be higher than that seen with claudication because a higher degree of vascular disease is present. In this setting, early graft failure occurs in 20% to 35% of all patients, with failures of 30% to 50% at 2 years after operation. Seven to ten percent come to amputation despite a patent graft, and less than 50% have significant palliation for 2 years after operation. For this reason, several vascular surgeons have asked whether amputation should be done primarily for impending limb loss, especially with the knowledge that a failed graft may convert a BKA to AKA.

BKA carries an 80% chance of eventual rehabilitation compared with a 50% chance that those with AKA will eventually be able to walk again with a prosthesis. Therefore, before undertaking a distal bypass procedure, the surgeon should consider the whole patient and base his decision upon the status of the limb to be salvaged and the ability of the patient to walk before and after the procedure, as well as his ability to walk if the graft fails. A painful and technically difficult operation should not be performed on a patient for whom there is little hope of ultimate functional recovery or limb salvage. Selection of patients and tailoring of the operation to the individual are of the utmost importance for better results in distal vascular reconstructive procedures.

BIBLIOGRAPHY

Boyd AM: The natural course of atherosclerosis of the lower extremities. Angiology 11:10, 1960

Brewster DC, Darling RC: Optional methods of aortoiliac reconstruction. Surgery 84:739, 1978

Ehrenfeld WK, Wilbur BG, Olcott CN et al: Autogenous tissue reconstruction in the management of infected prosthetic grafts. Surgery 85:82, 1979

Flinn WR, Flanigan D, Berta MJ et al: Sequential femoral tibial bypass for severe limb ischemia. Surgery 88:357, 1980

Fry WJ, Lindenauer SM: Infection complicating the use of plastic arterial implants. Arch Surg 94:190, 1967

Fuchs JCA, Mitchner JS, Hagen P: Postoperative change in autologous vein grafts. Ann Surg 188:1, 1978

Kinlough-Rathbone RL, Mustard JF: Atherosclerosis: Current concepts. Am J Surg 141:638, 1981

Kwann, JHM, Connolly JE: Successful management of prosthetic graft infections with continuous povidone-iodine irrigation. Arch Surg 116:716, 1981

Mitchell RA, Bone GE, Bridges R et al: Patient selection of isolated profundaplasty. Am J Surg 138:912, 1979

O'Mara CS, Neiman HL, Flinn WR et al: Hemodynamic assessment of the transluminal angioplasty for lower extremity ischemia. Surgery 89:106, 1981

Pitt AJ, Postier RG, MacGowan WA: Prophylactic antibiotics in vascular surgery, topical, systemic or both. Ann Surg 192:356, 1980

Reichle FA, Rankin KP, Tyson RR et al: Long-term results of 474 arterial reconstructions for severely ischemic limbs—14-year follow-up. Surgery 85:93, 1979

Rutherford RB: The surgical approach to vascular problems. In Rutherford RB (ed): Vascular Surgery. Philadelphia, W B Saunders, 1977

Spence RK, Freiman DB, Gatenby R et al: Long-term results of transluminal angioplasty of the iliac and femoral arteries. Arch Surg 116:1377, 1981

Stoney RJ: Ultimate salvage for the patient with limb-threatening ischemia: Realistic goals and surgical considerations. Am J Surg 136:228, 1978

Strandness DE: Collateral Circulation in Clinical Surgery. Philadelphia, W B Saunders, 1977

Szilagyi DE, Smith RF, Elliott JP et al: Anastomotic aneurysms after vascular reconstruction: Problems of incidence, etiology and treatment. Surgery 78:800, 1975

Towne JB, Bernhard VM, Rollins DL et al: Profundaplasty in perspective: Limitations in the long-term management of limb ischemia. Surgery 90:1037, 1981

Vollmar J: Reconstructive Surgery of the Arteries. New York, Georg Thieme Verlag, 1980

Whelan TJ: Popliteal entrapment. In Rutherford RB (ed): Vascular Surgery. Philadelphia, W B Saunders, 1977

Wyatt AB, Rothnie NG, Taylor GW: The vascularization of vein grafts. Br J Surg 51:378, 1964

Yao JST: Arterial survey with the Doppler ultrasonic velocity detector. In Rutherford RB (ed): Vascular Surgery. Philadelphia, W B Saunders, 1977

James D. Hardy

Aneurysms of the Aorta and Its Branches

Aneurysms may involve any and all arteries of significant size. The surgical management of large aneurysms represents one of the major success stories of the last 30 years. Beginning primarily with the replacement of an infrarenal aortic aneurysm with a homograft by Dubost in 1951, the treatment of these lesions was rapidly and enormously extended by many surgeons throughout the world and especially by DeBakey and Cooley and their associates. Now, almost every extracranial aneurysm can be resected successfully if the general condition of the patient will permit what at times is a prolonged operation.

Moreover, as the years have passed, the etiology of major true aneurysms has gradually shifted from a significant role of late syphilis to one largely due to atherosclerosis. Other conditions cause a small percentage of true aneurysms, including cystic medial necrosis (Marfan's syndrome), loss of elastic fibers (Ehlers-Danlos syndrome), and infective agents represented by bacteria, fungi, and, perhaps on occasion, viruses. Since atherosclerosis is by far the principal cause of true aneurysms, it is not surprising that the majority of major aneurysms occur in older persons, usually in the sixth or seventh decade of life. Therefore, the patient who needs an operation for aneurysm often has other medical problems, such as hypertension, coronary or cerebrovascular disease, renal impairment, diabetes mellitus, or emphysema due to smoking. These factors must be considered in the timing of any operation and in estimating the prognosis. There is no really effective nonoperative treatment for most aneurysms.

Whereas the true aneurysm, or aneurysm involving usually all layers of the vessel wall, is generally due to atherosclerosis, the false aneurysm, or "pulsating hematoma," has a hole in the arterial wall at some point and is usually caused by trauma or by a leak at an arterial anastomosis. The dissecting aneurysm represents blood forcing its way between layers of the arterial wall, and rupture with fatal hemorrhage is the rule.

The advent of the arterial homograft for clinical use gave great impetus to aneurysm surgery, but even greater dimensions were realized after use of the human allograft, which was always in limited supply, gave way to use of suitable fabric grafts. Dacron is probably by far the most commonly used material, and we have yet to see an aneurysm develop in the graft itself, although of course there will occasionally develop a false aneurysm at one of the anastomoses to the native aorta of the patient. A vein graft may be used to replace aneurysms of smaller arteries such as the arteries of the limbs and of the viscera in the abdomen when a fabric graft is not appropriate.

By and large, the approach to resection of any aneurysm, wherever it may be, is to support the patient adequately, gain adequate anatomical exposure, and then cross-clamp the artery proximal and distal to the aneurysm, open or resect the aneurysm, and place a suitable graft. Meanwhile, however, it may be necessary to provide perfusion of the artery to the involved organ by one means or another, using pump oxygenator, shunt or bypass (or both), or hypothermia temporarily. Otherwise, the concept of aneurysm resection is similar for all aneurysms, no matter what part of the body is involved. Temporary local or total-body heparinization is used on occasion to prevent clotting distally while there is almost static arterial inflow. Actually, there is at least some degree of collateral blood flow to most tissues and organs, and surgeons vary considerably regarding the frequency with which they employ heparinization in specific circumstances.

AORTIC ANEURYSMS

ANEURYSM OF THE SINUS OF VALSALVA

Aneurysm of the aortic sinuses of Valsalva is uncommon. Men are far more commonly involved than women, and the right coronary cusp is the one affected in 95% of cases. The lesion is usually congenital and is much more common in Japan than in Western countries (Fig. 36-37). However, not all aneurysms of the sinus of Valsalva are due to congenital weakness of the wall; some are due to bacterial endocarditis, tuberculosis, or syphilis. The aneurysm may eventually rupture into the right ventricle or right atrium.

CLINICAL MANIFESTATIONS

Unless the aneurysm of the sinus of Valsalva is ruptured, the patient is asymptomatic and has no disability. Diagnosis can be made only accidentally during aortography performed for other reasons. However, when the aortic sinus aneurysm protrudes into the right ventricle with no ventricular septal defect, there may be a systolic murmur produced from partial obstruction of the pulmonary outflow tract by the aneurysm, and this could be diagnosed as pulmonic stenosis.

Once rupture occurs, the symptoms become distinctive. The average age at rupture is 31 years, although a few such instances have been reported in childhood. Rupture usually occurs without known cause and is soon followed by congestive heart failure.

In almost all cases, rupture of the aneurysm is marked by acute right upper quadrant or anginalike pain. Vomiting usually occurs and may confuse diagnostic efforts. Following rupture, there is usually a period of dyspnea on exertion, chest pain, and a feeling of constriction. The symptoms disappear or abate after 24 hours. After the acute phase has passed, symptoms of congestive heart failure become in-

Fig. 36-37. Aneurysm of the sinus of Valsalva: type, frequency, and more common locations. *LCS*, left coronary sinus; *RCS*, right coronary sinus; *NCS*, noncoronary sinus; *vsd*, ventricular septal defect. (Suzuki A: Aneurysm of the sinus of Valsalva. In Hardy JD [ed]: Rhoads Textbook of Surgery, 5th ed. Philadelphia, J B Lippincott, 1977)

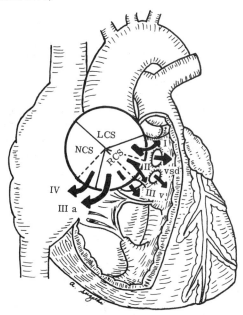

Type	No. of Cases	
	Japan	Western Countries
I	69	19
II	11	7
III a	1	8
III v	3	29
IV	2	29

creasingly severe until death. If the aneurysm ruptures into the right atrium, life expectancy after rupture is about 4 weeks. If the rupture is into the right ventricle, however, much longer survival is possible. In some cases, no acute symptoms are reported.

After rupture of an aneurysm of the sinus of Valsalva, a characteristic heart murmur develops. It may be a continuous murmur or a to-and-fro murmur. The murmur is best heard along the left parasternal border at the third or fourth intercostal space. The murmur is similar to that of the patent ductus arteriosus. However, it is often located somewhat lower than the usual murmur of a patent ductus arteriosus, and there is a somewhat louder component in diastole. Of course, the location of the murmur is greatly dependent upon the point of rupture of the aneurysm. The murmur is unusually superficial in location and is widely transmitted. The intensity of murmur is different from case to case but is usually over grade IV.

Other physical findings are a wide pulse pressure, cardiac enlargement, and pulmonary congestion.

DIFFERENTIAL DIAGNOSIS

The differential diagnosis must exclude patent ductus arteriosus, aortic pulmonary window, aortic valve incompetence, ventricular septal defect, and coronary arteriovenous fistula. Some of the fistulas attributed to rupture of an aortic sinus aneurysm may be formed by anomalous coronary arteries opening directly into an atrium or ventricle. The coronary fistula usually manifests itself soon after birth, whereas aortic sinus aneurysms usually produce symptoms only after rupture later in life.

LABORATORY FINDINGS

The chest roentgenogram may be normal or may give evidence of increased pulmonary blood flow. The right atrium, right ventricle, or left ventricle may appear enlarged, depending on the site of rupture.

A left ventricular hypertrophy or biventricular hypertrophy is seen on the electrocardiogram.

On cardiac catheterization, a left-to-right shunt can be identified at the atrial or ventricular level. In the latter case, there is often a small difference in systolic pressure in the inflow and outflow portions of right ventricle produced by the wind sock of the aneurysm.

Diagnosis is best established by selective aortography, demonstrating the aneurysm itself or the leakage of the dye from the aortic sinus of Valsalva into the involved cardiac chamber.

TREATMENT

Operative correction should be performed as soon as the diagnosis has been established. Without surgical correction, the disease is progressive and soon develops into cardiac failure; this is particularly true in the case of a large rupture of the aneurysm. It may require emergency surgery to cure the patient.

Surgical correction should be undertaken with the aid of extracorporeal circulation. A median sternotomy is the incision of choice. On palpation, the ruptured chamber has the strongest thrill. A right atriotomy or ventriculotomy is performed, avoiding injury to coronary arteries. The ruptured fistulous sac is excised and the opening sutured. The basic object of the operation is to close the defect in the aortic wall at the mouth of the aneurysm by attaching the aortic media superiorly to the aortic ring below. Some

ANEURYSMS IN GENERAL	
Etiology	*True aneurysm:* Atherosclerosis, cystic medial necrosis, and syphilis and other infective or mycotic agents (bacteria, fungi, possibly viruses) *False aneurysm:* (pulsating hematoma): Trauma or anastomotic leak, principally *Greatest hazard:* Rupture with fatal hemorrhage
Dx	History of pain, apparent compression of surrounding structures, possible blood loss, pulsating lump; often asymptomatic Physical examination Plain roentgenograms, sonography, CT scan, arteriography
Rx	Surgical excision with fabric-graft replacement in vast majority of patients; results generally excellent

surgeons prefer a transaortic approach, which permits more precise closure of the defect without injury to the aortic cusp.

However, Suzuki prefers both approaches at the same time. In this way, the complete picture of the ruptured sinus of Valsalva can be visualized and more precise repair performed. In the presence of a large ventricular septal defect, not only are excision and closure of the fistulous sac performed, but also a ventricular septal defect should be closed with a Teflon or Dacron patch (Fig. 36-38).

The hospital mortality, in cases in which the aneurysm ruptures into the right atrium or the right ventricle is in most centers less than 5%, and the results of operation are excellent.

ANEURYSMS OF THE ASCENDING AORTA AND TRANSVERSE ARCH

Aneurysms of the ascending aorta or transverse arch may be asymptomatic or may present with a variety of symptoms,

Fig. 36-38. Surgical repair of ruptured sinus of Valsalva with ventricular septal defect (vsd). *(A)* Ruptured sinus. *(B)* Direct closure of the ruptured sinus and vsd. *(C)* Closure of vsd with a Teflon patch. (Suzuki A: Aneurysm of the sinus of Valsalva. In Hardy JD [ed]: Rhoads Textbook of Surgery, 5th ed. Philadelphia, J B Lippincott, 1977)

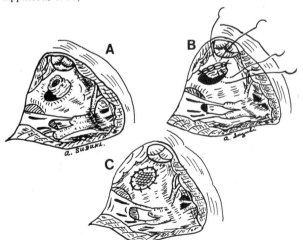

depending upon their etiology, size, location, and site of rupture. The goal of surgical intervention is to resect the aneurysm prior to the occurrence of life-threatening complications. With a combination of current surgical techniques and medical support, most patients can be successfully treated, thus avoiding the serious complications and death that eventually occur in the natural history of the aneurysm.

ETIOLOGY AND INCIDENCE

Atherosclerosis is the most common etiology of aneurysms of the ascending aorta and aortic arch. Their shape is usually fusiform. They occur most commonly in the sixth and seventh decades of life but are occasionally seen at earlier ages. Men are affected more frequently than women, with a ratio reported as high as 9:1. There may be concomitant atherosclerotic aneurysms or occlusive disease in other segments of the aorta or peripheral arterial tree.

Syphilis, reported to be the most common cause of aneurysms of the thoracic aorta in the past, is now seen only rarely. These aneurysms usually develop after 50 years of age and have a predilection for the ascending aorta. Most often the shape is fusiform; however, sacciform aneurysms are not uncommon.

CLINICAL MANIFESTATIONS

Signs and symptoms produced by aneurysms of the aortic arch are secondary to compression, distortion, or erosion of surrounding structures; intramural arterial dissection; and rupture. Aneurysms can become large without producing symptoms.

The most common symptom is pain. This may be sudden in onset, as with acute dissection or rupture, or may develop slowly as the aneurysm gradually expands. Pain or discomfort is usually located in the region of the aneurysm; however, it may radiate to the neck, shoulders, back, or abdomen. Increasing intensity of pain is an ominous sign usually associated with expansion or impending rupture of the aneurysm.

Aortic valvular insufficiency occurs commonly with aneurysms of the ascending aorta from distortion of the valve or annulus. Respiratory difficulty is caused by compression or distortion of the trachea or bronchi. This is sometimes associated with a "brassy" cough. Hoarseness from vocal cord paralysis is produced by stretching of the vagus or recurrent laryngeal nerves. Pressure on the esophagus produces dysphagia. Heart failure is usually associated with aortic valvular insufficiency or an aortointracardiac fistula from intracardiac rupture. Emboli and dissection can produce ischemia to vital organs and structures, resulting in a wide variety of symptoms.

Rupture of the aneurysm most often causes sudden death from hypovolemic shock or cardiac tamponade. Containment of a leaking aneurysm by surrounding structures or an intracardiac rupture occasionally allows time for emergency surgery and salvage of the patient. Patients with nonfatal ruptures may present with a variety of symptoms, depending upon the site of rupture and blood loss. There may be sudden onset of or increase in pain. Hemoptysis results from rupture into the lung or tracheobronchial tree. Hematemesis may occur from communication with the esophagus. Cardiac tamponade develops with intrapericardial rupture. Death from hypovolemic shock or cardiac tamponade will occur unless immediate surgical intervention is instituted. Congenital sinus of Valsalva aneurysms commonly rupture into a cardiac chamber, producing an aortointracardiac fistula and congestive heart failure, which rarely causes sudden death.

DIAGNOSIS

On physical examination, aneurysms of the ascending aorta and aortic arch are usually not detectable. Palpation is only possible if the aneurysm extends above the suprasternal notch or if there is erosion through the thoracic cage. Aortic valvular insufficiency occurs not uncommonly with aneurysms of the ascending aorta and sinus of Valsalva. It may develop acutely in dissecting aneurysms or slowly from progressive annular or valvular distortion. Sudden onset of a continuous murmur in the aortic area with congestive heart failure results from intracardiac rupture of a sinus of Valsalva aneurysm. Peripheral pulses are usually normal but may be delayed, diminished or absent because of distortion or dissection. Left vocal cord paralysis, tracheal deviation, or tug is not uncommon in transverse arch aneurysms.

Plain anteroposterior and lateral roentgenograms of the chest will demonstrate an enlargement of the involved segment of the aorta. If serial roentgenograms are available, one may observe progressive aortic enlargement. Calcification in the wall of the aneurysm may be seen, especially in syphilis and atherosclerosis. A cardiac series with barium swallow is often helpful in identifying and localizing the aneurysm. Ruptured and traumatic aneurysms produce widening of the mediastinum or hemothorax from hemorrhage.

Arteriography is used routinely to establish and confirm the diagnosis and to determine the location and the size of the aneurysm. The most precise method of arteriography is direct arterial catheterization. It provides the best radiologic contrast; in addition, cardiac catheterization and coronary arteriography may be performed when indicated. If proper facilities are not available or if difficulty is encountered in arterial catheterization, a venous angioaortogram may be performed. Arteriography demonstrates a dilated arterial lumen in most aneurysms; however, occasionally, the lumen may appear relatively normal because of laminated clot. When this occurs, one must determine the width of the arterial wall to ascertain whether or not there is an aneurysm. Computerized tomography (CT scan) can be useful. Calcification is helpful when present. In dissecting aneurysms, one looks for the characteristic double lumen, demonstrating the true and false channels. There may be distortion of the aorta and its branches from the dissection. On occasion with acute dissection, the aortogram may appear relatively normal because the false lumen has clotted, allowing no contrast medium to enter the dissection. In acute traumatic aneurysms, extravasation of contrast medium is noted along with distortion of the aorta from the hematoma or laceration. Chronic traumatic aneurysms are well encapsulated and localized. Echo studies are helpful in the diagnosis of dissecting aneurysm and in the estimation of the size of the aneurysm.

TREATMENT

Current methods of medical and surgical treatment of aneurysms of the ascending aorta and aortic arch have significantly altered their grave prognosis (DeBakey).

Medical treatment, except in patients with acute dissecting aneurysms, is limited to stabilization and control of associated illness in preparing the patient for surgery. In acute dissecting aneurysms, medical therpay is directed toward control of hypertension and reduction of the cardiac contractile force with drugs such as propranolol and trimethaphan camsylate (Arfonad). Many patients can be stabilized with this therapy during acute dissection so that surgical intervention may be delayed or avoided. Surgical resection of aneurysms of the ascending aorta and transverse arch is the treatment of choice, except in rare instances when the patient has an associated illness that would result in a prohibitive operative risk.

The timing of the operative intervention will vary with the status of the aneurysm and associated illnesses. In chronic aneurysms, emergency surgery is only necessary when rupture occurs or is suspected to be imminent.

Ascending Aorta

Aneurysms of the ascending aorta and aortic arch are primarily approached through a median sternotomy incision. Extracorporeal cardiopulmonary support is required in virtually all cases. Bypass with Dacron grafts or nonthrombogenic tubing can be employed occasionally, thus avoiding extracorporeal cardiopulmonary bypass. Partial aortic occlusion is possible in some sacciform aneurysms. In patients with ruptured, expanding, or very large aneurysms, the femoral artery and vein should be cannulated prior to performing the median sternotomy so that if rupture has occurred or if it results during dissection, the patient is ready for immediate support and collection of the blood lost while control is obtained.

Aneurysms localized in the ascending aorta are resected and replaced with a tube graft. Occasionally with sacciform and localized dissecting aneurysms, a patch graft is employed. Congenital sinus of Valsalva aneurysms can usually be obliterated with simple sutures through the aorta. When an intracardiac fistula has developed or concomitant aortic valvular insufficiency or ventricular septal defect is present, they are simultaneously repaired (Fig. 36-39).

Aortic Arch

Aneurysms of the transverse arch are preferably exposed through a median sternotomy incision, although occasionally a bilateral anterior thoracotomy through the fourth interspace or a left thoracotomy extension of the median sternotomy is required because of distal extension of the aneurysm into the descending thoracic aorta. Cardiopulmonary bypass and maintenance of cerebral perfusion during the procedure are performed as already outlined. Operative technique is shown in Figure 36-40.

Postoperative Problems

During the postoperative period, a variety of complications may be encountered. The most common include the following: bleeding, cardiac dysfunction from pump failure or arrhythmias, respiratory insufficiency, neurologic deficit (either localized or generalized from emboli or poor perfusion), and renal insufficiency. Postoperative bleeding results in blood loss through the drainage tubes and intrathoracic hematomas, producing an increase in size of the cardiac and mediastinal silhouette. Blood volume and clotting factors should be maintained by blood replacement and the use of specific blood components when indicated. Normothermia is maintained. Reoperation is indicated when there is persistent or massive blood loss.

Cardiac rhythm is controlled with drugs; maintenance of normal pH, Po_2, Pco_2, and electrolytes; and cardiac pacing. Pump failure is treated with cardiotonic drugs, regulation of blood volume, and circulatory assist devices.

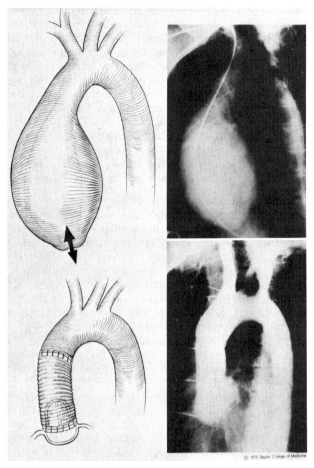

Fig. 36-39. *(Top)* Drawing and preoperative aortogram illustrate a fusiform aneurysm of the ascending aorta with aortic valvular insufficiency. *(Bottom)* Drawing and postoperative aortogram demonstrate a satisfactory appearance following resection of the aneurysm of the ascending aorta and aortic valve and replacement with a prosthetic aortic valve and Dacron graft. Cardiopulmonary bypass is required for replacement of the aortic valve and ascending aorta. (DeBakey ME, Noon GP: Aneurysms of the ascending aorta and transverse arch. In Hardy JD [ed]: Rhoads Textbook of Surgery, 5th ed. Philadelphia, J B Lippincott, 1977)

PROGNOSIS

The outlook for patients with aneurysms of the thoracic aorta has changed dramatically with the advances in surgical and medical management that have occurred in the past 20 years.

The natural history of aneurysms is eventual rupture and death. The average survival from the time of diagnosis in patients with thoracic aneurysms was 6.3 to 8.9 months in Kampmeier's study of 596 patients. Mortality rates in acute dissecting aneurysms in a study by Hirst was 75% within 2 weeks of onset and 93% after 1 year. Only about 20% of patients with traumatic aneurysms survive long enough to receive medical attention.

Surgical treatment of aneurysms of the thoracic aorta provides salvage for most patients who previously would have died of rupture of the aneurysm. There has been a marked reduction in operative mortality with refinement of surgical techniques and preoperative and postoperative management. The operative mortality rate is close to 10% for aneurysms of the ascending aorta and between 15% and 20% with transverse arch aneurysms. Operative risk is increased in those patients with hypertension and associated heart disease. The result of follow-up studies extending over 15 years in patients treated with operation is very gratifying. Postoperative complications such as false aneurysms and aneurysms of homografts can be avoided with the use of Dacron sutures and a Dacron arterial prosthesis. These patients should be examined at yearly intervals following surgery. Occasionally, a patient may develop a second aneurysm or occlusive disease in another segment of the arterial tree. Atherosclerotic coronary artery disease has been the most common cause of death during the follow-up period.

ANEURYSMS OF THE DESCENDING THORACIC AORTA

Aneurysms of the descending thoracic aorta are second only to infrarenal abdominal aneurysms in incidence. Such aneurysms are usually due to atherosclerosis, but they may be due to aortic dissection in association with hypertension, to trauma, or—rarely, in recent years—to syphilis. Cystic medial necrosis is an additional cause. This discussion centers upon atherosclerotic aneurysms.

Aneurysms of the thoracic aorta are found principally in the sixth, seventh, and eighth decades of life. Although they are found most commonly in men, they are not uncommon in women.

PATHOLOGY

The majority of these atherosclerotic aneurysms begin just distal to the left subclavian artery and may extend for only several centimeters, or they may involve the entire thoracic aorta and even enter the abdomen to involve the major visceral arteries of the abdominal aorta. They are usually fusiform, but they may be saccular. In contrast to abdominal aortic aneurysms, which most often cause death by rupture, thoracic aneurysms expand slowly and do not usually rupture as early in their course. Thus, thoracic aneurysms may cause symptoms or death by compression of surrounding structures such as the trachea and esophagus. In contrast to atherosclerotic aneurysms, syphilitic aneurysms are more often saccular and are more likely to enlarge rapidly and to cause death by rupture and exsanguination. Bone erosion is less common with fusiform atherosclerotic aneurysms than with syphilitic aneurysms.

DIAGNOSIS

Symptoms

The symptoms of an aneurysm of the descending thoracic aorta usually include pain or minor effects of compression of surrounding organs, or both. For example, the patient may complain of nonproductive brassy cough, stridor, and dyspnea due to compression of the bronchus, or to dysphagia caused by compression of the esophagus, or to hoarseness due to stretching of the left recurrent laryngeal nerve by enlargement of the aneurysm. However, the most common symptom is pain, due either to bone erosion or to stretching and compression of surrounding tissues. If the aneurysm erodes into a bronchus, hemoptysis may result. Hemoptysis may recur a number of times before a major hemorrhage results in massive blood loss and either drowning or exsanguination. At other times, the lung parenchyma may be eroded. In fact, it is common for the lung to be stuck tightly to the aneurysm and occasionally to form a portion of the wall of the aneurysm, buttressing the clot to prevent free

Fig. 36-40. Technique for resection and graft replacement of aneurysm of the transverse arch using temporary bypass with Dacron grafts to maintain cerebral and aortic perfusion. *(a)* Aneurysm of the transverse arch with normal proximal ascending aorta. *(b)* Bypass graft from the ascending aorta to the descending thoracic aorta and attachment of the bifurcation graft for perfusion of the innominate and left common carotid arteries. *(c)* Anastomosis to the innominate and left common carotid arteries illustrating a temporary shunt in the left common carotid artery. *(d)* The shunt is removed prior to completion of the anastomosis. *(e)* The aneurysm is resected and *(f)* replaced with a Dacron graft. *(g)* The innominate, left common carotid, and left subclavian arteries are anastomosed to the graft. *(h)* The bypass grafts are transected and oversewn when all anastomoses are completed. (DeBakey ME, Noon GP: Aneurysms of the ascending aorta and transverse arch. In Hardy JD [ed]: Rhoads Textbook of Surgery, 5th ed. Philadelphia, J B Lippincott, 1977)

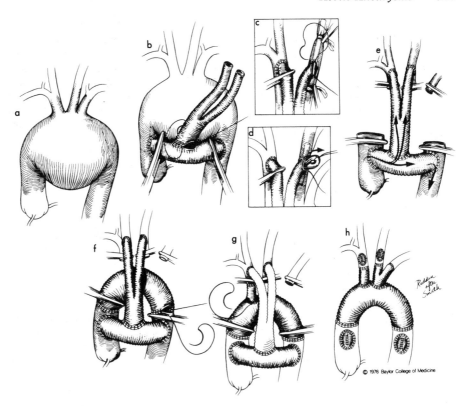

hemorrhage (Fig. 36-41). For this reason, it is always wise to gain control of the aorta both above and below the aneurysm prior to dissecting the lung free.

A considerable number of atherosclerotic aneurysms of the descending aorta are asymptomatic and are discovered on a routine chest roentgenogram. A wide variety of bizarre symptoms have occurred secondary to rupture of these aneurysms in various directions.

Fig. 36-41. Saccular aneurysm of the descending thoracic aorta. The aneurysm is readily visible on the lateral roentgenogram. This patient presented with intermittent hemoptysis, owing to aortobronchial fistula.

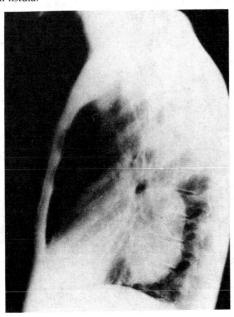

Physical Examination

The majority of aneurysms of the descending thoracic aorta do not produce changes that can be detected on physical examination. However, occasionally the aneurysm may produce a bruit, perhaps associated with thrombus within the aneurysm, and occasionally it may encroach on the left subclavian artery and cause a reduction in blood pressure in the left arm as compared with the right arm.

In most instances, however, an aneurysm of the descending thoracic aorta does not produce obvious physical signs, unless an element of dissection in a previously existing atherosclerotic aneurysm occurs. In such an instance, the dissection could extend all the way to the femoral arteries and result in diminished femoral pulses or, if proximal dissection occurs, in diminished pulses of the great vessels of the arch of the aorta. At times one may experience difficulty in determining at operation whether the aneurysm represents a chronic dissecting aneurysm or extensive dissection in a previously existing atherosclerotic aneurysm.

Laboratory Findings

The diagnosis of aneurysm of the descending thoracic aorta is usually apparent on plain anteroposterior and lateral roentgenograms of the chest. The diagnosis is facilitated if calcification is seen in the wall of the aneurysm; otherwise, the usual differential diagnosis of mediastinal masses must be considered. The diagnosis is usually made definitively with an aortogram, but the aortogram can be misleading if the aneurysm is partially filled with thrombus as it usually is. Not only does aortography disclose the presence of the aneurysm, but it also identifies the probable overall dimensions and especially whether or not the great vessels of the aortic arch are involved. Echo studies and CT scan can be helpful.

TREATMENT

The treatment of aneurysms of the descending thoracic aorta is surgical. Preoperative measures include a careful evaluation of the function of other organs, including the heart, lungs, and kidneys, since, as has been seen, atherosclerosis is a generalized disease and commonly has affected to varying degrees the arterial supply to most other organs. The aortogram itself would generally have disclosed the presence or absence of significant stenosis of the great vessels of the aortic arch and their major branches. Inasmuch as myocardial infarction, pulmonary dysfunction, and renal insufficiency represent the major postoperative complications, the decision in regard to operative intervention is of necessity influenced by the functional reserve of these important organs.

The operative technique employed in the resection of aneurysms of the descending thoracic aorta is shown in Figure 36-42.

Localized aneurysms of the descending thoracic aorta are now resected with much confidence and a high success rate. This current state of affairs has been achieved, first, through additional experience, second, through the use of a nonthrombogenic bypass shunt without heparinization, and third, by backing of the aortic side of the suture line with Teflon felt or some other suitable type of fabric. Crawford no longer uses a shunt, either external or internal, in the resection of thoracic and thoracoabdominal aneurysms, and he reports his results equal to or better than those achieved when he did use a shunt or bypass.

The postoperative complications are relatively few but involve the usual problems of pulmonary embolism, respiratory dysfunction, and myocardial infarction, as well as paraplegia and hepatic and renal failure. Other than respiratory insufficiency and myocardial infarction, complications are uncommon. In our experience, there is rarely any difficulty with the graft itself.

Fig. 36-42. Insertion of a woven Dacron graft within the sac of the thoracic aneurysm. Note suturing of intercostal arteries from within the aneurysm. The temporary bypass is readily removed after the aneurysm has been resected. Teflon felt backing of the aortic wall adds considerable strength to the suture line, and heparinization is not used except by those surgeons who still prefer to use a pump with left heart bypass. Other surgeons use no bypass.

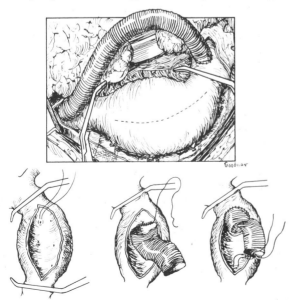

ANEURYSMS OF THE THORACOABDOMINAL AORTA

Thoracoabdominal aneurysms may arise anywhere in the thoracic aorta and extend into the abdomen to involve the various branches of the abdominal aorta. These aneurysms are rare; the overwhelming majority of aneurysms of the abdominal aorta arise below the renal arteries. In fact, no more than 5% of abdominal aortic aneurysms extend to involve the renal arteries. The majority of thoracoabdominal aneurysms are due to atherosclerosis, with the occurrence of syphilitic aneurysms now rare. The principal significance of the thoracoabdominal aneurysm, as opposed to the aneurysm of the descending thoracic aorta or of the infrarenal aorta, is that the thoracoabdominal aneurysm may involve some or all of the major visceral branches of the abdominal aorta, including the celiac, superior mesenteric, and both renal arteries. This presents technical difficulties in the resection of the aneurysm, with the concurrent risk of ischemic damage to the liver, intestine, kidneys, and spinal cord.

The largest experience with the excision of thoracoabdominal aneurysms has been that of Crawford and DeBakey and their associates. Atherosclerosis was the cause of the majority of the aneurysms in their patients. Men predominated over women in a ratio of 8:1.

We prefer a thoracoabdominal incision for exposure of the lower thoracic aorta and the upper abdominal aorta. A stepwise progression of vascular anastomoses is then carried out, either as shown in Figure 36-43 or by placing the fabric graft within the aneurysm sac, with the various vessels then sewn to the graft. Rob, in an early report of resections of

Fig. 36-43. Aortogram shows fabric graft and abdominal arteries. This study was made almost 2 years following resection of aneurysm. (Hardy JD, Timmis HH, Saleh SS et al: Thoraco-abdominal aortic aneurysm: Simplified surgical management with case report. Ann Surg 166:1008, 1967)

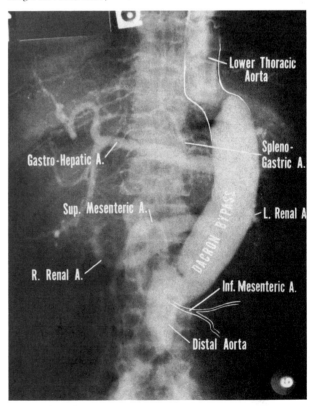

the abdominal aorta and its major branches, found three patients in whom the celiac axis and superior mesenteric artery were occluded prior to operation.

The multiple anastomoses required for the resection of a thoracoabdominal aneurysm that involves the major visceral branches of the abdominal aorta represent a significant surgical undertaking, but the operation may be fully justified. The thoracoabdominal aneurysm has the same propensity for complications as do aneurysms elsewhere: It may gradually enlarge, compress surrounding structures, and eventually rupture. However, in years past, when resectional therapy for these extensive lesions had not yet been developed, we observed that some patients with thoracoabdominal aneurysms remained relatively asymptomatic for several years. Therefore, although lesions of significance should be resected in most patients, we may temporize with an elderly and otherwise poor-risk patient whose aneurysm is asymptomatic, especially a patient with limited renal function.

The reported series of resected thoracoabdominal aneurysms are still not numerous, and it is somewhat difficult to state precisely the overall operative mortality rate. Crawford's operative mortality rate is now only about 10% to 15%, but it would be misleading to suggest that is the average operative mortality rate for the United States as a whole. This is a formidable operation and is not to be undertaken by the occasional vascular surgeon.

DISSECTING THORACIC ANEURYSM

PATHOLOGY

Dissecting aneurysm is a common vascular catastrophe in which blood escapes into the arterial media, usually through a readily discernible intimal fracture. The intramural hematoma, propelled by systemic arterial pressure, pursues a course within the vascular wall determined as to direction and extent by various factors that include the cohesive strength of the media, the level of arterial blood pressure, the rate of acceleration of arterial pulse pressure, and the tendency of the blood to clot. A useful classification scheme introduced by DeBakey is shown in Figure 36-44. Type 1 dissections originate in the ascending aorta, and the false lumen extends beyond the aortic arch, often to the femoral arteries or beyond. Type 2 aneurysms are similar in origin but do not extend beyond the origin of the head vessels. Type 3 dissections originate distal to the left subclavian artery. About 70% of dissections are type 1 or 2, 25% are type 3, and the remainder originate in the transverse arch or distal aorta. The splitting of the media necessary to the development of dissecting aneurysm is promoted by the degenerative changes called cystic medial necrosis. This process may occur as a congenital connective tissue defect in Marfan's syndrome, or it may be the result of vascular wall fatigue, becoming more noticeable with increasing age and under such circumstances of increased stress as poststenotic turbulence and severe hypertension. More recently, dissecting aneurysms of the aorta have often been referred to simply as ascending to the arch and descending beyond this level.

In susceptible persons, hypertension and rapid rise in systolic pressure are important precipitating causes. Intimal fractures tend to occur at areas of greatest intimal shear stress: in the ascending aorta and immediately distal to the left subclavian artery. The fracture is usually transverse but may be spiral or even linear in the longitudinal axis. As the

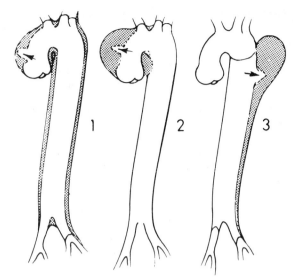

Fig. 36-44. Classification of dissecting aneurysms according to site of origin and extent of hematoma. Type 1 originates in the ascending aorta and extends beyond the arch. Type 2 has ascending aorta origin but does not extend beyond the arch. Type 3 begins in the descending thoracic aorta, usually quite near the left subclavian artery. (Collins JJ: Dissecting thoracic aneurysm. In Hardy JD [ed]: Rhoads Textbook of Surgery, 5th ed. Philadelphia, J B Lippincott, 1977)

hematoma progresses distally and proximally from the intimal tear, it rarely involves the entire aortic circumference but rather proceeds in a spiral column occupying 45 to 270 degrees. If the column intersects a branch origin, the hematoma may extend into the tributary or block it by intimal compression, thereby producing a complex of symptoms dependent upon the site and severity of the peripheral organ ischemia that results.

CLINICAL MANIFESTATIONS

Patients with acute dissecting aneurysm characteristically describe instantaneous onset of severe substernal or interscapular pain, sometimes perceived as a ripping or tearing sensation, which may radiate into the back, neck, abdomen, legs, or arms as the hematoma progresses. Although most victims are 40 to 60 years of age, the disease may occur from childhood to senility. Men are affected three times more frequently than women. Persistence of severe pain usually signifies extension of the hematoma. Manifestations of peripheral organ ischemia appear as the lumina of major arterial branches become narrowed by the expanding intramural blood column. Neurologic symptoms may occur in 20% to 40% of patients as a result of ischemia of the brain or spinal cord. Syncope, seizures, paresthesias, or paralysis may be noted. However, symptoms of limited dissection may be minimal.

Involvement of limb vessels may produce a pulseless extremity with coolness, pallor, and pain more often in the arms than in the legs. The mesenteric vessels may be compromised with severe abdominal pain and signs of ischemic ileus. Bilateral renal ischemia is uncommon, although one renal artery is often obstructed. If the hematoma proceeds proximally into the base of the aorta, additional problems may develop. The aortic valve attachments may be displaced, allowing prolapse of the cusps, thus causing moderate to massive aortic insufficiency. Either the coronary artery origins may be compressed as the hematoma surrounds them or the dissection may extend into these vessels, producing arrhythmias or the electrocardiographic signs of myocardial ischemia or infarction.

The high-pressure hematoma in the aortic base often extends into the subepicardial fat, particularly over the pulmonary outflow tract, and may rupture into the pericardial sac. A small leak produces a pericardial friction rub, while larger escaped quantities may result in fatal cardiac tamponade.

DIAGNOSIS

Although the diagnosis of dissecting aneurysm may be established on the basis of signs and symptoms, aortography is desirable in most cases for localizing the intimal tear and determining the extent of the hematoma. The chest roentgenogram will often demonstrate widening of the mediastinum, sometimes of remarkable degree. If widening is confined to the descending aorta, a type 3 dissection may be suspected, as shown in Figure 36-44. Contrast material may be introduced by intravenous injection as multiple films are obtained, to record the aortic contour during passage of the dye; more commonly, multiple films may be taken as dye is injected through a catheter passed retrograde in the aorta from a puncture in the femoral artery. The safety of retrograde arterial catheterization is satisfactory in expert hands. The films should demonstrate the site of origin and extent of the intimal tear, as well as the size of the intramural hematoma in some cases. CT scan may confirm.

TREATMENT

There are two approaches to the management of dissecting aneurysm that may favorably alter the dismal outlook of the natural history of this disease. These are surgical repair or resection of the intimal tear with reestablishment of aortic continuity and aortic valve competence, and hypotensive medical treatment directed toward limiting the extent of hematoma progression short of life-endangering complications (Fig. 36-45).

Medical

In 1965, Wheat and associates introduced the first carefully planned medical therapeutic protocol based upon alteration of the pathophysiological mechanisms responsible for progression of the hematoma. They reasoned that most acute deaths were caused by progression of the hematoma rather than the intimal tear and that pressure differentials along the vascular wall, as well as the contour of the pressure pulse, were the important factors determining the extent of dissection. A program of drug therapy for reduction of blood pressure and broadening the pressure pulse contour was devised as follows. The patient is placed in a surgical intensive care unit with monitoring of electrocardiogram, blood pressure, and urinary output. Intravenous infusion of 1 mg to 2 mg/minute of trimethaphan camsylate is used for initial blood pressure control and may be continued for 24 to 48 hours. Because of rapid tachyphylaxis and the need for prolonged blood pressure control, reserpine and propranolol are begun by intramuscular injection within a few hours. Guanethidine sulfate, 25 mg to 50 mg, is given orally twice each day. Propranolol is used to reduce the rate of rise of systolic pressure.

With this program, it should be possible to bring hypertension under control quite readily, achieving systolic levels of around 100 mm Hg if cerebral function and urine output are not adversely affected. A very important facet of phar-

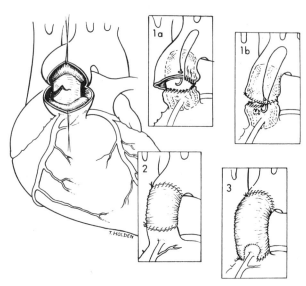

Fig. 36-45. The bulging adventitia is opened to show intima of normal diameter, as seen in many acute ascending dissections. *(1a)* Oversewing the "sandwich" of intima, cloth, and adventitia. *(1b)* Anastomosis of the reinforced aorta. *(2)* Sleeve replacement of ascending aorta above the coronary arteries. *(3)* Pedicled-patch coronary placement with proximal prosthetic graft aortic replacement. The aortic valve may have to be replaced if it cannot be repaired. (Collins JJ: Dissecting thoracic aneurysm. In Hardy JD [ed]: Rhoads Textbook of Surgery, 5th ed. Philadelphia, J B Lippincott, 1977)

macological management is periodic assessment of therapeutic success. The disappearance of pain is considered to indicate lack of progression of the hematoma. Frequent recording of peripheral pulses is extremely important, and a chest roentgenogram should be obtained every 12 hours until it is certain that the mediastinal width is stable.

If upon admission the patient shows no hypertension, Wheat recommends the use of reserpine or propranolol to reduce the cardiac contractile force and thereby flatten the aortic pressure pulse contour.

Failure of pharmacologic therapy is indicated by failure to control pain within 4 hours, development of significant aortic insufficiency, symptomatic compromise of aortic branches, adventitial rupture, or development of an acute saccular area in the aneurysm. In those patients who achieved a chronic phase, surgical intervention was necessary in about 25% for correction of aortic insufficiency, saccular aneurysm, or symptomatic compromise of a major arterial branch.

Contraindications to medical management of dissecting aneurysm include the signs of pharmacologic failure just described and which, in Collins' experience, precluded hypotensive therapy in 26 of 31 patients with ascending dissection seen since 1963. Recently reported results of early definitive surgical repair for ascending aorta dissection show a clear advantage over medical management.

Surgical

The goals of surgical treatment may be outlined as (1) resection of the intimal tear of origin, (2) restoration of aortic integrity to ensure visceral perfusion through normal channels, (3) restoration of aortic valve competence, and (4) reconstruction of the aortic root and sinuses of Valsalva to prevent late aneurysm formation (Figs. 36-45 and 36-46).

Patients with dissecting aneurysms have fragile aortic walls that tend to bleed rather easily, particularly from suture lines. It is well to use as few suture lines as possible and to keep all of them within easy view of the surgeon when cardiopulmonary bypass has been terminated.

Dissecting aneurysms involving the descending aorta most frequently originate at or just distal to the origin of the left subclavian artery. The surgical approach is through a left thoracotomy, and in most instances it is necessary to use venoarterial or left atrial femoral bypass to maintain flow in the distal aorta when the midportion of the aorta between the subclavian artery and the diaphragm is cross-clamped. A simple tubular shunt may occasionally suffice. The general principles of operation are the same as for the ascending aorta (Fig. 36-45). That is, the area of intimal tear should be resected or a cloth-lined repair with over-sewing of the cut ends of the aorta should be performed and aortic continuity reestablished. Because of the unhandy position of the origin of these aneurysms and because of the large size of the surrounding hematoma that may be often encountered, resection of dissecting aneurysm of the descending aorta may be in fact more difficult than operations of the ascending aorta, where the entire anatomy is more easily exposed. When necessary for increased exposure, the sternum may be transected to obtain a better view of the entire aortic arch and great vessels. Cloth-graft interposition after cloth lining of the false lumen and oversewing the aortic edges is usually required, although primary anastomosis of the reinforced oversewn edges may occasionally be possible.

An interesting new surgical technique for dissection aneurysms is that of Carpentier and co-workers (Fig. 36-46).

Care of patients following repair of dissecting aneurysms is entirely similar to that for patients after other major cardiac surgery, except that control of hypertension is of paramount importance. Bleeding is the most common complication and may be virtually uncontrollable from suture lines if hypertension is severe. Collins used the program advocated by Wheat for medical treatment of acute dissections and, with monitoring of left atrial and systemic arterial pressures, found it both safe and efficacious in postoperative management.

After discharge of the patient from the hospital, control of hypertension remains the cornerstone of successful management. In many patients, abnormal degeneration of the media is widespread and new dissection is a continuing threat. Recurrent dissection after surgery is less common than might be expected but may be devastating when it occurs. In Collins' series of 27 patients followed up to 12 years after surgery, only one recurrence was noted, and it occurred in the descending aorta 5 years after ascending aorta replacement in a patient with Marfan's syndrome.

PROGNOSIS

Untreated cases of dissecting aneurysm have an extremely poor prognosis. In a series of 963 collected cases reported by Anagnostopoulos and associates in 1972, 83% of the patients were dead within 1 month and only 8% survived 1 year after onset. Those who do survive often require later surgery for chronic aortic insufficiency or local saccular aneurysms as the adventitia expands. In unusual instances, the acute symptoms of dissection may pass unnoticed, and patients may present *de novo* with late complications. Chronic dissecting aneurysm must be suspected in the patient with noncalcific aortic insufficiency associated with gross aortic root dilatation.

TRAUMATIC RUPTURE OF THE THORACIC AORTA

The most characteristic traumatic rupture of the thoracic aorta is that which results from motor vehicle or other deceleration injury. The lesion is usually situated just distal to the left subclavian artery at the level of the ligamentum arteriosum. However, the aorta may be injured at any level, and the anatomical pathology may consist of free rupture, contained false aneurysm covered only by pleura, or even true aneurysm if the aortic wall or a portion thereof remains

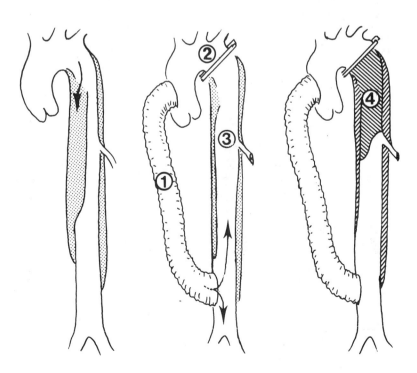

Fig. 36-46. Concept of flow reversal and thromboexclusion of aortic dissection. *(1)* A Dacron graft is placed so as to bypass the dissected aorta. *(2)* A permanent clamp is placed at the upper limit of the dissection. *(3)* Flow reversal in the descending aorta restores blood flow in the true lumen and reduces the size and extent of the false lumen. *(4)* Thrombosis in the false lumen and in the segment of the aorta devoid of major branches. (Carpentier A, Deloache A, Fabiani JN et al: New surgical approach to aortic dissection: Flow reversal and thromboexclusion. J Thorac Cardiovasc Surg 81:659, 1981)

intact. Other causes of aneurysms of the thoracic aorta include atherosclerosis, dissection (which usually occurs with hypertension, cystic medial necrosis, or Marfan's syndrome), and syphilis, which is becoming rare. Traumatic rupture and aneurysm formation in the thoracic aorta are being diagnosed with increasing frequency, perhaps the result of rapid transportation of the injured patient to a hospital and also of a high index of suspicion and immediate diagnosis of the lesion through chest roentgenography and aortography. It has been estimated that 10% to 15% of all automobile fatalities are associated with rupture of the aorta.

PATHOLOGY

Penetrating injuries to the aorta with associated true or false aneurysms are also considered in connection with arterial injuries. Moreover, the aorta or even more peripheral arteries may be ruptured by compression injury. Nevertheless, the substantial majority of deceleration injuries to the aorta result in the characteristic lesion just distal to the origin of the left subclavian artery, leaving a segment of normal aorta distal to the subclavian with which to complete a proximal anastomosis (Fig. 36-47). Multiple aneurysms are occasionally encountered.

The patient who reaches the hospital alive (20% of the total) will usually have an incomplete rupture of the aorta, at least initially. That is, the intima and media may be completely transected and retracted, with only the adventitia and parietal pleura preventing exsanguination into the left hemithorax. At times the intimal tear involves only a portion of the aortic wall and does not involve the entire circumference. When all layers except the adventitia have separated, it is apparent that only a very thin layer remains to prevent fatal hemorrhage. Thus, death will occur in the great majority of patients unless operative intervention is forthcoming. On the other hand, occasionally—and especially with a tear that involves only a portion of the

Fig. 36-47. Typical traumatic rupture of the aorta just distal to the left subclavian artery. The possibility of aortic or other great vessel intimal tear or free rupture should be suspected when the chest roentgenogram shows widening of the mediastinum, first-rib fracture, loss of aortic outline, pulse deficit, tracheal shift, loss of clear space between the aorta and pulmonary artery, or obliteration of the medial aspect of the left upper lobe. Diagnosis is established by aortogram.

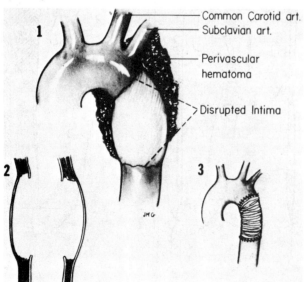

circumference of the aorta—an aneurysm may form and may actually persist for weeks, months, or years without rupture. In general, however, the blunt injury or deceleration traumatic rupture of the thoracic aorta represents an emergency of the first order, in which expeditious diagnosis and surgical management are required for routine salvage. Prompt operation does result in a successful outcome in most instances, if the patient is not already in deep shock due to bleeding into the thorax or to other traumatic injuries.

A major problem associated with blunt thoracic aortic rupture is various other injuries that may also have been sustained, among these being injury to the heart, head trauma, flail chest, intra-abdominal organ rupture, long-bone fractures, and still other problems. These other factors will influence the circumstances surrounding the diagnosis and repair of the aortic injury.

The accepted explanation for the fact that aortic rupture most commonly occurs at the level of the ligamentum arteriosum is that the aorta is fixed here, below which the aorta is more mobile and moves forward at the instant of impact. However, the aorta may be injured anywhere from the aortic valve to the aortic bifurcation. Moreover, the aortic tear may be asymptomatic at the time of injury, only to cause sudden death days later from hemorrhage into the thorax or pericardial tamponade.

Usually, the tear in the aorta is transverse; occasionally, it may take other forms. The transverse tear, especially if incomplete, lends itself readily to repair without graft replacement, and here Teflon-felt backing of the sutures may be useful. Since motor vehicle deceleration accidents most often involve younger persons, the aorta is readily repaired because atherosclerosis is essentially absent in this group. Aortic wall dissection can occur with traumatic injury as with other types of aortic disorders, but in our experience it has been rare.

NATURAL HISTORY

As has been indicated, rupture of the aorta represents an emergency of the first order, since death from exsanguination is the rule unless operative intervention is prompt. In a series of 275 aortic injury patients analyzed by Parmley and associates, 70% had associated heart injury. There was no correlation between the extent of aortic disruption—that is, partial versus complete transection of the intima and media—and the mortality rate. Fourteen percent of all patients survived the initial injury. Isolated rupture of the aorta was associated with a 20% initial survival rate, whereas combinations of heart and aortic injury were associated with only 4% initial survival rate. Thus, 90% of the patients died immediately of exsanguination, whereas in 10% to 20% the aortic tear was controlled temporarily by the aortic adventitia or the parietal pleura, as discussed previously. Parmley and co-workers found that 66% of the patients who survived the initial injury died within 2 weeks of aortic rupture, 82% died within 3 weeks, and 90% died within 10 weeks. Clearly, a high index of suspicion is essential for salvage of a significant proportion of patients with traumatic injury of the thoracic aorta.

It is rare that a patient with severe major transection injury of the aorta will survive to permit the formation of a false aneurysm, although this does occur. If weeks and months are permitted for the development of the false aneurysm, it may eventually cause symptoms due to compression of surrounding structures, distal embolization, or indeed from late rupture of the lesion.

DIAGNOSIS

The possibility of rupture of the thoracic aorta should be considered in every patient who has sustained major deceleration injury, as should cardiac and other injuries. The hallmark of injury to the aortic arch or the descending thoracic aorta is a widening of the mediastinal shadow. Some surgeons consider this finding to be pathognomonic of aortic rupture, and they perform operation without further study. However, in our experience, a widening of the mediastinum on x-ray film has not invariably indicated aortic injury. Therefore, since these patients commonly have serious injuries to other areas of the body, rendering them less than optimal operative risks to begin with, we prefer to accept the brief delay required for emergency aortography, to confirm the presence of aortic injury and also its location. Multiple sites of aortic injury may exist, and the aortographic evidence of aortic or great vessel injury can be very subtle. If an aortic tear is missed and thus not repaired, death will commonly ensue.

Suggestive evidence of aortic injury is to be found in a bloody pleural effusion, but this may well have come from rib or lung injuries. For a firm diagnosis, aortography is required.

TREATMENT

The possibility of aortic injury is suspected from the nature of the blunt trauma and further suggested by widening of the mediastinal shadow on chest roentgenogram. With this evidence at hand, it is wise to prevent hypertension by pharmacologic means in such a patient until the emergency aortography has been performed. Meanwhile, blood should be typed and cross-matched for operation and the operating room prepared, to which the patient is moved immediately after the aortogram has identified the presence and location of the aortic injury. The pump oxygenator should be available but will not usually be required.

Most surgeons prefer to use some type of perfusion of the lower portion of the body while the thoracic aorta is cross-clamped for the repair of the aortic injury. In 1957, Gerbode and co-workers first used extracorporeal left heart bypass for resection and grafting of the thoracic aneurysm. This technique required heparinization, but it represented a significant advance. Later, a simple bypass shunt from the aorta above to the aorta distally was used, without heparinization. The nonthrombogenic tubing is now widely employed. This modification avoided the use of both a pump, with its deleterious effect on blood clotting elements, and heparinization, and it resulted in a reduced mortality. At present, most surgeons prefer to use a bypass without heparin while the aorta is cross-clamped (see Fig. 36-42). Others, however, cross-clamp the aorta and proceed with repair, using neither shunt nor hypothermia; they maintain that the incidence of neurologic, renal, and hepatic complications due to ischemia is the same whether a shunt is used or not.

A transverse repair using Teflon felt backing and synthetic sutures is carried out; in the event that the entire intima and the media have been transected and have retracted over a distance of several centimeters, a Dacron graft is usually inserted, although this is not always required. The repair is straightforward and almost invariably satisfactory.

PROGNOSIS

If the patient reaches the operating room before significant shock has developed, the repair of the aortic injury is usually successful. With the use of a bypass, we have had no spinal cord damage, nor has there been any significant lasting dysfunction of the abdominal organs such as the liver, kidney, or intestine. The bypass must function well, however, and this is ensured by monitoring urine output and femoral artery pressure. We know of two instances of paraplegia in patients in whom a bypass shunt was not employed, but factors other than failure to use a bypass may, of course, have played a role in the causation of the paraplegia. Good results are achieved without a shunt. Teflon felt backing of the suture lines may be useful.

In general, late complications from the insertion of the fabric graft into the aorta have been rare, but all fabric materials are prone to some degree of eventual deterioration. Nevertheless, considering the dire emergency that exists at the time the graft is inserted when necessary, late fabric complications are a small price to pay, and reoperation is available although rarely required.

As mentioned, in the occasional patient the diagnosis is not made at the time of the accident, and calcium deposits may eventually form in the wall of the aneurysm. Such aneurysms should be managed in the same manner as any other chronic aneurysm of the descending aorta.

ANEURYSMS OF THE INFRARENAL AORTA AND ILIAC ARTERIES

The most important single aneurysm is the infrarenal abdominal aortic aneurysm. These lesions are now resected successfully in the vast majority of patients whose aneurysm has not ruptured. The modern management of this lesion began in 1951, when Dubost resected such an aneurysm and replaced it with an aortic homograft. Rapid contributions were reported by DeBakey and Cooley and others. It was soon found, however, that homografts were not only in short supply but also at times became aneurysmal. Thus, an intense search was mounted for synthetic fabrics that could be used instead of homografts. Many fabrics were variously investigated experimentally and clinically before the modern prostheses were developd. At present, either Dacron or, occasionally, Teflon is usually employed satisfactorily, but additional materials are under study. Silk sutures were originally used to sew in the prosthesis, but it was found that silk became frayed after several years; now one of the several strong synthetic materials is used. Since film cellular union between the fabric graft and the aorta is not to be anticipated, the suture material must serve permanently to secure the anastomosis. When the wall of the native aorta at the level of the suture line is thin or friable, fabric backing of the sutures affords additional security. Fortunately, while some late complications do occur, fabric grafts inserted for the replacement of abdominal aneurysms are now highly successful.

ETIOLOGY

The most common underlying cause of abdominal aortic or iliac artery aneurysm is atherosclerosis. As with aneurysms in other portions of the body, other factors may have an influence in the given patient; these include hypertension, hyperlipidemia, smoking, diabetes, sex, genetic influences, trauma, and still other causes. Infection may affect an abdominal aortic aneurysm but is rarely the primary cause. In the curious Ehlers-Danlos syndrome, there is a deficiency of elastic fibers in the media.

SPECIAL PROBLEMS THAT MAY BE ASSOCIATED WITH ABDOMINAL AORTIC ANEURYSM

1. *Occlusion disease* of cerebral, coronary, mesenteric, renal, or extremity arteries
2. Disease of other vital organs, such as those above plus the lungs and liver not due to arterial occlusive disease
3. Aneurysms of other arteries, such as the iliac, popliteal, femoral, and cerebral
4. Horseshoe kidney involved by aneurysm
5. Accessory renal arteries or predominant inferior mesenteric artery arising from the aortic aneurysm

PATHOLOGY

The abdominal aortic aneurysm may involve any portion of the abdominal aorta, but 90% to 95% occur below the renal arteries. Not infrequently, it involves one or both of the iliac arteries, but, in fact, isolated aneurysms of the iliac arteries are often encountered. Occasionally, only an internal iliac (hypogastric) artery is involved.

The fact that the overwhelming majority of abdominal aortic aneurysms begin below the renal arteries contributes heavily toward the low current operative mortality rate for resection of these lesions. The aorta can be cross-clamped below the renal arteries for a reasonable period without serious risk to tissues whose blood supply arises more distally, although it is a wise precaution to heparinize the patient systemically while the aorta is occluded, to prevent distal thrombosis in large or small vessels. The abdominal aneurysm may be either fusiform or saccular, but it is almost always fusiform. Initially, the aneurysm is small, and for some years, small to moderate-sized lesions were managed without operation, being watched carefully. In some patients, it is still appropriate to do this. However, in recent years, it has been increasingly appreciated that embolic material from the thrombus that occupies much of the aneurysm may embolize distally to occlude arteries in the legs, in addition to the fact that even small aneurysms may rupture into the retroperitoneal space, the peritoneal cavity, or the intestine. Therefore, most aneurysms of significant size in the good-risk patient are now resected when discovered.

In their fine monograph, Crisler and Bahnson summarized as follows: The risk of rupture of the aneurysm is approximately 50% (of all cases observed during a 10-year period), and the 5-year survival rate of patients with aneurysms 6 cm to 7 cm in diameter is about 5% to 10% without resection and about 50% with resection. One-year survival without resection is about 50%.

The risk of resecting an infrarenal aortic aneurysm depends largely on the presence or absence of associated heart, lung, or renal disease or ischemia of legs or brain. The majority of the patients will be in their 60s and 70s and frequently they represent less than optimal risks for any major operative procedure. However, resection of the aneurysm does not involve invasion of the chest or of the alimentary tract, and the resection of the aneurysm that is not huge, in an otherwise good-risk patient, by an experienced vascular surgeon, can be accomplished with a mortality rate of about 5%.

Therefore, it is clear that usually the risk from rupture of the aneurysm far exceeds the risk of the operation itself. In the occasional patient, however, risk of operation exceeds that of close observation of a small to moderate-sized

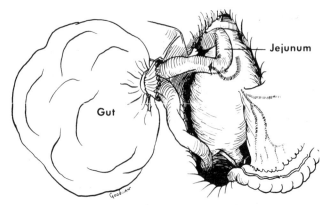

Fig. 36-48. Aortoenteric fistula at the usual site between the proximal jejunum and the aneurysm (the small bowel has been placed in a Lahey bag to facilitate exposure of the retroperitoneal aneurysm). Note the left renal vein crossing the aorta above the jejunum. The inferior mesenteric artery gives off branches to the sigmoid colon. An aortoenteric fistula may cause multiple sporadic episodes of gastrointestinal bleeding prior to diagnosis or fatal issue. (Hardy JD, Timmis HH: Abdominal aortic aneurysms: Special problems. Ann Surg 173:945, 1971)

asymptomatic aneurysm. In such circumstances, the patient may wisely be followed, operation being recommended only when the onset of pain suggests impending rupture of the lesion, although even small aneurysms may rupture occasionally.

It must always be remembered that the aneurysm is only one manifestation of generalized atherosclerotic disease, often in a heavy smoker. The patient whose abdominal aneurysm has been resected may well die within several years of a stroke, a myocardial infarction, or pulmonary disease, including obstructive emphysema and cancer.

NATURAL HISTORY

The natural history of the abdominal aortic aneurysm is important from the point of view of selection of management and comparison of results with and without operation. A classic modern study of the natural history of untreated abdominal aortic aneurysms was that of Estes, published in 1950 just before effective surgical treatment became available. In a series of 101 patients, only 18.9% survived 5 years after diagnosis, compared with the 79.1% expected 5-year survival rate in a normal population of the same mean age (65 years).

Special problems that may be associated with abdominal aortic aneurysm are shown in Figure 36-48. *Complications of the aneurysm* itself are displayed below.

SOME COMPLICATIONS OF THE ANEURYSM ITSELF

1. Rupture
2. Distal embolism
3. Infection in wall
4. Thrombosis of the aneurysm
5. Aortoenteric fistula
6. Aortocaval or left renal vein fistula
7. Compression of ureter, inferior vena cava, or small bowel
8. Dissection in wall of aneurysm (major dissection uncommon)
9. Colon ischemia causing abrupt but transient abdominal pain, or limited necrosis, especially of mucosa, or late stricture

DIAGNOSIS

Many abdominal aortic aneurysms are asymptomatic. In fact, perhaps the majority of such aneurysms are discovered accidentally by the patient himself, or in the course of a routine physical examination, or on x-ray films of the abdomen taken for other purposes. Approximately 50% of the aneurysms are sufficiently calcified that the outlines of the lesion can be seen on plain anteroposterior and lateral roentgenograms of the abdomen.

The first symptom noted may be severe pain due to abrupt rupture of the aneurysm, often accompanied by blood loss, a declining hematocrit level, and shock. Pain in the abdomen or flank may be severe. However, most aneurysms give rise to discomfort weeks or months prior to rupture. The most common symptom is back pain, because the aorta lies against the spine. Substantial enlargement of the aneurysm may cause erosion of the spine. Some causes of back pain are arthritis, aneurysm (lies against spine), metastasis, intervertebral lesions, pancreatic disease, penetrating peptic ulcer, gallbladder disease, spinal cord tumor, sacroiliac strain, and prostate carcinoma metastasis.

In the relatively thin patient, the aneurysm may be readily palpated or even seen on physical examination. However, in the obese patient whose aneurysm is not sufficiently calcified to be seen on plain reontgenograms of the abdomen, aortography may be required for diagnosis, and even with aortography the diagnosis may remain in doubt if the channel through the thrombus in the aneurysm is approximately the size of the normal aorta. Sonography and CT scan have added a further parameter to the accuracy of diagnosis, since ultrasound will identify the total dimensions of the mass even when most of the aneurysm is filled with thrombus. Occasionally, the pain in the aneurysm may be referred to the groin and may be interpreted as reflecting disease of the urinary tract. This is particularly likely when the lesion involves an internal iliac (hypogastric) artery, which lesion is especially difficult to diagnose prior to rupture, since it is not easy to palpate it in the pelvis; thus prompt arteriography or other special studies are necessary. Otherwise, the aneurysm may produce symptoms by compression of the intestine or elements of the urinary tract, erosion into the gut, abrupt thrombosis of the inferior mesenteric artery, and various other uncommon developments.

The importance of roentgenography has already been noted. Calcification in the wall of the aneurysm is best demonstrated on anteroposterior and lateral films of the lumbar spine. If neither physical examination nor plain films are diagnostic, aortography should be employed. Aortography is most often used when aneurysm is suspected in the obese patient in whom noninvasive measures have not been diagnostic, when visualization of the renal and leg arteries is required, when a small aneurysm may be the cause of distal embolism or alimentary tract hemorrhage, when a mass palpated may represent bucking of the iliac arteries instead of a true aneurysm, or after resection, when the presence of a false aneurysm at a suture line must be excluded. For example, if the femoral pulses are weak, the blood supply to the legs should be accurately assessed by angiography so that maneuvers to improve leg perfusion can be carried out at the time the aneurysm is resected. However, some surgeons request aortography in practically all cases. If the patient has had transient ischemic attacks, possibly due to vertebral or carotid artery occlusive disease, arteriography may be required to evaluate this problem prior to aneurysm resection; if so, the aneurysm can be assessed angiographically at the same time. Actually, the aortogram frequently provides useful and often unexpected information, but it is not without risk and discomfort. Again, ultrasonography is increasingly useful, as is CT scan.

TREATMENT

Operative Technique

The technique for resecting the infrarenal aortic or iliac aneurysm has now been standardized and is highly effective (Fig. 36-49). The abdomen is opened in the midline, and the small bowel is either packed away or (our preference) over the right side of the abdomen in a Lahey intestinal bag (Fig. 36-49, *A*). The posterior peritoneum overlying the aneurysm is then divided upward to the level where the left renal vein crosses the aorta and downward to just below the aortic bifurcation, as needed. If the jejunum is densely adherent, the aneurysm should be opened to the left of the jejunum, because the aneurysm can represent the posterior wall of an eroded jejunum (Fig. 36-49, *B*) and the risk of infection must be minimized. The ureters are protected throughout their course and especially where they cross the iliac arteries. Careful attention to colon blood supply is required, but this should be checked routinely in any case (Fig. 36-50).

Horseshoe kidney may require special maneuvers (Fig. 36-51).

Resection with Enteric or Biliary Tract Procedures

Occasionally, the surgeon is faced with strong indications for removal of an acutely inflamed gallbladder or for correction of gastric or small-bowel disease that otherwise might require another operation in the immediate future. While not specifically recommended, it is worth noting that the scrupulously careful completion of such additional procedures, in addition to resection of the aneurysm, has not been attended by an increased infection rate.

Postoperative heparinization is avoided, since hematomas may result.

Resection of Ruptured Abdominal Aortic Aneurysm

The management of the ruptured abdominal aortic aneurysm does not differ materially in principle from the management of the unruptured aneurysm, but there is a considerable difference both in the speed with which the patient must be taken to the operating room and in the overall mortality. Whereas the in-hospital mortality rate is only from 5% to 10% in good-risk patients, the mortality rate for freely ruptured aneurysm resection approaches 40%. In general, the first bleeding from a ruptured abdominal aneurysm need not be fatal. Often, the patient clearly has experienced pain from the initial rupture and bleeding into the retroperitoneal space some hours prior to the time that he reaches the hospital, as reflected in a declining blood hematocrit level preoperatively and in the character of the retroperitoneal hematoma found at operation. On the other hand, the patient in the hospital awaiting elective resection of an aneurysm may exhibit major rupture and die almost immediately. Therefore, once the diagnosis of possible rupture of an aneurysm has been made, the patient should be operated upon as quickly as possible. He should be taken immediately to the operating suite and the operation begun as soon as feasible. If properly typed and crossmatched

(Text continues on p. 927)

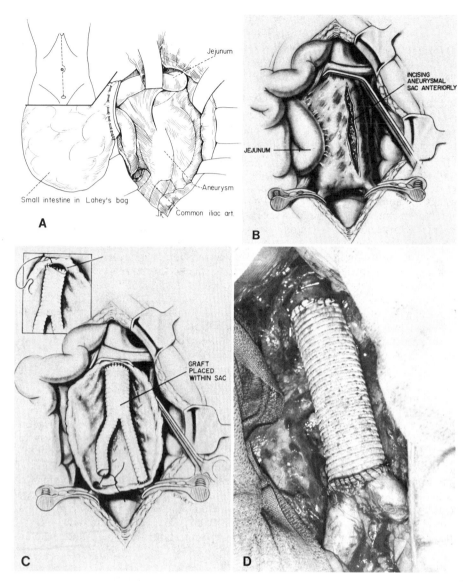

Fig. 36-49. Steps in aneurysm resection. *(A)* The abdomen is opened through the midline, all viscera are explored, the dimensions of the aneurysm are noted, including possible involvement of renal and iliac arteries, and the small intestine is placed in a Lahey bag over the right side of the abdomen to expose the posterior parietal peritoneum, which is then incised to expose the aneurysm. *(B)* The aneurysm is exposed, adherent jejunum is not molested, the patient is given 10,000 units (100 mg) heparin intravenously, the aorta is clamped just below the left renal vein crossing over to the vena cava, and noncrushing clamps are placed across the iliac arteries. The aneurysm sac is incised anteriorly, no effort being made to excise the sac itself. *(C)* A straight tube or bifurcation fabric graft, usually Dacron, is sutured inside the aneurysm after suture ligation to any bleeding lumbar arteries in the depths of the aneurysm posteriorly, with similar treatment of the inferior mesenteric artery if not already obliterated by old thrombus within the aneurysm. Fabric suture material is used, and a fragile aortic wall is "backed" with fabric (Teflon felt) if indicated. The aneurysm is usually largely filled with thrombus, and this is carefully removed to prevent distal embolism when flow through the graft is restored. As soon as the limb to one leg is anastomosed, this leg is perfused while the anastomosis involving the other leg is being completed. Heparinization is adjusted appropriately. *(D)* The Dacron tube graft is completed. The left renal vein lies just at the proximal depths of the wound and the aortic bifurcation just distal to the graft below. The aneurysmal sac or adjacent tissues are sutured over the fabric graft to prevent adherence of graft to intestine. *(A* from Hardy JD: Surgery of the Aorta and Its Branches. Philadelphia, J B Lippincott, 1960; *C* from Hardy JD: Abdominal aortic aneurysm. Am J Med Sci 254:221, 1967)

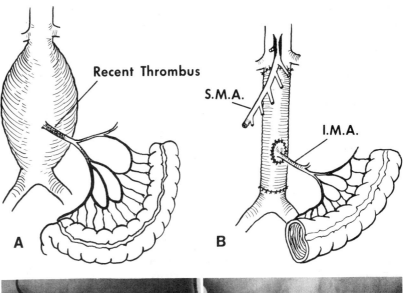

Fig. 36-50. Inferior mesenteric artery blood supply to the colon. *(A)* Abrupt and symptomatic thrombosis of the inferior mesenteric artery (IMA), which occurred in a man with aneurysm simulating pain of rupture. *(B)* Preservation of the IMA by its replantation into fabric graft. Preservation of the IMA is most likely to be required where severe stenosis of the superior mesenteric artery exists or hypogastric arteries are occluded. *(C)* Ischemic stricture of the sigmoid colon. The patient had the ruptured abdominal aortic aneurysm resected, with sacrifice of the IMA; colon stricture developed because of ischemia. *(D)* Aortogram of patient in *C.* Note severe stenosis of the right common iliac and left hypogastric arteries. Late resection of the colon stricture was uneventful. (Hardy JD, Timmis HH: Abdominal aortic aneurysms: Special problems. Ann Surg 173:945, 1971)

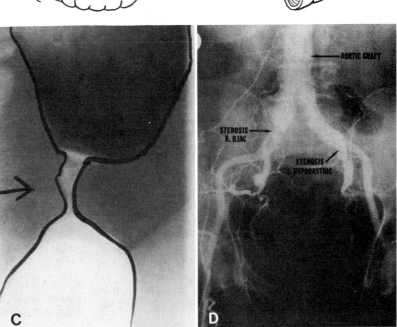

blood is not yet available, plasma and type O packed red cells should be used in dire emergency. Of course, Ringer's lactate is also useful. The important thing is to control the hemorrhage quickly, before irreversible shock, kidney or brain damage, or even cardiac arrest occurs.

Fig. 36-51. Management of aneurysm associated with horseshoe kidney. (Hardy JD, Timmis HH: Abdominal aortic aneurysms: Special problems. Ann Surg 173:945, 1971)

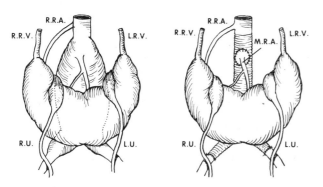

POSTOPERATIVE COMPLICATIONS

Early

The most common and the most serious immediate problems are continued oozing in the operative field leading to hypotension, respiratory insufficiency secondary to previous chronic lung disease from smoking, myocardial infarction, renal failure in the rare patient with unruptured aneurysm and in many patients with ruptured aneurysms, leg ischemia, and, occasionally, colon ischemia.

Hypotension in the recovery room is most often a reflection of inadequate circulating blood volume, and if so, additional blood transfusion is required. At times, the surgeon must decide whether or not reexploration is indicated, although usually it is not. Adequate blood transfusion is monitored with central venous pressure and intra-arterial recording of blood pressure and, when indicated, a Swan-Ganz catheter. It is usually known whether or not to suspect the possibility of continued diffuse oozing within the abdomen. We prefer to insert drains for 24 hours if we consider that additional postoperative oozing may occur despite all reasonable efforts to achieve perfect hemostasis in the field of dissection at operation. However, drains are not always indicated. If used, they always are removed in 24 hours.

Respiratory insufficiency is managed by appropriate continued endotracheal intubation, with assisted ventilation and modern monitoring.

Myocardial infarction is a major cause of death in elective operation for aneurysm, although respiratory insufficiency has often been a prominent factor. The risk of myocardial infarction is minimized by optimal respiratory and circulatory support of the patient before, during, and after operation.

Renal failure is rare following elective resection of aneurysm, but it is a common problem in patients who have sustained serious shock due to ruptured aneurysm. The management of acute renal failure is discussed elsewhere.

Leg ischemia can be a serious problem in the occasional patient. Leg ischemia can be due to preoperative atherosclerotic occlusive disease, thrombosis during aortic cross-clamping, or embolism. If the patient had good femoral and even better foot pulses preoperatively, the block is almost surely due to thrombosis or embolization of thrombotic material, and arteriography and use of a Fogarty catheter should be appropriately employed to remove this material, using a femoral artery exposure under local anesthesia. If some technical imperfection exists, it must be dealt with effectively. It is rare, at the present time, that the leg must be amputated for ischemia following aneurysm resection, since the overall operative technique and understanding of the requirements for this surgery have improved greatly over the past 20 years.

Stroke may occur but is uncommon.

Late

The principal late complications of abdominal aneurysm resection, although uncommon, are wound separation or hernia, infection in the wound or around the graft, and false aneurysm.

Infection about the graft constitutes a very serious problem, and for management the reader is referred to page 900. It carries a poor prognosis.

False aneurysm formation may occur weeks, months, or years following the insertion of the original fabric graft (Fig. 36-52). The false aneurysm may be due to inadequate suture material, such as silk, which fragments; to a weakening of the aortic wall due to ischemia or progressive disease; or to other factors. The false aneurysm may be secondary to infection, but often no infection is present and the condition can be suitably repaired, as necessary, following initial demonstration of the false aneurysm on aortography (although at times, aortography may fail to demonstrate the false aneurysm). False aneurysms occur fairly commonly in any large practice of vascular surgery. Should an aortoenteric fistula have developed, however, the prognosis will be very poor because of associated graft infection.

PROGNOSIS

The results of resection of otherwise uncomplicated abdominal aortic aneurysm are excellent; the mortality rate is less than 5%. In the patient who has disease of other organs, such as the heart, lungs, or kidney, the mortality rate for resection of the unruptured aneurysm is in the neighborhood of 10% to 15%. In contrast, the patient with a large abdominal aortic aneurysm has about a 50% chance of

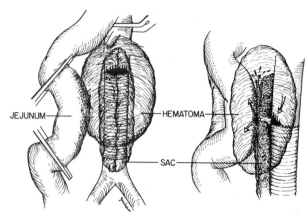

Fig. 36-52. Late disruption of the aortic fabric graft suture line. Free rupture of aortoenteric fistula may occur, as well as infection. A "normal" aortogram does not necessarily exclude an aortoenteric fistula. Exploratory laparotomy and actual exposure of the graft may be required.

rupture in 1 year, and this hazard is even greater in the patient whose aneurysm is already painful. The mortality rate of the resection of ruptured abdominal aneurysm is approximately 40%, due largely to the usual effects of shock due to blood loss. Of course, patients with aneurysms commonly have other complications of atherosclerosis, such as coronary, renal, and cerebral ischemia, all of which diminish overall longevity.

MISCELLANEOUS OTHER TRUE ANEURYSMS

The infrarenal abdominal aortic aneurysm represents by far the most important aneurysm in clinical practice, but thoracic, extremity, and visceral aneurysms are met occasionally.

ANEURYSMS OF THE INNOMINATE, SUBCLAVIAN, AND CAROTID ARTERIES

True aneurysms of the innominate, subclavian, and carotid arteries are relatively uncommon, each comprising less than 1% of all aneurysms. The majority of carotid aneurysms involve the common carotid artery and the bifurcation. Isolated internal carotid or external carotid aneurysms occur with great rarity. False aneurysms of the innominate, subclavian, and carotid arteries secondary to trauma are encountered with some frequency in hospitals that admit a large number of injured patients.

ETIOLOGY

Congenital weakness or absence of media, cystic medial necrosis, and fibromuscular dysplasia may occasionally result in innominate, subclavian, or carotid aneurysms. Acquired causes include arteriosclerotic aneurysms and mycotic infective aneurysms. Syphilitic aneurysms, once relatively common, have become practically nonexistent since the advent of penicillin. The thoracic outlet syndrome is sometimes associated with a subclavian aneurysm, which is often in the nature of a poststenotic dilatation. Trauma, both the penetrating and the nonpenetrating varieties, can lead to arterial rupture and false aneurysm formation, sometimes associated with an arteriovenous fistula.

CLINICAL MANIFESTATIONS

Aneurysms of extrathoracic parts of the carotid and subclavian arteries frequently present as visible or palpable pulsatile masses. Innominate aneurysms are concealed behind the sternum even though occasionally they may be palpable in the suprasternal notch on close examination. Moderate- and small-sized aneurysms of the subclavian artery may be difficult to palpate if the muscles around the root of the neck or the shoulder girdle are well developed. Internal carotid aneurysms may present as palpable masses in the tonsillar fossa or external auditory canal, where some have been mistaken in the past for an abscess and incised. Large aneurysms of the innominate, carotid, or subclavian artery, when situated at the narrow thoracic inlet, may produce pressure symptoms by encroachment on structures that pass through it. Such pressure symptoms may include tracheal compression, dysphagia, or recurrent laryngeal nerve palsy. Horner's syndrome may be produced by pressure on the ansa subclavia or the main sympathetic chain by subclavian aneurysms (Fig. 36-53). False aneurysms of the subclavian artery are especially likely to enlarge without detection and cause brachial plexus compression. An anomalous right subclavian artery arising from the descending aorta and passing behind the esophagus may become aneurysmal and produce dysphagia. Poststenotic aneurysms of the subclavian artery, associated with thoracic outlet syndrome, may present as distal ischemia due to multiple small emboli arising in the aneurysm.

Arteriography may be indicated with certain types of injury, such as first-rib fracture and avulsion injuries of the brachial plexus, which carry a significant incidence of arterial involvement. False aneurysms usually result from penetrating injuries, but blunt trauma can also occasionally cause false aneurysm. Small false aneurysms are seldom palpable and distal pulses are commonly present, either because the artery itself is patent despite the presence of the false aneurysm, or because of rich collateralization even when thrombosis has occurred. For the same reasons, signs of distal ischemia may be minimal or absent. If untreated, such traumatic aneurysms of these three important arteries may gradually enlarge and result in serious complications in the course of time. Because of special anatomical considerations, the usual complications associated with all aneurysms, such as enlargement, rupture, and thrombosis, assume additional manifestations and significance at these three locations. Innominate aneurysms may enlarge to very large size without being detected behind the sternum and may ultimately rupture, causing exsanguination, acute pressure effects on vital structures, or, rarely cardiac tamponade. Carotid aneurysms may undergo thrombosis, resulting in serious neurologic deficit. Subclavian aneurysms may also become large without being detected, causing recalcitrant brachial plexus palsy due to compression. Because of the seriousness of these complications and the ease with which small aneurysms can be missed, some centers carry out routine mandatory surgical exploration when penetrating or serious blunt trauma involves the neck. However, in the great majority of trauma centers in this country, routine arteriography is carried out first, exploration being reserved for those cases in which false aneurysms are either obvious clinically or detected on such arteriography. Premonitory signs such as the presence of a bruit or a thrill, a widened mediastinum on plain x-ray film, or an enlarging hematoma in the neck or axilla lend further urgency to arteriography.

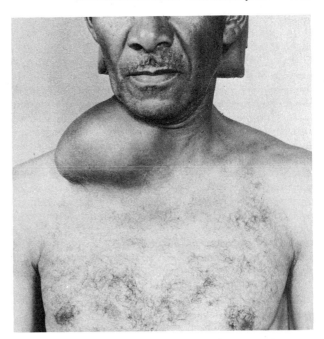

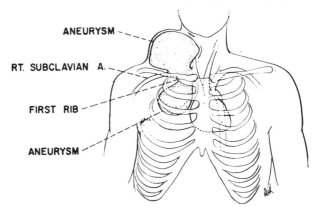

Fig. 36-53. *(Top)* Subclavian aneurysm. This patient had right-sided Horner's syndrome. *(Bottom)* Only the supraclavicular portion was visible. Outline reveals total dimensions of this subclavian aneurysm. (Hardy JD: Arterial lesions of the upper extremity: A clinical review with illustrative cases. Am Surg 26:525, 1960)

DIFFERENTIAL DIAGNOSIS

Carotid aneurysms should be differentiated from carotid body tumors, tortuosity of carotid vessels in hypertensive patients (which may be mistaken for a true aneurysm), lymph nodes, and other neck masses that may be closely applied to the carotid vessels resulting in transmitted pulsations. Thrombosed aneurysms are particularly difficult to distinguish from true solid neck tumors. True aneurysms of the carotid artery may be moved from side to side but not along the direction of the carotid vessels. Other neck masses may not possess this differential mobility. Innominate aneurysms should be differentiated from other upper mediastinal masses, such as lymphoma, teratoma, and thymoma. Subclavian aneurysms should be differentiated from neurofibroma, hamartoma of the lung, and lymphoreticular tumors that occur in the region. Arteriography will almost always provide a definitive diagnosis; however, if a true aneurysm is filled with thrombus through which passes a lumen of normal size, the presence of aneurysm must be established on physical examination, by ultrasound or CT scan, or even by surgical exploration.

TREATMENT

Because of the potential for serious complications, aneurysms in all the three locations should be excised as soon as feasible after diagnosis. Primary anastomosis without recourse to a graft is sometimes possible if the vessels are tortuous and length can be obtained by mobilization. Usually, however, a graft has been necessary to execute the repair without tension. When feasible, vein grafts are preferred to prosthetic grafts, especially in the relatively young person. Autogenous vein grafts are very useful for replacement of carotid and subclavian aneurysms but may not be large enough for replacement of an innominate aneurysm, where a synthetic fabric graft should be used. Vein grafts have the advantage that, unlike fabric grafts, they do not form a pseudointima, parts of which may rarely embolize distally. Of course, the internal jugular veins may be used to bridge arterial defects, and compound saphenous vein grafts may be constructed to a large enough diameter to accommodate a large carotid or subclavian artery.

Specificity of technique in excision of innominate, carotid, and subclavian aneurysms differs somewhat from the principles used in other aneurysms. Total excision of the aneurysmal sac is often readily feasible and, if so, no residual sac remains to disturb surrounding structures (Fig. 36-54). Meticulous proximal and distal control should be secured before the aneurysm is carefully dissected out. Several important nervous structures are encountered in the course of dissection of carotid and subclavian aneurysms. Injury to these structures should be avoided. Distal control may be difficult or impossible in internal carotid aneurysms extending to the base of the skull, in which rare instance proximal ligation may be the only procedure available to control the aneurysm. In the course of excising carotid aneurysms, some provision should be made for continued cerebral perfusion, even though on occasion this may not be necessary if the "stump" pressure is satisfactory. Satisfactory cerebral perfusion can be provided by employing a temporary carotid shunt of either the external or the internal type with heparinization. The internal shunt devised by Javid is convenient and widely employed, but several other types of shunts are satisfactory (see Fig. 36-54).

The innominate aneurysm is best approached by median sternotomy. As with carotid aneurysms, temporary devices for continued cerebral perfusion are necessary. A heparin-bonded external shunt has been used successfully for the purpose without systemic heparinization, but a temporary

fabric external bypass or an internal shunt where feasible will serve equally well.

A subclavian aneurysm, depending on its location, may be approached by a posterolateral thoracotomy, an anterior thoracotomy, an upper median sternotomy, a supraclavicular incision at the base of the neck, or another incision. Occasionally, two incisions or combinations of two or more incisions, such as a trapdoor incision or a supraclavicular–infraclavicular incision with division of the clavicle, may be required for adequate exposure. Because of the presence of rich collaterals in the area, vascular isolation of the subclavian aneurysm may not be achieved until numerous closely spaced branches have been carefully dissected out and controlled. The brachial plexus is closely applied to the distal subclavian artery, and this poses an additional problem in dissection. At times, it is advisable to open the aneurysm, after achieving proximal and distal control, and to oversew the collaterals from within the sac. The proximal subclavian artery is a delicate, thin-walled vessel that requires a meticulous and gentle technique. Of course, in the absence of anomalies, the right subclavian artery is extrathoracic, while much of the left subclavian artery is intrathoracic. The left subclavian artery aneurysm can usually be resected without concern for brain perfusion, but proximal control of the right subclavian artery can involve the right common carotid and require the use of a temporary shunt to provide adequate brain perfusion.

The long-term results of resection and repair of innominate, subclavian, and carotid aneurysms are excellent.

FEMORAL ARTERY ANEURYSMS

Femoral artery aneurysms are relatively common, and true aneurysms are almost always due to arteriosclerosis. The lesions are bilateral in about one third of patients so afflicted, and a femoral aneurysm is associated with an abdominal aortic aneurysm in 20% to 30% of patients. Moreover, as might be expected in patients who have generalized arteriosclerosis, hypertension is to be found in perhaps 50% of patients with femoral aneurysm. The age distribution is essentially the same as that for abdominal aortic aneurysms, the patients most commonly being in their 60s.

True arteriosclerotic aneurysms do not often rupture, as opposed to false aneurysms of the femoral artery due either to injury or to disruption of an aortofemoral bypass graft (Fig. 36-55). True aneurysms may rupture but usually produce their symptoms and complications by enlargement and compression of neighboring structures or by thrombosis or embolization to produce ischemia of the distal extremity.

Fig. 36-54. Steps in the resection of a carotid aneurysm, using an internal (Javid) shunt for brain perfusion. An autogenous saphenous vein graft is preferred, but a fabric graft will serve.

Fig. 36-55. Use of the Fogarty catheter balloon to control bleeding from the profunda femoris artery during repair of femoral false aneurysm.

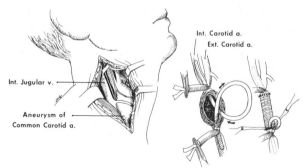

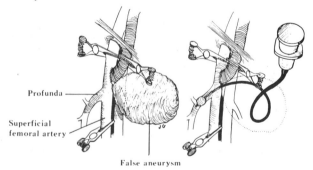

Thrombosis is the most common complication in femoral artery aneurysm, but is found somewhat less in popliteal arteries, where repeated embolization may so occlude the distal vessels that resection of the aneurysm with graft replacement may still be followed by gangrene and loss of the extremity. Of course, thrombosis of the femoral aneurysm may be associated with such propagation of distal and proximal thrombosis that the extremity can be lost from the femoral aneurysm as well. Either the common femoral or the superficial artery is most commonly involved, with the profunda being involved only rarely.

The clinical manifestations of femoral aneurysm are a pulsating mass below the inguinal ligament, pain due to pressure on surrounding sensory nerves if the aneurysm is large and expanding, or distal ischemia, if thrombosis or, more rarely, embolism occurs. Infection and associated inflammation may develop.

Physical examination discloses either a pulsatile mass or a firm solid mass if the aneurysm has become thrombosed. The diagnosis is usually easily made and is confirmed by arteriography if the aneurysm is still patent. However, as with a popliteal aneurysm, the arteriogram may be misleading regarding the presence of an aneurysm if the aneurysm is completely filled with thrombus except for a patent channel that is approximately normal in size. Further, complete occlusion of the vessel may exist, suggesting acute thrombosis or embolism. However, there is rarely any question of the diagnosis.

TREATMENT

The femoral artery aneurysm is easily resected in most patients. If the patient represents a poor operative risk because of the atherosclerotic coronary artery disease or emphysema that is commonly present in these patients, the operation can readily be performed under local anesthesia. Control of the femoral artery both above and below the aneurysm is achieved, with appropriate acknowledgment of the fact that the profunda artery may enter the posterior wall of the aneurysm (Fig. 36-56). Heparin is instilled either systemically or into the distal artery to prevent thrombosis while inflow stasis is maintained, and the aneurysm is resected and replaced with either a reversed saphenous vein graft or, preferably, a fabric graft to preserve the saphenous vein for some future use.

RESULTS

Long term results of resection of a femoral aneurysm are generally good, although occasionally continued deterioration of the wall of the femoral artery itself may permit disruption of the suture line, and a false aneurysm may appear at one end or the other of the fabric graft. However, this complication is readily corrected, again under local anesthesia if desired.

POPLITEAL ARTERY ANEURYSMS

The popliteal artery is a common site of peripheral arterial aneurysm formation. This lesion is especially interesting in that it may produce a variety of symptom complexes or it may be completely asymptomatic. The patient may present with chronic or abrupt swelling of the lower part of the leg, with venous distention due to chronic or acute enlargement of the popliteal aneurysm, or he may exhibit chronic or acute ischemia of the foot due to slow or acute thrombosis of the aneurysm, at times with distal embolism of small

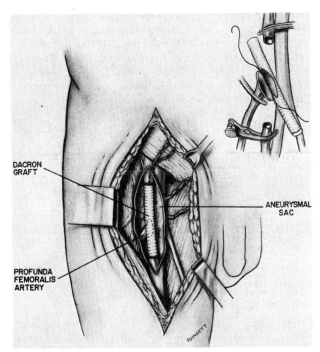

Fig. 36-56. Maneuver for preservation of the profunda femoris artery when resecting a femoral aneurysm. The profunda is anastomosed to the posterior wall of the graft. (Hardy JD: Preservation of accessory arterial supply in abdominal aneurysm resection. Surg Gynecol Obstet 123:1317, 1966)

particles of thrombus to occlude the smaller arterial branches. Pressure on elements of the sciatic nerve, which has branches stretched out over the aneurysm, may give rise to neurologic symptoms. The patient may have noted the aneurysm, pulsating or thrombosed, symptomatic or asymptomatic, as a mass behind the knee. Acute ruptures of the lesion may occur occasionally, giving rise to considerable pain, although rarely to sufficient blood loss to produce hypotension. This is because tissue pressure builds up and, eventually, bleeding ceases. Finally, the presence of a small thrombosed and thus essentially "cured" aneurysm may be completely unsuspected by the surgeon until discovered at exploration of the popliteal artery, perhaps in an effort to relieve ischemia of the foot by placing femoropopliteal bypass graft. Thus, the preoperative arteriograms may have merely shown an abrupt cutoff of the radiopaque medium at the level of the popliteal artery due to complete thrombosis of the aneurysm. In other instances, a patent channel through the thrombus in the aneurysm is smooth and essentially normal in diameter, and the presence of the aneurysm is detected only by palpation, by discovery at operation, or by noting calcification in the rim of the aneurysm on plain roentgenogram.

In a review of 31 true aneurysms of the popliteal artery, which occurred in 23 patients, we found an age range of 30 to 80 years, but the largest number were in their 50s and 60s. Men predominated over women 2:1. The aneurysm was located on the right in ten patients and on the left in five; it was bilateral in eight. It was concluded that virtually all the aneurysms were due to arteriosclerosis, and no aneurysm appeared to be due to syphilis or to other microbial agents. Fourteen of the 23 patients were hypertensive. The most common major symptom was rest pain in 11 patients, followed by intermittent claudication in ten patients. Five patients had noted a mass behind the knee, and tenderness in the popliteal area had been present in four. Four patients complained of pain due to compression of the elements of the sciatic nerve, and a steadily enlarging mass had been noted by two. Two patients exhibited evidence of popliteal vein compression, and two were asymptomatic. Twenty-five of the 31 aneurysms were palpable, and an absence of popliteal pulse was reported in four patients. Furthermore, the foot pulses were absent in 15 patients, and impending or frank gangrene was met in four. Ten patients had additional aneurysms elsewhere, the most common site being the abdominal aorta.

It was especially significant that 16 patients presented with some complication of the aneurysm: thrombosis in 11, definite embolism in three, and rupture in two. Of the 11 popliteal aneurysms that were thrombosed, immediate amputation was required in two. Nonoperative treatment rarely provided satisfactory relief of symptoms or rehabilitation, and nonoperative management of popliteal aneurysms is to be discouraged, since operative management is easily achieved and the results are generally good if irreversible distal ischemia has not occurred.

TREATMENT

The popliteal aneurysm should be resected and replaced with a reversed saphenous vein graft, if irreversible distal changes due to thrombosis of the aneurysm or embolism, which will necessitate amputation, have not occurred. Actually, severe ischemia of the distal extremity may exist but can be remedied by resection of a thrombosed aneurysm or by use of the balloon catheter to remove embolic particles from the anterior and posterior tibial arteries, with restoration of adequate arterial flow.

The actual surgical technique is shown in Figure 36-57. Although both the medial incision traversing the knee joint and the posterior or S-shaped incision across the popliteal space are available, we have abandoned the posterior approach in favor of the medial incision. The latter provides access to the superficial artery proximally and to the trifurcation of the popliteal artery distally in the event that the several branches must be individually cleared of embolic material under direct visualization. Furthermore, the ele-

ments of the sciatic nerve are at risk with the posterior incision, whereas these neural elements fall away posteriorly with the medial incision. Also, the aneurysm is exposed directly and entered immediately after control of the popliteal artery both proximally and distally, and the graft is placed within the aneurysm; this avoids the necessity for identifying and retracting the neural elements and avoids injury to the popliteal vein. Furthermore, the medial approach considerably expedites the speed of the operation and renders it essentially a very simple maneuver.

Inasmuch as the popliteal artery crosses a flexion crease, we prefer to use the saphenous vein graft instead of the fabric graft (Fig. 36-58); this is opposed to the situation that exists with aneurysms of the femoral artery, in which the fabric graft serves quite well and the saphenous vein is thus spared for other needs in the future.

RESULTS

The results of resection of the popliteal aneurysm are dependent upon the condition of the distal extremity and its arterial blood supply at the time of resection. If thrombosis of the vessels distal to the aneurysm has not occurred, or can be corrected by use of the Fogarty at operation, and adequate distal runoff thus achieved, the results of operation are quite satisfactory. We have rarely had secondary complications following resection of a popliteal aneurysm where distal runoff was excellent. On the other hand, if long-standing thrombosis of the aneurysm or distal embolization precludes the reestablishment of satisfactory distal runoff, the graft may well not remain patent and ultimately the leg may be lost.

VISCERAL ARTERY ANEURYSMS

Many authors have attempted to indicate the true incidence of aneurysms involving the visceral branches of the abdominal aorta. An interesting report on aneurysms in general presents an analysis of 10,600 necropsy reports from the Philadelphia General Hospital in the United States and the Queen Elizabeth Hospital in Birmingham, England (Farooki,

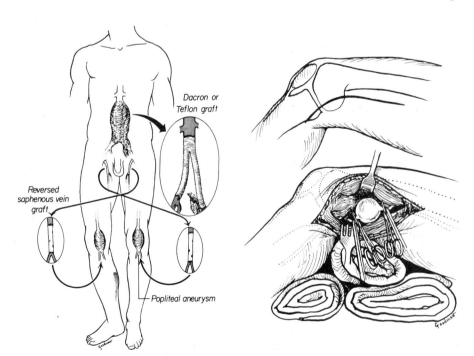

Dacron or Teflon graft

Reversed saphenous vein graft

Popliteal aneurysm

Fig. 36-57. *(Left)* Patient who had a large abdominal aneurysm involving the iliac arteries plus bilateral symptomatic popliteal aneurysms. These were resected. Several years later, he recovered from a mild stroke and later died from acute myocardial infarction. *(Right)* Medial approach to popliteal aneurysm. (Hardy JD, Tompkins WC, Jr, Hatten LE et al: Aneurysms of the popliteal artery. Surg Gynecol Obstet 140:401, 1975)

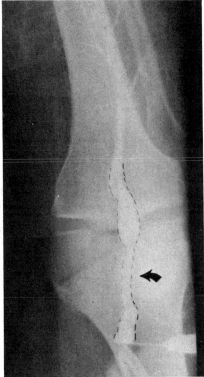 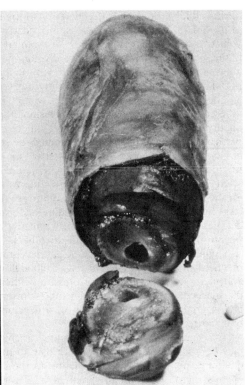

Fig. 36-58. *(Left)* Arteriogram shows replacement of a popliteal aneurysm with a reversed vein graft. *(Right)* A characteristic thrombus is seen in a popliteal aneurysm with only the central channel remaining. Most arterial aneurysms contain such a thrombus, particles of which may embolize occasionally.

1973). The overall incidence of aneurysms was 3.6% after correcting for patients with more than one lesion. Aneurysms of the visceral arteries appear to represent 1.5% of all aneurysms. The splenic artery is most commonly involved, followed by the renal artery and then the hepatic artery. Relatively few aneurysms have been described involving the celiac axis, left gastric artery or superior mesenteric artery and its branches. Aneurysmal involvement of the inferior mesenteric artery is exceedingly rare.

The peak incidence occurred in the seventh decade, which reflected a substantial difference from a peak in the fourth and fifth decades in a similar report by Lucke in 1921. This shift is believed to be due to a lessened incidence of untreated syphilis and to more effective medical management of subacute bacterial endocarditis.

The age range has been 14 to 96 years except for the renal artery, in which lesions have been found in infants. Aneurysms found in the second to fifth decades more frequently have been associated with trauma, serious cardiac disease such as rheumatic heart disease and subacute bacterial endocarditis, and various forms of arteritis such as seen with polyarteritis nodosa and with a number of unusual syndromes (Marfan's, Ehlers-Danlos). True congenital aneurysms appear to be uncommon. Aneurysms reported in the sixth decade and later have increased in number in recent years, and the majority are atherosclerotic, less likely to rupture than some others.

The threat of rupture varies depending on the artery involved, as does surgical risk. The likelihood of rupture also depends on the etiology of the aneurysm, as derived from analysis of 428 aneurysms (Farooki, 1973). The incidence of rupture as noted at necropsy was greatest with dissecting aneurysms (56%). In the saccular or fusiform type, congenital and arteritic aneurysms appeared very prone to rupture. Traumatic and mycotic aneurysms had ruptured in half those found, whereas atherosclerotic lesions had

ruptured in only 37%. In the visceral lesions, one third had ruptured at the time of necropsy, with more occurring in men. It is of interest that arterial hypertension was noted in half the patients in whom rupture had occurred.

In view of the fact that symptoms and signs may be absent, it is encouraging to see the greater application of selective arteriography in patients with unusual gastrointestinal bleeding or obstructive jaundice or with a painless, nonpulsatile mass in the abdomen.

As shown in Table 36-8, virtually any significant artery within the abdomen has been the site of aneurysm formation, but the most common aneurysms are splenic, renal, and hepatic.

SPLENIC ARTERY

The majority of the aneurysms in men are arteriosclerotic. On the other hand, in women the predominant etiology

TABLE 36-8 VISCERAL ARTERY ANEURYSMS

ARTERY	ESTIMATED LESIONS
Gastric	30
Celiac trunk	55
Splenic	715
Hepatic	270
Gastroduodenal or pancreaticoduodenal	40
Superior mesenteric	100
Jejunal, ileal, colic	35
Renal	420
Total	1665

(Deterling RA Jr: Visceral artery aneurysms. In Hardy JD [ed]: Rhoads Textbook of Surgery, 5th ed. Philadelphia, J B Lippincott, 1977)

during childbearing age is degeneration of the medial zone of the splenic artery. With increasing civilian violence and vehicular accidents, the incidence of traumatic aneurysms of the spleen has increased significantly. Rarely, intrasplenic aneurysms may follow splenic puncture in patients with portal hypertension. Congenital and mycotic types are rare.

The behavior of the splenic artery in women is sufficiently different to merit special mention. Inclusion of splenic artery aneurysms observed in women during childbearing age and particularly during pregnancy has shifted the sex incidence in favor of the woman by 2 or 3:1. Aneurysms encountered in elderly women and in men are predominantly atherosclerotic, whereas those observed in young women are due for the most part to medial necrosis of the arterial wall. The large number of aneurysms reported in the third and fourth decades associated with pregnancy greatly reduces the statistical average if included with the others.

Suggestions to explain aneurysmal development in the pregnant woman have been increased blood flow, shunting, and increased intra-abdominal pressure. Other factors are the markedly altered endocrine pattern during pregnancy and arterial hypertension, which may develop late in the pregnancy.

The signs and symptoms are quite variable, but there may be a vague discomfort to sharp pain in the left upper quadrant, occasionally with radiation to the left shoulder (Kehr's sign). Occasionally, nausea and vomiting have occurred, and a mass or systolic bruit is frequently detected. Splenomegaly has been noted in 45% and portal hypertension in 29% of reported cases. Arterial hypertension is also a factor.

Diagnosis may be aided by the presence of a concentric, calcific shadow on the axis of the splenic artery, not infrequently observed in patients over 50 years of age. Larger aneurysms may produce a filling defect in the posterior wall of the stomach, which is pulsatile when viewed by fluoroscopy. Intragastric rupture is not uncommon and is estimated as high as 10% by some authors. When rupture occurs, there may be an increase in the severity of pain. Most commonly, the aneurysm ruptures into the lesser sac. At this time, the patient may respond well to transfusion and other supportive measures only to have the "double rupture" take place into the free peritoneal space, with attendant severe hemorrhagic shock. The double rupture may occur from 1 to 55 days following the initial episode, with an average of 48 hours.

Many of the ruptures occurring during labor or in the postpartum period are the double rupture type, which has been estimated to occur in about 45% of those with ruptured aneurysms.

Selective arteriography of the celiac axis is most likely to demonstrate aneurysm of the splenic artery, and up to 25% have been discovered incidentally during a procedure performed for other reasons.

The surgical treatment of choice is bipolar ligation and excision with or without splenectomy or partial resection of the tail of the pancreas. Surgical results are good unless rupture of the aneurysm with massive blood loss has occurred.

RENAL ARTERY

Most renal aneurysms appear to be the result of atherosclerosis (Fig. 36-59). Trauma has been an increasing cause, from both penetrating and blunt injury. Rare aneurysms have resulted from closed needle biopsy. Congenital and

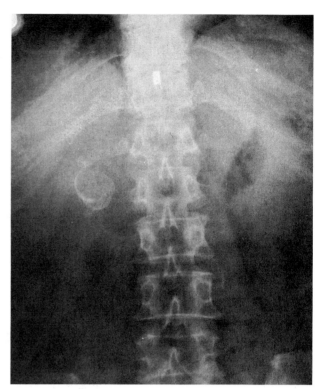

Fig. 36-59. There is a circular calcific shadow in the right upper abdomen. Arteriography revealed a saccular aneurysm involving the ventral branch of the right renal artery. No mass or bruit was noted. Atherosclerotic aneurysm of the hepatic or splenic artery may present a similar appearance. (Deterling RA Jr: Aneurysm of the visceral arteries. J Cardiovasc Surg 12:309, 1971)

mycotic forms have been reported. Periarteritis nodosa, which involves the renal artery in up to 80% of cases, can produce multiple small saccular intrarenal aneurysms bilaterally. Close observation of such patients suggests that these lesions may disappear or regress. Several authors have refuted the claim that these small peripheral saccular aneurysms are pathognomonic of polyarteritis nodosa and report patients with similar lesions in whom this collagen disorder could not be diagnosed. Recently, there has been a growing appreciation that generalized neurofibromatosis can produce multiple bilateral saccular aneurysms of the renal arteries or dissecting aneurysms with rupture. Kidneys used for homotransplantation and removed after loss of function have demonstrated many small intrarenal aneurysms.

Extrarenal aneurysms are usually located in the main artery; fewer are seen in the bifurcation and still fewer in the primary branches. Only about 20% of patients have bilateral lesions. Intrarenal aneurysms are found in about 30% of the patients, and rupture can occur in about 30%. Extrarenal aneurysms rupture in only about 15%. From approximately 420 cases reported to 1975, it appears that the sex incidence is about equal.

The signs and symptoms associated with renal aneurysm are often minimal or absent. In view of the fact that hypertension has been found in from 75% to 90% of patients with extrarenal aneurysms, some of the symptoms may be related to the elevation of blood pressure. Only about 15% of the patients with intrarenal aneurysms have hypertension. Between 20% and 35% of patients with renal aneurysms have hematuria, 20% have a bruit, and only about 5% note discomfort in the flank. A mass is not found, although systolic murmur has been detected in 25% of the extrarenal lesions. Since arteriosclerosis is a common etiology, these lesions may frequently be suggested by the calcification of the sac (see Fig. 36-59). Arteriography is usually confirmatory. Much younger persons are affected by renal aneurysms than by any other, and there is an age range from 9 months to 72 years (average 48 years).

In patients with solitary significant intrarenal aneurysms, partial or total nephrectomy is indicated. If hypertension is present in such patients, it is usually not benefited by removing the aneurysm. On the contrary, in a large number of patients with extrarenal aneurysm and associated hypertension, removal of the aneurysm often has reduced or eliminated the hypertension. Similar beneficial effect has been observed if nephrectomy was necessary (Deterling).

Efforts should be made to excise the aneurysm but maintain adequate arterial flow to the kidney. In a series of 21 patients with extrarenal aneurysms reported in 1973 by De Bakey and colleagues, nephrectomy was required in only 7%. Aneurysmectomy with patch was used in 26%, bypass in 22%, primary repair in 22%, end-to-end anastomosis after aneurysmectomy in 19%, and graft replacement in only 4%.

HEPATIC ARTERY

When signs and symptoms are absent, diagnosis of hepatic aneurysm may be virtually impossible without arteriography. Conversely, there may be a sufficiently well defined clinical picture to include the "classic triad" of epigastric or right upper quadrant pain, gastrointestinal hemorrhage, and obstructive jaundice. Regrettably, this combination may be observed in only one third of the patients. The presence of hemobilia following acute trauma involving the liver or cholecystectomy should suggest the presence of an aneurysm communicating with the common or hepatic duct. A mass is not often detected on physical examination and, if present, may not be pulsatile. Systolic bruit is infrequent and need not be associated with a palpable mass. Pain is a complaint in over two thirds of the patients, usually noted as steady or colicky in nature.

It is estimated that about 80% of these lesions are extrahepatic, 15% are intrahepatic, and only 5% involve both areas. About two thirds involve the common hepatic artery, one fourth the right branch, and the remainder the left branch or both branches. As with other visceral aneurysms, with the greater availability of selective arteriography since 1965, the majority of lesions have been detected in symptomatic patients prior to rupture. Previously, 85% were discovered after rupture had occurred. Because of the increased incidence of intact aneurysms diagnosed since 1960, the mortality rate of the entire group reported since then has been under 30% (Deterling).

In view of the great propensity of hepatic aneurysms to rupture or at least produce serious secondary effects, it is reasonable to employ selective arteriography in patients with unexplained epigastric or right upper quadrant symptoms and to seek competent surgical consultation for all those patients with a proved diagnosis of hepatic aneurysm for at least serious consideration of definitive surgical treatment.

In developing this section the author has drawn upon his own and the following material presented in Chapter 55 of Hardy JD (ed): *Rhoads Textbook of Surgery* (5th ed): Akio Suzuki, Aneurysm of the Sinus of Valsalva: Michael E. DeBakey and George P. Noon, Aneurysms of the Ascending Aorta and Transverse Arch; and Ralph A. Deterling, Jr., Visceral Artery Aneurysms.

BIBLIOGRAPHY

Aneurysm of the Sinus of Valsalva

ABBOTT ME: Clinical and developmental study of a case of ruptured aneurysm of the right anterior aortic sinus of Valsalva. Contrib Med Biol Res 2:899, 1919

LILLIHEI CW, STANLEY P, VARCO RL: Surgical treatment of ruptured aneurysm of the sinus of Valsalva. Ann Surg 146: 459, 1957

MORROW AG, BAKER RR, HANSEN HE et al: Successful repair of a ruptured aneurysm of the sinus of Valsalva. Circulation 16:533, 1957

SUZUKI A: Aneurysm of the sinus of Valsalva. In Hardy JD (ed): Rhoads Textbook of Surgery, 5th ed, p 1726. Philadelphia, J B Lippincott, 1977

Aneurysms of the Ascending Aorta and Transverse Arch

COOLEY DA, BLOODWELL RD, BEALL AC et al: Surgical management of aneurysms of the ascending aorta. Surg Clin North Am 46:1033, 1966

DEBAKEY ME, BEALL AC, COOLEY DA et al: Resection and graft replacement of aneurysms involving the transverse arch of the aorta. Surg Clin North Am 46:1057, 1966

DEBAKEY ME, DIETHRICH EB, NOON GP et al: Surgical management of aortic arch aneurysms. Circulation 38:64, 1968

HIRST AE, JONES VJ, KIME SW: Dissecting aneurysms of the aorta: Review of 505 cases. Medicine 37:217, 1958

KAMPMEIER RH: Saccular aneurysms of the thoracic aorta: A clinical study of 633 cases. Ann Intern Med 12:624, 1938

MOOTHART RW, SPANGLER RD, BLOUNT SG: Echocardiography in aortic root dissection and dilatation. Am J Cardiol 36:11, 1975

WHEAT MW JR: Treatment of dissecting aneurysms of the aorta: Current status. Prog Cardiovasc Dis 16:87, 1973

Aneurysms of the Descending Thoracic Aorta and the Thoracoabdominal Aorta

BAHNSON HT: Definitive treatment of saccular aneurysms of the aorta with excision of the sac and aortic suture. Surg Gynecol Obstet 96:382, 1953

CRAWFORD ES, RUBIO PA: Reappraisal of adjuncts to avoid ischemia in the treatment of aneurysms of the descending aorta. J Thorac Cardiovasc Surg 66:693, 1973

CRISLER C, BAHNSON HT: Aneurysms of the aorta. Curr Probl Surg 9:1, 1972

DEBAKEY ME, CRAWFORD ES, GARRETT HE et al: Surgical considerations in the treatment of aneurysms of the thoracoabdominal aorta. Ann Surg 162:650, 1965

DILLON ML, YOUNG WG, SEALY WC: Aneurysms of descending thoracic aorta. Ann Thorac Surg 3:430, 1967

GARRETT HE, CRAWFORD ES, BEALL AC, JR et al: Surgical treatment of aneurysm of the thoracoabdominal aorta. Surg Clin North Am 46:913, 1966

GOTT VL: Heparinized shunts for thoracic vascular operations. Ann Thorac Surg 14:219, 1972

Dissecting Thoracic Aneurysm

ANAGNOSTOPOULOS CE, PRABHAKER MJS, KITTLE CF: Aortic dissections and dissecting aneurysms. Am J Cardiol 30:263, 1972

CARLSON RG, LILLEHEI CW, EDWARDS JE: Cystic medial necrosis of the ascending aorta in relation to age and hypertension. Am J Cardiol 25:411, 1970

CARPENTIER A, DELOCHE A, FABIANI JN et al: New surgical approach to aortic dissection: Flow reversal and thromboexclusion. J Thorac Cardiovasc Surg 81:659, 1981

COLLINS JJ JR, COHN LH: Reconstruction of the aortic valve. Arch Surg 106:35, 1973

DAILY PO, TRUEBLOOD HE, STINSON EB et al: Management of acute aortic dissections. Ann Thorac Surg 10:237, 1970

WHEAT MW, JR, PALMER RF, BARTLEY TD, Treatment of dissecting aneurysms of the aorta without surgery. J Thorac Cardiovasc Surg 50:364, 1965

Traumatic Rupture of the Thoracic Aorta

ALLEY RD, VAN MIEROP LHS, LI EY et al: Traumatic aortic aneurysm: Four cases of graftless excision and anastomosis. Ann Thorac Surg 2:514, 1966

BENNETT DE, CHERRY JK: The natural history of traumatic aneurysms of the aorta. Surgery 61:516, 1967

CRAWFORD ES, RUBIO PA: Reappraisal of adjuncts to avoid ischemia in the treatment of aneurysms of descending thoracic aorta. J Thorac Cardiovasc Surg 66:693, 1973

GERBODE F, BRAIMBUDGE M, OSBORN J et al: Traumatic thoracic aneurysms: Treatment by resection and grafting with the use of an extracorporeal bypass. Surgery 42:6, 1957

JAHNKE EJ, JR, FISHER GW, JONES RC: Acute traumatic rupture of the thoracic aorta: A report of six consecutive cases of successful early repair. J Thorac Cardiovasc Surg 48:63, 1964

LIM RC, JR, SANDERSON RG, HALL AD et al: Multiple traumatic aneurysms after nonpenetrating chest injury. Ann Thorac Surg 6:4, 1968

Infrarenal Aortic and Iliac Artery Aneurysms

BEITA DS, MERENDINO KA: Abdominal aneurysm and horsehoe kidney: A review. Ann Surg 181:333, 1975

BIRNHAUM W, RUDY L, WYLIE EJ: Colonic and rectal ischemia following abdominal aortic aneurysm. Dis Colon Rectum 7:293, 1964

BRADBROOK RA, MARSHALL AJ, SPREADBURY PL: Hypertension with dissecting abdominal aortic aneurysm. Br Med J 4:23, 1974

CRISLER C, BAHNSON HT: Aneurysms of the aorta. Curr Prob Surg 9:1, 1972

DAVIS JT, HARDIN WJ, HARDY JD et al: Abdominal aneurysm and horseshoe kidney. South Med J 64:75, 1971

DEBAKEY ME, COOLEY DA: Surgical treatment of aneurysm of abdominal aorta by resection and restoration of continuity with homograft. Surg Gynecol Obstet 97:257, 1953

DEMUTH WE, MCCONAGHIE RJ: Salmonella infection in ruptured abdominal aortic aneurysm. Arch Surg 95:193, 1967

DONOVAN TJ, BUCKNAM CA: Aortoenteric fistula. Arch Surg 95:810, 1967

DUBOST C, ALLARY M, OECONOMOS N: Traitement chirurgical des aneurysmes artériels: Le rétablissement de la continuité après éxerèse par l'emploi de graffes artérielles. Sem Hop Paris 27:2678, 1951

ESTES JE: Abdominal aortic aneurysms: A study of 102 cases. Circulation 2:258, 1950

FRY WJ, LINDENAUER SM: Infection complicating the use of plastic arterial implants. Arch Surg 94:600, 1967

HARDY JD: Preservation of accessory arterial supply in abdominal aneurysm resection. Surg Gynecol Obstet 123:1317, 1966

HARDY JD, TIMMIS HH: Abdominal aortic aneurysms: Special problems. Ann Surg 173:945, 1971

OCHSNER J, COOLEY DA, DEBAKEY ME: Associated intra-abdominal lesions encountered during resection of aortic aneurysms: Surgical considerations. Dis Colon Rectum 3:485, 1960

TOMPKINS WC, CHAVEZ CM, CONN JH et al: Combining intra-abdominal arterial grafting with gastrointestinal or biliary tract procedures. Am J Surg 126:598, 1973

Aneurysms of the Innominate, Subclavian, and Carotid Arteries

BEALL AC, JR, CRAWFORD ES, COOLEY DA et al: Extracranial aneurysms of the carotid artery: Report of seven cases. Postgrad Med 32:93, 1962

CAMPBELL CF: Repair of an aneurysm of an aberrant retroesophageal right subclavian artery arising from Kommerell's diverticulum. J Thorac Cardiovasc Surg 62:330, 1971

HARDY JD, RAJU S, NEELY WA et al: Aortic and other arterial injuries. Ann Surg 181:640, 1975

RAPHAEL HA, BERNATZ PE, SPITTELL JA, JR et al: Cervical carotid aneurysms: Treatment of excision and restoration of arterial continuity. Am J Surg 105:771, 1963

SPENCER FC: Aneurysm of the common carotid artery treated by excision and primary anastomosis. Ann Surg 145:254, 1957

Femoral Artery Aneurysms

CHAVEZ CM: False aneurysms of the femoral artery: A challenge in management. Ann Surg 183:694, 1976

STONEY RJ, ALBO RJ, WYLIE EJ: False aneurysms occurring after arterial grafting operations. Am J Surg 110:153, 1965

Popliteal Artery Aneurysms

CRAWFORD ES, DEBAKEY ME: Popliteal artery atherosclerotic aneurysm. Circulation 32:515, 1965

HARDY JD, TOMPKINS WC, JR, HATTEN LE et al: Aneurysms of the popliteal artery. Surg Gynecol Obstet 140:401, 1975

HODGE L: Spontaneous cure of a popliteal aneurysm. Am J Med Sci 40:124, 1960

LINTON RR: The arteriosclerotic popliteal aneurysm: A report of 14 patients treated by preliminary lumbar sympathetic ganglionectomy and aneurysmectomy. Surgery 26:41, 1949

WYCHULIS AR, SPITTELL JA, JR, WALLACE RB: Popliteal aneurysms. Surgery 68:942, 1970

Visceral Artery Aneurysm

DETERLING RA JR: Aneurysm of the visceral arteries. J Cardiovasc Surg 12:309, 1971

FAROOKI MA: Aneurysms of the United States and the United Kingdom. Int Surg 58:7, 1973

GUTHRIE W, MACLEAN H: Dissecting aneurysms of arteries other than the aorta. J Pathol 108:219, 1972

STANLEY JC, THOMPSON NW, FRY WJ: Splanchnic artery aneurysms. Arch Surg 101:689, 1970

Perry M. Shoor/Thomas J. Fogarty

Arterial Embolism

CARDIOTHROMBOTIC EMBOLISM
  Diagnosis
    Acute Arterial Thrombosis
    Acute Aortic Dissection
    Acute Venous Thrombosis
  Treatment
    Preoperative Management
    Operative Therapy (Embolectomy)
    Postoperative Care
  Special Problems
    Advanced Ischemia
    Concomitant Occlusive Disease
  Prognosis

ATHEROMATOUS EMBOLISM
  Historical Background
  Pathophysiology
  Diagnosis
  Treatment

CARDIOTHROMBOTIC EMBOLISM

Thrombotic material dislodged from an intimal surface (usually within the heart) is carried through the arterial system until it lodges at a site of vessel narrowing, often severely obstructing arterial flow.

Harvey described the consequences of abrupt arterial

ARTERIAL EMBOLISM	
Etiology	Thrombotic material, dislodged usually from the heart, occludes an artery, resulting in circulatory stasis, propagation of thrombus, and with time, ischemic tissue damage
Dx	Abrupt onset of ischemia in a patient with atrial fibrillation or recent myocardial infarction suggests embolism
	Patient presents clinically with the "embolic syndrome" consisting of extremity pain, pulselessness, pallor, paresthesia, and finally, paralysis; coronary, cerebral, mesenteric, or renal embolism may also occur
Rx	Immediate anticoagulation with intravenous heparin; try fibrinolysis(?); surgical (balloon catheter) embolectomy after appropriate medical stabilization; postoperative anticoagulation with Coumadin; long-term prognosis guarded in atrial fibrillation (repeated embolism)

compromising collateral pathways and extending the ischemic process. It has long been recognized that the extent of distal thrombosis is the primary determinant of the clinical course following embolic arterial occlusion (Fig. 36-60).

The tissues deprived of oxygen by the embolic process undergo a shift to anaerobic cellular metabolism. Local acidosis in time proceeds to cellular death with neural and muscular necrosis. Intracellular enzymes (CPK and lysozymes) and ions (K^+) are released into the bloodstream and interstitial tissues under these conditions. Because neural tissue is most sensitive to ischemia, pain and paresthesia are usually the presenting symptoms and are confined to the ischemic area. Later, extension of the ischemic damage leads to muscle swelling and eventually rigor. Although local factors influence the rate at which ischemic cellular death occurs, tissue necrosis may occur within 6 hours and is common after 12 hours of profound ischemia. When the process of distal propagation of clot proceeds unchecked, blood flow may become so stagnant that concomitant venous thrombosis occurs. It should be remembered that smaller emboli must occasionally lodge in well-collateralized arterial beds, producing no significant ischemia or symptoms.

ETIOLOGY

In a previously reported series of 300 consecutive embolic occlusions, 94% of the emboli were thought to have originated from within the heart. About 2% came from an abdominal aortic aneurysm or atherosclerotic plaque, and the sources of the remaining 4% were not identified. The majority of patients have atrial fibrillation, and the remainder, except for the rare patient with an endocardial tumor (myxoma), have had a myocardial infarction. In atrial fibrillation, thrombus forms in relatively stagnant areas of the left atrium. Following myocardial infarction, thrombus may form along the damaged left ventricular endocardial surface, particularly when the infarction results in wall dyskinesia. Changes in circulatory dynamics or thrombus maturation may then result in dislodgement of the embolic material into the arterial tree.

blockage in the early seventeenth century, but it was not until 1911 that the first successful arterial embolectomy was carried out by Labey. In spite of treatment, acute major arterial occlusion was associated with extremely high morbidity and mortality rates through most of the first half of this century. However, the isolation of heparin by Murray and Best in 1938 and the development of the balloon embolectomy catheter by Fogarty in 1963 have greatly simplified and improved the treatment of arterial embolism.

PATHOPHYSIOLOGY

Acute arterial occlusion results in both distal and proximal stagnation of flow. In the absence of anticoagulation, a soft coagulum of blood forms in these areas, progressively

Fig. 36-60. Impaction of embolus. The associated distal and proximal propagation of thrombosis often greatly extends the primary effects of the embolus.

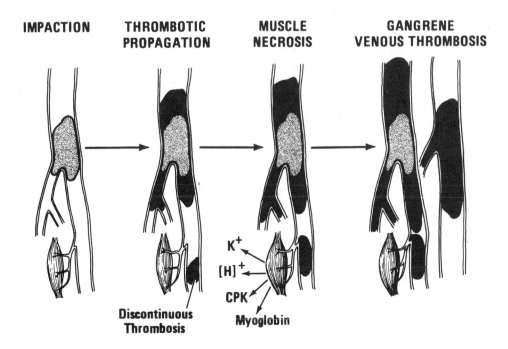

IMPACTION THROMBOTIC PROPAGATION MUSCLE NECROSIS GANGRENE VENOUS THROMBOSIS

Discontinuous Thrombosis

K^+
$[H]^+$
CPK
Myoglobin

Although emboli do occasionally lodge in the upper extremity and in the cerebral, mesenteric, and renal vascular beds, almost 90% of surgically treatable emboli are carried toward the lower extremities. In order of decreasing frequency, the common sites of impaction are the femoral (46%), iliac (18%), aortic (14%), and popliteal (11%) arterial bifurcations. Embolic occlusion of more than one vascular bed affects about 10% of patients and may be simultaneous or sequential.

DIAGNOSIS

The sudden presentation of an ischemic extremity, particularly in a patient with atrial fibrillation, should suggest the diagnosis of acute embolic arterial occlusion. A correct diagnosis should be made in more than 85% of patients on the basis of the clinical presentation and physical findings alone.

CLINICAL PRESENTATION

Without antecedent symptoms, the patient presents with most or all of the components of the "embolic syndrome." Pain in the affected extremity is followed in time by paresthesia and paralysis if flow is not reestablished; pulselessness and pallor are found on examination of the extremity. The pain is often severe, and the patient may be able to describe the exact instant it began. The patient should be questioned about the presence of any pre-existing cardiac or peripheral arterial disease.

PHYSICAL FINDINGS

The initial examination should be focused on an evaluation of the circulatory status and the viability of the affected limb. The color and temperature should be noted and compared with those of the opposite extremity, and the presence or absence of cutaneous sensation, proprioception, and motor movement are noted. A careful evaluation of all arterial pulsations must be performed.

The amplitude of pulsation may be increased just proximal to a major occlusion secondary to obstruction of the runoff bed. Distal to the occlusion, there is poor capillary filling and collapsed superficial veins, and with time, the muscles may become firm and doughy with loss of active ankle movement.

ADJUNCTIVE LABORATORY STUDIES

We have found noninvasive Doppler ultrasound techniques quite helpful in localizing the site of embolic occlusion and in differentiating between *in situ* thrombosis and embolic occlusion in patients with antecedent vascular disease. Because over 90% of these patients have associated cardiac disease, evaluation of the heart should proceed simultaneously with that of the extremity. Patients should have electrocardiography, chest x-ray, and muscle isoenzyme determination. In patients with no obvious source of emboli, echocardiography of the heart and abdomen and arteriography should be considered following embolectomy to rule out valvular heart disease, intracardiac mural thrombus, and aortic aneurysm or ulcerative atherosclerotic plaque. Initial laboratory evaluations of the coagulation, renal, and hepatic systems are also helpful and are easy to perform.

DIFFERENTIAL DIAGNOSIS

When there is acute ischemia of the extremity, it is imperative to make the correct diagnosis early because the natural history, threat to limb viability, and therapy (including surgical techniques) may differ markedly.

ACUTE ARTERIAL THROMBOSIS

The sudden onset of ischemia of the extremity in the absence of underlying cardiac pathology or other obvious source of embolism is likely to be the result of *in situ* arterial thrombosis, especially if the patient has a history of antecedent arterial insufficiency. The onset is frequently less abrupt, and the patient may complain of numbness (instead of pain) as the presenting symptom. Signs of chronic arterial insufficiency such as loss of toe hair, thickened nails, atrophic skin, and even ischemic ulceration are often found on the affected or opposite extremity.

Although the formation of atherosclerotic plaque usually proceeds gradually, acute arterial insufficiency may be brought about by hemorrhage within the plaque or *in situ* thrombosis on the narrowed irregular plaque surface. In many instances collateral pathways have already developed, preventing extensive distal propagation of the ischemic process. In the presence of adequate collateral circulation, progression to tissue damage is less frequent, and the initial discomfort often subsides over several days.

Management of the patient with acute arterial thrombosis is based on the degree of extremity ischemia present. When symptoms are mild and tissue viability is not in question, it is often appropriate to start the patient on an exercise (walking) program to stimulate maximal collateral development. However, when symptoms are severe (rest pain or paresthesia) or tissue viability is impaired, immediate arteriography and appropriate therapy must be instituted. Although it may be appropriate to treat certain lesions in especially high-risk patients with high-dose heparin therapy alone, the majority are best managed by operative revascularization. The specific operative approach is determined by the location and extent of the atherosclerotic involvement. Although endarterectomy may be indicated for patients with very localized disease, the usual patient requires bypass of the occluded arterial segment.

ACUTE AORTIC DISSECTION

The patient with acute arterial ischemia secondary to an aortic dissection usually presents with a brief history of excruciating chest or back pain. The expanding intramural dissection may lead to stenosis or occlusion of the aortic branch vessels. Involvement of the iliac arteries with lower extremity ischemia is not uncommon and is often associated with visceral artery involvement as well. A history of hypertension is frequently present. If the chest x-ray film suggests the diagnosis by demonstrating a widened mediastinal shadow, emergency aortography is mandatory to confirm the diagnosis and select the most appropriate therapeutic approach.

ACUTE VENOUS THROMBOSIS

The patient with acute venous thrombosis may also present with a painful, pulseless extremity. However, the presence of massive swelling and warm ruborous skin should rule out acute arterial embolism. Only if the process has progressed to "total" circulatory stasis with resultant rigor might there be difficulty in correctly identifying the primary underlying pathologic mechanism.

TREATMENT

The combination of immediate anticoagulation with early operative embolectomy is the most effective method of therapy for acute arterial embolic occlusion.

PREOPERATIVE MANAGEMENT

To prevent both propagation of thrombosis and further embolization, anticoagulation is instituted once the diagnosis is made. A loading dose of 5000 units of heparin is given intravenously and is followed by a constant infusion sufficient to prolong the partial thromboplastin time (PTT) to about 2.5 times the control time. Since virtually all of these patients have associated cardiac disease, part of the preoperative management should be aimed toward improving myocardial performance. Cardiac monitoring and judicious use of digitalis, diuretics, and antiarrhythmic agents are frequently indicated.

Beyond patient survival, the salvage of a viable and functional extremity is the goal of treatment. Although the degree of tissue damage is clearly related to the duration of ischemic insult, the absolute ischemic interval *per se* has been shown to be an unreliable predictor of the success of limb salvage and a poor criterion of operability. We feel that only the absence of both sensation and motor activity in association with muscle rigor contraindicates an attempt at embolectomy in an otherwise viable patient. Even in the presence of far advanced distal ischemia, a lower level of amputation may be possible following a successful embolectomy.

OPERATIVE THERAPY (EMBOLECTOMY)

The basic principles of embolectomy have remained essentially unchanged since the introduction of the Fogarty embolectomy catheter in 1963.

Instrumentation

The Fogarty embolectomy catheter consists of a hollow pliable body with a soft balloon at the tip. Each size catheter has been calibrated to produce an optimal degree of balloon distention, and overdistention increases pressure on the vessel intima and may produce injury. The deflated catheter is inserted into the lumen through an arteriotomy and is passed through the embolus. The balloon is inflated *by the surgeon* as the catheter is gently withdrawn, retrieving the embolic material and its associated thrombus (Fig. 36-61).

Technique

Once the diagnosis has been made, heparin has been given, and the patient's condition has been stabilized, he is brought to the operating room where a surgical preparation from the nipple line to the toes is performed. Although local anesthesia is frequently employed, an anesthesiologist must be present to monitor these critically ill patients and provide general anesthesia should a more extensive surgical procedure be required.

The most effective and flexible surgical approach to lower extremity ischemia due to emboli has been through a femoral incision, regardless of the anatomic location of the occlusion. The common femoral, superficial femoral, and profunda femoris arteries are isolated, and vascular clamps are applied. A transverse or oblique arteriotomy is made at the junction of the superficial and deep femoral arteries to allow visualization of both orifices and avoid significant narrowing at the time of arteriotomy closure (Fig. 36-62).

Distal exploration is carried out first with catheters inserted down the superficial and deep femoral arteries. An open deep femoral system is capable of maintaining limb viability in many patients with advanced ischemia and in patients with previous occlusion of the superficial femoral system. Recovery of embolic material from the deep femoral artery, even in the presence of a patent common femoral artery, has been frequent in our experience. The No. 3 and No. 4 French catheters are most commonly employed for exploration of the femoral and popliteal systems. If uncertainty exists concerning the adequacy of removal of the

Fig. 36-61. Technique for extraction of embolus with balloon catheter.

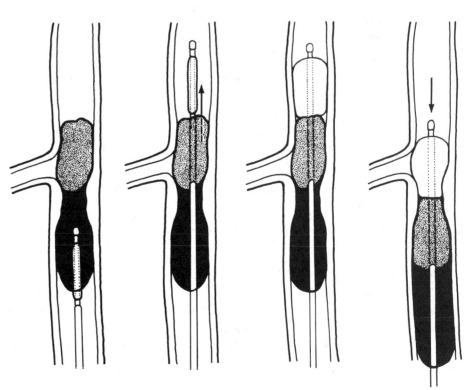

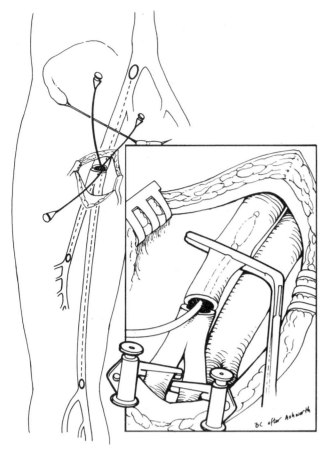

Fig. 36-62. Transverse arteriotomy, with fogartization of the several arterial branches, and *(inset)* technique of minimizing blood loss during fogartization of the opened vessel.

distal thrombus, operative arteriography is performed. The presence of additional distal thrombotic material that is unretrievable from the proximal arteriotomy is an indication for a second incision exposing the distal popliteal artery and the popliteal trifurcation. In this instance, a No. 2 or No. 3 Fogarty catheter should be introduced selectively in each of these vessels through a transverse popliteal arteriotomy. If these vessels were previously patent and are uninvolved with significant atherosclerosis, a No. 2 French catheter should pass beyond the ankle joint with ease. Following removal of the thrombotic material, irrigation of the distal arterial system should be carried out with heparinized saline solution. In all cases, the proximal arterial segment also should be explored with a catheter prior to closure of the arteriotomy. A No. 4 or No. 5 French catheter is inserted retrograde up the common femoral artery as far as the aortic bifurcation. The balloon is carefully inflated and withdrawn. Several gentle passes are made until forceful, pulsatile flow is obtained and no further embolic debris is seen. If an aortic (saddle) embolus is occluding both common iliac arteries, simultaneous operative exposure of both common femoral arteries is the preferred technique.*

POSTOPERATIVE CARE

Following successful reestablishment of arterial flow, the patient must be closely observed for the development of a

* The intra-arterial instillation of fibrinolysin as an alternative or adjunctive therapy shows some promise.—ED.

number of unique postoperative conditions. To prevent recurrent embolization, intravenous heparin therapy is continued uninterrupted or restarted several hours later, depending on the quantity of heparin already administered and the adequacy of hemostasis at wound closure. Unless contraindicated, the patient is later switched to oral anticoagulants (Coumadin). Early ambulation is encouraged, and prolonged sitting is prohibited. Frequent examination of peripheral pulses, skin color, and temperature is advised. When pulses are not readily palpated or venous patency is in question, the use of Doppler ultrasonic equipment is helpful.

Reocclusion following an apparently successful embolectomy is usually an indication for reoperation. Although the most common causes of such failures are technical (arterial perforation, intimal injury, or retained embolic material), the possibility of reembolization to the same extremity must not be overlooked.

Following the successful reestablishment of arterial circulation, further management should focus on the underlying causal pathologic condition. If the emboli were secondary to mitral stenosis or prosthetic valvular dysfunction, consideration must be given to valve replacement, and atrial fibrillation can be converted to sinus rhythm in some patients. If the emboli originated as mural thrombi resulting from a recent or old myocardial infarction, or if atrial fibrillation cannot be converted, oral anticoagulation is indicated indefinitely.

SPECIAL PROBLEMS

ADVANCED ISCHEMIA

In the setting of a prolonged ischemic period, specific adverse sequelae must be anticipated. Large quantities of potassium and myoglobin may be released from the injured muscle and flushed into the bloodstream upon reestablishment of arterial flow. The sudden return of the hyperkalemic, acidotic blood frequently results in cardiac arrhythmias and hypotension and, in conjunction with large quantities of myoglobin may result in acute renal tubular necrosis and renal failure. In this setting, removal of several hundred milliliters of blood through a small femoral venotomy as arterial flow is reestablished is beneficial. Judicious use of buffering agents and antiarrhythmic drugs is also appropriate at this time.

Following the reestablishment of circulation, swelling of the previously ischemic extremity can be severe and may lead to secondary compromise of arterial flow. Failure to recognize the situation, if severe, will lead to arterial reocclusion. Surgical decompression by fasciotomy is the appropriate treatment and has been required in about 10% of our patients with acute embolic occlusion.

If ischemia is far advanced, simultaneous major venous thrombosis is often found. The majority of these patients are found to have extensive distal arterial clot, and concomitant venous thrombectomy must be performed, using special venous thrombectomy balloon catheters.

CONCOMITANT OCCLUSIVE DISEASE

Arterial embolism in the presence of chronic peripheral vascular disease presents additional problems. A careful history and examination of the uninvolved extremity affords a reliable assessment of the peripheral circulation prior to the acute episode. In general, it is advisable initially to attempt only to return the circulation to its preocclusive status. Definitive reconstructive procedures are usually delayed until a more critical evaluation of the patient is possible; however, such procedures may be necessary initially if the viability of the extremity remains in question and the patient was relatively healthy and active prior to the acute episode.

PROGNOSIS

The goal of surgical embolectomy is to restore the peripheral circulation to its preocclusive state. Therefore, critical analysis of the results of embolectomy is best determined by consideration of the perioperative mortality and limb salvage rates. The probability of maintaining a viable, functional extremity following acute embolic arterial occlusion should exceed 90%; however, such success rates obviously are a function of patient selection and the gravity of the underlying pathologic conditions. The condition of the extremity, not the duration of arterial occlusion, is the primary determinant of operability and limb salvage.

In our series of 300 patients with acute embolic arterial occlusion, 16 amputations were required, yielding a limb salvage rate of 95%. Limb salvage is defined as maintaining a functional extremity without rest pain. Patients with claudication were subsequently evaluated on an elective basis, and further reconstructive surgery was carried out if necessary. Even in the presence of established gangrene, amputation can be performed at a more distal level if successful embolectomy is feasible and successful.

The hospital mortality of these patients was 16%. All deaths were due to cardiopulmonary dysfunction and in about 75% of cases were the direct result of the patients' underlying cardiac pathology. Recognition and treatment of the underlying cardiovascular condition must be a part of the management of these patients, and just under 10% of our patients underwent subsequent corrective cardiovascular procedures (valve replacement, ventricular and aortic aneurysmectomy).

In an attempt to reduce the disappointingly high mortality associated with acute arterial ischemia (25% in some series), "conservative" approaches have been advocated by some. One recent approach advocates the use of high-dose heparin therapy in all patients, reserving surgical intervention only for those patients with containdications to or complications from anticoagulation. Fifty-four patients were treated using this approach; a 67% limb salvage rate and a 7.5% mortality rate were reported. Although promising, three potential areas of concern exist. First, no distinction was made between acute embolic and thrombotic occlusions; second, the series reported was small; and finally, although the reported mortality rate is excellent, the limb salvage rate was substantially inferior to that currently expected following surgical treatment of acute embolic arterial occlusion. Although this approach may be appropriate for poor-risk patients with acute arterial thrombosis, it is our opinion that patients with acute embolic occlusion can be most effectively managed using the strategy described in this chapter coupled with adjunctive heparin anticoagulation.

ATHEROMATOUS EMBOLISM

Spontaneous peripheral embolization of atheromatous debris is a less common entity than embolism of thrombotic material and usually presents with a unique clinical syndrome.

HISTORICAL BACKGROUND

Although peripheral atheromatous embolization was first described by Flory over three decades ago, it has been only in the last 10 to 15 years that the importance of this syndrome has been recognized and specific management formulated.

PATHOPHYSIOLOGY

Atheromatous emboli may be composed of cholesterol crystals, fibrin and platelet aggregates, or larger pieces of more mature calcific plaque. This material may be released from the atherosclerotic arterial wall owing to hemodynamic changes or plaque maturation. Larger pieces of debris may produce obstruction of major segments of the peripheral arterial tree and similar sequelae as cardiothrombotic emboli. More commonly, numerous small embolic fragments are released and "shower" the peripheral arterial bed. These microemboli obstruct the smaller vessels, usually of the feet and toes, producing small areas of cyanosis or gangrene. If these showers are extensive or recurrent, large confluent areas of tissue necrosis may occur.

DIAGNOSIS

The diagnosis may be especially perplexing in that the majority of patiens have no outward signs of the underlying embolic source and appear to have adequate peripheral circulation.

The patient with microembolization presents with small painful areas of cyanosis or gangrene usually on the feet and toes. Peripheral pulses are almost always present and commonly are of normal intensity. In extensive microembolization from a more proximal source, the visceral vessels may be affected and the patient may present with renal or gastrointestinal complaints. The diagnosis may be obscure and is frequently mistaken for diabetes, collagen vascular disease, or various angiospastic disorders. Once clinically recognized, the diagnosis may be confirmed by angiography and, in appropriate instances, by skin biopsy.

The patient with large vessel atheromatous emboli presents a syndrome similar to that of the patient with cardiothrombotic embolism, but at embolectomy the material retrieved may be recognized as atheromatous plaque, and the embolic source may be sought by angiography.

TREATMENT

The mainstay of treatment is the removal of the embolic source to prevent further embolization. There is often an understandable reluctance to perform major vascular reconstructive surgery on patients with relatively mild symptoms. However, unless appropriate treatment is carried out, subsequent embolization frequently leads to progressive arterial occlusion and irreversible tissue necrosis. Either endarterectomy or exclusion with bypass of the embolic source is an appropriate procedure. When tissue necrosis is present, sympathectomy should be added to the procedure. Unfortunately, anticoagulants have not proved particularly helpful in preventing recurrent atheroembolism and are not commonly employed.

BIBLIOGRAPHY

BLAISDELL FW, STEELE M, ALLEN RE: Management of acute lower extremity arterial ischemia due to embolism and thrombosis. Surgery 84:822, 1978

FISCHER RD, FOGARTY TJ, MORROW AG: Clinical and biochemical observations of the effect of transient femoral artery occlusion in man. Surgery 68:323, 1970

FOGARTY TJ: Complications of arterial embolectomy. In Beebe HG (ed): Complications in Vascular Surgery. Philadelphia, J B Lippincott, 1973

FOGARTY TJ, CRANLEY JJ, KRAUSE RJ et al: A method for extraction of arterial emboli and thrombi. Surg Gynecol Obstet 116:241, 1963

FOGARTY TJ, DAILY PO, SHUMWAY NE et al: Experience with balloon catheter technique for arterial embolectomy. Am J Surg 122:321, 1971

PATMAN RD, THOMPSON JE: Fasciotomy in peripheral vascular surgery. Arch Surg 101:663, 1970

SAMUELS PB, KATZ DJ: Diagnosis and management of arterial mural emboli. Am J Surg 134:209, 1977

James D. Hardy

Arterial Injuries

Arterial injuries have challenged the best efforts of surgeons through the ages. An important segment of the medical history of each war has been devoted to an analysis of the incidence and types of arterial injuries and to the amputation rates associated with the interruption of various arteries of the extremities. But although the records of the successive major conflicts reflected an increasing preoccupation with the study and improvement of methods designed to treat arterial trauma more effectively by restorative surgery, it was not until the Korean War that immediate repair by direct suture was widely performed under field conditions. The success achieved with this prompt restitution of arterial continuity revolutionized the management of arterial injuries, not only in battle casualties but in civilian life as well. It is now possible, by one means or another, to repair injury to virtually any accessible artery, and all significant arteries are readily accessible except those within the skull. However, there are circumstances in which it may not be appropriate to repair an artery by primary anastomosis or grafting with vein or fabric. Such circumstances might include massive soft tissue injury to the extremity, major bacterial contamination and infection, the need to preserve the patient's life in critical circumstances, and still other factors. Civilian arterial injuries are usually not associated with the massive explosive tissue damage often produced in war wounds, but close-range shotgun blasts and severe crushing injury can cause major soft tissue destruction.

TYPES OF ARTERIAL INJURIES

The types of arterial injuries that may occur following different types of wounds are shown in Figure 36-63, and the incidence in one series is given in Table 36-9. The anatomic defect may represent a simple laceration, perforation, transsection, at times a loss of arterial substance,

Fig. 36-63. Types and management of arterial injuries. (Hardy JD, Raju S, Neely WA et al: Aortic and other arterial injuries. Ann Surg 181:640, 1975)

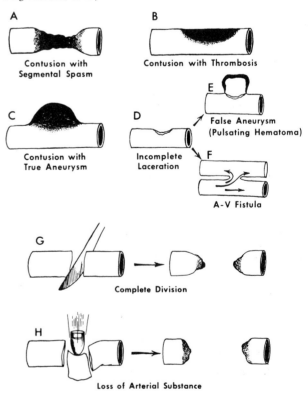

TABLE 36-9 BREAKDOWN BY TYPE OF 360 ARTERIAL INJURIES

TYPE OF INJURY	NO. OF CASES
Laceration	111
Perforation, transection, and loss of arterial substance	140
False aneurysm	39
Arteriovenous fistula	38
Contusion and thrombosis	21
Missile embolism	5
True aneurysm	3
Vasospasm	2
Burn	1

(Hardy JD, Raju S, Neely WA et al: Aortic and other arterial injuries. Ann Surg 181:640, 1975)

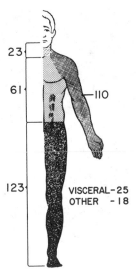

Fig. 36-64. Anatomic distribution of 360 arterial injuries. (Hardy JD, Raju S, Neely WA et al: Aortic and other arterial injuries. Ann Surg 181:640, 1975)

false aneurysm ("pulsating hematoma"), arteriovenous fistula, contusion or thrombosis, vasospasm, causalgia, or missile embolism. Blunt trauma may produce incomplete or even complete division of the arteries, but in these cases a frequent operative finding is that all layers except the adventitia have separated. Iatrogenic arterial injuries are common and are caused by cardiac catheters, intra-arterial blood pressure monitoring, and injection of irritating substances, among many other causes.

It is useful to the surgeon to formulate preoperatively a mental image of the anatomic defect he is likely to encounter, and for this purpose an arteriogram may provide invaluable assistance. This study should be performed initially in almost every instance of possible arterial injury, since it will usually demonstrate the precise site of injury and the probable anatomic defect. Once the nature of the injury has been disclosed by arteriography, operative correction should be performed as soon as possible, other factors being appropriate. The longer a serious arterial injury is left unrepaired, the greater the risk to the part of the body supplied by the artery, not to mention the continued risk of massive hemorrhage that might cost the patient his life. Delay in the presence of arterial thrombosis may preclude success; the sooner an arterial injury in the extremity is repaired, the lower the amputation rate. The extremities are injured more often than any other part of the body (Fig. 36-64), and the majority of civilian injuries are caused by gunshot or knife (Table 36-10).

In general, knife wounds are usually relatively simple and are readily managed, whereas crushing and gunshot injuries frequently cause not only severe vascular damage but injury to many other organs as well. Civilian gunshot injuries are usually inflicted by low-velocity missiles, and thus the soft tissue and bone damage is not nearly so extensive as it is in war wounds caused by high-velocity missiles, which are often multiple and penetrate several areas of the body.

DIAGNOSIS OF ARTERIAL INJURIES

The first important consideration is to suspect that arterial injury may have occurred. Arterial injury should always be considered in the presence of obvious major blood loss. In an extremity, the most prominent feature of arterial injury,

other than bright red bleeding, is distal coldness or pallor, with weak or absent pedal or foot pulses if arterial flow has been impaired. Of course, the distal pulse may have been absent prior to the injury, or a previously narrowed atherosclerotic vessel may have been completely occluded by blunt injury or may have thrombosed during shock due to blood loss. However, it is younger people who are most often injured in a conflict, and in such patients the absence of a distal pulse usually indicates arterial damage, if other clinical findings agree. Excessive localized swelling also may indicate arterial injury because the arterial pressure may cause extensive blood loss into the deep muscle planes (Fig. 36-65). In contrast, venous injury above may produce swelling of the entire distal leg from edema due to venous occlusion, but because of the low venous pressure the volume of blood loss into the tissues following venous injury is not as great as that accompanying arterial injury (though, of course, external venous bleeding can be massive). If a localized swelling is pulsatile, a false aneurysm ("pulsating hematoma") should be suspected. A thrill may be palpated, caused by partial arterial occlusion or by an arteriovenous

TABLE 36-10 CAUSE OF ARTERIAL INJURY IN 360 CASES

CAUSE	NO. OF CASES
Firearms	
Gunshot	155
Shotgun	37
	(192)
Stab wounds and lacerations	91
Blunt trauma	
Automobile	29
Other	19
	(48)
Iatrogenic	20
Miscellaneous, unknown	9

(Hardy JD, Raju S, Neely WA et al: Aortic and other arterial injuries. Ann Surg 181:640, 1975)

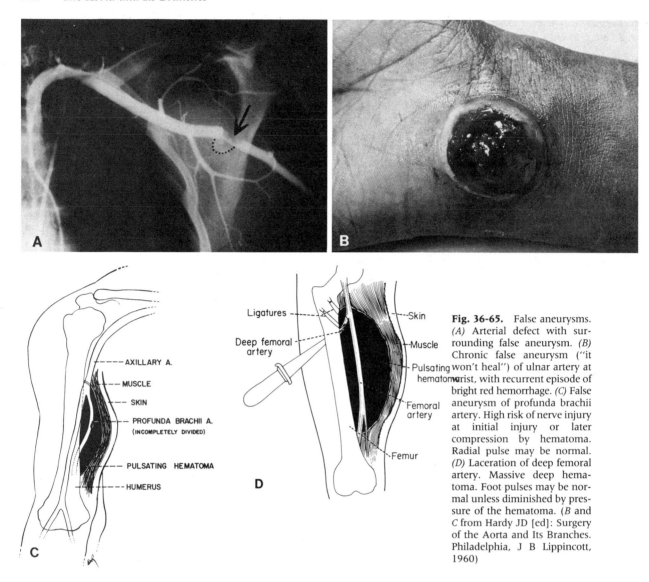

Fig. 36-65. False aneurysms. *(A)* Arterial defect with surrounding false aneurysm. *(B)* Chronic false aneurysm ("it won't heal") of ulnar artery at wrist, with recurrent episode of bright red hemorrhage. *(C)* False aneurysm of profunda brachii artery. High risk of nerve injury at initial injury or later compression by hematoma. Radial pulse may be normal. *(D)* Laceration of deep femoral artery. Massive deep hematoma. Foot pulses may be normal unless diminished by pressure of the hematoma. (*B* and *C* from Hardy JD [ed]: Surgery of the Aorta and Its Branches. Philadelphia, J B Lippincott, 1960)

fistula. Auscultation may reveal a systolic bruit if significant arterial stenosis exists, or a continuous bruit if an arteriovenous fistula is present. Neurologic changes may be due to ischemia, nerve transsection, blast effect, or nerve compression. Distal causalgia is in some way related to injury to the sympathetic innervation of the artery or adjacent nerves, and it is commonly relieved by sympathetic block or lumbar sympathectomy.

Symptomatically, arterial injury with vastly reduced distal flow first results in pain due to ischemia, then numbness progressing to anesthesia, and then to progressive loss of motor power and ultimately complete paralysis and tissue necrosis. Severe ischemia may prove irreversible unless corrected within 6 hours or so, but success will at times be achieved by operation performed even later.

Finally, *arteriography* represents the most specific diagnostic modality, and it should be employed for the complete evaluation of virtually every suspected arterial injury. Again, this study will usually delineate the site of arterial injury and the anatomic pathology that must be corrected at operation. Arteriography is also valuable in excluding arterial injury, to obviate the need for extensive dissection. Of course, if the injury occurred weeks or months before the patient is seen, the more chronic types of post-traumatic arterial problems (*e.g.,* relative ischemia, false aneurysm, A-V fistula) may be observed long after evidence of hemorrhage has subsided.

MANAGEMENT OF SPECIFIC TYPES OF ARTERIAL INJURIES

The accurate repair of an arterial injury requires adequate diagnosis and localization, appropriate instruments, general metabolic support of the patient, and a knowledge of the technical requirements of arterial surgery. The maneuvers to be employed in correcting the arterial defect or defects will be determined on the basis of the type of arterial injury likely to be encountered as well as the region of the body to which the injury has occurred. It is to be remembered that arteries are adjacent to veins and often to nerves, and these other anatomic elements may require appropriate management as well. Extensive muscle or visceral damage may have occurred, including bacterial contamination. Arterial repair is more successful when restoration of venous outflow has also been achieved.

ARTERIAL LACERATIONS

An arterial laceration is commonly produced by some sharp instrument or by a bullet. In Figure 36-65 are shown several types of pathologic defects that may result from arterial laceration. The injury may have been produced by a simple slash with a knife, which is usually a clean wound with little soft tissue damage and in which arterial repair can usually be achieved without the use of a graft of either autogenous saphenous vein or fabric. The ends of an artery may retract over a distance of several centimeters if the vessel has been completely severed, and the hemorrhage may have ceased under these circumstances of pronounced arterial retraction and spasm closing the vessel. On the other hand, if the artery has been incompletely divided by the laceration, prolonged hemorrhage may occur and may continue because retraction of the ends of the artery has not been possible. Not infrequently the injury has occurred to a branch of a major artery, in which circumstances the main artery will exhibit normal pulsations (Fig. 36-65). However, swelling of the part will suggest arterial hemor-

rhage, and an arteriogram will usually prove diagnostic. Again, the dissection of the hematoma along muscle planes can be quite extensive, and a sufficient volume of blood can be lost into the thigh to cause shock. This may seriously compress the arterial inflow and the venous outflow of the extremity, and this severe pressure that develops from the hematoma may compress surrounding nerves, which otherwise may have escaped damage at the time of the original injury. If the injury is superficial, as in the wrist, the possibility of arterial laceration should be immediately suspected if the patient gives a history of significant bright red hemorrhage (Fig. 36-65). Occasionally, the inexperienced physician may cut into the warm skin overlying a *false aneurysm* (pulsating hematoma), in the belief that he is draining an abscess. This can, of course, result in severe hemorrhage, especially in a situation where appropriate instruments and knowledge are not available. A laceration that penetrates an artery or extends into the adjacent vein or vice versa, may result in an arteriovenous fistula, which will be discussed separately. If a bullet has produced the laceration, it may actually enter a vein and embolize either into the heart from a peripheral vein or from the heart into a peripheral artery (Fig. 36-66).

Most arterial lacerations are produced by hostile action with a sharp instrument, a gunshot, or blunt trauma, but a considerable number of arterial lacerations are produced by physicians in the course of their work. We have met a wide variety of such injuries, including injury to the aorta or iliac artery during operation for lumbar disc, to the femoral artery by sharp self-retaining retractors in hip operations, to various arteries in the course of sharp dissection at operation, and to arteries with large-bore needles that resulted in hemorrhage or thrombosis. Injuries occur also to the brachial or femoral arteries in the course of diagnostic heart catheterization and to the radial artery from intra-arterial pressure monitoring and from a wide variety of other circumstances. Hospital-incurred arterial injuries constitute a distinct segment of the vascular surgeon's practice.

The management of arterial laceration is usually relatively simple if the laceration has occurred in a part of the body where the artery is readily accessible, which is almost invariably the case with arm and leg injuries. However,

Fig. 36-66. Bullet embolism with subclavian steal. *(Left)* Bullet arrested in left subclavian artery following embolism from left ventricle. *(Right)* Left subclavian artery distal to bullet is shown filling via left vertebral artery from circle of Willis.

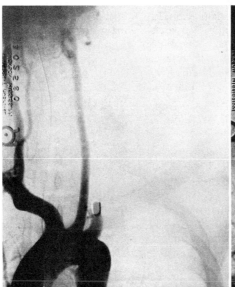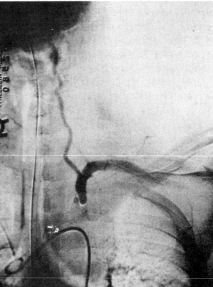

injuries to the thoracic or abdominal aorta can require major mobilization of facilities and expertise simply to save the patient's life. Injury to a subclavian artery is not necessarily associated with massive uncontained hemorrhage, though it may be; however, this artery can be difficult to expose rapidly and safely without injury to the brachial plexus. Here the proximity of the brachial plexus precludes indiscriminate clamping of poorly visualized bleeding vessels. Furthermore, there are multiple important branches of the subclavian and axillary arteries, and thus the vessel must be controlled virtually at the site of injury to prevent excessive bleeding from the rich collaterals. Furthermore, the left subclavian artery emerges from the thorax, and the operative exposure frequently requires division of the clavicle and perhaps even the first rib unless formal thoracotomy is used. Nonetheless, one should not hesitate to divide whatever portion of the upper thorax is required to expose the bleeding vessel adequately. The bony structures can all be repaired and stabilized satisfactorily once the emergency posed by hemorrhage has passed.

Injuries to the large vessels arising from the aortic arch are frequently associated with other problems, notably injury to the trachea or the esophagus, or occasionally to the spinal cord. A false aneurysm may develop that over the months produces such a dense fibrous reaction that repair is difficult. For this reason arterial injuries should be repaired promptly. Compression of surrounding nerves by the aneurysm can result in serious and often permanent neurologic deficits, especially in the arm.

Once the defect in the artery has been exposed and adequate proximal and distal control of the vessel has been achieved, it can usually be repaired transversely with a simple continuous suture using a permanent suture material, if the injury is due to a knife wound. If the laceration is due to a bullet wound, not only may *blast effect* have damaged the adjacent portions of the artery, but there may have been gross *loss of arterial substance*. The ends of the artery can usually be mobilized and brought together without undue tension over a distance of perhaps 2 cm, especially if the injury was recently inflicted, so there is less opportunity for mobilization in the scar tissue of a chronic arterial injury. However, if a gunshot wound has resulted in substantial loss of arterial substance, it will usually be preferable to bridge the defect with a saphenous vein graft or, should such a vein not be available, with a suitable fabric graft. In general it is preferable to employ an autogenous vein graft to bridge defects following acute injury when possible because there is always the probability of bacterial contamination of the wound. However, if a vein graft is not feasible, a fabric graft will have to be employed. The margins of laceration should be debrided prior to suturing.

ARTERIOVENOUS FISTULA

An arteriovenous (A-V) fistula (see Fig. 36-63) may develop anywhere in the body when the injury involves both the artery and an adjacent vein (Fig. 36-67). As a rule, simultaneous injury to both vessels is sustained at the initial wounding, but occasionally a chronic aneurysm or pulsating hematoma of the artery may eventually rupture into the adjacent vein and thus produce a true A-V fistula if in fact the fistula was not produced immediately at the time of injury. The reason for this belief is that, whereas one may hear the characteristic continuous bruit over the site of the fistula immediately after injury, in some instances no such

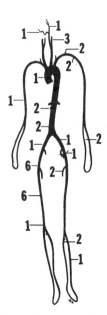

Fig. 36-67. Distribution of 38 traumatic arteriovenous fistulas. (Hardy JD, Raju S, Neely WA et al: Aortic and other arterial injuries. Ann Surg 181:640, 1975)

bruit is audible for weeks or even several months following the injury. If the bullet completely traverses the artery and vein and emerges on the opposite side, the defect in the vein on the side away from the artery will eventually close due to the pressure of the surrounding hematoma. However, a significant defect between the wall of the vein adjacent to the artery and the arterial lumen will usually not close because the pressure in the artery will tend to maintain patency of the aperture. In addition to this A-V fistula, a false aneurysm may develop adjacent to the arterial injury on the side away from the vein, or indeed between the artery and the vein (Fig. 36-68). The term arteriovenous aneurysm is often used instead of arteriovenous fistula, but this term can be misleading. Actually, there commonly is no true aneurysm of the artery immediately after the formation of the fistula. However, if a fistula of large size persists for weeks, months, or years, there will usually develop an enormous collateral circulation consisting of dilated veins and, ultimately, dilated arteries. Moreover, the main artery that is feeding the fistula may become quite

ARTERIOVENOUS FISTULA	
Etiology	Penetrating injury most commonly caused by bullet or knife wounds
	Large fistulas may cause tachycardia, left ventricular enlargement, and eventual left heart failure; rarely, subacute bacterial endocarditis; and occasionally aneurysm
Dx	History and physical findings, especially a continuous bruit or "machinery murmur"
	Arteriography
Rx	Surgical correction with repair of major arteries and, when possible, the accompanying vein

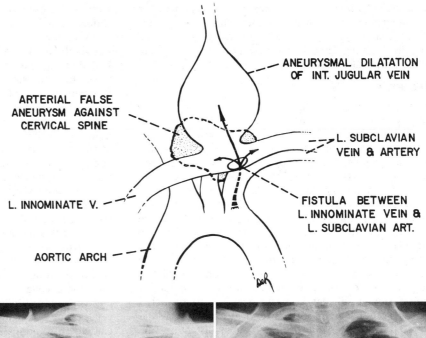

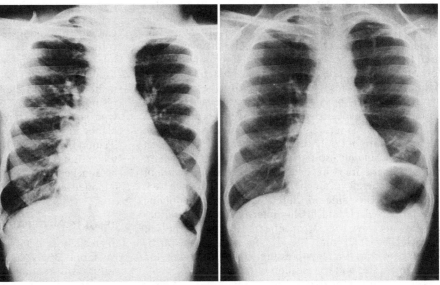

Fig. 36-68. Chronic traumatic arteriovenous fistula. *(Top)* Note fistula between left subclavian artery and left innominate vein, with huge dilatation of left internal jugular vein. False aneurysm was present. *(Bottom)* On the left, the chest roentgenogram discloses marked cardiac enlargement due to this arteriovenous fistula, which had been present for over 10 years. The chest roentgenogram on the right shows marked reduction of heart size 6 months after repair of arteriovenous fistula. (Hardy JD [ed]: Surgery of the Aorta and Its Branches. Philadelphia, J B Lippincott, 1960)

enlarged and aneurysmal, especially proximally, and may in fact eventually rupture as a true aneurysm. Furthermore, the collateral circulation may become so massive that the uninitiated surgeon may have difficulty at operation in deciding just where the fistula is located. In earlier days, when experience with arterial surgery was less extensive, it was by no means uncommon to fail to excise the true fistula, and thus it was said to have recurred postoperatively when in fact it had never been dealt with adequately during the operative procedure. There is occasionally the mistaken impression that the channel between the artery and the vein may represent a considerable distance (*e.g.*, as patent ductus arteriosus extends between the aorta and the pulmonary artery); however, this is very rarely the case, and only when a false aneurysm is located between the vein and the artery. The vein and the artery are almost invariably closely adherent to each other, surrounding the common aperture represented by the fistula itself.

All these pathologic anatomic considerations are important to the surgeon as he approaches correction of the fistula because it is a great advantage to have a clear mental picture of what pathology he can expect to find; this makes for

expeditious and complete correction of the lesion. Much of this information is derived from the preoperative arteriograms.

One special problem is associated with shotgun injuries, in which multiple A-V fistulas may have been produced. Unless one uses a *sterile stethoscope* at the time of operation, it is easy to miss a fistula, which may then require a second operation for its correction.

COMPLICATIONS

The reason that A-V fistula has always been of much interest to surgeons is that a considerable range of pathophysiologic complications may develop early with large fistulas and late with moderate size fistulas. A large acute fistula, such as that between the aorta and the inferior vena cava, can result in acute *cardiac decompensation* due to left ventricular failure and thus require early repair. This high output failure may develop with a fistula of less magnitude if a sufficient number of months or years pass for development of left ventricular failure. Another interesting complication of A-V fistula is bacterial endocarditis, which may affect the heart valves or may occasionally be found at the site of the fistula itself. Positive blood cultures may be obtained. If a false aneurysm is associated with the fistula, its continued enlargement may compress surrounding structures and cause distal paralysis in a limb from compression of adjacent nerves. It may also rupture.

DIAGNOSIS

The diagnosis of an A-V fistula is not difficult. The history of injury, usually a penetrating injury as by bullet, knife or needle, should suggest the possibility of arterial injury. Bright hemorrhage may have occurred at the time of the injury, and a pulsating mass representing a false aneurysm may be present. However, it is by palpation, auscultation, and arteriography that the diagnosis is made. If one places a hand over the pulsating area or over the site of a fistula in the absence of a pulsating mass, a thrill will usually be felt. Following this, a stethoscope may be applied to the skin adjacent to the injury, and a continuous bruit ("machinery murmur") can be heard throughout the cardiac cycle. This sound is very characteristic and, once heard, can rarely be confused with any other diagnosis. Incidentally, a purely systolic bruit may be heard over any artery that is partially occluded from any cause. If an extremity fistula has persisted for a period of time, venous distention surrounding the site may be noted. The pulse may be weaker distal to the fistula because a considerable amount of blood flow through the artery is being diverted through the diminished area of resistance into the vein. These days, the commonest cause of A-V fistula is a surgical operation performed to provide access for chronic renal hemodialysis.

The diagnosis is securely established with arteriography. The arteriogram not only will disclose the site of the defect in the artery but will also show that the radiopaque medium injected into the artery has entered the adjacent vein without passing peripherally through the capillaries and thence back up the vein. The same principle is involved in identifying intracardiac defects and finding interventricular septal defects by injecting the radiopaque medium into the left ventricle or left atrium. The dye flows from the high-pressure area to the low-pressure area, identifying the approximate size and the location of the fistula.

Another important physical finding with A-V fistula is the fact that when firm point pressure is exerted over the fistula, preventing blood flow through the fistula, the cardiac rate will usually decline abruptly if the fistula is of significant size (Branham's sign).

MANAGEMENT

The management of A-V fistula is invariably surgical unless the fistula is quite small or other circumstances dictate that the patient should not have the operation. The principal indications for operation include the complications given previously, such as enlargement of an associated false aneurysm, compression of surrounding nerves, aneurysmal dilatation of the artery that may eventually rupture, and most especially the development of left heart failure and, rarely, subacute bacterial endocarditis.

The timing of operative intervention has changed radically over the past thirty years. Prior to the rapid forward movement of direct arterial surgery as a result of the Korean War, the fistula was usually allowed to persist for weeks or even months to permit collateral circulation to develop. Following this, the artery and vein were both excised by quadruple ligation and excision, and the segments of the two vessels containing the fistula were delivered to the pathologist. Both ends of the artery and of the vein were simply ligated. Obviously this often meant ligation of the main supply to a part, and ischemia and even gangrene frequently developed. Incidentally, the pathologist at times had difficulty in determining which was the artery and which the vein, since "arterialization" or thickening of the vein with hypertrophy of its musculature had often occurred.

At present, however, A-V fistulas and almost all other traumatic arterial defects are corrected as soon after the injury as feasible. In almost all instances when an artery of significant size is involved, the continuity of the artery and the vein is restored by the separation of the two vessels from one another and direct transverse suture where feasible. At times, however, the scar tissue and dense inflammatory reaction are so great that the vessels cannot be satisfactorily mobilized proximally and distally to permit direct anastomosis; in this instance the defect in the artery is bridged with a portion of a reversed autogenous saphenous vein graft or with a fabric prosthesis. If the ends of the vein cannot be brought together, the vein is usually ligated, since the venous collateral circulation is usually sufficiently extensive to drain the part. However, a graft of autogenous vein may be inserted with successful maintenance of venous patency in some instances. If the fistula is associated with contamination or overt infection, it is preferable to treat the infection, allow the wound to heal, and then attack the fistula through a clean operative field. If there should be hemorrhage from the fistula or from associated false aneurysm in the presence of infection, a bypass graft of suitable type should be employed, passing through clean tissue planes and diverting the flow around the site of injury, with ligation of the artery both above and below this level. Once the graft has been placed and is functioning, the fistula can be attacked directly and the vessel ligated. However, such a maneuver is not often required.

RESULTS OF REPAIR OF ARTERIOVENOUS FISTULAS

In an analysis of 360 arterial injuries treated in our hospital, we found 38 A-V fistulas (Fig. 36-67). Repair of these fistulas with restoration of arterial flow (and usually venous flow as well) was almost invariably successful. Although the surgeon may prefer to obtain both proximal and distal control of both the artery and the vein at a site away from the dense reaction at the site of a chronic fistula, the experienced operator will frequently find it preferable to enter the fistula directly, control hemorrhage as necessary and repair the defect expeditiously. Intraluminal inflation of the balloon of a Fogarty catheter will provide sufficient temporary hemostasis if required. In the extremities, the inflation of a pneumatic tourniquet proximally may expedite the operation.

POSTOPERATIVE CONSIDERATIONS IN ARTERIAL INJURIES

1. Palpable pulse? If not, prompt arteriogram. Reexplore.
2. Antibiotics.
3. Dextran? Avoid heparin.
4. Neurologic status? Fasciotomy?
5. Sympathetic blocks are of little help.
6. Maintain blood volume.

BLUNT ARTERIAL INJURIES WITH OR WITHOUT THROMBOSIS

The discussion thus far has been devoted primarily to arterial injuries resulting from penetrating injuries, usually with knife or gunshot. Another important group of arterial injuries are those that are secondary to blunt trauma. An injury may be associated with a long bone fracture, but it can occur without a fracture. The vessel may be completely divided with possibly fatal hemorrhage, or the adventitia may remain intact. Serious venous injury may also occur.

Perhaps the most classic arterial injury due to blunt trauma is that of traumatic aneurysm of the thoracic aorta at the level of the ligamentum arteriosum. This injury, which was discussed in some detail in the section on aneurysms of the aorta, should always be suspected when there is a widening of the mediastinum following a deceleration accident. Arteries anywhere in the body can be injured by severe blunt trauma. Accurate arteriography and prompt surgical intervention are commonly required for the salvage of life or limb.

OTHER CAUSES AND CONSIDERATIONS IN ARTERIAL INJURIES

In addition to these major types of arterial injuries, a wide range of other sources of injuries may be encountered.

INJURY BY BONE FRAGMENTS

It is by no means uncommon for an artery to be injured by the fragments of bones themselves, even if the artery escaped injury at the original trauma. If the distal pulses, present on admission, disappear after the application of a plaster cast, the situation is serious, and usually the cast must be removed and reapplied. Arteriography should always be done when indicated.

SHOTGUN INJURIES

Another type of injury that can be particularly severe and extensive is that caused by a shotgun blast, especially at close range (Fig. 36-69). The large number of pellets may produce multiple wounds in one artery or in several arteries, even in different extremities. The single pellet may go through the vessel and leave no lasting injury. However, an A-V fistula, false aneurysm or thrombosis can occur. On the other hand, if the full blast is taken at close range, or if several pellets enter the artery at the same site, major arterial damage can result. Frequently there are so many pellet holes in the artery, over a distance, that the wise course is simply to excise the most damaged portion of the artery and to restore continuity with primary anastomosis or with a saphenous vein graft. A fabric graft is avoided here if possible because of the possible contamination.

A pellet injury may result in no gross external evidence of injury but may have caused dissection beneath the intima with subintimal hemorrhage and occlusion of the lumen (Fig. 36-69). Again, whatever measures are required to restore pulsatile flow in the artery are employed. In our experience shotgun blasts more frequently result in the loss of the extremity than do bullet injuries, largely because of the extensiveness of the injury with massive soft tissue loss. The remaining soft tissue may be inadequate to cover and thus to protect the arterial and venous repairs. Severe bone damage may be present. Furthermore, contamination may exist even if sufficient skin coverage remains.

IATROGENIC ARTERIAL INJURIES

A remarkable range of arterial injuries occur in the course of patient diagnosis and treatment (Fig. 36-70), and a number of these have been cited. Prompt and appropriate surgical intervention will permit removal of clots and other maneuvers to restore satisfactory blood flow through the injured vessel.

ARTERIAL SPASM WITH OR WITHOUT THROMBOSIS

There has been much interest and controversy over the years about the clinical significance of arteriospasm, which was once thought to be severe enough to result in arterial thrombosis. Actually, we believe that the diagnosis of arterial spasm should rarely be accepted until appropriate diagnostic studies, including arteriography, have excluded the more likely diagnosis of organic occlusion. This is especially true following injury, for thrombosis within the otherwise unremarkable vessel may have occurred. If occlusion has

Fig. 36-69. Multiple perforations from shotgun injury. The extensive bone and soft tissue damage inflicted by a close-range shotgun blast may preclude ultimate salvage of the extremity. (Hardy JD, Raju S, Neely WA et al: Aortic and other arterial injuries. Ann Surg 181:640, 1975)

SHOTGUN INJURY

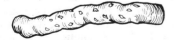

LIMITED DISSECTION

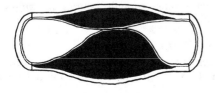

Fig. 36-70. Finger necrosis secondary to indwelling radial artery catheters for continuous blood pressure monitoring. Such injuries are apt to occur in desperately ill patients with a low cardiac output. Preventive measures include verification of both radial and ulnar arterial arches in the hand prior to insertion of the catheter, as well as removal of the catheter at the first evidence that the hand is becoming significantly ischemic. Once injury has occurred, no tissue should be amputated until it becomes obligatory, because a remarkable degree of recovery of the involved digits may occur.

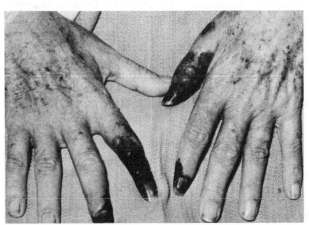

occurred, the appropriate therapy should be carried out. On the other hand, severe arteriospasm certainly can occur with the use of certain medications, especially those containing ergot derivatives. We have observed this in a number of patients, two of whom suffered distal gangrene of an extremity and required amputation. One patient had such severe arterial spasm, visualized by us on arteriogram and directly at operation, that neither common femoral artery contained a significant amount of blood. This spasm was so protracted, despite bilateral lumbar sympathectomy at the time, that the patient developed ischemic neuritis in the legs distally and suffered for several years from the atrophic appearance of the slick and shiny skin that is seen at times following severe ischemia and is associated especially with causalgia.

REGIONAL CONSIDERATIONS IN ARTERIAL EXPOSURE AND REPAIR

CAROTID INJURIES

Carotid injuries are diagnosed by physical examination, possible neurologic changes, and arteriography. The carotid artery is readily exposed in the neck. An internal shunt should be used during repair when indicated and feasible. If end-to-end continuity cannot be restored, a saphenous vein graft or even a fabric graft may be used. In some patients a hemiplegia present preoperatively may disappear during the postoperative period. The possibility of intracranial hemorrhage and infarction secondary to restoration of flow through the previously occluded internal carotid has been emphasized in some quarters, but we did not meet this complication following restoration of flow in traumatized patients.

SUBCLAVIAN ARTERY INJURIES

The subclavian artery presents special problems, primarily because it is not easily exposed, especially on the left, but also because of its proximity to the brachial plexus. Further, the subclavian artery has multiple sizeable collaterals, and control proximal and distal to the site of injury can represent a problem (Fig. 36-71), especially in chronic injury with dense surrounding fibrosis.

The first requirement in subclavian artery injury with continuing hemorrhage is to stop the bleeding. On the left, this may require a thoracotomy in order to approach the intrathoracic portion of the left subclavian artery. Otherwise, on either side, any of the other incisions shown in Fig. 36-71 may be employed to afford access to the artery. The important consideration, in the face of rapid hemorrhage from the subclavian artery, is to expose the site of bleeding by any necessary incision and maneuver to permit firm point pressure at the site of hemorrhage. Following this, with normal blood volume restored, the defect in the vessel can be carefully exposed and sutured, with protection of the brachial plexus. The bony structures that were hastily divided to gain access to the bleeding vessel can then be managed satisfactorily, regardless of what incision was employed.

Chronic false aneurysm of the subclavian artery may compress the brachial plexus and cause permanent neurologic deficit. Thus, false aneurysms should usually be repaired promptly, and in fact most arterial injuries are more easily exposed soon after injury than they are later when scarring has occurred.

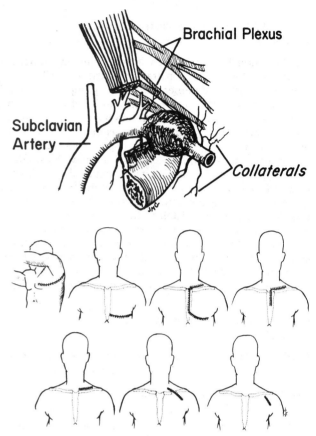

Fig. 36-71. Injury to subclavian artery. *(Top)* The proximity of the brachial plexus requires meticulous exposure and the multiple collaterals of the subclavian and axillary arteries can render precise hemostasis difficult. *(Bottom)* Incisions for approach to left subclavian artery. The right subclavian artery can usually be exposed adequately using a transverse incision in supraclavicular fossa. *(Top,* Hardy JD, Raju S, Neely WA et al; Aortic and other arterial injuries. Ann Surg 181:640, 1975)

ARTERIAL INJURIES IN THE ARM

Figures 36-72 and 36-73 present some of the problems met in the management of arterial injuries in the arm. A knife wound may readily produce both nerve and arterial injury in the arm, whereas serious nerve injury is less likely in the thigh because the femoral nerve anteriorly gives off its important muscle branches high, and the sciatic nerve is situated posteriorly. If the arm injury represents an essentially clean wound, it may be advisable to repair the artery and the nerve at the same time, but frequently neurologic surgeons prefer to "tag" the ends of the nerve and to effect formal repair at a later date.

A close-range shotgun wound of the forearm can require the collaboration of the orthopaedist, the vascular surgeon, and perhaps the neurosurgeon and the plastic surgeon. Figure 36-73 shows such a wound in which the ulna has been stabilized with an intramedullary pin, the ulnar artery grafted with saphenous vein, and the false aneurysm of the radial artery (see arrow) subsequently excised with primary end-to-end anastomosis. The soft tissue loss may be so massive in close-range shotgun injuries that amputation is unavoidable.

AORTIC INJURIES

The management of blunt thoracic aortic injuries is also considered elsewhere (p. 921). Aortic injuries are usually

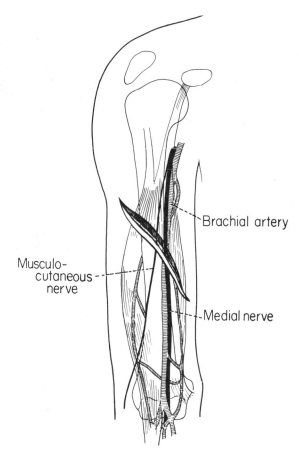

Fig. 36-72. Laceration with division of brachial artery, medial nerve, and musculocutaneous nerve. Arterial injuries in the arm are readily repaired, but nerve damage may severely limit the overall functional result.

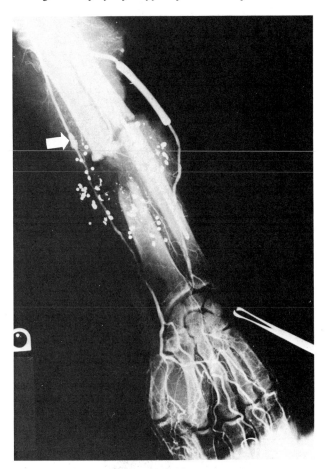

Fig. 36-73. Close-range shotgun injury to forearm. The ulna was stabilized with an intramedullary pin. The ulnar artery was repaired with a vein graft, and the small false aneurysm of the radial artery (*arrow*) was resected, with primary end-to-end anastomosis.

serious and the overall mortality rate in a series of 36 such patients who reached our emergency ward was 58%. The major cause of death was hemorrhagic shock and its complications. Many patients with aortic injury do not survive to reach the hospital. Penetration injury must be appropriately exposed, bleeding controlled, and the aorta repaired.

In our experience in patients who survived to reach the hospital, injuries to the abdominal aorta were more common than those involving the thoracic aorta. The upper abdominal aorta is more difficult to expose and control than is the thoracic aorta owing to its position behind the stomach and pancreas, plus the fact that the celiac, superior mesenteric, and renal arteries arise close together. Considerable experience and poise can be required to successfully manage an injury to the infradiaphragmatic aorta.

A common problem with penetrating injuries to the abdominal aorta is that of associated injuries, such as injuries to the bowel with contamination and the questionable importance of a retroperitoneal hematoma without obvious continuing hemorrhage. In brief, the known aortic injury should be excluded with appropriate vascular clamps and repaired without fabric grafts when possible if contamination has occurred. Retroperitoneal hematomas should be routinely explored to identify or exclude injury to the aorta or renal arteries or the vena cava. Otherwise, a high-risk reoperation may be required, either early for renewed hemorrhage or late for false aneurysm or A-V fistula.

THE MAJOR ARTERIES TO THE LEGS

The major arteries to the legs, beginning at the aorta, are usually readily exposed, and a simple injury can be readily repaired if the patient presents soon after injury. Unfortunately, there may have been a delay of many hours by the time the patient arrives at the hospital. Furthermore, extensive soft tissue loss, contamination, fractures, and neurologic deficits may seriously limit the success to be achieved by repair of the injured artery and vein. In Figure 36-74 is shown a long saphenous vein bypass that was used to carry blood from the right common femoral artery, beneath the subscrotal skin, to the left popliteal artery. This procedure was used to save the left leg when a massive and grossly infected shotgun injury to the left thigh and buttock had necessitated ligation of the left external iliac, internal iliac, common femoral, and profunda femoral arteries. The reversed saphenous vein is widely used as an autogenous graft, generally with gratifying results. Loss of flow through the popliteal artery results in a high amputation rate, and early repair is mandatory.

A prolonged period of ischemia often results in marked edematous swelling of the part. This is not uncommonly met in lower leg ischemia, and *fasciotomy* may be required to relieve compression of the neurovascular elements in both the anterior tibial compartment and in the posterior tibial compartment, where fibulectomy may be necessary for adequate decompression (Fig. 36-75).

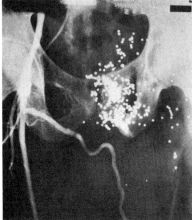
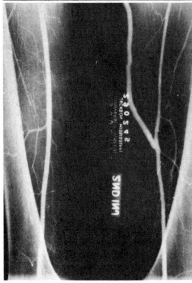

Fig. 36-74. Femoro-subscrotal-femoral saphenous vein graft. Massive close-range shotgun blast to thigh and buttock with obligatory ligation of major arterial supply to left leg. (Hardy JD, Bane JW: Arterial injury and massive blood loss: A case report of management of pelvic gunshot injury with femoro-subscrotal-femoral bypass and 116 units of blood. Ann Surg 181:245, 1975)

Fig. 36-75. Technique of fasciotomy.

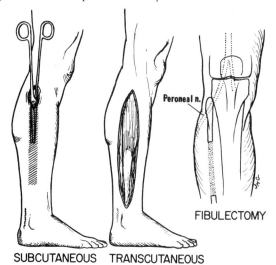

SUBCUTANEOUS   TRANSCUTANEOUS   FIBULECTOMY

Peroneal n.

CAUSALGIA

Causalgia is a peculiar type of pain in a part that may follow traumatic injury. The artery may not have been demonstrably injured, and the nerves may appear to be intact. The condition was first described by S. Weir Mitchell in 1878, and the mechanism by which the pain is produced has still not been fully explained. Nonetheless, it is usually intimately associated with injury to the artery or an adjacent nerve. If this results from a bullet wound in the leg, for example, the skin of the distal portion of the extremity and especially the foot may take on a slick, shiny, erythematous, and atrophic appearance, and the skin may be exquisitely sensitive to touch. Excessive sweating of the part may be observed.

Whereas the exact mechanism of injury from which the pain results is still uncertain, almost by definition the condition should be relieved by sympathetic nerve block or by division of the sympathetic nerves to the part.

Causalgia should not be confused with *ischemic neuritis,* which can occur in the nerves of a part that has been subjected to prolonged ischemia. This, too, may result in atrophic changes in the skin of the part. Unfortunately, ischemic neuritis will not respond so readily to sympathectomy and may be the cause of prolonged disability.

BIBLIOGRAPHY

COHEN A, BRIEF D, MATHEWSON C JR: Carotid artery injuries: An analysis of eighty-five cases. Am J Surg 120:210, 1970

CONN JH, HARDY JD, CHAVEZ CM et al: Challenging arterial injuries. J Trauma 11:167, 1971

FLETCHER JP, LITTLE JM: Vascular trauma. Aust NZ J Surg 51:333, 1981

FLINT LM, SNYDER WH, PERRY MO et al: Management of major vascular injuries in the base of the neck: An 11-year experience with 146 cases. Arch Surg 106:409, 1973

GASPAR MR: Arterial trauma. In Gaspar MR, Barker WF (eds): Peripheral Arterial Disease, 3rd ed. Major Problems Clinical Surgery, Vol. 4. Philadelphia, W B Saunders, 1981

HARDY JD, RAJU S, NEELY WA et al: Aortic and other arterial injuries. Ann Surg 181:640, 1975

HUGHES CW: Arterial repair during the Korean War. Ann Surg 147:555, 1958

JACOBSON JH II: Microsurgery. Curr Probl Surg 8:3, 1971

MITCHELL SW: On a rare vaso-motor neurosis of the extremities and on the maladies with which it may be compounded. Am J Med Sci 76:17, 1878

OCHSNER JL, CRAWFORD ES, DEBAKEY ME: Injuries of the vena cava caused by external trauma. Surgery 49:397, 1961

PATMAN RD, THOMPSON JE: Fasciotomy in peripheral vascular surgery: Report of 164 patients. Arch Surg 101:663, 1970

PERRY MO, THAL ER, SHIRES GT: Management of arterial injuries. Ann Surg 173:403, 1971

REUL GJ JR, RUBIO PA, BEALL AC JR: The surgical management of acute injury to the thoracic aorta. J Thorac Cardiovasc Surg 67:272, 1974

RICH NM, BAUGH JH, HUGHES CW: Acute arterial injuries in Vietnam: 1000 cases. J Trauma 10:359, 1970

SMITH PL, LIM WN, FERRIS EJ et al: Emergency arteriography in extremity trauma: Assessment of indications. AJR 137:803, 1981

SMITH RF, SZILAGYI DE, ELLIOTT JP JR: Fracture of long bones with arterial injury due to blunt trauma. Arch Surg 99:315, 1969

SPENCER FC, GREWE RF: The management of arterial injuries in battle casualties. Ann Surg 141:304, 1955

WARD PA, SUZUKI A: Gunshot wound of the heart with peripheral embolization: A case report with review of literature. J Thorac Cardiovasc Surg 68:440, 1974

R. E. Zierler/D. E. Strandness, Jr.

Diseases of the Small Arteries of the Extremities

ANATOMY AND FUNCTION

Any definition of what constitutes a small artery is somewhat arbitrary. The aorta and its major branches in the thorax, abdomen, and neck are considered large arteries. The medium-sized arteries arise as branches of these vessels, either within the thorax and abdomen or in the extremities. The term "small artery" is used to refer to those vessels without proper names which arise as branches of the medium-sized arteries. For the purpose of the following discussion, this includes the arteries distal to the wrist and ankle: the plantar and palmar arches, the digital arteries, and the arterioles. The point of transition between artery and arteriole is not precisely defined; however, vessels with diameters in the range of 30μ to 40μ can be classified as arterioles.

The small arteries down to and including the terminal digital vessels are primarily distributing conduits; they have little influence on vasomotor tone. Moving distally in the arterial tree from the large arteries to the arterioles, the relative amount of elastic tissue decreases as the amount of smooth muscle increases. At the level of the arterioles, the arterial wall consists almost entirely of smooth muscle. The total cross-sectional area of the arterial tree increases by a factor of approximately 125 between the aorta and the level of the arterioles.

The small muscular arterioles are responsible for control of vasomotor tone and consequently are important in maintaining blood pressure, regulating body temperature, and partitioning blood flow among various tissues. Arterioles within the skin of the hands and feet are abundantly supplied with sympathetic vasoconstrictor fibers. Marked changes in sympathetic tone occur in response to alterations in ambient temperature, emotional states, and blood volume shifts such as those resulting from a rapid change in body position or hemorrhage. Therefore, the amount of blood flowing through the distal portion of a limb is extremely variable, even in the normal state. This is particularly true in the digits of the hand, where slight changes in ambient temperature cause large alterations in digit blood flow.

An important feature of the microcirculation in the skin is the presence of direct arteriovenous shunts. Since shunt flow bypasses the capillaries and is not nutritive, it probably plays a role in temperature regulation. Sympathectomy causes a loss of vascular tone in those vessels supplied by vasoconstrictor fibers and results in increased blood flow to the skin. Muscle blood flow is not affected, since arterioles in skeletal muscle are regulated primarily by locally produced metabolites. The increased skin blood flow after sympathectomy is largely through the arteriovenous shunts, although nutritive capillary flow may also be augmented to a moderate degree.

OCCLUSIVE ARTERIAL DISEASE

Arteriosclerosis obliterans is a chronic progressive disease characterized by the presence of intimal plaques which results in stenosis or occlusion of large and medium-sized arteries. For some unknown reason, this disorder does not

DISEASES OF THE SMALL ARTERIES OF THE EXTREMITIES	
Etiology	Microembolism, thromboangiitis obliterans (Buerger's disease), vasospastic disease including the Raynaud's type, erythromelalgia, vasculitis including various collagen diseases, and cryoglobulinemia and polycythemia vera
Dx	History and physical examination; digital plethysmography; angiography (Fig. 36-76); skin, muscle, nerve biopsy
Rx	Appropriate to diagnosis Modification of occupation or other aspects of life-style Steroids Available drug therapy Consider sympathectomy

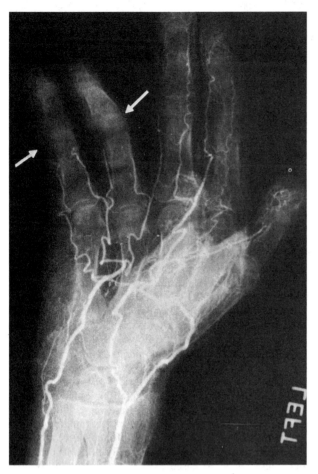

Fig. 36-76. Arteriogram of obliterative small-artery disease. (Haimovici H: Diseases of small arteries of the extremities. In Hardy JD [ed]: Rhoads Textbook of Surgery, 5th ed. Philadelphia, J B Lippincott, 1977)

affect the small arteries, so it need not be considered further here. Another potential source of confusion is the arterial lesion associated with diabetes mellitus. Arteriosclerotic lesions involving the large and medium-sized arteries of diabetic patients are indistinguishable from those observed in nondiabetic patients. Although diabetics and nondiabetics have the same incidence of occlusion in the femoral-popliteal segment, there is a higher incidence of involvement in the tibial and peroneal arteries among diabetics. This relative increase in the extent of disease, combined with earlier age at onset and the frequent occurrence of peripheral neuropathy, is sufficient to explain the higher incidence of gangrene and tissue loss in the diabetic patient. A specific lesion of small arteries and arterioles that is unique to the diabetic state has not been observed. Thickening of capillary basement membranes in the diabetic patient has been described, and it is possible that such lesions could interfere with nutrient exchange at the cellular level. However, the contribution of this microcirculatory lesion to the clinical presentation of diabetic peripheral vascular disease is uncertain.

MICROEMBOLISM

Microembolism to the small arteries of the extremities requires the presence of a proximal embolic source and a patent distal arterial tree. Also called atheroemboli, these embolic particles range in size from 50μ to 900μ in diameter and consist of either cholesterol fragments or fibrinoplatelet material. The most commonly described source for microemboli is the stenotic or ulcerated atheromatous plaque located at the aorto-iliac or superficial femoral level. Microemboli have also occurred in association with abdominal aortic and popliteal artery aneurysms. Rarely, emboli may originate from an intrathoracic source such as a plaque in the thoracic aorta or a left atrial myxoma. Exactly what stimulates a plaque to become an active embolic source is not known; however, ulceration appears to be important, since it allows shedding of plaque contents and initiates formation of platelet thrombi.

CLINICAL PRESENTATION

The microemboli lodge in the arteries of the distal limb and produce acute focal ischemic symptoms. Simultaneous involvement of both lower extremities indicates an embolic source proximal to the aortic bifurcation. Unilateral symptoms suggest emboli originating from iliac or femoral-popliteal lesions.

The cutaneous lesion of microembolism consists of a sharply demarcated red to blue or black area with an irregular border. There may be a zone of inflammation around the periphery of the lesion. The toes are the most commonly involved site, although lesions can also be found on the skin of the foot; this presentation has given rise to the term "blue-toe syndrome." The cutaneous lesions are generally quite painful, and impaired sensation may also be noted in the ischemic area.

Microembolism to the distal limb is somewhat analogous to the transient ischemic attacks of the brain, since the underlying mechanism appears to be the same. Like transient brain ischemia, the symptoms of peripheral microembolism may be repetitive and reversible; however, there is also the same potential for infarction and tissue loss.

DIAGNOSIS

The diagnosis of microembolism is based on the finding of typical cutaneous lesions in a patient with patent distal arteries and an otherwise well perfused foot. A history and physical examination emphasizing the symptoms and signs of peripheral vascular disease is mandatory. In addition to palpation of pulses and auscultation for bruits, segmental leg pressures measured with the Doppler ultrasonic velocity detector may indicate the level of the occlusive arterial lesions. The degree of change in the ankle/arm pressure index after treadmill exercise reflects the hemodynamic severity of the proximal lesions. B-mode scanning is the technique of choice for confirming the presence of abdominal aortic or popliteal artery aneurysms. Echocardiography may be indicated to rule out a cardiac source for microemboli.

Contrast arteriography of all segments from the aorta down to the lower leg and foot is the definitive diagnostic test. In addition to noting the location and severity of ulcerated atherosclerotic plaques and stenoses, study of the distal arteries may reveal one or more sites of embolic occlusion.

Although not strictly required for diagnosis, a characteristic microembolic lesion has been observed in skin biopsy specimens. This consists of a slitlike space in the arterial lumen called a *cholesterol cleft*, which results when a cholesterol crystal dissolves during histologic preparation.

TREATMENT AND PROGNOSIS

Although the natural history of microembolism due to ulcerated atheromatous plaques is not known in detail, the available evidence suggests that embolic events are often repetitive and may lead to tissue loss. An aggressive surgical approach is therefore indicated whenever the embolic source is surgically accessible and the patient is an acceptable operative risk.

The principles of treatment are removal or exclusion of the embolic source and restoration of arterial continuity. Aortic lesions, either aneurysms or plaques, generally require aortobifemoral bypass grafts. Localized lesions in the femoral-popliteal segment may be suitable for endarterectomy and vein patch angioplasty, while more extensive involvement requires bypass grafting. Whenever the bypass technique is used, the main segmental artery must be interrupted to prevent further embolization.

If the entire aorta is diffusely ulcerated, or there are multiple scattered ulcerated lesions throughout the limb, surgical correction may not be possible. The similarity between peripheral microembolism and transient ischemic attacks suggests that antiplatelet agents, such as aspirin and dipyridamole, may be of benefit. Although there are as yet no data to support the use of these agents, they are well tolerated and worthy of a clinical trial.

THROMBOANGIITIS OBLITERANS (TAO)

In 1908 Leo Buerger of New York described a specific nonatheromatous lesion involving arteries, veins, and nerves that frequently led to the development of nonhealing ulcers and gangrene of the digits. He observed an inflammatory and thrombotic process involving the distal vessels of the extremities with sparing of the more proximal vessels. The condition was described in young men, and it was often accompanied by cold sensitivity of the Raynaud type. He proposed the term "obliterating thrombo-angiitis," and the disorder is now known as thromboangiitis obliterans, or Buerger's disease. There has been some controversy concerning the existence of a specific lesion of the type described by Buerger; however, there is now sufficient clinical, epidemiologic, and pathologic evidence to continue to recognize it as a separate entity.

ETIOLOGY AND PATHOGENESIS

Although the pathogenesis of TAO is unknown, there is a definite relationship with the smoking or chewing of tobacco. The condition is virtually unheard of in nonsmokers, and the clinical progression of disease in patients who continue to smoke and improvement in those who stop are well recognized. While there are several reports of cutaneous sensitivity to tobacco extracts in patients with TAO, the concept of vascular allergy has not been established.

The disease is uncommon, with an estimated incidence of 12 per 100,000 population per year. It affects men primarily; the proportion of women in reported series varies from less than 1% to 10%. In spite of sporadic reports, no consistent association has been found between TAO and race, occupation, socioeconomic class, geographic location, or coagulation abnormalities.

The pathologic features of TAO are distinct from those of other vascular lesions such as arteriosclerosis obliterans. The process involves small and medium-sized arteries of the extremities, including the tibial, peroneal, radial, ulnar, plantar, palmar, and digital arteries. Involvement is generally bilateral and symmetrical, with the lower limbs more commonly affected. The lesions tend to be focal rather than diffuse, and the border between normal and diseased vessel is quite distinct. Although the disease causes venous as well as arterial occlusion, its major effects are due to ischemia of distal tissues.

The lesion of TAO is an inflammatory, nonsuppurative panangiitis with thrombosis but without necrosis of the vessel wall. Early in the disease, the lesion is characterized by multiple microabscesses in a fresh thrombus and a chronic inflammatory infiltrate in the adjacent vessel wall. In the more advanced lesion, the thrombus becomes organized by a proliferation of endothelial cells and fibroblasts. Recanalization of the thrombus may occur, along with periarterial fibrosis that binds together artery, vein, and nerve. Throughout this process the general architecture of the vessel wall is preserved, and the internal elastic lamina remains intact. The arterial lesions of atherosclerosis are characteristically absent.

CLINICAL PRESENTATION

TAO typically occurs in young men who are heavy cigarette smokers. The initial symptoms usually appear between the ages of 25 to 40 years. A migratory, nodular, superficial phlebitis can occur and may be the first manifestation of the disease. Cold sensitivity of the Raynaud type is seen in about one-half of patients and is frequently confined to the hands.

Instep claudication, pain in the foot resulting from exercise and relieved by rest, is one of the characteristic symptoms of TAO. Calf claudication is rare, since the arterial occlusion does not usually extend into the femoral-popliteal segment. When the upper extremity is involved, hand claudication may occur. The symptoms, like the pathologic lesions, are generally bilateral and symmetrical. As the disease progresses, ischemic rest pain develops in the digits. Ulceration and gangrene of the digits are common, and these lesions are exquisitely painful and difficult to heal (Fig. 36-77). Ulcers often result from minor trauma and are located on the digit tips or around the margins of the nails. Gangrene occasionally involves the foot, but involvement of the leg, arm, or hand itself is extremely rare.

DIAGNOSIS

The presence of the typical clinical picture just described is the strongest evidence for a diagnosis of TAO. Physical findings include intense rubor of the feet and absent pedal pulses with normal femoral and popliteal pulses. The radial or ulnar pulses may also be absent or diminished. Noninvasive measurement of segmental leg pressures demonstrates the distal location of the occlusive lesions. Strain-gauge plethysmography has been used to document the location and severity of isolated digital artery disease.

Contrast arteriography is required to precisely outline the pathologic anatomy. The arteriographic features of TAO were described in detail by McKusick. These include absence of atheromatous changes in large arteries, smooth vessels of uniform caliber down to an abrupt point of obstruction, segmental rather than diffuse involvement, earliest lesions in arteries of the feet and lower legs, and striking bilateral symmetry.

TREATMENT AND PROGNOSIS

Because of the distal location of the occlusive lesions, direct arterial surgery is generally not possible in TAO. The only effective means to arrest progression of the disease is complete and permanent abstinence from tobacco. However, clinical experience has shown that very few patients are able to comply with this simple measure. In those who can refrain from smoking, exacerbations do not occur and the disease may remain relatively stable. For the majority of patients who continue to smoke, the course is one of slow episodic progression to ulceration and gangrene.

Anticoagulants, steroids, and vasodilating drugs have all been tried, but no consistent benefit has been observed. Avoidance of vasoconstriction by keeping the affected extremity warm is desirable. The response to surgical sympathectomy has been variable. While some beneficial results have been reported, sympathectomy does not influence the underlying occlusive arterial lesion. Once the stage of rest pain is reached, amputation is almost inevitable. Treatment of ulceration and gangrene is directed toward minimizing infection and conservative débridement of necrotic tissue. Formal amputation is offered as a last resort.

VASOSPASTIC DISEASE

The term *vasospasm* implies a reversible constriction of blood vessels. This constriction reduces blood flow and results in varying degrees of ischemia in the peripheral tissues. Vasospasm may be episodic or persistent and initiated by local effects on peripheral vessels or by the sympathetic nervous system. The hands and feet, which are abundantly supplied with sympathetic vasoconstrictor fibers, are the areas most commonly affected. Primary and secondary forms of vasospastic diseases are recognized. Distinguishing between them is important, since the primary forms tend to be benign and self-limiting, while the secondary forms are associated with significant morbidity and mortality.

COLD SENSITIVITY OF THE RAYNAUD TYPE

Episodic color changes involving the digits of the hands and feet resulting from exposure to cold or emotional stimuli were first described by Maurice Raynaud in 1862. The observation by Hutchinson in 1893 that any one of several underlying causes could be responsible for the condition described by Raynaud resulted in an improved understanding of the vasospastic diseases. This led to the classification of episodic vasospasm as either primary or secondary.

Raynaud's phenomenon is used as a general term to designate the symptom complex of digital cold sensitivity. Classically, the digits of an affected patient respond to cold or emotional stimuli by first becoming pale and waxy; later, as warming begins, they assume a cyanotic hue and finally take on the rubor of hyperemia. Variations in this "triphasic" color response are common; however, the most important element from a diagnostic standpoint is the stage of pallor. The primary form is referred to as Raynaud's phenomenon—etiology unknown, or idiopathic Raynaud's disease. This category includes those patients with true primary Raynaud's disease as well as some whose underlying diagnosis has not yet been established. In the secondary form, Raynaud's phenomenon—etiology known, one of the conditions associated with cold sensitivity is present.

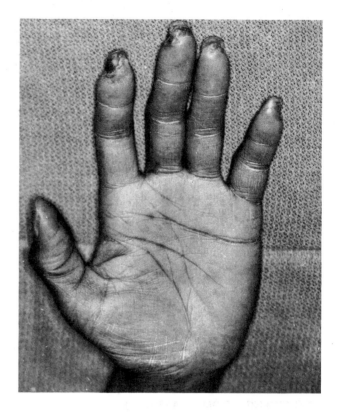

Fig. 36-77. Ischemic ulcers of left 2nd, 3rd, and 4th fingers of a 40-year-old patient with TAO. The patient was a heavy smoker and had involvement of all four extremities. The arteriogram disclosed occlusion of the radial and ulnar arteries just proximal to the wrist joint and involvement of the distal portions of the digital arteries. A left upper thoracic sympathectomy was carried out, followed later by amputation of the distal phalanx of the index finger. Microscopic study of the small vessels of the digit showed narrowed lumina by proliferative endothelial lesions. (Haimovici H: Diseases of small arteries of the extremities. In Hardy JD [ed]: Rhoads Textbook of Surgery, 5th ed. Philadelphia, J B Lippincott, 1977)

A detailed classification of cold sensitivity of the Raynaud type follows.

I. Raynaud's phenomenon—etiology unknown (primary)
   A. Idiopathic Raynaud's disease
   B. Undiagnosed (later reclassified as secondary)
II. Raynaud's phenomenon—etiology known (secondary)
   A. Collagen-vascular diseases
      1. Scleroderma
      2. Rheumatoid arthritis
      3. Systemic lupus erythematosus
      4. Periarteritis nodosa
   B. Organic vascular diseases
      1. Thromboangiitis obliterans
      2. Arteriosclerosis obliterans
      3. Thrombotic or embolic arterial occlusion
   C. Trauma
      1. Vibration injury (pneumatic tools)
      2. Percussion injury (pianist, typist)
   D. Neurovascular syndromes
      1. Thoracic outlet syndrome
      2. Causalgia
   E. Cold injury
      1. Frostbite
      2. Nonfreezing cold injury (immersion foot)

F. Hematological disorders
   1. Cold agglutinins
   2. Cryoglobulinemia
   3. Polycythemia vera
G. Intoxication
   1. Ergot
   2. Propranolol
   3. Heavy metals (lead)

ETIOLOGY AND PATHOGENESIS

Theoretically, peripheral vasospasm could be produced by local effects on digital vessels, alterations in sympathetic tone, or both. Although the exact mechanism of primary Raynaud's disease is unknown, the basic defect appears to reside in the digital arteries themselves. Anatomic changes in the digital arteries are generally absent, although they have been observed in cases of long duration. The major abnormality seems to be a local hypersensitivity of the digital arteries to cold. Vasospastic episodes can be provoked in susceptible patients by local cold exposure regardless of the state of sympathetic outflow. It is quite possible, however, that increased sympathetic tone could intensify cold-induced digital artery constriction. Thus, patients with Raynaud's disease may simply have an exaggeration of the normal response to cold.

The conditions associated with secondary Raynaud's phenomenon all involve some form of obstruction, trauma, or inflammation of the arteries in the affected extremity. This underlying lesion, together with the normal increase in sympathetic tone that occurs in response to cold, is generally sufficient to produce recurrent episodes of digital ischemia.

CLINICAL PRESENTATION AND DIAGNOSIS

A history of digital cold sensitivity with the "triphasic" color response or some variant of it suggests the diagnosis of Raynaud's phenomenon. The diagnosis of primary Raynaud's disease is based on the exclusion of known associated conditions. It is well recognized, however, that Raynaud's phenomenon may precede the other manifestations of an underlying disease process by many years. True Raynaud's disease is more common in women, often starting in the late teens. The involvement is usually bilateral and symmetrical, with the hands more commonly involved than the feet. Digital gangrene and ulceration are extremely rare and, when present, are confined to the superficial aspects of the digit tips.

In secondary Raynaud's phenomenon, cold sensitivity may be overshadowed by the more severe symptoms of the underlying disease. Secondary Raynaud's phenomenon is also characterized by onset later in life (over age 50), particularly in men. The onset tends to be sudden, with rapid progression to severe pain, ulceration, and tissue loss. Involvement is typically not bilateral or symmetrical and may be confined to only one or two digits.

TREATMENT AND PROGNOSIS

When symptoms and signs fit the criteria for primary Raynaud's disease, the prognosis is favorable and the course is generally benign. The disease disappears or becomes less severe in a high proportion of patients. Therapy of mild cases involves simple reassurance and avoidance of cold exposure. As in all peripheral vascular diseases, smoking should be vigorously discouraged. For more severe cases, sympathectomy and a variety of drugs have been advocated.

The results of surgical sympathectomy have been variable, although a more consistent benefit has been observed in the lower limb than the upper. This is owing to the higher probability of permanent denervation after lumbar sympathectomy compared to the cervicodorsal approach. Reserpine, administered either orally or intra-arterially, has been reported to promote healing of ulcerations and reduce the severity of vasospastic symptoms. A similar benefit has been described for α-methyldopa.

In secondary Raynaud's phenomenon the treatment is directed at the underlying disease. Due to the presence of an anatomic arterial lesion, measures designed simply to relieve vasoconstriction, such as drugs or sympathectomy, are rarely effective. It is generally accepted that sympathectomy should be avoided in all patients with collagen-vascular disease. The clinical course of patients with secondary Raynaud's phenomenon is usually unfavorable, with digital ischemia progressing to ulceration and tissue loss. The ultimate prognosis is determined by the systemic complications of the underlying disorder.

LIVEDO RETICULARIS

Livedo reticularis is a vasospastic disease characterized by a persistent cyanotic mottling of the skin that produces a typical "fishnet" appearance. This cutaneous pattern may be accentuated by exposure to cold. Unlike Raynaud's phenomenon, which is confined to the digits, livedo reticularis may involve an entire extremity and extend over the trunk.

The primary or idiopathic form is most common in young women but may be seen at any age. Progression to skin ulceration has been described but is extremely rare. Secondary livedo reticularis is a cutaneous manifestation of a more serious underlying disease. The list of associated conditions is similar to that for Raynaud's phenomenon and includes collagen-vascular diseases, particularly systemic lupus erythematosus; hematologic disorders such as the dysproteinemias; microembolism arising from proximal atherosclerotic or aneurysmal lesions; Cushing's syndrome; prolonged dependency or immobilization; and the late result of cold injury. As would be expected, the secondary forms are more likely to result in cutaneous necrosis, and the clinical course is determined by the associated condition.

The principles of treatment for livedo reticularis are as outlined for Raynaud's phenomenon. From the surgical point of view, the diagnosis and treatment of microembolism, as previously discussed, are particularly important.

ACROCYANOSIS

The least common of the vasospastic diseases is acrocyanosis. This presents as a persistent and diffuse cyanotic discoloration of the fingers, hands, toes, and feet. The cyanosis may be intensified by cold or emotional stimuli. The involved extremities are usually cool, and excessive perspiration is commonly noted. Acrocyanosis is seen more frequently in women, and a familial tendency has been reported. It is a benign condition not associated with an underlying disorder, and digital necrosis does not occur. Treatment is conservative and involves reassurance and avoidance of cold exposure.

ERYTHROMELALGIA

This rare disorder is sometimes considered as one of the vasospastic diseases, but it really belongs in a category by itself. The term erythromelalgia was first used by Mitchell in 1872 to describe a red, painful extremity. In 1938 Smith and Allen suggested the more descriptive term "erythermalgia" to emphasize the increased temperature of the skin in the affected area.

ETIOLOGY AND PATHOGENESIS

Although the detailed pathophysiology is not understood, it is clear that the skin of patients with erythromelalgia is abnormally sensitive to warmth. While vasodilatation undoubtedly contributes to the clinical manifestations, plethysmographic studies have shown that symptoms are related to local heating and not to increased blood flow.

Both primary (idiopathic) and secondary forms are recognized. Primary erythromelalgia occurs in otherwise healthy persons without any detectable evidence of systemic or peripheral vascular disease. The conditions associated with the secondary form include the myeloproliferative disorders, particularly polycythemia vera, and the collagen-vascular diseases.

CLINICAL PRESENTATION AND DIAGNOSIS

The condition presents as an unpleasant burning, tingling, or itching sensation of the foot and lower leg, which appears as the ambient temperature increases. During an attack the affected areas become bright red and hot. The critical temperature above which symptoms appear varies from patient to patient; however, it usually falls within the range of 37.1° to 36.1°C (89° to 97°F).

The diagnosis of erythromelalgia is based on a history that relates the typical symptoms to an increase in skin temperature. Episodes of distress may be exacerbated by dependency and relieved by elevation, a response opposite to that seen in patients with arterial occlusive disease. Examination of the peripheral vascular system is generally normal, particularly in the primary form. This observation, together with the unique nature of the symptoms, should prevent confusion with ischemic rest pain. Specific tests to detect conditions associated with the secondary form may be indicated.

Primary erythromelalgia is rare in childhood, the onset being most common in middle age. It is more often bilateral than the secondary form. Both men and women are affected, and a familial tendency has been reported. Symptoms last from minutes to hours and may involve both the feet and hands. Patients quickly discover that their symptoms are related to increased temperature and learn to avoid heating the extremities. They will often obtain relief by immersing the affected areas in cold water or cooling their skin with fans. Symptoms may be prevented by wearing sandals, avoiding stockings, and sleeping with the feet outside the bedcovers. The diagnosis can be confirmed by provocative tests using either reflex vasodilatation or direct application of heat.

TREATMENT AND PROGNOSIS

Treatment of primary erythromelalgia is often unsuccessful. Keeping the feet as cool as possible offers some symptomatic relief. Favorable results have been reported with aspirin, phenoxybenzamine, and methysergide maleate. In the secondary form, treatment of the underlying disorder is the main objective. The primary form appears to be benign, the only complications being of an emotional nature due to the recurrent episodes of distress. Ulceration and gangrene have been described with secondary erythromelalgia, and the poor prognosis in such cases is related to the associated disease.

VASCULITIS

Inflammation of the small arteries occurs in a variety of diseases. The cellular infiltrate in the vessel wall and perivascular area is generally nonspecific and is accompanied by necrosis and fibrin deposition. Endothelial edema and proliferation, together with destruction of the vessel wall, finally result in vascular occlusion or hemorrhage, with subsequent ischemia of distal tissues (Fig. 36-78). Most forms of vasculitis (or arteritis) are thought to be due to immune complex disease. Although a detailed discussion of the vasculitides is beyond the scope of this chapter, several examples will be given that affect the small arteries of the extremities.

SCLERODERMA

Although the cutaneous manifestations of scleroderma are most easily observed, the disease affects multiple organ systems. As previously mentioned, cold sensitivity of the Raynaud type is common and may be the initial symptom. Arteriographic studies of patients with scleroderma have shown a characteristic pattern of occlusive disease in the arteries of the hand, with involvement of the proper digital arteries in approximately 90% of patients. Histological changes include medial hypertrophy and intimal proliferation, which result in narrowing and occlusion of the vessel lumen. Perivascular fibrosis may compress the vessel and contribute to the occlusive process.

SYSTEMIC LUPUS ERYTHEMATOSUS (SLE)

Several peripheral vascular syndromes have been associated with SLE, including secondary Raynaud's phenomenon, livedo reticularis, and erythromelalgia. The vascular lesions in SLE are of the nonspecific inflammatory and proliferative type, and immunologic studies have shown that they contain DNA, antibodies to DNA, and complement components. The small arteries, particularly the digital vessels, are most commonly involved, and gangrene is usually confined to the digits. When livedo reticularis is present, it is often associated with recurrent painful ulcerations around the ankle.

PERIARTERITIS NODOSA

The characteristic pathologic feature of periarteritis nodosa is necrotizing inflammation of small and medium-sized arteries. The lesions are segmental and give rise to small aneurysms that may rupture. As in the other collagen-vascular diseases, the lesions are present throughout the body. When they involve the digital vessels, ulceration and gangrene occur. Livedo reticularis and secondary Raynaud's phenomenon have also been described.

HEMATOLOGIC DISORDERS RESULTING IN LIMB ISCHEMIA

CRYOGLOBULINEMIA

The presence in the bloodstream of increased amounts of cold-precipitable protein has been noted in multiple mye-

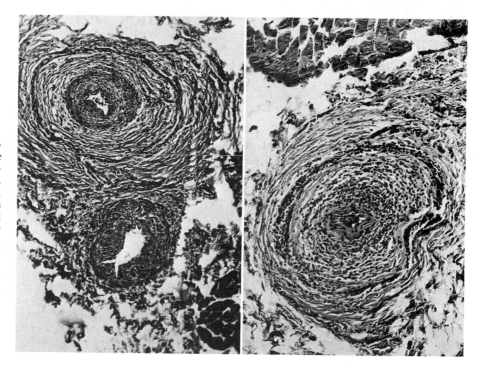

Fig. 36-78. *(Left)* Cross section of a small artery in the gastrocnemius muscle, displaying lesions of panarteritis. (Elastica Van-Gieson stain. × 30) *(Right)* Small arteriole in the gastrocnemius muscle and adjacent venule. The arteriole is almost completely occluded, displaying less inflammatory changes than that in the picture at left. (Elastica Van-Gieson stain. × 30) (Haimovici H: Diseases of small arteries of the extremities. In Hardy JD [ed]: Rhoads Textbook of Surgery, 5th ed. Philadelphia, J B Lippincott, 1977)

loma, Waldenström's macroglobulinemia, lymphoproliferative disorders, collagen-vascular diseases, and the acute phase of some infectious diseases. Although cryoglobulins are normally present in amounts less than 25 mg/dl, clinical symptoms are associated with concentrations in excess of 1 g/dl of plasma. When exposed to cold these proteins cause blood in the small arteries to lose its fluidity, resulting in an interruption of flow. The major cutaneous manifestations are petechiae, purpura, livedo reticularis, and secondary Raynaud's phenomenon. Chronic ulcers may form in areas of skin infarction.

The diagnosis is made by demonstrating significant amounts of cold-precipitable protein in the plasma. Treatment and prognosis are determined by the underlying disease.

POLYCYTHEMIA VERA

Polycythemia vera is one of the myeloproliferative disorders and is characterized by a markedly increased red blood cell mass. Clinical symptoms are related to increased blood volume and blood viscosity. Peripheral vascular complications result from both arterial and venous thrombosis and hemorrhage. Secondary erythromelalgia and Raynaud's phenomenon may also occur. Control of polycythemia by periodic phlebotomy, radiotherapy, or chemotherapy often reduces the frequency of thrombotic episodes.

BIBLIOGRAPHY

ALLEN EV, BROWN GE: Raynaud's disease: A critical review of minimal requisites for diagnosis. Am J Med Sci 183:187, 1932

BUERGER L: Thrombo-angiitis obliterans: A study of the vascular lesions leading to presenile spontaneous gangrene. Am J Med Sci 136:567, 1908

COFFMAN JD, DAVIES WT: Vasospastic disease: A review. Prog Cardiovasc Dis 18:123, 1975

DABICH L, BOOKSTEIN JJ, SWEIFLER A et al: Digital arteries in patients with scleroderma—arteriographic and plethysmographic study. Arch Int Med 130:708, 1972

FROHNERT PP, SHEPS SG: Long term follow-up study of periarteritis nodosa. Am J Med 43:8, 1967

HUTCHINSON J: Inherited liability to Raynaud's phenomenon, with great proneness to chilblains—gradual increase of liability to paroxysmal local asphyxia—acrosphacelus with scleroderma—cheeks affected. Arch Surg 4:312, 1893

JUERGENS JL, SPITTELL JA, FAIRBAIRN FJ (eds): Peripheral Vascular Diseases. 5th ed. Philadelphia, W B Saunders, 1980

KARMODY AM, POWERS SR, MONACO VJ et al: "Blue-toe" syndrome—an indication for limb salvage surgery. Arch Surg 111:1263, 1976

McKUSICK VA, HARRIS WS, OTTESEN OE et al: Buerger's disease: A distinct clinical and pathophysiological entity. JAMA 181:93, 1962

MEHIGAN JT, STONEY RJ: Lower extremity atheromatous embolization. Am J Surg 132:163, 1976

MITCHELL SW: Clinical lecture on certain painful affections of the feet. Philadelphia Med. Times 3:81; 113, 1872

RAYNAUD AGM: De l'asphyxie locale et de la gangrène symétrique des extrémités (On local asphyxia and symmetrical gangrene of the extremities). Paris, Rignoux, 1862

SMITH LA, ALLEN EV: Erythermalgia (erythromelalgia) of the extremities: A syndrome characterized by redness, heat, and pain. Am Heart J 16:175, 1938

STRANDNESS DE, PRIEST RE, GIBBONS GE: Combined clinical and pathologic study of diabetic and nondiabetic peripheral arterial disease. Diabetes 13:366, 1964

STRANDNESS DE, SUMNER DS: Hemodynamics for Surgeons. New York, Grune & Stratton, 1975

THIEME WT, STRANDNESS DE, BELL JW: Buerger's disease—further support for the entity. Northwest Med 64:264, 1965

James D. Hardy

Vascular Tumors: Hemangiomas and Related Disorders

HEMANGIOMAS
    Hemangioendothelioma (Immature Hemangioma,
        Strawberry Mark)
    Capillary Hemangioma (Port-Wine Spot)
    Sclerosing Hemangioma
    Cavernous Hemangioma (Mature Hemangioma)
GLOMUS TUMOR (GLOMANGIOMA)
KAPOSI'S SARCOMA

The congenital malformation or indeed the proliferation of small vascular conduits can result in a wide variety of lesions, ranging from the very minor superficial skin "strawberry mark" of the newborn to the very serious Kaposi's angiosarcoma. In between lie a remarkably varied group of disorders, a number of which are considered here.

HEMANGIOMAS

Hemangiomas, or benign tumors of blood vessel origin, along with pigmented nevi are the commonest of tumors found in man. The majority of hemangiomas are found in the skin, where they often appear at birth or during the early postnatal months or years and can assume a bewildering variety of appearances, many of which have been descriptively named by dermatologists. The etiology is uncertain, though most are thought to be congenital. Although these lesions are best catalogued by histologic appearance, perhaps the simplest classification method is by gross appearance.

The hemangiomas that are clinically important include hemangioendotheliomas, capillary hemangiomas, sclerosing hemangiomas, and cavernous hemangiomas (discrete and diffuse).

HEMANGIOENDOTHELIOMA (IMMATURE HEMANGIOMA, STRAWBERRY MARK)

This harmless birthmark lesion is named immature hemangioma because of its unpredictable growth pattern. The lesion usually appears at birth and may undergo alarming increase in size during the subsequent few months, only to regress spontaneously at about 1 year of age and almost certainly before school age. Rarely, the lesion will persist, and excision or other measures may be indicated. It may begin as a large lesion, decrease in size, then grow rapidly, and again usually regress spontaneously after the age of 1 year. Clinically it is a raised, compressible, irregularly outlined bright red lesion that can ulcerate easily, particularly if located in easily traumatized areas. Bleeding is not usually a problem, however, and direct pressure easily controls the ooze. Recurrent episodes of trauma, ulceration, bleeding, and superficial infection are thought to actually hasten the involution of the tumor, and treatment consists of reassuring the parents that the lesion will ultimately disappear. Otherwise, the concerned parents may insist on active intervention, such as dry ice (solid CO_2) applications, sclerosing injections, laser treatments, or even excision. Unfortunately, each of these modalities may leave a permanent scar that prolonged observation would have avoided.

CAPILLARY HEMANGIOMA (PORT-WINE SPOT)

Commonly referred to as a birthmark, the capillary hemangioma is harmless. Microscopically it is composed of dilated, capillary-size, thin-walled blood vessels in the dermal or subdermal area of the skin. Grossly the involved area is reddish-purple and not elevated from the surrounding normal skin. The clinical importance of capillary hemangioma consists predominantly of its cosmetic effect; it should be remembered, however, that the visible "birthmark" may represent the superficial element of a deeper cavernous hemangioma.

Treatment consists of surgical excision of small lesions and the application of cosmetic preparations to larger lesions. Tattooing has been employed to modify the discoloration but is not widely used.

SCLEROSING HEMANGIOMA

Sclerosing hemangioma, often called histiocytoma, denotes those lesions undergoing regressive changes, including fibrosis, vascular obliteration, and phagocytosis of lipid or iron pigment or both. Some reserve the term *sclerosing hemangioma* for a subdermal fibrotic lesion related to trauma. Usually located in the extremities, the subdermal nodules are associated with deposition of pigment in the overlying skin, thus making their distinction from melanoma difficult. The treatment is surgical excision.

CAVERNOUS HEMANGIOMA (MATURE HEMANGIOMA)

The result of arrest at the retiform stage of vascular development, cavernous hemangioma consists microscopically of thin-walled vessels larger than capillary size, and sinuses lined with endothelium and filled with blood. Cavernous hemangiomas are thought to be present at birth, are usually full size in relation to the patient's size, and usually do not exhibit either rapid growth nor spontaneous regression but may grow slowly throughout life and attain considerable size. There are two types of cavernous hemangiomas, discrete and diffuse, the former fortunately being more common than the latter.

Discrete cavernous hemangiomas may be found in the face, neck, oral mucosa, extremities, bones, liver, and GI tract. In the skin the lesion appears as an elevated, soft, spongy mass, with multiple bluish swellings resembling dilated veins (Fig. 36-79). If located in an extremity, there is usually no associated limb hypertrophy; concomitant varicose veins, particularly in the lower extremities, do occur and predispose to ulceration and hemorrhage.

In the GI tract, discrete cavernous hemangioma can be

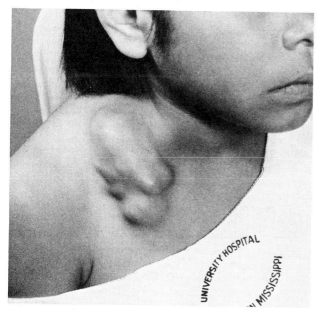

Fig. 36-79. Discrete cavernous hemangioma involving right supraclavicular fossa and right upper anterior chest wall. (University of Mississippi Hospital series)

an uncommon cause of lower GI hemorrhage. Treatment of discrete lesions, when feasible, consists of wide surgical excision. However, the rare lesion can be so extensive, as for example of the cheek through to the buccal mucosa, that it cannot be excised, and repeated episodes of ulceration and hemorrhage can be life-threatening.

Diffuse cavernous hemangioma is, fortunately, a relatively rare lesion. It involves all or part of an extremity either with or without involvement of the contiguous portion of the trunk. It may involve all layers even including the bone. It usually cannot be totally excised, and even amputation will not suffice if the lesion also extends to the trunk. There may be limb hypertrophy and elongation with circumferential swelling that increases slowly with age. In time the affected limb becomes enlarged and discolored and the cavernous lesions may break down, ulcerate, and bleed (Fig. 36-80). There is no adequate surgical treatment, short of amputation, and blood vessel tumors are resistant to radiation. Local complications are treated as they arise.

An interesting and sometimes helpful phenomenon is the radiographic finding of phleboliths on plain x-ray films of the suspected area. Giant hemangiomas (either discrete or diffuse) can cause hemangioma-thrombocytopenia (Kasabach-Merritt) syndrome.

GLOMUS TUMOR (GLOMANGIOMA)

Glomus tumor is a benign, small, exquisitely painful neoplasm of subcutaneous tissue in the extremities, and particularly the digits. The lesion is also known as angioneuroma, angioneuromyoma, tumor of neuromyoarterial glomus, painful subcutaneous tubercle, and Popoff tumor.

The glomus is an arteriovenous shunt abundantly supplied with nonmyelinated nerve fibers (hence the exquisite pain associated with a glomangioma). The normal glomus is a neuromyoarterial receptor that regulates blood flow and is very sensitive to changes in temperature. It may be located anywhere in the skin but is more commonly found in the

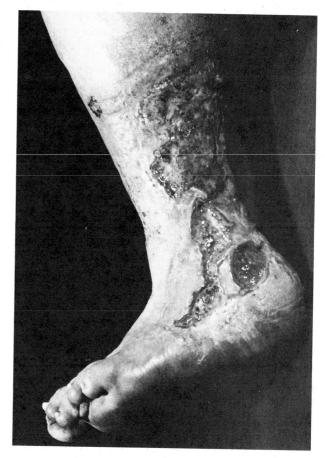

Fig. 36-80. Diffuse cavernous hemangioma of left leg with overlying ulceration and chronic infection. (University of Mississippi Hospital series)

tips of the fingers and toes, particularly under the nails. Glomangiomas, then, are benign tumors of the glomic end organ and, in addition to their most common location under the nails, have been described as occurring at the flexor surfaces of the arms and around the knee. The tumors are usually small (less than 5 mm) and solitary and are first manifested by sharply localized pain exacerbated by pressure or by acute changes in ambient temperature. Subungual lesions are far more common in females.

Clinically the patient presents with a long history of an undiagnosed painful spot, usually subungual, and anxiously protects it from any contact. Physical examination reveals a very small bluish tumefaction beneath the nail which is extremely sensitive to pressure, the *sine qua non* of this lesion. More often than not, the patient will show the physician the offending spot—but not let him dare to touch it.

Treatment is complete excision of the tumor, best accomplished with a tourniquet, in order to assure a bloodless field, and magnifying lenses with microsurgical technique.

KAPOSI'S SARCOMA

Included here because it is generally thought to be a form of angiosarcoma, Kaposi's sarcoma still has an unresolved etiology and pathogenesis. However, an increased reported incidence in active homosexual males suggests an infective agent, and a viral etiology has been proposed. The condition

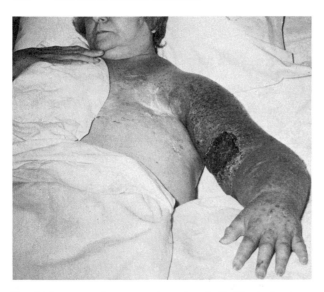

Fig. 36-81. Kaposi's sarcoma in a chronically lymphedematous arm, years after radical mastectomy. (University of Mississippi Hospital series; Shands WC: Soft tissue sarcomas in children and adults. Am Surg 29:811, 1963)

may occur in a lymphedematous arm years following a radical mastectomy (Fig. 36-81).

The tumor arises from undifferentiated mesenchymal cells arranged along vessels in a sheathlike manner. These cells are pluripotential and can give rise to endothelial cells, pericytes, reticulum cells, fibroblasts, and histiocytes. This helps explain the characteristic admixture of fibrous and vascular elements in the lesion and, perhaps, its multicen-tricity. Kaposi's sarcoma is uncommon; the peak incidence is the fifth to seventh decades, and over 90% of cases have been reported in males.

The disease usually begins in the skin of the lower extremities, but may arise in the hands or arms as well. It presents as bluish, red, or purple macules or papules that have no characteristic shape but are usually small. The lesions may coalesce or remain single, and they spread proximally along the veins and lymphatics. Edema of the involved extremity is not uncommon secondary to obstruction of lymph nodes.

As the disease progresses proximally one sees visceral involvement, with the GI tract, liver, spleen, lymph nodes, and lungs as the most common sites of metastases. Gastrointestinal hemorrhage is perhaps the most common cause of death late in the disease.

Confusion exists as to the precise nature of this lesion primarily because of the variable histologic picture. Whether Kaposi's sarcoma represents a well-vascularized fibrosarcoma or a sclerosing angiosarcoma remains to be established.

Treatment consists of irradiation of the involved extremity. Recurrences are common. Wide surgical excision, including amputation, offers more promise. Recent experience has shown that actinomycin-D is helpful in far advanced cases. In general, however, the prognosis is poor.

BIBLIOGRAPHY

Hill GJ II, Longino LA: Giant hemangioma with thrombocytopenia. Surg Gynecol Obstet 114:304, 1962

Landing BH, Farber S: Tumors of the cardiovascular system. Atlas of Tumor Pathology, Sec. 3, Fasc. 7, pp 46–57, 103, 1956

Vogel CL, Templeton CJ, Templeton AC et al: Treatment of Kaposi's sarcoma with actinomycin-D and cyclophosphamide: Results of a randomized clinical trial. Int J Cancer 8:136, 1971

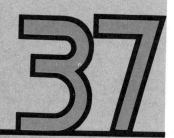

Veins and Lymphatics

Robert L. Kistner

Venous System of the Lower Extremity: An Overview

The veins and lymphatics in the lower extremity drain blood and extravascular fluid from the extremity. Compared to the arterial side of the circulation, relatively little investigation has been devoted to the venous circulation and to the lymphatics. This overview is designed to point out the anatomic and physiologic basis for understanding the venous system in the lower extremity and the lines of investigation that may be fruitful in managing venous disease states during the next decade.

The anatomy and physiology of venous return in the erect human is complex in the normal state and more complicated in disease states. It is apparent that blood is driven through the arteries by the pumping action of the heart and is further aided by the erect position in its distribution to the distal lower extremity. On the venous side of the circulation, the main forces driving the circulation are the *vis a tergo* (onward flow) of the arterial blood, the pumping action of the calf and thigh muscles, and the unidirectional flow created by valves in the veins and the lymphatics. The multiple connections, too numerous to know in detail, between veins of the deep, perforator, and saphenous veins, as well as between muscular and other unnamed venous tributaries, permit collateral flow patterns to develop that compensate for venous disease states.

Pathologic states in the veins produce obstruction or incompetence. *Obstruction* is due to phlebitis or tumor or extrinsic inflammatory compression; *incompetence* is due to congenital or acquired deformity of valves. The clinical effect in the leg depends upon the site and nature of venous disease and upon the collateral channels available in a given patient.

After acute thrombophlebitis, the emergence of chronic disease states depends upon the severity and site of the acute venous disease. Destruction of valves by the phlebitic process renders the later occurrence of recanalization a far less effective compensatory mechanism than one might expect it to be. Because valve destruction after phlebitis is a permanent change, the best treatment available for chronic venous insufficiency is to limit the extent of the acute phlebitis through early diagnosis and effective management of the phlebitic process.

ANATOMY

Knowledge of the anatomy of the venous system in the lower extremity is important in understanding the patho-

---

VENOUS SYSTEM OF THE LOWER EXTREMITY

Anatomy	Division of veins into superficial, deep, and perforator channels
Physiology	Importance of the valves and muscular pump
	Detailed examination of the "gating" function of the valves in various states of valve dysfunction
	Reaction of the venous system to obstruction, with attention to collateral flow and recanalization
Disease States	Description of primary valve incompetence as a recently recognized cause of chronic venous insufficiency (CVI)
	Discussion of relationship between acute venous thrombosis and CVI
	When CVI occurs, medical measures help
	New developments in surgical treatment of CVI provide ways to improve venous dynamics but require accurate diagnosis of the specific abnormality in each patient

---

physiology of complicated venous disease states and the potentials of collateral circulation.

As discussed by Linton, the veins of the lower extremity are artificially separable into three systems: superficial, deep, and perforator. This classification is useful in studying disease states and planning surgical therapy.

SUPERFICIAL VEINS

The superficial system consists of the greater saphenous vein (GSV) and the lesser saphenous vein and their tributaries. These are the veins involved in varicose vein problems, and it is usually their secondary and tertiary branchings that become the varicosities. Telangiectases of the skin, or spider nevi, represent dilated arterial and venular channels in the dermis that can be shown to drain directly into subcutaneous varicose channels. The proximal ends of the greater and lesser saphenous veins empty directly into the deep venous system at the popliteal and the femoral level. Multiple pathways between the saphenous and deep system occur through connections of saphenous branches with perforating veins of the calf and thigh. In the foot, dorsal foot veins drain directly into both the deep and the superficial veins of the ankle and calf. Through all these channels, and others unnamed, the superficial venous system connects the veins of the skin and subcutaneous layers to the deep veins of the leg.

DEEP VEINS

The deep system is the main venous drainage channel of the extremity. Beginning in the foot and ankle, it forms anterior and posterior tibial and peroneal veins, typically paired, in the calf. These veins join to form the popliteal at the knee, and this ascends through the thigh as the superficial femoral vein (SFV). The transition from popliteal to SFV occurs at the level of the adductor hiatus. It is to be noted that the SFV is actually a part of the deep venous system; it is only superficial in its relation to the profunda femoris vein (PFV) in the thigh. In the thigh, the PFV drains the deepest musculoskeletal tissues and joins with the SFV below the lesser tubercle of the femur to form the common femoral vein (CFV).

The CFV crosses behind the inguinal ligament and continues into the pelvis as the external iliac vein. The CFV is a central terminus for most of the drainage of the leg, since it receives the profunda and superficial femoral, the greater saphenous, and medial and lateral collateral channels of the thigh and pelvis. Because of this we regard the CFV as the neck of the funnel of veins draining the lower extremity and believe that a patent CFV is of utmost importance in maintaining a healthy venous outflow for the extremity.

Just as the profunda vein in the thigh drains venous flow from muscles and skeletal parts, so in the calf the muscular veins drain into tibial and popliteal veins. The muscular veins are important as a storage site for venous blood and represent a large part of the capacitance function of the leg. When the calf muscle contracts, a large volume of blood is forcibly ejected toward the heart, emptying the venous sinuses and making room for new flow from the arterial side of the circulation.

PERFORATOR VEINS

The third system of veins is the perforator system, which connects the deep and superficial veins in the lower extremity. Rather than forming a longitudinal (vertical) drainage channel, perforator veins are a horizontal conduit between deep and superficial veins. Strictly speaking, greater and lesser saphenous veins are perforators because they traverse the deep fascia and connect superficial and deep veins, but they are arbitrarily excluded in the discussion of perforator veins. Perforator veins are more numerous below the knee than above it. Typically, they are direct branches of a deep vein, such as the tibial vein, that travel horizontally beneath the deep fascia and receive tributaries, then pierce the deep fascia and divide above the fascia. The perforator usually connects with the saphenous vein by one or more branches, rather than directly. Many small perforators are identifiable by dissection in the leg, but typically half a dozen on the medial side of the calf and half that number on the lateral side are grossly identifiable and surgically important.

This artificial division of veins into three anatomic systems is useful in understanding disease states and the potential collateral flow patterns that provide compensatory outflow for the leg. Although the rest of this discussion will speak of these anatomic divisions as separate entities, it is to be understood that the veins of the extremity function as a single system to provide total outflow for the extremity, and pathologic states that affect one part of the venous tree have an immediate effect on the rest of the system. It is probably accurate to state that we as physicians have erred by considering the venous system as a single passive pathway rather than a complex mechanism governed by multiple physiological forces, and in doing so have neglected the thorough study required to understand these forces.

VENOUS VALVES

All major veins in the lower extremity contain valves. The presence of valves is essential for proper function of the lower extremity veins, since they act as "gates" to direct the unidirectional flow of blood toward the heart. Several studies have reported the position and frequency of valves in the lower extremity veins.

In general, valves are more frequent distally and more widely spaced proximally. A valve is usually found at the site of branching of a major vein, and valves are also spaced along the course of long veins. Valves do not occur in the inferior vena cava or common iliac veins. The external iliac vein may have a single valve, but often this is absent. A valve is almost always present in the common femoral vein, and one or more valves will be found in each of the branches of the common femoral. Typically, the SFV contains one to three valves as it traverses the thigh, the popliteal has one or more valves, and each tibial vein has multiple valves. Greater saphenous veins contain from 3 to 15 valves between groin and ankle. The profunda femoris vein contains multiple valves. Perforator veins contain one or more valves.

The lower extremity venous valve is a bicuspid structure. Each cusp is a thin, diaphanous fibroelastic membrane covered by endothelium. It has a semilunar shape and inserts into the vein wall in semicircular fashion, with the convexity pointing distally. The vein wall is thinned and forms a sinus at the level of the valve.

The importance of the valves is to produce unidirectional flow of blood returning to the heart. They direct flow from superficial to deep and from distal to proximal.

The valve mechanism is highly efficient in preventing backflow when it functions normally. When the human is in the horizontal position, the valve cusps lie open and blood flows through easily in its course to the heart. When the human stands erect, the valves lie open while blood flows through. However, when stress is placed on the valve by retrograde flow of blood, as in a Valsalva maneuver or a cough, the valve sinus fills with blood and the cusp leaflets abut in the midline, producing an amazingly efficient valve mechanism.

COLLATERAL PATHWAYS

Venous collateral pathways are too numerous and complex to appreciate in detail. To illustrate some examples where collaterals work well, we know that the superficial system can easily tolerate removal of both greater and lesser saphenous veins with no apparent ill effects. Likewise, large segments of the deep system, such as the superficial femoral vein or multiple tibial veins, can be obliterated and the individual will have little or no disability. The perforator veins can be interrupted throughout the calf and the saphenous veins stripped, and still the venous drainage can function well. Detailed venographic study of venous patterns in disease states reveals every possible combination of occlusion in the deep, perforator, and superficial veins, and still the venous drainage may remain more or less compensated in the individual case.

These examples illustrate the great capacity of the veins to compensate for the loss of normal anatomic channels by rerouting the venous return through unnamed muscular and subcutaneous vessels. Gross patterns of compensation, such as the saphenous compensating for deep vein occlusion, or vice versa, are recognizable. Precise details of small vessel flow patterns through long segments of muscle or an entire calf or thigh are too minute to delineate.

A curious fact of the venous system is that the efficient patterns of collateral flow which become established soon after acute occlusion, such as occurs in deep phlebitis, become less efficient as time passes. Within 3 to 6 months after extensive deep vein occlusion due to phlebitis, the patient's leg may function very well, but 3 to 5 years later that same leg may be severely incapacitated with the findings of chronic venous insufficiency, even though there has been no recognizable intercurrent thrombosis. This "fatigue" of the collateral circulation is ascribed to the long-term effects that follow upon loss of effective valves in the system. Dilated collateral veins lack efficient valves. Veins that become recanalized also lack valve integrity. Without valves, the venous return channels that are present are unable to provide adequate compensation because they are functionally inefficient. There exists a threshold between the number of channels available for venous return and their valvular efficiency that must be reached to provide a fully compensated lower-extremity venous return. Appreciation of both anatomic channels and functional integrity is needed to analyze the specific problem in a given clinical condition. Because of this relationship, study of the physiological mechanisms in venous return is necessary.

PHYSIOLOGY OF VENOUS RETURN

MUSCLE PUMP

The major driving force for venous return in the lower extremity is the pumping action of the muscles of the calf and thigh (Fig. 37-1). Within the investing deep fascial compartments, muscular contraction literally squeezes blood

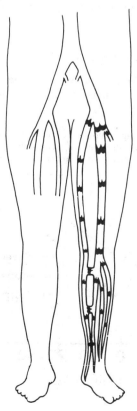

Fig. 37-1. Lower extremity veins. Valves are situated so that blood flows only from distal to proximal in the deep and superficial systems. Perforator veins contain valves that direct flow from superficial to deep.

out of the veins within that compartment. Since the muscular veins serve a major capacitance function, large amounts of blood flow are generated. The muscular contraction creates a great force analogous to the pumping action of the heart, capable of generating pressures over 100 torr, and it is this force that allows the venous circulation to overcome the effects of gravity in the erect position.

As the muscles contract, blood contained in the deep veins is propelled centrally and the venous channels are emptied. When the muscles relax, the newly emptied venous channels are refilled by flow from the arterial side to the venous side by the *vis a tergo,* or forward force, of the arterial flow through the capillary bed. Since this flow is occurring at a low pressure head of 25 to 35 torr, it is essential that the resistance on the venous side remain low.

Gravity in the erect human results in a pressure gradient that impedes return flow to the heart. Resting ankle pressure in both health and disease is equal to the weight of a column of blood from the heart to the ankle, amounting to a resting ankle pressure of 90 to 100 torr in the normal-sized adult. This pressure gradient severely impedes flow from the arterial to the venous side and requires the pumping action of the muscles to empty out the venous system. With exercise of the muscular pump, the venous pressure at the ankle falls to 30 torr or lower. When exercise ceases and the individual returns to the resting erect state, ankle pressure requires 20 seconds or longer to return to the baseline level of 100 torr (Fig. 37-2).

This pumping action of the muscles to empty the veins, followed by refill through onward force of the arteriovenous system, requires that the valves in the veins remain intact to direct flow centrally to the heart. The valves in the deep and superficial veins direct flow from distal to proximal, and the valves in the perforators direct flow from superficial to deep. The valves act as a system of gates in the venous pathway, preventing distalward or outward flow of blood. The direction of flow when valves are intact is depicted in Figure 37-3.

AMBULATORY VENOUS PRESSURE

To understand the need for valves in the leg, consider the situation where all valves are incompetent (Fig. 37-4). In

Fig. 37-2. Walking venous pressures: normal and abnormal curves as obtained with walking venous pressure test. Note the sharp contrast between normal and severely abnormal curves.

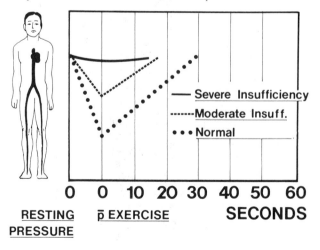

RESTING PRESSURE — $\bar{p}$ EXERCISE — SECONDS

— Severe Insufficiency
---- Moderate Insuff.
••• Normal

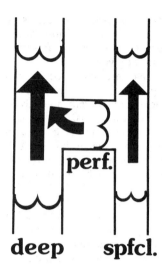

Fig. 37-3. Venous flow with intact valves. Direction of flow is from distal to proximal and from superficial to deep through the system.

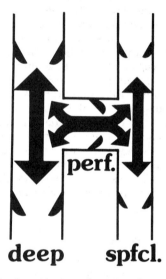

Fig. 37-4. All valves (deep, perforator, and superficial) incompetent. Blood flows in all directions with the action of the calf muscle pump, similar to squeezing a sponge.

Any one or all valves of the superficial, deep, or perforating veins may be incompetent—with appropriate changes in venous dynamics and general pathophysiology. Competent perforator valves protect the superficial tissues from high pressures generated by the muscle pump, even when both deep vein and superficial vein valves are incompetent.

this instance blood will squirt in all directions when the muscle contracts—flow will proceed proximally, distally, and surfaceward. This is analogous to squeezing a sponge and produces random and inefficient flow patterns. Pressure relationships are severely altered so that the force generated by muscle contraction is transmitted throughout the leg. In this case the ambulatory venous pressure (AVP) will show no fall in ankle pressure with exercise, and there is sustained venous hypertension throughout the lower leg. This is depicted in Figure 37-2 by the line marked "severe insufficiency." This state of sustained high pressure in the lower leg prevents efficient emptying of the venous blood from the leg and leads to impaired nutrition in the tissues of the ankle region.

VENOUS FLOW PATTERNS IN STATES OF VALVE INCOMPETENCE

To depict the altered patterns of venous flow under pathologic conditions, we will consider the various patterns that emerge when one system or another becomes incompetent.

PERFORATOR INCOMPETENCE

If perforator valves are incompetent but both the deep and superficial valves are intact, flow will proceed abnormally from deep to superficial with calf contraction but will ascend toward the heart in both superficial and deep veins. This forcible transmission of flow and pressures from deep to superficial throws a heavy load on the unsupported superficial veins and can lead to valve breakdown or stasis in the superficial veins. The long-term effect may be stasis in superficial veins and secondary changes of swelling, induration, and poor nutrition of subcutaneous tissues and skin in the lower leg or ankle region. Ultimately, small vessel circulation will be impaired and ulceration of the skin may follow.

DEEP VEIN INCOMPETENCE

In isolated deep valve incompetence where perforator and superficial venous valves remain intact, flow and pressure in the deep veins will be transmitted both proximally and distally at the time of muscle contraction. Intact perforator valves protect the subcutaneous tissues. The clinical effect may be aching or swelling or both, but subcutaneous induration and ulceration will not occur.

SUPERFICIAL VEIN INCOMPETENCE

When only the superficial valves are incompetent and the deep and perforator valves are functional, the calf muscle contraction does not seriously alter the dynamics in the subcutaneous tissues and major flow proceeds in its proper direction toward the heart. During muscle relaxation, flow still can occur from superficial to deep, as in the normal state. Because of this, the clinical state is mild and is limited to varicose veins. Induration and ulceration should not occur.

COMBINED SUPERFICIAL AND PERFORATOR INCOMPETENCE

When the superficial and perforator valves are incompetent and the deep valves retain their competence, severe changes in the lower leg can occur. With each calf contraction, flow and pressure erupt into the subcutaneous tissue, where flow proceeds both proximally and distally. This leads to swelling, induration, and ulceration.

COMBINED DEEP AND PERFORATOR INCOMPETENCE

When the deep and perforator valves are incompetent but the superficial valves remain competent, inappropriate transmission of flow and pressure occurs in the deep system and also from deep to superficial. Aching and swelling in the leg are likely to follow. The additional load placed on the superficial system can lead to secondary subcutaneous changes over the long run, but the ability of the superficial system to direct all flow centrally may be enough to overcome this tendency. The clinical state may vary from mild to severe disability. Induration and ulceration can develop in the late stages.

COMBINED DEEP AND SUPERFICIAL INCOMPETENCE

When the deep and superficial valves are incompetent but the perforators remain competent, flow and pressure dynamics are altered but the transmission of muscular contraction forces remains largely confined to its proper subfascial plane. The clinical effects on the subcutaneous tissues may be quite mild. Varicose veins would be expected, and deep leg aching or swelling might occur. Severe clinical changes of the subcutaneous tissues may or may not occur.

ALL SYSTEMS INCOMPETENT

When all systems are incompetent (see Fig. 37-4), flow and pressure patterns are most severely deranged. Muscular contraction can send flow in all directions—upward, downward, and outward. The clinical state that follows may include aching, swelling, induration, and ulceration. Compensatory mechanisms are negated, and the clinical syndrome is likely to be severe.

VARIATIONS IN EFFICIENCY OF THE CALF MUSCLE PUMP

Clinical states that alter the efficiency of the calf muscle pump produce changes in the venous return. Swelling of the extremities in the paraplegic who sits with the legs dependent is an example leading to the very high frequency of postparalytic deep venous thrombosis. Older individuals who lose muscle tone become prone to dependent edema and to phlebitis. Riding on an airplane when one sits for long periods with minimal leg activity causes swelling in healthy adults. There is no accurate test for the efficiency of the calf muscle pump at this time.

FLOW PATTERNS IN STATES OF VENOUS OBSTRUCTION

EARLY COLLATERAL CIRCULATION

Obstruction of venous outflow occurs most often in the form of thrombophlebitis, but other factors such as tumors, arteriovenous fistulas, and congenital webs are seen from time to time. The immediate physiological effect of an acute venous occlusion is the sudden appearance of venous hypertension distal to the point of occlusion. Experimentally, if one clamps the common femoral vein and measures the venous pressure just distal to the clamp, the pressure will rise immediately to 80 to 90 torr. This sudden rise of pressure becomes clinically evident in the form of swelling and discomfort. Over a period of 48 to 72 hours, collateral channels open and reroute venous return around the obstruction, and swelling comes under control. This sequence is seen in the patient with acute phlebitis who improves dramatically when placed at bed rest and given anticoagulants to prevent further extension of the thrombosing process.

During the ensuing weeks after deep venous thrombosis, improved patterns of collateral flow develop that are usually sufficient to compensate for the area of obstruction. The level of obstruction is important, because collateral flow capacity varies at different sites in the leg. In the inferior vena cava, obstruction is usually well compensated. Common iliac and hypogastric occlusions are also well compensated, but external iliac and common femoral occlusions may be poorly tolerated.

Occlusion in the superficial femoral vein is usually well tolerated if the common femoral and profunda femoral veins are patent. Isolated popliteal and tibial vein occlusions are usually well tolerated. Saphenous vein occlusions cause no symptoms over the long run.

Long occlusions cause more symptoms than short ones. Not infrequently, one finds occlusion from the ankle all the way to the iliac veins, and this creates greater problems than shorter blockages.

ROLE OF RECANALIZATION

Recanalization following venous occlusion is a frequent but not universal occurrence. The precise cause of recanalization in the venous system is not known. It appears to be a maturing process in which the thrombus retracts and shrinks from the vein wall itself, leaving randomly arranged septae and threads that occupy the lumen of the vessel. These septae become endothelialized, and flow is reestablished through the vein. Valves are destroyed by the original inflammatory process, and the patient develops a partially patent but totally incompetent segment of vein.

In many areas of the body, such as in the pulmonary vessels, recanalization is physiologically helpful, but lower extremity recanalization can be more of a detriment than a help because it produces an incompetent segment of vein. This newly patent vein becomes a site for inappropriate transmission of flow and pressure relationships in the leg because it is incompetent. A close temporal relationship between recanalization and onset of chronic venous insufficiency syndromes occurs so frequently in clinical practice that a cause-and-effect relationship seems likely. It has been shown that restoration of competence in such a recanalized segment results in dramatic improvement of the clinical syndrome of venous insufficiency, further supporting the observation that recanalization without valvular competence is detrimental in the lower extremity.

The combination of proximal obstruction in the iliac and common femoral veins with distal incompetence in the thigh and leg veins is the worst circumstance for venous drainage of the leg. Typically, this occurs as a result of extensive iliofemoral thrombophlebitis involving the deep veins from ankle to pelvis. Compensatory mechanisms are at a minimum, and the erect position is poorly tolerated. Those veins in the thigh and leg that are patent are incompetent, and the blood that courses through them has to follow a circuitous route around iliac and common femoral obstructions to reach the vena cava. Patients with this combination of destruction and incompetence present with severe swelling, aching, induration, and ulceration in the leg and ankle.

ROLE OF PRIMARY VALVE INCOMPETENCE IN CHRONIC VENOUS DISEASE

The venous valve is critical to proper function of the lower extremity venous system, as discussed earlier in this section. In chronic venous insufficiency states, incompetence of part of the venous system is invariable. Incompetence occurs as a result of recanalization in a postphlebitic vein, it occurs in collateral veins that are devoid of valves, and it occurs as a primary problem in which the venous valve cusp becomes stretched and prolapses, resulting in incompetence.

The occurrence of primary valve incompetence was described by Bauer in 1948 in patients who were studied by descending venography. Interest in the problem has been rekindled since 1975, when direct surgical repair of primary valve incompetence was described.

The clinical syndrome of primary valve incompetence is similar to that of any other cause of venous insufficiency. When the deep veins in the thigh and calf are involved, aching and swelling are the main symptoms. When the perforator veins are incompetent as well, subcutaneous induration and ankle ulceration also occur. The morphologic finding in primary valve incompetence is stretching of the valve cusp, which allows prolapse of the cusp under pressure and produces incompetence of the valve. The cause of the stretched valve may be congenital weakness of the valve tissue or wear and tear due to chronic stress. The stretched cusp is analogous to the stretching of the peritoneum in a hernia sac. Similar to the hernia, repair is effected by shortening the cusp.

Through study of a large series of descending venograms, mild incompetence is found frequently enough that it alone should not be considered a pathologic process. Incompetence becomes a clinical problem when it is severe in degree and when it involves the deep system from the common femoral vein all the way into the calf. Clinically, the otherwise normal leg can compensate for certain amounts of incompetence, but when the degree of incompetence in the deep system is severe, the compensatory mechanisms will be overcome.

RELATIONSHIP OF ACUTE THROMBOPHLEBITIS TO CHRONIC VENOUS INSUFFICIENCY (CVI)

There is common agreement that CVI is most frequently a result of previous phlebitis and that CVI is a major cause of disability in the working force of the United States and other countries. This cause-and-effect relationship between the acute event of phlebitis and the chronic state plays itself out over a period of 5 to 20 years, rendering it difficult for a single physician to personally observe the transition from a healthy extremity to one crippled by CVI symptoms.

Because of the remote time relationship between acute event and chronic effect, rather little definitive study has been devoted to the critical elements in the acute stage of phlebitis that contribute to a poor late result. It would be generally agreed that an extensive deep vein phlebitis is more likely to cause long-term CVI sequelae than a localized process. This is to say that thrombosis of all deep veins from ankle to iliac level will cause greater late sequelae than local phlebitis of the tibial veins. From our study of venograms in patients who have postphlebitic venous insufficiency, it appears that permanent occlusion of the common femoral and external iliac veins is a worse problem than permanent occlusion of more distal segments, such as the superficial femoral vein or the popliteal vein. Destruction of valve integrity in the perforator veins is a particularly critical occurrence, which leads to long-term skin and subcutaneous changes in the lower leg and ankle.

Definitive information about the relationship between the site of acute phlebitis in the leg and later development of CVI is limited partly because there has been slow acceptance of venography to define the extent of thrombosis in acute DVT. It will require many years of accurate study of venograms in the acute phase of DVT, coupled with follow-up venograms of the same patients 5, 10, and 20 years later, to really know the important relationships between acute DVT and CVI.

TREATMENT OF CVI

MEDICAL MEASURES

Treatment of CVI is usually a matter of judicious use of elastic support and elevation of the feet at needed intervals. Ambulatory care of ulcers is best managed by constant compression with a bootlike dressing that is kept on throughout the 24-hour period.

SURGICAL PROCEDURES

Surgical treatment of the saphenous and perforator veins in chronic venous disease is achieved by conventional ablative techniques. Ligation and stripping of the incompetent saphenous system is successful. Subfascial interruption of perforator veins is an excellent procedure when the perforator veins are demonstrably incompetent (see p. 985).

In patients with CVI who experience recurrent or unrelenting ulceration or severe pain in spite of medical management, surgical reconstructive procedures should be considered. Important advances have been made in applying surgical techniques to both obstructive and incompetent deep vein abnormalities. Reconstructive techniques for obstruction include bypass of chronically occluded segments utilizing the saphenous vein. The best example of this is the femoral-vein to femoral-vein bypass of an obstructed iliac vein using the saphenous vein. In this instance, the contralateral saphenous vein is transected at the popliteal level, and the distal end of the divided segment is placed across the front of the pubis to anastomose to the ipsilateral femoral vein below an occluded iliac vein. The proximal end of the transplanted saphenous vein remains in its normal position.

Reconstructive techniques for deep vein incompetence consist of valve reconstruction for the valve afflicted with primary incompetence or anastomosis of an incompetent vein to an adjacent vein that has a competent proximal valve. These procedures have been reported since 1975 and are presently under investigation for their long-term effectiveness.

The femoral vein valve was first repaired in 1968 and reported in 1975. This procedure is used in patients with primary valve incompetence, where it has been successful in restoring the deep venous system to a compensated state. When combined with appropriate interruptions of incompetent saphenous or perforator veins, the CVI syndrome has been reversed in 80% of patients with follow-up of 5 to 10 years.

In the patient whose valves have been destroyed by previous phlebitis it is not possible to repair the valve, but it has been shown possible to transfer the incompetent segment to an adjacent vein that still has a competent

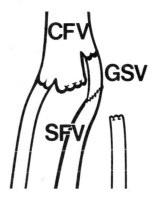

Fig. 37-5. Vein transposition. Reconstructive technique restores competence in postphlebitic disease by anastomosing incompetent superficial femoral vein (SFV) to competent greater saphenous vein (GSV). The distal end of the GSV is ligated in this example. (CFV, common femoral vein)

proximal valve (Fig. 37-5). As long as a proximal competent valve at the femoral end of the GSV, SFV, or PFV is present, other segments that are incompetent can be anastomosed end–end or end–side below the competent valve. This achieves the same result as repair of the femoral valve and can be used to help restore the leg to a compensated clinical state.

The success of these procedures in the past decade demonstrates that intravenous surgery can be done successfully and that a single competent valve in the femoral-popliteal segment is of great importance.

BIBLIOGRAPHY

CRANLEY JJ, CANOS AJ, SULL WJ et al: Phleborheographic technique for diagnosing deep venous thrombosis of the lower extremities. Surg Gynecol Obstet 141:331, 1975

DALE WA, HARRIS J: Cross-over vein grafts for iliac and femoral venous occlusion. J Cardiovasc Surg 10:458, 1969

DeCAMP PT, SCHRAMEL RJ, RAY CJ et al: Ambulatory venous pressure determinations in postphlebitic and related syndromes. Surgery 29:44, 1951

EDWARDS WH, SAWYERS JL, FOSTER JH: Iliofemoral venous thrombosis: Reappraisal of thrombectomy. Ann Surg 171:961, 1970

KISTNER RL: Primary venous valve incompetence of the leg. Am J Surg 140:218, 1980

KISTNER RL, FERRIS EB: Technique of surgical reconstruction of femoral vein valves. In Bergan JJ, Yao JST (eds): Operative Techniques in Vascular Surgery. New York, Grune & Stratton, 1980

KISTNER RL, SPARKUHL MD: Surgery in acute and chronic venous disease. Surgery 85:31, 1979

LANSING AM, DAVIS WM: Five-year follow-up study of iliofemoral venous thrombectomy. Ann Surg 168:620, 1968

LINTON RR: The communicating veins of the lower leg and the operative technic for their ligation. Ann Surg 197:582, 1938

LINTON RR: The post-thrombotic ulceration of the lower extremity: Its etiology and surgical treatment. Ann Surg 138:415, 1953

MAHORNER H, CASTLEBERRY JW, COLEMAN WO: Attempts to restore function in major veins which are the site of massive thrombosis. Ann Surg 146:510, 1957

MULLARKY RE: Valves of the iliac and femoral veins. Northwest Med 63:230, 1964

Lazar J. Greenfield

Acute Venous Thrombosis and Pulmonary Embolism

ACUTE DEEP VENOUS THROMBOSIS IN LEG

ETIOLOGY

Historically, deep venous thrombosis was considered by John Hunter to be a response to an inflammatory change in the lining layer of the veins. This concept persisted until 1856, when Virchow introduced the term thrombosis, emphasizing an intrinsic disorder of coagulation. He suggested the three possible mechanisms for thrombosis that remain the foundation of our understanding of the disorder—stasis, endothelial damage, and hypercoagulability.

Stasis is the most important factor for surgical patients, who are especially vulnerable to venous thrombosis. There is a significant reduction in venous flow in the lower extremities following induction of general anesthesia that persists throughout the procedure. There is also a relationship between the duration of bed rest and the incidence of venous thrombosis that provides the stimulus for early ambulation. Stasis alone, however, is not sufficient to induce thrombosis, which is promoted by coexisting disorders such as trauma, shock, congestive heart failure, and infection. Aging, obesity, and malignancy are also recognized as contributing factors.

Vessel wall injury can occur in collapsed vessels when the intimal walls are in contact, and some intimal injury can be demonstrated after hypoxemia. Although routine histologic examination of veins containing thrombi fails to show an inflammatory response consistent with vessel wall injury, ultrastructural study shows leukocytic attachment between endothelial intercellular junctions in areas of venous stasis after trauma at a remote site. These changes can be the nidus for the formation of a propagating thrombus (Fig. 37-6).

Hypercoagulability has assumed increased importance as a causative factor with the recognition that women who use oral contraceptive anovulatory agents develop thrombotic disorders 3 to 6 times more frequently than those who do not take these agents. Earlier efforts to find differences in coagulation factors among patients with or without deep venous thrombosis were unrewarding, but it was possible to identify a naturally occurring inhibitor of activated Factor X called antithrombin III. This factor was thought to be reduced by oral contraceptives, but subsequent studies have shown that it is more likely to be related to a reduction in the inhibitory activity of Factor Xa. Congenital deficiency in antithrombin III levels has been found to be a predisposing factor in venous thrombosis and pulmonary embolism. Other unexplained hypercoagulable states seem to be associated with recent trauma, major surgical procedures, and sepsis. When stasis enters the picture, the substances that promote platelet aggregation, including activated Factor X, thrombin, fibrin, and catecholamines, remain at high concentrations in a given area. This leads to platelet aggregation, which initiates coagulation and thrombin generation with release of ADP, further aggregating platelets as the fibrin complex propagates. Opposing this process is the fibrinolytic system of the blood and vein walls. The endothelium of the vein wall contains an activator that converts plasminogen to plasmin, which lyses fibrin. As might be expected, however, the fibrinolytic system is inhibited after surgery and trauma, and there is less activity in the veins of the lower extremity than in those of the upper extremity.

PATHOPHYSIOLOGY

Our present level of understanding of venous thrombosis evolved from autopsy data that were limited to *in vivo* studies of the dynamics of the venous circulation by means of radiographic contrast injections and noninvasive flow

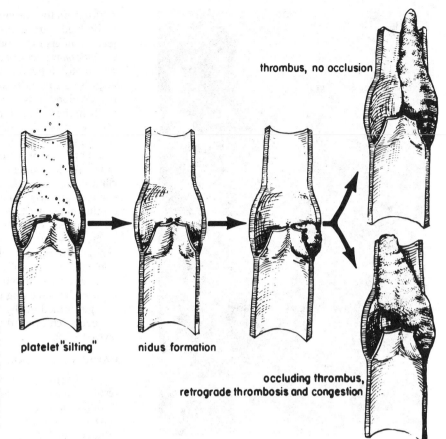

Fig. 37-6. The evolution of venous thrombosis begins with stagnant flow that permits silting of platelets, which form a nidus in the venous valvular sinus. The cycle of fibrin retraction and thrombin release aggregates more platelets as the thrombus enlarges and usually extends into the stream without occlusion, or it may occlude the vein with retrograde thrombosis.

studies. When contrast medium is injected in supine immobilized patients, it may remain in venous valve sinuses for as long as an hour, confirming the stasis existing in the soleal sinuses. This is the favored location for the formation of a nidus of thrombus, as has been described. Successive layering of platelets, fibrin, and leukocytes produces an organized white thrombus, which is more adherent to the vein wall than the propagating red thrombus that extends into the venous stream (Fig. 37-6) and is more likely to embolize. The original thrombus may become attached to the opposite wall, causing interruption of flow, retrograde thrombosis, and signs of venous stasis in the extremity. Subsequent formation of edema within the confines of the deep muscular fascia produces pain and the characteristic Homans' sign elicited by forcible dorsiflexion of the foot. More commonly, however, in about 60% of patients the thrombus propagates without interrupting flow and develops a long floating "tail" that is more susceptible to breaking loose from its tenuous anchor within the valvular sinus. It is this latter sequence of events that is the most dangerous aspect of the disorder, because major pulmonary embolism can and does occur without premonitory signs or symptoms at its point of origin.

The site of venous obstruction determines the level at which swelling is observed clinically. Swelling at the thigh level always implies obstruction at the level of the iliofemoral system, whereas swelling of the calf or foot suggests obstruction at the femoropopliteal level (Fig. 37-7). Autopsies suggest that it is more common for thrombi to originate in the veins of the soleus and then propagate proximally, but there is evidence that primary thrombosis of the femoral and iliac venous tributaries occurs as well (Fig. 37-8).

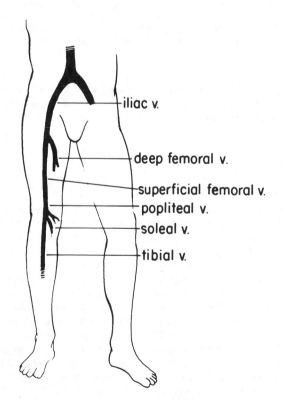

Fig. 37-7. The location of venous obstruction determines the clinical picture; most thrombi originate silently in the soleal veins. With occlusion of femoropopliteal veins, edema of the lower leg occurs, and further involvement of the iliofemoral system results in massive swelling of the thigh.

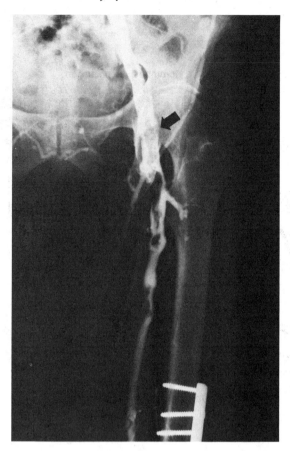

Fig. 37-8. Contrast venogram showing a thrombus originating in a femoral vein tributary (*screws*) and extending to the level of the groin (*arrow*). Such a patient might have no signs of deep vein thrombosis on physical or Doppler examination.

Resolution of deep venous thrombosis will affect the competence of the valves within the veins and can result in the postphlebitic syndrome, which is discussed in another section.

DIAGNOSIS

CLINICAL PRESENTATION

Major venous thrombosis involving the deep venous system of the thigh and pelvis produces a characteristic clinical picture of pain, extensive pitting edema, and blanching that has been termed *phlegmasia alba dolens* or *milk leg*. Association with pregnancy may be related to hormonal effects on blood, relaxation of vessel walls, or mechanical compression of the left iliac vein at the pelvic brim, resulting in the term "milk leg of pregnancy." It was originally believed that the blanching was due to spasm and compromise of arterial flow, but arteriograms fail to confirm this, and efforts to achieve sympatholysis to overcome "vasospasm" are ill advised because the subcutaneous edema is responsible for the blanching. In addition to pregnancy, other mechanical factors that can affect the left iliac vein include compression from the right iliac artery and an overdistended bladder and congenital webs within the vein. These factors are responsible for the observed 4:1 preponderance of left versus right iliac vein involvement.

As venous thrombosis impeding most of the venous

return from the extremity progresses further, there is danger of limb loss from cessation of arterial flow. The clinical picture differs from milk leg, with more congestion producing *phlegmasia cerulea dolens* (blue leg), which loses sensory and motor function. Venous gangrene is likely unless an aggressive approach is utilized to remove the thrombus and restore blood flow. A variant of this disorder occurs peripherally in the leg and is associated with concurrent malignant disease and a high mortality rate.

As indicated earlier, these major complications occur in less than 10% of patients with venous thrombosis. In fact, only 40% of patients with venous thrombosis have any clinical signs of the disorder. In addition, false positive clinical signs occur in up to 30% of patients studied. Because of this there has been a great deal of interest in the development of screening tests that can reveal thrombi before they become evident clinically. Of course, contrast venography provides direct evidence of both occlusive and nonocclusive thrombi, but it is an invasive procedure and usually requires moving the patient to a radiographic suite. Ideally, the screening test would be accurate, noninvasive, and performed at the bedside. Although the ideal has not yet been achieved, there are a number of tests that have proved useful.

RADIOACTIVE-LABELED FIBRINOGEN

In 1957 Ambrus et al showed that radioactive thrombi resulted from injection of radio-labeled fibrinogen and thrombin into an occluded vessel, and in 1960 Hobbs and Davies demonstrated preferential uptake of ^{131}I-labeled fibrinogen in formation of a thrombus. Clinical application of this finding required simplification of the test by development of portable scintillation counters for bedside use. After iodine blockage of the thyroid gland, the counts are obtained from marked locations on the lower extremities and expressed as a percentage of the radioactivity measured by counting over the heart. An increase of 20% or more in one area indicates the presence of an underlying thrombus. The test permits sequential scanning of the extremities over a period of days and is most sensitive to thrombi forming in the veins of the calves shortly after an operative procedure. It does not permit detection of thrombi in pelvic veins, and it cannot be used in an extremity in which there is a healing wound, fracture, cellulitis, arthritis, edema, ulceration, or superficial thrombophlebitis. It is also contraindicated in patients under 30 years of age and in women of childbearing age. Apart from these conditions it is quite accurate, however, and has a 90% positive correlation with contrast venograms. A negative correlation usually is explained by cessation of active thrombosis and failure to incorporate the tagged fibrinogen, making the test useful in discriminating between old and new venous thrombi.

ULTRASOUND

The Doppler ultrasound probe can be used to advantage to detect major venous thrombi with a high degree of accuracy, but it is a subjective form of testing dependent on the examiner's experience. The principle is straightforward and is based on the change in flow signal produced by intraluminal thrombi. The examination begins at the ankle with identification of the posterior tibial vein signal adjacent to the artery. The flow signal should be altered by distal and proximal compression, producing augmentation and interruption of flow, respectively, which can also be produced by the Valsalva maneuver. The same maneuvers are repeated

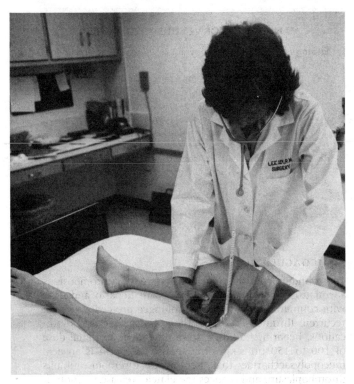

Fig. 37-9. Use of the Doppler probe to examine the popliteal vein. The technician is compressing the thigh to detect reflux and then the increased velocity signal that follows release of occlusion.

over the superficial and deep femoral veins and can be done over the popliteal vein as well (Fig. 37-9). Failure of augmentation of flow on compression below the probe or release of interruption of flow above the probe suggests a venous thrombus. The sensitivity of the test exceeds 90%, but the specificity is 5% to 10% lower owing to the possibility of other mechanical problems (*e.g.*, Baker's cyst, hematoma) interfering with venous flow. A negative Doppler ultrasound examination is reassuring, but a positive or equivocal test should be confirmed by contrast venography. A negative test is *not* reassuring when thromboembolism is suspected, because the thrombus may have been evacuated from the extremity.

IMPEDANCE PLETHYSMOGRAPHY

The impedance method measures the volume response of the extremity to temporary occlusion of the venous system. The diagnosis of venous thrombosis depends on the changes in venous capacitance and rate of emptying after release of the occlusion. A proximal thigh cuff is inflated to 45 cm H_2O pressure for 56 seconds or until maximum filling has occurred by plateau of the electrical signal. The cuff is then rapidly deflated, allowing rapid outflow and reduction of volume in a normal limb. Prolongation of the outflow wave suggests major venous thrombosis with 95% accuracy and is much more reliable than any voluntary technique of venous occlusion. The deficiency of this technique, as with all noninvasive methods, is the lack of detection of calf vein thrombosis or old post-thrombotic sequelae. The strain gauge plethysmograph can be used in a similar fashion.

VENOGRAPHY

The injection of contrast material for direct visualization of the venous system of the extremity is the most accurate

method of confirming the diagnosis of venous thrombosis and the extent of the involvement. Injection is usually made into the foot while the superficial veins are occluded by tourniquet, and a supplemental injection into the femoral veins may be required to visualize the iliofemoral system. Both filling defects and nonvisualization occur. An additional sign of the potential gravity of a thrombus is when it is floating free and extending into the iliofemoral system (Fig. 37-10). Potential false positive examinations may result from external compression of a vein or washout of the contrast material from collateral veins. The procedure can also be performed with isotope injection using a gamma scintillation counter to record flow of the isotope. Delayed imaging of persistent "hot spots" may also reflect isotope retention at the sites of thrombus formation. A perfusion lung scan can also be obtained for baseline comparison and for detection of silent embolism. There is less definition of deep vein thrombi with this technique than with contrast venography, but it is a valuable technique for sequential study of patients and avoids the potential thrombogenesis associated with the injection of contrast medium.

PROPHYLAXIS

Theoretically it should be possible to prevent formation of venous thrombi either by eliminating or reducing venous stasis or by altering blood coagulability. The belief that early ambulation prevents stasis and reduces the formation of

Fig. 37-10. Large free-floating thrombus within the femoral vein seen on contrast venogram (*arrow*). Such a thrombus can become detached during movement or straining to produce pulmonary embolism.

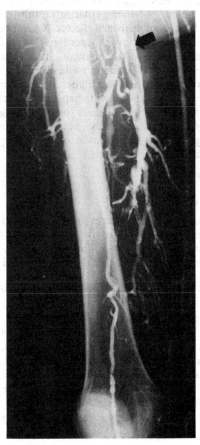

thrombi has been controversial, and studies using tagged fibrinogen have not supported this assumption. One explanation for this is that early ambulation usually involves having the patient walk to a chair and sit, whereupon the legs are subjected to even more stasis. Other efforts, including electrical stimulation of calf muscles, pneumatic compression of the calves, and passive motor-driven flexion of the foot, are under investigation, but discomfort, type of operative procedure, and cost remain obvious limitations.

There has been considerably more interest in the prophylactic use of anticoagulant drugs and, more recently, in drugs that inhibit platelets such as aspirin and dipyridamole. These drugs are under evaluation for this role, but preliminary reports have not shown that they provide much protection. However, there are good data to support the use of preoperative oral anticoagulant therapy with warfarin derivatives in high-risk patients. Unfortunately, this procedure increases the risk of hemorrhage, and, because of the added difficulties of laboratory control of prothrombin time, there has not been widespread acceptance of this approach. The administration of dextran, which produces a variety of effects on platelets and clotting factors, has been demonstrated to reduce the incidence of detectable thrombi, but it too can produce hemorrhagic problems as well as allergic reactions and, in older patients, congestive failure.

There has been renewed interest in minimizing the problems associated with anticoagulant prophylaxis by administration of heparin prior to and following surgery in low ("mini") doses that do not alter the laboratory clotting profile. Generally, a 5000 unit dose is given subcutaneously 2 hr preoperatively and then every 12 hr postoperatively for 6 days. This apparently provides protection for most high-risk groups with the exception of those undergoing orthopedic procedures. The beneficial effect may be due to the enhancement of heparin cofactor (antithrombin III), a natural inhibitor of activated Factor X. Although some studies have failed to show a protective effect, Kakkar et al, in a randomized series of 4121 patients, showed that heparin protected against fatal pulmonary embolism as well as deep venous thrombosis. There is a higher incidence of bleeding and wound complications with heparin prophylaxis, and because its major benefit appears to be reducing the incidence of calf vein thrombosis, which is of questionable clinical significance, the question of optimal prophylaxis remains unresolved.

TREATMENT

The approach to management of the patient with deep venous thrombosis is based on minimizing the risk of pulmonary embolism, limiting further thrombosis, and facilitating resolution of existing thrombi to avoid the post-phlebitic syndrome.

Initially, the patient is placed at bed rest with the foot of the bed elevated 8 to 10 inches. Further improvement in venous return can be obtained by application of elastic bandages, which must be reapplied twice daily to avoid a tourniquet effect as they loosen. Generally, pain, swelling, and tenderness resolve over a 5- to 7-day period, at which time ambulation can be permitted with continued elastic support. Warm, moist compresses also have been used to improve blood flow and can provide symptomatic improvement. Standing still and sitting should be prohibited to avoid increased venous pressure and stasis.

MANAGEMENT OF VENOUS THROMBOSIS	
Etiology	Stasis, vessel wall injury, hypercoagulability
Dx	Symptoms: pain, edema, pallor, cyanosis Noninvasive testing: radio-labeled fibrinogen, Doppler ultrasound examination, impedance plethysmography; definitive diagnosis by venography
Rx	Prophylactic measures, bed rest with continuous infusion anticoagulation followed by oral coumarin derivatives Vena caval interruption (?) or thrombectomy (?)

ANTICOAGULATION

The foundation of therapy for deep venous thrombosis is adequate anticoagulation, initially with heparin and then with coumarin derivatives for prolonged protection against recurrent thrombosis. Unless there are specific contraindications, heparin should be administered in an initial dose of 100 to 150 units/kg intravenously. Heparin is an acid mucopolysaccharide that neutralizes thrombin, inhibits thromboplastin, and reduces the platelet release reaction. It may be administered by continuous or intermittent intravenous doses regulated by whole blood clotting time. Bleeding complications can be minimized by doses of heparin that prolong the laboratory clotting determinations by about twice the normal time with no loss of effectiveness. Continuous intravenous infusion regulated by an infusion pump seems to minimize the total dose required for control and is associated with a lower incidence of complications.

Oral administration of anticoagulants is begun shortly after initiation of heparin therapy, because several days are usually required to bring the prothrombin time within the therapeutic range of 2 to 2.5 times the control value. The coumarin derivatives block the synthesis of several clotting factors, and prolongation of the prothrombin time beyond the range suggested is associated with a high incidence of bleeding complications. Fortunately, administration of vitamin K can usually restore the prothrombin time rapidly. After an episode of acute deep venous thrombosis, anticoagulation therapy should be maintained for a minimum of 3 months; some investigators favor 6 months for treatment of thrombi in the larger veins. Many drugs interact with coumarin derivatives (*e.g.*, barbiturates), and therefore it is essential to establish a routine for regular monitoring of prothrombin time after the patient leaves the hospital.

FIBRINOLYSIS

There has been great interest in the use of fibrinolytic agents to activate the intrinsic plasmin system. Both streptokinase and urokinase have been used and found to be effective, although they are associated with a high incidence of hemorrhagic complications. These agents have no advantage over heparin in the treatment of recurrent venous thrombosis or thrombosis that has existed for over 72 hr, and they are contraindicated in postoperative or post-traumatic patients. Another interesting agent under investigation, derived from the venom of the Malayan pit viper, produces reversible defibrination.

SURGICAL APPROACHES

Operative Thrombectomy

A direct surgical approach to remove thrombi from the deep veins of the leg by way of the common femoral vein is facilitated by the use of Fogarty venous balloon catheters and an elastic wrap for milking the extremity. Although the operative results are impressive, venograms obtained prior to discharge from the hospital show rethrombosis in the majority of patients, and there does not seem to be any lesser incidence of the postphlebitic syndrome. Consequently, the procedure is now usually reserved for limb salvage in the presence of phlegmasia cerulea dolens and impending venous gangrene.

Vena Caval Interruption

Adequate anticoagulation is usually effective in managing deep venous thrombosis, but if recurrent pulmonary embolism occurs during anticoagulant therapy or if there is a contraindication to anticoagulation, a surgical approach is necessary. Operation is also indicated as prophylaxis against recurrence of embolism for the patient who has required pulmonary embolectomy and in some high-risk patients who cannot tolerate recurrence.

Early surgical efforts to prevent recurrence of pulmonary embolism were directed to the common femoral vein, which was ligated bilaterally. This resulted in a high incidence of sequelae due to stasis in the lower extremity and an unacceptable rate of pulmonary embolism. The next approach tried was ligation of the inferior vena cava below the renal veins, which added the adverse effect of a sudden reduction in cardiac output. This effect, coupled with stasis sequelae and recurrent embolism through dilated collateral veins, led to efforts to compartmentalize the vena cava by means of sutures, staples, and external clips in order to provide filtration without occlusion.

Because these procedures required general anesthesia and laparotomy, the next logical step was to devise a transvenous approach that could be performed under local anesthesia. The Mobin-Uddin "umbrella" unit is inserted from the jugular vein and positioned under fluoroscopic control below the renal veins, where it usually produces (in 70% of cases) thrombosis of the vena cava (Fig. 37-11).

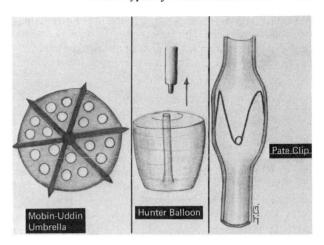

Fig. 37-11. Several devices have been developed for permanent implantation in the inferior vena cava to prevent passage of emboli. The Mobin-Uddin umbrella (*left*) has been widely used, with generally favorable results.

The Greenfield cone-shaped filter was developed to maintain patency after trapping emboli and to permit continued flow to avoid stasis and to facilitate lysis of the embolus (Fig. 37-12). It can be inserted from either the jugular vein or the femoral vein, the latter insertion being reserved for inadequate size or technical problems with the jugular vein or open wound of the neck. The rate of recurrent embolism with this device has been less than 3%, and its long-term patency rate of 95% allows it to be placed above the renal veins when necessary for embolism control, such as when there is a thrombus within the renal veins or vena cava. Another device, the Hunter balloon, occludes the vena cava after it is positioned below the renal veins and only contributes to stasis sequelae.

OTHER TYPES OF VENOUS THROMBOSIS

The term thrombophlebitis should be restricted to the disorder of the superficial veins characterized by a local inflammatory process that is usually aseptic. The cause of thrombophlebitis in the upper limb is usually acidic fluid

Fig. 37-12. The most recent development in transvenous filter devices, because of the geometry of the cone, permits trapping of emboli without loss of patency. A thrombus is shown trapped in the filter, and flow can continue around it to facilitate lysis and avoid the stasis sequelae of complete vena caval occlusion.

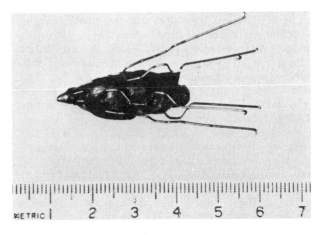

INDICATIONS FOR INSERTION OF A VENA CAVAL FILTER

1. Recurrent thromboembolism in spite of adequate anticoagulation
2. Documented thromboembolism in a patient who has a contraindication to anticoagulation
3. Complication of anticoagulation that forces therapy to be discontinued
4. Chronic pulmonary embolism with associated pulmonary hypertension and cor pulmonale (class V)
5. Immediate insertion following pulmonary embolectomy
6. Septic pulmonary embolism
7. Relative indications—patient with more than 50% of the pulmonary vascular bed occluded (class III) who cannot tolerate any additional embolism; patient wih a propagating iliofemoral thrombus despite anticoagulation; patient with a large free-floating iliofemoral thrombus on venogram

infusion or prolonged cannulation. In the lower extremities it is usually associated with varicose veins and may coexist with deep vein thrombosis. Its association with the injection of contrast material can be minimized by washout of the contrast material with heparinized saline.

THROMBOPHLEBITIS MIGRANS

Thrombophlebitis migrans, a condition of recurrent episodes of superficial thrombophlebitis, has been associated with visceral malignancy, systemic collagen vascular disease, and blood dyscrasias. Involvement of the deep veins and the visceral veins has also been described.

SUBCLAVIAN VEIN THROMBOSIS

Thrombosis of the subclavian vein is most likely to be secondary to an indwelling catheter and can occur in the pediatric age group. It may also occur as a primary event in a young athletic person (*effort thrombosis*), presumably as a result of injury at the thoracic inlet. It usually responds well to elevation of the limb and anticoagulation, although some venous insufficiency and discomfort with exercise may persist.

ABDOMINAL VEIN THROMBOSIS

Thrombosis of the inferior vena cava can result from tumor invasion or propagating thrombus from the iliac veins. Most commonly, however, it results from ligation, plication, or insertion of partially occluding caval devices such as the Mobin-Uddin umbrella. Any caval filtration device can become totally occluded by a trapped massive thrombus, causing sudden reduction in venous return and cardiac output. In the patient with known prior pulmonary embolism it is a grave error to ascribe the resulting hypotension to recurrent embolism. Thrombosis of the renal vein is most likely to occur in association with the nephrotic syndrome. It can be a source of thromboembolism and has been treated successfully by suprarenal placement of the Greenfield filter.

Portal vein thrombosis can occur in the neonate, usually secondary to propagating septic thrombophlebitis of the umbilical vein. Collateral development leads to the occurrence of esophageal varices. Thrombosis of the portal, hepatic, splenic, or superior mesenteric vein in the adult can occur spontaneously but usually is associated with hepatic cirrhosis. Thrombosis of mesenteric or omental veins can simulate an acute condition of the abdomen but usually results in prolonged ileus rather than intestinal infarction.

Hepatic vein thrombosis (Budd-Chiari syndrome) usually produces massive hepatomegaly, ascites, and liver failure. It can occur in association with a congenital web, endophlebitis, or polycythemia vera. Although some success has been reported using a direct approach to the congenital webs, the usual treatment is a side-to-side portacaval shunt to allow decompression of the liver.

The development of pelvic sepsis after abortion, tubal infection, or puerperal sepsis can lead to *septic thrombophlebitis* of the pelvic veins and septic thromboembolism. Ligation of the ovarian vein and vena cava has been the traditional treatment, but the emphasis should be on drainage or excision of the abscesses and appropriate antibiotic therapy. We have also used the Greenfield filter in this

situation because it is inert stainless steel and avoids the development of an intraluminal abscess that can occur after ligation of the vena cava.

PULMONARY THROMBOEMBOLISM

The clinical significance of major pulmonary embolism can be appreciated by referring to the annual mortality attributed to it, which has been estimated to be 90,000 deaths in the United States alone. It is estimated that 5 of every 1000 adults undergoing major surgery will die from massive pulmonary embolism. Because it represents the most important complication of deep venous thrombosis, it is of particular concern to surgeons whose patients are prone to develop deep vein thrombosis in the immediate postoperative period.

Just as with deep vein thrombosis, our understanding of the pathophysiology of pulmonary embolism dates back to Virchow, who first recognized the association between the two findings. It also became obvious in the early reports by pathologists that pulmonary embolism could be well tolerated by some patients who then died of other causes. In fact, the full spectrum of the disorder ranges from asymptomatic minor embolism to sudden death from massive embolism.

DIAGNOSIS

CLINICAL PRESENTATION

The signs and symptoms of an embolic episode obviously depend primarily on the quantity of embolus involved and, to a lesser extent, on the cardiopulmonary status of the patient. In the classic presentation, the patient suddenly develops chest pain, cough, dyspnea, tachypnea, and marked anxiety (Table 37-1). Although hemoptysis has traditionally been associated with pulmonary embolism, it is actually an uncommon sign; when present it usually occurs late in the course of disease and probably represents pulmonary infarction. Objectively, the patient with major embolism usually shows tachycardia, an increased pulmonary second sound, cyanosis, prominent jugular veins, and varying degrees of collapse. Less commonly there may be wheezing, a pleural friction rub, splinting of the chest wall, rales, low-grade fever, ventricular gallop, and wide splitting of the pulmonic second sound. The incidence of these findings is shown in Table 37-1.

The differential diagnosis includes esophageal perforation, pneumonia, septic shock, and myocardial infarction. Since all of these entities are life-threatening, it is mandatory that an orderly approach be formulated to confirm or reject

TABLE 37-1   CLINICAL MANIFESTATIONS OF MAJOR PULMONARY EMBOLISM

SYMPTOMS	INCIDENCE (%)	SIGNS	INCIDENCE (%)
Dyspnea	80	Tachypnea	88
Apprehension	60	Tachycardia	63
Pleural pain	60	Accentuated P_2	60
Cough	50	Rales	51
Hemoptysis	27	S_3 or S_4	47
Syncope	22	Pleural rub	17

TABLE 37-2 CLASSIFICATION OF PULMONARY THROMBOEMBOLISM

CLASS	SYMPTOMS	GASES	PA OCCLUSION (%)	HEMODYNAMICS
I	None	Normal	<20	Normal
II	Anxiety, hyperventilation	$PaO_2 < 80$ torr $PaCO_2 < 35$ torr	20–30	Tachycardia
III	Dyspnea, collapse	$PaO_2 < 65$ torr $PaCO_2 < 30$ torr	30–50	CVP elevated, $\overline{PA} > 20$ torr
IV	Shock, dyspnea	$PaO_2 < 50$ torr $PaCO_2 < 30$ torr	>50	CVP elevated, $\overline{PA} > 25$ torr BP < 100 torr
V	Dyspnea, syncope	$PaO_2 < 50$ torr $PaCO_2$ 30–40 torr	>50	CVP elevated, $\overline{PA} > 40$ torr CO low, no shock

the working diagnosis. Laboratory studies in general are not very helpful in the differential diagnosis, although a white blood cell count of less than 15,000/mm³ may be suggestive when a pulmonary infiltrate is present to help rule out pneumonitis. The following determinations are particularly useful in the evaluation of suspected major embolism.

ELECTROCARDIOGRAPHY

The most common electrocardiographic change associated with pulmonary embolism is nonspecific ST and T wave changes (66% of patients). More specific signs of right ventricular overload such as the often quoted S_1, Q_3, T_3 pattern are seldom seen. Consequently, the primary value of the electrocardiogram is to exclude the presence of a myocardial infarction. Unfortunately, the finding of a myocardial infarction does not exclude the diagnosis of pulmonary embolism, and in some cases a lung scan or pulmonary angiogram may be required to clarify the problem.

CHEST RADIOGRAPHY

Although the chest radiograph may suggest the diagnosis of pulmonary embolism because of central vascular enlarge-

	PULMONARY EMBOLISM
Etiology	Pulmonary arterial occlusion by clot from deep venous system
Dx	Symptoms: chest pain, cough, dyspnea, anxiety EKG: nonspecific ST-T wave change Chest x-ray: nonspecific; arterial blood gases: hypoxia, hypocarbia; elevated CVP Role of lung scan, definitive treatment with heparin, pulmonary arteriography
Rx	Anticoagulation—parenteral then oral (coumarin derivatives) Mechanical: catheter suction devices; vena cava interruption; pulmonary embolectomy (rarely necessary in patients not responding to vascular drug and intravenous heparinization)

ment, asymmetry of the vascular markings with segmental or lobar ischemia (Westermark's sign), or pleural effusion, these signs are nonspecific. The chest radiograph then serves to exclude other diagnostic possibilities such as pneumonia, pneumothorax, esophageal perforation, or congestive heart failure. It also is critical in the interpretation of a lung scan, because any radiographic density or evidence of chronic lung disease makes a perfusion defect in that area less likely to represent pulmonary embolism. Chronic lung disease also reduces the applicability of lung scanning to the diagnosis.

ARTERIAL BLOOD GASES

The more widespread availability of blood gas and pH determinations has improved the assessment of all critically ill patients and provides important support for the diagnosis of pulmonary embolism. Hypoxemia with PaO_2 of less than 60 torr is found in the majority of patients and is felt to be due to shunting by overperfusion of nonembolized lung and a widened alveolar arterial oxygen gradient due to reduced cardiac output. The reduction in arterial Pco_2 that follows major embolism is the most discriminating finding, because hypoxemia is present in several disorders likely to be misdiagnosed as massive embolism (e.g., septic shock). If hypoxemia and hypocarbia are not present, the diagnosis of major embolism in the severely ill patient can be excluded with a high level of confidence, and an alternate diagnosis should be sought.

CENTRAL VENOUS PRESSURE

In the patient with systemic hypotension, the central venous pressure can supply valuable information, and the line provides access for administration of drugs and fluids as well. Low central venous pressure virtually excludes pulmonary embolism as the primary cause of the hypotension because massive embolism almost always is accompanied by right ventricular overload and elevated right atrial pressures. Elevated right ventricular filling pressures may be transient, however, as hemodynamic accommodation occurs, and in subacute or chronic embolism the central venous pressure may be normal.

LUNG SCAN

The availability and widespread usage of lung photoscanning have led to overemphasis on this test and a tendency to overdiagnose pulmonary embolism. In a nonhypotensive patient with a normal chest radiograph, the lung scan is a valuable screening test that has increasing validity as the size of the perfusion defect approaches lobar distribution. Smaller peripheral perfusion defects are much more difficult to interpret because pneumonitis, atelectasis, or other ventilation abnormalities alter pulmonary perfusion. A normal lung scan, on the other hand, usually excludes the diagnosis of pulmonary embolism. Adding a ventilation scan for combined ventilation–perfusion imaging increases the accuracy of the diagnosis of thromboembolism, provided that there are at least two moderate size areas or one large area of ventilation–perfusion mismatch. The assumption that the underperfused regions of the lung after embolism will remain normally ventilated, producing the mismatch in the scans, is clouded by the known physiological effect of bronchoconstriction produced by embolism. When the additional variable of wide variance in scan interpretation among observers is considered, the diagnosis is much more reliable when it is based on arteriography.

PULMONARY ARTERIOGRAPHY

Selective pulmonary arteriography is the most accurate method of confirming the presence, size, and distribution of pulmonary emboli. The procedure is invasive, requiring passage of a cardiac catheter into the main pulmonary artery for injection of a bolus of contrast medium. A rapid film changer produces a series of radiographs that outline areas of decreased perfusion and usually show filling defects or the rounded trailing edge of impacted emboli (Fig. 37-13). Straight cutoffs of the smaller pulmonary arteries are more difficult to interpret, particularly if there is associated chronic lung disease that tends to obliterate pulmonary vessels. The

procedure can be performed with low risk, although this particular group of patients is at highest risk for this type of study, which usually carries a 0.3% to 0.5% mortality rate. Avoidance of injection of contrast medium into the main pulmonary artery minimizes the complications. Additional useful information is obtained prior to contrast injection by measurement of pulmonary arterial pressures. A normal pulmonary angiogram excludes the diagnosis of pulmonary embolism in acutely ill patients.

PATHOPHYSIOLOGY

Although deep vein thrombosis precedes pulmonary embolism, less than 33% of patients with documented pulmonary embolism show signs of venous thrombosis. Despite this, it is estimated that 85% to 90% of all pulmonary emboli originate from the veins of the lower extremity, and the remainder arise from the right side of the heart or other veins. In addition, the emboli tend to be multiple, fragmenting either in the right side of the heart or during impaction into the pulmonary vascular bed. Older thrombi, however, contain laminated fibrin layers that make them more solid and more difficult to lyse.

Once the embolus has lodged and interrupted pulmonary blood flow, the ratio of regional ventilation to perfusion increases, and the lung responds by bronchoconstriction to reduce wasted ventilation. This response is mediated by local reduction in CO_2 output, since it can be prevented by ventilation with increased concentration of CO_2. Some experimental studies also suggest a generalized neural reflex vasoconstriction, but even if this occurs in humans, it is not likely to be as significant a factor in survival as the me-

Fig. 37-13. Selective pulmonary arteriograms showing embolus occluding right upper lobe branches (*left*) and trailing into the lower lobe branches. Distal focal occlusions are seen in the selective left arteriogram (*right*).

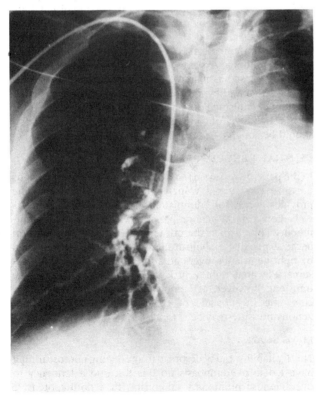
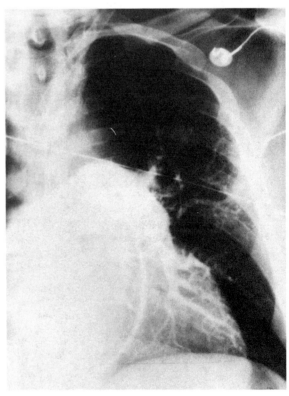

chanical effect of major vascular occlusion. Similarly, the effects of vasoactive humoral agents can be demonstrated in animals, and there is good documentation that serotonin is elaborated from platelets adherent to the embolus, which also contributes to the bronchoconstriction. The ability of heparin to inhibit the release of serotonin adds further weight to the early use of this drug. Other vasoactive agents such as histamine and prostaglandins may play a role in humans, but the net effect is a reduction in size of peripheral airways, reduced lung volume, and reduced static pulmonary compliance.

The hypoxemia that characterizes major embolism is thought to be due to a ventilation–perfusion imbalance secondary to the ventilation changes described above, although the findings in some patients resemble true arteriovenous shunting. Such shunting is anatomically possible if there is an unobliterated foramen ovale that opens in the presence of elevated right atrial pressures. Such an opening can allow passage of a venous embolus into the systemic circulation; it then is termed paradoxical embolism. Although there may be some improvement in PaO$_2$ after supplemental oxygen is administered, the effects usually are minimal. The return of pulmonary blood flow effected by embolectomy restores respiratory gas exchange, but the ischemia appears to result in loss of capillary integrity, causing interstitial pulmonary edema or overt pulmonary hemorrhage.

Pulmonary infarction as a consequence of embolism is relatively rare and is associated clinically with problems of poor systemic perfusion such as shock and congestive heart failure. In these patients the symptoms include pleuritic chest pain, dyspnea, cough, and hemoptysis. The signs include fever, tachycardia, splinting, and occasionally friction rub. There is usually prominent leukocytosis, an elevated lactic dehydrogenase level, and bilirubinemia. A wedge-shaped density usually is seen on chest radiography.

The pulmonary vascular and cardiac effects of embolism are a direct consequence of the degree of filling of the pulmonary vascular bed. Occlusion of more than 30% of the vascular tree is required to begin to elevate mean PA pressure, and usually more than 50% occlusion is required to reduce systemic pressure. The degree of pulmonary hypertension produced is proportional to the extent of angiographic vascular occlusion, but in a previously normal patient the limit of pressure elevation observed is approxi-

mately 40 torr. The fate of pulmonary emboli in human patients is not easy to predict, although a great deal of experimental work in animals has been reported. Injection of autologous thrombi into the pulmonary circulation of dogs is followed by relatively rapid recovery of pulmonary function and objective evidence of lysis over a period of weeks. Activation of plasminogen to plasmin, which is found in high concentration in the pulmonary circulation, promotes this fibrinolytic effect. Unfortunately, the resolution of aged thrombi proceeds more slowly and is hampered further by impaction of the embolus and isolation from pulmonary blood flow. Consequently, resolution after massive embolism in patients is unpredictable and often incomplete. It is not unusual to find residual fibrin strands or webs in the pulmonary arteries at autopsy as remnants of prior embolism.

CLASSIFICATION AND MANAGEMENT

ANTICOAGULATION

The hemodynamic variables mentioned above provide a means of classification of patients that employs five grades of severity and is a useful guide to therapy and prognosis (Table 37-2). The minor degrees of embolism (classes I and II) can usually be managed by anticoagulants alone with a satisfactory outcome (Fig. 37-14). Heparin is selected for initial treatment in a dosage designed to prolong the partial thromboplastin time to at least twice normal. At this dosage of approximately 150 units/kg there is adequate protection against further attachment of thrombi and platelets to the embolus. Heparin should be administered intravenously by pump-regulated continuous infusion. Many clinicians also begin oral anticoagulation therapy with warfarin derivatives shortly after starting heparin administration to allow several days' overlap of the drugs as prothrombin time is extended into the therapeutic range.

VENA CAVAL INTERRUPTION: SPECIFIC INDICATIONS

In some patients, however, anticoagulants cannot be used because of associated problems (*e.g.,* peptic ulcer disease), and management must be directed toward a mechanical means of protection against recurrent embolism as outlined previously. Other patients, in whom anticoagulation appears to be adequate, sustain recurrent embolism and become

Fig. 37-14. Management process for patients with documented pulmonary embolism for each class of patients. The foundation of treatment is anticoagulation as indicated; for major embolism (classes III and IV), both findings at arteriography and hemodynamic status influence the choice of surgical procedures undertaken. For example, the patient with more than 50% occlusion of the pulmonary vascular bed who needs vasopressors may require partial bypass for support during transvenous embolectomy and insertion of a transvenous filter to prevent re-embolism, as well as long-term anticoagulation for underlying venous thrombosis.

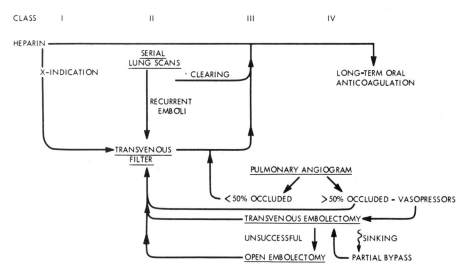

candidates for surgical intervention. The third indication for a surgical procedure is protection against recurrent embolism in a patient who has sustained massive pulmonary embolism requiring open or catheter embolectomy. In these patients, in spite of a satisfactory embolectomy of the pulmonary circulation, the original focus of venous thrombosis remains untreated, and recurrent embolism is likely.

There are two additional relative indications for vena caval procedures to prevent embolism. One is the high-risk patient over 40 years of age who is obese and has a serious associated medical illness (*e.g.,* heart disease), malignant disease, or a history of previous embolism and who undergoes a major abdominal or vascular procedure. The final relative indication is the patient in whom 40% to 50% of the vascular bed has been occluded (class III) and who would most likely not be able to tolerate additional emboli, particularly if there is associated cardiac or pulmonary disease.

Pulmonary emboli may accumulate gradually over a prolonged period if they are small enough to produce microembolism rather than macroembolism. The clinical picture in this case is one of chronic cor pulmonale because significant pulmonary hypertension results from changes in the pulmonary vascular bed (class V). The presentation may be subtle with only dyspnea or syncope on exertion, but there is a loud P_2 and right-sided strain on the EKG. The sequence may also occur unaccompanied by significant respiratory symptoms, and this may explain the etiology in some of the patients considered to have primary pulmonary hypertension. When the diagnosis is made, there is a very limited life expectancy, and the patient may benefit from a vena caval procedure to prevent further embolism even if the disorder is primary pulmonary hypertension. The rationale for this is that otherwise they will develop right heart failure, predisposing to pulmonary embolism that is lethal even if small. When acute cardiopulmonary decompensation occurs in these patients after embolism, they are not good candidates for embolectomy because of fixation of the older thrombi to the pulmonary arterial wall. They should be classified separately (class V) and managed by long-term anticoagulation therapy.

When the emboli originate from a septic focus, usually the pelvis in a female, the classic treatment has been vena caval ligation with ligation of the ovarian or spermatic veins. It must be recognized, however, that large collateral veins develop as a consequence of vena caval occlusion, that may then become the avenue of recurrent embolism.

The methods of vena caval protection are reviewed in the preceding section on acute deep venous thrombosis. It is worth repeating that the current interest in transvenous methods of permanent implantation of devices in the inferior vena cava will probably be greatly enhanced by further technological improvements.

PULMONARY EMBOLECTOMY

In patients who sustain massive embolism (classes III and IV), management must be a coordinated and rapidly responsive effort, since survival may be only a matter of minutes. As indicated earlier, it is critical to document the presence of massive pulmonary embolism by pulmonary arteriography because the clinical diagnosis, regardless of "classic" appearance, often is in error. The initial approach to patients who have either transient collapse (class III) or persistent systemic hypotension (class IV) should include full heparinization and administration of inotropic drugs if

necessary to support the circulation while the diagnosis is confirmed. Isoproterenol (4 mg in 1000 ml of 5% dextrose in water) is useful initially because of its bronchodilating and vasodilating effects as well as its positive inotropic cardiac effect. It may provoke arrhythmias, however, and necessitate use of dopamine. In the class II patient who responds to heparin and does not require vasopressors for systemic pressure or urine output, careful monitoring is essential to determine whether anticoagulation alone will control the disorder (see Fig. 37-14). In most circumstances the spontaneous lysis of pulmonary emboli will proceed over a period of days and can be documented by serial lung scans performed at weekly intervals. The rate of clearing may be prolonged for weeks, particularly after a sizable embolism, and may be incomplete, as indicated previously. The latter condition has been observed in association with persistent pulmonary hypertension even after additional lytic drugs (*e.g.,* urokinase) were administered. Lytic agents, however, may become a useful adjunct in management in the future.

The direct surgical approach to pulmonary embolism can be traced back to Trendelenburg (1908), who demonstrated the feasibility of pulmonary embolectomy experimentally but had no successes clinically. It remained for his pupil Kirschner (1924) to confirm the possibility of embolectomy by a successful clinical outcome. Because this procedure was attempted without circulatory support by direct approach to the pulmonary artery at thoracotomy, the number of survivors was very small, and the first successful case in the United States was not reported until 1958 by Steenburg. A modification of this technique using hypothermia to occlude the circulation temporarily was reported by Allison et al in 1960. The very high mortality rate associated with the Trendelenburg procedure prompted Gibbon to consider the use of extracorporeal circulation to bypass the impacted pulmonary circulation. The first successful open embolectomy during cardiopulmonary bypass was reported by Sharp in 1962. Since then partial bypass support has also been utilized. Local anesthesia is used, and the femoral artery and vein are cannulated for venoarterial bypass. The equipment is fully portable (Fig. 37-15), and the patient can be supported during pulmonary arteriography and then transported to the operating room where he can tolerate general anesthesia and thoracotomy much better while being maintained on partial cardiopulmonary bypass. Once the sternotomy is performed, the partial bypass can be converted to total bypass by insertion of a superior vena caval catheter; the pulmonary emboli are then removed through a pulmonary arteriotomy.

Open pulmonary embolectomy still carries a high mortality rate, however, and uncontrollable pulmonary hemorrhage may follow restoration of pulmonary perfusion. Consequently, an alternative approach utilizing local anesthesia has been suggested by Greenfield et al for transvenous removal of pulmonary emboli. A cup device attached to a steerable catheter is inserted in the femoral vein, and the cup is positioned adjacent to the embolus seen on arteriography. The position is verified by injection of contrast medium through the catheter (Fig. 37-16). Then syringe suction is applied to aspirate the embolus into the cup, where it is held by suction vacuum as the catheter and captured embolus are withdrawn. Clinical experience with the technique reported in 1979 in 15 patients showed that emboli could be extracted in 13 of them (87%) with an overall survival of 73%. Emboli could not be removed when

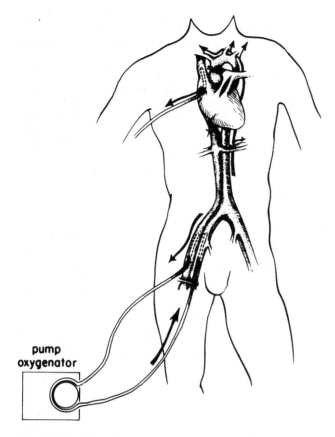

Fig. 37-15. The patient who sustains massive pulmonary embolism with shock (class IV) and fails to respond to resuscitation must be supported by partial bypass and considered for open pulmonary embolectomy. This is accomplished by cannulation of the femoral artery and vein under local anesthesia. After general anesthesia and median sternotomy, insertion of a cannula into the superior vena cava and connection to the pump permit conversion to total bypass by snare of the inferior vena cava. The main pulmonary artery is opened, and the emboli are extracted by forceps and suction.

they had been impacted for more than 72 hours or if the patient suffered cardiac arrest at the time of angiography, in which case open embolectomy was required. Placement of a Greenfield vena caval filter after removal of sufficient emboli to produce near normal hemodynamics protected the patients from recurrent embolism.

CHRONIC PULMONARY EMBOLISM AND PULMONARY HYPERTENSION

Recurrent thromboembolism may lead to progressive obliteration of the pulmonary vascular bed if the thrombi fail to undergo lysis. The resultant pulmonary hypertension produces exertional dyspnea and signs of right heart strain with cor pulmonale. With further progression of right heart overload tricuspid insufficiency may develop. This disorder may be difficult to distinguish from primary pulmonary hypertension, although the latter is more likely to be found in women under 20 years of age without a history of deep venous thrombosis. Severe pulmonary hypertension is a serious problem and usually limits the life expectancy to less than 2 years from diagnosis.

Open thrombectomy for chronic occlusion was first performed by Allison et al in 1958 and remains a possibility for improving pulmonary blood flow. Unfortunately, to be eligible for this procedure the occlusion must involve the proximal portion of the pulmonary arterial tree and the distal bed must be patent. The physiological basis for continued distal patency after proximal occlusion is bronchial arterial collateral flow. The procedure also has a significant mortality, reported at 38% by Cabrol et al in a series of 16 patients. For the majority of patients with severe pulmonary hypertension, however, the outlook is poor unless they receive maximum protection from recurrent embolism, which in our experience has required both anticoagulation therapy and vena caval filter placement.

BIBLIOGRAPHY

ABERNATHY EA, HARTSUCK JM: Postoperative pulmonary embolism. A prospective study utilizing low dose heparin. Am J Surg 128:739, 1974

Fig. 37-16. Transvenous catheter embolectomy is performed through the common femoral vein (*A*), where the cup device is inserted and steered into the pulmonary artery. Partial venoarterial bypass may be necessary for resuscitation and can be applied to the opposite femoral artery and vein during angiography and embolectomy (*B*). The cup is positioned according to the angiogram (*C*), and the proximity to the embolus is verified by injection of contrast medium (*D*).

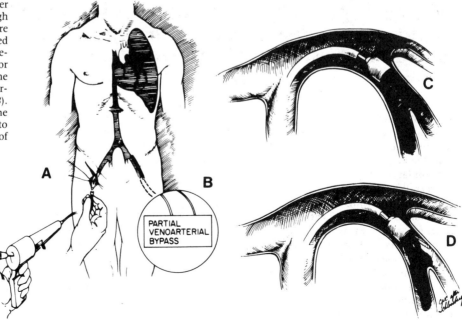

ALLISON PR, DUNHILL MS, MARSHALL R: Pulmonary embolism. Thorax 15:273, 1960

AMBRUS JS, AMBRUS CM, BOCK M et al: Clinical and experimental studies of fibrinolytic enzymes. Ann NY Acad Sci 68:97, 1957

ATKINS P, HAWKINS LA: The diagnosis of deep vein thrombosis in the legs using 125I-fibrinogen test. Lancet II:1217, 1965

BONNAR J, WALSH J: Prevention of thrombosis after pelvic surgery by British dextran 70. Lancet I:614, 1972

BRENNER O: Pathology of the vessels of the pulmonary circulation. Arch Int Med 56:1189, 1935

BROWN S, MUDLER D, BUCKBERG G: Massive pulmonary hemorrhagic infarction following revascularization of ischemic lungs. Arch Surg 108:795, 1974

CABROL C, CABROL A, ACAR J et al: Surgical correction of chronic postembolic obstruction of the pulmonary arteries. J Thorac Cardiovasc Surg 76:620, 1978

FLANC C, KAKKER VV, CLARKE MB: The detection of venous thrombosis of the legs using 125I-labelled fibrinogen. Br J Surg 55:742, 1968

GOODALL RJR, GREENFIELD LJ: Clinical correlations in the diagnosis of pulmonary embolism. Ann Surg 191:219, 1980

GREENFIELD LJ: Pulmonary embolism: Diagnosis and management. Curr Probl Surg 13:1, 1976

GREENFIELD LJ: Intraluminal techniques for vena caval interruption and pulmonary embolectomy. World J Surg 2:4559, 1978

GREENFIELD LJ: Technical considerations for insertion of vena caval filters. Surg Gynecol Obstet 148:422, 1979

GREENFIELD LJ, BRUCE TA, NICHOLS NB: Transvenous pulmonary embolectomy by catheter device. Ann Surg 174:881, 1971

GREENFIELD LJ, CRUTE SL: Retrieval of the Kimray-Greenfield^R vena caval filter. Surgery 88:719, 1980

GREENFIELD LJ, PEYTON MD, BROWN PP et al: Transvenous management of pulmonary embolic disease. Ann Surg 180:461, 1974

GREENFIELD LJ, SCHER LA, ELKINS RC: KMA-Greenfield^R filter placement for chronic pulmonary hypertension. Ann Surg 189:560, 1979

GREENFIELD LJ, ZOCCO J, WILK JD et al: Clinical experience with the Kimray-Greenfield vena caval filter. Ann Surg 185:692, 1977

HARTSUCK JM, GREENFIELD LJ: Postoperative thromboembolism: A clinical study using 125I-fibrinogen and pulmonary scanning. Arch Surg 107:733, 1973

HOBBS JT, DAVIES JWL: Detection of venous thrombosis with 131I-labelled fibrinogen in the rabbit. Lancet II:134, 1960

HUNTER JR: Observations on the Inflammation of the Intimal Layer of Veins. London, Transactions of a Society for the Improvement of Medical and Chirurgical Knowledge, 1793

INNES D, SEVITT S: Coagulation and fibrinolysis in injured patients. J Clin Pathol 17:1, 1964

JARRELL BE, MENDEZ-PICON G, SZENTPETERY S et al: Greenfield filter in renal transplant patients. Arch Surg 116:930, 1981

KAKKAR VV, CARRIGAN TP, FOSSARD DP: Prevention of fatal pulmonary embolism by low doses of heparin. Lancet II:45, 1975

KAKKAR VV, CARRIGAN TP, SPINDLER JR et al: Efficacy of low doses of heparin in prevention of deep vein thrombosis after major surgery: A double blind, randomized trial. Lancet II:101, 1972

McINTYRE KM, SASAHARA AA: Determinants of cardiovascular responses to pulmonary embolism. In Moser KM, Stein M (eds): Pulmonary Thromboembolism. Chicago, Year Book Medical Publishers, 1973

MOSER KM, STEIN M (eds): Pulmonary Thromboembolism. Chicago, Year Book Medical Publishers, 1973

SABISTON DC JR, WOLFE WG: Experimental and clinical observations on the natural history of pulmonary embolism. Ann Surg 168:1, 1968

SALZMAN EW, HARRIS WH, DESANCTIS RW: Anticoagulation for prevention of thromboembolism following fractures of the hip. N Engl J Med 275:122, 1966

SONNENBLICK EH (ed): Current problems in pulmonary embolism, I–III. Prog Cardiovasc Dis 17 (3–5): 1974–1975

STEENBURG RW, WARREN R, WILSON RE et al: A new look at pulmonary embolectomy. Surg Gynecol Obstet 107:214, 1958

STRANDNESS DE JR, SCHULTZ RD, SUMMER DA et al: Ultrasonic flow detection. A useful technique in the evaluation of peripheral vascular disease. Am J Surg 113:311, 1967

STRANDNESS DE JR, THIELE BL: Selected Topics in Venous Disorders. Pathophysiology, Diagnosis and Treatment, Mount Kisco, Futura Publishing, 1981

The Urokinase Pulmonary Embolism Trial (American Heart Association Monograph No. 39). Circulation 47 (Suppl 2) April 1973.

VIRCHOW R: Ressmelte Abhoudlungen zur wissenschaftchen Medicin. Frankfurt am Main, Meidinger, Sahn, 1856

WESTERMARK N: On the roentgen diagnosis of lung embolism. Acta Radiol 19:357, 1938

WOLFE WG, SABISTON DC JR: Pulmonary Embolism (Major Problems in Clinical Surgery, Vol XXV). Philadelphia, W B Saunders, 1980

Seshadri Raju

Varicose Veins, Thrombophlebitis, Postphlebitic Syndrome, Vena Caval Syndromes, and Superior Mesenteric Vein Occlusion

VARICOSE VEINS

PATHOPHYSIOLOGY AND GENERAL ASSESSMENT

Varicosity of the lower limb has been known since biblical times. Yet the cause of varicose veins is not known. Often, a family history can be obtained indicating a genetic predisposition for this condition. The term *varicosity* has been loosely applied to a variety of clinical conditions. This term should probably be reserved for the tortuous dilated veins distributed along the long saphenous or the short saphenous system. Not infrequently a mass of dilated veins fed by an incompetent perforator may be found in an ectopic location outside the distribution of either the short or the long saphenous system. Over the years, some confusion has occurred by applying the term *varicose ulcer* to stasis dermatitis, when in fact the ulceration is only infrequently caused by or even associated with superficial varicosities.

Patients with long saphenous varicosities should undergo the Trendelenburg test to determine the function of the saphenofemoral valve. After emptying the vein by elevation, digital pressure is applied to the saphenofemoral junction and the patient is made to stand. Rapid filling of the system from the leg region indicates perforator incompetence. When the pressure on the saphenofemoral junction is released, additional retrograde filling of the varicosities will take place in the presence of an incompetent saphenofemoral valve (this denotes a positive Trendelenburg test). The saphenofemoral valve and perforator valves may be incompetent independent of each other. Percussion of the saphenous vein in the upper thigh will frequently transmit a fluid wave to the ankle in the presence of a dilated saphenous vein obscured by thick subcutaneous fat.

The approximate location of incompetent perforator veins can be localized by the "three-tourniquet test." After the varicosities are emptied by elevation of the leg, Penrose tourniquets are applied above the ankle, below the knee, and at the lower thigh level. On the assumption of erect posture, superficial varicosities fed by incompetent perforators will rapidly fill with the tourniquets still in place.

Perthe's test is used to determine the patency of the deep venous system. With a tourniquet applied to the upper calf to occlude the superficial venous system, the patient is asked to exercise for a few minutes. Increasing pain and discomfort in the calf region is indicative of an obliterated deep venous system.

Besides the bedside examination of the patient with venous disease, a number of flow detection devices aid in the management of patients with venous disease. The discussion in this chapter centers on those devices useful in management of the patient with venous varicosities, postphlebitic syndrome, and incompetent perforators. Further discussion of deep venous thrombosis, with its diagnosis and management, can be found in the preceding section of this chapter.

NONINVASIVE INVESTIGATION OF THE VENOUS SYSTEM

Noninvasive investigation of the venous system is gaining steadily in importance. The venous Doppler, impedance plethysmography (Fig. 37-17), and photoplethysmography all give indirect data regarding venous flow and venous obstruction. By their use, invasive studies may be avoided.

INVASIVE MEANS OF ASSESSING VENOUS COMPETENCE

AMBULATORY VENOUS PRESSURE MEASUREMENTS

With the help of a minitransducer affixed to the foot, the venous pressure in a dorsal vein of the foot may be measured by venipuncture. The resting level is usually between 75 and 90 mm Hg. The patient is asked to raise his heel off the floor, exercising the calf muscle, several times. Within a few seconds, the venous pressure should fall to 40% to

Fig. 37-17. Impedance plethysmography tracings in an abnormal limb (deep venous thrombosis) and a normal limb. Nomograms are available to determine whether venous outflow in a given limb falls within the normal range.

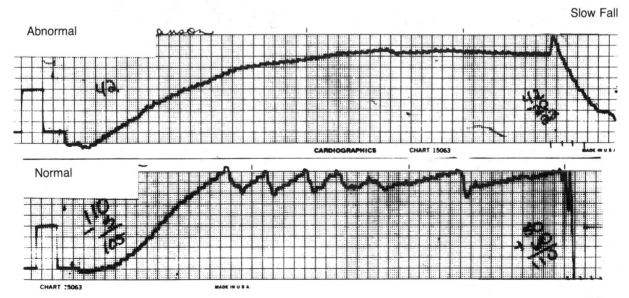

Slow Fall

Abnormal

Normal

Rapid Fall

50% of the original value. A less substantial reduction is considered to represent ambulatory venous hypertension. In some patients with severe deep venous obstruction, postexercise venous levels may in fact be higher than the resting level, resulting in venous claudication and discomfort. In most patients, however, abnormal venous dynamics are represented by a return of the postexercise venous pressure level back to the resting level in less than 20 seconds. This is usually due to rapid retrograde reflux through incompetent valves in the deep venous system.

ASCENDING VENOGRAPHY

Contrast venography by introduction of dye into a dorsal foot vein to delineate the deep venous system is routinely practiced in all major medical centers. A tourniquet lightly applied above the ankle is used to direct the contrast material into the deep venous system by occluding the superficial veins. Contrast ascending venography is usually resorted to in order to determine the patency of the deep venous system and to demonstrate the extent and location of suspected venous thrombi. When this technique is properly performed, the number and location of perforator veins can also be detected.

DESCENDING VENOGRAPHY

Descending venography has been popularized recently by Kistner to demonstrate the extent of deep venous reflux and to ascertain the location of venous valves. A bolus of contrast material is placed in the iliac veins with the patient in a semirecumbent position. With intact venous valves, almost all contrast material usually flows in a cephalad direction (Fig. 37-18). When valve incompetence is present, however, a variable amount of dye will reflux in a retrograde direction. In patients with severe reflux disease, almost all the dye placed in the iliac vein will be seen to reflux down as far as the popliteal veins. With the Valsalva maneuver, the amount of refluxing dye is considerably increased.

SIGNS AND SYMPTOMS OF VARICOSE VEINS

The great majority of patients, especially women in the younger age-group, approach the physician with complaints of varicosities primarily from a cosmetic viewpoint. True varicosities, if present, are invariably asymptomatic in this group of patients. In some patients with long-standing and extensive varicosities, symptoms such as ankle swelling and vague lower limb pain on prolonged standing or walking may be described. Relief of these symptoms on elevation is a clue to their venous origin. It is not clear, however, whether ankle swelling and venous pain are caused by pure superficial varicosities or by associated deep venous insufficiency. In some patients, spontaneous thrombosis of some segments of varicosities may occur, resulting in painful subcutaneous nodules that gradually disappear over a period of weeks or months. Spontaneous pinpoint ulceration into varicose legs, resulting in bleeding, also occurs.

DIAGNOSIS AND TREATMENT

Young patients with mild to moderate varicosities who approach physicians primarily for reassurance seldom require surgical therapy. However, surgery should not be withheld from otherwise asymptomatic patients who have an overwhelming concern for the cosmetic aspects of varicose veins, provided complete surgical extirpation appears

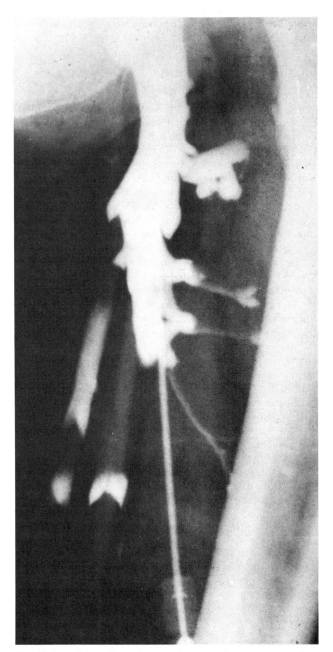

Fig. 37-18.   Descending venogram demonstrating competent valves. The contrast has outlined valves in the femoral and saphenous veins.

possible. Symptomatic patients with varicose veins, who suffer from complications of superficial phlebitis, bleeding, swelling, and venous-type pain, should be offered surgical therapy. A careful physical examination should be carried out in this group of patients, followed by ascending venography, primarily to demonstrate a patent deep venous system. When varicosities are secondary to a compromised deep venous system, surgical treatment is contraindicated.

OPERATIONS FOR VENOUS VARICOSITIES

The traditional surgical approach for treatment of varicose veins has always focused on the saphenofemoral junction, which is extirpated or ligated in some fashion. It is important to perform a high ligation of the saphenous vein to prevent recurrence (Fig. 37-19). The focus on the saphenofemoral

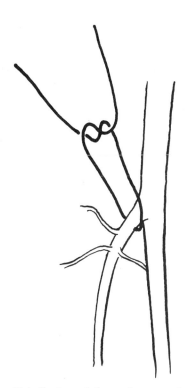

Fig. 37-19. High ligation of the saphenous vein. The ligature should be placed proximal to the vein's highest tributaries.

junction has been fostered by the conviction that incompetence of the saphenofemoral valve is a major etiologic mechanism in the cause of varicose veins. The procedure of long saphenous vein stripping popularized by Mayo is now invariably used in conjunction with ligation and division of the saphenofemoral junction. Such perforators as may drain into the long saphenous vein are sheared off by the stripping procedure; any others draining into the posterior arch vein or elsewhere are ignored, owing to the conviction that perforator incompetence is secondary to perforator dilatation or increased retrograde flow through the saphenofemoral junction. In this view, obliteration of the saphenofemoral valve will ultimately result in resolution of perforator incompetence by removing the primary causative mechanism. A group led by Linton in this country and Cockett in England have placed the primary focus on the perforator veins. According to these authors, incompetent perforator veins initiate the vicious cycle of varicose dilatation of the long saphenous vein, which thereby secondarily affects the competence of the saphenofemoral valve by dilatation. Subcutaneous or subfascial ligation of the perforator veins is used as a primary surgical procedure for varicosities and is often combined with stripping of the long saphenous vein. It should be stressed that there have been few experimental or hemodynamic studies available to support either of these two views. In reality, both these theories subscribe to venous valve incompetence in an isolated anatomic location to explain what is probably an extensive and uniformly distributed defect in the entire venous system. Varicosities along the short saphenous system are primarily treated with ligation of the saphenopopliteal vein junction. The segment of short saphenous vein is seldom stripped, as neural complications due to traction on the accompanying sural nerve frequently result from this procedure. Groups of varicosities in ectopic loca-

tions can safely be excised *en masse*, with ligation of the underlying perforator vein. Spider varicosities may be treated with sclerotherapy.

Saphenous Vein Stripping

Under general anesthesia, the patient is placed supine and the lower limb is prepared, including the lower part of the abdomen. A transverse groin incision is made approximately three fingerbreadths outwards and three fingerbreadths below the pubic tubercle. The saphenous vein is usually identified by following one of the subcutaneous tributaries. When difficulties are encountered in identification of the vein, especially in obese patients, the femoral vein may be exposed for a length of 2 inches to help identify the saphenofemoral junction. Once the saphenofemoral junction is identified, it is important to dissect out and ligate the tributaries of the saphenous vein of this location (see Fig. 37-19). The saphenofemoral junction is suture ligated flush with the femoral vein, and the saphenous vein is divided free.

A small transverse incision is made anterior to the medial malleolus after distal ligation division, and a Myers stripper is passed up the vein easily and allowed to exit through the upper end of the vein in the groin incision. Intermediate incisions may be necessary to guide the stripper or separately to ligate prominent perforator veins. For all incisions made below the knee, it is important to be cognizant of the adjoining saphenous nerve, since saphenous neuralgia is a well-recognized complication of this surgical procedure. To avoid injury to the saphenous nerve, a small "acorn," rather than a large one, is attached to the stripper. To avoid traction on the nerve, some surgeons prefer to strip the vein up rather than down. Once the stripping is completed, compression is applied to the saphenous vein tract for a few minutes before closure of the wound. A firm Ace bandage is applied from the toe to the groin to secure hemostasis and to provide elastic support in the immediate postoperative period. With an intact elastic support, ambulation may be started the next day. Prolonged elastic support is usually advisable, switching from bandage to a stocking type of support once the incisions are well healed.

The short saphenous vein is identified through a transverse incision in the popliteal fossa. The saphenopopliteal junction should be ligated flush with the popliteal vein and divided. Stripping of the short saphenous vein is usually not advocated because of the danger of injury to the adjoining sural nerve.

Subfascial Ligation of Perforators (Modified Linton's Procedure)

While some authors have advocated subfascial ligation of perforators as a primary procedure, the general practice is to reserve this rather extensive operation for recurrent varicosities or for prominent perforator incompetence that persists after saphenous vein stripping. In selected cases of stasis ulceration secondary to the postphlebitic syndrome, this procedure (see later in this chapter) may be of value in providing symptomatic relief of the recalcitrant nonhealing ulcer.

A long incision, 1.5 cm posterior to the medial border of the tibia, is preferred. The incision extends from the medial malleolus to the junction of the upper and middle thirds of the leg. The deep fascia is split along the entire incision, and the underlying musculature is separated from the deep aspect of the fascia by a combination of blunt and sharp dissection. Large perforator connections traversing the space are palpated, ligated, and divided. Smaller perforators may be torn digitally and hemostasis secured by firm compression for a few minutes. After all perforators are ligated subfascially, hemostasis is secured by applying a firm Ace bandage to the leg. The fascia is usually left open to accommodate the postoperative swelling that occurs. Metal staples or other nonreactive skin closure should be used as this incision usually heals slowly and sutures may have to be retained for weeks. Continued postoperative elastic support is mandatory.

SCLEROTHERAPY

Obliteration of varicose veins by injecting sclerosing material intraluminally is popular in some vein clinics in Europe, but this method is not widely used in the United States. Injection sclerotherapy is usually reserved for obliterating small segments of veins, usually perforators in the lower leg. Multiple injections at sequential visits are often necessary, with sodium tetradecyl sulfate injected intraluminally into varicosities with a fine hypodermic needle. The leg should be elevated, and the varicosities emptied before injection. Soon after injection, a compression dressing is applied to leave the injected vein collapsed. Recurrences are common with this technique.

CONDITIONS ASSOCIATED WITH VARICOSE VEINS

Patients with congenital arteriovenous fistulas and more extensive arteriovenous malformations frequently present with varicose veins. Extensive varicosities presenting at an unusually young age (Klippel-Trenaunay syndrome) are often due to congenital arteriovenous malformations. The arteriovenous connections may be limited or, more commonly, extensive, involving skin, subcutaneous tissue, muscle, and bone. A bruit is not usually present, since the fistulas are small. An arteriogram frequently reveals early opacification of the venous system without direct visualization of the fistula itself. Unless the arteriovenous connections are limited in number and can be identified and ligated, surgical treatment is usually ineffective and unjustified. Disproportionate limb growth may be present, which may require orthopaedic procedures to improve gait.

Patients with a traumatic arteriovenous fistula will also present with prominent superficial veins, which may be mistaken for varicosities. On careful examination, a bruit can almost always be heard over the fistula, and stasis ulceration may be present due to chronic venous hypertension. Ligation of the arteriovenous fistula in this case is curative.

THROMBOPHLEBITIS

SUPERFICIAL

Superficial thrombophlebitis is a relatively common condition that develops secondary to a variety of minor insults to the superficial veins. It is common in hospital practice following venipuncture or infusion of irritant solutions such as for chemotherapy. Minor trauma or adjoining infection predisposes to it. The clinical presentation is a "knot" with variable pain and tenderness. Management consists in ruling out associated deep venous thrombosis and assurance to allay patient anxiety. When pain is severe, analgesics and, occasionally, anti-inflammatory agents (indomethacin) may be of value. Some patients seem to benefit from warm compresses. When varicose veins are present, elastic support is advised. Limb rest is unnecessary and, in fact, may lead to progression of the thrombotic process from stasis.

MIGRATORY

Recurrent superficial thrombophlebitis occurring in different parts of the limb successively has been associated with neoplastic conditions and certain vasospastic disorders, such as Buerger's disease. The condition, however, is a rare one; more commonly, deep venous thrombosis of the ileofemoral system is associated with malignant conditions, due to hypercoagulability of blood. For this reason, spontaneous development of ileofemoral thrombosis in the cancer age-group should lead to a thorough examination of the patient with this possibility in mind.

SEPTIC

For the most part, deep venous thrombosis is noninfective in origin; however, an infective thrombophlebitis develops occasionally secondary to an infected venipuncture site or other source of infection in the extremity. This type of phlebitis is being described more and more in the patient population that makes a habit of "mainlining" drugs by venipuncture. The septic thrombophlebitis that results may involve both the superficial and the deep venous system. Fluctuant abscesslike areas may develop over the course of the vein, and elsewhere the vein may present as thrombotic cords. The patient runs a septic course with high fever, chills, and a positive blood culture. Septic pulmonary emboli with cavitating lesions of the lung may eventually develop. Persistence of a septic course despite adequate eradication of the primary focus of infection in the extremity should arouse the suspicion of septic thrombophlebitis. Purulent material can often be expressed along with liquifying thrombus from a vein adjacent to the septic focus in such instances. Along with adequate antibiotic therapy, excision of an extensive segment of the involved vein may be necessary to control the infective process. Abscesses along the course of the vein must be drained.

POSTPHLEBITIC SYNDROME

Every major hospital has a complement of patients with postphlebitic syndrome. Patients fall into two broad categories, those with chronic limb pain and those with stasis ulceration. There is considerable overlap of symptomatology, with both ulceration and pain occurring in some patients. The pain described by patients with this syndrome is often vague, appearing to intensify with prolonged standing or work. Some patients admit to relief of pain with elevation of the limb, while in others the pain is persistent. In one group of patients, the pain appears to occur at night, forcing the patients to constantly move the limb to achieve a comfortable position (restless leg syndrome). Patients with stasis ulceration present with an indolent ulcer, usually on the medial portion of the leg above the malleolus. Ectopic locations do occur. The ulcer is characteristically shallow, seldom penetrating the deep fascia. The superficial scars where previous ulcers have healed may be evident. There is often brawny induration of the lower limb due to chronic edema and discoloration of skin due to intradermal hemorrhage and hemosiderin deposits.

The etiology of postphlebitic syndrome is uncertain. It is not uncommon to have patients undergo vein stripping operations, even though varicosities are not often a prominent feature. In this class of patients, there is almost always underlying deep venous insufficiency which is etiologically significant. The deep venous insufficiency may be obstructive or due to reflux from destruction of venous valves.

DIAGNOSIS

Since there has been considerable recanalization of the previously thrombosed venous system, impedance plethysmography is usually within normal limits. Doppler venous examination reveals considerable reflux. There is ambulatory venous hypertension, with postexercise venous pressures at the ankle level remaining abnormally high. Return of postexercise venous pressure to resting level occurs very rapidly due to reflux. Ascending venography usually reveals a valveless deep venous system with recanalization and abnormally large venous collaterals, which are also usually valveless (Fig. 37-20). Multiple channels may be seen along the course of the femoral-popliteal veins as a result of inadequate recanalization. Descending venography will reveal reflux of contrast injected into the femoral vein to at least the popliteal vein and often lower.

TREATMENT

Currently, there is no accepted surgical treatment of postphlebitic syndrome; patients are treated conservatively, with elevation of the limb when possible, elastic support, and generalized foot care. Anticoagulation should be pursued only if there is evidence of recent fresh or recurrent venous thrombosis. Change of occupation to facilitate elevation of the limb and reduce the period of standing may be of help.

Stasis ulcers are treated by rest, elevation of the foot, and skin grafting in selected instances. Most patients can be treated in an ambulatory fashion with medicated gelatinized pressure dressings (Unna boot). An exciting new area of research into the management of deep venous insufficiency has been described with the use of direct repair of venous valves or venous valve interposition (see the first section of this chapter).

VENA CAVAL SYNDROMES

SUPERIOR VENA CAVA

Acute superior vena caval syndrome is most often due to a malignant neoplasm compressing the structure in the superior mediastinum. Bronchogenic carcinoma of the right upper lobe is the most common malignancy encountered. Other types, such as lymphosarcoma, Hodgkin's disease, and thymic and thyroid neoplasms, may also result in superior vena caval compression. In a small group of patients (approximately 10%), benign lesions such as aortic aneurysms, thyroid goiters, or mediastinal benign cysts may result in superior vena caval syndrome. Mediastinal fibrosis, often secondary to mediastinal histoplasmosis infection, is also a well-recognized cause of this obstruction.

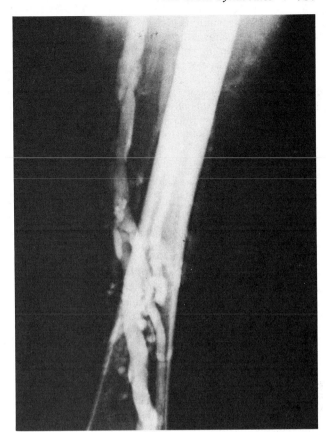

Fig. 37-20. Ascending venogram in the postphlebitic syndrome. The vein is irregular due to recanalization with multiple channels. Valves are absent. Several abnormal tributaries have developed since thrombosis.

CLINICAL FEATURES

Patients with acute superior vena caval syndrome present with sudden onset of swelling localized to the head and neck, upper portion of the trunk, and arms. Their eyelids are puffy, and they frequently tear uncontrollably. Markedly dilated veins tense with elevated venous pressure may be visible prior to the onset of edema. The face and upper portion of the trunk assume a characteristic dusky and cyanotic appearance. Patients may develop voice change and breathing difficulty due to edema of the larynx and the tracheobronchial tree.

Chronic superior vena caval syndrome is more insidious in onset, and there may be only a slight amount of edema or none at all. Dilated veins in the neck and prominent venous collaterals along the pectoral folds coursing down the thorax are, however, visible.

MANAGEMENT

Every effort should be made to reach a diagnosis of the underlying pathology, because some benign clinical conditions present with superior vena caval syndrome as outlined above. This small group of patients may achieve long-lasting relief by excision of the underlying benign lesion. The possibility of malignant origin should be confirmed by needle biopsy or supraclavicular node biopsy if possible. In many instances, diagnostic maneuvers cannot be used and the presumptive diagnosis of malignancy must be assumed; intravenous chemotherapy or mediastinal irradiation is then given on an emergency basis. This is especially true in patients who present with acute respiratory disease secondary to vena caval syndrome. Usually with emergency treatment as outlined above, there is dramatic resolution of the compression syndrome within 48 to 72 hours.

Bronchogenic carcinoma resulting in superior vena caval obstruction is invariably inoperable for cure. Attempts to bypass the obstructed superior vena cava have been reported in the literature, and the most successful of these have been with a modified widened-diameter reconstructed saphenous vein connecting the right atrium to the innominate vein. Short-term results and patency rate have been good, but long-term follow-up is available only in a small number of patients.

INFERIOR VENA CAVA

Occlusion of the infrarenal vena cava is surprisingly well tolerated. Occlusion of the suprarenal inferior vena cava may occur due to thrombosis or compression by tumor masses in the retroperitoneum. Hypernephroma may actually invade the vena cava and extend intraluminally to the right atrium. Primary sarcoma of the inferior vena cava is a rare but well-recognized entity that may compress the vena cava in this location. Likewise, benign causes of inferior vena caval compression include retroperitoneal fibrosis, benign tumors, and cysts of the caudate lobe of the liver. The Budd-Chiari syndrome, sometimes caused by congenital membranous occlusion of the suprahepatic inferior vena cava, may also cause inferior vena caval syndrome. Patients with inferior vena caval compression syndrome develop collaterals along the side of the trunk in which the flow can be demonstrated to be cephalad. Periumbilical collaterals with a similar type of flow direction can be detected in these persons. When renal vein drainage is affected, a nephrotic type of syndrome, with hematuria, proteinuria, and hypertension, may be present. The site and nature of caval compression can usually be demonstrated by a contrast study. While extrinsic compression by tumor masses may sometimes be relieved by resection, the results of treatment of inferior vena caval syndrome continue to be disappointing.

SUPERIOR MESENTERIC VEIN OCCLUSION

Chronic superior mesenteric vein occlusion may occur in association with chronic volvulus, congenital bands, or malrotation of the gut and as a part of the syndrome of cavernous transformation of the portal vein. Acute superior mesenteric vein occlusion occurs without any obvious cause in the great majority of instances. It may occur with administration of oral contraceptives or with polycythemia, carcinomatosis, or reduced fibrinolytic activity resulting in a hypercoagulable state. Other factors believed to be impli-

cated include trauma; venous stasis secondary to cirrhosis, heart failure, or dehydration; previous irradiation; and intra-abdominal sepsis.

CLINICAL FEATURES

Acute thrombosis of the superior mesenteric vein characteristically has an insidious onset with symptoms that may have persisted for days or weeks before the patient seeks medical consultation. Initially, symptoms are vague; later, unremitting abdominal pain is characteristic of the condition. Objective physical findings may be disproportionately mild despite severity of the pain. Rebound tenderness may not be present during the early stages, and roentgenographic findings are often nonspecific. Occasionally, submucosal hemorrhage may present as "thumbprinting" or pseudo-polyposis on x-ray contrast study. Bloody diarrhea and malabsorption may present in some patients.

TREATMENT

Correct preoperative diagnosis is rare, and exploratory laparotomy is invariably undertaken for diagnosis. When gangrenous bowel is encountered, it should be resected. An adequate margin of normal mesentery and bowel should also be resected. Continued propagation of thrombus and recurrence of thrombosis have been documented, and this may be prevented by using anticoagulation with heparin. Venous thrombectomy is usually not feasible; however, if the thrombus is fresh, this may be attempted with concomitant removal of necrotic gut. In instances of extensive resection in which the viability of remaining bowel is in doubt, a second-look operation at 24 hours may be desirable. In some instances, surgeons resort to a temporary double-barreled enterostomy, which allows inspection of the enteric mucosa for adequacy of bowel perfusion. Conservatively treated acute superior mesenteric vein thrombosis is fatal in nearly 100% of the cases. The mortality rate following surgical treatment ranges from 11% to 21%.

BIBLIOGRAPHY

BAUER G: The etiology of leg ulcers and their treatment by resection of the popliteal vein. J Int Chir 8:937, 1948

BERGAN JJ, YAO JST (eds): Venous Problems. Chicago, Year Book Medical Publishers, 1978

HOBBS JT: The Treatment of Venous Disorders. Philadelphia, J B Lippincott, 1977

KAKKAR VV, CORRIGAN TP: Detection of deep vein thrombosis: Survey and current status. Prog Cardiovasc Dis 17:207, 1974

KISTNER RL: Surgical repair of the incompetent femoral vein valve. Arch Surg 110:1336, 1975

NAITOVE A, WEISMANN RE: Primary mesenteric venous thrombosis. Ann Surg 161:516, 1965

STRANDNESS DE JR, THIELD BL: Selected Topics in Venous Disorders. Mount Kisco, NY, Futura Publishing, 1981

Carlos M. Chavez

Disorders of the Lymphatic System

The first anatomic recognition of lymphatic structures is credited to Peiresc, who in 1628 described the presence of lacteal ducts in the human body. This was followed by the first illustration of the human lymphatic vessels by Vesling. In 1647, Jean Pecquet identified the ductus thoracicus in the dog and described what later was called the cisterna chyli. These same structures were later described by Jan van Horne in the human body in 1652. It was, however, Cruikshank and Mascagni who provided the most complete description of the lymphatic system and detailed the presence and distribution of the lymph nodes, which they called lymphatic or round glands (Fig. 37-21).

Radiologic demonstration of the lymphatic vessels and lymph nodes was not practical until 1955, when Kinmonth of England described a rather simple method for visualization of the lymphatic vessels and lymph nodes by direct injection of contrast medium into a peripheral lymphatic vessel. Several modifications of this procedure were subsequently introduced using oily contrast media, which allowed clearer visualization and follow-up of the progression of the opaque material through the lymphatic system.

Despite the tremendous progress made in the study of the arterial and venous systems, the lymphatic system has remained neglected apart from the great progress made in the radiologic study of the lymphatics. Although lymphatic transport of hormones and other metabolites is well known, the significance of this phenomenon is not well understood. Under normal conditions, the lymphatic system transports to the bloodstream the large molecules that leak from the blood as well as some of the other substances secreted by various body tissues. The composition of the lymph varies according to the organs or tissues with which the lymphatics are connected, but in general, the basic composition of lymph is similar to that of venous plasma. The transfer of

material and fluid from the interstitial spaces or tissues to the lymphatic vessels is determined by the amount of fluid in the tissues, the concentration of the molecules, and the pressure within the interstitial space. The migration of the molecules from within the lymphatic vessels to the outside varies in turn with the size of the molecule. Under normal conditions only a very small number of larger or medium-sized particles leave the lymphatic vessels. However, under abnormal conditions, such as an increase in resistance to the lymph flow or injury to the capillary wall, such particles may leave and accumulate in the interstitial space, impairing the drainage of fluid. Among the factors affecting the flow of lymph from the interstitial space to the capillary are variations in the composition of the interstitial fluid, active contraction of the muscles, changes in pressure around the lymphatic vessels that affect the propulsion of the lymph, and changes in pressure of the interstitial tissues as a result of alterations in venous drainage. Intrathoracic and intra-abdominal pressures have also been shown to contribute to variations in the flow of lymph.

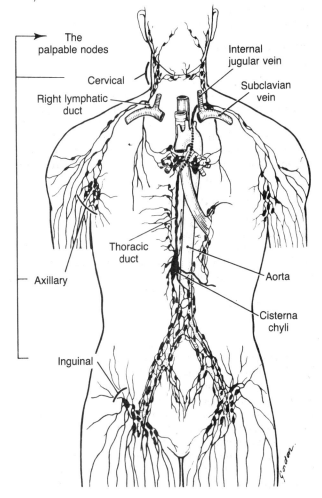

Fig. 37-21. Schematic drawing of lymphatic channels. (Basmajian JV: Primary Anatomy, 7th ed. Baltimore, Williams & Wilkins, 1976)

CAUSES OF LYMPHATIC DISEASE

Because of the complicated and not well-defined nature of the diseases affecting the lymphatic system, it is difficult to establish clear-cut distinctions for diseases affecting the lymphatic system that can be considered within the scope of surgical treatment. However, most conditions that can be managed by surgical means fall into three categories.

CONGENITAL ABNORMALITIES

Congenital diseases can be the result of hypoplasia or dysplasia of any of the structures that form part of the lymphatic system. In this group are primary or idiopathic lymphedema that most frequently affects the extremities and less commonly the visceral areas. Involvement of the head and neck has been described but is found only rarely. Other pathologic conditions include cavernous lymphangiomas, congenital lymphatic cysts, and possibly other lymphatic abnormalities responsible for protein-losing gastroenteropathy.

TUMORS

Benign and malignant tumors involve the lymph nodes as well as the lymphatic vessels. These can occur as primary neoplasms or as part of tumor spread from adjacent areas. In certain instances, isolated lymphatic tumors are amenable to surgical excision, whether they involve the lymph nodes or the lymphatic vessels. We will review in more detail the cystic lesions of the lymphatic system that fall into the surgeon's domain when they occur in isolation.

CYSTIC HYGROMA

Fluid-filled cystic lesions are found in many locations, but by and large they occur most frequently in the neck (80% to 90%) and are present at birth, demonstrating a slow growth rate. They are usually asymptomatic but represent a cosmetic and psychological problem to the child. The lesion consists of large cavities lined with endothelial cells; neurovascular elements and lymphatic tissue are present in the trabeculae of the cyst. Surgical excision is the treatment of choice, and the recurrence rate is very low.

CAVERNOUS LYMPHANGIOMA

Cavernous lymphangiomas are considered a variant of cystic hygromas and are composed of multiple endothelium-lined cavities surrounded by connective tissue. The cavities contain a clear fluid similar to lymph, although sometimes blood cells and other debris are present. These lesions may be superficial or deep and are often found in the head and neck, axilla, and groin.

TRAUMA

Blunt or penetrating trauma involving the large collecting lymphatic ducts as well as iatrogenic injuries to these vessels are not at all uncommon. They are in many instances associated with development of pseudocysts (lymphocysts), fistulas (internal or external), and accumulation of lymph in the interstitital tissues (lymphedema) or body cavities such as the pleura, peritoneum, and pericardium. The seriousness of the resultant trauma depends upon the extensiveness of the injury, the size of the ruptured vessel, and the presence of obstruction beyond the injured area.

POST-TRAUMATIC LYMPHATIC CYSTS

Sometimes called lymphocysts, post-traumatic lymphatic cysts are in reality pseudocysts and are formed by traumatic rupture of the lymphatic vessels (usually the larger collecting vessels) with extravasation of the lymph into the interstitial tissues. The interstitial tissues will form a wall around the accumulated lymph, creating a cystic cavity. Rarely, these cysts may attain large proportions and produce pressure symptoms. The injury can be either blunt or penetrating or may follow certain surgical procedures, particularly those involving extensive dissections near or through the lymphatic structures. The occurrence of these lymphocysts following radical node dissections is well recognized.

DISORDERS INVOLVING THE THORACIC DUCT

The thoracic duct is the largest lymphatic vessel in the body and originates from the confluence of the collecting lymphatic vessels of the abdomen and the lower extremities. These collectors empty into a large sac, the cisterna chyli (Pecquet), and the thoracic duct originates from this sac. From this point, the duct proceeds toward the chest, traversing the diaphragm through the aortic hiatus and thence through the posterior mediastinum between the aorta and the azygos vein. Opposite the fifth thoracic vertebra the duct crosses to the left side of the thoracic cavity to enter the superior mediastinum and ascends dorsal to the aortic arch, emptying into the subclavian vein at the confluence with the left internal jugular vein. The thoracic duct varies in length from 35 cm to 40 cm with a diameter of between 3 mm and 5 mm before it empties into the subclavian vein.

The right lymphatic duct, which measures approximately 1.25 cm in length, receives the lymph from the right side of the head and neck, right upper extremity, right side of the thorax, right lung, right side of the heart, and part of the liver. This structure courses along the medial border of the scalenus anticus in the neck, emptying into the right subclavian vein at the level of its junction with the right internal jugular vein.

By far the most common pathologic conditions associated with the thoracic duct are obstruction and perforation.

TRAUMATIC LESIONS OF THE THORACIC DUCT AND THORACIC DUCT FISTULA

Rupture or laceration of the thoracic duct will result in extravasation of large amounts of lymphatic fluid. This may occur in the abdomen or retroperitoneal space but is most frequently found within the thoracic cavity. Less commonly, extravasation of lymph has been found inside the pericardium as part of a traumatic, neoplastic, or inflammatory process. Extravasation or fistula formation in the neck usually follows operations in this region. Here, treatment is easily accomplished by identification and suture of the point of leakage of the thoracic duct, if in fact it has not closed spontaneously in a few days, perhaps hastened by application of a pressure dressing.

LACERATION OR PERFORATION OF THE THORACIC DUCT WITHIN THE CHEST CAVITY (Fig. 37-22)

Although some patients may develop extravasation of lymph within the chest or pericardium because of neoplastic or inflammatory infiltration of the thoracic duct or any of its major branches, for the most part this problem develops following trauma to the thoracic duct. By far the most common nontraumatic lesion associated with lymph extravasation within the chest is a mediastinal lymphoma. With the successful control of tuberculosis in this country, the incidence of chylothorax secondary to this type of infection has been drastically reduced.

CHYLOTHORAX

In a recent review of spontaneous, postoperative, and traumatic chylothorax, Servelle described 13 cases of spontaneous chylothorax in youngsters. In these cases, malformations of the lymphatic vessels were found inside the chest, and the extravasation of lymph was not necessarily related to the rupture of the thoracic duct. In most instances the point of leakage was found in the area of abnormal lymphatic vessels of the lung or diaphragmatic pleura. The treatment of choice was suture ligation of the area of leakage. No attempt was made to ligate the thoracic duct for the control of lymph drainage. Abnormalities of the thoracic duct in the upper chest or neck have also been described as determining factors in the occurrence of spontaneous chylothorax in adults.

Chylothorax has been found following a variety of intrathoracic operations. However, laceration of lymphatic structures with subsequent development of chylothorax has also been described in operations of the neck. We have seen this in one instance following a carotid–subclavian bypass operation on the left side. Chylothorax has been described following cardiovascular surgery, esophageal operations, pleuropulmonary surgery, mediastinal surgery, and operations involving the diaphragm. Chylous effusion may result from a variety of cardiac operations as well as from those involving the great vessels such as coarctation of the aorta, patent ductus arteriosus, and aneurysms of the aortic arch and descending aorta. It has been estimated that approximately 0.5% of patients having operations for cardiovascular disease develop chylothorax in the postoperative period. The proximity of the thoracic duct to the cardiovascular structures, particularly on the left side, makes this vessel susceptible to surgical injuries. In the past most of these cases were treated by ligation of the duct through a formal thoracotomy. The point of leakage inside the chest can be identified readily by injection of a supravital dye into the diaphragm or esophagus. The blue dye will easily be seen flowing through the area of the thoracic duct injury. External drainage with a pericardial tube has been sufficient in many cases to decompress the pericardial sac with no further accumulation of lymph drainage. In recent reports, treatment of this complication by talc suspension introduced through a thoracostomy tube has been used successfully to prevent a second thoracotomy.

The most common operations associated with chylothorax are thoracoplasty, lobectomy, and pneumonectomy. Resections of lung tumors or other lesions with firm adhesions to the mediastinum and to the lower part of the chest have been the most likely procedures associated with injuries of the thoracic duct. In one of our cases, a mycotic lesion of the right lower lobe was found firmly attached to the lower esophagus. Following lobectomy, this patient developed a chylothorax on the right side that required subsequent surgical ligation of the thoracic duct at this point. Resection of mediastinal tumors has also been associated with development of chylothorax. Operations for intrathoracic goiters, cervicomediastinal lymphangiomas, and malignant tumors of the lung with mediastinal node metastasis are commonly associated with chylothorax in connection with mediastinal lesions.

Because of the close proximity of the thoracic duct to the base of the diaphragm, operations at this level requiring extensive dissection are sometimes followed by extravasation of chyle into the pleural space in the postoperative period.

Extensive neck operations may be followed in some cases by development of postoperative chylothorax. The number of cases reported, which amount to no more than a dozen, probably does not reflect the true incidence of this complication. As stated before, we have seen this complication without the development of pneumothorax in a patient who had a vascular operation in the neck. Chylothorax has also been found following operations on the sympathetic nerve system, particularly those performed through an open thoracotomy.

The treatment of chylothorax varies with the etiologic factor. For spontaneous chylothorax, a direct approach is preferable because the exact point of rupture is not known preoperatively. Because most of these cases are associated with congenital malformations of the lymphatic vessels, these vessels can be resected at the time of thoracotomy, but if the malformation is diffuse, suture ligation of the leaking point will be all that is necessary. As recommended by Servelle, no attempt should be made to identify and ligate the thoracic duct because in most cases of rupture of a lymphatic malformation the malformation is supplied by collateral lymphatic vessels.

Penetrating, blunt, and surgical injuries of the thoracic duct can be treated by infusion of talc as recommended by Adler; in cases of malignant lesions such as lymphomas or for patients in poor general condition, the use of an elemental diet and medium-chain triglyceride administration will markedly reduce the volume of chyle leak and in some cases will stop the drainage of lymph. This will be a temporizing measure until the patient is in better condition for a thoracotomy or until radiotherapy or chemotherapy becomes effective and seals the area of lymphatic involvement. Tube thoracostomy will be required to drain the accumulated fluid and allow reexpansion of the collapsed lung. When a traumatic injury has been documented, thoracotomy is the preferred approach because it will permit exploration of the chest for other injuries at the same time that the thoracic duct is ligated. Surgical exploration and ligature of the thoracic duct is by far the most common procedure in the treatment of chylothorax secondary to rupture of the thoracic duct.

CHYLOPERICARDIUM

Chylopericardium is found in an isolated form or associated with other lymphatic effusions, the most common of which is chylothorax. Isolated chylopericardium can be associated with malignant tumors such as lymphoma or may follow cardiovascular surgical procedures. However, this condition can also occur spontaneously without apparent etiology. In this instance, abnormal lymphatic structures may be responsible for the problem as they are in idiopathic chylothorax. Lymphatic abnormalities were found in a case described by us in which a lymphogram was performed. This was a 27-year-old man with isolated chylopericardium in whom no history of trauma, infection, or neoplasm was found.

Congenital lymphatic abnormalities, lymphangiomatous

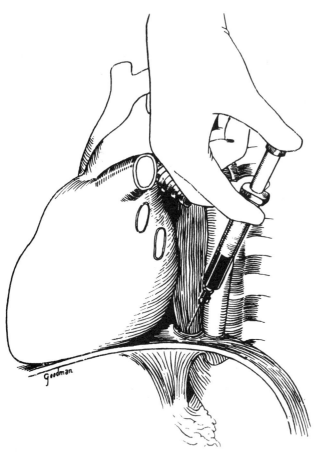

Fig. 37-22. Injection of blue dye into wall of the lower esophagus at left thoracotomy. The dye will flow retrograde, to enter the thoracic duct below the diaphragm and then ascend, revealing the site of the thoracic duct fistula leakage in the thorax. The duct is then simply ligated above and below the fistula. (Hardy JD, Walker GR Jr, DeGuzman VC: Thoracic duct fistula in infant; blue dye localization and operative closure. JAMA 182:187, 1962)

and nonlymphatic tumors, infection, blunt or penetrating trauma, and radiation injuries are listed as some of the causes of chylopericardium. A variety of cardiac operations associated with a chylopericardium have been described. The ages of the patients have varied from a few months to adults. Operations for both congenital anomalies and acquired cardiac diseases were performed in these patients. Two patients in whom chylopericardium was complicated by acute cardiac tamponade after cardiovascular surgery were reported; in one of these, the diagnosis was made promptly and the effusion was drained by tube pericardiostomy. The second patient, in whom the diagnosis was delayed, died despite an urgent thoracotomy.

In the large majority of patients, external drainage controlled the chyle extravasation and in others the institution of a diet with medium-chain triglycerides reduced or eliminated the pericardial effusion. Only in one exceptional case were thoracotomy and ligation of the thoracic duct necessary after failure of external drainage to control the chylous effusion.

OTHER LYMPHATIC PROBLEMS

Chyle may extravasate to the various body cavities or spaces as well as to the outside of the body. Congenital malformation of the lymphatic vessels, malignant tumors, and

other inflammatory conditions are determining factors in the origin and persistence of lymph extravasation. Superimposed trauma with extensive laceration or surgical dissection in otherwise normal territory can lead to formation of lymphatic or chylous fistulas with subsequent accumulation of lymph in the body cavities or interstitial spaces or to persistent drainage through the skin.

We have reviewed some of these problems that result in formation of lymphocysts, chylothorax, and chylopericardium. In other body regions, extravasation of lymph results in chylous ascites when it drains into the peritoneal cavity, chyluria when the communication is to the genitourinary tract, and lymphoenteric fistulas when the extravasation empties into the gastrointestinal tract. External communications between the lymphatic vessels and the exterior of the body are commonly seen whenever there is extensive damage of the collecting vessels caused by either blunt or penetrating trauma or surgical intervention. Lymphatic drainage in these cases is temporary and almost invariably ceases spontaneously. When a fistulous communication, commonly secondary to external trauma, is established through the skin in patients with underlying lymphedema, the lymph drainage may persist for long periods of time. This condition can also occur without any apparent lymphedema. In this instance, abnormal lymphatic structures may be responsible for the problem as they are in idiopathic chylothorax.

CHYLOUS ASCITES

A variety of conditions affecting the lymphatic structures are responsible for the production of chylous ascites. Malignant tumors in the retroperitoneal area and congenital abnormalities of the lymphatic vessels in the abdominal cavity are in most cases responsible for extravasation of chyle into the peritoneal cavity. Surgical trauma to the lymphatic collectors in the retroperitoneal area of the upper abdomen may occur, but in such cases the extravasation of chyle is temporary and does not become a significant problem. The presence of an extensive blockage of the thoracic duct, on the other hand, may lead to lymphangiectasis proximal to the level of obstruction. Trauma to these vessels will lead to continuous leakage of chyle into the peritoneal cavity. Specific infections such as tuberculosis were commonly associated in the past with development of chylous ascites. Clinically, the presence of abdominal distention resulting from accumulation of chyle in the peritoneal cavity strongly suggests this condition. A definitive diagnosis is made by paracentesis or laparotomy. The prognosis of ascites is related to that of the disease causing the chylous effusion. Medical therapy of an infectious process or treatment for a malignant disease will lead to cessation of the extravasation of chyle. The presence of a malignant condition usually carries a serious prognosis. In congenital abnormalities, lymphography offers great help in localizing the point of extravasation; treatment consisting of suture ligation of this point of leakage will thus be greatly facilitated. Unfortunately, no other therapeutic measure is available for the prevention of a recurrence.

CHYLURIA

Chyluria, or elimination of chyle through the urine, is a rare condition resulting from abnormal communications between the lymphatics and the urinary tract. The most common condition associated with this disease is that of parasitic infestation by filaria; less commonly, other types of infections or congenital malformations of the lymphatic vessels may be responsible.

The diagnosis is suspected by the presence of chyle in the urine. The urine becomes milky and thick; these characteristics vary during the day and according to the amount of fat ingestion. The diagnosis can be supported by noninvasive methods such as the ingestion of ^{131}I-labeled Triolein or a mixture of butter with Sudan-3. The latter will cause a characteristic change of color in the urine. The two most specific diagnostic tools are retrograde pyelography, which in some cases demonstrates reflux of the contrast medium into the perirenal lymphatics, and lymphangiography, which permits a more specific diagnosis. The first lymphangiographic demonstration of lymphatic abnormalities associated with chyluria was reported in 1962 by Turiaf.

Dietary therapy with medium-chain triglycerides has been reported to effect considerable improvement in the control of chyluria. This type of therapy is suited for patients with malignant conditions and nonoperable tumors and for those in poor clinical condition. By and large, the definitive treatment is surgical ablation of the lymphatics and multiple ligation of the abnormal communications previously demonstrated by lymphography. The results with this therapy have been excellent, and a high rate of cure has been reported. In rare cases, the chyluria ceases spontaneously and remains latent for many years.

CHYLOUS DIARRHEA

Chylous diarrhea is an uncommon condition that in some cases has been ascribed to the presence of lymphatic malformations in the gut. These patients have a tendency to lose large amounts of proteins in the stools owing to the extravasation of protein-rich chyle through the intestinal mucosa. When localized, these lesions can be treated successfully by ligation of the lymphatics at that point or by a limited intestinal resection.

PRIMARY LYMPHEDEMA

The nature of the lymphedematous fluid makes this type of edema considerably different from other types. The fluid accumulated in the interstitial spaces is a protein-rich fluid that gives a rubbery consistency to the tissues. Resorption of the lymphedematous fluid thus depends upon the mobilization of the proteins back into the systemic circulation.

According to the etiology, there are two forms of lymphedema, primary and secondary. In general, there is no known cause for primary lymphedema (Fig. 37-23), and there is a general consensus that this form is mainly the result of congenital abnormalities of the lymphatic vessels and glands. This type of edema usually appears during the early years of life and may be classified according to the time of appearance as congenital, praecox, or tarda. Some of these abnormalities are familiar, such as those seen in Milroy's disease. Other classifications are based upon the lymphographic findings and are grouped according to the number and appearance of the lymphatic vessels into aplastic, hypoplastic, and hyperplastic forms. Secondary lymphedema, on the other hand, is classified according to the many etiologic factors, which fall into the general categories of traumatic, neoplastic, or inflammatory factors. Treatment of primary lymphedema is not very satisfactory,

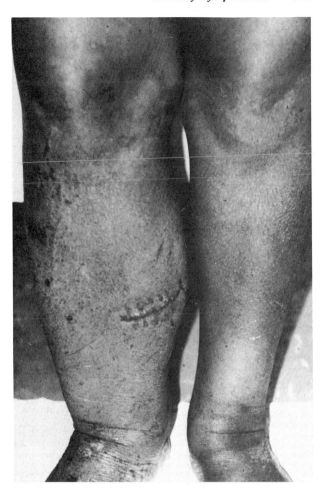

Fig. 37-23. Primary lymphedema in a 17-year-old girl. Note the swelling in both legs, which is more marked on the right. Repeated episodes of cellulitis aggravated the edema.

but surgical palliation has been employed occasionally (Fig. 37-24).

The term primary lymphedema was introduced by Allen of the Mayo Clinic. This condition is also described as spontaneous or idiopathic. The etiology is obscure but is basically related to congenital alterations—mainly underdevelopment of the lymphatic vessels causing impaired lymphatic drainage. In primary lymphedema, there is an alteration in not only the number but also the characteristics

THE SWOLLEN EXTREMITY—CAUSES

1. Trauma
   Bites and stings
   Fracture
2. Infection
3. Acute arterial occlusion
4. Venous occlusion
5. Lymphatic disease
   Primary
      Praecox
      Tarda
   Secondary
6. Radiation therapy
7. Tumor

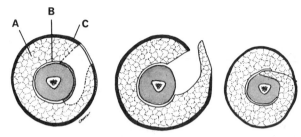

Fig. 37-24. The Thompson flap operation for the treatment of lymphedema. (*A*) Lymphedematous subcutaneous tissue. (*B*) Muscular compartment and aponeurosis. (*C*) Skin after removal of a strip of subcutaneous tissue. A "shaved" flap is buried in the muscle. A segment of fascia also is removed, to allow possible establishment of communication between the deep and the superficial vessels.

of the vessels and lymph nodes. The lymphographic pattern also varies from patient to patient, but the main feature is a decreased number of lymphatic vessels with abnormal appearance. In other patients there is an extensive proliferation of the small lymphatic vessels, reflecting perhaps an obstructive factor during intrauterine life. The term aplasia, referring to absence of lymphatic vessels, is probably improper because lymphatic vessels have been demonstrated by one method or another in every patient with primary lymphedema. A combination of the above described patterns can be found in the majority of patients. In some patients venous obstruction is associated with primary lymphedema; however, this obstruction is an aggravating factor and not a determining cause of the edema.

According to the time of clinical appearance of the swelling, the lymphedema is classified as praecox (early) or tarda (late). This rather subjective labeling is arbitrary because the lymphedema may have been present in a mild stage but was not noticed by the patient or the family. My impression is that these abnormalities are present from birth and either progress slowly until they become clinically evident or suddenly become obvious by superimposed trauma or infection. The lymphographic findings in these two forms are interchangeable with no specific picture for each type. From the standpoint of treatment, the presence of a traumatic or inflammatory process superimposed upon the lymphedema is an indication for bed rest and anti-inflammatory agents, which are of great help in the palliative treatment of this condition. Such a traumatic or inflammatory process may explain also the presence in some patients of "unilateral" lymphedema of the lower extremities. In fact, the performance of bilateral lymphograms in patients with so-called unilateral lymphedema will show definite abnormalities in the apparently healthy extremity also.

Primary lymphedema of the upper extremities is infrequent; it is usually associated with lymphatic abnormalities such as those described above or as part of a diffuse lymphedematous process.

SECONDARY LYMPHEDEMA

Lymphedema in this particular group of patients develops as a result of several conditions affecting the circulation and the drainage of the lymph from the involved or affected territory.

Impairment in the lymphatic drainage of a region that results in lymphedema has several causes but is most commonly due to surgical interruption of the lymphatic drainage in both the upper and the lower extremities. In general, the interruption of the lymphatic drainage must be extensive to interfere with the lymphatic circulation. It is well known that the lymphatic system has a tremendous capacity to regenerate and to develop collateral channels and open venous–lymphatic communications that are normally closed. This fact is demonstrated by the difficulty of producing secondary lymphedema in the laboratory. This is possible only by extensive interruption of the lymphatic structures in dogs, creating appreciable gaps between the divided ends of the extremities, as reported by several investigators. In the clinical setting, this interruption, although not as extensive as the one produced in the laboratory, is reinforced by radiotherapy and infection, and in some cases, by the added factor of venous thrombosis.

Massive interruption of lymphatic drainage, such as that seen during extensive radical node dissection procedures, is considered one of the main factors in the production of secondary lymphedema following surgery. Among the most common operations associated with this problem are radical mastectomy and radical node dissections of the groin for malignant tumors of the extremities. Lymphedema of the lower extremities is infrequent following lumbar node dissection in patients with testicular tumors. This is due in part to the extensive collateral drainage through other parts of the abdominal and pelvic walls. The occurrence of infection and hematomas and the addition of radiotherapy to these procedures are significant contributing factors in the occurrence or aggravation of edema following these operations. Some investigators have also found that venous thrombosis or stenosis secondary to radiotherapy, venous injury, or fibrosis is a determining factor in the development of postmastectomy lymphedema.

It has been estimated that from 7% to 25% of all patients undergoing radical mastectomy will develop lymphedema. Radiotherapy increases the possibility of this complication in these patients. Lesser degrees of edema are found in an additional number of patients following radical mastectomy, but these patients are not significantly affected either cosmetically or clinically by this degree of swelling. An estimated 50% of patients undergoing radical mastectomy develop mild degrees of lymphedema. The growing number of surgeons using procedures less extensive than a radical mastectomy for carcinoma of the breast may contribute to a significant decrease of this complication in the future.

ANGIOSARCOMA POSTMASTECTOMY

The serious complication of postmastectomy angiosarcoma has been related to the duration of lymphedema in patients who have had radical mastectomy. The estimated incidence is 0.45% of patients surviving 5 or more years after radical mastectomy for carcinoma of the breast. It is infrequent to find this complication in patients with lymphedema of less than 5 years' duration.

Contrast medium injected into a peripheral lymphatic vessel in patients with lymphedema of the extremities will show a considerable delay in the flow through the lymphatic system of the affected territory. The appearance of the lymphatic vessels is dramatic, and in most patients there is massive proliferation of collateral vessels with great distortion of the normal pattern. Preservation of the main collecting channels is found in some of these patients, and, as will be seen later, this represents a favorable condition for direct surgical correction of lymphatic stasis. The obstruction may be so extensive in some patients that dermal backflow of the contrast medium appears in the lymphangiogram.

SURGICAL MANAGEMENT OF LYMPHEDEMA

In contrast to the significant advances seen in the treatment of arterial and venous disorders, treatment of lymphedema has remained rather at a standstill. In general, this lack of progress is related to the anatomy of the lymphatic system and the nature of the disease. Many procedures were devised in the past for the treatment of symptomatic lymphedema, but most were of questionable effectiveness. Most of them have been abandoned, and only a few procedures remain that are relatively effective in the treatment of this troublesome condition. In the past few years, a new upsurge in interest in the treatment of this disease has developed, and we will analyze these procedures briefly.

The procedures still in use at present are as follows.

1. Silk threads are implanted subcutaneously to drain the lymph around them into territories that are anatomically and functionally intact. Other materials used for this purpose include nylon threads and, more recently, Teflon wicks. Degni and associates have described their initial results with this technique, which at best are partially effective and of temporary duration.

2. Pedicles containing normal lymphatics are used to bridge obstructed areas of lymphatic drainage (Gillis and Fraser, 1935). Although theoretically sound, these procedures have not been successful in the clinical setting.

3. Omental transposition (Goldsmith, 1967) involves bridging the obstructed area of lymphatic drainage with the greater omentum, which is left attached to its vascular pedicle with the distal portion placed at the area of lymphatic stasis; the purpose is to create or promote the establishment of anastomosis, thus enhancing the drainage of the lymphedematous territory. The large number of complications with this technique led to its abandonment. Reduction of lymphedema was accomplished in some patients.

4. The lymphedematous tissue is excised in combination with skin grafting (Charles, 1912). The cosmetic results are unpleasant, and in some patients there is recurrence of the lymphedema.

5. Lymphovenous anastomosis is performed between lymph nodes and veins (Rivero, 1967; Nielubowicz, 1968). Decompression of the lymphatic stasis through the anastomosis between a lymph node and an adjacent vein was attempted in patients with lower extremity lymphedema. Although the principle was sound and the initial results were encouraging, recurrence of the lymphedema was seen in a significant number of patients after 1 year. This was due to fibrosis of the area of the lymph node exposed to the venous flow.

6. Lymphatic transposition using "shaved" subcutaneous skin flaps, described by Thompson in 1962, has remained as the procedure of choice for most patients with moderate and advanced stages of lymphedema of the extremities. This operation combines the removal of the lymphedematous tissue with the establishment of communications between the superficial and deep lymphatic vessels. The transposition of the shaved subcutaneous flap into the deep muscle compartment prevents the regeneration of the fascia of the muscles, thus maintaining the communication between the superficial and deep lymphatic vessels. The cosmetic results as well as the reduction of the lymphedema are acceptable.

The significant complications reported have been related to inadequate shaving of the skin from the flaps. The incidence of infection in the series of Kinmonth was approximately 42%, and most of these cases were related to improper technique and therefore were subject to improvement.

The introduction of microsurgical techniques has opened a new field in the treatment of lymphedema. The pioneer work of Degni and Cordeiro in Brazil has stimulated other investigators to use direct lymphaticovenous anastomosis for the treatment of lymphedema. Ingenious techniques have allowed Degni to anastomose one or several lymphatics to the same vein. The initial reports are encouraging, but long-term observation will be necessary to assess the true effectiveness of this procedure. A recent report by Baumeister and associates in West Germany described the experimental and clinical application of lymph vessel transplantation for the treatment of secondary lymphedema. Although their patient sample was small (two patients), this report demonstrates the feasibility of lymphatic transplantation in a manner similar to that of a femoropopliteal bypass performed by microsurgical techniques.

CONSERVATIVE MANAGEMENT OF LYMPHEDEMA

In lieu of a surgical procedure, intermittent pneumatic compression of the affected extremity can be used for the treatment of lymphedema. This technique employs external compression to force the return of edematous fluid from the interstitial space into the systemic circulation. Reduction of limb size is thus accomplished and maintained by continuous use of this equipment and the addition of elastic stockings or sleeves. This procedure at least offers an alternative to surgical treatment with acceptable cosmetic results.

BIBLIOGRAPHY

ADLER RH, LEVINSKY L: Persistent chylothorax. Treatment by talc pleurodeses. J Thorac Cardiovasc Surg 76:859, 1978

BAUMEISTER RGM, SEIFERT J, WIEBECK B et al: Experimental and clinical lymph vessel transplantation for the treatment of secondary lymphedema. World J Surg 5:401, 1981

BEAHRS OH: Complications of surgery of the head and neck. Surg Clin North Am 57:823, 1977

BURIHAN E: Quilotorax uma complicacao rara da aortografia translombar com comprovacao linfografica. Rev Bras Cardiovasc 10:19, 1974

CAVALLO CA, HIRATA RM, JAQUES DA: Chylothorax complicating radical neck dissection. Am Surg 41:266, 1975

CEVESE PG, VECCHIONI R, D'AMICO DR et al: Postoperative chylothorax. J Thorac Cardiovasc Surg 69:966, 1975

CHAVEZ CM: The clinical significance of lymphaticovenous anastomosis. Vasc Dis 5:35, 1968

CHAVEZ CM, RODRIGUEZ GR, CONN JH: Isolated chylopericardium. Am J Cardiovasc Surg 32:352, 1973

DEGNI M: New technique of lymphatic-venous anastomosis (buried type) for the treatment of lymphedema. Rev Argent Angiol 8:38, 1974

DELANEY AL, DAICOFF GR, HESS PJ et al: Chylopericardium with cardiac tamponade after cardiovascular surgery in two patients. Chest 69:381, 1976

HARDY JD, WALKER GR, DEGUZMAN VC: Thoracic duct fistula in infants. Blue dye localization and operative closure. JAMA 182:187, 1962

SERVELLE M, NOGUES CI, SOULIE J et al: Spontaneous, postoperative and traumatic chylothorax. J Cardiovasc Surg 21:475, 1980

SILVER D, PUCKETT CL: Lymphangioplasty: A ten-year evaluation. Surgery 80:748, 1976

J. Kent Trinkle/Michael H. Crawford

38

The Heart: Anatomy, Diagnostic Modalities, and the Pump Oxygenator

ANATOMY

THORACIC RELATIONSHIPS

The approximate positions of the major cardiovascular structures in relation to the bony skeleton are depicted in Figure 38-1. These relationships will vary slightly with body build, respiration, and chamber enlargement.

The sternal notch is at the level of the second thoracic vertebral body. The sternal angle, the junction of the manubrium and the body of the sternum, is at the level of the second costal cartilage and the fourth thoracic vertebral body. The area between the notch and the angle is the manubrium, and posterior to this structure lie the major branches of the aortic arch: the innominate, left carotid, and left subclavian arteries. The innominate artery bifurcates into the subclavian and right carotid arteries at the junction of the right clavicle and the manubrium. The pericardium extends from the level of the sternal angle to the xiphisternal junction. The right pericardial border is 2 cm lateral to the sternum. The left margin angles from a point 2 cm lateral to the left sternal margin, at the level of the second costal cartilage, to the midclavicular line at the level of the fifth rib anteriorly. The pulmonary valve is at the level of the left third costal cartilage, and the aortic valve is at the third left interspace. The orifice of the mitral valve lies one half interspace inferior and slightly lateral to the aortic valve. The orifice of the tricuspid valve is immediately retrosternal in the midline at the level of the fifth costal cartilage. The anterior surface of the pericardium is a "bare area" in

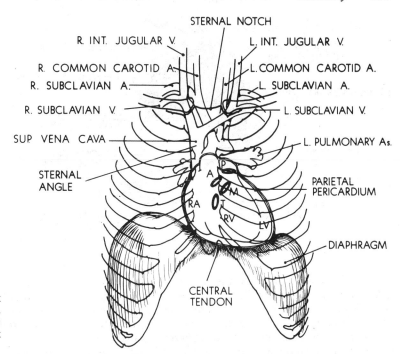

Fig. 38-1. The anterior relationships of the heart and great vessels to the overlying thoracic skeleton. (*A*, aortic valve; *LV*, left ventricle; *M*, mitral valve; *P*, pulmonary valve; *RA*, right atrium; *RV*, right ventricle; *T*, tricuspid valve)

intimate contact with the posterior aspect of the sternum and left costal cartilages with no interposed pleura. This bare area may be entered surgically without violating either pleural space.

The anterior surface of the pericardium is separated from the sternum only by a potential space. This is an avascular plane that allows blind dissection in preparation for a median sternotomy.

There are three surgical approaches to the heart: median sternotomy, right anterolateral thoracotomy, and left anterolateral thoracotomy. Median sternotomy, used in most cardiovascular procedures, provides excellent exposure of all anterior intrapericardial structures. The right anterolateral incision in the fourth intercostal space provides exposure of the right atrium, left atrium, mitral valve, and both venae cavae. The left anterolateral thoracotomy exposes the left atrium and appendage in the fourth intercostal space and the left ventricular apex in the fifth intercostal space. A very short left anterolateral incision will expose the pericardium for biopsy without violating the pleura.

PERICARDIUM

The heart and proximal great vessels are enclosed in a two-layered sac of pericardium (Fig. 38-2). A thin inner layer of serous or visceral pericardium coats the heart and great vessels. The outer fibrous or parietal pericardium is continuous with the visceral layer as it reflects off the great vessels. Thus, the heart swings like a pendulum within the parietal pericardium while suspended by the great vessels. This relationship allows the surgeon to displace the heart for various posterior and lateral exposures from an anterior median sternotomy approach. Each of the great vessels is suspended from the parietal pericardium by a two-layered mesentery of visceral pericardium. Because of the additional layer of visceral pericardium, the great vessels are less fragile within the pericardium. Thus, various surgical maneuvers,

such as clamping, suturing, and cannulation, should be performed inside the pericardium whenever possible.

RIGHT ATRIUM

The free anterolateral wall of the right atrium is lined by pectinate muscles. The precise size and contour of the appendage will vary considerably in both the normal and the diseased heart. This area contracts and contributes to cardiac output by augmenting ventricular filling. The pectinate line and crista terminalis mark the posterior limit of the right atrium derived from the primitive cardiac tube.

The interatrial septum is shaped like a triangle with blunt angles. The base of the triangle is located along the right side, and there is a blunt angle under the orifice of each vena cava. The rounded apex of the triangle is to the left. The septum lies in a plane almost horizontal to the sternum but inclining approximately 10° to the right. The septum is smooth except for a horseshoe-shaped rim of tissue, the limbus of the fossa ovalis. The floor of the fossa ovalis and the inferior portion of the interatrial septum is formed only by the septum primum. The superior and lateral areas are thicker and formed by fusion of the septum secundum with the septum primum.

The coronary sinus, located immediately superior to the tricuspid valve annulus, is a remnant of the left common cardinal vein. The superior vena cava developed from the right common and anterior cardinal veins.

RIGHT VENTRICLE

The right ventricle is retrosternal and vulnerable to both blunt and penetrating anterior trauma. Blood supply is through the right coronary artery in the right atrioventricular groove. The branches of this vessel run transversely, except for a conal branch, which may run vertically along the outflow tract. The muscle fibers are also transverse. The anterior wall is free of important structures on its deep

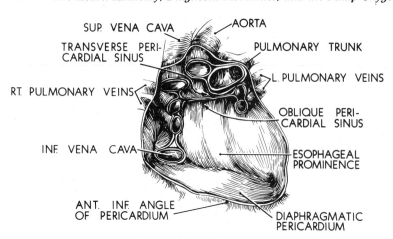

Fig. 38-2. The posterior pericardium is shown with the heart removed, illustrating the pericardial recesses and attachments of the great vessels.

surface. The crista terminalis, the inferior margin of the bulbar septum, marks the dividing line between the right ventricle and its outflow tract. The aortic valve annulus and sinuses lie deep to the outflow tract, since the aortic valve is approximately 2 cm inferior to the pulmonary valve. The parietal bands bind the anterior to the posterior wall in the outflow tract. The left margin of the crista terminalis extends onto the septum as the septal band. The septal band then gives rise to the moderator band, which traverses the cavity of the right ventricle to the right anterolateral free wall. The anterior papillary muscle to the tricuspid valve arises from the moderator band, and the posterior papillary muscle arises from the right posterior wall.

LEFT ATRIUM

The left atrium lies posteriorly in the midline. It is fixed superiorly and laterally on each side by the pulmonary veins. The posterior, inferior, and left lateral areas of the left atrium are free within the pericardial cavity. The left atrium can be divided into the following three components on the basis of its embryologic origin: (1) The smooth posterior wall of the left atrium, adjacent to the pulmonary veins, derives from the primitive pulmonary venous plexus and becomes adherent to the cardiac tube to form a single chamber. (2) The primitive cardiac tube is the anlage of the inferior and lateral margin of the left atrium, which is lined with contractile pectinate muscles and contains the left atrial appendage. (3) The interatrial septum from the left side is composed almost entirely of septum primum except for the area of the fossa ovalis, a defect in the septum primum, which is covered only by the septum secundum.

Surgical access to the interior of the left atrium can be obtained on the right side with an incision anterior to the right pulmonary veins, superiorly between the superior vena cava and the aorta; access along the left side can be obtained through either the left atrial appendage or an incision above the left atrioventricular groove.

LEFT VENTRICLE

The left ventricle is less trabeculated and thicker than the right ventricle. There are two papillary muscles, anterior and posterior, each of which gives chordae tendineae to both leaflets of the mitral valve. The septum of the left ventricle is relatively smooth, allowing easy visualization of

muscular ventricular septal defects. The muscle fibers are concentric. The membranous portion of the interventricular septum is inferior to the aortic valve annulus. Note that the annuli of the aortic and mitral valves are adjacent.

INTRAPERICARDIAL GREAT VESSELS

The superior vena cava is formed by the confluence of the right and left innominate veins. Just before entering the pericardium, it is joined by the azygos vein, a remnant of the right posterior cardinal vein. The anterior and lateral walls of the 5-cm intrapericardial portion are free and suspended posteriorly by a mesentery. The superior vena cava crosses anterior to the right pulmonary artery.

The inferior vena cava has a very short intrapericardial course. It angles rather sharply posteroanteriorly as it penetrates the diaphragm and parietal pericardium to enter the right atrium. A thin, two-layered mesentery of visceral pericardium attaches the right lateral wall of the inferior vena cava to the parietal pericardium.

The intrapericardial ascending aorta is approximately 8 cm in length. The annulus of the aortic valve and the posterior aortic sinus can be visualized in the transverse sinus. However, the anterior portion of the aortic annulus is covered by the outflow tract of the right ventricle and the main pulmonary artery. The ascending aorta is adherent along its left posterior margin to the main pulmonary artery. The space between these vessels is avascular, with a common coating of visceral pericardium and a variable amount of fat.

The proximal portion of the pulmonary artery is anterior and slightly to the left of the midline. The main pulmonary artery angles posteriorly and to the left before it bifurcates. The left pulmonary artery has a short intrapericardial course and passes almost directly posteriorly. The right pulmonary artery has a long intrapericardial course and passes posterior to both the ascending aorta and the superior vena cava. The apical anterior branch of the right pulmonary artery arises at the point where it leaves the parietal pericardium.

There are four pulmonary veins, two left and two right. The right superior pulmonary vein drains the right upper and right middle lobes. The left superior pulmonary vein drains the left upper lobe and lingula. The inferior pulmonary veins drain the corresponding lower lobes. Each of the four pulmonary veins enters the left atrium as a separate structure (see Fig. 38-2).

FIBROUS SKELETON OF THE HEART

The fibrous skeleton of the heart is comprised of the annuli of the four cardiac valves and the interposed fibrous trigones. The annuli of the aortic and pulmonary valves are complete and of constant thickness. However, the annulus of the mitral valve is frequently deficient in the left posterolateral aspect adjacent to the posterior leaflet. Likewise, the annulus of the tricuspid valve is a very thin structure except anteromedially, adjacent to the trigone.

CARDIAC VALVES

The cardiac valves promote unobstructed, unidirectional blood flow. They are thin, fibrous tissue with a mesothelial covering. The atrioventricular valves are supported by papillary muscles and chordae tendineae arising in the ventricles. The aortic and pulmonary valves are supported by commissures arising from the corresponding great artery.

The aortic valve has three cup-shaped leaflets, the right and left coronary and the noncoronary cusps. There is a corresponding sinus of Valsalva above each valve leaflet. The commissures are attached to the aortic wall and suspend the cusps, thus preventing prolapse during diastole. The coronary artery orifices are immediately above the right and left cusps. The right coronary artery passes to the right and anteriorly at an acute angle to the aorta. The left coronary artery passes to the left and slightly anteriorly at a less acute angle.

The pulmonary valve is comprised of three cup-shaped leaflets with supporting commissures attached to the pulmonary artery. This valve lies approximately 2 cm cranial to the aortic valve except in certain congenital anomalies such as transposition of the great vessels.

The tricuspid valve is comprised of three leaflets, a large anterior and a small posterior leaflet and a septal leaflet. The anterior leaflet occupies approximately 50% of both the circumference and surface area. The three leaflets are supported by papillary muscles and chordae tendineae arising within the ventricle. The anterior papillary muscle has origin from the moderator band, and the posterior papillary muscle arises from the right lateral posterior wall of the right ventricle. The medial papillary muscle arises from the junction of the crista terminalis and the septal band. Exposure of the tricuspid valve is through a right atrial incision parallel to the atrioventricular groove.

The mitral valve has two leaflets. The anterior leaflet is considerably larger in surface area than the posterior leaflet but occupies approximately the same circumference of the valve annulus. The commissures between the two leaflets are located left, anterolaterally, and right, posteromedially, adjacent to the aortic valve annulus. The commissures are not complete, and there is a small cusp of tissue interposed between the normal valve orifice and the annulus. The anterior and posterior papillary muscles arise in the left ventricle, and each papillary muscle supplies chordae tendineae to both leaflets. The mitral valve may be approached surgically through an incision in the right side of the left atrium, superiorly between the superior vena cava and the ascending aorta, or from the left through the atrial appendage or an incision in the left atrioventricular groove.

CORONARY CIRCULATION

The recent evolution of coronary angiography and the direct approach in surgery of the coronary artery has increased the importance of a thorough knowledge of coronary artery anatomy (Fig. 38-3). There are two coronary arteries, left and right, which arise approximately 5 mm above the corresponding aortic valve cusp. However, the left coronary artery branches within 1 cm into the left circumflex and the left anterior descending arteries. Coronary artery anatomy is somewhat variable with respect to which vessel supplies the posterior wall of the left ventricle and is thus declared the "dominant" coronary artery. The right coronary

Fig. 38-3. Anterior (*left*) and posterior (*right*) views of the heart, demonstrating the coronary arteries and veins.

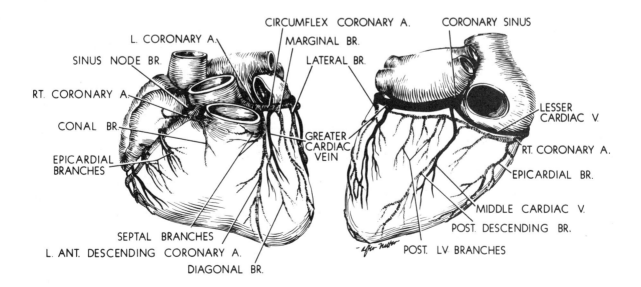

artery is dominant in approximately 60% of patients and the left circumflex in 20%. In the remaining 20%, the blood supply to the posterior wall of the left ventricle is through a combination of right coronary and left circumflex arteries and the left anterior descending branches passing around the apex.

The right coronary artery passes to the right at an acute angle with the ascending aorta. It traverses the right atrioventricular groove until reaching the posterior interventricular septum. A nondominant vessel will terminate at this point. A dominant vessel will give rise to a posterior descending branch, overlying the posterior interventricular septum, and will continue for a variable distance in the left posterior atrioventricular groove. In addition, there is a proximal nodal branch passing to the posterior surface of the right atrium near the junction of the superior vena cava. A conal branch passes vertically down the outflow tract of the right ventricle for a variable distance. There are multiple epicardial branches to the right ventricle and atrium arising in the right atrioventricular groove.

The left coronary artery arises from the left posterolateral aspect of the aorta above the left coronary cusp. It passes to the left and anteriorly around the base of the pulmonary artery at the level of the pulmonary valve annulus. Before emerging anteriorly, it divides into the anterior descending and circumflex coronary arteries. The left anterior descending coronary artery passes down the anterior surface of the heart in the interventricular groove to the apex. Multiple septal branches emerge from the deep surface of this vessel to supply the interventricular septum. At the junction of the proximal and middle thirds, a large diagonal branch is visible on the anterior surface of the left ventricle. Proximal occlusion of this vessel can give rise to infarction of the anterior left ventricle and the interventricular septum.

The circumflex coronary artery occupies the left atrioventricular groove and passes for a varying distance to the posterior aspect of the left ventricle. In approximately 20% of patients, this vessel is dominant and gives rise to the posterior descending coronary artery in the posterior interventricular groove. The first branch of the circumflex is the obtuse marginal, which passes obliquely down the anterolateral wall of the left ventricle. There are a variable number of smaller lateral and posterior marginal branches passing more or less vertically along the surface of the left ventricle. Multiple small branches supply the left atrium.

The great coronary vein arises in the distal end of the anterior interventricular septum parallel to the anterior descending coronary artery. It passes into the left atrioventricular groove and ultimately empties posteriorly into the coronary sinus. This vein receives multiple tributaries from the left ventricle. The middle cardiac vein parallels the posterior descending coronary artery in the posterior interventricular groove and empties into the great cardiac vein just prior to its entrance into the coronary sinus. The lesser cardiac vein is parallel to the right coronary artery in the right atrioventricular groove and enters the great cardiac vein at its junction with the coronary sinus.

Lymphatic drainage of the myocardium is from inside out. A subendocardial lymphatic plexus traverses the myocardium to the epicardium. From this point, several vessels pass along the aorta and pulmonary artery, and their intervening areolar tissue, to drain into lymph nodes in the middle mediastinum. Obliteration of the epicardial lymphatics by irradiation, inflammation, or neoplasm leads to pericardial effusion.

INTRINSIC CONDUCTION

Cardiac muscle possesses its own automatic rhythmicity. The tissues derived from the sinus venosus, the right atrium, and the ventricles have a decreasing rate of contraction. Thus, the cardiac impulse normally originates in the sinoatrial node at the junction of the superior vena cava and the right atrium. The atrioventricular node is located immediately anterior to the orifice of the coronary sinus and superior to the tricuspid valve annulus. When the sinoatrial node is not functioning, the atrioventricular node will initiate cardiac contraction at a rate of approximately 60/minute. From the atrioventricular node, the bundle of His passes immediately deep to the tricuspid annulus and along the posteroinferior margin of the membranous interventricular septum. At the lower margin of the septum, the bundle divides into a right and a left bundle branch. The left bundle branch penetrates the septum and divides into an anterior and a posterior division. The right bundle branch travels through the septal and moderator bands to reach the right ventricle.

DIAGNOSTIC MODALITIES

HISTORY

The cornerstone of clinical evaluation is the history, which guides the physician toward more specific tests to confirm the diagnosis and establish the extent of the disease.

CHEST PAIN

Chest pain may be caused by a variety of diseases. Chest pain due to myocardial ischemia, or angina pectoris, is more of a discomfort or unpleasant sensation often described as pressing, squeezing, choking, or sometimes, burning. This discomfort is usually located substernally but may be felt to the left or right side of the chest; extension to the neck, jaw, arms, or back is not uncommon. Other symptoms are shortness of breath, abdominal pain, diaphoresis, lightheadedness, and occasionally, nausea and vomiting. Untreated angina pectoris usually lasts less than 10 minutes. Pain lasting longer than 30 minutes is indicative of myocardial infarction. Angina pectoris is due to an increase in myocardial oxygen demands, especially those that raise the heart rate or the blood pressure, such as exercise, emotional stress, and eating a large meal. Sublingual nitroglycerin usually relieves the pain within 2 minutes but is nonspecific.

DYSPNEA

Dyspnea is an uncomfortable awareness of breathing and occurs in a wide variety of cardiopulmonary diseases. Slowly developing dyspnea is typical of congestive heart failure and begins as dyspnea on exertion and progresses to paroxysmal nocturnal dyspnea and finally orthopnea. Paroxysmal nocturnal dyspnea also occurs in patients with chronic lung disease. In addition, many patients routinely sleep on two or three pillows for comfort because of musculoskeletal, pulmonary, or sinus problems. Thus, the elicitation of a history of orthopnea alone is not evidence of cardiac or pulmonary disease.

COUGH

Cough is a common symptom associated with bronchopulmonary disease. A dry, hacking cough can occur in cardiac

CARDIAC SURGICAL ASSESSMENT

History	Angina, dyspnea, palpitation, syncope?
Physical	Murmur, sounds, prominent apical impulse
Noninvasive Dx	Chest film: cardiomegaly, calcification; electrocardiogram: ischemia vs. old infarct; echo: cardiac dimension, morphological picture; radionuclide angiography: ejection fraction; ischemia with thallium scanning; new infarct by pyrophosphate scan
Invasive Dx	Right and left heart catheterization, coronary cineangiograph
Decision	Disease amenable to surgery?

disorders that lead to accumulation of fluid in the lungs, such as pulmonary venous hypertension, interstitial and alveolar pulmonary edema, and pulmonary infarction.

HEMOPTYSIS

The expectoration of blood may be due to nasal bleeding, tuberculosis, bronchiectasis, pulmonary infarction, bronchogenic carcinoma, and pulmonary arteriovenous fistula. The most common cardiac causes are mitral stenosis with severe pulmonary venous hypertension and acute pulmonary edema.

EDEMA

Edema is subcutaneous fluid accumulation in dependent areas such as the feet or over the sacrum. It may be due to right heart failure, local obstructions to venous or lymph flow, local inflammation, renal failure, and hepatic cirrhosis.

PALPITATION

Palpitation is an abnormal awareness of heart action due to rapid, forceful beating of the heart or irregularities of the rhythm and force of contraction.

SYNCOPE

Syncope is a sudden loss of consciousness that is often associated with severe disorders of cardiac rhythm with inadequate central nervous system blood flow. Syncope also may be due to seizures, cerebrovascular disease, aortic stenosis, orthostatic hypotension, and prolonged coughing.

PHYSICAL EXAMINATION

ARTERIAL PULSE

A weak carotid pulse indicates diminished left ventricular stroke volume due to hypovolemia or left ventricular failure. A bounding pulse is associated with an increased left ventricular stroke volume with a hyperkinetic circulation that may be due to anemia or fever. Aortic regurgitation causes a rapidly rising, bounding arterial pulse because of a large stroke volume. A delayed upstroke of the carotid pulse is associated with mechanical obstruction of the left ventricle, such as aortic stenosis.

JUGULAR VENOUS PULSE

The jugular venous pulse may be used to estimate the central venous pressure and to assess cardiac function by observing the wave form. The patient's upper body is elevated while the pulsating column in the right internal jugular vein is observed. The sternal angle is roughly 5 cm above the right atrium, and jugular venous pulsations above this angle give a rough estimate of the central venous pressure in centimeters of blood.

The normal jugular venous pulse has two dominant positive waves. The presystolic wave, or *a* wave, is caused by right atrial contraction. The late systolic *v* wave results from ventricular systole when the tricuspid valve is closed. The *a* wave is accentuated with increased right atrial pressure and is absent in patients with atrial fibrillation. The *v* wave increases in patients with tricuspid regurgitation and atrial septal defect.

PRECORDIAL PALPATION

Precordial palpation assesses the character of the left ventricular apical impulse. The normal left ventricular apical impulse is to the right of the midclavicular line in either the fourth or fifth intercostal space. It is of brief duration and is not more than 3 cm in diameter. Left ventricular hypertrophy increases the amplitude and duration of this impulse, and left ventricular enlargement results in lateral and downward displacement and an increase in size. Right ventricular hypertrophy causes a sustained systolic lift in the lower left parasternal area. A pulsation in the right second intercostal space suggests an aortic aneurysm, and pulsations in the second left intercostal space indicate pulmonary hypertension. Systolic thrills are frequent in patients with aortic stenosis or ventricular septal defect. A diastolic thrill suggests mitral stenosis.

CARDIAC AUSCULTATION

Heart sounds are created by the opening and closing of cardiac valves and the associated acceleration and deceleration of blood. The first sound is coincident with closing of the atrioventricular valves and is heard best at the lower left sternal border. Splitting of the first heart sound by 10 msec to 30 msec often occurs in normal persons due to separate closure of the mitral and tricuspid valves. Splitting is widened in right bundle-branch block, which delays tricuspid valve closure. However, the absence of splitting of the first heart sound is not abnormal. The first heart sound is accentuated in mitral stenosis, in which the leaflets are thickened.

The second heart sound is due to closure of the aortic and pulmonary valves and is normally split during inspiration. Splitting is normally heard during inspiration, with merging of the sounds during expiration, due to increased blood flow into the right ventricle and lungs during inspiration. Persistent, fixed splitting of the second heart sound is due to chronic volume overload of the right ventricle; this occurs in conditions such as atrial septal defect.

The third heart sound is low pitched and best heard at the apex. It occurs in early diastole, approximately 15 msec after the second sound. This sound is frequent in normal children. However, in older adults, it usually indicates either volume overload of the left ventricle or left ventricular decompensation.

The fourth heart sound is a low-pitched presystolic sound, heard best at the apex. This sound occurs when the ventricle is stiffened due to such diseases as left ventricular hypertrophy or coronary artery disease. It is produced by atrial contraction.

A systolic ejection sound is a sharp, high-pitched sound occurring in early systole and closely following the first heart sound. These sounds occur in the presence of aortic or pulmonary stenosis. Variable midsystolic clicks are associated with mitral valve prolapse.

Heart murmurs are caused by vibrations that result from turbulent blood flow. The intensity of murmurs is usually graded from 1 to 6. The grade 1 murmur is so faint that it can be heard only with special effort. The grade 2 murmur is usually audible but soft. A grade 3 murmur is louder. A grade 4 murmur is one that is associated with a palpable thrill. A grade 5 murmur can be heard with only part of the stethoscope touching the chest, and a grade 6 murmur is audible with the stethoscope removed from the chest. The pitch and character of murmurs depend on their origin and can be altered by altering the hemodynamic condition of the patient.

The most common heart murmur is early systolic, crescendo–decrescendo, and medium frequency. This usually is due to normal aortic outflow. Such murmurs are heard in up to 80% of children and may be as loud as grade 3. It is also heard with high-output states such as fever and anemia in older persons. A lower pitched murmur peaking in midsystole is often associated with valvular aortic stenosis and may be accompanied by an ejection sound and a fourth heart sound.

Pansystolic high-frequency murmurs are generated when there is abnormal systolic flow between two chambers with markedly different pressures, such as the left ventricle and the left atrium. The murmur of mitral regurgitation begins at the onset of systole, persists until the second heart sound, and is loudest over the apex and radiates to the axilla. The murmur of ventricular septal defect is loudest at the left sternal border and is often accompanied by a thrill. The murmur of tricuspid regurgitation is loudest at the lower left sternal border and is augmented by inspiration.

High-pitched early diastolic murmurs are usually due to aortic or pulmonary regurgitation and are best heard at the base. These murmurs are decrescendo, since there is a decreasing gradient during diastole between the great vessel and the respective cardiac chamber. Mid-diastolic murmurs are generated by flow across the atrioventricular valves and may be accentuated by atrial contraction at the end of diastole.

Continuous murmurs are those that begin in systole and persist into diastole. These murmurs signify continuous flow due to a communication between a high and a low pressure area which persists throughout the cardiac cycle. Usually, this means the connection between an artery and a vein, such as occurs in ductus arteriosus and systemic arteriovenous fistula. These murmurs must be differentiated from friction rubs, which are scratchy sounds that may be accentuated by having the patient lean forward.

CHEST FILM

There are two important features of the chest film. One is the cardiac silhouette, which indicates the size of the heart and its various chambers. The second is the pulmonary vasculature, which reveals the physiological state of the pulmonary circulation.

CARDIAC SILHOUETTE

The cardiac silhouette is created where the heart borders with the more radiolucent lung. The right border of the posteroanterior projection is composed of four basic curves: the innominate artery, the superior vena cava, the right atrium, and the inferior vena cava. The normal left heart border is composed of six curves, starting superiorly with the left subclavian artery, the aortic arch, the main pulmonary artery, the left atrial appendage, the left ventricular apex, and the apical fat pad. In the lateral projection, the anterior border of the heart is the right ventricle and the posterior border is composed of the left atrium, left ventricle, and inferior vena cava. Abnormalities in cardiac size are deduced from alterations of these basic curves. The ratio of the normal cardiac-to-thoracic diameter, or the cardiothoracic ratio, is usually less than 0.5 on a posteroanterior radiograph.

CARDIAC CALCIFICATIONS

The lateral projection is usually best for visualization of calcium. However, the best roentgenographic method for assessing cardiac calcification is image-intensified fluoroscopy. Calcification of the coronary arteries almost always signifies coronary artery disease. Calcium may occur in organized atrial or ventricular mural thrombi. Valvular calcifications most often occur in the mitral and aortic valves.

PULMONARY VASCULATURE

The normal right and left pulmonary arteries are seen at the hilus and then taper toward the periphery, appearing more prominent at the bases than at the apex. Pulmonary venous hypertension leads to a progressive basilar pulmonary vessel constriction, such that the superior pulmonary veins become more prominent. This occurs at a mean pulmonary capillary pressure of approximately 20 torr. With further elevations in pulmonary venous pressure, pulmonary edema occurs, with leakage of fluid into the alveolar spaces resulting in rosette formation and generalized haziness in a butterfly-wing pattern.

With pulmonary arterial hypertension, there is central pulmonary artery dilatation and constriction of peripheral arteries, giving a pruned-tree appearance. With increased pulmonary blood flow, the arteries and veins throughout the lung become enlarged and more prominent. Patients with decreased pulmonary flow may demonstrate small pulmonary arteries and relative oligemia of the lung fields.

ELECTROCARDIOGRAPHY

The electrocardiogram (ECG) is a graphic recording of the electrical activity of the heart. There are two basic diagnostic considerations on the ECG: The first is an assessment of the cardiac rhythm; the second is an analysis of the characteristics of the various wave forms as they reflect cardiac structural pathology.

CARDIAC RHYTHM

When atrial activity precedes ventricular activity, normal sinus rhythm is inferred at a rate between 60 and 100 beats per minute. Sinus tachycardia is a similar configuration, with rates greater than 100 but less than 180. Sinus bradycardia occurs at rates less than 60 but usually greater than 40. Atrial tachydysrhythmias are present when the atrial rate exceeds 180 beats per minute. In paroxysmal atrial tachycardia, there is still a 1:1 relationship between the atrium and the ventricle, but in atrial flutter or fibrillation, there are fewer ventricular depolarizations than atrial.

The most common ventricular rhythm disturbance is the premature ventricular depolarization. Two such consecutive beats at a rapid rate are a couplet, and three or more are ventricular tachycardia. Persistent ventricular tachycardia can result in reduced blood pressure and syncope. The bradyarrhythmias can be either normal mechanisms at slow rates or heart block, in which there is interruption between atrial and ventricular conduction. This condition also may lead to hypotension and syncope.

STRUCTURAL PATHOLOGY

Disease of the electrical conduction system will prolong the duration of the ventricular depolarization wave and alter its configuration. Chamber hypertrophy will alter the amplitude and configuration of the ECG deflections. Ischemic heart disease can produce specific changes in the ECG. Intermittent ischemia often produces alterations in the ventricular repolarization deflections as manifested by changes in ST-T wave segments. Myocardial infarction causes alterations in the configuration of the ventricular depolarization wave over the infarcted area, with the Q wave reflecting areas of previous infarction.

TREADMILL ECG TESTING

Exercise ECG testing was developed to study patients during the systematic application of stress. Such tests have become a standard technique for evaluating patients with overt or suspected ischemic heart disease. They are also useful for assessing functional capacity or provoking dysrhythmias in patients with other cardiac diseases. When a patient is allowed to exercise, as on a treadmill, change in the ECG with ST segment depression, with or without associated chest pain, will confirm the presence of ischemic heart disease and serve as an indication for angiography.

ECHOCARDIOGRAPHY

Echocardiography employs ultrasound to create representations of cardiac anatomy. Currently, there are two predominant types of systems: time-motion, or M-mode, and real-time, or two-dimensional, echocardiographs.

M-MODE

A small hand-held transducer is used to transmit ultrasound through the heart at 1000 pulses per second. Between pulses, the transducer functions as a receiver for the returning echo. The returning echoes are displayed on an oscilloscope screen in the order of their depth in the chest from the transducer face. The echo signals are transmitted onto light-sensitive paper by a cathode ray tube, which results in a linear printout of the moving cardiac echoes.

M-mode has excellent resolution, and the distances between various echo signals are very accurate. Therefore, one use of M-mode echocardiography is to measure the dimensions of various cardiac chambers. Hypertrophy of the walls of the chambers, especially the left ventricle, can be readily detected. The technique will also detect any separation between the epicardium and pericardium due to pericardial effusion. M-mode echocardiography can assess valvular anatomy and function.

TWO-DIMENSIONAL

M-mode echocardiography has a narrow beam width that results in poor lateral resolution. Two-dimensional echocardiography provides an image of large segments of the heart in real-time. These tomographic-type images are produced by a fan-shaped ultrasound beam that can be angled through the heart from a number of planes. This technique provides a true anatomical picture of the heart along the tomographic planes cut by the broad ultrasound beam (Fig. 38-4). Thus, both the size and the shape of various cardiac chambers can be appreciated. Most new instruments combine both two-dimensional and M-mode

Fig. 38-4. Two-dimensional echocardiograph of all four cardiac chambers taken from an apical transducer position (*top*) and demonstrating the diastolic position of the mitral valve leaflets. Note the intraventricular septum separating the two ventricles. (*LA*, left atrium; *LV*, left ventricle; *mv*, mitral valve (*arrow* on anterior leaflet); *RA*, right atrium; *RV*, right ventricle.)

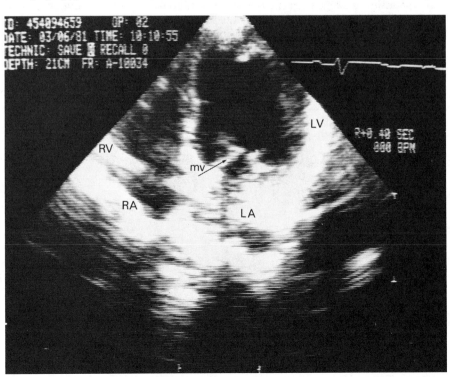

echocardiography into one unit because of the separate advantages and disadvantages of each system. Besides providing a representative picture of cardiac anatomy with respect to its overall structure, two-dimensional echocardiography is useful in detecting abnormalities of the valves, structure, and motion; monitoring prosthetic valve performance after surgery; detecting intracardiac shunting; and evaluating overall ventricular functional performance.

NUCLEAR MEDICINE TECHNIQUES

Recent advances in radiopharmaceuticals, instrumentation, and computer technology have resulted in the development of nuclear medicine techniques that may be applied to a large number of clinical problems. Currently, there are three major areas of cardiac nuclear imaging: radionuclide angiography, myocardial perfusion imaging, and myocardial infarction imaging.

RADIONUCLIDE ANGIOGRAPHY

After the intravenous administration of a radioisotope that is designed to stay in the blood pool, a gamma camera detects the radiation emitted from the isotope within the cardiac chambers (Fig. 38-5). A computer generates time—activity curves for each cardiac structure, and these curves show the change in counts that occurs with each cardiac cycle. From this change in counts, the ejection fraction of the chamber can be calculated. By using an ECG gating technique, images can be built up for end-diastole and end-systole, allowing an analysis of segmental wall motion. Radionuclide angiography can be performed during exercise to detect wall motion abnormalities induced by myocardial ischemia. Valvular regurgitation and pulmonary/systemic flow ratios can be quantitated.

MYOCARDIAL PERFUSION IMAGING

The preferred agent for myocardial perfusion imaging is ^{201}Tl, a potassium analogue that enters viable cells. Coronary artery perfusion defects can be demonstrated by a lack of uptake of isotope. A defect on thallium scanning occurs in myocardial infarction. Exercise-induced ischemia is demonstrated by injecting the isotope during exercise and imaging immediately afterward. Exercise thallium augments the diagnostic value of the exercise ECG test. When the

exercise ECG is combined with thallium perfusion studies, sensitivity for the detection of coronary artery disease is approximately 90%.

MYOCARDIAL INFARCTION IMAGING

Technetium-labeled pyrophosphate administered intravenously concentrates in areas of recent myocardial infarction. This concentration is maximum at 24 to 48 hours and diminishes after 5 to 7 days. This agent will accumulate in the bony thorax and calcified areas of the heart. Therefore, a positive pyrophosphate image is not specific for myocardial infarction. The technique is also useful for detecting myocardial contusion due to trauma.

CARDIAC CATHETERIZATION AND ANGIOGRAPHY

Cardiac catheterization provides information about the pressures and oxygen content of the blood in different chambers and can be used to deliver indicators for calculation of cardiac output. Angiography provides visualization of structural detail. Therefore, catheterization and angiography define the functional status and anatomy of the heart and great vessels.

CARDIAC CATHETERIZATION

Cardiac catheterization is performed under local anesthesia using either an arm or leg artery and vein. This may be done either percutaneously or by a cutdown. The catheters are guided under fluoroscopic control with continuous pressure monitoring. The right heart can be catheterized without fluoroscopic guidance using a balloon-tipped catheter and continuous pressure monitoring. This type catheter will lodge in a pulmonary artery and give the pulmonary capillary wedge pressure, which reflects left atrial pressure. When the balloon is deflated, pulmonary artery pressure is measured and blood can be sampled from the pulmonary artery. Also, an indicator can be delivered for measuring cardiac output by the indicator dilution technique. This procedure can be done at the bedside or in the operating room. Complications of right heart catheterization are rare but include dysrhythmias; clots on the catheter, which cause pulmonary embolization; and perforation of thin right-sided cardiac chambers. The catheters have multiple ports for pressure or blood sampling and include a pacing electrode.

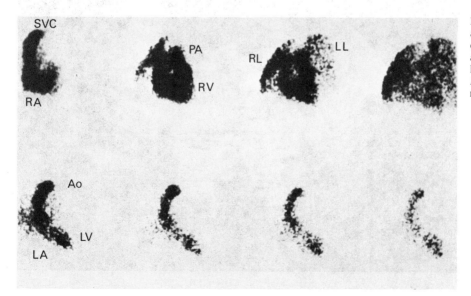

Fig. 38-5. Sequential radionuclide angiogram of the heart from a peripheral venous injection of isotope (*Ao,* aorta; *LA* left atrium; *LL,* left lung; *LV,* left ventricle; *PA,* pulmonary artery; *RA,* right atrium; *RL,* right lung; *RV,* right ventricle; *SVC,* superior vena cava)

Left heart catheterization usually is performed by a retrograde catheter from the aorta across the aortic valve into the left ventricle. The complications of left heart catheterization include dysrhythmias and systemic emboli.

Derivative of Pressure Pulses
The first derivative of ventricular pressure (dP/dt) from the early part of systole, before the semilunar valves open, is a measure of the contractile state of the myocardium. Patients with left ventricular disease have values below 1200 torr/second. This is elevated by agents that improve contractility.

Cardiac Output
The two most common methods used to measure cardiac output are the Fick and indicator dilution methods. The Fick principle states that the rate at which a substance distributed in a fluid is delivered by a moving stream is equal to the product of the flow rate and the concentration difference of the substance at the proximal and distal sampling sites. The direct Fick technique uses oxygen as the substance and assumes that at rest the oxygen uptake in the lungs is equal to that used by the body tissues. A completely mixed venous sample is used from the pulmonary artery and is compared with systemic arterial oxygen content. Oxygen uptake (qO_2) is measured by analysis of a 3-minute collection of expired air, and cardiac output (co) is calculated as follows:

$$co = \frac{qO_2}{Ca - Cv}$$

where Ca equals arterial oxygen content and Cv equals venous content.

With the indicator dilution method, a substance is injected and its concentration measured downstream. The two most commonly used agents are indocyanine green and cold sterile fluids. A balloon-tipped catheter with a proximal port in the right atrium and a thermistor for measuring temperature change at the distal tip is used for thermal dilution cardiac outputs. This method can be used in the operating room or intensive care unit.

Resistance Calculation
From flow measurements and the pressure difference across a vascular bed, resistance can be estimated by a simple formula that ignores vessel length and blood viscosity. Since resistance is directly proportional to the pressure drop and inversely proportional to the rate of flow, pulmonary vascular resistance (PVR) would be calculated as follows:

$$PVR = \frac{PAP - LAP}{co}$$

where PAP equals mean pulmonary artery pressure, LAP equals mean left atrial pressure (pulmonary capillary wedge pressure), and co equals cardiac output.

Valve Orifice Calculation
The severity of a stenotic lesion can be estimated from the pressure gradient. When cardiac output is elevated or reduced, this relationship is altered. Also, heart rate is important because the length of systole in relation to diastole increases as heart rate increases. The hydraulic formula of Gorlin states that the orifice area is directly proportional to the rate of flow and inversely proportional to the square root of the pressure gradient. This relationship is different from the resistance formula because of kinetic energy losses across a stenotic orifice.

Circulatory Shunts
Angiography detects circulatory shunts, but indicator techniques are useful for quantitating their magnitude. Oxygen content is sampled in various chambers (upstream method), or an indicator dye is injected in selected chambers (downstream sampling method); the Fick principle can then be used to calculate the pulmonary and systemic flow (not equal in this situation) and derive their flow ratio.

CARDIAC ANGIOGRAPHY

Once catheters have been positioned, radiopaque contrast material can be delivered to any chamber and the images recorded on x-ray still frames or cine film. Left ventricular cineangiography is used to assess size and performance. The left ventricular volumes at end-diastole and end-systole are calculated, and their difference is the stroke volume. Stroke volume divided by end-diastolic volume is the systolic ejection fraction, an index of ventricular performance. Ejection fraction values greater than 0.5 are normal. Angiographic stroke volume minus forward stroke volume (cardiac output divided by heart rate) equals the amount of aortic or mitral regurgitation. An end-diastolic volume measurement greater than 170 ml or 90 ml/M² body surface area indicates left ventricular dilatation.

Selective coronary artery angiography has provided the ability to accurately define the pathologic anatomy of the coronary arteries. A catheter is advanced retrograde into the orifice of the coronary artery for contrast injection (Fig. 38-6). The mortality rate of coronary arteriography is less than 0.005%, and the morbidity rate is approximately 4%. Coronary arteriography provides accurate anatomical information but very little functional data. For this purpose, ECG exercise testing, with or without thallium imaging, is more useful. Also, an analysis of segmental wall motion on radionuclide or contrast angiography during exercise often is helpful. Perfusion defects or abnormalities in segmental wall motion during exercise, in areas supplied by the diseased coronary artery, would attest to the functional significance of the coronary lesion.

PUMP OXYGENATOR

During cardiopulmonary bypass, all venous blood returning to the heart is diverted into the pump oxygenator by cannulas in the right atrium or venae cavae. There it is oxygenated, cooled or rewarmed, filtered, and pumped back into the arterial tree through a cannula in the ascending aorta or femoral artery. This allows the surgeon to work inside a quiet, bloodless heart. The first successful clinical use of a pump oxygenator for cardiopulmonary bypass was by Gibbon on May 6, 1953. His patient had an atrial septal defect and survived this historical first operation. As with many advances, this was only the final application of knowledge and techniques developed by many other investigators. Individual organs had already been sustained outside of the body by external perfusion techniques before the turn of the century. Others had performed experiments to prove that blood could be oxygenated by foaming techniques and, later, by coating a rotating cylinder with a fine film of blood. Perhaps the most significant advance was the discovery of heparin by Howell and Holt in 1918, without which no form of extracorporeal circulation would be possible. The development of the pump oxygenator for cardiopulmonary bypass has made possible a wide variety of intracardiac operations that are performed routinely in thousands of

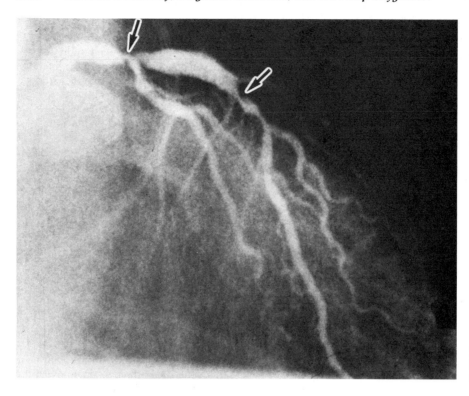

Fig. 38-6. Selective left coronary artery cineangiogram demonstrating two severe obstructions (*arrows*).

hospitals around the world. The following paragraphs outline the individual components of the pump oxygenator and the problems in operative and postoperative care. The state of the art is evolving rapidly.

PUMPS

Almost all heart–lung machines use a roller pump that was first described by DeBakey in 1934. A constantly rotating arm, with a roller on either end, compresses a large-caliber plastic tube to propel blood. Blood flow is dependent upon the diameter of the tubing, which remains constant, and the rate of revolution of the rotating arm. The roller pump is used in almost all modern heart–lung machines for unidirectional blood flow. It has the advantage of simplicity and safety but the disadvantage of nonpulsatile flow. Attempts have been made to provide pulsatile flow from the

heart–lung machine generally using a piston-driven diaphragm or cylinder to propel blood in and out of a ventricle. Unidirectional flow is provided by inlet and outlet mechanical valves. Pulsatile pumps have the advantage of providing a more physiologic flow but in general are mechanically complex and less reliable than roller pumps. The physiological benefits of pulsatile flow are chiefly in maintaining a normal peripheral vascular resistance. This advantage is generally not significant when the patient is on cardiopulmonary bypass for less than 2 hours.

OXYGENATORS

The purpose of an oxygenator is to oxygenate the blood and expel carbon dioxide to physiologic levels. All oxygenators require that a large surface area of blood be exposed to oxygen. This promotes gas exchange much as the capillary bed in contact with the pulmonary alveoli performs the same function. In the initial oxygenator used by Gibbon, blood flowed over a series of screens while oxygen was forced over the surface of the screens. Next came the rotating drums and helix configuration of Dewall, which also created a thin film of blood exposed to oxygen. Subsequently, a series of rapidly rotating discs were used to increase the blood–oxygen surface area. Most oxygenators today are either of the bubble or of the membrane variety. In a membrane oxygenator, blood is separated from oxygen by thin sheets of plastic. Ideally, the film of blood should be equal to the diameter of the pulmonary capillaries. Theoretically, the membrane equilibrates oxygen and carbon dioxide tension between the gas and blood. The advantage is less hemolysis due to the lack of direct blood and oxygen contact. The disadvantages are its complexity and the fact that blood has to be pumped under pressure across most membrane oxygenators rather than allowing gravity flow. The majority of oxygenators in use today are of the disposable bubble type. Millions of fine bubbles of oxygen are

PUMP OXYGENATOR	
Purpose	Perfuse the body with oxygenated blood during open heart procedures
Components	Roller pump Oxygenator 　Membrane 　Bubble Heat Exchanger Cannulas 　Arterial 　Venous Anticoagulant
Complications	Hemolysis, coagulopathy, respiratory problems

forced through the venous blood returning from the patient, thereby providing a large surface area for gas exchange. One problem is the "foaming" effect, which has required the use of various types of filters to "defoam" the blood before it is returned to the patient. This appears to be relatively well corrected in present oxygenators.

HEAT EXCHANGER

During extracorporeal circulation, blood cools in the tubing exposed to room air temperature. In some ways this is desirable, since total body oxygen consumption decreases approximately 10% for each 1°C decline in body temperature. Thus, hypothermia decreases metabolic needs and minimizes the need for high-velocity blood flow. Today, most open heart operations are performed at 30°C or lower and the blood is rewarmed at the conclusion of the operation. This requires a conduction-type heat exchanger in the extracorporeal circuit to initially cool and then rewarm the blood. A conducting metal is interposed between the blood and a moving column of water that is circulated from a water bath with a controlled temperature. The temperature gradient between the blood and the water should not exceed 10°C, since too-rapid cooling or rewarming will result in peripheral vascular resistance changes, which lead to poor microcirculation flow and arteriovenous shunting. Today, most heat exchangers are built into the oxygenator and require only a water bath for cooling and rewarming the constantly circulating water.

PRIMING SOLUTIONS

Initially, the heart–lung machine was voluminous and required as much as 3 liters to fill the oxygenator, heat exchanger, and tubing. The first attempts at extracorporeal circulation used only fresh heparinized blood to "prime the pump." Subsequently, various combinations of plasma, mannitol, low-molecular-weight dextran, and crystalloid solutions were used. It was soon learned that hemodilution with a balanced saline solution had considerable advantages, such as simplicity, availability, and increased flow in the microcirculation. As the pump oxygenator was further perfected, a priming volume of 1000 ml or less was required and the use of blood in the circuit became unnecessary. Today, virtually all open heart surgery is done with a balanced saline solution prime. Blood components, such as packed red blood cells and fresh frozen plasma, are used as needed at the conclusion of the operation.

TECHNIQUE OF PERFUSION

During cardiopulmonary bypass, all venous blood is diverted from the right side of the heart into the pump oxygenator and returned to the arterial circulation (Fig. 38-7). Typically, two venous cannulas are inserted, using purse-string sutures into the right atrium and then positioned in the inferior and superior venae cavae. The cannulas drain blood into the oxygenator by gravity. Direct suction is not applied to the venous line because of increased hemolysis with negative pressure. Suction is used only to remove blood in the operative field. Following oxygenation, filtering, and heat exchange, the blood is pumped back into the aorta or femoral artery by a roller pump. Both venous and arterial cannulas are connected to the heart–lung machine by clear plastic tubing that has been sterilized in ethylene oxide. All tubing must be scrupulously clean and sterile to prevent infection and pyrogenic reactions. It is essential that all surfaces of the cannulas and the tubing are smooth and have no positive charges that might lead to platelet or fibrin deposition. Stainless steel, glass, silicone rubber, and various nonwettable plastics meet these criteria.

Suction is available to remove excess blood from the operating field and return it to a cardiotomy reservoir and then to the oxygenator, so little or no exogenous blood is needed. This has caused a marked reduction in transfusion reactions and the risk of serum hepatitis. During cardio-

Fig. 38-7. The extracorporeal circulation of blood through the pump oxygenator during cardiopulmonary bypass. All systemic venous blood is diverted from the heart by two cannulas in the venae cavae into the oxygenator. Blood in the operative field is removed by suction and is filtered in a cardiotomy reservoir before passing into the oxygenator. Blood is oxygenated by millions of small bubbles and is cooled or warmed by water circulating through metal tubing in contact with the blood. Blood then flows through a filter, to remove the bubbles, and is propelled by a roller-type arterial pump into the ascending aorta.

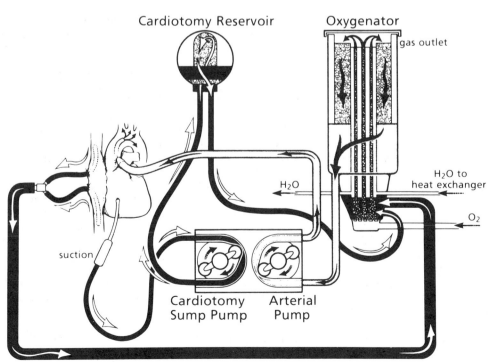

pulmonary bypass, the flow from the pump is maintained in the range of 60 ml/kg in adults and 100 ml to 120 ml/kg in infants and children. Hypothermia reduces the need for these relatively high flows as body temperature declines. Body temperature is measured with temperature probes in various sites, such as the esophagus, nasopharynx, and rectum. Rectal temperature is the best estimate of peripheral tissue temperature and is noted to decline and rise less rapidly than the blood and nasopharyngeal temperature. Coarse filters are used in the cardiotomy reservoir and in the oxygenator to remove microscopic bubbles and particulate matter. The use of filters in the arterial line is debatable, and it is not clear whether the fibrin and platelet aggregates on these filters are created by the filter or removed from the circulation. Prior to inserting the cannulas into the heart, the patient must receive intravenous heparin, 2 or 3 mg/kg. After 1 hour of bypass, 50% of the dose of heparin is repeated. The patient's clotting time is repeatedly checked during the operation.

A great advance in open heart surgery is the use of cold potassium cardioplegic solutions to preserve myocardial function. After total cardiopulmonary bypass has been started, iced saline with 20 mEq to 30 mEq potassium per liter is infused into the ascending aorta to arrest and cool the myocardium. Repeated doses of cardioplegic solution are infused to maintain the myocardial temperature below 20°C and to maintain asystole. This has been shown to preserve the energy substrates and function of the myocardium much better than ventricular fibrillation or anoxic arrest. When the cardiac portion of the operation is finished, the clamp is removed from the ascending aorta so that the heart is once again perfused with blood and myocardial contraction resumes.

TERMINATION OF PERFUSION

At the completion of the cardiac operation, the flow from the heart–lung machine is gradually decreased by partially occluding the gravity flow of blood in the venous line. The lungs are ventilated, and a portion of the venous return then bypasses through the lungs and into the left heart. A brief period of partial bypass is important, to allow the myocardium to slowly recover and to provide pulsatile flow once again to the peripheral circulation. This decreases peripheral vascular resistance and improves the completeness of rewarming peripheral tissues. All flow through the venous cannulas is finally stopped, and the myocardium then carries the full load of the circulation. After all cannulas are removed, the heparin is neutralized with protamine.

Frequently, the myocardium is transiently weakened by the operation and various cardiotonic agents are needed. One or 2 g intravenous calcium chloride is given to neutralize the effects of citrated blood products. Intravenous atropine is used for bradycardia, particularly in patients with coronary artery disease who have been receiving large doses of propranolol. If further stimulation is needed, the drug of choice is dopamine, which provides a β-adrenergic stimulus with little or no increase in peripheral vascular resistance or decrease in renal blood flow. If this is insufficient, a dilute drip of epinephrine, 1 mg to 5 mg/500 ml. is slowly infused for its cardiotonic effect and nitroprusside, 50mg/250 ml, is given to decrease peripheral vascular resistance. Unless there has been a major intraoperative accident or inadequate cooling of the myocardium, these measures are usually sufficient.

Physiological monitoring consists of an arterial pressure line plus a Swan–Ganz catheter to measure pulmonary artery and wedge pressures and cardiac output by thermodilution. With the use of intravenous cardiotonic agents such as dopamine and epinephrine and the unloading agents such as nitroprusside or nitroglycerin, it is possible to "fine tune" the cardiac output. If further circulatory support is needed, an intra-aortic balloon is inserted through a femoral artery or the ascending aorta and positioned so that the balloon is in the descending aorta. The balloon is alternately inflated and deflated, as triggered by the ECG, so that it inflates during diastole and deflates during systole. Deflation of the balloon allows myocardial contraction to occur during a low resistance phase, and inflation maintains an increased diastolic pressure, which promotes coronary blood flow. Finally, pacemaker wires may be attached to the heart. Direct ventricular stimulation is reliable, but the lack of atrial synchronous contraction causes a 20% to 25% loss of cardiac output. An atrial pacemaker wire increases the heart rate and provides atrioventricular sequential contraction with an improved cardiac output.

SPECIFIC COMPLICATIONS

The risk of cardiopulmonary bypass alone is minimal. The mortality and morbidity are related almost entirely to the underlying disease and the operation. Cardiopulmonary bypass *per se* results in some hemolysis due to red blood cell trauma. This is rarely significant, and the free hemoglobin is rapidly cleared by the kidneys. With too-rapid cooling by the heat exchanger, there is an increase in peripheral vascular resistance and arteriovenous shunting, which results in inadequate perfusion of the peripheral tissues and metabolic acidosis. Excessive perfusion flow may result in cerebral edema. Rarely, the arterial cannulation may result in an acute aortic dissection. There is invariably some decrease in the serum oncotic pressure due to hemodilution, leading to mild pulmonary edema and respiratory insufficiency; this is treated with diuretics and mechanical ventilation.

Postoperative bleeding is a frequent problem. Heparin is a small molecule that freely equilibrates with the extracellular fluid and remains active for several hours. Protamine has a short duration of action and is a large molecule that remains in the vascular tree. Thus, the protamine neutralizes only the heparin that is in the vascular tree, and repeated small doses or a drip of protamine may be required for several hours to neutralize the heparin that slowly leeches back into the circulation. Due to hemodilution and defibrination, the plasma clotting factors are frequently reduced. This is treated with fresh frozen plasma and, occasionally, with platelets.

Arrhythmias are also frequent and troublesome. Ventricular irritability is counteracted by maintaining high levels of serum potassium and with intravenous lidocaine (Xylocaine) or procainamide (Pronestyl). Sinus bradycardia is treated first with atropine and then with either isoproterenol (Isuprel) or dopamine. Refractory bradycardia may require the use of external atrial or ventricular pacing wires. Tachyarrhythmias may be diagnosed by use of the atrial electrodes left on the right atrium, and specific arrhythmias may be terminated by use of rapid atrial pacing.

Respiratory insufficiency is generally transient and may be treated with small doses of intravenous furosemide (Lasix). All postoperative patients are on mechanical ventilation with at least 5 cm of positive end-expiratory pressure to maintain an adequate functional residual volume and to reduce pulmonary edema due to a low serum oncotic pressure. Renal failure is uncommon when adequate cardiac output and renal blood flow are maintained. Occasionally, small doses of intravenous Lasix or mannitol may be used to correct fluid overload caused by hemodilution from the priming solution. If the patient is oliguric, a small sample of urine is analyzed for sodium and urea content. If tubular function is intact and the oliguria is due to low cardiac output, the urine sodium should be below 40 mEq/liter and the urine/blood urea ratio should be above 10.

Temperature elevation in the postoperative period is undesirable because of the increase in total-body oxygen consumption, particularly when accompanied by shivering. This is treated vigorously with steroids, a cooling mattress, and sedation to block shivering. Patients occasionally have cerebral dysfunction postoperatively. During cardiopulmonary bypass, it is important to maintain not only blood oxygenation but also adequate levels of carbon dioxide, since a pCO_2 below 20 torr may lead to inadequate cerebral perfusion. Other cerebral insults include air bubbles from the oxygenator or air that has been left inside the heart during the operative procedure. Occasionally, flecks of calcium from a badly calcified valve may remain in the heart to embolize later. Postoperative convulsions, although rare, should be treated vigorously with intravenous diazepam (Valium), barbiturates, or phenytoin (Dilantin) to prevent further cerebral insult and hypoxia. Occasionally, patients will undergo a postoperative psychosis, or "ICU syndrome," due to disorientation. The precise etiology of this syndrome is obscure but may be related to sleep deprivation and lack of orientation as to time and place in an environment without windows in which there is constant light and noise.

Upper gastrointestinal tract bleeding occurs periodically but is usually associated only with systemic sepsis. Patients who are suspected of being septic or who have been on the ventilator for prolonged periods should be treated with hourly antacids through a nasogastric tube. Some degree of anemia is common in the postoperative period, due to hemodilution, hemolysis, and a decreased red blood cell survival time. Since the reticuloendothelial system is overwhelmed with iron stores from hemolysis during cardiopulmonary bypass, this is generally self-correcting. Rebound hypertension may occur and is treated with intravenous nitroprusside, trinitroglycerin, or methyldopa (Aldomet) to decrease the workload on the recovering heart.

Today, the above complications of cardiopulmonary bypass are rare. Those of us who grew up with the evolution of the pump oxygenator became more adept at treating complications than performing the operations. The speed and simplicity of setting up the heart–lung machine for cardiopulmonary bypass are such that the risk is minimal. The postoperative monitoring techniques are likewise sophisticated.

BIBLIOGRAPHY

ANSON BJ, MCVAY CB: Surgical Anatomy, Vol 1. Philadelphia, W B Saunders, 1971

AREY LB: Developmental Anatomy. Philadelphia, W B Saunders, 1954

BRASH JC: Cunningham's Manual of Practical Anatomy, Vol 2, Thorax and Abdomen. New York, Oxford University Press, 1952

BRAUNWALD E (ed): Heart Disease: A Textbook of Cardiovascular Medicine. Philadelphia, W B Saunders, 1980

FAVALORA RG, EFFLER DR: Surgical Treatment of Coronary Arteriosclerosis. Baltimore, Williams & Wilkins, 1970

GIBBON JH, JR, SABISTON DC, JR, SPENCER FC (eds): Surgery of the Chest. Philadelphia, W B Saunders, 1969

GRAY SW, SKANDALAKIS JE: Embryology for Surgeons. Philadelphia, W B Saunders, 1972

HOLLINSHEAD WH: Anatomy for Surgeons, Vol 2. New York, Harper & Row, 1971

ISSELBADRER KJ, ADAMS RD, BRAUNWALD E et al: Harrison's Principles of Internal Medicine. New York, McGraw-Hill, 1980

KUBIIK S: Surgical Anatomy of the Thorax. Philadelphia, W B Saunders, 1970

MARRIOTT HJL: Practical Electrocardiography. Baltimore, Williams & Wilkins, 1977

NETTER FH: The CIBA Collection of Medical Illustrations, Vol 5, Heart. Summit, NJ, Ciba Pharmaceutical, 1969

Fred A. Crawford, Jr./John W. Hammon, Jr.

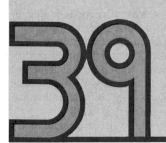

Congenital Heart Disease

Surgical correction of congenital heart defects began in 1938 with the ligation of a patent ductus arteriosus (PDA) by Robert Gross. While simple intracardiac defects could be approached with other techniques, the development of the pump oxygenator by Gibbon in 1953 made possible correction of more complex defects. Since that time, congenital heart surgery has continually evolved, and, at present, there are only a few defects that cannot be either palliated or totally corrected.

Congenital heart defects are present in approximately 8 of 1000 live births. If untreated, more than one third of these may be fatal in the first year of life. The relatively stable incidence makes it possible to predict, for a given population, the number of children requiring catheterization and surgery, thus making long-range planning for appropriate care more feasible than with many other problems.

The etiology of most congenital heart defects is unknown. Most seem to be multifactorial (*i.e.,* a combination of genetic and environmental influences). Some chromosomal abnormalities have a high incidence of associated heart defects, such as atrioventricular canal in Down's syndrome, coarctation in Turner's syndrome, and pulmonary stenosis and atrial septal defect in Noonan's syndrome. Maternal rubella is known to result in an increased incidence of congenital heart disease, primarily PDA and pulmonary stenosis. Infants with other congenital defects tend to have an increased incidence of cardiac defects.

The diagnosis of congenital heart disease is based on a careful history and physical examination, chest film, electrocardiogram, echocardiogram, and cardiac catheterization. Obviously, the presentation of congenital heart disease may vary tremendously in each of the above categories. Some infants with congenital heart disease are obviously abnormal at birth. In others, including some with severe complex defects, the abnormality may not be discovered until the time of routine examination as adolescents or even adults. Careful physical examination is extremely useful in diagnosis. Chest film will demonstrate abnormal size, shape, and position of the heart, along with normal, increased, or decreased pulmonary blood flow. Electrocardiography is particularly helpful in many defects. The most recent improvement in diagnostic technique involves echocardiography, both M-mode and two-dimensional. The use of this technique allows for determination of size, shape, and function of the different cardiac chambers; the relationship of the great vessels; and valve anatomy and function and allows for delineation of specific defects such as ventricular septal defect (VSD). In the near future, echocardiography may permit appropriate surgical therapy in some patients without the need for catheterization. Cardiac catheterization permits measurement of pressures and oxygen saturation in each cardiac chamber and in the great vessels. Thus, pressure gradients between chambers may be determined. By using standard formulas and this information, the magnitude of shunts may be determined, as well as cardiac index and systemic and pulmonary vascular resistance. The latter is particularly important when predicting operability in children with pulmonary vascular disease. Cineangiocardiography permits definition of the anatomy of the cardiac chambers and valves as well as the location and specific anatomy of particular defects.

The medical management of congenital heart disease depends upon the defect and the degree of symptoms. Some children may require no specific therapy initially (*e.g.*, those with atrial septal defect), while others with severe congenital heart failure in infancy may require intense management with diuretics, digitalis, and afterload reduction. The most significant recent change in medical management has been the knowledge of the relationship between the ductus arteriosus and prostaglandins. In neonates with PDA and congestive heart failure, the use of prostaglandin inhibitors such as indomethacin has resulted in a significant number of ductal closures. Indomethacin has certain toxic side-effects, so this method of treatment must be compared with standard surgical therapy. The infusion of prostaglandin E_1 has been extremely valuable in maintaining or restoring ductal patency in infants with cyanotic congenital heart disease and severely restricted pulmonary blood flow and in those in whom perfusion of the lower body depends upon ductal patency. Frequently, a tentative diagnosis can be made by two-dimensional echocardiography and prostaglandins can be started. This improves peripheral perfusion and tissue oxygenation and prevents progressive metabolic acidosis. The infant can then be catheterized when he is more stable and subsequently referred for surgery under a more elective circumstance and when the patient is in much better overall physical condition. This technique will improve results in newborns with such severe defects.

The surgical management of congenital heart disease may be considered either palliative or corrective. Palliative procedures are generally designed to increase (systemic–pulmonary shunts) or decrease (pulmonary artery banding) pulmonary blood flow. Such procedures may allow one to postpone corrective surgery until the infant is older or may, in some cases, be the only type of surgical help that is available for a particular defect. In general, because of improvement in surgical and anesthetic techniques, the tendency has been in favorable situations to avoid initial palliative procedures and to go ahead with corrective pro-

cedures in infancy. This is discussed further under each defect.

Corrective procedures are designed to return anatomy and function to normal (PDA) or more normal (tetralogy of Fallot) conditions. Some procedures for congenital cardiac problems may be performed without cardiopulmonary bypass (*e.g.*, PDA, coarctation, pulmonary artery banding); these are termed "closed" procedures. Intracardiac defects, on the other hand, require the use of the pump oxygenator and extracorporeal circulation and are termed "open" procedures.

Corrective surgery using cardiopulmonary bypass may be performed at moderate (28°C–32°C) hypothermia or deep (18°C–22°C) hypothermia. The latter technique permits low-flow perfusion or even total circulatory arrest. Total circulatory arrest and profound hypothermia permit better visualization of complex defects in tiny infants but should be used only when necessary. Periods of up to 50 minutes of circulatory arrest are safe at 20°.

Anesthesia for congenital heart surgery is extremely important, especially in infants. Careful attention to detail, insofar as fluid management, temperature, and drugs are concerned, is imperative to obtain good results.

Careful attention to detail is also necessary in the postoperative management of the cardiovascular, respiratory, and renal systems of these patients. Arterial and venous pressures are routinely monitored by indwelling catheters. We frequently leave catheters in the left atrium and pulmonary artery for pressure monitoring and cardiac output determination in the postoperative period. Atrial and ventricular pacing wires may be useful in the diagnosis of various arrhythmias or in the atrial, ventricular, or atrioventricular sequential pacing postoperatively. Cardiac output is routinely monitored and optimized by controlling preload (volume), contractility (inotropic agents), heart rate (pacing), and afterload (vasodilators). Urine output is monitored by an indwelling catheter, which is removed as soon as possible. Residual shunts may be demonstrated by indicator dilution studies in the operating room or intensive care unit. Most patients are maintained on respirators for several hours or overnight and are monitored with arterial blood gases. Patients are extubated as soon as they are awake and hemodynamically stable, with good ventilatory mechanics. While the major contribution to the patient's future welfare is made in the operating room, a dedicated team of physicians and nurses in a specialized care area is necessary to achieve optimal results.

There are several possible classifications of congenital heart defects. We have chosen to present the more common defects in detail, and the less common defects are summarized briefly.

PATENT DUCTUS ARTERIOSUS

The ductus arteriosus is derived from the dorsal portion of the sixth branchial arch. The ductus is almost always on the left side and extends from the ventral portion of the aorta just distal to the left subclavian to the pulmonary artery near its bifurcation (Fig. 39-1, *A*). Even when the aortic arch is on the right, the ductus is usually on the left, joining the innominate artery to the pulmonary artery. The recurrent laryngeal nerve loops around the typical ductus, aiding in its identification. Following spontaneous closure, the ductus persists as a fibrous cord, the ligamentum arteriosum.

PATENT DUCTUS ARTERIOSUS	
History	Harvey described, 1628; Gross surgically corrected, 1938
Incidence	12% to 15% of congenital heart defects
Anatomy	Communication between thoracic aorta and pulmonary artery
Pathophysiology	L → R shunt produces ↑ pulmonary blood flow, pulmonary hypertension
Dx	History: Some patients asymptomatic; congestive heart failure (CHF) in neonates
	Physical exam: Continuous machinery murmur in left chest; bounding peripheral pulses
	ECG: ± left ventricular hypertrophy (LVH)
	Chest film: ↑ heart size; ↑ pulmonary artery; ↑ pulmonary vascularity
	Echo: ↑ left atrium/aorta ratio
	Catheterization: L → R shunt; ± pulmonary hypertension
Rx	Surgical ligation or division
Results	Operative mortality rate < 1%, higher in adults; long-term results excellent

PATHOPHYSIOLOGY

In the fetus, the ductus shunts blood from the pulmonary artery to the aorta, since circulation through the lungs is unnecessary. At birth and following expansion of the lungs, pulmonary vascular resistance falls. In most cases, the ductus begins to close shortly following birth but may not be completely closed for several weeks. Anatomically, the ductus is different from the pulmonary artery and aorta and is responsive to a variety of stimuli, including hypoxia and prostaglandins. In some children with other severe cyanotic congenital heart defects, the resulting hypoxia keeps the ductus open and the duct may, in fact, be the only source of pulmonary blood flow. In premature neonates with immature lungs and respiratory distress, the resulting hypoxia may also keep the ductus open. Finally, in some children—for reasons that are poorly understood—the duct simply remains patent. The net result in all cases is a flow across the ductus from aorta to pulmonary artery creating a left-to-right shunt of variable magnitude, depending upon both the size of the duct and the pulmonary vascular resistance. While this shunt is important to those with cyanotic congenital heart disease, its presence in otherwise normal persons is deleterious. It may well be tolerated for years, but in some it may produce overwhelming congestive heart failure early in life. If a sizable shunt is allowed to persist, pulmonary vascular obstructive changes may result. In time, this will cause progressive pulmonary hypertension and eventually a balanced or net right-to-left shunt that cannot be surgically corrected. Because of this, Shipyro and Keyes estimated that the life expectancy of those with PDA who are alive at age 17 years is approximately one half of the normal expectancy.

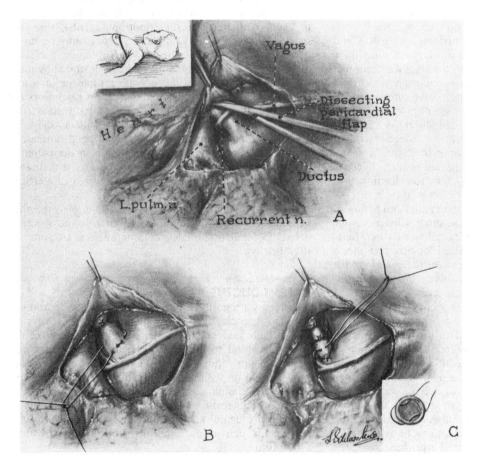

Fig. 39-1. Operative treatment of ductus arteriosus by ligation. (Bahnson HT: In Sabiston DC, Spencer FC (eds): Gibbon's Surgery of the Chest, p 890. Philadelphia, W B Saunders, 1976)

DIAGNOSIS

The history is quite variable. Many patients with uncomplicated PDA are relatively asymptomatic, and the murmur may be first heard at the time of a preschool or some other routine physical examination. However, other children may have significant congestive heart failure early in life. Several years ago this was particularly common in low-birth-weight premature neonates. It still occurs in this group but is much less common because of current vigorous treatment with fluid restriction, digitalis, and diuretics.

PHYSICAL EXAMINATION

The characteristic physical finding in PDA is a continuous, harsh, "machinery" murmur of varying intensity in the second left intercostal space. The diastolic blood pressure may be low due to "runoff" into the pulmonary artery. In neonates, the murmur may be softer and heard only in systole. However, the wide pulse pressure noted above produces bounding peripheral pulses in these children. Other defects that may be confused with PDA because of the continuous murmur include aortopulmonary window (see below); pulmonary, coronary, or other types of arteriovenous communications; and ventricular septal defect with aortic insufficiency.

ELECTROCARDIOGRAPHY

The electrocardiogram may be normal in asymptomatic children with small shunts or may show left ventricular hypertrophy if the shunt is large.

CHEST FILM

The chest film may also be normal in patients with small shunts. If the shunt is large, the heart may be somewhat enlarged and the pulmonary artery will be prominent. There will be increased pulmonary vascularity and, possibly, left ventricular hypertrophy.

ECHOCARDIOGRAPHY

M-mode echocardiography may show left ventricular hypertrophy if present. In larger shunts, the left atrium will be enlarged compared with the aorta. This comparison is frequently useful in attempting to decide if the shunt is increasing or decreasing in neonates. Two-dimensional echocardiography is of little help in the diagnosis of a routine PDA.

CARDIAC CATHETERIZATION

Cardiac catheterization is not mandatory. We do not catheterize those patients whose physical findings and noninvasive workup is typical of PDA, nor do we catheterize premature infants for simple PDA. Catheterization is carried out in any child in whom the findings are atypical or in those in whom other heart defects are suspected in addition to the PDA. A diagnosis can frequently be made by passing the catheter out the pulmonary artery, across the patent ductus, and into the descending aorta. The magnitude of the shunt can be determined by the degree of the step-up in oxygen saturation at the pulmonary artery level. Finally, if dye is injected and cineangiograms are performed, the exact anatomy of the defect can be ascertained.

TREATMENT

In those patients in whom the ductus is the only source of pulmonary blood flow, interruption is obviously not indi-

cated. As mentioned, the ductus arteriosus is responsive to prostaglandins. It has been found that indomethacin may cause ductal closure in a significant number of premature infants, especially if administered in the first few days of life. For the past few years, a nationwide, randomized, prospective trial of indomethacin in these patients has been carried out. Until the data from this study are available, the exact indications for the use of indomethacin in these patients will not be known. If properly performed, surgery in these small infants can be done quite safely. In all other patients, surgery is recommended when a significant ductus is present and when the net shunt is left to right. Surgery may be necessary very early in neonates or in others with severe congestive heart failure. In the asymptomatic patient, we now go ahead with surgery at about age 2 or at the time of diagnosis if it is made at a later age.

In most patients, a small posterolateral thoracotomy in the fourth intercostal space provides adequate exposure. In the adult or if pulmonary artery pressure is elevated or bacterial endocarditis has been documented, a more extensive thoracotomy is preferred because of better exposure of the aorta. The ductus may also be ligated through a median sternotomy incision when repair of an intracardiac defect is being performed simultaneously. Once the chest is opened, the duct is identified and dissected; care is taken to avoid injury to the phrenic and recurrent laryngeal nerves. Meticulous care must be taken to precisely identify the ductus because ligation of the left pulmonary artery and the descending thoracic aorta has been mistakenly carried out at the time of ductal ligation.

The ductus may be obliterated with multiple suture ligatures or divided between appropriate vascular clamps with oversewing of the aorta and pulmonary ends (Figs. 39-1, *B* and *C* and 39-2). Simple ligation is satisfactory in the neonate and may be effectively performed with a

Fig. 39-2. Operative technique for division and suture of the patent ductus. (Hardy JD, Webb WR, Timmis HH, et al: Patent ductus arteriosus: Operative treatment of 100 consecutive patients with isolated lesions without mortality. Ann Surg 164:877, 1966)

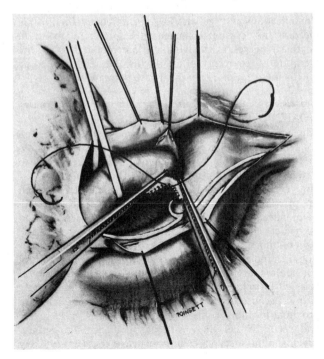

hemoclip. If the ductus is part of a vascular ring, division of the ductus is mandatory to interrupt the ring. A trial occlusion of the ductus may be indicated when the pulmonary artery pressure is elevated. A decrease in pulmonary artery pressure with a simultaneous increase in systemic pressure during trial occlusion indicates that the interruption may be safely performed. It may also be helpful at times to temporarily reduce the arterial pressure with sodium nitroprusside or other agents as the vascular clamps are applied or as the ductus is ligated. Meticulous attention to detail is necessary to achieve results in the premature infant comparable to those in other patients. While some have advocated carrying out the operation in the neonatal intensive care unit, we have routinely performed the operation in the standard operating room. During transportation and surgery, the temperature must be carefully regulated. Careful anesthetic management, especially in regard to fluid administration, is extremely important. The operation should be performed as rapidly as is safely possible. Continuing attention to detail in the postoperative period with regard to respiratory and fluid management is equally important.

RESULTS

In the uncomplicated patient, the operative risk should be less than 1%. In the adult or the patient with pulmonary hypertension, the risk may be somewhat greater. Several recent series have indicated that ductus interruption can be performed in the premature infant with a very low operative mortality. However, a significant number of these small infants are not long-term survivors because of problems related to prematurity, such as continued respiratory failure, necrotizing enterocolitis, and intracerebral bleeding. In those with congestive heart failure, there may be a dramatic improvement almost immediately, with a decrease in pulmonary vascularity and heart size. When the reason for surgery is continued respiratory distress, a good response may also be seen. While some infants maintained on prolonged respiratory support may promptly be weaned from the respirator, the overall results are not as good in this group of infants as in those with congestive heart failure. Complications of surgery for PDA are infrequent but include bleeding and occasional damage to the phrenic and recurrent laryngeal nerves. Although there are rare reports in the literature of recurrence of the ductus, the relief granted by ductus interruption is nearly always permanent.

AORTOPULMONARY WINDOW

The aortopulmonary window or septal defect is a rare congenital defect. Since the first surgical correction by Gross in 1952, approximately 50 patients have been reported to have undergone surgical correction. The defect exists as a large communication, 1 cm to 3 cm in diameter, between the proximal portion of the ascending aorta and the main pulmonary artery. A second type has been described to occur between the more distal aorta and the origin of the right pulmonary artery (Fig. 39-3). The defect is felt to result from incomplete fusion of the conotruncal ridge in the distal aortopulmonary septum. The result of this communication is a left-to-right shunt from the aorta to the pulmonary artery. Because of the large size of the defect and its more proximal location, congestive heart failure is more severe and occurs earlier than with patent ductus. For similar reasons, pulmonary vascular obstructive changes are likely

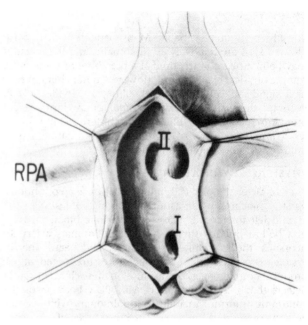

Fig. 39-3. Classification of aortopulmonary septal defects. Type I defects are located superior to the sinus of Valsalva and in close proximity to the left coronary artery. Type II defects are located more distal in the ascending aorta and open into the origin of the right pulmonary artery (*RPA*). (Doty DB et al: Aortopulmonary septal defect: Hemodynamics, angiography, and operation. Ann Thorac Surg 32:244, 1981)

to develop earlier. Doty found such changes in seven of nine patients before the age of 2. Physical examination will reveal a loud continuous murmur over the precordium and wide pulse pressures. The electrocardiogram is more likely to show left ventricular hypertrophy. Heart size may be enlarged on x-ray, and there will be evidence of increased pulmonary blood flow. Two-dimensional echocardiography may show the communication, but this is demonstrated most conclusively by cardiac catheterization. Because of the severity of congestive heart failure and pulmonary vascular changes, surgery should be recommended for all patients with this defect. Gross's first patient was treated with ligation, but this is impossible in all but the smallest of defects. Early surgical attempts also included division of the communication between vascular clamps. Currently, correction is best carried out using cardiopulmonary bypass with closure of the defect using a prosthetic patch from within the aorta. In a unique combined series of 25 patients from the United States and the USSR, Doty reported an overall survival rate of 80%.

COARCTATION OF THE AORTA

Coarctation occurs most often in the thoracic aorta but rarely is present in the abdominal aorta. The opening may be quite small, and in as many as 25% of patients, the aorta may be atretic at the point of coarctation. In more severe forms, the aortic arch may be completely interrupted and flow to the lower half of the body is by way of a PDA.

Coarctations have been classified as infant, or preductal, and adult, or postductal (Fig. 39-4). It has been suggested, however, that these terms are overlapping and not precise and that a more accurate division would be discrete coarctation (corresponding to adult or postductal) and diffuse

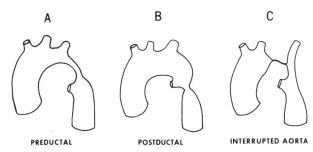

Fig. 39-4. Representative anatomical types of coarctation of the aorta. (Hardy JD: Coarctation of the aorta. In Hardy JD [ed]: Rhoads Textbook of Surgery, 5th ed. Philadelphia, J B Lippincott, 1977)

coarctation (corresponding to infant or preductal). Discrete coarctations are well localized just distal to the left subclavian artery near the entrance of the ductus arteriosus and are not commonly associated with other intracardiac defects except bicuspid aortic valves, which may occur in 50%. Discrete coarctations may give difficulty with heart failure in infancy, but this is uncommon. When heart failure does occur, it usually responds well to medical therapy and does

COARCTATION	
History	Morgagni described, 1760; Gross and Huffnagel, Craaford and Nylin corrected, 1945
Incidence	6% of all congenital heart disease
Anatomy	Discrete (adult, postductal): localized narrowing of descending aorta; diffuse (infant, preductal): may involve entire aortic arch and descending aorta
Pathophysiology	Produces obstruction to blood flow and left ventricular pressure overload; upper extremity hypertension results
Dx	History: May be asymptomatic; headaches; ↑ fatigability; ↓ growth; CHF Physical exam: upper extremity hypertension; ↓ lower extremity pulses; ± CHF; ± differential cyanosis ECG: Right ventricular hypertrophy (RVH) in infants; LVH in older children Chest film: LVH; "3" sign; ± rib notching Echo: bicuspid aortic valve; LVH Catheterization: gradient across coarct; location and type of coarct; associated cardiac defects
Rx	Repair by end-to-end anastomosis, patch aortoplasty, or subclavian flap technique
Results	Operative mortality rate <5% in older children; may be 25% in infants with associated defects; long-term results good but hypertension not always relieved

not require urgent surgery. Diffuse coarctations may result in a narrowing of the entire aortic arch (tubular hypoplasia) as well as a narrowing distal to the left subclavian artery. Sixty percent of patients with diffuse coarctation will have other intracardiac defects. Approximately half of these will be simple (ventricular septal defect, PDA), and half will be more complex. As a result, diffuse coarctations are more likely to cause severe congestive heart failure in infancy, which in turn may not respond well to medical therapy.

As a result of the obstruction produced by the coarctation, collateral vessels around the coarctation are well developed. The collateral flow occurs through enlarged internal mammary, intercostal, subscapular, and other arteries. These vessels may be markedly enlarged and thin walled and may form aneurysms. Such aneurysms may rupture spontaneously, and even in the absence of aneurysm formation, these large, thin-walled vessels are easily damaged at the time of surgical correction of the coarctation.

The etiology of coarctation is unknown. One theory holds that closure of the ductus arteriosus may extend into the aorta and result in localized narrowing. Another theory suggests that coarctation is related to patterns of blood flow in the fetus. Evidence exists to support both of these concepts, and in fact both may be operative in the development of coarctation.

PATHOPHYSIOLOGY

The net effect of coarctation, either diffuse or discrete, is to produce obstruction to blood flow out of the left ventricle and to the lower half of the body. Upper extremity hypertension develops, but again the exact etiology is unclear. The hypertension is in part due to obstruction to blood flow, but it also appears to be related to renal factors, perhaps because of the changes in flow characteristics to the kidney produced by the obstruction. Experimental data related to the etiology of hypertension in coarctation have recently been summarized by Scott, one of the original investigators in this area. It should be noted that coarctation represents one of the surgically correctable forms of hypertension and that surgery appears to be more successful when the coarctation is repaired at an early age.

As indicated, discrete coarctation usually does not produce difficulty in infancy and may be discovered in asymptomatic persons on routine examinations later in life. Hypertension is common in these patients. Despite the fact that the persons are asymptomatic early in life, overall life span is significantly reduced to an average of approximately 34 years in one study. Common causes of death include complications of bicuspid aortic valves, bacterial endocarditis, and bleeding from intrathoracic or intracerebral aneurysms. Diffuse coarctations usually produce severe congestive heart failure shortly following birth and may not respond to the usual medical measures. Mortality is extremely high in infancy in this group of patients, particularly those with associated defects.

DIAGNOSIS: THORACIC AORTA

Some patients with coarctation are completely asymptomatic. Others complain of headaches, lower extremity weakness (particularly with exercise), chest pain, and fatigability. As indicated, infants with diffuse coarctation may present shortly following birth with manifestations of severe congestive heart failure, including tachypnea, poor growth, and respiratory infection.

PHYSICAL EXAMINATION

The hallmark of the physical examination for coarctation is upper extremity hypertension associated with absent or diminished lower extremity pulses and lower extremity hypotension. In the older child with discrete coarctation, a systolic murmur may be present over the back and a thrill may be palpable in the suprasternal notch. In the infant with diffuse coarctation, these murmurs may be absent and the physical findings consistent with other associated defects may predominate. The usual findings of congestive heart failure, tachypnea, hepatomegaly, and ventricular gallop may be present. In patients in whom the origin of the left subclavian artery is involved in the coarctation, there may be no difference between left arm and lower extremity blood pressure. In patients with complete interruption of the aorta at the site of coarctation and in whom lower extremity flow is by way of a patent ductus, there may be differential cyanosis, with the head and upper extremities appearing pink and well perfused and the abdomen and lower extremities appearing cyanotic.

ELECTROCARDIOGRAPHY

In infants with diffuse coarctation and congestive heart failure, right ventricular hypertrophy dominates. In older children with long-standing hypertension, left ventricular hypertrophy is more common.

CHEST FILM

In infants with diffuse coarctation and congestive heart failure, the heart is enlarged and the lung fields are congested. In the older patient, concentric left ventricular hypertrophy is apparent. Because of the hourglass configuration of the aorta in the region of the coarctation, a "3" sign may be apparent on routine chest film, and a reverse "3" sign may be apparent on barium swallow. In children over the age of 8 or 10 years, rib notching, particularly in the third through eighth ribs, may be apparent.

ECHOCARDIOGRAPHY

M-mode echocardiography may not be useful except for defining other defects such as bicuspid aortic valves. Two-dimensional echocardiography will demonstrate the bicuspid aortic valve, other associated defects, and left ventricular function and in some cases may be successful in defining the anatomy of the coarctation.

CARDIAC CATHETERIZATION

Cardiac catheterization is necessary in all patients to define precisely the location of the coarctation, involvement of other vessels such as the left subclavian, and any other intracardiac defects. The gradient across the coarctation can be determined. The adequacy of the collateral circulation around the coarctation can also be determined.

TREATMENT

A true coarctation in a child or adult is an indication for surgery, because of the markedly diminished life span of those patients who go untreated. In past years, surgery was delayed somewhat in asymptomatic children until they reached the age of 10 or 12 years, so that an end-to-end anastomosis might be performed with less chance of resten-osis. It has recently been pointed out that the successful relief of hypertension is more likely to occur in patients treated prior to the age of 6, and accordingly we are currently recommending surgical correction in asymptomatic patients just prior to beginning school. On the other hand, in infants with severe congestive heart failure secondary to coarctation, surgery may be necessary as an emergency lifesaving measure.

At the present time, several techniques are available for surgical correction of coarctation. All of these techniques require excellent exposure of the thoracic aorta; this is best obtained through a generous posterolateral thoracotomy incision through the fourth intercostal space. In making this incision, meticulous care must be paid to hemostasis; bleeding from enlarged collateral vessels can be quite profuse. Until recently, most coarctations were repaired by resection and end-to-end anastomosis. In this technique, the ligamentum arteriosum (or patent ductus) is divided, and the aorta and coarctation are mobilized. Vascular clamps are applied proximal and distal to the coarctation, and the area of involvement is completely resected. An end-to-end anastomosis is then performed without tension, using either interrupted or continuous sutures (Fig. 39-5). If the area of coarctation is long, or in adults or older children with a less mobile aorta, it may be necessary to insert a prosthetic graft to bridge the gap between the ascending aorta and the descending aorta (Fig. 39-6). While this technique seems to work perfectly well in older children and adults, it does appear to be associated with a higher incidence of restenosis or recoarctation, particularly when it is used in infants and younger children.

Two additional approaches to coarctation repair have been advocated because of these problems with residual gradients and recurrent coarctation, particularly when the operation is done in infants. Waldhausen and others have advocated the subclavian flap approach. In this technique, the subclavian artery is divided distally, split along its inferior margin, and sutured down to an incision through the coarctation as a patch graft. Because this is a living patch, it continues to grow, and it is felt that this technique results in a decreased incidence of restenosis. The second technique is somewhat similar in that an incision is made through the anterior wall of the coarctation and into the aorta above and below it. Any residual webs or membranes within the aorta are resected, and then an overly generous patch of prosthetic material is sutured into place with continuous sutures. It is obvious that such prosthetic material will not grow, but by making the patch larger than necessary, it is felt that no gradient will occur across it as the child grows. An advantage of the latter technique is that the subclavian artery is not sacrificed. At the present time, both of the two

Fig. 39-5. Repair of coarctation by resection and end-to-end anastomosis. (Hardy JD: Coarctation of the aorta. In Hardy JD [ed]: Rhoads Textbook of Surgery, 5th ed. Philadelphia, J B Lippincott, 1977)

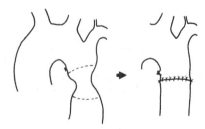

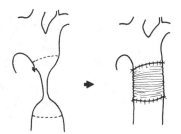

Fig. 39-6. Repair of coarctation by resection and insertion of a prosthetic graft. (Hardy JD: Coarctation of the aorta. In Hardy JD [ed]: Rhoads Textbook of Surgery, 5th ed. Philadelphia, J B Lippincott, 1977)

latter techniques are being used in infants, and it is unclear which of the methods is better.

Excellent anesthesia support is necessary for the surgical correction of coarctations, particularly in the small infant. During the period of aortic occlusion, the blood pressure is maintained at or near preoperative levels to maintain collateral flow. Severe hypertension during cross-clamping may be controlled by infusion of sodium nitroprusside. Some have advocated measuring pressures in the distal aorta after aortic cross-clamping, with consideration of some type of bypass if the distal pressure is low to reduce the risk of spinal cord injury. Others use moderate hypothermia to decrease this risk. Intraoperative pressure measurement may be obtained to demonstrate any residual gradient that might indicate an inadequate repair.

RESULTS

The operative risk should be less than 5% in children and may be slightly higher in adults. If surgery is necessary in the first few months of life, the risk may be much higher due to the severity of congestive heart failure and to the associated congenital heart defects. In these patients, operative risk may approach 20% to 30%.

Complications that may occur during or after surgery include bleeding secondary to hypertension or damage to enlarged collateral vessels and spinal cord injury. The latter is a rare but devastating complication that may result in weakness or paralysis of the lower extremities. In a review of 12,532 cases, Brewer and associates found the incidence to be 0.41%. The etiology is unclear, and since it may not be preventable, the patient and family must be made aware of this potential hazard when obtaining informed consent. Indeed, this complication has been reported to occur prior to operation.

Most patients will obtain satisfactory relief from hypertension following the surgery, but hypertension in the immediate postoperative period may occur as a well-recognized complication and is best controlled with sodium nitroprusside and propranolol therapy. Some patients require antihypertensives for a variable period following the surgery, and a few remain hypertensive even with appropriate medication. As indicated previously, it appears that the incidence of residual hypertension is less if corrective surgery is performed prior to 6 years of age. The mechanism for residual hypertension is not well understood but may be due in part to residual gradients, especially during exercise. Postoperative gradients or restenosis may occur with any of the techniques described and may be as related to the age of the patient at the time of surgery as to the

particular operative technique. Such gradients may not be apparent at rest but may be frequently demonstrated with exercise. Rarely, a syndrome manifested by abdominal pain and hypertension may occur immediately after surgery. This is thought to be due to vasculitis and is best treated with sympatholytic agents.

Surgical correction of coarctation can be accomplished in most patients with satisfactory improvement in hypertension and in long-term prognosis. While the results are not as favorable in infancy, steady improvement has occurred in recent years.

COARCTATION OF THE ABDOMINAL AORTA

Coarctation of the abdominal aorta is rare and may occur in several forms and locations (Fig. 39-7). Treatment depends upon the exact anatomy but usually consists of some type of bypass graft.

INTERRUPTED AORTIC ARCH

Interrupted aortic arch is a rare congenital lesion in which there is complete discontinuity between the ascending aorta and the descending aorta. In type A, the interruption occurs distal to the left subclavian artery, and in type B, the interruption is just distal to the left carotid artery. In both types, blood flow to the lower body is by way of a PDA. This lesion accounts for less than 1% of all congenital heart defects but is highly lethal, with 80% of the infants dying within 1 month of birth. Associated defects occur frequently: Ventricular septal defect is present in some 90% of these patients. Since blood flow to the lower body is by way of the patent ductus, ductal constriction and closure result in oliguria, progressive acidosis, and death.

In the past, a few of these critically ill infants have been

Fig. 39-7. Types of coarctation of the abdominal aorta. (Ben-Shoshan M, Rossi NP, Korns ME: Coarctation of the abdominal aorta. Arch Pathol 95:224, 1973)

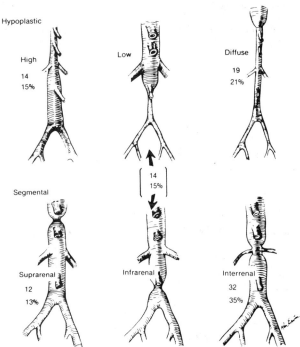

salvaged by various palliative or reconstructive techniques, but operative mortality was extremely high, partially because of the necessity for operating on these children when they were critically ill and deteriorating. The recent advent of prostaglandin infusion to maintain ductal patency has resulted in significant temporary palliation in these infants. This allows time for more thorough diagnostic procedures. As a result, more careful operative procedures may be planned and carried out on infants whose overall condition is much better than in previous years. Using these concepts, Moulton and Bowman have recently reported successful one-stage correction of interrupted aortic arch and closure of ventricular septal defect with survival in four of five patients. The combination of temporary palliation with prostaglandin infusion and one-stage surgical correction appears to offer significant hope for this group of patients in whom the outlook was previously so dismal.

AORTIC ARCH ANOMALIES (VASCULAR RINGS)

It is necessary to understand the embryology of the aortic arch to understand the development of these anomalies. This has been best described by Edwards. In the embryo, six primitive aortic arches connect the dorsal and ventral aortic roots. As development proceeds, certain portions of these primitive arches regress and others persist to form the normal adult anatomy (Fig. 39-8). The carotid arteries are formed from portions of the third pair of arches, the normal aortic arch is formed from the left fourth arch, and the pulmonary arteries and ductus arteriosus are derived from the sixth pair of arches. Abnormal regression or persistence of other parts of these primitive arches results in the anomalies under discussion.

PATHOPHYSIOLOGY

Certain of these anomalies produce true complete vascular rings: double aortic arch and right aortic arch with left

AORTIC ARCH ANOMALIES (VASCULAR RINGS)	
History	Hommel described, 1737; Gross corrected double aortic arch in 1945
Incidence	<1% of all congenital heart defects
Anatomy	Abnormal development of embryonic aortic arches produces vascular ring around esophagus and trachea
Pathophysiology	Vascular rings may produce tracheal and esophageal compression
Dx	History: respiratory distress; dysphagia; respiratory infections Physical exam: tachypnea; stridor; wheezing; ± pneumonia ECG: normal Chest film: tracheal compression; esophageal compression with barium swallow Echo: No specific findings Catheterization: rarely indicated; aortogram confirms diagnosis
Rx	Appropriate division of vascular ring
Results	Operative mortality rate 3% in infants, less in adults; long-term results good

ductus arteriosus or aberrant left subclavian artery (Fig. 39-9). Because of compression of the trachea and esophagus in these patients, the ring may produce difficulty with breathing and swallowing. In other forms of the anomaly, the vascular ring may be incomplete (left arch with aberrant right subclavian artery and right arch with aberrant left

Fig. 39-8. (*Left*) Hypothetical depiction of the simultaneous presence of all six aortic arches. In actuality, the regular arches I, II, and V shown here will have disappeared before arches III, IV, and VI are well developed. (*Right*) Striped arches shown are the final segments to retrogress and disappear. in addition, note the pulmonary artery buds developing from the sixth arches. (Hufnagel CA: Vascular rings of the aortic arch. In Hardy JD [ed]: Rhoads Textbook of Surgery, 5th ed. Philadelphia, J B Lippincott, 1977)

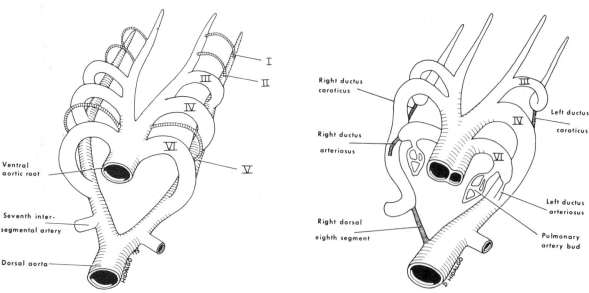

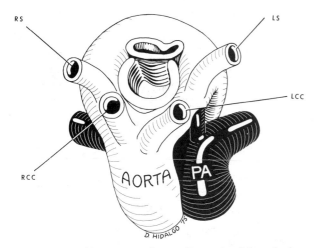

Fig. 39-9. Double aortic arch. Small anterior left arch, large posterior right arch, and left ductus arteriosus. *LCC,* left common carotid, *LS,* left subclavian; *PA,* pulmonary artery; *RCC,* right common carotid; *RS,* right subclavian. (Hufnagel CA: Vascular rings of the aortic arch. In Hardy JD [ed]: Rhoads Textbook of Surgery, 5th ed. Philadelphia, J B Lippincott, 1977)

subclavian artery), but symptoms are related to breathing and swallowing, particularly the latter. In abnormal origin of the innominate artery, there is no vascular ring but the abnormal position of the innominate vessel may produce anterior compression of the trachea.

DIAGNOSIS

The diagnosis should be suspected in all newborns with symptoms of airway obstruction and no other obvious etiology. Symptoms will vary depending upon the particular anomaly and the degree of obstruction but are frequently severe in those with complete vascular rings. In these patients, severe respiratory distress and difficulty in swallowing may occur shortly after birth. In older children and adults, dysphagia may be a more prominent symptom, particularly dysphagia with solid food.

PHYSICAL EXAMINATION

Tachypnea, intercostal retractions, nasal flaring, stridor, wheezing, cyanosis, and other findings of respiratory distress may be apparent, and all may be accentuated with feeding. Physical findings of pneumonia may be also present, since aspiration is common. Hyperextension of the neck may reduce the degree of obstruction and relieve the symptoms, whereas flexion may aggravate them.

ELECTROCARDIOGRAPHY

The electrocardiogram is usually normal except in the rare patient with an associated cardiac anomaly.

CHEST FILM

Plain chest film may demonstrate hyperlucent lung fields and flat diaphragms along with tracheal compression. In persons in whom the diagnosis is suspected, a carefully performed barium esophagogram is the most useful diagnostic tool. By carefully noting the pattern of tracheal and esophageal compression, the skillful pediatric radiologist can almost always make the correct diagnosis. Arch aortograms provide little additional information and are rarely indicated.

ECHOCARDIOGRAPHY

There are no specific findings of vascular rings.

CARDIAC CATHETERIZATION

Catheterization is rarely indicated, but an aortogram will confirm the diagnosis made on barium swallow.

TREATMENT

Patients with demonstrated arch anomalies who have manifestations due to compression, including repeated respiratory infections, stridor, wheezing, and dysphagia, are candidates for surgery. With few exceptions, the various arch anomalies can best be approached through a left thoracotomy in the fourth intercostal space. In all cases, meticulous dissection of the aortic arch and its branches is necessary for positive identification of each vessel. Occasionally, a trial occlusion of the vessel to be divided is useful. In general, the vascular ring must be divided at some point so as to completely relieve esophageal and tracheal compression and at the same time maintain normal perfusion. In all patients, the ligamentum arteriosum or ductus arteriosus must be divided together with all other fascial attachments and bands. The divided ends should be widely separated to completely free the constricting ring.

The double aortic arch must be interrupted at some point so as to relieve the vascular ring and yet preserve normal perfusion. In the usual case of the smaller anterior arch and larger posterior arch, there is frequently an atretic area distal to the origin of the left subclavian on the anterior arch, and the ring is divided at that point. If no atretic area exists, a smaller anterior arch may be divided between the origin of the left common carotid and the left subclavian or between the origin of the left subclavian and the insertion of the anterior arch into the descending thoracic aorta. If the posterior arch is smaller, it is divided just proximal to its junction with the descending thoracic aorta. Again, the ligamentum arteriosum or ductus arteriosus is divided, and the ring is completely interrupted.

In the right aortic arch with a left ductus arteriosus, the ductus or ligament is divided. If an aberrant left subclavian is also present, it is usually also divided to completely interrupt the ring. In the left aortic arch with an aberrant right subclavian, the right subclavian is divided at its origin from the aorta. The presence of a rich collateral network makes reanastomosis of the subclavian unnecessary, although some have advocated this. In the case of the anomalous innominate artery producing anterior tracheal compression, good results can usually be obtained by tacking the vessel anteriorly to the sternum, thus relieving the tracheal compression.

RESULTS

The risk of operation in this group of malformations is generally quite low. In the largest reported series, Binet recorded seven deaths in 150 patients with no deaths in the past 8 years. Complications include postoperative bleeding and infrequent injuries to the recurrent laryngeal and phrenic nerves and, rarely, to the thoracic duct. These may each be avoided by careful surgical technique. Meticulous attention must be paid to respiratory care in the postoperative period. While respiratory difficulty, stridor, and wheezing may be immediately relieved when tracheal compression is relieved, some patients, particularly infants, may have significant tracheomalacia and postoperative tracheal edema due to prolonged tracheal compression. At the time of tracheal extubation, the patient should be carefully observed for signs of respiratory obstruction, and prompt reintubation may be necessary if it occurs. Long-term results are generally good, with complete relief of respiratory and gastrointestinal symptoms.

ORIGIN OF LEFT PULMONARY ARTERY FROM RIGHT PULMONARY ARTERY

Rarely, the left pulmonary artery may originate from the right pulmonary artery, cross over the right main stem bronchus, and then course between the trachea and the esophagus to reach the left lung. This may result in compression of the right main stem bronchus and has been termed a vascular sling. Associated cardiovascular anomalies are common. Most infants with this anomaly are symptomatic early in life with respiratory obstruction. The diagnosis is usually made from plain chest film and fluoroscopy but may be confirmed by angiography. Operative therapy entails division of the left pulmonary artery at its origin from the right pulmonary artery, mobilization of the segment between the trachea and the esophagus, and reanastomosis of the then normally located left pulmonary artery to the main pulmonary artery. Mortality for this procedure has been quite high until recently, and the long-term outlook is not as good as for other vascular rings.

ATRIAL SEPTAL DEFECTS

The exact etiology of atrial septal defects is unknown, but it is probably related to both genetic and environmental influences. A definite familial incidence has been described. The defect results from a failure of the septum secundum to completely cover the ostium secundum.

Ostium secundum defects may vary in size and location but generally are located in the midportion of the atrial septum. Occasionally, they may be quite large and extend to the orifice of the superior or inferior vena cava (Fig. 39-10). In approximately 10% to 15%, anomalous drainage of one or both right pulmonary veins into the right atrium will be associated with the defect. Sinus venosus–type defects occur high in the atrial septum at the point of entry of the superior vena cava into the right atrium. In these defects, the right superior pulmonary vein will almost always enter directly into the superior vena cava or right atrium. Ostium primum atrial septal defects occur low in the atrial septum just above the atrioventricular valves. Because their embryology is more related to that of the endocardial cushion defects, they are considered in the discussion of these defects.

PATHOPHYSIOLOGY

The net result of an uncomplicated defect in the atrial septum is to produce a flow of blood from the left atrium to the right atrium, thus producing an overall increase in pulmonary blood flow. Early in life, the magnitude of this shunt is dependent upon the size of the defect and the difference in left and right atrial pressures, because left and right ventricular compliance is nearly equal. After several months, as pulmonary vascular resistance falls, right ventricular compliance increases and the left-to-right shunt may increase, particularly if the defect is large. The development of pulmonary hypertension occurs more slowly in

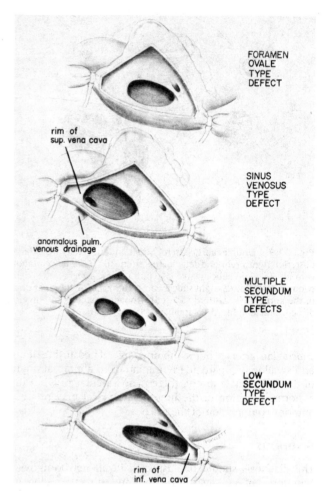

Fig. 39-10. Representative types of atrial ostium secundum defects. (Hardy JD, Timmis HH, Watson DG, et al: Secundum type atrial septal defect: Operation in 31 patients using cardiopulmonary bypass. South Med J 61:288, 1968)

atrial sepal defects than in ventricular septal defects, but if and when it occurs, right ventricular compliance will decrease and the left-to-right shunt may decrease. If the atrial septal defect is not closed, progressive pulmonary hypertension may develop, ultimately causing a reversal of the shunt, cyanosis, and right ventricular failure. As a group, patients with untreated atrial septal defect have a significantly decreased life span: The average age at death is about 50 years. However, as noted, it is not unusual for persons with an atrial septal defect to live a completely normal life span.

DIAGNOSIS

Patients with isolated atrial septal defect are rarely symptomatic in infancy or early childhood. Occasionally, mild growth retardation may occur, and dyspnea on exertion and easy fatigability may be noted. These latter two symptoms increase in frequency and severity with age. Arrhythmias such as atrial fibrillation become more common after 30 years of age.

PHYSICAL EXAMINATION

Examination of the chest may demonstrate a right ventricular lift. Auscultation usually reveals a soft systolic murmur along the upper left sternal border and "fixed splitting" of the second heart sound. Both of these findings are related

ATRIAL SEPTAL DEFECTS	
History	Rokitansky described, 1875; Lewis and Swann corrected (hypothermia), 1953; Gibbon corrected (extracorporeal circulation), 1953
Incidence	8% to 10% of all congenital heart defects
Anatomy	Ostium secundum type in midatrial septum; sinus venosus type at junction of superior vena cava and right atrium
Pathophysiology	L → R shunt through atrial septal defect produces increased pulmonary blood flow
Dx	History: Some patients asymptomatic; dyspnea on exertion; palpitations Physical exam: Soft systolic murmur; fixed splitting of S_2 ECG: right atrial enlargement; RVH Chest film: ↑ right atrium, right ventricle, and pulmonary artery; ↑ pulmonary blood flow Echo: may show the defect Catheterization: L → R shunt at atrial level; ± pulmonary hypertension
Rx	Surgical closure
Results	Operative mortality rate <1% in children; long-term results excellent

to the increased flow through the right ventricle and across the pulmonary valve.

ELECTROCARDIOGRAPHY

The electrocardiogram demonstrates features of right ventricular volume overload and right ventricular hypertrophy.

CHEST FILM

The chest film usually demonstrates moderate enlargement of the right atrium, right ventricle, and pulmonary artery. The pulmonary vasculature is increased consistent with a left-to-right shunt.

ECHOCARDIOGRAPHY

M-mode echocardiography will demonstrate increased right atrial, right ventricular, and pulmonary artery size. Two-dimensional echocardiography will confirm these findings as well as demonstrate ventricular function and valvular anatomy. It also will demonstrate an intact ventricular septum and frequently will show the exact location and size of the defect in the atrial septum. Contrast echocardiography will show the left-to-right shunt across the atrial septum.

CARDIAC CATHETERIZATION

Cardiac catheterization will show the diagnostic findings of a step-up in oxygen saturation at the right atrial level. By using standard formulas, oxygen saturation, and pressures, it is possible to calculate the magnitude of the left-to-right

shunt and also the systemic and pulmonary vascular resistance. Right atrial, right ventricular, and pulmonary artery pressures are usually mildly elevated but may be severely increased in those patients with advanced pulmonary vascular changes. Cineangiograms may aid in demonstrating the level of the shunt in the atrium and in detecting possible anomalous pulmonary venous return but do little to define the exact anatomy of the defect. They are useful in excluding other associated abnormalities.

TREATMENT

In general, the presence of an atrial septal defect with a left-to-right shunt greater than 1.5 to 2.0:1 is indication for surgery. Patients with pulmonary artery pressures equal to systemic or greater than systemic and who have significantly increased pulmonary vascular resistance (Rp > 7) should be considered carefully for surgery and may be inoperable. Most atrial septal defects are approached through a standard median sternotomy incision, although a right anterolateral thoracotomy provides adequate exposure in most patients and provides a much superior cosmetic result in the female. The aorta and both venae cavae are cannulated, and the patient is placed on cardiopulmonary bypass. The heart is electrically fibrillated to prevent air embolus. Many secundum atrial septal defects can be closed primarily with suture only. If the defect is quite large or if the closure appears to be under some tension, it may be closed using a patch of autogenous pericardium, various synthetic materials (Dacron), or, more recently, glutaraldehyde-preserved bovine pericardium. If there is anomalous pulmonary venous return, the patch is placed in such a fashion that the anomalous veins are diverted to the left atrium (Fig. 39-11). The sinus venosus defects almost always require the use of some type of patch to close the defect and baffle the anomalous pulmonary veins to the left atrium. Care must be taken at the time the defect is closed and at the conclusion of cardiopulmonary bypass to avoid air embolization. Meticulous care must also be taken to avoid injury to the sinus node in sinus venosus defects and to the atrioventricular node in large inferior atrial septal defects that extend down to the coronary sinus and inferior vena cava.

RESULTS

The operative risk is less than 1% in uncomplicated atrial septal defects but may be considerably higher in adults, especially those with pulmonary hypertension and increased pulmonary vascular resistance. Those patients operated on as children or in early adolescence recover rapidly. Some may have a growth spurt within months of their surgery. Their long-term outlook is nearly the same as for patients without congenital heart defects. For adult patients with large defects, recovery may be slow, and it may be several months to a year before the patient receives the full benefits of operation. Most often, pulmonary hypertension will regress following correction; however, if pulmonary resistance is markedly elevated, it may not regress. There is some debate about the effectiveness of the operation in the obliteration of atrial arrhythmias.

VENTRICULAR SEPTAL DEFECTS

The pathologic anatomy of ventricular septal defect is illustrated in Figure 39-12. The most common defect (80%) seen in surgical series is the perimembranous or infracristal

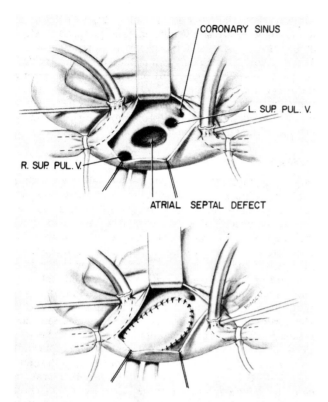

TEFLON BAFFLE INCORPORATING ANOMALOUS VEINS AND SEPTAL DEFECT

Fig. 39-11. Anomalous pulmonary venous drainage associated with foramen ovale ostium secundum atrial septal defect. A new atrial septum was constructed with Teflon to return the anomalous pulmonary venous drainage through the foramen ovale into the left atrium. (Hardy JD, Timmis HH, Watson DG, et al: Secundum type atrial septal defect: Operation in 31 patients using cardiopulmonary bypass. South Med J 61:288, 1968)

ventricular septal defect. This defect is related to the aortic and tricuspid valves. The bundle of His passes along the posterior and cephalad portions of the defect before branching into the left and right bundle branches. The supracristal and posteroinferior (atrioventricular canal) ventricular septal defects are seen infrequently (5%–10%). Muscular defects may be multiple and are seen infrequently in surgical reports.

PATHOPHYSIOLOGY

The size and direction of the shunt across a ventricular septal defect depends upon the size of the defect and the pulmonary vascular resistance. When the defect is small, it offers considerable obstruction to flow, and slight variations in size of the defect are accompanied by large variations in interventricular shunting. Thus, only a large pressure difference, which commonly occurs during mid-to-late systole, results in significant flow across small defects. Large defects offer little resistance to flow, and small pressure differences that exist late in systole and during diastole determine the magnitude of the interventricular shunt. These complex interrelationships include the relative compliance of the two ventricles and the relative pressures in the two atria. Anatomical obstruction by muscle bands or fibrous tissue may limit flow through an apparently large ventricular septal defect.

In the presence of large defects, the major determinant

of blood flow across the defect is pulmonary vascular resistance. This resistance is elevated for the first 7 to 14 days of life; thus, infants with large ventricular septal defects rarely present before this time, because the elevated vascular resistance limits left-to-right shunting across the defect. As vascular resistance drops, infants with large ventricular septal defects will have torrential pulmonary blood flow, which soon increases left ventricular preload to the point that the ventricle fails and left atrial pressure begins to rise. At this point, pulmonary arterial pressure rises with a consequent moderate elevation in vascular resistance. This is termed hyperdynamic pulmonary hypertension. Prolonged exposure to high blood flow and pressure causes anatomical changes in the pulmonary circulation, which in turn results in fixed elevations of pulmonary vascular resistance. When the resistance is severely elevated, usually above 10 resistance units per square meter of body surface, pulmonary and systemic blood flow are usually approximately equal.

The natural history of ventricular septal defect is extremely interesting. Small ventricular defects rarely produce symptoms in infancy or in adult life. Some infants with

Fig. 39-12. Ventricular septal defects, classified according to location. Type 1 defects occur superior to the crista supraventricularis and immediately below the pulmonic valve. Defects in this location are far removed from the bundle of His and are relatively simple to repair. Type 2 defects are the most frequent, occurring in 85% to 90% of all patients with ventricular septal defect. These defects are located in the region of the membranous septum. They are below the crista supraventricularis and are adjacent to the junction of the septal and anterior leaflets of the tricuspid valve. These defects are also immediately adjacent to the aortic annulus in their superior margin. Type 3 defects may be called defects of the atrioventricular canal. They are located beneath the septal leaflet of the tricuspid valve. They are further removed from the aortic valve than type 2 defects. Type 4 defects are in the muscular septum, surrounded completely by muscle, and may be multiple in their location. (Hollingsworth JF: Interventricular septal defect without pulmonic stenosis. In Hardy JD [ed]: Rhoads Textbook of Surgery, 5th ed. Philadelphia, J B Lippincott, 1977)

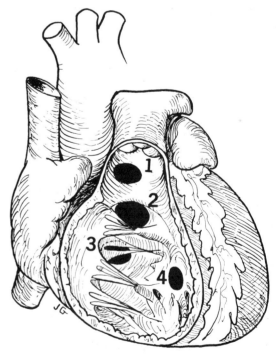

VENTRICULAR SEPTAL DEFECTS	
History	Roger described, 1879; Lillehei first corrected, 1954
Incidence	20% of congenital heart defects
Anatomy	Defect in membranous ventricular septum most common; also muscular defects
Pathophysiology	L → R shunt increases with size of defect; produces heart failure in infancy; can cause irreversible pulmonary hypertension later
Dx	History: poor feeding in infancy; growth failure in older patients Physical exam: holosystolic murmur in left chest; thready pulses ECG: ±LVH; RVH late Chest film: ↑ heart size; ↑ pulmonary vascularity early; "pruning" of pulmonary vessels late Echo: ↑ left atrium and left ventricle Catheterization: location of defect; ± ↑ pulmonary vascular resistance
Rx	Surgical closure through right atriotomy in infants; transventricular closure in older patients if defect is large
Results	Operative mortality 5%; late results excellent

ventricular septal defect follow a course characterized by failure of the defect to enlarge as the heart grows or by obstruction to blood flow by muscular hypertrophy of the right ventricle. These infants may develop heart failure in infancy but, because of the increased resistance to flow, shunting gradually decreases, and these children are usually asymptomatic by the age of 2 years. This type of defect has a propensity for spontaneous closure, and it has been estimated that of all children born with ventricular septal defects, approximately 20% will undergo spontaneous closure, usually before the age of 2 years.

If the ventricular septal defect is large and blood flow is torrential in infancy, heart failure rapidly develops. Such infants present with failure to thrive, since they are unable to nurse satisfactorily because of dyspnea complicating their ability to suck. In the majority of these children, treatment with digitalis and diuretics offers symptomatic improvement. If large defects are not closed surgically, at some period during the first few years of life hypertensive pulmonary vascular disease will become a problem. Pulmonary blood vessels undergo rapid muscular hypertrophy and then develop full-blown pulmonary atheroscleroticlike lesions. At this point, the pulmonary vascular resistance becomes fixed and the patients will have bidirectional shunting across the ventricular defect. Such patients are said to have the Eisenmenger complex, and they then gradually die of the complications of cyanosis and polycythemia. This complication can almost uniformly be prevented by operative closure of the defect within the first 2 years of life.

DIAGNOSIS

Patients with small ventricular septal defects rarely have symptoms. Bacterial endocarditis occurs infrequently, usually after the age of 2 years. Patients with moderate or large ventricular septal defects, with only moderate left-to-right shunting, may in childhood or adult life have limitations in exercise tolerance and show some growth failure. Infants with large ventricular septal defects usually do not have symptoms until the age of 6 weeks to 3 months, when pulmonary vascular resistance has fallen. Then growth failure with tachypnea and sweating during feeding is a common complaint. Repeated respiratory infections may appear, especially in the winter months.

PHYSICAL EXAMINATION

Small ventricular septal defects are characterized by a harsh short systolic murmur heard best in the second or third left intercostal space. The heart is not enlarged, and there is usually no systolic thrill. A diastolic murmur is not heard, and a right ventricular lift is not present. The infant with a large ventricular septal defect and markedly increased pulmonary blood flow and heart failure presents a classic picture. The infant is usually wasted, with a very small amount of subcutaneous fat. The complexion is waxen and there is marked evidence of sympathetic hyperactivity. There is constant sweating, tachycardia, and tachypnea. The jugular venous pulses are prominent in both the erect and the supine posture. The precordium is bulging, and a rapid, overactive heart is evident. A thrill is usually palpated in the third to fifth intercostal spaces on the left. There is a loud holosystolic murmur, maximal in the same area, usually coupled with a short mid-diastolic murmur heard best at the apex. The second heart sound at the base is usually loud and may be slightly split. The liver and spleen are usually enlarged, and the peripheral pulses are rapid and thready.

In older patients with large ventricular septal defects, the left chest is ordinarily deformed due to the enlarged right ventricle. A systolic thrill over the entire left precordium is evident. The characteristic harsh holosystolic murmur is heard best in the second, third, and (maximally) fourth left intercostal spaces in the midclavicular line. In patients with a large ventricular septal defect and significant elevation of pulmonary vascular resistance, the precordium is quiet to examination. The systolic murmur is soft and short or may be nearly absent. The second sound at the base is markedly accentuated but is not split. When the pulmonary vascular resistance has risen above the systemic vascular resistance (Eisenmenger complex), cyanosis with clubbing of the nail beds may be evident.

ELECTROCARDIOGRAPHY

The electrocardiogram helps to accurately define the pathophysiology. If the defect is large and pulmonary vascular resistance is only mildly elevated with large pulmonary blood flows, electrocardiographic evidence of both left and right ventricular hypertrophy and in some cases strain is apparent. Evidence of left atrial hypertrophy with tall notched P waves in the left precordial leads is present. When the ventricular septal defect is large and the pulmonary vascular resistance is severely elevated, right axis deviation is usually present. The right precordial leads show the typical RSR' of right ventricular hypertrophy.

CHEST FILM

The chest film in many cases also accurately predicts the pathophysiology. In large defects, the pulmonary arteries are enlarged both centrally and peripherally, reflecting the increased pulmonary blood flow. There is usually evidence of an enlarged left atrium with marked enlargement of the left ventricle. If the pulmonary vascular resistance is markedly elevated, the chest film assumes a different configuration. The main pulmonary artery segments are often markedly enlarged, but the peripheral pulmonary arteries are normal in size and there is no evidence of increased pulmonary blood flow.

ECHOCARDIOGRAPHY

The size of the ventricular septal defect cannot adequately be established by current echocardiographic techniques. However, this modality is extremely useful in detecting abnormalities of the atrioventricular and semilunar valves, abnormalities of the great vessels, and the presence of a single ventricle. Echocardiography can provide a valuable estimate of the left-to-right shunt by quantitation of left atrial and left ventricular dimensions.

CARDIAC CATHETERIZATION

The purposes of the cardiac catheterization in ventricular septal defect are primarily to document the presence of the defect or defects, evaluate the magnitude of shunting across the defect, estimate pulmonary vascular resistance, estimate the work load of the two ventricles, demonstrate associated defects, if present, and provide the surgeon with a clear anatomical picture of the location of the defect or defects in those patients in whom operation is required. In the typical ventricular septal defect, right ventricular and pulmonary artery pressures will be elevated. There is a step-up in oxygen saturation in the right ventricle and pulmonary artery. Cineangiography will demonstrate the location of the defect as well as other abnormalities.

TREATMENT

A small ventricular septal defect with no hemodynamic alteration does not require operation. The risk of bacterial endocarditis is very small, and if the defect is present in a small growing infant or a child, there is a good likelihood that the defect will close. The older infant with a persistent modest but important shunt and normal pulmonary pressure dictates watchful conservatism. These children with a small to moderate left-to-right shunt and low pulmonary artery pressure run almost no risk of pulmonary vascular disease and have little added left ventricular work. The ventricular septal defect in such a patient is quite likely to close or become smaller, but if closure has not occurred when the child reaches the immediate preschool years, we recommend elective closure at that time if the pulmonary/systemic flow ratio is approximately 2:1 or greater.

Symptomatic infants with ventricular septal defects require the most skill and judgment for correct and timely therapy. Intensive medical treatment is tried for the infant who experiences symptoms of congestive heart failure during the first 24 months of life. If the infant improves with medical treatment, operation is delayed. In many of these infants who respond to treatment, the defect may close or become smaller spontaneously in coming months. If the congestive failure persists or worsens, primary operative closure of the defect is performed at this early age. Although delayed operation seems desirable in the early months of life if at all possible, we do not advocate delay in primary closure of the defect in the infant with persistent refractory congestive failure. Repeat catheterization is mandatory by 12 months of age in the infant with pulmonary hypertension who does not have operative closure, and closure is indicated if pulmonary hypertension persists.

Pulmonary artery banding for the treatment of isolated ventricular septal defect is rarely performed today and is usually indicated only if there are serious other associated defects, most commonly coarctation of the aorta. Pulmonary banding has also been used by some surgeons when multiple muscular defects are present causing symptomatic heart failure in infancy. Definitive repair through a left ventricular approach is delayed until the child grows larger.

Intracardiac repair is performed through a midline sternotomy in all cases. In small infants, the technique of profound hypothermia and circulatory arrest is preferred. The majority of ventricular septal defects presenting in infancy can be repaired through a right atriotomy with retraction of the tricuspid valve (Fig. 39-13). In the inferior and caudal portions of the defect, sutures are placed through the annulus of the tricuspid valve and well away from the rim of the defect to avoid the conduction system. In the cephalad portion of the defect, great care must be taken to avoid damage to the aortic valve.

In older children, standard cardiopulmonary bypass techniques with moderate systemic hypothermia to 25°C to 28°C are used. Cold, potassium-induced cardioplegia facilitates exposure and myocardial protection during the intracardiac portion of the repair. Most high defects can be repaired through a right atrial approach, although supracristal defects and most defects in the muscular septum must be repaired through a right or left ventriculotomy. If the pulmonary artery has been previously banded, the band is released during the cooling period prior to circulatory arrest or aortic closs-clamping. If the band has been in place for 6 months or less, the pulmonary artery will usually regain its normal configuration. If the band has been in place for

Fig. 39-13. Technique for surgical correction of ventricular septal defects. Right atriotomy (the right ventricular approach) has also been commonly used. (Hollingsworth JF: Interventricular septal defect without pulmonic stenosis. In Hardy JD [ed]: Rhoads Textbook of Surgery, 5th ed. Philadelphia, J B Lippincott, 1977)

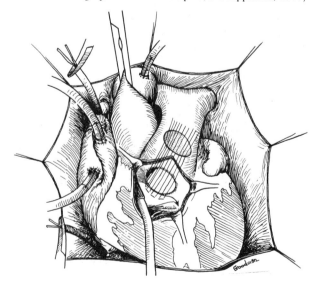

longer, the pulmonary artery can be progressively dilated to an acceptable size or be reconstructed with a diamond-shaped patch of pericardium to regain normal configuration.

RESULTS

Hospital mortality and complications are related to the nature of the defect and the degree of preexisting pulmonary vascular disease. In most institutions doing large volumes of infant cardiac surgery, the operative mortality rate is 5% or less. Multiple muscular ventricular septal defects are associated with a greater risk of repair in infancy. Late mortality is extremely rare, and it is generally recognized that complete closure of ventricular septal defects at an early age affords a nearly normal life expectancy.

Complications of operation are usually related to damage to the conduction system, which occurs in 1% to 2% of patients. With large ventricular septal defects and especially multiple ventricular defects, incomplete repair is more common and is usually present in 5% to 10% of the patients. Preoperatively elevated pulmonary vascular resistance will usually resolve, especially if the child is younger than 2 years of age. Older patients with elevated pulmonary vascular resistance preoperatively should be followed closely in the postoperative period. In approximately half of these patients, pulmonary vascular resistance will stabilize or regress, thus affording a good long-term prognosis.

ENDOCARDIAL CUSHION DEFECTS

Endocardial cushion defects or atrioventricular canals were described as early as 1700 by Méry. Successful correction of the complete form of atrioventricular canal was reported in 1955 by Lillehei, but operative results remained poor until the anatomy was more clearly defined by Rastelli and others and this new knowledge incorporated into surgical techniques in the early 1970s.

Endocardial cushion defects make up 3% to 5% of all congenital heart defects. The incomplete forms are approximately twice as common as the complete forms. Complete atrioventricular canal is the most common cardiac defect occurring in children with Down's syndrome, and most series of complete atrioventricular canals will include 30% to 50% Down's syndrome patients. The incomplete form rarely occurs in children with Down's syndrome.

ANATOMY AND EMBRYOLOGY

Endocardial cushion defects result from incomplete development of the embryonic endocardial cushions. The incomplete form of this defect (also called ostium primum atrial septal defect) occurs when the developing endocardial cushions fail to meet the septum primum. Although the defect is primarily due to a deficiency in the ventricular septum, the atrioventricular valves are downwardly displaced and are fused to the top of the ventricular septum. As a result, there is no communication between the ventricles beneath the atrioventricular valves (*i.e.*, no ventricular septal defect). The defect that occurs is low in the atrial septum in the region of the septum primum and adjacent to the atrioventricular valves. There is usually a cleft in the anterior leaflet of the mitral valve. As a result of the downward displacement of the atrioventricular valves, the left ventricular outflow tract is narrowed and elongated, producing

the so-called goose-neck deformity seen on cineangiograms of both the complete and the incomplete form of this defect.

Further maldevelopment of the endocardial cushions may result in a ventricular septal defect and more extensive deficiency of the atrioventricular valves. Rastelli classified complete atrioventricular canals into three types. In type A, the anterior common leaflet is divided into mitral and tricuspid components and is attached to the ventricular septum by short chordae. In type B, the anterior common leaflet may or may not be divided but is attached to a papillary muscle that inserts into the right ventricle. In type C, the anterior common leaflet is completely undivided and not attached to the ventricular septum in any way. These descriptions contributed enormously to the understanding of complete endocardial cushion defects, but it is generally agreed that there is considerably more variability in the anatomy than present in this classification. Although the anatomy and the development of both complete and incomplete atrioventricular canals are similar, the subsequent course of patients with the two defects is quite different and is considered separately.

INCOMPLETE ATRIOVENTRICULAR CANAL (OSTIUM PRIMUM ATRIAL SEPTAL DEFECT)

The end result of the defect in the atrial septum in incomplete atrioventricular canals is nearly the same as in secundum atrial septal defects. A net left-to-right shunt is produced causing right ventricular overload and increased pulmonary

INCOMPLETE ATRIOVENTRICULAR CANAL (OSTIUM PRIMUM ATRIAL SEPTAL DEFECT)	
History	Méry described, 1700
Incidence	2% to 3% of congenital heart defects
Anatomy	Failure of developing endocardial cushion to meet septum primum produces defect low in atrial septum; cleft mitral valve.
Pathophysiology	L → R shunt; ± mitral regurgitation
Dx	History: depends upon degree of mitral regurgitation; from asymptomatic to severe CHF Physical exam: soft systolic murmur over upper left chest; split S_2; ± systolic murmur of mitral regurgitation ECG: left axis deviation Chest film: mild cardiomegaly; ↑ pulmonary blood flow Echo: defect in low atrial septum; abnormal AV valves Catheterization: L → R shunt; ± mitral regurgitation; goose-neck deformity of left ventricular outflow tract
Rx	Surgical closure
Results	Operative mortality rate 3% to 4%; long-term results good but depend on residual mitral regurgitation

blood flow. The natural history is similar to secundum atrial septal defect, with pulmonary hypertension being a late development. This course is likely if mitral regurgitation through the cleft mitral valve is absent or minimal. On the other hand, if mitral regurgitation is severe, then early congestive heart failure results and the outlook is much worse.

DIAGNOSIS

The history will depend upon the presence or absence of mitral regurgitation. If absent, the patients may be asymptomatic or have mild dyspnea and growth retardation. If mitral regurgitation is severe, symptoms of congestive heart failure occur early along with frequent respiratory infections.

Physical Examination
In the absence of mitral regurgitation, physical findings are similar to secundum atrial septal defect with a soft systolic murmur in the left intercostal space due to increased flow across the pulmonary valve. The second heart sound is widely split. In the patient with significant mitral regurgitation, the above findings may be accentuated, and the systolic murmur of mitral regurgitation will be apparent along with other signs of congestive heart failure.

Electrocardiography
The electrocardiogram in endocardial cushion defects typically shows left axis deviation. In the frontal plane, the vectorcardiogram will show a counterclockwise loop shifted superiorly and leftward. Although not diagnostic of atrioventricular canal defects, these findings help distinguish between incomplete atrioventricular canal and secundum atrial septal defect.

Echocardiography
M-mode echocardiography will show abnormal displacement of the mitral and tricuspid valves with the mitral valve appearing to move through the ventricular septum. Two-dimensional echocardiography is most helpful in confirming these atrioventricular valve abnormalities. In addition, it may demonstrate the low-lying defect in the atrial septum, thus distinguishing it from a secundum atrial septal defect.

Cardiac Catheterization
Catheterization will quantitate the left-to-right shunt at the atrial level as well as the presence or absence of pulmonary hypertension. Cineangiography demonstrates the absence of a ventricular septal defect, the typical goose-neck deformity of the left ventricular outflow tract, the cleft in the mitral valve, and the presence and magnitude of mitral regurgitation.

TREATMENT

Surgery is recommended for all patients with this defect if there is a significant left-to-right shunt or mitral regurgitation. Surgery can be performed at any age but may be required as soon as significant mitral regurgitation is present. The heart is exposed through a median sternotomy, and standard complete cardiopulmonary bypass and moderate hypothermia are used. In the past, this repair has been performed with the heart beating, to detect any injury to the conduction system. We prefer the improved visibility and exposure provided by aortic cross-clamping and potassium-induced cardioplegia. The defect is exposed through

the right atrium, and the anatomy is carefully inspected. The cleft in the mitral valve is repaired with several interrupted nonabsorbable sutures if mitral regurgitation is present. Care must be taken not to produce mitral stenosis. The septal defect may then be closed with a pericardial patch or one of some other prosthetic material. We prefer to place interrupted sutures across the rim of tissue separating the mitral and tricuspid valves and to use a continuous suture to close the remaining portion of the defect. Care must be taken to avoid injury to the conduction system.

RESULTS

The overall operative mortality rate has been reduced to 3% to 4%. Long-term prognosis is related to the mitral valve. In the absence of mitral regurgitation postoperatively, the postoperative course is similar to that following repair of secundum atrial septal defect. Approximately 3% to 5% of patients will subsequently develop mitral insufficiency of sufficient severity to require mitral valve replacement.

COMPLETE ATRIOVENTRICULAR CANAL

The combination of defects in the complete atrioventricular canal produces a much more severe hemodynamic alteration than is present in incomplete canal. The degree of severity is determined by the size of the atrial and ventricular communications, the amount of mitral incompetence, and the degree of pulmonary hypertension. The net result early in life is a left-to-right shunt at the atrial and ventricular level. Because the ventricular communication is usually large, left and right ventricular pressures are equal, and this is transmitted directly to the pulmonary arteries. Pulmonary hypertension develops very early in these infants and is frequently present before the age of 2. Because of the large left-to-right shunt and the mitral regurgitation, severe congestive heart failure is frequently present early in infancy.

DIAGNOSIS

Infants with complete atrioventricular canals usually present early with difficulty feeding, tachypnea, respiratory infection, and other features of severe congestive heart failure. There is usually severe growth retardation, even in infants who are being optimally treated for heart failure. Some of these problems, such as respiratory infections, are accentuated in children with Down's syndrome.

Physical Examination
The infants are frequently acutely ill and markedly undersized. Tachypnea is generally present, and mild cyanosis may be apparent. The latter may be due to mixing produced by the large defects and atrioventricular valve insufficiency and does not necessarily represent fixed pulmonary hypertension and inoperability. The precordium is active, and a systolic thrill is usually present. A loud systolic murmur is present and is due both to the ventricular septal defect and to the mitral regurgitation. The second heart sound will be increased if pulmonary hypertension is present. Hepatomegaly, cool extremities, and other signs of poor perfusion may be present.

Electrocardiography
First-degree heart block along with right and, frequently, left ventricular hypertrophy is present. Again, there is left

COMPLETE ATRIOVENTRICULAR CANAL

History	Méry described, 1700; Lillehei first repaired, 1955
Incidence	About 1% of congenital heart defects; much higher in Down's syndrome
Anatomy	Incomplete development of the endocardial cushions produce common AV valve, VSD, low-lying atrial septal defect
Pathophysiology	Large L → R shunt; pulmonary hypertension; mitral or tricuspid regurgitation
Dx	History: severe CHF at early age with tachypnea, respiratory infections, poor growth Physical exam: systolic thrill and murmur; ↑ S₂; hepatomegaly; ± cyanosis ECG: left axis deviation; RVH and ± LVH Chest film: marked cardiomegaly; pulmonary congestion Echo: single AV valve; atrial septal defect; VSD Catheterization: L → R shunt; ↑ right ventricular and pulmonary artery pressures; ↑ pulmonary vascular resistance; mitral regurgitation; gooseneck deformity of left ventricular outflow tract
Rx	Surgical correction
Results	Operative mortality rate 10% to 15%; short- and long-term results related to degree of mitral regurgitation

axis deviation, and the frontal plane vectorcardiogram shows a counterclockwise loop deviated superiorly and to the left.

Chest Film

There is usually marked cardiomegaly on chest film, with enlargement of all four cardiac chambers. The pulmonary artery is enlarged, and there is evidence of both increased pulmonary blood flow and pulmonary venous congestion.

Echocardiography

M-mode echocardiography will depict abnormalities in the atrioventricular valve. Two-dimensional echocardiography is extremely useful and shows the downward displacement of the atrioventricular valves and the presence of a common atrioventricular valve instead of two separate valves. The defects in the atrial and ventricular septum are usually well outlined.

Cardiac Catheterization

Cardiac catheterization will demonstrate the degree of left-to-right shunt. Right ventricular and pulmonary artery pressures are markedly elevated, and the pulmonary vas-

cular resistance can be calculated and the absolute value, as well as its relation to systemic vascular resistance, used to determine operability. Cineangiography will demonstrate the communication between the left and right ventricles, thus distinguishing the complete form of the defect from the incomplete. The typical goose-neck deformity of left ventricular outflow tract will be demonstrated and the degree of mitral and tricuspid insufficiency estimated. In addition, other cardiac anomalies will be demonstrated.

TREATMENT

Complete atrioventricular canal is a particularly severe form of congenital heart disease, and most of these children if not treated will die in the first year or two of life, particularly if there are associated defects. Until recently, surgery carried an extremely high operative risk. Because of better understanding of the anatomy and especially that of the atrioventricular valves as described by Rastelli, recent surgical results have improved significantly. Current results depend upon surgery being performed before the development of irreversible pulmonary hypertension and also upon the ability to adequately reconstruct the atrioventricular valves. Surgery may be performed at any age, but in very small infants under 6 months old, there is still a significant risk. Palliation of these tiny infants by pulmonary artery banding has not been successful in most centers, and it is estimated to carry an operative risk in excess of 20% to 30%. This is most likely due to the associated mitral insufficiency, which may be made worse by pulmonary artery banding.

Currently, it is our practice to recommend surgical correction for complete atrioventricular canals before age 2 if heart failure is well controlled and earlier if uncontrolled. The presence at catheterization of pulmonary vascular resistance greater than 10 units or of pulmonary vascular resistance greater than 75% of systemic vascular resistance is indication of inoperability in most cases.

Surgery may be carried out through a median sternotomy using standard cardiopulmonary bypass with moderate hypothermia and periods of low flow. Surgical exposure is facilitated in very small infants by the use of profound hypothermia and circulatory arrest. The defect is exposed through the right atrium. The method of repair will depend upon the exact anatomy of the atrioventricular valves. In general, the initial part of the repair consists in dividing the common anterior and common posterior leaflets of the single atrioventricular valve into mitral and tricuspid components. This always should involve giving more tissue to the mitral valve than to the tricuspid valve, since mitral insufficiency is tolerated much more poorly than tricuspid insufficiency. The cleft in the anterior mitral valve leaflet is repaired using several interrupted sutures. The ventricular portion of the defect is then closed by approximating a prosthetic patch to the right ventricular side of the septum with multiple interrupted sutures. The septal components of the newly formed mitral and tricuspid valves are resuspended at the proper level from the prosthetic patch. The atrial septal portion of the defect can then be closed using the remaining patch and a continuous suture. Because of the reported complication of hemolysis occurring secondary to a jet of blood striking the "raw" prosthetic patch if residual mitral insufficiency is present, we currently amputate the patch just above the level of the atrioventricular valve resuspension and close the atrial septal portion of the defect with a pericardial patch. Meticulous care must be taken in the repair of both the atrial septal and the ventricular septal portions of the defect to avoid injury to the conduction system, thus producing complete heart block.

In some patients, there is inadequate tissue for mitral valve reconstruction, and a mitral valve replacement must be carried out at the time of initial repair. In a small percentage, mitral insufficiency develops immediately post-operatively or at a later date and may require mitral valve replacement.

RESULTS

The operative mortality for complete correction of complete atrioventricular canal depends upon the adequacy of mitral valve repair, the presence of pulmonary hypertension, and surgically induced heart block. In children, complete correction can be performed with an operative risk of 10% to 20%, but the risk is clearly higher in infants if surgery is necessary prior to the age of 6 months. The long-term results depend upon the presence of residual mitral regurgitation.

TETRALOGY OF FALLOT

Tetralogy of Fallot is a complex of four related defects: (1) large ventricular septal defect, (2) obstruction of the outflow tract of the right ventricle, (3) "overriding" of the aorta so that it originates in part from the right ventricle, and (4) right ventricular hypertrophy (Fig. 39-14). The first two of these are most important, and the second two are more or

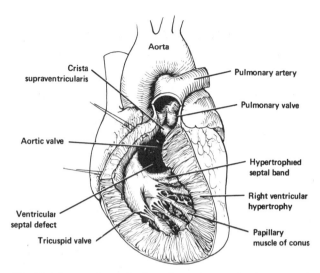

Fig. 39-14.   Tetralogy of Fallot. The aorta overrides the ventricular septum. A large ventricular septal defect is present, and the hypoplastic infundibulum with hypertrophied parietal and septal muscle bands obstruct blood flow to the pulmonary arteries. (Dunphy JE, Way LW: Current Surgical Diagnosis and Treatment. Los Altos, CA, Lange Medical Publications, 1973)

less secondary to the others. The ventricular septal defect is always large, usually equal to the size of the aortic valve orifice, and located high in the septum just beneath the aortic valve. The obstruction to right ventricular outflow usually occurs in the infundibular region and is secondary to hypertrophied septal and parietal muscle bands, which obstruct the underdeveloped infundibulum. Obstruction can also be localized to the pulmonary valve in some patients, or it may be both infundibular and valvular in location. The overriding of the aorta is variable and is related to the ventricular septal defect. Right ventricular hypertrophy is secondary to the outflow tract obstruction. The entire complex is felt to be secondary to underdevelopment of the right ventricular infundibulum.

Associated defects are common in tetralogy of Fallot. Atrial septal defect or patent foramen ovale occurs frequently, and a right aortic arch is present in 25% to 30% of these patients. The pulmonary valve may be atretic, or the leaflets may be absent (absent pulmonary valve syndrome). There may be stenosis of either the right or the left pulmonary artery, or the left pulmonary artery may be entirely absent. Coronary artery anomalies occur in approximately 10% of patients. The most significant of these is origin of the left anterior descending coronary artery from the right coronary artery with the course of the left anterior descending artery being across the right ventricular outflow tract to reach the left ventricle.

PATHOPHYSIOLOGY

These defects combine to produce obstruction to blood flow to the lungs with an associated right-to-left shunt across the ventricular septal defect and into the aorta. The net result of this is cyanosis, the severity of which is variable depending upon the anatomy, particularly the degree of right ventricular outflow tract obstruction. Usually, cyanosis is not severe at birth because blood flow to the lungs across the partially obstructed right ventricular outflow tract is supplemented by flow through the ductus. If right ventricular outflow tract obstruction is severe, then as the duct closes

TETRALOGY OF FALLOT	
History	Fallot described, 1888; Blalock palliated, 1944; Scott and Lillehei corrected, 1955
Incidence	12% of congenital heart defects
Anatomy	VSD; right ventricular outflow tract obstruction; overriding aorta; RVH
Pathophysiology	Obstruction to blood flow to lungs; R → L shunt; cyanosis
Dx	History: cyanosis; squatting; poor growth; "tet" spells Physical exam: cyanosis; clubbing; systolic murmur ECG: RVH Chest film: boot-shaped heart (RVH, ↓ pulmonary artery); ↓ pulmonary vascularity; right aortic arch in 30% Echo: large overriding aorta; small pulmonary artery, VSD Catheterization: ↑ right ventricular pressure; right ventricle → pulmonary artery gradient; R → L shunt; VSD; coronary artery anomalies
Rx	Total correction if anatomy and size favorable; palliative shunt if anatomy unfavorable
Results	Operative mortality rate 5%; long-term results usually good

in several days to weeks following birth, cyanosis might become apparent and increase. If the pulmonary valve is atretic, then pulmonary flow will be totally derived from the ductus and other collaterals and cyanosis will be severe at birth. If right ventricular outflow tract obstruction is not severe, then cyanosis may be mild or absent for some time. As the child grows, in most cases cyanosis becomes more severe as right ventricular hypertrophy increases and right ventricular outflow tract obstruction progresses. Occasionally, associated defects prevent immediate development of apparent cyanosis. While patients may occasionally remain asymptomatic indefinitely, most do not, and most studies indicate that fewer than 10% of untreated patients with tetralogy of Fallot survive to age 20.

DIAGNOSIS

The symptoms will depend upon the severity of the lesion, specifically the degree of obstruction to pulmonary blood flow. Depending upon the severity of the lesion, the patient may present with cyanosis at birth or a history of the gradual development of cyanosis and dyspnea. Characteristically, there is a history of "squatting," which is felt to increase pulmonary blood flow. Growth is generally retarded, and exercise tolerance is decreased. As the cyanosis progresses, hypoxic episodes may occur and are characterized by severe cyanosis, tachypnea, and even unconsciousness.

PHYSICAL EXAMINATION

These children are frequently small, and cyanosis may be apparent around the lips or in the nail beds. Clubbing of the fingers and toes may be apparent. Auscultation reveals a systolic murmur of varying intensity along the left sternal border. In the presence of severe right ventricular outflow tract obstruction or during a hypoxic episode, the murmur may be less apparent or absent. The systolic murmur is absent in pulmonary atresia, but a continuous murmur may be present indicating ductal or collateral flow.

ELECTROCARDIOGRAPHY

The electrocardiogram will show moderate to severe right ventricular hypertrophy.

CHEST FILM

In those patients with typical tetralogy of Fallot, the chest film will demonstrate diminished pulmonary vascularity, absent or decreased pulmonary artery, and right ventricular

hypertrophy. These combine to produce the typical "boot-shaped" heart. In 30%, there may be a right aortic arch.

ECHOCARDIOGRAPHY

M-mode echocardiography will demonstrate the large overriding aorta, small pulmonary artery, and right ventricular hypertrophy. These findings are confirmed by two-dimensional echocardiography, and the ventricular septal defect may also be demonstrated by this method.

CARDIAC CATHETERIZATION

Cardiac catheterization will demonstrate elevation of right atrial and right ventricular pressures, with the right ventricle being equal to the left ventricle. The degree of right-to-left shunt can be determined. Pull-back pressure tracings from pulmonary artery to right ventricle will demonstrate the point of right ventricular outflow tract obstruction. Cineangiograms will demonstrate size and anatomy of the right ventricle and left ventricle, the points of obstruction of the right ventricular outflow tract, and the anatomy of the right ventricle, the main pulmonary artery, and the left and right pulmonary arteries. Coronary artery abnormalities will also be seen.

TREATMENT

The management of patients with tetralogy of Fallot remains quite variable, depending upon the anatomy of the defect, the size and age of the child, and the surgeon and cardiologist involved. Initial treatment for tetralogy was directed at improving pulmonary blood flow by way of various palliative systemic–pulmonary shunts. The first of these, the Blalock–Taussig shunt, involves division of the subclavian artery and end-to-side anastomosis of the proximal subclavian artery to the pulmonary artery on the side opposite the aortic arch (Fig. 39-15). This operation is performed through a thoracotomy without the need for cardiopulmonary bypass. When carried out with meticulous technique, it results in significant improvement in pulmonary blood flow and no distortion of the pulmonary artery; pulmonary hypertension or congestive heart failure almost never develops. The operation is also applicable to other forms of cyanotic congenital heart disease. Because of difficulty with long-term patency of the Blalock–Taussig shunt in small infants, other surgeons turned to other palliative shunts. The Waterston–Cooley shunt involves side-to-side anastomosis of the right pulmonary artery to

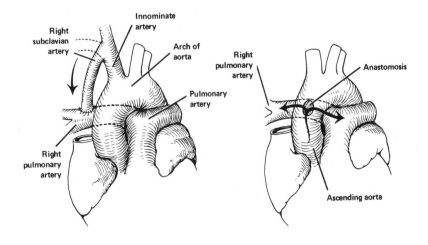

Fig. 39-15. Palliative operations to increase pulmonary arterial blood flow. (*Left*) Blalock–Taussig subclavian–pulmonary arterial anastomosis. (*Right*) Waterston aortic-to-right pulmonary arterial anastomosis. (Dunphy JE, Way LW: Current Surgical Diagnosis and Treatment. Los Altos, CA, Lange Medical Publications, 1973)

the ascending aorta (see Fig. 39-15). It is easier to perform, particularly in the smaller infant. However, the size of the anastomosis is more difficult to control, and, as a result, pulmonary hypertension and congestive heart failure are more common following this procedure. In addition, it has been shown to produce distortion of the right pulmonary artery, thus making subsequent total correction of the underlying defect much more difficult. While some centers continue to advocate its use because of good results, it is being used less frequently today than in the past. The Potts shunt involves a side-to-side anastomosis between the descending aorta and the left pulmonary artery. Again, it is more likely to result in pulmonary hypertension or congestive heart failure than is a Blalock shunt, but its major drawback is the difficulty in closing it at the time of subsequent total correction, thus increasing morbidity and mortality of total correction. It is rarely used today. The Glenn shunt involves anastomosis of the superior vena cava to the right pulmonary artery, thus bypassing the right atrium and right ventricle. This shunt becomes less effective with time and is rarely used except in some forms of tricuspid atresia. Modifications of the Blalock–Taussig shunt have become popular in the past several years and consist of placing a microporous polytetrafluoroethylene graft from either the subclavian artery or the aorta to the pulmonary artery. Some authors have reported excellent results with this form of palliation. Recent improvements in microvascular surgical techniques, probably derived from extensive experience with coronary artery surgery, have improved the results obtained with standard Blalock–Taussig shunts, and today it is the most frequently used palliative procedure to increase pulmonary blood flow.

At present, most would agree that patients over the age of 2 who have favorable anatomy should undergo total correction of tetralogy of Fallot as the initial operative procedure. This operation is performed through a median sternotomy using standard cardiopulmonary bypass and moderate hypothermia. An incision is made in the right ventricular outflow tract, and the hypertrophied septal and parietal bands and other obstructing muscle bundles are resected (Fig. 39-16, *A* and *B*). The pulmonary valvotomy, if necessary, may be performed through the same incision. The ventricular septal defect is closed with a prosthetic patch, with care being taken to avoid injury to the conduction system (Fig. 39-16, *C* and *D*). If present, an atrial septal defect or patent foramen ovale may be closed through the tricuspid valve or directly through the right atrium. The incision in the right ventricle is closed either primarily or, more often, with an oval prosthetic patch. If the pulmonary valve annulus is severely hypoplastic, the incision in the right ventricle is extended across the pulmonary valve annulus and the prosthetic patch carried out onto the main pulmonary artery. Occasionally, it will be necessary to extend the patch out onto the right or left pulmonary artery because of obstruction at the bifurcation. After cardiopulmonary bypass has been discontinued, right and left ventricular pressures are measured. It is our feeling that a ratio of right ventricular to left ventricular pressure (PRV/LV) less than 0.8 is satisfactory because it will usually decrease somewhat more in the first few postoperative days. A PRV/LV greater than 0.8 usually indicates inadequate relief of right ventricular outflow tract obstruction and may be an indication to extend the ventriculotomy across the pulmonary valve annulus or to patch the outflow tract if this has not been done initially. Intraoperative dye curves are useful

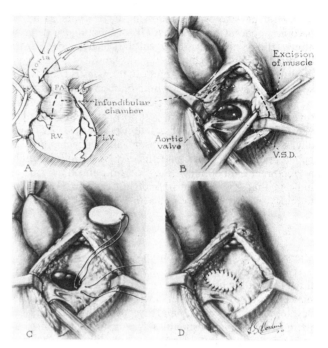

Fig. 39-16. Illustration of method employed for a complete correction of tetralogy of Fallot. (*A*) Diagram showing cannulation of the superior and inferior venae cavae for extracorporeal circulation. The infundibular chamber of the right ventricle is illustrated. (*B*) The outflow tract of the right ventricle has been opened. The hypertrophied muscle characteristic of the infundibular stenosis is seen and is being excised. The ventricular septal defect is shown, and the proximity of the aortic valvular leaflets may be seen. (*C*) The prosthetic patch is being placed to close the ventricular septal defect. The aorta is temporarily occluded to provide a bloodless operative field. (*D*) Completion of the placement of the prosthesis. (Sabiston DC: Cardiovascular surgery. In Wilkinson AW: Recent Advances in Pediatric Surgery. London, JA Churchill, 1964)

in demonstrating the absence of residual shunts at the completion of the procedure. In those patients with pulmonary atresia or anomalous origin of the left anterior descending coronary artery from the right coronary artery, it may be necessary to reconstruct the right ventricular outflow tract by placing a valved conduit from the right ventricle to the pulmonary artery.

The controversy in the surgery for tetralogy of Fallot surrounds those children less than 2 years old, particularly those under 1 year of age who are symptomatic with increasing hypoxic episodes. While operative mortality is increased in this group, some authors maintain that these infants can be corrected in one stage with an operative risk less than that of an initial shunt procedure followed by total correction at a later date (two stage). Others have indicated that the two-stage approach is best in these small infants. In a very carefully documented series of publications, Kirklin and associates have demonstrated that age, body surface area, and the necessity for a transannular patch affect the operative mortality. Because some studies indicate that transannular patches are associated with an increase in operative risk and poor long-term results, they have reverted to using transannular patches only when necessary, preferring instead to accept a slightly higher PRV/LV. In their hands, if a transannular patch is not necessary (and this can be predicted reasonably well preoperatively), then one-stage total correction is safer unless the body surface area is less than 0.36 M². If a transannular patch will be necessary, and if the patient is less than 24 months old or if body surface area is less than 0.48 M², then the two-stage procedure (*i.e.,* initial palliation followed by total correction at a later date) is safer. We have in general adopted this approach to correction of tetralogy of Fallot in infants and have been pleased with our results.

RESULTS

In those patients over 2 years of age who have favorable anatomy and who undergo total correction, the operative mortality rate is now less than 5%. In good hands, the risk of those patients who require initial shunt because of unfavorable anatomy or other reasons and who then undergo total correction is only slightly increased. The risk for total correction in infants under 2 years of age is also increased. Complete heart block is unusual now following total correction of tetralogy, but some degree of right ventricular failure is not uncommon, particularly in the immediate postoperative period. Some degree of pulmonary insufficiency is common, especially in those in whom a patch across the pulmonary valve annulus is necessary. Pulmonary insufficiency is usually well tolerated, but more recent studies have indicated that long-term prognosis might not be as good in those patients with significant residual pulmonary insufficiency.

A recent report indicated that excellent long-term results were obtained in 87% of 396 patients. Of the 13% with less than excellent results, 7% were due to postoperative death, 4% to necessity for reoperation, and 2% to residual symptoms. Despite the complexity of this lesion, excellent surgical therapy results in a good long-term outlook for most of these patients.

PULMONARY VALVULAR STENOSIS AND PULMONARY ATRESIA

In pulmonary valvular stenosis, the basic problem resides in abnormal formation of the pulmonary valve. In its classic, severe form, the pulmonary valve takes the shape of a conical fibrous funnel, which projects superiorly into the pulmonary trunk and is formed by the fusion of the valve leaflets. In extremely severe cases, the opening of the valve may be only 1 mm to 2 mm in diameter. In moderate stenosis, only a partial peripheral fusion of the cusps occurs, leaving the central portion of each leaflet relatively free. In pulmonary valve atresia, the pulmonary cusps are fused and form a diaphragmlike membrane with two or three well-discernible raphe. In the majority of instances of pulmonary atresia, the pulmonary valve ring as well as the main pulmonary artery is hypoplastic.

Secondary changes due to valvular obstruction occur in the right ventricle and pulmonary arteries with typical pulmonary valvular stenosis. The right ventricle may be markedly hypertrophied. This hypertrophy is particularly noticeable in the infundibular region, producing narrowing of the outlet of the right ventricle. When pulmonary atresia with an intact ventricular system is present, the right ventricle is small and may be severely hypoplastic. The pulmonary arterial trunk is usually dilated, except in cases of pulmonary atresia, and a "jet" lesion may be found in its wall. The dilatation begins with the pulmonary ring, which in some cases may be smaller than normal. A distinctive type of familial pulmonary valvular stenosis called pulmonary valvular dysplasia has been described. It is

PULMONARY STENOSIS AND PULMONARY ATRESIA	
History	Morgagni described, 1761; Brock valvotomy, 1948
Incidence	10% of congenital heart defects
Pathophysiology	Obstruction to pulmonary blood flow → RVH In pulmonary atresia, pulmonary flow through PDA
Dx	History: symptoms mild to moderate with pulmonary stenosis; severe cyanosis with pulmonary atresia Physical exam: systolic murmur and right ventricular lift with pulmonary stenosis; cyanosis with atresia ECG: RVH Echo: abnormal pulmonary valve in pulmonary stenosis; absent valve in pulmonary atresia Catheterization: gradient from right ventricle → pulmonary artery and "domed" pulmonary valve with pulmonary stenosis; hypoplastic right ventricle with pulmonary atresia and intact septum; ± VSD
Rx	Pulmonary valvotomy for pulmonary stenosis; systemic pulmonary shunt for pulmonary atresia with subsequent correction through right ventricle–pulmonary artery conduit
Results	Mortality rate <1% and good long-term results with pulmonary stenosis; results with pulmonary atresia and VSD similar to tetralogy of Fallot; long-term results for pulmonary atresia and intact septum not as good

characterized by dysplastic stenosis of the valve without fusion of the cusps. If a ventricular septal defect is present with pulmonary valvular stenosis, the lesion is often termed tetralogy of Fallot, although the relationship of the aorta to the ventricular septal defect is important in classifying this lesion.

PATHOPHYSIOLOGY

In pulmonary valvular stenosis, the physiologic aberrations are directly related to the amount of stenosis present. If the stenosis is mild, the ventricle is enlarged but functions well and the patient is asymptomatic. If the stenosis is moderate, the right ventricle gradually hypertrophies and later in life may demonstrate reduced function. If the obstruction is severe from birth, the lesion may simulate pulmonary atresia with intact ventricular septum with severe cyanosis occurring with ductal closure. In these patients, the right ventricle functions poorly, probably due to right ventricular subendocardial ischemia resulting in part from the very high right ventricular end-diastolic pressures. In older patients with severe pulmonary stenosis, cyanosis during exercise may be caused by high right ventricular end-diastolic pressures, with diastolic right-to-left shunting through a patent foramen ovale. Pulmonary atresia with intact ventricular septum in infancy is associated with extreme cyanosis and marked diminution in pulmonary blood flow when the ductus arteriosus closes. Pulmonary atresia associated with a ventricular septal defect produces similar symptoms; however, the right ventricle in pulmonary atresia with ventricular septal defect is usually quite large and possesses good function, whereas the right ventricle in pulmonary atresia with an intact ventricular septum is usually markedly abnormal. The chamber size is very small unless there is significant tricuspid regurgitation. The function of this ventricle is usually markedly impaired, and there are often direct communications between the right ventricular cavity and the epicardial coronary arteries, especially when tricuspid regurgitation is not present.

DIAGNOSIS

Patients with pulmonary atresia or severe pulmonary valve stenosis with or without ventricular septal defect present early in life with cyanosis. If pulmonary stenosis is not severe, pulmonary blood flow may be adequate until secondary right ventricular obstructive changes cause the gradual development of cyanosis within the first year of life. Patients with moderate to severe pulmonary valve stenosis with intact ventricular septum may be asymptomatic until later in childhood and early adulthood, when exercise produces some dyspnea. Mild pulmonary stenosis may be well tolerated for a normal life expectancy.

PHYSICAL EXAMINATION

Physical examination is remarkable for extreme cyanosis in the case of pulmonary atresia and cyanosis in cases of pulmonary valve stenosis in which there is right-to-left shunting across the foramen ovale. When the right ventricle is enlarged, there is usually a marked substernal lift. A loud left parasternal murmur is heard, and there is often an ejection click if the valve leaflets are pliable.

ELECTROCARDIOGRAPHY

The electrocardiogram demonstrates right axis deviation, right ventricular hypertrophy, and, in some cases, right atrial enlargement.

CHEST FILM

The chest film in most cases of pulmonary atresia demonstrates the typical boot-shaped heart described in tetralogy of Fallot. In pulmonary valve stenosis, there is usually marked enlargement of the pulmonary artery (poststenotic dilatation). Right ventricular enlargement is seen on the lateral projection.

ECHOCARDIOGRAPHY

In pulmonary stenosis, the echocardiogram will show the abnormal pulmonary valve. In cases of pulmonary atresia, the echocardiogram may demonstrate absence of the pulmonary valve.

CARDIAC CATHETERIZATION

Cardiac catheterization reveals the essential features of the lesions. With simple pulmonary valve stenosis, a gradient between the right ventricle and pulmonary artery is iden-

tified and the "domed" abnormal valve is seen. In cases of pulmonary atresia with intact ventricular septum, it may be very difficult to enter the hypoplastic right ventricle, and a mistaken diagnosis of tricuspid atresia may be made. If the ductus arteriosus is patent, an injection into the aorta usually discloses the main pulmonary artery and pulmonary valve, if present. A left ventricular angiocardiogram will identify the presence or absence of a ventricular septal defect.

TREATMENT

In older children with simple pulmonary valve stenosis, open division of the fused commissures using cardiopulmonary bypass will give excellent results (Fig. 39-17). In infants with critical cyanosis due to pulmonary atresia or severe pulmonary valvular stenosis, infusion of prostaglandin E$_1$ to maintain ductal patency may be lifesaving. This allows the infant to be stabilized, the acidosis to be corrected, and the child to be made ready for urgent operation. In cases of critical pulmonary stenosis associated with relatively normal right ventricular size and function, a pulmonary valvotomy, usually performed in a closed fashion through the right ventricular outflow tract or through the pulmonary artery with inflow occlusion, often produces good results (Fig. 39-18). In cases of critical pulmonary stenosis associated with poor right ventricular function or pulmonary atresia with an intact ventricular septum, it is often necessary to construct a systemic pulmonary artery shunt to improve pulmonary blood flow in addition to establishing some continuity between the right ventricle and the pulmonary arteries. Patients with pulmonary atresia and ventricular septal defect are best treated with a systemic pulmonary artery shunt until later in life when repair of the ventricular septal defect and conduit replacement of the main pulmo-

Fig. 39-17. A fused commissure is incised. The incision is made into the wall of the pulmonary artery and then carried inferiorly into the right ventricle. This maneuver allows retraction of the valve leaflets, which are fused at the commissure level. (Ochsner JL: Isolated pulmonary stenosis and atresia. In Hardy JD [ed]: Rhoads Textbook of Surgery, 5th ed. Philadelphia, J B Lippincott, 1977)

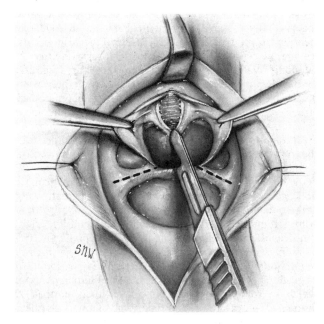

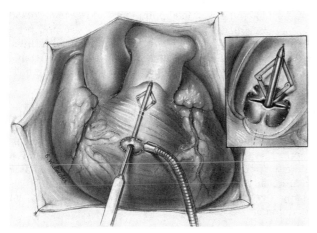

Fig. 39-18. Valvulotome knife is passed through the domed valve and the leaflets are incised. This maneuver is repeated with the knife at right angles to first passage. Dilators are then passed through the incised valve to ensure an adequate opening. (Ochsner JL: Isolated pulmonary stenosis and atresia. In Hardy JD [ed]: Rhoads Textbook of Surgery, 5th ed. Philadelphia, J B Lippincott, 1977)

nary artery and valve will be necessary using standard cardiopulmonary bypass techniques. If patients with pulmonary atresia and intact ventricular septum survive the critical period during infancy, several options are open for treatment. If the right ventricle enlarges, it is sometimes possible to open completely the pulmonary outflow tract with a patch or valve containing conduit. If, however, the right ventricle fails to grow, it is probably desirable to perform several shunting procedures with the ultimate goal of performing an anastomosis of the right atrium to the pulmonary artery (Fontan operation) later in life if the left ventricle is still functioning well and the pulmonary vascular resistance is low.

TRANSPOSITION OF THE GREAT ARTERIES

Transposition means, quite literally, that the aorta arises from the right ventricle and the pulmonary artery arises from the left ventricle. The term *transposition of the great arteries* refers to an abnormal ventriculoarterial relationship but represents only one of several forms of abnormal positioning of the great arteries. The most frequent type of transposition abnormality is called complete d-transposition of the great arteries. The modifying *d* (dextro) applied to a ventriculoarterial connection indicates that the aortic valve is spatially positioned to the right of the left ventricle, suggesting that the embryologic rotation of the heart has been in the rightward (or dextro) direction. Transposition of the great arteries is also present in association with other forms of cardiac malposition and abnormal atrioventricular relationships. These are unusual and are not covered in this section. Approximately one half of patients with d-transposition of the great arteries will have simple transposition, indicating that no additional significant malformations (other than a PDA) are present. Approximately one half of the remaining patients will have a significant ventricular septal defect in association with subvalvular pulmonary stenosis. The small remaining group will have transposition associated with other more complicated forms of congenital heart disease, the most common being tricuspid atresia.

TRANSPOSITION OF THE GREAT ARTERIES	
History	Ballie described, 1797; Blalock and Hanlon palliated, 1950; first complete correction by Senning, 1959
Incidence	10% to 12% of congenital heart defects
Anatomy	Ventriculoarterial discordance; 50% have "simple" d-transposition; of remaining, 50% will have a VSD and the rest will have complicated anatomy
Pathophysiology	Parallel circulations which require a communication at some level to permit survival beyond infancy; increased incidence of pulmonary hypertension especially with associated PDA or VSD
Dx	History: extreme cyanosis in infancy; heart failure with VSD Physical exam: no murmur in simple transposition; loud murmur with VSD and pulmonary stenosis ECG: RVH with simple transposition, LVH with VSD or PDA Chest film: normal heart size in simple transposition; ↑ heart size with complicated disease Echo: reversed systolic time intervals Catheterization: ventriculoarterial discordance; ± VSD; ± PDA; ± pulmonic stenosis
Rx	Balloon atrial septostomy in infancy; Senning or Mustard repair at 3 to 6 months
Results	Operative mortality ~ 5% in "simple" transposition; late results generally good

PATHOPHYSIOLOGY

The physiologic aberrations of this lesion result in the circulation being altered from its conventional "series" connection between the pulmonary and systemic circulation to a complete "parallel" circulation, in which oxygenated blood circulates through the lungs and the left side of the heart and unoxygenated blood circulates through the systemic circulation and the right side of the heart (Fig. 39-19). The only opportunity for oxygenated blood to enter the systemic circulation is through intracardiac communications such as in atrial or ventricular septal defects or a PDA. Because of this abnormal relationship, it is easy to see why infants born with transposition immediately become quite ill when the ductus arteriosus closes.

The other physiologic aberration that plays a great role in the clinical course of patients with transposition of the great arteries is the physiologic prerequisite of increased pulmonary blood flow. With an atrial septal defect or PDA, it is necessary for the pulmonary blood flow to be greater

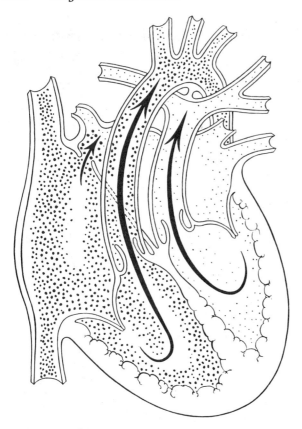

Fig. 39-19. Transposition of the great arteries. The aorta arises from the right ventricle, and the pulmonary artery arises from the left ventricle. Except for minimal shunting through the patent foramen ovale, there is no mixing of the systemic and the pulmonary circulation. (Waldhausen JA, Pierce WS: Transposition of the great arteries. In Hardy JD [ed]: Rhoads Textbook of Surgery, 5th ed. Philadelphia, J B Lippincott, 1977)

than the systemic blood flow for effective oxygenation of systemic blood. This greater pulmonary blood flow may explain the rather rapid and accelerated development of pulmonary vascular obstructive disease in patients with transposition, especially when transposition is combined with persistent PDA or ventricular septal defect.

Because the anatomical right ventricle is required to pump blood through the systemic circulation and to oppose systemic vascular resistance, it is not surprising that measured indices of ventricular function in infants and children with tranposition demonstrate that right ventricular function is depressed. The causes of this dysfunction remain unclear but are possibly related to the relatively prolonged early myocardial hypoxia. The angiographic and echocardiographic findings of depressed right ventricular function are usually in contrast to the clinical appearance of these children, who, when palliated or corrected by an interatrial transposition of blood flow, appear to grow and behave normally.

DIAGNOSIS

Cyanosis, hypoxic deterioration, or congestive heart failure with early death summarizes the usual clinical course in the untreated infant. Because the circulation is so abnormal in transposition of the great arteries, the clinical manifestations and course are influenced by the extent of communications between the two circulations. Because of the

minimal aberrations of fetal pulmonary and systemic blood flow, these infants are usually of normal size and body weight and rarely are victims of intrauterine fetal distress. Extreme cyanosis without alteration with oxygen therapy, grunting respiration, and progressive acidosis are the hallmark features.

ELECTROCARDIOGRAPHY

There are no findings specific to transposition of the great arteries on the electrocardiogram. If the main communication between the two circulations is at the atrial level, there is often right ventricular hypertrophy. If a large ventricular septal defect or PDA is present, left ventricular changes consistent with left ventricular hypertrophy will predominate.

CHEST FILM

The chest film does not demonstrate any specific changes strongly suggestive of transposition of the great arteries other than a very narrow vascular pedicle in the superior mediastinum. The appearance of the heart and superior mediastinum in transposition has often been likened to an "egg on a string."

ECHOCARDIOGRAPHY

The echocardiogram can be quite specific for the diagnosis of transposition of the great arteries. Systolic time intervals recorded over both ventricles will show a reversal of the normal ratio, with the left ventricular systolic time interval being prolonged over the right. The semilunar valves appear to lie side by side without an intervening crista. These features may not be present if a large PDA or ventricular septal defect is present or if there is pulmonary hypertension.

CARDIAC CATHETERIZATION

Cardiac catheterization is carried out on an emergent basis in the neonate with poor intercirculatory mixing. Ordinarily, the diagnosis at cardiac catheterization is very obvious when the catheter passes from the right atrium into the right ventricle, which is at systemic pressure, and thence into the aorta. Entrance into the pulmonary artery and measurement of pulmonary artery flow are often difficult. Cineangiocardiography is useful in detecting other associated anomalies, in quantitating ventricular function, and in more carefully investigating the presence of subvalvular or valvular pulmonary stenosis. Cardiac catheterization is therapeutic in the neonate when balloon atrial septostomy, first described by Rashkind in 1966, is performed. By rupturing the thin atrial septum in the area of the fossa ovalis, intercirculatory mixing at the atrial level is greatly facilitated. This often allows delay of any operative procedures until 6 months of age or later.

TREATMENT

PALLIATIVE PROCEDURE

The Blalock–Hanlon atrial septectomy is an ingenious technique by which a portion of the atrial septum may be resected (thus increasing "mixing" at the atrial level) without the need for cardiopulmonary bypass. Currently, the Blalock–Hanlon atrial septectomy is rarely needed for the palliation of infants with transposition of the great arteries. This technique is necessary only if balloon atrial septostomy is repeatedly unsuccessful or cannot be performed because of anatomical variations in the atrium, such as absence of the fossa ovalis (commonly seen with persistent left superior vena cava draining to the coronary sinus). This procedure may also be performed to create a large atrial septal defect if there are other associated malformations precluding early corrective operation.

The procedure is carried out through a right thoracotomy. The pericardium is opened at the junction of the pulmonary veins with the left atrium, and the phrenic nerve is retracted upward. The oblique pericardial sinus is dissected such that it communicates with the transverse pericardial sinus, allowing a partial-occlusion vascular clamp to be placed underneath the left pulmonary veins, including both the rightward portions of the right and left atria. The right pulmonary artery and right pulmonary veins are occluded, and an incision is made in the right atrium and left atrium paralleling the septum. A portion of atrial septum, which includes the fossa ovalis, is excised, and the clamp is then reapplied to allow the newly created atrial septal defect to slip backward into the nonclamped portion of the atria. The atrial incision is then closed. Great care must be taken during the operation to maintain stable acid–base balance and to avoid major hemorrhage, which are the most frequent causes of poor results.

CORRECTIVE OPERATIONS

At this time, operations to transpose venous inflow into the heart are the most commonly performed operations for correction of transposition of the great arteries. These operations can be carried out in infancy without significant additional risk. The goal of these operations is to transpose systemic venous inflow to the mitral valve and pulmonary venous flow to the tricuspid valve. The operation that has been performed in greatest numbers is the Mustard procedure, which employs a pericardial baffle to direct systemic venous flow through the mitral valve and pulmonary venous return through the tricuspid valve. Using this operation, it is often necessary to use additional pericardium to enlarge the new pulmonary venous atrium so that unobstructed flow from the pulmonary veins to the tricuspid valve is achieved. In the past few years, a resurgence in the use of the Senning operation has come about. In the Senning operation, flaps of atrial tissue are used to create baffles to redirect systemic and pulmonary venous flow. The interest in this operation has been prompted by the rather high incidence of caval obstruction with the Mustard operation and the disturbing number of atrial dysrhythmias following this procedure.

Deep hypothermia and circulatory arrest greatly facilitate creation of an atrial transposition procedure. Infants are cooled to 18°C with a combination of surface cooling and pump-induced hypothermia. The dry, motionless field afforded by this technique greatly increases the likelihood of the creation of an accurate, nontraumatic suture line in creating the various baffles. If a ventricular septal defect is to be closed, great care must be taken not to damage the tricuspid valve, as this is the systemic atrioventricular valve. Systemic atrioventricular valve incompetence is one of the most common causes for failure after the combination of ventricular septal defect repair and atrial transposition procedures.

If severe subpulmonic stenosis is present, the Rastelli procedure is preferred. Since this procedure requires the use of a Dacron valve containing conduit, this operation should be carried out later in life, usually at 2 to 3 years of age.

Standard cardiopulmonary bypass techniques are used, and a large intracardiac baffle redirects left ventricular blood flow through the ventricular septal defect into the aorta, and the conduit bypasses the stenotic subpulmonic obstruction by directing flow from the anterior right ventricle to the bifurcation of the pulmonary arteries.

The disadvantage to both the Mustard and the Senning operation is that the tricuspid valve becomes the systemic atrioventricular valve and the right ventricle becomes the systemic ventricle. A more ideal procedure would involve switching the aorta and pulmonary arteries ("anatomical correction"). This procedure was first successfully performed by Jatene and co-workers in 1977. Anatomical correction for transposition of the great arteries has been carried out in several centers throughout the world. Suffice it to say that at this time it is classified as an experimental procedure that is applicable to only certain types of transposition, and the rather high operative mortality rate (10%–50%) in reported series precludes its use on a routine basis.

RESULTS

Results with the Mustard and Senning operations are usually quite good, with an operative mortality rate less than 5% and a very low late mortality. A feature of both atrial transposition operations is that the right ventricle must act as the systemic ventricle. Most patients who have repeat cardiac catheterization after atrial transposition operations demonstrate poor right ventricular function. This leads to the inevitable speculation that the right ventricle will not support the systemic circulation over a normal life span.

DOUBLE OUTLET RIGHT VENTRICLE

Both great arteries arise from the anatomical right ventricle, and a variety of associated defects can be present (Fig. 39-20). Although double outlet right ventricle has been classified in several ways, a useful classification is presented in Table 39-1. This classification emphasizes the relationship of the ventricular septal defect and the great arteries, since this is an important determinant of the technique for surgical repair. In patients with this lesion, subpulmonic obstruction may be present in a few cases.

PATHOPHYSIOLOGY

The pathophysiology is primarily determined by the presence or absence of pulmonic stenosis, the relationship of the great arteries to the ventricles, and the presence or absence of ventricular inversion. In patients without significant pulmonic stenosis and normally related great arteries, the pathophysiology is similar to that of ventricular septal defect. The pulmonary blood flow will be high and congestive heart failure will be present in most cases. If the great arteries are transposed or if the ventricles are inverted and pulmonic stenosis is not present, a combination of arterial desaturation causing cyanosis and high pulmonary blood flow will simulate transposition of the great arteries and ventricular septal defect. Obstructive pulmonary vascular disease may occur early. If pulmonic stenosis is present with any of the above combinations of situations, cyanosis will be prominent and its complications, polycythemia and dyspnea with growth failure, will be evident early in infancy. A few patients with relatively balanced pulmonary and systemic

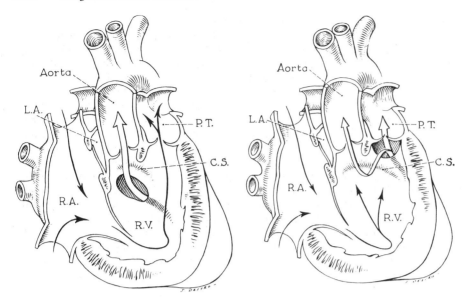

Fig. 39-20. (*Left*) Origin of both great vessels from the right ventricle without pulmonary stenosis, type I. Characteristically, the defect lies posteroinferiorly to the crista supraventricularis (*C.S.*). (*Right*) Origin of both great vessels from the right ventricle without pulmonary stenosis, type II. The defect lies anterosuperiorly to the crista supraventricularis and is closely applied to the origin of the pulmonary trunk (*P.T.*). This type is synonymous with the Taussig–Bing complex. *R.A.*, right atrium; *L.A.*, left atrium; *R.V.*, right ventricle. (Waldhausen JA, Pierce WS: Double-outlet right ventricle. In Hardy JD [ed]: Rhoads Textbook of Surgery, 5th ed. Philadelphia, J B Lippincott, 1977)

DOUBLE OUTLET RIGHT VENTRICLE

History	Peacock first reported, 1866; McGoon first repaired, 1957
Incidence	1%–2% of congenital heart defects
Anatomy	Both great vessels arise from the anatomical right ventricle; VSD
Pathophysiology	↑ pulmonary blood flow if pulmonary outflow obstruction is absent ↓ pulmonary flow with pulmonary obstruction; cyanosis and ↑ flow if transposition of great arteries (TGA) is associated with no pulmonary obstruction
Dx	History: heart failure, cyanosis, or both Physical exam: cardiac enlargement and prominent murmur in most ECG: RVH Chest film: cardiac enlargement, cardiac malposition in some Echo: lack of aortic–mitral continuity Catheterization: VSD, lack of aortic–mitral continuity
Rx	Operative repair by baffling left ventricular blood into the aorta and closing VSD
Results	Operative risk ~ 10%, late results guarded

circulations will experience normal growth and development.

DIAGNOSIS

When pulmonary blood flow is increased, a history of congestive failure with dyspnea on exertion, poor feeding,

sweating, and growth failure will be prominent. If pulmonary obstruction is present, cyanosis will be prominent with its attendant difficulties.

PHYSICAL EXAMINATION

In most cases, the heart will be enlarged and there will be a parasternal murmur. If pulmonic stenosis is present, cyanosis will be obvious.

ELECTROCARDIOGRAPHY

Evidence of right ventricular hypertrophy and a counter-clockwise vector loop in the frontal plane are present in most cases of double outlet right ventricle.

CHEST FILM

There is no characteristic radiographic appearance. The heart is most often enlarged and evidence of increased blood flow is present in cases without pulmonic stenosis. Cardiac malposition is present in some cases of ventricular inversion.

ECHOCARDIOGRAPHY

There are no consistently characteristic features on echocardiography that establish this diagnosis. In some cases, absence of direct aortic valve–mitral valve continuity suggests the diagnosis.

CARDIAC CATHETERIZATION

The passage of the cardiac catheter from the aorta into the right ventricle and from the right ventricle into the pul-

TABLE 39-1   CLASSIFICATION OF DOUBLE OUTLET RIGHT VENTRICLE

I. Situs solitus of atria and ventricles
  A. Normally related great arteries
    1. Subaortic VSD
    2. Subpulmonary VSD
  B. Abnormally related great arteries
    1. Subpulmonary VSD
    2. Subaortic VSD
II. Situs solitus of atria, situs inversus of ventricles
  A. Normally related great arteries
  B. Abnormally related great arteries

monary artery suggests the diagnosis. Careful angiocardiographic examination reveals a lack of angiographic continuity between the aortic and the mitral annulus and is the characteristic feature in this lesion. The other associated angiographic patterns are based on the specific type of double outlet right ventricle present.

TREATMENT

The treatment in this lesion is primarily surgical. If cyanosis is prominent in infancy, systemic pulmonary artery shunting is indicated to improve arterial oxygen saturation. If excessive pulmonary blood flow is present in infancy and congestive heart failure is severe, and if the lesion is associated with other anomalies that would make complete repair difficult, pulmonary artery banding may be indicated.

Complete repair in infancy may be possible in the other types of this lesion. All are performed using cardiopulmonary bypass with or without the use of profound hypothermia and circulatory arrest. In type IA, the repair is carried out through a right ventriculotomy with direction of the left ventricular blood flow through the ventricular septal defect into the aorta by an interventricular baffle. In type IB, it is often necessary to perform an interatrial transposition of venous return by the Senning or Mustard technique and repair the ventricular septal defect through the atrium, if possible. Other repairs are based upon the specific anatomy of each individual patient, which may be quite variable. The location of the ventricular septal defect in relation to the aorta and pulmonary artery is extremely important in determining the specific operation to be performed.

RESULTS

The operative mortality for the treatment of this lesion has declined in recent years. Currently, the operative risk is about 10%, but this depends upon the specific anatomy. The presence of associated anomalies increases the risk. Long-term results of these operations will be determined by careful follow-up of operated patients.

TRICUSPID ATRESIA

The spectrum of tricuspid atresia consists of failure of formation of the right atrioventricular (tricuspid) valve, varying degrees of hypoplasia of the right ventricle and infundibulum, and a defect in the atrial septum. In addition to the above abnormalities, there may be transposition of the great arteries and a ventricular septal defect with or without pulmonary outflow tract stenosis. A simplified classification of the anatomical types of tricuspid atresia is presented in Table 39-2. This classification divides tricuspid atresia according to associated lesions. In type I, the great arteries are normally related and subtypes involve the presence of a small or large ventricular septal defect and related pulmonary stenosis or atresia. In type II, there is d-transposition of the great arteries associated with a ventricular septal defect with or without pulmonary stenosis. In type III, there is l-transposition of the great arteries.

In all forms of tricuspid atresia, there is a dimple in the right atrium at the usual anatomical position of the tricuspid valve. The right atrium is invariably enlarged, with thickened muscular walls. There is always an interatrial communication, which is usually a patent foramen ovale, but a true secundum atrial septal defect may be present. The right ventricle is hypoplastic, especially in its inflow portion.

TABLE 39-2   TRICUSPID ATRESIA: ANATOMIC TYPES AND FREQUENCY

TYPE	INCIDENCE FROM CLINICAL SERIES (%)

I. Normally related great arteries
   Intact ventricular septum with pulmonary atresia
   Small ventricular septal defect and pulmonary stenosis
   Large ventricular septal defect without pulmonary stenosis
	69–75

II. d-Transposition of the great arteries
   Ventricular septal defect with pulmonary atresia
   Ventricular septal defect with pulmonary stenosis
   Ventricular septal defect without pulmonary stenosis
	20–28

III. l-Transposition of the great arteries	3–7

TRICUSPID ATRESIA	
History	Holmes described, 1824; Blalock palliated, 1945; Fontan corrected, 1968
Incidence	1%–3% of congenital heart defects
Anatomy	Tricuspid valvular atresia; hypoplasia of the right ventricle; associated with pulmonary outflow tract stenosis, VSD, TGA
Pathophysiology	Cyanosis in 75%; the rest a mixture of cyanosis and heart failure
Dx	History: extreme cyanosis with dyspnea is most common; also congestive heart failure in some, and a few may be asymptomatic Physical exam: cyanosis, systolic murmur common; few with systemic venous congestion ECG: left axis deviation; notched P waves Chest film: normal heart size in most Echo: absent tricuspid valve; ↓ right ventricle Catheterization: catheter cannot traverse tricuspid valve
Rx	Palliative shunt procedure or pulmonary artery band in infancy depending on physiology; right ventricular bypass (Fontan procedure) to be considered later in life
Results	75% survive to the second decade

PATHOPHYSIOLOGY

There are two distinct physiological variants associated with different anatomical atresia. The largest subtype (75%) has reduced pulmonary blood flow due to the absence of a ventricular septal defect or varying degrees of pulmonary outflow tract obstruction. These patients usually have moderate to severe clinical cyanosis. The small pulmonary flow also results in reduced volume presented to the left ventricle, resulting in normal heart size and no heart failure.

The opposite physiology is associated with the other types; there is little or no obstruction to pulmonary blood flow associated with a ventricular septal defect. In these patients, only mild to moderate clinical cyanosis is present, and then usually present with congestive heart failure that may be quite severe. In patients with associated transposition of the great arteries, pulmonary vascular obstructive disease can develop quite early. In types associated with normally related great arteries, pulmonary blood flow gradually decreases from infancy, probably due to increasing muscular obstruction to flow through the ventricular septal defect or to actual closure of the muscular walls of the defect itself.

DIAGNOSIS

Three fourths of the patients with tricuspid atresia present with a history of cyanosis, usually from birth. Infants with decreased pulmonary blood flow and no ventricular septal defect or pulmonary outflow tract obstruction will become deeply cyanotic upon closure of the ductus arteriosus. They present with grunty respirations, hypoxemia, and acidosis, and their treatment is emergent. When increased pulmonary blood flow is moderate, associated with ventricular septal defect and some obstruction to pulmonary blood flow, cyanosis may be mild, but these patients may present later in infancy or early childhood with gradually deepening cyanosis, clubbing, and squatting. Increased pulmonary blood flow in this tricuspid atresia usually is indicated by a history of mild cyanosis and pulmonary congestion associated with poor feeding, dyspnea, and growth retardation.

PHYSICAL EXAMINATION

A systolic murmur is heard in 75% of the patients with diminished pulmonary blood flow. This is usually associated with a small ventricular septal defect or severe pulmonary outflow tract obstruction. In patients with increased pulmonary blood flow, there is always a relatively loud systolic murmur along the left sternal border or at the apex. The characteristic murmur of a PDA suggests pulmonary atresia. If the atrial septal defect is small, the signs of systemic venous congestion, including hepatomegaly, pulsation of jugular veins and liver, and peripheral edema, may be prominent.

ELECTROCARDIOGRAPHY

Extreme left axis deviation in a cyanotic child should raise a strong suspicion of the presence of tricuspid atresia. Right axis deviation occurs with transposition of the great arteries in which a large pulmonary artery is present. A notched P wave suggestive of right atrial enlargement is quite common.

CHEST FILM

In most patients, the heart size is either normal or only slightly increased. Cardiomegaly may be quite marked in those types with torrential pulmonary blood flow. The cardiac configuration usually resembles the boot-shaped heart seen in tetralogy of Fallot or the egg-shaped heart with a narrow superior mediastinal vascular pedicle typical of transposition of the great arteries. The pulmonary vascular markings are usually reduced but may be quite marked in patients with large pulmonary blood flows.

ECHOCARDIOGRAPHY

The echocardiogram is helpful in making the initial diagnosis of tricuspid atresia. The absence of tricuspid valve echoes in association with reduced right ventricular dimensions is strong presumptive evidence of tricuspid atresia. The echocardiographic features closely resemble those of single ventricle.

CARDIAC CATHETERIZATION

Cardiac catheterization data are characteristic. The right ventricle cannot be entered through the tricuspid valve. There is a very prominent A wave in the right atrium, a right-to-left shunt at the atrial level, and, in some cases, a gradient across the atrial septum. Angiocardiography discloses a typical sequence of appearance of contrast material in the cardiac chambers after a venous-to-right atrial injection. The contrast material appears first in the left atrium, then the left ventricle, and finally in the great arteries. There is typically a triangular area within the heart shadow that fails to fill with contrast medium early in the ventricular phase. That shadow is due to the absence of the inflow portion of the right ventricle. Angiocardiography gives valuable information about the size of cardiac chambers and relationships of the great arteries to the ventricles.

TREATMENT

All surgical treatment for patients with tricuspid atresia has been considered palliative. In the cyanotic infant, augmentation of pulmonary blood flow is required. This is accomplished by one of three types of shunts: aortopulmonary artery shunts, subclavian-to-pulmonary artery shunts, or superior vena cava-to-pulmonary artery shunts. The Blalock–Taussig shunt using the subclavian branch of the innominate artery to the side of the pulmonary artery is now becoming widely used in infancy. In some cases, the use of a prosthetic graft in the ascending aorta to the main pulmonary artery has offered good results in very tiny infants. Other types of systemic pulmonary artery shunts, including the Potts and Waterston operations, are becoming less popular because of significant late complications, specifically the development of pulmonary vascular disease, since this may prevent later "correction" by the Fontan procedure. In older children, the Blalock–Taussig shunt or a Glenn operation (superior vena cava-to-pulmonary artery shunt) will provide long-term relief of cyanosis.

In infants or children with increased pulmonary blood flow, medical management with digitalis and diuretics should be undertaken. If this treatment regimen fails, banding of the pulmonary artery may be necessary. In all groups, a large interatrial communication is necessary. If a large atrial septal defect is not present, a balloon atrial septostomy or Blalock–Hanlon atrial septectomy is required.

In many centers throughout the world, various modifications of the right ventricle bypass operation reported in 1971 by Fontan and Baudet have been performed. In this procedure, a connection is made between the right atrium and the pulmonary artery and the atrial septal defect is closed. Initially, the connection between the right atrium and right ventricle involved the use of a synthetic graft (conduit) containing a porcine valve. More recently, the necessity of a valve in the conduit has been questioned and direct communication between the right atrium and the pulmonary artery has been advocated, thus deleting both the conduit and the valve. If there is sufficient size to the hypoplastic right ventricle, some have reported direct communication from the right atrium to this portion of the right ventricle, allowing it to act as an auxiliary pump. The performance of this operation is dependent upon a condition of adequate left ventricular function and low pulmonary vascular resistance.

Postoperative care in these patients usually involves a period of systemic venous congestion, which usually subsides if a sinus rhythm is maintained. The presence of atrial dysrhythmias in the postoperative period is a disabling complication.

RESULTS

The overall survival in patients with tricuspid atresia is much less than normal. With appropriate management, 75% of the patients survive to the second decade of life. This compares with less than 10% without surgical therapy. With further follow-up, the results of the various newer modifications of the Fontan operation should allow a better understanding of the surgical therapy of this condition.

TRUNCUS ARTERIOSUS

Truncus arteriosus has its embryologic derivation in the first few weeks of fetal life. This defect is due to a lack of partitioning of the embryonic conus and is almost always associated with a ventricular septal defect. The large truncal valve may have from two to six cusps, although most valves have three cusps. Truncal valvular insufficiency is present in approximately 30% of patients. One quarter of the patients will demonstrate a right aortic arch, and an interruption of the aortic arch occurs in 10% to 15%.

The Collett–Edwards classification of persistent truncus arteriosus divides the defect into four types, based on the origin of the pulmonary arteries. In type I, a single arterial trunk gives rise to the aorta and main pulmonary artery. In type II, the right and left pulmonary arteries arise immediately adjacent to one another from the dorsal wall of the truncus. In type III, the right and left pulmonary arteries arise from either side of the truncus, and in type IV, the proximal pulmonary arteries are absent and pulmonary blood flow is by way of bronchial arteries. For practical purposes, most clinical cases of truncus arteriosus will be classified as either type I or II of the Collett–Edwards classification. These types comprise more than 75% of all cases in autopsy series.

PATHOPHYSIOLOGY

Blood from both the left and the right ventricle is ejected into the truncus. The systemic and pulmonary venous blood mix, and the degree of arterial oxygen unsaturation is dependent on the amount of pulmonary blood flow. Although pulmonary blood flow may be limited by stenosis of the pulmonary arteries, this is uncommonly present. In the great majority of patients, pulmonary blood flow (and thus arterial oxygen saturation) is determined by the re-

TRUNCUS ARTERIOSUS	
History	Taruffi first described, 1875; McGoon first successfully repaired, 1968
Incidence	1% to 4% of congenital heart defects
Anatomy	Large single vessel (truncus) overlying the septum and VSD receives blood from both ventricles; pulmonary artery arises from aorta
Pathophysiology	Pulmonary blood flow determined by pulmonary vascular resistance (PVR); cyanosis present if PVR ↑
Dx	History: severe heart failure in infancy, cyanosis later Physical exam: systolic murmur; cardiomegaly ECG: biventricular hypertrophy Chest film: biventricular enlargement; 25% with right aortic arch Echo: large single semilunar valve; large single vessel (truncus) arising from heart and overlying both ventricles Catheterization: equal pressures in both ventricles; large L → R shunt in infancy; pulmonary artery arises from aorta; ± truncal valve insufficiency
Rx	Operation in infancy before PVR ↑; remove pulmonary artery from aorta; close VSD; right ventricle–pulmonary artery continuity by valved conduit
Results	Operative mortality rate ~ 10% to 20%; late results guarded

sistance of flow in the pulmonary vascular bed. In infants with low pulmonary vascular resistance, pulmonary blood flow is torrential and heart failure is extremely common. If the infant survives this period, the high-pressure, high-flow lesion rapidly leads to the development of obstructive pulmonary vascular disease. There is a significant correlation between pulmonary vascular resistance and arterial oxygen saturation in truncus arteriosus. Patients with no anatomical pulmonary artery obstruction who have arterial oxygen saturation less than 85% in most instances have pronounced increases in pulmonary vascular resistance and advanced pulmonary vascular obstructive disease.

DIAGNOSIS

Symptoms of truncus arteriosus are dependent upon the level of pulmonary vascular resistance. During the first few weeks of life, when pulmonary vascular resistance is normally increased, symptoms are usually mild, unless there is associated significant truncal valve incompetence. With maturation of the fetal pulmonary vascular bed associated with a decrease in pulmonary vascular resistance and an increase in pulmonary blood flow, symptoms of congestive heart failure may develop. These include dyspnea, excessive sweating, and failure to thrive. Cyanosis is usually not present at this stage. With the progressive development of pulmonary vascular obstructive disease as the infant grows, cyanosis becomes more evident and heart failure decreases.

PHYSICAL EXAMINATION

Infants with heart failure will be thin and malnourished and have an extremely active precordium. There is a systolic thrill and murmur over the left third and fourth intercostal spaces. The apical impulse is prominent, and there are signs of cardiomegaly. When truncal valve incompetence is present, a diastolic murmur follows the second heart sound. In older children, the heart remains enlarged but is less active. The second heart sound is accentuated as pulmonary vascular resistance is increased.

ELECTROCARDIOGRAPHY

The electrocardiogram is nonspecific in this lesion and usually demonstrates biventricular hypertrophy.

CHEST FILM

The chest film demonstrates cardiomegaly with biventricular enlargement. The aortic arch is to the right in 15% of the patients, and the left pulmonary artery may be elevated from the normal position. The peripheral pulmonary vasculature is increased unless there is advanced pulmonary vascular obstructive disease.

ECHOCARDIOGRAPHY

The echocardiogram is useful in establishing the diagnosis of truncus arteriosus. Characteristic findings are those of a larger than normal aortic (truncal) root, which overrides the ventricular septum. The pulmonary valve will be absent. These findings are similar to those in patients with pulmonary atresia.

CARDIAC CATHETERIZATION

Right and left heart catheterization and angiocardiographic studies are indicated in all patients suspected of having truncus arteriosus, to establish the diagnosis, define the anatomy, and determine the pulmonary vascular resistance. Ventricular pressures will be equal, and in the absence of pulmonary artery stenosis, there are equal pressures in the ventricles, aorta, and pulmonary arteries. Oxygen saturation studies indicate bidirectional shunting at the ventricular level, the predominant shunt being left to right. Pulmonary flow and resistance should be determined by measurement of pressures and oxygen saturations in both pulmonary arteries. Angiocardiography outlines the ventricular septal defect beneath the truncal valve. Both ventricles eject into a single arterial trunk. Injection of the truncus reveals the origin of the pulmonary arteries and allows assessment of truncal valve incompetence.

TREATMENT

Due to the extremely high mortality of infants treated medically for this lesion, surgical therapy constitutes the most practical alternative (Fig. 39-21). Palliative therapy consisting of pulmonary artery banding of the main pulmonary artery in type I lesions or of both branch pulmonary arteries in type II lesions has been used in the past but with a very high mortality. With anatomical pulmonary artery obstruction, systemic pulmonary artery shunting allows good palliation leading to later complete repair.

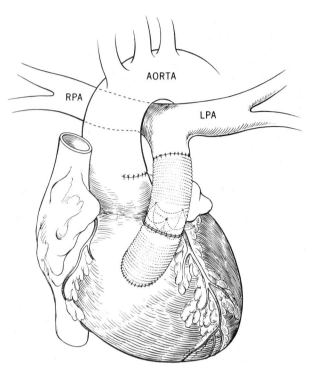

Fig. 39-21. Operative correction of a type A, subtype 1, common aorticopulmonary trunk. *LPA*, left pulmonary artery; *RPA*, right pulmonary artery. (Waldhausen JA, Tyers GFD: Common aorticopulmonary trunk. In Hardy JD [ed]: Rhoads Textbook of Surgery, 5th ed. Philadelphia, J B Lippincott, 1977)

Recent series indicate the superiority of early complete repair in truncus arteriosus not associated with anatomical pulmonary artery obstruction. The operation is performed through a median sternotomy incision, and repair in small infants may be facilitated by the use of profound hypothermia and circulatory arrest. In older children, standard cardiopulmonary bypass techniques with local myocardial hypothermia with or without the use of cardioplegia are used. The pulmonary arteries usually can be excised from the truncus as a single segment, even in type II defects. The site of pulmonary artery origin from the aorta is repaired with simple suture. An incision in the right ventricle is made high in the ventricle in the planned direction of the conduit. A patch is used to close the ventricular septal defect. A Dacron conduit of appropriate size containing a porcine valve is cut to proper length and used to establish continuity between the right ventricle and the pulmonary arteries. The course of the conduit should be such that kinking is avoided and the closed sternum does not compress the conduit.

RESULTS

Operative mortality is low in patients over 2 years of age who have complete repair of truncus arteriosus. Unfortunately, this experience is biased in that a large number of infants with this lesion will have died due to the high mortality of medical treatment and palliative procedures. Recent experience suggests that the proper management of patients with truncus arteriosus and high pulmonary blood flow is complete correction when fetal pulmonary changes begin to regress and pulmonary blood flow increases. A hospital mortality rate of 10% to 20% can be expected with this approach and is related to the type of anatomical lesions, the degree of pulmonary vascular resistance, and the clinical condition of the infant prior to operation. The prognosis for long survival is guarded due to the need for reoperation to replace the conduit with larger sizes as the child grows.

TOTAL ANOMALOUS PULMONARY VENOUS CONNECTION

Total anomalous pulmonary venous connection (TAPVC) defines the anomaly in which the pulmonary veins have no direct communication with the left atrium. Instead, they connect to the right atrium or one of the systemic veins. The left atrium has no tributaries and receives all blood by an atrial septal defect. In this condition, the valves and ventricles are usually normal and a successful repair should lead to an excellent long-term result. The most common

TOTAL ANOMALOUS PULMONARY VENOUS CONNECTION	
History	Wilson first described, 1798; Lewis first corrected, 1956
Incidence	1% of congenital heart defects
Anatomy	Pulmonary veins have no connection with left atrium but instead connect to a systemic vein or right atrium.
Pathophysiology	Obstruction of anomalous connection produces severe pulmonary congestion and hypertension.
Dx	History: moribund in infancy if obstruction is severe; poor growth, dyspnea if partial or no obstruction Physical exam: stiff lungs and poor myocardial function with obstruction; right ventricular lift, left parasternal flow murmur, and split second sound in older patients ECG: right axis deviation; RVH Chest film: normal heart size and congested lungs with obstruction; snowman-shaped heart produced by anomalous vertical vein; enlarged heart and pulmonary arteries without obstruction Echo: right ventricular diastolic volume overload; may identify anomalous drainage, especially coronary sinus Catheterization: elevated pulmonary artery pressure in most; pulmonary angiogram demonstrates the anomalous connection
Rx	Urgent operation in infancy; anastomosis between common venous chamber and left atrium
Results	Higher operative mortality in infants with obstruction; excellent long-term results in survivors

classification of TAPVC was first described by Darling in 1957. This classification divides the anomaly into four subtypes that conveniently describe the anatomical connections of the pulmonary venous circulation to the systemic venous circulation. Type I, or supracardiac, anomalies result when a common pulmonary vein connects with the remnants of the cardinal venous system to form an ascending ("vertical") vein that usually connects with the innominate vein or superior vena cava. In type II, or cardiac, TAPVC, the common pulmonary venous sinus most commonly connects to the coronary sinus. In a second major subgroup, the pulmonary veins drain individually or collectively into a sinus in the posterior right atrium. In type III, or infracardiac, connections, a common venous chamber connects to an inferior vein that passes through the diaphragm, where it then connects to the portal vein, ductus venous, or other systemic veins in the upper abdomen. Type IV, mixed TAPVC, is an uncommon condition in which the pulmonary venous connections are divided such that one lung drains to one of the systemic veins and pulmonary veins from the opposite side usually join one of the cardiac chambers, usually the coronary sinus.

PATHOPHYSIOLOGY

The factors that influence the pathophysiology of TAPVC include obligatory mixing of pulmonary and systemic blood upstream to or at the right atrium, the presence of obstruction of the anomalous connection, the size of the atrial septal defect, and associated anomalies. The presence or absence of obstruction of the anomalous connection is the most significant factor that influences the patient's clinical condition. The pathophysiological consequences of an obstructive anomalous pulmonary venous connection are pulmonary edema, pulmonary hypertension, and poor myocardial function. Infants born with obstructive connections often retain ductal patency. This serves to decompress the pulmonary artery and thus unload the right ventricle.

DIAGNOSIS

The severity of the clinical manifestations of TAPVC is directly related to the presence or absence of obstruction of the anomalous connection. With obstruction, the infant usually becomes symptomatic, with mild to moderate cyanosis, tachypnea, and low cardiac output in the first hours or days after birth. Children with partially obstructed connections, or those with hyperkinetic pulmonary hypertension, usually present within the first 1 to 2 years of life. The history of dyspnea on exertion, poor feeding, and failure to thrive is common. Ten to 20% of children with TAPVC will be relatively asymptomatic until young adulthood. Their history is similar to that of patients with atrial septal defect.

PHYSICAL EXAMINATION

Infants with obstructive connections appear very ill and are sometimes moribund shortly after birth. Extreme difficulty in breathing is present, with evidence of stiff lungs and poor cardiac function. Infants and children with partially obstructed connections or pulmonary hypertension demonstrate a very prominent right ventricular impulse and a left parasternal flow murmur. There is a very loud and widely split and fixed second heart sound. Older children and adults with nonobstructed TAPVC will have a prominent, hyperactive precordium. The second cardiac sound is split and fixed; however, the pulmonary component is not loud. A parasternal systolic flow murmur is present and is similar to that in those patients with atrial septal defects.

ELECTROCARDIOGRAPHY

The electrocardiogram is least helpful in diagnosing TAPVC. Right axis deviation and other electrocardiographic changes indicative of right ventricular hypertrophy are common. If the condition has been present for more than several years, first-degree heart block and right bundle-branch block may be evident.

CHEST FILM

Infants with obstructed TAPVC will have the appearance of pulmonary venous congestion in the lung fields but no evident cardiomegaly. Older children with partially obstructed connections will have increased pulmonary vascularity and cardiomegaly. In these patients and also in older patients with TAPVC, a characteristic mediastinal silhouette representing the dilated vertical vein may be evident (''snowman'' heart).

ECHOCARDIOGRAPHY

Echocardiographic signs of right ventricular diastolic volume overload predominate in TAPVC. A highly reliable sign appears to be the finding of an echo-free space posterior to the left atrium representing the pulmonary venous confluence.

CARDIAC CATHETERIZATION

As soon as the diagnosis of TAPVC is considered in an infant, cardiac catheterization should be carried out. Severe pulmonary hypertension is present, usually with a right-to-left ductal shunt. Visualization of the anomalous connection may be possible only with an injection of individual pulmonary arteries or occlusion of the ductus arteriosus with a balloon catheter and injection of contrast material through a proximal port or separate catheter. Older patients with TAPVC demonstrate moderate to severe elevations in pulmonary artery pressure, high pulmonary blood flow, and low pulmonary vascular resistance. The right ventricle is greatly dilated on cineangiography, and anomalous connections can easily be visualized with a pulmonary artery injection.

TREATMENT

Current practice indicates that cardiopulmonary bypass be used for all operations involving the correction of total anomalous pulmonary venous connection. The defect is best approached through a median sternotomy incision, and the type of perfusion support is dependent on the age of the patient. In infants, the avoidance of pulmonary venous distention and myocardial injury is facilitated by the use of profound hypothermia and circulatory arrest. Standard cardiopulmonary bypass techniques with the use of cardioplegia are preferred in older children and adults.

Supracardiac connections can be repaired using a direct anastomosis of the common venous chamber to the posterior surface of the left atrium with fine running sutures. Cardiac connections are repaired using a large baffle, which directs blood from the coronary sinus or malplaced pulmonary veins through the atrial septal defect into the left atrium. Infracardiac connections are repaired in a similar manner to supracardiac anomalies, and great care is taken not to

place tension upon the anastomosis. Type IV anomalies are repaired using a combination of the above techniques. The atrial septal defect is repaired in all cases.

Postoperative care may be difficult in these patients because of high pulmonary artery pressures and very stiff, edematous lungs present preoperatively. Long-term ventilatory management using positive end-expiratory pressure facilitates care of these very sick infants.

RESULTS

The results of operations for total anomalous pulmonary venous connection are directly related to the presence of obstruction and thus indirectly related to the type of connection present. Operative mortality is highest in the very young infant and approaches that of the repair of atrial septal defect in older patients. Successful repair in infants and in older patients is usually associated with an excellent long-term prognosis with few late symptoms or major sequelae.

CONGENITAL VALVULAR LESIONS

CONGENITAL AORTIC STENOSIS

Congenital aortic stenosis is produced by a group of malformations that cause obstruction to the flow of blood from the left ventricle to the aorta. These lesions account for 5% to 10% of all congenital heart defects. In 1844, Padgett described the tendency of congenitally bicuspid aortic valves to cause obstruction. Tuffier, in 1913, successfully dilated

AORTIC STENOSIS	
History	Padgett described bicuspid valve, 1844; Swan and Lewis performed aortic valvotomy, 1955
Incidence	5% of congenital heart defects
Pathophysiology	Obstruction to outflow from left ventricle by subaortic membrane, valvular stenosis, or supravalvular stenosis produces LVH
Dx	History: CHF in infancy if obstruction is severe Physical exam: systolic murmur; ↓ pulses Chest film: LVH ECG: LVH + strain Echo: subaortic membrane; bicuspid or abnormal aortic valve; LVH Catheterization: gradient from left ventricle to aorta identifies specific type of obstruction
Rx	Resection of subaortic membrane or aortic valvotomy; patch widening of ascending aorta
Results	Operative risk high in infancy, 5% in children; long-term results usually good but may need AVR later

an aortic valve as a palliative procedure. In 1955, Swan and Lewis independently performed aortic valvulotomy using hypothermia.

The four types of obstruction that occur between the left ventricle and the aorta are supravalvular, valvular, discrete subvalvular, and hypertrophic muscular subaortic stenosis. The stenosis is usually confined to one site but may be a combination of the above. One quarter of the patients have other associated cardiovascular defects, principally coarctation of the aorta, PDA, ventricular septal defect or pulmonary stenosis.

PATHOPHYSIOLOGY

The basic hemodynamic alteration produced by obstruction of left ventricular outflow is an increase in left ventricular pressure and therefore left ventricular work. The increased left ventricular wall tension produced by this lesion causes the development of left ventricular hypertrophy. An increased systolic ejection period required in this lesion results in a decrease in the length of diastole and therefore reduces coronary perfusion. Increased myocardial energy requirements coupled with the relative decrease in coronary flow ultimately result in left ventricular ischemia or failure. The development of subendocardial ischemia either during exercise or with severe defects at rest produces the electrocardiographic abnormality of left ventricular strain.

DIAGNOSIS

Infants with congenital aortic stenosis of a critical nature often present with severe cardiac decompensation associated with absent peripheral pulses and marked pulmonary congestion. Aortic stenosis in older children is usually asymptomatic, and there is the finding of a harsh systolic murmur in the right parasternal area radiating to the carotids, associated with electrocardiographic changes of hypertrophy and, in some cases, left ventricular strain. With severe aortic stenosis in children and young adults, angina, syncope, and, ultimately, heart failure may result. The echocardiogram may demonstrate a subaortic membrane; a thickened, abnormal aortic valve; or supravalvular narrowing. Cardiac catheterization discloses a gradient across the area of stenosis that may be from the aortic outflow tract to just above the aortic valve. A gradient greater than 50 torr is considered extremely significant, especially when coupled with resting or exercise electrocardiographic abnormalities. The specific type of obstruction is defined by angiocardiography.

TREATMENT

The preferred treatment for symptomatic patients with aortic stenosis or patients with resting or exercise electrocardiographic abnormalities is surgical. The type of operation is dependent upon the type of obstruction present. Valvular aortic stenosis is best treated in infants and children with aortic valvotomy. These operations are performed on cardiopulmonary bypass, and myocardial protection is best afforded with the use of profound myocardial hypothermia and cardioplegia. The fused commissures of a bicuspid valve are sharply divided, and any dysplastic material is removed. Supravalvular aortic stenosis is treated with a prosthetic graft to widen the aorta just above the aortic annulus. Discrete subvalvular aortic stenosis is treated with resection of the subvalvular membrane causing obstruction to the left ventricle. Hypertrophic subaortic stenosis is treated with the removal of a bar of hypertrophied muscle on the septal

portion of the left ventricular outflow tract. In the most severe forms of this lesion, with fibrous hypoplasia of the entire aortic outflow tract, an operation in which the entire aortic outflow tract is widened using a prosthetic graft and valve prosthesis may have to be performed. An alternative operation, in which a valved conduit is placed from the apex of the left ventricle to the aorta, has been performed with good results in older children and young adults.

RESULTS

Infants presenting with aortic outflow obstruction of any etiology represent the most severe risk. Operations in older children and young adults can usually be performed with low mortality (2% to 5%). In the case of valvotomy for valvular stenosis and resection of muscle in hypertrophic subaortic stenosis, long-term results will be influenced by the appearance of late sequelae due to calcification of the aortic valve in the former and recurrence of the lesion in the latter. A significant number of patients who undergo aortic valvotomy as infants or children may require valve replacement in later years.

AORTIC VALVE INSUFFICIENCY

Aortic valve insufficiency as an isolated lesion is usually very uncommon and primarily associated with other malformations, such as ventricular septal defect and truncus arteriosus. Congenital primary aortic valve incompetence is ordinarily associated with congenital malformations resulting in a defect in collagen formation. Indications for valve replacement are similar to those in adults.

CONGENITAL MITRAL STENOSIS OR ATRESIA

Congenital mitral stenosis is a rare cardiac lesion; it is highly lethal. Only 20% of the patients survive to 3 years of age or older without surgery.

In congenital mitral stenosis, the mitral valve may be one of three types: a funnel-shaped, elongated-cone type of congenital stenosis; the ballooning type of valve with short chordae and hypertrophic papillary muscles obstructing the annulus of the mitral valve; and parachute valve, in which all of the chordae of both malformed leaflets are connected to a single large papillary muscle. Very rarely, a membrane or shelflike structure with one or two orifices is located close to the mitral valve and obstructs flow from the left atrium. In congenital mitral atresia, there is only a dimple in the area of the left atrium where the mitral valve is usually present.

PATHOPHYSIOLOGY

The pathophysiology of these lesions resembles mitral stenosis in the adult unless associated anomalies are present. Obstruction of flow through the mitral valve causes an increased pulmonary venous pressure with transudation of fluid into the lungs causing difficulty breathing. Secondary changes in pulmonary arterioles result in increased pulmonary vascular resistance and an increase in right ventricular size and wall thickness. In mitral atresia, the presence of a patent foramen ovale or atrial septal defect is necessary for the maintenance of life. In addition, there must be a communication between the right and left ventricles for an operable situation to result.

DIAGNOSIS

Symptoms of pulmonary congestion occur in 75% of patients prior to 1 year of age. An infant or child with congenital mitral stenosis usually has a heart murmur that is discovered early in life. In mitral atresia, the diagnosis becomes apparent early in life. Chest film and electrocardiogram demonstrate the classic changes of mitral valve obstruction with cardiomegaly, especially involving the left atrium and right ventricle. Echocardiography may reveal abnormalities of the mitral valve. Cardiac catheterization reveals pulmonary hypertension with elevated pulmonary capillary wedge pressure. Angiocardiography often reveals the etiology of the mitral valve obstruction. In mitral valve atresia, the presence of associated lesions is also revealed at cardiac catheterization.

TREATMENT

Operative procedures for congenital mitral stenosis are associated with a very high mortality due to the difficulty of replacing the mitral valve in the infant or young child. In general, mitral valve replacement is extremely difficult in children under 1 year of age who have congenital mitral stenosis. Often, replacement of the mitral valve in children is complicated by a small mitral annulus that restricts the size of prostheses used for the operation. Calcification of porcine valve prostheses early after replacement in children makes it preferable to use a low-profile mechanical prosthesis. The problems of anticoagulation in young children are formidable and therefore the late results, which include multiple reoperations for valve replacement, will be poor. In mitral atresia associated with an intraventricular communication, a Blalock–Hanlon procedure is sometimes necessary to enlarge a patent foramen ovale. Pulmonary artery banding is also necessary if the intraventricular communication causes increased pulmonary blood flow.

CONGENITAL MITRAL REGURGITATION

Congenital mitral regurgitation is an isolated entity occurring very rarely and is usually associated with dysplastic mitral valve leaflets. Most children with this anomaly can be treated medically with digitalis and diuretics for some time before valve replacement is necessary.

EBSTEIN'S ANOMALY

Ebstein's anomaly consists of an abnormal attachment of the tricuspid valve leaflets. The anatomy can be highly variable, and the defect exists as a wide spectrum of abnormalities as described by Anderson. In the most typical form, the anterior leaflet of the tricuspid valve is enlarged and may be normally attached, but the septal and posterior leaflets are more or less atretic and do not attach to the normal tricuspid valve annulus; instead, the lines of attachment spiral down into the right ventricle. As a result, the right heart may have three chambers: the enlarged right atrium, a small functional right ventricle, and an abnormal thin-walled "atrialized" portion of right ventricle created by the abnormally low attachment of the tricuspid valve leaflets. The degree of this abnormal attachment is highly variable, and either severe tricuspid insufficiency or tricuspid stenosis may be the result. There is usually an atrial septal defect or a patent foramen ovale.

EBSTEIN'S ANOMALY	
History	Ebstein described, 1866; Barnard corrected surgically, 1962
Incidence	<1% of congenital heart defects
Anatomy	Downward displacement of tricuspid valve leaflets; atrial septal defect
Pathophysiology	Tricuspid stenosis or insufficiency; inefficient right ventricle; R → L shunt; cyanosis
Dx	History: congestive heart failure; dyspnea; cyanosis Physical exam: systolic murmur of tricuspid insufficiency; cardiomegaly ECG: right atrial enlargement; Wolf–Parkinson–White in 20% Chest film: cardiomegaly; decreased pulmonary vascularity Echo: ↑ right atrium; ↓ right ventricle; displacement of tricuspid valve Catheterization: R → L shunt: displacement of tricuspid valve; atrialized right ventricle; tricuspid insufficiency
Rx	Annuloplasty technique or tricuspid valve replacement; closure of atrial septal defect
Results	Operative mortality rate 10% to 15%; long-term results good

PATHOPHYSIOLOGY

The alteration in hemodynamics depends upon the extent of anatomical abnormality and ranges from quite mild to extremely severe. In some, the anterior leaflet may be so enlarged as to cause tricuspid stenosis and right ventricular outflow tract obstruction. In most, the hemodynamic alteration is secondary to the tricuspid insufficiency, the atrialized right ventricle, and the atrial septal defect. Displacement of the tricuspid valve leaflets into the right ventricle will decrease the size and effectiveness of the right ventricle as a pump. The efficiency of the right ventricle is further impaired by the sometimes huge, thin-walled atrialized portion of the right ventricle, and the abnormalities produced by these two problems are further accentuated by the usually severe tricuspid valve insufficiency. The net result of this is to impair blood flow through the right ventricle to the lungs. Because of the elevated right-sided pressures and the defect in the atrial septum, blood then shunts right to left across the atrial septum and produces arterial desaturation and cyanosis. These problems may be particularly severe in the infant who at birth has elevated pulmonary vascular resistance, and mortality is extremely high in this group.

DIAGNOSIS

Signs and symptoms are related to the degree of tricuspid insufficiency, the size of the atrial septal defect, and the degree of impairment of right ventricular function. The infant may present with severe congestive heart failure and cyanosis, but these may improve as pulmonary vascular resistance decreases. The older patient will usually present with dyspnea, variable cyanosis, and sometimes a history of arrhythmias or palpitations.

PHYSICAL EXAMINATION

Cyanosis is usually present in varying degrees along with clubbing. Cardiac examination will demonstrate cardiomegaly, a gallop rhythm, a systolic murmur of tricuspid insufficiency, and usually a widely split second heart sound. Growth and development are usually normal.

ELECTROCARDIOGRAPHY

The electrocardiogram usually demonstrates sinus rhythm. Approximately 10% to 20% of these patients will have conduction abnormalities of a Wolf–Parkinson–White preexcitation type. Right atrial enlargement is also present.

CHEST FILM

The chest film may demonstrate marked cardiomegaly not unlike that seen with pericardial effusion, which is usually due to right atrial enlargement. If cyanosis is severe, there may be decreased pulmonary vascularity due to the right-to-left shunt.

ECHOCARDIOGRAPHY

Echocardiography plays an important role in the diagnosis of Ebstein's anomaly. M-mode echocardiography will demonstrate delayed closure of the tricuspid valve compared with the mitral valve. Two-dimensional echocardiography demonstrates nicely the overall anatomy, with downward displacement of the tricuspid valve, small right ventricle, atrialized right ventricle, and enlarged right atrium. The atrial septal defect may be seen.

CARDIAC CATHETERIZATION

The definitive diagnosis of Ebstein's anomaly is made at cardiac catheterization either by cineangiography or by intracardiac electrocardiography. Right atrial pressures are increased with large v waves present when tricuspid insufficiency is severe. Arterial desaturation may be present, and the degree of right-to-left shunt can be quantitated. Cineangiography demonstrates the downward displacement of the tricuspid valve, a small and abnormally functioning right ventricle, and tricuspid insufficiency. Recordings from the atrialized right ventricle will show a right ventricular electrogram at the same time that the pressure recordings show a right atrial contour, thus making the diagnosis Ebstein's anomaly.

TREATMENT

The natural history of Ebstein's anomaly is quite variable, depending upon the anatomy. From the review of Watson in 1974 and Giuliani in 1979, there appear to be three groups of patients. One group will have mild forms of the abnormality, may remain asymptomatic or nearly so, and will require no surgical therapy. Another group will have severe deformity of the valve, will be profoundly symptomatic in infancy, and will frequently die of their disease with or without surgical intervention. The third group of patients present later in life with progressive symptoms of congestive heart failure and deteriorating cardiac status. The indications

for surgery include functional class III or IV, deteriorating cardiac status, moderate to severe cyanosis, paradoxical emboli, right ventricular outflow tract obstruction, and Wolf–Parkinson–White type of intractable arrhythmias.

Initial surgical attempts involved different systemic–pulmonary shunts and were unsuccessful. Current surgical techniques include relocation of the tricuspid valve to its normal position along with plication of the atrialized right ventricle (Hunter, Lillehei, 1958; Hardy, 1964), valve replacement with plication of the atrialized right ventricle (Timmis, 1968), and valve replacement alone without plication (Barnard, 1962) (Fig. 39-22). Each of these procedures is performed through a median sternotomy using standard cardiopulmonary bypass. Each attempts to correct the disorder by obliterating the tricuspid insufficiency and improving the efficiency of the right ventricle. The atrial septal defect is closed in all instances. Each technique has a significant incidence of danger to the conduction system with possible production of heart block. When Wolf–Parkinson–White preexcitation abnormalities are present (10% to 20%), simultaneous obliteration of these anomalous conduction pathways should also be carried out; in fact, surgery in patients with Ebstein's anomaly and associated Wolf-Parkinson-White abnormalities should not be undertaken unless facilities are available for intraoperative mapping and obliteration of these pathways.

Comparison of these techniques is difficult because of the highly variable anatomy in different patients and the relatively small experience of any one person or institution. Sealy indicated that up to 1979, a total of 34 patients had undergone valve replacement with or without plication, for an overall survival rate of 53%; 16 had undergone plastic-type repairs of the valve without replacement, for a survival rate of 69%. A more recent review indicates that since 1979, 78 additional patients have undergone valve replacement, with an overall survival rate of 82.1%. Whether or not the right ventricle was plicated appeared to have no influence on survival. A recent report from the Mayo Clinic indicates an overall survival rate of 87.5% in their series of 16 patients undergoing tricuspid annuloplasty without valve replace-

Fig. 39-22. Tricuspid valve replacement with a frame-mounted heterograft. (Blondeau P: Traité de Technique Chirurgicale, Vol 4. Paris, Masson, 1972)

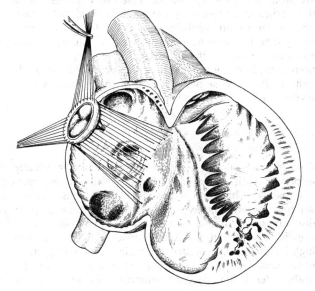

ment. Operative deaths in all types of repair are frequently related to arrhythmias.

It appears that surgical correction of Ebstein's anomaly can now be carried out successfully by several different techniques, and because of variable anatomy, different techniques may be appropriate in different patients. When repair is successful, marked improvement in heart failure occurs and long-term prognosis is significantly improved.

OTHER MISCELLANEOUS CONGENITAL CARDIAC LESIONS

INTERRUPTED AORTIC ARCH

Interruption of the aortic arch is usually associated with a ventricular septal defect or truncus arteriosus. It is a highly lethal lesion, and infants rarely survive to 6 months of age. In most centers treating infants for congenital heart disease, an early reparative operation using hypothermia or circulatory arrest is preferred. The operative mortality rate is high and is probably in excess of 20%.

DOUBLE-CHAMBERED RIGHT VENTRICLE

The double-chambered right ventricle is a very rare lesion producing pulmonary stenosis; the obstruction occurs at the junction between the inflow and outflow portions of the right ventricle and is caused by a very large muscular band that subdivides the ventricle into two chambers. In many cases, there is a small ventricular septal defect, usually entering the upper chamber. Operation is carried out with the standard indications of pulmonary stenosis. Cardiopulmonary bypass and a right ventriculotomy usually reveal the lesion, which can be directly excised.

CONGENITAL ABSENCE OF THE PULMONARY VALVE

Congenital absence of the pulmonary valve is a very uncommon lesion associated with massive dilatation of the main pulmonary artery and usually associated with a ventricular septal defect, infundibular pulmonary stenosis, and hypoplasia of the pulmonary annulus. The predominant symptom is respiratory distress caused by compression of the trachea and bronchi by the greatly dilated pulmonary arteries. Operation consisting of closure of the ventricular septal defect, widening of the pulmonary annulus, and reduction in size of the very large pulmonary artery has been carried out successfully, but the operative mortality is quite high and postoperative care of these patients with severe respiratory distress is often difficult.

CORRECTED TRANSPOSITION (L-TRANSPOSITION) OF THE GREAT ARTERIES

Corrected transposition of the great arteries is usually associated with one of the splenic syndromes (asplenia, polysplenia). This anomaly results when there is transposition of the great arteries associated with atrioventricular discordance. With this as an isolated entity, patients are usually asymptomatic, but unfortunately there is a very high incidence of associated anomalies, usually congenital heart block, ventricular septal defect, and pulmonary stenosis. Later in life, systemic atrioventricular valve incom-

petence results in cardiac failure. Operation or pacemaker implantation is performed for standard indications.

DOUBLE OUTLET LEFT VENTRICLE

Double outlet left ventricle is present when both great arteries arise from the morphological left ventricle. Operation can be entertained when a ventricular septal defect is present. Most patients have some form of pulmonary outflow obstruction that must be contended with at the time of operation.

SINGLE VENTRICLE

Single ventricle is present in several forms. Most are associated with increased pulmonary blood flow, and pulmonary banding is the preferred palliative operation. Occasionally, pulmonary atresia is associated and a palliative systemic pulmonary shunt is required. In cases in which systemic or pulmonary blood flow is restricted by a closing bulboventricular foramen, surgical relief of this obstruction may provide dramatic relief of symptoms. At this time, complete operative repair of single ventricle, either by septation or a modification of the Fontan procedure, has been performed at several centers. Operative mortality is high, and there is no clear indication that this form of therapy is better than palliative therapy alone.

COR TRIATRIATUM

Cor triatriatum is a rare defect in which a membrane, localized in the left atrium usually just above the mitral valve, effectively divides the left atrium into two parts and produces obstruction to pulmonary venous return. Diagnosis is suspected by echocardiography and confirmed by cineangiocardiography. Correction is carried out by excising the membrane with the use of cardiopulmonary bypass.

HYPOPLASTIC LEFT HEART SYNDROME

Hypoplastic left heart syndrome includes a spectrum of diseases ranging from mild to severe underdevelopment of the left heart. It makes up about 1% of congenital heart disease but is highly lethal and is responsible for a large number of the deaths from heart disease in the neonatal period. In its severe form, the aortic valve is atretic, the left ventricle is severely hypoplastic, and aortic flow is dependent upon flow across the ductus. These infants develop severe distress shortly after birth, and the majority die within several days. Although there have been isolated reports of palliation by surgery, this is not practical in most such infants at this time.

CORONARY ARTERY ANOMALIES

Anomalies of the coronary arteries include anomalous origins of the left or right coronary artery, coronary fistulas, and aneurysms. Coronary artery fistulas most frequently involve the right coronary artery and terminate in the right ventricle, right atrium, or pulmonary artery. If the fistula is large, congestive heart failure may result. Such fistulas can usually be surgically interrupted. Anomalous origin of the left coronary artery from the pulmonary artery may be a cause of heart failure in infants, and surgical correction of this lesion is more difficult.

BIBLIOGRAPHY

Patent Ductus Arteriosus

BRANT B, MARVIN WJ, EHRENHAFT JL et al: Ligation of patent ductus arteriosus in premature infants. Ann Thorac Surg 32:167, 1981

DOTY DB, RICHARDSON J, FACKOVSKY G et al: Aortopulmonary septal defect: Hemodynamics, angiography and operation. Ann Thorac Surg 32:255, 1981

EDMUNDS LH: Operation or indomethacin for the premature ductus. Ann Thorac Surg 26:586, 1978

GROSS RE: Surgical closure of an aortic septal defect. Circulation 5:858, 1952

GROSS RE, HUBBARD JP: Surgical ligation of a patent ductus arteriosus. JAMA 112:729, 1939

JOHN S, MUWALIDHARAN S, JAIRAJ PS et al: The adult ductus. J Thorac Cardiovasc Surg 82:314, 1981

JONES JC: Twenty-five years' experience with the surgery of patent ductus arteriosus. J Thorac Cardiovasc Surg 50:149, 1965

PONTIUS RG, DANIELSON GK, NOONAN JA et al: Illusions leading to surgical closure of the distal left pulmonary artery, instead of the ductus arteriosus. J Thorac Cardiovasc Surg 87:107, 1981

WRIGHT JS, NEWMAN CC: Ligation of the patent ductus: Technical considerations at different ages. J Thorac Cardiovasc Surg 75:695, 1978

Coarctation of the Aorta

ABBOTT ME: Coarctation of the adult type. Am Heart J 35:74, 1928

BREWER LA III, FOSBURG RG, MULDER GA et al: Spinal cord complications following surgery for coarctation of the aorta. J Thorac Cardiovasc Surg 64:368, 1972

CAMPBELL J, DELORENZ R, BROWN J et al: Improved results in newborn undergoing coarctation repair. Ann Thorac Surg 30:273, 1980

CAMPBELL M: Natural history of coarctation of the aorta. Br Heart J 32:633, 1970

CRAAFORD C, NYLIN G: Congenital coarctation of the aorta and its surgical treatment. J Thorac Surg 13:347, 1945

FERGUSON J, BARRIE W, SCHENK W: Hypertension of aortic coarctation: The role of renal and other factors. Ann Surg 185:423, 1977

FISHMAN NH, BRONSTEIN MH, BERMAN W et al: Surgical management of severe aortic coarctation and interrupted aortic arch in neonates. J Thorac Cardiovasc Surg 71:35, 1976

FREED M, HEYMAN M, LEWIS A et al: Prostaglandin E in infants with ductus arteriosus. Circulation 64:899, 1981

FREED M, ROCCHINI A, ROSENTHAN A et al: Exercise induced hypertension after surgery: Repair of coarctation of the aorta. Am J Cardiol 143:253, 1979

GROSS RE: Surgical correction for coarctation of the aorta. Surgery 18:673, 1945

HESSLEIN PS, MCNAMARA DG, MORRISS MJ et al: Comparison of resection versus patch aortoplasty for repair of coarctation in infants and children. Circulation 64:164, 1981

KAMAN P, MILES V, TOEWS W et al: Surgical repair of coarctation of the aorta in infants less than six months of age. J Thorac Cardiovasc Surg 81:171, 1981

SADE RM, TAYLOR AB, CHARRIKER EP: Aortoplasty compared with resection for coarctation of the aorta in young children. Ann Thorac Surg 28:346, 1979

SCOTT HW, DEAN RH, BOERTH R et al: Coarctation of the abdominal aorta. Ann Surg 189:746, 1979

SCOTT HW JR, BAHNSON HT: Evidence for a renal factor in the hypertension of experimental coarctation of the aorta. Surgery 30:206, 1951

SEALY WC: Coarctation of the aorta and hypertension. Ann Thorac Surg 3:15, 1967

WALDHAUSEN JA, WHITMAN V, WERNER JC et al: Surgical intervention in infants with coarctation of the aorta. J Thorac Cardiovasc Surg 81:323, 1981

Aortic Arch Anomalies

ARCINIEGAS E, HAKIMI M, HERTZLER JH et al: Surgical management of congenital vascular ring. J Thorac Cardiovasc Surg 77:721, 1979

BINET JP, LONGLOIS J: Aortic arch anomalies in children and infants. J Thorac Cardiovasc Surg 73:248, 1977

EDWARDS JE: Malformations of the aortic arch system manifested as "vascular rings." Lab Invest 2:56, 1953

ERICSSON NO, SODERLUND S: Compression of the trachea by an anomalous innominate artery. J Pediatr Surg 4:427, 1979

GROSS RE: Surgical relief for tracheal obstruction from a vascular ring. N Engl J Med 233:586, 1945

STEWART JR, KINCAID OW, EDWARDS JC: An Atlas of Vascular Rings and Related Malformations of the Aortic Arch Systems. Springfield, IL, Charles C Thomas, 1964

WOLMAN IJ: Syndrome of constricting double aortic arch in infancy: Report of a case. J Pediatr 14:527, 1939

Atrial Septal Defects

GIBBON JH JR: Application of a mechanical heart and lung apparatus to cardiac surgery. Minn Med 37:171, 1954

GROSS RE, WATKINS E, POMERANZ AA et al: A method for surgical closure of interauricular septal defects. Surg Gynecol Obstet 96:1, 1953

KYGER ER, FRAZIER OH, COOLEY DA et al: Sinus venous atrial septum defect: Early and late results following closure in 109 patients. Ann Thorac Surg 25:44, 1978

LEWIS FJ, TAUFFIC M, VARCO RL et al: The surgical anatomy of atrial septal defects: Experiences with repair under direct vision. Ann Surg 142:401, 1955

ROKITANSKY CF: Die Defekte der Scheidewande des Herzens. Vienna, Braumuller, 1875

SELBY JH, CRAWFORD FA, WATSON DG et al: Familial occurrences of atrial septal defect. J Miss State Med Assoc 18:167, 1977

SUTTON MG, TAJIK AJ, McGOON DC: Atrial septal defect in patients ages 60 years or older: Operative results and long-term postoperative followup. Circulation 64:402, 1981

Ventricular Septal Defects

CORDELL D, GRAHAM TP, ATWOOD GF et al: Left heart volume characteristics following ventricular septal defect closure in infancy. Circulation 54:294, 1976

FISHER RD, FAULKNER SL, SELL CG et al: Operative closure of isolated defects of the ventricular septum: Planned delay. Ann Thorac Surg 26:351, 1978

HOFFMAN JIE, RUDOLPH AM: Natural history of ventricular septal defect in infancy. Am J Cardiol 16:634, 1965

LILLEHEI CW, COHEN M, WARDEN HE et al: The results of direct vision closure of ventricular septal defects in 8 patients by means of controlled cross circulation. Surg Gynecol Obstet 101:446, 1955

MULLER WH, DAMMANN JF: The treatment of certain congenital malformations of the heart by the creation of pulmonic stenosis to reduce pulmonary hypertension and excessive pulmonary blood flow. Surg Gynecol Obstet 95:213, 1952

RICHARDSON JV, SCHICKEN RM, LAVER RM et al: Repair of large ventricular septal defects in infants and small children. Ann Surg 195:318, 1982

SUBRAMANIAN S: Primary definitive intracardiac operation in infants: Ventricular septal defect. In Kirklin JW (ed): Advances in Cardiovascular Surgery. New York, Grune & Stratton, 1973

Endocardial Cushion Defects

BERGER TJ, BLACKSTONE EH, KIRKLIN JW et al: Survival and probability of cure without and with operation in complete atrioventricular canal. Ann Thorac Surg 27:104, 1979

BERGER TJ, KIRKLIN JW, BLACKSTONE EH et al: Primary repair of complete atrioventricular canal in patients less than two years old. Am J Cardiol 41:906, 1978

CULPEPPER W, KOLFF J, LIN C et al: Complete common atrioventricular canal in infancy: Surgical repair and postoperative hemodynamics. Circulation 58:550, 1978

KIRKLIN JW: Management of the infant with complete atrioventricular canal. J Thorac Cardiovasc Surg 78:32, 1979

McCABE JC, ENGLE MA, GARY WA et al: Surgical treatment of endocardial cushion defect. Am J Cardiol 39:72, 1977

McMULLAN MF, WALLACE RB, WEIDMAN WH et al: Surgical treatment of complete atrioventricular canal. Surgery 72:95, 1972

WARD R, ANDERSON R, GOLDBERG S et al: Septum primum defect repair. Ann Thorac Surg 24:291, 1977

Tetralogy of Fallot

ARCINIEGAS E, FAROOKI I, HAKIMI M et al: Results of two stage surgical treatment of tetralogy of Fallot. J Thorac Cardiovasc Surg 79:876, 1980

BLACKSTONE E, KIRKLIN J, PACIFICO A: Decision making in repair of tetralogy of Fallot based on intraoperative measurements of pulmonary arterial outflow tract. J Thorac Cardiovasc Surg 77:26, 1979

BLALOCK A, TAUSSIG HB: Surgical treatment of malformations of the heart in which there is pulmonary stenosis or pulmonary atresia. JAMA 128:189, 1945

DABIZZI R, CAPRIOLO G, AIAZZI L et al: Distribution and anomalies of coronary arteries in tetralogy of Fallot. Circulation 61:95, 1980

DONAHOO J, GARDNER T, ZAHKAK K et al: Systemic-pulmonary shunts in neonates and infants using microporous expanded polytetrafluoroethylene: Immediate and life results. Ann Thorac Surg 30:146, 1980

FUSTER V, McGOON D, KENNEDY M et al: Long-term evaluations (12–22 years) of open heart surgery for tetralogy of Fallot. Am J Cardiol 46:635, 1980

GLENN WWL, PATINO JF: Circulatory bypass of the right heart: I. Preliminary observation on direct delivery of vena caval blood into pulmonary arterial circulation: Azygos vein–pulmonary artery shunt. Yale J Biol Med 27:147, 1954

KIRKLIN J, BLACKSTONE E, PACIFICO A et al: Routine primary repair versus two stage repair of tetralogy of Fallot. Circulation 60:373, 1979

LILLEHEI CW, COHEN M, WARDEN HE et al: Vision intracardiac surgical correction of the tetralogy of Fallot, pentalogy of Fallot, and pulmonary atresia defects. Ann Surg 142:418, 1955

PARENZAW L, ALFIERI O, VANINI V et al: Waterston anastomosis for initial palliation of tetralogy of Fallot. J Thorac Cardiovasc Surg 82:176, 1981

POTTS WF, SMITH S, GIBSON S: Anastomosis of the aorta to a pulmonary artery for certain types of congenital heart disease. JAMA 132:629, 1946

SABISTON DC: Role of the Blalock-Taussig operation in the hypoxic infant with tetralogy of Fallot. Ann Thorac Surg 22:303, 1976

SADE RM, WILLIAMS RG, CASTANEDA AR: Corrective surgery for congenital cardiovascular defects in early infancy. Am Heart J 90:656, 1975

TUCKER W, TURLEY K, OLLGOT D et al: Management of symptomatic tetralogy of Fallot in the first year of life. J Thorac Cardiovasc Surg 78:494, 1979

Pulmonary Valvular Stenosis and Pulmonary Atresia

DOBELL A, GRIGON A: Early and late results in pulmonary atresia. Ann Thorac Surg 24:264, 1977

GRIFFITH B, HARDESTY R, SIEWERS R et al: Pulmonary valvulotomy alone for pulmonary stenosis: Results in children with and without muscular infundibular hypertrophy. J Thorac Cardiovasc Surg 83:577, 1982

MOULTON A, BONMAN F, EDIE R et al: Pulmonary atresia with intact ventricular septum. J Thorac Cardiovasc Surg 78:527, 1979

Transposition of the Great Arteries

BLALOCK A, HANLON CR: The surgical treatment of complete transposition of the aorta and pulmonary artery. Surg Gynecol Obstet 90:1, 1950

COTO E, NORWOOD W, LAND P et al: Modified Senning operation for treatment of transposition of the great vessels. J Thorac Cardiovasc Surg 78:721, 1979

JATENE A, FONTES V, SOUZA L et al: Anatomic correction of transposition of the great arteries. J Thorac Cardiovasc Surg 83:20, 1982

OLDHAM H: Arterial repair of transposition. Ann Thorac Surg 32:1, 1981

TAUSSIG HB: Complete transposition of the great vessels. Am Heart J 16:728, 1938

TRUSLER G, WILLIAMS W, IZUKAWA T et al: Current results with the Mustard operation in isolated transposition of the great arteries. J Thorac Cardiovasc Surg 80:381, 1980

Double Outlet Right Ventricle

DANIELSON GK, RITTER DG, COLEMAN HN III et al: Successful repair of double outlet right ventricle with transposition of the great arteries (aorta anterior and to the left), pulmonary stenosis and subaortic ventricular septal defect. J Thorac Cardiovasc Surg 63:741, 1972

KIRKLIN JW, HARP RA, McGOON DC: Surgical treatment of origin of both vessels from right ventricle, including cases of pulmonary stenosis. J Thorac Cardiovasc Surg 48:1026, 1964

STEWART R, KIRKLIN J, PACIFICO A et al: Repair of double outlet right ventricle. J Thorac Cardiovasc Surg 78:502, 1979

Tricuspid Atresia

DOTY D, MARVIN W, LAUER R: Modified Fontan procedure. J Thorac Cardiovasc Surg 81:470, 1981

FONTAN F, BAUDET E: Surgical repair of tricuspid atresia. Thorax 26:240, 1971

MARCELETTI C, MAZZERA E, OLTHO FH et al: Fontan's operation: An expanded horizon, J Thorac Cardiovasc Surg 80:764, 1980

MATHUR M, GLENN WWL: Long-term evaluation of cavapulmonary artery anastomosis. Surgery 53:899, 1973

NEVEUX J, DREYFUS G, LECA F et al: Modified technique for correction of tricuspid atresia. J Thoracic Cardiovasc Surg 82:457, 1981

WALKER DR, SBOKOS CG, LENNOX SC: Correction of tricuspid atresia. Br Heart J 37:282, 1975

WILLIAMS WG, RUBIS L, TRUSLER GA et al: Palliation of tricuspid atresia. Arch Surg 110:1383, 1975

Truncus Arteriosus

BHARATI S, McALLISTER HA JR, ROSENQUIST GC et al: The surgical anatomy of truncus arteriosus communis. J Thorac Cardiovasc Surg 67:501, 1974

COLLETT RW, EDWARDS JE: Persistent truncus arteriosus: A classification according to anatomic types. Surg Clin North Am 29:1245, 1949

EBERT PA, ROBINSON SJ, STANGER P et al: Pulmonary artery conduits in infants younger than six months of age. J Thorac Cardiovasc Surg 72:351, 1976

MARCELLI HC, McGOON D, DANIELSON G et al: Early and late results of surgical repair of truncus arteriosus. Circulation 55:636, 1977

Total Anomalous Pulmonary Venous Connection

BENDER HW, FISHER RD, WALKER WE et al: Reparative cardiac surgery in infants and small children: Five years' experience with profound hypothermia and circulatory arrest. Ann Surg 190:437, 1979

DARLING RC, ROTHNEY WB, CRAIG JM: Total pulmonary venous drainage into the right side of the heart. Lab Invest 6:44, 1957

HAMMON JW, BENDER HW, GRAHAM TP et al: Total anomalous pulmonary venous connection in infancy. J Thorac Cardiovasc Surg 80:544, 1980

IVEMARK BI: Implications of agenesis of the spleen on the pathogenesis of conotruncus anomalies in childhood: An analysis of the heart malformations in the splenic agenesis syndrome with fourteen new cases. Acta Paediatr Scand (Suppl) 104:1, 1955

KATZ NM, KIRKLIN JW, PACIFICO AD: Concepts and practices in surgery for total anomalous pulmonary venous connection. Ann Thorac Surg 25:479, 1978

NEILL CA: Development of the pulmonary veins: With reference to the embryology of anomalies of pulmonary venous return. Pediatrics 18:880, 1956

Congenital Valvular Lesions

BRAUNWALD E, GOLDBLATT A, AYGEN MM et al: Congenital aortic stenosis: I. Clinical and hemodynamic findings in 100 patients. Circulation 27:426, 1962

COLLINS-NAKAI R, ROSENTHAL A, CASTANEDA A et al: Congenital mitral stenosis. Circulation 56:1039, 1977

DAVACHI F, MOLLER J, EDWARDS J: Diseases of the mitral valve in infancy. Circulation 43:565, 1971

DOBELL A, BLOSS R, GIBBONS J et al: Congenital valvular aortic stenosis. J Thorac Cardiovasc Surg 81:916, 1981

DOTY D, POLANSKY D, JENSON C: Supravalvular aortic stenosis. J Thorac Cardiovasc Surg 74:362, 1977

DUNN J: Porcine valve durability in children. Ann Thorac Surg 32:357, 1981

HARDESTY R, GRIFFITH B, MATHEWS R et al: Discrete subvalvular aortic stenosis. J Thorac Cardiovasc Surg 74:352, 1977

Ebstein's Anomaly

BARNARD CN, SCHRIRE SV: Surgical correction of Ebstein's malformation with prosthetic tricuspid valve. Surgery 54:302, 1963

DANIELSON GK, FUSTER V: Surgical repair of Ebstein's anomaly. Ann Surg (in press)

EBSTEIN W: Ueber einen sehr seltenen Fall von insufficienz der Valvula Tricuspidalis, beding durch eine Angeborene hochgradige Miss Gildung derselben. Arch Anat Physiol, pp 238–254, 1866

HARDY KL, MAY IA, WEBSTER CA et al: Ebstein's anomaly: A functional concept and successful definitive repair. J Thorac Surg 48:927, 1964

HUNTER SW, LILLEHEI CW: Ebstein's malformations of the tricuspid valve. Dis Chest 33:297, 1958

TIMMIS HH, HARDY J, WATSON DG: The surgical management of Ebstein's anomaly: The combined use of tricuspid valve replacement, atrioventricular plication and atrioplasty. J Thorac Cardiovasc Surg 53:85, 1967

WATSON H: Natural history of Ebstein's anomaly of tricuspid valve in childhood and adolescence: An international co-operative study of 505 cases. Br Heart J 36:417, 1974

ZUBERBUHLER J, ALLWORK S, ANDERSON R: The spectrum of Ebstein's anomaly of the tricuspid valve. J Thorac Cardiovasc Surg 77:202, 1979

Miscellaneous Cardiac Lesions

ALLWORK S, BENTAL H, BECKER A et al: Congenitally corrected transposition of the great arteries: Morphologic study of 32 cases. Am J Cardiol 38:910, 1976

ARCINIEGAS E, FAROOKI Z, HAKIMI M et al: Surgical treatment of cor triatriatum. Ann Thorac Surg 32:571, 1981

DRISCOLL D, NIHILL M, MULLINS C et al: Management of symptomatic infants with anomalous origin of the left coronary artery from the pulmonary artery. Am J Cardiol 47:642, 1981

DUNNIGAN A, OLDHAM H, BENSON D: Absent pulmonary valve syndrome in infancy: Surgery reconsidered. Am J Cardiol 48:117, 1981

FELDT R, MAIR D, DANIELSON G, WALLACE R, MCGOON D: Current status of the septation procedure for univentricular heart. J Thorac Cardiovasc Surg 82:93, 1981

GALE A, DANIELSON G, MCGOON D et al: Modified Fontan operation for univentricular heart and complicated congenital lesion. J Thorac Cardiovasc Surg 78:831, 1979

LOWE J, OLDHAM H, SABISTON DC: Surgical management of congenital coronary artery fistula. Ann Surg 194:373, 1981

NORWOOD W, LANG P, CASTANEDA A et al: Experiences with operations for hypoplastic left heart syndrome. J Thorac Cardiovasc Surg 82:511, 1981

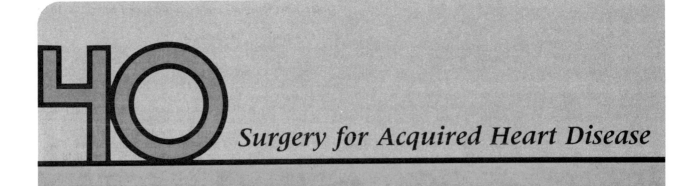

40 Surgery for Acquired Heart Disease

John J. Collins, Jr.

Cardiac Lesions

In this chapter, surgery for complications of acquired heart disease is considered under anatomic headings with the addition of discussions of pre- and postoperative care, tumors, cardiac transplantation, and artificial hearts and circulatory assist devices. The performance of cardiac surgery requires a thorough basic education in general surgical principles and practice. One important difference that the general surgeon will encounter in learning the specialty of cardiac surgery is the importance of time. There was an era in general surgery, particularly before the utilization of general anesthesia, when quickness was an important, if not the principal, virtue in the performance of surgical operations. With the development of anesthetic techniques and physiological support mechanisms it became possible for surgeons to approach their work in a less hasty and more meticulous fashion. As in most changes, the pendulum swung perhaps too far, and some prominent surgical teachers lost sight of the importance of an organized and expeditious approach. Advances in preoperative and postoperative care made great differences in the eligibility of patients for surgery and in the ability of persons to withstand the trauma of operative manipulation. There was even a tendency among some to denigrate the importance of the operation itself in favor of excellent postoperative management. This was a great mistake. Careful preoperative preparation, competent intraoperative care, and skillful postoperative management including prolonged follow-up are all necessary and important. It should be remembered, however, that the one characteristic that distinguishes surgeons from other physicians is the ability to perform operations. It is, therefore, necessary as well as desirable that medical practitioners desiring to perform operations take the time and effort necessary to achieve a high degree of technical skill, and this is the essential characteristic of surgical specialization.

The instruments must be carefully studied. The concepts and practice of antisepsis and asepsis must be thoroughly understood and carefully followed. Techniques of gaining exposure must be mastered. In fact, no aspect of surgery is more difficult or more important. It has been said, "if you can see it, you can sew it," and this simple aphorism should never be forgotten.

No surgeon works alone. As the sophistication of surgical practice increases, its breadth becomes narrowed, and in this process the surgeon becomes more dependent upon consultants and advisors from other areas of special knowledge. Preeminent among persons with special skills with whom the surgeon will always work closely are nurses. Within the nursing profession a variety of areas of special interest in cardiovascular disease have developed. Specialists in operating room technique, preoperative care including psychological preparation of patients for surgery, and postoperative care have developed. These dedicated men and women deserve respect and understanding. They are an integral part of the surgical team, and without them no progress is possible. The cardiac surgeon will also require consultation from time to time from multiple specialty groups and will work very closely with colleagues in medical cardiology and cardiac radiology. Skillfully managed interpersonal relationships with knowledgeable consultants are an integral part of providing optimal care.

In the final analysis, the cardiac surgeon must court certain virtues if he is to make a maximal contribution. These include knowledge, technical skill, physical stamina, strength of character, humility, and kindness.

Table 40-1 shows some milestones in the development of surgery for acquired heart disease. As in other surgical specialties, cardiac surgery began with the management of trauma and has progressed to the transplantation of organs.

PREOPERATIVE CARE FOR CARDIAC SURGICAL PATIENTS

Preoperative preparation for cardiac surgical patients should include the establishment of a complete and accurate diagnosis, achievement of optimal metabolic balance, and attention to proper psychological preparation. Judgment as well as skill and experience is necessary to recognize when these requirements have been satisfactorily met. There are a vast number of diagnostic studies that might be performed on any given patient. The experienced surgeon should choose only those that are essential to avoid unwarranted risks and undue costs in preliminary investigations. The number of interventions that may be possible to achieve optimal metabolic balance in various patients is nearly

TABLE 40-1 SOME MILESTONES IN SURGERY FOR ACQUIRED HEART DISEASE

YEAR	SURGEON	PROCEDURE
1897	Rehn	Suture of cardiac laceration
1923	Cutler	Transventricular mitral valvulotomy
1925	Souttar	Transatrial mitral commissurotomy
1948	Harken, Bailey, Brock	Transatrial closed mitral valvuloplasty
1953	Hufnagel	Ball valve in descending aorta for aortic insufficiency
1954	Gibbon	First clinical use of a heart–lung machine
1958	Vineberg	Internal mammary artery implantation
1960	Harken	Resection and total replacement of aortic valve with a prosthetic device
1962	Starr	Mitral valve replacement
1964	DeBakey	Saphenous vein coronary bypass graft for acute coronary artery disruption
1964	Hardy	First human cardiac transplant
1967	Barnard	First successful human cardiac transplant
1969	Favaloro, Effler	Saphenous vein coronary bypass for arteriosclerotic obstruction

impossible to count. Again, judgment is necessary. In particular, the patient's best interest must always be kept in mind, and the urgency of intervention must be carefully considered.

For patients with some types of urgent cardiovascular problems a short history and physical examination provide sufficient information for operation. This may often be the case in emergency operations performed for penetrating trauma of the chest. In less urgent situations a wide variety of tests are available. The following common diagnostic techniques are of specific interest in cardiac surgery:

1. History
2. Physical examination
3. Blood chemistries
4. Roentgenography and fluoroscopy
5. Electrocardiography
6. Echocardiography
7. Cardiac catheterization
8. Angiography
9. Nuclear imaging
10. Pulmonary function studies

In addition to the history and physical examination, certain blood studies are often of specific interest to the cardiac surgeon. For example, it may be important to know that serum enzymes indicate recent myocardial damage or that there is chemical evidence of increasing renal failure before operation. Virtually every patient should have routine posteroanterior and lateral chest roentgenograms a few days prior to cardiac surgery. It is not uncommon to discover the presence of a new pulmonary lesion that may require a change in operative planning. Fluoroscopy as a separate diagnostic study is rarely used today. As a technique for discovering whether calcification is present in the cardiac valves, fluoroscopy has been largely replaced by echocardiographic techniques.

A resting electrocardiogram should be obtained in virtually every patient before surgery. Electrocardiograms obtained during exercise need not be universally obtained even in patients with coronary artery disease. The principal utility of an exercise stress test is to assist in ascertaining the need for coronary angiography. If the need for angiography can be established without a positive stress test, then such a study should not be performed unless it is needed for comparison after surgery. For example, patients with unstable angina pectoris need not undergo a stress test to determine the need for coronary angiography.

The development of M-mode and two-dimensional echocardiographic techniques has enormously simplified the accurate diagnosis of the variety of cardiac diseases. Pericardial effusions can be accurately measured, and the hemodynamic significance of intrapericardial fluid can be closely estimated in many instances. The presence or absence of valvular heart disease may often be definitively established and even the severity of obstruction or insufficiency predicted. In idiopathic, hypertrophic subaortic stenosis echocardiography may be a very useful diagnostic tool. Conspicuous advantages of echocardiographic techniques include their noninvasiveness, portability, easy availability, and lack of expense by comparison with catheterization. A complete study can often be done at the bedside without time-consuming preparations. Echocardiography may also be a useful and effective screening procedure for patients suspected of having valvular or congenital heart disease.

Cardiac catheterization continues to occupy a prominent place in the diagnostic armamentarium of a cardiac surgeon. This is not to say that every patient undergoing open heart surgery needs preliminary catheterization. When accurate measurement of intracardiac pressures is needed or when it is necessary to resolve a question of the presence or absence of coronary artery obstruction, catheterization with angiography provides otherwise unobtainable information. Ventricular angiography as well as pulmonary artery or aortic angiography may often add valuable information as well.

Nuclear imaging is a relatively new and rapidly developing diagnostic technique. Functional significance of coronary artery obstructions may be estimated in many instances and the presence or absence of myocardial infarction established in others. In the future, visualization of the coronary circulation may be possible without the utilization of direct injection coronary angiography.

Pulmonary function studies need not be obtained in most patients before cardiac surgery. A proper history and physical examination usually are sufficient to establish the presence of adequate pulmonary function. In patients with respiratory problems suspected to be caused by noncardiac dysfunction, pulmonary function studies may be extremely valuable in preparing the patient and the surgeon for possible complications in postoperative recovery.

The surgeon must balance urgency of operation with the need for preliminary information. Certain studies may best be considered "routine" and others used only after judicious consideration.

The achievement of optimal metabolic balance needs some comment. Although uncontrolled heart failure or unstable angina pectoris may increase surgical risk, undue delay may also be detrimental. Only by careful observation and analysis of complications and results can the surgeon hope to recognize when the benefits of preoperative preparation are maximal and further manipulations are likely to be futile or harmful. Remember that all too commonly "perfect is the enemy of good."

Psychological preparation is important in all areas of surgical preparation but especially in cardiac surgery. For most persons the operation is the most serious event they have ever encountered, and the threat in even a "safe" operation cannot be overestimated. Nurse-specialists are used in many units with great success for pre- and postoperative teaching and support. Their contribution has been remarkable. Nowhere in surgery is the aphorism of Francis Peabody more apt: "The secret of the care of the patient is caring for the patient."

PERICARDIUM

The pericardium surrounds the heart in much the same manner that the pleura surrounds the lung (see Chapter 34). The pericardium, like the pleura, has extensive sensory innervation, and interference with the normal smooth passage of one layer on the other may be exquisitely painful. The basic response of the pericardium to injury is an increased fluid production and perhaps decreased absorption as well. Gradual accumulation of fluid within the pericardium will produce stretching and distention of the pericardium to a very great size. Rapid accumulation exceeds the compliance of the pericardium very quickly, and volumes as small as 50 ml to 100 ml may cause significant tamponade. Compression of the heart by the pericardium, whether from fluid accumulation or direct constriction, impedes ventricular filling and results in a rise in atrial pressure. In advanced cases the diastolic pressure in all chambers is raised and equalized, and ventricular pressure contour tracings show a characteristic "square root" configuration. There is also a marked increase in the normal respiratory variation of systemic arterial pressure that has been called *pulsus paradoxus*. To support the diagnosis of tamponade, inspiratory reduction of systolic pressure should be 10 or more mmHg. For practical purposes, easily palpable respiratory variation in peripheral pulse amplitude should be considered significant until proved otherwise. Additional signs include elevation of systemic venous pressure, reduction of pulse amplitude, and reduction of systolic blood pressure. Diminished intensity of heart sounds is irregularly present. Patients with tamponade due to constrictive pericarditis may often have a characteristic diastolic filling sound called "pericardial knock."

Definitive diagnosis of significant pericardial effusion can usually be established by M-mode or two-dimensional echocardiography. The older technique of contrast visualization of atrial cavities for measurement of pericardial thickness is now rarely needed. Cardiac catheterization is required for most patients with constrictive pericarditis.

ACUTE PERICARDITIS

Inflammatory lesions of the pericardium may be caused by a number of injurious influences including infection with bacteria or viruses, uremia, immunologic disturbances, trauma, tumors, and a variety of uncertain causes. The characteristic clinical presentation includes pain, friction rub, and electrocardiographic abnormalities. It has been said that the development of sufficient pleural fluid to cause tamponade will also cause disappearance of a pericardial friction rub. This is a myth. Tamponade may frequently be seen in viral, idiopathic, and uremic pericarditis in the presence of a loud friction rub. Pain is sometimes ameliorated by the presence of fluid, sometimes not. The large majority of patients with acute pericarditis will not require surgical drainage of the pericardium. However, any patient with the characteristic signs and symptoms of cardiac tamponade should undergo pericardiocentesis without delay. The technique of pericardiocentesis is illustrated in Figure 40-1. After making a 2-mm or 3-mm skin incision into the subcutaneous tissue just beneath the most proximal left costal margin, a large bore, Teflon-sheath needle is introduced and advanced through the properitoneal fat to the undersurface of the diaphragm. This is the area of the fibrous trigone, and the parietal pericardium is intimately applied to the upper surface of the diaphragm in this area. Cardiac pulsation is transmitted through the long axis of the needle and can be felt by the fingertip of the operating surgeon. Most persons expert in pericardiocentesis do not presently use electrocardiographic aids. The needle is advanced a few millimeters through the diaphragm. A characteristic sensation is produced as the needle pops through the tough fibrous diaphragmatic tissue. The trocar may then be retracted several millimeters into the interior of the Teflon sheath and the sheath advanced approximately 1 cm. The trocar is then withdrawn. The custom of attaching an electrode from an

Fig. 40-1. For pericardiocentesis, a 16-gauge plastic-sheathed needle is introduced beneath the costal margin and passed through the properitoneal fat and into the pericardial cavity through the tendinous part of the diaphragm. (Edwards EA, Malone PD, Collins JJ Jr: Operative Anatomy of the Thorax. Philadelphia, Lea & Febiger, 1972)

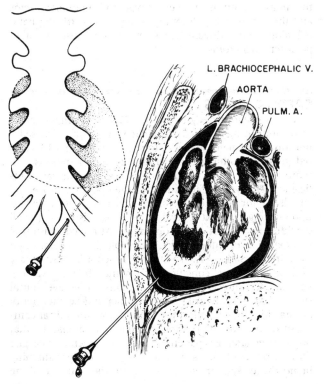

electrocardiograph to the base of the needle to detect an injury potential when the myocardium is touched by the needle is hazardous unless the electrocardiograph is isolated from line current or has battery power.

If the trocar is properly positioned in the pericardium, there will be immediate flow of pericardial fluid from the trocar. Aspiration using a three-way stopcock is then easily accomplished. More than 1 liter of fluid may be removed from some patients in whom the pericardium has become enormously distended. On the other hand, patients with acute pericardial tamponade may be substantially improved by the removal of only 30 or 40 ml of blood or fluid. With the catheter in place the patient may be moved from one position to another in order to facilitate complete drainage. In patients who have more than 250 ml of fluid, it is possible to inject air during or following pericardiocentesis in a volume of up to approximately one half that of the fluid removed. Air in the pericardium provides an excellent contrast medium for roentgenograms that, if taken in multiple projections, may then show the surface contour of the myocardium. It is obviously necessary for the operator to be absolutely certain that the open tip of the plastic catheter is in the pericardium and not within one of the cardiac chambers before introduction of air. This is usually quite easy, but if there is doubt, no air should be injected. It may be suggested that perhaps carbon dioxide would be a safer gas to inject, and this is indeed true. However, carbon dioxide disappears so quickly from the pericardial cavity that adequate visualization is often not obtained. In addition, because air may remain in the pericardium for several days, the extent of fluid reaccumulation may be ascertained simply by watching the air–fluid level on daily chest roentgenograms.

Following removal of as much fluid as possible, the catheter is usually withdrawn. In persons who are expected to reaccumulate fluid, there may be a temptation to leave the catheter in place for continued drainage. Although probably not specifically harmful, this procedure is often not very helpful because the catheter quickly becomes obstructed by fibrinous debris. In patients taking immunosuppressive drugs, the risk of infection is increased if the catheter is left in place for a prolonged period. A better course in patients requiring prolonged pericardial drainage is open operation with partial pericardiectomy and drainage into a pleural space.

Pericardiocentesis performed by aspiration through the left fourth or fifth intercostal space, in the "bare area" of the pericardium, is very hazardous unless the effusion is very large. The anterior descending coronary artery may be easily lacerated by the needle point if the effusion has not separated the heart sufficiently from the anterior chest wall. It is probably best to avoid this approach altogether.

Most patients with idiopathic pericarditis, viral pericarditis, and pericarditis of uremia respond to one or several pericardiocenteses. Pericardial effusion due to the presence of tumor on the myocardial surface or in the pericardium itself tends to recur unless the tumor is specifically treated by radiation, chemotherapy, or other techniques.

A useful technique for partial pericardiectomy involves removing portions of pericardium anterior and posterior to the phrenic nerve, leaving a strip of pericardium along the phrenic nerve to protect the nerve and its accompanying blood vessels. This type of limited drainage of the pericardium is usually adequate but does not ensure that pericardial effusion will never recur. The edges of the cut pericardium rather soon become adherent to the epicardium (visceral pericardium), and the apertures may be sealed. Accumulation may then occur in other areas. If troublesome reaccumulation occurs, a more extensive pericardiectomy through a median sternotomy may be necessary. The usual partial pericardiectomy required for drainage of pericardial effusion can be nicely accomplished through an anterior left thoracotomy.

Most cases of idiopathic, viral, and uremic pericarditis are self-limited and will disappear without specific surgical therapy other than prevention of pericardial tamponade. Use of antiinflammatory drugs and, in uremics, more intense dialysis is usually sufficient. Bacterial pericarditis, like the pericarditic response to the presence of tumor, requires specific therapy, however. Administration of systemic antibiotics, usually by an intravenous route, is the preferred treatment. In most instances 7 to 10 days of treatment should be sufficient. Purulent bacterial pericarditis is an unusual occurrence in patients free of other systemic illness. Patients lacking adequate immunologic response capability are more likely to suffer from bacterial pericarditis, and these patients require a judicious combination of chemotherapy and surgical drainage. Most instances of bacterial pericarditis result from blood-borne deposition of bacterial colonies. In some cases, however, direct extension from a pneumonitic process in the right middle lobe or lingula may produce purulent pericarditis. Pericarditis has rarely been observed as a result of esophageal perforation into the pericardium posteriorly. In such instances, open drainage of the pericardium into the left pleural space with esophageal repair is mandatory. Most cases of acute pericarditis resolve with neither recurrence nor significant residual disability, although adhesions may be persistent and extensive. Some cases may progress to chronic recurring or constrictive pericarditis.

CHRONIC PERICARDITIS

Chronic pericarditis may be a recurrent process with pain, fever, and sometimes effusion continuing for a period of months or even years. The precise etiology of such a disease process is often difficult or impossible to establish. When a nonspecific inflammatory disturbance is present or when a collagen disease is either proved or suspected, steroid therapy may be beneficial. If further recurrence is evident after cessation of a course of steroid therapy or if it is difficult to discontinue the steroids, "total" pericardiectomy may be necessary.

A more common type of chronic pericarditis is that which in most instances produces no pain or other symptoms until chronic progressive tamponade develops. This entity, called chronic constrictive pericarditis, may occur following any type of acute pericarditis. In the more remote past, tuberculosis was the commonest cause of constrictive pericarditis, producing a thickened pericardium with extensive calcification and total loss of compliance. The scarring process eventually caused the pericardium to shrink also, producing tamponade even in patients with normal heart size. Chronic constrictive pericarditis today is more often caused by agents other than the tubercle bacillus, although tuberculosis may still be suspected in every case. Frequently, patients may have no history of a previous episode of acute pericarditis. In these instances, it is probable that a viral or perhaps idiopathic episode of pericarditis has occurred, and chronic inflammation has continued to the point of constriction.

Uremic pericarditis may progress to chronic constrictive pericarditis, but this is relatively uncommon.

A particularly vexing form of pericarditis may follow radiation therapy to the mediastinal structures. During the past several decades, mediastinal lymphomas, particularly Hodgkin's disease, have been managed by a combination of radiation and chemotherapy that has proved remarkably beneficial in eradicating the disease. Patients who were treated early in the course of development of radiation therapy protocols often developed chronic pericardial inflammation. This process produced remarkable thickening of the pericardium, which in some instances reached several centimeters. In such patients the parietal and visceral pericardial layers become densely adherent, and careful surgical dissection is necessary to free the heart.

Radiation pericarditis is usually not accompanied by severe calcification. On the other hand, chronic constrictive pericarditis from other causes may be accompanied by such remarkably heavy calcification that the heart appears to be ensheathed in a concrete corset. Calcification often may involve the superficial layers of the myocardium as well as the epicardial surface. The dissection is tedious, bloody, and remarkably difficult in such patients.

A significant advance in the technique of pericardiectomy for chronic constrictive pericarditis came with the introduction of cardiopulmonary bypass. Using the heart–lung machine, the heart may be conveniently collapsed and the boundaries between myocardium and pericardium much more readily identified than in the era when the pericardium had to be dissected with the heart beating and bulging where the constricting covering had been recently removed. Pericardiectomy may produce a dramatic initial result, but in some patients the early improvement may not be so marked, and a number of months may elapse during which the patient feels gradually better and myocardial function slowly improves. If the pericardium has been removed thoroughly and completely, recurrence is rare. Care must be taken to free not only the ventricular surfaces but also the areas of entry of the vena cavae and pulmonary veins and the exit of the pulmonary artery. A constricting band left along the atrioventricular groove may also result in persistent symptoms.

CARDIAC VALVES

Elective cardiac surgery began in 1923, when Elliot Cutler of Boston, using a transventricular valvulotome, excised a portion of the major leaflet of the mitral valve in a 14-year-old girl, attempting to convert severe mitral stenosis into more tolerable mild mitral stenosis and mild mitral insufficiency. This young lady survived the operative procedure and lived for another 4 years. Seven patients operated upon during the next several years using this technique all died during or shortly after operation. At the conclusion of this experience, Cutler and his cardiologic consultant and close friend, Samuel A. Levine, published a final summary of their experience, concluding sadly that the time was not yet ripe for direct surgical operations to relieve mitral stenosis. Apparently unknown to Cutler and Levine, Henry Souttar in London performed a finger fracture mitral commissurotomy in 1925 using a technique similar to that popularized later. His patient also survived operation despite the occurrence of a left atrial tear and temporarily frightening hemorrhage. Souttar was pleased with the outcome of the surgery but remarked in correspondence some years later that his medical colleagues never would send him another patient, and so this early attempt did not result in a sustained effort to repair the mechanical defect of mitral stenosis surgically. In 1948, after animal experimentation and experience gained in removing foreign bodies from the heart and great vessels in Allied servicemen during World War II, Dwight E. Harken of Boston, nearly simultaneously with Charles H. Bailey of Philadelphia, reintroduced the concept and technique of closed mitral commissurotomy, or valvuloplasty, as Harken preferred to call the operation. These two pioneers persisted in their efforts, and the result was the development of the technique of transatrial finger fracture valvuloplasty. A number of ingenious knives were devised to aid the surgeon in initiating fracture of the often leather-tough commissures of the rheumatically damaged mitral valve. The technique for this operation spread rapidly around the world owing to improved communication and the burgeoning number of thoracic surgeons who were prepared to begin the difficult task of developing intracardiac surgery. These operations were technically difficult and, although possible to learn, were nearly impossible to teach because the surgical manipulation was performed with the operator's finger completely hidden within the left atrium. A significant modification of the technique of closed mitral valvuloplasty came with the introduction of the transventricular dilator. This instrument could be introduced in the closed position through a relatively small aperture in the left ventricular apex, positioned between the stenosed leaflets, and opened to a predetermined diameter, thus fracturing the fused commissures. For most surgeons this provided an easier and more reproducible technique for treatment of mitral stenosis. Although closed mitral valvuloplasty is now uncommonly performed in the United States because of the simplicity, safety, and ease of performance of open mitral valve repair, the operation remains very common in countries where cardiopulmonary bypass is still too expensive for widespread utilization and where mitral stenosis remains a common problem.

Although mitral stenosis was peculiarly adapted to closed manipulative therapy because the leaflets tend to open under stress along the commissures, rheumatic and congenital fusion of the aortic leaflets was more difficult. In the aortic valve an anatomically acceptable cleavage plane often did not develop, and the valve was either simply dilated, producing only temporary benefit if any, or tears might occur in the substance of the leaflets, producing unacceptable valvular insufficiency. With the advent of cardiopulmonary bypass in 1954, the pace of progress in open operations upon the cardiac valves accelerated. The placement of valves in the descending aorta to relieve aortic insufficiency, as described by Murray, Heimbecker, and Bigelow of Toronto and Hufnagel of Washington, DC, was soon abandoned in favor of replacing diseased valves with prosthetic devices placed in the normal anatomic position of the aortic, mitral, and tricuspid valves. The first aortic valve replacement was performed by Dwight Harken on March 10, 1960, at the Peter Bent Brigham Hospital using a caged ball prosthesis. Mitral valve replacement was introduced in 1962 by Albert Starr. The Starr-Edwards caged ball valve became within a few years the standard cardiac valve prosthesis throughout the United States and much of the world. This and other valves are shown in Figure 40-2.

The caged ball valve, although conceptually simple, had significant mechanical disadvantages. As shown in Figure

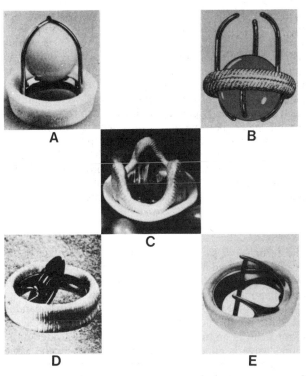

Fig. 40-2. Cardiac valve prostheses. (*A*) Starr-Edwards, model 1200. (*B*) Cutler-Smeloff. (*C*) Hancock porcine valve. (*D*) Bjork-Shiley. (*E*) Lillehei-Kaster. (Braunwald E [ed]: Heart Disease: A Textbook of Cardiovascular Medicine. Philadelphia, W B Saunders, 1980)

40-3, there were actually three separate orifices through which blood leaving the left ventricle had to pass. Restriction of any orifice could produce significant obstruction. In the atrioventricular position the size of the cage projecting into a small ventricular cavity was also potentially harmful. Low profile valves with a central flow orifice using a discoid occluder were developed. Improvements in prosthetic valve design and fabrication occurred simultaneously with devel-

Fig. 40-3. The complex orifice of a ball valve in the aortic position has potential obstruction at planes *A*, *B*, and *C*. (Roschke EJ, Harrison EC: Size comparisons of commercial prosthetic heart valves. Med Instr 7:281, 1973)

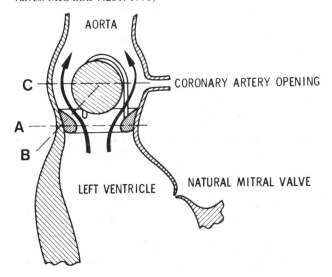

opment of biologic and bioprosthetic valves. Human homograft valves, used fresh or following preservation with various techniques, provided adequate mechanical performance with minimal thrombogenicity but were difficult to implant perfectly and had limited durability. Bioprosthetic valves, especially those employing stent-mounted, glutaraldehyde-preserved, porcine aortic valves, were commercially refined and widely utilized. Although they were less thrombogenic than the purely prosthetic valves, some patients still required anticoagulation therapy, notably those with atrioventricular valve replacement who had large atria or atrial fibrillation. A comparison of prosthetic and bioprosthetic valves in regard to mechanical function, thrombogenicity, and durability is shown in Table 40-2.

AORTIC VALVE

The aortic valve, situated rather deeply in the center of the heart, is supported by fibrous commissures. The three cusps, one anterior and two posterior, are supported by their commissural attachments to the fibrous arches of the aortic "annulus." It should be noted that the suspensory apparatus for the aortic valve leaflets is attached to the fibrous skeleton of the heart in an intimate fashion. The major leaflet of the mitral valve is attached to the undersurface of the same fibrous tissue that tethers the noncoronary leaflet of the aortic valve, and the bundle of His travels through an aperture just beneath the junction of the right coronary and noncoronary (anterior and right posterior) cusps.

AORTIC INSUFFICIENCY

The aortic valve is occasionally damaged by blunt external trauma. Rupture of the aortic leaflets may occur from an extremely severe blow to the chest during cardiac diastole when the leaflets are normally in the closed position. It will be remembered that cardiac diastole occupies more time in the sequence of cardiac contraction than does systole, and it is more likely that the heart will be in diastole at the moment of impact in any given traumatic occurrence. Nonetheless, aortic cusp rupture is uncommon, and when it occurs it is nearly always associated with such severe chest trauma so that patients rarely survive. Some do, however, and such patients may have a characteristic diastolic murmur along the left sternal border and in the aortic valve area. Congestive heart failure in these patients may be early in onset and rapidly progressive, or the course may be benign for up to several years. Careful observation is in order with early operation if necessary. Penetrating trauma to the aortic valve in the form of knife or bullet wounds may also occur. Significant traumatic damage to the aortic valve demands aortic valve replacement.

AORTIC VALVE DISEASE	
Etiology	Rheumatic disease, dissecting aneurysm, congenital malformation, Marfan's syndrome, trauma (external and operative), bacterial endocarditis
Dx	Symptoms: Congestive heart failure, angina pectoris, arrhythmia, syncope, sudden death EKG: Hypertrophy Chest x-ray: Calcification in valve, left ventricular dilatation vs hypertrophy Echocardiography Angiography: 50 mm gradient, ejection fraction
Rx	Surgical replacement with mechanical prosthesis or bioprosthesis
Special Considerations	Good myocardial protection with avoidance of left ventricular dilatation, necessity for coronary vascularization, avoidance of heart block

A more common cause of traumatic injury to the aortic valve leaflets, although also uncommon, is surgical manipulation through the aortic valve of structures within the left ventricular cavity. Transaortic resection of hypertrophic subaortic stenosis is an example of an operation in which aortic valve leaflet injury may occur. If laceration involves more than 1 or 2 mm of the aortic valve attachment or if the belly of the leaflet is torn or incised, aortic valve replacement is advisable. The normal aortic valve is a diaphanous structure that is nearly impossible to repair without subsequent dissolution of the repair or distortion of the leaflets that prevents adequate closure.

Other causes of aortic insufficiency more commonly encountered are rheumatic heart disease and bacterial endocarditis. Rheumatic heart disease may at times be difficult to distinguish in its late phases from deformities of the valve due to congenital anatomic abnormalities. The aortic valve is involved by rheumatic heart disease less commonly than the mitral valve but more commonly than the tricuspid or pulmonic valves. The valve leaflets become thickened and scarred. Some fusion of the commissures nearly always occurs, but this varies considerably in extent. If commissural fusion is extensive, aortic stenosis will result. If commissural fusion is less extensive and the principal process is thickening and rolling backwards of the edges of the valve leaflets, aortic insufficiency will be the predominant critical entity. Bacterial endocarditis is more common in patients who have a previously damaged or deformed aortic valve, but occasionally an apparently normal valve may become infected.

Gradually developing aortic insufficiency produces a quite different clinical picture from that seen in the acute onset of significant aortic valve leakage. Aortic insufficiency produces a volume overload defect that, if it develops gradually, is accompanied by both hypertrophy and dila-

---

TABLE 40-2 **COMPARISON OF PROSTHETIC AND BIOPROSTHETIC VALVES***

	MECHANICAL FUNCTION	THROMBO-GENICITY	DURA-BILITY
Prosthetic	4	0	3 to 4
Bioprosthetic	Large—4 Small—0 to 2	0 to 4	2 to 3

* Comparison of excellence graded 0 (poor) to 4 (best) of prosthetic and bioprosthetic valves

tation of the left ventricle. As time passes, dilatation becomes predominant, and not only does the left ventricular cavity enlarge but the configuration becomes radically altered. The normal left ventricular cavity is an elongated cylinder with a closed ellipsoid at one end and the aortic valve at the other. Such a configuration, surrounded by the thick walls of the left ventricle, has a relatively short radius of curvature and is therefore well designed to pump normal volumes of blood at high pressure. When the stroke volume must be increased to compensate for retrograde leak through an incompetent aortic valve, the ventricular cavity must enlarge. The left ventricular myocardium becomes stretched, and the interior of the left ventricular cavity gradually assumes a more spherical shape, which, for hydrodynamic reasons, is an inefficient configuration for a high-pressure contractile pump. The initial clinically discoverable abnormality in cardiac deterioration due to aortic insufficiency is left ventricular enlargement. This may be found by physical examination in advanced cases, by chest roentgenography, or by more sophisticated techniques involving measurement of left ventricular cavity dimensions. Whether discovered or undiscovered, left ventricular dilatation is a harbinger of left ventricular mechanical failure. Unfortunately, the onset of symptoms in patients with gradually developing left ventricular failure due to aortic insufficiency is often delayed to a point where mechanical damage from long-standing stretching of the left ventricular musculature is no longer entirely reversible. Indeed, in some persons the restoration of normal valve function may not produce sufficient improvement in myocardial contractility to allow a patient with advanced left ventricular dilatation to enjoy much benefit from cardiac surgery.

The principal symptoms of significant aortic insufficiency are congestive heart failure, angina pectoris, and arrhythmias. The principal manifestation of congestive heart failure in these patients is exertional dyspnea that at first may be mild but becomes progressively more severe. Angina pectoris may occur in the absence of coronary artery disease and is a significant manifestation of progressive disease. A dichotomy between the myocardial oxygen requirement and coronary blood flow in these patients is produced not only by hypertrophy and dilatation of the left ventricular musculature with a higher oxygen requirement per unit of external work obtained but also by the diminished diastolic aortic pressure, which causes a reduction in coronary artery perfusion pressure. Survival without surgery averages about 4 years after onset of angina and about 2 years with congestive heart failure. Arrhythmias, usually ventricular premature beats, most commonly occur late in the course of aortic insufficiency. If aortic insufficiency is caused by a disease process that also affects the myocardium, somewhat earlier onset of ventricular arrhythmias may be observed. Syncope may occur with repetitive ventricular premature beats and may be fatal in these patients. Acute stretching of the myocardium, whether from a normal or already stretched configuration, may produce increased automaticity of myocardial muscle fibers that in turn results in an increased hazard of sustained ventricular tachyarrhythmias. This may occur with exertion in patients with otherwise reasonably well compensated aortic insufficiency. For this reason, it is probably unwise for patients with aortic insufficiency to engage in activities requiring severe or prolonged exertion.

Acute aortic insufficiency is a far more urgent clinical problem than chronic aortic insufficiency. When a previously normal aortic valve undergoes dissolution for any reason, most commonly bacterial endocarditis, the left ventricle has difficulty accommodating the sudden increase in diastolic volume required to sustain an adequate cardiac output. In addition, the influence of sudden stretching of the systemic diastolic pressure on the left ventricular myocardium produces a marked hazard of sudden development of intractable ventricular arrhythmias. Angina pectoris is usually not a significant clinical problem in these patients. Deterioration in acute aortic insufficiency may be so rapid that a change in cardiac size is detectable at hourly intervals. The onset of ventricular ectopic rhythms is an ominous sign and is an indication for urgent surgical intervention.

AORTIC STENOSIS

Calcific aortic stenosis is probably the most common valvular lesion encountered in adults. Whereas rheumatic carditis is the most common cause of mitral stenosis, most cases of aortic stenosis are probably either congenital or degenerative. At autopsy or at the time of surgery the damaged valve is often so deformed that a precise differentiation between congenital and acquired disease is not possible. In rheumatic aortic stenosis, there is usually a readily identifiable tricuspid configuration with fusion of the commissures and heavy scarring and calcification of the valve leaflets. Because the edges of the leaflets are rolled backward, a fixed central orifice often occurs, producing both stenosis and regurgitation. For obvious reasons, it is impossible to have severe stenosis and severe regurgitation in the same patient. In patients with congenital deformity of the aortic valve there often is heavier calcification in the central portion of the valve leaflets, leaving the edge relatively spared. These patients may have very severe aortic stenosis with virtually no aortic insufficiency. Whatever the etiology, the pathophysiological consequences of progressive aortic stenosis are similar. The principal physiological response of the left ventricle is concentric hypertrophy. This may reach dramatic proportions, with the left ventricular mass increasing to as much as four times normal.

The classic triad of symptoms in aortic stenosis includes congestive heart failure, angina, and syncope. Congestive heart failure is a relatively late stage in aortic stenosis, and at this point there is usually significant left ventricular dilatation as well as concentric hypertrophy. There is increased diastolic "stiffness" of the heart (decreased compliance), which impedes left ventricular filling. The atrial A wave becomes larger as left ventricular end diastolic pressure rises. Loss of the normal cardiac rhythm has a particularly marked effect on cardiac output in persons with poorly compliant ventricles. With sudden onset of atrial fibrillation, diastolic filling abruptly declines, and mean left atrial pressure rises dramatically. A similar problem may develop with other supraventricular tachycardias even though the sequence of chamber contraction remains normal because the time allowable for ventricular filling has been substantially reduced. Myocardial oxygen requirements for performance of increased pressure work are progressively raised as hypertrophy continues. In addition, the intramyocardial distribution of coronary arterial blood flow is disturbed, and those areas with the highest tension development may squeeze off the blood supply to the point of symptomatic myocardial ischemia or even myocardial infarction. The subendocardial myocardium is most vulnerable, and subendocardial scarring is very common in these patients even when coronary obstructive disease is not present.

Syncope and its close relative, sudden death, always hang over persons with aortic stenosis as an ominous cloud. There are probably at least two mechanisms for syncope in these patients. The occurrence of sudden tachyarrhythmias is one, and disproportionate loss of peripheral vascular tone is the other. The syncope of aortic stenosis characteristically is related to exertion, and in many patients a combination of arrhythmias and a change in peripheral vascular resistance may be responsible. In many instances, spontaneous resolution of arrhythmias may occur, and repeated syncopal attacks are possible. In other instances, ventricular fibrillation supervenes, and resuscitation may be difficult or impossible. Ross and Braunwald found that the characteristic natural history of patients with aortic stenosis included a very long latent period during which increasingly severe valvular obstruction developed as well as increasing myocardial hypertrophy. The average age at the onset of symptoms was just short of 60 years. Following the onset of symptoms, maximum survival was about 5 years for those with angina, 3 years for those with syncope, and 2 years for those with congestive heart failure. A diagrammatic illustration of the course of patients with aortic stenosis is shown in Figure 40-4.

MEDICAL AND SURGICAL MANAGEMENT FOR AORTIC VALVE DISEASE

The medical management of most patients with aortic valve disease consists primarily of watchful waiting. This may sound simple enough, but in fact it is not because the critical problem in these patients is to choose the most propitious time for surgical intervention. In both aortic insufficiency and aortic stenosis, patients may live comfortably for many years despite severe anatomic valve abnormalities; however, ventricular decompensation will begin during this time. If this is allowed to progress to its end stage, hypertrophy and dilatation may be complicated by functional or anatomic changes in the left ventricle that are irreversible. The onset of clinical symptoms is often late, and complete recovery cannot be expected even though functional integrity of the valve is restored by a replacement operation. There has been a great deal of interest in the utilization of left ventricular size as a criterion for choosing an optimal time

for surgery. Measurements include those made with serial roentgenograms and estimates of ventricular volume made by echocardiography or radionuclide ventriculography. The significance of left ventricular enlargement in aortic regurgitation has been especially emphasized, but cardiac enlargement with aortic stenosis also cannot be overlooked even though the patient remains asymptomatic.

Because of the ominous prognosis following the onset of symptoms, patients with angina, syncope, or congestive heart failure due to either aortic stenosis or regurgitation should be considered candidates for aortic valve replacement. Temporary symptomatic relief may often be obtained with digitalis, diuretics, and pharmacologic rate and rhythm control. However, persistent use of medical measures simply prolongs existence to a point where mechanical correction is no longer effective. One question that arises from time to time is whether there should be some age beyond which patients are not considered suitable candidates for valve replacement surgery. Experience has shown that elderly persons may do quite well with surgery. Patients in the ninth and even tenth decades of life have been successfully operated upon and usefully rehabilitated following aortic valve replacement. The decision should be based upon whether aortic valve dysfunction is the principal debilitating disease present and whether other diseases are likely to limit either longevity or comfort in such a fashion that the prolongation of life no longer represents a kindness.

EVALUATION OF PATIENTS FOR AORTIC VALVE SURGERY

Preoperative evaluation of patients being considered for aortic valve replacement should answer two critical questions. First, is aortic valve dysfunction the principal cause of cardiac disability? Second, are there other contributing cardiac factors that should be either considered or corrected at the time of surgery? In patients with aortic insufficiency, estimation of the volume of regurgitant flow is both difficult and unreliable. More to the point are measurements of mean left atrial pressure as an index of the degree of left ventricular failure and ejection fraction as an index of the potential for rehabilitation following valve replacement. The ideal candidate for surgery among persons with aortic valve

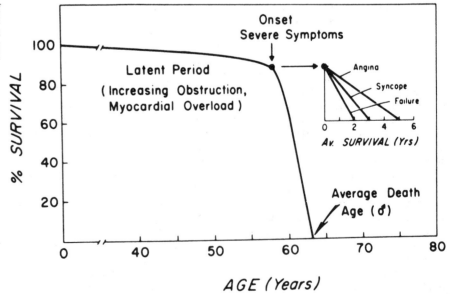

Fig. 40-4. The ominous significance of symptoms of angina, syncope, and congestive heart failure in patients with aortic stenosis. (Ross J Jr, Braunwald E: Aortic stenosis. Circulation 38 [Suppl 5]:61, 1968)

regurgitation has an ejection fraction of 40% or better. Often this may not be the case, and a judgment must then be made as to the likelihood of recovery following valve replacement. Because of the difficulties involved in such a decision, it is often better to replace the valve when in doubt than to refuse surgery to a potentially rehabilitatable person.

In the presence of aortic stenosis, a peak systolic pressure gradient of 50 mmHg or more at rest or a measured valve area of 0.5 cm² or less in the adult constitutes reliable evidence of critical aortic stenosis. A very high pressure gradient across the aortic valve usually indicates excellent capability of the left ventricle to maintain the cardiac output after surgery. The gradient may decline as the disease progresses to a point where the left ventricle is unable to generate enough force to demonstrate significant aortic stenosis by pressure measurements. When the gradient falls below 35 mmHg, the probability of operative survival and rehabilitation must be questioned. With very low gradients the anatomic deformity of the valve is probably no longer the most critical factor, and left ventricular decompensation is the principal limiting factor for cardiac output generation. Under these circumstances, correction of the valvular abnormality is not likely to produce an overall functional improvement.

OPERATIVE TECHNIQUE FOR AORTIC VALVE REPLACEMENT

Patients should be transported to the operating room with the head elevated to approximately 30 degrees to avoid hypoxia or pulmonary edema. In addition, preoperative narcosis and sedation should be minimal.

Following the induction of general anesthesia, the usual skin preparation and drapes are applied. The heart is exposed gently and quickly. Although it is possible to accomplish institution of cardiopulmonary bypass within 5 to 8 minutes after the beginning of a median sternotomy, this portion of the operation usually takes about 30 minutes using aortic and right atrial cannulation.

Following establishment of cardiopulmonary bypass, the surgeon's major responsibility should be to ensure that no further myocardial damage occurs. Perfusion techniques and ischemic techniques have been utilized to accomplish adequate myocardial protection. Most surgeons presently use "hypothermic cardioplegia" for myocardial preservation. A cold solution of balanced electrolyte buffered to *p*H 7.4, containing 15 to 30 mEq potassium per liter, is infused into the aortic root after distal clamping of the ascending aorta, as shown in Figure 40-5, or directly infused into the coronary ostia after opening the aorta. The heart is arrested, and cellular metabolism is slowed by cooling and biochemical paralysis.

In the presence of significant aortic insufficiency adequate coronary artery perfusion may be achieved by the infusion of cardioplegic solution into the root of the aorta. Great care must be taken not to injure the orifices of the coronary arteries nor to perfuse the coronary arteries with such high pressures that intramyocardial edema is produced when solutions are directly perfused into them.

When myocardial protection has been accomplished, the aortic valve is resected. In many cases the valve leaflets may be simply excised using a knife or scissors. In patients with severe calcification, however, more skill and experience are required. Sufficient calcium must be removed to allow adequate positioning of the base of the prosthetic device.

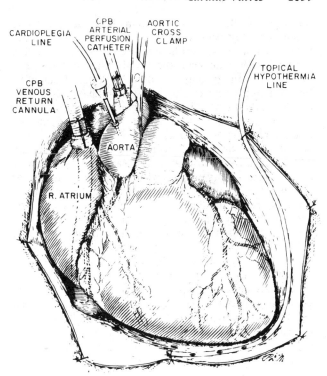

Fig. 40-5. Technique of using hypothermic cardioplegia for myocardial preservation during cardiac surgery. (Cohn LH [ed]: The Treatment of Acute Myocardial Ischemia: An Integrated Medical/Surgical Approach. Mt. Kisco, Futura Publishing, 1979)

On the other hand, dissection must not produce irreparable dissolution of the attachments of the base of the aorta to the left ventricular outflow tract, and if possible the conduction system should be preserved.

A suitable aortic prosthesis or bioprosthetic device is sutured in place using braided sutures of synthetic fiber. The sutures are passed around the fibrous annular arch. Some care must be taken to ensure a proper fit of the replacement device within the aorta. Calibrated obturators are available for this purpose.

When the valve has been seated and the sutures tied, the aortotomy is closed with running suture. The patient is rewarmed and defibrillated with a direct current defibrillator. Recovery of normal myocardial contractility requires a few minutes to a half hour or longer. Cardiopulmonary bypass is discontinued, but monitoring of ventricular filling pressures and systemic arterial blood pressure continues. A temporary pacemaker may be necessary for some patients. Intravenous inotropic agents may often be required in the operating room or intensive care area soon after surgery. When the patient is in a stable condition and is adequately maintaining blood pressure independent of the heart–lung apparatus, the cardiopulmonary bypass cannulae should be removed and protamine given to counteract the anticoagulant effect of the heparin that is necessary during operation of the heart–lung apparatus. When bleeding has been brought under control, the incision is closed with drainage of the pericardium by suction.

POSTOPERATIVE CARE

Following aortic valve replacement, patients should be removed to a specialized cardiac intensive care unit. Systemic arterial blood pressure, venous pressure, left atrial filling pressure, and the electrocardiogram should be constantly monitored. Most patients will require respiratory assistance for ventilation for several hours to several days depending upon the anesthetic technique and the clinical status prior to surgery. Urinary output should be watched carefully. Intravenous prophylactic therapy with antibiotics is continued for several days. The most important areas of clinical concern in the immediate postoperative period include respiratory function, maintenance of an adequate cardiac output, and elimination of postoperative bleeding. By 24 hr after surgery, most patients are capable of maintaining their own respiratory function without the aid of a respirator and their hemodynamic function without the aid of pressor drugs or arterial monitoring, and many may often be well enough to sit on the edge of the bed or briefly in a chair. Postoperative discomfort will be maximal during the first 2 or 3 days but diminishes rapidly thereafter in most patients. The median sternotomy incision is less painful than an intercostal incision, and, if the sternum is stable, most patients are quite comfortable by 5 or 6 days after surgery. They can expect to spend about 10 days in the hospital following surgery, of which 1 or 2 days will be in the intensive care area.

MITRAL VALVE

MITRAL STENOSIS

Mitral stenosis is most commonly caused by rheumatic fever but may occasionally be congenital. The time between an acute episode of rheumatic fever and the occurrence of mitral stenosis is quite variable but in the United States averages 15 to 25 or more years. For reasons that are not entirely clear, the interval appears to be longer in highly developed countries where acute rheumatic illnesses are less prevalent. The basic pathologic feature initially involves inflammatory changes and vascularization of the valve leaflets, apparently as an autoimmune reaction. Later, fibrosis with severe contraction of the leaflet structure and chordae tendineae occurs, with leaflet fusion as well as fusion of the chordae. Calcification is a late and progressive feature in many cases.

Variations

There are three important variations in pathologic anatomy that may affect the outcome of surgical repair. In the simplest, there is a fusion of the leaflets with diminution of the effective orifice to a fishmouth slit. If the leaflets remain pliable without significant calcification and the length of the chordae tendineae is preserved without significant fusion, surgical repair involves simply division of the fused commissures of the valve leaflets with excellent hope for long-term amelioration of symptoms. A second pathophysiologic variety of mitral stenosis occurs when there is not only fusion of the commissures but shortening of the chordae tendineae. The chordae pull the valve leaflets deep into the left ventricular chamber, producing a funnel-type valvular deformity. Simple division of the adherent commissures may not result in sufficient mobility of the leaflets to allow total correction of mitral stenosis. These patients may be expected to do significantly less well following reparative surgery even when special effort is made to split the papillary muscles. The third variety of mitral stenosis, for which surgical repair is even more difficult, is a combination of commissural fusion, leaflet deformity, and fusion of the chordae tendineae. In this type of mitral stenosis, there may actually be two separate areas of anatomic obstruction. One of these is the narrowed orifice between the fused leaflets, and the second is the reduced aggregate orifice between the chordae tendineae, which may have assumed the configuration of a loosely woven basket. Reparative surgery in these cases involves not only freeing the commissural adherence but also restructuring the chordae tendineae to a considerable extent. In some instances, the chordae may have virtually disappeared, resulting in adherence of the papillary muscles to the undersurface of the valve leaflets. In such instances repair is impossible, and valve replacement is necessary.

As the heart increases in size during normal growth, so do the effective orifice areas of the various cardiac valves. In adults the normal mitral valve orifice is approximately 4 cm² to 6 cm². Reduction of this area to approximately 2 cm² may be expected to produce a pressure gradient across the mitral valve during diastole. Reduction to 1 cm² is considered to constitute "critical" mitral stenosis because left atrial pressures required for adequate ventricular filling through such a small orifice must rise to a mean of 15 torr or more, placing the patient on the verge of pulmonary edema at rest. Under such circumstances, exertional dyspnea comes on rapidly and with minimal effort. In the presence of long-standing mitral stenosis, chronically elevated left atrial and pulmonary venous pressure results in pulmonary arterial hypertension and a slowly progressive form of pulmonary arterial obstruction that has both an organic and a functional component. The pulmonary arterial branches may show considerable endothelial proliferation with a reduction of effective cross-sectional area in the pulmonary vascular bed. In contrast to the situation observed in pulmonary vascular obstruction with congenital defects

MITRAL VALVE DISEASE	
Etiology	Rheumatic disease, dysfunction due to coronary insufficiency, trauma, endocarditis
Dx	*Symptoms* of congestive heart failure, arrhythmia (atrial fibrillation), angina pectoris *Signs:* Pulmonary edema, rales, embolization, murmur, hemoptysis *Evaluation:* Echocardiography, chest x-ray, ECG, angiography
Rx	*Mitral stenosis:* Valvulotomy, chordae splitting, valve replacement with mechanical or bioprosthesis *Mitral insufficiency:* Carpentier ring, valve replacement
Other Considerations	Presence or absence of urinary disease, need for anticoagulation, management of left atrial thrombus, necessity of concomitant tricuspid valve replacement

causing high pulmonary blood flow, the functional component of pulmonary vascular obstruction in patients with mitral stenosis appears to be more predominant than the irreversible structural alteration. In severe instances, the pulmonary arterial blood pressure may approach systemic levels. In these patients, right ventricular failure often supervenes and may become a dominant factor in determining the risk of surgical repair or valve replacement.

Chronically elevated left atrial pressure results in distention of the left atrium. In time the muscle fibers become severely stretched with enhanced automaticity, resulting in a tendency toward development of supraventricular arrhythmias, particularly atrial fibrillation. In patients with mitral stenosis, augmentation of left ventricular filling due to atrial contraction contributes significantly to cardiac output as well as enabling the mean left atrial pressure to remain significantly lower. Sudden development of atrial fibrillation in the presence of significant mitral stenosis reduces the cardiac output by about 20% and is accompanied by an immediate and significant rise in mean left atrial pressure. In some patients this rise in pulmonary venous pressure may result in rapid onset of intractable pulmonary edema, occasionally with a fatal outcome. The severity of pulmonary edema appears to be greater in patients with less severe pulmonary arterial changes.

Signs and symptoms in mitral stenosis are related to the usual cardiac triad of congestive heart failure, angina pectoris, and arrhythmias. Of earliest onset in patients with mitral stenosis are symptoms of congestive heart failure, principally those related to pulmonary venous hypertension and manifested by dyspnea. Initially, dyspnea may occur only on severe exertion. Then there will be a gradual reduction of exercise tolerance, and eventually dyspnea will occur on minimal exertion or at rest. The occurrence of atrial fibrillation in the course of development of mitral stenosis may significantly aggravate and accelerate the course of congestive heart failure. Angina pectoris is an unusual symptom in patients with mitral stenosis but may occur with advanced illness and very low cardiac output. Another type of pain may be related to distention of the pulmonary artery in patients with marked pulmonary hypertension. Cough and hemoptysis may occur. Severe, exsanguinating hemoptysis is a rare complication of mitral stenosis that may require emergency valvuloplasty or valve replacement.

Patients with mitral stenosis may suffer systemic arterial embolization with devastating strokes or other vascular occlusions. Atrial fibrillation increases the risk of embolization, and patients with chronic fibrillation are best maintained on anticoagulant drugs. Emboli may come from large clots within the atrium or from fibrin or calcific debris formed on the valve leaflets. At operation, about 50% of patients with a history of embolism have an identifiable intra-atrial clot. Embolization in the absence of significant symptoms of congestive heart failure is an indication for anticoagulation but not necessarily for surgery. At one time closed valvuloplasty with amputation of the atrial appendage was advocated, but anticoagulation alone is more commonly used at present unless multiple episodes occur.

Diagnosis of Mitral Stenosis

Characteristic abnormalities are found on physical examination and on roentgenograms, on echocardiography, and at cardiac catheterization. The usual patient with mitral stenosis is slender and may be cachectic. One may occa-

sionally see well nourished or even obese patients with mitral stenosis, but this is distinctly unusual and should alert the observant surgeon to the possibility of other abnormalities. Auscultatory findings in mitral stenosis are diagnostic. An opening snap is heard in patients with a flexible anterior leaflet. The temporal proximity of the opening snap to the second heart sound is related to the level of left atrial hypertension and to the flexibility of the anterior leaflet. In the presence of high left atrial pressures, the opening snap occurs closer to the second sound. Similarly, stiffness of the anterior leaflet tends to move the opening snap toward the second sound. Patients with a loud opening snap well removed from the second heart sound are often excellent candidates for valvuloplasty or commissurotomy. Following the opening snap, if it is present, is a diagnostic low-pitched diastolic murmur often described as a rumble. In patients with advanced heart failure and reduced cardiac output, it may be difficult or impossible to hear the murmur of mitral stenosis. Even in these patients, there is often a characteristic rhythm that gives the impression of mitral stenosis to the experienced observer. A blowing diastolic murmur due to pulmonic insufficiency may be heard in some patients, but a more frequent cause of a soft diastolic murmur is the presence of mild aortic insufficiency.

The chest roentgenogram in mitral stenosis shows abnormalities of both the pulmonary vasculature and the cardiac contour as shown in Figure 40-6. There is often redistribution of pulmonary blood flow, resulting in a more prominent vascular pattern toward the apices than is normal, and there may be evidence of pulmonary interstitial edema in the lower lobes. The cardiac silhouette may show the heart to be of overall normal size or perhaps slightly enlarged. The pulmonary outflow tract is prominent, and the pul-

Fig. 40-6. Chest roentgenogram in mitral stenosis. The left atrium and pulmonary outflow tract are enlarged and the pulmonary venous pattern is accentuated.

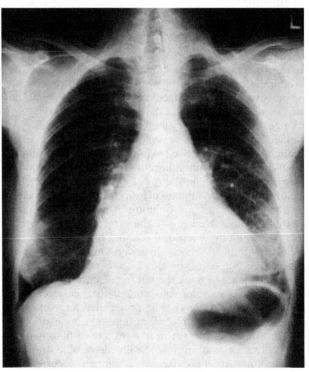

monary arteries may be enlarged as well. A diagnostic sign is a double density caused by the enlarged left atrium. In the lateral roentgenogram, the right ventricle may intrude upon the usual empty space anterior to the heart, and the enlarged left atrium may cause posterior or posterolateral deviation of the esophagus.

The introduction of M-mode and two-dimensional echocardiography during the past decade has greatly simplified the precise diagnosis of mitral stenosis without cardiac catheterization. Cardiac catheterization also yields characteristic findings in the presence of mitral stenosis, but the information is not additionally beneficial in most cases unless the catheterization is accompanied by coronary arteriography. Patients with angina pectoris or a history of myocardial ischemic events should undergo coronary angiography prior to any contemplated cardiac surgery. Appropriate preparations and plans for coronary bypass can then be made.

MITRAL INSUFFICIENCY

Mitral insufficiency, like mitral stenosis, is most commonly caused by rheumatic fever. Primary mitral insufficiency due to rheumatic heart disease is more common in men than in women. A secondary form of mitral insufficiency that occurs late in the course of disease after surgical correction of mitral stenosis is more common in women because mitral stenosis is more frequent in women. Mitral insufficiency may also result from bacterial endocarditis superimposed upon a previously abnormal or even a normal valve. Certain degenerative diseases, including Marfan's syndrome and Hurler's syndrome, involve premature deterioration of connective tissue in the cardiac valves, and mitral insufficiency due to annular dilatation, eccentricity of cusps, or rupture of chordae tendineae may occur. Other causes of ruptured chordae tendineae include rheumatic heart disease (possibly the most common cause) and papillary muscle necrosis due to myocardial infarction.

Symptoms

Clinical syndromes in mitral insufficiency, like those in aortic insufficiency, vary according to the suddenness and severity of the mitral valve leak. Most commonly, the degree of mitral regurgitation gradually increases. There may be an interval of many years during which a murmur of mitral insufficiency may be heard without onset of symptoms or progressive cardiac enlargement. Eventually, cardiac enlargement will occur, and the left ventricular cavity will change from the normal cylindroid shape to a more spherical configuration. Progressive enlargement and particularly change in shape of the left ventricular cavity are ominous prognostic signs in mitral insufficiency. Onset of symptoms may occur quite late in the course of cardiac deterioration. Among the classic symptoms of heart failure, angina pectoris and arrhythmia that are common to nearly every cardiac disability, congestive heart failure is by far the most prominent and striking. Exertional dyspnea brought on by progressive pulmonary venous hypertension is usually slowly progressive but is inexorable. Late in the course of this disease, fatigue and weakness due to reduction of the cardiac output become more prominent. Left atrial enlargement is invariably seen in the chronic progressive form of mitral insufficiency. The atrium may at times reach gigantic proportions and may consist nearly entirely of fibrous tissue with only occasional microscopically identifiable strands of myocardium. Atrial fibrillation is a common occurrence. It

has been popularly assumed that the risk of systemic embolization in the presence of mitral insufficiency is less than that with mitral stenosis. Published reports, however, indicate that the frequency of arterial embolization in the presence of atrial fibrillation is approximately the same in both types of mitral valve dysfunction.

Medical Treatment of Mitral Insufficiency

Medical management of symptomatic mitral insufficiency includes utilization of digitalis for its inotropic effect as well as for slowing the ventricular response rate in the presence of atrial fibrillation. Fluid retention is a prominent problem for many patients, and diuretics may provide symptomatic relief for a prolonged interval. Recently, use of systemic vasodilator agents to reduce left ventricular afterload has provided dramatic, if temporary, relief for some patients. The rationale for vasodilator therapy is very simple. In the presence of severe mitral insufficiency there is no isovolumic contraction period for the left ventricle. Mitral insufficiency occurs instantaneously with the onset of rise of left ventricular wall tension even at low intracavitary left ventricular pressures. As the velocity of circumferential fiber shortening increases, intracavitary tension rises high enough to effect opening of the aortic valve, and left ventricular ejection into the systemic circulation occurs. With reduction of systemic vascular resistance, the opening of the aortic valve occurs earlier in the contractile sequence, and the proportion of blood leaving the left ventricle into the aorta increases. There is, thus, both a reduction in the volume of mitral regurgitant flow and an increase in systemic cardiac output.

With improvements in surgical technique and improvements in the prosthetic and biologic devices available to replace the natural mitral valve, the threshold of surgical referral by physicians and of acceptance by patients has become progressively lower.

EVALUATION AND SELECTION OF PATIENTS FOR MITRAL VALVE REPAIR OR REPLACEMENT FOR MITRAL REGURGITATION

Mitral valve surgery is indicated in the management of mitral insufficiency in the following circumstances: (1) symptomatic patients exhibiting progressive congestive heart failure, (2) patients with stable symptoms exhibiting progressive cardiac enlargement, (3) patients with combined aortic and mitral valve disease in whom the degree of mitral insufficiency might not, if occurring alone, constitute an indication for valve replacement, and (4) patients with abrupt onset of severe mitral insufficiency as a result of ruptured chordae tendineae or active bacterial endocarditis.

Exposure of the mitral valve for mitral insufficiency is technically similar to but often easier than that for mitral stenosis. In the presence of mitral insufficiency, the larger left atrium makes visualization of the mitral valve easier in most instances.

Several techniques are available for the correction of mitral insufficiency depending upon the nature of the lesion, the integrity of the mitral leaflets and chordae tendineae, and the experience of the operating surgeon. Reparative techniques (mitral annuloplasty) have been utilized with variable success in several centers throughout the world. When mitral insufficiency is a result of annulus stretching with intact leaflet structure and intact chordae tendineae, a reduction of the annulus diameter may be effective in limiting or abolishing mitral insufficiency. It should be kept in mind that the mitral "annulus" is really a semiannulus. The fila coronaria are incomplete posteriorly in the mitral valve and posterolaterally in the tricuspid valve rings. In the presence of a stretching force, such as the chronic increased intracavitary pressure that may occur in chronic mitral insufficiency, the posterior circumference of the valve annulus becomes progressively longer. A rigid ring for reinforcement of the circumference of the mitral valve was introduced by Carpentier, and in his hands excellent results have been obtained for the control of mitral insufficiency. Valvuloplastic procedures using reinforcement of the annulus for management of mitral insufficiency have had greater success outside the United States. The precise explanation is not clear, but it may be that this operation has its greatest chance for success in patients with a somewhat more virulent form of early rheumatic mitral insufficiency than is commonly seen in this country.

In the presence of a limited number of ruptured chordae, particularly those involving the posterior leaflet of the mitral valve, partial excision or plication of the leaflet may be accomplished in some patients with quite acceptable long-term results.

More sophisticated operations, including reimplantation of ruptured chordae into the papillary muscles, have been advocated and successfully utilized by some surgeons, but because of the greater complexity of the operative maneuvers and the hazard of early recurrence of severe mitral insufficiency, such operations have not found widespread acceptance.

Mitral valve replacement remains the commonest and most successful treatment for mitral regurgitation regardless of the cause. Either prosthetic or bioprosthetic valves may be used.

SURGICAL TECHNIQUE FOR MITRAL VALVE REPLACEMENT

The technique of mitral valve replacement is basically similar whether it is done for mitral insufficiency or for mitral stenosis. Major points are shown in Figures 40-7 and 40-8. After induction of general anesthesia, the chest is prepared and draped for median sternotomy. The heart is exposed in the usual manner. Although cannulation of the right atrium with a single catheter is acceptable for operations involving the aortic valve or coronary arteries, it is usually necessary to use both a superior vena caval and an inferior vena caval cannula because of the distortion produced by introduction of a retractor into the left atrium on the right side of the heart. Aortic cannulation for arterial return from the pump is usually used.

Patients are cooled to 29° or 30°C. With the ascending aorta clamped, the heart is protected with cold cardioplegia and topical hypothermia. The mitral valve is visualized through an incision made in the left atrium on the right side of the heart, posterior to the interatrial groove and anterior to the entry of the pulmonary veins. The mitral valve including the chordae tendineae is carefully resected. Most surgeons resect only the tips of the papillary muscles if any muscle at all. The mitral valve replacement device is fixed in place with braided synthetic sutures.

Any thrombus encountered within the left atrium is removed. Very often a plane of dissection can be established

Fig. 40-7. Resection of mitral valve in preparation for replacement with a prosthetic or bioprosthetic valve. (Cohn LH [ed]: Modern Techniques in Surgery. Mt. Kisco, Futura Publishing, 1979)

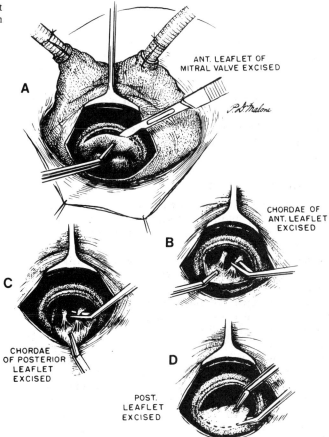

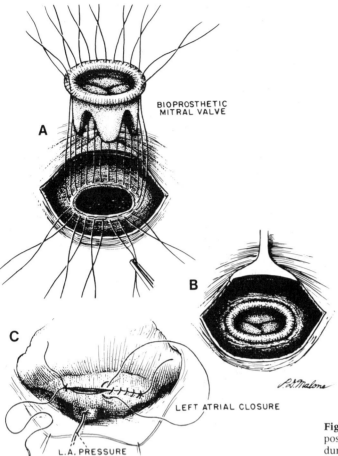

A

BIOPROSTHETIC
MITRAL VALVE

B

C

LEFT ATRIAL CLOSURE

L.A. PRESSURE
MONITOR

Fig. 40-8. Placement of a porcine bioprosthetic valve in the mitral position. A plastic catheter is used for monitoring left atrial pressure during the early postoperative period. (Cohn LH [ed]: Modern Techniques in Surgery. Mt. Kisco, Futura Publishing, 1979)

in which the thrombus is readily shelled out. Following closure of the left atrium, the heart is refilled with blood, taking care to remove all residual air through the left ventricular apex, the ascending aorta, and the left atrium itself. As with aortic valve replacement, cardiopulmonary bypass is gradually discontinued with monitoring of atrial and arterial pressures when the patient has been totally rewarmed and shows evidence of strong organized cardiac contractility.

POSTOPERATIVE CARE

Care after mitral valve replacement or multiple valve replacement does not differ markedly in most respects from care after aortic valve replacement. It should be remembered, however, that many patients requiring mitral valve replacement have a poorer nutritional status than patients requiring aortic valve replacement. In these persons, every phase of recovery may be significantly slowed. Patients with severely elevated pulmonary arterial pressure at the time of mitral or multiple valve replacement may also be expected to have a slower and more difficult postoperative recovery. As will be mentioned subsequently in the section on artificial hearts and circulatory assist devices, reversal of the normal relationships between right and left atrial pressures is a signal that the overall cardiac output is dependent upon right ventricular function. This is undesirable, and special attention must be given to the contractile state of the right ventricle as well as the outflow resistance in the pulmonary circulation.

TRICUSPID VALVE

The tricuspid valve may be involved in rheumatic heart disease, resulting in either stenosis or insufficiency. Tricuspid stenosis is the less common entity. Tricuspid insufficiency in the presence of rheumatic heart disease may be a combination of functional and organic incompetence. Functional incompetence occurs when there is dilatation of the atrioventricular ring in the presence of chronic pressure overload of the right ventricle.

Less common acquired diseases of the tricuspid valve include sclerosis as part of the carcinoid heart syndrome, primary bacterial endocarditis (seen especially in drug addicts), and, rarely, disease from injury from blunt or penetrating trauma.

SYMPTOMS

The signs and symptoms of tricuspid stenosis and tricuspid insufficiency are similar. Both produce chronic increase in systemic venous pressure with edema, hepatomegaly, and ascites. Predominant tricuspid stenosis is usually not accompanied by severe respiratory symptoms of congestive heart failure, whereas tricuspid insufficiency, which is usually caused by left-sided heart failure, is most often accompanied by significant symptoms of pulmonary venous hypertension.

SURGICAL TREATMENT OF TRICUSPID STENOSIS AND INSUFFICIENCY

Tricuspid stenosis may be treated by either tricuspid valvuloplasty or by tricuspid valve replacement. If the valve leaflets have retained pliability and the primary problem is one of commissural fusion, the commissures between the septal leaflet and the anterior and posterior leaflets may be sharply divided with a high expectation of a good functional result. Only these two commissures should be incised. Incision of the commissure between the anterior and the posterior tricuspid leaflets in addition to mobilization of the septal leaflet will often result in significant mitral insufficiency.

Tricuspid insufficiency caused by organic disease due to rheumatic fever or bacterial endocarditis usually requires valve replacement. In patients with mitral insufficiency due to dilatation of the tricuspid annulus, a variety of valvuloplastic techniques have given good functional results in many patients. Suture techniques to reduce the circumference of the tricuspid annulus as well as implantation of a flexible or rigid ring to stabilize the circumference of the annulus have been successfully utilized. Patients with basically normal myocardial function who are afflicted with active bacterial endocarditis involving the tricuspid valve may tolerate resection of the tricuspid valve without replacement. Following completion of antibiotic therapy, such patients can subsequently undergo tricuspid valve replacement to achieve improved maximal cardiac function.

In all operations on the tricuspid valve, care must be taken to avoid injury to the bundle of His as it passes close beneath the endocardium adjacent to the attachment of the septal leaflet.

The indications for surgical treatment of tricuspid valve disease include significant venous hypertension due to stenosis or insufficiency that does not resolve or is not likely to resolve after repair of left-sided mechanical lesions. This deceptively simple recommendation requires surgical judgment. For patients with tricuspid stenosis there usually is no problem. The stenosis should be relieved in a fashion that does not produce significant insufficiency, or the valve should be replaced. In patients with organic damage to the tricuspid valve resulting in tricuspid insufficiency, valve replacement should likewise be performed. Questions about surgical treatment may arise in patients with predominantly functional tricuspid insufficiency in the presence of severe left-sided valvular lesions. A useful general rule is as follows. If patients with cardiac failure due to left-sided valvular lesions have clinical evidence of tricuspid insufficiency that resolves during preoperative bed rest, tricuspid valve replacement is usually unnecessary. In patients for whom medical management does not result in significant amelioration of tricuspid insufficiency, the decision for tricuspid valve replacement or surgical repair may be based upon the presence or absence of significant right ventricular hypertension and the response of the right ventricle to correction of lesions on the left side of the heart. For example, a patient with continuing tricuspid insufficiency despite maximal medical management undergoes cardiac catheterization. If the pressures in the right ventricle are only mildly elevated and tricuspid insufficiency continues to be present, there is a very high likelihood that such valvular incompetence will not spontaneously improve later. However, if pulmonary pressures are high, there is a real possibility that amelioration of left-sided valvular defects will result in a fall of right ventricular pressure with restoration of competence of the unaltered tricuspid valve. It is useful at the time of operation in such patients to measure right and left atrial filling pressures upon completion of repair of the left-sided valvular abnormalities. If the left atrial pressure is higher than the right atrial pressure, the right side of the heart does not constitute a critical limiting factor for maintenance of the cardiac output, and these patients will generally do very well without further tricuspid manipulation. When the right atrial filling pressure is higher than the left, correction of tricuspid insufficiency is indicated.

PULMONARY VALVE

Acquired lesions of the pulmonary valve are uncommon. Pulmonary artery stenosis may occasionally be seen as part of the carcinoid heart syndrome. Bacterial endocarditis may uncommonly involve the pulmonary valve and should be suspected, particularly in patients with septic lesions who have indwelling balloon catheters through the pulmonary valve. Particularly in burn patients, there seems to be a susceptibility to pulmonary valve endocarditis from this cause.

Significant pulmonary artery stenosis should be surgically corrected. In most instances, it is possible simply to incise the stenotic valve to reduce or abolish the gradient. Resection of the pulmonary valve is well tolerated in patients with otherwise normal cardiovascular function. In patients with significant pulmonary arterial hypertension, a competent pulmonary valve is desirable, and valve replacement may be necessary on rare occasions.

MULTIPLE VALVE DISEASE

Particularly in patients with rheumatic heart disease, two or more valves may be significantly abnormal. Although the symptoms and signs of congestive heart failure, arrhythmia, and angina pectoris are similar to those found in single valve disease, additional considerations must be given in surgical management to achieve an optimal result with the least complex operation. The most commonly damaged valve in rheumatic heart disease is the mitral valve, followed in frequency by the aortic, tricuspid, and pulmonic valves. The most common multiple valve combination is that of the aortic and mitral valves. Mitral and tricuspid combinations are less common but are not rare, especially when including functional tricuspid insufficiency. Involvement of the aortic, mitral, and tricuspid valves may also be seen. Significant involvement of the pulmonic valve in multiple valve disease is rare if it ever occurs.

Several facts are of interest in multiple valve disease. One is that functional abnormalities may be additive, producing symptoms at an earlier stage of anatomic abnormality than would be expected for the same level of disability if only a single valve were involved. The technical difficulty of replacement of the individual valves is thus usually less than when only one valve causes severe symptoms. A combination of aortic stenosis and mitral insufficiency causes severe reduction of maximal cardiac ouput and an increase in pulmonary venous pressure early in its course. Very severe aortic valve obstruction accompanied by left ventricular dilatation may cause mild to moderate mitral insufficiency that may resolve after successful aortic valve replacement. A combination of aortic and mitral stenosis is better tolerated for a longer interval, and therefore the individual valves may be more severely damaged and more difficult to replace. Additionally, the left ventricular cavity may be small due to severe myocardial hypertrophy, and left ventricular compliance may be significantly impaired, necessitating high filling pressures in the postoperative interval.

The variety of combinations of possible anatomic and functional abnormalities in multiple valve disease is both diagnostically and therapeutically challenging. A good rule in deciding how many valves should be replaced or repaired is the sicker the patient, the more important is a perfect immediate functional result. Thus, a patient with moderate functional tricuspid insufficiency after mitral valve replacement may be allowed to recover gradually if the cardiac output is reasonably maintained early after surgery. In the presence of severe myocardial decompensation, however, the same measured quantity of tricuspid insufficiency may be intolerable, and tricuspid valve replacement is needed to ensure early survival, regardless of the fact that late functional improvement might have occurred without replacement.

MULTIPLE VALVE REPLACEMENT

When multiple valve replacement is necessary, the technique does not vary significantly from that used for replacement of individual valves. However, some planning is necessary to ensure the shortest ischemic interval. A convenient technique involves initial excision of the aortic valve followed by excision and replacement of the mitral valve, followed by replacement of the aortic valve, reconstitution of the ascending aorta, and restoration of myocardial blood flow. It is usually inconvenient or even unwise to replace the aortic valve before completing the mitral valve replacement because the torsion of the base of the heart necessary to obtain mitral valve exposure may cause tearing if a rigid prosthetic device is placed in the subcoronary aortic position before completion of mitral valve replacement. The tricuspid valve may be conveniently replaced after blood flow is restored to the heart in the presence of a competent aortic valve prosthesis. During replacement of the tricuspid valve, rewarming may be completed and the beating heart allowed to recover from an interval of ischemic cardioplegic arrest.

BACTERIAL ENDOCARDITIS

Bacterial endocarditis was an incurable disease with a uniformly fatal issue until the advent of antibiotic therapy. Since 1943, when the first report of cure using penicillin was reported, a large number of patients have been successfully treated, usually by prolonged administration of intravenous antibiotics. More recently, and particularly within the past 5 to 10 years, it has become recognized that surgical resection of cardiac valves involved with active bacterial infection followed by prosthetic replacement may result in a cure of the infection otherwise unobtainable even with intensive antibiotic therapy.

Bacterial endocarditis may be acute or subacute. Although the clinical course of acute or subacute bacterial endocarditis may be more rapid or somewhat slower, respectively, the principal differentiation is made by the infecting organism. Endocarditis caused by *Staphylococcus aureus*, *Streptococcus pyogenes*, *Haemophilus influenzae*, and *Neisseria gonorrheae* are usually considered acute infections. When α-hemolytic streptococci or *Staphylococcus epidermidis* are the causative agents, the infection is considered subacute. Whether acute or subacute, untreated bacterial endocarditis results in a massive destruction of the valve leaflets and may cause burrowing abscesses within the myocardium and dissolution of the fibrous skeleton of the heart. Embolization of septic particles may cause widespread abscess formation, which is especially serious in the central nervous system. Patients are seriously ill and appear so. Fever is universal, and the toxic effects of bacteremia and septicemia are usually readily apparent. Blood cultures in the absence of preliminary antibiotic therapy are nearly always positive. Patients with valves damaged by congenital anomalies or by preceding rheumatic fever or other cause are particularly susceptible to bacterial infection, as are patients with prosthetic valves. An episode of bacteremia results in the seeding of bacteria on a valve, and infection proceeds. Such an event may or may not be definable in a patient's history. The most common cause of bacteremia resulting in endocarditis is probably dental manipulation, which may be as mundane as daily toothbrushing. Other accidental or surgical trauma may also be responsible, as may the occurrence of casual infections elsewhere in the body. Bacteremia has been observed after colonic manipulation such as that used in barium enema examination or sigmoidoscopy.

Chemotherapy with antibiotics selected specifically to combat the infecting organism is always the first line of therapy. Patients who fail to respond to specific antibiotic therapy for a week or more, or patients exhibiting hemodynamic deterioration despite otherwise successful antibiotic chemotherapy, should be considered candidates for urgent valve replacement surgery. Progressive hemodynamic deterioration in a patient with active bacterial endocarditis indicates approaching mortality without valve replacement. The risk for aortic or mitral valve replacement in the presence of active endocarditis is higher than that for elective valve replacement and may approach 20%. This risk is the product of several variables, including the extent of destruction of the valve annulus, the presence or absence of intramyocardial abscesses, the presence of other foci of sepsis, and the degree of devastation produced by previous embolic episodes, particularly those involving the brain. Early endocarditis is often confined entirely to the resectable portion of the valve leaflets, and total surgical cure is readily achievable in such patients. The usual practice in most centers includes utilization of organism-specific antibiotic therapy during the course of operation and for 3 to 6 weeks following surgery. Recurrence or persistence of bacterial infection in patients so treated is remarkably uncommon.

RISKS AND COMPLICATIONS OF CARDIAC VALVE SURGERY

Mortality risks for patients undergoing cardiac valve replacement are shown in Table 40-3. These are necesssarily approximate but fairly accurately portray the results to be expected in good surgical hands. Patients with severe disability have a somewhat higher risk for every operation, principally because the additional disability is usually related to myocardial dysfunction superimposed on abnormalities of valve function. Although valvular adequacy is instantaneously improved by surgery, myocardial dysfunction recovers much more slowly and sometimes not at all. Also there is the possibility that some degree of additional myocardial dysfunction may be experienced during the first several days after operation. If patients do not have sufficient reserve to withstand the operative trauma, they will not survive. It is, therefore, important that operative intervention not be delayed until myocardial dysfunction is so severe that the probability of surgical survival and eventual rehabilitation is compromised severely.

Patients surviving operation must contend with a variety of possible complications following cardiac valve replacement. Albert Starr has observed that the operation of valve replacement consists in exchanging one disease for another.

TABLE 40-3 REPRESENTATIVE OPERATIVE RISKS IN CARDIAC VALVE SURGERY

	CLASS I–III (%)	CLASS IV (%)
AVR	2 to 5	5 to 15
MVR	3 to 6	10 to 20
AVR and MVR	5 to 8	10 to 20
MVR and TVR	5 to 15	15 to 25
AVR, MVR, TVR	5 to 15	20 or more

(AVR, aortic valve replacement; MVR, mitral valve replacement; TVR, tricuspid valve replacement)

It is certainly true that the presence of an artificial valve constitutes a significant cardiac abnormality even when that valve is functioning properly. The criteria by which proper function of a prosthetic or bioprosthetic valve must be judged include mechanical performance, thrombogenicity, and durability. The mechanical performance of a valve is judged by its ability to allow flow of blood in the open phase without pressure drop or undue turbulence. The ideal valve should be nonthrombogenic even without utilization of anticoagulant drugs. Some of the tissue valves, particularly in the aortic position, come close to this ideal performance, but at present all replacement devices have a higher thrombogenic potential than normal valves. In the atrioventricular positions there is a greater hazard of thrombotic or embolic events than there is in the aortic position. Durability, or resistance to degeneration as a result of wear and tear, is a significant consideration in all replacement valves. Normal living valves are constructed primarily of collagen but have sufficient living tissue that replacement and repair of the collagen takes place continuously. Such characteristics do not exist in any replacement valves available. The valve begins to wear immediately after implantation, and the length of satisfactory service expected from such a device varies according to the rapidity of deterioration. Advances in production of biomaterials has resulted in the availability of prosthetic cardiac valves with a very low potential for wear. Tissue valves, on the other hand, probably deteriorate somewhat more rapidly. Factors contributing to premature deterioration of biologic valves include uncertainties in the process of fixation and unequal distribution of stress as a result of imperfections in fixation of tissue to the stent and alterations in stent flexibility.

Possible valve-related complications following cardiac valve replacement include hemodynamic inadequacy, thromboembolism, mechanical wear, hemolysis, perivalvular leak, and infection. *Hemodynamic inadequacy* may result from selection of too large or too small a valve, alteration of valve function by entanglement in some other intracardiac structure, or deposition of clot or incursion of tissue after implantation. All replacement valves must be considered subject to deposition of platelet thrombi as well as other forms of blood clot. The utilization of anticoagulant drugs to reduce the *thromboembolic potential*, particularly of purely prosthetic devices, is commonly employed but is used less often than it once was. *Mechanical wear and tear* occurs in all devices but as mentioned, appears most serious in bioprosthetic valves. Some degree of *hemolysis* occurs with virtually all replacement valves. The mechanical or purely prosthetic valves have a higher potential for hemolysis than tissue valves. The extent of hemolysis in the absence of

perivalvular leak appears to be a linear function of the exposed valvular surface. Patients with a single valve replacement thus have a lower level of hemolysis than those with two valves, and patients with triple valve replacement have the highest levels of hemolysis. *Perivalvular leak* often produces sufficient turbulence to damage red cells, and rapid serious hemolysis may be observed in some of these patients. An additional risk of perivalvular leak is the occurrence of congestive heart failure, which at times may appear disproportionate to the degree of observable leak. This is a common phenomenon, and the surgeon would be unwise to rely upon an angiographic estimate of mild insufficiency in these patients if they are symptomatic. All prosthetic and bioprosthetic valves represent an increased hazard for *bacterial endocarditis*. These patients should have prophylactic antibiotic therapy at times of invasive manipulation, particularly when that manipulation may involve contaminated structures.

RESULTS OF VALVULAR SURGERY

Patients who have recovered from cardiac valve replacement surgery may resume a normal and functional life or, in some instances, may continue with some residual disability. Prognosis for life expectancy is closely related to the extent of left ventricular dysfunction at the time of valve surgery, the nature of the valvular abnormality (whether stenosis or insufficiency and whether caused by rheumatic heart disease, endocarditis, or coronary heart disease), and the adequacy of the valve replacement device. Representative actuarial survival curves are shown in Figures 40-9, 40-10, and 40-11 for patients with aortic valve replacement, mitral valve replacement, and multiple valve replacement, respectively. Patients with normal heart size and normal sinus rhythm have a remarkably better prognosis than do patients with cardiac enlargement and atrial fibrillation. In general, patients with distention of ventricular cavities as a result of long-standing cardiac failure also have a compromised prognosis compared with those with a more normal size and shape of the left ventricular cavity at the time of operation. Although there is considerable variation among reported surgical results, there is no question that the prognosis for longevity following valve replacement surgery vastly exceeds what could be expected if such surgery were not available.

THE CORONARY ARTERIES AND VEINS

A diagrammatic representation of the coronary vascular system is seen in Figure 40-12. There are normally two coronary arteries, the left arising from the left posterior sinus of Valsalva and the right arising from the anterior sinus of Valsalva. The left coronary artery branches after a few millimeters to 2 cm and travels behind the pulmonary artery into the anterior descending and circumflex branches. By convention, disease of the coronary arteries, particularly atherosclerotic obstructive disease, has been referred to as one-vessel, two-vessel, or three-vessel disease, considering the right, anterior descending, and circumflex arteries as the principal coronary arterial circulation. The right coronary artery travels in the atrioventricular groove around the acute margin of the heart on its right lateral aspect to the area of the junction of the right and left ventricles with the atrioventricular groove. This area of the heart is called the crux.

(Text continues on page 1070)

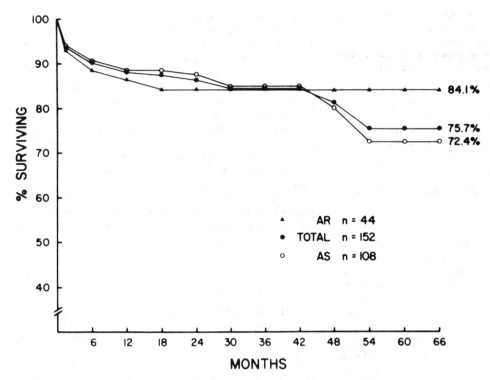

Fig. 40-9. Actuarial survival, including operative mortality, after aortic valve replacement using a porcine bioprosthesis. AR = aortic regurgitation; AS = aortic stenosis. (Cohn LH, Mudge G: Five to eight-year follow-up of patients undergoing porcine bioprosthetic valve replacement. N Engl J Med 304:258, 1981)

Fig. 40-10. Actuarial survival following replacement of mitral valve with porcine bioprosthetic valve in patients with mitral stenosis and mitral insufficiency. MR = mitral regurgitation; MS = mitral stenosis. (Cohn LH, Mudge G: Five to eight-year follow-up of patients undergoing porcine bioprosthetic valve replacement. N Engl J Med 304:258, 1981)

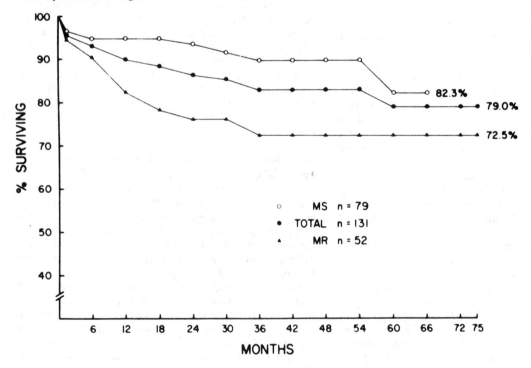

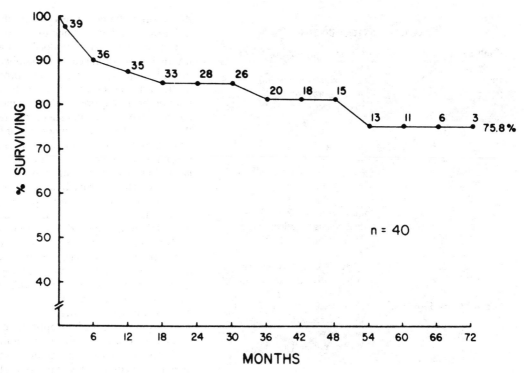

Fig. 40-11. Actuarial survival following multiple valve replacement with porcine valves. (Cohn LH, Mudge G: Five to eight-year follow-up of patients undergoing porcine bioprosthetic valve replacement. N Engl J Med 304:258, 1981)

Fig. 40-12. Anterior view of the coronary arterial circulation. (Edwards EA, Malone PD, Collins JJ Jr: Operative Anatomy of the Thorax. Philadelphia, Lea & Febiger, 1972)

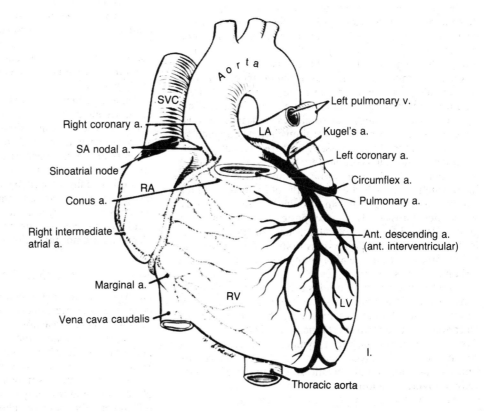

CORONARY ARTERY DISEASE	
Etiology	Atherosclerosis, trauma, arteritis
Dx	Angina pectoris, congestive heart failure, arrhythmia EKG: Evidence of ischemia vs infarct Echocardiography: Left ventricular function Stress testing Angiography: Presence of significant lesions
Rx	*Medical:* Beta blockade, calcium antagonists, vasodilators, balloon dilatation of stenotic proximal lesions *Surgical:* Reverse saphenous vein coronary revascularization
Special Considerations	Early revascularization of "left main" disease or equivalent, management of postinfarction VSD and aneurysm

In approximately 60% of patients, the right coronary artery makes an abrupt turn at the crux and continues downward in the posterior interventricular groove as the posterior descending coronary artery. This is called a right dominant circulatory pattern. A left dominant pattern occurs when the circumflex coronary supplies the posterior descending artery. When both the distal right coronary and the circumflex supply branches to the area of the posterior interventricular sulcus, the result is said to be a "balanced" circulation. The extent of distribution of the circumflex and distal right coronary arteries is of surgical significance because quite extensive areas of myocardium may be supplied by one or the other of these vessels. In these cases of "superdominant" right or left coronary arteries, loss of one posterior artery may be a fatal event. The venous circulation of the heart roughly parallels the arterial distribution with a final pathway into the right atrium through the coronary sinus, which lies transversely in the posterior atrioventricular groove. There is a series of valves, more or less complete, in the coronary sinus. Some veins from the atrioventricular groove area and from the atria empty directly into the right atrium as thebesian veins.

Both the arteries and the veins generally lie immediately beneath the epicardium. In some instances, the principal coronary arterial branches may lie rather deeply in the epicardial fat or beneath substantial bridges of myocardium. Occasional patients may have symptoms of coronary obstruction caused by myocardial bridges. Such instances are unusual, but occasional operations are performed specifically to divide such muscular bundles.

TRAUMA TO THE CORONARY VASCULATURE

Traumatic injuries to the arteries and veins supplying the myocardium are uncommon. Blunt trauma may result in myocardial infarction with thrombosis of the anterior descending coronary artery. This is a rare event. Rupture of the coronary blood vessels due to blunt trauma is virtually unknown, but hemorrhage from laceration of the coronary arteries or veins may often occur in association with penetrating injuries of the cardiac chambers due to knife wounds or bullet injuries. Injury to the coronary arterial system is particularly hazardous because the resultant hemorrhage may be brisk, causing cardiac tamponade, and emergency ligation, even if accomplished, may result in distal ischemia that causes significant myocardial infarction. The coronary veins may be safely ligated in virtually all areas except the coronary sinus near its entry into the right atrium. Traumatic laceration of large coronary arterial vessels is best treated by immediate coronary bypass if possible.

Trauma to the coronary arteries may occur during the performance of coronary angiography. Precautions are always taken to inject dye at relatively low velocity and pressure into the coronary ostia, but accidents may still occur in diseased vessels. The most common manifestation of coronary arterial trauma from angiography is dissecting hematoma. For some reason, this seems to occur more commonly in the right than in the left coronary artery. The usual sequence of events following dissection of the right coronary is the immediate appearance of a current of injury in the electrocardiographic monitor indicating inferior myocardial ischemia. In most instances, ischemic changes regress over a period of minutes or hours, and myocardial infarction may not occur. In some instances, the injury will be followed by inferior myocardial infarction. If the injury occurs in the presence of a superdominant right coronary not previously severely obstructed, a very large posterior myocardial infarction with possible fatal outcome may be expected, and immediate emergency coronary bypass surgery is indicated. If the injury occurs in a previously tightly obstructed coronary artery, the probability of significant additional distal myocardial ischemia is small, and the patient may be safely watched.

Dissecting hematomas of the coronary arteries may also occur secondary to a dissecting aneurysm of the ascending aorta. Most commonly, these dissections also involve the right coronary artery, and therefore one may expect to see patients in the coronary care unit from time to time with an electrocardiographic pattern of inferior myocardial infarction actually caused by unsuspected ascending aortic dissection. This possibility must be kept in mind when a patient's history suggests aortic dissection but the electrocardiogram suggests acute myocardial infarction. These two diagnoses are not mutually exclusive.

INFLAMMATORY DISEASE OF THE CORONARY ARTERIES

The coronary arteries are subject to damage by vasculitis occurring in a variety of disease states, including the collagen diseases, allergic reaction to certain drugs, and radiation injury. It is estimated that 50% to 60% of patients with periarteritis nodosa have significant coronary arterial lesions. Lesions of an inflammatory nature are surgically germane because these patients may also have local coronary artery obstruction, and coronary bypass surgery is technically more difficult and the prognosis perhaps less optimistic in patients with such lesions. They are, fortunately, rare.

DEGENERATIVE DISEASES OF THE CORONARY ARTERIES

Atherosclerotic obstruction of the coronary arteries constitutes the most common surgically significant abnormality of the coronary circulation. Indeed, coronary obstructive disease is the most common cause of death in adults living in developed countries. Surgical operations for the relief of ischemia resulting from atherosclerotic obstructions of the coronary arteries began in 1935 with the work of Claude Beck, who advocated pericardial irritation to improve collateral blood supply. Several operative procedures designed to enhance the probability of development of significant collateral channels between the parietal pericardium and the native coronary arterial circulation were developed subsequently. Pericardial poudrage using talc was one of these operations. In 1946, Vineberg reported the production of significant collateral blood flow between an internal mammary artery pedicle introduced into the myocardium and native branches of the coronary arterial system. This work became the focus of much controversy. Saphenous vein bypass surgery was introduced by Favaloro and his associates in 1969. This new technique of direct revascularization of the native coronary arterial circulation quickly swept mammary implantation into the background and became itself the focus of widespread argument.

At present it is generally agreed that persons with angina pectoris who have significant (greater than 50% luminal area) obstruction of the main left coronary artery or significant proximal obstruction of the three major coronary arterial branches are likely to live longer with surgery than without. The vast number of other combinations of symptoms, extents of arterial obstruction, and left ventricular dysfunction are not clearly defined. An additional perturbing factor is the frequent introduction into clinical practice of new medications that promise to improve medical management results. As a result of this continually changing mix of variables, careful tabulation of clinical results and comparison of various modes of therapy remain important and useful.

EVALUATION AND SELECTION OF PATIENTS FOR CORONARY BYPASS SURGERY

Principal indications for direct coronary artery revascularization are shown in Table 40-4. Hemodynamically significant obstruction of the main left coronary artery, proximal branches of all three major coronary arterial divisions, and proximal obstruction of the anterior descending and dominant posterior coronary artery are generally accepted throughout the cardiologic community as indications for prompt revascularization in the presence of angina pectoris. Whether the prognosis of coronary obstructive disease is different in persons with no significant angina pectoris and whether noninvasive studies such as stress electrocardiography and radionuclide scans may serve to identify groups in which the hazard of infarction or death is particularly great remain to be seen.

Preoperative evaluation of patients with chronic stable angina pectoris usually includes stress electrocardiography. If the angina pectoris has been present for more than 1 year, is stable, and the stress test produces no significant electrocardiographic abnormality when criteria for significant exertion are met, most cardiologists favor medical management. If angina pectoris is unstable or progressive or intractable to medical management, stress electrocardiography has a more limited role, and many cardiologists would recommend direct progression to coronary angiography as a prelude to revascularization surgery if left main,

TABLE 40-4   INDICATIONS FOR CORONARY BYPASS SURGERY

GENERALLY AGREED

Intractable angina pectoris
Main left coronary obstruction with angina
Proximal three-vessel obstruction with angina
Left main "equivalent" states
Intermittent severe LV dysfunction

SOMEWHAT CONTROVERSIAL

Two-vessel obstruction including LAD with angina
Proximal partial obstruction of superdominant posterior artery
Proximal obstructions accompanying significant valve disease
Unstable angina syndromes

VERY CONTROVERSIAL

Asymptomatic two- or three-vessel obstruction with positive exercise test
Asymptomatic patients after myocardial infarction
Acute myocardial infarction

three-vessel, or significant two-vessel obstruction is found. Single-vessel obstruction is usually not considered an adequate threat to justify revascularization surgery. There are exceptions, however. Significant partial obstruction of a superdominant posterior coronary artery or of the anterior coronary artery proximal to any branching is regarded as an ominous finding by most cardiologists and cardiac surgeons. A totally obstructed coronary artery probably represents less hazard for myocardial infarction and death than a partially obstructed vessel. Data to support this, however, are sadly lacking. In fact, data to document the prognosis in both medically and surgically managed patients with significant coronary obstructive disease are difficult to interpret because most series use the simple classification of left main, three-vessel, two-vessel, or one-vessel obstruction without specifying whether the obstructions are all proximal or may perhaps occur in distal branches. There is a considerable difference, for example, in the prognostic significance of three proximal obstructions as opposed to three lesions in small distal branches of the same arteries. The present classification system does not differentiate this.

CORONARY BYPASS: SURGICAL TECHNIQUE

Coronary bypass surgery requires expert anesthesia delivered by experienced cardiac anesthesiologists. Careful selection of anesthetic technique and judicious utilization of intravenous drugs are requisite.

The heart is approached through a median sternotomy incision. The saphenous vein is harvested gently and carefully and irrigated with heparinized blood or saline solution.

There are various techniques of anastomosis of saphenous vein segments to the coronary arteries. The vein may be attached to the recipient artery by an end-to-side or side-to-side anastomosis. The anastomosis may be performed with continuous or interrupted sutures. Exaggerated differ-

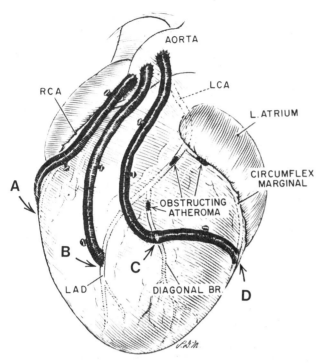

Fig. 40-13. A combination of end-to-side and side-to-side anastomoses provides capability for extensive revascularization for diffuse coronary obstructive disease. (Cohn LH [ed]: The Treatment of Acute Myocardial Ischemia: An Integrated Medical/Surgical Approach. Mt. Kisco, Futura Publishers, 1979)

ences between the internal diameter of the vein and that of the recipient artery are to be avoided if possible. All anastomoses should be performed with great care under direct vision to ensure that a minimal number of sutures are placed carefully and symmetrically. Care must be taken to place the anastomosis distal to significant obstructive lesions in the recipient coronary artery. A second or third anastomosis may be necessary in some large vessels with multiple obstructions. Possible configurations of multiple anastomoses are shown in Figure 40-13. The proximal anastomosis of vein grafts is as important and as technically demanding as the distal. The majority of surgeons favor anastomosis to the ascending aorta after completion of distal anastomoses. It is important that the ascending aortic wall not be damaged during the application of clamps to achieve hemostasis or by the suturing technique. The vein graft should lie loosely but not redundantly on the surface of the heart at the completion of all anastomoses. Too short a graft produces tension in the vein with narrowing and allows no provision for elongation of the graft if cardiac dilatation occurs in the immediate postoperative period. Too long a vein graft may result in kinking.

Other conduits have been used for direct coronary revascularization in addition to vein grafts. The most common is the left internal mammary artery. The internal mammary artery may be mobilized by careful dissection from its usual position lateral to the sternum. Using microsurgical technique, the left internal mammary artery may be conveniently anastomosed to the anterior descending coronary artery, diagonal branches of the anterior descending, or marginal branches of the circumflex coronary artery. Initial experience suggested that the patency rate at 1 year after surgery of internal mammary artery anastomoses

approached 95%, whereas that of saphenous vein to coronary artery anastomosis was closer to 85%. Improvements in technique have probably narrowed this difference. Disadvantages of the internal mammary graft technique include the following: (1) it adds 30 to 60 minutes to operation time; (2) a saphenous vein must also be harvested for additional grafts in multivessel obstruction; and (3) in many instances, the maximum available blood flow through the internal mammary artery is less than could be obtained through the usual saphenous vein.

RESULTS OF CORONARY ARTERY REVASCULARIZATION SURGERY

The risk of mortality in coronary revascularization surgery depends primarily upon the adequacy of coronary arteries beyond the obstruction, the integrity of left ventricular contractile function, and the absence of other severe systemic illnesses. Age and the absolute number of proximal coronary obstructions are not as significant. In most centers, patients with stable angina pectoris can be operated upon with an expected surgical mortality of about 1%. The presence of unstable angina pectoris raises the operative mortality somewhat because there is an increased risk in these patients of perioperative myocardial infarction. The most hazardous combination appears to be the presence of both unstable angina pectoris and significant left main coronary artery obstruction. Patients with very recent preoperative myocardial infarction, acute evolving myocardial infarction, cardiogenic shock, and congestive heart failure and those requiring additional surgical manipulation have a higher risk. Approximate risks in patients requiring coronary bypass surgery are shown in Table 40-5. Figures 40-14 through 40-16 show actuarial tables depicting the probability of longevity, occurrence of myocardial infarction, and recurrence of angina pectoris in patients operated upon at the Peter Bent Brigham Hospital from July, 1970 through June, 1978. The longevity data are similar to those reported from other major institutions in the recent past. Few data have been published to document the expected rate of occurrence of myocardial infarction after revascularization surgery. The data on recurrence of angina pectoris are somewhat less optimistic than those occasionally reported. Documentation of recurrent angina after coronary bypass surgery may be difficult in some patients. In the data depicted in Figure 40-16, all patients with chest pain syndromes are included whether typical or not for angina pectoris. These data, therefore, represent the "worst possible case" technique of reporting.

TABLE 40-5 OPERATIVE RISK IN CORONARY BYPASS SURGERY

	STABLE (%)	UNSTABLE (%)
CABG (good LV function)	0.5–1	1–2
CABG (poor LV function)	2–5	3–10
CABG + valve	5–10	10–50
CABG + aneurysm	2–10	5–50
Evolving myocardial infarction	2–5	5–25
Cardiogenic shock		20–60

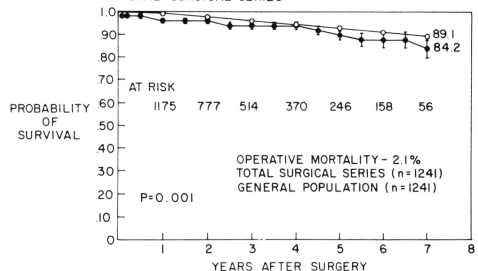

Fig. 40-14. Probability of survival (including operative mortality) in 1241 patients followed up to 7 years after coronary bypass surgery at Peter Bent Brigham Hospital, Boston.

Fig. 40-15. Probability of occurrence of myocardial infarction was less than 20%, including 2% perioperative infarction rate, up to 7 years after coronary bypass surgery.

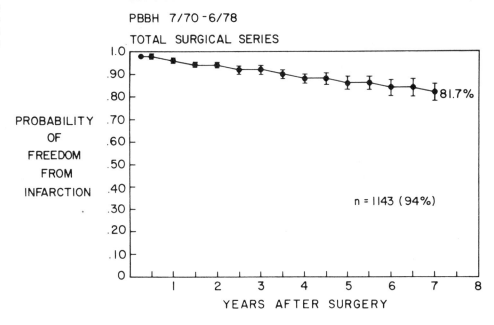

SURGERY FOR COMPLICATIONS OF MYOCARDIAL INFARCTION

Cardiac complications of surgical interest following myocardial infarction include ischemic power failure, myocardial disruption, electrophysiological instability, and late scarring. These abnormalities produce a clinical picture predominantly of either congestive heart failure or arrhythmias.

Ischemic left ventricular power failure may occur very early after acute coronary occlusion when 30% to 40% or more of the ventricular myocardium has insufficient blood supply. The earliest mechanical derangement of the myocardium is loss of diastolic compliance followed by loss of capability for systolic power generation. Extensive functional derangement of myocardial fibers results in cardiogenic shock. Possible therapeutic approaches to patients with cardiogenic shock due to left ventricular power failure include balloon counterpulsation to reduce left ventricular oxygen consumption and increased diastolic coronary perfusion pressure and emergency revascularization to restore adequate myocardial blood flow. Early excision of acute myocardial infarcts has proved hemodynamically beneficial in laboratory animals but has not been widely utilized clinically.

Many coronary care units utilize a protocol to assist in decision-making for patients with extensive early myocardial infarction and threatened or present left ventricular power failure. A typical schematic is shown in Figure 40-17. If

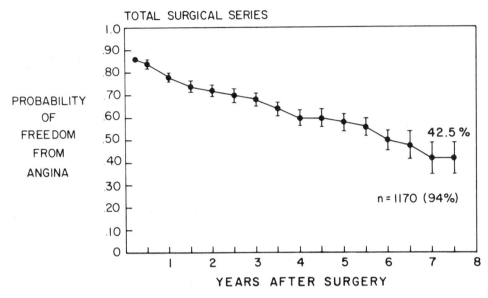

CORONARY BYPASS SURGERY

PBBH 7/70 - 6/78

TOTAL SURGICAL SERIES

PROBABILITY OF FREEDOM FROM ANGINA

42.5%

n = 1170 (94%)

YEARS AFTER SURGERY

Fig. 40-16. Recurrence rate of angina pectoris (or any repetitive chest discomfort) up to 7.5 years after coronary bypass surgery.

restoration of intravascular volumes does not adequately restore systemic perfusion pressure, mechanical circulatory assistance is indicated. Most commonly, this involves the utilization of intra-aortic balloon counterpulsation. A typical intra-aortic balloon is shown in Figure 40-18. Early expectations that the mortality of left ventricular power failure with cardiogenic shock might be reduced from the 90% or more common with pharmacologic management alone were soon dashed. A few patients survived who probably would not have otherwise, but it became evident that balloon counterpulsation provided primarily a temporary means for

left ventricular support. The addition of myocardial revascularization for patients with left ventricular power failure was an additional but not dramatic improvement. Despite advances in hemodynamic monitoring, new inotropic drugs, and mechanical circulatory assistance, the mortality for patients in shock with massive established myocardial infarction still exceeds 75%. Clinical experimentation with early revascularization (within 6 hours) of patients with electrocardiographic evidence of evolving myocardial infarction has been undertaken by a few groups. The experience of Berg and associates, confirmed by several later studies, showed that patients with "evolving acute myocardial infarction" who were operated upon within a few hours after the onset of symptoms had a mortality of only about 5%. Many of these patients did not ultimately show

Fig. 40-17. Decision-making protocol for acute myocardial infarction.

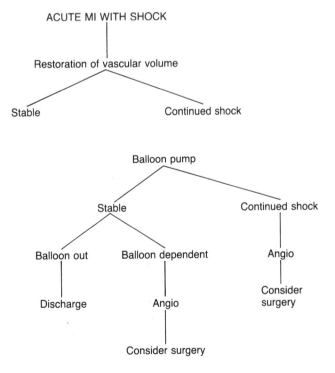

ACUTE MI WITH SHOCK

Restoration of vascular volume

Stable — Continued shock

Balloon pump

Stable — Continued shock

Balloon out — Balloon dependent — Angio

Discharge — Angio — Consider surgery

Consider surgery

Fig. 40-18. Schematic drawing of intra-aortic counterpulsation balloon in the descending aorta.

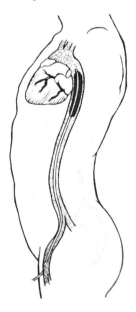

electrocardiographic or enzyme evidence of myocardial necrosis. This experience cannot be directly applied to the management of patients with early established myocardial infarction, but it certainly suggests that revascularization with coronary reperfusion prior to the onset of irreversible necrosis in patients with widely distributed myocardial ischemia may be both theoretically and practically advantageous.

MYOCARDIAL DISRUPTION FOLLOWING INFARCTION: DIAGNOSIS AND MANAGEMENT

Areas of myocardium weakened by infarction are subject to rupture. There are three relatively separate syndromes of surgical importance.

1. Rupture of the free wall of the left ventricle may produce instantaneous tamponade and death. Although it might seem that this is a simplistic statement of a foregone conclusion, several factors may alter the circumstances. Rupture always occurs following transmural myocardial infarction. In the presence of transmural infarction, virtually all patients develop pericarditis over the site of the infarction, and there may be relatively well developed fibrinous adhesion of the epicardium to the parietal pericardium in the area of infarction. When rupture occurs, bleeding may not always be rapid. The typical clinical syndrome suggesting external myocardial rupture includes the presence of transmural myocardial infarction with a friction rub followed by sudden development of hypotension with signs of tamponade progressing to electromechanical dissociation. The time between the onset of hypotension and the development of electromechanical dissociation may vary from a few moments to several hours. Patients exhibiting this complex of clinical events should be removed immediately to the operating room without hesitating for more sophisticated diagnostic tests if surgical repair is to be accomplished.

2. Transmural infarction of the interventricular septum may be complicated by septal rupture. Although not as rapidly fatal in most instances as rupture of the free left ventricular wall, septal rupture has a very high eventual mortality. The site of rupture may be anterior or posterior, high or low. The clinical setting includes presence of transmural myocardial infarction involving the interventricular septum and sudden hemodynamic deterioration accompanied by the development of a loud systolic murmur. The diagnosis is confirmed by observing a step-up in oxygen saturation at the right ventricular or pulmonary arterial level. This can be ascertained at the bedside by the passage of a balloon tip catheter into the pulmonary artery with appropriate sampling. Hemodynamic deterioration of patients with septal rupture may be sudden and irretrievable or gradual with time available for accurate diagnosis. Patients who show early deterioration should be operated upon with the intent of closing the ventricular septal defect and revascularizing threatened but not infarcted areas of myocardium. A coronary arteriogram is very helpful in these persons but in extreme emergencies should not be regarded as essential. Because of the surrounding necrotic myocardium, the closure of acute ventricular septal defects is more difficult technically than the closure of congenital septal defects. A useful technique, shown in Figure 40-19, utilizes the apposition of two layers of patch material in order to place the least possible strain on the suture line. Even with the most careful technique, recurrence of such defects in survivors is not uncommon. When ventricular septal rupture occurs near the cardiac apex, the apex may be simply amputated and both the right and left ventricles repaired. This technique, while not frequently applicable, may be very successful. Septal defects occurring toward the base of the heart or those involving a large portion of the interventricular septum have a very high surgical mortality.

3. Papillary muscle rupture most frequently involves the posterior papillary muscle. Rupture may occur without transmural myocardial infarction. The characteristic clinical syndrome includes the presence of a posterior or inferior acute myocardial infarction (which may be subendocardial) followed in 3 to 10 days by development of a systolic murmur and often by impairment of forward cardiac output and development of congestive heart failure. The diagnosis may be established directly by the use of bedside echocardiography, which will usually show extensive prolapse of the mitral valve and may actually depict a ruptured portion of papillary muscle tip prolapsing into the left atrium. The diagnosis may also be made by exclusion if sampling of blood from the

Fig. 40-19. A useful technique for patch closure of postinfarction ventricular septal defect. (Cohn LH [ed]: The Treatment of Acute Myocardial Ischemia: An Integrated Medical/Surgical Approach. Mt. Kisco, Futura Publishing, 1979)

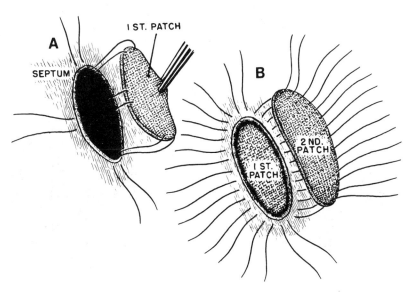

right ventricle and pulmonary artery fails to show a step-up in oxygen saturation in the presence of sudden development of new systolic murmur.

The clinical course may be one of rapid deterioration, or clinical stabilization may occur with later progressive congestive heart failure. Early emergency or later elective mitral valve replacement is usually required for rehabilitation. Longevity following mitral valve replacement is substantially impaired in these patients compared with patients undergoing mitral valve replacement for rheumatic abnormalities. Revascularization surgery, when indicated, should accompany mitral valve replacement whether early or late.

VENTRICULAR ANEURYSM

After myocardial infarction there will be a residual scar that is often recognizable in the left ventricular angiogram as an area of akinesis (no motion) or dyskinesis (abnormal motion with systolic expansion). When large enough, such an area may be called an aneurysm. In the aneurysm, myocardial fibers may be entirely absent or separated by means of fibrotic scar. When myocardium is absent, the scar often becomes progressively thinned, and the area stretches to dampen more and more the force of left ventricular con-

traction. Such aneurysms rarely rupture but commonly produce congestive heart failure that becomes worse with time even without new infarctions. In some patients, significant ventricular arrhythmias may originate in the border zone between scar and functional myocardium. Most aneurysms have some clot on the endocardial surface, and systemic embolization may occur.

Indications for surgery for ventricular aneurysm are primarily progressive heart failure and poorly controlled arrhythmias. Systemic embolization, in the absence of other complications, can usually be controlled by anticoagulation. Additionally, aneurysmectomy does not confer total protection against subsequent embolization. Heart failure is rarely a significant problem unless the aneurysm is large. Small stable areas of scar need not be resected.

The technique of aneurysm resection varies according to whether the principal indication is heart failure or arrhythmia. For management of heart failure, it is sufficient to resect the major portion of the scar, leaving a rim of about 1 cm of scar to be everted in the closure as shown in Figure 40-20. Although some patients with arrhythmias may benefit from simple aneurysm resection, many may show little or no improvement. Using a computerized electrographic analysis system, it is possible to define accurately the focus of origin of repetitive tachycardias in most patients by

Fig. 40-20. Technique for resection of ventricular aneurysm. (Cohn LH [ed]: The Treatment of Acute Myocardial Ischemia: An Integrated Medical/Surgical Approach, Mt. Kisco, Futura Publishing, 1979)

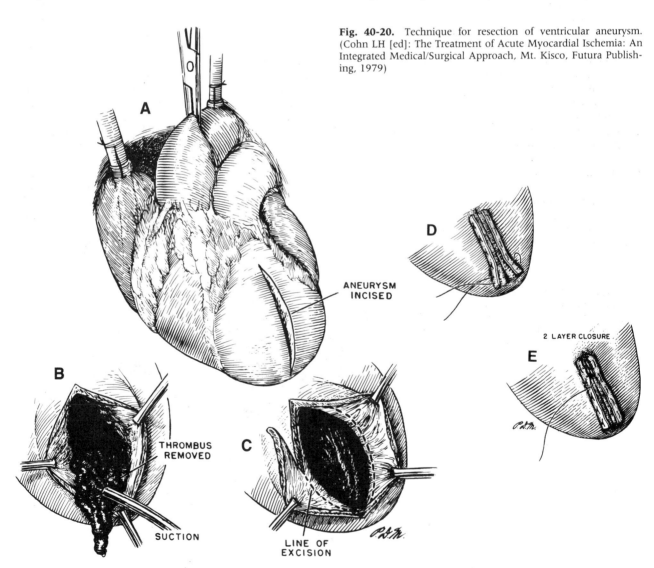

intraoperative epicardial and subendocardial mapping. Specific ablation of the area of origin seems to be much more effective in relieving attacks of ventricular tachycardia. An approach intermediate between blind aneurysmectomy and endoepicardial mapping is that of encircling endomyocardial incision as suggested by Guiradon. In this operation, a deep endomyocardial incision is made between the area of visible endocardial sclerosis and the surrounding viable myocardium and is carried around the entire circumference of the ventricular cavity. Endocardial scarring is often much more extensive than transmural damage, and the Guiradon operation may isolate a very large portion of the left ventricle. Complications include worsened left ventricular dysfunction and false aneurysms of the ventricular wall.

Late results of mapping with endocardial ablation seem favorable, but the technique is still relatively new. Rehabilitation after resection of left ventricular aneurysm for congestive heart failure depends upon the vigor of residual contractile function and the avoidance of further infarction. Compromised blood supply to functioning myocardium should be corrected when possible by coronary bypass. Five-year survival ranges from about 50% in patients with extensive coronary artery obstruction to nearly 90% in those having an intact blood supply to residual muscle. The influence of coronary bypass has been favorable in some reports and inconsequential in others. The apparent lack of influence in some studies of revascularization is probably more a reflection of the classification of patients than of the ineffectiveness of revascularization.

POSTOPERATIVE CARE

Patients who have had cardiac surgical operations should be removed from the operating room to a specialized intensive care area with highly trained personnel. Certain physiological variables should be monitored continuously while others need to be measured only intermittently. The organ systems most critical to recovery include the cardiovascular system, respiratory system, and kidneys. The great majority of patients following operations for acquired heart disease should recover without difficulty provided homeostasis is maintained.

Adequate and safe respiratory function may be provided by controlled respiration for a number of hours following surgery. Many cardiac surgical units provide controlled respiration for all patients who undergo cardiopulmonary bypass, whereas in other units patients are awakened more quickly and extubated even in the operating room.

Maintenance of adequate cardiac output is probably the single most critical requirement for early postoperative care. Direct measurement of the cardiac output using thermodilution techniques is both simple and accurate. Criteria indicating that the cardiac output is satisfactory for a smooth postoperative course without actually providing a numerical value include (1) mean arterial pressure above 70 mmHg, (2) urine output of 25 ml or more per hour, (3) extremities warm and dry with easily palpable pulses, and (4) mental alertness.

Limitation of cardiac output may occur owing to a failure of either the right or the left ventricle. The earliest measurable sign of ventricular failure is a rise in filling pressure. When both atrial pressures are measured, the ventricle that determines the maximum available cardiac output is identified as the one having the higher filling pressure. All efforts to improve the cardiac output should be directed toward

improving the performance of the less effective ventricle, which may be called the "critical" ventricle.

The determinants of cardiac output include the heart rate and end-diastolic fiber length, contractile state, and output resistance of the critical ventricle. The only available means for altering the cardiac output is alteration of one or more of these factors.

For most patients an optimal heart rate is between 70 and 110 beats per minute. If the rate is slower, a pacemaker may be used. If the rate is too rapid, medication or possibly countershock may be used. End-diastolic fiber length in either ventricle may be most readily altered by changing the intravascular blood volume with transfusion. The contractile state of the myocardium may be altered by the administration of inotropic drugs. Side-effects, including an increase in the cardiac rate or the occurrence of arrhythmias, must be kept in mind.

A useful therapeutic adjunct may be to decrease ventricular output resistance (commonly referred to as ventricular after-load). A number of agents are available for reduction of left ventricular output resistance by reducing peripheral arterial resistance. Nitroprusside is commonly used for this purpose. Right ventricular output resistance is not easily altered by medication, but attention to mechanical clearance of the airway may improve the cardiac output in patients with right ventricular failure.

If these measures fail to provide adequate improvement of the cardiac output, right or left ventricular assist devices including balloon counterpulsation and a mechanical auxiliary ventricle may be used.

Routinely monitored variables after cardiac surgery should include (1) electrocardiogram, (2) right and left atrial pressures, (3) arterial blood pressure, (4) urine output, (5) chest tube drainage, (6) arterial blood gas tension, and (7) serum potassium level. Not all need be measured in every patient, and the frequency of measurements may vary according to the degree of illness present.

Interventions most commonly required in the care of postoperative cardiac surgical patients include blood transfusion, administration of drugs to improve myocardial contractility and maintain renal function, elimination of hemorrhage from the perioperative site, maintenance of adequate respiratory gas exchange, and elimination of arrhythmias.

If a patient shows continued bleeding early after cardiac surgery, the most likely cause is an open blood vessel of significant size. In patients who have had uncomplicated operations and who are not suspected to have a specific bleeding diathesis, reoperation is probably advisable. In subsequent hours, the signals for reoperation include (1) significant rise in the hourly bleeding rate, (2) failure of hourly bleeding to fall below 200 ml/hr in the first 6 postoperative hr, and (3) a total volume of bleeding exceeding 2000 ml in the first 12 hr after surgery. If bleeding continues or is excessively troublesome, the usual tests for adequate hemostatic capability should be obtained. If necessary, a hematologist should be consulted. In some patients with diffuse capillary bleeding, the addition of 3- to 5-cm H_2O end-expiratory pressure may occasionally prove useful.

When a patient is stable and awake, the endotracheal tube can usually be removed. Simple tests of respiratory volumes and inspiratory pressure may provide guidelines for recognition of patients likely to have respiratory problems after extubation. Tidal volume of more than 350 ml and inspiratory pressure of more than 15 cm H_2O are usually adequate.

After extubation coughing should be encouraged to keep the airway clear and reduce the risk of atelectasis or pneumonia. Specially trained pulmonary physiotherapists are a useful addition to respiratory management.

Many patients may sit up for short periods on the day following surgery with gradual ambulation until on the fourth or fifth day they may be walking alone in the hallways. Prolonged sitting with the legs dependent should not be allowed because of the risk of venous stasis leading to clots and pulmonary embolism. Most surgeons do not advocate routine use of anticoagulants for all patients after cardiac surgery. Patients with a particular risk for thromboembolic complications should be started on warfarin when they are able to take medication by mouth.

Prophylactic antibiotic therapy is usually administered intravenously beginning just before operation and continuing for 2 to 5 days. Prolonged antibiotic administration is not appropriate.

Digitalis and other cardiac drugs may have undesirable side-effects and should be administered only for a specific purpose. Daily medication review is wise to prevent prolonged use of an unnecessary drug.

THE CONDUCTION SYSTEM AND PACEMAKERS

The cardiac conduction system of specialized myocardial fibers is shown diagrammatically in Figure 40-21. There are two principal situations in which surgical therapy may be beneficial for patients suffering from abnormalities of the cardiac conduction system. These are (1) failure of normal electrical impulse passage through proper anatomic pathways, and (2) conduction of electrical impulses through aberrant anatomic pathways.

Failure of normal electrical impulse passage through proper anatomic pathways may occur because of abnormalities in the initiation of electrical impulses or in their

Fig. 40-21. Schematic representation of the cardiac conduction system. (Edwards EA, Malone PD, Collins JJ Jr: Operative Anatomy of the Thorax. Philadelphia, Lea & Febiger, 1972)

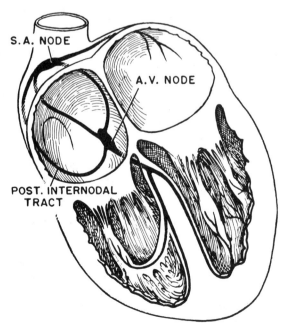

transmission. The normal cardiac conduction system includes the sinoatrial node, three internodal tracts traversing the right atrial wall, a tract from the sinoatrial node to the left atrial musculature (Bachman's bundle), the atrioventricular node, a common atrioventricular bundle (bundle of His), the right and left bundle branches to the respective ventricles, and the Purkinje network. For an anatomic-physiological system that occupies such a small volume of tissue, the cardiac conduction system has received an inordinate amount of attention. This is best understood when the consequences of failure are considered. The first direct attempt to introduce an external power source for the initiation of cardiac electrical impulses seems to be that of Albert Hyman in 1930. His device was hand operated and very primitive. Its use met with little enthusiasm and little success. In 1952, Paul Zoll reported the utilization of transthoracic cardiac stimulation to prevent asystole in patients with failure of adequate impulse initiation. The expected storm of controversy followed, but the course was inexorably set for the development of the modern pacemaking system. Transvenous pacing was introduced by Seymour Furman in 1958, and in the same year Ake Senning used the first totally implantable pacemaker. Subsequent developments included improvements in the pulse generator and wire connectors to the point where today many thousands of pacemaking units are in use throughout the world with a very high degree of success and a low risk of failure.

The pacemaker pulse generator consists of a battery power source, electronic circuitry to regulate the timing of impulse delivery, an encapsulating case to prevent exposure of the delicate mechanism to body fluids, and an electrode connection to the myocardium. Several basic types of pacemaker are available. The simplest is a device that delivers a preset electrical impulse at regular intervals independent of the native cardiac rhythm. This is a fixed-rate pacemaker. Because of concern that fixed-rate pacemakers might precipitate malignant arrhythmias if the impulse fell during a vulnerable period in the native electrical cycle, such devices are uncommonly used today. Demand pacemakers have incorporated within their electronic circuitry a system for monitoring the production of native electrical impulses with a delaying circuit to ensure that the impulses generated by the pacemaker fall within an acceptable portion of the cardiac electrical sequence. Most pacemaking systems are designed to deliver an impulse to the ventricular musculature, which then is transmitted to initiate cardiac contraction without regard to the atrial rhythm. More complex pacemaking circuitry is available, and with proper electrodes, sequential atrioventricular pacing can be accomplished. One variation of this system monitors the naturally occurring P wave and delivers a ventricular impulse at a proper interval following recognition of the P wave. In another system, active stimulation of the atria is followed by active stimulation of the ventricles. As may be expected, the rate of failure of the more complex systems is higher than that of the simpler ones.

The most common indication for cardiac pacing is complete heart block with a slow ventricular response. However, a variety of other arrhythmias may also be successfully treated by electrical pacing. In patients with brady–tachycardia syndromes, medication may be used to suppress the maximum rate of ventricular response during tachycardias and a pacemaking system may be used to increase the minimal rate during bradycardia episodes. Some persons with paroxysmal tachycardias may require so much medication that there is a hazard of inordinate slowing. Pacemaking may be very effective in combatting this possibility.

More recently pacemakers have been used for the control of supraventricular tachycardias by rapid atrial pacing. This may be particularly effective in atrial flutter. The pacing rate of an atrial electrode is increased to the point of atrial capture, and pacing is then suddenly stopped. The heart may often return to a more acceptable type of sinus rhythm, particularly with a background of antiarrhythmic medication. The most common configurations used today for pacemaking systems are shown in Figure 40-22, which depicts both a transvenous and an epicardial electrode system with the pulse generator located either on the anterior thoracic wall or in the upper abdominal wall. Placement of a transvenous electrode requires fluoroscopic control whereas direct placement of an epicardial lead does not. The transvenous operation is usually quicker and simpler but does require that an adequate vein be found for introduction of the pacing lead into the systemic venous circulation. The usual indication for epicardial placement of pacing electrodes is failure of transvenous system or the need for a pacing system at the time of surgical cardiac exposure. Of course, patients with prosthetic or bioprosthetic valves in the tricuspid position should not have electrodes traversing these valves.

Complications of pacemakers include (1) failure of pacing, (2) perforation of the right ventricular myocardium (tamponade is very rare), and (3) infection.

Pacemaker monitoring systems have been developed that allow frequent evaluation of the function of pacemakers even by telephone from the patient's home. In addition, battery failure in most modern units is predictable on the basis of a rate change well in advance of loss of pacing. With these safety maneuvers, catastrophic pacemaker failure is quite unusual.

The problem of electrical impulse conduction through aberrant anatomic pathways is an infrequent but important disease state. Such abnormal atrioventricular communications may be located by endocardial mapping in the cardiac catheterization laboratory or in the operating room. Precise location of such bundles allows surgical interruption, which has met with a high degree of success in these patients. The aberrant bundles are most frequently found near the atrio-

ventricular node or in the perimeter around the mitral and tricuspid rings.

TUMORS OF THE HEART AND PERICARDIUM

A large variety of primary and secondary tumors may involve the heart and pericardium. Autopsy studies have shown that the heart is involved in approximately 10% of patients dying of malignant neoplasms. The pericardium is involved in up to 85% of these patients. Malignant tumors most frequently metastasizing to the heart are melanoma, lymphoma, and leukemia. Because of the higher overall incidence, the absolute number of patients having pericardial or cardiac metastases are those with breast cancer (women) and bronchogenic carcinoma (men). Cardiac and pericardial metastases most commonly occur in the presence of far advanced metastatic disease to other organs and locations. The principal clinical response to metastatic tumor is the development of pericardial effusion, often with tamponade. Pericardiocentesis together with specific antitumor therapy is usually successful in averting recurrent episodes. The limited survival potential of many of these patients makes most surgeons reluctant to undertake major operative procedures to relieve recurring pericardial effusion. Careful judgment is needed to achieve a balance between overenthusiastic surgical extension of hopeless existence and failure to achieve possible temporary rehabilitation.

Primary pericardial tumors most commonly are mesothelioma, sarcoma, teratoma, fibroma, and lipoma. Primary cardiac tumors may additionally include rhabdomyoma or rhabdomyosarcoma and a variety of angiomas and lymphangiomas as well as other uncommon tumors. The most common primary cardiac tumor is myxoma.

Signs and symptoms of cardiac and pericardial tumors include primarily the spectrum of problems associated with pericardial effusion and tamponade as well as arrhythmias, congestive heart failure, and a variety of nonspecific systemic abnormalities including fever, thrombocytopenia, hemolytic anemia, polycythemia, joint pain, elevation of the sedimentation rate, and immunoglobulin abnormalities.

Although somewhat controversial for a time, myxomas are now regarded as true neoplasms. Grossly, they appear smooth and often almost gelatinous in consistency with

Fig. 40-22. Schematic representation of electrode configuration for permanent epicardial pacing and perivenous endocardial pacing. (Courtesy of Medtronic Corporation)

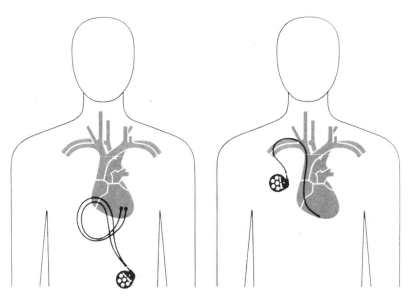

numerous frondlike appendages. They are usually pedunculated and are attached to the endocardial surface by a relatively short stalk. Most occur in the atria with about 75% lying in the left atrium after originating from the limbus of the fossa ovalis. Only about 5% of myxomas originate in the ventricles. They may occur at virtually any age. Although benign, myxomas may recur following inadequate excision.

The most frequent clinical presentation of myxoma includes the systemic symptoms mentioned above as well as a hemodynamic symptom complex suggesting mitral or tricuspid stenosis. Positional variation of a murmur of mitral or tricuspid stenosis should strongly suggest the possibility of myxoma.

The management of pericardial and cardiac tumors depends upon whether the tumor is benign or malignant and on the location and clinical complex of symptoms accompanying the disease. Patients with malignant pericardial effusion represent a difficult therapeutic challenge, and success is often only temporary. Benign tumors can usually be totally excised but sometimes involve vital structures, and less than total excision must be tolerated in such cases.

The surgical management of intracavitary myxomas consists primarily in total surgical removal. This can usually be readily accomplished in atrial tumors and in most ventricular ones as well. Careful removal of the attachment of the tumor to the endocardial surface is an absolute necessity if recurrence is to be avoided. Excellent results are usually obtained.

CARDIAC TRANSPLANTATION

The first human-to-human cardiac transplantation was carried out in 1967 by Barnard. Reports of cardiac transplants performed in a variety of institutions around the world soon followed. Of these, only about 12 programs remain active today with the most successful being at Stanford under the direction of Shumway.

Specific contraindications to cardiac transplantation that have become evident include (1) significant irreversibly elevated pulmonary vascular resistance, (2) active infection, (3) recent or unresolved pulmonary embolus or infarction, (4) insulin-dependent diabetes mellitus, (5) systemic illness that independently limits survival or may be exacerbated by immunosuppressant drugs, (6) age over 55 years, and (7) psychological abnormalities that may interfere with progress under the stress of convalescence.

Patients who are candidates for cardiac transplantation include primarily those with acquired heart disease, but occasional patients with severe congenital disease have also had transplants (see also Chapter 13).

Preoperative studies include cardiac catheterization with ventriculography and coronary angiography, and cardiac biopsy in certain cases. When a donor heart becomes available, a potential recipient is selected by consideration of height, weight, and ABO blood type compatibility. There should also be a negative lymphocytotoxic cross match. Evidence has accumulated that mismatch at the HL-A–A2 locus correlates with an increased rate of development of coronary atherosclerosis, and mismatching of this antigen should be avoided where possible.

The technique of cardiac transplantation includes preservation of the donor atrioventricular conduction system. Anastomoses are made between the donor and recipient right and left atria, aorta, and pulmonary artery.

Immunosuppressant treatment usually includes azathio-

prine with rabbit antithymocyte globulin (RATG) and methylprednisolone. More recently, cyclosporin A has been used rather than azathioprine and appears to offer some advantage.

Results of cardiac transplantation have improved progressively. Figure 40-23 shows the experience at Stanford with cardiac transplantation. It is evident that survival following cardiac transplantation in patients operated upon after January, 1974 is considerably better than that for those operated upon between 1968 and 1973.

The most common cause of death in patients following cardiac transplantation is infection, and the most common site is the lung. The second most common cause of death is rejection.

A more recent innovation in cardiac transplantation has been the clinical utilization of combined heart and lung transplantation. This experimental operation has also been pioneered at Stanford. As of this writing, only four patients have undergone heart and lung transplantation with one death.

Heterotopic auxiliary cardiac transplantation has been done infrequently but probably offers some promise for palliation of severe myocardial dysfunction. Experience in this field is so limited that it is impossible to comment on its eventual utility.

THE ARTIFICIAL HEART AND LEFT VENTRICULAR ASSIST DEVICES

The only left ventricular assist device in common use is the intra-aortic counterpulsating balloon, which has already been discussed in conjunction with management of coronary heart disease. The concept of counterpulsation or phase reversal diastolic augmentation originated early in the 1960s with the work of Harken, Birtwell, Soroff, and associates. The original device was a blind ventricle into which blood was sucked during systole (reducing left ventricular afterload) and from which blood was expelled forcefully during

Fig. 40-23. Improvement in results of cardiac transplantation at Stanford compared with course of patients selected but not operated upon. (Jamieson SW, Oyer PE: Cardiac transplantation at Stanford. Heart Transplantation 1:86, 1981)

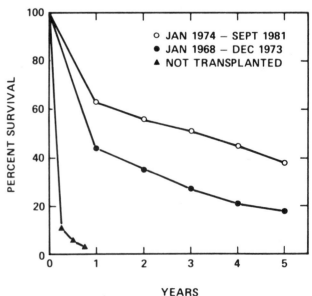

diastole. Within a few years after description of this concept, the intra-aortic counterpulsating balloon was introduced to perform virtually the same function with much less complex apparatus. A variety of balloons have been developed, and the consoles for the operation of intra-aortic balloons have become so sophisticated that present devices are capable of following arrhythmias and monitoring their own function.

For patients in whom intra-aortic balloon counterpulsation is an inadequate form of left ventricular assistance, there are other devices that partially or totally bypass the left ventricle. Perhaps the simplest concept is the left atrial to aorta bypass introduced by Litwak. Because oxygenated blood is present already in the left atrium, no artificial oxygenator need be included in the circuit. Blood is simply removed by a large-bore catheter from the left atrium, passed through a reservoir and roller pump, and returned to the aorta. This device does require heparinization but is tolerable over a period of several days for most patients.

The left ventricular assist device (LVAD), which really is half an artificial heart, is a more complicated device. It consists of a pumping chamber with two valves, one for ingress and the other for egress of blood. The pumping chamber consists of a compressible bladder that is alternately emptied and filled by compressed gas supplied from a control console. The LVAD is positioned in the chest or abdomen and connected to the left ventricle through a large bore supply cannula and to the aorta through a slightly smaller valved conduit. This unit depends upon an external power source and not only requires anticoagulation but is more likely to cause platelet damage and fibrinolysis than the counterpulsating balloon or Litwak bypass.

An even more complex device is the total artificial heart (TAH). The total artificial heart includes two pumping chambers and four valves (one operation has already been remarkably successful at this writing.—ED) Experience in animals has shown the possibility of long-term maintenance with a total artificial heart. The greatest disadvantage is continued reliance upon an external power source, which makes the machine incompatible with a return to "normal" life during the interval of its utilization. Major stumbling blocks to the development of a totally implantable artificial heart are difficulties with power supply and with obtaining biologically acceptable surfaces compatible with the stresses exerted on a pumping chamber.

The future of a totally implantable artificial heart seems rather dim at present, but the achievements of the past must encourage the view that such a thing is possible.

BIBLIOGRAPHY

BAILEY CP: The surgical treatment of mitral stenosis (mitral commissurotomy). Dis Chest 15:377, 1949

BARNARD C: The operation. A human cardiac transplantation: An interim report of the succeful operation performed at Groote Schuur Hospital, Cape Town. S Afr Med J 41:1271, 1967

BECK CS: The development of a new blood supply to the heart by operation. Ann Surg 102:801, 1935

BERNHARD WF, POIRIER V, LaFARGE CG et al: A new method for temporary left ventricular bypass: Preclinical appraisal. J Thorac Cardiovasc Surg 70:880, 1975

BIRTWELL W, GIRON F, SOROFF H et al: Support of the systemic circulation and left ventricular assist by synchronous pulsation of extramural pressure. Trans Am Soc Artif Intern Organs 11:43, 1965

BREGMAN D: Mechanical support of the failing heart. Curr Probl Surg 13:1, 1976

CARPENTIER A, DUBOST C: From xenograft to bioprothesis: Evolution of concepts and techniques of valvular xenografts. In Ionescu MI, Ross DN, Wooler GH (eds). Biological Tissue in Heart Valve Replacement, p 515. London, Butterworth, 1972

CARPENTIER A, LEMAIGRE G, ROBERT L et al: Biological factors affecting long-term results of valvular heterografts. J Thorac Cardiovasc Surg 58:467, 1969

CUTLER EC, LEVINE SA: Cardiotomy and valvulotomy for mitral stenosis. N Engl J Med 188:1023, 1923

DIMOND EG, KITTLE CF, CROCKET JE: Comparison of internal mammary artery ligation and sham operation for angina pectoris. Am J Cardiol 5:483, 1960

FAVALORO RG: Saphenous vein graft in the surgical treatment of coronary artery disease. Operative technique. J Thorac Cardiovasc Surg 58:178, 1969

FURMAN S, ROBINSON G: Use of intracardiac pacemakers in correction of total heart block. Surg Forum 9:245, 1958

GUIRAUDON G, FONTAINE G, FRANK R et al: Encircling endocardial ventriculotomy: A new surgical treatment for life-threatening ventricular tachycardias resistant to medical treatment following myocardial infarction. Ann Thorac Surg 26:438, 1978

HARKEN DE, ELLIS LB, WARE PF et al: The surgical treatment of mitral stenosis. N Engl J Med 239:802, 1948

HARKEN DE, LEFEMINE AA, BEATTY AC JR: Assisted circulation by counterpulsation. Nat Conf Cardiov Dis 2:643, 1964

HARKEN DE, SOROFF HS, TAYLOR WJ et al: Partial and complete prostheses in aortic insufficiency. J Thorac Cardiovasc Surg 40:744, 1960

HUFNAGEL CA, HARVEY WP: The surgical correction of aortic regurgitation. Preliminary report. Bull Georgetown Univ Med Cen 6:3, 1953

HURST JW (ed): Bypass Surgery for Obstructive Coronary Disease. New York, McGraw-Hill, 1980

HYMAN AS: Resuscitation of the stopped heart by intracardial therapy. Arch Int Med 46:553, 1930

JONES JW, OCHSNER JL, MILLS NL et al: Impact of multiple variables on operative and extended survival following coronary artery surgery. Surgery 83:20, 1978

LITWAK RS, KOFFSKY RM, SILVAY G et al: Early clinical experiences with a heart assist device. Langenbecks Arch Chir Suppl: 81, 1975

LOWER RR, STOFER RC, SHUMWAY NE: Homovital transplantation of the heart. J Thorac Cardiovasc Surg 41:196, 1961

MURRAY G: Homologous aortic valve segment transplants as surgical treatment for aortic and mitral insufficiency. Angiology 7:446, 1956

SAMET P, EL-SHERIF N: Cardiac Pacing, 2nd ed. New York, Grune & Stratton, 1980

SENNING A: Discussion of paper by Stephenson et al. J Thorac Surg 38:639, 1959

SOUTTAR PW: The surgical treatment of mitral stenosis. Br Med J 2:603, 1925

STARR A, EDWARDS ML: Mitral replacement: Clinical experience with a ball valve prosthesis. Ann Surg 154:726, 1961

VERREL D: Cardiac Catheterization and Angiocardiography. New York, Churchill Livingstone, 1978

VINEBERG AM: Development of an anastomosis between the coronary vessels and a transplanted internal mammary artery. Can Med Assoc J 55:117, 1946

ZOLL PM: Resuscitation of the heart in ventricular standstill by external electric stimulation. N Engl J Med 274:768, 1953

James D. Hardy

Cardiac Injuries

GROSS PATHOLOGY OF CARDIAC INJURY
DIAGNOSIS OF CARDIAC INJURY
MANAGEMENT OF CARDIAC INJURY
General Procedures
Specific Cardiac Injuries
Simple Cardiac Laceration by Knife or Bullet;
Pericardial Tamponade
Injury to Heart Valves
Blunt Injury with Rupture of Various Elements of
the Heart: Further Comment
Arrhythmias
THE RETAINED FOREIGN BODY FOLLOWING CARDIAC
INJURY
LEGAL CONSIDERATIONS

Cardiac injuries are common and represent a significant segment of surgical heart disease. The causes of such injuries are legion. They represent the entire spectrum from simple penetration by a flying object, bullet, or knife, to devastating blunt deceleration injury, as in an automobile or airplane accident. The injury may be iatrogenic, caused by cardiac catheterization, placement of central venous catheters, excessive cardiac massage, and still other modalities. For classification purposes cardiac injuries are usually divided into penetrating injuries and blunt injuries. The damage caused by penetrating injuries is frequently less extensive and more easily managed than that produced by blunt injuries. In either penetrating or blunt trauma, however, blood may escape into the fibrous pericardium, producing pericardial tamponade, reduced cardiac output, and shock. Massive blood loss into the thorax may occur.

GROSS PATHOLOGY OF CARDIAC INJURY

Either penetrating or blunt injury can result in damage to any portion of the heart (Table 40-6). Blunt or penetrating injury may produce contusion, immediate or late rupture, aneurysm, or intracardiac septal defects. The conduction mechanism may sustain damage that results in various types of arrhythmias, includng bundle branch block, complete heart block, "sick sinus" syndrome, or other rhythm disturbances. The heart valve leaflets may be lacerated or perforated, subluxation may occur, or papillary muscles or chordae tendineae may be disrupted. Any of these may produce serious valvular insufficiency with attendant heart failure. Intracardiac bullets may embolize. Coronary arteries and veins may be lacerated or divided, may undergo thrombosis caused by blunt trauma, or may become the site of an arteriovenous fistula or a fistula into one of the cardiac chambers. Gunshot wounds have increased in incidence and now approximate the incidence of knife wounds.

Pericardial tamponade has been mentioned. The pericardium itself may be opened sufficiently wide by knife wounds to permit herniation of the heart through the defect, with embarrassment of venous flow into the heart and immediate shock, leading to cardiac arrest if not corrected. Late after injury, constrictive pericarditis may develop. Although aspiration of blood from the pericardium is frequently life-saving in the extreme emergency, the pericardium is rarely emptied completely by aspiration, and the residual blood may eventually clot and embarrass cardiac

activity. Furthermore, diagnostic pericardiocentesis is plagued with a substantial incidence of both false positive and false negative diagnoses. Electrocardiographic guidance can be misleading. To exclude the possibility that the aspirating needle is in a cardiac chamber, Stone and Martin suggested that indocyanine green be injected through the needle and checked with earpiece densitometry.

The great vessels may also be injured by penetrating or blunt trauma, resulting in hemorrhage, pericardial tampon-

---

CAUSES OF CARDIAC INJURY

Penetrating Injury
Stab and gunshot wounds
Pins, needles, wires, icepicks, etc.
Cardiac catheters and pacemaker leads
Central venous pressure catheters
Rib fracture fragments
Miscellaneous

Blunt Injury
Motor vehicle accidents
Cardiac massage injury
Any blow over chest

TABLE 40-6 TYPES OF CARDIAC INJURIES

Myocardium
Musculature—contusion, rupture
Septal defect
Rupture of atrium
Late necrosis

Conduction Mechanism
Arrhythmias (other than below)
Bundle branch block
Complete heart block
Sick sinus syndrome

Valves
Perforation or laceration
Subluxation
Papillary muscle or chordae tendineae damage

Coronary Vessels
Laceration or division
Thrombosis
A-V fistula
Fistula into right atrium or ventricle

Pericardium
Pericardial tamponade (fluid or viscera)
Constrictive pericarditis
Rupture or laceration with heart herniation

Great Vessels
Aneurysm of aorta from blunt trauma
Penetrating injuries
A-V fistula

ade, false aneurysm, aortopulmonary or aortoatrial fistula and many other anatomic defects.

DIAGNOSIS OF CARDIAC INJURY

A first requirement for the diagnosis of cardiac injury is to suspect that it may have occurred. The possibility of cardiac damage should always be excluded when an object has penetrated the chest and may have traversed the mediastinum. In stab wounds, most physicians are likely to consider the possibility of cardiac injury if the site of penetration is in the region of the heart. However, when a bullet has entered at a distance from the chest—for example, through the lower back or the abdomen—the cardiac injury may not be so readily suspected. Moreover, a bullet may richochet off the spine and emerge from the body at a site much different from that which might be imagined.

Any patient who has sustained severe blunt trauma to the chest may have sustained cardiac injury, and the resilient ribs or sternum of a young person need not have been fractured for severe cardiac injury to have occurred. However, the presence of a fracture of the sternum or of a first rib usually indicates severe trauma, and cardiac or great vessel injury may well have occurred.

If the patient is dyspneic and shows other evidence of cardiopulmonary embarrassment, especially if the chest roentgenogram reveals essentially normal lung fields, the possibility of cardiac injury should always be considered, regardless of whether the trauma was penetrating or blunt. Distended neck veins, with a diminished blood pressure and perhaps pulsus paradoxus, should suggest pericardial tamponade. Of 45 patients operated on by Trinkle et al for wounds that had penetrated the pericardium, the preoperative diagnosis was pericardial tamponade in 36 and hemorrhagic shock in nine. Pericardial tamponade can be difficult to identify with certainty, and pericardiocentesis, isotopic scans, and echocardiography are all helpful. At times it may be necessary to make a short subxiphoid incision and open the pericardium to establish the diagnosis. If there is significant ecchymosis over the sternum, again the possibility of compression injury of the heart should be considered.

A varying cardiac rhythm, recorded by serial electrocardiograms or cardiac monitor, may reflect significant damage. The heart sounds may be abnormal at once, owing to intracardiac injury, or they may be normal initially only to change later as necrosis due to ischemic change progresses. When murmurs appear after cardiac injury, the anatomic defect should be identified with appropriate studies, which may include electrocardiograms, phonocardiograms, echocardiograms, and especially right- and left- heart catheterization with angiocardiography. Widening of the mediastinum may represent damage to the great vessels, especially traumatic rupture of the aorta.

The possibility of cardiac injury will usually be suspected and established, but at other times the injury may appear minor. In one such instance the heart of a young boy had been penetrated by a piece of wire thrown by a rotary lawnmower from a considerable distance. The possibility of penetrating injury to the heart was suspected only after examination of the chest x-ray film. Another patient complained of a "sticking pain" in his heart on repeated visits to an emergency room. No recent injury had occurred, though the patient had been in various altercations in the past. The anterior–posterior chest film was nonrevealing, but eventually when a lateral film was taken, an ice pick was seen to lie within the left ventricle.

Finally, the cardiac injury may not be apparent on any of the initial diagnostic studies but may develop weeks later owing to ischemic necrosis of a septum or papillary muscle. Of course, the trauma may be so massive that the chambers of the heart are simply ruptured immediately (Fig. 40-24), and in some instances not enough useful cardiac muscle remains to effect a satisfactory result, even if the patient survives to reach the hospital. We had a car wreck victim in whom all four chambers were ruptured. Patients who may have sustained cardiac injury should be monitored for several weeks and even months.

MANAGEMENT OF CARDIAC INJURY

GENERAL PROCEDURES

The presence of hemothorax should prompt the immediate insertion of closed thoracotomy tube drainage. Recurrent hemorrhage must be taken very seriously, and surgical exploration is usually advisable.

Once the possibility of cardiac damage has been suspected, the patient should be moved either to the operating room or to the adjacent intensive care unit. If pericardial tamponade appears probable, as evidenced by increased central venous pressure and low arterial blood pressure and especially if pulsus parodoxus is manifest, aspiration of the pericardium may permit withdrawal of nonclotted blood, with prompt improvement in the patient's cardiorespiratory parameters (see Fig. 40-1). Unfortunately, pericardiocentesis is not always successful, even when the pericardium contains liquid blood. Furthermore, much of the blood may have clotted, or it may lie posteriorly. If evidence of significant cardiac compression exists, and if pericardiocentesis is not satisfactory, the patient should be moved promptly to the operating suite because cardiac arrest could occur at any time. Before moving the patient, however, we prefer to

Fig. 40-24. Rupture of cardiac chambers in blunt injury. Any or most of the anatomic elements of the heart may be injured in either blunt or penetrating trauma. (Hardy JD: Cardiac injuries. In Hardy JD [ed]: Rhoads Textbook of Surgery, 5th ed. Philadelphia, J B Lippincott, 1977)

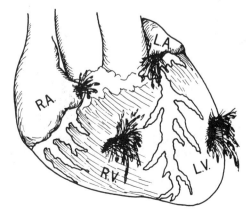

DIAGNOSIS OF CARDIAC INJURY
History and physical examinations (serial)
Electrocardiograms (serial)
Chest x-ray studies (serial)
Echocardiograms (serial)
Cardiac catheterization
Angiocardiograms

EMERGENCY OPERATIVE MANAGEMENT OF CARDIAC INJURIES

Insert closed thoracotomy tube drainage if indicated
Aspirate pericardium as indicated
Prep chest before anesthesia
Intubate patient while he is awake
Have blood for transfusion at hand
Assemble necessary instruments, sutures, drugs, defibrillator,
    pump oxygenator
Control hemorrhage with finger
Use Teflon felt backing of sutures if indicated

---

insert a nasotracheal tube under topical anesthesia, to provide a dependable airway in case abrupt deterioration in the patient's condition should necessitate immediate thoracotomy. Blood is transfused as indicated.

Whereas in former years we often performed pericardiocentesis several times before resorting to thoracotomy, early operation is now advised in most patients—first, because of the immediate risk of nonoperative management, and second, because a considerable number of patients not operated on immediately eventually require operation anyway. Certainly, it is a simple matter to expose the pericardium with the subxiphoid incision and exclude hemopericardium and tamponade (Fig. 40-25). General endotracheal anesthesia is preferable to permit extension of the incision, although local anesthesia can be used for the pericardial window if severe head injury renders local anesthesia advisable and particularly when the diagnosis is in doubt. Of course, if life-threatening pericardial tamponade is not a consideration, adequate diagnostic studies should be performed to permit accurate correction of all cardiac injuries present. Facilities for cardiopulmonary bypass should always be immediately available.

It may not be necessary to divide the sternum all the way to the manubrium, and, if complete division of the sternum can be avoided, major sternal separation problems will not occur, and the quality of postoperative respiration, in a patient who may have sustained multiple rib injuries, will be that much better.

If formal exposure of the heart becomes advisable, we simply extend the subxiphoid incision made for diagnosis. We have largely abandoned the left thoracotomy approach for the management of cardiac injuries, except in extreme

Fig. 40-25. Mini-pericardiotomy. Approach to pericardium for diagnostic purposes. The sternum may be split upward if hemopericardium identifies the need for additional surgical exposure. (Hardy JD: Cardiac injuries. In Hardy JD [ed]: Rhoads Textbook of Surgery, 5th ed. Philadelphia, J B Lippincott, 1977)

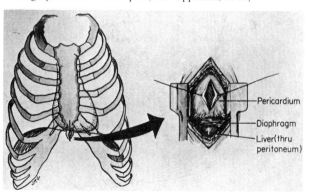

emergencies in which haste is essential. The median sternotomy incision permits access to all vessels and chambers, and it facilitates the institution of cardiopulmonary bypass. However, in extreme emergencies, or where the surgeon is unfamiliar with the median sternotomy approach, a left lateral incision in the fourth or fifth intercostal space is easily and rapidly performed and is often adequate. The pericardium should be left widely open to minimize pericardial tamponade.

If cardiac murmurs have developed, the patient's condition should be allowed to stabilize, if possible, and appropriate cardiac diagnostic studies should be performed to determine the nature of the injury prior to operative intervention (Fig. 40-26). Then, with complete diagnosis available, in a patient who is now stabilized from other injuries frequently associated with blunt trauma, one can operate with precision and correct appropriately the cardiac pathology that exists.

SPECIFIC CARDIAC INJURIES

SIMPLE CARDIAC LACERATION BY KNIFE OR BULLET; PERICARDIAL TAMPONADE

The most common type of cardiac injury that the general surgeon is required to manage in an emergency is cardiac

Fig. 40-26. (*Top*) Bullet wound causing aorto–right atrial fistula and aorto–right ventricular fistula. The defects were closed with fabric sutures and Teflon felt backing (see drawing at right). (*Bottom*) At *left* is shown the marked enlargement of the cardiac silhouette. This enlargement was due to both ventricular enlargement and pericardial effusion. At *right* is shown a normal heart silhouette 7 months later, following surgical repair of the intracardiac fistulas noted above. (Hardy JD, Timmis HH: Repair of intracardiac gunshot injuries: Report of three cases. Ann Surg 169:906, 1969)

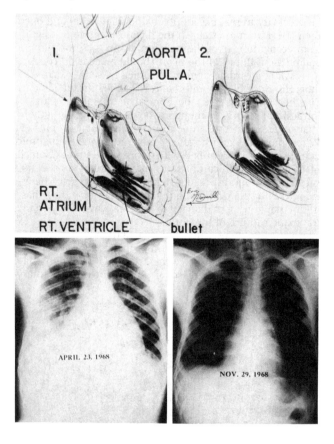

laceration due to stab wound or bullet wound. As noted above, we have moved toward almost routine exploration of the pericardial cavity through a short subxiphoid incision whenever we believe a significant cardiac injury may have occurred. This is because often one cannot be certain whether or not cardiac damage has been inflicted. Theoretically, the diagnosis of pericardial tamponade should be a simple matter, but in the multiple-injury patient who may be drunk and who may have lost blood from other wounds, it is not always easy to make a definite diagnosis of cardiac injury.

The first requirement is that the patient be placed where continuous intensive monitoring and observation can be carried out. As long as the patient's condition remains stable and there is no significant evidence of cardiorespiratory embarrassment, nonoperative management may be justified, at least on a temporary basis. On the other hand, if the classic signs of pericardial tamponade develop and if the patient's overall condition begins to deteriorate, previously typed and cross-matched blood for transfusion should be made immediately available, and the pericardium should be explored. Once all is in readiness, and the pericardium is incised vertically, the blood in the pericardium may escape under considerable pressure, followed by fresh hemorrhage from the laceration in one of the various cardiac chambers or in the aorta or pulmonary artery. Here, the first requirement is to employ finger compression to control the bleeding from the laceration in the heart or great vessel. The defect is then closed appropriately, often with mattress sutures using Teflon felt backing (Fig. 40-27).

In the course of suturing the laceration, finger pressure should be applied to diminish hemorrhage while the mattress sutures with Teflon felt backing are being placed. If the injury is immediately adjacent to a coronary artery, the sutures should be placed so that they pass beneath the coronary artery. Rehn was the first to suture a laceration of the heart successfully.

Fig. 40-27. Management of stab wound of heart. Bleeding from the stab wound (*A*) is controlled with firm finger pressure (*B*) while the defect is undersewn with mattress sutures using Teflon felt backing. When bleeding has been thus controlled, an additional row of fine sutures can be used to approximate the margins of the divided heart muscle (*B, C*). (Hardy JD: Cardiac injuries. In Hardy JD [ed]: Rhoads Textbook of Surgery, 5th ed. Philadelphia, J B Lippincott, 1977)

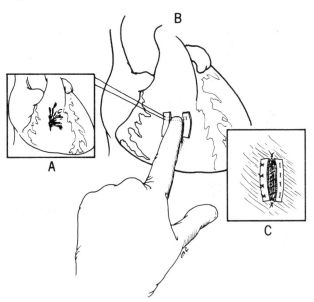

It is easier to suture lacerations on the anterior surface of the heart than on the posterior surface because elevation of the heart embarrasses cardiac function and there are additional difficulties of exposure. If the injury on the posterior surface appears to be a formidable one and is not readily amenable to simple suture using Teflon felt backing, one should occlude the injury with the finger, maintain adequate blood volume with blood transfusion, and meanwhile place the patient on cardiopulmonary bypass, following which the repair of most cardiac stab or bullet wounds becomes a relatively simple matter. If a coronary artery has been severed, it should be anastomosed using 6–0 or 7–0 sutures. Fistula between a coronary artery and a cardiac chamber may occur.

There is no substitute for poise and experience in the management of cardiac injuries, but many patients' lives have been saved by prompt intervention by surgeons of limited experience with cardiac surgery. If it appears that serious cardiac injury has occurred, the most experienced surgeon available should proceed with operation. A number of patients have reached our emergency room "dead," only to have the chest opened by a resident, the cardiac laceration sutured, adequate circulation restored, and the chest then closed in the operating room—with discharge from the hospital in 10 days. Decisiveness and speed are essential if the patient's condition is deteriorating rapidly.

INJURY TO HEART VALVES

In addition to laceration of the heart with hemorrhage and pericardial tamponade, the penetrating object may have injured various heart valves, either cusps or such supporting structures as chordae tendineae or papillary muscles. Such injuries are usually signaled by the presence of a murmur preoperatively. It has been our policy to avoid immediate operation on patients with murmurs if they are otherwise stable. We prefer to treat acute heart failure with digitalis and other appropriate measures until emergency diagnostic studies have identified the specific intracardiac pathology. Even so, if pericardial tamponade develops, operation is necessary if this problem is not manageable by pericardial aspiration.

BLUNT INJURY WITH RUPTURE OF VARIOUS ELEMENTS OF THE HEART: FURTHER COMMENT

Akenside is credited with the first autopsy-confirmed case of myocardial contusion due to nonpenetrating chest trauma. As noted above, blunt injury to the heart can produce a wide range of serious injuries. The fact is that the human body is simply not capable of withstanding the tremendous force of certain deceleration accidents. Steering wheel injuries, for example, may result in sternal compression and injury to the heart. Severe blunt injuries with rupture of the heart may be immediately fatal, but lesser degrees of damage may be readily tolerated, permitting appropriate diagnosis and repair.

Major clinical features met in 25 consecutive patients with blunt injury reported by Madoff and Desforges were fractured sternum, variable cardiac rhythm, tachycardia, changing EKG, new cardiac murmur, recurrent hemothorax, widening mediastinum, and hemopericardium. Rupture of the heart may also be caused by external cardiac massage.

ARRHYTHMIAS

Arrhythmias following cardiac injury may be missed unless continuous cardiac monitoring is employed. The treatment of arrhythmia consists of maintaining good respiratory function, antiarrhythmic drugs when indicated, optimal electrolyte balance, pacemakers where required, and long-term follow-up.

THE RETAINED FOREIGN BODY FOLLOWING CARDIAC INJURY

A question of importance is whether or not to operate for removal of foreign bodies such as bullets, needles, and other radiopaque objects when no other compelling indication for operation exists. The possible late complications of such foreign bodies include embolism, formation of aneurysm, infection, erosion, and hemorrhage. Also, anxiety neurosis may develop in a susceptible patient who becomes increasingly concerned about the thought that his heart harbors a foreign body. In a review of 35 patients with missiles in the heart, Bland and Beebe found that 21 patients had an abnormal electrocardiogram, but late complications from leaving the missiles *in situ* were not observed. However, 5 of the 35 patients were emotionally incapacitated by the knowledge that they harbored a foreign body in the heart.

The problem also obviously has significant legal implications for both the assailant and the physician. If the object appears to be embedded in the wall of the left ventricle or the right ventricle or even the septum and is small, we have not routinely advised its removal. Bullets free in a cardiac chamber often embolize early, to the lungs from the right ventricle or to a peripheral artery from the left ventricle. On at least three occasions we have observed peripheral arterial embolism of a bullet from the left ventricle prior to the time when a decision about operative removal would have had to be made. Of course, there is always the risk that a small missile may embolize to the brain or a coronary artery. Each case must be decided on its own merits.

LEGAL CONSIDERATIONS

Cardiac injuries are often surrounded by circumstances that invite litigation. This is true whether the damage was inflicted by knife or gunshot, by blunt injury, or, indeed, by the physician himself in the course of diagnostic or therapeutic measures. One legal expert has classified cardiac injury from a litigation standpoint as that due to penetrating trauma, nonpenetrating trauma, heart disease arising from physical exertion that produces injury, heart disease caused by psychic trauma associated with the accident, and aggravation of pre-existing heart disease. The physician who manages the patient with cardiac injury will almost invariably be called on to supply information and testimony and to complete the documentation of the case from start to finish, including the long-term follow-up, which is most important.

BIBLIOGRAPHY

AKENSIDE M: An account of a blow upon the heart and its effects. Philosophical Transact, 1764, p. 353. Cited by Chung EK, Renn J: Electrocardiographic changes in nonpenetrating trauma to the chest. Acta Cardiol 25:418, 1970

BARRETT NR: Foreign bodies in the cardiovascular system. Br J Surg 37:416, 1950

BEALL AC JR, PATRICK TA, OKIES JE et al: Penetrating wounds of the heart: Changing patterns of surgical management. J Trauma 12:468, 1972

BHARATI S, NHERVONY A, GRUHN J et al: Atrial arrhythmias related to trauma to sinoatrial node. Chest 61:331, 1972

BRAVO AJ, GLANCY DL, EPSTEIN SE et al: Traumatic coronary arteriovenous fistula: A twenty-year follow-up with serial hemodynamic and angiographic studies. Am J Cardiol 27:673, 1971

CHENG TO, ADKINS PC: Traumatic aneurysm of left anterior descending coronary artery with fistulous opening into left ventricle and left ventricular aneurysm after stab wound of chest. Am J Cardiol 31:384, 1973

CLEVELAND JC, CLEVELAND RJ: Successful repair of aortic root and aortic valve injury caused by blunt chest trauma in a patient with prior aortic dissection. Chest 66:447, 1974

DECKER HR: Foreign bodies in the heart and pericardium. Should they be removed? J Thorac Surg 9:62, 1939

DEMUTH WE, BAUE AE, ODON JA: Contusions of the heart. J Trauma 7:443, 1965

DOLARA A, MORANDO P, PAMPALONI M: Electrocardiographic findings in 98 consecutive non-penetrating chest injuries. Dis Chest 52:50, 1969

ESPADA R, WHISENNAND HH, MATTOX KL et al: Surgical management of penetrating injuries to the coronary arteries. Surgery 78:755, 1975

FITTS CT, BARNETT LT, WEBB CM et al: Penetrating wounds of the heart caused by central venous catheters. J Trauma 10:764, 1970

GILLANDERS AD: Traumatic aorto-pulmonary fistula. Br Heart J 17:411, 1955

GLANCY DJ, ITSCOITZ SB, McINTOSH CL et al: Successful operative correction of intrapulmonary rupture of a posttraumatic left ventricular aneurysm. Documentation of complete spontaneous closure of an associated ventricular septal defect. Am J Cardiol 30:914, 1972

GOGGIN MJ, THOMPSON FD, JACKSON JW: Deceleration trauma to the heart and great vessels after road traffic accidents. Br Med J 2:767, 1970

GOLDSTEIN S, YU PN: Constrictive pericarditis after blunt chest trauma. Am Heart J 69:544, 1965

HARDY JD, TIMMIS HH: Repair of intracardiac gunshot injuries: Report of three cases. Ann Surg 169:906, 1969

HARKEN DE: Surgical removal of foreign bodies from the heart. Surgery 21:150, 1947

HARVEY JC, PACIFICO AD: Primary operative management: Method of choice for stab wounds to the heart. South Med J 68:149, 1975

IVATURY RR et al: Emergency room thoracotomy for the resuscitation of patients with "fatal" penetrating injuries of the heart. Ann Thorac Surg 32:377, 1981

JONES JW, HEWITT RL, DRAPANAS T: Cardiac contusion: A capricious syndrome. Ann Surg 181:567, 1975

LEVINE RJ, ROBERTS WC, MORROW AG: Traumatic aortic regurgitation. Am J Cardiol 10:752, 1962

O'SULLIVAN MJ, SPAGNA PM, BELLINGER SB et al: Rupture of the right atrium due to blunt trauma. J Trauma 12:208, 1972

PATE JW, RICHARDSON RL JR: Penetrating wounds of cardiac valves. JAMA 207:309, 1969

RAVITCH MM, BLALOCK A: Aspiration of blood from pericardium in treatment of acute cardiac tamponade after injury. Arch Surg 58:463, 1949

REHN H: Ueber penetrirende Herzwunden und Herznaht. Arch Klin Chir 55:315, 1897

SIMS BA, GEDDES JS: Traumatic heart block. Br Heart J 31:140, 1969

SUGG WL, REA WJ, ECKER RR et al: Penetrating wounds of the heart: An analysis of 459 cases. J Thorac Cardiovasc Surg 56:4, 1968

SYMBAS PN: Residual or delayed lesions from penetrating cardiac wounds. Chest 66:408, 1974

TRIMBLE C: Arterial bullet embolism following thoracic gunshot wounds. Ann Surg 168:911, 1968

TRINKLE JK, MARCOS J, GLOVER FL et al: Management of the wounded heart. Ann Thorac Surg 17:230, 1973

WATANABE T et al: Ruptured chordae tendineae of the tricuspid valve due to non-penetrating trauma. Echocardiographic findings. Chest 80:751, 1981

YAMADA EY, FUKUNGA FH: Cardiopulmonary complications of external cardiac massage. Hawaii Med J 29:114, 1969

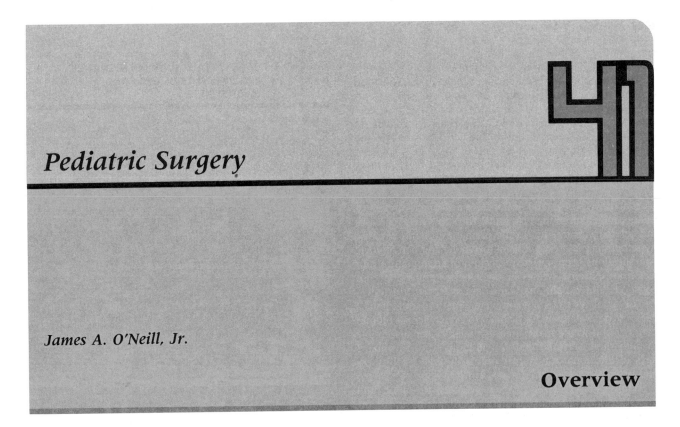

Pediatric Surgery

James A. O'Neill, Jr.

Overview

PHYSIOLOGICAL CONSIDERATIONS
PREOPERATIVE AND POSTOPERATIVE CARE
  Acid Base, Blood, and Fluid Management
  Infection
  Monitoring

Pediatric surgery has developed as a specialized area of general surgical care, since the problems of children are so different from the day-to-day surgical problems seen in adults. Additionally, the body of knowledge within the field of children's surgery has increased so much over the last 20 years that it is appropriate for individuals to devote their entire professional efforts to infants and children.

The three main causes of death in childhood are traumatic injuries, malignancies, and congenital malformations. Improvements in the management of these entities have come from individuals working in institutions where there has been an opportunity for concentration of experience and evaluation of results in large numbers of patients.

PHYSIOLOGICAL CONSIDERATIONS

Children with surgical problems differ in every respect from their adult counterparts. Metabolic rate, water turnover, and calorie and protein needs are all clearly higher in infants and children than in adults. The rate of growth and development varies with the age group involved. Any surgical procedure must be designed to take these factors into consideration. Not only is the patient different but pathology is also widely variable, requiring a thorough understanding of endless variations in teratogenesis and malignancy. With respect to traumatic injuries, blunt trauma is more common in children than are penetrating injuries, and scald burns are encountered more than flame burns. Surgical approaches to children's problems are often modified in terms of timing and whether staged approaches or primary repairs should

be considered. Finally, depending upon the age of the child involved, psychological considerations are clearly important with regard to the timing of elective surgical procedures. The purpose of this section is to cover fundamental information regarding the common disorders of infancy and childhood, with the exception of trauma, which is covered in Chapter 10.

PREOPERATIVE AND POSTOPERATIVE CARE

The goal of pre- and postoperative care is to maintain normal physiological function and avoid complications. The principles of care are related to understanding the normal function of various organ systems, their response to stress, and precise therapy based on frequent monitoring.

While individual responses to the same stress may differ, organ systems respond in predictable patterns. Various organ systems are first in the process of transition from the intrauterine to the external state and then in the long process of maturation. Since different systems mature at different rates, their response to stress varies in time as well.

Unless an infant or child has cardiac pathology, cardiovascular response to stress is adequate. Generally the myocardium functions very well, but peripheral circulation may be labile in those less than 1 year of age, since most of the blood volume is in the relatively large splanchnic circulation. This may make it difficult to judge the adequacy of cardiac output on the basis of the quality of peripheral circulation.

While gas exchange and ventilation are generally efficient in all infants and children, the low-birth-weight infant will frequently have impaired function related to immaturity, hyaline membrane disease, or meconium aspiration. Even in mature infants with healthy lungs, high metabolic demands may occasionally exceed pulmonary reserve. The respiratory system usually matures by 1 year of age as well, so while avoidance of atelectasis, thoracic restriction, airway compromise, and pneumonia is important in all age groups, it is particularly important in the infant under 1 year of age.

The integumentary system and temperature regulation do not mature until puberty. Until then, the skin is thin and the dermal glands and hair follicles are less concentrated. Infants less than 6 months old compensate for cold stress by nonshivering thermogenesis. The younger the child the more labile temperature regulation is, and the greater the disparity in the ratio of surface area to body weight. This disparity results in rapid shifts in core temperature with a tendency to equilibration with ambient temperature. Rates of evaporative heat and water loss are much higher in infants and children than in adults. The stress state increases this tendency markedly. In the premature infant, extreme hypothermia may result in fatal metabolic and hematologic complications. Appropriate protection of an immature subject from extreme swings in body temperature may also conserve limited pulmonary and cardiovascular function.

The renal system is not completely mature until about 2 years of age. Relatively fixed ability to excrete large volumes of water and solute makes infants under 1 year susceptible to both fluid overload and dehydration. After the first 2 days of life, renal function is ordinarily well established, and normal output approximates 1 ml/Kg/hour.

While many differences exist between the adult and immature gastrointestinal systems, perhaps the most important consideration in children is the tendency to gastric dilatation. All patients with intestinal obstruction or abdominal distention or those in whom gastric dilatation would further limit respirations should have a nasogastric tube passed and left in place until peristalsis is firmly established. Passage of a nasogastric tube is particularly important in patients who are to be transferred from one hospital facility to another. Frequently gastrostomy is used postoperatively in infants when prolonged nasogastric drainage is anticipated or as a method of facilitating feedings in small weak patients, since sucking on a bottle requires so much energy.

ACID BASE, BLOOD, AND FLUID MANAGEMENT

As a basic principle, all patients should be treated to be as near normal as possible before operation is undertaken. Postoperative fluid therapy is a continuation of that process (Table 41-1). Before operation it is necessary to provide maintenance needs and to correct preexisting losses resulting from vomiting or diarrhea. In patients with losses from the proximal gastrointestinal tract, as with pyloric stenosis, the tendency is toward hypochloremic hypokalemic alkalosis. In distal gastrointestinal obstructions, loss of intestinal secretions tends to produce acidosis. Under these circumstances, one should calculate the estimated degree of dehydration representing the preexisting deficit and then provide additional fluid therapy to provide for maintenance needs and continuing losses. Careful observation of the response to fluid therapy in the form of urine output, general circulation, and measurements of electrolytes and pH indicates whether the deficits have been replaced adequately. Basal maintenance needs for water are approximately 1500 ml/m²/24 hours. Newborn infants require only half this much fluid for the first 24 hours, while older patients may require more if they have increased metabolic activity. Maintenance requirements may ordinarily be met with 5% glucose in 0.2 normal saline with added potassium according to need. Replacement of losses must be adjusted according to the electrolyte content of the body fluid being lost. Infants

TABLE 41-1   TWENTY-FOUR-HOUR MAINTENANCE REQUIREMENTS OF FLUID AND ELECTROLYTES

Water	Newborn first 24 hours	750 ml/m²
	Thereafter	1500 ml/m²
Electrolytes	Sodium	3–4mEq/Kg
	Chloride	2–3mEq/Kg
	Potassium	2–3mEq/Kg
Calories	Newborn	120 Cal/Kg
	Children	60–80 Cal/Kg
Replacement	Gastric losses	D₅0.45NS plus 30mEq KCl/ liter
	Enteric losses	D₅R. lactate plus 30mEq KCl/ liter
Normal urine flow		1 ml/Kg/hr

tend to lose more sodium in gastric juice than adults. In addition to clinical observation of the patient and measurement of serum electrolytes, pH, and blood gases, daily measurement of body weight and careful monitoring of intake and output ordinarily provide sufficient information for accurate management of fluid and electrolyte balance. Patients who present in shock must be treated initially with intravenous infusions designed to restore circulation before the above-mentioned methods of fluid therapy can apply. Ringer's lactate administered in increments of 10 ml/Kg until circulation is restored is usually effective. Packed red cells are given as well in patients who are anemic.

The transfusion needs of infants and children differ from those of adults. While most normal infants and children tolerate hematocrits from 25 to 30 ml/dl without difficulty, those with respiratory or circulatory impairment may require a higher than normal level; this is particularly true of low-birth-weight infants. Intraoperative losses of less than 10% of blood volume are ordinarily well tolerated provided adequate amounts of crystalloid have been administered.

Infants and children are prone to disorders of coagulation, particularly thrombocytopenia and disseminated intravascular coagulation. Thrombocytopenia is an early indication of sepsis. All infants should receive 1 mg of vitamin K preoperatively and weekly postoperatively if oral feedings are withheld in patients on long-term parenteral nutrition.

Hypoglycemia is commonly seen in newborn infants and in depleted patients subjected to stress. Severe hypoglycemia may result in seizures and brain damage. Consequently, glucose determinations on heel-stick blood should be performed at frequent intervals. Sudden hyperglycemia in the stable postoperative patients is a sign of potential sepsis, as is sudden unexplained thrombocytopenia.

Hyperbilirubinemia in the newborn period may be dangerous to the central nervous system, particularly in those infants with hypoxia, acidosis, or hypoalbuminemia. Unconjugated bilirubin is not completely bound to albumin, and the free portion is toxic and may produce kernicterus. As a general rule, unconjugated bilirubin levels should not exceed 15 mg/dl in low-birth-weight infants or 20 mg/dl in full-term infants. Since phototherapy diminishes the obvious visual signs of jaundice, frequent measurements of serum bilirubin must be performed in order to maintain awareness of a rapidly rising bilirubin level so that exchange transfusion may be performed if necessary.

Hypocalcemia from inadequate maternal transfer, from reduction of acidosis with sodium bicarbonate administration, or from gastrointestinal losses may cause tremors or seizures. Replacement of calcium deficits must be given gradually. Maintenance requirements are approximately 1 g/24 hours. Magnesium deficiency should also be considered in patients who have large gastrointestinal losses.

INFECTION

Patients with infection should be treated with specific antibiotic therapy guided by culture information. Young patients who are seriously ill usually have defective immune defenses. Since newborns are particularly prone to septicemia when exposed to pathogens, antibiotics are ordinarily indicated preoperatively. Ampicillin and gentamicin or tobramycin are frequently used prophylactically and for the treatment of most infections seen in the infant age group. Other antibiotics are used as indicated.

MONITORING

In addition to laboratory monitoring of serum electrolytes, osmolality, hemogram, glucose, bilirubin, calcium, *p*H, and blood gases, proteins and liver functions are monitored as indicated as well. Physiological monitoring with a transcutaneous oxygen electrode may supplement that information. Central venous pressure measured via a catheter placed in the superior vena cava either by means of a subclavian puncture or through a common facial vein cutdown provides the ability to measure central venous pressure on a serial basis, and the levels should approximate normal adult levels. Larger subjects who require determination of cardiac output or pulmonary wedge pressure may have Swan–Ganz catheters placed in a distal pulmonary artery. This is ordinarily not now possible in children under the age of 4 years. More commonly, radial artery catheters are placed for the purpose of monitoring arterial blood pressure and for frequent blood gas determinations.

BIBLIOGRAPHY

ADAMS JM, RUDOLPH AJ: The use of indwelling radial artery catheters in neonates. Pediatrics 55:261, 1975.

COEN R, GRUSH O, KAUDER E: Studies of bacteriocidal activity and metabolism of the leucocyte in full-term neonates. J Pediatr 75:400, 1969

GODFREY S, BAUM, JD (ed); Clinical Pediatric Physiology. London, Blackwell Scientific Publications, 1979

KLAUS MH, FANAROFF AA (ed): Care of the High-Risk Neonate. Philadelphia, W B Saunders, 1973

SINCLAIR JC (ed): Temperature Regulation and Energy Metabolism in the Newborn. New York, Grune & Stratton, 1978

James A. O'Neill, Jr.

Thoracic Problems of Infancy and Childhood

RESPIRATORY DISTRESS OF THE NEWBORN
PNEUMOTHORAX
UPPER AIRWAY OBSTRUCTION
POSTEROLATERAL DIAPHRAGMATIC HERNIA
ESOPHAGEAL ATRESIA
PULMONARY MALFORMATIONS (SEE ALSO CHAPTER 34)
VASCULAR RING
CHRONIC PULMONARY INFECTION
PULMONARY SEQUESTRATION (SEE ALSO CHAPTER 34)
MEDIASTINAL MASSES
DEFORMITIES OF THE CHEST WALL

RESPIRATORY DISTRESS OF THE NEWBORN

Respiratory distress characterized by tachypnea, retractions, nasal flaring, and acidosis may be related to pulmonary disease, cyanotic heart disease, disorders of the central nervous system, restriction of diaphragmatic motion by marked abdominal distention related to intestinal obstruction, or metabolic problems related to impairment of renal function. The diagnosis of most of the surgically correctable causes of respiratory distress of the newborn may be made by two simple maneuvers: chest film and passage of a nasogastric tube into the stomach to check the patency of the upper airway and the esophagus. At times, bronchoscopy, esophagoscopy, barium swallow, and special radiologic imaging techniques such as angiography or computed tomography will be needed.

PNEUMOTHORAX

The most common problem seen in the newborn, particularly of low birth weight, is pneumomediastinum and pneumothorax related to the air-block syndrome, sometimes accentuated by assisted ventilation. Alveolar rupture in this age-group results in dissection of air along interbronchial planes into the mediastinum with caval compression, pneumopericardium, or, most commonly, pneumothorax. Since the diseased lung is characteristically hyperinflated, dangerous tension pneumothorax may exist even when the chest film appears to show only a limited amount of free air within the thorax. Tube thoracostomy drainage, rather than aspiration, is always the safest route to follow in these instances. At times, drainage of the pericardium will be required. Pneumoperitoneum may be seen as a result of pneumomediastinum under extreme tension, a condition that must be differentiated from perforated viscus.

UPPER AIRWAY OBSTRUCTION

Passage of a nasogastric tube into the stomach provides information regarding the patency of the nasal passages. Posterior choanal atresia will result in life-threatening respiratory distress in the newborn if it is bilateral. Emergency management includes positioning the infant prone and insertion of an airway or orogastric tube to hold the tongue forward and facilitate mouth breathing. Many of these infants may be treated expectantly as they adapt to mouth breathing, while others will require intubation, operative relief of the choanal obstruction, and gastrostomy. The same is true of micrognathia or the Pierre Robin syndrome. In this condition, a normal-sized tongue is relatively too large for the pharynx when the mandible is underdeveloped. A cleft palate may coexist. Emergency management is the same as for choanal atresia, and operative relief is frequently required in the form of glossopexy and gastrostomy.

POSTEROLATERAL DIAPHRAGMATIC HERNIA

Another entity that is easily recognized on chest film is congenital posterolateral diaphragmatic hernia, which presents clinically as cyanosis, dyspnea, and apparent dextrocardia, since over 80% occur on the left side. This is probably the most emergent condition in the newborn period, although occasionally patients are not symptomatic for several days or even weeks of life. Those infants who are cyanotic at birth or shortly thereafter have a 60% mortality rate, and the defect is relatively common. Once the diagnosis has been established, an endotracheal tube should be passed for assisted ventilation, as well as a nasogastric tube to minimize the degree of intestinal distention within the chest. Since most of the viscera have been developing within the thorax during the fetal period, pulmonary hypoplasia on the affected side is common, and the degree of mediastinal shift also impairs the function of the contralateral lung. Most feel it is preferable to treat these infants with assisted ventilation and sodium bicarbonate until they can be made physiologically stable prior to operation, but clearly operation cannot be delayed very long. Abdominal repair of the diaphragmatic defect is ordinarily performed, and no extreme efforts are made to expand the hypoplastic lung except to place a tube within the chest. Too-rapid expansion of the lung results in rupture. Despite remarkable improvements in perinatal care, persistent fetal circulation resistant to therapy is still a significant problem in patients with this disorder symptomatic at birth.

ESOPHAGEAL ATRESIA

Choking and copious secretions are characteristic of proximal esophageal atresia with distal tracheoesophageal fistula (Figs. 41-1 and 41-2). As more mucus is inhaled and aspirated, respiratory distress worsens. Passage of air through the tracheoesophageal fistula into the stomach, causing distention, further interferes with respiratory excursion, since the newborn's mechanism of breathing is primarily diaphragmatic. Additionally, reflux of gastric juice into the lungs produces pneumonia. Passage of a relatively stiff

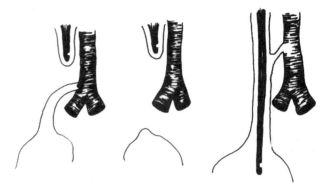

Fig. 41-1. This drawing depicts the common forms of esophageal anomalies and how the nasogastric tube is used for diagnosis. Air is seen in the gastrointestinal tract if a fistula is present, but not otherwise. An intact esophagus with an H-type tracheoesophageal fistula is best diagnosed by endoscopy.

nasogastric tube through the nose or mouth, followed by chest film, is ordinarily sufficient to make the diagnosis, although instillation of a small amount of contrast material with the infant in the upright position is helpful. If an infant is to be transferred from one hospital to another, repeated suctioning of the pharynx must be performed en route to minimize pulmonary aspiration, and the infant should be nursed in the upright position to avoid reflux. Following preoperative preparation, gastrostomy and right retropleural thoracotomy with division of the fistula and primary anastomosis of the two esophageal segments are in order (see

Fig. 41-2. (*Top*) The usual combinations of esophageal atresia and tracheoesophageal fistula are shown with their relative frequency. (*Bottom*) Before thoracotomy for definitive repair, while the atelectasis and pneumonia are being treated, the infant is propped up. A sump suction catheter decompresses the proximal pouch, and a gastrostomy empties the stomach of gas and gastric secretions. (Holder TM, Ashcraft KW: Esophageal atresia and tracheoesophageal fistula. In Hardy JD [ed]: Rhoads Textbook of Surgery, 5th ed. Philadelphia, J B Lippincott, 1977)

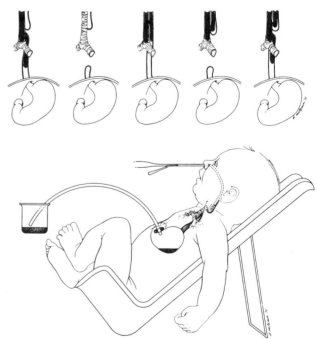

Fig. 41-2). Occasionally, low-birth-weight infants, particularly if there are associated life-threatening anomalies, will require either delayed or staged anastomosis. Overall survival rates are in the range of 90%.

Infants with isolated esophageal atresia may be treated either by initial gastrostomy and cervical esophagostomy, followed by interposition of colon or a reversed gastric tube after 1 year of age, or by gastrostomy, bougienage of the two esophageal segments, and delayed anastomosis. The results are generally good, and mortality is low in this form of the disorder.

Infants with intact esophagus and an H-type fistula frequently do not present for several days or even weeks of life, and the characteristic symptoms are recurrent bouts of aspiration pneumonia. The diagnosis is best made by endoscopy; since most of these fistulas occur at the level of the thoracic inlet, a cervical approach for division of the fistula is indicated. Unless pulmonary impairment is severe, the results with this form of the anomaly are uniformly good.

PULMONARY MALFORMATIONS

Congenital lobar emphysema is probably the result of absence of bronchial cartilages causing valvular obstruction, and overaccumulation of air within the affected lobe with compression of the remaining lungs results in progressive respiratory distress. In most instances, the diagnosis is easily made on clinical and radiologic grounds, and lobectomy is curative.

Congenital lung cysts and cystic adenomatoid malformations may also occur in the newborn presenting with respiratory distress. The radiologic picture is characteristic. These cysts become progressively larger and frequently become infected, so lobectomy is necessary.

VASCULAR RING

Abnormalities in the development of the aortic arches may result in persistence of a vascular ring that surrounds the esophagus and trachea, causing obstruction and tracheomalacia. While the anatomy of the vascular ring is variable, the common forms noted on angiography are right aortic arch with a left-sided ductus arteriosus, double aortic arch, and anomalous subclavian, innominate, or carotid arteries. Anomalous origin of the arch vessels does not constitute a complete ring and does not ordinarily cause acute respiratory distress, but it may cause dysphagia. Operative division of the involved vessel and anterior aortopexy performed through the left side of the chest ordinarily provide relief, but tracheomalacia takes some time to correct itself (see Chapter 39).

CHRONIC PULMONARY INFECTION

Since respiratory passages are small and the cough reflex is frequently ineffectual in young patients, chronic pulmonary infection and atelectasis are common. Occasionally, pneumonia will result in infected pleural effusion and empyema. The most common organisms involved are *Staphylococcus,* pneumococcus, *Hemophilus influenzae,* and *Streptococcus.* In most instances, tube thoracostomy drainage will result in gradual resolution of the process. However, in some cases of persistent bronchopleural fistula or chronic restrictive processes, decortication, sometimes with pulmonary resec-

tion, is required. Long-term specific antibiotic therapy is required. Patients with acute bacterial empyema ordinarily present with a septic course and severe respiratory distress. Mortality is low with expeditious diagnosis and institution of therapy.

While efforts should be made to conserve functioning pulmonary tissue, lobectomy may be required in patients with chronic pulmonary infection associated with bronchiectasis. Appropriate antibiotic therapy has reduced the need for lobectomy in instances of chronic pulmonary infection except in patients with immune deficiencies.

While aspirated foreign bodies may ordinarily be removed safely by bronchoscopy, missed foreign bodies or those that cannot be extracted occasionally result in chronic pulmonary infection. Bronchotomy with removal of the foreign body is the most desirable approach, but occasionally lobectomy is required in these instances.

PULMONARY SEQUESTRATION

Certain congenital malformations of the lung also result in chronic pulmonary infection and require resection. The characteristic picture of recurrent respiratory infections located in the same lobe on chest film suggests sequestration. The most common form is intralobar sequestration, in which case the abnormal tissue is contiguous with the related lobe, which is virtually always the right or left lower lobe. All these patients have systemic arterial supply, and aortography will clearly show the location of these vessels preoperatively. Lobectomy is indicated. Occasionally, extralobar sequestration will occur; in these instances, complete resection may be performed without ablating normal lung.

MEDIASTINAL MASSES

Tumors of the mediastinum are common (Fig. 41-3). Most are asymptomatic and diagnosed as incidental findings on chest film taken for some other reason. Mediastinal teratomas and lymphomas are the most common tumors found in the anterior mediastinum. Tumors related to the neural crest are the most common ones found in the posterior mediastinum, while bronchogenic cysts and esophageal duplications constitute the remainder and are seen in the middle mediastinum. Tumors of the lymphoma group and thymoma are ordinarily best treated by nonoperative means in children, although occasionally a surgical approach is required for diagnosis or relief of life-threatening compression of the airway. Paravertebral neuroblastomas frequently present in the immediate newborn period and are best treated by operation. Occasionally, a young child will present with spinal cord compression under which circumstance there is intraspinal as well as intrathoracic tumor; a dual approach to surgical removal is required. X-ray therapy and chemotherapy are frequently indicated postoperatively, except in the newborn period. The benign masses, including duplication cysts of the esophagus, bronchogenic cysts, and most of the teratomas, should be removed on an elective basis.

DEFORMITIES OF THE CHEST WALL

A depression abnormality of the sternum, referred to as *pectus excavatum,* can range from mild to severe. They are usually isolated defects not associated with cardiac disease. The usual clinical course is one of deformity noted soon

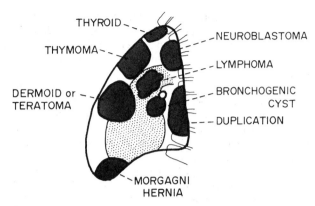

Fig. 41-3. Usual locations of various forms of mediastinal masses.

after birth increasing in severity until about 4 years of age, when the chest wall appears to stabilize. The defect may further worsen at the time of puberty and rapid growth. Most patients are not symptomatic, but some have diminished exercise tolerance, chest pain, and impairment of cardiac function on exercise. Most patients do not require operation. The abnormality can be corrected successfully by operation, but it should not be performed until the chest wall stabilizes. Improvement in cardiac and respiratory function following operation has been reported.

Less commonly, a protrusion abnormality of the chest may be seen, called *pectus carinatum.* These may be congenital

or acquired, particularly following sternotomy for repair of cardiac malformations that frequently coexist. Since these deformities are frequently extreme, repair is often indicated.

Occasionally, deficiencies in the formation of various components of the chest wall occur. Delayed repair by means of rib implants, prostheses, and large muscle flaps is often corrective.

BIBLIOGRAPHY

ADELMAN S, BENSON CD: Bochdalek hernias in infants: Factors determining mortality. J Pediatr Surg 11:569, 1976

AVERY ME: The Lung and Its Disorders in the Newborn Infant. Philadelphia, W B Saunders, 1964

DEPAREDES CG, PIERCE WS, JOHNSON DG et al: Pulmonary sequestration in infants and children. J Pediatr Surg 5:136, 1970

GROSFELD JL, BALLANTINE TVN: Esophageal atresia and tracheoesophageal fistula: Effect of delayed thoracotomy on survival. Surgery 84:394, 1978

HALLER JA, MAZUR DO, MORGAN WW: Diagnosis and management of mediastinal masses in children. J Thorac Cardiovasc Surg 59:385, 1969

HALLER JA, PETERS GN, MAZUR D et al: Pectus excavatum: A 20 year surgical experience. J Thorac Cardiovasc Surg 60:375, 1970

HALLORAN LG, SILVERBERG SC, SALZBERG AM: Congenital cystic adenomatoid malformation of the lung. Arch Surg 104:615, 1972

NIKAIDOH H, RIKER WL, IDRISS FS: Surgical management of "vascular rings." Arch Surg 105:327, 1972

SANDERSON JM, KENNEDY MCS, JOHNSON MF et al: Bronchiectasis: Results of surgical and conservative management: A review of 393 cases. Thorax 29:406, 1974

WELCH KJ, VOS A: Surgical correction of pectus carinatum (pigeon breast). J Pediatr Surg 5:659,1973

John M. Templeton, Jr.

Intestinal Obstruction and Other Intestinal Disorders in the Newborn

OBSTRUCTION
    Duodenal Atresia and Stenosis
    Malrotation
    Jejunoileal Atresia
    Colon Atresia
    Meconium Ileus
    Meconium Peritonitis
    Meconium Plug Syndrome
DUPLICATIONS
NECROTIZING ENTEROCOLITIS

OBSTRUCTION

The cardinal signs of congenital intestinal obstruction are maternal polyhydramnios, bilious vomiting, abdominal distention, and failure to pass normal meconium within the first 48 hours of life (Table 41-2). Because all signs are not routinely present, any one of them is an indication for roentgenography of the chest and abdomen. Barium enema is indicated in patients with distal intestinal obstruction because it is not possible to distinguish colon from small bowel in the newborn.

Atresia is complete obstruction of the bowel, whereas

stenosis indicates that a small and usually inadequate opening is present.

DUODENAL ATRESIA AND STENOSIS

Duodenal obstruction is complete in 90% of cases and occasionally is associated with an annular pancreas (Fig. 41-4). Because the site of obstruction is distal to the ampulla of Vater in 85% of cases, bilious vomiting is usually seen as well as maternal polyhydramnios. One third of patients also have Down's syndrome. The abdomen is usually scaphoid, and meconium will be passed. Diagnosis is best made on the basis of plain x-ray films of the abdomen. Only the stomach and duodenum will contain air, the so-called double bubble sign, unless stenosis is present and small amounts of air pass distally. In the latter situation it is best to obtain a barium enema or upper GI series to rule out malrotation with volvulus, which may be confused with duodenal stenosis and is more serious.

Significant metabolic alkalosis should be corrected preoperatively. Operative correction is accomplished by duodenoplasty or duodenojejunostomy. Annular pancreas should be bypassed and not divided to avoid postoperative fistula.

Gastrostomy and parenteral nutrition are helpful. Mortality is 5% or less, and long-term gastrointestinal function is normal.

MALROTATION

Incomplete rotation and lack of fixation of the midgut may result in either partial obstruction of the duodenum due to restrictive peritoneal folds called Ladd's bands or complete obstruction due to clockwise volvulus of the midgut, a true emergency. Patients with duodenal obstruction due to Ladd's bands appear healthy but have intermittent bilious vomiting; severe electrolyte disturbances are uncommon. Patients with midgut volvulus usually look ill and may have mild abdominal distention. Upper gastrointestinal contrast x-ray films and barium enema are diagnostic. Operative division of Ladd's bands, derotation of the volvulus, and appendectomy are curative. If operative intervention for volvulus is too late, bowel necrosis may result in short bowel syndrome.

JEJUNOILEAL ATRESIA

Atresias of the jejunum and ileum are common forms of newborn intestinal obstruction and probably result from intrauterine mesenteric vascular accidents. The signs of small bowel atresia are bilious vomiting, various degrees of abdominal distention depending on whether the jejunum or ileum is involved, and lack of meconium passage, particularly in distal obstructions. Polyhydramnios is not present. Low birth weight is common. In all forms of small bowel atresia there are dilated loops of bowel with air–fluid levels on plain x-ray film of the abdomen. Sometimes there is calcification, suggesting intrauterine bowel perforation. If distal bowel obstruction is suspected, a contrast enema is indicated to rule out other disorders such as meconium ileus and various forms of colon obstruction.

Surgical management depends upon the pathology encountered. In most instances resection of a short segment of proximal dilated bowel followed by end-to-end anastomosis is preferable. At times, complicated distal obstructions are best managed by Mikulicz resection or exteriorization of

NEONATAL INTESTINAL OBSTRUCTION	
History	Maternal polyhydramnios, bilious or nonbilious vomiting, no meconium passage
Physical Examination	Flat or distended abdomen, tender erythematous abdomen, shock
Dx	Electrolyte imbalance; abdominal x-ray shows quantity and location of distended loops; calcification; alkalosis vs. acidosis; sonography; CT scan
Rx—Surgical	Duodenal obstruction: duodeno-duodenostomy Annular pancreas: duodenoduodenostomy Malrotation: derotation, division of bands, appendectomy Jejunoileal atresia: exteriorization or anastomosis Colon atresia: colostomy Meconeum ileus: Conray enema or staged resection Necrotizing enterocolitis: bowel rest, hyperalimentation, anastomosis or resection and exteriorization
Rx—Supportive Measures	Nasogastric suction, appropriate fluid replacement and maintenance, antibiotics if indicated

the distal intestine with proximal-to-distal end-to-side anastomosis by the method of Bishop-Koop. Side-to-side anastomosis is not used because it will result in a blind loop syndrome. Prolonged postoperative gastrointestinal dysfunction is common, and many patients have deficiencies of bowel length. Many patients with as little as one third the normal length of intestine are capable of adaptation, particularly if the ileocecal valve is present and provided that nutritional support is given. It is in such patients that intravenous nutrition has provided an opportunity for survival not previously available. Various forms of elemental enteral diets are helpful also. Overall mortality is in the range of 15%.

COLON ATRESIA

Colon atresia is uncommon. It is characterized by slowly progressive abdominal distention, small amounts of bilious vomiting, failure to pass any meconium, and an x-ray film that demonstrates many dilated loops of bowel and one or two extraordinarily dilated loops of bowel. A few patients with colon atresia have other complicated deformities such as abdominal wall defects and bladder exstrophy. Because most of these patients, however, do not have a rectum, they are more properly viewed as having partial or total absence of the hindgut.

Because all of the small bowel as well as the ileocecal valve is usually intact, and because a primary anastomosis

TABLE 41-2 GASTROINTESTINAL OBSTRUCTION IN THE NEONATE

	PROXIMAL	DISTAL*
Vomit		
Character	Bile—yes or no	Bile—yes
Volume	Large	Small
Timing	Early	Later
Distention	Mild	Great
Meconium	Adequate	Scanty
Number of dilated loops of bowel seen on x-ray	Few	Many
Polyhydramnios	Yes	No
Impact on patient prior to resuscitation	Early prostration	Late prostration
Microcolon	No	Yes

* Consider a contrast enema (e.g., Gastrografin, barium) in all infants with a "low" (distal) obstruction.

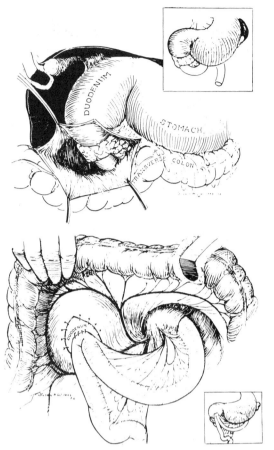

Fig. 41-4. Annular pancreas and its management. To avoid possible common duct injury and pancreatic fistula, it is usually better not to try to resect the obstructing pancreatic annulus but to perform duodenojejunostomy. (Wilson H, Bushart JH: Annular pancreas producing duodenal obstruction. Ann Surg 137:818, 1953)

is so technically difficult, it is usually safest to perform colostomy with anastomosis at a later time. Early and long-term results are good.

MECONIUM ILEUS

Meconium ileus is a form of newborn intestinal obstruction caused by inspissation of small bowel contents that are very tenacious and that produce an intraluminal obstruction, usually in the mid- to distal ileum. Mucoviscidosis or cystic fibrosis is a hereditary recessive disorder in which a deficiency of pancreatic enzymes causes the meconium to tend to obstruct the bowel, and in fact all exocrine glands are affected. Inspissation of respiratory mucus causes severe pulmonary disease. Approximately 15% of patients with cystic fibrosis have meconium ileus as the first clinical sign of the disorder. Also, approximately 15% of newborns with intestinal obstruction have meconium ileus. Meconium ileus typically presents as a distal form of newborn intestinal obstruction with bilious vomiting, abdominal distention, and no passage of meconium. Plain films of the abdomen tend to show varying sized loops of dilated bowel, relative absence of air–fluid levels, and large areas of opacity. If prenatal volvulus and perforation have occurred, a fine pattern of calcification will be evident. Contrast enema with dilute Conray or Gastrografin shows the characteristic pattern of meconium plugs. Sometimes patients with simple forms of obturation obstruction may be relieved without operation by this technique. However, patients with extensive plugs or complicated forms of meconium ileus associated with atresia require operation.

If operation is required, the best approach is some variation of staged resection and later anastomosis either by the Mikulicz or the Bishop-Koop technique. Generally, primary anastomosis is not possible because of the presence of obstructing plugs. Although early mortality is now only 10% to 15%, patients with mucoviscidosis rarely live beyond the second decade of life.

MECONIUM PERITONITIS

Meconium peritonitis is the result of prenatal intestinal perforation from any cause. Patients have a discolored, tender, massively distended abdomen due to the spillage of meconium into the free peritoneal cavity, which results in a marked chemical peritonitis and formation of large, fluid-containing spaces. Following birth, the ongoing chemical inflammatory insult to the peritoneal cavity results in further rapid fluid shifts out of the vascular tree into the abdomen. Furthermore, there is steadily increasing pressure on the diaphragm, resulting in respiratory compromise.

Diagnosis and surgical management depend on the exact cause of the obstruction, but physiological management of these infants is difficult and mortality is high. Staged resection, late anastomosis, and prolonged intravenous hyperalimentation are helpful.

MECONIUM PLUG SYNDROME

Meconium plug syndrome is a form of obturation obstruction of the colon in the newborn that is not due to meconium ileus. In approximately 15% to 20% of patients Hirschsprung's disease is the cause. Infants with meconium plug syndrome usually have a long continuous cast of meconium that is adherent to the colon wall and produces obstruction.

In patients with classic meconium plug syndrome, Conray or Gastrografin enema is both diagnostic and therapeutic. Operation is rarely required unless perforation has resulted from delay in diagnosis.

DUPLICATIONS

Duplications of the gastrointestinal tract can occur at one or more locations along its length beginning at the mouth and extending to the anus. Duplicated portions may contain one or all of the tissue layers found in the parent bowel. If gastric mucosa is present, bleeding may occur. Owing to both anatomy and presumed embryologic development, duplications above the diaphragm are different from those in the abdomen. Most duplications in the thorax are cystic, do not communicate with the adjacent bowel, and cause symptoms related to pressure on adjacent structures. Cystic duplications in the abdomen are usually noticed because partial intestinal obstruction is present or because a mass is felt. Tubular duplications may produce obstruction, but often bleeding due to uleration occurs. Diagnosis is usually made on clinical grounds, although conventional x-ray films, contrast studies, and abdominal ultrasound studies may be helpful.

Surgical management varies. Most esophageal duplications can be excised completely and the esophagus repaired primarily. In the abdomen cystic duplications can usually be resected along with the involved adjacent bowel with appropriate anastomosis. In some instances, such as in the stomach or duodenum, resection is not feasible, so these lesions are best managed by excision of the common wall between the duplication and the adjacent normal viscus. Tubular duplications are managed either in this fashion or by resection, depending on the location and the length of bowel involved. If gastric mucosa is present in a long tubular duplication, mucosal stripping is a possible method of treatment. At times, staged resections are indicated to preserve bowel function.

NECROTIZING ENTEROCOLITIS

Necrotizing enterocolitis has become a major clinical problem only in the last 15 to 20 years as increasing numbers of premature infants have survived in neonatal care centers. The typical subject is a low-birth-weight newborn who has suffered intrauterine sepsis, perinatal shock, asphyxia, or prolonged hypoxemia. Early feeding of hyperosmolar formulas, infection, exchange transfusion, and patent ductus arteriosus are additional risk factors. All these influences may result potentially in splanchnic ischemia associated with redistribution of the circulation when there is decreased cardiac output.

Clinical signs include gastric retention, bilious vomitus, intestinal bleeding, and abdominal distention and tenderness early, followed by lethargy, apnea, and shock. The typical x-ray findings are intestinal distention associated with collections of intramural gas. Gas may be seen in the portal tree, and there may be free air in the abdomen. Barium contrast studies are contraindicated in this disorder. Anemia,

hyponatremia, and acidosis resistant to therapy are signs of patient deterioration, and progressive thrombocytopenia is particularly important in this respect.

Three fourths of patients will recover with aggressive supportive therapy, antibiotics, intravenous hyperalimentation, and prolonged bowel rest. The remaining one fourth will require operation. Exteriorization resection of gangrenous bowel and delayed anastomosis is the standard method of surgical therapy. A few patients who appear to have recovered with medical therapy will later develop obstruction due to colon or small bowel stenoses, and resection with anastomosis is indicated in these circumstances. Long-term results are excellent in the 60% to 70% of patients who survive operation unless intestinal length is inadequate.

BIBLIOGRAPHY

BOLES ET, VASSY LE, RALSTON M: Atresia of the colon. J Pediatr Surg 11:69, 1976

CLATWORTHY HW, HOWARD WHR, LLOYD J: The meconium plug syndrome. Surgery 39:131, 1956

DOTT NM: Anomalies of intestinal rotation: Their embryology and surgical aspects with report of 5 cases. Br J Surg 11:251, 1923

GROSFELD JL, O'NEILL JA, CLATWORTHY HW: Enteric duplications in infancy and childhood: An 18 year review. Ann Surg 172:82, 1970

JONA JZ, BELIN RP: Duodenal anomalies and the ampulla of Vater. Surg Gynecol Obstet 143:565, 1976

LOUW JH: Jejunoileal atresia and stenosis. J Pediatr Surg 1:8, 1966

O'NEILL JA: Neonatal necrotizing enterocolitis. Surg Clin North Am 61:1013, 1981

O'NEILL JA, GROSFELD JL, BOLES ET et al: Surgical treatment of meconium ileus. Am J Surg 119:99, 1970

WILMORE DW: Factors correlating with a successful outcome following extensive intestinal resection in the newborn infant. J Pediatr 80:88, 1972

John M. Templeton, Jr.

Anorectal Malformations and Disorders of Function in Infancy and Childhood

HIRSCHSPRUNG'S DISEASE
CHRONIC CONSTIPATION
IMPERFORATE ANUS
RECTAL PROLAPSE (SEE ALSO CHAPTER 26)

The colorectal complex has storage and control functions that, if deranged, lead to disability. The balance between effective defecation of stool and the attainment of social continence involves the intrinsic function of the bowel and its mucosa, the ability of the bowel to relax distally, and the ability to relax voluntary muscles of fecal control in the sphincter mechanism in association with the use of voluntary muscles of defecation such as the abdominal musculature. Any defect, either functional or anatomic, in this complex sequence can lead to major problems in stooling or even to intestinal obstruction.

HIRSCHSPRUNG'S DISEASE

Hirschsprung's disease is caused by an absence of ganglion cells in the myenteric plexus, involving anywhere from 2 cm to 3 cm of distal rectum to the entire colon and small bowel. In most cases, the rectosigmoid is involved. The absence of these parasympathetic ganglion cells is associated with apparent overactivity of sympathetic nerve supply, resulting in failure to transmit normal propulsive waves downward so that stooling is impeded or prevented. The involved bowel tends to remain contracted.

Symptoms are variable and do not necessarily correlate with the length of the aganglionic segment. Hirschsprung's disease is now the most common single cause of alimentary tract obstruction in the newborn. Other newborns will stool initially but develop progressive obstipation. In most instances, history will reveal that some abnormality of stooling

HIRSCHSPRUNG'S DISEASE	
Etiology	Absence of ganglion cells in myenteric plexus of rectum or colon causing intestinal obstruction
Symptoms	Constipation alternating with diarrhea; toxemia from enterocolitis
Dx	Barium enema; rectal biopsy; manometrics
Rx	Initial colostomy, followed late by pull-through procedure

or a need for rectal stimulation was present from birth. As time progresses, older children develop an intermittent pattern of constipation and diarrhea that suggests the presence of impacted stool above the area of Hirschsprung's disease. Colitis may intervene and growth retardation may occur.

If the diagnosis of Hirschsprung's disease is suspected, a short-segment barium enema is indicated, but no rectal stimulation should be performed for 48 hours prior to the study in order to prevent confusion from an overstretched internal sphincter muscle. If a narrow distal segment is seen with a transition into a dilated proximal portion of the colon, the contrast enema does not need to be continued. The presence of a transition zone is highly suggestive of Hirschsprung's disease; if the child fails to evacuate this after 24 hours, the evidence is stronger but still not necessarily proof positive. While this evidence may be sufficient indication for colostomy in an infant with obstruction, definitive biopsy is required before a corrective pull-through operation is done. On the other hand, some infants with colitis may not demonstrate a clear-cut transition zone on x-ray film and evacuation may be prompt.

The most serious form of Hirschsprung's disease is enterocolitis, which probably results from a combination of partial intestinal obstruction, fortuitously unfavorable bacterial overgrowth, and colonic ischemia related to overdistention. This results in toxemia and a fulminant secretory diarrhea. These infants present with impressive abdominal distention, prostration, acidosis, and hypernatremic, hyperosmolar dehydration. Mortality ranges from 20% to 50% in a variety of series. Aggressive supportive therapy, immediate colostomy, and bowel rest with intravenous nutritional support are essential for survival. Enterocolitis may recur in some patients, particularly following corrective operations. Under these circumstances rectal washouts, antibiotics, and bowel rest may be sufficient to reverse the process.

Rectal biopsy is the most definitive diagnostic approach, but in a neonate older than one month it is possible to obtain anorectal manometrics that will confirm the inability of the internal sphincter area to relax in the presence of a proximal bolus of simulated stool. While manometry is considered definitive by some, most prefer to obtain a biopsy. Multiple suction biopsies of the muscularis mucosa may demonstrate the absence of ganglion cells in Meissner's plexus. However, the absence of ganglion cells in the intermyenteric plexus on rectal biopsy 2 cm to 3 cm above the dentate line is the most definitive study. The latter study requires an anesthetic but involves little risk.

Although an occasional patient will have a true short-segment Hirschsprung's disease lending itself to a transanal anorectal myomectomy, most patients with Hirschsprung's disease will ultimately require some form of pull-through procedure. Colostomy is advisable as a preliminary measure in most instances, either just above the transition zone or in the transverse colon but definitely in ganglionated colon. This allows the proximal dilated colon to return to a normal caliber and provides a period of improved nutrition. Definitive pull-through operation may ordinarily be performed at 6 to 18 months of age.

At least three corrective operations are available. The Swenson procedure involves rectosigmoidectomy with a low anastomosis performed by the pull-through technique. While this provides good results, the procedure is technically demanding and is used less now than previously. The Duhamel procedure involves a limited resection with creation of a window between the proximal normal colon and a short segment of retained rectal pouch. The Soave or endorectal pull-through involves passage of normal proximal colon through a seromuscular cuff of rectum that has had the mucosa stripped away with a low anastomosis. The Duhamel and Soave procedures are most popular today and appear to provide excellent functional results with low mortality.

CHRONIC CONSTIPATION

A large number of children have complaints of difficulty stooling with a pattern suggestive of Hirschsprung's disease. The usual subject is 4 years of age or older, but some are much younger. Barium enema studies may even suggest Hirschsprung's disease of a short-segment type. In these cases, biopsy of megacolon will usually demonstrate the presence of ganglion cells. Dietary causes, hypothyroidism, mental retardation, neurologic syndromes, and psychogenic causes are all involved, but in most instances the etiology is unclear. Treatment is nonoperative, and long-term function improves as the children mature.

IMPERFORATE ANUS

Anorectal malformations are common and vary widely in type depending upon whether the defect has its origin early or late in fetal life. Common to all forms of the anomaly are varying degrees of intestinal obstruction. Associated malformations are common. Since the process of pelvic maturation involves both the hindgut and the urinary system, associated genitourinary anomalies are noted in 30% of patients with imperforate anus. Half of these are incompatible with life. Other major anomalies in children with imperforate anus include cardiac anomalies in 7% and esophageal atresia in 10%

The most accurate classification of imperforate anus defects relates each defect to the appropriate stage in embryologic development. From a clinical viewpoint it is more practical to classify imperforate anus based on sex and on whether the defect is supra- or infralevator in location (Fig. 41-5). From a surgical viewpoint, low defects are ones that lend themselves to surgical correction through the perineum shortly following birth, while high-lying anomalies are best treated by colostomy followed 6 to 12 months later by sacroperineal or abdomino-sacroperineal pull-through of the proximal colon. Three fourths of female infants with

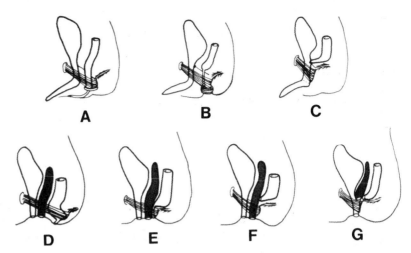

Fig. 41-5. Some common variations of imperforate anus of the supra- and infralevator types in males and females. (*A*) Anal atresia with rectoperineal fistula. (*B*) Anorectal atresia with rectoperineal fistula. (*C*) Anorectal atresia with rectourethral fistula. (*D*) Anal atresia with rectoperineal fistula. (*E*) Anorectal atresia with rectovestibular fistula. (*F*) Anorectal atresia with high rectovaginal fistula. (*G*) Anorectal atresia with rectocloacal fistula.

imperforate anus have some form of infralevator defect, while that is true of only 40% of male infants.

Imperforate anus is evident at birth in most cases, but sometimes only subtle differences from normal exist. In both male and female infants careful evaluation is required when no anal opening is identified. Chest films should be obtained to evaluate any possible cardiac or intrathoracic defects. Routine films of the abdomen also help to evaluate any defects of the vertebral column. A nasogastric tube should be passed to rule out the possibility of esophageal atresia. It is often helpful to obtain an inverted lateral x-ray film that includes the pelvis, with a lead marker at the presumed site of the external sphincter. If air is seen in the rectum below the pubococcygeal or ischial lines, the defect is probably infralevator. If the air column is higher, if air is seen in the bladder on x-ray film, if meconium is noted in the urine, or if one is uncertain, diverting colostomy is in order.

In all patients with imperforate anus one should look for a fistula arising from the apex of the atretic rectum. Male infants with low imperforate anus usually have a discernible fistula in the perineum along the midline, while in females the opening may be in the perineum or distal vagina. Often these patients will begin to pass meconium within the first 24 hours of life. In the latter instance it is useful to pass a catheter into the opening and to perform a contrast x-ray study. For patients with a high imperforate anus, the presence of an associated fistula can be confirmed by the passage of meconium from some point high in the vagina, the identification of air in the bladder by x-ray film, or the passage of meconium in the urine. Any patient with a urinary tract fistula has a supralevator malformation. Although it is not usually required in the immediate newborn period, an eventual formal urinary tract workup should be conducted. All patients with either a high or low imperforate anus should have an excretory urogram and a more extensive urinary workup if indicated.

Patients found to have infralevator defects can usually have definitive repair performed by the perineal approach in the neonatal period by one of the many variations of anoplasty, depending upon the location of the fistula and its relationship to the external sphincter. This may range from simple perforation of a membrane to a complicated relocation procedure. Patients with supralevator defects treated initially by either diverting sigmoid or transverse colostomy should have contrast injection x-ray studies performed prior to definitive repair in order to be certain of the level of the rectal pouch and where rectourinary and rectovaginal fistulas communicate. This is the best guide to selection of the appropriate surgical approach.

The ultimate relationship of the rectum to the puborectalis sling is the major determinant of long-term fecal continence. Most repairs for low-lying defects result in satisfactory continence. However, despite the fact that procedures designed to preserve the relationship of the puborectalis to the rectum in supralevator repairs have been devised, the results still leave a 20% incidence of incontinence. Other factors are involved, such as the association of sacral anomalies and other conditions that result in deficient innervation of the levator mechanism.

RECTAL PROLAPSE

Rectal prolapse is a condition usually seen in the extremes of life. It involves the extrusion of one or more coats of the rectum. In 90% of children with this condition, prolapse is complete in that all layers of the bowel are involved.

Usually prolapse first presents in children between the first and third birthdays and is idiopathic. However, there are some physiological and anatomic reasons for prolapse to occur in this age group. As toddlers, children assume the erect position most of the time, often before pelvic and perineal structures have obtained full development. Also, there are some conditions which predispose to rectal prolapse, such as marked ascites in infants, sustained coughing, and excessive straining at stooling (as in children with constipation, parasites, colitis, or rectal polyps). Other disorders associated with rectal prolapse include meningomyelocele, exstrophy of the bladder, and such malabsorption disorders as untreated cystic fibrosis and celiac disease.

Initially, rectal prolapse presents as a painless protrusion of the distal rectum during defecation. When the child relaxes, the prolapse usually reduces spontaneously. In time, however, the prolapse may become more pronounced and require manual reduction. When the prolapse becomes severe or prolonged, marked edema and congestion may occur in the exposed rectal bud and hospitalization may be required.

Nonoperative therapy is usually all that is required. In rare, severe, and unrelenting situations, perianal injection of hypertonic saline or a modified Thiersch suture procedure may be necessary. Major operative correction is almost never required.

BIBLIOGRAPHY

DUHAMEL B: Retrorectal and transanal pull-through procedure for treatment of Hirschsprung's disease. Dis Colon Rectum 7:455, 1964

KIESEWETTER WB, CHANG JHT: Imperforate anus: A five to thirty year follow-up perspective. Progr Pediatr Surg 10:111, 1977

SOAVE F: Hirschsprung's disease: A new surgical technique. Arch Dis Child 39:116, 1964

STEPHENS FD, SMITH ED: Anorectal Malformations in Children. Chicago, Year Book Medical Publishers, 1971

SWENSON O, BILL AH: Resection of rectum and rectosigmoid with preservation of the sphincter for benign spastic lesions producing megacolon: An experimental study. Surgery 24:212, 1948

Moritz M. Ziegler

Gastrointestinal Problems After the First Month of Life

VOMITING
    Hypertrophic Pyloric Stenosis
    Gastroesophageal Reflux
    Other Causes
GASTROINTESTINAL BLEEDING
    Fissure in Ano
    Meckel's Diverticulum
    Intussusception
    Polyps
    Peptic Ulcer
    Portal Hypertension
    Other Causes
ABDOMINAL PAIN
    Acute Appendicitis
    Inflammatory Bowel Disease

VOMITING

Vomiting in infancy is common and is usually related to excessive feeding as suggested by the history, but surgical conditions must be excluded. Vomiting must be characterized as to frequency, volume, temporal and positional relationship to previous feedings, and color. Bilious vomiting should be assumed to be related to intestinal obstruction.

The physical examination of a vomiting child may reveal a normal, scaphoid, or distended abdominal contour. Palpation may demonstrate a mass, but most often physical findings are absent. Radiography is the primary means of evaluation. The use of barium contrast facilitates radiographic diagnosis, since one can evaluate esophageal motility, gastroesophageal reflux, the presence or absence of delayed gastric emptying, and the patency and position of the duodenum.

HYPERTROPHIC PYLORIC STENOSIS

Pyloric stenosis is a common disorder. More than 80% of infants with pyloric stenosis are males, 40% being the firstborn; the majority of patients are white. A familiar history of pyloric stenosis may be present. The onset of symptoms varies from the first week to the fourth month of life; the peak occurs between 4 to 6 weeks of life. Weight loss, constipation, and dehydration are common, but the diagnosis of pyloric stenosis is usually made on the basis of a history of projectile nonbilious vomiting, the presence of visible gastric waves on observation of the patient's abdomen, and the presence of a palpable pyloric "olive" or "tumor" on abdominal examination. Detection of the hypertrophied pylorus on examination is difficult in a child who is resisting and crying. In about 15% of patients, or those with an atypical presentation, an upper gastrointestinal tract x-ray series will be required to confirm the diagnosis (Fig. 41-6).

Prior to operation, metabolic alkalosis (see first section of this chapter) must be corrected with appropriate intravenous fluids, including potassium, as guided by serum electrolytes. Operative correction by the Fredet–Ramstedt pyloromyotomy is highly successful and associated with little or no morbidity or mortality, provided acid–base balance is normal preoperatively and any mucosal tear that might have occurred during operation does not go unnoticed.

GASTROESOPHAGEAL REFLUX

The incidence of gastroesophageal reflux in children is apparently increasing in the United States. This disorder may be closely linked to the normal maturation process in childhood in which the lower esophageal sphincter is poorly developed in the neonate and gradually matures at 1 or 2 years of age. Such patients present with varying degrees of regurgitation of feedings and vomiting immediately following feeding or sometimes several hours after eating. Patients with significant gastroesophageal reflux may present with failure to thrive, recurrent aspiration pneumonia, apnea, neurologic symptoms secondary to esophagitis and posturing of the head (Sandifer's syndrome), anemia secondary to chronic blood loss from esophagitis, and esophageal stricture.

The evaluation of the patient with esophageal reflux requires several studies. A barium contrast film is valuable in assessing esophageal motility as well as gastroesophageal reflux; however, the false-negative incidence approaches 50%. A radionuclide milk scan is a more sensitive study for assessing reflux, pulmonary aspiration, and rate of gastric

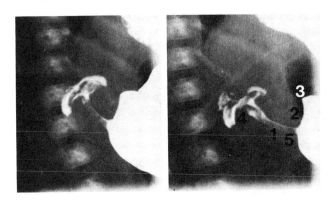

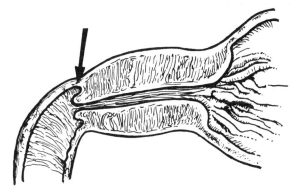

Fig. 41-6. (*Above, left*) Barium in stomach, showing long narrow pyloric canal emptying into the duodenum. (*Right*) (1) Unchanging elongated pyloric canal (note "railroad tracks" due to mucosal folds in flattened canal). (2) Impression of the hypertrophied muscle ("shoulder sign") is commonly seen on the lesser curvature and less commonly seen on the greater curvature. (3) Pylorus "tit" (junction of the lesser curvature with the hypertrophied muscle). This is exaggerated with peristalsis. (4) The base of the poorly filled duodenal bulb. (5) "Beak" sign, which is the beginning of the antral side of the pyloric canal and sometimes is seen without visualization of the remainder of the canal. (*Below*) Arrow indicates superficial position of the duodenal lumen. (Lynn HB: Hypertrophic pyloric stenosis. In Hardy JD [ed]: Rhoads Textbook of Surgery, 5th ed. Philadelphia, J B Lippincott, 1977)

emptying. Esophageal manometry measures both esophageal motility and lower esophageal sphincter pressure. Midesophageal *p*H monitoring may be the most sensitive index for determining the presence of reflux; *p*H scores are based on the frequency, duration, and degree of reflux episodes. Endoscopic analysis of gastroesophageal reflux includes visualization of reflux episodes and assessment of stricture and the degree of esophagitis present.

Only those infants with recurrent apneic spells or severe pulmonary soiling should be treated with primary operative intervention. All other patients should first be given a vigorous and prolonged trial of medical management, including use of thickened, more frequent, small-volume feedings and constant positioning in the 30° upright position. Hospital care should be tried for those who fail at home on a conservative regimen. Administration of antacids, cimetidine, and bethanechol is sometimes helpful also. If the medical management fails, Nissen fundoplication is the preferred operative approach along with gastrostomy in infants. Patients with neurologic problems are likely to require operative intervention more frequently than others. The results of operation are excellent in over 95% of patients, and mortality is rare.

OTHER CAUSES

Malrotation, duodenal stenosis, preduodenal portal vein, duodenal duplications, and other lesions that usually cause proximal intestinal obstruction in the neonate may present at several weeks or months of age if lesser degrees of obstruction are present. These conditions are described in the third section of this chapter.

GASTROINTESTINAL BLEEDING

The team approach to the bleeding child is required, and aggressive resuscitation in the presence of significant bleeding is urgent because of a limited reserve and a smaller circulating blood volume. The level of blood loss should first be assessed by noting stool color and volume and by placement of a nasogastric tube.

The etiology of gastrointestinal bleeding in childhood is age related (Tables 41-3 and 41-4). In the neonate, the major cause of bleeding is swallowed maternal blood, a formula allergy, or a colitis secondary to an infectious problem. Only in the sick child should such things as necrotizing enterocolitis, midgut volvulus, coagulation profile deficits, and intussusception be considered. Following the first month of life, fissure in ano is a common cause of bleeding, and Meckel's diverticulum and bleeding due to intussusception become significantly more frequent. It is only the older child in whom more serious causes of bleeding occur with greater frequency, specifically, peptic ulcer disease, vascular malformations, and portal hypertension with varices. It is also the older child who will have occult bleeding secondary to polyps.

TABLE 41-3 AGE-RELATED ETIOLOGY OF UPPER GASTROINTESTINAL TRACT BLEEDING

AGE	ETIOLOGY
Neonatal period	Swallowed maternal blood
	Hemorrhagic disease
	Esophagitis
	Hemorrhagic gastritis
	Stress ulcer
	Foreign-body irritation (nasogastric tube)
	Vascular malformations
Infancy	Esophagitis
	Mallory–Weiss tears
	Acute ulcer, gastritis
	Pyloric stenosis
	Vascular malformations
	Duplication
Preschool	Esophageal varices
	Esophagitis
	Foreign body
	Mallory–Weiss tears
	Acute ulcer, gastritis
	Vascular malformation
	Hemobilia
School age	Esophageal varices
	Esophagitis
	Mallory–Weiss tears
	Acute ulcer, gastritis
	Peptic disease
	Inflammatory bowel disease
	Hemobilia

TABLE 41-4   **AGE-RELATED ETIOLOGY OF LOWER GASTROINTESTINAL TRACT BLEEDING**

AGE	WELL INFANT	SICK INFANT
Neonatal period	Swallowed maternal blood	Necrotizing enterocolitis
	Infectious colitis	Infectious colitis
	Milk allergy	Disseminated coagulopathy
	Hemorrhagic disease	Midgut volvulus
	Duplication of bowel	Intussusception
	Meckel's diverticulum	Congestive heart failure
Infancy	Anal fissure	
	Infectious colitis	
	Milk allergy	
	Nonspecific colitis	
	Juvenile polyps	
	Intussusception	
	Meckel's diverticulum	
	Duplication	
	Hemolytic uremic syndrome	
	Inflammatory bowel disease	
Preschool	Infectious colitis	
	Juvenile polyps	
	Anal fissure	
	Intussusception	
	Meckel's diverticulum	
	Angiodysplasia	
	Henoch–Schönlein purpura	
	Hemolytic uremia	
	Inflammatory bowel disease	
School age	Infectious colitis	
	Inflammatory bowel disease	
	Polyps	
	Angiodysplasia	
	Hemolytic uremic syndrome	
	Hemorrhoids	

FISSURE IN ANO

An anal fissure is a split in the surface of the anocutaneous junction most commonly occurring in a patient several weeks to months of age who presents with bright-red blood on the stool surface or in the diaper. Such infants often have a history of constipation and intermittent episodes of pain on stooling. Diagnosis is by anoscopy. Treatment is conservative, in the form of anal dilatation, stool softeners, diet, and glycerine suppositories. Operation is rarely required.

MECKEL'S DIVERTICULUM

A Meckel's diverticulum occurs in 2% of children, and most are not symptomatic. Patients occasionally present with bleeding secondary to ectopic gastric mucosa and adjacent ileal ulceration, obstruction secondary to intussusception or volvulus of bowel around a persistent omphalomesenteric remnant extending to the umbilicus, or signs of peritonitis secondary to Meckel's diverticulitis. More than half of the symptomatic patients present before 2 years of age, and most have painless rectal bleeding.

The diagnosis of a Meckel's diverticulum is best made with a ^{99m}Tc scan, an isotope primarily concentrated by the ectopic gastric mucosa in the diverticulum. Such scans are positive in 85% of patients; the incidence of false-positive scans is rare, and such results usually demonstrate other significant pathology, including duplications, intussusception, hemangioma, and ulcers.

Operative indications for Meckel's diverticulectomy include recurrent severe lower gastrointestinal tract bleeding of unknown cause even in patients who have a negative scan and all the above-mentioned conditions as well. Operative management includes diverticulectomy or segmental resection of ileum with primary anastomosis. Whether it is prudent to do incidental Meckel's diverticulectomy during laparotomy done for other reasons is a matter of individual judgment at the time.

INTUSSUSCEPTION

Idiopathic intussusception occurs between 2 and 24 months of age, is more common in males, and seems to be seasonal (Fig. 41-7). Often there is a history of a recent upper respiratory tract infection or gastroenteritis, but the classic mode of presentation includes abdominal pain, an abdominal mass, passage of "currant jelly" stools, and vomiting.

Idiopathic intussusception is usually ileocolic, subsequently telescoping into the ascending and more distal colon. A progressive intussusception will eventually result in ischemic necrosis of the intussuscepted bowel, with potential perforation and peritonitis.

While history and physical findings are suggestive, x-ray films are confirmatory. A plain abdominal film may show a pattern of obstruction or may even be normal. A barium

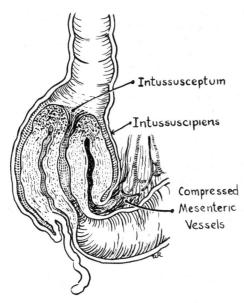

Fig. 41-7. An early ileocolic intussusception. (Courtesy of Dr William R Richardson; from Rosenkrantz JG: Ileocolic intussusception. In Hardy JD [ed]: Rhoads Textbook of Surgery, 5th ed. Philadelphia, J B Lippincott, 1977)

contrast study is essential to secure the diagnosis, but such patients should be prepared with a nasogastric tube, intravenous fluids, and morphine sedation beforehand. If the barium enema confirms the presence of an intussusception, and if the patient is free of peritoneal signs, systemic toxicity, or high-grade intestinal obstruction, hydrostatic reduction should be attempted. The barium column should not be elevated above 3 feet, no manual palpation or manipulation of the abdomen should be performed, and the child should be observed closely under fluoroscopy as the contrast column slowly reduces the intussusceptum back into its normal position. Successful hydrostatic reduction requires visualization of free reflux of barium into the distal ileum.

Indications for operation include failure of hydrostatic reduction, recurrence of ''idiopathic'' intussusception on two or three occasions, and signs of peritonitis, a long history and advanced obstruction. Preoperative administration of antibiotics is indicated. Manual reduction should be attempted at operation; if unsuccessful, resection with either primary anastomosis or temporary exteriorization is indicated. If a potential lead point is coincidentally found at the operating table, it should be resected and an appendectomy performed.

The recurrence rate is 12% following successful hydrostatic reduction and 3% following operative reduction. Approximately 5% of all patients with intussusception will have a lead point, the most common being a Meckel's diverticulum. Most will be older children. Other potential lead points include gastrointestinal polyps, duplications, vascular malformations, and ileocecal lymphoma.

POLYPS

Juvenile or inflammatory polyps are benign lesions that comprise the majority of polyps of the gastrointestinal tract. Most are solitary and colonic, 80% being in the rectosigmoid and 30% being palpable on rectal examination. Juvenile polyps present beginning at age 4 or 5; they rarely present after age 15. They present with intermittent, bright-red, painless rectal bleeding; prolapse through the anal canal; or as lead points for intussusception. Endoscopic removal is indicated for symptomatic patients.

Peutz-Jeghers syndrome in children is associated with gastric, colonic, and small-intestinal polyps. This hamartomatous lesion of the intestinal tract has a dominant inheritance and occurs predominantly in the muscularis mucosa; such patients present with classic findings of pigmentation of their lips or buccal mucosa. Polyps in the small bowel can serve as lead points for intussusception or can cause intermittent bleeding. Malignancy rarely occurs in these patients.

Gardner's syndrome also has a dominant inheritance; this lesion presents as colonic and small-bowel polyps, soft-tissue tumors, and osteomas. The polyps are adenomatous and have malignant potential.

Malignancy is most commonly associated with familial polyposis of the colon, in which adenomatous polyps are present and are inherited on a dominant basis.

PEPTIC ULCER

Peptic ulcer disease occurs occasionally in childhood, usually after the age of 6. Infants tend to develop acute gastric or duodenal ulcers, but the older child presents with chronic duodenal ulcer more commonly. Chronic ulcer disease occurs three times more frequently in males than in females, and as many as 25% of children have a positive family history of peptic ulcer disease. Pain and upper gastrointestinal tract bleeding are the most common presenting symptoms.

Definitive diagnostic studies include upper gastrointestinal tract x-ray series and gastroduodenoscopy. Medical and surgical management is similar to that described for adults. Those children who present with chronic duodenal ulcer disease early in life require definitive operation more often than adults.

PORTAL HYPERTENSION

Portal hypertension with bleeding esophageal and gastric varices is the most common cause of massive upper gastrointestinal tract hemorrhage in the child beyond the first month of life. The essentials of this disorder and its variations are covered in the first section of Chapter 27.

OTHER CAUSES

Intestinal duplications as previously described, irritation from foreign bodies, Mallory–Weiss tears from forceful vomiting, and a variety of vascular malformations may be associated with significant bleeding also. Henoch–Schönlein purpura and small-bowel intussusception may cause mild bleeding.

ABDOMINAL PAIN

Abdominal pain may be due to a wide variety of acute and chronic organic and psychological disorders. Pertinent history includes nature, duration, intensity, and location of the pain; diet and feeding habits; stooling pattern; growth patterns; associated illnesses; and medication history.

The physical examination must be done in a quiet area on a cooperative person if masses or subtle degrees of peritoneal irritation are to be detected. Sedation and patience are often required. Repeated examination is frequently the key to establishing the need for operation. Percussion is usually more helpful than rebound palpation in the evaluation of tenderness. While routine laboratory tests and abdominal films are decidedly helpful, physical examination is usually the most help in evaluation of the child with abdominal pain.

Many of the same entities that cause bleeding, such as Henoch–Schönlein purpura, may cause pain. Additionally, a number of medical disorders, such as sickle-cell disease, hemophilia, nephrosis, and diabetes, may have abdominal pain associated with acute episodes of illness. The most common problems are infectious. In fact, distinguishing bacterial gastroenteritis from acute appendicitis is the major problem in evaluation of abdominal pain in childhood.

ACUTE APPENDICITIS

Acute appendicitis is covered in Chapter 25. Certain additional considerations relative to children are worthy of mention. The incidence of perforation is much higher in childhood than later in life, as high as 80% in those under the age of 4 years. The clinical course tends to progress more rapidly in the younger patient, since mechanisms for localizing intra-abdominal perforation are less efficient in infants and young children. In this sense, operative management is more emergent than in the adult age-group.

Operative intervention in childhood appendicitis is comparable to techniques used in the adult. In the face of perforative appendicitis, antibiotics should be administered preoperatively. Appendectomy should always be the goal of operation, and abandoning this goal with subsequent interval appendectomy should be considered only if the child's life would be jeopardized otherwise.

INFLAMMATORY BOWEL DISEASE

Noninfectious inflammatory bowel disease usually implies the diagnosis of either ulcerative colitis or Crohn's disease,

disease entities that are uncommon in the young child but that become progressively more common with age. Other painful inflammatory bowel conditions include hemolytic uremic syndrome, radiation enterocolitis, ischemic colitis, graft-versus-host disease in bone marrow transplant patients, and various types of vasculitis.

The treatment of all these various forms of inflammatory bowel disease is supportive medical therapy. In Crohn's disease, those patients who require operation for complications should have total resection of involved bowel if possible. Every effort should be made to conserve bowel length, because the recurrence rate is 50%. Classic surgical approaches to ulcerative colitis are in order, except that there is recent evidence to suggest that endorectal pull-through and sphincter preservation may be a useful alternative to standard ileostomy.

BIBLIOGRAPHY

ABRAMS R, LYNN HB: Rectal bleeding in children. Am J Surg 104:831, 1962

EIN SH, STEPHENS CA: Intussusception: 354 Cases in 10 years. J Pediatr Surg 6:16, 1971

FONKALSRUD EW: Surgical management of portal hypertension in childhood: Long-term results. Arch Surg 115:1042, 1980

GELLIS SS (ed): Gastroesophageal Reflux: Report of the Seventy-sixth Ross Conference on Pediatric Research. Columbus, Ross Laboratories, 1979

HOLGERSON LO, MILLER RE, ZINTEL HA: Juvenile polyps of the colon. Surgery 69:288, 1971

RAFFENSBERGER JG, LUCK SR: Gastrointestinal bleeding in children. Surg Clin North Am 56:413, 1976

SAVRIN RA, CLATWORTHY HW: Appendiceal rupture: A continuing diagnostic problem. Pediatrics 63:37, 1979

SCHARLI AF, SIEBER WK, KIESEWETTER WB: Hypertrophic pyloric stenosis at the Children's Hospital of Pittsburgh from 1912–1967: A critical review of current problems and complications. J Pediatr Surg 4:108, 1969

SHERMAN NJ, SWANSON V, FLEISCHER D et al: Regional enteritis in childhood, J Pediatr Surg 7:585, 1972

WERLIN SL, GRAND RJ: Severe colitis in children and adolescents: Diagnosis, course and treatment. Gastroenterology 73:828, 1977

Louise Schnaufer

Disorders of the Liver, Biliary Tree, and Pancreas

BILIARY ATRESIA
MANAGEMENT OF INFANTS WITH OBSTRUCTIVE
      JAUNDICE
  Surgical Management
CHOLEDOCHAL CYST
CHOLECYSTITIS AND CHOLELITHIASIS
PANCREATITIS

In evaluating the infant with protracted hyperbilirubinemia, the goal is to rule out specific treatable diseases in order to define the infant who may benefit from surgical treatment. The differentiation between unconjugated hyperbilirubinemia and the conjugated form is not difficult, and the diagnosis of physiological jaundice of the premature

or full-term neonate can easily be made. However, jaundice persisting after 3 to 4 weeks of age implies conjugated hyperbilirubinemia of the cholestatic type. Cholestasis is the result of either a mechanical obstruction to bile flow or a functional disturbance with failure to generate bile flow.

A definitive diagnosis can be made in the majority of instances by appropriate studies to determine hemolytic, metabolic, toxic, or septic causes of biliary secretory failure. Appropriate cultures, both bacterial and viral, Coombs' test, coagulation profile, TORCH titers, α_1-antitrypsin, and lipoprotein determinations are required to differentiate cholestatic jaundice from obstructive jaundice.

Although 90% of jaundiced babies can be diagnosed and treated, the remainder who have obstructive cholangiopathy present a diagnostic dilemma. In spite of radionuclide scanning of the liver, ultrasonography, and liver biopsy, the differentiation between neonatal hepatitis and biliary atresia often requires a laparotomy and cholangiogram.

BILIARY ATRESIA

Biliary atresia is a congenital anomaly of the intrahepatic and extrahepatic biliary systems in which an ongoing sclerotic or inflammatory process leads to fibrosis and obliteration of the ducts. Two types of biliary atresia are described based on the gross appearance of the extrahepatic biliary system observed at operation. The so-called correctable type is quite rare, accounting for only 5% of children with biliary atresia. In this form, there is an isolated atresia of the common bile duct with patency proximal to the obstruction. Drainage can be accomplished by a Roux-en-Y jejunal anastomosis to the proximal patent duct. Although one would expect the salvage rate of infants with this correctable form to be high, as many as 90% may succumb to ongoing cirrhosis and liver failure, indicating that this correctable type of biliary atresia is only a variation of the ongoing obliteration of intrahepatic ducts that occurs in the noncorrectable type.

More than 90% of children with biliary atresia have noncorrectable anatomy. Although the etiology has never been identified, an intrauterine viral infection of the fetal liver has long been thought to be the most likely cause. There is a 10% to 15% incidence of associated intra-abdominal anomalies.

From the recent results of operating on these infants before the age of 3 months there is considerable evidence that this is an ongoing process. A baby operated on within the first 4 weeks of life may have a patent distal extrahepatic system with a patent gallbladder but fibrosis of the common hepatic duct at the hilum of the liver. In older infants the extrahepatic system may be completely fibrotic with an atretic gallbladder, or both may be absent.

MANAGEMENT OF INFANTS WITH OBSTRUCTIVE JAUNDICE

When the initial screening of infants with cholestatic jaundice has ruled out metabolic, septic, or genetic diseases, the differentiation between neonatal hepatitis and biliary atresia always presents a problem. Although occasionally the diagnosis may be made on clinical grounds, it is more often necessary to resort to laparotomy and cholangiography.

Most preoperative tests, including needle biopsy of the liver, are ambiguous in differentiating the two diseases. Alkaline phosphatase levels are higher in biliary atresia than in neonatal hepatitis, whereas elevated SGPT and SGOT

ATRESIA OF THE BILE DUCTS	
Etiology	Congenital abnormality
Dx	Jaundice appears during first 2 weeks of life; progressive, dark urine, acholic stools. Exclude neonatal jaundice and hepatitis
Rx	Operate 4 to 5 weeks after birth to prevent permanent liver damage

levels may indicate neonatal hepatitis. An elevated serum α-fetoprotein level may also suggest neonatal hepatitis. Radionuclide ^{99}Tc-PIPIDA studies are useful in determining hepatobiliary secretion with low radiation, fine definition, and rapid excretion of the isotope. However, lack of excretion does not necessarily rule out neonatal hepatitis if cholestasis is so severe that the biliary ductules are mechanically obstructed. Twenty-four hour duodenal drainage for visible bile is another useful screening study.

Screening for α$_1$-antitrypsin deficiency has separated out a large segment of infants who previously were thought to have neonatal hepatitis.

SURGICAL MANAGEMENT

Operation is best done before the age of 3 months and is ideally performed between the ages of 3 and 6 weeks if further obliteration of the intrahepatic ductal system is to be avoided. Liver biopsy and an operative cholangiogram are done initially if a gallbladder with a lumen is present. The presence of bile in the gallbladder suggests a patent system, and if this is confirmed on cholangiography, the diagnosis of neonatal hepatitis or hypoplasia of the bile ducts is made and the procedure is terminated. On the other hand, if the gallbladder is atretic or if there is no reflux of dye into the liver, further exploration is done.

In 1955 Kasai reported that although no visible external ducts may be evident, microscopic ductules may exist in the fibrotic mass at the hilum. After excising the entire extrahepatic biliary tree and transecting it directly at the hilum, a portoenterostomy is done with a Roux-en-Y segment of jejunum. Postoperative cholangitis is a serious problem, but the incidence appears to decrease after the age of 1 year, and during this time the children should be maintained on antibiotics. Biliary cirrhosis and portal hypertension are the eventual outcome in at least 50% of long-term survivors.

The major factors affecting the survival of these patients seem to be primarily the age of the child at the time of portoenterostomy, operative technique, and the avoidance of cholangitis; one third of patients with biliary atresia now survive 5 years or more.

CHOLEDOCHAL CYST

A choledochal cyst is a rounded dilatation of the common bile duct between the junction of the cystic duct and its duodenal outlet. The distal portion of the common duct is partially obstructed, and generally the proximal ducts and liver parenchyma are normal. The wall of the cyst is fibrous with no epithelial lining, and inflammation is noted.

In infancy the most common sign is jaundice, but in older children a right upper quadrant mass, vague abdominal pain, and occasional mild episodes of jaundice are more useful.

Liver function tests and bilirubin determinations during the acute episode will indicate obstructive jaundice, and signs of pancreatitis may also be present. An upper gastrointestinal barium study may demonstrate an indentation of the duodenum. Smaller cysts are easily found by ultrasonography, and dilatation of intrahepatic ducts can also be demonstrated by this technique.

After operative drainage of the cyst into the duodenum or into a Roux-en-Y limb of jejunum, long-term follow-up may show failure of the cyst to decrease in size, stricture of the anastomosis, progressive dilatation of the intrahepatic ducts, continuing episodes of ascending cholangitis with resultant hepatic fibrosis, and development of portal hypertension. Results from Japan suggest that excision of the choledochal cyst with Roux-en-Y drainage of the proximal hepatic ducts is the treatment of choice.

CHOLECYSTITIS AND CHOLELITHIASIS

The causes of cholecystitis and cholelithiasis in children differ from those in adults in that children have a higher incidence of an associated disease such as hereditary hemolytic anemia; the incidence of biliary tract calculi in children with spherocytosis is as high as 60%. Of children with sickle cell disease and thalassemia major 10% to 20% develop stones. Children with chronic renal disease or ileal loops for urinary diversion may also develop cholelithiasis.

Acalculous cholecystitis is usually associated with dehydration, sepsis, or a severe burn. It is often seen in children with *Salmonella* infections and some viremias.

Symptoms of gallbladder disease in children are similar to those in adults including fatty food intolerance, abdominal pain, and febrile episodes with or without jaundice. Cholecystectomy is the treatment of choice with exploration of the common duct and cholangiography if indicated. In children with cholelithiasis and spherocytosis, cholecystostomy with removal of stones may be done rather than cholecystectomy at the time of splenectomy.

PANCREATITIS

Pancreatitis occurs in childhood more frequently than is generally recognized and may be associated with a mortality of as high as 30%. The pathology of acute pancreatitis is autodigestion, which may present as hemorrhagic fat necrosis or simply as an edematous pancreas. The pathogenesis is unclear, with 50% of cases classified as idiopathic. Anomalies of ductal drainage and familial metabolic abnormalities explain many cases. Pancreatitis frequently oc-

curs in a severely ill child who may be septic, traumatized, or very dehydrated and who has severe acute abdominal pain. Although trauma and infection seem to cause pancreatitis most frequently, its association with drugs such as steroids and valproic acid is recognized. Pseudocyst may follow blunt trauma.

The diagnosis of acute pancreatitis is made by determination of an elevated serum amylase. Confirmation of chronic pancreatitis depends upon history, notation of calcification on plain x-rays, or demonstration of ductal deformity on endoscopic retrograde pancreatography.

Treatment of acute pancreatitis is directed toward the prevention of vascular collapse due to third space sequestration by the inflamed pancreas, correction of dehydration and electrolyte imbalance, and control of pain. Nasogastric suction, intravenous fluids, and antibiotics are indicated. In more severe cases, ventilatory assistance, central venous monitoring, and peritoneal lavage may be necessary. Surgery is rarely needed but exploratory surgery with another diagnosis in mind is often performed because acute pancreatitis is rarely thought of in childhood. If acute pancreatitis is encountered, the biliary tree need not be explored. The peritoneal cavity should be thoroughly lavaged and the lesser sac drained. Nutritional support is extremely important. Patients with chronic pancreatitis may require sphincteroplasty for jaundice or pancreatic ductal drainage into the intestine.

BIBLIOGRAPHY

BUNTAIN WL, WOOD JB, WOOLLEY MM: Pancreatitis in childhood, J Pediatr Surg, 1978

GREENE HL, HELINEK GL, MORAN R et al: A diagnostic approach to prolonged obstructive jaundice by 24-hour collection of duodenal fluid. J Pediatr 95:412, 1979

HOLCOMB GW, O'NEILL JA, HOLCOMB G: Cholecystitis, cholelithiasis, and common duct stenosis in children and adolescence. Ann Surg 191:626, 1980

KASAI M, SUZUKI H, OHASHI E et al: Technique and results of operative management of biliary atresia. World J Surg 2:571, 1978

O'NEILL JA, CLATWORTHY HW: Management of choledochal cysts: A 14 year followup. Am Surg 37:230, 1971

Harry C. Bishop

Disorders of Abdominal Wall and Inguinal Canal in Infants and Children

DISORDERS OF THE ABDOMINAL WALL

DIASTASIS RECTUS ABDOMINIS

A midline separation of the two rectus abdominis muscles occurs in infancy and is demonstrated by a symmetrical bulging from the xyphoid to the umbilicus when the infant or child increases his intra-abdominal pressure. This is a self-limiting weakness and becomes less prominent or disappears when the infant matures. It does not require surgical correction.

EPIPLOCELE (EPIGASTRIC HERNIA)

This is a small defect of the linea alba fascia that occurs in the midline anywhere from the xyphoid to the umbilicus but is found most frequently a third of the way up from the umbilicus toward the xyphoid. With increasing intra-abdominal pressure, properitoneal fat bulges out through the defect and produces a visible and palpable mass that may cause abdominal pain and may be tender to palpation. If the properitoneal fat becomes incarcerated, the mass is irreducible. Surgical repair is indicated.

OMPHALOCELE

An omphalocele is a persistence of the normal extracoelomic stage of development with herniation of bowel and liver into the umbilical cord region. The intact amnion and peritoneum forming the sac that covers the herniated, nonrotated viscera are transparent but rapidly become dried and eventually will become permeable to bacteria or will rupture. Such an infant should be operated on without delay, and the sac should be kept covered with a sterile dressing until operation is accomplished. Nasogastric suction should be used early to avoid distention of the intestinal tract, which will make primary reduction more difficult. Small omphaloceles are easily repaired by excising the omphalocele sac and cord, closing the defect primarily. Medium-sized omphaloceles may be handled by inverting the intact sac into the abdominal cavity and closing the anterior rectus fascia in the midline over it. Very large intact omphalocele sacs frequently contain the liver and the intestinal tract. These have been successfully handled by mobilizing the skin laterally and inferiorly and converting the sac into a large ventral hernia by the method of Gross. Recently some surgeons have preferred excision of the sac with construction of a Silastic silo (see next section on gastroschisis), which allows time to enlarge the abdominal cavity. Occasionally the omphalocele sac ruptures *in utero,* allowing evisceration of the intestinal tract out in the amniotic cavity, which produces a thickening and apparent shortening. Following either primary or staged repair with a prosthesis, prolonged intravenous nutrition is necessary, but eventually the bowel improves and peristalsis returns. Occasionally atresia of the intestinal tract is associated with omphalocele, and in such cases failure of normal rotation and fixation is usually present but rarely leads to secondary volvulus of the midgut. Associated anomalies, particularly cardiac anomalies, are common and adversely affect survival in patients with large omphalocele defects.

GASTROSCHISIS

Gastroschisis is a complicated anomaly in which a major portion of the intestinal tract herniates out through a small defect to the right of the umbilical cord in the area of the umbilicus. This probably results from an *in utero* rupture of an umbilical hernia, allowing the intestinal tract to eviscerate through a relatively small defect of the abdominal wall and producing thickening and foreshortening of the intestinal

tract due to chronic exposure to amniotic fluid. Sometimes an acquired atresia of the intestinal tract is present or a portion of the intestinal tract may become gangrenous due to constriction of the mesentery at the level of the defect.

These infants should be transported to a special care center with nasogastric suction and the eviscerated intestinal tract placed in a plastic bag or covered with sterile gauze to protect the bowel and to avoid hypothermia during transfer.

At the time of surgery the intestinal tract is cleansed, and the abdominal wall defect is enlarged in the midline. An effort is made to stretch the intra-abdominal cavity in order to replace the enlarged intestinal tract in the general abdominal cavity with primary closure of the midline defect if possible. If a primary closure cannot be accomplished without producing intolerable elevation of the diaphragms or venous engorgement from pressure on the vena cava, a Silastic silo is used, and staged reduction is performed. Postoperatively, these infants require endotracheal respiratory support for a variable period of time as well as intravenous hyperalimentation for a period of weeks until the intestinal tract improves, peristalsis returns, and oral alimentation is possible. These measures have improved survival to over 90%.

PERSISTENCE OF OMPHALOMESENTERIC DUCT

Persistence of an intact omphalomesenteric duct (Fig. 41-8) with drainage of intestinal contents at the umbilicus

Fig. 41-8. This drawing depicts the variations in persistence of the omphalomesenteric duct. (*A*) Open, draining omphalomesenteric remnant. (*B*) Fibrotic band remnant, which frequently serves as a point of volvulus. (*C*) Omphalomesenteric duct cyst. (*D*) Meckel's diverticulum.

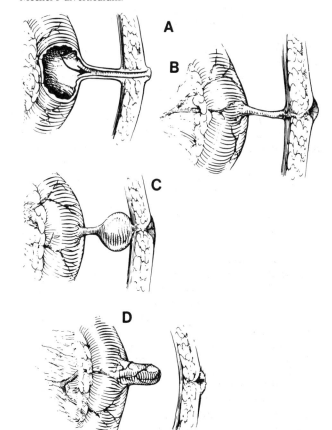

is a very rare anomaly. More frequently, only the proximal end persists as a Meckel's diverticulum with or without a connection to the underside of the umbilicus as a fibrous stalk or cyst. Although the surgery for a patent omphalomesenteric duct is not urgent, it is well to perform surgical correction before complications occur or chronic infection of the skin around the umbilicus becomes troublesome.

UMBILICAL GRANULOMA

Granulation tissue in the base of the umbilicus after most of the umbilical cord sloughs away is a common problem. These granulomas should be cauterized with silver nitrate followed by alcohol, and general good hygiene of the area should be maintained. If silver nitrate treatment does not eliminate the polyp of granulation tissue, this should be excised.

PATENT URACHUS

A patent urachus will allow leakage of urine onto the umbilical area owing to the persistence of the congenital fistula to the dome of the bladder. It is a rare anomaly and is frequently seen in infants when there is a congenital deficiency of the abdominal musculature, the so-called prune belly. All patients with a patent urachus develop irritation around the umbilicus. Before surgical correction, attention must be directed to the bladder and urethra to be certain there is no obstruction that is producing back pressure and causing the persistence of the draining urachus.

UMBILICAL HERNIA

Weakness of the umbilical area, although present from birth, usually does not become apparent until a few weeks after birth when the umbilical scar has completely healed. The defect may gradually enlarge and become a marked protuberance, even though the ring through the abdominal wall may be small.

Umbilical hernias are common, are frequently familial, and are especially common in the black race. Incarceration rarely occurs, and spontaneous obliteration of the defect occurs in 80% to 90% of patients, so surgical correction is not indicated in infancy or early childhood unless there has been a history of incarceration or other complications. Because defects that have a supraumbilical component do not tend to correct themselves, they may be repaired early.

Adhesive strapping is not effective therapy and causes skin problems. Surgical repair is indicated by 5 or 6 years of age if the hernia has stabilized and shows no regression in the size of the ring.

INGUINAL HERNIA AND HYDROCELES

Congenital inguinal hernia is the most common congenital anomaly occurring in humans. Familial incidence is high, and it is found 10 times more frequently in males than in females. It is more frequent in prematurely born infants than in full-term infants, undoubtedly because of an arrest of the normal obliteration of the processus vaginalis at the time of birth. Embryologically, the processus vaginalis opens through the internal and external rings and descends into the scrotum at about 3 months of gestation. By 7 months of gestation the processus vaginalis still persists, and the testicle descends extraperitoneally from its origin near the

kidney. By 9 months of gestation the testicle has made its full descent into the scrotum, and the processus vaginalis is obliterated, leaving a patent tunica vaginalis around the testicle. If there is an arrest of completion of this normal process, many variations can result.

As seen in Figure 41-9, if the processus vaginalis has not been obliterated, a long indirect inguinal hernia sac descends and surrounds the testicle. If a portion of the hernia distally has been obliterated, there is a normal tunica vaginalis and a shorter length of hernia sac leading part way down the cord. If obliteration has started but has not been completed, the sac may be narrowed, leading to a collection of fluid around the testicle and communicating with the abdominal cavity, producing a so-called communicating hydrocele. If the distal portion of the sac above the tunica has obliterated and another portion has narrowed, a hydrocele of the cord may result. A hydrocele of the cord usually indicates the presence of a communicating hernia sac above the hydrocele opening into the general peritoneal cavity at the internal ring.

The presence of an indirect inguinal hernia may become apparent in the first few days of life or any time through infancy, childhood, or adolescence. Frequently there is a bulge as a loop of intestine distends the hernia sac intermittently, or there may be a varied amount of fluid in a hydrocele of the tunica vaginalis or a hydrocele of the cord in which a detectable thickness of the cord suggests the presence of an empty hernia sac. When there is a suspicion of a hernia in an infant or child, the presence of the hernia sac can frequently be detected either by the thickness of the spermatic cord just distal to the internal ring or by the so-called silk glove sign, by which one examining hand holds a slight amount of tension on the testicle in the scrotum while an examining finger of the opposite hand runs back and forth across the cord. The two smooth anterior and posterior peritoneal membranes crossing over one another produce a characteristic feel. This is the best way of determining the presence of a hernia in an infant or a child and is better than inverting the scrotum and having the patient cough against a finger at the external ring. Although this method is used in adults, it is painful and unreliable in children.

PHYSIOLOGICAL HYDROCELE

During the spontaneous closure of the processus vaginalis, there may be an extra amount of peritoneal fluid trapped in the tunica vaginalis around the testicle. This may persist for 6 months or more without change. Frequently there is difficulty in determining whether such a hydrocele is physiological and will spontaneously resolve, or whether there is communication and thus a potential risk of an associated inguinal hernia. Such infants should be observed in order to detect a variation in the amount of fluid in the tunica vaginalis that suggests a communication to the abdominal cavity or a bulging in a hernia along the inguinal canal.

TIMING OF HERNIA REPAIR

Ideally, all hernias should be repaired prior to incarceration because this can lead to strangulation of a loop of intestine or can damage the spermatic cord, leading to atrophy of the testicle. Unlike management of incarceration in adults, management of infants and children who present with incarceration usually involves reduction in the emergency

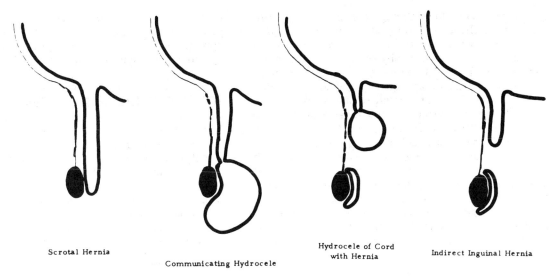

Scrotal Hernia Communicating Hydrocele Hydrocele of Cord with Hernia Indirect Inguinal Hernia

Fig. 41-9. The variants of incomplete development of the inguinal canal structures.

room or the physician's office and elective repair a day or two later, but such patients should be admitted to the hospital for observation to be sure that bowel damage has not occurred.

Unfortunately, differentiation of an incarcerated hernia from an acute hydrocele of the cord with the small empty hernia sac above it is often difficult. If there is doubt about this differential diagnosis, emergency surgery should be performed.

INCIDENCE OF BILATERALITY

Many infants and children have bilateral hernias. Such hernias are particularly common in infants born prematurely and occur in 50% of infants under 1 year of age, so many pediatric surgeons routinely perform bilateral exploration in this age group. In infants more than 1 year of age, the surgeon should be selective and should operate on the opposite side only if there is evidence that a hernia is present. Children with hernias that present on the left have a statistically greater chance of having an associated one on the right; bilateral exploration and repair may be advised if the surgeon is anxious to avoid a second operative procedure with its anesthetic risks because of cardiac or other associated disorders.

OPERATIVE REPAIR

The surgeon's role is to eliminate the surgical remnant that failed to obliterate. These young patients require a careful dissection of the hernia sac away from the spermatic cord and a high ligation of the sac at the level of the internal ring. The internal ring need not be narrowed, and the cord should not be transplanted to an abnormal location. The external oblique aponeurosis is opened, but the external ring may be left intact (see also Chapter 32).

HERNIAS IN THE FEMALE

In the female the processus vaginalis goes down through the same internal and external rings as it does in the male but adjacent to the round ligament. This processus is more likely to be obliterated in the female. The female, however,

frequently will have the fallopian tube as a sliding component of the hernia sac and might present with an ovary in the sac that is felt as a small rounded mass, loosely trapped beyond the external ring. Surgical repair is straightforward if there is no sliding component; but if there is a sliding fallopian tube, the hernia sac should be doubly ligated distal to the sliding component and then the closed hernia sac inverted into the abdominal cavity through a purse-string suture taken around the neck of the sac with closure of the internal ring.

RECURRENCE AND AFTER CARE

Because these are embryologic remnants that have been excised at the time of surgery, the recurrence rate is low and is generally considered to be about 1 in 300. Because there is no weakness of the area, there is no need for postoperative restriction of activity or prolonged hospitalization.

CONGENITAL UNDESCENDED TESTICLE

Unilateral congenital undescended testicle is a relatively common anomaly, but bilateral nondescent is rare. Like inguinal hernias, congenital undescended testicle is caused by an arrest of the embryologic descent of the testis outside the processus on its way to the scrotum, so persistence of the processus vaginalis as a hernia is commonly associated with undescended testis.

The *retractile testis* is due to an overactive cremasteric response. The true retractile testis can be differentiated by obtaining the youngster's confidence and examining him in a warm room in the supine position. It will be found that the testicle can be milked gently down into the scrotum, where it remains until stroking on the medial side of the thigh produces the cremaster response, causing the testicle to rise up in the inguinal canal. This is a self-limiting problem and needs no therapy. When the testicle becomes heavier by its own maturation, it will remain in the scrotum. Much of the confusion about the success of exogenous hormone treatment for youngsters with "undescended testicles" is based on the error of diagnosis of retractile testis.

In patients with true embryologic nondescent, the testicle

cannot be pushed down through the inguinal canal into the scrotum. The associated inguinal hernia that occurs in 90% of cases may or may not be symptomatic. If the hernia is symptomatic, a herniorrhaphy and orchidopexy must be done earlier than would be ideal. In experienced hands, elective herniorrhaphy and orchidopexy should be done around 1 year of age but certainly should be accomplished before the age of 5 because there are damaging histologic changes in testicles operated upon past that age. The operation frees the inguinal hernia from the spermatic cord so that the latter may be freed upward and lengthened. The testicle characteristically is more spherical in shape and has a very loosely attached epididymis. Care must be taken not to damage the epididymis, particularly since it may have an inferior segment considerably lower than the gonad. Prostheses may be required for children who have no testes or for those who have intra-abdominal testes that cannot be brought down.

TORSION OF THE TESTIS

Acute torsion of the testis can occur unexpectedly in children who appear normal and is particularly frequent in youngsters with embryologically undescended testicles. There is need for early diagnosis because torsion will rapidly lead to devascularization of the gonad. Epididymitis is confused with torsion, and examination of the urine for infection and use of the Doppler ultrasound equipment to determine vascularity of the testicle can be helpful in this differentiation. When in doubt, the testicle should be explored through a scrotal incision, and even if its viability is questioned after release of the torsion, the testicle should probably be fixed in the scrotum with the hope that it will survive. The opposite side should be examined and fixed at the same operation because the condition is usually bilateral.

TORSION OF THE APPENDIX TESTIS

The appendix testis is a prominent structure in many males who are prone to torsion. This structure is at the top of the testicle close to the epididymis and on occasion it can volvulize, producing acute scrotal pain with some hydrocele fluid and exquisite point tenderness at the local site. Although these signs are not damaging to the rest of the structures in the area, they do produce prolonged symptoms. It is relatively simple to open the scrotum and excise the gangrenous appendix testis, which immediately relieves the uncomfortable symptoms.

BIBLIOGRAPHY

ALLEN RG, WRENN EL: Silon as a sac in the treatment of omphalocele and gastroschisis. J Pediatr Surg 4:3, 1969

JACKSON DJ, MOGLEN LH: Umbilical hernia: A retrospective study. Calif Med 113:8, 1970

JONES P: Torsion of testis and its appendages during childhood. Arch Dis Child 37:214, 1962

KIESEWETTER WB: Undescended testes: Surgery and its results. Am Surg 37:20, 1971

ROWE MI, COPELSON LW, CLATWORTHY HW: The patent processus vaginalis and the inguinal hernia. J Pediatr Surg 4:102, 1969

SCHUSTER SR: A new method for the staged repair of large omphaloceles. Surg Gynecol Obstet 125:837, 1967

SONDERLUND S: Meckel's diverticulum, a clinical and histologic study. Acta Chir Scand (Suppl) 248:1, 1959

Harry C. Bishop

Sinuses, Cysts, and Benign Tumors of Childhood

PREAURICULAR SINUSES
FISTULAS AND CARTILAGE REMNANTS
  First Branchial Cleft Fistula
  Second Branchial Cleft Fistula
  Branchial Cartilage Remnants
CYSTS
  Branchial Cleft Cyst
  Thyroglossal Duct Cyst
  Dermoid Cysts
BENIGN TUMORS
  Torticollis
  Lymphangioma—Cystic Hygroma
  Hemangioma
  Juvenile Breast Hypertrophy
  Fibroadenoma of the Breast
  Teratoma

Benign masses are common in childhood and are most frequently congenital. All unexplained tumors must be viewed with suspicion because unusual malignancies can occur throughout the body. Biopsy or excision is usually necessary for precise diagnosis. Congenital lesions require an understanding of the embryology involved for appropriate surgical management.

PREAURICULAR SINUSES

Preauricular sinuses occur unilaterally or bilaterally and are often familial. These sinuses have an external opening on the tragus of the ear and can be probed. The tract descends anteriorly superficial to the parotid gland and may have branching of the sinus below the skin level.

Preauricular sinuses are prone to infection. Once infection has occurred they frequently require incision and drainage and then later removal. Occasionally a buried cyst will form without obvious infection. These are best removed by injecting a small amount of methylene blue through the external opening and then adequately removing all involved tissue.

FISTULAS AND CARTILAGE REMNANTS

FIRST BRANCHIAL CLEFT FISTULA

The first branchial cleft, with either a cyst or a fistula, is rare and is dangerously located just below the ear, frequently with a connection to the external auditory canal and close approximation with the facial nerve. Surgical excision is indicated.

SECOND BRANCHIAL CLEFT FISTULA

A fistula of the second branchial cleft has an external opening in the lower neck along the anterior border of the sternocleidomastoid muscle and runs subcutaneously external to the deep fascia for a variable distance superiorly before it makes a right angle bend, descending through the deeper neck structures between the internal and external carotid arteries to an internal opening at the tonsillar fossa. These lesions can occur unilaterally or bilaterally and may be familial.

Elective surgical excision is recommended before infection occurs in the tract, which complicates the surgical removal. Occasionally an incision and drainage of an abscess followed by later excision must be done. Excision must be as complete as possible if recurrence is to be avoided.

BRANCHIAL CARTILAGE REMNANTS

Buried segments of cartilage, usually with an associated skin tag, occur in front of the ear and along the lateral neck without an associated fistula. These are excised for cosmetic reasons, and the cartilage is completely removed from the deeper neck.

CYSTS

BRANCHIAL CLEFT CYST

A branchial cleft cyst is a rare anomaly that does not have an external opening and gradually enlarges. It is most commonly seen in the midlateral neck and should be totally excised before it becomes infected.

THYROGLOSSAL DUCT CYST

The thyroid gland originates at the foramen caecum at the base of the tongue and descends, perforating the midportion of the hyoid bone, to its normal location on either side of the trachea. Remnants may be left anywhere from the foramen caecum area of the tongue to the pyramidal lobe of the thyroid either in the midline or slightly to the left. The most common presentation is a relatively superficial mass just to the left of the midline either directly over or slightly inferior to the hyoid bone. This cystic remnant frequently becomes infected and may require incision and drainage. Ideally, the cyst and its proximal tract should be excised before infection occurs. Along with excision of the cyst, the midportion of the hyoid bone should be excised, and any tract leading back to the base of the tongue should be excised and securely ligated. If the entire tract is not excised, recurrence is frequent.

In very rare instances a presumed cyst is found to be solid thyroid tissue. It should be bivalved and a biopsy should be done. A scan is done later to determine if there is a thyroid gland in the normal location. Occasionally, the only thyroid gland that is present occurs in the base of the tongue, and care should be taken to determine the presence of thyroid tissue elsewhere before the presumed cyst is removed.

DERMOID CYSTS

Dermoid cysts are lined with skin epithelium that degenerates and gradually enlarges. They occur subcutaneously beneath the scalp and on the neck, usually at the site of congenital cleft closures. Those that occur in the midline along the scalp and posterior neck must be studied to determine whether they have deeper components that go through the bone as dumbbell lesions, which have neurosurgical implications.

The most frequent site is just above the lateral end of the eyebrow. Simple excision is sufficient.

BENIGN TUMORS

TORTICOLLIS

Torticollis is a congenital fibrous shortening of the sternocleidomastoid on one side that frequently produces a palpable mass in the lower neck involving one or both heads of the muscle. The etiology is unknown but involves muscle degeneration and not hemorrhage as previously thought.

Mild shortening of the muscle can be relieved by appropriate exercises, and the accompanying mass will spontaneously disappear. Cervical spine films may be required to rule out vertebral anomalies as a cause of torticollis. If exercises are ineffective, the facial asymmetry will become worse, and diplopia may occur. In these severe cases the sternocleidomastoid muscle should be transected, allowing the cut ends to spring apart. After the wound is healed, the exercises should be continued to assure complete rotation to the involved side.

LYMPHANGIOMA—CYSTIC HYGROMA

Congenital abnormalities of the lymphatic system can lead to multiple small dilated lymphatics or very large multilocular cysts containing lymphatic fluid. Frequently, when the lymphatics are small there is considerable fibrous tissue around them that produces a firm rather than a cystic mass. These lesions can occur anywhere in the body but are most frequently found in the neck, floor of the mouth and tongue, axilla, extremities, and occasionally mediastinum. An intraabdominal lymphangioma presents as an asymptomatic mass, usually in the mesentery or retroperitoneum.

Although these lesions frequently are recognized at birth or in the early newborn period, they can appear later in childhood as lymphatic fluid accumulations in a previously unrecognized area of involvement. Sudden enlargement can occur if there is bleeding within a cyst. Lymphangiomas are prone to infection, particularly in the floor of the mouth, which produces signs of sepsis and rapid enlargement.

Small lymphangiomas and hygromas can be excised in early infancy or later, but it should be remembered that because they are benign lesions, important nerves and other structures should be preserved. Multiple excisions may be required, and recurrence is common.

HEMANGIOMA

Hemangioma is a congenital abnormality of the blood vessels that usually involves just the capillaries and is referred to as a capillary hemangioma or hemangioendothelioma. A rare lesion contains larger vascular channels and is referred to as cavernous hemangioma. The most common capillary hemangioma is the "strawberry birthmark" on the skin with a variable degree of involvement of the subcutaneous tissue. These lesions most frequently occur on the head and face or genitalia but can occur anywhere and are best treated expectantly. Occasionally such a lesion will ulcerate, but good local care results in healing. Most hemangiomas regress spontaneously by the time the child is of school age, and they should not be treated with carbon dioxide ice, irradiation, or sclerosing injections. Occasionally, after the active hemangioma has disappeared redundant tissue may remain that will require plastic revision.

Hemangiomas can involve the parotid gland, producing a small or somewhat larger tumor. If there is skin involvement, one can be quite sure of the diagnosis, and surgery should be avoided. In uncertain cases, a small posterior biopsy can confirm the diagnosis. The exposed tissue has the appearance of thyroid tissue and is characteristic of hemangioendothelioma on biopsy. Because these lesions subside spontaneously, surgical removal is unnecessary and is dangerous to the facial nerve.

Cavernous hemangiomas and venous lakes do occur. They are variable in size and location and should be treated individually. They occasionally develop areas of thrombosis. Usually excisional surgery is eventually needed.

JUVENILE BREAST HYPERTROPHY

Both males and females can develop unilateral or bilateral enlargement of a nubbin of breast tissue beneath the areola. These occur without any other signs of sexual precocity. Very frequently they are self-limiting, and therefore biopsies should be avoided. A small biopsy of a girl's breast lesion may lead to a major deformity of the adult breast in later life.

The endocrinologic explanation of juvenile hypertrophy is unknown, although innumerable children have been studied. It can occur if the child accidentally is given exogenous estrogens, either orally or in the form of cutaneous ointments.

FIBROADENOMA OF THE BREAST

Adolescent girls can develop single or multiple breast masses. In black girls this frequently is a fibroadenoma, and usually surgical excision is needed to determine the benignity of the lesion.

TERATOMA

Abnormal differentiation of embryonal tissue producing a teratoma is found in a number of organs of the body. The most common is a sacrococcygeal teratoma, which involves the coccyx and usually produces an obvious external mass protruding from the lower spinal area. Intrapelvic teratomas occasionally are not recognized unless a rectal examination is done because of rectal or urinary symptoms. They should be excised early because they may contain malignant elements or undergo malignant change.

A teratoma of the ovary usually presents as a palpable abdominal mass. Occasionally these lesions are large enough to produce pressure symptoms on the urinary tract, and x-ray films frequently show the presence of teeth or other bony structures. Such teratomas are usually unilateral and should be excised and carefully examined for possible malignant elements.

Teratomas in the neck and mediastinum are often large and cause symptoms by compression and deviation of other important structures in the area. Surgical excision is indicated.

BIBLIOGRAPHY

EDGERTON MT: The treatment of hemangiomas with special reference to the role of steroid therapy. Ann Surg 183:517, 1976

FONKALSRUD EW: Surgical management of congenital malformations of the lymphatic system. Am J Surg 128:152, 1974

GROSFELD JL, BALLANTINE TVN, LOWE D et al: Benign and malignant teratomas in children: Analysis of 85 patients. Surgery 80:297, 1976

LING CM: The influence of age on the results of open sternomastoid tenotomy in muscular torticollis. Clin Orthop 116:142, 1976

MCAVOY JM, ZUCKERBRAUN L: Dermoid cysts of the head and neck in children. Arch Otolaryngol 102:529, 1976

SEASHORE JH: Breast enlargements in infants and children. Pediatr Ann 4:7, 1975

TELANDER RL, DEANE SA: Thyroglossal and branchial cleft cysts and sinuses. Surg Clin North Am 56:779, 1977

Louise Schnaufer

Malignant Tumors in Childhood

WILMS' TUMOR
NEUROBLASTOMA
RHABDOMYOSARCOMA
LYMPHOMAS
OVARIAN TUMORS
TESTICULAR TUMORS
LIVER TUMORS

Malignancy is second only to trauma as the leading cause of death in childhood. Tumors of the central nervous system and eye account for 20% of the total; the lymphoma group including the leukemias account for about 30%; and Wilms' tumor and neuroblastoma are responsible for 20%. The remaining 30% comprise the rhabdomyosarcomas, teratomas, liver, bone, and testicular tumors. Childhood tumors are predominantly sarcomas that are distinctly different from adult lesions.

WILMS' TUMOR

Wilms' tumor is the most common intrarenal malignancy of childhood and may be associated with other congenital anomalies, the most common of which are hemihypertrophy and aniridia. These tumors usually present as large, asymptomatic abdominal masses. Abdominal pain, fever, weight loss, and hematuria may also be present. About 80% of Wilms' tumors occur in children under the age of 5 years.

The diagnosis is confirmed by intravenous pyelogram, which will show calyceal distortion indicating an intrarenal tumor. Ultrasound has replaced inferior vena cavagrams to determine invasion by the tumor into the renal vein and inferior vena cava. Chest films will determine the presence of pulmonary metastatic lesions, which occur in approximately 25% of children with Wilms' tumors.

The initial management of these tumors is nephrectomy. Staging is determined by extent or by spread of tumor beyond the kidney capsule into adjacent organs or regional lymph nodes. Wilms' tumors are highly sensitive to chemotherapeutic drugs and to irradiation, and multiple protocols utilizing these agents in various combinations are indicated, depending on the stage of the disease. Three important prognostic indicators for survival are the histologic designation (either favorable or unfavorable) of cell type, lymph node involvement, and age.

NEUROBLASTOMA

Neuroblastoma is the most common solid tumor of childhood, comprising about one half of all malignant solid tumors in children. It can occur at any site where neural crest tissue is found and is derived from migration of neuroblasts from the developing spinal cord. Seventy-five percent of neuroblastomas arise in the abdomen; one half of these originate in the adrenal gland. About 15% occur in the thorax; other common sites include the pelvis and the neck.

The majority of children with neuroblastoma have large abdominal masses but have more associated symptoms than children with Wilms' tumors. Weight loss, abdominal pain, fever, anemia, and symptoms mimicking arthritis or rheumatic fever are common. On physical examination these tumors are more nodular than Wilms' tumors, frequently cross the midline, or may present in the pelvis. Diagnostic studies should include an intravenous pyelogram, a 24-hr urine study for catecholamine excretion, chest film, bone scan, and bone marrow aspiration. Neuroblastomas frequently show some calcification, which is usually central within the tumor and is finely stippled. An adrenal neuroblastoma will depress the kidney downward, but there will be no distortion of the calyceal system. Metastases may occur in the retroperitoneal space by direct extension with distant spread to regional lymph nodes, liver, and bones. Pulmonary metastases are relatively uncommon. Elevated vanillylmandelic acid (VMA) levels are found in about 90% of neuroblastoma patients, and this determination is useful not only in the diagnosis but also for indication of recurrence and for assessment of the response to therapy.

Therapy is determined by tumor location and clinical staging. Tumors in the neck, chest, and pelvis can usually be excised, but most of the large retroperitoneal neuroblastomas are not resectable. Since so many of these tumors cannot be removed and metastases are present at the time of diagnosis, chemotherapy and irradiation are indicated in most cases. The prognosis of children with advanced disease is poor, and the survival rate of 20% to 25% for patients with all stages of neuroblastoma has not changed significantly in the last 20 years.

RHABDOMYOSARCOMA

Rhabdomyosarcoma is the third most frequent malignant tumor found in childhood. These are tumors of striated muscle and are found in the nasopharynx, auditory canal, bladder, vagina, prostate, head and neck, trunk, and extremities. They are rapidly growing, infiltrating lesions, and treatment depends on the staging of the disease as well as the site of origin and its extent of growth.

In the past, mutilating surgical procedures were done for total extirpation of these tumors, but this has been replaced by less radical excision followed by aggressive chemotherapy and irradiation.

LYMPHOMAS

Hodgkin's disease and non-Hodgkin's lymphoma comprise the group of lymphomas. The most common finding in children with Hodgkin's disease is enlarged, nontender cervical nodes or a mediastinal mass on chest x-ray. Biopsy of the cervical nodes will confirm the diagnosis, and staging of the disease is determined by bone marrow aspiration, ultrasound to determine the presence of the intra-abdominal nodes, the presence of systemic symptoms, and staging laparotomy to determine the need for radiation to the liver, spleen, or lymph nodes.

Non-Hodgkin's lymphomas are classified as lymphocytic, Burkitt's, and histiocytic. Diagnosis is made by biopsy of an involved lymph node or by excision of an abdominal or mediastinal mass. Frequently the diagnosis can be made by bone marrow aspiration alone.

OVARIAN TUMORS

The most common ovarian tumors are benign, simple cysts or cystic teratomas. Solid ovarian tumors are more frequently malignant and are classified as granulosa cell tumor, malignant teratoma, embryonal carcinoma, and dysgerminoma. Symptoms and signs often depend on the size of the tumor and the presence of hormonal activity. A palpable mass is the most frequent finding. Sudden onset of pain may indicate a torsion or rupture of the ovarian mass.

Treatment consists of a salpingo-oophorectomy and biopsy of regional lymph nodes. Removal of the opposite ovary or a radical pelvic exenteration is not indicated in children.

TESTICULAR TUMORS

Testicular tumors are uncommon in childhood, occurring in only 1.5% of all malignancies. In postpubertal males, the adult type of tumor is generally found including seminoma, choriocarcinoma, and teratocarcinoma. The incidence of tumors of germ cell origin and non–germ cell origin is much higher in prepubertal males. Eighty-five percent of germ cell tumors are yolk sac or embryonal cell carcinomas. The remainder are benign teratomas. Non–germ cell tumors include Sertoli cell tumors, Leydig cell tumors, rhabdomyosarcomas, and lymphomas.

Treatment consists of radical orchiectomy through an inguinal crease incision; transcrotal biopsy should never be done. In the younger age group radical retroperitoneal lymphadenectomy is not indicated because of the infrequency of lymph node metastases. The use of chemotherapy and irradiation is based on the type of tumor, stage of disease, and age of the patient.

LIVER TUMORS

The most common malignant hepatic tumors are hepatoblastoma, which is usually seen in children under 2 years of age, and hepatocellular carcinoma, seen in older children. Malignant tumors of the bile duct or vascular origin are rare. The most common presenting sign is an abdominal mass of an intraperitoneal nature. Anemia, anorexia, and weakness are common. These lesions may be in only one lobe of the liver or they may be multifocal. Spread is by extension to adjacent lymph nodes or metastasis to lung. In addition to routine assessment of the patient, serum α-fetoprotein determination, ultrasound examination of the abdomen, liver scan, and hepatic arteriography are helpful.

Surgical resection is the treatment of choice, because survival is rare otherwise. Following adequate resection, chemotherapy and sometimes irradiation may improve the survival rate, which averages 30% to 40% for all stages of lesions.

BIBLIOGRAPHY

BILL AH: Immune aspects of neuroblastoma. Am J Surg 122:143, 1971

EVANS AE, D'ANGIO GJ, RANDOLPH J: A proposed staging for children with neuroblastoma. Cancer 27:374, 1971

KOOP CE: The neuroblastoma. In Progress in Pediatric Surgery. Baltimore, University Park Press, 1972

LEAPE LL, BRESLOW NE, BISHOP HC: The surgical treatment of Wilms' tumor: Results of the National Wilms' Tumor Study. Ann Surg 187:351, 1978

MOSTOFI FK: Testicular tumors. Cancer 32:1186, 1973

TOWNE BH, MALOUR GH, WOOLLEY MM: Ovarian cysts and tumors in infancy and childhood. J Pediatr Surg 10:311, 1975

YOUNG JL, MILLER R: Incidence of malignant tumors in U.S. children. J Pediatr 86:254, 1975

Michael E. Jabaley

42

The Hand

OVERVIEW

Sixteen million Americans suffered hand and extremity injuries in 1980. They comprised 40% of all emergency room trauma. Cost of treatment of injuries, arthritis, and birth defects of the upper extremity is estimated at $10 billion annually. Regardless of specialty, most physicians will be challenged by the patient whose hand hurts or is numb, cold, stiff, or deformed. The physician must understand the workings of the hand and recognize the common conditions that affect it.

HISTORY

Hand surgery began after World War I through the efforts of Sterling Bunnell and reached specialty status under the tremendous demands of the injuries produced by World War II. The surgical veterans of the military hand centers which Bunnell helped develop during that war formed the American Society for Surgery of the Hand in 1946, and the specialty has spread throughout the world from that beginning. The International Federation of Hand Societies now numbers 22 national societies in its membership. A hand surgeon may be a general, orthopaedic, or plastic surgeon, and he frequently will have taken additional fellowship training in the field after completing the requirements for certification in his primary specialty. Nevertheless, the majority of hand conditions are still treated by primary-care physicians or surgical specialists whose training in hand surgery may have been brief.

FUNCTIONAL ANATOMY

The hand functions as a gripping tool and as a sensory organ. Power grip is accomplished by wrapping the fingers and thumb about an object; pinch grip occurs when small objects are manipulated between the tips of the fingers and thumb. Pinch may involve pulp-to-pulp contact, lateral or "key" pinch, or thumb and fingers "chuck" pinch. Both gripping functions require sensation and motion. Consequently, joint stiffness, numbness, or pain will severely retard function. The highly developed sensation of touch permits the hand to explore, evaluate, and provide a constant flow of information about the environment (and exposes it to a host of potentially noxious stimuli). Touch is mediated primarily by the median and ulnar nerves (Fig. 42-1). Motion requires supple joints and a tendon system to motor them, which is described later.

Hand function depends on a highly developed and integrated system of bones, tendons, nerves, and muscles. The upper arm and forearm serve primarily to position and stabilize the hand in space. The eight carpal bones allow precise hand motion independent of the forearm. The hand itself consists of three units: a central fixed unit, comprised of the second and third rays, an ulnar component, comprised of the fourth and fifth rays, and a radial component, the first ray (thumb). A ray consists of the metacarpal and phalanges of a finger. The radial and ulnar units rotate

Fig. 42-1. Territories of sensory nerves. (*Left*) Dorsal branches of radial and ulnar nerves supply all except index-, middle-, and ring-finger tips. Nerves are subcutaneous and easily injured. Failure to recognize injury results in loss of sensation. Painful neuromas may form and may be disabling. (*Right*) Volar surface of hand. Median and ulnar nerves supply nearly all areas, although division line on ring finger may vary. In fingers, digital branches are subcutaneous and easily injured. In the palm, they are covered by palmar fascia. A territory must be carefully examined whenever a laceration lies over the course of its nerve trunk. (Peacock EE Jr: The hand. In Hardy JD [ed]: Rhoads Textbook of Surgery, 5th ed. Philadelphia, J B Lippincott, 1977)

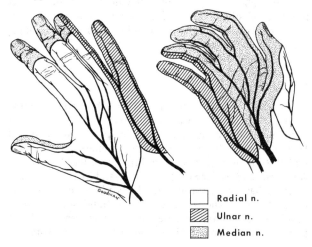

	Radial n.
	Ulnar n.
	Median n.

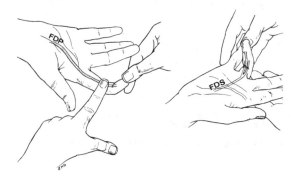

Fig. 42-2. (*Left*) The flexor digitorum profundus (FDP) is the sole flexor of the distal interphalangeal joint. It is tested by immobilizing the middle phalanx and asking the patient to bend the tip. (*Right*) The flexor digitorum superficialis (FDS) is the primary flexor of the proximal interphalangeal joint, but an intact profundus plays a secondary role. Forced extension of the other three fingers inactivates the FDP and allows detection of an isolated superficialis tendon injury. (Jabaley ME, Curtis RM: Hand injuries. In Hardy JD [ed]: Rhoads Textbook of Surgery, 5th ed. Philadelphia, J B Lippincott, 1977)

around the fixed central portion. These motions form a transverse arch in both the proximal and the distal palm and allow the important cupping function of the palm. The saddle joint at the base of the thumb is extremely mobile and permits this digit to assume the all-important position of opposition.

The design of the hand is such that the linkage of bones in each finger is both mobile and stable. Stability and motion are accomplished by a system of intrinsic and extrinsic tendons that work both independently and in concert. They are vulnerable to injury and may be transected, avulsed, or torn from their attachments.

The wrist is directly motored and fixed by a combination of three flexor and three extensor tendons. The flexor carpi radialis and flexor carpi ulnaris tendons are the prime wrist flexors and are assisted by the palmaris longus. The extensor carpi radialis longus and extensor carpi radialis brevis, as well as the extensor carpi ulnaris, are all primary wrist extensors and may work in concert with appropriate flexors to deviate the wrist in either an ulnar or a radial direction.

The fingers are flexed, in order, at the distal interphalangeal (DIP) joint by the flexor digitorum profundus tendon, at the proximal interphalangeal (PIP) joint by the flexor digitorum superficialis, and at the metacarpophalangeal (MP) joint by the lumbrical muscle (Fig. 42-2). Each primary flexor tendon is also a secondary flexor of the joints more proximal to its insertion. Extension is accomplished by an elaborate system of extrinsic tendons (extensor digitorum communis, indicis, and digiti minimi) and intrinsic tendons (interossei and lumbrical). The thumb enjoys a different arrangement, in that all its extensors are extrinsic and there is only one extrinsic flexor, the flexor pollicis longus. Its versatility derives from the fact that the carpometacarpal joint is a biconcave saddle joint that is augmented and motored by the four intrinsic muscles that comprise the thenar eminence. The little finger is the most mobile of the four fingers, and the muscles of the hypothenar eminence mimic, to an extent, the movements of the thenar muscles. The little and ring fingers are most important for power grip. while the index and middle fingers are most important for the various pinch maneuvers.

DIAGNOSTIC AIDS

A plain film of the hand or fingers may be extremely helpful in the diagnosis of fractures, bone tumors, arthritic changes, systemic diseases, calcifications, and foreign bodies. It is a mainstay of diagnosis. Tomograms can be used to demonstrate joint instability or subtle fractures. Nerve conduction studies and electromyography can confirm suspected nerve compression or neuropathy but is limited in value because positive tests frequently lag behind symptoms. A normal study does not rule out disease. Skin temperature studies, stellate blocks, and diagnostic blocks of specific nerves should be performed when evaluating patients with vasomotor complaints or sympathetic dystrophies. Arteriograms and isotope scans provide useful information about vascular occlusions, spasm, or injuries. Now that small-vessel (1 mm) microsurgery is a reality, these studies are more important than ever and should be considered more often, particularly in heretofore poorly understood ailments such as Raynaud's disease and Buerger's disease and other vasospastic problems.

ELECTIVE INCISIONS

There is no area where ill-planned incisions cause more trouble than the volar surface of the fingers and palm. Elective incisions have three goals: exposure of critical structures, minimal denervation and diminution of blood supply, and primary healing without crippling contracture (Fig. 42-3). Certain principles are important, whether one

Fig. 42-3. Standard hand incisions. Incisions are based on the flexion diamonds, as shown in the index finger. Longitudinal incisions in these areas will heal with contracting scars. Such areas must be crossed transversely. Diagonal incisions, illustrated in the ring finger, heal more kindly and are preferred. Short longitudinal incisions, as shown in the middle finger, are acceptable and may be useful for drainage of tendon sheaths. If a laceration is already present, it can be incorporated into an incision by following these principles, as shown in the little finger. The midaxial incision (*insert*) does not contract and gives the best exposure of neurovascular bundles. The curvilinear incision parallel and ulnar to the thenar crease gives best exposure of the carpal canal and avoids injury to important skin nerves.

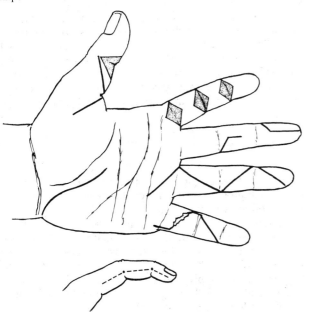

chooses the midaxial incision, the volar zigzag incision, or combinations of these: (1) Several small incisions are usually better than one large one. (2) Incisions must respect the flexion diamonds of the fingers and palm and be designed transversely in these areas. (3) The blood supply is perpendicular to the skin surface; if one undermines very far, flap tips will be devascularized. (4) Incisions in the palm that parallel and are slightly out of the flexion creases will be safe. (5) Straight midline incisions on the dorsum of the hand and fingers are satisfactory; they do not contract in normal skin.

POSTOPERATIVE CARE

The goals of early postoperative care are relief of pain and restoration of function. Immobilization for at least a short period is nearly always indicated to decrease pain and prevent swelling. Either plaster or synthetic materials can be molded to the hand and fingers to control position. If tendons or nerves have been repaired, the position should be one to relieve tension on these repairs. Otherwise, an excellent position is slight extension of the wrist with the MP joints flexed 45° to 50°, the interphalangeal (IP) joints nearly straight, and the thumb abducted and opposed. Elevation best prevents edema. Early motion is indicated when possible and appropriate splinting when not. A reasonable compromise, even in some fractures, is to use early protected motion with such devices as buddy straps, dynamic splinting, and passive motion by the surgeon or therapist.

ANESTHESIA

Most hand operations can be performed as well with local or regional anesthesia as with general anesthesia. With a monitor and an intravenous line in place, a well-sedated patient can be effectively treated by specific nerve block, field block, or intravenous block (Bier block). A healthy adult can be premedicated with 10 mg diazepam (Valium) and 75 mg meperidine (Demerol) intramuscularly. This can be supplemented during the case with 1.25-mg increments of diazepam sufficient to produce sedation. Nerve blocks may be performed using lidocaine or bupivacaine (Marcaine). Metacarpal-level blocks are preferred to digital blocks because of the danger of thrombosis and subsequent skin slough with digital blocks. Epinephrine-containing solutions are contraindicated in blocks at the hand level. If one elects to use a field block on the palm or digits, it is helpful to spray with ethyl chloride prior to inserting the needle. Freezing temporarily anesthetizes the skin and makes needle pricks more tolerable.

TOURNIQUET ISCHEMIA

Practically all hand operations are better and more safely performed with tourniquet ischemia. Interruption of flow prevents troublesome bleeding and allows visualization of small structures. It is important that tourniquets be well padded and placed over the large portion of the muscle mass of the upper arm. The gauge should be calibrated prior to use, and tourniquet duration should be limited to the shortest time necessary to dissect and identify structures. For example, tendon ends, once found, can be easily sutured with the tourniquet deflated. Nerve-compression injuries have been reported from tourniquet use and are probably due more to excessive pressure than to excessive time. An appropriate setting to stop bleeding is 100 mm above the systolic pressure, and a suggested time is 90 to 120 minutes. These should always be modified for each specific situation.

MAGNIFICATION

Magnification is helpful in hand surgery. Loupes worn on the eyes which magnify $2 \times$ to $4 \times$ are satisfactory for most procedures. Microsurgical operations on nerves and blood vessels are usually better performed with a microscope and magnification of $6 \times$ to $25 \times$.

INJURY

Wounds may be tidy or untidy. Tidy wounds can be closed safely and primary repair of injured structures performed. Untidy wounds or wounds with a major crush component are best left open, with delay of definitive repair. This approach reduces the likelihood of infection, decompresses the wound, and improves patient comfort. Wounds repaired before scar forms (*i.e.*, within 7–10 days) are considered delayed primary repairs. It is less important *when* a wound is closed than that it heals once closed (Fig. 42-4).

INJURIES WITH NO LOSS OF SKIN

Wounds usually can be anesthetized, vigorously scrubbed with gauze and saline, and then sutured. Nylon (4-0 or 5-0) on a cutting needle is an acceptable material. Wounds can be splinted satisfactorily with a soft dressing, and sutures should be removed in 5 to 7 days.

HAND INJURY	
Etiology	Crush, cut, shear, missile, or puncture causes tissue disruption and death Ischemia from dissipation of energy, increased pressure from swelling
Dx	Careful history, examination, and a high index of suspicion Inspection of posture of the hand Functional testing of specific tendons and nerve territories for precise diagnosis. X-ray film to confirm status of bony skeleton
Rx	Simple suture of open wounds and repair of wounds which require no dissection can frequently be performed in emergency room or physician's office; deep structures best treated in operating room setting, although not necessarily in a hospital
Caveats	Deep wounds and structures such as tendons best not explored in emergency room Injudicious clamping may injure a nerve. Decide whether the injury justifies treatment in an operating room setting When in doubt, *don't* close wounds; delayed primary closure is frequently preferred

INJURIES WITH SKIN LOSS

Closure with mild tension is acceptable if skin loss is slight. Undermining is usually of no value and further decreases critical blood supply. With greater skin loss and no exposure of critical structures, a small graft can be applied immediately. Favored sites are the wrist crease and thenar or hypothenar areas, taking care to stay in the "silent" areas (those not used in gripping). If more skin is needed, it is better taken from the trunk or an unexposed area than from the forearm. Such cosmetically damaging donor sites should be avoided. If important structures such as tendon or bone are exposed, a flap may be necessary. Local flaps can sometimes be used to cover IP joints, and rotation flaps will cover tendons in the dorsum of the hand. Major areas of skin loss requires distant flaps from the abdomen, groin, chest, or opposite upper arm.

SUBUNGUAL HEMATOMA

Subungual hematoma frequently occurs when the fingertip is crushed and the hightly vascular nail bed bleeds into the space beneath the nail. The throbbing pain can be relieved instantly by drilling a hole through the nail with a heated paper clip or small drill and draining the blood. The nail will usually be lost weeks later.

FINGERTIP INJURIES OR AMPUTATIONS

All fingertip injuries or amputations produce tissue loss. It must first be decided whether the amount of loss is acceptable or unacceptable. If it is a small loss, the wound can be dressed and daily washing and antibiotic ointment applications begun in 48 hours. Healing by contracture and epithelialization will take place over 2 to 3 weeks, producing a scar that is frequently excellent from the standpoint of function and appearance. If the wound is too large or is in a position where this technique seems inappropriate, a small skin graft may result in early healing. If the area of loss is major, if bone is exposed, or if there has been major injury to the nail bed, a flap is indicated. If tissue loss is not excessive, advancement flaps from the sides or volar portion of the finger are helpful. Such flaps redistribute remaining skin but add no additional tissue to the tip. If more tissue is needed, a regional flap, such as the cross-finger flap or thenar flap, is a better choice. Distant flaps from the trunk are indicated only when none of the lesser procedures will do. The main causes of deformity after fingertip injuries are nail bed trauma with resultant nail deformity and pain. These can be minimized by careful repair of the nail matrix at the time of injury and thoughtful management of the digital nerves.

TENDON INJURIES

Tendon injuries pose a special challenge in wound healing. One must effect a rigid bond of scar between the tendon ends while producing mobile scar between the tendon and the surrounding tissue so that the repaired tendon will glide. Adhesion problems unique to the sheath of the flexor tendons gave rise to the name "no man's land." Primary repair was not advised for many years because of poor results in this area. Tendon healing now appears related to intrinsic blood supply and tenocytes as well as extrinsic factors, and tendon healing can sometimes occur without crippling adhesions to surrounding sheath.

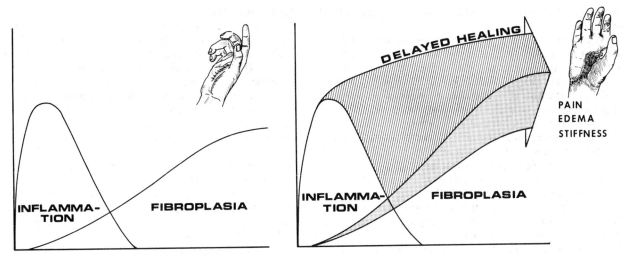

Fig. 42-4. Normal and abnormal wound healing. (*Left*) The inflammatory response is immediate in onset and subsides rapidly. Resolution of inflammation is accompanied by decrease in swelling and pain. Fibroplasia results in collagen formation and bonding of the wound edges by scar. (*Right*) The result of a chronically open wound. The inflammatory response (*lined*) is heightened and prolonged. Increased fibroplasia (*stippled*) results in more scar production. The outcome is a swollen, sore wound granulating on its surface and scarred in its depth. All joints are stiff, and the patient does not move the hand. The primary objective in treating hand injuries is a healed wound. (Jabaley ME, Curtis RM: Hand injuries. In Hardy JD [ed]: Rhoads Textbook of Surgery, 5th ed. Philadelphia, J B Lippincott, 1977)

FLEXOR TENDONS

No man's land extends from the mid-portion of the middle phalanx to the proximal palmar crease. It corresponds to the sheath that encircles the flexor digitorum superficialis and flexor digitorum profundus tendons. There is no paratenon in this area, and blood supply is through the vincula. Wound cleansing, skin closure, and secondary tendon grafting was once the recommended treatment, but primary repairs can yield superior results if done carefully. The first repair is the best opportunity for a successful outcome in this demanding area and should be performed by a physician skilled in hand surgery.

Diagnosis

A wound in the appropriate location and inability to flex a digit are usually sufficient to make the diagnosis. X-ray films are helpful if a fracture or foreign body is suspected, and other laboratory data are useful only in assuring the safety of surgery. It is unnecessary to explore wounds containing injured tendons in the emergency room; in fact, this is contraindicated. The only judgment to be made is whether or not the patient needs to be operated upon.

Technique of Repair

Tendons can be located by extending the laceration proximally or distally and flexing the wrist and digit. A second incision in the palm may occasionally be necessary. The sheath should be opened carefully so that it can be repaired later. The tendon ends are stitched with a permanent nonreactive suture such as nylon or Prolene. A modification of the Mason–Allen–Kessler suture technique is used (Fig. 42-5). If both flexor tendons are injured, both are repaired. An intact tendon should never be cut. The sheath is closed and the skin is closed. A suture through the fingernail is used for early protected motion in the postoperative period, beginning at 24 to 36 hours. A dorsal plaster splint prevents extension for 3 weeks.

Transections of the flexor digitorum profundus distal to the sheath are sometimes treated with excision of the distal end and advancement and reinsertion of the proximal end into bone. Advancements up to 10 mm to 15 mm have been reported, but direct tendon suture without excision is the preferable technique when possible.

Partial injuries of a tendon are best left unsutured unless over 50% of the tendon is involved. They should be treated

Fig. 42-5. Technique of tendon suture. (*Top*) A 5-0 synthetic or wire suture on a tapered needle is used. Suture is begun and completed so that the single knot lies between the cut edges. (*Bottom left*) An unsatisfactory repair results if bites are too far from the edge, producing bunching of the tendon and a bolus. Heavy, reactive suture with exposed knots and inaccurate alignment are also to be avoided. (*Bottom right*) A proper repair does not strangulate, includes only enough tendon for strength, and exposes a minimal amount of suture material. Knots are buried. No. 6-0 monofilament continuous suture may be used to improve alignment. (Jabaley ME, Curtis RM: Hand injuries. In Hardy JD [ed]: Rhoads Textbook of Surgery, 5th ed. Philadelphia, J B Lippincott, 1977)

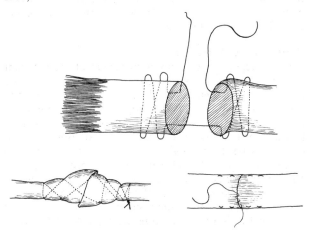

with wound closure and protected motion in a splint for 3 weeks.

When repair is not carried out as an immediate or delayed procedure, finger flexion can still be recovered by tendon grafting. In this procedure, the damaged tendon is excised from the level of the lumbrical muscle to its insertion and replaced with a graft. Preferred donor grafts are palmaris longus, plantaris, toe extensors, and supplemental finger extensors. Flexor tendon grafting is a more difficult procedure than repair. Judgment of graft length and tension can be tricky, adhesion formation is mandatory, and postoperative management is more demanding.

Flexor tendon ruptures represent a small percent of tendon injuries. They are usually athletic injuries involving the long and ring fingers of young men who have their fingers forcibly extended while they are grasping and flexing. The most common site of rupture is at the insertion of the flexor digitorum profundus. Patients usually note pain and swelling over the volar aspect of the proximal phalanges, a tender mass, and inability to flex the tip. Treatment consists in exploration, retrieval, and reinsertion of the profundus tendon into the distal phalanx.

Severely injured and previously treated digits can still be salvaged by the use of a two-stage flexor tendon grafting technique. At the first stage, the old tendon is excised and a silicone rod implanted beneath the remaining pulleys. The wound is closed, and the finger is passively exercised for several weeks while the finger forms a new sheath in response to the silicone. At a second operation, the skin is opened at the proximal and distal ends of the rod, which is then removed and replaced with a tendon graft. Although less than perfect, functioning fingers can sometimes be obtained by this method.

EXTENSOR TENDONS

Extensor tendons differ from flexors in many ways. Their blood supply is by a paratenon, not vincula. They do not pass through a sheath, and, when cut, they do not retract as far. There is no such thing as no man's land on the dorsum of the hand or fingers. Thus, they are more amenable to repair and results are usually better. Each joint has a specific extensor and a recognized clinical picture with injury.

Mallet Finger

A "dropped tip" occurs when the extensor of the distal phalanx is transected. After repair, the phalanx must be maintained in extension by a Kirschner wire or external splint for 4 weeks to permit healing. The greater strength of the flexor digitorum profundus almost always assure good flexion of the tip ultimately.

Boutonnière Deformity

This characteristic deformity with flexion of the PIP joint and hyperextension of the DIP joint occurs when the insertion of the central band of the extensor digitorum communis is ruptured or transected at its insertion into the middle phalanx. The skin may or may not be cut. Attempts to straighten the finger by contracting the extensor digitorum communis result in secondary hyperextension of the tip through the intact lateral bands. Again, early recognition and repair results in good function. The repair should be protected by a transarticular Kirschner wire for 4 weeks. Secondary repairs can be successful if a full range of passive motion exists, but these are considerably more difficult.

Other Injuries

Injuries of the extensor digitorum communis, extensor indicis, and extensor digiti minimi result in inability to extend the MP joint and can be repaired by simple direct suture. The tendon ends do not retract and can usually be identified in the wound. They can be stitched with a combination suture, which includes both skin and tendon ends, or they can be closed with buried sutures. A disadvantage of the latter technique at the MP joint level is that tender red granulomas sometimes form beneath the skin. The combination suture technique avoids this problem. MP joints must be splinted in full extension or even hyperextension for about 4 weeks to assure adequate healing. The most common disability postoperatively is the inability to fully extend the fingers. Before the skin is closed, one should examine the repair site and select a position for joints that reduces tension on the repair.

Untreated or unrecognized injuries of the extrinsic extensors can frequently be managed by transfer of an intact tendon from an adjacent finger. For the long or ring finger, the extensor indicis is a satisfactory tendon for transfer. If several tendons are injured, grafting is also effective. On occasion, a two-stage reconstruction with silicone rods may be necessary.

NERVE INJURIES

Peripheral nerves can be injured by crush, stretch, avulsion, or transection. Whatever the cause, significant injury produces Wallerian degeneration distal to the injury and proximally to the first node of Ranvier. The goals of nerve suture are (1) primary healing of the nerve ends with as little scar as possible so as to permit (2) regeneration of axons across the suture line and down the distal stump.

The results of nerve repair have always been relatively poor and have not improved as much as in some types of hand surgery. Since axons tolerate trauma and handling so poorly, it now seems obvious that results will improve only as technique improves. The important features of successful nerve repair are meticulous handling of the nerve ends to prevent further injury, use of magnification, and appreciation for the cross-sectional anatomy of each nerve so that the subunits can be correctly matched (Fig. 42-6). This can best be done in the acute phase by primary or early delayed primary repair. These techniques are not applicable in missile wounds, in which the degree of damage may not be apparent on first inspection; early secondary repair is indicated in such cases.

Nerve grafting is a salvage procedure for gaps that are too great to overcome by direct suture. Tension is one of the main anatomical causes of poor results, since it causes stretching of the repair, a thick scar, and loss of many axons because of their inability to bridge the thick scar interface. A graft is preferable to a repair under excessive tension. The most frequent nerve donor sites are the sural, the cutaneus antebrachii lateralis, the cutaneus femoris lateralis, the dorsal sensory branch of the ulnar nerve, and the superficial radial nerve. Successful grafts must lie in a well-vascularized bed to acquire circulation at the new site. All damaged nerve must be trimmed away. The proximal and distal ends must be inspected and mapped. Appropriate bundles are matched and then joined with lengths of graft that are held in place with only one or two 10-0 nylon stitches. Successful nerve grafting requires precise microsurgical technique, correct

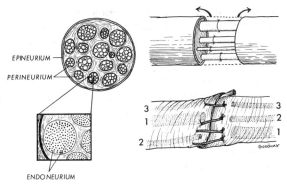

Fig. 42-6. Peripheral nerve repair. (*Left*) Cross section of a nerve. Fascicles of axons and endoneurium are surrounded by perineurium. All fascicles together are invested by a thicker connective tissue, the epineurium. (*Right, top*) Interfascicular repair is performed with magnification. Epineurium has been trimmed back. Individual fascicles are matched and sutured with 10-0 nylon. (*Right, bottom*) Epineurial repair is simpler but produces more scar, retraction, and misalignment of fascicles. (1,2,3) Axonal regeneration is less likely to reach fingertips and intrinsic muscles, owing to mechanical barrier of scar at the point of repair. (Jabaley ME, Curtis RM: Hand injuries. In Hardy JD [ed]: Rhoads Textbook of Surgery, 5th ed. Philadelphia, J B Lippincott, 1977)

matching of appropriate subunits, and absolute avoidance of tension.

INJURY TO NERVES AT SPECIFIC LEVELS

Digital nerves at finger levels are pure sensory nerves and offer the best potential result. Sutures should be placed with microsurgical technique and magnification. An epineurial suture is adequate. Slight flexion of the digit is acceptable to overcome tension. Digital nerves in the palm and common digital nerves are still pure sensory nerves, but tension may be more difficult to overcome because there are no joints

NERVE INJURIES	
Etiology	Nerve may be acutely crushed or stretched, avulsed or cut, or chronically compressed. Early effect is to block conduction and limit functions. Distal wallerian degeneration and secondary atrophy may occur.
Dx	Subjective numbness, muscle weakness, or pain; muscle wasting and electro-diagnostic change come later. In acute cases, a significant wound or injury over a nerve and altered sensation are diagnostic if no improvement in a week
Rx	In sharp transections, best results from primary or secondary microsurgical repair. Blast, missile, or avulsion wounds better treated with initial joining of ends with suture to prevent retraction and early secondary repair. Successful repair requires accurate matching of component bundles of fasciculi and a tension-free nerve juncture: if impossible resort to a graft

to flex. Small grafts can be inserted if tension is excessive. The cutaneus antebrachii lateralis is approximately the same diameter and is a good donor nerve. Median and ulnar nerves at the wrist and proximal palm are both motor and sensory, but the branches are well formed and separate within the epineurium. They should be separated for direct suture to be certain that correct matching of motor and sensory components occurs. With median and ulnar nerves in the distal two thirds of the forearm, quadrants containing motor and sensory fibers can still be identified and should be repaired by group fascicular suture. Match ups with the same degree of accuracy seen in the wrist may be more difficult but should be attempted. With injuries in the proximal forearm, interconnecting branches between bundles are such that specific representation no longer exists and fiber distribution is more diffuse. Cross-sectional maps may be used in the secondary case, and one should still match "according to his best guess."

COMPRESSION

Direct pressure on any peripheral nerve can result in either intermittent or continuous loss of function. Minimal amounts of compression first appear as sensory loss because sensation is most easily perceived by the patient. Motor loss occurs only after more pronounced injury and may be associated with muscle atrophy. Electrical studies may be helpful in corroborating the diagnosis but findings frequently are normal in some patients with symptomatic compression. A careful history and examination are the keys to a correct diagnosis. Pain or numbness in the sensory distribution of a nerve, occurring episodically and either waking the patient at night or developing in association with specific tasks, is usually diagnostic. First-degree lesions (Sunderland classification) may respond to splinting, diuretics, and thiamine. Steroid injections of triamcinolone acetonide (Kenalog), 10 mg/ml into inflamed synovium, may also be helpful. Persistent symptoms require surgery. This consists of decompression of the nerve by dividing the offending structures about it. In cases with first- and second-degree injury, response will be prompt. Third-degree lesions are demyelinated and may have peripheral degeneration; recovery may require many months and patients should be forewarned.

Carpal Tunnel Syndrome

One of the most common and best known compression neuropathies involves the median nerve at the carpal tunnel. It may follow synovitis, trauma, sprains, or fractures that may reduce the size of the canal, but antecedent causes frequently cannot be found. The syndrome consists in sensory loss in the median nerve territory and signs of nerve irritation at the wrist. There may also be thenar motor weakness and retrograde forearm pain. Division of the transverse carpal ligament is curative in a high percent of cases.

Bowler's Thumb

Persistent trauma to the digital nerves by a tool or bowling ball can result in numbness of the thumb. Symptoms have been seen after gripping pliers, surgical scissors, or other instruments. Many patients improve spontaneously if the offending agent is removed. A few require surgery to lyse the scar tissue that forms around the nerve.

Pronator Teres Syndrome

A hypertrophic or tight pronator teres may compress the median nerve in the proximal forearm and result in a total or partial compression. If the anterior interosseous nerve is nonfunctional, a characteristic pinch deformity between the thumb and index finger results. There may be point tenderness or Tinel's sign over the proximal edge of the muscle where the nerve goes underneath.

Guyon's Canal

The ulnar nerve can be compressed at the level of Guyon's canal by the same causes mentioned for the median nerve. Both motor and sensory changes may result. Occasionally, a ganglion can cause symptoms.

Tardy Ulnar Palsy

A common site for compression of the ulnar nerve is at the elbow, where any of a number of structures may produce symptoms. The intermuscular septum of the upper arm, the medial epicondyle of the humerus, and the flexor carpi ulnaris muscle origin can all be causative. If conservative measures fail, surgery may be necessary. In some instances, it is sufficient to decompress the nerve in its bed. More severe cases require translocation anterior to the medial epicondyle of the humerus. A key diagnostic point is that ulnar nerve compression at the elbow involves the dorsal cutaneous branch and produces numbness on the dorsum of the hand. This is not present with compression at Guyon's canal.

Radial Nerve at the Arcade of Frohse

The radial nerve may be compressed in the forearm and a partial radial paralysis may occur owing to the anatomical configuration of the tissues through which the nerve travels as it enters the supinator muscle. This causes a motor paralysis of the extensors of the fingers, thumb, and wrist (with the exception of extensor carpi radialis longus, which originates more proximally).

Caveats

The surgical treatment of any pain syndrome is challenging, and nerve compression is no exception. Surgical judgment will be tested; one must decide such things as whether to simply decompress a nerve, whether to translocate it, or whether to perform an internal neurolysis. If incorrectly selected and applied, any of these maneuvers may worsen rather than improve the patient's condition. Lastly, incisions must always be planned which do not further injure cutaneous nerves. A common source of complaint is a transected palmar cutaneous branch of the median nerve while treating a carpal tunnel syndrome. Such surgical errors result in unhappy patients at best and, at worst, in litigation.

IRREPARABLE NERVE INJURY

Irreparable nerve injury leads to distal muscle atrophy that will not recover with any form of treatment. In such cases, other techniques must be applied to restore balance and motor function. Proximal joints can be stabilized by tenodesis or arthrodesis. Those remaining functional muscle–tendon units can be transferred to other areas to restore balance. There are many available motors that can be spared without great loss to improve a partially paralyzed hand.

In *radial nerve palsy*, the inability to extend the wrist to a functional position is a disabling feature. It can be corrected by transferring the pronator teres from its insertion into the radius to the extensor carpi radialis brevis. This is an ideal transfer because it is synergistic with the planned motion (wrist extension) and the pronator teres retains its original function (pronator of the forearm). Other transfers for finger and thumb extensors will be necessary.

A common feature of *median nerve paralysis* is the inability to abduct and rotate the thumb to a position opposite the fingers. Any of several muscles may be transferred to correct this deformity. A common transfer is the flexor digitorum superficialis of the ring finger into the insertion of the abductor pollicis brevis so that the thumb opposes as the fingers flex.

In *ulnar nerve paralysis,* the little and ring fingers frequently go into the "claw" position with hyperextension of the MP joints and a flexion contracture of the PIP joints. A direct transfer of the flexor digitorum superficialis or a wrist extensor into the paralyzed intrinsics can be effective. A simpler approach is to insert the flexor digitorum superficialis at a more proximal level so that it becomes a flexor of the MP joint rather than the PIP joint. This is accomplished by looping the flexor digitorium superficialis around the first annular pulley, which arises from the proximal phalanges. By flexing the MP joints, the IP joints are extended by the extensor digitorum communis. An added bonus of this transfer is that grip strength is also increased.

PAIN PROBLEMS

Painful Neuroma

Neuroma formation is the natural consequence of nerve injury, and it occurs in all patients. Most neuromas are not tender or painful, but occasionally a patient develops a painful neuroma after division of a peripheral nerve. If a nerve has been transected, the best preventative for a painful neuroma is to restore continuity by performing a secondary repair. This is not always possible, and one must sometimes resort to a nerve graft. If a graft is impossible (*e.g.,* in amputations), other approaches are available. In some cases, a skilled hand therapist may be able to reduce the symptoms by a program of skin desensitization. Injection of triamcinolone acetonide, 10 mg/ml, directly into the neuroma may help. Its collagenase effect may soften the scar enough to relieve symptoms. If surgery becomes necessary, one should either relocate the peripheral nerve to a more proximal and protected location or select one of a number of available procedures. Capping, burning, injection, oversewing, or burying in bone have all been advocated. The likelihood of success postoperatively can be increased by ancillary techniques such as biofeedback, transcutaneous stimulation, and well-managed therapy.

Causalgia

Causalgia, which literally means "burning pain," is a sequela of injury to a mixed peripheral nerve. This poorly understood disability frequently follows a gunshot wound and is characterized by hypersensitivity, sweating, vasomotor instability, and secondary atrophy of soft tissue and osteoporosis of bone (Sudeck's atrophy). Because of the lack of a clear understanding of etiology or pathogenesis, these and other such afflictions are broadly classified as reflex sympathetic dystrophies. Treatment is directed toward manipulation of the sympathetic nervous system by physical, pharmacologic, and surgical maneuvers, or combinations of all three.

SPECIAL INJURIES

INJECTION INJURIES

Workers who use high-pressure injection tools are susceptible to accidental injection of foreign material such as paint, grease, and other petroleum products into the hand. Such injuries may appear deceptively trivial on first inspection, but they progress rapidly to severe pain, tissue ischemia, and necrosis. Treatment consists in opening the involved area widely and removing as much foreign material as possible. More than one procedure may be required, and skin loss or amputation is common after major injection injuries.

Intra-arterial injections may be self-inflicted in addicts or iatrogenic with diagnostic studies or intra-arterial monitoring devices. In both instances, spasm, distal thrombosis, or embolization of the arterial tree may occur and may be accompanied by ischemia or frank tissue necrosis. Advice and treatment by a hand surgeon should be obtained early because amputation is a frequent aspect of care.

Intravenous extravasation is a recognized complication of parenteral therapy. Many drugs have been implicated in tissue slough, resulting in painful, indolent ulcers that persist for long periods with no inclination to heal. Cytotoxic drugs and hypertonic solutions are the common offenders. Treatment may be indicated even in terminal cancer patients because of pain. Excision of sloughs with closure by either flaps or grafts heals the wound and relieves the pain. Local steroid or streptokinase/streptodornase injections early in the course may minimize tissue loss.

REPLANTATION

The ultimate injury, of course, is amputation of a part. Microsurgical capability has made replantation of digits and hands a reality, and successfully replanted parts are often superior in function and appearance to amputation stumps and prostheses. Replantation is indicated in thumb amputations at any level, multiple digits through the middle or proximal phalanges, and any palmar or more proximal amputations. It is ordinarily not indicated in single-digit amputations or distal phalangeal amputations. Amputated parts should be wrapped in saline-moistened gauze sponges, placed in a plastic bag, and transported in ice. They need not be perfused. Patients should have bleeding controlled by pressure and elevation; clamping and ligature should be specifically avoided. General resuscitative measures should be taken prior to transportation of the patient. Time is important, but successful replantation can be accomplished as long as 12 to 15 hours after injury.

Replantation is best performed by a microsurgery team working with magnification, microinstruments, and suture. The general rule is to fix bone, repair tendons and nerves, and then repair arteries and veins, all at the initial procedure. Sharp amputations under ideal conditions should yield 80% to 90% success rates. Technique is described in the section on microsurgery.

CONGENITAL DEFORMITIES

The upper limb bud appears about 26 days after fertilization, when the embryo is 4 mm in length. It lengthens in a proximal-to-distal fashion, and the hand forms last. By day 31, the hand segment is recognizable; by day 36, digital rays and fissures are formed. Within another 12 days, the cartilaginous skeleton has formed, and the entire process is complete by day 50. Developmental defect may result from vascular accidents, heredity, teratogens, infections, or spontaneous mutations.

CLASSIFICATION

I. Failure of formation of parts
  A. Transverse deficiencies—amputation-type stumps of fingers, ranging from aphalangia to amelia (absence of arms)
  B. Longitudinal deficiencies—all other skeletal limb absences, such as phocomelia and radial club hand
II. Failure of differentiation (separation) of parts. Syndactyly is the most common type.
III. Duplication of digits or a part. Polydactyly is the most common type (*e.g.*, supernumerary digits).
IV. Overgrowth (gigantism). May involve an entire limb or be limited to a single digit
V. Undergrowth (hypoplasia). Defective or incomplete development of a part. May be small but function normally
VI. Congenital constriction ring syndrome. Etiology is unknown, but ''amniotic bands'' may involve digits or the entire extremity.

TREATMENT

Malformed parts will never look normal and may never function completely; nevertheless, children have a remarkable ability to adapt to such anomalies and may be capable of excellent function. Treatment is based on recognition of this fact, and surgery is designed toward positioning of parts to permit the child to use them to maximum advantage (*i.e.*, to ''give an assist,'' not make a new hand). Similarly, objectionable parts or those that are impediments can be deleted. Preservation of sensation is extremely important, and corrective surgery, when indicated, should be performed early so that the child develops cerebral cortical representation of the part in the reconstructed position.

Transverse deficiencies, such as digital amputations, may require removal of small nubbins for improvement in appearance or, sometimes, no surgery. Major deficiencies can be improved with appropriate prostheses. Longitudinal deficiencies, such as radial club hand, can be treated by surgical repositioning of the hand on the limb and frequently will require a prosthesis as well.

Differentiation failure, such as syndactyly of the fingers, varies in complexity. Soft-tissue webbing can be separated and flaps and skin grafts used to avoid contracture and place sensate skin in the most useful position. Complex syndactylies involving bone and nail with absence of joints are less satisfactory because fusion is often required. Polydactylies are treated either by amputation of a supernumerary digit or by combination of parts. Supernumerary digits may be amputated in the nursery by ligature. Those that contain bone require surgical excision, and the cosmetic result is superior by this technique. Bifid digits such as thumbs are treated with removal of the central portion and union of the halves.

Overgrowths, such as gigantism, are difficult to treat and maintain function. Minor abnormalities can be managed successfully by defatting and selective osteotomy of bone. Major deformities may be best treated by amputation if the remainder of the hand is normal. Hypoplasias rarely require surgery, but congenital constriction bands or rings almost always do. In more severe forms, the distal structures may become chronically edematous because of the tourniquet effect, and peripheral nerves may be compressed. Excision of the band and Z-plasty closure is effective.

Camptodactyly, or congenital flexion, most commonly of the little fingers, is frequently bilateral and hereditary. Many adults have enjoyed near-normal function without treatment. Surgical correction is sometimes successful but may require lengthening of all soft-tissue parts and release of the PIP joint. Many surgeons feel this is unjustified on the basis of the deformity that is present. Evaluation at an early age by a hand surgeon is advisable.

TUMORS, CYSTS, AND MASSES

A mass may develop in any structure in the hand. Fortunately, the vast majority of these are benign and can be treated by simple means. Only in rare cases are major surgery and ablation necessary. The initial complaint is usually the presence of an otherwise asymptomatic "lump." Radiographs and other special studies are helpful in some instances.

BENIGN CONDITIONS

Ganglia comprise over half of all hand masses. The moderately firm, multiloculated tumor is fixed to the joint on its deep surface but otherwise movable. Diagnosis can be confirmed by aspiration. A ganglion occurs when a weakness develops in the capsular portions of a joint and is accompanied by a one-way valve mechanism so that joint fluid may be pumped into the ganglia but may not return. As water is absorbed, a characteristic thick, clear gelatin residue is produced. Not all ganglia require treatment. Aspiration and instillation of corticosteroids or subcutaneous rupture is occasionally effective, but surgical excision may be indicated if symptoms persist. To prevent recurrence, excision must be complete and must include a portion of the joint capsule. The most common sites are the dorsal and volar wrist, the flexor sheath of tendons, and the distal IP joint (mucous cyst).

Verruca vulgaris are viral warts that occur on the hand. They can be difficult to treat in areas such as the nail bed. They respond begrudgingly to keratolytic compounds and are best treated by hyfrecation and curettage.

Actinic keratoses are benign, slightly raised, scaly, and frequently abraded skin lesions. They appear in sun-exposed areas in whites and are often familial. They can be controlled with 5-fluorouracil or surgical planing and cauterization of their base. Surgical excision is a last resort. They sometimes progress to low-grade squamous cancer.

Epidermoid inclusion cysts are hard, movable, and painful and are found in the subcutaneous area. They can usually be shelled out easily through a small incision and contain typical cystic contents.

Pyogenic granuloma is a highly vascular lesion with a thin epithelial cover; it runs a course of rapid explosive growth. They are friable and may bleed, and their appearance may be suggestive of tumor. They are benign, and simple excision or even curettage is usually curative. Fingertips are the most common site.

Lipomas occur in the hand, as elsewhere. Excision may be treacherous if they happen to arise beneath the thenar or hypothenar muscles. A tourniquet should be used to allow visualization and protection of the nearby branches of nerves.

Giant cell tumors follow ganglia and epithelial cysts in frequency and occur on the fingers. They may grow relatively large, are multilobular, are firmer than a ganglion, and are less movable. They do not appear on x-ray film and are rarely ever malignant. They dissect out easily, but their origin is frequently from the underside of a tendon or the edge of a joint capsule.

Glomus tumors arise from the normal glomus, a neuro-myoarterial apparatus. They may arise in the nail bed and have a translucent appearance. They are exquisitely painful and may be subtle to diagnose. Excision produces dramatic relief.

Enchondromas comprise nearly 90% of the skeletal tumors of the hand. They are usually diagnosed radiographically following a pathologic fracture of the phalanges. They appear as a multiloculated oval lesion that expands the cortex. To treat, one must heal the fracture and then curet the tumor and bone graft the defect.

Osteochondromas are benign bony exostoses that usually occur near a zone of growth such as the metaphysis or the tuft of the distal phalanx. On x-ray film, they may appear pedunculated and have a covering of thin sclerotic bone. The tumor proper appears comprised of normal bony elements. Simple excision only is necessary.

Solitary bone cyst is a defect usually found in the distal metacarpal or proximal phalanges. It frequently appears as a painless swelling and, unlike enchondromas, is rarely seen in pathologic fractures. X-ray film demonstrates an asymmetrical mass that may be uniloculated or multiloculated with a sclerotic surface. Surgery is usually curative.

Osteoid osteoma is a rare tumor of young adults, which usually presents as pain in one of the phalanges. It appears as a sclerotic patch of bone on x-ray film and can be removed, with subsequent relief of pain.

Aneurysmal bone cysts are expanding lesions of the metacarpal and proximal phalanx which usually present as painless masses. On x-ray film, one sees a thin-shelled mass with faint trabeculations. At operation, the tumor is quite vascular but can be cured by curettage and bone grafting.

Giant cell tumors of the bone must be considered in the differential diagnosis of a mass in the region of the MP joint, but they are extremely rare.

Hemangiomas of the hand are similar to those of other parts of the body. In skin, they are easily diagnosed, and treatment usually poses no problem. They can be excised. A skin graft may sometimes be necessary.

Arteriovenous fistulas are frequently associated with enlargement of a digit or a larger component of the hand. There may be bony overgrowth, and an arteriogram illustrates the complex nature of the communications. The outlook may be poor, and amputation of parts is sometimes necessary.

Lymphangioma is a rarely seen benign tumor of the hand. It appears as a multiloculated mass with cutaneous excrescences. Surgical excision is the treatment of choice.

MALIGNANT TUMORS

Squamous cell carcinoma is by far the most common malignant tumor. Fortunately, they are usually low grade. They occur most often in the skin of keratotic persons who have had frequent tumors before. Local excision is curative in most cases. In a rare instance, the tumor will appear as an enlarging mass or will involve bone. Destructive changes are demonstrated radiographically, and the tumor should be treated more aggressively, usually with amputation of the digit. Metastases to regional nodes are possible but rarely seen. They should always be sought.

Basal cell carcinoma may appear as a rodent ulcer or a cutaneous mass on the hand as it does in other sun-exposed areas. Excision with primary closure or skin graft is adequate treatment, because they practically never metastasize.

Melanoma is the most malignant skin tumor and may arise on the palm or beneath the nails. Pigmentation is not always present, and the diagnosis may be a subtle one. It should be considered in an unusually located and aggressively behaving tumor. Treatment requires more radical excision, and regional lymphadenectomy may be necessary.

Sarcomas such as chondrosarcoma, liposarcoma, osteogenic sarcoma, and fibrosarcoma of the hand have all been reported but are extremely rare. Low-grade tumors respond to local excision, but aggressive tumors have a high mortality, and treatment should combine chemotherapy and surgery. Malignant vascular tumors such as hemangioepitheliomas and hemangiosarcomas may also be quite aggressive, and treatment is frequently only palliative.

INFECTION

Hand infection is common, but with the advent of the antibiotic era the condition has changed from one of grave consequence to one that is readily treatable. Nevertheless, delays in treatment by either patient or physician can still result in great functional disability. Tendons and joints tolerate suppuration poorly, and stiffness and pain are inevitable results (For hand incisions, see Figure 42-3.)

PARONYCHIA

Paronychia (runaround, hangnail) is the most common infection, and it occurs in nail biters or pullers. Swelling, redness, and pain at the nail edge confirm the diagnosis. Most are staphylococcal, and early cases respond to soaks and the administration of penicillin. The tip of a needle beneath the nail edge will usually evacuate a drop of pus. Advanced cases require incision of the eponychium and removal of part of the nail to effect adequate drainage.

FELON

Felon is a deep closed-space infection of the fingertip pulp that occurs when organisms are seeded between the fibrous septa that fix skin to bone. Early redness and throbbing pain progress to ashen gray numbness unless treatment is begun early. Felons must be distinguished from the exquisitely painful vesicular eruption of herpetic viral infections, which, of course, do not require incision and drainage. Early felons can be cured with antibiotics, elevation, and warm soaks but must be observed closely.

TENOSYNOVITIS

Tenosynovitis, infection within the flexor sheath, has potentially high morbidity because of the closed space (tendon sheath) and relatively avascular structures (flexor tendons) involved. The cardinal signs of fixed position in slight flexion, pain on passive extension of the tip (similar to rebound

HAND INFECTION	
Etiology	Mostly bacterial, sometimes viral and fungal
	Penetrating wounds are frequent antecedents, but cause may be unknown
	Staph and strep the most common organisms in home and workplace; gram-negative organisms more frequent in soiled wounds
Dx	Diagnosis presumptive until appropriate culture and sensitivity are available; special culture media and temperature indicated in unusual cases
	Viral infections can be distinguished by appearance and history
	Suspect human bite wounds around knuckles and tips
Rx	Early infection usually cured by antibiotics, rest of part, elevation, and warm soaks
	If pus is suspected, early incision and drainage to limit necrosis and preserve function
	Appropriate and multiple small incisions preferred
	Catheter irrigation with antibiotic solution and splinting helpful
	Cleanse, dress, and perform delayed closure of wounds suspected of human bite or other contaminated source

tenderness), uniform swelling, and redness, plus an appropriate history, are usually diagnostic. One must rule out nonbacterial tenosynovitis resulting from rheumatoid arthritis, osteoarthritis, or acute gouty arthritis before instituting surgical treatment.

Treatment of early tenosynovitis is application of local heat, rest, and administration of a staphicidal antibiotic. Early surgical drainage is indicated if pus is suspected, because frank pus in the tendon sheath almost certainly results in necrosis of the tendon and a disabled finger. If patient reliability is questionable, hospitalization is advised.

DEEP SPACE INFECTIONS

Deep space infections of the palm occur by direct inoculation or extension from undrained tenosynovitis into either the thenar space or the midpalmar space (these lie deep to the flexor tendons and are separated by a longitudinal septum). One must be aware of this possibility, since these spaces may otherwise be overlooked. Similarly, extensions from the tendon sheaths of the thumb and little finger to the radial and ulnar bursae proximal to the wrist crease may require drainage in the lower forearm. In advanced cases, extension may even continue to Parona's space at the level of the pronator quadratus muscle.

COLLAR-BUTTON ABSCESS

Collar-button abscess is an anachronistic name for the shape of a continuous infection that appears on both the dorsal and the volar aspect of the digital web space; the central portion is limited in size by the palmar fascia and lumbrical canal. Treatment is surgical drainage from both sides.

VARIOUS SUBCUTANEOUS INFECTIONS

Various subcutaneous infections may occur anywhere on the hand and are to be distinguished from deep infections of specific spaces. These may arise in a variety of dermatologic conditions, such as rashes or folliculitis, as well as from puncture wounds, foreign bodies, or cuts.

RARE INFECTIONS

In addition to common bacterial infections, mycobacterium infections are sometimes seen. Tuberculosis is becoming rarer but may still occur in bones, synovium, and joints. Surgical synovectomy is helpful in both treatment and diagnosis, but cure requires long-term antituberculous drug therapy. In addition, *Mycobacterium marinum* is sometimes encountered. A history of exposure to an aquatic environment or to nautical equipment is helpful. The bacteriologist must be told that the diagnosis is suspected, because cultures must be incubated at a lower temperature. Again, treatment is with surgery and antituberculous drugs.

A number of fungal infections occur, particularly around the nails. These are usually chronic and indolent, with resulting nail deformity. Cures are possible with antifungal drugs, but treatment must continue for many months.

SPECIAL TYPES

HUMAN BITE INFECTIONS

The diagnosis of human bite infection should be suspected in patients with lacerations over the MP joint that might have occurred by striking a tooth. They may be several hours old or a few days old, profusely swollen, and tender. The patient may be febrile. This usually means that the joint has been inoculated with oral organisms. Treatment frequently requires hospitalization, open drainage, and intravenous antibiotics. When seen early, such injuries should be suspected and the wounds should not be closed.

INFECTIONS IN DIABETICS

Infected hands, like other infections in diabetes, are more serious and respond less well to treatment. When infection occurs in a typical location or the course seems inappropriate, the patient should be screened carefully for diabetes. Whether the poor response is due to the diabetes itself or to the associated small-vessel disease is not known. Patients should be warned that major infections sometimes result in amputation.

INFECTIONS IN IMMUNOSUPPRESSED PATIENTS

Immunosuppressed patients, for whatever reason, tolerate infection poorly. An otherwise minor problem in such patients requires close supervision and aggressive treatment.

BURNS

ACUTE BURN TREATMENT

The goal of acute burn treatment is to heal the wound and preserve function. In treating burned hands, the techniques are not unlike those of burn care in general, *with this exception:* Inattention to splinting and range-of-motion exercises during the healing period may result in a healed

BURNS OF THE HAND	
Etiology	Usually heat induced; frostbite and radiation may produce similar change
Dx	Assess as minimal, partial, or full thickness of skin; deep structures may be burned also Trained eye is only available tool, although vital dyes may be used Look for signs of ischemia in circumferential burns of hand or arm
Rx	Burn creams and motion to prevent infection and restore function Tangential excision and immediate grafting for partial-thickness burn and full-thickness excision and grafting for deeper burns Early escharotomy for sensory changes or signs of ischemia

wound with stiff joints and contractures—a treatment failure.

Deep dermal burns should yield uniformly good results if infection does not supervene and convert the depth of injury to full thickness and if healing is completed by 3 weeks. This can often be accomplished by frequent dressings, antibiotic ointment, and exercises. Alternatively, tangential excision of the burned elements while preserving the unburned deep dermal layer permits skin grafting and earlier wound closure, thereby hastening the healing process.

Full-thickness burns of skin are best treated with early excision and skin grafting, either immediately or after a 1- to 2-day delay. Motion in the grafted hand can then be started a few days later and function preserved.

Deeper burns, which involve subcutaneous fat, tendon, and joint capsule, are notoriously difficult to treat and practically guarantee some functional loss. If the burn is limited to the hand or extremity, aggressive measures are justified to try and save functioning structures, but deep burns frequently accompany other major injuries, and one may have to compromise treatment of the hands to save life. Simple maneuvers such as splinting or Kirschner wire fixation of joints will buy time and will be worthwhile if the patient survives.

Circumferential burns of digits, hand, or arm should be measured and observed frequently for signs of vascular compromise. If increased pressure is suspected, early escharotomy is indicated. Subeschar pressure measurements by the method of Whitesides are helpful if doubt exists.

LATE BURN RECONSTRUCTION

Secondary joint deformity with stiffness and malposition may occur despite one's best effort. Although such hands are rarely returned to full function, they can be improved by secondary reconstructive procedures. Hypertrophic scars and mild contractures respond to custom-fitted elastic compression garments. Major skin contractures are best treated with surgical release and Z-plasty with local skin or with excision and skin graft. The characteristic post-burn deformity of MP joint extension, IP joint flexion, and thumb adduction requires appropriate capsulectomy and skin graft.

Tenotomy of the adductor pollicis and other intrinsic tendons may be necessary. In more severe deformities of all joints, it may be necessary to resort to IP joint fusion in slight flexion and to concentrate on MP joint motion. If IP joint motion can be preserved in the little or ring finger, grip strength will be significantly greater. When bone and joint are burned, the outlook is for limited function only, but silicone joint replacement is occasionally helpful in selected cases.

Amputation of gangrenous digits or even hands may be necessary in the acute phase of burn care, but this is virtually never indicated in reconstructive situations, because the sensation remaining in the part makes it more valuable than a prosthesis. Viable digits are always best preserved.

ARTHRITIS, CONTRACTURES, FIBROMATOSES

ARTHRITIS

Osteoarthritis, degenerative arthritis, and rheumatoid arthritis are the three most common of the many types of arthritis. Of these three types, rheumatoid disease is easily the most deforming, but all may be quite painful and disabling. The basic pathologic process in rheumatoid arthritis is a proliferation of synovium and subsynovial fibrous tissue, which results in destruction of hyaline cartilage and subchondral bone along with stretching, attenuation, and actual rupture of ligaments and tendons. Although medical management is the mainstay of the systemic illness, surgery can be valuable in pain relief and rehabilitation of crippled hands.

A variety of procedures are available, and treatment is based on the needs of each patient. These may include arthrodesis of joints for stability, arthroplasty with silicone implants for mobility, tendon transfer for ruptures or rebalancing, synovectomy for pain relief, and decompression of nerves or tendons rendered nonfunctional by the proliferative synovitis. All such procedures can be performed with minimal risk using regional or local anesthesia and can improve function substantially. They may be extremely valuable in improving the quality of life for the patient afflicted with arthritis.

DUPUYTREN'S DISEASE

Dupuytren's disease may present with cutaneous nodules or contracting bands. In either case, the underlying process is the same: thickening and shortening of the palmar fascia. Frequently bilateral, the disease occurs most often in males of European extraction and is hereditary. The treatment is excision of the diseased fascia.

DE QUERVAIN'S DISEASE

De Quervain's disease and trigger finger have in common that both occur where synovium-wrapped tendons pass through fibrous tunnels. Why de Quervain's disease occurs at the first dorsal compartment of the wrist and trigger finger occurs in the ring finger is not known. Both cause pain and tenderness, and the tendon may "lock." Fortunately, both respond to a relatively innocuous operation. Division of the overlying fascia is curative.

BIBLIOGRAPHY

BEASLEY RW: Hand Injuries. Philadelphia, W B Saunders, 1981

CHANG WHJ (ed): Fundamentals of Plastic and Reconstructive Surgery. Baltimore, Williams & Wilkins, 1980

FLATT AE: The Care of Congenital Hand Anomalies. St. Louis, C V Mosby, 1977

FLYNN JE (ed): Hand Surgery, 3rd ed. Baltimore, Williams & Wilkins, 1982

JABALEY ME: Current concepts of nerve repair. Clin Plast Surg 8:33, 1981

LISTER G: The Hand: Diagnosis and Indications. Edinburgh, Churchill Livingstone, 1977

SPINNER M: Injuries to the Major Branches of Peripheral Nerves of the Forearm. Philadelphia, W B Saunders, 1978

WOLFERT FG (ed): Acute Hand Injuries: A Multispecialty Approach. Boston, Little, Brown & Co, 1980

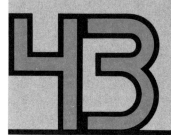

Frederick R. Heckler

Principles of Plastic and Reconstructive Surgery

The term plastic surgery is derived from the Greek *plastikos*, meaning to shape, mold, or form, and signifies a discipline whose primary objectives and special abilities center around the repair and reconstruction of acquired and congenital deformities and tissue defects. These surgical efforts may be oriented toward restoring or improving appearance, function, or both, and may be directed toward the surface tissues or deeper structures in almost any anatomic region of the body.

The plastic surgeon himself typically possesses broad-based training in general surgery as well as advanced training in plastic and reconstructive surgery. This broad-based background and extensive training enable the board-certified plastic and reconstructive surgeon to apply the general principles of wound healing and tissue transfer to all areas of the body in multiple and varied pathophysiologic situations.

GENERAL PRINCIPLES

WOUND MANAGEMENT AND REPAIR

General principles of wound management and wound repair are applicable to all surgical situations whether elective or traumatic. The goals of these techniques are to obtain primary wound healing without infection or prolonged inflammation and to produce a scar that is favorable, both in functional stability and cosmetic appearance.

ELECTIVE SURGICAL INCISIONS

Elective incisions, particularly those on the face, neck, and extremities should be placed in or parallel to the natural skin creases and folds (Fig. 43-1A). In the head and neck these lines are normally perpendicular to the pull of the underlying muscles of facial expression. In the extremities they are perpendicular to the axis of motion of the joints. Scars from incision lines that do not conform to these guidelines tend to hypertrophy in unsightly fashion and, following normal scar contraction, may distort the adjacent facial features or limit joint motion.

Elective surgical incisions should be made perpendicular to the skin plane and should not be beveled, except in hair-bearing areas where bevelling in the direction of hair follicles will avoid damage to these underlying structures and prevent subsequent hair loss (Fig. 43-1B, C). Emphasis on gentle tissue handling and the use of fine instruments will minimize local surgical trauma and encourage favorable wound healing. Hemostasis should be absolute.

Wound closure should be accomplished with the finest suture that is adequate for existing wound tension. Generally the subcutaneous tissues are approximated with fine absorbable material incorporating a small dermal bite in each suture. If done properly, this subcutaneous-dermal closure will closely approximate and slightly evert the skin edges,

Fig. 43-1. Elective incisions and skin closure technique. (*A*) Elective incisions should be placed in or parallel to natural skin creases and folds. (*B*) Subcutaneous-dermal absorbable suture approximates the skin and takes up all wound tension. Fine, nonabsorbable skin suture everts and aligns the epidermis (*arrows*). (*C*) In hair-bearing areas, elective incisions are beveled to avoid damaging hair roots with subsequent hair loss. Perpendicular incisions, proper in other areas of the body, will permanently damage hair roots (*arrow*).

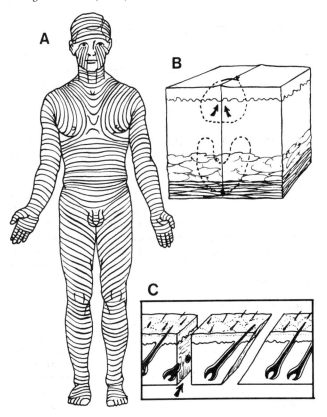

allowing the role of the final skin suture to be simple alignment of the epidermal margins of the already approximated wound. Extremely fine suture material may then be employed (usually 5–0 or 6–0 nylon or silk), resulting in less wound edge trauma and scar formation. If skin tension is too great to allow the use of such fine materials, then it is probably also too great for ideal wound healing and favorable scarring. In such situations, consideration should be given to some of the various surgical maneuvers available to reduce wound tension such as skin undermining and advancement, local flap rotation, and skin grafting.

Sutures should be removed at the earliest possible time consistent with the development of adequate tensile strength to avoid wound disruption. The key to safe, early suture removal is proper use of the absorbable subcutaneous-dermal suture. This layer takes up most of the tension of the wound closure and permits early skin suture removal. Sutures that are left in place longer than necessary often result in the cosmetically undesirable "railroad track" appearance of punctate suture scars along the central surgical scar.

TRAUMATIC INCISIONS AND WOUNDS

The importance of proper wound management is magnified in the treatment of traumatic lacerations. Such wounds by their nature are bacterially contaminated in varying degrees and in addition often contain contused, ragged, completely or partially devitalized bits of tissue. Surgical creation of a wound environment favorable to primary wound healing will promote cosmetically acceptable scarring and avoid the negative effects of infection and poor healing.

Cleaning and Débridement

Thorough irrigation of the wound with isotonic saline, removal of all dirt and foreign matter, and sharp débridement of devitalized or hopelessly contaminated soft tissues should be the first order of business. Primary wound closure, even of unfavorable wounds, will usually be successful in the head and neck area and is most likely to result in the best scar. The key to this successful result, however, lies in meticulous initial cleansing and débridement. The actual suturing then proceeds as in elective incisions. A short course of antibiotics is also usually advisable when the wound is compromised. The status of tetanus immunization should be checked and additional prophylaxis provided if indicated.

Timing of Repair

Traumatic wounds in areas outside the head and neck generally can also safely be repaired primarily after vigorous cleansing and débridement. Extremely heavily contaminated wounds in these anatomic areas are less favorable, and surgical judgment in assessing the local wound conditions must be exercised before deciding if primary wound repair is indicated. In such compromised situations, it is often wisest to cleanse, debride, and pack the wound at the initial surgical effort, and consider delayed primary repair after several days.

FLAPS AND GRAFTS: WHAT THEY ARE, WHERE THEY ARE USED

Flaps and grafts in various forms are the main tools in the reconstructive surgeon's armamentarium. They provide the means of transferring living tissue from one area of the body to another and are used to repair difficult wounds that do not permit direct approximation and suture or to reconstruct absent, malformed, or malfunctioning body parts.

DEFINITIONS AND TERMINOLOGY

The term graft means that the tissue transferred is completely detached from its donor site during transfer to the recipient site. Inherent in the grafting of the living tissue, therefore, is the fact that the transferred tissue is completely cut off from its normal sources of oxygen and nutrients and within a finite time span must acquire a new source of such supply at the recipient site in order to maintain viability.

Flaps fundamentally differ from grafts in that during transfer they remain attached to the body by a pedicle through which blood supply is maintained. Much of the normal quantity of skin blood flow is interrupted during flap elevation and transfer, but because adequate nutrition is maintained through the pedicle, early revascularization from the recipient bed, mandatory for grafts, is *not* necessary to maintain flap viability.

SPLIT-THICKNESS SKIN GRAFTS

Split-thickness skin grafts (Fig. 43-2), depending on particular reconstructive requirements, include the epidermis and varying thicknesses of dermis. Thin split-thickness skin grafts are 10 to 12 thousandths of an inch in thickness, and thick split-thickness grafts are 18 to 20 thousandths of a inch thick. The graft is removed from the donor site as a sheet of tissue by using either a long razorlike free-hand knife or one of several types of mechanical dermatomes. These instruments facilitate the cutting of large sheets of split-thickness skin of uniform thickness.

The skin graft is transferred to the recipient site and secured in position. The donor site re-epithelializes its surface with cells derived from the surrounding intact skin and also from the remaining intradermal epithelium-lined appendages such as sweat glands and hair follicles. The length of time required for donor site healing depends upon the thickness of the graft taken but is usually completed within 2 or 3 weeks.

Successful grafting requires the presence of a recipient bed capable of revascularizing the graft by capillary sprouting and ingrowth into the transferred tissue. Indeed, the presence or absence of such an adequate recipient bed is the most important criterion in choosing whether a graft or a flap is the best reconstructive modality for the situation at hand.

Initially, the graft survives on diffusion of oxygen and nutrients across the graft-bed interface. Within 24 hr, capillaries from the recipient bed begin invading the raw dermal undersurface of the graft and reestablish blood circulation. Failure or delay of such revascularization may be caused by infection or by prevention of intimate contact between graft and recipient bed by hematoma or seroma. Mechanical disruption of the newly formed capillary ingrowths may result from inadequate immobilization of the graft or of the grafted part. Any of these factors, if not appropriately prevented, will result in graft necrosis.

FULL-THICKNESS SKIN GRAFTS

Full-thickness skin grafts consist of all skin layers but not the underlying subcutaneous fat. Their survival after transfer also depends upon revascularization by capillary ingrowth at the recipient site. Such revascularization, however, is less reliable than with a split-thickness graft simply because of

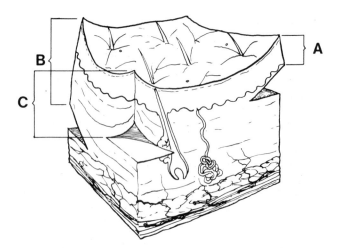

Fig. 43-2. Types of skin grafts. (*A*) Thin split-thickness skin graft transfers all epidermis and a small amount of dermis. (*B*) Full-thickness skin graft transfers epidermis and all of the dermal layer, leaving subcutaneous fat exposed. (*C*) Medium split-thickness graft transfers epidermis and approximately half of the dermis.

the greater volume of tissue requiring reestablishment of blood flow and the limited time in which this process must occur.

OTHER TYPES OF GRAFTS

Other free grafts used by the reconstructive surgeon include cartilage (from nasal septum, costal cartilage, or auricle), bone, mucous membrane, nerve, and composite grafts such as skin and hair follicle, dermis and fat, or skin combined with underlying cartilage. The basic biology of the grafting of each of these follows the same principles described for skin grafting with minor variations.

FLAPS

In contrast to grafts, flaps maintain an attachment to the body so that some portion of the usual quantity of blood supplied to the flap while in its native anatomic position is maintained. During flap elevation and transfer, a considerable proportion of the usual vascular supply of the flap must be divided, and the volume of tissue that can safely be moved is limited by this fact. Despite this inherent diminution in blood flow, the fact that flaps carry with them their own blood supply makes them relatively independent of the condition of the recipient bed and allows transfer of greater volumes of tissue than is possible with grafts.

As the transferred flap heals to the recipient site, vascular connections are established with the surrounding tissues. It takes 2 to 3 weeks for sufficient recipient-site connections to be established to allow detachment of the umbilical cordlike pedicle. The transferred tissue will then survive on this new blood supply derived from the tissues surrounding the recipient site.

Basic Physiology

Blood Supply of Skin. It is self-evident that success in flap surgery requires proper planning and thoughtful insight into the normal anatomy of skin vasculature (Fig. 43-3*A*).

Skin blood flow is principally distributed through a ubiquitous and diffuse microvascular network in the subdermal plexus. This vascular plexus in turn is generally fed by small vertical perforating vessels from the underlying

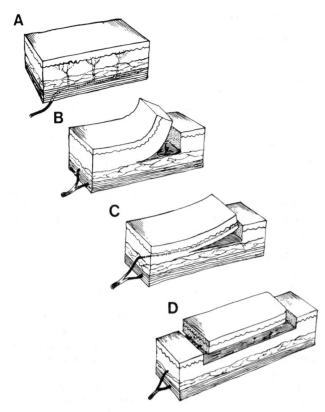

Fig. 43-3. Categories of flaps. (*A*) Normal skin vascular supply. Major blood vessel enters muscle. Small vertical perforating vessels pass through fascia and subcutaneous tissue to subdermal plexus where blood supply is distributed to skin.

(*B*) Random pattern flap. Flap is elevated through subcutaneous tissue. Vertical perforating vessels are therefore divided during flap elevation, leaving skin blood supply only through flap base.

(*C*) Axial pattern flap. Flap is elevated at extrafascial level but includes a major longitudinal vessel running in subcutaneous tissues.

(*D*) Island pedicle flap. Flap is elevated at the same level as an axial flap but the skin is divided at the base, leaving the flap dependent on the arteriovenous pedicle alone.

musculature. In certain anatomic areas, larger, longitudinally oriented vessels penetrate the underlying muscular fascia and run in the subcutaneous tissues, giving off multiple branches to the subdermal plexus. These vessels are termed *axial or direct cutaneous vessels.* Some examples of axial vessels include the superficial temporal, dorsalis pedis, and superficial circumflex iliac arteries. Application of this understanding of skin vascular anatomy and of the anatomic alterations in blood supply engendered by flap elevation has given rise to the modern categorization of flaps by their blood supply and patterns of vascularity.

Nomenclature and Categories of Flaps

Skin flaps that depend for their blood supply upon musculocutaneous perforating vessels alone are termed *random pattern flaps* (Fig. 43-3*B*). The length of flap and quantity of tissue that can be transferred are limited by the perfusion pressure transmitted to the base of the flap through these musculocutaneous perforators. In the head and neck area, experience has taught that the random pattern flap dimensions that are safe can be 2:1 or 3:1 in length-width ratios, whereas in the trunk and lower extremity length-width

ratios of $1\frac{1}{2}$:1 or 1:1 are the most that can be tolerated without risking distal necrosis of the flap.

If a known longitudinal axial vessel running in the subcutaneous tissues is elevated and included with the flap, it is termed an *axial pattern flap* (Fig. 43-3*C*). Because such axial flaps carry their own major blood vessel with them, long narrow flaps with considerable length-width ratios may be safely constructed and transferred. If the skin and soft tissues of the axial pedicle are removed leaving the flap tissues attached only by the vessels themselves, the term *island pedicle flap* is applied (Fig. 43-3*D*).

With the realization that the limiting factor in size and length of random pattern flaps was that the skin flap was separated in large part from the underlying muscle from which its feeding musculocutaneous perforator vessels derived, another concept of flap reconstruction was developed. It was reasoned that the skin and underlying muscle might be elevated and shifted into a new position as a composite unit based upon a single major muscular vascular branch. This was termed a *musculocutaneous flap* and has proved to be feasible and successful in many anatomic areas. *Muscle flaps* alone, without their overlying skin, are also widely used. The muscle is shifted to the recipient site, and a split-thickness skin graft is applied.

Other Categories and Classifications of Flaps

Through the years a number of other classifications and nomenclature systems for flaps have been utilized. These systems have had various bases, including site of flap origin, geometric construction and pattern, types of tissues included in the flap, and surgical maneuvers required to construct and transfer the flap.

Probably the most useful current system other than those described in preceding sections is the nomenclature based on site of origin. Flaps derived from tissues adjacent to the defect to be reconstructed are called *local flaps.* These flaps usually provide skin that closely matches the color and consistency of the skin previously present in the defect being reconstructed. The residual local skin available for flap reconstruction may, however, be somewhat limited, and the resulting donor scar may be undesirable, particularly in exposed areas such as the head, neck, and distal extremities. On the plus side, the proximity of donor to recipient locations usually allows the flap's pedicle to be incorporated into the repair. The pedicle can then remain permanently in place, obviating the need for a second surgical procedure for pedicle division.

Distant flaps are derived, as the name implies, from tissues at a distance from the defect. In practice, distant flaps are most often derived from the trunk and lower extremity. Large quantities of skin are available, and donor scars are concealed by clothing. Color and texture match are not as good as with local flaps, and the nutrient pedicle, which temporarily maintains flap viability while vascular connections are being established at the recipient site, usually must be detached at a second surgical procedure.

MICROSURGERY AND FREE FLAP TRANSFER

Recently another modality has been added to the armamentarium of the plastic and reconstructive surgeon. Reconstructive efforts were somewhat limited previously by the length of flap pedicle that could practically be developed while still maintaining enough blood flow to avoid flap necrosis. The development of the operating microscope, appropriately fine-sized microneedles and suture, and microinstruments have allowed successful anastomosis of vessels in the range of 0.5 mm to 2.0 mm in diameter. Concomitantly, advancements in the understanding of the blood supply to the skin and superficial muscles have allowed the detachment of large areas of skin and soft tissue that are dependent upon a single arterial–venous axial pedicle. These tissue segments may now be reliably completely detached from the donor site, transferred to a recipient site, and sutured to the recipient vascular pedicle using microtechnique. These microtechniques have been used for the free transfer of skin, muscles, and compound musculocutaneous and osteomusculocutaneous flaps as well as for free vascularized bone grafts.

The same microtechniques have allowed considerable success in the replantation of traumatically amputated body parts including fingers and toes, scalp, ear, extremities, and the penis.

CHOICE OF RECONSTRUCTIVE MODALITY

In determining whether or not the reconstructive problem at hand requires a skin graft, a flap, or both, the reconstructive surgeon must consider a large number of variables. First, the needs of the injured or malformed part are considered including whether or not skin or both skin and underlying bulk are required to effect an ideal reconstruction. The surgeon assesses whether or not bony or cartilaginous architecture must be rebuilt, whether bulk is required to repair a contour defect, and what color, texture, and quality of skin are needed to best repair the tissue deficit present.

The vascularizing potential of the recipient bed is of prime importance. Damaged, heavily scarred, or irradiated tissue beds will not support free grafts, and flaps are usually required. Likewise, injuries or defects that expose bone devoid of periosteum, cartilage devoid of perichondrium, or open joints will not support skin grafts and require flap coverage. The reconstructive surgeon must also consider the donor site deformity that will be created and must choose the reconstructive technique that will best reconstruct the problem at hand while minimizing the attendant donor deformity.

FACIAL TRAUMA

The incidence of major facial trauma continues to rise in our modern era of high-speed vehicular travel. These injuries may endanger life, threaten function, and leave aesthetically undesirable consequences. An organized approach to early management will minimize these adverse effects and maximize chances for a favorable outcome.

LIFE-THREATENING VS. NON–LIFE-THREATENING INJURIES

Major facial injuries may threaten life in several ways:
1. Upper airway obstruction
2. Profuse hemorrhage
3. Direct damage to adjacent intracranial structures
4. Injury to the cervical spinal cord

Early acute management should, therefore, be directed toward these entities. A suggested order of approach follows.

AIRWAY OBSTRUCTION

Airway obstruction may result from aspirated blood clots, teeth, bone, or soft tissue fragments. With severe facial fractures, skeletal support of the tongue or facial soft tissues is lost, and these structures may prolapse posteriorly, occluding the airway. Upon arrival in the emergency room, inspection for adequate respiration is performed. If cyanosis, cervicothoracic retractions, or labored respirations are present, the oropharynx should be inspected and cleared of debris. Positioning the patient face down will encourage drainage of foreign matter, secretion, and blood and will allow the tongue and soft tissues to drop forward out of the pharynx. If these measures are inadequate, endotracheal intubation through oral or nasal routes should be performed. Emergency tracheotomy is implemented as a last resort but is rarely needed unless intubation cannot be accomplished.

HEMORRHAGE

Hemorrhage in facial trauma frequently appears to be life-threatening owing to the copious bleeding that occurs from the highly vascular facial structures. Most bleeding from facial injuries will be well controlled by the application of pressure alone. Blind attempts at clamping and ligating bleeding vessels deep in facial wounds are strongly discouraged owing to the danger of inadvertently injuring other important structures within the wound such as branches of the facial nerve. Once pressure has controlled major hemorrhage, specific hemostasis can be accomplished under more ideal conditions with adequate light, instruments, and assistance.

INTRACRANIAL AND CERVICAL SPINE INJURIES

Intracranial and cervical spine injuries should always be suspected in patients with major facial trauma. A brief evaluation of the level of consciousness, cranial nerve functions, spinal cord reflexes, and peripheral sensation and motor function should be an early part of the initial examination. Abnormal findings call for appropriate skull x-ray films and neurosurgical consultation. Any patient sustaining trauma severe enough to fracture the facial skeleton may have sustained enough force to result in cervical spine fractures. Cervical spine x-ray films should therefore be strongly considered for all patients suffering severe facial trauma, particularly deceleration-type injuries such as those occurring in high-speed vehicular crashes.

NON–LIFE-THREATENING SOFT TISSUE INJURIES

Soft tissue injuries, while not life-threatening, are nevertheless serious in that they threaten important facial functions, appearance, or both. Following the initial efforts to deal with life-threatening injuries, a more leisurely and detailed evaluation, including close physical examination and evocative tests for neuromuscular function, is carried out.

Functional soft tissue units at risk include the eyelids, nasal airway, lips and perioral musculature, facial nerve, and parotid gland and duct.

EYELID INJURIES

Simple lid lacerations are cleansed, débrided, and repaired in layers, using absorbable suture or a continuous pull-out type suture on the tarsal plate and 6–0 nylon for skin closure. Great care must be taken to accurately align the lid margins, thus avoiding lid notching.

If actual loss of the eyelid tissue has occurred, reconstructive measures will be required. Simple skin loss is replaced by a local flap or a skin graft. Wide undermining of skin with closure under tension is *not* done because tension will distort the lid and interfere with normal lid mobility and function. A large number of procedures have been described to replace full-thickness loss of lid tissue. Up to 30% of the horizontal length of the lid may be lost and still allow suture repair without undue tension. Losses of greater magnitude are managed with regional cheek flaps or flaps from the opposing undamaged lid.

Lacerations of the lid that are medial to the lacrimal punctum should lead to suspicion of injury to the lacrimal canaliculus. A lacrimal probe placed through the punctum will appear in the wound if such injury has occurred. Continuity of the tear duct is reestablished using magnification and extremely fine suture material. Failure to diagnose such an injury will result in chronic tearing due to blockage of the lacrimal drainage system.

PAROTID GLAND AND FACIAL NERVE INJURIES

The seventh cranial nerve exits from the stylomastoid foramen and enters the substance of the parotid gland in the preauricular area. Within the parotid, the nerve divides into its major subdivisions with each major trunk proceeding toward its focal muscles of innervation. Considerable interchange and interconnections exist between the more peripheral branches of the facial nerve.

Facial lacerations in the areas of distribution of the facial nerve are always suspect for nerve injury. Evocative tests for facial motor nerve function should always be performed *prior* to the injection of any local anesthetics. In sequence, the patient is asked to elevate the eyebrows wrinkling the forehead, squeeze the eyes tightly shut, raise the upper lip showing the upper teeth, depress the lower lip showing the lower teeth, form the lips into an O, and puff out the cheeks. This easily performed sequence will demonstrate voluntary action of each of the important facial mimetic groups innervated by major facial nerve trunks. Failure of any group to contract in symmetry with the opposite side is diagnostic.

Nerve repair is always performed in the major operating theatre under optimal conditions, never in the emergency room. The distal nerve endings remain sensitive to electrical stimulation for 48 hr to 72 hr following nerve division. Repair carried out within this time frame allows easier identification of the distal cut ends using the nerve stimulator. Repair is performed with the aid of the operating microscope using microsurgical techniques. Groups of fascicles within the cut nerve ends are matched and lined up with each other, and repair is accomplished with 9–0 or 10–0 nylon.

PAROTID INJURIES

Lacerations of the cheek that injure the facial nerve also of necessity penetrate the parotid salivary gland. These injuries are of modest significance as long as the major parotid duct remains patent. In such instances, local cleansing and débridement followed by suture closure of the parotid capsule and repair of the skin laceration are all that are required. Some temporary leakage of saliva into the subcutaneous tissues may ensue but will be reabsorbed without untoward results in the absence of infection.

Lacerations of the parotid duct itself, however, do require repair. Failure to do so will result in continued major leakage of saliva into the soft tissues, inadequate drainage of the parotid parenchyma proximal to the injury, and eventual infection, abscess, salivary fistula, or cyst formation.

Topographically, the parotid duct lies deep to a line drawn on the face between the auricular tragus and the midportion of the upper lip. If a laceration crosses this line, parotid duct laceration must be considered. A small metal probe or a narrow diameter polyethylene tube is passed transorally through the parotid duct orifice. The probe will appear in the wound if a ductal laceration is present.

The lacerated parotid duct should be repaired with fine absorbable sutures over a tube stent that is led out through the parotid duct orifice into the mouth and sutured to the buccal mucosa. This stent will maintain ductal patency during the healing period.

AURICULAR INJURIES

The external ear is structurally unique in that the delicately folded and sculpted cartilaginous framework is covered on both sides with thin skin with little or no intervening subcutaneous tissue. Blunt trauma, lacerations, and avulsive injuries thus readily involve both the cutaneous cover and the underlying cartilaginous framework of the ear.

Blunt trauma may be either direct or shearing in nature. Shearing forces are particularly apt to produce subperichondrial hematoma. Calcification, fibrosis, and scarring of these hematomas lead to permanent deformity commonly called cauliflower ear. Treatment is directed toward prevention and consists of draining the hematoma and preventing its recurrence with a carefully molded pressure dressing that holds the soft tissues in close apposition to the underlying cartilage.

Lacerations of the ear most often involve both skin and cartilage. Repair consists of judicial débridement of skin and cartilage, trimming back 1 mm to 2 mm of cartilage and following this by suture repair. A few absorbable sutures are placed to align the cartilage, and fine nylon repairs the skin. Antibiotics should be considered because the relatively avascular cartilage is prone to infection in contaminated wounds.

PERIORAL INJURIES

Lacerations of the lips are often seen after blunt external blows that drive the perioral soft tissues onto the teeth. Such wounds, as well as lip lacerations from other sources, may generally be repaired primarily despite the obvious contaminations with local oral bacterial flora. Good healing is the general rule, due in great part to the superb blood supply of the facial region.

After vigorous cleansing and careful débridement, lip repair proceeds in layers (Fig. 43-4). The initial suture should precisely align the mucocutaneous junction or "white roll border." Absorbable sutures then repair the oral mucosa and the orbicularis oris muscle, and the skin is sutured last.

Major avulsive injuries with extensive loss of tissue require replacement, generally with local flaps. The extensive dissection required to deliver new tissue into the lip after major avulsive loss may encourage infection if done immediately after contaminated and traumatic injury and is best deferred to a later elective time.

FACIAL FRACTURES

The initial management of patients with facial fractures is identical to that previously outlined for treatment of any

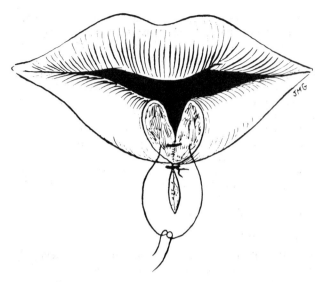

Fig. 43-4. Technique of suture of lip laceration. Initial suture precisely aligns mucocutaneous junction. Orbicularis oris, mucosa, and vermilion are then separately sutured in layers. (Heckler FR, Jabaley ME: Maxillofacial injuries. In Chang WHJ [ed]: Fundamentals of Plastic and Reconstructive Surgery. Copyright © 1980, The Williams & Wilkins Co, Baltimore)

major facial trauma: primary attention is given to life-threatening entities such as airway obstruction or uncontrolled hemorrhage. Careful evaluation of the entire patient is mandatory because the more dramatic facial lacerations and injuries may distract attention from coexisting intra-abdominal or intrathoracic injury. Facial fractures in themselves are not life-threatening, and therapy may be deferred if required.

There may be obvious deformity of the normal facial contour in terms of depressions, angulations, or prominences. These observational findings will be more obvious soon after injury before massive edema obscures local landmarks. Palpation will also reveal bony irregularities, fracture lines, motion, or crepitance. Since the teeth are rigidly attached to the facial skeleton, displaced facial fractures frequently result in abnormal interdigitation of the maxillary and mandibular dentition (malocclusion). The majority of facial fractures can be diagnosed using bedside clinical techniques, but radiologic confirmation should always be obtained to outline more specifically fracture location and severity.

NASAL FRACTURES

Isolated nasal fractures are quite common and require surgical reduction only if bony displacement is present. The mere presence of a fracture line seen on x-ray film of the nasal skeleton does not require specific therapy.

Diagnosis

Examination of the fractured nose may reveal contour deformity with the nasal pyramid displaced on either side, or flattening and broadening of the nasal dorsum if the blow was directly anterior. The fracture and displacement may involve the bony nasal skeleton, cartilaginous skeleton, or both. Careful intranasal inspection with a nasal speculum and adequate light is required and will reveal septal deformities or septal submucous hematomas not suspected from external stimulation.

Treatment

Nondisplaced nasal fractures require only mild analgesics and cold compresses for comfort. Displaced nasal fractures are treated by closed manipulation and repositioning of the fractured structures, usually under local anesthesia. A lubricated gauze nasal pack and external taping and splinting are used to maintain proper position and contour. Reduction and manipulation of nasal fractures may be deferred a few days to allow diminution of soft tissue swelling. This will permit more accurate replacement of the fracture fragments. Late attempts at fracture reduction are very difficult owing to fixation and early healing of the fracture fragments, and patients should be informed that under such conditions surgical osteotomies may be necessary to mobilize the fractured bones and return them to their normal positions.

ZYGOMATIC FRACTURES

The zygoma makes up the "cheekbone" prominence and in this exposed position often suffers direct trauma. Zygomatic fractures (Fig. 43-5) usually do not occur through the thick body of the zygoma itself but through its junctures with the surrounding bones—the zygomaticofrontal, zygomaticotemporal, and zygomaticomaxillary bony suture lines. Because all three suture lines are usually involved, this fracture is often termed a trimalar fracture.

Diagnosis

Clinical findings include tenderness and swelling over the cheekbone. The malar prominence will be depressed, giving a sunken appearance to the cheek. Palpation of the orbital rims may reveal irregularities or "step-offs" at the fracture sites. Often the medial fracture line will traverse the infraorbital foramen, and the infraorbital nerve will be contused

Fig. 43-5. Zygomatic fractures. Fracture usually occurs through junctions of zygoma with maxilla, frontal, and temporal bones (*a*). Repair includes reduction of bone into normal position and stabilization with stainless steel wires (*b*). (Heckler FR, Jabaley ME: Maxillofacial injuries. In Chang WHJ [ed]: Fundamentals of Plastic and Reconstructive Surgery. Copyright © 1980, The Williams & Wilkins Co, Baltimore)

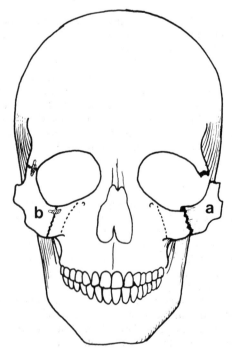

or torn. In these cases there will be hypesthesia or anesthesia over the infraorbital nerve sensory distribution on the anterior cheek.

Radiographic evidence is best sought using the standard Water's view and will demonstrate fracture lines at the sites previously noted. Clouding of the maxillary antrum will also frequently be present due to edema or hemorrhage in the maxillary sinus.

Treatment

Nondisplaced stable zygomatic fractures require no treatment other than analgesics and local cold packs for comfort. Displaced and unstable fractures require surgical repair. Incisions are placed just inside the brow to approach the frontozygomatic fracture and along the infraciliary margin to approach the infraorbital rim. The zygoma is manipulated back into normal position and wired into place using drill holes made adjacent to the fracture sites.

ZYGOMATIC ARCH FRACTURES

Diagnosis

Diagnosis is again made clinically by palpation and observation of a depression in the lateral portion of the cheek. Occasionally the patient will complain of pain on opening the mouth. This is caused by impingement of the depressed zygomatic arch onto the underlying coronoid process of the mandible. The most useful radiologic view is the submentovertex view, which throws the zygomatic arch into relief, allowing easy visualization.

Treatment

The depressed zygomatic arch is elevated into position using a percutaneous bone hook, a metal elevator passed deep to the arch through an incision in the temporal hairline, or direct pressure applied with finger or instrument through the gingivobuccal sulcus. Most zygomatic arch fractures are stable following reduction. The occasional unstable fracture

may be maintained in position with percutaneous metal pins or suspension wires.

MAXILLARY FRACTURES

Midfacial fractures (Fig. 43-6) tend to occur in one of three distinct patterns, first described by the French surgeon René Le Fort. All are the result of direct force applied to the maxillary skeleton. Fractures in this area tend to produce respiratory obstruction, and careful attention must be paid to the patency of the upper airway during the initial management.

LeFort I fractures extend transversely across the lower maxilla through the pyriform aperture. A LeFort II fracture is pyramidal in configuration, extending upward across the root of the nose. LeFort III fractures are often termed craniofacial dysjunction because all of the facial skeletal components, including the maxillae, nasal bones, and zygomas are separated from the cranial base.

Diagnosis

When any major maxillary or midfacial fracture is suspected, the key diagnostic maneuver is to grasp the upper alveolus and test for mobility of the midfacial skeleton. From clinical examination alone, it will often be possible to state only that abnormal mobility exists. Radiologic examination will then permit precise characterization of the fracture. Another helpful diagnostic sign in midfacial fractures is malocclusion. The maxillary teeth bear a normal and constant relationship to their mandibular partners. Since the teeth are rigidly fixed to the underlying skeleton, displaced fractures of the maxilla are accompanied by changes in normal interdental relationships. Patients will often voluntarily state that their teeth "don't fit together as they used to."

Treatment

General anesthesia is required. Wires are affixed to the teeth, and proper occlusion is reestablished by wiring the upper teeth to the lower in normal alignment. The fracture

Fig. 43-6. Maxillary fractures. (*I*) LeFort I (transverse maxillary) fracture. Repair by reduction of fracture to normal anatomic position, intermaxillary wiring to ensure normal occlusion, and suspension of fracture fragment with stainless steel wires.

(*II*) LeFort II fracture (pyramidal type fracture). Repair with reduction, intermaxillary fixation in normal occlusion, and suspension to frontal bones with stainless steel wires.

(*III*) LeFort III fracture (craniofacial dysjunction). Repair with intermaxillary fixation in normal occlusion and suspension to frontal bones with stainless steel wires. (Heckler FR, Jabaley ME: Maxillofacial injuries. In Chang WHJ [ed]: Fundamentals of Plastic and Reconstructive Surgery. Copyright © 1980, The Williams & Wilkins Co, Baltimore)

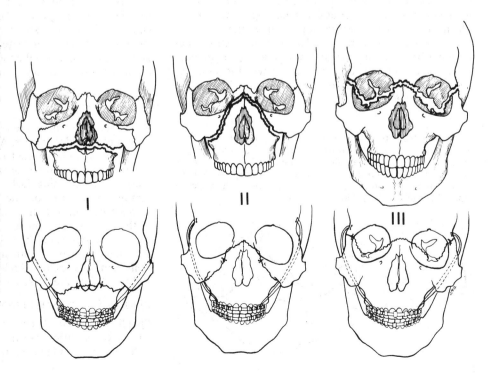

fragments are reduced into proper anatomic position and suspended with stainless steel wires to the intact bony structures above, usually the zygomas in LeFort I fractures and the frontal bones in LeFort II and III fractures.

MANDIBULAR FRACTURES

Diagnosis

The medical history will indicate direct trauma to the mandibular area, and the patient will complain of localized pain, particularly with mastication.

Examination will reveal local swelling and tenderness. The inferior alveolar nerve traverses the mandibular medullary canal, emerging from the mental foramen to innervate the lower lip. Mandibular fractures may impinge upon or even lacerate this nerve, and numbness of the lip will then be a prominent symptom. Stress applied to the mandible across the tender area may reveal bony instability or crepitance.

It is important to remember that the mandible, a rigid structure, may transmit force delivered onto one location to more distant and structurally weaker sites. This may produce fractures at loci distant from the actual site of the blow. Such fractures commonly result from trauma to the chin, where force delivered to the symphyseal area is transmitted to the weaker condylar region, producing fractures at either or both sites (Fig. 43-7).

If there is displacement of the fracture segments, malocclusion of the mandibular dentition with the maxillary teeth will be evident. Malalignment of the mandibular arch itself may also be seen. The degree and extent of displacement of the fracture segments depend upon the magnitude and direction of the injuring force and upon the location of the fracture line in relation to the pull of the various muscle groups acting upon the mandible as a whole (Fig. 43-8). Helpful radiologic studies include standard mandibular views and specialized panoramic and occlusal radiographs.

Treatment

The goals of treatment are to reestablish normal bony alignment and dental occlusal relationships while immobilizing the mandible to allow proper bony healing. Fixation of the maxillary to the mandibular teeth with dental wires accomplishes both purposes and will suffice in the presence of adequate dentition. The jaws remain wired together for 4 to 6 weeks while nutrition is maintained with a liquid blenderized diet.

Fig. 43-7. Mandibular fractures. Force on point of chin (*large arrow*) may be transmitted to weaker areas such as the condylar necks with fractures at sites distant to the actual injury. (Heckler FR, Jabaley ME: Maxillofacial injuries. In Chang WHJ [ed]: Fundamentals of Plastic and Reconstructive Surgery. Copyright © 1980, The Williams & Wilkins Co, Baltimore)

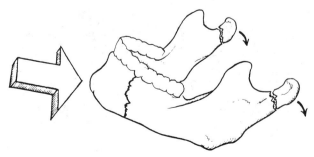

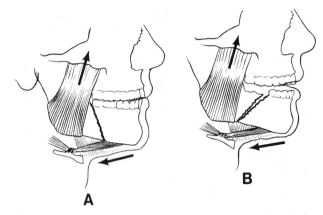

Fig. 43-8. Displacement of mandibular fractures. (*A*) Favorable fracture angle—muscles acting on fracture fragments tend to impact and approximate fracture fragments if fracture angle is favorable. (*B*) Unfavorable fracture angle combined with normal muscle pull causes distraction and separation of fracture fragments. (Heckler FR, Jabaley ME: Maxillofacial injuries. In Chang WHJ [ed]: Fundamentals of Plastic and Reconstructive Surgery. Copyright © 1980, The Williams & Wilkins Co, Baltimore)

Open surgical manipulation of the fracture fragments with direct wiring of the fracture is indicated when not enough teeth are present for adequate immobilization or when fracture displacement is so great that simple closed reduction and interdental wiring will not suffice. Often a combination of open and closed techniques is called for.

CONGENITAL ANOMALIES OF THE HEAD AND NECK

Congenital anomalies of the head and neck constitute some of the most distressing deformities for both patients and their families. Society seems to tolerate and adapt less well to birth defects than to deformities secondary to trauma or surgery. Consequently, the congenitally deformed child frequently suffers great social and emotional stress during childhood and adolescence. Fortunately, modern plastic surgical techniques allow reconstruction of most of these anomalies so that social acceptance and a normal outlook on life are now the norm for the great majority.

CLEFT LIP AND CLEFT PALATE

Facial clefts are among the most common of the congenital head and neck deformities. Approximately 1 in 800 infants is born with cleft lip, cleft palate, or both. The cleft may involve those structures derived from the embryologic primary palate, including the lip, premaxilla, columella, caudal septum, and nose, or the structures derived from the secondary palate including the hard and soft palates posterior to the incisive foramen. Of all patients with cleft lip and palate, approximately 25% have a cleft of the lip alone, 50% have defects of both lip and palate, and 25% have clefts of the palate alone. Males are more frequently affected, and the defects are more common on the left side.

GENETICS AND INHERITANCE PATTERNS

Cleft lip and palate are considered to be congenital disorders with a genetic predisposition in families with histories of cleft deformities. Clefts are more common in Orientals than

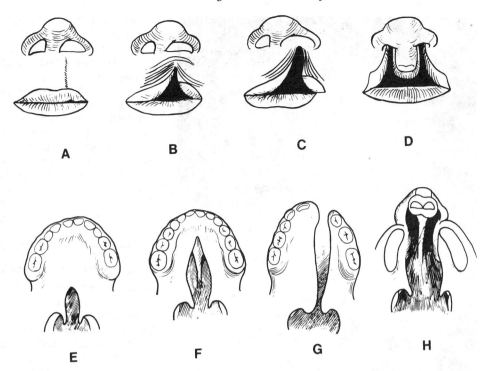

Fig. 43-9. Classification of cleft lip and cleft palate. (*A*) Minimal cleft lip. Slight notching of the vermilion border, a ridge or depression along the philtral column, and a minimal deformity of nostril sill. (*B*) Incomplete cleft lip. Cleft extends part way through the lip to the nose with partial interruption of the orbicularis muscle fibers and more severe nostril deformity. (*C*) Complete unilateral cleft lip. Cleft extends from vermilion border through nostril floor. Orbicularis fibers are completely interrupted and turned in a cephalic direction to parallel the cleft. Major nostril deformity including lateral displacement of ala, displacement of lower lateral cartilage, and shortening of columella on cleft side. (*D*) Complete bilateral cleft lip. (*E*) Cleft of the secondary palate. Cleft involves soft palate only, with disruption of normal levator muscular sling. (*F*) Complete cleft of secondary palate with incomplete cleft of primary palate. Cleft extends completely through the soft palate and partially through the hard palate anterior to the incisive foramen. Vomer and perpendicular plate of the ethmoid are seen in the midline of the cleft. Alveolus is intact. (*G*) Complete unilateral cleft palate. Cleft extends all the way through soft and hard palates. (*H*) Complete bilateral cleft of primary and secondary palate.

in Caucasians but are less commonly seen in blacks. Genetic counseling should be offered to affected families.

CLASSIFICATION OF CLEFTS

Clefts of the primary palate are termed *complete* if the cleft extends all the way from the vermilion of the lip through the nostril floor (Fig. 43-9). Lesser lip clefts are termed minimal or *incomplete* depending upon their severity. These clefts may or may not extend through the alveolar bone and always include some degree of nostril and caudal nasal deformity. Primary palatal clefts may also be bilateral, with either side being complete or incomplete. Clefts of the secondary palate that extend through the soft palate only are likewise termed incomplete, and those extending all the way through the soft and hard palates are called complete clefts.

TREATMENT

Cleft Lip Repair

The goals of cleft lip treatment are to return the cleft portions of the upper lip to a normal relationship with each other, restoring a normal appearing vermilion, Cupid's bow, and philtrum and reconstituting the normal orbicularis oris muscle sphincter. Symmetry of nostril position and form is likewise desired (Fig. 43-10, *A,B*).

Lip surgery is usually performed when the child is 3 months old. Many types of repair have been proposed. The techniques generally applied in modern practice all involve a surgical relocation of the cleft parts, differing mainly in the location of final scar placement. The nasal deformity, although considerably corrected at the initial procedure, frequently requires further reconstruction at a later age after the facial contours are more mature. Dental orthodontic management of the cleft alveolus is essential in obtaining appropriate dental alignment and arch form.

Cleft Palate Repair

The most important goal of cleft palate repair is the attainment of normal speech. Children with unrepaired or inadequately repaired clefts develop nasal-sounding speech patterns termed rhinolalia. Cleft palate repair is therefore usually done when the child is 12 to 18 months old, before consequential speech development. In addition to closing the cleft itself, an important goal of palate repair is approximation in normal alignment of the levator palati muscles, which are responsible for oronasal valving in speech and swallowing.

The cleft palate is closed by loosening the palatal mucoperiosteum from the underlying bone and either approximating it in the midline (Langenbeck technique) or using a V–Y type of retrodisplacement and closure (Wardill–Kilner

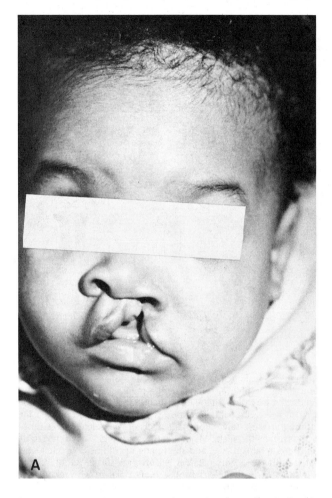

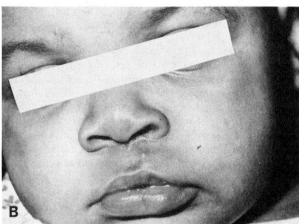

Fig. 43-10. Cleft lip repair. (*A*) Complete unilateral cleft lip displaying cleft extending from vermilion through nostril floor, and complete cleft lip nasal deformity. (*B*) Millard-type repair restoring lip anatomy and function as well as nasal symmetry.

techniques). In either method the levator muscles are specifically dissected, and the levator sling is reconstructed.

Other Problems

All children with cleft palate deformities have abnormal and inadequate drainage of the eustachian tube of the middle ear. This causes a high frequency of recurrent middle ear infections, which, if untreated, lead to eventual hearing

impairment. These children should be closely monitored, and surgical middle ear drainage should be instituted when necessary to prevent such complications.

A small percentage of patients with repaired clefts of the palate will not attain adequately intelligible speech even with intensive speech therapy. Their speech is nasal in character due to an inability of the repaired palate to close off the nasopharynx adequately from the oropharynx during phonation. If this problem is persistent, correction can be accomplished by surgical measures that will assist in obtaining normal velopharyngeal competence. This usually is done by developing a flap of pharyngeal tissue and suturing it to the palate, leaving adequate space for nasal respiration but effectively narrowing the aperture requiring closure to avoid nasal air escape during speech.

CONGENITAL DEFORMITIES OF THE EAR

PROMINENT OR LOP EARS

Abnormal prominence of the ears is caused by excessive development of the concha, inadequate development of the antihelical fold, or both. The ears stand out from the side of the head and may be a considerable source of embarrassment and social discomfort for the patient.

Correction is accomplished by contouring and bending the ear cartilage to recreate the normal antihelical fold and by resecting a portion of the excessive conchal cartilage. Excellent correction and appearance can be obtained, and patient gratification is considerable. Surgery is usually performed when the child becomes discomfited by his appearance but not before 4 to 5 years of age.

CONGENITAL MICROTIA

The term microtia refers to underdevelopment of the external ear. The deformity may range from an external ear that is only moderately misshapen to near complete absence of the auricle. Because the problem is only one manifestation of the broader spectrum of problems seen with maldevelopment of structures derived from the first and second branchial arches, there may also be coexisting deformities of the external and internal ear, maxilla, zygoma, mandible, cheek, and facial nerve. (The most severe complete expression of the syndrome is therefore often called *hemifacial microsomia.*) Microtia is usually unilateral but rarely may be bilateral.

Treatment

Early investigation and middle ear surgery are indicated in children with the bilateral deformity because they may have bilateral deafness. Middle ear surgery in the unilateral cases is not mandatory because adequate hearing will be present on the normal side.

The external ear deformity may be corrected by subcutaneous implantation of a carved cartilaginous framework using costal cartilage grafts. Surgery is not done before the opposite ear has reached near-adult size and configuration to avoid later disparity in appearance with continued growth. Corrective surgery for microtia involves multiple staged procedures and is not done without first apprising the patient and the family of other less complicated alternatives, such as prosthetic ears and simple alteration of hairstyle to conceal the deformity.

CONGENITAL BRANCHIAL ANOMALIES

The embryologic branchial clefts and arches normally coalesce and evolve into the mature structures of the external ear, maxillomandibular complex, and neck. Abnormalities in maturational development of the branchial arches will lead to malformation or absence of the structures derived from them. Persistence of the intervening branchial clefts results in cysts or sinuses in the head and neck. These lesions are most commonly derived from either the first or second branchial cleft.

First branchial cleft sinuses run between the external ear canal and the submandibular area, whereas the more common second branchial cleft sinus originates in the tonsillar fossa and has a fistulous opening along the anterior border of the sternocleidomastoid muscle. Both types of sinuses present as chronically draining sinus tracts with intermittent secondary infection. If the branchial cleft remnant does not connect with the skin or does not drain well, a branchial cleft cyst may be formed instead.

Treatment consists of excision of the sinus tract or cyst. Great care must be taken to excise the sinus tract completely all the way from its external to its internal orifice. If excision is incomplete, recurrence is common. This dissection may be difficult owing to the close proximity of other important anatomic structures derived from the first and second branchial arches including the facial nerve.

CONGENITAL CRANIOFACIAL ANOMALIES

A number of other less common craniofacial anomalies may be encountered. These include Treacher-Collins syndrome, Crouzon's deformity, and Apert's deformities. Each is characterized by a constellation of bony and soft tissue abnormalities involving both facial maxillary–mandibular complexes and cranial structures, particularly those around the orbits and the cranial base.

Until recent years, surgeons have concentrated primarily on corrections of the soft tissue problems using local and distant skin flaps to augment deficient areas and add contour bulk where needed. Onlay bone and cartilage grafts were similarly applied.

More modern techniques, championed primarily by Tessier of France, have emphasized the importance of total corrective surgery in the early years to allow a proper growth matrix environment for normal craniofacial maturation. Techniques used involve combined intracranial and extracranial approaches, with complete osteotomies and repositioning of malpositioned orbits, maxillae, and mandible. Extensive bone grafting helps maintain the new bony configurations. Fears that such extensive surgical manipulation would retard and interfere with later growth have not been borne out by long-term follow-up. The improvement in both physical and social outlook for these deformed children has been dramatic.

DISTORTED MAXILLARY–MANDIBULAR RELATIONSHIPS

The maxilla and mandible normally have a harmonious relationship with regard to size, shape, and rates of growth. Similarly, the maxillary and mandibular teeth fit together in a relationship called *normal occlusion.* Abnormalities in these relationships due to trauma, congenital malformations, surgical manipulation, or growth abnormality may occur. Minor distortions cause minimal problems and may often be adequately corrected with orthodontic measures. More major disproportions may seriously alter the facial aesthetic harmony and form as well as jeopardize normal masticatory function.

Diagnosis is established by physical examination, the use of dental casts and models, and specific radiographic studies called cephalometrics. These studies are particularly useful in that they permit accurate, quantitative evaluation and measurement of the size and development of the facial bones in relation to each other and to the overall craniofacial complex. Various deformities exist either independently or in combination. In the mandible these include mandibular protrusion (prognathism) and mandibular underdevelopment and retrusion (micrognathia). Maxillary retrusion ("dish face" deformity) is also seen. Once appropriate diagnoses are made, correction is accomplished by appropriately placed osteotomies, movement of the bones into normal, harmonious relationships, and either bone grafting or removal of excess bone, depending upon the situation.

COSMETIC SURGERY

Cosmetic surgery may be defined as surgery performed to alter the appearance of a body part that might otherwise be considered within the limits of normal according to the usual aesthetic standards of the society in which the patient lives. Inherent in this definition is the fact that cosmetic surgery should be surgery requested by the patient, not recommended by the doctor. Cosmetic surgery, therefore, is done to help the patient to be happier with his own body image. The surgeon must carefully assess preoperatively not only the physical characteristics of the feature to be changed but also the actual expectations of the patient. Realistic expectations of surgical results pertain to realism in terms of the expected physical alterations and also to the expected or imagined effect this physical change will have on the psychosocial relationships within the environment in which the patient lives. Patients with unreal expectations will be dissatisfied with the surgical result, no matter how good the physical result may actually be.

SURGERY OF THE AGING FACE

With aging, facial and neck skin gradually loses its elasticity, and sags downward in response to gravity. The resulting baggy eyelids, and sagging neck and jowl areas can be most distressing in terms of the patient's self confidence in social and business interactions.

Correction of these problems (Fig. 43-11) is accomplished by incisions placed in the hairline, in the natural skin creases, and adjacent to the lash margins to make them inconspicuous after healing. Facial or eyelid skin is undermined to allow it to be drawn up and tightened, and excess skin is trimmed away.

Proper patient selection in terms of realistic expectations and appropriate physical indications for surgery combined with meticulous surgical technique lead to a high degree of patient satisfaction following these operations.

RHINOPLASTY

The nose is a major aesthetic focal point of the face. As such, real or perceived deformities of the nose may cause considerable embarrassment and may be psychosocially crippling. Many patients, if properly selected in terms of emotional stability and realistic expectations of surgical results, will benefit greatly from cosmetic rhinoplasty.

The shape and external appearance of the nose depend to a great extent on the underlying bony and cartilaginous

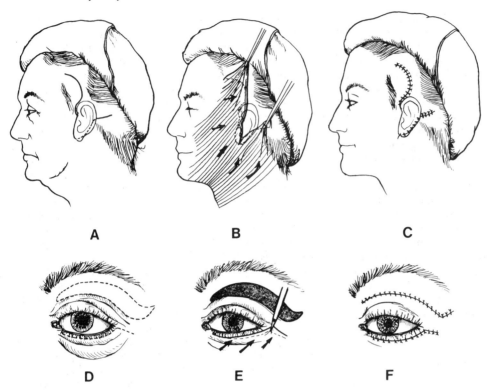

Fig. 43-11. Surgery of the aging face. (*A*) Incision line for facelift extends from temporal hairline, into a preauricular natural crease, around the lobule onto the concha, and then into the mastoid hairline. (*B*) Skin undermining accomplished and redundant skin advanced superiorly and posteriorly. (*C*) Excess skin excised and suturing accomplished. Scar placement is mostly hidden postoperatively by hair regrowth. (*D*) Blepharoplasty incision lines. Excess skin of upper eyelid will be excised; lower eyelid skin will be undermined, advanced, and excised. (*E*) Shaded area indicates upper eyelid skin excision. Arrows indicate advancement of redundant lower lid skin, which will then be excised. Excess orbital fat pads will be removed simultaneously. (*F*) Incisions are sutured. Scars will be concealed within natural eyelid creases.

supporting structures. These include the nasal bones, the upper and lower lateral nasal cartilages, and the nasal septum. Cosmetic rhinoplasty is most frequently performed through an endonasal approach by way of the nostrils, thereby leaving no external scars. The nasal skin and soft tissues are freed from the underlying support structures. Bony and cartilaginous architecture is reshaped using scalpel, chisels, and rasps. When septal deformities create concomitant respiratory difficulties, the septum is surgically straightened or a portion of it is removed to clear the nasal airway.

BREAST SURGERY

AUGMENTATION MAMMAPLASTY

Breast enlargement for cosmetic purposes has been increasingly popular among women who have either never developed adequate mammary tissue or who have undergone postpartum mammary involution.

A Silastic rubber prosthesis is used, consisting of an outer envelope filled either with Silastic gel, which has the consistency and feel of normal breast tissue when implanted, or with isotonic saline when an inflatable type of implant is used. A small incision is made either in the inframammary crease, along the inferior margin of the areola, or adjacent to the anterior axillary fold. A pocket is dissected between

the pectoral musculature and the overlying breast, and the prosthesis is inserted (Fig. 43-12). Alternatively, in patients with very thin skin or very hypoplastic breasts, a submuscular pocket will be used to better conceal the prosthesis and provide a more aesthetic result.

REDUCTION MAMMAPLASTY

Massive hypertrophy of the female breast is distressing not only in terms of physical appearance but also because of the many physical problems that may result. These problems are caused by the large weight and size of the hypertrophied glands and include chronic neckache and backache, postural problems, irritation and shoulder pain from brassiere straps, and recurrent skin irritation in the redundant inframammary skin folds.

Resection of excess breast tissue, relocation of the nipple–areolar complex on the smaller breast mound, and redistribution of excess skin will relieve the physical problem and free the patient from the social and psychologic stress imposed by the condition.

POSTMASTECTOMY BREAST RECONSTRUCTION

Surgical reconstruction of the female breast following ablation for malignant disease has become more widely used in recent years. This probably reflects the better and more reliable results obtainable with modern reconstructive techniques, greater public awareness of the availability of re-

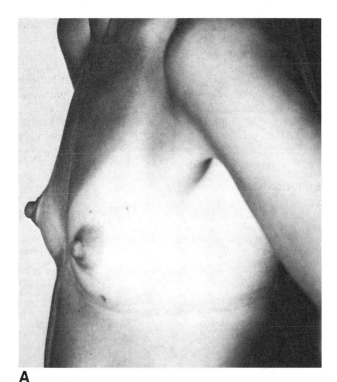

A

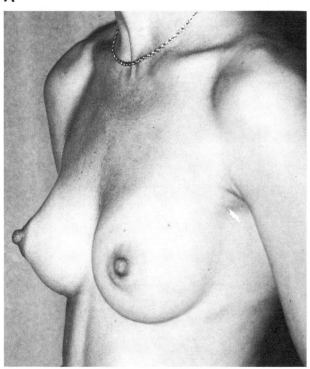

B

Fig. 43-12. Cosmetic augmentation mammoplasty. (*A*) Patient requesting surgical breast enlargement. (*B*) Silicon-gel subcutaneous breast prostheses have been inserted. Periareolar incisions are scarcely discernible.

constructive surgery, and the emphasis on the breast as an important secondary sexual characteristic in our society.

Indications for surgical reconstruction are based primarily upon the patient's own desires and attitudes toward the amputated breast. Many patients find that they are quite able emotionally and physically to cope with the absence of the breast and are satisfied with wearing an artificial prosthesis contained within a brassiere to provide an adequate contour under clothes. Other patients find that they feel "castrated" and robbed of their female identity by the loss of a breast, and are constantly troubled by the potential or actual movement and accidental displacement of an external prosthesis. These patients, after proper counseling about the need for additional surgery, hospitalization, expense, and scarring, are the patients generally considered appropriate candidates.

A second important criterion in patient selection is the prognosis in terms of the patient's malignant disease for which the mastectomy was performed. Patients with small primary tumors and no nodal metastases are generally considered to be the best candidates for reconstruction. Patients with more advanced Stage II breast carcinomas may also be appropriate candidates following consultation both with the plastic surgeon and the ablative surgeon about prognosis and the advisability of proceeding with further surgery. Sometimes in such situations an interval of several years is allowed to elapse between mastectomy and reconstruction.

The goals of treatment include an improved appearance in clothing and an enhanced self-image for the patient. The extent of reconstruction required will depend upon the type of mastectomy that was performed. Modified radical mastectomies that leave the pectoralis musculature in place require only reconstruction of the breast mound and nipple–areolar complex. True radical mastectomies with removal of the pectoralis require not only breast mound and nipple–areolar reconstruction but also reconstruction of the anterior axillary fold and filling in the infraclavicular hollow.

Treatment

The breast mound is rebuilt using a Silastic breast prosthesis. This is placed behind the pectoralis major muscle, a technique that provides more durable, reliable soft tissue cover for the prosthesis and minimizes postoperative complications of implant erosion through skin and wound breakdown. If the pectoralis is surgically absent or if skin cover is inadequate and too tight due to surgical resection, additional tissue must be introduced using flap transfer.

A large number of flap designs have been used for this purpose. Currently, the most successful and widely used is the latissimus dorsi musculocutaneous flap. This flap is based upon the thoracodorsal vascular pedicle and is swung from the back to the anterior chest. The transferred muscle supplies the bulk required to replace the anterior axillary fold and to fill the infraclavicular hollow. The skin portion of the flap adds enough tissue to provide an adequate envelope to contain the simultaneously placed breast prosthesis.

Nipple and Areolar Reconstruction

Nipple and areolar reconstruction is accomplished by adding a free graft to the apex of the reconstructed breast mound. Donor sites used have included a portion of the opposite nipple and areola, pigmented tissue from the vaginal labia minora, and skin from the upper medial thigh, which is somewhat more deeply pigmented than skin from other areas. The donor tissue is transferred as a free full-thickness graft to a recipient site prepared by excising a partial thickness of skin on the reconstructed breast mound.

MALE GYNECOMASTIA

A small percentage of males develop prominent breasts in adolescence. The great majority of these regress after a few years. For those that persist, resection of excess tissue may be performed through a small periareolar incision. Results are uniformly satisfactory with a negligible recurrence rate as long as any major underlying causative endocrine abnormality is investigated and ruled out prior to excision.

BODY SCULPTURE

Skin that is markedly stretched by obesity or during pregnancy may not have enough elasticity to adjust to the new body habitus following massive weight loss. In such situations, large excess folds and rolls of skin may be unpleasantly apparent over the abdomen, buttocks and thighs, or upper arms. Patients with such a problem may find it embarrassing to appear in bathing attire, have difficulty wearing some clothing styles such as form-fitting slacks, and suffer from repeated bouts of skin irritation in areas where redundant skin folds promote moisture retention in warm weather.

Corrective surgery in such situations involves placement of the necessarily long incisions where they will be least apparent and covered by shorts or bathing attire, and resection of redundant skin and subcutaneous tissue.

It should be emphasized that such surgery should *not* be undertaken to correct problems with obesity *per se* but rather to correct the excessive stretched-out skin remaining after the desired weight loss.

BIBLIOGRAPHY

CHANG WH (ed): Fundamentals of Plastic and Reconstructive Surgery. Baltimore, Williams & Wilkins, 1980

CONVERSE JM (ed): Reconstructive Plastic Surgery, 2nd ed. Philadelphia, W B Saunders, 1977

GRABB WC, SMITH JW (eds): Plastic Surgery, 3rd ed. Boston, Little, Brown & Co, 1979

Orthopaedic Surgery

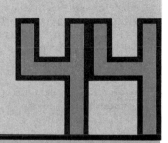

Alan E. Freeland/E. Thomas James

Common Fractures and Dislocations

The goals of fracture treatment are to achieve healing without infection and to restore the injured part to normal or as near to normal function as possible. This should be done in the shortest possible time and with the least possible amount of risk to the patient. Guidelines are presented in this chapter for fracture management according to fracture configuration and region, but treatment must also take into consideration any associated injuries, including other fractures, the age of the patient, associated medical illnesses, the job or avocation of the patient, the desires and needs of the patient and the family, and the skill of the surgeon.

The best treatment for complications is prevention. Those complications that are not preventable must be anticipated, identified early, and treated aggressively. In the early post-injury period, the mnemonic "AVOID complications" is useful:

*Arterial and neurologic injury
*Volkmann's ischemic contracture
*Open fracture
*Intra-articular fracture
*Dislocation

A comprehensive physical and radiographic examination to identify vascular injury and neurologic damage must be performed as soon as possible. Compartment syndromes can lead to Volkmann's ischemic contracture and must be identified early. Open skeletal injuries require immediate attention. Displaced intra-articular fractures have the best results if there is early congruent restoration of joint surfaces

and stable internal fixation. Dislocations should be reduced as quickly as possible to relieve pain, to relieve pressure on adjacent neurovascular structures, to prevent adjacent skin necrosis, and to restore normal physiology and function to the joint.

A particular emphasis is placed on getting the patient vertical and mobilized as soon as possible. This is a tremendous adjunct to restoring normal pulmonary physiology and preventing pulmonary insufficiency, particularly in the elderly patient and in the polytraumatized and polyfractured patient. For the individual fracture or dislocation, early joint motion and muscle rehabilitation are important for functional recovery.

This chapter is an overview of the treatment and complications of common fractures and dislocations. The principal objective of treatment in fractures and dislocations of the upper extremity is to ensure proper hand function. In the lower extremity it is to ensure painless and stable ambulation.

FIRST AID AND TRANSPORTATION

First aid at the scene of the accident for a patient with an injured extremity includes control of hemorrhage, placement of a sterile dressing on any open wound, and splinting of the injured part. Hemorrhage is controlled by direct pressure at the site of bleeding. Tourniquets are not used as first aid measures because of the risk of peripheral nerve injury or permanent damage distal to the site of application due to ischemia. Clamps are not used because they damage the ends of blood vessels, thereby precluding repair, and because of the risk that indiscriminate application would damage other vital structures. Sterile dressings are applied to open wounds to protect them from further contamination. Splinting prevents conversion of a closed fracture to an open fracture and minimizes pain, further tissue damage, and blood loss at the fracture site, thereby combating shock. A spinal board is used to transport patients with spinal injuries to and within the hospital until the extent of injury is determined. For the patient with an unstable fracture or dislocation of the spine, the spinal board should be used until an alternative method of stabilization is established. After initial stabilization and application of first aid at the scene of the accident, the patient is transported as expeditiously as possible to a facility for definitive medical care.

PRIORITIES IN POLYTRAUMA

Priorities in the severely injured patient are first life-saving and then limb-saving. The catastrophic result of focusing on an apparent and overt severe extremity injury while ignoring a more occult but life-threatening injury must be avoided. This is accomplished by first resuscitating and stabilizing the patient and then by performing a disciplined systematic evaluation of the patient's injuries; the patient's clothing must be removed for adequate examination. Establishing an adequate airway for breathing is the highest priority. An inadequate airway should be suspected in patients who are unconscious or who have facial fractures, and if present, endotracheal intubation or tracheostomy must be performed. Hemorrhage must be controlled. For the patient in shock, volume is corrected first with Ringer's lactate solution and later with whole blood when it becomes available.

Once the patient is resuscitated and stabilized, the mneumonic "CRASH PLAN" is used to ensure a complete and reproducible examination that becomes reflex in a crisis situation:

Cardiac	includes resuscitative efforts for establishing an airway, breathing and peripheral vascular support, and treatment of shock
Respiratory	
Abdomen	
Spine	
Head—	includes evaluation for increased intracranial pressure, particularly in the patient with an altered state of consciousness
Pelvis	
Limbs	
Arteries	
Nerves	

DIAGNOSIS OF FRACTURES AND DISLOCATIONS

Extremities must be thoroughly and systematically examined in turn, again with caution to detect the inapparent injury. The location and appearance of a wound may be misleading in regard to the extent of subfascial injury. In addition, the presence of a wound does not exclude the possibility of injury proximal or distal to this site.

Clinical signs of fracture or dislocation include deformity, pain, local tenderness, crepitus, swelling, ecchymosis, abnormal motion, and loss of function. In many instances, the diagnosis will be apparent on the basis of results of the physical examination. In such cases it is unnecessary, and even contraindicated, to demonstrate the physical signs of fracture. To do so may cause extreme discomfort to the patient and increase local soft tissue damage. Prompt radiographic examination is of much greater value in determining the extent of the injury. At least two views, an anteroposterior and a lateral, should be taken of the injured extremity and should include the joints proximal and distal to the injury site. In cases of intra-articular fractures, oblique views should be taken. Views of the opposite extremity may be useful for comparison.

All fractures and dislocations are either open or closed. This is determined clinically by examination of the patient. In open fractures, there is a break in the overlying skin or mucous membrane and, consequently, the fracture communicates with the outside air. In closed fractures, there is no break in the overlying skin or mucous membrane.

A fracture is a break in the continuity of a bone. Fractures are evaluated clinically and also roentgenographically. First, the examiner determines which bone is fractured and whether the fracture is in the epiphysis, the metaphysis, or the diaphysis or a combination of these (Fig. 44-1, *A*). A diaphyseal fracture may be described as being in the proximal, middle, or distal third of the bone. A fracture may also be described by designating the particular bony prominence through which the fracture occurs (*e.g.,* lateral malleolus, medial malleolus, tibial spine, tibial tuberosity, greater trochanter). Fractures that extend into joints are designated as intra-articular fractures (Fig. 44-1, *B*). A fracture may be complete (Fig. 44-1, *C* and *D*), involving the entire cross section of a bone, or incomplete (Fig. 44-1, *E*), involving only a portion of the cross section of a

bone. A fracture is undisplaced (Fig. 44-1, *C*) when the normal anatomy of the bone is undisturbed and displaced (Fig. 44-1, *D*) when the normal anatomy of the bone is disrupted. A description of the fracture also includes the fracture pattern. A transverse fracture is a straight fracture perpendicular to the long axis of the bone (Fig. 44-1, *F*). A short oblique fracture makes an angle of 45° or less to the long axis of the bone (Fig. 44-1, *G*). A long oblique fracture makes an angle of more than 45° to the long axis of the bone (Fig. 44-1, *H*). A spiral fracture winds around the long axis of the bone (Fig. 44-1, *I*). A comminuted fracture has more than two fragments with two or more distinct fracture lines (Fig. 44-1, *J*). A comminuted fracture may have a butterfly fragment (Fig. 44-1, *K*). A segmental fracture has two levels of fracture without communicating fracture lines (Fig. 44-1, *L*). Segmental loss occurs when the bone between two levels of fracture is missing (Fig. 44-1, *M*). An impacted fracture has one fragment of the bone driven into the other (Fig. 44-1, *N*). A greenstick fracture is a type of incomplete fracture seen almost entirely in children in which the cortex is broken on the concave side but is only bent or angulated on the convex side (Fig. 44-1, *O*); this is a type of incomplete fracture. An avulsion fracture is caused by a ligamentous or tendinous attachment pulling away a fragment of bone (Fig. 44-1, *P*). In a compression fracture, a bone loses height by being compressed by an adjacent bone or bones (Fig. 44-1, *Q*). Compression fractures are commonly seen in the spine.

Overriding is another term for shortening (Fig. 44-1, *R*). It indicates the distance that one fragment overlaps the other. *Apposition* and *alignment* are terms used in describing the position of fractures. Apposition is said to exist when the fragment ends are abutting; alignment occurs when the fragments are parallel to each other (Fig. 44-1, *S*). When the long axis of the two fragments are not in alignment, they are said to be angulated and the amount of the angulation is specified both in degrees and by direction. The direction of the angulation is named according to the direction of the apex of the angle formed. The angulation may also be designated as varus, with the distal fragment angulated laterally (Fig. 44-1, *T*), or valgus, with the distal fragment angulated medially (Fig. 44-1, *U*).

Pathologic fractures occur through an area of abnormal bone (Fig. 44-1, *V*). The bone may be abnormal because of generalized osteopenia from a variety of causes, primary benign or malignant bone tumor, or because of metastatic bone tumor.

A stress fracture (march or fatigue fracture) usually results from bone being exposed to unaccustomed cyclic activities. The most common locations for these fractures are the second metatarsal neck, the posteromedial border of the proximal third of the tibia, and the femoral neck (see Fig. 44-1, *E*). These fractures may often be discovered before they are complete or at least before they are displaced.

Dislocation means a complete loss of continuity of a joint so that the articular surfaces are no longer in contact (Fig. 44-1, *W*). Subluxation is a less severe disruption of a joint in which the articular surfaces remain in partial contact (Fig. 44-1, *X*).

An epiphyseal fracture is a fracture that involves all or a portion of the epiphyseal line. Epiphyseal fractures are classified into five types; the higher the number, the greater is the chance of disturbance in terms of growth arrest or angular deformity (Fig. 44-2).

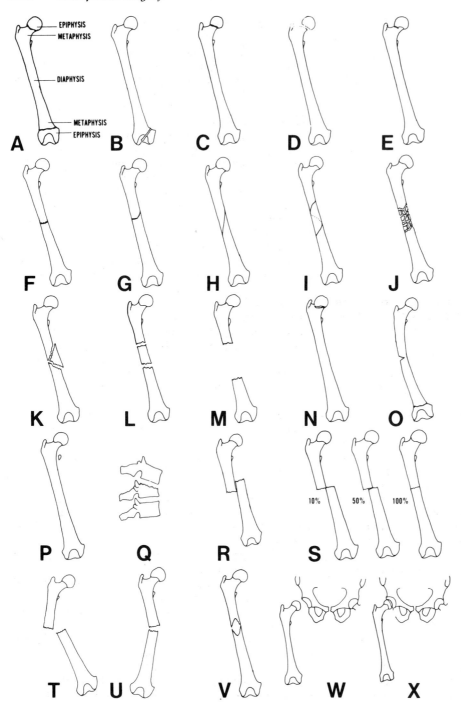

Fig. 44-1. Fractures and dislocations. (*A*) The regions of a long bone labeled on the femur. (*B*) Minimally displaced intra-articular fracture of the medial femoral condyle. (*C*) Complete undisplaced subcapital femoral fracture. (*D*) Complete displaced subcapital femoral fracture. (*E*) Incomplete undisplaced subcapital femoral stress fracture. (*F*) Undisplaced transverse midshaft femoral diaphyseal fracture. (*G*) Undisplaced short oblique midshaft femoral diaphyseal fracture. (*H*) Undisplaced long oblique midshaft femoral diaphyseal fracture. (*I*) Undisplaced spiral midshaft femoral diaphyseal fracture. (*J*) Comminuted midshaft femoral diaphyseal fracture. (*K*) Comminuted midshaft femoral diaphyseal fracture with minimally displaced butterfly fragment. (*L*) Segmental femoral diaphyseal fracture. (*M*) Segmental femoral diaphyseal bone loss. (*N*) Impacted subcapital femoral fracture. (*O*) Greenstick femoral diaphyseal fracture. (*P*) Minimally displaced avulsion fracture of the lesser trochanter of the femur. (*Q*) Vertebral compression fracture. (*R*) Overriding transverse midshaft femoral diaphyseal fracture. (*S*) Aligned and 10%, 50%, and 100% apposed transverse midshaft femoral diaphyseal fractures. (*T*) Varus deformity. (*U*) Valgus deformity. (*V*) Undisplaced pathologic midshaft femoral diaphyseal fracture. (*W*) Femoral head dislocation. (*X*) Femoral head subluxation.

METHODS OF FRACTURE MANAGEMENT

CLOSED REDUCTION AND PLASTER IMMOBILIZATION

Closed reduction and plaster immobilization is well suited for many fractures of the distal radius in adults, for most fractures of the shaft of the tibia and fibula (Fig. 44-3), and for almost all fractures of the shafts of long bones in children, with the possible exception of the femur. Adequate anesthesia and muscle relaxation are usually necessary. The proximal fracture fragment is stabilized, and countertraction is applied while the distal fragment is brought into apposition and alignment with the proximal fragment by means of traction and manipulation. The reduction is then maintained by plaster immobilization and confirmed by roentgenograms in at least two planes.

CONTINUOUS TRACTION

Continuous traction is exerted through the distal fracture fragment to bring it into proper apposition and alignment with the proximal fragment. Traction is applied to the skin or the skeleton through a system of ropes, pulleys, and weights attached to an overhead traction frame on the bed. The injured extremity is often supported by special traction

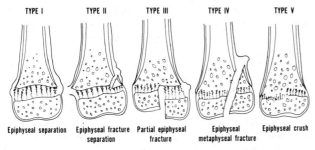

TYPE I   TYPE II   TYPE III   TYPE IV   TYPE V

Epiphyseal separation | Epiphyseal fracture separation | Partial epiphyseal fracture | Epiphyseal metaphyseal fracture | Epiphyseal crush

Fig. 44-2. The Salter-Harris epiphyseal fracture classification. (After Salter R, Harris W: Injuries involving the epiphyseal plate. J Bone Joint Surg [Am] 45:587, 1963)

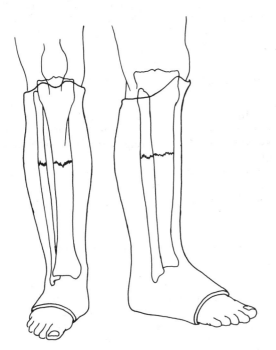

Fig. 44-3. Patellar weight-bearing plaster cast for ambulatory treatment of aligned and apposed fractures of the tibia and fibula.

splints or slings. Continuous traction is often used as a provisional means of fracture stabilization until more suitable definitive stabilization can be applied.

Skin traction is used in the treatment of femoral shaft fractures in children prior to immobilization in plaster and for fractures of the hip in adults prior to internal fixation. Only limited weight can be used with skin traction, or the adhesive tape or moleskin through which the traction is applied will pull loose from the skin and cause skin burns.

Skeletal traction is often used for early provisional stabilization of femoral fractures. It may also be used for some severely comminuted tibial plateau fractures and intra-articular fractures of the distal tibia, as well as for displaced supracondylar fractures of the humerus in children. A Kirschner wire or Steinman pin is drilled transversely through the distal fragment or through a bone distal to the one that is fractured using aseptic technique. The skin about the wire or pin is relieved by incision and cleaned and dressed daily as a precaution against pin tract infection.

INTERNAL FIXATION

The principles of internal fixation of fractures include anatomical reduction of the fracture fragments, preservation of

the blood supply to the fracture fragments, stable internal fixation, and early active pain-free mobilization of muscles and joints adjacent to the fracture. Compression, when applied, is an important adjunct in achieving fracture stability and primary osseous healing. Kirschner wires (Fig. 44-4, *A*), Steinman pins (Fig. 44-4, *B*), screws (Fig. 44-4, *C*), plates and screws (Fig. 44-4, *D*), and intramedullary nails (Fig. 44-4, *E*) and pins (Fig. 44-4, *F*) are among the most commonly used metallic fixation devices. Malleable wire can be used in tension band (Fig. 44-4, *G*) and circumferential wiring techniques (Fig. 44-4, *H*). Implants used for fracture fixation are made from strong but non-reactive metals such as stainless steel or vitallium. Reduction of the fracture may be by either open or closed methods

Fig. 44-4. Types of internal fixation. (*A*) Smooth Kirschner wire fixation of a Salter-Harris type IV fracture of the lateral humeral condyle. (*B*) Smooth Steinman pin fixation of a supracondylar fracture. (*C*) Compression lag screw fixation of the medial tibial malleolus. (*D*) Dynamic compression plate fixation of transverse diaphyseal fractures of both forearm bones. (*E*) Küntscher type intramedullary rod fixation of a transverse midshaft femoral diaphyseal fracture. (*F*) Enders intramedullary pin fixation of a stable subtrochanteric femoral fracture. (*G*) Tension band wire fixation of a transverse olecranon fracture. (*H*) Circumferential wire fixation of a transverse midpatellar fracture.

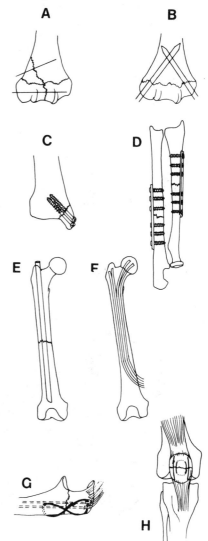

and must be as anatomical as possible prior to application of the implant. At the conclusion of a procedure, roentgenograms must be made in at least two planes to check the precision of the reduction and the precision of implant application. The quality of the bone is a key factor in internal fixation. Internal fixation is more likely to fail when bone is osteopenic.

Good indications for internal fixation include displaced intra-articular fractures, displaced Salter-Harris type III and IV epiphyseal fractures, and fractures that either cannot be reduced or cannot be maintained by closed methods, such as both forearm bone fractures, hip fractures, fractures of the distal third of the radial shaft, and Monteggia fracture-dislocations. Internal fixation is important in reducing mortality and morbidity from prolonged bed immobilization in hip fractures in the elderly and in the polytraumatized or polyfractured patient, particularly one with a fractured femur. In these patients the ability to get at least the upper body into a vertical position is an extremely important deterrent to pulmonary insufficiency and its sequelae. Other indications for internal fixation include many nonunions, pathologic fractures, and fractures in brain-injured patients. Internal fixation is usually used to stabilize the bone in replantation procedures.

The scourge of internal fixation is infection, and every precaution must be taken against it. Aseptic technique, gentle handling of tissues, evacuation of hematoma, hemostasis, and elimination of dead space are critical factors. The surgeon must not use internal fixation if he has to incise skin where there is active soft tissue infection, where there are abrasions or lacerations more than 8 hours old in the operative field, or when there are severe burns. Appropriate preventive perioperative antibiotics are often used in major fracture reconstructions.

EXTERNAL FIXATION

In external fixation, pins are drilled into the proximal and distal fracture fragments and are connected and stabilized by one or more frames external to the skin. External fixator systems can be made rigid, and in some systems compression can be applied. It is important to incise the skin about the pins so that the skin does not impinge on the pins and to provide daily pin care by cleaning and dressing the area about each pin; this usually prevents pin tract infection. External fixators are a type of portable traction that may allow patients to sit, stand, walk, and exercise when they otherwise could not do these activities. External fixators allow simultaneous fracture treatment and wound access in severe open fractures, especially when there is bone loss and severe soft tissue damage and skin loss (Fig. 44-5). External fixators also are particularly effective in managing displaced fractures of the hemipelvis, fractures associated with severe burns, fractures associated with vascular injuries, segmental fractures of the tibia, and severely comminuted and displaced fractures of the distal radius. External fixators are useful for rapid stabilization of fractures associated with polytrauma, especially femoral fractures.

RESECTION OR REPLACEMENT ARTHROPLASTY

Displaced comminuted fractures of the radial head in adults must be removed and the bone smoothed off just proximal to the radial tuberosity or the fragments will act as loose bodies and cause joint locking and early posttraumatic arthritis.

In certain femoral neck fractures, prosthetic replacement or total joint arthroplasty of the femoral head is the procedure of choice. Specific indications are discussed in the section on femoral neck fractures.

PROTECTION AND EARLY INITIATION OF RANGE OF MOTION EXERCISES

In patients with impacted fractures in which displacement is unlikely, protection and the early initiation of range of motion exercises are advised. Impacted fractures of the radial head are protected for 2 to 3 weeks with a sling. At 10 to 14 days after injury, gentle progressive active range of motion exercises are initiated at the elbow and forearm. Impacted fractures of the neck of the humerus are protected by a shoulder immobilizer or sling for 6 weeks. At 2 to 3

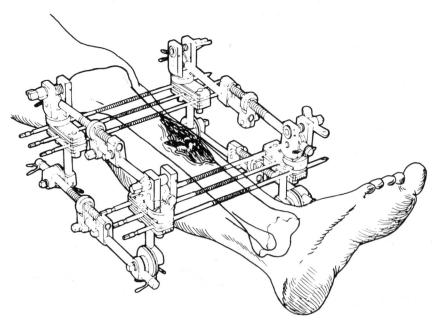

Fig. 44-5. Hoffman-Vidal external fixation of an open tibial fracture with severe skin and soft tissue loss.

weeks after injury, gentle progressive active range of motion exercises of the shoulder are started. Undisplaced fractures of the distal radius may be protected in a plaster cast for 3 weeks and then in a volar splint; the splint is removed several times daily for active range of motion exercises of the wrist. An undisplaced fracture of the tibial plateau may be protected in a cast brace, which will allow simultaneous gentle progressive active range of motion exercises.

FRACTURE HEALING

Fracture healing has three overlapping phases: (1) the inflammatory phase, (2) the reparative phase, and (3) the remodeling phase.

The inflammatory phase begins immediately after the fracture and lasts several days. The endosteal and periosteal blood supply is disrupted, causing hemorrhage and hematoma formation. Muscles surrounding the fracture are damaged. There is swelling and edema. The environment about the fracture is hypoxic and acidic. Many inflammatory cells, including polymorphonuclear leukocytes and macrophages, migrate into the area. Lysosomal enzymes are released. Osteoclasts mobilize to resorb dead bone at the fracture ends. The reparative phase may develop in response to some or all of these factors.

Repair in the incompletely immobilized fracture includes the formation of an external callus, which is supported by the periosteal blood supply. Multipotential mesenchymal cells from the periosteum, endosteum, endothelium of small vessels, and adjacent muscles invade the fracture hematoma, along with capillaries and fibroblasts, and move toward the fracture site from either side. Cartilage is formed, and as stability increases blood supply improves, oxygenation improves, and acidity decreases in a centripetal fashion about the fracture, the cartilage of the external callus is solidified by a process of enchondral ossification (Fig. 44-6). As this collar of external callus stabilizes the fracture, further enchondral ossification or gap healing occurs between the cortical ends of the bone and across the medullary canal. The endosteal blood supply is instrumental in achieving intracortical and intramedullary healing. This is the way fracture healing occurs with treatment in plaster or in traction. If the patient is ambulatory in a plaster cast brace, the controlled motion and intermittent compression stimulate the proliferation and healing of the external callus. With intramedullary fixation, the periosteal circulation and external callus are critical for fracture healing.

Fig. 44-6. Enchondral ossification of periosteal callus with gap healing of the cortices. The central wedge of hyaline cartilage in the periosteal callus is converted into immature trabecular bone.

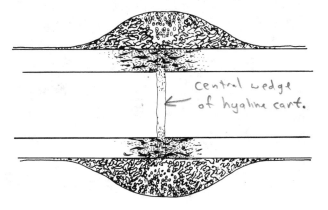

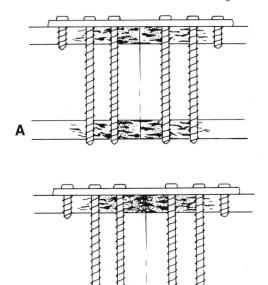

Fig. 44-7. Contact healing of cortical bone. (*A*) The fracture is anatomically reduced and compressed by plate fixation. (*B*) Osteons cross the fracture site and are followed by bone-producing osteoblasts, which solidify the fracture.

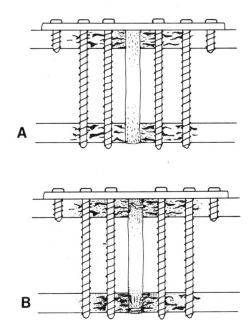

Fig. 44-8. Gap healing of cortical bone. (*A*) The fracture is reduced with a gap of less than 2 or 3 mm and rigidly held by plate and screw fixation. (*B*) Osteons invade the gap and are followed by bone-producing osteoblasts, which solidify the gap and thus the fracture.

If a fracture is rigidly immobilized in contact in the anatomical position by a plate and screws, the plate and screws take the place of the external callus and no external callus forms. Intracortical and intramedullary healing occurs primarily by contact healing, by the direct formation of bone across the fracture site without a cartilaginous phase, and without enchondral ossification (Fig. 44-7). If there is a gap between the bone ends rigidly held by a plate and screws and the gap is no more than 2 mm to 3 mm, gap healing can occur (Fig. 44-8). In such instances, osteoblasts migrate into the gap from the periphery of the fracture and synthesize bone directly to fill the gap. If a gap is greater than 2 mm to 3 mm, it exceeds the critical distance for gap healing and either replating and compression of the bone ends or bone grafting will be necessary to achieve healing.

The third phase of fracture healing is remodeling, which takes place over many months and even years. Primary woven bone is transformed to lamellar bone along the lines of stress applied to the bone. New cortical bone is formed to give the bone the greatest strength and callus and is resorbed in places where it is not needed for functional strength. Children with open epiphyses have the greatest potential for remodeling. The remodeling process in children helps the bone to return to its original shape. Remodeling will help to correct angular deformities but will not correct rotational malalignment.

FRACTURES IN CHILDREN

Nonunion is rare in diaphyseal fractures in children because of the tremendous osteogenic potential of the cambium layer of the periosteum. Almost all diaphyseal fractures in children can be treated by closed methods and tolerate some angular deformity due to the ability of the bone to remodel through epiphyseal growth. Rotational deformity will not remodel and must be corrected by reduction. A less than perfect reduction of a Salter-Harris type II epiphyseal fracture is also usually tolerated due to the remodeling capability in the child. Remodeling capability in the child is inversely proportional to age, so that the older the child, the more precise the reduction must be.

There is always the potential for growth disturbance after epiphyseal fractures (Fig. 44-2). The prognosis for growth disturbance worsens as the Salter-Harris classification progresses. Displaced Salter-Harris type III and IV epiphyseal fractures require open reduction and internal fixation, usually with Kirschner wires, to avoid joint incongruity and consequent posttraumatic arthritis and also to avoid bony bridge formation between the epiphysis and the metaphysis that will lead to angular deformity with growth. Salter-Harris type V epiphyseal injuries are almost always followed by growth disturbance. This growth disturbance can be either a complete cessation of growth at the involved physis or a partial cessation of growth, with continued growth in the remainder of the physis leading to progressive angular deformity.

The parents of children with epiphyseal fractures should be counseled regarding the possibility of growth disturbance. These children must be monitored carefully for cessation of growth or angular deformity at their fracture sites.

COMPLICATIONS OF FRACTURES

EARLY COMPLICATIONS

ARTERIAL AND NEUROLOGIC INJURY

A good neurovascular examination of the extremity is mandatory prior to and following fracture treatment.

Arterial Injury

Arterial injuries caused by fractures or dislocations tend to occur where vessels pass adjacent or are fixed to bone.

The brachial artery is particularly vulnerable where it is adjacent to the humerus and in the antecubital space (Fig. 44-9). The superficial femoral artery is particularly vulnerable in the adductor canal, where it is adjacent to the femur. The popliteal artery is vulnerable because it is tethered in the popliteal fossa.

Major arterial injuries must be recognized for optimal limb salvage. In cases of arterial insufficiency following fracture or dislocation, either arteriography should be done or the patient can be taken directly to the operating room for arterial exploration and arteriography, if necessary, can be performed during the operation. Adequate fasciotomies must be done after arterial repair or reconstruction. The fracture may be immobilized with continuous traction, with an external fixator, or with rigid internal fixation. The surgeon must remember that intimal injuries can present with good pulses, pink color, good capillary filling, and a warm extremity, all of which disappear over a period of hours as a thrombus forms.

Peripheral Nerve Injury

Nerves, like arteries, are more vulnerable to injury from fractures when they are in close approximation to bone and from dislocations in areas where they are tethered adjacent to joints. A careful motor and sensory neurologic examination should be carried out and the results recorded for every injured extremity prior to any treatment. This examination should be repeated after reduction of the fracture or dislocation. A nerve deficit that was not present prior to reduction is reason for immediate exploration of the involved nerve. Otherwise, in contrast to arterial injuries, peripheral nerve injuries in association with fractures and dislocations usually do not demand prompt corrective measures. A majority of these nerve injuries are only contusion neuropraxias, and approximately 85% of the nerve injuries associated with fractures of shafts of long bones will recover spontaneously within 4 months. Nerve injuries due to a dislocation or fracture-dislocation are often stretch or trac-

Fig. 44-9. Arteriogram shows disruption of the brachial artery following a dislocation of the elbow. Arterial disruption was suspected because of massive swelling in the antecubital area. The collateral circulation about the elbow carries blood flow to the radial and ulnar arteries. Radial and ulnar pulses were present but diminished compared with the uninvolved forearm, and the hand was pink and warm and had good capillary filling. The brachial artery was subsequently surgically repaired.

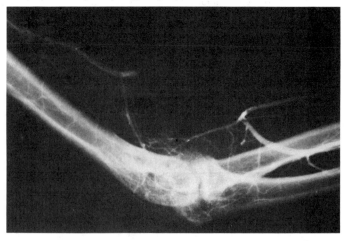

tion injuries to a nerve tethered across a joint. These types of injuries are less likely to have a spontaneous return of function than those nerve injuries associated with a shaft fracture. Recovery of function of a contused nerve may be rapid, but it may be slow if the neurons have been killed and have undergone peripheral degeneration. In cases in which the nerve is in continuity and the neurons distal to the injury have undergone peripheral degeneration, regeneration of the nerve occurs from proximal to distal at a rate of about 1 mm/day. An estimate of the approximate time of recovery can hereby be made by measuring the distance from the site of injury to the level of the first muscle innervated distal to the injury.

If internal fixation is used to treat a fracture, an associated nerve injury can be explored and treated at the same time. Otherwise, if the nerve has been severed, end-to-end nerve sutures should be performed after healing of the fracture. Intrafascicular nerve grafting may be done in preference to end-to-end suturing under undue tension and in instances of segmental nerve loss. Nerve deficits that have shown no sign of return within 6 months should be explored, since the chances for successful nerve suturing or grafting decline after that time.

Spinal Cord Injury

In the presence of a known or possible injury to the spine, an immediate careful neurologic examination is mandatory to determine the function of the spinal cord. It is extremely important to distinguish a complete from an incomplete lesion of the spinal cord. The prognosis for a complete spinal cord lesion lasting 48 hours is hopeless. Conversely, a partial spinal cord lesion, particularly a minimal lesion that shows early and rapid spontaneous recovery, has a good prognosis. The level and degree of spinal cord injury should be determined. In distinguishing a complete from an incomplete spinal cord lesion it is extremely important to evaluate the sacral segments since perianal sensation, toe flexion, and sphincter control may be the only areas where sparing exists. If the patient has no sensation below the level of the lesion and cannot feel pin prick on the anal skin or the gloved finger in the rectum, there is a complete sensory lesion. If there is no motor function below the level of the lesions including lack of toe flexion and sphincter control, complete motor paralysis is present. In serious spinal cord injuries, a generalized sympathectomy of the trunk and lower extremities can occur for 24 to 48 hours. The patient is also areflexic beyond the level of the lesion. The blood pressure is often lowered in the range of 90 torr systolic and 50 torr diastolic. This syndrome of spinal shock is distinguished from hemorrhagic shock by a knowledge of the lesion and by a pulse that is within normal limits. The bulbocavernous reflex and anal wink are normal cord-mediated reflexes, and their return signifies the termination of spinal shock. If complete paralysis and anesthesia persist below the level of the lesion after the return of the bulbocavernous reflex and the anal wink, the diagnosis of a complete lesion is confirmed.

Many incomplete spinal cord lesions will be a central cord syndrome, a Brown-Séquard syndrome, or an anterior cord syndrome. Cauda equina deficit is more likely to return than spinal cord deficit. The peripheral nerves in the lumbar area are less susceptible to injury in a fracture or dislocation than the spinal cord or cauda equina.

Laminectomy is contraindicated in spinal cord injuries unless there is a progressive neurologic deficit because it is an ineffective method for decompression and is often harmful by causing or increasing spinal instability. Early reduction of spinal fractures, dislocations, or fracture-dislocations is the best method of decompression of the spinal cord. After reduction, unstable fractures should be stabilized early. Stability of the cervical spine is achieved by means of a halo and jacket or by internal fixation and arthrodesis. The thoracolumbar spine is best stabilized by open reduction, internal fixation, and arthrodesis. Reduction and stabilization of the spine in all cord-injured patients avoid further cord injury and improve pulmonary function, rehabilitation, mental outlook, and skin care. Reduction and stabilization also safeguard against the delayed complications of pain and deformity due to progressive gibbus.

VOLKMANN'S ISCHEMIC CONTRACTURE

Compartment syndromes are caused by increased pressure in a closed subfascial space and may be due to increased volume in the noncompliant compartment due to bleeding from fracture fragments; muscular, venous, or arterial bleeding; and edema secondary to soft tissue trauma. Later, postischemic edema can add to the volume. Compartment syndromes can also be caused by tight external dressings, such as plaster casts. An uninterrupted compartment syndrome can lead to progressive muscle and nerve ischemia, necrosis, and fibrosis. This is followed by muscle contracture and deformity. Compartment syndromes occur soon after injury and must be recognized and treated early to avoid catastrophic consequences. Adequate fasciotomy is the treatment for compartment syndromes. When compartment syndrome is due to a tight cast, the cast is bivalved and the anterior half is removed while all dressings and padding are cut down to the skin for the full length of the cast. If this does not relieve the compartment syndrome, adequate fasciotomies are done. Fractures and dislocations about the elbow and distal to the elbow in the upper extremity and about the knee and distal to the knee in the lower extremity are particularly vulnerable to development of a compartment syndrome.

The four Ps, *p*ain, *p*allor, *p*ulselessness, and *p*aralysis, classically associated with Volkmann's ischemic contracture are unreliable. Pain occurs in any traumatized extremity, varies in degree, and is difficult to quantitate and evaluate. Furthermore, anesthesia may occur in later stages of ischemia and may be misinterpreted, leading to dire consequences. Since most compartment syndromes occur between 30 and 60 torr pressure and the normal systolic arterial pressure is 120 torr, pallor and pulselessness almost never occur, particularly if the radial pulse, which is extracompartmental, is monitored. Paralysis is such a late finding that it loses its value as an early diagnostic tool. The old four Ps should therefore be revised to eight Ps: *p*ain referred to the compartment in question on passive stretch of the fingers or toes (this is the earliest sign of a compartment syndrome); decreased two-*p*oint sensory appreciation (the earliest sensory sign in a compartment syndrome); increased *p*ressure in the involved portion of the extremity with swelling and tenseness; flexed *p*osture of the fingers or toes in the involved extremity; *p*ulses present; *p*ink color; *p*aresthesia; and *p*aresis. There are accurate methods for measuring interstitial tissue pressure to aid in diagnosis and decision making. The prime indications for surgical decompression of the fascia are clinical signs and symptoms of a compartment syndrome and interstitial fluid pressure of 30 torr or above or both.

OPEN FRACTURES

Open fractures are classified according to the extent of the wound, the amount of devitalized or avascular tissue, the amount of foreign material present, and the degree of injury to the bone. The value of this classification lies in the fact that the more serious the soft tissue and bony injury, the more difficulty there is in obtaining fracture union and the greater is the risk of infection. A type I open fracture is a low energy open fracture that is relatively clean and has a skin laceration of less than 2 cm. This is generally considered to occur as a result of the bone passing from inside out or from a low velocity bullet passing inward. There is minimal soft tissue damage. A type II open fracture results from moderate energy forces and causes comminution or displacement of the bone with skin laceration of more than 2 cm and moderate adjacent skin contusion and muscle damage. A type III open fracture is caused by high-energy forces and results in a significantly displaced fracture pattern with severe comminution, segmental fracture, or bone defect. There may be extensive skin loss, muscle damage, and further damage to other deep structures.

In open fractures there are two problems, the wound and the fracture.

Management of the Wound

The first goal of wound management is to avoid tetanus. Tetanus primarily threatens only wounded persons not previously immunized. All patients with open fractures must be appropriately immunized. The patient's immunization history must be established, and the physician must determine what is required for adequate prophylaxis against tetanus for each patient with an open fracture.

The next goal of wound treatment is to avoid infection, both clostridial and pyogenic. This goal is achieved by adequate irrigation and débridement of the wound and by good judgment in timing the closure or coverage of the wound. The wound is extended by incising the skin and deep fascia parallel to the long axis of the extremity from normal tissue proximally to normal tissue distally so that all foreign material and devitalized or necrotic tissue can be removed. Color, consistency, contractility, and capillary bleeding assist the surgeon in determining muscle viability. Contractility is the most reliable of these parameters and clearly establishes viability when present.

A culture is taken of the wound of an open fracture in the emergency room. Preventive intravenous antibiotics are started after culture of the wound. The antibiotic administered should be bacteriocidal and should be a broad-spectrum agent effective against both gram-positive and gram-negative organisms as well as against coagulase-positive *Staphylococcus aureus* organisms. Cephalosporins are currently preferred. A therapeutically effective concentration of the antibiotic should be achieved in the tissues. Antibiotics are discontinued 48 hours after débridement unless there are specific indications for their continuation, in which case any adjustments should be made to reflect the results of cultures and sensitivities. Antibiotics should never be substituted for adequate cleansing and débridement of the wound of an open fracture nor for adequate immunization for tetanus.

Wound closure or coverage is elective. Primary closure of the wound in open fractures is controversial. If the wound is less than 12 hours old, it is considered contaminated, whereas if it is more than 12 hours old, it is considered infected. Some surgeons believe that if the wound is less than 12 hours old and there is no gross soilage, no devitalized or necrotic tissue, and no foreign body that primary closure may be performed. When the wound is more than 12 hours old, when there is gross soilage, or when there is difficulty ascertaining tissue viability at the initial débridement, the wound should be left open and staged wound care should be instituted. The key to wound closure or coverage is not so much the time that the wound is closed but that the wound is controlled when closure or coverage is performed. A wound is considered controlled when there is no infection, minimal contamination, no devitalized or necrotic tissue, and all foreign, particularly organic, material is removed. Whenever there is any question about meeting these criteria, it is safest to leave the wound open and to delay closure or coverage. Wounds should never be closed under excessive tension. Hemostasis should be excellent at the time of closure or coverage, all hematoma should be evacuated, and any dead space should be eliminated or drained.

Management of the Fracture

The fracture fragments should be cleaned with great care so as not to disturb the periosteal blood supply. Bone ends may be trimmed when this is necessary to remove gross soilage. Small devascularized pieces of cortical bone should be removed from the wound. Large fragments of cortical bone with soft tissue connection may be retained. Large cortical fragments with tenuous or no soft tissue connection have a real potential value in reconstituting a defect as an *in situ* bone graft but are also a potential sequestrum. There are no absolutely clear criteria about retaining such a fragment. The degree of contamination of the fragment and of the wound and the vascularity of the adjacent soft tissue influence the surgeon's judgment. If the fragment is retained, it is a calculated risk.

Open fractures require stabilization. If satisfactory apposition and alignment are present or can be obtained by manipulation, stabilization with a plaster cast may be sufficient to permit bone healing. However, certain open fractures will require fixation to provide ideal management for the wound, the fracture, or both.

External fixation devices are used effectively for provisional as well as definitive fixation of open fractures. They can be used provisionally until the wound is controlled, closed, or covered and is suitable for internal fixation. In instances of more severe wounds, external fixators can provide the stability necessary for optimal wound management. When internal fixation is not suitable, external fixators can be used for definitive fracture management.

Internal fixation may be necessary for optimal treatment of some open fractures. In such instances, strict standards must be applied. Classically, open fractures are converted to closed fractures by closure or coverage of the wound. Successful closure or coverage of the wound of an open fracture constitutes *prima facie* evidence that the wound is not infected. Internal fixation may be performed then with minimal risk. Internal fixation must be rigidly stable. Otherwise, motion at the fracture site or at interfaces with metallic fixation devices can lead to micronecrosis of tissue, which may then act as a nidus for infection. Motion at the fracture site can also lead to nonunion by interrupting the circulation at the fracture site.

A more modern understanding of wound and fracture healing indicates that type I and some type II open fractures seen within 12 hours of injury may be stabilized with internal fixation at the time of initial surgery. In addition, open fractures may be stabilized with internal fixation as a delayed primary or secondary procedure. In such cases, the wound must be adequately decompressed as well as surgically clean and controlled. Again, it is essential that the fracture be rigidly fixed. Metallic fixation devices must be covered with soft tissues in order to prevent desiccation necrosis of underlying bone. Minimal osteosynthesis (*i.e.*, the least amount of metal that will rigidly stabilize the bone) should be used in open fractures. Wound closure or coverage is elective and should be performed only when it is certain that the wound is surgically clean and controlled and will remain adequately decompressed. Thus the wound may be closed primarily if, in the opinion of the surgeon, these criteria are met at that time. Otherwise, the wound may be left open and staged closure or coverage carried out later as a precautionary measure. Excellent judgment and technique are necessary in treating open fractures with internal fixation and in choosing the timing of wound closure or coverage. The concepts of anatomic reduction and stable internal fixation of the fracture fragments and preservation of the blood supply to the bone fragments and soft tissue, followed by early active pain-free mobilization of muscles and joints adjacent to the fracture, are critical prerequisites for successful treatment of open fractures.

Intermedullary devices do not provide rigid bony fixation and should be used with caution in open fractures of the diaphyseal shafts of major long bones. Ordinarily, intermedullary devices should only be used for fracture fixation in those open fractures that have successfully been converted to closed fractures.

INTRA-ARTICULAR FRACTURES

Patients with intra-articular fractures may develop posttraumatic arthritis as a late complication. Displacement and comminution increase this risk. Displaced intra-articular fractures have the best results with early congruent joint surface restoration, stable internal fixation, and early joint motion. Some intra-articular fractures may be too comminuted to fix internally and may require alternative methods of treatment, such as continuous traction with early joint motion. Arthroplasty or arthrodesis may be necessary if severe posttraumatic arthritis develops.

DISLOCATIONS

Dislocations should be reduced as early as possible to relieve pain, to relieve pressure on adjacent neurovascular structures, to prevent adjacent skin necrosis, and to restore normal physiology and function to the joint as quickly as possible.

ILEUS

Patients with thoracolumbar vertebral body fractures, transverse process fractures of the lumbar vertebrae, or pelvic fractures may develop ileus due to retroperitoneal hemorrhage and should be admitted to the hospital and observed. Ileus usually develops within the first 24 hours after injury. It is treated with nasogastric suction and intravenous fluid and electrolyte replacement and usually resolves within 3 to 5 days.

FAT EMBOLISM SYNDROME

Fat embolism syndrome is a form of posttraumatic respiratory distress syndrome that is seen after severe or multiple trauma with one or more fractures, multiple fractures, and even isolated fractures, principally those of the pelvis, hip, and long bones of the lower extremity. The changes in the lung parenchyma are both simple mechanical blocking of capillaries by fat droplets and interstitial hemorrhagic pneumonitis. Eighty-five percent of patients who develop fat embolism syndrome do so within the first 48 hours after injury. The clinical signs of fat embolism syndrome are fever, tachycardia, tachypnea, and progressive changes of cerebral anoxia, including, in sequence, restlessness, disorientation, confusion, stupor, and coma. Petechiae are found on the conjunctivae, root of the neck, chest, trunk, axillae, groin, and anterior thighs and clinch the diagnosis. The critical laboratory finding is an arterial blood oxygen pressure of less than 60 torr in the presence of respiratory distress. Pulmonary edema may be present on the chest roentgenogram.

Fat embolism syndrome is treated with oxygen by nasal cannula or mask, provided the arterial oxygen remains above 70 torr. Failure to maintain the arterial oxygen above 70 torr, progressive hypoxia with clinical manifestations of pulmonary distress or change in the level of consciousness, or an arterial oxygen below 50 torr for any reason requires endotracheal intubation and mechanical assistance of ventilation with a volume-cycled respirator and positive end-expiratory pressure. If continued ventilation is necessary at 4 days, a tracheostomy is done to prevent tracheal necrosis and permanent vocal cord damage by the endotracheal tube. Diuresis, fluid restriction, and corticosteroids are an important part of the treatment of fat embolism syndrome. Early fixation of long bone fractures, particularly those of the femur, so that the patient may assume a vertical posture is an important adjunct in treating fat embolism syndrome and avoiding prolonged cardiopulmonary failure that leads to death. Mortality varies with the extent of the syndrome and is minimized by early recognition and aggressive treatment.

INFECTION

Infection is heralded by rubor, calor, dolor, and tumor (*i.e.*, redness, heat, pain, and swelling). Fluctuance is found in abscess formation. Purulent drainage from a postoperative incision or drain site is a definite sign of infection. Cellulitic infection is treated by rest, immobilization, elevation, and intravenous antibiotics. Purulent infection is incised, drained, cultured, and debrided of septic necrotic and granulation tissue. The wound is left open to heal by secondary intention or to be closed or covered electively when wound control is achieved. Antibiotics are used and are adjusted according to culture and sensitivity results. Purulent infections are either superficial or deep, depending on their position in relation to the deep fascia. Incision, drainage, and débridement of superficial infections need not extend beyond the deep fascia; but for deep infections, incision, drainage, and débridement must be carried out to the source of infection, usually at the site of open reduction and internal fixation. If the fixation is rigidly stable, it is left in place; if not, it is replaced with internal fixation that is rigidly stable. Many of these fractures will proceed to union. After union, metal fixation can be removed and any residual infection treated, again, by incision, drainage, débridement, and open wound care. Again, the wound may be allowed to heal by secondary intention or may be closed or covered electively when wound control is achieved.

REFLEX SYMPATHETIC DYSTROPHY

Although it is poorly understood, the pathophysiology of reflex sympathetic dystrophy seems to include a painful lesion, a susceptible patient, and an abnnormal autonomic reflex. Reflex sympathetic dystrophy should be suspected when pain, swelling, and stiffness are out of proportion to the severity of the injury and when there are color, temperature, or pseudomotor changes, muscle and skin atrophy, and osteopenia. Prophylactic measures include early and precise reduction of a fracture, avoiding edema, and early institution of active range of motion exercises. The key to treatment of a reflex sympathetic dystrophy is early recognition. Although the etiology is an enigma, it is well established that the condition is a result of sympathetic overactivity; therefore, therapy must be directed at the sympathetic nervous system. One or a series of sympathetic blocks may be both diagnostic and therapeutic. If blocks give only temporary relief, surgical sympathectomy should be considered. If there is a specific operable lesion causing the reflex sympathetic dystrophy, this should be corrected. Otherwise, elective surgery should not be done until the dystrophy is resolved.

THROMBOEMBOLIC DISEASE

There is an increased incidence of thromboembolic disease in fractures of the thoracolumbar spine, pelvis, and hip. These patients should be carefully monitored for deep vein thrombosis. Preventive anticoagulation is controversial, as is selection of the anticoagulating agent to be used. Low-dose heparin, coumadin, low molecular weight dextran, and aspirin each have their advocates. Preventive anticoagulation does not serve to prevent deep venous thrombosis or pulmonary embolism in patients with fractures but may prevent mortality when pulmonary embolism occurs. Patients with the above fractures who are at high risk for thromboembolic disease may be considered for preventive anticoagulation after fracture bleeding has been controlled unless there are specific contraindications. Patients who are at high risk include patients with prior thromboembolic disease, prior lower extremity venous surgery or venous insufficiency, obesity, diabetes, malignancy, or paraplegia; women taking estrogens; and patients with conditions requiring prolonged bed rest. The use of preventive anticoagulation is tempered by its complications, including an increased incidence of hematoma at fracture sites and a subsequent increased infection rate as well as delayed fracture healing. When preventive anticoagulation is used, it is continued for 2 weeks or until the patient is ambulatory. Early rigid fracture stabilization, decreased blood loss at surgery, good hemostasis, decreased operative time, good postoperative wound drainage, compression dressings, elevation of the affected extremity, use of antiembolic stockings, and early mobilization of the patient are measures that may help to decrease the incidence of thromboembolic disease. If deep vein thrombosis or pulmonary embolism occurs, the patient should be given anticoagulants unless there are specific contraindications.

LATE COMPLICATIONS

FAILURE OF PROGRESSION TOWARD UNION

Disruption of local blood supply at the fracture site is an important cause of failure of a fracture to progress toward union. There is an increased injury to the blood supply at the fracture site in open fractures. The more severe the fracture, the displacement of the fracture, the bone loss, and the soft tissue loss, the greater is the risk of nonunion. Some areas of bone, such as the carpal scaphoid and the

femoral head, have an inherently poor blood supply and are therefore at higher risk for nonunion. Other causes of failure of normal progression toward union that can result in delayed union, nonunion, or pseudarthrosis include soft tissue interposition at the fracture site, repeated manipulation of the fracture, inadequate reduction or immobilization, insufficient length of time of immobilization, persistent separation or distraction at the fracture site, and infection.

Delayed Union

Delayed union is the prolongation of the healing time of a fracture beyond a theoretical average for the location and configuration of a given fracture in a patient in a particular age-group. Healing of the fragments is taking place but is progressing more slowly than anticipated. A delayed union is generally said to exist if any fracture has not united at 4 months after injury. Continued treatment is indicated with the hope that union will follow. Delayed union may precede nonunion.

Nonunion

Nonunion occurs when a fracture fails to unite in the anticipated time for the location and configuration of a given fracture in a patient in a particular age-group and when three consecutive monthly roentgenograms thereafter show no further evidence of progression of fracture healing and one or more radiographic signs of nonunion. Roengenographic signs of nonunion include a persistent radiolucent fracture line extending from outer cortex to outer cortex; sclerosis of the fracture margins; submarginal cyst formation; linear osteoporosis of disuse; medullary sealing with cortical bone; increased width of the ununited radiolucent fracture line; progressive rounding, molding, or mushrooming of the fracture margins; or a complete absence of any bony reaction of one or both fracture ends. Clinical signs of nonunion are pain, tenderness, swelling, erythema, increased heat, and motion at the fracture site. In the lower extremity, the patient may either walk with an antalgic gait or be unable to bear weight owing to pain and instability at the fracture site. Nonunions are classified as noninfected or infected. Noninfected nonunions are either hypertrophic or atrophic. Hypertrophic nonunions are reactive, are vascular, have molding or mushrooming at the ends, and have the potential to heal without bone grafting if their ends are apposed, aligned, and compressed, usually with a plate and screws and sometimes with a medullary nail followed by ambulation in the lower extremity. If a gap persists after alignment and stabilization of a hypertrophic nonunion, bone grafting is performed. Atrophic nonunions are avascular and have a complete absence of any bone reaction at the fracture ends. These nonunions require stable fixation and a bone graft (Fig. 44-10). Classically, infected nonunions are converted to noninfected nonunions by débridement of all infected and devitalized bone and soft tissue, thus obtaining wound control. At a second stage, closure is performed or coverage is applied. Bone stabilization and grafting are done after control of the infection is ensured. A more aggressive, but equally effective approach to selected infected nonunions obtains wound control by débridement of all infected and devitalized bone and soft tissue, stabilization of the bone, and bone grafting simultaneously. This is only done when the surgeon is certain that all infected and necrotic tissue has been removed. The wound is then allowed to heal by secondary intention or is closed or covered electively.

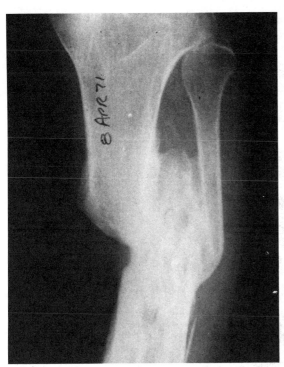

Fig. 44-10. There is some hypertrophic proliferative molding of the proximal tibial fragment, but the distal tibial fragment is tapered and shows no reaction or effort at bone formation.

Pseudarthrosis

A pseudarthrosis is the end stage of a nonunion in which a false joint occurs with sealing of the medullary cavity and formation of a fluid-filled cavity lined with pseudosynovial cells. A pseudarthrosis will generally exist if a fracture is not united within 2 years. For all practical purposes, the terms *nonunion* and *pseudarthrosis* are synonymous.

MALUNION

A fracture is malunited when it unites along with a deformity that results in an impairment in function, cosmesis, or both (Fig. 44-11, *A*). The deformity may be a result of displacement, malalignment, malrotation, or shortening. In many fractures, some degree of deformity is acceptable because there is no adverse effect in function or appearance. Good fracture reduction, good stabilization of the fracture, good follow-up, and good patient compliance with the treatment program will prevent malunion. When malunion does occur, surgery, usually osteotomy, is necessary to correct it (Fig. 44-11, *B* through *D*). The functional loss must justify the operative risk. Operation is rarely justified for cosmetic reasons alone. Arthrodesis or arthroplasty may be performed for some cases of painful arthritis resulting from malunion involving joint surfaces.

CAST DISEASE

Cast disease is joint stiffness, muscle atrophy, edema, and generalized osteopenia resulting in an extremity after a fracture. It is common after prolonged treatment in a plaster cast that immobilized the joints above and below the fracture. Modern casting techniques, such as with a patellar weight-bearing cast with a free polypropylene ankle and heel cup, tend to allow at least some mobility in the joints above and below a fracture. Cast disease is commonly associated with nonunions. Edema causes a proteinaceous

exudate that can organize with fibrous tissue about joints, causing stiffness, contracture, and even ankylosis. This can be compounded by posttraumatic intra-articular arthrofibrosis, which can occur after intra-articular fractures. Cast disease is prevented by stable fixation of the fracture, by elevation, and by range of motion, isometric, and muscle-strengthening exercises as part of a well-supervised rehabilitation program.

MYOSITIS OSSIFICANS

Myositis ossificans is the heterotopic formation of bone in soft tissues that can occur after fractures or dislocations. This lesion most commonly occurs about the elbow and hip and can cause an extra-articular ankylosis (Fig. 44-12). It also can occur in fractures of the forearm, resulting in a loss of rotation. The cause is not known, but there is some relation to the severity of the injury.

AVASCULAR NECROSIS OF BONE

Posttraumatic avascular necrosis of bone occurs when a fracture, a dislocation, or a combination of the two disrupts the blood supply to a region of the bone or to one or more of the fracture fragments. This may take some time to become apparent on roentgenograms; the avascular bone eventually becomes relatively denser than the vascularized bone. The femoral head, carpal scaphoid, humeral head, and talus are particularly predisposed to avascular necrosis owing to their precarious blood supply. The more severe the displacement of the fracture and the longer a dislocation remains unreduced, the greater is the likelihood of avascular necrosis. Avascular necrosis is generally apparent on a radioisotope bone scan prior to its manifestation on roentgenograms. Delayed union or nonunion is more frequent in patients with avascular necrosis of bone since the healing process depends entirely on the vascularized segment. A particularly devastating complication of avascular necrosis, especially in the weight-bearing hip and ankle joints, is subchondral bone collapse of the femoral head and talus, respectively, leading to severe posttraumatic arthritis. Arthroplasty or arthrodesis is usually required.

REHABILITATION

Nicholas André, the father of orthopaedics, said, "I operate, God heals." The orthopaedic surgeon's job is not completed after closed or open reduction and stabilization of the fracture or dislocation. The rehabilitation of each patient must be planned and supervised. Occupational and physical therapists play an instrumental role in rehabilitation, and contact between the therapist and the patient should occur at the earliest possible moment after injury. Therapists execute the rehabilitation plan, and under the physician's guidance they motivate the patient, encourage him, and support his morale while directing him in techniques designed to regain function and prevent cast disease.

The first important goal of rehabilitation is to get the patient in a vertical position. This is particularly important in patients whose cardiorespiratory function may be compromised (*e.g.*, in patients with hip fractures and in polytraumatized patients). The vertical or near-vertical position significantly improves pulmonary function by allowing the abdominal contents to become dependent in the abdomen, leading to increased diaphragmatic excursion and increased ease of respiration. The first step in achieving the vertical

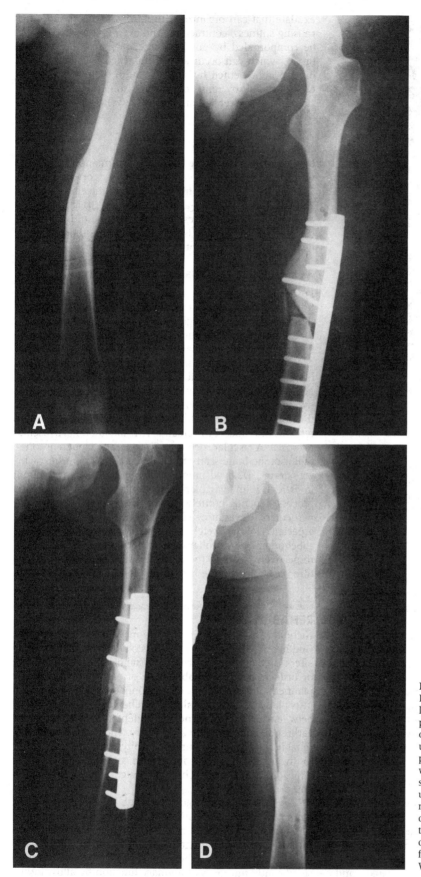

Fig. 44-11. Malunion of the left femur. (*A*) Roentgenogram of a malunion of the midshaft left femur in valgus deformity that caused the patient to walk with a limp. (*B*) A surgical osteotomy was performed to correct the malunion, and stability was achieved in the corrected position with a plate and screws. A bone graft was added at the medial side at the osteotomy site. (*C*) The bone graft has incorporated, and union has occurred at the osteotomy site at the midshaft femur. (*D*) Eighteen months after the osteotomy and bone grafting were performed the plate and screws were removed. The osteotomy is united, and the valgus malunion deformity is corrected. (Courtesy of Dr. E. Frazier Ward)

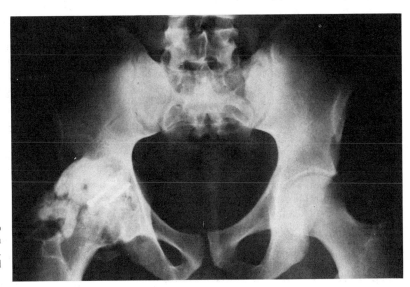

Fig. 44-12. Myositis ossificans of the right hip occurred following a posterior dislocation with fracture of the posterior rim of the acetabulum. The posterior acetabular rim had been reduced and fixed with two screws.

position is reduction and stabilization of the fracture or dislocation. The vertical position may then be achieved by sitting the patient in a chair or by using a circle electric bed. In some cases it is necessary to gradually reaccustom the patient to the vertical position by the use of the tilt table. Of course, the ultimate vertical position is achieved when the patient can stand and ambulate.

The second important goal is to regain motion in the joints and strength and excursion in the musculotendinous units adjacent to each fracture or dislocation. This is achieved by active, active-assisted, and passive range of motion exercises and by graduated strengthening exercises. These exercises are initiated and increased as stability of the fracture will allow. Modern functional casting and cast bracing no longer always immobilize the joint above and the joint below a fracture, so that these joints may often undergo early rehabilitation even when plaster casting is the primary means of fracture stabilization.

The third important goal of rehabilitation is to get patients with lower extremity injuries ambulatory. This goal also is dictated by the degree of fracture stability as well as by the method chosen to achieve this stability. Parallel bars are often used to initiate ambulation, followed by training in the use of a cane, crutches, or a walker as assistive devices. Ambulatory casts or cast braces are often used for lower extremity fractures. Weight bearing is initiated in accordance with the type and location of the fracture, the method of stabilization, and the degree of fracture consolidation. The goal is to achieve full independent weight bearing. This is not always possible, and sometimes a patient may require the continued use of a brace, cane, crutches, or walker to achieve the highest level of ambulation possible for him.

Mobilization of the patient through exercises and ambulation is an important deterrent to thromboembolic disease.

FRACTURES AND DISLOCATIONS OF THE UPPER EXTREMITY

FRACTURES AND DISLOCATIONS ABOUT THE SHOULDER

DISLOCATIONS OF THE STERNOCLAVICULAR JOINT

Dislocations of the sternoclavicular joint are either anterior or posterior and are of about equal frequency. The injury results from a fall on the outstretched upper extremity, with the force being transmitted to the sternoclavicular joint. In the anterior dislocation there is a prominence at this joint, and in the posterior dislocation there is an indentation. Both types of dislocations are reduced by closed methods, with the use of posterior and lateral traction for the anterior dislocation and a sandbag between the scapulae and downward pressure on both shoulders for the posterior dislocation. Anterior dislocations are usually unstable. However, stabilization with pins is contraindicated because of the proximity of vital structures in the mediastinum. Smooth pins, even if properly placed initially, have been notorious for migration into the mediastinum, with disastrous consequences. Many recurrent anterior sternoclavicular dislocations can be left unreduced and ignored. In athletes and manual laborers in whom stability is preferred, stabilization may be achieved by a fascial sling to the second rib. In these instances, all dissection should be carried out close to bone and the points of entrance and exit of all drill holes placed in bone should be visible. Alternatively, resection of the medial 2 cm to 3 cm of clavicle is appropriate treatment, particularly if there is persistent pain in or about the joint. Posterior dislocations are dangerous because of the proximity of vital mediastinal structures. Severe dyspnea can occur as a result of tracheal or bronchial compression. Stability of the reduction is the rule in posterior dislocations. A chest roentgenogram and admission to the hospital for observation are prudent for these injuries. In all injuries about the shoulder, early initiation of range of motion exercises is important. Flexion and external rotation are concentrated on, and gravity may be eliminated for these exercises.

FRACTURES OF THE CLAVICLE

Fractures of the diaphysis of the clavicle, even though not anatomically reduced, are usually best treated nonoperatively with the shoulders in hyperextension and immobilized by a figure-eight clavicle strap. Even when the fragments heal with some overlap with bony prominence, this will resorb and decrease in size with time and the functional and cosmetic results are quite predictably acceptable. Open reduction is associated with an increased incidence of nonunion and with scars that often spread, occasionally develop keloids, and are unsightly. Open reduction of clavicular shaft fractures therefore should be reserved for specific indications. Indications for open reduction and internal fixation of the clavicle include neurovascular compromise due to posterior displacement and impingement of the bony fragments on the brachial plexus, subclavian vessels, or the carotid artery; fracture of the distal third of the clavicle with disruption of the coracoclavicular ligaments and marked displacement of the fragments; severe angulation or comminution of a fracture in the middle third of the clavicle, especially with wide separation of the fragments and interposition of soft tissue, and also if the fragments impinge on and threaten the integrity of the overlying skin; the patient's inability to tolerate prolonged immobilization required by closed treatment because of Parkinson's disease, a seizure disorder, or other neuromuscular disease; and symptomatic nonunion following treatment by closed methods. Fixation is by a contoured one-third semitubular plate or by an intermedullary pin. When internal fixation is performed, autogenous cancellous bone grafting is done in instances of defect, severe comminution, and nonunion.

DISLOCATIONS OF THE ACROMIOCLAVICULAR JOINT

Dislocations of the acromioclavicular joint are the result of a downward force on the acromion, such as a fall on the point of the shoulder. Stress anteroposterior roentgenograms taken of both shoulders with the patient erect, holding weights, are necessary to determine the grade of injury with certainty. Nondisplaced injuries are treated symptomatically with a sling, ice, analgesic medication, and early initiation of shoulder range of motion exercises, with strengthening exercises and the resumption of activities as pain will permit. Partial separations are treated in the same manner or may be treated with a Kenny-Howard splint for 3 to 6 weeks to maintain the reduction. Complete dislocations may be treated symptomatically in older, inactive individuals, but in young, active patients the reduction should be maintained by a Kenny-Howard splint for 8 weeks. In a patient with a significant athletic commitment or in a manual worker open reduction and internal fixation are advised. The lateral end of any pins across the acromioclavicular joint should be bent to prevent migration. For chronic symptomatic complete dislocation, in older and inactive patients, the distal clavicle may be resected, while in active patients, athletes, and manual laborers the distal 1 cm of the clavicle is resected, the fibrocartilaginous acromioclavicular disk is removed, and the coracoclavicular relationship is reestablished. Posttraumatic arthritis can occur as a later complication of these injuries.

DISLOCATIONS OF THE GLENOHUMERAL JOINT

The glenohumeral joint has little inherent stability and is the most commonly dislocated joint in the body. Anterior dislocation occurs far more frequently than posterior dislocation, which constitutes only 1% to 4% of glenohumeral dislocations.

The mechanism of anterior dislocation is abduction and external rotation with a posterior force. The shoulder then locks in this position, and adduction and internal rotation are impossible. The coracoid process is more prominent than usual. The humeral head is more prominent in the subacromial region anteriorly while losing its anterior prominence at the shoulder.

Anteroposterior and lateral axillary roentgenograms are important in confirming the dislocation and in determining if there are any associated fractures. The axillary lateral view demonstrates the exact relationship of the humeral head to the glenoid fossa, (*i.e.,* anterior or posterior), and is particularly important in detecting a posterior dislocation, which may not be apparent on anteroposterior view alone.

The treatment of both anterior and posterior acute glenohumeral dislocation is by closed manipulation. Although intravenous analgesia may suffice for anterior dislocations, patients with posterior dislocations nearly always require general anesthesia for reduction.

Reduction must be confirmed by anteroposterior and lateral axillary roentgenograms. A Velpeau dressing or shoulder immobilizer is maintained for 3 weeks in patients under 50 years of age and for 2 weeks in patients over 50 years of age. Pendulum exercises are then initiated. Active abduction and external rotation are permitted at 6 weeks after injury.

Axillary nerve injury may occur in dislocations of the glenohumeral joint. Motor and sensory examination should be performed before and after closed manipulation because this deficit is frequently missed.

If anterior dislocation is more than 4 weeks old or if posterior dislocation is more than 2 weeks old, open reduction will usually be necessary because of scarring and contracture and since rapidly developing osteoporosis greatly increases the risk of humeral neck fracture with the increased forces necessary to reduce an old dislocation. If the dislocation has been present for a long period of time and the patient is elderly and not significantly impaired by pain or loss of motion, surgery will not improve the condition and should not be performed. If the patient is young or symptomatic, open reduction and often internal fixation should be performed. Arthrodesis, arthroplasty, or total shoulder replacement may be necessary to stabilize the joint or if the articular surface is badly damaged.

Recurrent dislocation is the most common complication of dislocation of the glenohumeral joint. This is age related, occurring in as many as 70% to 80% of males under 30 but in only 10% to 15% of those over 30. Three or more dislocations are an indication for a surgical reconstructive procedure.

FRACTURES OF THE PROXIMAL HUMERUS

Fractures about the proximal humerus in adults may be classified as avulsion fractures of the tuberosities, impacted fractures of the surgical or anatomical neck, displaced fractures, and fracture-dislocations.

Avulsion fractures of the tuberosities of the humerus may occur from direct trauma, from seizure disorders, or with glenohumeral dislocations. When the avulsed tuberosity remains displaced more than 1 cm, even after reduction of a glenohumeral dislocation, open reduction and internal fixation with either a lag screw technique or a tension band wire is indicated. When a tuberosity has been displaced and retracted, a significant tear has occurred in the rotator cuff and must be repaired for optimal results.

Impacted fractures occur almost exclusively in older patients (Fig. 44-13). The mechanism of injury is either a direct fall on the shoulder with the arm at the side or a fall on the outstretched arm. The fracture may occur at either the anatomical or surgical neck, although the surgical neck is by far the more frequent site. As much as 30° to 40° of angulation may be accepted. A Velpeau dressing is used for 7 to 10 days. Pendulum exercises are then initiated, and a sling or shoulder immobilizer is used between exercise periods. Early motion is the key to a good result. Fractures without displacement are best treated as outlined for impacted fractures.

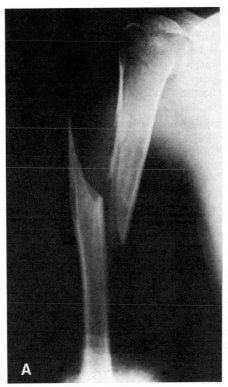 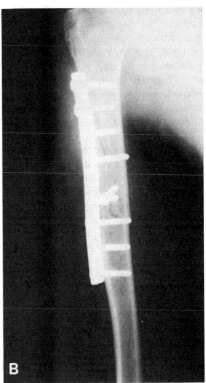

Fig. 44-13. Impacted fracture of the humeral neck and irreducible long oblique fracture of the proximal humeral diaphysis. (*A*) Roentgenogram of an impacted fracture of the humeral neck associated with a long oblique fracture of the proximal humeral shaft that could not be reduced by closed manipulation because the long spike of the distal fragment was impaled into the substance of the deltoid muscle. (*B*) An open reduction of the humeral shaft fracture was performed, and the fracture was stabilized with a plate and screws. The humeral neck fracture was then treated in a shoulder immobilizer.

Displaced fractures of the anatomical neck render the articular fragment avascular. If reduction and union can be achieved, many patients will not be sufficiently symptomatic to require prosthetic replacement. If satisfactory reduction cannot be achieved by closed methods, prosthetic replacement is indicated. Fractures of the surgical neck can usually be managed by closed manipulation and either a hanging cast or Velpeau dressing. When open reduction is required, stabilization is provided by a T-buttress plate.

Fractures of the surgical neck of the humerus and either the greater or the lesser tuberosity can rarely be reduced by closed methods. When the greater tuberosity is displaced, the articular segment has an adequate blood supply through the lesser tuberosity but is internally rotated by the unopposed pull of the subscapularis. When the lesser tuberosity is displaced, the articular segment has an adequate blood supply through the greater tuberosity but is externally rotated by the unopposed pull of the rotator cuff muscles. In these fractures, the displaced tuberosity should be fixed to the remaining metaphysis by lag screw or wiring technique. The reconstructed metaphysis is then fixed to the diaphysis with a T-buttress plate. Three-part anterior and posterior fracture-dislocations require early open reduction and internal fixation. If not approached early, contracture and scar may impede reduction while osteopenia may compromise fixation.

Fractures of the surgical neck and both tuberosities and head-splitting fractures result in avascular necrosis of the humeral head. Therefore, these fractures are best treated by primary prosthetic replacement, as are impression fractures of the articular surface involving greater than 50% of the humeral head. The tuberosities should be carefully retained and should be reassembled and wired beneath the prosthetic replacement. These fractures also should be surgically approached as early as the patient's condition will allow.

Epiphyseal separations of the proximal humerus are usually seen in adolescent children when the epiphysis is growing most rapidly and is therefore the weakest. It usually is a Salter-Harris type II epiphyseal fracture, is rarely impacted, and is angulated anteriorly and laterally. Considerable deformity may be accepted since the remodeling potential of the proximal humerus is so great and since the mobility of the glenohumeral joint compensates for some deformity. Treatment is by Velpeau immobilization, with gradual progressive mobilization starting at 3 weeks after injury. Premature closure of the physis occurs in 10% of undisplaced and up to 40% of displaced fractures, but the resulting discrepancy in length in the upper extremity is seldom noticed by the patient. Open reduction is rarely indicated.

FRACTURES OF THE SHAFT OF THE HUMERUS

Fractures of the shaft of the humerus result from both direct and indirect trauma. Most are complete, displaced, shortened, and angulated. Closed treatment methods are preferred for most humeral shaft fractures. The neurovascular status of the extremity, especially of the radial nerve, must be examined both prior to and after reduction of the fracture. Reduction is achieved by longitudinal traction. Gravity assists this reduction. Immobilization is provided by coaptation splints and a Velpeau bandage, sling and swathe or shoulder immobilizer. A hanging cast or a functional cast brace may be used as an alternative method of treatment.

Open reduction and internal fixation may be indicated when satisfactory position and alignment cannot be achieved by closed methods, when associated injuries in the extremity require early mobilization, when there are other fractures in the same extremity, when there is associated major vascular injury, when open fractures of the humerus present with a radial nerve palsy, when a radial nerve palsy develops after manipulation of a humeral shaft fracture, for transverse fractures, in displaced segmental humeral shaft fractures that cannot be adequately reduced or maintained by closed methods, in pathologic fractures, for bilateral humeral shaft fractures, in the polytraumatized or polyfractured patient when optimal respiratory care and nursing care require an unencumbered patient with a stabilized fracture, and in nonunions. When internal fixation is used, a wide dynamic compression plate is preferred, with screws securing at least eight cortices in each of the main fragments on either side of the fracture when length of the fragments will permit. This provides the most rigid fixation (Fig. 44-13). Intramedullary devices do not control rotation well and if inserted proximally may interfere with shoulder function. Their main use is in stabilizing both pathologic fractures due to malignant tumors and displaced segmental fractures. External fixators are used as provisional and sometimes definitive fixation in patients with severe open fractures.

In children, closed reduction and the use of a U-shaped plaster coaptation splint and a Velpeau dressing for 3 to 6 weeks provide satisfactory immobilization. Up to 1 cm of overlap of the bone ends may be accepted in children.

Radial nerve injuries associated with humeral fractures and present prior to manipulation are observed for 6 months. The vast majority return within this time. If there is no evidence of return 6 months after injury, the radial nerve is explored and neurolysis, suture, or nerve grafting is performed.

FRACTURES AND DISLOCATIONS ABOUT THE ELBOW

FRACTURES OF THE DISTAL HUMERUS

Supracondylar fractures without an intra-articular component may be treated by closed methods much the same as a humeral shaft fracture. If closed manipulation does not produce a satisfactory reduction, open reduction and internal fixation is performed. Intercondylar fractures may be displaced or undisplaced. Undisplaced intercondylar fractures are treated with a long arm posterior plaster splint and gentle progressive active range of motion exercises as healing permits. Displaced intercondylar fractures are treated by early open reduction and internal fixation whenever possible, with great care being taken to restore the congruity of the articular surface. The ulnar nerve must be identified and protected. Some intercondylar fractures may be so comminuted as to preclude fixation. In these patients, continuous skeletal traction through an olecranon pin followed by early motion may produce the best results. Isolated fractures of the medial or lateral condyle are uncommon in adults. If these fractures are displaced, open reduction and internal fixation is performed, usually with one or more interfragmentary lag screws. Fractures of the capitellum in adults are best treated by excision, followed by gentle progressive active range of motion exercise of the elbow and forearm.

SUPRACONDYLAR FRACTURES IN CHILDREN

Supracondylar fracture of the humerus is the most common fracture about the elbow in children. It usually occurs between the ages of 3 and 10 from a fall on the outstretched hand with the elbow partially extended.

Undisplaced supracondylar fractures are treated in a posterior splint or cuff and collar with the elbow flexed to 100° for 3 to 4 weeks.

Displaced supracondylar fractures are either flexion or extension types. The vast majority are extension type with the distal fragment displaced posteriorly. There is marked deformity and swelling at the elbow related to the severity of the trauma and the length of time from the injury. The supracondylar fracture can be distinguished from a posterior dislocation of the elbow on physical examination because the bony prominences of the medial and lateral epicondyles and the olecranon maintain their normal triangular relationship. Physical examination should include a careful evaluation for compartment syndrome, vascular injury, and peripheral nerve function. The radial nerve is the most commonly injured nerve in supracondylar fractures.

Compartment syndrome, if unrelieved, can lead to Volkmann's ischemic contracture, the most severe complication of supracondylar fractures. The most important initial step in avoiding compartment syndrome is to relieve venous congestion by early complete and accurate reduction. Good relaxation is necessary and is best achieved by general anesthesia. In the majority of posterior dislocations, the distal fragment is displaced posteriorly and medially with medial rotation. In this type of fracture, traction is applied to the forearm and wrist, with the elbow in extension and the forearm supinated. Medial displacement is corrected first, and then posterior displacement is corrected by pushing the distal fragment of the humerus anteriorly. The intact soft tissue hinge is medial. Thus the elbow is flexed and the forearm is pronated to achieve the position of stability. When displacement is posterior and lateral with lateral rotation, the same steps are taken, except lateral displacement is corrected first with the forearm pronated; after correcting posterior displacement, the elbow is flexed and supinated to achieve the position of stability. A posterior plaster splint is applied with no pressure in the antecubital fossa for 4 to 5 weeks. Thereafter, a sling is used for 7 to 10 days, and gentle progressive active range of motion exercises are begun. Passive exercises are never used in the elbow because they can lead to myositis ossificans and stiffness.

Skeletal traction with a percutaneous olecranon pin or eye hook in the proximal olecranon or percutaneous pinning is appropriate when swelling is so marked that the elbow cannot be flexed more than 90° without endangering the circulation or when reduction is difficult and unstable. Care must be taken to avoid the ulnar nerve and olecranon epiphysis with the pins. In cases in which the distal fragment is displaced posteriorly and medially, overhead traction is used with the forearm in pronation. In instances when the distal fragment is displaced posteriorly and laterally, side arm lateral traction is used and the forearm is supinated.

Lateral angulation cannot be accepted because it leads to cubitus varus, a loss of normal carrying angle, and a "gunstock deformity." Similarly, medial angulation can lead to cubitus valgus. In addition to anteroposterior and true lateral views, oblique postreduction films should be taken for better assessment of medial and lateral angulation. If there is any gap or opening on oblique views, medial or lateral angulation has not been corrected adequately.

Percutaneous pinning is preferred in flexion type supracondylar fractures with anterior displacement of the distal fragment and in supracondylar fractures with associated displaced forearm fractures. When there is an associated displaced forearm fracture, the supracondylar fracture is reduced and pinned first and then the forearm fracture is reduced; the elbow now can be flexed to 90° and a cast for the forearm fracture is applied.

Open reduction followed by internal fixation with Kirschner wires is indicated when the fracture cannot be reduced satisfactorily by closed methods, when the brachial artery has been lacerated or caught between the fragments, when there are signs of impending Volkmann's contracture, as an alternative to skeletal traction when swelling is so marked that the elbow cannot be flexed more than 90° without endangering the circulation, or when reduction is difficult and unstable.

FRACTURES OF THE LATERAL CONDYLE IN CHILDREN

Fractures of the lateral condyle result from a fall on the outstretched arm with a varus force, generally in children in the 4- to 10-year age range. This usually results in a Salter-Harris type IV epiphyseal fracture. Undisplaced fractures are treated in a posterior splint with the elbow joint flexed 90°, the forearm in a neutral position, and the wrist in extension. Even the slightest displacement demands early open reduction and internal fixation, with pins fixing the lateral condyle to the remaining distal humerus for 6 weeks. A long arm posterior plaster splint is also used for 6 weeks. On removal of the pins and discontinuation of the splint, the arm may be placed in a sling for 7 to 10 days while gentle progressive active range of motion exercises are initiated. In cases of malunion or nonunion, a loss of growth in the lateral portion of the epiphysis may result in a cubitus valgus and in gradual increase in the carrying angle. A tardy ulnar nerve palsy may be a late complication. Growth disturbance is the rule when there is 3 or 4 weeks or more of delay between the time of displaced fracture and open reduction and internal fixation.

FRACTURES OF THE MEDIAL EPICONDYLE IN CHILDREN

Avulsion of the medial epicondyle may occur from valgus forces acting on the forearm or from sudden violent contracture of the pronator and flexor muscles and is frequently associated with a dislocation of the elbow. The medial epicondyle is a traction epiphysis that does not contribute to the longitudinal growth of the humerus and is not a part of the articular surface. Therefore, deformity as a result of growth disturbance does not occur and anatomical reduction is not as important as in fractures of the humeral condyles. Most fractures of the medial epicondyle are displaced less than 1 cm and are best treated with immobilization in a posterior plaster splint with the elbow flexed to 90° for a period of 2 weeks. A valgus stress roentgenogram with the elbow flexed 30° determines stability. Open reduction and internal fixation with sutures or transfixing pins or screws is performed when displacement is greater than 1 cm, when there is valgus instability on the stress roentgenogram, when the epicondyle is caught within the joint after dislocation of the elbow, and in cases of ulnar nerve palsy. When the epicondyle is caught within the elbow joint, severe joint damage will occur if it is not removed. The fragment may be either excised or replaced. When late ulnar nerve palsy results from callus formation or scar contracture, anterior transposition of the ulnar nerve should be performed.

DISLOCATIONS OF THE ELBOW

Dislocations of the elbow occur in both children and adults. Associated fractures frequently accompany elbow dislocations and should be suspected. The most commonly associated lesions are fractures of the medial epicondyle, the radial head, and the coronoid process. In most elbow dislocations, the forearm bones are displaced posteriorly to the humerus with some element of either medial or lateral displacement. The mechanism of injury is a fall on the outstretched arm with the elbow extended. On physical examination, the normal triangular relationship between the bony prominences of the medial and lateral epicondyles and the olecranon is lost. The olecranon and radial head can be palpated posteriorly to the distal humerus, the triceps tendon is more prominent than normal, and the distal humerus can be palpated in the antecubital fossa. Reduction is achieved by the application of downward pressure by the surgeon on the forearm just below the elbow with one hand while applying distal traction with the other. An assistant applies countertraction to the anterior surface of the lower arm. The coronoid process is brought beneath the trochlea, and the forearm is then flexed to 110°. A plaster splint is applied for 3 weeks. Thereafter, a sling is worn for 2 to 3 weeks, and gentle progressive active range of motion exercises are initiated. Treatment of associated fractures of the medial epicondyle and of the radial head is the same as when they occur as isolated fractures. If a fracture of the coronoid process is small, it may be disregarded; however, if it is large and there is instability following reduction, open reduction and internal fixation are necessary.

MONTEGGIA'S FRACTURE-DISLOCATIONS

Monteggia's fracture-dislocations are fractures of the ulna with radial head dislocation. There are probably several mechanisms of injury, including a direct blow to the ulnar aspect of the forearm or a fall with hyperpronation or hyperextension with the strong supinating force of the biceps pulling the radial head anteriorly as the fracture of the ulna is produced by the compression forces of the fall. This lesion is generally best treated by closed manipulation in children but routinely requires open reduction in the adult. The ulna is best rigidly, internally fixed by a compression plate. Closed manipulation is then performed on the radial head. Open reduction of the radial head and repair or reconstruction of the annular ligament is reserved for those instances when satisfactory reduction cannot be achieved by closed manipulation due to interposition of the annular ligament or capsule. The elbow is immobilized for 6 weeks in a position of flexion greater than 90° with the forearm supinated. In injuries in which the radial head dislocation has not been reduced for 6 weeks or more and in cases in which insufficient fixation of the fractured ulna has allowed angulation of this fracture and redislocation of the radial head, the radial head is excised. Many of these fractures are complicated by one or more of the following problems: limitation of elbow motion or forearm rotation, synostosis of the radius and ulna, and nonunions of the ulna. Wrist injuries are common with Monteggia's fracture-dislocations, and it is particularly important to obtain a roentgenogram of the joint below the fracture.

FRACTURES OF THE OLECRANON

Fractures of the olecranon are caused by direct trauma and by avulsion due to violent forceful contraction of the triceps. There is swelling and tenderness about the point of the elbow, and in displaced fractures a defect can be palpated where the olecranon is separated from the remainder of the ulna. In complete and displaced fractures, active extension is impossible. Fractures of the olecranon are uncommon in children and are rarely displaced. Fractures are classified as avulsion fractures, transverse or oblique fractures, fracture-dislocation (Monteggia group), and comminuted fractures. If the fracture is undisplaced and the triceps insertion is intact, active extension, although painful, is possible. Undisplaced fractures are treated in a posterior splint for 3 to 4 weeks. The patient is then converted to a sling, and gentle active range of motion exercises are started with no effort to reach full flexion for several weeks. Displaced fractures are treated by open reduction and internal fixation using two intramedullary Kirschner wires and a figure-of-eight tension band wire or by excision. When the tension band wiring technique is used, early active range of motion exercises are initiated both to regain motion and to create compression across the fracture line. Reduction of the fracture must be exact and the olecranon sulcus preserved, or limited motion, delayed recovery, and posttraumatic arthritis may result. Excision of the proximal fragment provides equally good results. Excision should not be carried past the coronoid process since this would not leave a stable base for the trochlea and elbow instability could occur. The olecranon may also be excised in an effort to regain motion in a healed comminuted olecranon fracture with narrowing of the olecranon sulcus and limited elbow motion.

FRACTURES OF THE RADIAL HEAD AND NECK

Fractures of the radial head and neck are the result of a fall on the outstretched hand with the radial head being driven against the capitellum. On physical examination there is distention of the elbow joint capsule laterally, tenderness over the radial head, and limitation of elbow joint motion and forearm rotation. These fractures are undisplaced, marginal, comminuted, or associated with dislocation of the elbow (Fig. 44-14, *A*). Undisplaced fractures are usually stable and are treated by aspiration of the elbow joint and use of a posterior plaster splint for 10 to 14 days. Active range of motion exercises are then initiated, and the patient is provided with a sling until the elbow is asymptomatic without it. Displaced marginal fractures of one third of the

joint surface or more are treated by open reduction and internal fixation with one or more small fragment lag screws. Care then proceeds much the same as that for undisplaced fractures. In displaced marginal fractures involving less than one third of the joint surface, the radiohumeral joint is aspirated and injected with a local anesthetic. If 70° of active pronation and 70° of active supination can be achieved, these lesions are treated like undisplaced fractures. If not, either early open reduction and internal fixation or excision of the radial head may be performed. In comminuted fractures of the radial head, early excision of the radial head is performed (Fig. 44-14, *B*). The radial head should be reconstructed on a towel as the pieces are removed to ensure removal of the entire head and all of its constituent pieces; no piece must be inadvertently left free in the joint (Fig. 44-14, *C*). Fractures with loose fragments in the joint should be operated on early, the fragments removed, and the fracture treated according to the above precepts. Usually, this will involve radial head excision. If radial head excision is delayed when indicated, arthritic changes and limitation of motion may result. When comminuted fracture of the radial head exists in concert with dislocation of the elbow and fracture of the coronoid process of the ulna, excision of the radial head should be delayed 3 to 6 months until the coronoid fracture and soft tissue have healed. Otherwise, early excision of the radial head will result in extreme elbow instability and redislocation.

Fractures through the articular surface of the radial head are rare in children; the usual site is through the physis with a metaphyseal fragment, a Salter-Harris type II epiphyseal fracture. Injuries that are commonly associated with fractures of the proximal end of the radius are medial epicondylar fracture, rupture of the medial collateral ligament, and olecranon fractures. Open reduction is necessary only for completely displaced fractures and for the rare fracture that cannot be reduced to an acceptable angulation of 45° or less. Internal fixation may be used for completely displaced fractures and should consist of oblique Kirschner wires inserted from the lateral side of the radial head and

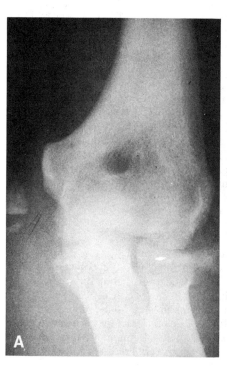

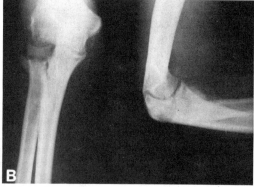

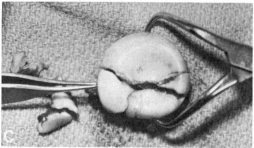

Fig. 44-14. Comminuted fracture of the radial head with an associated posterior elbow dislocation. (*A*) The elbow dislocation has been reduced. One fragment of radial head remains on the medial side of the elbow, and there is a second major fragment of bone on the lateral side of the elbow adjacent to the proximal radius. (*B*) The radial head is excised and replaced by a Swanson Silastic spacer. (*C*) The radial head is reconstructed on a towel to ensure that all of the fragments have been recovered.

not crossing the radiocapitellar joint. The prognosis is worse in older children. Decreased capacity for remodeling may explain this, and there may be enough residual angulation of the neck of the radius to interfere with forearm rotation. Removal of the head of the radius is contraindicated in a child and may result in cubitus valgus and functional disturbance at both the wrist and the elbow. Avascular necrosis of the radial head often occurs in completely displaced fractures after open reduction and may be associated with a poor result. Growth arrest of the proximal radial epiphysis can occur.

FRACTURES OF THE SHAFT OF THE RADIUS AND ULNA IN ADULTS

Fractures of the radius and ulna occur from direct trauma or indirectly, such as from a fall on the outstretched hand. These fractures are usually complete and displaced with overriding, angulation, and rotation. If good results are to be achieved and good function preserved, reduction must be anatomical, restoring length, axial alignment, rotational alignment, and the radial bow. This is best achieved by using dynamic compression plating. The ulna is plated on its medial border. The distal two thirds of the radius are either plated volarly or on its lateral side. The proximal one third of the radius may be plated using a lateral approach by dividing the seam between the extensor carpi radialis brevis and the extensor digitorum communis. If this approach is used, the posterior interosseous branch of the radial nerve must be identified and protected. Some surgeons prefer not to use this approach because of concern for injuring the posterior interosseous nerve when reentering a scarred area if they should ever have to remove the plate. An alternative is to use a volar approach for fractures of the proximal one third of the radius. In using this approach, the radial fracture must be plated with the forearm in full pronation or pronation can be blocked by the plate. Usually plates placed in the forearm are not removed because of the high incidence of refracture through the screw holes. When more than one third of the circumference of either the radius or ulna is comminuted, autogenous cancellous bone graft is added. Bone grafts should not be placed on the interosseous border of the bone to avoid synostosis and limitation of rotation. With good fixation, early active range of motion exercises of the elbow, forearm, and wrist can be instituted and will contribute toward a good result.

FRACTURES OF THE SHAFT OF THE RADIUS AND ULNA IN CHILDREN

Fractures of the shaft of the radius and ulna in children may be of the greenstick type or may be complete and displaced. Greenstick fractures should be completed or the fracture will reangulate. Care is taken not to displace greenstick fractures. They are then treated in a long arm plaster cast with a well-molded interosseous space. Complete and displaced fractures are difficult to reduce. If the patient is under the age of 10, closed reduction is carried out whenever possible. If the fracture cannot be anatomically reduced, bayonet apposition with slight shortening can be accepted, provided axial and rotational alignment is achieved. A long arm plaster cast with three-point pressure and well-molded interosseous space is then applied. The rotational position of the forearm is dictated by the level of the radial fracture. The biceps and the supinator muscles exert supi-

nation forces on the proximal one third of the radius. Fractures proximal to the insertion of the pronator teres are held in a position of full supination. The pronator teres inserting onto the midshaft and the pronator quadratus inserting onto the distal fourth of the radius exert pronation and ulnar angulary forces on the distal two thirds of the radius. Fractures at the mid third of the radius are held in slight supination or in neutral rotation, while fractures of the distal one third of the radius are held in slight to full pronation. A loop wire is incorporated into the cast proximal to the level of the fracture, and the cast is suspended from a sling through this loop. Placing the pull of the sling proximal to the fracture prevents ulnar angulation. Six to 8 weeks of immobilization are required. In children 10 years of age and older, compression plating is permissible when satisfactory reduction cannot be achieved by closed means.

FRACTURES OF THE DISTAL RADIAL SHAFT

Fractures of the distal third of the radius are usually shortened, ulnarly angulated, pronated, and often associated with a derangement of the distal radioulnar joint. This fracture is called a "fracture of necessity" in adults, indicating that an open reduction and internal fixation with a dynamic compression plate is necessary to obtain a good result. In contrast, in children this fracture is best treated by closed methods.

FRACTURES OF THE ULNAR SHAFT

Fractures of the shaft of the ulna are often the result of direct blunt trauma. One must look for Monteggia fracture-dislocations, which were discussed previously. Open reduction and internal fixation of associated ulnar shaft fractures are performed using a dynamic compression plate and the principles outlined in the treatment of fractures of both bones of the forearm. Nonunion of the ulna is common when treated by closed methods even when the fracture is not comminuted or displaced.

FRACTURES AND DISLOCATIONS ABOUT THE WRIST

FRACTURES OF THE DISTAL RADIUS

In undisplaced fractures of the distal radius, immobilization in a short arm plaster cast for from 4 to 6 weeks is sufficient to allow healing. Early motion of the digits, elbow, and shoulder is encouraged.

Colles' Fracture

Colles' fracture results from a force on the outstretched hand with the wrist in extension. In a Colles' fracture of the distal radius, the principal fracture line runs transversely, 1 cm to 2 cm proximal to the articular surface of the distal radius. There is volar angulation and dorsal displacement of the distal fracture fragment, producing a "silver fork deformity." Comminution into the radiocarpal joint, the radioulnar joint, or both may occur. Most Colles' fractures can be reduced by distraction and closed manipulation. The reduction is held by a short arm plaster cast or plaster sugar-tong splint with three-point pressure for 6 weeks. Unstable Colles' fractures may be recognized by the presence of severe comminution, severe dorsal angulation, or extensive intra-articular involvement and may have a propensity for short-ening, loss of reduction, or both. If adequate reduction cannot be achieved or maintained by closed methods, operative intervention is indicated, usually employing external fixation. Early digital, elbow, and shoulder motion is encouraged. The external fixator is discontinued after 10 weeks. Consideration should be given to inserting a cancellous bone graft for any dorsal bone defect.

Dorsal Barton's fractures involve the dorsal articular margin of the distal radius and are associated with subluxation or dislocation of the carpus dorsally. These fractures are characteristically unstable and are best treated by open reduction and internal fixation with Kirschner wires or with a small T-buttress plate.

Smith's Fracture

Smith's fractures of the distal radius have dorsal angulation and volar displacement. They are treated by closed manipulation. Open reduction and internal fixation is indicated if reduction in extension fails. A type II Smith fracture is the same as a volar Barton fracture and has a fracture of the volar articular margin of the radius with volar subluxation or dislocation of the carpus. These fractures are inherently unstable because of the obliquity of the fracture and are best treated by open reduction and internal fixation by a small T-buttress plate.

FRACTURES OF THE SCAPHOID

Fractures of the scaphoid are usually seen in young adult males as a result of a fall on the outstretched hand with the wrist dorsiflexed 90° or more at the time of maximum impact. Either the radial styloid or the capitellum can act as a fulcrum to fracture the scaphoid. On physical examination, there is swelling about the wrist and tenderness in the anatomical snuff box. Fractures of the scaphoid may be difficult to demonstrate on ordinary anteroposterior and lateral roentgenograms due to overlapping shadows cast by the other bones about the wrist. Additional oblique views, air gap magnification technique, and trispiral tomography are helpful in diagnosing these fractures when they are undisplaced. If a patient presents with the typical clinical findings of a fractured scaphoid and no fracture is visualized on the roentgenogram, it is prudent to treat the patient as though he has an undisplaced scaphoid fracture for 3 weeks and then repeat the roentgenographic studies. Most fractures of the scaphoid are undisplaced and will unite in 3 to 6 months of treatment in a short arm plaster cast with a thumb gauntlet. The more proximal the fracture of the scaphoid, the higher is the incidence of the complication of avascular necrosis of the proximal fragment. This is a result of interruption of the blood supply to the proximal fragment when that blood supply enters the scaphoid in its distal half on the dorsolateral surface. Union is delayed and in some instances does not occur in cases of scaphoid fracture with avascular necrosis of the proximal fragment. Delay in diagnosis and treatment is another frequent cause of delayed union or nonunion. Displaced scaphoid fractures should alert the examiner to the possibility of an associated perilunate or lunate dislocation. If displaced scaphoid fractures can be reduced and mainstayed by closed methods, they may be treated as undisplaced scaphoid fractures. If reduction cannot be achieved by closed methods or if reduction is not stable, then open reduction and internal fixation with a small cancellous bone screw, a scaphoid staple, or Kirschner wires should be done.

DISLOCATION OF THE CARPAL BONES

Perilunar Dislocations

Perilunar dislocations are the result of the combined forces of hyperextension, ulnar deviation and pronation at the wrist. All of the volar ligaments connecting the carpal bones to the lunate are ruptured. While the lunate remains in its normal position, the remainder of the carpus dislocates dorsally around the lunate (Fig. 44-15, *A*). In this injury, either rotatory subluxation or fracture of the scaphoid must occur. In instances of transscaphoid-perilunar fracture-dislocation, the proximal portion of the scaphoid remains in normal relationship to the distal radius and lunate, while the distal portion of the scaphoid and the remainder of the carpus dislocate dorsally.

Fig. 44-15. Carpal dislocations. (*A*) Perilunate dislocation. (*B*) Stabilization of a carpal dislocation in the anatomic position with Kirschner wires.

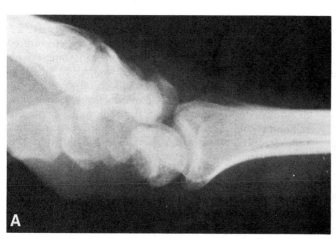

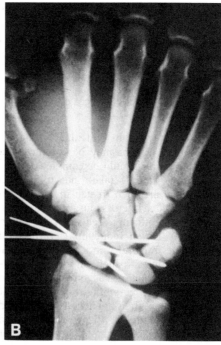

Closed reduction of perilunar dislocations should be attempted with the patient under general anesthesia. If a perfect reduction is achieved in perilunar dislocations, it should be stabilized by percutaneous Kirschner wire fixation from the scaphoid to the capitate and from the scaphoid to the lunate (Fig. 44-15, *B*). When a perfect reduction of a perilunar dislocation cannot be achieved by closed methods, open reduction, ligament repairs, and internal fixation with Kirschner wires are indicated. Primary ligamentous reconstruction is indicated in instances in which ligament repair cannot be accomplished. The wrist is then held in neutral position for 8 weeks in a short arm plaster cast. The Kirschner wires are then removed, and the wrist is protected in a short arm volar splint for 4 more weeks while active range of motion exercises are initiated. In cases of transscaphoid-perilunar fracture dislocation, if a perfect reduction is achieved, the wrist is held in 30° of flexion and a short arm plaster cast with a thumb gauntlet is applied. Immobilization is maintained until the scaphoid fracture is radiographically united. In most cases of transscaphoid-perilunar fracture-dislocations, it is impossible to obtain a good closed reduction of the fracture of the two scaphoid fragments and, in these cases, open reduction and internal fixation of the scaphoid fracture should be performed with a small cancellous bone screw, a scaphoid staple, or Kirschner wires.

Lunate Dislocations

In lunate dislocations the mechanism of injury, the ligamentous injuries, and the injuries to the scaphoid are the same as in a perilunar dislocation. One additional injury occurs—rupture of the dorsal radiolunate ligament. The volar radiolunate ligament remains intact, and the lunate pivots 60° to 90° anteriorly about this intact ligament, through the space between this ligament and the volar radiocapitate ligament into the carpal tunnel (Fig. 44-16). There may be signs of median nerve compression. To avoid further injury to the median nerve and in order to repair the rent between the volar radiolunate and radiocapitate ligaments, open reduction of the lunate is carried out through a volar approach. If the reduction is perfect, percutaneous Kirschner wires are applied between the scaphoid and capitate and between the scaphoid and lunate. Further care is then the same as for perilunar dislocation. If the reduction is not satisfactory, a dorsal wrist incision is used to assist in aligning the carpal bones and in either repairing or primarily

Fig. 44-16. Lunate dislocation.

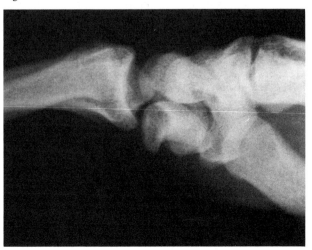

reconstructing the ligaments. Again, the reduction is transfixed with Kirschner wires as above and further care is the same as for perilunar dislocations.

FRACTURES AND DISLOCATIONS OF THE SPINE

CERVICAL FRACTURES AND DISLOCATIONS

Fractures and dislocations of the cervical spine most commonly result from automobile or motorcycle accidents, diving accidents, and gunshot wounds. Fracture, dislocation, or a combination of the two should be suspected in patients complaining of neck pain after injury. Cervical spine roentgenograms should be obtained in an unconscious patient or a patient with a significant injury above the clavicles.

Fractures of the cervical spine are notoriously difficult to diagnose. Overlapping bony processes make roentgenograms difficult to interpret. Good quality roentgenograms, including anteroposterior, lateral, oblique, and odontoid views, are mandatory. The lower cervical spine, including the seventh cervical vertebra, must be visualized. This is where many diagnoses are missed because of lack of adequate visualization. If this cannot be done by pulling the shoulders down, a swimmer's view may be helpful. If conventional or swimmer's views do not adequately visualize the spine, tomograms must be done, and if the results of all these views are negative, flexion and extension films should be made, with the physician wearing lead gloves and apron and holding the patient's head himself to be sure that there is no ligamentous instability of the cervical spine. Unstable fractures and dislocations have a much higher incidence of spinal cord injury than those that are stable.

Compression fractures are the most common cervical spine fractures and result from flexion injuries of the neck. Compression fractures of the vertebral body without dislocation of the posterior facets or the intervertebral disk joints and without comminution of the body usually have no neurologic deficit, are stable, and heal without problem with treatment in a cervical spine brace for 10 to 12 weeks. Spinous process avulsion fractures, fractures of the lateral mass, and most fractures from low velocity gunshot wounds are stable.

Teardrop fractures of the cervical spine are unstable and may cause cord damage from retropulsed fragments of the vertebral body into the spinal canal as may burst fractures of the vertebral body. In instances of cord injury, these fractures are decompressed from an anterior approach and an anterior interbody fusion is performed for stability. In teardrop fractures without cord injury, a posterior arthrodesis and wiring is performed to prevent the frequent complication of late instability and collapse about this fracture.

Unilateral and bilateral facet dislocations are unstable and must be reduced either by traction and manipulation or by open reduction. Healing of ligaments cannot be relied on to provide adequate stability after reduction, and so posterior wiring and arthrodesis must be performed on these injuries.

Fractures of the odontoid above its junction with the second cervical vertebral body may be treated supportively with a cervical brace and symptomatic treatment. Fractures of the odontoid at its junction with the second cervical vertebral body should be treated with arthrodesis and posterior wiring of C1 to C2 because of the high incidence of nonunion and later instability. Odontoid fractures extending into the second cervical vertebral body are treated in a halo jacket until union occurs. Burst fractures of the ring of C1 are treated in a halo jacket until they are united.

THORACOLUMBAR FRACTURES AND DISLOCATIONS

Anterior wedge, lateral wedge, and compression fractures of the dorsal and lumbar spine are common and are caused by flexion, axial compression, or both. These are usually stable, provided there is no disruption of the posterior ligaments or arch. An anterior wedge fracture of less than 50% of the vertebral body height may be treated first by bed rest and then by mobilization of the patient within the patient's pain tolerance. Range of motion exercises of the lower extremity should be started early, and hyperextension exercises of the back are initiated. A body jacket or hyperextension brace is applied, and sitting, tilt-table exercises, use of the parallel bars, and ambulation are undertaken in keeping with the patient's tolerance. If the anterior wedge fracture is greater than 50% of the vertebral body height, posterior arthrodesis is performed to prevent further late progressive painful gibbus and the development of late spasticity from such a gibbus.

Compression fractures are stable and are treated much the same as anterior wedge fractures, but if they are so severe that a burst effect occurs, the posterior portion of the vertebral body may retropulse into the spinal canal and cause cord injury. If this occurs, anterior decompression and arthrodesis are undertaken.

It is common to see more than one compression fracture, particularly in older individuals. Cases with generalized osteopenia should be evaluated for cause, particularly in instances of spontaneous fractures and of a single intervertebral body collapse. Metastatic tumor and plasma cell myeloma should be considered in these patients.

Transverse process fractures are seen in the lumbar spine and are the result of a direct blow or avulsion force from the muscle attached to them. These fractures are treated supportively and symptomatically.

All other spinal injuries are considered unstable until proved otherwise. It is most unusual to see an unstable fracture of the dorsal spine because of the attachments of the thoracic cage. Unstable injuries and dislocations of the lumbar spine may be purely ligamentous, primarily osseous, or a combination of the two. Spontaneous reduction of an unstable injury may occur in either the supine or the prone position and a careful roentgenographic examination is essential. Any degree of malalignment, however small, in either the anteroposterior or the lateral view should make the physician suspect instability. A majority of vertebral body fractures and spinal cord injuries occur at the thoracolumbar junction, and dangerous patterns such as the slice fracture and seat-belt type injuries should be identified. Comminution or displacement of the posterior cortex of the vertebral body, transverse translation displacement, and disruption of the posterior neural arch are all radiographic signs of spinal instability, as are combined injuries of the anterior and posterior columns. All dislocations and fracture-dislocations of the thoracolumbar spine are unstable. Tomograms and flexion-extension views are helpful in determining stability. All unstable fractures of the thoracolumbar spine should be reduced, stabilized by Harrington rods two levels above and below the level of instability, and arthrodesed.

PELVIC FRACTURES AND DISLOCATIONS

Pelvic fractures without a break in the pelvic ring include avulsion fractures of the anterior-superior iliac spine, the anterior-inferior iliac spine, and the ischial tuberosity; undisplaced fractures of one or both pubic rami on the same side of the pelvis; fractures of the iliac wing; fractures of the sacrum; and fractures of the coccyx. These fractures are usually treated symptomatically. Range of motion and muscle strengthening exercises are initiated early in the lower extremities and progressed according to the patient's pain tolerance. Ambulation is started early and a walker or crutches may be used until the patient is comfortable and strong enough to walk without them.

Dangerous fractures of the pelvis include those with double breaks in the pelvic ring. The anterior lesion may be through the symphysis pubis or through the pubic rami, while the posterior lesion may be through the sacrum; through the sacroiliac joint, usually with a marginal fracture of the ilium; or through the ilium itself. These fractures or fracture-dislocations have an increase in morbidity and mortality commensurate with their degree of disruption. Complications include hemorrhage, genitourinary tract injuries, injuries to the lumbosacral plexus, ileus, fat embolism syndrome, and thromboembolic disease.

Hemorrhagic shock and resultant renal failure are the most serious complications of pelvic fractures and are responsible for at least half of the deaths attributed to this injury. Approximately 40% of all patients with pelvic fractures require blood transfusions. While the average blood loss in a pelvic fracture is 3 units, the surgeon should be prepared to transfuse as much as 15 units or more of whole blood in patients with more severe injuries.

Early reduction and stabilization are important in treating hemorrhage from pelvic fractures, but the critical therapeutic measure for treatment of the blood loss is transfusion in quantities sufficient to correct the estimated loss. Ordinarily, tamponade controls the bleeding. External counterpressure suits have been useful as adjuncts in controlling bleeding from pelvic fractures. Laparotomy is dangerous by virtue of disrupting the tamponade effect and risking infection, is usually unsuccessful, and is an absolute last resort.

Hemorrhage and shock uncontrolled by massive transfusion and external pressure suits may indicate major arterial or venous injury. In such instances venography and arteriography are performed to identify the site of injury. Major arterial injuries are treated with the standard precepts of surgical repair or reconstruction. More often, the injury is located in the obturator or internal pudendal arteries or their branches and can be controlled by embolization of autologous clot or insertion of Gelfoam into the injured artery through a selectively placed angiographic catheter.

Approximately 13% of all patients with pelvic fractures have a major urinary tract complication. All patients with a double break in the pelvic ring must be considered to have a urinary tract injury until proved otherwise and therefore must undergo cystography. Although patients with displaced pelvic fractures have a higher incidence of urinary tract injury, these injuries can occur in instances of undisplaced fractures of the pelvis, such as in the case of rupture of a distended bladder by sudden compression. Bladder rupture occurs in about 4% of pelvic fractures and may be extraperitoneal or intraperitoneal.

Rupture of the urethra associated with fractures of the

pelvis is virtually limited to the male and is extraperitoneal. Rupture of the anterior urethra may be seen with straddle fractures and is accompanied by contusion and ecchymosis of the perineum and penis as well as by extrapelvic extravasation of urine. Rupture of the posterior urethra is usually in the membranous rather than the prostatic portion and is the most common lower urinary tract injury seen with pelvic fractures in the male. This injury is most commonly seen in pelvic crushes with severe anteroposterior pelvic displacement. The patient is unable to void despite the desire to do so. Bleeding at the external urethral meatus is commonly seen but is not pathognomonic. Usually, a catheter cannot be passed into the bladder. Rectal examination discloses cephalad retraction of the prostate from its normal position and is pathognomonic. The urethrogram confirms the diagnosis of urethral tears. Since both the cystogram and the urethrogram may show extraperitoneal extravasation of dye, the cystogram is done before the urethrogram in males except in straddle fractures and when it is impossible to pass a catheter into the bladder. Cystostomy should be performed in virtually all instances in which urinary extravasation is present.

Following evaluation of the lower urinary tract, intravenous pyelography should be done in patients with gross hematuria or microscopic hematuria in the amount of 10 or more red blood cells per high-powered field to evaluate the kidneys and upper urinary tract. Results of the intravenous pyelogram will prove unsuccessful if the patient is in shock, and they may be delayed until systolic blood pressure is restored to at least 100 torr; if necessary, pyelography may be done intraoperatively.

On physical examination, extremity shortening may be present owing to superior displacement of a hemipelvis. Internal or external rotation of the leg may result from internal or external rotation of the disrupted hemipelvis. There may be ecchymosis and swelling about the pelvis or in the perineal region. The pelvis may exhibit instability to manual compression of the iliac crests.

The pelvis should be investigated roentgenographically in patients with multiple trauma because of the frequency and severity of this injury in the multiply injured patient. The basic roentgenogram for evaluation of the pelvis is an anteroposterior view. Inlet and outlet anteroposterior views taken 45° to either side of a perpendicular axis to the pelvis complete the evaluation.

One type of pelvic fracture with a double break in the pelvic ring is the straddle or butterfly fracture. In this fracture, both pubic rami are disrupted on one side and either the symphysis pubis or both pubic rami on the other side are disrupted. Patients with these fractures have a high incidence of severe hemorrhage and of lower urinary tract injury. The mechanism is either anteroposterior or lateral compression. These fractures are treated symptomatically since they do not involve the main weight-bearing arch of the pelvis.

Displaced fractures of the hemipelvis are treated by closed manipulation, and the reduction is stabilized by external fixators (Fig. 44-17). This enhances skin care, toilet, and care of associated injuries. Pulmonary function is improved since fracture stability is sufficient to allow early use of the tilt table, early sitting in a chair, and early ambulation.

FRACTURES OF THE ACETABULUM

Fractures of the acetabulum may be defined by their anatomical location, by any displacement of the fracture fragments, and by subluxation or dislocation of the femoral head when it occurs. The anatomical location has been variously defined. One classification divides the anatomical sites of the fracture into inner wall, superior weight-bearing dome, and posterior acetabular fractures. This parallels the divisions of the acetabulum in the skeletally immature patient by the triradiate cartilage. Acetabular fractures have also been classified as anterior lip, anterior or iliopubic column, posterior or ilioischial column, posterior lip, transverse, or combinations of the above. Knowledge of the extent and precise anatomical location of the fracture is

Fig. 44-17. Treatment of Malgaigne type fractures of the hemipelvis. (*A*) Unstable fracture of the left hemipelvis with downward displacement and external rotational displacement. (*B*) Closed manipulation is performed, and the reduction is stabilized with an external fixator.

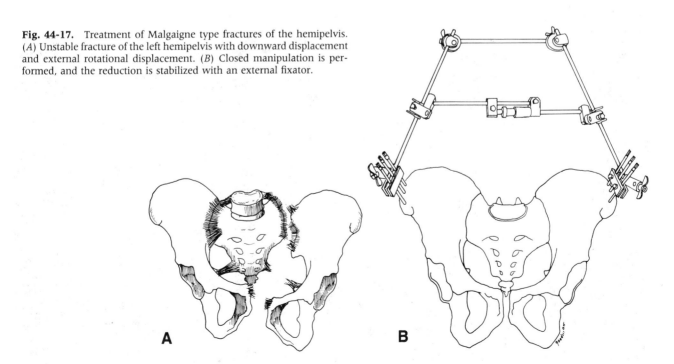

A　　　　**B**

essential in planning treatment, particularly when operative intervention is necessary. Anterior lip and column fractures should be approached by an anterior iliofemoral approach; posterior lip and column fractures should be approached posteriorly; and transverse fractures may be approached by an anterior, a posterior, or a combined approach.

The basic roentgenograms are an anteroposterior view of the pelvis and a lateral view of the involved hip. Oblique views of the acetabulum are helpful. Tomograms, computed axial tomography, or both are extremely useful in cataloging the extent and site of the fracture as well as in identifying any intra-articular fragments.

Intra-articular fragments demand operative intervention and removal. Just as in other intra-articular fractures, displacement of the fragments justifies open reduction, provided the fragments are large enough to hold fixation. In cases of displacement with severe comminution, continuous skeletal traction may be the only alternative. In all methods of treatment it is important to reestablish joint continuity and congruity as much as possible.

Undisplaced acetabular fractures without intra-articular fragments can be treated by Buck's traction and early range of motion exercises for 3 to 4 weeks, followed by crutch walking with no weight-bearing on the involved extremity until 12 weeks following injury. Gradual progressive weight-bearing is then instituted. Good results may generally be expected.

Displaced acetabular fractures without intra-articular fragments in which the femoral head maintains a normal relationship with the superior weight-bearing dome with the joint space preserved and in which the superior weight-bearing dome is intact are treated with either open reduction and internal fixation or with continuous skeletal traction along with range of motion exercises for 3 to 4 weeks. The involved extremity is protected by the use of crutches until 12 weeks post injury. Progressive weight-bearing is then instituted in accordance with the patient's strength, range of motion, pain tolerance, ability to walk without a limp, and radiographic evidence of healing. The key to a good result in acetabular fractures is maintaining a normal congruent relationship between the femoral head and the superior dome of the acetabulum.

CENTRAL DISLOCATION OF THE HIP

Central fracture dislocations of the hip are produced by a force applied through the greater trochanter or by a force in line with the shaft of the femur with the femur in abduction. Serious hemorrhage or injury to the pelvic viscera can occur and is lethal. Bowel incarceration has been reported in the fracture site and can be masked by ileus.

To achieve a good result, it is critical to restore the continuity of the superior weight-bearing dome of the acetabulum and to restore the relationship between the superior weight-bearing dome of the acetabulum and the weight-bearing surface of the femoral head. When the skill of the surgeon is sufficient and the size of the fragments are large enough to hold fixation, this may be done by open reduction and internal fixation. Alternatively, continuous skeletal traction may be applied, particularly in very comminuted fracture-dislocations. Longitudinal traction is applied through the distal femur. If this does not bring the femoral head into a proper relationship with the superior weight-bearing dome of the acetabulum, lateral traction must be applied through an eye-bolt or pins at the level of the lesser trochanter (Fig. 44-18). The combination of longitudinal and lateral traction results in a traction vector parallel to the long axis of the neck of the femur. If skeletal

Fig. 44-18. Central dislocation of the hip. (*A*) Roentgenogram shows central dislocation of the hip with comminution of the inner wall of the acetabulum. (*B*) Reduction of the central dislocation of the hip has been accomplished with skeletal traction through the distal femur and through an eye bolt at the level of the lesser trochanter. (*C*) One year after injury the joint space is well maintained and there is a good congruent relationship between the weight-bearing portion of the femoral head and the superior weight-bearing dome of the acetabulum. The patient has no pain and walks without a limp.

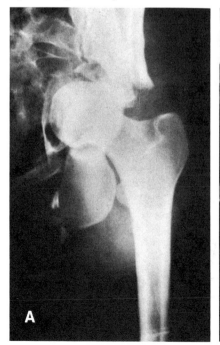
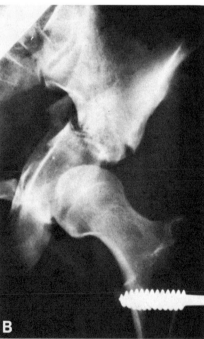
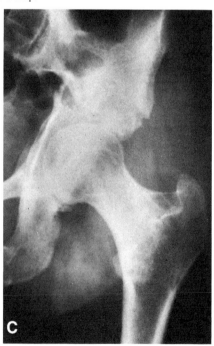

traction does not result in a satisfactory reduction and the patient's condition permits, closed manipulation should be carried out, preferably within 48 hours after injury. If this restores the proper relationship between the superior weight-bearing dome of the acetabulum and the weight-bearing portion of the femoral head, continuous skeletal traction is continued. There is a marked tendency for these fractures to redisplace medially if traction is not continued long enough. Lateral traction may often be discontinued after 4 weeks but longitudinal traction should be continued for 12 weeks or until roentgenograms reveal solid union of fractures of the acetabulum.

If skeletal traction or closed reduction and skeletal traction do not restore the relationship between the femoral head and the superior weight-bearing dome, open reduction and internal fixation should be considered. Primary arthroplasty should be considered when a congruent relationship cannot be restored between the acetabular dome and the femoral head by any means.

Rehabilitation includes isometric exercises while in traction, with active range of motion exercises and strengthening exercises about the ipsilateral knee and ankle. Range of motion exercises and strengthening exercises cannot be instituted about the hip until stability of the fracture dislocation is ensured but should certainly be initiated at that point and increased within the patient's tolerance. No weight should be borne on the injured extremity for at least 12 weeks after injury. Progressive partial weight-bearing with crutches is started only when clinical and radiographic union are certain and is increased to full weight-bearing without crutches in accordance with the patient's tolerance.

The functional results after central fracture dislocation of the hip are often much better than would be expected from the appearance of the roentgenogram. If posttraumatic arthritis is going to be a problem after central fracture dislocation of the acetabulum, it will usually be clinically manifest within a year after injury.

FRACTURES AND DISLOCATIONS OF THE LOWER EXTREMITY

FRACTURES AND DISLOCATIONS OF THE HIP

DISLOCATIONS OF THE HIP

Most hip dislocations are posterior and may be associated with fractures of the posterior acetabular rim, femoral head, femoral neck, or femoral shaft. The mechanism of injury is usually a force in line with the shaft of the femur with the hip in a flexed and often adducted position. Many of these injuries result from motor vehicle accidents when the patient's knee strikes the dashboard, and they often could be prevented by wearing a seat belt.

The position of the hip when dislocated posteriorly is classic and clinically diagnostic. It is fixed in a shortened, flexed, adducted, and internally rotated position. An anteroposterior roentgenogram of the pelvis and a posterior acetabular view of the involved hip should be taken to confirm the posterior dislocation and to determine the presence and extent of a fracture of the posterior acetabular wall and of any intra-articular fracture fragments. Tomograms, computed tomography, or both are extremely helpful in delineating the extent of any associated fracture and in spotting intra-articular fragments.

Sciatic nerve injury occurs in approximately 10% of posterior hip dislocations and fracture-dislocations. Careful neurologic examination should be carried out and recorded at initial examination before and after reduction. When open reduction is employed, the sciatic nerve should be explored and its condition documented. When closed reduction is performed, exploration of the sciatic nerve should be considered 4 weeks after injury if the signs and symptoms of nerve injury fail to improve.

The treatment of a posterior dislocation or fracture-dislocation of the hip is a true orthopaedic emergency. Unreduced dislocation of the hip may contribute to refractory shock. Early reduction relieves pain, prevents additional trauma to the sciatic nerve, may reduce or limit the incidence of ectopic ossification, and prevents avascular necrosis of the femoral head following posterior hip dislocation. Avascular necrosis of the femoral head is directly related to the time elapsed between dislocation and reduction. If the dislocation is reduced within 3 to 4 hours, avascular necrosis of the femoral head seldom occurs. Conversely, if reduction is delayed more than 24 hours, avascular necrosis of the femoral head is the rule. In all posterior hip dislocations, the patient should be followed for a sufficient length of time to be sure that avascular necrosis does not develop or that if it does develop, it is detected. Avascular necrosis of the femoral head following posterior hip dislocation will usually become manifest within 18 months, but sometimes is not apparent for up to 3 years. Patients with posterior hip dislocations should have roentgenograms at 6-month intervals during this period. Patients with hip pain, particularly deep inguinal pain, and normal results of roentgenography should have a bone scan. The bone scan can detect avascular necrosis of the femoral head prior to its radiographic appearance.

General anesthesia and muscle-relaxing agents are ordinarily preferred in reducing hip dislocations to lessen the risk of injury or fracture to the femoral head and neck. The hip is reduced by flexing the hip and knee to 90° and then applying traction while stabilizing the pelvis and gently rotating the hip until it reduces with a definite thump. The hip is then fully extended.

If there is no fracture of the posterior acetabulum or only a chip fracture so minor as to be of no consequence, the hip is usually stable once reduced. To test this, the hip is gently flexed to 90° to make sure redislocation does not occur. Balanced suspension without skeletal traction for 2 weeks is sufficient management, along with early range of motion exercises. Walking supported by crutches is then allowed with progressive partial weight-bearing. Crutches are discontinued when full weight-bearing is achieved 6 to 8 weeks after injury.

If there is a fracture of the posterior acetabulum, instability of the hip may be present and is usually related to the size of the fragment. If the fragment is small and the hip can be flexed to 70° without tendency to redislocate, the patient is treated in balanced suspension with skeletal traction of 10 pounds through a pin in the tibial tubercle for 6 weeks. Early active range of motion exercises are initiated. After 6 weeks, traction is discontinued and crutch walking with progressive partial weight-bearing is started. At 12 weeks after injury, full weight-bearing is allowed and crutches are then discarded.

If the hip redislocates as it is flexed to less than 70° and the posterior acetabular fracture is large, open reduction and internal fixation of this fragment should be done. The patient is then kept in skeletal traction for 6 weeks and nonweight-bearing is allowed for 12 weeks. Range of motion exercises are started early while the patient is in traction. If the patient's condition does not permit surgery or if the posterior acetabulum is so comminuted as to preclude fixation, skeletal traction is continued for at least 12 weeks or until there is radiographic union of the fracture.

Free intra-articular osteochondral fracture fragments demand early operative removal.

In a posterior hip dislocation with fracture of the femoral head, the fracture is usually in the inferior quadrant of the head. If the fracture is undisplaced, this is acceptable. If the osteochondral fracture fragment is displaced, surgery is necessary. If soft tissue is attached to the fragment, it may be restored to the femoral head with pins or screws; it may heal or it may undergo avascular necrosis. If the fragment is free in the joint, it must be removed; if it is a large fragment, this is an indication to consider primary hip arthrodesis or arthroplasty since posttraumatic arthritis is likely. Primary hip arthrodesis or arthroplasty in such instances avoids a second operation and shortens the disability period, and the muscles about the hip will not have undergone atrophy.

When posterior hip dislocation occurs with femoral neck fracture, the femoral head lies as a free fragment posterior to the acetabulum and avascular necrosis is inevitable. Excision of the femoral head and total hip arthroplasty are best advised.

The prognosis of posterior dislocation and fracture-dislocation of the hip in children is better than in adults, and there is a lower incidence of both avascular necrosis of the femoral head and posttraumatic arthritis of the hip.

Anterior dislocation of the hip represents about 10% of hip dislocations. The femoral vessels and nerve may be injured. Anterior dislocations are classified according to the position of the femoral head and are iliac, pubic, obturator, or perineal. In an obturator or perineal dislocation, the hip is usually fixed in flexion, abduction, and external rotation. Most anterior dislocations can be reduced by closed manipulation. If closed manipulation is unsuccessful, an anterior iliofemoral approach is used. If there are osteochondral fragments in the joint, they are treated just as described for posterior hip dislocations. Hip reduction is followed by treatment in balanced suspension without skeletal traction for 2 weeks. The hip is usually stable after reduction, and prolonged immobilization and protection from weight-bearing after anterior hip dislocations is unnecessary. Crutch walking with graduated weight-bearing may be started after the second week.

FRACTURES OF THE HIP

Fractures of the hip may be divided into three large categories: (1) intracapsular fractures of the neck, (2) intertrochanteric fractures, and (3) subtrochanteric fractures. These fractures tend to occur in the sixth decade and beyond and are becoming more common because people are living longer. They are seen more frequently in women than in men. Osteopenia is a common factor. Minor falls are associated with many of these fractures.

The patients have an increased incidence of associated medical illnesses, usually pulmonary, cardiac, or renal, or the potential to develop these illnesses. This accounts for an increased morbidity and mortality among these patients. These patients tolerate bed confinement poorly, usually for cardiopulmonary reasons, and their fractures should be reduced and fixed within 24 to 36 hours after injury. Spending the first 12 to 24 hours in medical evaluation and treatment should decrease anesthetic and operative risks as well as decrease postoperative complications. Waiting longer than 24 to 36 hours after injury to operate usually adds little to the medical management and may significantly increase the mortality rates.

The patient has the usual clinical signs of fracture, and the extremity is often shortened and externally rotated. In an older patient without deformity but with hip pain after a fall, it is a pitfall not to suspect a fracture. An impacted fracture of the femoral neck can occur without deformity and must be searched for carefully.

Intracapsular Fractures of the Femoral Neck

Nonunion and avascular necrosis are the principal complications of femoral neck fractures. Both are due to the precarious retinacular blood supply of the femoral head. Their incidence is influenced by the amount of displacement of the fracture, the occurrence and degree of posterior neck comminution, the time elapsed between injury and reduction and stabilization, and the rigidity of fixation. Bony continuity should be reestablished between the fracture fragments so that the distal fragment assumes the loading forces at the hip joint.

Impacted femoral neck fractures will almost always unite if stabilized with long cancellous screws (*e.g.*, Knowles' or similar pins) and have an incidence of avascular necrosis of the femoral head of only about 10%. If not fixed, about 15% of these fractures will disimpact and displace.

Undisplaced femoral neck fractures are not stable and will displace. They should be impacted anatomically or in slight valgus and rigidly fixed. The sliding hip compression lag screw with a side plate and an ancillary cancellous lag screw to control the rotation of the femoral head provide an excellent method of rigid internal fixation.

Displaced intracapsular fractures of the femoral neck have a nonunion rate as high as 20% to 30% and an incidence of avascular necrosis of about 35%. These fractures should be reduced and impacted anatomically or in slight valgus and then treated as undisplaced fractures as outlined above. Some surgeons recommend a muscle pedicle bone graft for all displaced femoral neck fractures to help stabilize the fracture and to bring in a blood supply.

Functional capacity after a successful closed reduction and internal fixation is usually better than that following a successful endoprosthesis or primary total hip arthroplasty. However, endoprosthetic or primary total hip arthroplasty may be considered for displaced intracapsular femoral neck fractures in cases of failed closed reduction, prolonged delay in reduction, pathologic fractures due to metastatic disease, subcapital fractures that show no vascularity on technetium 99m sulfur colloid scan, femoral neck fractures associated with femoral head dislocation, and femoral neck fractures in patients with Paget's disease or significant hip arthritis. An endoprosthesis should be considered only in an inactive sedentary individual since, otherwise, acetabular wear will lead to hip pain and the early need for revision. Total hip arthroplasty is preferred in active individuals with the above indications as well as for reconstruction of the failed femoral neck fixation and in instances of avascular necrosis that becomes sufficiently symptomatic to require treatment.

Femoral neck fractures in young adults are particularly pernicious, with a combined incidence of nonunion and avascular necrosis of 90% or more. The only chance for success with these fractures is early anatomical reduction with compression and rigid fixation.

Following internal fixation, the patient is sitting in a chair the day following surgery. Range of motion and strengthening exercises are initiated early. The tilt table is used to accustom the patient to a vertical position. Parallel bars are used to initiate ambulation. Ambulation with the assistance of crutches or a walker is started with progressive partial weight-bearing to tolerance. Union generally requires at least 3 months. Full weight-bearing is not allowed until union is solid. A cane is used permanently to improve balance and confidence and to prevent another fall.

Nonoperative treatment in femoral neck fractures may be justified in patients with severe mental illness or retardation, in patients with a bed–chair existence, and in patients with deep pressure sores that prevent a safe surgical incision. These patients should be up in a chair immediately if possible. Their fracture is then untreated while attention is directed to avoiding medical illness.

Intertrochanteric Fractures

Intertrochanteric fractures start in the extracapsular area at the base of the neck of the femur and extend across the intertrochanteric region of the femur to the inferior border of the lesser trochanter. Practically, intertrochanteric fractures are either stable or unstable. Stability is determined by the ability to reestablish cortical bone continuity or medial buttress on the medial side of the fracture. Stable fractures may be reduced anatomically and rigidly fixed with a sliding hip compression lag screw with a side plate. In a patient with an intertrochanteric fracture that is stable in configuration but who is a very poor operative risk, Enders pins may be used for fixation. This decreases the operative time, the blood loss, and the infection rate with some compromise in rigidity of fixation.

Unstable intertrochanteric fractures are converted to stable fractures by osteotomy or by osteotomy and medial displacement of the distal fragment and then are stabilized by a sliding hip compression lag screw with a side plate. Enders pins are not suited for fixation of unstable intertrochanteric fractures.

Nonunion of these fractures and avascular necrosis of the femoral head are rare. Mortality during the first 3 months after fracture is as high as 15%, about twice the morbidity of patients with subcapital fractures.

Rehabilitation is similar to that in patients with femoral neck fractures.

Subtrochanteric Fractures

Subtrochanteric fractures extend from the superior border of the lesser trochanter to a level 4 cm below the inferior border of the lesser trochanter. Fractures that start distal to this region are considered femoral shaft fractures and are treated accordingly. Like intertrochanteric fractures, subtrochanteric fractures are either stable or unstable depending on whether or not medial cortical continuity can be reestablished by anatomical fracture reduction.

Stable subtrochanteric fractures should be rigidly fixed with either an angle blade plate or a Zickle nail. Again, in poor operative risks, Enders pins may be used for stable fractures (Fig. 44-19).

Unstable fractures are reduced as anatomically as possible and rigidly fixed. Autogenous cancellous bone graft is applied to the medial border of the fracture.

These fractures are rehabilitated much like subcapital

and intertrochanteric fractures except that weight-bearing is not allowed until union is ensured.

FRACTURES OF THE FEMORAL SHAFT

Fractures of the femoral shaft are often the result of high energy trauma, such as falls, motor vehicle accidents, and gunshot wounds, and frequently are associated with multiple trauma. Femoral shaft fractures are located from an area 4 cm below the inferior border of the lesser trochanter to the distal femoral metaphysis at the flare of the femoral condyles. Several methods of treatment are available, and the surgeon must be aware of their advantages and limitations.

Most femoral shaft fractures are initially treated with continuous skeletal traction applied through a pin in the tibial tuberosity. Care must be taken to align the fracture and to bring it to length but not to overdistract it. If the fracture is in the distal half of the femoral shaft, skeletal traction may be continued for a few days to a few weeks. A femoral cast brace is then applied and ambulation is allowed. Ambulation stimulates external callus formation and maturation and allows knee motion to be regained. Treatment by this method is predictable in obtaining union, has few complications and little morbidity, mobilizes the patient and his knee early, and requires a reasonable length of hospitalization. The method cannot be used above the midshaft of the femur because above this level the control of angulation is unpredictable. Femoral shortening is the principal complication of this method of treatment.

When internal fixation is chosen for definitive treatment, it should be applied 5 to 14 days after injury. This allows the fat emboli syndrome to declare itself if it is going to occur and to be treated, other system injuries to be treated or controlled, and blood loss and electrolyte imbalance to be corrected. Local conditions at the fracture site are also better inclined to favor union.

Intramedullary fixation is particularly suitable for transverse and short oblique fractures of the isthmus of the femur. It is important that the intramedullary rod circumferentially engages bone on both sides of the fracture in order to control rotation. Intramedullary rods are best applied by closed methods with the patient on a fracture table. Closed technique, inserting the intramedullary rod into the proximal end of the femur through a small incision in the buttocks, markedly decreases the risk of infection. The proper length and diameter of the rod should be selected. The diameter should be at least 13 mm whenever possible so that the bending strength of the rod is at least the bending strength of bone.

Metal plates and screws may be used for fractures of the upper or lower thirds of the femoral shaft and for some comminuted fractures of the isthmus that are not suitable for intramedullary fixation. When anatomical reduction with medial cortical continuity under compression cannot be reestablished, the plate and screws should be supplemented by a medial autogenous cancellous bone graft.

External fixators are used in some instances of open femoral fractures and in cases of extreme comminution.

Rehabilitation efforts should be directed at getting the patient ambulatory and, in particular, at regaining knee motion. Patients in femoral cast braces and those with intramedullary fixation can ambulate with crutches and progressively increase their weight-bearing within their pain tolerance. In patients with femoral shaft fractures treated with plates and screws, weight-bearing on the injured extremity is not permitted for 3 months for fear that the cyclic stresses of ambulation would loosen or break the fixation before fracture healing occurs.

Fractures of the femoral shaft in children past the age of 12 are treated much as those of adults except that intramedullary rods should not be used while the femoral epiphyses are open.

For children under the age of 3 most femoral shaft fractures can be treated by closed manipulation and the application of a spica cast until union is ensured. Children between the ages of 3 and 12 may be treated in either skin or skeletal traction initially. For most fractures Russell's traction will suffice, but for more proximal fractures a pin may be placed in the distal femur and the extremity placed in 90°-90° traction, with the hip flexed 90° and the knee flexed 90°. The fracture fragments are allowed to override 1 cm to compensate for the overgrowth of the femur in children's femoral shaft fractures. After early fracture consolidation, the child is placed in a one-half spica cast until union is complete. Knee stiffness is not a problem in children's fractures as it is in adult femoral shaft fractures.

FRACTURES AND DISLOCATIONS ABOUT THE KNEE

FRACTURES OF THE DISTAL FEMUR

Fractures of the distal femur are called supracondylar fractures and may extend into the knee joint. They are initially treated with continuous skeletal traction applied through a proximal tibial pin. Supracondylar fractures that extend into the knee joint must be anatomically reduced and rigidly fixed to prevent posttraumatic arthritis. The metaphyseal fragments are first reduced and provisionally fixed with Kirschner wires. Roentgenograms are then taken to ensure reestablishment of joint congruity. Definitive fixation is provided with transfixing cancellous screws. The reconstructed metaphysis can then be secured to the diaphysis of the femur with an angle blade plate or with a Burri plate.

In cases without an intra-articular fracture, the metaphysis is reconstructed to the diaphysis with either an angle blade plate or a Burri plate. Continuous traction may be followed by the application of a femoral cast brace in these fractures.

Patients treated in a femoral cast brace are rehabilitated similarly to patients with femoral shaft fractures treated in a cast brace. Patients with supracondylar femoral fractures are rehabilitated similarly to patients with femoral shaft fractures treated with a plate and screws.

Fractures of the distal femur in children usually are Salter-Harris type II fractures and occur between the ages of 12 and 16. Stress roentgenograms distinguish these fractures from ligament tears about the knee joint. These fractures are treated by closed reduction and immobilization in a molded long leg plaster cast for approximately 6 weeks. There may be a crush injury to the physeal plate in these fractures, causing premature closure of the growth plate and consequent femoral shortening.

KNEE DISLOCATIONS

Dislocations of the knee are true orthopaedic emergencies. The overriding concern with these injuries is to identify or exclude a popliteal artery injury. Knee dislocations are reportedly uncommon but the incidence may be higher than reported since many are reduced at the scene of the injury and never accurately documented later. For the same reason, the position of the knee joint first seen by the physician may not accurately represent the extent of the injury. The physician must not be complacent. Popliteal artery injuries occur in up to 40% of knee dislocations. The popliteal artery collateral branches are also vulnerable in these injuries. The neurovascular status of the extremity must be evaluated carefully as soon as these patients are seen. Time should not be taken for initial radiographs. Knee dislocations are designated according to the displacement of the tibia relative to the femur. Anterior dislocation is most common. A clinical assessment of this displacement

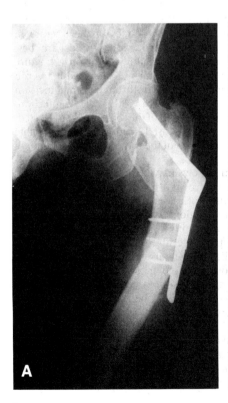
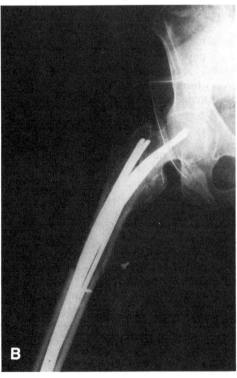

Fig. 44-19. Stabilization of a subtrochanteric fracture with Enders pins. (*A*) This patient had a previous pathologic intertrochanteric fracture secondary to metastatic breast carcinoma stabilized with a Jewett nail 6 months prior to this roentgenogram. The intertrochanteric fracture healed, but, unfortunately, the metastatic disease progressed distally in the femur, causing this second pathologic fracture at the subtrochanteric region. (*B*) The patient's life expectancy and general health were sufficient to justify surgical stabilization of her subtrochanteric fracture. The Jewett nail and screws were removed, although the broken screw head seen in this view could not be recovered. Enders pins were then used to stabilize the fracture.

should be made when possible; then, if the knee joint is not already reduced, closed reduction should be performed by using longitudinal traction on the knee and gently manipulating the proximal tibia into the reduced position. Then, if there is no sign of arterial injury or ischemia, anteroposterior, lateral, and oblique views of the knee should be taken to evaluate the dislocation for an associated fracture. If there is any sign of arterial injury or peripheral ischemia, the patient should be taken directly to the operating room for popliteal artery exploration. An arteriogram may be done in the operating room. Thrombectomy, repair, or reconstruction of the popliteal artery may be necessary. The best results are obtained within 6 to 8 hours of injury. The seriousness of arterial injury is attested to by the fact that up to 50% of reported knee dislocations with popliteal artery injuries have resulted in above-knee amputations. The posterior capsule and the tibial attachment of the posterior cruciate ligament can be repaired at the time of popliteal artery exploration and treatment. All other ligament repairs or reconstruction should be deferred for 5 to 7 days until viability of the extremity and adequacy of the circulation are ensured. The extremity is treated in a well-padded posterior splint with the knee joint flexed 15° to 20° until this time.

Other reasons for immediate operation are an open dislocation, which requires irrigation and débridement, and an irreducible knee dislocation, usually a posterolateral dislocation, which requires extrication of the medial femoral condyle from a buttonhole defect in the capsule, the medial collateral ligament from the joint, or both from a medial surgical approach. Ligament repairs are delayed in the open injury, whereas they should be done concurrently with open reduction in the otherwise irreducible dislocation unless precluded by popliteal artery injury.

If there is no indication for immediate operative intervention, the knee may be aspirated using sterile technique. Testing for instability must be gentle, avoiding hyperextension that will injure the popliteal artery and avoiding more than a few degrees of varus stress that may injure the peroneal nerve. Nerve injury occurs in 25% to 35% of patients with knee dislocations, usually involving the peroneal nerve by traction injury or rupture. The prognosis of a peroneal nerve injury is uncertain: if a traction injury, function returns gradually in some instances; if ruptured, return of peroneal nerve function is nearly hopeless. In either case, immediate exploration of the peroneal nerve is not indicated.

Neurovascular injury occurs in up to 54% of patients with knee dislocations. In these cases it is important to distinguish the sensory changes of nerve injury from those of ischemia. After examination, the extremity is immobilized in a well-padded posterior splint and the circulatory status is observed for 5 to 7 days. Intimal injury can result in thrombosis, which may take several hours or a few days to occur. In 5 to 7 days, after which one can be sure about the circulation, repair, or repair with reconstruction, of all the torn ligaments is indicated. The lower extremity is then immobilized in a plaster cast for 6 weeks, with the position of the knee joint dictated by which ligaments were operated on. Knee rehabilitation is then undertaken.

FRACTURES OF THE PATELLA

The patella is an important fulcrum in achieving knee extension and maintaining quadriceps strength. Fractures of the patella occur by sudden violent contraction of the quadriceps muscle, resulting in an avulsion type fracture that is usually transverse, or by direct violence to the anterior surface of the patella, usually from a car dashboard, resulting in a comminuted fracture. Fractures of the patella occur in all age-groups but are much more common in adults than in children. These fractures, when displaced, should be reconstructed and joint congruity restored whenever possible. Three millimeters to 4 mm of separation and 2 mm to 3 mm of incongruity may be accepted for closed treatment. When operation is necessary, it should be done as soon as possible. If superficial skin abrasions or lacerations are present, open reduction should be done within the golden period of 12 hours or delayed for 7 to 10 days until the potential for contamination is controlled.

Fractures of the patella may be classified as undisplaced fractures, linear displaced fractures, displaced fractures of the superior or inferior pole of the patella, and displaced comminuted fractures.

Undisplaced fractures of the patella have the retinaculum of the knee joint intact and need only to be protected while healing. They should be immobilized in a cylinder cast with the knee in full extension. The patient walks on crutches, with partial weight-bearing progressing to full weight-bearing over a 4- to 6-week period. The cast is then removed, and gentle progressive range of motion exercises are started; the quadriceps and hamstrings are rehabilitated.

Linear displaced fractures may be vertical or oblique but are usually transverse. If transverse and displaced, this fracture is associated with retinacular disruption of the extensor mechanism of the knee. This disruption must be repaired to restore knee extension, and the fracture must be accurately reduced and fixed to restore joint congruity, which can be done by using lag screws and the lag screw principle or by tension band wire technique. This reduction and fixation can be performed when the fracture is transverse regardless of whether it is in the proximal third, middle third, or distal third of the patella.

In some instances of displaced comminuted fractures of the patella, it may be possible to reduce and fix the patella with lag screws, with Kirschner wires and tension band, with circumferential wiring techniques, or with combinations of these. This is more likely possible when the fragments are few and large. When it is impossible to restore a congruent articular surface, the patellar fragments must be excised and a strong circumferential suture of wire or 5-mm Mersilene is placed about the margin of the tendon and tightened as a pursestring to restore the normal length to the extensor mechanism. If the proximal or distal pole of the patella is comminuted, it is excised and the quadriceps or patellar tendon is approximated to the remaining patella.

FRACTURES OF THE PROXIMAL TIBIA

Fractures of the proximal tibia may be of the lateral plateau, medial plateau, or both. These fractures may be undisplaced, split, depressed, or, in more osteopenic bone, comminuted. Split fractures of the lateral plateau result from a valgus force at the knee. Fractures of the medial plateau, which are less common, result from a varus force. Fractures of both plateaus result from an axial compression. An axial compression component also causes depressed plateau fractures (Fig. 44-20, *A*).

These fractures are evaluated by anteroposterior, lateral, and oblique films. An anteroposterior film directed parallel with the proximal tibial joint surface, 10° superior to the perpendicular to the tibia, is especially helpful in determining

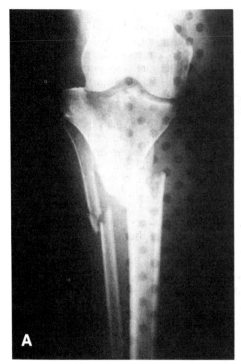
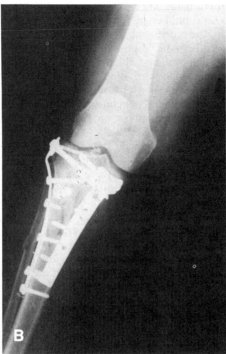

Fig. 44-20. Fracture of the proximal tibia. (*A*) Fracture of both tibial plateaus with a comminution and a depressed fragment on the lateral side. (*B*) The depressed fragment has been elevated and held with Kirschner wires. The underlying defect has been bone grafted. The plateau fractures are reduced and fixed with medial and lateral T-buttress plates and screws.

the amount of depression in a tibial plateau fracture. Tomograms are extremely helpful in evaluating these fractures. Stress films should be taken at 0° and 30° of knee flexion, particularly in undisplaced and depressed fractures in which collateral ligament injury is most common. If the knee joint is unstable and opens up 1 mm more than on the uninvolved opposite side, the collateral ligament should be explored and repaired. Stress films are best made under anesthesia. Since lateral plateau fractures are more common than medial plateau fractures, injuries to the medial ligament complex are more frequent than injuries to the lateral ligament complex.

The goals of proximal tibia fracture treatment are joint congruity and function. A range of motion from full extension to at least 110° of flexion is desirable.

Undisplaced fractures may be protected with a cast brace for 5 to 6 weeks. Roentgenograms should be taken weekly for the first 3 weeks to be sure that these fractures do not displace and require further treatment. Weight-bearing should be deferred for 12 weeks or until union of the fracture is ensured to prevent late valgus or varus deformity.

If displacement occurs in single plateau fractures, 4 mm or more separation requires open reduction and internal fixation with either lag screws or a buttress plate. Eight millimeters or more of depression requires elevation of a depressed fracture and bone grafting of the underlying defect and stabilization with a buttress plate. A fracture that is unstable to stress testing and in which this instability is due to the fracture and not ligamentous disruption should be reduced and fixed. Any displaced intracondylar eminence fracture should be reduced and incorporated into the fixation. If fixation is rigid, range of motion exercises should be instituted within 3 weeks of fixation but weight-bearing should be deferred for 12 weeks or until union of the fractures is ensured.

The meniscus should always be preserved whenever possible. Peripheral meniscus tears should be repaired. Only

menisci with tears in the substance likely to lead to internal knee derangement should be removed.

Fractures of the medial tibial plateau have been associated with knee dislocation. A most careful evaluation of the circulatory status is therefore important in medial tibial plateau fractures.

When both tibial condyles are fractured and displaced, open reduction, internal fixation with buttress plates on both sides and bone grafting, or skeletal traction with early knee exercises will restore joint congruity (Fig. 44-20, *B*). The method chosen will vary with the experience and skill of the surgeon as well as with the degree of comminution. If open reduction is chosen, the fixation must be sufficiently rigid to allow early range of motion or a stiff knee will result. If traction is chosen, motion is usually well restored, but there may be a problem restoring joint congruity and stability.

FRACTURES OF THE SHAFT OF THE TIBIA AND FIBULA

Fractures of the shaft of the tibia and fibula can result from direct and indirect trauma. Fractures of all configurations are seen. Anteroposterior and lateral roentgenograms showing both the knee joint and the ankle joint on the same film should be taken initially and at each follow-up evaluation. When a fracture of the fibular shaft occurs alone, the knee and ankle should be examined with care for ligamentous injury. Such a fracture without ligamentous injury requires only symptomatic treatment with crutches or a walking cast. These are stable fractures, and even if they fail to unite, it is of no consequence.

Fractures of the tibial shaft with an intact fibula can be managed by ambulatory treatment in a plaster cast provided there is good alignment. If good alignment cannot be obtained by closed methods, open reduction and internal fixation may be necessary.

Fractures of the shafts of the tibia and fibula should

almost always be treated by closed reduction and plaster cast immobilization in children. Older children often can be taught to ambulate on crutches and to progress from partial to full weight-bearing in a long-leg plaster cast with the knee position from 0° to 5° of flexion. The cast is removed when the fracture is united, usually about 12 weeks after injury.

In closed fractures of the tibia and fibula in adults, the best results in terms of union without infection are usually achieved by closed reduction and ambulatory treatment in a plaster cast. A long leg plaster cast is used initially with the knee flexed between 0° and 5° of flexion. Ordinarily, this long leg cast can be changed to a patellar weight-bearing cast 2 to 6 weeks after injury so that knee motion can be regained and the quadriceps and hamstring muscles can be rehabilitated. The cast is maintained until clinical and radiographic union have occurred. In open fractures of the tibial and fibular shafts, the wound is incised, irrigated, and débrided. The fracture is then reduced and treated like a closed fracture as outlined above. Wound closure or coverage is elective when the wound is clean and controlled. Open reduction and internal or external fixation of tibial shaft fractures should be done only for specific indications, such as when closed reduction is impossible, perhaps due to soft tissue interposition between the fragments; for open fractures requiring complicated procedures for coverage, such as local or distant flaps; for some cases in which there is associated polytrauma or polyfractures; in paraplegics with sensory loss; in segmental fractures with displaced central fragments; when there are gaps resulting from missing bone fragments; and when vascular injuries are associated. External fixators are generally preferred to internal fixation because they are less likely to be complicated by infection. External fixators allow a rigid fixation of the fracture and wound access and permit plastic procedures. Reconstructive procedures should be done early so that the external fixators can be removed within 6 weeks after injury and the patient can be converted to ambulatory treatment in a plaster cast as outlined above.

The important prognostic factors in tibial shaft fractures are the amount of initial displacement, the degree of comminution, the presence or absence of infection, and the severity of the soft tissue injury excluding infection.

FRACTURES AND DISLOCATIONS ABOUT THE ANKLE

INTRA-ARTICULAR FRACTURES OF THE DISTAL TIBIA

Intra-articular fractures of the distal tibia are also called pilon fractures. There are three types of pilon fractures: (1) undisplaced, (2) displaced with articular incongruity, and (3) displaced with articular incongruity and depression.

The undisplaced pilon fracture is placed in a patellar weight-bearing type of plaster cast. This allows knee motion while protecting the fracture from rotatory forces. Weight-bearing is not allowed until the fracture unites, which usually occurs from 14 to 20 weeks after the fracture was sustained.

Displaced fractures can be treated with skeletal traction through a calcaneal pin and with early initiation of active range of motion exercises of the ankle while in this traction. Better results are obtained with open reduction and internal fixation provided that the fragments are of sufficient size to stabilize and that joint congruity is restored. Any depressed fragments are elevated and restored anatomically, and the

resulting bony defect is grafted with autogenous cancellous bone. Fixation should be rigid so that active range of ankle motion exercises may be initiated early. Displacement of the fibular fracture that occurs with this injury is a relative indication to consider open reduction and internal fixation. Anteroposterior and lateral tomograms are most helpful in preoperative evaluation and planning. The principles of open reduction and internal fixation in displaced pilon fractures are, in sequence: (1) reconstruction of the correct length of the fibula, (2) reconstruction of the articular surface of the distal tibia, (3) application of a cancellous bone autograft to any tibial metaphyseal defect, and (4) stabilization of the medial aspect of the tibia by a cloverleaf-shaped plate. A spoon-shaped plate may be used when the tibial fracture must be stabilized anteriorly. Early range of ankle motion is encouraged when stabilization is rigid, but, again, weight-bearing is not allowed until the fracture has healed, usually 14 to 20 weeks after injury. Post-traumatic ankle joint arthritis is a frequent complication of these fractures and may require ankle arthrodesis.

UNDISPLACED FRACTURES OF THE ANKLE

Undisplaced fractures of the ankle are usually of the lateral malleolus and result from an external rotation force insufficient to cause displacement. If there is tenderness over the medial malleolus and no fracture there, a tear of the deltoid ligament should be suspected in association with a lateral malleolar fracture that has undergone spontaneous reduction. In such cases, a stress film should be taken to evaluate whether or not the deltoid ligament is intact. If there is no significant swelling or tenderness about the medial malleolus, and the only injury is the undisplaced fracture of the lateral malleolus, simple immobilization in a short leg walking cast for 6 weeks is sufficient. If the fracture is unstable on stress films, it must be treated like a displaced fracture.

Undisplaced fractures of the medial malleolus are rare and result from direct trauma. They usually heal after 4 to 6 weeks of protection in a short leg plaster cast.

Most bimalleolar and trimalleolar fractures are displaced, but an occasional undisplaced fracture of this type is seen. These undisplaced fractures may be treated by immobilization in a long leg cast with the knee flexed 30° to 40° to prevent torsion forces on the ankle that might cause displacement. After 4 weeks of treatment, the long leg cast is converted to a short leg walking cast for an additional 4 weeks. These fractures must be monitored very carefully, and if they displace during treatment they must be managed accordingly.

DISPLACED FRACTURES ABOUT THE ANKLE

Fractures of the Lateral Malleolus
In single fractures of the lateral malleolus with displacement of the talus there is almost always an associated tear of the deltoid ligament. Some surgeons prefer closed reduction and external immobilization for these fractures and reserve open reduction only for those in which the deltoid ligament is trapped between the talus and medial malleolus and thus prevents reduction. On the other hand, in recent years, many surgeons have used open reduction and internal fixation of the fracture of the lateral malleolus and open repair of the deltoid ligament. In any case, anatomical reduction of the lateral malleolus is necessary. Otherwise, lateral shift of the talus will distort the tibiotalar weight-

bearing area and this can lead to posttraumatic arthritis. In displaced lateral malleolar fractures, anatomical or near anatomical reduction must be achieved when using closed methods or the lateral malleolus should be openly reduced and internally fixed. An additional benefit of open reduction in all displaced ankle fractures is the ability to remove osteochondral fragments and treat their source. These occur in up to 20% of ankle fractures and if untreated can lead to arthritis. Better healing of the deltoid ligament is possible if it is accurately sutured, and this should be strongly considered in younger patients with an active life-style and in patients with a significant athletic commitment. If the displaced lateral malleolar fracture is treated by closed methods, management and aftercare are similar to those outlined previously for an undisplaced bimalleolar fracture. After open repair, a well-padded stirrup-type plaster splint is applied and the leg is elevated. The patient is mobilized on crutches early and is not allowed to place weight on the affected extremity. The stirrup splint is removed 5 days after surgery, and active range of motion exercises are initiated. Four weeks after surgery the patient is placed in a short leg walking cast for 4 additional weeks.

If the displaced fracture of the fibula is in the shaft above the distal tibiofibular syndesmosis with lateral displacement of the talus, then there is a tear of the distal tibiofibular syndesmosis as well as the deltoid ligament. These fractures require a lag screw just above the syndesmosis to hold the distal fibula in a proper relationship to the tibia, in addition to an open repair of the deltoid ligament. The lag screw may be placed through an appropriate screw hole in a plate used to fix the fibular fracture and should be tightened with the ankle in maximum dorsiflexion to avoid later restriction of dorsiflexion. The postoperative management is the same as for open repairs of the lateral malleolus except that the patient must not bear weight until the lag screw holding the distal tibiofibular syndesmosis is removed. This is done 8 weeks after open reduction and internal fixation.

Displaced fractures of the medial malleolus are openly reduced and fixed with either one or two malleolar screws or by tension band wiring technique. If there is medial displacement of the talus with the medial malleolar fracture, there is a tear of the lateral capsule and ligaments of the ankle, and these should be repaired. Aftercare is similar to that outlined previously for displaced fractures of the lateral malleolus.

Bimalleolar Fractures

If a displaced bimalleolar fracture can be reduced accurately and maintained in satisfactory position, closed treatment is permissible and the fracture can be treated like an undisplaced bimalleolar fracture except that immobilization is maintained for 12 weeks. Because this is an intra-articular fracture, because there is little forgiveness for lateral talar shift, and because closed anatomical reduction is difficult to achieve and hold, most surgeons choose open reduction and internal fixation for these fractures. An intra-articular osteochondral fragment demands removal, and open reduction and internal fixation can be done concurrently. A patellar weight-bearing type of cast is used to allow knee motion while protecting the ankle from rotational forces. This may be converted to a short leg walking cast 6 to 8 weeks after injury. If a screw has been used to stabilize the distal tibiofibular syndesmosis, it is removed at this time. Progressive partial weight-bearing is then initiated. The plaster cast is removed at 12 weeks after injury. Crutches

may be discarded when the patient is able to bear full unsupported weight on his injured extremity.

Trimalleolar Fractures

Trimalleolar fractures are treated just like bimalleolar fractures except for the fracture of the posterior malleolus. If the fracture of the posterior malleolus is undisplaced or if it is displaced but involves less than 30% of the articular surface of the distal tibia on lateral roentgenogram, no reduction or fixation is necessary. If the fracture of the posterior malleolus is displaced and involves more than 30% of the articular surface of the distal tibia on lateral roentgenogram, it must be reduced and fixed with pins, screws, or a combination of the two to prevent posterior subluxation or dislocation of the talus.

FRACTURES AND DISLOCATIONS ABOUT THE FOOT

PERITALAR DISLOCATION

Peritalar dislocation may be anterior, posterior, or lateral but is usually medial. Medial peritalar dislocation is a result of combined plantar flexion and inversion forces. Pressure necrosis of the overlying skin is a particular concern in unreduced peritalar dislocations. Manipulative reduction should be performed as soon as possible under regional or general anesthesia. One or more tendons may be caught between the bones and prevent closed reduction. Open reduction is then performed, preferably through a lateral incision to prevent medial skin slough. A short leg cast is then applied with the foot and ankle in a neutral position and is worn for 6 weeks. During this time, the patient may ambulate on crutches but should not bear weight on the injured extremity. The cast is then removed and active range of motion and muscle-strengthening exercises are initiated. When there is no pain in the foot, progressive weight-bearing is started and increased according to the patient's pain tolerance. Results with this injury are generally good, although avascular necrosis of the talus and subtalar post-traumatic arthritis can occur.

FRACTURES OF THE TALUS

Most fractures of the talus result from a dorsiflexion force at the ankle that drives the neck of the talus against the anterior lip of the distal tibia and fractures the talus at the junction of the neck and the body.

Undisplaced fractures of the neck of the talus are treated by non-weight-bearing and placement in a short leg cast with the foot and ankle in a neutral position for 8 weeks. Union without complications is the rule.

Displaced fractures of the neck of the talus must be reduced anatomically. Usually this requires open reduction, and the fracture should be fixed and compressed by inter-fragmentary cancellous bone lag screws. Displaced fractures of the neck of the talus may be complicated by avascular necrosis of the talus. The incidence of avascular necrosis of the talus is proportional to the degree of fracture displacement. Delayed union or nonunion is rare if the fracture is properly reduced and stabilized.

Displaced fractures of the neck of the talus can be complicated by posterior medial dislocation of the body of the talus from the ankle mortise. The body of the talus must be promptly reduced or pressure necrosis of the overlying skin, gangrene of the foot from pressure occluding the posterior tibial vessels, or both may occur. This requires open reduction, and osteostomy of the medial malleolus is often necessary. The displaced fracture of the neck of the talus is treated as outlined above. Dislocation of the body of the talus increases the incidence of avascular necrosis of the talus and of delayed union and nonunion.

Fractures of the body of the talus are associated with a high level of avascular necrosis. Avascular necrosis can occur in undisplaced fractures of the body of the talus, but, again, its incidence parallels the degree of displacement. Undisplaced fractures are protected in a short leg plaster cast without weight-bearing until they unite, usually 6 to 8 weeks after injury. Displaced fractures of the body of the talus require open reduction, usually with osteotomy of the medial malleolus and fixation with interfragmentary cancellous bone lag screws, pins, or both. Displaced fractures are then protected in a short leg cast without weight-bearing until they heal, usually for a period of 3 to 4 months. Posttraumatic arthritis of the ankle, subtalar joint, or both can be a late complication of displaced fractures of the body of the talus.

FRACTURES OF THE CALCANEUS

Fractures of the calcaneus are usually the result of a jump or a fall from a height with the patient landing on his heel. They are often associated with severe hemorrhage, swelling, pain, and ecchymosis; occasionally ischemic fracture blisters occur. Definitive treatment often must be deferred for several days until the skin and soft tissues are in better condition. All calcaneal fractures should be treated initially by application of ice, elevation, and use of a compression dressing protected by a short leg posterior plaster splint. Vertebral fractures frequently accompany calcaneal fractures and should either be identified or excluded.

Whether or not they extend into the subtalar joint, undisplaced and minimally displaced calcaneal fractures are treated nonoperatively. The patient is ambulated early but is fitted with a short leg elastic stocking and advised to keep his foot elevated whenever he is not ambulating. Range of motion exercises are started early, but weight-bearing is not permitted on the injured extremity until union is solid, which usually is evident 2 to 3 months after the fracture occurs. Good results are generally obtained.

In displaced calcaneal fractures that extend into the subtalar joint, the lateral process of the talus acts as a wedge to burst the superior articular surface of the calcaneus. Neither closed nor open reduction with internal fixation produces a predictably good result in these fractures. The surgeon should use that method with which he is most skilled and familiar. A pin may be placed in the posterior calcaneus to assist closed manipulation and is then incorporated into a short leg cast that is worn for 1 month. The pin is then removed and a short leg cast is worn for 3 months. The patient is ambulatory on crutches during this time but keeps his foot elevated whenever he is not ambulating. When the cast is removed 3 months after injury, progressive weight-bearing is initiated within the patient's pain tolerance. There is a high incidence of subtalar arthritis after displaced calcaneal fractures, and subtalar arthrodesis may be required in the patients with significant symptoms. The peroneal tendons are occasionally entrapped as a result of displaced calcaneal fractures, and release of these tendons may be necessary.

TRANSMETATARSAL DISLOCATIONS

Transmetatarsal dislocations result from strong rotational forces and may be dorsal, plantar, medial, lateral, or a combination of these. Avulsion fractures may be present. Prompt recognition and early stable reduction are necessary to prevent painful and impaired weight-bearing. Reduction of the base of the second metatarsal into its mortiselike joint is the key to the reduction. Usually the reduction can be accomplished by closed manipulation with the patient under general or regional anesthesia. If closed reduction is complete but unstable, percutaneous pins may be used to stabilize the second metatarsal tarsal joint. If closed reduction is unsuccessful, open reduction is performed and the second metatarsal tarsal joint is stabilized with pins. A short leg cast is worn for 6 weeks, at which time the pins are removed and graduated weight-bearing is initiated.

FRACTURES OF THE METATARSALS

Fractures of the metatarsals occur at the base, shaft, or neck. Fractures of the base of the metatarsals usually result from blunt trauma and are often undisplaced or minimally displaced. They can be treated in a short leg walking cast with progressive ambulation within the patient's pain tolerance. The cast can be removed in 6 weeks. Crutches and progressive partial weight-bearing are continued until the patient can bear his full unsupported weight on the injured extremity.

A fracture of the base of the fifth metatarsal can occur as an avulsion of bone at the insertion of the peroneus brevis tendon due to forceful inversion of the forefoot. If undisplaced or minimally displaced, these fractures are treated as outlined above for fractures of the metatarsal base. If they are displaced, open reduction and stabilization with one or more pins or screws is indicated.

Fractures of the metatarsal shaft can result from blunt trauma or torsional stresses. If there is minimal or no displacement, these fractures are treated like undisplaced fractures of the metatarsal base. If there is displacement, open reduction and internal fixation with pins, screws, or small fragment plates and screws is indicated. When more than one metatarsal shaft is fractured, displacement is more likely.

Fractures of the metatarsal neck can result from vertical forces acting on the forefoot. If undisplaced, they are treated just as other undisplaced metatarsal fractures. If they are displaced, open reduction and internal fixation with pins, screws, or small fragment T- or L-shaped plates is carried out. If a metatarsal head is allowed to remain inferiorly displaced into the plantar surface of the foot, painful metatarsalgia can result. Stress fractures most commonly occur at the second metatarsal neck owing to cyclic stresses of increased ambulation or running in a person not accustomed to these activities. They present with pain, tenderness, swelling, heat, and redness. The roentgenogram may initially prove negative, but periosteal callus formation and a radiolucent line usually appear 2 to 3 weeks after the onset of symptoms. These fractures are often seen in military recruits and are therefore called march fractures. They need only to be protected until they are asymptomatic.

BIBLIOGRAPHY

Anderson LD: Common fractures and dislocations. In Hardy JD (ed): Rhoads Textbook of Surgery. Philadelphia, J B Lippincott, 1977

Brooker AF, Edwards CC: External Fixation. Baltimore, Williams & Wilkins, 1979

Brooker AF, Schmeisser G, Jr: Orthopedic Traction Manual. Baltimore, Williams & Wilkins, 1980

Burri C: Post Traumatic Osteomyelitis. Bern, Hans Huber, 1975

CHARNLEY J: The Closed Treatment of Common Fractures. New York, Churchill-Livingstone, 1974

EPPS CH, JR: Complications in Orthopedic Surgery. Philadelphia, J B Lippincott, 1978

FREELAND AE: Complications of common fractures and dislocations. In Hardy JD (ed): Complications in Surgery and Their Management. Philadelphia, W B Saunders, 1981

FREELAND AE, HUGHES JL: Early management of the severely injured extremity. In Hardy JD (ed): Critical Surgical Illness. Philadelphia, W B Saunders, 1980

HEIM V, PFEIFFER KM: Small Fragment Set Manual. New York, Springer-Verlag, 1974

HEPPENSTALL RB: Fracture Treatment and Healing. Philadelphia, W B Saunders, 1980

HOOPES JE, JABALEY ME: Soft tissue injuries of the extremities. In Ballinger WF, II, Rutherford RB, Zuidema GD (eds): The Management of Trauma. Philadelphia, W B Saunders, 1973

JOHNSON RM: Advances in External Fixation. Chicago, Year Book Medical Publishers, 1980

MATSEN FA III: Compartmental Syndromes. New York, Grune & Stratton, 1980

MATTER P, RITTMAN WW: The Open Fracture. Bern, Hans Huber Publishers, 1977

MUBARAK SJ, HARGENS AR: Compartment Syndromes and Volkmann's Contracture. Philadelphia, W B Saunders, 1981

MÜLLER ME, ALLGÖWER M, SCHNEIDER R, WILLENEGGER H: Manual of Internal Fixation. New York, Springer-Verlag, 1979

RANG M: Children's Fractures. Philadelphia, J B Lippincott, 1974

ROCKWOOD CA, GREEN DP: Fractures. Philadelphia, J B Lippincott, 1975

SARMIENTO A, LATTA LL: Closed Functional Treatment of Fractures. New York, Spring-Verlag, 1981

SISK TD: Fractures. In Edmonson AS, Grenshaw AH (eds): Campbell's Operative Orthopedics. St. Louis, C V Mosby, 1980

WEBER BG, BRUNNER C, FREULER F: Treatment of Fractures in Children and Adolescents. New York, Springer-Verlag, 1980

WEBER BG, CECH O: Pseudoarthrosis, Pathology, Biomechanics, Therapy, Results. Bern, Hans Huber Publishers, 1976

WRIGHT PE: Dislocations. In Edmonson AS, Grenshaw AH (eds): Campbell's Operative Orthopedics. St. Louis, C V Mosby, 1980

Raymond R. White/James L. Hughes

Adult Orthopaedic Disorders

Orthopaedics may seem vastly different from other fields of medicine. When one looks more closely, however, the eight basic forms of disease are the same in orthopaedics as in all areas of medicine. These include inflammatory, degenerative, infectious, neoplastic, metabolic, traumatic, iatrogenic, and congenital disorders. In this section the more common forms of orthopaedic disorders that affect adults will be discussed. Each of these areas will be broadly covered and then confined to more specific problems, area by area. Some of the newer advances in orthopaedics will be discussed briefly.

The basis for formulating any good treatment plan begins with the history and physical examination. Many students and physicians are often confused about how to take an orthopaedic history; yet the orthopaedic history is fundamentally no different than a history obtained from a person with abdominal, chest, or head pain. The basic components of the history from any patient, especially one presenting with pain, are the same. These include the location, duration, onset, severity, quality, quantity, radiation, and course of the pain. Also important are factors that aggravate the discomfort, factors that relieve the discomfort, associated symptoms, any disability caused by it, past treatments for the disorder, constitutional symptoms, and a broad area of general negatives that are specific for each area of the body. To leave any of these factors out is to take an incomplete history, thus making diagnosis more difficult.

The orthopaedic physical examination is similar to that of any general examination. First, the examiner must simply observe the manner in which the patient moves his affected extremity or spine as well as his overall alignment, symmetry, size, shape, color, and swellings. One advantage that the examiner has when performing an orthopaedic examination is that in most patients one side is normal. This affords the opportunity to compare range of motion, alignment, ligamentous laxity, size, shape, motor strength, sensation, and deep tendon reflexes of the affected and normal sides.

As in most fields of medicine, it is often possible to make an accurate assessment of the patient from the history and physical examination alone. In some patients, the diagnosis is more difficult. To this end, the orthopaedist uses the radiograph as his next most common modality for investigation. In obtaining radiographs of affected areas it is mandatory to have two views obtained 90° apart. This is very difficult in some instances, such as in the shoulder where special views are needed. When taking joint radiographs, it is often best to obtain a third or fourth (most often oblique) view. Radiographs of the feet are especially useful if taken in the weight-bearing position. For most orthopaedic work, the standard radiographs are satisfactory. For more difficult problems tomograms in either anteroposterior or lateral planes are used, and more recently the computed tomographic (CT) scan has become quite useful. Other useful modalities include the technetium 99m bone scan for bone lesions and arthrography for specific joint problems. The uses of tomograms, bone scans, and CT scans are shown in Figure 44-21.

Useful laboratory studies include the complete blood cell count (CBC); the erythrocyte sedimentation rate (ESR); and serum levels of calcium, phosphorus, and alkaline phosphatase. The CBC may reveal anemia or leukocyte elevations that can indicate infection. The ESR is often elevated in infectious, inflammatory, or neoplastic processes. The more specific screening tests such as calcium, phosphorus, and alkaline phosphatase determinations are useful for metabolic disorders related to the skeleton. When ordered judiciously with specific problems in mind, these tests can be quite helpful in sorting out orthopaedic problems.

BASIC DISEASE PROCESSES

INFLAMMATORY DISORDERS

RHEUMATOID ARTHRITIS

Etiology. Rheumatoid arthritis is a disease of the synovial joint lining. Its exact etiology is uncertain, but it is currently thought to be an immune reaction type disease. The synovium becomes inflamed and thickened, resulting in mechanical obstruction of the joint by pannus formation and poor production of lubricating fluid by the inflamed synovium.

History. Rheumatoid arthritis is usually a polyarticular disease and is often symmetrical. The classic symptoms are pain, swelling, malaise, stiffness, and effusion. The stiffness is generally noted in the morning and lasts for an hour or more. The onset is variable and various combinations of the above symptoms may exist. The course is likewise variable; a waxing and waning course is common. Symptoms are aggravated by joint use and relieved with rest and anti-inflammatory medications.

Physical Examination. The early signs include swelling of the synovium, muscle weakness, and flexion contractures. The synovium may feel boggy. Other signs include effusion, deformities, rheumatoid nodules, tendon ruptures, and ligamentous laxity.

Other Studies. Generally, the diagnosis of rheumatoid arthritis is made from the history and physical findings. Studies that are helpful include the CBC, which may show normocytic normochromic low-grade anemia; the ESR, which is elevated; and the rheumatoid factor or antinuclear antibody test, which proves positive. The radiographic

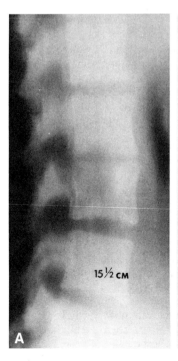

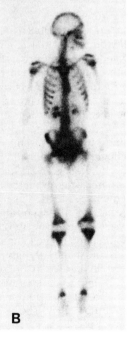

15½ CM

A **B**

Fig. 44-21. Standard anteroposterior and lateral radiographs of a 19-year-old man with persistent back pain showed only a slight abnormality. (*A*) Tomograms show a large defect in L1. (*B*) The bone scan shows increased uptake. (*C*) The CT scan shows this lesion and a smaller lesion in the anterior portion of the vertebral body. By adjusting the computer for better soft-tissue visualization, a psoas abscess could be appreciated. Diagnosis: tuberculous osteomyelitis.

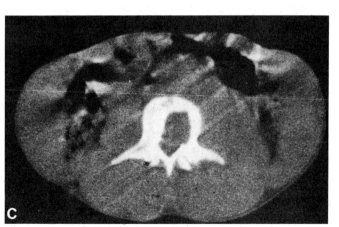

C

findings are dependent on the state of disease. Initially, there may be only soft tissue swelling followed by effusion, periarticular erosions, osteopenia (bone loss), and joint destruction of various degrees. Aspirated synovial fluid is most useful for the differential diagnosis, and rheumatoid factor studies can be performed on the fluid.

Treatment. The major goal of treatment is to maintain function. This is accomplished by using a combination of anti-inflammatory agents, physical therapy, and splinting. When anti-inflammatory agents are not effective, the physician can use corticosteroids, gold injection, or immunosuppressive drugs such as azathioprine (Imuran). These latter agents should be used only by rheumatologists. Surgical management is to control the active disease that has proved uncontrollable by medical means. For the knee and wrist, this often means a synovectomy. In older patients and in those with severe deformities, total joint replacement may be the treatment of choice.

CRYSTALLINE ARTHROPATHIES

Gout and pseudogout are characterized by the formation of crystals within the joint space that causes an acute inflammatory reaction by the synovium.

Gout

Etiology. Gout is a crystalline-induced arthropathy that results from either the overproduction or underexcretion of uric acid. Uric acid is produced via the following pathway:

Nucleic acids → Purines → Urate.

The urate produced is mainly excreted by the kidneys via tubular secretion. Primary gout is a defect in this pathway, leading to increased urate production or decreased excretion of urate. Secondary gout can be caused by the treatment of myeloma or lymphoma in which there is a sudden release of nucleic acids into the system.

Gouty attacks are generally secondary to sudden changes in the level of urate in the body. These changes can be triggered by fasting, ingestion of alcohol, surgery, trauma, or ingestion of drugs such as diuretics. A supersaturated urate solution in the joint fluid exists in people predisposed to gout. When such a solution is disturbed by the above sudden changes, crystallization of urate occurs. Biomechanically, these crystals are needle shaped and elicit a terrific inflammatory response from the synovium. This starts a vicious cycle (Fig. 44-22), which leads to cartilage destruction and further crystal production.

History. Gout generally affects older men and is associated with diabetes, heart disease, elevated triglyceride levels, hypertension, poor renal function, and a positive family history. Attacks are characterized by sudden onset of pain that rapidly escalates over the course of a few hours. These patients have a warm, excruciatingly painful joint that cannot tolerate even the touch of covers or socks. Most often affected is the metatarsophalangeal joint of the great toe, with other joints in the foot and ankle next most commonly affected.

Physical Examination. The patient is in acute distress with an exquisitely tender, erythematous joint, usually in the foot. Masses that may appear about the joint are called tophi. The radiograph may show swelling, joint destruction, or periarticular masses. There may be an elevated level of uric acid, which is helpful but not absolutely necessary for

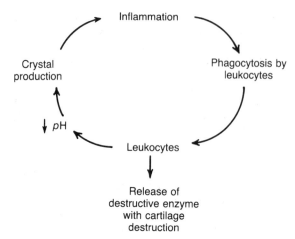

Fig. 44-22. Graphic representation of how crystal production leads to joint destruction. Anti-inflammatory agents block the cycle at the inflammation step. Colchicine blocks the cycle by inhibiting leukocyte activity.

the diagnosis. The diagnosis is confirmed when negatively birefringent crystals are seen on polarized microscopy.

Treatment. Treatment of gout has two phases: (1) to stop the acute attack and (2) to control the urate level in the blood. In the acute phase the disease is treated with colchicine; 1 mg is given orally every hour until the pain is relieved, gastrointestinal symptoms intervene (*e.g.,* nausea, vomiting, or diarrhea), or a maximum 7-mg dose is given. It is also possible to give colchicine intravenously, but its effectiveness when given orally is such that this route is seldom used. Also, in the acute episode phenylbutazone (Butazolidin), indomethacin (Indocin), naproxen (Naprosyn), or oral corticosteroids may be used. Long-term control of gout can be accomplished with allopurinol, a xanthine-oxidase inhibitor, or with uricosuric drugs such as probenecid. Both allopurinol and probenecid should be used with caution because they sometimes, in the early stages, initiate a gouty attack. The purpose of using these drugs is to reduce the level of uric acid in the blood.

Pseudogout

Etiology. Pseudogout is also a crystalline-induced arthropathy but the crystals are calcium pyrophosphate instead of urate. This disease occurs in older men and is often associated with osteoarthritis, hyperparathyroidism, ochronosis, Wilson's disease, hemachromatosis, acromegaly, gout, and diabetes. It is present mainly in the larger joints, especially the knee.

Clinical Presentation. Pseudogout presents with nearly the same history and similar objective findings as gout. The radiographic examination is useful in differentiating pseudogout from gout, in that pseudogout may present with chondrocalcinosis on the radiographs of the wrist and knee. In the knee the triangular shape of the menisci are outlined because of the deposition of the calcium pyrophosphate crystals. The single most important study is microscopic examination of the joint fluid with the polarizing light. One finds rod-shaped crystals that are positively birefringent and generally located in leukocytes.

Treatment. The treatment of pseudogout is aspiration of the affected joint and administration of anti-inflammatory medication for a short duration. There is no long-term control of the calcium pyrophosphate.

TENDINITIS AND TENOSYNOVITIS

Tendinitis and tenosynovitis are inflammations of the tendons and their synovial sheaths, respectively. The terms are sometimes used interchangeably because if the tenosynovitis is severe enough, it can affect the tendon and vice versa.

Etiology. Both diseases are generally caused by an irritative process, usually at a point where the tendon either attaches to the bone or goes around a bony prominence. There are numerous sites in the body for these to occur; some of the more common sites are shown in Figure 44-23. When the synovium becomes inflamed it does not produce thin synovial fluid but instead a thicker, more exudative type fluid that does not lubricate as well. This aggravates the situation and makes gliding of the tendons even more difficult. Tendinitis is often seen at the site where a tendon attaches to bone and is caused by microruptures in the tendon; the inflammatory process is the body's attempt to repair these ruptures.

History. Patients generally present with an overuse type syndrome; that is, they have initiated a new activity or increased a standard activity. As an example, one might see a tendinitis in the wrist of a fisherman after the opening day of fishing season. There is usually an area of localized, acute tenderness that is aggravated by motion of any kind. The pain is generally relieved by aspirin and rest.

Physical Examination. On examination swelling, erythema, edema, pain with motion, and often crepitation over the affected area (especially with tenosynovitis) are noted. There is generally pain at a well-localized area. The possibility of infection, fracture, and systemic disease such as rheumatoid arthritis must be excluded. Radiographs are often helpful in ruling out the fracture, and a good history is probably most useful for ruling out infection.

Treatment. Treatment of these lesions consists of resting the affected part. In the case of the wrist and upper extremity, this is best accomplished with a splint and/or sling. For the lower extremity, this is often aided by crutches. Antiinflammatory agents, ranging from aspirin to phenylbutazone, depending on the severity of the inflammation, also are used. Rarely it is necessary to inject a small amount of local anesthesia mixed with long-acting corticosteroid into the tendon sheath. This procedure can be both diagnostic and therapeutic. If the pain is relieved completely at the time of injection, it is indicative that this is the site of pathology. If the patient gets long-term relief of the discomfort and then the identical pain recurs, surgical intervention must be strongly considered.

Operative treatment is reserved for those in whom nonoperative methods have failed. Operation generally consists of releasing hypertrophied synovium and stenosing bands of tissue, such as in the case of DeQuervain's tenosynovitis. The operative intervention for tendinitis involves release of the tendon from its bony attachment at the painful spot if there is a large attachment. Such is the case with operative intervention for tennis elbow. Sometimes a small degenerative portion of the tendon is removed to allow a more physiological scar to form in the area.

BURSITIS

Etiology. Bursal cavities are formed wherever two surfaces in the body rub against one another. This may be in areas such as the extensor surfaces of the knee and elbow where the skin must glide freely over the underlying bony prominences. Other examples are where muscles and tendons must pass around bony prominences. An example of this would be the shoulder area where the supraspinatus tendon runs underneath the acromium. There are multiple other spots in the body where bursae exist (Fig. 44-24). Bursitis is generally the result of either trauma to the area or an overuse problem in which the bursal surfaces are subjected to more wear and tear than the bursal fluid and surfaces can accommodate comfortably. When such is the case, the

Fig. 44-23. Common sites of tendon and tendon sheath inflammation.

Fig. 44-24. Common sites of bursitis.

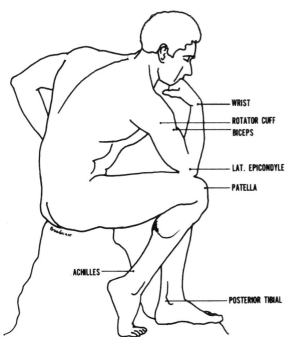

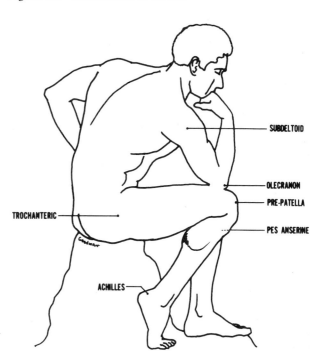

bursal tissues become inflamed and produce more fluid, which is often of a reactive type and has poor lubricating properties. The more superficial bursae are generally affected when they are traumatized. The deep bursae, such as those between muscles or between muscles and bones, generally become inflamed with overuse.

Clinical Presentation. The discomfort that these patients notice is well-localized aching or burning, usually of gradual onset, which is aggravated by striking or moving the affected area. The inflammation is relieved by rest, by use of anti-inflammatory agents and usually by application of ice. On physical examination, there is swelling, erythema, tenderness, and pain with motion, especially if it is a deep bursa. A differential diagnosis must include the possibility of a septic bursitis, especially in olecranon or prepatellar areas. Presentation of septic bursitis might include more constitutional symptoms, no diminution of the pain with rest, a history of puncture, systemic disease, lowered resistance, a large area of induration about the inflamed area, or local skin lesions. If there is doubt about the diagnosis, these superficial bursae should be aspirated and the fluid should be sent for Gram stain and culture.

Treatment. The hallmark of therapy with these lesions is, as in most cases of inflammatory disease, putting the affected part to rest. This is best accomplished with some form of splint, sling, or immobilizer. In addition to this, patients are started on a regimen of anti-inflammatory medication. Aspirin or one of the many nonsteroidal anti-inflammatory agents is chosen. Corticosteroids are rarely used but may be considered in cases in which there is no infection and anti-inflammatory agents have not provided relief. On rare occasion, it is necessary to excise recurrent, chronic bursae about the knee or elbow.

INFECTIONS

SEPTIC ARTHRITIS

History. In adults, there is generally some underlying process (*e.g.,* diabetes, rheumatoid arthritis, immunosuppression) that makes the patient susceptible to septic arthritis. The infecting organism generally enters the joint from a pre-existing infection in the body, either local or distant (*e.g.,* gallbladder, intestinal, bladder, or superficial skin infections). In the young adult, the most common cause of monoarticular arthritis is gonococcal infection. Penetrating injuries to a joint may lead to infection.

Physical Examination. On physical examination, the standard signs of infection about the joint (redness, heat, pain, and swelling) are found. The patient may voluntarily splint the extremity, and this is confirmed when range of motion is evaluated. Generally, any range of motion is painful for a patient with a septic joint. Lymphatic streaking, nodes proximal to the affected joint, or a rash may be found. Radiographic findings may range from soft tissue swelling or mild effusion to destructive changes of the articular surface or the metaphyseal bone. Laboratory studies should include a CBC to check for leukocytosis or anemia. The ESR may be a guide for treatment efficacy. The most definitive procedure is a joint aspiration. Joint aspirant should be evaluated for leukocyte count, Gram stain, culture and sensitivity, crystal analysis, and glucose. In general, in infective arthritis the leukocyte count is elevated (usually over 50,000/cu mm); the Gram stain may identify the infecting organism; the glucose is lowered (usually to about half the serum level); and crystal analysis is negative (unless the patient has associated crystalline arthropathy).

Treatment. Treatment of the septic joint is controversial. The internist's point of view is that multiple aspirations will suffice; however, most surgeons believe that formal arthrotomy is the best way to completely cleanse the joint. We believe that if septic arthritis is detected very early (less than 1 week), repeated aspirations and appropriate antibiotics given intravenously may provide adequate therapy. If there is any doubt whatsoever, we do not hesitate to perform an arthrotomy. Certain large weight-bearing joints such as the hip and the knee should be opened without question, especially if the process is chronic. Also, one should not hesitate to open the joint if repeated aspirations have failed to show satisfactory response.

Following irrigation and débridement, the patient's knee should be closed over a drain; in severe cases a suction-irrigation type drainage system may be required. The patient should be continued on intravenous antibiotics for at least 2 weeks. If the patient is clinically improved and the ESR begins to fall to half the pretreatment level, intravenous antibiotics should be discontinued and oral antibiotics are prescribed for 3 to 6 months.

OSTEOMYELITIS

Bone infections are a potentially devastating problem because they are very difficult, if not impossible, to eradicate. There is almost always an underlying problem or insult that contributes to the infection. These factors include open fracture, surgery, traction or fixator pins, systemic infection such as endocarditis or tuberculosis, and a compromised host. The site of infection is in bone where vascular sludging occurs, that is, in the watershed area of the distal diaphysis and in the vertebrae.

History. The symptoms of osteomyelitis are often insidious in onset and include pain, redness, swelling, disability, fever, chills, and malaise. The history should include an extensive search for underlying disorders that cause or contribute to the infection.

Physical Examination. The signs of osteomyelitis are those of infection, pain, redness, heat, swelling, fluctuance, and drainage. These signs are more difficult, if not impossible, to detect if in the vertebral column.

Diagnostic Tests. Blood studies may show anemia, leukocytosis with a left shift, an elevated ESR, and positive results of culture. Any drainage should be sent for Gram stain and culture. Soft tissue swelling and lytic lesions may be evident on the radiograph. In the case of chronic osteomyelitis, there may be a sequestrum (*i.e.,* an area of dead, dense bone) or an involucrum (*i.e.,* new bone formed around the infected area).

Treatment. The hallmark of treatment is drainage and débridement. Adequate débridement should be followed by appropriate intravenous antibiotics for at least 4 weeks. Then, if the infection is clearing rapidly and the ESR is falling, the patient can be placed on a chronic regimen of oral antibiotics.

DEGENERATIVE JOINT DISEASE

Osteoarthritis is perhaps the most common orthopaedic problem facing the adult population, and some people feel that it is the most common joint problem. It affects almost one half of the population over 60 years of age. Common sites are the lumbosacral spine, hip, knee, and hand.

Etiology. The exact etiology of osteoarthritis is the subject of heated debate. Many theories are being proposed, but it is generally regarded that osteoarthritis is secondary to altered mechanics. Suggested causes include incongruency of the joint surfaces secondary to trauma; poor lubrication of the joint by supporting structures that are fibrosed due to age or vascular insufficiency; and repeated trauma, causing hardening of the subchondral plate of bone and reduction of its capacity as a shock absorber. The first theory is supported by the high incidence of posttraumatic arthritis (especially intra-articular fractures). The second theory is supported by the fact that osteoarthritis is seen in the older age-group. The theory of repeated microtrauma causing osteoarthritis is supported by the findings of osteoarthritis in weight-bearing joints and in the elbow and shoulders of those using pneumatic drills, which subject these non-weight-bearing joints to repeated microtrauma. All of these processes are the result of demand exceeding the capacity of the joint and surrounding tissues to meet the joint's needs. As a result of altered mechanics, the articular surface is damaged and sloughed from the surface in much the same manner as wood dust is produced with sanding. It is through the synovium that this particulate matter is cleared, and these particles represent irritative foci to the synovium. Once the cartilage destruction begins, the mechanical properties of the joint are changed so that in addition to the initial insult, further degeneration of the joint occurs. When the synovium is irritated, it does a poorer job of lubricating. Another joint response is one of osteophyte production, which some believe is an effort by the joint to expand its surface area so as to spread out the stress. Further discussion will be confined to what is commonly known as osteoarthritis or hypertrophic arthritis.

History. The usual presenting symptom of osteoarthritis is pain or stiffness in the affected joint. Pain is generally aching in quality and has an insiduous onset, although a single incidence of excessive trauma may exacerbate the underlying problem. Such is the case with low back pain that has osteoarthritis as its underlying etiology. The pain is aggravated by motion of the joint and relieved by rest. Some people with this problem have what is called a warmup phenomenon. Initially, they have a painful, stiff joint that is improved in a few minutes after the joint is "warmed up." This is different from a joint with rheumatoid arthritis, which may be stiff for an hour in the morning. The pain in osteoarthritic joints is often relieved by salicylate or other anti-inflammatory medication.

Physical Examination. Physical examination of the patient with osteoarthritis often shows bony enlargement about the affected joint. This is especially evident in the knee, which is a subcutaneous joint. Another characteristic finding of osteoarthritis is Heberden's nodes, which are located at the distal interphalangeal joints in the fingers. At the knee, there may be genu varum (bow legs). These people have an antalgic, painful gait. One of the first signs of osteoarthritis is a limitation of range of motion. It should also be noted that the osteoarthritic patient uses every bit of his limited range of motion but will voluntarily limit himself to a smaller arc of motion. It is extremely painful to move beyond a certain endpoint regardless of whether the joint is moved actively or passively. Crepitation, effusion, and boggy synovium may be present.

Diagnostic Tests. Serum laboratory studies are generally not useful in the diagnosis of osteoarthritis; however, they may be useful in ruling out inflammatory processes. The radiographic examination is most helpful, with the findings generally being loss of joint space, representing loss of the articular cartilage; osteophytes, which are bony spurs at the margin of the joint; increased density at the subchondral plate, representing reactive bone laid down in response to microtrauma; and subchondral cystic lesions.

Treatment. Treatment of early stages of osteoarthritis consists mainly of salicylate therapy and judicious use of range of motion exercises as well as moderate exercise. Patients should be instructed not to exercise to the point of discomfort and to avoid any repetitive activity that aggravates the symptoms. Deep heat therapy is sometimes of use. When the affected joint is in a weight-bearing extremity, use of a cane will unload the joint sufficiently to decrease the destructive process on the joint surface. The next line of therapy should include the stronger anti-inflammatory agents such as nonsteroidal anti-inflammatory drugs. Corticosteroids are not given orally and are rarely given intra-articularly; if used, injections should not be done repeatedly. In more advanced cases of osteoarthritis in people who have already begun to limit their activities, a total joint replacement may be considered. The criteria for a total joint replacement vary from surgeon to surgeon, but it is generally believed that for a cemented total joint arthroplasty the patient should be over the age of 60, have a diminished activity demand, have rest pain such that sleep is severely limited at night, have failed nonoperative treatment, be cooperative, and understand the limitations of the total joint.

METABOLIC DISEASES

Bone is mineralized connective tissue. The components of the connective tissue matrix of bone are collagen and ground substances, which are chondroitin sulfate and keratosulfate. This matrix, which has some physical integrity of its own, is reinforced by calcium hydroxyapatite crystals. The mineralization process takes place while the collagen fibers and ground substance are being formed by the osteoblast. The crystals are deposited in and on the collagen fibers. Calcium ions on the surface are essentially tissue fluid ions and are readily accessible. The ions within the fibers are inaccessible until the collagen fibers are digested by enzymes produced by the osteoclast.

The formation and destruction of bone is a complex interaction of osteoblasts, which produce the matrix; osteoclasts, which degrade the matrix; and mechanical and physiological factors that control the mineralization process. The formation of bone requires the presence of matrix, oxygen, mechanical factors (*e.g.*, compression), hormones (especially parathormone), minerals (calcium and phosphorus), vitamins C and D, and alkaline phosphatase. These latter four are interrelated, and disorders involving these elements of bone formation are the basis of metabolic bone disease.

These diseases result in osteopenia, which is a total decrease in bone mass, and can be divided into two broad classes depending on the affected process. Osteoporosis is a matrix defect, and osteomalacia is an alteration in mineralization.

OSTEOPOROSIS

Osteoporosis plagues the elderly, especially women, and is responsible for many of the fractures in this group. The defect of osteoid synthesis in this disorder may be congenital or secondary to dietary deficiencies, endocrine imbalances, trauma, or lack of stress. Lack of vitamin C results in scurvy, and a diet deficient in protein may cause osteoporosis. Endocrine causes include lack of estrogen or androgen, hyperthyroidism, cortisone administration, or diabetes. In the latter three, the bone proteins are broken down to supply a source of energy (*e.g.,* gluconeogenesis in diabetes). Posttraumatic osteoporosis may be seen following even relatively minor trauma. The exact mechanism is uncertain but may be a neurogenic increase in blood flow or disuse. If the skeleton does not experience stress, the osteoblast will not be stimulated to produce osteoid. This is seen in patients with casted bones, those with bones under rigid plates (see section on fractures), patients placed at bed rest, and astronauts. The best example of congenital osteoporosis is osteogenesis imperfecta.

Clinical Presentation. The bone is mechanically weaker in osteoporosis, and these patients present with fractures of the femoral neck or compression fractures of the spine. The radiograph shows there is less bone and less density. The cortex is thinned and less dense, and the medullary cavity is widened. Laboratory studies are useful in the differential diagnosis. A biopsy is sometimes needed. Treatment consists of reversing the underlying cause, if possible. In addition, fluoride can be used; it replaces calcium in the crystals and makes them less resistant to resorption, but it also tends to make the bone more brittle.

OSTEOMALACIA

In osteomalacia the underlying disorder is mineralization of bone. This process requires calcium, phosphorus, and alkaline phosphatase. Only the disorders that affect calcium and phosphorus balance will be discussed.

The body maintains the serum calcium level at the expense of the bone. The level of calcium is dependent on levels of vitamin D, thyrocalcitonin, and phosphorus and on renal function, dietary intake, and gastrointestinal loss. This regulation is mediated through parathyroid hormone (PTH), and derangements of PTH can mimic metabolic bone disease.

Vitamin D is a fat-soluble vitamin that undergoes changes at the level of the skin, liver, and kidney, before reaching its fully active state. Its main function is to control serum calcium, which it does mainly by increasing gastrointestinal absorption and also by increasing release of calcium from the bone. (Hypervitaminosis D can cause widespread bone resorption.) Vitamin D deficiency can be the result of decreased intake, increased loss via steatorrhea or sprue, and lack of sunlight. In children, lack of vitamin D may result in rickets. In adults, lack of vitamin D leads to decreased absorption of calcium with resultant decreased serum calcium and increased bone loss.

Renal-induced osteomalacia is usually due to increased calcium loss. This leads to increased PTH production and increased loss from bone to maintain serum levels. Dietary deficiencies leading to osteomalacia are rare in people in developed nations due to the availability of foods high in calcium, such as dairy products. Pregnancy can lead to a calcium-deficient state, especially in the breast-feeding mother, when the pregnancies are multiple and closely spaced.

Clinical Presentation. Patients with osteomalacia may have pain in the back, pelvis, or hips that may be the result of pathologic fractures or microfractures. They may have deformities due to the decreased structural integrity of the bones. The radiograph may show increased lucency, coarse trabeculae, a focal lucent area, or deformities in weight-bearing bones. Biopsy is sometimes necessary to make a definite diagnosis. Treatment of osteomalacia is correction of the underlying disorder.

IATROGENIC DISEASES

In adult orthopaedics iatrogenic diseases, fortunately, are few in number. They are often the result of a necessary treatment for other systemic disorders. An example would be avascular necrosis of the femoral head caused by the use of corticosteroids as immunosuppression in the control of severe rheumatoid arthritis. Another example is radiation therapy for metastatic disease. Given in large enough doses, the radiation can cause a weakening in the structural aspects of the bone and thereby lead to pathologic fracture.

AFFLICTIONS OF SPECIFIC JOINTS

ELBOW

The elbow is a hinge joint with two major articulations: radiohumeral and ulnohumeral. In addition, there is a radioulnar joint that allows supination and pronation of the hand. Since the elbow is a non-weight-bearing joint, it is not usually affected by osteoarthritis. This joint is not a common site of orthopaedic pathology, so only one disorder, lateral epicondylitis (tennis elbow), will be discussed.

Although referred to as tennis elbow, this disorder is more commonly seen in people who do not play tennis. The disorder may be found in any person involved with gripping and wrist extension activities such as raking. The underlying problem is irritation at the site of the common extensor attachment.

Clinical Presentation. The patient presents with lateral elbow or forearm pain that is increased by gripping activities. There is usually the history of overuse or injury to the area. On examination, tenderness is evident just anterior to the lateral epicondyle of the humerus, which is increased by gripping and wrist dorsiflexion. Two good tests are as follows: (1) ask the patient to lift a chair by grasping it by the back with his palm upward, then downward; if the latter action is painful, the test is positive; (2) with the patient holding his fingers and wrist in neutral, push down on each finger individually. If pushing the middle finger reproduces the pain, this is correlative. Radiographs are of no help unless they show an avulsion of the lateral epicondyle.

Treatment. Treatment consists of rest and administration of anti-inflammatory agents, followed by a strengthening program and changing the factors that aggravate this area. It may be necessary to splint the wrist for a week or so. Usually aspirin is satisfactory for relief of pain. Rarely are corticosteroids injected into the area, and even more rarely is the common extensor attachment of the lateral epicondyle released. Another treatment program consists of administration of anti-inflammatory drugs and of wrist extension exercises. With the patient's hand over the edge of the table, he holds a small can and lifts the can up as many times as he can. This is done beginning with light cans and progressing to increasingly heavier ones. Tennis players can be helped by decreasing string tension of the racket, selecting the proper grip size, using the correct techniques, and using an arm band just distal to the elbow.

SHOULDER

The shoulder is the combination of three joints: glenohumeral, acromioclavicular, and scapulothoracic. Its main functions are lifting and positioning the hand. The glenohumeral joint is a non-weight-bearing, modified ball-and-socket joint that depends on muscles, ligaments, and capsule for its structural integrity. It is for these reasons that the shoulder is rarely affected by degenerative joint disease but is often affected by inflammatory diseases of the supporting structures (Fig. 44-25). The acromioclavicular joint is a rigid joint with close approximation of the joint surfaces; the major pathologic process in this joint is degenerative disease. The scapulothoracic joint is seldom symptomatic.

The history should include any injury, painful motion or limitation, dislocation, or subluxation. It is useful to know if the patient can sleep on the affected side; the answer may indicate a rotator cuff tear, bursitis, or acromioclavicular joint problems.

Physical examination should specifically note active and passive range of motion, motor power, and specific tests for problem areas. In treating shoulder disorders, rest can be accomplished with a sling or with a sling and a swathe. Prolonged use of immobilization, especially in older people, may lead to restricted motion and should be avoided.

ROTATOR CUFF TEAR

The rotator cuff is made up of the conjoined tendons of the subscapularis, supraspinatus, infraspinatus, and teres minor. In general, the defect is in the supraspinatus tendon portion. This injury may be a degenerative tear seen in older people or may be traumatic in a young person who has fallen on an abducted shoulder. On examination, there is weak or no abduction, weak external rotation, and tenderness over the insertion of the supraspinatus tendon (see Fig. 44-25). In partial tears the torn portion may impinge on the

Fig. 44-25. Common sites of shoulder pain. (*1*, acromioclavicular joint; *2*, subacromial bursa; *3*, greater tuberosity (site of rotator cuff attachment); *4*, bicipital groove; *5*, anterior capsule)

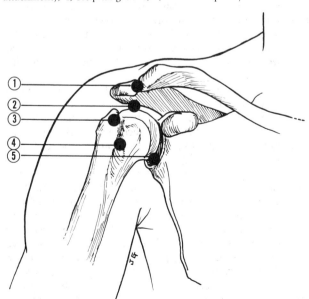

acromion or acromial clavicular ligament. Full abduction can be attained actively once the examiner passively moves the shoulder beyond this point of impingement. With the arm abducted 90°, this impingement can be noted as the arm is internally and externally rotated. Standard radiographs may show an avulsion of the supraspinatus attachment. The most definitive study is the arthrogram, which shows extravasation of the dye from the joint into the subacromial bursa. Treatment consists of primary repair, especially in young people. In the elderly physical therapy is recommended to teach ways of using the shoulder without the use of the supraspinatus.

BURSITIS

Bursitis in the shoulder usually refers to the subacromial bursa, which separates the supraspinatus tendon from the acromion. Patients generally have acute or subacute onset of severe pain following overuse of the shoulder. The pain is increased with motion and decreased by rest and administration of anti-inflammatory drugs. On examination, there are the signs of bursitis at or near the acromion. There is pain with active and passive motion. Amorphous calcification in the bursa may be seen on the radiograph. Treatment consists of rest (best accomplished with a sling) and administration of anti-inflammatory agents. Aspiration and injection of corticosteroids can be used if the shoulder does not respond. If calcification is present, aspiration can be attempted with a large-bore needle. Milky fluid will be obtained (*i.e.,* amorphous calcium). Aspiration is followed by injection of a small amount of corticosteroid.

BICIPITAL TENDINITIS

Inflammation of the synovial lining of the tendon as it passes through the bicipital groove in the anterior aspect of the humerus is an overuse problem with an acute or subacute onset. The signs of tenosynovitis in the bicipital groove are evident on physical examination. The motion that is most painful is shoulder flexion with the elbow extended and hand supinated (Speed's test). Treatment of this condition consists of rest and administration of anti-inflammatory agents; if this is not successful, corticosteroid injection may be necessary. Injections of corticosteroids should not be repeated more than once or twice. If severe problems persist, tenodesis (attachment of the tendon to the groove) should be considered.

ACROMIOCLAVICULAR ARTHRITIS

Disorders of the small acromioclavicular joint are a common cause of shoulder pain. The mechanics of the joint are altered by clavicle fractures and by partial acromioclavicular joint separation. Although almost anyone may have this problem, it seems to be more common in people engaged in strenuous labor. There is usually more pain with overhead activity, and the pain is often more chronic, with the patient complaining of crepitance. On physical examination, tenderness is generally present over the acromioclavicular joint. The pain is increased by compression of the joint, which is best done by bringing the arm across the chest with the shoulder partially abducted so that the elbow comes at least to the midline. Swelling and crepitation may or may not be present. Treatment is rest and administration of anti-inflammatory drugs, followed by injection of corticosteroids if there is no improvement. Results of the injection of a corticosteroid mixed with a local anesthetic are both diagnostic and therapeutic. If pain is relieved by this measure and then returns within a short time, excision of the distal clavicle, a procedure that affords relief of pain without any functional loss, should be strongly considered.

ADHESIVE CAPSULITIS

Sometimes called "frozen shoulder," adhesive capsulitis is the result of chronic restriction of shoulder motion. It is often the result of one of the above inflammatory processes, fractures, or dislocation. The patient may voluntarily limit shoulder motion, and this will lead to fibrosis and adhesions in the capsule of the glenohumeral joint. A vicious cycle may result. Any motion hurts, so the patient avoids any motion. The best treatment is prevention, and this is accomplished by putting the joint through a range of motion at least once a day. This is why patients, especially older ones, are begun on a program of physical therapy as soon as the inflammation has subsided. The findings of adhesive capsulitis are restricted active and passive shoulder motion in all planes, with diffuse pain in the shoulder. Sometimes the underlying inflammatory process can be determined and treated. The arthrogram shows reduced joint space as a result of adhesions. Treatment consists of administration of anti-inflammatory agents and intensive physical therapy. Occasionally, manipulation under anesthesia, injection of saline into the joint, or surgical release of the capsule is required.

LUMBAR SPINE

The lower spine is a complex area made up of a bony column through which pass the nerve roots to the lower extremities. Each bony segment meets its neighbor with three articulations: the intervertebral joint (disk space) and two facets posteriorly, which are synovial joints lined with articular cartilage. These joints are closely related and move as a unit. Each nerve root must pass by the disk and the facet joint on that side. Sources of pain include nerve roots, viscera, vascular structures, psychogenic problems, joints, capsule, and muscles. The last three are structural elements of the spine, and pain from these areas is called spondylogenic. These structures, not the disk, cause the majority of back pain.

Low back pain is perhaps the most common orthopaedic disorder. It affects nearly everyone at one time or another. It is the leading cause of lost work in younger workers and is a major cause of disability in the work force. Most physicians prefer not to see patients with back pain because they think the problem is chronic, diagnosis is difficult, treatment is complex, and results are only satisfactory at best. This need not be the case at all. Not all back pain is chronic. If back pain persisted indefinitely, nearly 100% of the adult population would be under treatment. With proper diagnosis and treatment the vast majority of patients who want improvement will get it. Diagnosis is based mainly on the history and physical examination. Because the back is hard to rest, the treatment response is slow.

History. The patient's history is very important in dealing with lumbar spine problems; the more information there is, the better. In addition to items mentioned earlier in this section, it is important to know the activity level of the patient and if any litigation is pending. If the patient has two pains or if the radiating pain is different, the history must be repeated for these as well. It is sometimes helpful to go through a day's activities with a patient to see what does and does not cause pain.

For example, spondylogenic back pain may be of slow or sudden onset; related to overuse or improper use; aching in nature; and located in the back or buttocks; with some radiating pain to the back of the legs but not to the feet. The pain is increased by bending and lifting and decreased by lying (often on one side with spine flexed) and anti-inflammatory agents. There is no lower extremity numbness or weakness. This is usually not the first episode. It is commonly seen in laborers and heavy machinery operators, and often legal claims surround it.

Nerve root pain may or may not be of sudden onset. The pain is sharp, burning, and strange (*e.g.,* tingling, knifelike) and radiates in a lancinating fashion along the course of the sciatic nerve to the leg and often to the foot. It is increased by standing or sitting (especially in low car seats). There may be associated numbness and weakness. Medication is of little benefit. These people are usually concerned about one thing: getting rid of the pain.

Physical Examination. The examination begins when the patient enters the room and continues during the history. How uncomfortable does the patient look? Formal examination begins with the gait, watching for limp, weakness, and walking posture. While the patient is standing, he is evaluated for posture alignment, abnormal skin creases, hair patterns in the back, and scars. Range of motion testing is carried out. It is important to know which motion causes the most pain. The muscles are also tested with the patient standing on one leg, on one tiptoe, and step-walking. The painful area is localized by the patient by touching the area with one finger only. The back, pelvis, and the course of the sciatic nerve are then palpated.

The patient is then asked to lie down, and this motion is observed. With the patient supine, the abdomen and pulses are palpated. Range of motion, sensation, deep tendon reflexes, and motor strength of the lower extremities are checked. The neurologic examination of the lower extremity becomes easy when you know that each joint is innervated by four nerve root levels; thus the hip is supplied by L2, L3, L4, and L5. Innervation of the next distal joint begins with the next lower level; thus the knee is supplied by L3, L4, L5, and S1, and the ankle, by L4, L5, S1, and S2. The upper two nerve roots to each joint supply the muscles that bring the joint into the anterior plane (*i.e.,* hip flexion, knee extension, and ankle dorsiflexion). The lower two nerve roots move the limb posteriorly (Fig. 44-26). Sensory levels are shown in Figure 44-27. One only has to remember "3 at the knee" to know the sensory level and motor level; then work up one root level for the hip and down one for the foot and ankle.

The straight leg raising test is next. To be indicative of a nerve root problem, it must be positive at 30° or less for the same pain described in the history. A bilateral leg lift test is performed to check for mechanical back pain (*e.g.,* facet joints). A rectal examination should be done if neurologic problems are suggested.

A patient with facet joint arthritis will move slowly and stiffly and be hunched over with the lumbar spine held rigid. There will be decreased motion; extension and twisting will cause pain, as may lying flat on the back. Usually there is no motor weakness or neurologic defects. The results of the straight leg raising test are negative and those of active bilateral straight leg lifting are positive for back pain. There is tenderness on manipulation of the spinous processes.

Patients with nerve root lesions vary with regard to mobility, muscle spasm, and posture. The best signs are presence of a neurologic defect, positive results of straight leg raising at 30° or less, and positive results of contralateral straight leg raising (raising one leg reproduces pain in the other).

Diagnostic Tests. In general, radiographs add little to a good history and physical. They may show degenerative joint disease (Fig. 44-28), congenital defects, or compression fractures. These findings must correlate with the history and physical findings or they are of no meaning. Laboratory studies are not generally required but may include CBC, ESR, calcium and phosphorus determinations, and urinalysis. Myelography is done on patients who have the picture of a diskogenic problem and are possible surgical candidates. Bone scans may be of help in identifying occult lesions such as tumors or myeloma.

Treatment. The hallmark of such therapy for mechanical or spondylogenic problems is rest and administration of anti-inflammatory agents, followed by learning proper me-

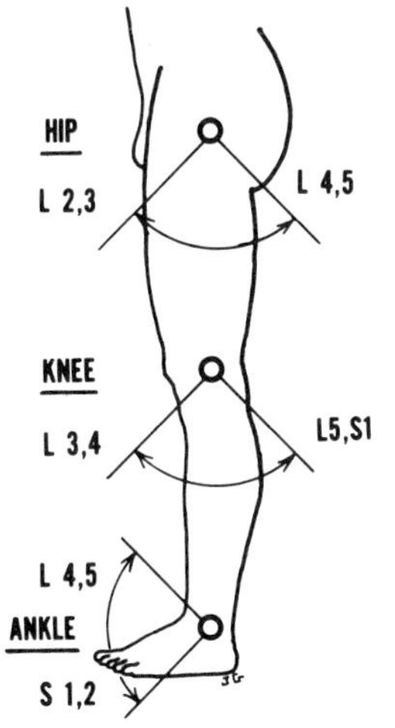

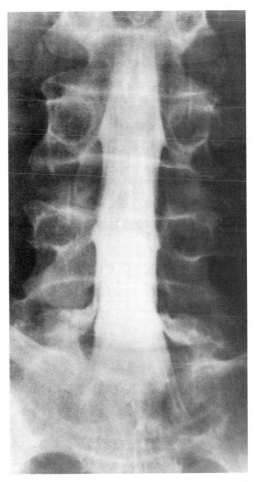

Fig. 44-28. Degenerative arthritis of the spine. The severe lipping at the facet joints at the L5–S1 junction in comparison to the level above can cause a defect in the dye column of this myelogram.

chanics. The latter is most important for preventing further problems. Rest is difficult to accomplish because the spine is weight bearing and in nearly constant motion. Bed rest in a comfortable position is the best form of rest for the spine. In some very active patients, bed rest is not an option; the patients are told that a cure will be delayed and are placed in a corset, which thus acts as a reminder and increases the abdominal muscle tone, which in turn helps support the spine. For patients with severe pain that does not respond, facet joint injections with corticosteroids and local anesthetics are considered as both diagnostic and therapeutic measures. If pain is relieved and then returns, surgical fusion is strongly advised.

If there is strong evidence of nerve root entrapment, the treatment is strict bed rest for 2 to 4 weeks, in a hospital if necessary. If the patient's condition is still unimproved, an electromyogram (EMG), bone scan, and myelogram are obtained. If the EMG shows changes and the myelogram is positive for a herniated disk, the option of surgery is offered to the patient. It should be noted that most patients will improve with nonoperative therapy.

HIP

The hip is a large weight-bearing ball-and-socket joint that is quite stable owing to its bony configuration. There are

Fig. 44-26. Innervation of lower extremity movement. Each joint is innervated by four root levels. At each joint the upper two levels bring the leg into a more anterior position (the same motion used in kicking a field goal!). L3 is the uppermost root to the knee.

Fig. 44-27. Sensory innervation of the lower extremity. L3 innervates the knee.

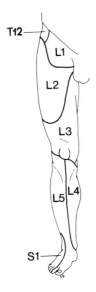

tremendous forces across the joint due to weight-bearing and muscular balancing forces. For this reason, the hip is a joint that is prone to osteoarthritis and fractures in older patients. It should be noted that hip problems present as groin pain, medial thigh pain, or knee pain. Pain from the hip is seldom referred to the buttock.

OSTEOARTHRITIS

Osteoarthritis of the hip is relatively common in the older age-group. The onset is usually gradual, beginning as an aching pain with weight-bearing. The patient may complain of limitation in motion, usually internal rotation and abduction. The pain is relieved by sitting and lying. Positive physical findings may include painful gait, weakness, decreased range of motion, and limb shortening. Radiographic findings include decreased joint space, increased subchondral bone density, osteophytes, and subchondral cysts.

Treatment consists of exercises to maintain range of motion, administration of anti-inflammatory agents, and use of a cane (to reduce the forces across the joint). Osteotomy or total hip relacement is considered in the older patient who is not helped by nonoperative therapy. Severe rest pain and decreased mobility are primary indications for arthroplasty.

SEPTIC ARTHRITIS

Septic arthritis is a difficult problem because the joint is deep and the usual signs of erythema and swelling are absent or not appreciated. For this reason, considerable damage is done by the time the diagnosis is made. The examiner should be wary of sudden onset of pain in compromised patients with any constitutional symptoms. The signs of septic arthritis are present, and there is pain with any motion, not just at the ends of motion. The ESR should be elevated. Anemia and leukocytosis may be present.

Definitive diagnosis consists of aspiration with synovial fluid analysis and culture. Treatment must include arthrotomy for drainage and removal of any necrotic material. This often leaves the patient with massive bone loss and what is called a girdlestone-type hip, which may be converted at a future time to a fusion or total hip replacement if the infection is completely cleared.

AVASCULAR NECROSIS

Avascular necrosis is due to the disruption of vascular supply to a section of bone and is most commonly seen in the head of the femur. It can be caused by trauma, embolism (caisson worker disease), radiation, systemic diseases (polycythemia, lupus, Gaucher's disease, sickle cell, and gout), idiopathic factors (seen in alcohol abusers), and iatrogenic factors (high dose of corticosteroids). There are three stages of disease: initial insult and early repair, delayed repair and pathological fracture, and late collapse. Stage I is painless and may show only a rim of reactive bone (dense bone) around the area. In stage II, there is pain due to the fracture and there is a depression type fracture below the subchondral bone. In stage III, the collapse increases and the support for the articular cartilage is lost.

Aseptic necrosis is treated initially by avoidance of weight-bearing, by drilling multiple holes into the infarcted area, or by placing bone pegs to support the subchondral bone. Once collapse has occurred, these measures are usually unsuccessful and the treatment is similar to that of osteoarthritis.

KNEE

The knee is a large joint that is actually two joints: the tibiofemoral and the patellofemoral. The tibial-femoral joint is a hinged weight-bearing joint with menisci aiding in distributing the weight-bearing forces across the joint. Like the shoulder and unlike the hip, the knee joint has little inherent stability and depends on ligamentous support for stability. The patellar femoral joint is a gliding joint whose function is to increase the mechnical advantage of the quadriceps.

The history should include injury, tricking (subluxation), giving way, locking, swelling, noises heard at the time of injury (*i.e.,* "pops") and results of previous aspiration (*i.e.,* blood, crystals, infection). The specifics of the physical examination will be covered below.

PATELLAR DISORDERS

The three major disorders of the patella (chondromalacia, subluxation, and plicas) are difficult to distinguish and often require arthroscopy to diagnose.

Chondromalacia is a softening of the articular cartilage of patella and is characterized by a vague aching pain around or under the knee cap. The patient may note grinding. The pain is increased by stair climbing and squatting, and decreased by rest, ingestion of aspirin, and straight-legged walking. On physical examination, there is subpatellar pain, crepitation, pain with patellar compression against the femur, and quadriceps atrophy (especially the vastus medialis). Treatment consists of quadriceps strengthening in the form of short-arc quadriceps exercises (from 0° to 20° of flexion) and administration of aspirin and vitamin C. Activities that aggravate symptoms are to be avoided. This therapy should be maintained for 3 months. If the patient is not improving, arthroscopy of the knee is done to make a definitive diagnosis and treatment is provided as necessary.

Patellar subluxation may be confused with chondromalacia or a cause of it. The physician must check for any history of subluxation or injury that may have caused an occult subluxation without actual dislocation. This could include blows from the medial side and sudden forcible extension of the leg with the foot externally rotated. The examiner must check for medial retinacular pain, abnormal tracking of the patella, high Q-angle, and pain with attempts to sublux the patella. Acute treatment consists of extension splinting with straight-leg raising exercises for 4 weeks, followed by gentle range of motion and short-arc quadriceps exercises. If symptoms persist, a lateral retinacular release can be done; if this is unsuccessful, formal extensor mechanism realignment is done.

Another disorder confused with chondromalacia is the symptomatic plica. This is the presence of a rudimentary band of tissue or synovium that may attach to the patella. If this becomes inflamed from trauma or overuse, it can cause patellar pain. There is tenderness along the edge of the medial femoral condyle and sometimes a distinct snapping can be felt. Treatment consists of rest, administration of anti-inflammatory agents (beginning with aspirin), and avoidance of activities that aggravate the symptoms. If this is unsuccessful, the plica is excised arthroscopically.

MENISCAL PROBLEMS

The menisci increase the joint congruency, thereby assisting in weight distribution and acting as secondary stabilizers (after the ligaments and capsule). They are at high risk for injury if the primary stabilizers (*i.e.*, the ligaments) are deficient. Injury usually occurs when the knee is flexed, bearing weight, and rotated. The most reliable symptom is locking, meaning that the patient is unable to straighten his leg without manipulation. There is often tenderness over the meniscus or clicking felt at the edge of meniscus. Double-contrast arthrography is very useful for the diagnosis of medial lesions, with results being positive about 95% of the time; it is less useful for lateral lesions. The combination of arthrography and arthroscopy is nearly 100% accurate in the diagnosis of meniscal lesions. Treatment of the meniscal lesion depends on symptoms experienced by the patient, on the skill of the surgeon, and on what equipment is available. For example, a bucket handle tear that cannot be reduced (*i.e.*, knee remains locked) could be treated by arthroscopic excision of the displaced portion or by arthrotomy and meniscectomy.

ARTHRITIS

The knee is commonly affected by both degenerative and inflammatory arthritis. Synovial involvement in rheumatoid arthritis affects the intra-articular ligamentous structures as well as the joint surface, leaving the patient with an unstable, painful knee. The instability can be reduced with the use of braces, and the pain should respond to standard rheumatoid arthritis management. If the patient is losing mobility and experiencing unrelenting pain, then total knee arthroplasty should be considered in the older patient and synovectomy, in the younger patient.

Degenerative arthritis of the knee can be due to ligamentous instability, loss of menisci, improper alignment (usually genu varus), or previous joint fracture or is idiopathic. Basic treatment is described in the section on degenerative joint disease. When conservative methods have failed, one of the following is considered: fusion, usually for the young worker with normal alignment when a total knee replacement would surely fail; osteotomy in the patient with alignment deformity; total knee replacement for the older, less active patient; and arthroscopic or open débridement in any of the above patients in order to achieve 1 to 3 years of relief before a definitive procedure is needed. An example of the latter case is a 63-year-old teacher without angular deformity who is planning to retire in 2 years and whose activity demands at that time will be compatible with those obtained by way of a total knee arthroplasty. This patient underwent arthroscopic débridement in order to postpone the eventual arthroplasty until he could retire.

FOOT

The foot (Fig. 44-29) is a complex structure that supports and propels the entire body. The foot is made up of 26 bones, supporting ligamentous structures, and musculotendinous units that originate in the lower leg and the foot itself. The overall design of the foot is similar to the hand, with adaptations made to withstand the large stresses at the sacrifice of dexterity.

The foot is prone to problems that the other parts of the body are not. The reasons for these problems are many. First, the foot is more prone to vascular and healing problems because of lower arterial pressures and poor venous return owing to dependency. Next, civilized people are hard on their feet; walking on hard surfaces and in hot, poorly fitting shoes leads to many problems. Many of today's foot problems are a result of this abuse.

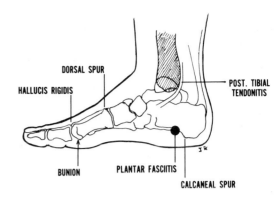

Fig. 44-29. Painful areas of the medial foot.

When a history is obtained from a patient with foot disorders, it is important to know whether there is any previous history of foot trouble and how it was treated; the type of work the person does; the amount of time spent on the feet; the type of footwear; the presence of any systemic or vascular disease; and the presence of any neuromuscular disorders. The physical examination of the person with foot pain should consist of the basic examination as well as special attention to the patient's gait, stance, basic foot type (*i.e.*, flat foot or highly arched foot), skin condition, calluses, and nail problems. Equally as important is the examination of the patient's shoes to determine the wear pattern.

STRUCTURAL DEFORMITIES

Normal architecture varies widely in the foot, ranging from wide, flexible flat feet (pes planus) to narrow, rigid, highly arched feet (pes cavus). These abnormalities are not generally problematic unless subjected to additional stress. When subjected to excessive stress, the rigid foot is susceptible to stress fractures of the metatarsals. The flat foot tends to have more muscular/ligamentous problems since these are the structures that offer support to the flat foot. Treatment for both is rest. For the patient with a planus foot, this may mean rigid arch supports; for those with a cavus foot, use of crutches or soft arch supports is recommended.

JOINT DISORDERS

Hallux valgus (bunions) is a disorder of the first metatarsophalangeal joint. It may be congenital (the result of a widened angle between the first and second metatarsal) or acquired (the result of narrow shoes, often with high heels).

The presenting complaint is pain, deformity, or both. The feet are generally supple and often splay type (*i.e.*, they become much wider when weight bearing). Treatment consists of improved footwear with low heel and wide toe box and stretch. Splinting may be of help, and surgery is indicated if nonoperative methods fail. Surgery is more aggressive in the symptomatic young adult. A bunionette is similar to a bunion, but it is located at the fifth metatarsophalangeal joint. Treatment is the same as for bunions.

Hallux rigidus is the result of arthritic spurs on the first metatarsal at the metatarsophalangeal joint with block extension at this joint. When extension is blocked at 20° or less, the patient is unable to walk normally and must roll the foot to one side or the other. This painful condition can be treated nonoperatively with a metatarsal bar placed on the shoes just proximal to the metatarsal heads. This substitutes for the loss of extension. Operative management consists of excising the spurs in younger patients with an otherwise normal joint or of a prosthetic implant for older patients with more severe joint involvement.

Dorsal spurs are also seen at the first metatarsal cuneiform joint. These are often painful and may have an inflamed bursa overlying the spur. These are best treated with pads to relieve the affected area and by excision of the spur if symptoms persist.

Metatarsalgia is a term used to describe pain in the area of the metatarsal heads. If it occurs in the area of the first metatarsal, it could be due to hallux valgus, hallux rigidus, or sesamoiditis. If in the area of the second toe, it could be due to a Morton's toe (abnormally long second ray). Other causes of metatarsalgia are avascular necrosis (Frieberg's disease) of the metatarsal head, stress fracture, rheumatoid arthritis, inflammation, and hammertoes that cause undue pressure to be placed on the metatarsal heads.

HIND FOOT SOFT TISSUE INFLAMMATION

Three soft tissue inflammatory processes found in the hind part of the foot are posterior tibial tendinitis, Achilles tendinitis, and plantar fasciitis. As in most soft tissue inflammations, these processes are usually the result of overuse. Treatment consists of rest and administration of anti-inflammatory drugs. Posterior tibial tendinitis is often seen in people with flat feet, and the pain is along the course of the tendon from behind the medial malleolus to the attachment on the inferomedial aspect of the navicular bone. Partial rest can be accomplished with the use of arch supports. Achilles tendinitis is located along the tendon and at its attachment to the calcaneus. A small heel lift will decrease the strain on the tendon attachment. Plantar fasciitis is manifested by pain on the medial distal calcaneus and along the plantar fascia. This is to be distinguished from heel pain (policeman's heel), which is directly on the bottom of the calcaneus (see Fig. 44-29). Plantar fascia pain is increased by placing the arch under stress by pushing up on the metatarsal heads and dorsiflexing the toes. Treatment is aided by firm arch supports. Anti-inflammatory medication is used in conjunction with the above devices. Corticosteroid injection is avoided, especially into the Achilles area. Surgery is rarely needed.

MORTON'S NEUROMA

Morton's neuroma is fibrosis of the common digital nerve to the toes (usually the third and fourth toes) and is generally caused by pressure from the metatarsal heads where the nerve passes between them. Patients complain of pain on weight-bearing and may have decreased sensation. A mass can often be palpated. Nonoperative treatment consists of proper width shoes and a metatarsal pad. Operative management consists of removal of the neuroma and at least 1 cm of nerve proximally.

NEW ADVANCES

TOTAL JOINT REPLACEMENT

Total joints are a relatively new advance in orthopaedics and have been constantly improved as a result of better design and materials. Almost any joint can be replaced; the more common are the hip, knee, and elbow. In the larger joints, the components are made of a combination of high-density polyethylene and metal and are usually held in

place with methyl methacrylate cement; this is not glue but is more like grouting. The smaller joints are usually made of special Silastic material and not cemented.

If the indications and limitations are understood, the patients can benefit tremendously. The major indication for total joint replacement is pain or marked impairment of mobility. Pain relief is dramatic, and function is often improved after replacement owing to improved alignment and increased range of motion.

Total joints fail because the implants fatigue with stress (breakage), the interface between implants and bone fails (loosening), and the joint can become infected (with resultant loosening). If breakage, loosening, or infection occurs, the prosthesis must be replaced. This is not always possible owing to loss of bone stock (a result of the original procedure or débridement to remove the implant or infected tissue). If it cannot be replaced, the patient faces a fusion, flail joint, or amputation. Therefore older, less active patients with severe pain are chosen as suitable candidates. For the younger, more active patients fusion is recommended.

Newer developments include improved design, materials, and methods. Work is progressing on prostheses that do not require cement for fixation. Other investigators are using antibiotics in the cement to reduce infection.

ARTHROSCOPY

Arthroscopy is not a new concept, but it has gained increasing popularity with recent advances in instrumentation and techniques. Scopes are now sophisticated fiber-optic instruments and can be connected to tiny television cameras. New instruments and techniques now allow the skilled arthroscopist to perform many procedures that previously required arthrotomy (*e.g.,* meniscectomy).

Used mainly in the knee, arthroscopy enables the surgeon to make accurate diagnosis of intra-articular lesions such as meniscal tears, ligament damage, and loose bodies. With the proper equipment, the following procedures are possible: meniscectomy, removal of loose bodies, débridement, biopsy, and retinacular releases. Indications for knee arthroscopy include any of the leg diagnoses listed above, vague persistent knee problems, and locking wih negative results of arthrography.

Arthroscopy has many advantages and few disadvantages. Advantages include negligible chance of infection (no reported cases of infection when arthroscopy alone is performed), small incisions, and decreased rehabilitation. Disadvantages are the need for special tools and the mastery of difficult techniques.

BIBLIOGRAPHY

Aegerter E, Kilpatrick JA Jr: Orthopedic Diseases, 4th ed. Philadelphia, W B Saunders, 1975

Cailliet R: Shoulder Pain. Philadelphia, F A Davis, 1975

Cailliet R: Foot and Ankle Pain. Philadelphia, F A Davis, 1978

Enneking WF: Clinical Musculoskeletal Pathology. Gainesville, FL, W F Enneking, 1977

Ficat RP, Hungerford DS: Disorders of the Patellar Femoral Joint. Baltimore, Williams & Wilkins, 1977

Hoppenfeld S: Physical Examination of the Spine and Extremities. New York, Appleton-Century-Crofts, 1976

Mann RA: Duvrie's Surgery of the Foot, 4th ed. St. Louis, C V Mosby, 1978

O'Connor RL: Arthroscopy. Philadelphia, J B Lippincott, 1977

Rodnam GP (ed): Primer on rheumatic diseases. JAMA 224 (suppl):1, 1973

Squire LF: Fundamentals of Radiology. Cambridge, MA, Harvard University Press, 1975

Luther C. Fisher III

Orthopaedic Disorders in Children

Some of the more common orthopaedic conditions of the growing child are discussed in this section. It is important to remember that these conditions may have their beginnings in one or more of a variety of different sources, including congenital, perinatal, developmental, metabolic, or traumatic etiologic factors. The uniqueness of pediatric orthopaedics, as opposed to adult orthopaedics, lies partially in the fact that the pediatric skeleton and other tissues are still in the developmental state and that growth and maturation are powerful forces for the improvement or deterioration of the condition. Before considering a particular problem in this field, it is necessary to look at the problem, not only as it stands now, but as it was in the past and as it will be in the future, modified by the future growth and development.

CEREBRAL PALSY

Cerebral palsy is a nonprogressive disorder of the immature central nervous system (CNS) that is caused by an irreparable lesion and is characterized by disorders of movement and posture. The term *cerebral palsy* is slightly misleading because it does not designate a specific disease in the normal sense of the word. It is a useful term, in that it covers a group of individuals handicapped by motor disorders of the brain that are not progressive. In addition to the motor disorders, it may include many other abnormalities, including mental retardation, eye problems, seizure disorders, and speech and hearing abnormalities.

INCIDENCE

The incidence of cerebral palsy has been estimated in various studies to range between 0.6 and 5.9 per 1,000 births. Approximately 25,000 affected children are born each year.

ETIOLOGY AND PATHOGENESIS

Cerebral palsy is caused by a nonprogressive brain lesion arising from prenatal, natal, or postnatal causes.

DIAGNOSIS

The diagnosis of cerebral palsy is often difficult in the first months of life. On the other hand, it is quite important to recognize this condition as early as possible for several reasons. The earlier the diagnosis is made, the earlier the treatment can begin and, therefore, the better the ultimate prognosis will generally be. Also, the sooner the family is made aware that the child is not normal, the better they will be able to deal with the reality of it and to modify their life accordingly. It is not uncommon for the child's mother to recognize within the first 2 to 4 months that the child is not developing normally and to take the child from physician to physician before a definitive diagnosis is established and a treatment program is begun.

In the first few months of life, the child frequently does appear normal. The earlier manifestations are often abnormal muscle tone or the failure of the infant to meet the usual developmental milestones at the proper time. Parents with older children are quite aware of the ages that infants should turn over, sit up, or say their first few words, and when their infant does not respond accordingly, the parents and physicians are alerted. The infant may demonstrate abnormal muscle tone or, less commonly, a dystonic type movement. Occasionally, the hypotonic or "floppy baby" syndrome will evolve to another type of abnormal muscle tone. Adventitious movements are sometimes present.

Normal flexor tone diminishes by 4 months of age, and if this persists to any great extent beyond this time, this is abnormal. Persistent primitive reflexes such as Moro, tonic neck, rooting, or sucking reflexes and others present after 6 months of age would suggest further examination.

Spasticity is manifested by increased stretch reflexes, hyperreflexia, clonus, a positive Babinski sign, and esotropia or exotropia. In athetosis of the tension type, the tension or tightness may be "shaken out" of the limb by the examiner. There is usually an extensor pattern, with normal or depressed deep tendon reflexes. Athetosis without the superimposed tension response consists of dystonic movements of the extremities, trunk, and head. Chorea is manifested by spontaneous jerking of the distal joints, whereas ataxia is seen as a lack of balance, uncoordinated movements, dysmetria, dysarthria, wide-based gait, and commonly pes valgus. The mixed types are frequently a mixture of spasticity and athetosis and often consist of total body involvement.

Monoplegia refers to the involvement of only one extremity. It is rare and usually is accompanied by spasticity. Hemiplegia involves spasticity of the upper and lower extremities on the same side of the body, and in order to exclude it the patient should be asked to run. Paraplegia is involvement of only the lower extremities and is rare. It is more common in patients with the familial type spasticity. Diplegia consists of minor involvement of upper extremities and of major involvement of the lower extremities, consisting of spasticity. Triplegia consists of involvement of three extremities, and quadriplegia is manifested by total body involvement (all four limbs, head, neck, and trunk); it may be spastic, athetoid, or mixed.

Many patients with cerebral palsy have other neurologic abnormalities due to the CNS lesions, which may be major determinants of the overall prognosis. In 1970 Tablan reported that 11.7% of patients had two disabilities, 40% had three disabilities, 32% had four disabilities, 11.7% had five disabilities, 3% had six disabilities, and 1.6% had seven disabilities. Eighty-two percent had speech problems, 34% had visual defects, 32% demonstrated hyperkinetic behavior, 19% were mentally retarded, 15% had some deafness, and 13.6% had perceptual difficulties. In 1961 Henderson reported that 25% had speech problems, 25% had epilepsy, 58% had visual defects, 50% were mentally retarded, and 33% demonstrated some deafness (Table 44-1).

DIFFERENTIAL DIAGNOSIS

The differential diagnosis is quite extensive. For that reason, it is very important to have as a member of the treatment team a pediatric neurologist or a pediatrician who is knowledgeable and interested in this area of pediatric practice. Because of the extensive nature of the differential diagnosis, it is impossible to go into much detail here. It is important to remember that this heterogeneous group of entities lumped under the general term *cerebral palsy* is nonprogressive. As the motor manifestations of the disability mature, they sometimes change, and further deformities and contractures are manifested with growth. On the other hand, if deterioration of the condition occurs, it is mandatory that the diagnosis be reviewed. Jones provided an extensive differential diagnosis in 1975.

TREATMENT

The treatment of the cerebral-palsied child is a multidisciplinary endeavor requiring a large team of specialists. Communication among this team is extremely important to ensure continuity of care, appropriate treatment of all of the aspects of the disease, appropriate communication with the parents, and setting of valid goals. After 12 to 18 months, it is usually possible to begin setting tentative goals for the patient's treatment. It is to be understood that as time goes on, the manifestations of the central lesion may be altered somewhat and the peripheral response may appear to be different. The goals can always be changed, but it is important to think in terms of the individual patient's possibilities. If it appears as though the patient will never walk, it is necessary to help the parents begin to accept this. It is not good to unduly discourage the parents or the patients, but it is helpful to begin early to concentrate therapeutic energies in directions that will be most productive. It is only natural for a parent to concentrate heavily on their child's ambulation; but if the patient's potential for walking is minimal, this wastes valuable time that can be put into work on the other developmental aspects. On the other hand, some parents are content to carry the child around and perform every function for the child at the expense of that patient's own personal development. Occasionally, it is necessary to encourage the parents to recognize their full responsibility in maximizing the potential that the patient does have. It is sometimes necessary to point out to parents that their child is easy to take care of while young and relatively small but that the child is growing bigger and heavier while the parent is also getting older.

TABLE 44-1 **COMMON CAUSES OF CEREBRAL PALSY WITH VARIOUS MOTOR MANIFESTATIONS**

MOTOR INVOLVEMENT	COMMON CAUSES
Spasticity	Prenatal hypoxia, prematurity, cerebral trauma, maternal rubella, and familial causes
Athetosis	Kernicterus due to Rh incompatibility
Chorea	Neonatal jaundice, hyperbilirubinemia, cerebral anoxia, encephalitis, and meningitis
Ataxia	Head injury and cerebral maldevelopment, encephalitis, cerebral anoxia, and birth trauma

Therefore, one of their prime functions as a parent is to help and encourage the patient to become as independent as possible.

PHYSICAL THERAPY

Following a thorough evaluation and diagnosis, physical therapy treatment should begin promptly. It is the first line of defense in the therapeutic program for the cerebral-palsied child, and it continues throughout the growing period and often into adult life. The physical therapist develops an exercise program to stretch the tight muscles, thereby maintaining normal ranges of motion of the involved joints. The patient's parents are drawn into the treatment program as early as possible and will continue the exercises on a daily basis with a periodic review by the physical therapist.

Another important effort of the physical therapy program is to encourage and guide the patient in the "developmental sequence." The normal child undergoes a sequential development of gross motor skills, fine motor skills, social skills, language skills, and cognitive skills, which seem to be the result of interaction of the child and his environment. When the child is delayed in both motor and mental development this process is slowed. The physical therapist directs the patient through a sequence of "play-like" activities to aid in this process of stepwise development. These activities will also help to break up or discourage persistent primitive reflexes and to develop the more mature reflexes necessary for sitting and walking.

In watching normal children develop, it appears as though balance is almost an automatic response to growth. In the young child with a disorder in motor development, balance, at times, must be a learned behavior. The child first learns to roll over and eventually to control the head, to sit up, and then to control the trunk. Head balance and trunk balance must first precede the development of standing balance. The process sometimes includes teaching the child to put the appropriate hand out to catch himself if he begins to lean in one direction or the other. The simple, more basic maneuvers must be learned before the patient will be able to walk.

In the earlier days of bracing for cerebral palsy, it was not uncommon to see patients with braces from the toes to the upper spine. These were full control braces with long leg braces, hip joints, pelvic bands, and spinal supports attached. In recent years, with the advent of a more functional, dynamic approach to the treatment of cerebral palsy, bracing has been reduced to a minimum, with the most common type of support being below-knee braces. The basic purposes of braces are to provide stability, prevent deformities, and inhibit primitive reflexes.

Seating devices are used basically for two reasons. One is in the developmental sequence program in order to learn head and trunk control and to be supported in the upright position to improve gross motor and fine motor control of the upper extremities. Second, seating devices are necessary for those patients who will not be independent ambulators. A wide variety of seating devices are available, depending on the age and size of the person, the need of the patient, and the degree that the patient is handicapped. These range all of the way from the simple umbrella stroller used for normal infants to the modular plastic insert (MPI) system (Fig. 44-30).

As a patient continues to improve, developmentally, and to gain head and eventually trunk control, the different

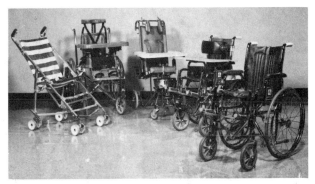

Fig. 44-30. Types of mobile seating devices used for patients with cerebral palsy.

supports added to the seating device can be removed in order to allow greater freedom of mobility and development for the child.

Standing supports are used in conjunction with the developmental sequence program to develop trunk control and to help develop balance and strength of the lower extremities. These basically include the prone stander and the standing table (Fig. 44-31).

SURGERY

Most of the surgery outlined below is performed in those patients with spasticity. Operative treatment is seldom indicated in patients with athetoid or ataxic cerebral palsy. They do not respond in the same way as patients with spasticity, and the common operations are often destructive to function. Occasionally, stabilization surgery on the feet is helpful, as well as spinal instrumentation and arthrodesis for severe scoliosis.

In the musculoskeletal realm, development of proper motor mechanisms is the basic aim of therapy. From the onset of treatment, efforts should be directed toward developing controlled function and preventing fixed deformity. Surgical treatment is a very important part of the overall rehabilitative process in that it can affect reduction of deformity, establish better balance of muscle power between flexors and extensors, and decrease the spasticity of muscles, thereby simplifying the problems of control. The timing and coordination of surgical procedures are also very important considerations. It is helpful to do most of the necessary procedures between the ages of 2 and 5 to help the child reach his maximum capabilities prior to school age. It is also wise to do several different operations at one time to decrease the period of recumbency and rehabilitation that might be necessary for multiple procedures.

Lower Extremity

Preoperative Considerations. The typical gait in spasticity is a "crouched" gait with flexion of the hips and knees and equinus of the feet and ankles; the patient ends up walking on his toes or, more accurately, the metatarsal heads (Fig. 44-32). Opinion is divided as to the most appropriate joint with which to begin the surgical releases. There seems to be little evidence to support an approach that begins with lengthening the achilles tendon, except in mild cases with only gastrocnemius-soleus muscle contractures. Either the knees or hips are released first, or both are released simultaneously. Once this is done, it is not uncommon to find the patient walking with his feet flat on the floor.

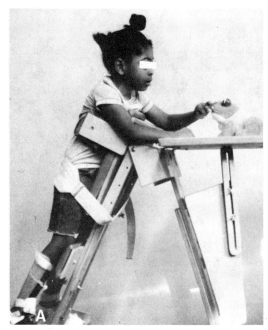
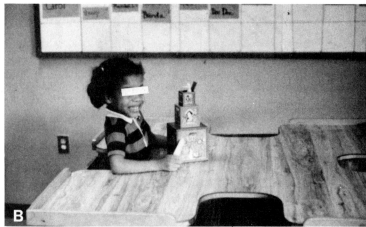

Fig. 44-31. (*A*) Prone stander. (*B*) Standing table.

Hip subluxation and dislocation needs to be diagnosed quite early and treated appropriately. There is a tendency to view hip displacement as having lesser importance, particularly in patients who will not ambulate. Hip displacement should be treated vigorously in all patients because of the complications of an uneven sitting posture and subsequent scoliosis or constant pain as the child grows into young adulthood.

Common Operations. *Hamstring lengthening.* Eggers introduced a procedure calling for a transfer of the insertion of the hamstrings from the tibias to the femurs in 1952. This procedure helped the knee flexion contracture quite well but not uncommonly tended to produce genu recurvatum. Z-lengthening of the hamstring tendons or fractional lengthening in the area of the musculotendinous junction has

Fig. 44-32. Spastic diplegic patient with crouched gait.

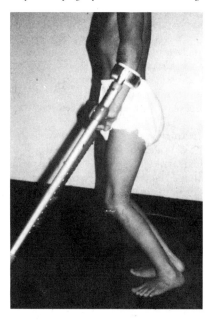

produced more consistent results with less complication. This is carried out with the patient prone through a transverse incision at the junction of the middle and distal thirds of the thigh or through medial and lateral longitudinal incisions.

Iliopsoas recession. The iliopsoas tendon is functionally lengthened or recessed in patients with flexion contractures of the hips due to this muscle. This is approached anteriorly through transverse incisions parallel to and 1 inch below the inguinal ligaments. The iliacus muscle is divided, and the psoas tendon is divided from the lesser trochanter and sutured to the anterior capsule of the hip joint. This usually produces lengthening of 1 to 2 inches.

Adductor tenotomy and neurectomy of the anterior branch of the obturator nerve. These procedures are performed through medial incisions directly over the origin of the adductor tendons. The adductor longus and brevis and sometimes the gracilis are tenotomized. The anterior branch of the obturator nerve is divided to prevent recurrence of the deformity. This operation is often done to allow abduction of the hips and better perineal care but also to prevent subsequent hip dislocations. It must be noted, however, that dislocations cannot always be prevented with this procedure alone. The iliopsoas tendon must be lengthened or recessed to ensure hip stability.

Tendo Achillis lengthening. The gastrocnemius, the soleus, or both may be tight, with the latter being the most common situation. If contracture is still present following thorough release of the knees and hips and the patient is still walking on his toes, it is often helpful to cautiously lengthen the Achilles tendon either by the Hoke method or by Z-lengthening. Excessive lengthening of the Achilles tendon produces a functional disability much more severe than the original equinus contracture.

Tibialis posterior lengthening. This type of lengthening is performed generally in younger patients who have a dynamic varus deformity of the foot with no fixed bony structural changes.

Grice-Green subtalar extra-articular arthrodesis. This arthrodesis uses a block bone graft from the tibia or fibula between the neck of the talus and the anterior portion of the calcaneus. Thus solid stability can be provided in a patient with a severe valgus deformity without interfering with subsequent growth.

Dwyer osteotomy. Older patients with a structural varus deformity will sometimes require a Dwyer calcaneal osteotomy. Also in older children who have completed their growth, a triple arthrodesis is sometimes useful for those patients with severe varus or valgus deformities with bony adaptation.

Upper Extremity

The common position of the upper extremity in a cerebral-palsied patient with spasticity consists of adduction and internal rotation of the shoulder; flexion of the elbow; supination of the forearm; flexion of the wrist and fingers; and flexion and adduction of the thumb, with a thumb-in-palm deformity. In order to determine if the patient will have useful function following reconstructive surgery, it is necessary to splint the patient's wrist in a functional position prior to surgery. If in a more functional position the patient begins to manifest more useful activities with the extremity, then surgery may well be indicated. On the other hand, if function is not improved even by splinting in a better position, then surgery should be delayed.

Common operations to correct wrist flexion include the Green transfer of the flexor carpi ulnaris around the ulnar border of the forearm to the extensor carpi radialis brevis. This corrects the flexor overpull and the ulnar deviation tendency that is often present. Also, routing the tendon around the ulnar border of the hand will counteract a tight pronator teres tendon. Another option, if the patient has very strong and deforming pronation, is to release the pronator teres and use this muscle to stabilize the wrist by transferring it into the extensor carpi radialis brevis. To overcome contracted finger and wrist flexors, the technique of fractional lengthening of the tendons is sometimes carried out. A thumb-in-palm deformity can be corrected by releasing the adductor pollicis from its origin and by lengthening of the flexor pollicis longus tendon. The brachioradialis can be transferred into the abductor pollicis longus and the extensor pollicis brevis to restore thumb abduction and extension.

Spine

It is important to examine the spine carefully on every medical visit of the cerebral-palsied patient. If the spine is not normal, then radiographic monitoring is necessary on a regular basis every 6 to 12 months. Progressive curves in younger children can often be controlled by bracing. A curve that is progressive and causing decompensation of the spine can potentially hamper sitting and standing balance and must be surgically stabilized. Instrumentation with Harrington rods and fusion has been the standard. More recently, segmental fixation using Lueke rods has shown great promise and probably will be more effective in the future since this allows rapid mobilization of the patient without a constricting cast.

MYELOMENINGOCELE

Myelomeningocele is a complex congenital condition of devastating proportions. In the past, these children usually succumbed early to the effects of hydrocephalus, sepsis from the open spine defect, or urinary tract infection. Today, the fatal complications can often be controlled by medical care: the hydrocephalus is controlled by shunting; the sepsis is controlled by early closure of the defect and by administration of antibiotics; and the upper urinary tract damage is prevented by early and vigorous urologic treatment. Because of the increasing survival of these children, the orthopaedic surgeon is being challenged to prevent and correct deformities of the spine and lower extremities.

INCIDENCE

Myelodysplasia occurs in 2 to 4 per 1,000 live births in Great Britain, approximately 1 per 1,000 live births in the United States, and less than that in most other countries. The risk for a child with myelodysplasia in a family jumps from 0.1% for the first child to 5% for the second. The risk of having a third child with this disorder goes up to 10%. The mode of inheritance is not known, but it appears to be multifactorial with some modification by the environment.

ETIOLOGY AND PATHOGENESIS

Myelomeningocele is a severe form of incomplete closure of the primary neural tube (dysrhaphism). The least disabling form is a simple failure of closure of the posterior bony elements of the spinal canal called spina bifida occulta. A meningocele is an outpouching of the coverings of the spinal cord through the defect in the bony structure with no neural elements involved. A myelomeningocele is an outpouching of the dural elements that contains neural tissue. It may occur at any level of the spinal cord or brain, in which case the appropriate terminology is encephalocele. More commonly, the lesion is located between the midthoracic region of the spine and the upper sacrum. The neural elements involved in the myelomeningocele may be cauda equina, spinal cord, or undifferentiated flattened tissue called the neural plate. Many theories regarding the etiology have been presented but can basically be condensed into two categories: (1) failure of fusion of the neural elements, posteriorly, in the normal embryologic development and (2) reopening of the neural elements due to increase in the hydrostatic pressure of the cerebrospinal fluid in the central canal. At the moment, the latter theory seems to be the most logical and have the most support.

DIAGNOSIS

The patient is often paraplegic, occasionally with some muscle groups spared. The actual motor and sensory level is determined by the level of the myelomeningocele, which may not be symmetrical bilaterally (Table 44-2). The prognosis for future ambulation will depend more on the level of the lesion than on any other single factor. Associated conditions can be numerous; these include hydrocephalus, which greatly complicates the overall rehabilitation of the child, particularly if it has caused cerebral damage. Hydromyelia, Arnold-Chiari malformation, and scoliosis can also be associated with myelomeningocele.

Patients with relatively poor prognosis can usually be identified in the newborn nursery. These criteria include a grossly enlarged head, lumbar kyphosis at the time of birth, paralysis above L3, and other general anomalies. Another criterion frequently associated with mental retardation is the lacunar skull deformity.

TABLE 44-2	FUNCTION REMAINING RELATED TO CORD LEVEL IN MYELOMENINGOCELE	
CORD LEVEL	**MUSCLES ACTIVE**	**FUNCTION**
L1	Psoas minor	Hip flexion
L2	Psoas minor, psoas major, and sartorius	Hip flexion
	Adductor longus	Hip adduction
L3	Rectus femoris	Hip flexion
	Adductor brevis, magnus gracilis	Hip adduction
	Quadriceps	Knee extension
L4	Gluteus medius	Hip abduction
	Tibialis anterior, extensor digitorum longus, extensor hallucis longus, peroneals	Ankle dorsiflexion and eversion
L5	Gluteus maximus	Hip extension
	Semitendinosus, semimembranosus, biceps	Knee flexion

The basic defect of the bony elements of the spine is separation of the posterior structures at the level of the myelomeningocele and below. The dysplastic posterior elements may be entirely absent, or they may form bony plates, rotated laterally 180° from their usual position. This alone causes sufficient instability to allow the spine to progress to severe kyphosis or scoliosis. The tendency to deviation of the spine is compounded by varying degrees of paralysis secondary to the neural damage. At least 20% of the children have other congenital anomalies of the spine that may be in the area of the neural defect or more cephalad to it. Another group of these patients have progressive hydromyelia, which further compounds the problem by manifesting even more proximal trunk muscular weakness or paralysis.

The level of disruption of the spinal cord dictates the functional capacity of the lower extremity. Hip stability is an early and constant consideration for the orthopaedic surgeon. In a patient with paralysis from T12 down, there are no active muscles around the hip joints so dislocation is unlikely. Likewise, from L5 down the muscles around the hips are well balanced in all quadrants and dislocation, again, is unlikely. From L3, however, with good hip flexion and adduction but no hip abduction or extension, the hip is extremely vulnerable to dislocation. In the knee, function of the quadriceps muscle is a good prognostic sign when considering future ambulation. With an L3 level function, the quadriceps muscle should be active and future ambulation is quite likely. The foot may manifest deformities secondary to congenital influences or due to muscle imbalance from paralysis. Talipes equinovarus is not uncommon and congenital vertical talus is occasionally seen. In function that includes the L4 nerve roots, ankle dorsiflexion is active through the tibialis anterior and the toe extensors. This results in a calcaneus or calcaneovalgus position of the foot and ankle with subsequent weight-bearing on the small

surface area of the heel; this is frequently associated with insensitivity of the plantar surface of the foot. The combination of high concentrations of pressures over a limited surface area with insensitivity almost certainly means skin breakdown if corrective efforts are not made.

TREATMENT

In 1974, Lorber, a British physician, published a set of criteria recommending that some patients with myelomeningoceles not be treated at all or only minimally. The result of this is to allow the severely disabled patients to die at a very early age. This received partial acceptance in the United States until recently. The general trend in this country at this time is to view this type of judgment on the part of the physician as inappropriate. The physician, therefore, must render the best available medical care indicated to each patient. The treatment is initiated in the neonatal intensive care unit as supportive care by the pediatricians and neonatologist and as early closure of the defect by the neurosurgeons with possible assistance from the plastic surgeons. Orthopaedic treatment is also begun in the nursery. The overall treatment program is first, last, and always a unified team effort. This team includes neurosurgeons, pediatricians, plastic surgeons, urologists, orthopaedic surgeons, social workers, public health nurses and coordinators, and others.

SPINE

When the child begins to sit and eventually to stand in a standing frame or braces, the instability of the spine will begin to manifest itself in scoliosis or kyphosis. When this occurs, it is necessary to provide added support for the spine with a molded body corset. As the child grows, if the trunk orthosis is not able to control the curvature, then an arthrodesis (anterior, posterior, or both) is required at an early age. If the curve can be controlled with an orthosis, then the fusion of the spine can be delayed until the spine is closer to maturity. Posterior fusions are difficult because of the loss or distortion of the posterior elements over a wide section. Stabilization can be accomplished with Harrington rod instrumentation and fusion. The newer segmental instrumentation using Luque rods has some advantage because they are transfixed to each segment of the spine. This allows postoperative mobilization without external support. For severe curves, an anterior release is necessary to gain correction and then a fusion to maintain it. This is done in a two-stage procedure, performing the anterior release fusion first and then the posterior fusion 1 to 2 weeks later.

Those patients with a recognizable lumbar kyphosis at birth are a special problem. The kyphosis can seldom be corrected with an orthosis and usually requires surgical stabilization. Vertebral resection followed by anterior and posterior fusion with instrumentation is usually necessary.

LOWER EXTREMITIES

Treatment in the hips in the first months of life requires positioning and splinting to maintain their reduction. Proper positioning can be accomplished in one of several different manners: foam cutout for legs and trunk (Fisher), cut off mattress with wedge between, and incline positioner. If the hips can be maintained in a reduced position for the first 9 to 12 months, then this position is usually maintained thereafter with the braces used for standing and ambulation. If the tendency to subluxation and dislocation continues in the older child, then surgical procedures are required to redirect the femoral heads into the acetabulum. A subtrochanteric, varus, derotation osteotomy is often necessary. The Sharrard transfer of the iliopsoas through the posterior ilium to the greater trochanter is sometimes helpful to increase the lateral stability of the joint.

Foot deformities require initiation of treatment in the newborn nursery. Congenital talipes equinovarus and congenital vertical tali are treated with serial casting as in a patient without the added burden of the myelomeningocele. Some of these patients will eventually need posterior, or posterior and medial, release of the soft tissues at 9 to 12 months of age. Bracing must be pursued vigorously to prevent recurrence of the contractures. In those patients with foot deformities secondary to muscle imbalance, splinting and bracing must be carried out aggressively until such time that tendon transfers can be done to properly balance the foot. This is best accomplished if postponed until 18 months to 3 years of age. The patient who has strong dorsiflexion and weak or no plantar flexion can be helped a great deal by transferring the tibialis anterior posteriorly into the calcaneus. It is important to produce plantigrade feet as early as possible in order to avoid unnecessary delays in standing and walking.

STANDING AND AMBULATION

Patients with an intact quadriceps mechanism will frequently be successful ambulators. Patients with less function will be able to walk with full control braces, provided they are blessed with an aggressive rehabilitative team and cooperative, determined parents. This ambulation will be somewhat limited, with the patients depending on a wheelchair to a varying extent while young. As these more disabled patients get into their teen years with increasing weight and increasing functional demands, they often find it more efficient to depend more on the wheelchair. In spite of the fact that many of these young ambulators (with spinal lesions of L2 and above) will not be effective walkers when they reach their teens, it still seems reasonable from phys-

iologic, emotional, and psychological perspectives to encourage them in standing and walking while in their early developmental years.

The general approach consists of starting with a trunk corset when they begin to sit and demonstrate spine instability. At 12 to 15 months of age, they are fitted with a standing frame to experience the upright position and develop strength in the muscles that are available (Fig. 44-33). At 18 months, they are fitted with the appropriate braces, which often means full control braces. These are long leg braces with joints at the hips and a pelvic band attached to the trunk corset. As the patient becomes stronger and more independent, the bracing can be diminished or locks at particular joints can be left unlocked, if function appears to be adequate to support the involved joints.

Throughout the growth period, the monitoring for progressive deformity continues. The spine is observed for scoliosis, the hips are checked for subluxation or dislocation, and the feet are observed for continuing deformities. As the patient grows into the teen years, the need for neurosurgical and orthopaedic treatment begins to take a back seat to the need for psychological, psychosocial, sexual, and occupational counseling.

SCOLIOSIS

Deformities of the spine are classified according to the direction of the deformity, the level of the spine involved, the etiology of the deformity, and the severity of the deformity. Lateral curvatures of the spine are referred to as scoliosis, and the direction of the convexity of the curve determines whether it is classified as right or left. Curves with the convexity posterior are termed *kyphosis,* and those with the convexity anterior are termed *lordosis.* A normal kyphosis is present in the thoracic spine, and a normal lordosis is present in the lumbar spine. The curve may be cervical, thoracic, lumbar, cervicothoracic, thoracolumbar, or lumbosacral, depending on the level of the apex of the curve.

INCIDENCE

The incidence of scoliosis in the general population is stated to be anywhere between less than 1% and 14% by different studies. Older studies have set the incidence quite low, but newer, prospective studies using school screening studies have recognized the incidence to be somewhat higher, the highest being about 14% of those people between 12 and 14 years of age. School screening has changed the perspective somewhat because smaller curves are being recognized. The occurrence of curves less than 10% is about equal in male and female, but for curves greater than 20%, the female-to-male ratio is approximately 5.4:1.

ETIOLOGY

Deformities of the spine can be produced by a wide variety of diseases. Idiopathic scoliosis is the most common type, accounting for over 80% of the deformities. Studies have indicated the high probability of scoliosis being an inherited disease, with the mode of inheritance to be multifactorial. On the other hand, however, congenital spine deformities are rarely caused by genetic influences.

Fig. 44-33. Myelomeningocele patient in standing frame.

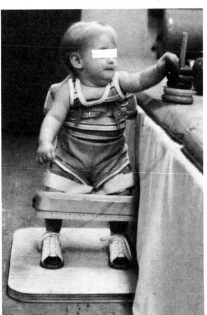

DIAGNOSIS

SCHOOL SCREENING

The early diagnosis and treatment of scoliosis is extremely important in preventing severe deformities of the spine. School screening has become an invaluable tool in the past decade to help accomplish this goal. Children are screened on a yearly basis during the seventh through ninth grades because this is a time of rapid growth and, therefore, a time for rapid increase of the scoliotic curve. The initial screening examination is carried out by a public health nurse, and the second screening of those children with questionable curves is then performed by a physician. If the physician confirms the presence of a spine deformity, the child is then referred to his family physician for examination and a confirmatory radiograph. Each child is examined from the back, front, and side and then from the back while bending forward (Fig. 44-34). While viewing the patient from the back, it is sometimes possible to detect a difference in the height of the shoulders, even if a minimal curve is present. From the front, rib cage asymmetry may be apparent. From the side, kyphosis or lordosis will become more evident. The real key to early detection, however, is the view from the rear with the patient bending forward. Subtle, lateral deviations of the spine are more apparent, as are posterior prominences of the thoracic cavity on the side of the convexity of the curve. When several vertebrae are displaced laterally, there is almost always rotation of the vertebra to the side of the convexity. This produces the posterior rib hump that is evident on the forward bending examination.

CLINICAL MANIFESTATIONS

Idiopathic scoliosis is divided into three types: (1) infantile, which occurs between birth and 4 years of age, (2) juvenile, which occurs between 4 years of age and puberty, and (3) adolescent idiopathic scoliosis, which occurs from the beginning of puberty until the cessation of growth. Juvenile and idiopathic scoliosis are roughly the same disease and respond similarly. Infantile scoliosis, on the other hand, appears to be a separate type of problem, with 50% or more of the curves either resolving or stabilizing. The remainder, however, can be progressive and cause severe deformity at a very early age.

School screening studies indicate that approximately 20% of the adolescent idiopathic curves under 10° resolve spontaneously. The behavior of the remainder of the curves is somewhat varied, and the patients need to be observed carefully throughout their growth period. Curves that progress beyond 50° frequently produce symptoms such as back pain and subsequent limitation of activities when the patients reach their late 20s or early 30s. Degenerative arthrosis is a frequent finding on the radiograph of these adult patients. Patients with curves between 40° and 50° will less commonly have symptoms as an adult. The progression of idiopathic curves will usually cease when the patient's growth is completed. Curves over 60°, however, will often continue to progress after maturity. In addition, patients with curves over 60° have a much higher incidence of degenerative arthritis and back pain and their mortality rate over 45 years of age is much higher than that of the general population, with death often coming from right heart failure and cor pulmonale.

Congenital curves are divided into those caused by defects of segmentation, those resulting from defects of formation, and those that are mixed or a combination of the above. These curves often become apparent in the first few years and will occasionally progress steadily year by year and become quite severe at a very early age.

The severity of the curve is determined by measurement in degrees according to Cobb's method. This measurement is obtained by determining the end vertebrae of a single curve and by drawing lines perpendicular to the end plates of these vertebrae. The angle of intersection that these two perpendicular lines make, away from a straight line, represents the angle of the curve (Fig. 44-35).

The curves are divided into major and minor curves. A major curve is the most deforming, with the most structural changes in the vertebrae involved. The minor curve is less

Fig. 44-34. Examination of scoliosis patient from the back with the patient standing (*A*) and bending forward to 90° (*B*). On bending the right posterior rib hump is revealed.

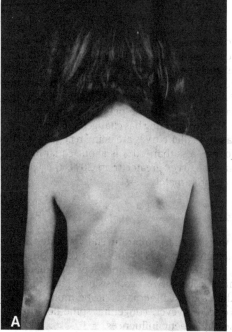

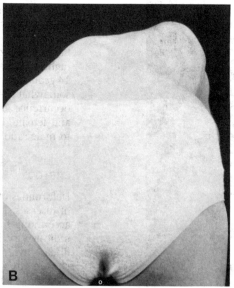

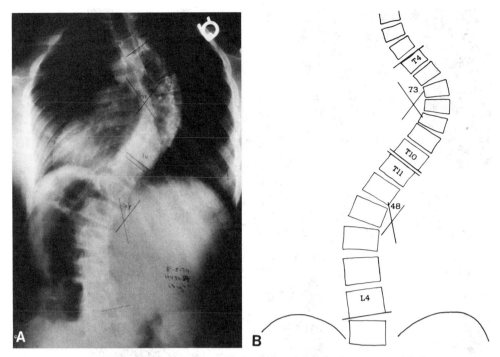

Fig. 44-35. Patient with scoliosis. (*A*) Right thoracic and left lumbar curves. (*B*) Same curve demonstrating Cobb's method of measurement.

deforming, with less structurally altered vertebrae. The longer a curve has been present and the more severe the curve, the more structural changes will be seen in the vertebrae included. These changes include wedging of the vertebrae and later degenerative arthritic changes.

TREATMENT

Nonoperative. Any child who is still growing with a curve under 20° must be observed at regular intervals from 3 to 6 months, depending on the rate of progression of the curve. An anteroposterior roentgenogram should be made of the entire spine with the patient standing. This should be compared with the previous roentgenogram, as well as the one made at the time of the initial examination. Any patient with a progressive curve over 20° must be treated with bracing. In the past, the Milwaukee brace was the universally accepted brace but, more recently, an underarm type orthosis of a lighter and less bulky material is used to correct and hold most curves (Fig. 44-36). It must be emphasized that the final result with brace treatment will not include much correction but the brace will stop the progress of the curvature.

Operative. Adolescent patients with curves over 50° require surgical stabilization and fusion. Correction and stabilization are usually accomplished with Harrington or Lueke rods, and the fusion is completed with autogenous bone graft from the patient's iliac crest. Patients with curves over 90° will often need some preliminary correction with traction or casting (Fig. 44-37).

Younger patients with idiopathic juvenile scoliosis should also be fused if the curve cannot be controlled with bracing. On the other hand, fusion should be deferred as long as possible in order to allow maximum growth in height of the trunk. Spine fusion will effectively stop the growth of the spine.

Postoperatively, the patients are placed in a body cast 1 week after surgery and allowed to be ambulatory. The cast is maintained for 6 to 9 months until the fusion is solid.

SLIPPED CAPITAL FEMORAL EPIPHYSIS

INCIDENCE

Slipped capital femoral epiphysis is a disturbance of the proximal femur that occurs during the period of rapid

Fig. 44-36. Scoliosis patient in thoracolumbar sacral orthosis.

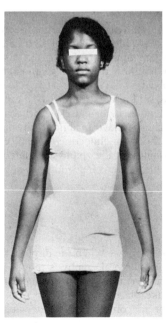

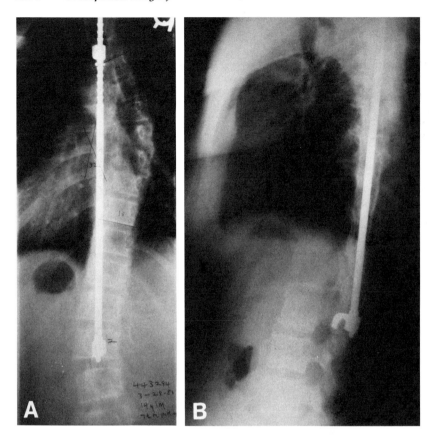

Fig. 44-37. Anteroposterior (*A*) and lateral (*B*) views of same patient in Figure 44-35 following stabilization and fusion.

growth in preadolescence and adolescence and that results in the displacement of the proximal epiphysis of the femur. The incidence has been reported to range from 0.71 to 3.41 per 100,000 population. The age range in males is from 10 to 17 years, with the highest occurrence from 11 to 12 years. It generally occurs 1 to 2 years earlier in females. It is more common in blacks than whites and the male-to-female ratio is roughly 2:1. Thirty percent of the patients have bilateral involvement.

ETIOLOGY

The etiology is unknown, but numerous theories have been proposed. These include mechanical, traumatic, endocrine, metabolic, and inflammatory factors. In addition, it has been reported that the risk of a second family member becoming involved is 7%. Approximately 50% of the patients are overweight, and a large number of the patients are in the upper percentiles in height. The fact that a high percentage of the patients have an abnormality of growth lends support to the theory of endocrine imbalance. The mechanism for final failure of the epiphyseal plate is simply that the strength of the plate is inadequate to support the load borne across it.

PATHOLOGY

It has been shown that synovitis is present in the hip joint in the preslippage phase. When the displacement begins to occur, the capital femoral epiphysis moves inferiorly and posteriorly. If this occurs over a long period of time, adaptive changes will take place in the femoral neck to allow the proximal femur to conform to the new position of the

femoral head. New bone is laid down on the inferior and posterior aspects of the femoral neck to provide support for the head in this position. The superior and anterior portion of the femoral neck that has become exposed by the displacement of the femoral head will be rounded off at the same time. Because of the new position of the femoral head in the acetabulum, joint motion will be severely limited.

DIAGNOSIS

CLINICAL MANIFESTATIONS

The displacement of the proximal femoral epiphysis may present itself in one of three different ways. It may present acutely, following significant trauma, in which case the patient had no pain or limitation prior to this incident. Somewhat more common is the situation in which the patient has had chronic pain in the involved hip for some time with limitation of motion and some difficulty walking or running. The patient then has a sudden acute episode in which further slippage takes place. There are significant increases in the patient's pain and limitation of motion so that he seeks medical treatment. The third and most common presentation is when the patient has chronic, often low-grade pain over an extended period of time. The pain is often in the hip, but it may be along the medial aspect of the thigh or knee. Approximately 20% of the patients experience medial distal thigh and knee pain alone. If the pain is located predominantly in the knee area, it is not uncommon to discover that the patient has been to one or more physicians for an examination of the knee and that the real pathologic process was not uncovered.

The displacement of the capital femoral epiphysis is

posterior and inferior; therefore, the leg is externally rotated, adducted, and somewhat short. Internal rotation is limited, and full extension may be lacking. With the patient in the supine position, flexion of the hip produces simultaneous external rotation. Abduction is limited or absent, and any of these motions may be painful. The patient walks with an antalgic gait, shifting his center of gravity over the right hip and, at the same time, shortening the period of weight-bearing on the involved leg as much as possible because of pain.

ROENTGENOGRAPHIC FINDINGS

One system of grading the severity of displacement is based on the amount of displacement relative to the width of the metaphysis of the femoral neck (Fig. 44-38). Grade I indicates that there has been 0 to 33% displacement; grade II indicates there has been 33% to 50% displacement; and grade III indicates displacement of greater than 50% of the width of the metaphysis of the femoral neck. These determinations are based on an anteroposterior roentgenographic projection. In an acute slip, there are no indications of healing or remodeling of the femoral neck. In a chronic slip, new bone formation is apparent on the interior and posterior aspects of the metaphysis, as the femoral neck is molding itself to conform to the new position of the femoral head. At the same time there is resorption of bone in the superior and anterior areas of the femoral neck that have been uncovered by the displaced epiphysis. Narrowing of the articular cartilage space may indicate destruction of the articular cartilage or chondrolysis. Increased density or collapse of the femoral head would signify avascular necrosis of the femoral head. These latter changes are almost always complications of treatment (Fig. 44-39).

TREATMENT

The goals of treatment are to prevent further displacement to avoid the complications of treatment mentioned above, to maintain motion as near to normal as possible, and to prevent degenerative arthritis in later years. Treatment of the patient with a grade I slip is simply pinning the femoral head *in situ*. Further slippage is prevented, and major complications of treatment are rare.

Opinions vary considerably as to the appropriate treatment for grades II and III. Formerly, an osteotomy of the femoral neck was used by some orthopaedic surgeons to replace the femoral head in a more anatomical position in relation to the neck and the acetabulum. This procedure is almost universally condemned now because of the high incidence of avascular necrosis of the femoral head. Pinning will prevent further migration of the head and avoid avascular necrosis. Following complete closure of the epiphyseal plate, the pins can be removed and a subtrochanteric osteotomy is performed. The osteotomy should be designed to rotate the proximal femur in such a manner so as to replace the articular surface of the head in a more appropriate relationship with the acetabulum. This will help to avoid the long-term complication of degenerative arthritis of the hip.

COMPLICATIONS

The major complications of a slipped capital femoral epiphysis or its treatment consist of avascular necrosis of the femoral head and chondrolysis, as stated previously. Chondrolysis may occur prior to treatment but more often is a result of treatment. The incidence of avascular necrosis is much higher in black children, so extreme caution must be

Fig. 44-38. Classification of slipped capital femoral epiphysis. (*A*) The three grades are divided by the amount of displacement of the femoral head on the neck. (MacEwen G, Ramsey PL: Congenital dislocation of the hip. In Lovell WW, Winter RB [eds]: Pediatric Orthopaedics. Philadelphia, J B Lippincott, 1978) (*B*) Distinguishing minimal slip: In the normal hip a line drawn along the top of the femoral neck should transect a small portion of femoral head. If no portion of the femoral head extends above the line, then the femoral head has been displaced.

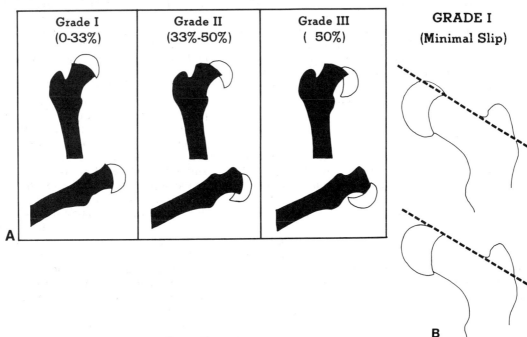

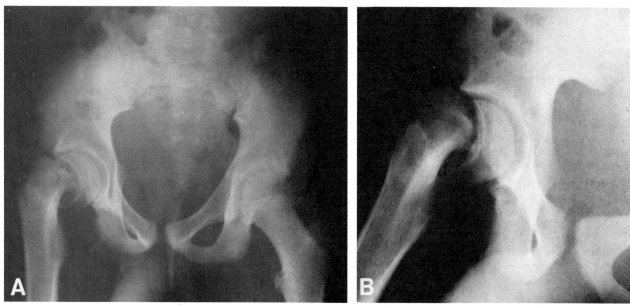

Fig. 44-39.   Grade II slipped capital femoral epiphysis on the right with almost 50% displacement of femoral head. (*A*) Anteroposterior projection. (*B*) Lateral projection.

taken in these patients. As stated, osteotomies through the femoral neck are to be avoided at all costs. Subtrochanteric osteotomies at the time of initial treatment are also associated with a higher incidence of avascular necrosis. Forceful reduction of the femoral head is also to be avoided because of its association with a higher incidence of avascular necrosis.

LEGG-CALVÉ-PERTHES DISEASE

INCIDENCE

Legg-Calvé-Perthes disease results from avascular necrosis of the femoral head in growing children. It is seen in children from 2 to 12 years of age, but most cases occur between 4 and 8 years of age. It is bilateral in approximately 12% of the children and occurs in males four times more often than in females. Some races have very few reported cases, such as Australians, Native Americans, Polynesians, and blacks. Higher incidences of the syndrome occur in Japanese, Mongoloid, Eskimo, and Central European people.

ETIOLOGY AND PATHOLOGY

The basic mechanism for production of the syndrome is loss of blood supply to the proximal femoral epiphysis. The etiology of this is still in question. A number of theories have been expounded that relate to thrombosis or trauma, for example, but none of these is universally accepted.

During the early avascular stage, there is death of the bone in all or a part of the femoral head. In the stage of fragmentation, new bone is laid down on the dead bone and the marrow elements are restored. Also, as time passes the bone is reabsorbed by osteoclastic activity and, even in this state, the femoral head is regaining a considerable amount of its inherent strength. In the healing or regeneration stage, the final bony architecture is being reestablished. The overall contour of the femoral head was altered during

the weakened phase early on in the course of the syndrome. Its distorted shape is maintained, and concentricity of the head is not reestablished.

DIAGNOSIS

CLINICAL MANIFESTATIONS

A limp is one of the most common early findings to be observed. It is often intermittent and painless in the beginning but, after continued activities, the limp will become constant and painful. The pain may be over the hip joint, over the medial proximal thigh, or over the medial distal thigh and knee joint. The involved leg is slightly short, and the gait will be antalgic owing to pain much like that described in the section on slipped capital femoral epiphysis. On further examination, muscle spasm and limitation of motion of the joint will be found with a flexion contracture of the hip. At this stage, motion is painful.

ROENTGENOGRAPHIC FINDINGS

The radiographic picture is a changing one throughout the process of the bone death and subsequent fragmentation and revascularization. It is necessary to use both anteroposterior and frogleg lateral views to follow the course of events. The earliest sign is often the crescent sign of Caffey. This is a radiolucent line just under the subchondral bone in the superolateral portion of the femoral head that is thought to represent a fracture. Also, the ossific nucleus of the femoral head may appear slightly smaller on the involved side. The changes are at times limited to the anterior portion of the head and, therefore, are seen more readily on the frogleg view. Subsequently, the femoral head appears to be fragmented with areas of increased density and areas of relative radiolucency. When revascularization and reossification become complete, the bone takes on the appearance of normal bony structure. As stated, if the shape of the femoral head is distorted during the weakened period, the misshapened condition persists. The total process from

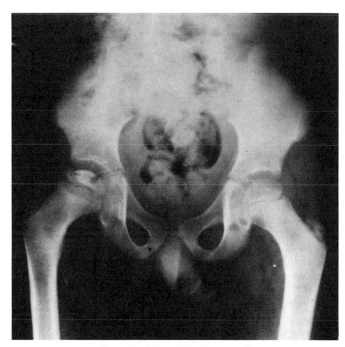

Fig. 44-40. Legg-Calvé-Perthes disease. Flattening and necrosis of femoral head with fragmentation are evident.

beginning to complete bony restoration may take 3 to 4 years (Figs. 44-40 and 44-41).

CATTERALL'S CLASSIFICATION

Catterall classified the patients according to the amount of femoral head involved. In group I, the anterior part of the head alone is involved and there is no collapse of the segment. In group II, there is slightly more anterior and superior involvement. There is still very little collapse, and the regeneration potential is still good. Group III includes those patients with up to 75% of the femoral epiphysis involved. The metaphysis is also involved, and collapse of the head may be severe. The prognosis of this group is extremely poor. In group IV, the entire epiphysis is affected and collapse occurs relatively early and is severe. The prognosis in this type is much worse.

TREATMENT

The initial treatment consists of bed rest (usually in the hospital) with traction to eliminate the muscle spasm and synovitis and improve the range of motion of the hip joint. When all symptoms have subsided and the range of motion is near normal, one may proceed with more definitive treatment. This is aimed at maintaining a femoral head concentric with the acetabulum. The accepted treatment in the past was either prolonged bed rest or ambulation in an ischial weight-bearing brace or a sling to prevent the involved leg from bearing weight. Because of the muscle action across the hip joint and frequent occurrence of muscle spasm, the compression of the femoral head on the acetabulum was not relieved by most of these methods. It is generally agreed now that weight-bearing is acceptable if the hip is in an abducted position, well contained in the acetabulum. The shape of the acetabulum maintains the normal shape of the femoral head and prevents uneven depression of the anterior and lateral rim of the epiphysis. This is best accomplished by an abduction orthosis, with the patient ambulating in marked abduction with crutches (Fig. 44-42). If this "containment" treatment cannot be accomplished with an abduction orthosis alone and the femoral head is not completely covered by the acetabulum, then surgical procedures are necessary to complete the containment. If there is excessive valgus of the femoral

Fig. 44-41. Legg-Calvé-Perthes disease. Slipped capital femoral epiphysis residual stage with flattening of the femoral head and projection of one third of the femoral head lateral to the acetabulum. (*A*) Anteroposterior radiograph. (*B*) Arthrogram outlining joint space and articular cartilage.

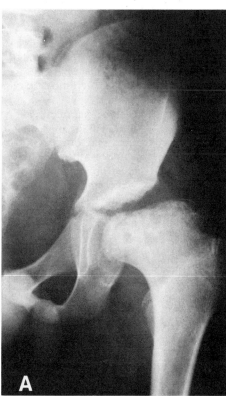

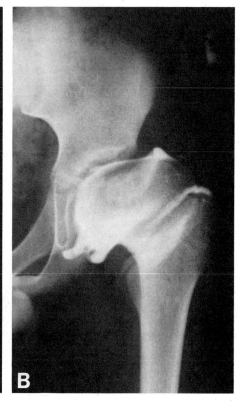

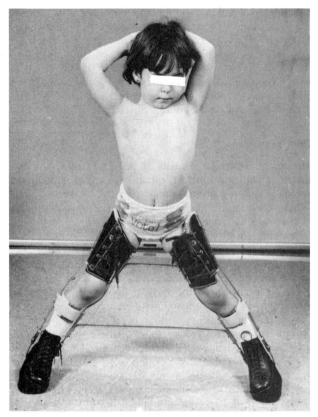

Fig. 44-42. Legg-Calvé-Perthes disease patient in abduction braces.

neck, then a varus-producing osteotomy of the proximal femur is performed. If the acetabulum is somewhat shallow, then an acetabular redirecting procedure can be performed to get better acetabular coverage. The femoral head is contained in the acetabulum until the bone of the femoral head is remodeled and strong.

TALIPES EQUINOVARUS (CLUBFOOT)

INCIDENCE

Congenital talipes equinovarus is a complex deformity of the foot that occurs in approximately 1 per 1,000 live births. It is two times more common in males than females and does have some familial occurrence. With normal parents and a child with congenital talipes equinovarus, the risk of a second child in the same family with this condition is about 3%. With parents who also have the condition, the risk increases to approximately 25%.

ETIOLOGY

The cause of talipes equinovarus has not been determined, but numerous theories have been advanced. Wynn-Davies concluded that the condition was partly genetic with a multifactorial inheritance pattern and partly environmental, due to forces acting on the fetus *in utero*. Irani and Sherman, following their dissections in 1963, felt that the deformity was a primary germ plasm defect with its origins in the early weeks of pregnancy. Palmer did a genetic study on patients with clubfoot and identified two basic groups; one group had a family history of talipes equinovarus and the other had no family history. Those with a positive family history had a 10% chance of additional children having the deformity. In the families he studied, this appeared to be an autosomal dominant trait with about 40% penetrance. In those families with no previous history of this deformity, subsequent children had the same chance of getting it as did the general population.

PATHOLOGY

The position of the foot consists of adduction of the forefoot, inversion or varus of the entire foot, and equinus, or plantar flexion, at the ankle and subtalar joints. There is sometimes a cavus deformity of the foot, with the forefoot being plantar flexed on the already plantar-flexed hindfoot.

The head and neck of the talus are directed plantarward and medially, with the articular surface facing this direction. The navicular bone is displaced even further medially and may be completely dislocated, resting against the neck of the talus and the medial malleous. The calcaneus is rolled medially underneath the talus, and the varus deformity of the heel may be fixed in this position, with extremely tight soft tissue structures. The metatarsals are directed medially and plantarward. Internal tibial torsion and rotation of the talus in the ankle mortise do not seem to be major components. The soft tissue structures are thought to be basically normal but changed in adaptation to the altered position of the bony skeleton. The musculotendinous units, capsular structures, and ligaments on the medial, plantar, and posterior aspects of the foot and ankle are short and may be extremely tight.

DIAGNOSIS

CLINICAL MANIFESTATIONS

Two basic categories of the talipes equinovarus are recognized. In the first group, the deformity is not rigid, the feet are similar in size, and the foot can generally be corrected by conservative means. These patients constitute about 75% of the total number. The second type is one in which the foot is short, is stiff, and often has a vertical crease on the medial side of the foot in the area of the arch (Fig. 44-43). This foot is difficult to correct and usually requires surgical release.

If the deformities are not treated early, even the flexible ones will become stiff and rigid, with severe adaptive shortening of the soft tissue structures on the medial and posterior aspects of the foot. The patient will walk on the lateral border of his foot and further aggravate the deformity. Talipes equinovarus is associated with a number of other conditions, including arthrogryposis multiplex congenita, myelomeningocele, cerebral palsy, Charcot-Marie-Tooth disease, and others.

ROENTGENOGRAPHIC FINDINGS

Appropriate roentgenograms for evaluating talipes include an anteroposterior view of both feet, lateral views of both feet, and forced dorsiflexion views of both feet in the lateral projection. Normally, the talus and calcaneus diverge anteriorly, with the talus pointing down the line of the first metatarsal. In a clubfoot, the talus and calcaneus approach being parallel, with the long axis of these two bones pointing down the line of the fifth metatarsal or even further laterally. Lines may be drawn down the axes of the talus and calcaneus, and the angle of intersection is the talocalcaneal

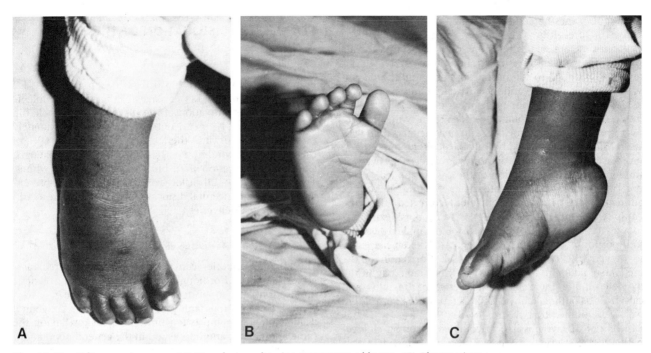

Fig. 44-43. Talipes equinovarus. (*A*) Dorsal view showing metatarsus adductus. (*B*) Plantar view showing adductus. (*C*) Lateral view showing equinus with medial and plantar crease in the midfoot.

angle of Kite. The angle may vary between 20° and 35°; over 35° indicates a valgus deformity and under 20° indicates a varus deformity.

On the lateral view, there is normally convergence of the anterior ends of the talus and calcaneus with some overlapping of the anterior ends of these two bones. On the forced dorsiflexion lateral view in talipes equinovarus, there is a more parallel relationship between the two bones and there is no overlapping of the anterior ends. There is also no dorsiflexion of the calcaneus. One line is drawn through the long axis of the calcaneus parallel to its inferior border

and another through the long axis of the talus. The angle formed at the junction of these two lines should be 35° or greater. If the angle is less than 35°, the deformity has not been corrected (Fig. 44-44).

TREATMENT

The majority of patients with clubfeet can be successfully treated by conservative management. This consists of repeated manipulations and casting at intervals of a week or less. The manipulation is a very gentle maneuver that does

Fig. 44-44. Talipes equinovarus. (*A*) Anteroposterior view shows parallelism of talus and calcaneus and narrowed Kite's angle of only 14°. (*B*) Lateral view shows parallelism of talus and calcaneus, with talocalcaneal angle of only 18°. This is uncorrected talipes equinovarus.

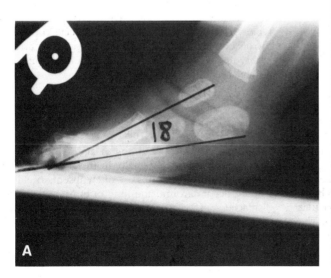

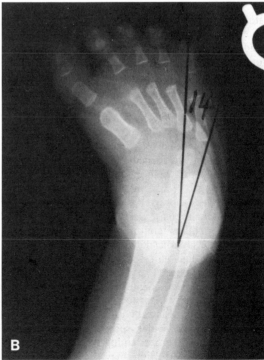

not require anesthesia nor cause injury to soft tissue or bony structures. It involves first traction along the long axis of the first metatarsal to stretch the soft tissues on the medial side of the foot and reduce the talonavicular joint. This traction is applied to the medial forefoot until the talonavicular joint is reduced and the varus deformity is corrected as much as possible. The first segment of the cast is applied just to the foot to maintain this correction, with pressure over the medial side of the heel and first metatarsal and the lateral side of the cuboid and calcanealcuboid joint area to provide fixation. The varus deformity is corrected by everting the foot as the upper portion of the cast is applied, incorporating the foot cast. At a later date, when the matatarsus adductus and varus are completely corrected, then the equinus deformity is corrected slowly by dorsiflexing the foot as the upper half of the cast is being applied over the foot portion of the cast. A long leg cast is often necessary to prevent the cast from slipping off. Correction of the metatarsus adductus and varus is confirmed radiographically by determining the relationship between the talus and calcaneus as outlined above. This "serial casting" procedure was well outlined by Lovell in 1978.

It is not always possible to completely correct clubfeet with these conservative means, especially those feet that are markedly deformed and rigid. In those instances, operative treatment is indicated to complete the correction. Surgery is also required in the occasional patient who has a recurrence of the deformity following previous correction. Surgical procedures are aimed at correcting the three basic deformities.

Residual forefoot adduction can be corrected by capsulotomies and mobilization of the tarsometatarsal joint. Tendon transfers have been advocated for correction or maintenance of correction for forefoot adduction or the varus deformity of the foot. Metatarsal osteotomies are occasionally needed for the older child with persistent forefoot adduction.

Dwyer has recommended osteotomies of the calcaneus for correction of the residual deformities of a clubfoot. Evans has used a wedge resection of the cuboid to shorten the lateral border of the foot and correct this aspect of a resistant clubfoot deformity. Children over 12 years of age with residual deformities often require a triple arthrodesis to correct the alignment of the foot and to stabilize it by fusing the talocalcaneal, the talonavicular, and the calcaneocuboid joints.

The most commonly used procedure today for the correction of an incompletely corrected or a recurrent clubfoot is the combination of a posterior and medial soft tissue release as advocated by Turco and Lovell. The age range for performing this procedure is from 6 months to 7 years. Correction of the three major deformities is accomplished at one sitting by releasing all of the contracted ligaments and shortened tendons. Posteriorly, the posterior capsule of the ankle joint is released as is the capsule of the talocalcaneal joint. The Achilles tendon is also lengthened by a Z-cut. Medially, the superficial deltoid ligament is released but the deep deltoid ligament securing the talus to the medial malleolus is retained. The tibialis posterior tendon is lengthened, as is the flexor digitorum longus and flexor hallucis longus, if necessary. The medial capsule of the talonavicular joint is released, as are the calcaneocuboid ligaments. The plantar calcaneonavicular (spring ligament) is also released, along with any other restraining structures. Overcorrection, as well as undercorrection, may be a complication.

CONGENITAL DISLOCATION OF THE HIP

INCIDENCE

Frank dislocation of the hip occurs in approximately 1.2 per 1,000 live births. Lesser stages of the same pathologic entity such as subluxation of the hip or a dislocatable hip occur in up to 11.7 per 1,000 live births. Approximately 80% occur in girls, and the left hip is involved in 60% of the cases. The condition is bilateral in 20% of patients. Congenital dislocation of the hip is more common in whites. Twenty percent of all dislocations occur in breech presentations, while congenital dislocation of the hip is present in 22% of breech deliveries.

ETIOLOGY AND PATHOGENESIS

The etiologic theories can be subdivided into three categories: Genetic, hormonal, and mechanical. The genetic implications are supported by the fact that the risk to a second child in the family of a patient with congenital dislocation of the hip is ten times as great for having the same anomaly as another person in the general population. The hormonal contribution to the etiology of congenital hip dislocation is supported by the observation of an increased mobility in the joints of newborns due to maternal estrogens. Studies seem to indicate that estrogen is a predisposing factor. The mechanical theories gain support from the fact that there is a much higher incidence of congenital hip dislocation in patients carried *in utero* in the breech position. It has also been observed that in societies where the infants are traditionally carried on the mother's back with the legs bound together congenital dislocation of the hip is much more of a problem. In contrast, in societies in which the infant is allowed to straddle the mother's back, with the legs abducted, the incidence is very low.

Congenital dislocation of the hip may also be divided according to the basic underlying pathologic stage or process. The first is the common or typical type of congenital dislocation of the hip, which appears to be partly positional, partly mechanical, and partly hormonally related. This group constitutes by far the largest majority, and the dislocation is thought to occur either just before or just after birth. The second type is the neuromuscular type from paralysis or abnormal muscle tone. This type is usually easily reducible but is also easily dislocatable because of the basic nature of the musculature inadequacy. The third type is the teratogenic type, which is a basic germ plasm defect. In this situation, the dislocated hip has been present since the early stages of embryologic development *in utero* and treatment is quite difficult.

DIAGNOSIS

CLINICAL MANIFESTATIONS

Between birth and 3 months of age, clinical diagnosis is often quite difficult, especially in the neonatal period. The "standard" manifestations are often absent. The dislocation usually occurs around the time of birth so the hip is only displaced somewhat laterally and has not had time, as yet, to ride proximally. Because of this, there is no femoral shortening and no asymmetrical folds. Asymmetrical gluteal folds are a well-publicized diagnostic criterion but are unreliable at any age. The Ortolani manuever and the

Barlow test are the most sensitive and reliable in the newborn period, and the newborn should have these tests as a part of his examination. In the Ortolani manuever, the thigh and hip are very gently abducted to the point where a dislocated hip will be reduced (Fig. 44-45). The movement of the femoral head over the acetabular rim will be detected by a faint palpable click. In the Barlow test, the hip is first adducted and gently pushed posteriorly to dislocate a dislocatable hip. The thigh is then very gently abducted in order to re-reduce the hip and feel the palpable click. It must be emphasized again that this manuever must be extremely gentle and the quality of sounds and vibrations produced by dislocation and reduction of this relaxed hip are extremely faint. Testing for limited abduction in order to diagnose a dislocated hip in a newborn is also inconclusive because all newborns have some stiffness in their hips and are limited in extension and abduction.

In the period between 3 and 12 months of age, some of the more standard manifestations of congenital dislocation of the hip are present and useful in making a diagnosis. Normal hips by this time have a good range of motion so that the limited abduction and femoral shortening will be apparent. Femoral shortening is best shown by Galeazzi's sign, which is detected by examining the patient in the supine position with the hips flexed to 90° and the knees maximally flexed. The knee of the dislocated hip will not extend as far anteriorly as the normal knee. Over 3 months of age, Ortolani's manuever will more likely reduce the hip with a definite click, but over 6 months of age it may not, because the hip may not be reducible at that point owing to shortening and contractures of the muscles.

Over a year of age, the diagnosis is made by the fact that the involved leg is somewhat shorter and the patient's ability to walk is usually delayed until 15 to 18 months of age. The gait will be abnormal because of the instability of the hip and the shortening of the leg. The patient will lean his trunk over the involved hip in order to shift the center of gravity in that direction. If the hip dislocation is bilateral, the movement of the trunk will be first to one side and next to the other, producing a waddling type gait. This gait may be extremely subtle and difficult to detect.

ROENTGENOGRAPHIC FINDINGS

The radiologic findings in the newborn are not always helpful. The reasons for this are basically twofold: (1) the secondary ossification center of the capital femoral epiphysis is not present at birth and does not appear until the eighth month or later and (2) as stated before, the proximal femur is not displaced widely but only slightly laterally. In the older child, there is lateral displacement as well as proximal migration of the femoral head with an increasingly sloping acetabular roof. In the teratologic dislocation, the sloped acetabular roof or "false acetabulum" with proximal migration of the femoral head may already be present at the time of birth. The radiologic indexes useful in diagnosing congenital dislocation of the hip are shown in Figure 44-46. In Figure 44-47, *A*, there is a roentgenogram of a 1-year-old with congenital dislocation of the hip and the same roentgenogram with the indexes drawn in is shown in Figure 44-47, *B*.

TREATMENT

The treatment consists of reduction of the hip and maintenance of the reduction, usually in flexion, abduction, and external rotation. Reduction in the newborn is simple and is maintained with one of a number of devices. The most common device used today is the Pavlek harness. A spica cast is necessary to maintain reduction in an older child.

Over 3 months of age, traction is always required preliminary to reduction. Reduction may be possible with force, but this same force will cause damage to the joint, consisting of avascular necrosis of the femoral head and possibly cartilage necrosis. Skin traction for 1 to 2 weeks is required to overcome the adaptive muscle shortening. When the femoral head has been pulled down to the level of the acetabulum, then reduction may be accomplished safely.

If a complete concentric reduction is not possible or if the reduction is not stable, then an open reduction is required. This is best accomplished through an anterior iliofemoral incision, using a T-incision in the capsule, with the base of the T being along the anterosuperior rim of the

Fig. 44-45. Examination of an infant for congenital dislocation of the hip by Ortolani's method. (*A*) Hips adducted. (*B*) Hips abducted to feel movement of the femoral head back into the acetabulum.

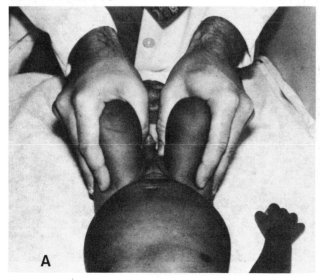
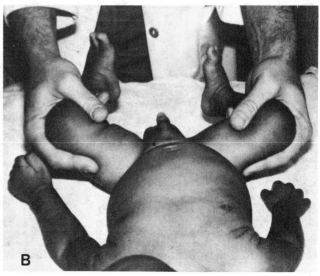

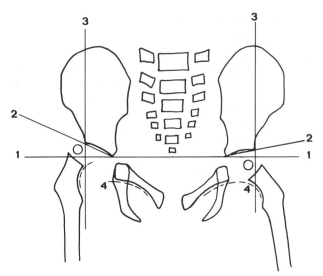

Fig. 44-46. Radiographic indexes of congenital dislocation of the hip. Hilgenreiner's line (*1*) is the horizontal line through the triradiate cartilage. Acetabular index angle line (*2*). The average acetabular index at birth is 27.5°. An acetabular index over 30° implies a dislocated hip. The index gradually decreases to 20° at 2 years of age. Perkins' line (*3*) is a vertical line through the outer lip of the acetabulum. In a normal hip the femoral head ossification center is in the medial inferior quadrant of the intersection between Hilgenreiner's line and Perkins' line, as in the left hip. The right femoral head ossification center is in the upper outer quadrant indicating dislocation. Shenton's line (*4*) is an imaginary smooth arc formed medially by the superior border of the obturator foramen and laterally by the inferior margin of the neck of the femur. The left hip is normal with a smooth Shenton's line; the right hip is dislocated with a broken Shenton's line.

acetabulum. In order to obtain a stable reduction, it is necessary to clean fibrofatty tissue from the depths of the acetabulum and to incise completely the transverse ligament of the acetabulum on its inferior aspect. Failure to completely transect this ligament is probably one of the most common causes of failure of open reduction. Following reduction, the capsule is closed in a double-breasted fashion and the

patient is maintained in a spica cast for a minimum of 8 to 12 weeks. Open reduction is seldom necessary under 1 year of age. An arthrogram is often helpful in determining the completeness of reduction.

The longer the hip is dislocated, the more secondary adaptive changes will occur in the femoral head, neck, and acetabulum. When a stable reduction is accomplished under 2 years of age, then further surgical reconstructive procedures are not usually necessary. If reduction is delayed until after 2 years of age, however, the resulting high acetabular index and valgus position of the femoral neck will not always correct itself. In this situation, an osteotomy of the pelvis to correct the position of the acetabulum or a trochanteric osteotomy of the femur may be necessary to correct the coxa valga excess anteversion.

BIBLIOGRAPHY

General

LOVELL WW, WINTER RB: Pediatric Orthopaedics. Philadelphia, J B Lippincott, 1978

OZONOSS MB: Pediatric Orthopedic Radiology. Philadelphia, W B Saunders, 1979

TACHDJIAN MO: Pediatric Orthopedics. Philadelphia, W B Saunders, 1979

Cerebral Palsy

BAKER LD, DODELIN RA: Extra-articular arthrodesis of the subtalar joint (Grice procedure). JAMA 168:1005, 1958

BALMER GA, MACEWEN GD: The incidence and treatment of scoliosis and cerebral palsy. J Bone Joint Surg [Br] 52:134, 1970

BANKS HH, PANAGAKOS P: Orthopaedic evaluation of the lower extremity in cerebral palsy. Clin Orthop 47:117, 1966

BLECK EE: Deformities of the spine and pelvis in cerebral palsy. Clin Dev Med 52/53:124, 1957

BLECK EE: Orthopaedic Management of Cerebral Palsy. Philadelphia, W B Saunders, 1979

DENHOFF E: Pre and post operative medical management of the cerebral palsy child. Clin Dev Med 52/53:112, 1975

EGGERS GWN: Transplantation of the hamstring tendons to femoral condyles in order to improve hip extension and to decrease knee flexion in cerebral spastic paralysis. J Bone Joint Surg [Am] 34:827, 1952

Fig. 44-47. Congenital dislocation of the left hip in a 1-year-old. (*A*) The left femoral head is displaced superiorly and laterally, with a false acetabulum present above the original acetabulum. (*B*) Index lines are drawn on the radiograph. The right acetabular index is 17° and the left acetabular index is 42°. The left femoral ossification center is present in the superior outer quadrant.

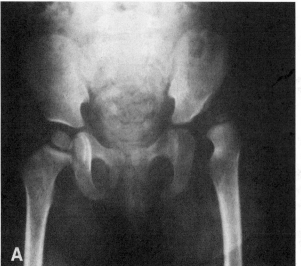 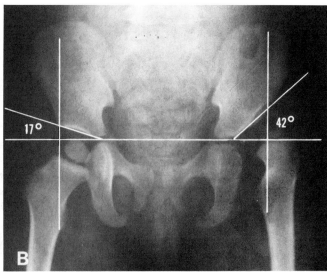

JONES MH: Differential diagnoses and natural history of the cerebral palsied child. Clin Dev Med 52/53:5, 1975

LITTLE WJ: On the influence of abnormal parturition, difficult papers, premature birth and neonatorum on the mental and physical condition of the child, especially in relation to deformities. Trans Obstet Soc London 3:293, 1862

PAINE RS: Cerebral palsy: Symptoms and signs of diagnostic and prognostic significance. In Adams JP (ed): Current Practice in Orthopaedic Surgery, vol III, pp 39–58. St. Louis, C V Mosby, 1966

SAMILSON RL: Orthopaedic Aspects of Cerebral Palsy. Philadelphia, J B Lippincott, 1975

SAMILSON RL, HOFFER MM: Problems and complications in orthopaedic management of cerebral palsy. Clin Dev Med 52/53:258, 1975

SAMILSON RL, PERRY J: The orthopaedic assessment in cerebral palsy. Clin Dev Med 52/53:35, 1975

THOMPSON SB: The nonoperative aspects of orthopaedic management of cerebral palsy. Clin Dev Med 52/53:89, 1975

Myelomeningocele

BUNCH WH: Myelomeningocele. Pediatr Orthop 1:406, 1973

CURTIS BH: The hip in the myelomeningocele child. Clin Orthop 90:11, 1973

GARDNER WJ: Myelomeningocele result of rupture of the embryonic neurotube. Cleve Clin Q 27:88, 1960

HALL JE, BOBECHAO WP: Advancement in the management of spine deformities and myelodysplasia. Clin Neurosurg 20:164, 1973

HOSTLER SL: The adolescent with myelomeningocele. AAOS Instructional Course Lecture 25:90, 1975

LINDSETH RE: Treatment of the lower extremity in children paralyzed with myelomeningocele. AAOS Instructional Course Lecture 25:76, 1976

LORBER J: Selective treatment of myelomeningocele: To treat or not to treat? Pediatrics 53:307, 1974

PATTEN BM: Embryological stages in the establishing of myeloschisis spina bifida. Am J Anat 93:365, 1953

ROSENBERGER R, STEWARD M, BUNCH WH: A standing frame for paraplegic children. Int Clin Inform Bul 14:13, 1975

Scoliosis

BJURE J, NACHEMSON A: Non-treated scoliosis. Clin Orthop 93:44, 1973

COBB JR: Outline for the Study of Scoliosis in Instructional Course Lectures, the American Academy of Orthopaedic Surgeons, vol 5. Ann Arbor, MI, W J Edwards, 1948

DRUMMOND DS, ROGALA E, GURR J: Spinal deformity: Natural history of the role of school screening. Orthop Clin 10:4, 751, 1979

HARRINGTON PR: Treatment of scoliosis: Correction and internal fixation by spine instrumentation. J Bone Joint Surg [Am] 44:591, 1962

LONSTEIN JE, WINTER RB, MOE JH, BIANCO AJ, CAMPBELL RG: School screening for the early detection of spinal deformities: Progress and pitfalls. Minn Med 59:51, 1976

MOE JH, WINTER RB, BRADFORD DS, LONSTEIN JE: Scoliosis and Other Spinal Deformities. Philadelphia, W B Saunders, 1978

Slipped Capital Femoral Epiphysis

BOYD HB: Treatment of acute slipped upper femoral epiphysis. AAOS Instructional Course Lecture 21:222, 1972

HERNDON CH: Treatment of minimally slipped upper femoral epiphysis. AAOS Instructional Course Lecture 21:188, 1972

HOWORTH MB: Pathology: Slipping of the capital femoral epiphysis. Clin Orthop 48:33, 1966

PONSETI IV, McCLINTOCK R: The pathology of slipping of the upper femoral epiphysis. J Bone Joint Surg [Am] 38:71, 1956

SOUTHWICK WO: Osteotomy through the lesser trochanter for slipped capital femoral epiphysis. J Bone Joint Surg [Am] 49:807, 1967

Legg-Calvé-Perthes Disease

CAFFEY J: The early roentgenographic changes in essential coxa plana: Their significance in pathogenesis. Am J Roentgenol Rad Ther Nucl Med 103:620, 1968

CATTERALL A: The natural history of Perthes disease. J Bone Joint Surg [Br] 53:37, 1971

EATON GO: Long-term results of treatment in coxa plana. J Bone Joint Surg [Am] 49:1031, 1967

PONSETI IV, COTTON RL: Legg-Calvé-Perthes disease: Pathogenesis in evolution. J Bone Joint Surg [Am] 43:261, 1961

Talipes Equinovarus

DUNN N: Stabilizing operations in the treatment of paralytic deformities of the foot. Proc R Soc Med 15:15, 1922

DWYER FC: Osteotomy of the calcaneous for pes cavus. J Bone Joint Surg [Br] 41:80, 1959

EVANS D: Relapsed clubfoot by the insertion of a wedge into the calcaneous. J Bone Joint Surg [Br] 43:722, 1961

HEYMAN CH, HERNDON CH, STRONG JM: Mobilization of the tarsal, metatarsal, and intermetatarsal joints for the correction for the resistent adduction of the fore part of the foot in congenital clubfoot or congenital metatarsus varus. J Bone Joint Surg [Am] 48:299, 1958

HOKE M: An operation for stabilizing paralytic feet. Orthop Surg 3:494, 1921

IRANI RN, SHERMAN MS: The pathological anatomy of clubfoot. J Bone Joint Surg [Am] 45:45, 1963

KITE JH: Conservative treatment of the resistant recurrent clubfoot. Clin Orthop 70:93, 1970

LOVELL WW, HANCOCK CI: Treatment of congenital talipes equinovarus. Clin Orthop 70:79, 1970

PALMER RM: The genetics of talipes equinovarus. J Bone Joint Surg [Am] 46:542, 1964

TURCO VJ: Surgical correction of the resistant clubfoot: One-stage posteriormedial release with internal fixation: A preliminary report. J Bone Joint Surg [Am] 53:477, 1971

WYNNE-DAVIES R: Family studies and the cause of congenital clubfoot. J Bone Joint Surg [Br] 46:445, 1964

Congenital Dislocation of the Hip

BARLOW TG: Early diagnosis and treatment of congenital dislocation of the hip. J Bone Joint Surg [Br] 44:292, 1962

CHUNG SMK: Hip Disorders in Infants and Children. Philadelphia, Lea & Febiger, 1981

COLEMAN SS: Treatment of congenital dislocation of the hip in the older child. Curr Pract Orthop Surg 6:99, 1975

MacEWEN GD, RAMSEY PL: Congenital dislocation of the hip. Pediatr Orthop 2:721, 1978

SALTER RB, DUBOS J: The first fifteen years personal experience with innominate osteotomy in the treatment of the congenital dislocation and subluxation of the hip. Clin Orthop 98:72, 1974

E. Frazier Ward

Amputations

Amputations are among the oldest of surgical procedures. There is evidence that amputees existed among prehistoric men as a result of trauma or congenital loss of limb. The earliest amputations were undoubtedly crude procedures in which a limb was rapidly separated from an unanesthetized patient and hemostasis was obtained by crushing the tissue or with boiling oil. Early prostheses, which were poorly suited for fitting amputation stumps, date from the time of the early Roman Empire. In the 16th century Paré introduced ligature control of bleeding vessels and attempted to create more functional stumps. Later, development of the tourniquet, anesthetic agents, and aseptic techniques permitted the fashioning of more functional amputation stumps and stimulated improvement in prosthetic devices. Most recently, as a result of the injuries sustained in modern warfare, progress has been made in developing improved surgical amputation techniques that have afforded better surgical prosthetic fitting and improvement of ultimate limb function.

Clearly the performance of an amputation should be viewed as the first step in a rehabilitative process for the patient that will eventually return him to a more normal and productive place in his environment. Negative emotional reactions to loss of limb are far less formidable when physician and patient discuss the amputation as an early stage of rehabilitation rather than as the end of treatment for a disease process. When an amputation is undertaken by a skilled surgeon with careful planning and knowledge of limb anatomy and greater prosthetic utilization, the procedure can be correctly perceived by patient and physician with the optimism of any reconstructive operation.

Amputation, by definition, is a procedure that removes the distal part of an extremity. Disarticulation is a procedure in which the distal part of an extremity is removed through a joint.

There are an estimated 500,000 amputees in the United States with 25,000 to 30,000 added each year. More amputees are found among older age-groups for whom vascular disease is the primary indication for amputation. Young and middle-aged adults require amputation primarily for trauma. In children, amputations for malignant disease are more commonly performed, particularly among teenagers. Seventy to 80% of all amputations involve the lower limbs, and about 75% of all new amputees are men.

INDICATIONS

PERIPHERAL VASCULAR DISEASE

Irreparable loss of blood supply to a limb is probably the most common indication for amputation. Arteriosclerosis and arteriosclerotic vascular disease, particularly when associated with diabetes and progressive vascular occlusion, are the most common underlying diseases among vascular amputees. The majority of amputations for vascular disease involve the lower extremities.

Solo studies have indicated that amputations of the lower extremity performed for peripheral vascular disease, with or without associated diabetes, will usually heal when the level of amputation is below the knee. Preservation of the knee joint, which controls the swing phase of gait, is of utmost importance in the patient with peripheral disease, owing to the improved ambulation afforded by a below-knee prosthesis when compared with an above-knee prosthesis in the patient at risk for sustaining a later amputation of the contralateral extremity, or suffering limitation from weakness of the contralateral limb because of previous musculoskeletal deficiencies or cerebrovascular accidents.

TRAUMA

Traumatic injuries are the second most common cause of amputation and frequently affect young adults in the productive years of life. Irreparable traumatic destruction of the blood supply to a limb or a crush injury sufficient to preclude reasonable reconstruction of an extremity are the chief indications for traumatic amputation. In most cases the indications for such amputation are immediately obvious, but occasionally the degree of injury to skin, muscle and tendon, bone, nerve, and artery cannot be ascertained for several days or even months. In such cases, initial débridement followed by delayed amputation is preferable to a hasty early initial amputation.

Other types of injury that may destroy tissue and necessitate amputation include electrical burns, thermal burns, and frostbite. In electrical or thermal burns, initial treatment should be conservative because the extent of injury is difficult to ascertain until several days or weeks of observation have elapsed. Early attempts to determine a proper level of amputation in such injuries may be in error owing to coagulation necrosis in areas removed from the site of initial injury.

INFECTION

Acute or chronic infection in an extremity that is uncontrolled by surgical or medical therapy is an indication for amputation. Most dangerous of such infections is fulminating gas gangrene, which requires immediate amputation proximal to the infection through clean, normal, viable tissue planes. In amputations performed in the presence of sepsis or overwhelming gas gangrene, the wounds are not closed and the tissues are left open and loosely dressed. Chronic osteomyelitis may necessitate amputation when the infection has sufficiently impaired the extremity because of loss of motion at a joint or loss of bone stability through an infected nonunited fracture. Infection occurring in a neurologically deprived extremity, such as occurs with myelomeningocele, is an occasional indication for amputation. A carcinoma arising in a draining sinus tract (which usually occurs after 20 to 25 years) may necessitate amputation.

TUMORS

Amputation is performed for benign tumors only when they are exceptionally large and have destroyed a majority of the bone or when surgical excision of an exceptionally large tumor would produce a functionless limb.

Malignant tumors are more often an indication for amputation to remove the malignancy before it metastasizes, for palliation of a fungating lesion which is ulcerated or bleeding, or to relieve pain due to the tumor itself or its resultant deformity.

NERVE INJURIES

Amputations in the presence of nerve injuries are usually indicated after the development of ulcers in an anesthetic limb that has become secondarily infected.

CONGENITAL ANOMALIES

A congenitally abnormal limb whose function would be improved by a prosthesis is an indication for amputation. When treating congenital anomalies, a disarticulation at the most distal joint that will provide a more functional gait when fitted with a prosthesis is preferable to an amputation through the midshaft or diaphyseal region of a leg. Amputation surgery for congenital anomalies is a highly specialized undertaking and must be carefully individualized for each patient.

BASIC PRINCIPLES

The application of sound surgical principles is as important in performing the amputation as in any other operation. These principles encompass consideration of the level of amputation and the use of the tourniquet.

The level of amputation should provide an adequate length of stump for fitting of a prosthesis that will be as functional and pain free as possible. There must be good bleeding skin edges to allow for satisfactory early healing of the soft tissues. The level of amputation may affect the adequacy of postoperative range of motion of the joint closest to the amputation. Very short below-knee and above-knee amputation stumps are prone to cause flexion contractures of the joint above them. The level of amputation should allow and preserve as much muscle strength as possible to be applied to the stump for moving the prosthesis when fitted. The level of amputation should eliminate the presence of infection or malignancy.

Exsanguination of a limb by an elastic bandage followed by inflation of a tourniquet makes amputation easier and more rapid with less blood loss. Elastic wrapping of the limb should not be performed in the presence of infection or malignant tumors. Instead, the limb should be elevated for 5 to 10 minutes followed by inflation of the tourniquet.

OPERATIVE TECHNIQUE

The line of the skin incision for an amputation should be chosen to enable sufficient blood supply to skin edges, thus allowing optimal primary healing in the postoperative period. The skin that will eventually cover the end of the stump should be mobile, should not be adherent to bone, and should have good vascular and sensory supply. Length and size of skin flaps may be varied in order to avoid areas of compromised blood supply or to locate the enclosure line in the areas of pressure as, for example, on the end of a bone or on a pressure-bearing surface that will contact the prosthesis. The skin edges should always be handled with meticulous care, especially in patients with peripheral vascular disease, so as to avoid further damage to the vascular supply that might endanger healing of the suture line. There must be no undermining of subcutaneous tissue at the line of the skin flap so that similar compromise to the arterial circulation is avoided. Tension at the skin closure suture line should be sufficient to hold the skin edges together without the danger of further tension leading to ischemia and necrosis of the wound edges. Adherence of the skin to the end of the bone after healing causes considerable difficulty with prosthesis fitting and may lead to skin breakdown after use of the prosthetic device. The flaps and skin closure should be designed to interpose muscle or subcutaneous fat between the bone and skin flap closure line to prevent this problem.

FACTORS IN TECHNIQUE

MUSCLE

A surgeon should decide prior to performing any amputation whether to perform a conventional muscle transection allowing the muscles to retract; a myodesis, which is contraindicated in peripheral vascular disease or ischemia; or a myoplasty.

In a conventional muscle dissection the muscles are cut in a guillotine fashion and allowed to retract. In a myodesis the muscles are divided 2 to 5 inches distal to the level of the transected bone and the transected muscles are then sutured to the bone. In a myoplasty the fascia and muscles are beveled to produce a rounded stump and opposing muscle groups and fascia are sutured together over the end of the transected bone.

Myodesis and myoplasty afford increased muscle and

soft tissue coverage of the transected bone surface, increased proprioception of the stump, reduced phantom limb pain, and an opportunity for improved prosthesis fitting.

Generally, it is preferable to obtain apposition of posterior and anterior muscle groups and fascia over the bone ends, which enable greater skin flap and stump mobility.

TENDONS

Tendons are cut at the level of the amputated bone and are allowed to retract. No attempt should be made to attach the ends of the tendons directly to bone.

NERVES

Although the treatment of peripheral nerves in order to prevent neuromas in amputations has been controversial, the best evidence indicates that nerves should be pulled gently distally for several centimeters and cut with a fresh scalpel at right angles to the nerve. This treatment allows the nerve to retract into a soft muscle mass that reduces potential pressure irritation after a neuroma has formed. Peripheral nerves should never be ligated, coagulated, or injected in a surgical amputation. If a large artery or vein lies within the nerve or on its surface, the vessel should be dissected free and ligated before the nerve is cut and allowed to retract.

BLOOD VESSELS

Larger blood vessels in any amputation should be isolated and doubly ligated before they are divided. If a tourniquet is used during the performance of an amputation, it should be released before closure of the stump so that all bleeding points can be coagulated or ligated.

BONE AND PERIOSTEUM

In an amputation, the periosteum should not be stripped excessively from the bone. Formation of a sequestrum, excessive bony spur formation, and irregular bone ends are likely to occur if the periosteum is stripped proximally. In a below-knee amputation the bone should be cut at the level at which the skin retracts. The periosteum should be cut with a sharp knife at this level, and a power oscillating saw should be used to cut the bone. The power oscillating saw can then be used to bevel the edges of the bone to a smooth surface, avoiding the use of a rasp, which can damage surrounding tissue and strip the periosteum from the bone. A smooth bone surface is desirable at all points in order to prevent bony prominences that may later cause pressure necrosis of the overlying skin.

DRAINS

Drains are generally placed in the subcutaneous soft tissue at the end of an amputation in order to prevent blood and fluid collection and are never a substitute for prior obtaining of meticulous hemostasis. Closed suction drainage using Hemovac drains placed so that they emerge from the skin 1 to 2 inches proximal to the incision is preferred. Suction drains are preferable to rubber capillary drains since the suction drains are more efficient at removing fluid and can be removed when placed through a rigid dressing without removing the entire rigid dressing in 48 to 72 hours.

CLOSED AMPUTATION VS. OPEN AMPUTATION

CLOSED AMPUTATION

In a closed amputation the stump wound is closed entirely at the primary surgical procedure. Such amputations are performed most often in clean amputations or for patients with clean traumatic injury. Most amputations for peripheral vascular disease should be closed primarily and performed at a level with adequate vascular supply to promote primary healing in preference to an open amputation wound, which may be slow to heal.

OPEN AMPUTATION

In an open amputation the skin and muscle fascia are not closed over the end of the stump at the primary procedure. An open amputation can be closed later by skin foreclosure traction in a stockinette dressing with 2 to 5 pounds of attached weights and with skin dressing changes performed at least daily or a secondary operative soft tissue closure. An open amputation generally requires a later revision, reamputation, or plastic repair to obtain a stump satisfactory for prosthesis fitting. Open amputations are generally performed when severe infection, severe contaminated traumatic wounds, foreign body contamination, or gas gangrene is present. Preoperative antibiotics are required in performing open amputations. The purpose of open amputations is to eliminate spreading infection so that final closure of the stump can be performed in the absence of chronic or invasive tissue infection.

POSTOPERATIVE CARE

The postoperative care of the amputee from the time of wound closure and prosthetic fitting is one of the most important phases in the rehabilitation of the patient. In our experience, immediate postoperative prosthesis fitting performed in the operating room with prolonged anesthesia has not been as effective as the application of a rigid dressing, particularly on the below-knee amputee.

For the below-knee amputee a well-molded rigid plaster cast should be applied to the extremity in full extension, with the cast extending well above the knee and molded above the patella and adductor tubercles. If this cast is well molded, it should not slip from the stump. The skin adjacent to the drains should be well padded under the cast to avoid pressure injury, and these drains should be removed in 48 to 72 hours without the necessity for cutting or splitting the cast. Unless the patient has inordinate pain or fever, the cast is usually not removed until the first postoperative week when the wound is carefully inspected and another well-molded rigid dressing is applied with elastic plaster to further remodel the stump. At the end of 2 weeks, if wound healing is satisfactory, the sutures are removed and a temporary plaster cast or temporary molded clear socket is applied in order to enable the patient use of a temporary leg.

The below-elbow amputee is treated with a compression dressing and a padded rigid plaster cast or posterior plaster splint. Above-elbow and above-knee amputees are satisfactorily treated with compression dressings alone and do not require a rigid dressing.

Postoperatively, the physical therapist should begin to see the patient within 24 hours and begin instructions in stump care, exercise, and progressive ambulation with crutches. The patient immediately preoperatively should not be positioned in such a manner that the joints proximal to the amputation stump develop flexion contractures. Active and passive range of motion exercises are helpful in this regard.

In the above-elbow and above-knee amputations daily

elastic bandage wrapping of the stump hastens healing, shrinkage, and the development of good stump tissue with little edema. At the end of 2 weeks when the sutures are removed in the below-elbow, above-elbow, or above-knee amputation, if the wound permits, the stump can be placed in a stump shrinker and preparations made for initial fitting of a prosthesis at 4 to 6 weeks. The amputee is completely rehabilitated only when he has been evaluated for possible prosthetic fitting, is capable of handling a prosthesis, and has been sufficiently trained in the use of a prosthesis.

POSTOPERATIVE COMPLICATIONS

NECROSIS

Skin necrosis can be minimal or extensive. It is usually noted about the suture line. The known factors contributing to skin necrosis include tension on the suture line at the time of closure, extensive peripheral vascular disease, inadequate level of surgical débridement and too distal an amputation level, lack of bleeding skin edges at the level of incision and closure, and previous radiation damage to the extremity.

If there is minimal skin necrosis, often it can be excised and treated with dressing changes, although ultimate healing might be delayed. Severe deep necrosis mandates reamputation at a more proximal level without delay.

POSTOPERATIVE BLEEDING AND HEMATOMA

If a tourniquet is used during an amputation, it must be released prior to stump closure. This allows for inspection of all bleeding and meticulous hemostasis. Further hematoma formation is prevented by the use of adequate suction drainage. Healing is often delayed in the presence of a hematoma, and infection is likely. If a hematoma is minimal, the stump can be wrapped to decrease bleeding and the hematoma may resorb. If there is a massive hematoma and continued evidence of bleeding, the stump should be reexplored for hemostasis and redrained and wrapped to control the bleeding.

INFECTION

The incidence of infection after amputation should be no more severe or frequent than following other elective orthopaedic procedures. Infection is most often seen in the patient with peripheral vascular disease, especially when associated with diabetes. Purulent material arising in an amputation stump should be adequately drained even if it requires removing the sutures and returning the patient to the surgical suite for débridement. Antibiotics should be started appropriate for the Gram stain and culture of the infected material. A higher amputation level should be obtained promptly if the infection is severe with a considerable destruction of soft tissue.

Superficial wound infections in the amputation stump can often be treated with drainage and warm moist dressing changes along with systemic antibiotic therapy. If no improvement occurs in a wound treated in this fashion within 2 to 4 days, a deeper infection may be present, and the patient should be returned for débridement or reamputation in the operating suite.

CONTRACTURES

Contractures can be prevented by correct positioning of the stump and by an exercise program to strengthen muscle and mobilize joints. Contractures are least likely to occur when the patient has been seen by a physical therapist and all modalities of physical therapy pertaining to the amputee can be applied. Unfortunately, many patients are discharged from hospitals without adequate physical therapy and prosthetic rehabilitation following amputation. Severe contractures may ensue, necessitating extensive physical therapy or causing ultimate failure of rehabilitation. Small contractures should be treated by general passive stretching of the joint after the stump wound is healed, but early active physical therapy is most important in preventing contractures of the joints closest to the level of amputation.

NEUROMAS

Neuroma formation at the end of a nerve cut during performance of an amputation is a normal occurrence. Pain from neuromas may result when the nerve is bound to scar tissue undergoing retraction in the postoperative period or during rehabilitation or when the neuroma is superficial and is not protected by adjacent soft tissues from repeated trauma by pressure. When conservative treatment consisting of analgesics, injections, and nerve blocks fails, the neuroma should be removed surgically as far away from the stump end, scar tissue, and areas of bony prominence as possible and the nerve should be allowed to retract deep within higher muscle.

PRESSURE SORES AND CYSTS OF THE RESIDUAL LIMB

Pressure sores and infected cysts in the residual limb are most often due either to a poorly fitting prosthesis or to a prosthesis that is much too large for the patient because the residual limb has shrunk. If detected early enough, pressure sores can be treated conservatively, and then a new prosthesis can be fashioned. If severe or serious infection is present, then drainage, administration of antibiotics, and local care of the pressure sore or cyst are indicated. When healing occurs, a new prosthesis providing relief over the area of pressure can be fitted.

PHANTOM SENSATIONS

Every amputee has a sensation that the amputated part is present. This sensation is usually very painful but has a tendency to disappear over a period of time, especially if a prosthesis is worn on a regular basis. Phantom pain can often be relieved by local therapy in the region of the stump, but occasionally the patient requires intense psychological therapy. The treatment for "phantom limb" includes massage to the extremity, nerve block, drug therapy, psychotherapy, and transcutaneous electrical stimulation of nerves. Amputation at a higher level is not indicated for treatment of "phantom disorders."

UPPER EXTREMITY AMPUTATIONS

Upper-limb amputations are much less frequently performed than lower-limb amputations. Indications for upper-extremity amputations include malignant disease, trauma, severe or uncontrollable infection, and dysvascular disease. If amputation is to be performed in the upper extremity, every effort must be made to preserve as much limb length as possible for fitting with an appropriate prosthesis. The longer stump enables more muscle and joint motion to the extremity when fitted to a prosthesis and allows greater muscular power transfer to the prosthesis. For this reason, wrist disarticulations and partial hand amputations are performed much more frequently now than previously in order to allow for pronation and supination.

The levels of upper-extremity amputation include partial hand amputation, wrist disarticulation, below-elbow amputation (Fig. 44-48), elbow disarticulation, above-elbow amputation (Fig. 44-49), shoulder disarticulation, and forequarter amputation. Prosthetic devices are available for each level of amputation. Less ultimate function is obtainable as the level of amputation approaches the trunk. Shoulder disarticulation and forequarter amputation do not allow any substantial motor rehabilitation of the upper extremity.

LOWER EXTREMITY AMPUTATIONS

Approximately 90% of amputations involve the lower extremity, with the most common being the below-knee and above-knee types. Whereas above-knee amputation was most common in many hospitals previously, over the past 2 decades increasing use has been made of the below-knee amputation. The importance of preservation of the knee in lower-extremity amputations has been due to the recognition of its importance in control of the swing phase of gait, which can be more effectively preserved when the knee joint is available in the amputated limb.

Indications for amputation of the lower extremity include the following: peripheral vascular disease, trauma, infection, and malignant tumors. The most common levels of amputation in the lower extremity include toe or phalangeal amputations, transmetatarsal and partial foot amputations, metatarsal amputations, Syme amputations, below-knee

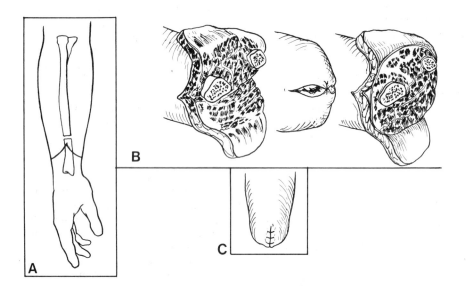

Fig. 44-48. Below-elbow amputation. (*A*) Skin incision with level of bone section. (*B*) Formation of skin flaps with bone and muscle section. (*C*) Completed amputation.

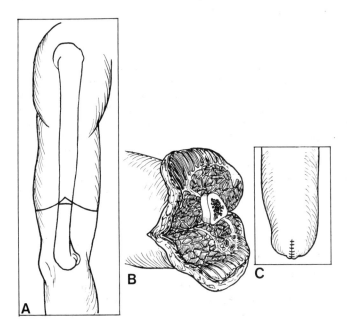

Fig. 44-49. Above-elbow amputation. (*A*) Position of skin incision with level of bone section. (*B*) Formation of skin and muscle flaps. (*C*) Completed procedure with skin closure.

amputations, knee disarticulation, above-knee amputations, hip disarticulation, and hindquarter amputations (hemipelvectomy).

Transmetatarsal and partial foot amputations are best suited for traumatic injuries in younger patients without peripheral vascular disease. Nonhealing and the necessity for higher levels of amputation occur in the majority of patients with vascular disease treated with transmetatarsal or partial foot amputation. Toe and phalangeal amputations are most commonly performed for trauma in young patients for similar reasons but they also are used to correct congenital deformity or acquired anomalies of the toes causing pain. Metatarsal amputations are well suited for traumatic injuries in younger patients unless bony deformity and infection, particularly associated with diabetic vascular disease, are present.

Syme amputation is useful for treating infection in the distal forefoot as well as crush and traumatic injuries to this area. It may be successful in patients with peripheral vascular disease who have a posterior tibial pulse of adequate pressure. Advantages of the Syme amputation include preservation of the heel flap, which provides a durable weight-bearing surface that can be carried out without the necessity of a prosthesis, allowing 80% to 100% of the body to be borne on the end of the stump. This ability can be valuable to the patient if he is required to ambulate for short periods of time. For these reasons the Syme amputation is generally preferred to a below-knee amputation on a functional basis. Women patients may object to the bulbous prosthesis required for a Syme amputation and may prefer a below-knee amputation and prosthesis for improved cosmetic appearance.

Below-knee amputation in conjunction with a proper-fitting prosthesis enables the patient to approach a normal gait pattern (Fig. 44-50 and 44-51). In addition to trauma, infection, and gangrene of the foot, the below-knee amputation is indicated for peripheral vascular disease of the lower extremity. In patients with peripheral vascular disease who are properly selected, 85% to 90% primary healing can be obtained. The importance of documentation of adequate popliteal blood flow has been of paramount importance in the prediction of successful primary healing in below-knee amputations. The helpful rule in deciding the

Fig. 44-50. Below-knee amputation. (*A*) Formation of long posterior skin flap and bevel of anterior crest of tibia. (*B*) Completed amputation with skin closure.

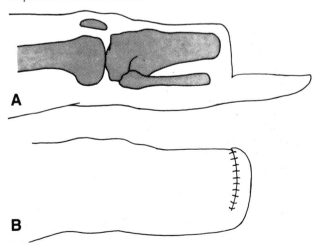

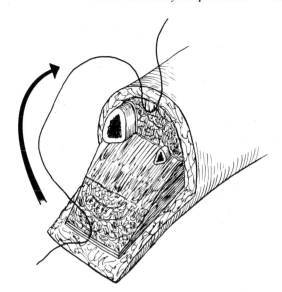

Fig. 44-51. Below-knee amputation. Formation of osteomyoplastic amputation.

length of tibia to be preserved below the knee in performing a below-knee amputation is to provide an inch of length for each foot in height of the patient. When such a length cannot be obtained due to technical problems or associated gangrene or infection, a shorter below-knee stump can be created that is preferable to an above-knee amputation. A longer posterior flap is preferable in a below-knee amputation; however, equal anterior posterior flaps may be used in preference to an above-knee amputation.

Knee disarticulations are being performed more commonly than before, especially in patients with peripheral disease in whom loss of the contralateral leg is imminent. A knee disarticulation provides an excellent weight-bearing stump on its end surface and is preferable to an above-knee amputation. Improved prosthetic devices enable excellent ambulation for patients with knee disarticulations.

Above-knee amputation (Fig. 44-52) is performed for the following indications: peripheral vascular disease, congenital limb abnormalities, severe uncontrollable infection, trauma, and malignant tumors. Whenever an above-knee amputation is performed, it is important that as much stump length be preserved as possible in order to provide a strong lever arm to power the above-knee prosthesis. It has been shown that an above-knee amputation, depending on its level, increases the patient's energy expenditure from 60% to 100% during ambulation. This inefficiency and abnormal appearance of gait in a patient with an above-knee prosthesis mandates that below-knee amputation should be performed in preference to above-knee amputation if possible. This consideration is particularly important in patients with peripheral vascular disease, since 12% of such patients lose the contralateral extremity within 2 years and 60% lose the contralateral extremity within 5 years. Whenever the level of above-knee amputation is more distal than the supracondylar region of the femur, the prosthetic knee joint may be displaced more distally than the knee of the normal side, which is cosmetically undesirable to the amputee in the sitting position.

Hip disarticulation is performed in patients with malignant tumors involving the shaft of the femur in the proximal and middle thirds, for severe chronic osteomyelitis of the entire femur not amenable to routine surgery, and for failed

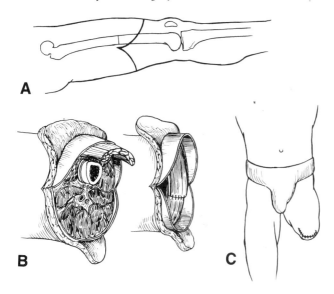

Fig. 44-52. Above-knee amputation. (*A*) Outline of skin incision. (*B*) Formation of skin flaps, bone and muscle section, and fascial closure. (*C*) Completed amputation with closure.

and chronically infected total joint replacement. Rarely, hip disarticulation is required for myonecrosis or severe gas infections of the thigh with progression to the joint capsule. These patients usually have associated peripheral vascular disease.

Hemipelvectomy is indicated for malignant disease of the proximal femur that involves the joint, malignant disease

of the soft tissues about the hip that extend across the joint into the pubic areas, metastatic and primary bone tumors that involve the pubic area and ilium, and progressive gangrene of the leg extending to areas proximal to the hip joint. Prosthetic fitting after hemipelvectomy is very difficult owing to the lack of bony support for ambulatory weight-bearing stability.

BIBLIOGRAPHY

AITKEN GT et al: Atlas of Limb Prosthetics—Prosthetic Principles. St. Lous, C V Mosby, 1981
BURGESS EM: Sites of amputation election according to modern practice. Clin Orthop 37:17, 1964
COMPERE C: Early fitting of prosthesis after amputation. Surg Clin North Am 48:215, 1968
CRENSHAW E et al: Campbell's Operative Orthopaedics, 6th ed. St. Louis, C V Mosby, 1980
FRIEDMANN LW: The Surgical Rehabilitation of the Amputee. Springfield, IL, Charles C Thomas, 1978
KANE WJ: Lower limb amputation in peripheral vascular disease. Minn Med 59:179, 1968
MASTRO BA, ROBERT T: Selected reading: A review of orthotics and prosthetics. American Orthotic and Prosthetic Association, Washington, DC, 1980
SCHMEISSER G, SEAMONE W: Upper limb prosthesis-orthosis power and control system with multi-level potential. J Bone Joint Surg [Am] 55:1493, 1973
SCOTT RN: Myoelectric control of prosthesis. Arch Phys Med Rehabil 47:174, 1966
SLOCUM DB: An Atlas of Amputations. St. Louis, C V Mosby, 1949
SPRANGER JW, LANGER LO, WIEDEMANN HR: Bone Dysplasias: An Atlas of Constitutional Disorders of Skeletal Development. Philadelphia, W B Saunders, 1974
WEISS M: Myoplastic Amputation: Immediate Prosthesis and Early Ambulation. Washington, DC, US Government Printing Office, 1971

E. Frazier Ward

Bone Tumors

DIAGNOSTIC APPROACHES TO BENIGN AND MALIGNANT BONE TUMORS
Roentgenograms
Isotopes
Arteriograms
Biopsy
Frozen Sections
Serum Alkaline Phosphatase Determinations
REPRESENTATIVE BONE TUMORS
Chondroblastoma
Osteoid Osteoma
Osteomas
Benign Osteoblastomas
Giant Cell Tumors
Unicameral Bone Cysts
Aneurysmal Bone Cysts
FIBROUS DISEASES OF BONE
Nonossifying Fibroma
Fibrous Dysplasia

Osteochondromas
Enchondroma
Chondrosarcoma
Secondary Chondrosarcomas
Osteogenic Sarcoma
Parosteal Osteosarcoma
Ewing's Sarcoma
Reticulum Cell Sarcoma—Lymphoma of Bone
Multiple Myeloma
Fibrosarcoma
Malignant Fibrous Histiocytoma
Synovial Sarcoma
Rhabdomyosarcomas
Liposarcoma

In addition to osteogenic tissues, bone also contains many other tissues that may give rise to tumors, such as hematopoietic tissue, fat, nerves, and blood vessels (Table 44-3).

TABLE 44-3   TUMORS CAUSED BY BONE TISSUES

CELL	BASIC TISSUE	LESION Benign	Low-Grade Malignancy	High-Grade Malignancy
Fibroblast	Fibrous	Fibrous cortical defect Nonossifying fibroma	Fibrosarcoma (grade I)	Fibrosarcoma (grades II–III)
Fibrocartilage	Fibrous chondroid	Chondromyxofibroma		
Fiber-bone	Fibrous bone	Fibrous dysplasia	Fibrosarcoma	
Chondroblast	Cartilage	Enchondroma Chondroblastoma Osteochondroma	Chondrosarcoma (grade I)	Chondrosarcoma (grades II–III)
Osteoblast	Bone	Osteoid osteoma Osteoblastoma Osteoma	Parosteal osteosarcoma	Intramedullary osteosarcoma
Osteoclast	Osteoclastic	Giant cell tumor Hyperparathyroid	Giant cell tumor	Giant cell sarcoma
Lipoblast	Fat-lipid	Lipoma	Liposarcoma	Liposarcoma
Endothelial	Vascular	Hemangioma	Hemangioendothelioma	Angiosarcoma
Leiomyomal	Smooth muscle	Leiomyoma	Leiomyosarcoma	Leiomyosarcoma
Physaliphorous	Notochord		Chordoma	
Leukocyte	Inflammatory	Osteomyelitis	Lymphoma, leukemia	
Inflammatory	Hematopoietic	Gout, sarcoid	Myeloma	
Histiocyte	Histiocytic	Eosinophilic granuloma Gaucher's disease	Hand-Schüller-Christian disease	Letterer-Siwe disease
Epithelial	Skin epithelium	Epidermoid inclusion cyst	Adamantinoma	Melanoma Squamous cell carcinoma
Neuronal	Nerve	Neurofibroma	Neurofibrosarcoma	Neurofibrosarcoma
Synovial	Synovium	Pigmented villonodular synovitis	Synovioma	Synovioma

New bone formation seen both microscopically and radiologically may be classified as either malignant ossification, in which the bone is formed by malignant osteoblasts, or benign ossification, in which the bone is formed by normal osteoblastic activity (Table 44-4).

Destruction or resorption of bone may result from either decreased or increased vascularity, from pressure of the tumor, or from mechanical compression of blood vessels with consequent ischemic necrosis and sequestrum formation.

On reviewing roentgenograms of patients with either malignant or benign bone tumors, it is important to determine the effects of the lesion on the bone and the response of the skeleton to the lesion. In the evaluation of a patient with a bone tumor a working differential diagnosis can be devised in many cases from the following four determinants in reading the roentgenograms:

1. Age. The type of lesion seen in the patient may depend on whether there is mature or immature skeletal development.
2. Location of the lesion. Frequently the location determines the type of tumor present; the parameters involving the location include type of bone involved, area of bone involved, and position in the bone (*e.g.*, whether it is eccentric or central).
3. Tissue types of tumors. Are they cartilage? If they are, do they have calcification or do they have a thick cartilaginous cap? Does the bone exhibit a marked blastic or lytic change? Are there fluid or fat-filled areas indicating cystic changes in the bony tissue itself?
4. Other determinants. Is there soft tissue involvement around the lesion? Are the tissue planes present? Are

TABLE 44-4   MALIGNANT LESIONS THAT MAY ARISE FROM BENIGN OR LOW-GRADE MALIGNANT LESIONS

MALIGNANT	BENIGN
Fibrosarcoma	Postradiation { Osteitis Giant cell tumor }
Malignant fibrous histiocytoma	Nonossifying fibroma Fibrous dysplasia Chronic osteomyelitis
Osteosarcoma	Paget's disease Postradiation osteitis Bone infarction Giant cell tumor Osteoblastoma
Chondrosarcoma	Enchondroma Osteochondroma Chondroblastoma Chondromyxofibroma

muscles displaced? Is there extensive edema? Are tissue muscle planes obliterated, which may occur in infection?

DIAGNOSTIC APPROACHES TO BENIGN AND MALIGNANT BONE TUMORS

ROENTGENOGRAMS

When a bone lesion is suspected, conventional anterior, posterior, and lateral roentgenographic views are obtained of the involved area. These basic views show the location and position of the lesion as well as its size and outline and are useful in determining whether the lesion is osteolytic, osteoblastic, expansile, indolent, deforming, or infiltrative.

An impression as to the type of bone lesion can often be obtained by its position in the bone (Table 44-5). Bony resolution or proliferation also may help to define the nature of the lesion. Osteolytic lesions include the following:

I. Primary sarcoma
   A. Osteosarcoma
   B. Chondrosarcoma
   C. Fibrosarcoma
   D. Liposarcoma
II. Round cell tumors
   A. Myeloma
   B. Lymphoma of bone
   C. Neuroblastoma
III. Metastatic lesions
   A. Hyponephroma
   B. Thyroid
   C. Breast (may be osteolytic or osteoblastic; the breast tumors have a tendency to become more osteoblastic following chemotherapy)
   D. Lung (may be osteoblastic or osteolytic)
   E. Colon
   F. Prostate (2% to 5% are osteolytic)
IV. Infection

The growth characteristics of the lesion may be useful and include the following:

I. Expansile
   A. Solitary bone cyst
   B. Aneurysmal bone cyst
   C. Giant cell tumor
   D. Enchondroma
   E. Some fibrous lesions
II. Indolent
   A. Nonossifying fibroma
   B. Benign lesions of metaphyseal fibrous cortical defect
   C. Brodie's infection
III. Deforming
   A. Paget's disease
   B. Ollier's disease
   C. Fibrous dysplasia
   D. Multiple hereditary exostoses
IV. Infiltrative
   A. Round cell
      1. Ewing's sarcoma
      2. Reticulum cell sarcoma
      3. Neuroblastomas

TABLE 44-5   POSITION IN BONE

CENTRALLY LOCATED	ECCENTRICALLY LOCATED	PERIPHERAL
Unicameral bone cyst	Aneurysmal bone cyst	Subperiosteal chondroma
Fibrous dysplasia	Giant cell tumor	Periosteal osteosarcoma
Round cell tumors	Nonossifying fibroma	Osteochondroma
Enchondroma	Osteoid osteoma	Osteoid osteoma
	Fibrous dysplasia	
	Chondromyxoid fibroma	

B. Leukemia
C. Lymphomas
D. Certain metastatic diseases
E. Infection

Routine roentgenograms may also indicate the skeleton's reaction to a lesion:

I. Endosteal reaction
   A. Minimal to no reaction may indicate a malignant lesion.
   B. Large to small margination is a consideration of malignant lesion.
   C. A well-contained lesion that is scalloped with a sclerotic border is often considered to be a benign process.
II. Periosteal reaction
   A. An onionskin appearance is shown by infection and Ewing's sarcoma.
   B. Codman's triangle reveals cortical breakthrough with the bone's response to rapidly growing tumor. Codman's triangle does not contain malignant tissue but is periosteal new bone in response to rapid tumor growth.
   C. The sunburst appearance in which tumor bone is formed at 45° to 90° to the shaft is seen primarily in osteosarcomas (Fig. 44-53).

The roentgenographic examination of involved soft tissue may be helpful in establishing the diagnosis. Swollen and blurred tissue planes are characteristic of inflammation and trauma. Present but displaced tissue planes indicate benign or malignant tumors. Tissue planes that are completely replaced are seen in myositis ossificans and tumoral calcinosis.

Further study of routine roentgenograms should define the area of involved bone as epiphyseal, diaphyseal, or metaphyseal. This information can impart a consideration to different types of bone tumor:

I. Epiphyseal
   A. Epiphyseal plates open: chondroblastoma
   B. Epiphyseal plates closed: giant cell tumor
   C. Pigmented villonodular synovitis and synovioma
II. Diaphyseal
   A. Fibrous dysplasia
   B. Round cell tumors
   C. Histiocytosis X (*e.g.,* eosinophilic granuloma)
   D. Osteoid osteomas
   E. Adamantinoma
   F. Metastatic tumors
III. Metaphyseal: remainder of lesions (60% to 80%)

Infection must be considered in the light of the patient's history. It can involve all types of bone, occur in all positions of the bone, and occur in all areas of the body.

Additional diagnostic tools or special procedures include tomograms of the chest and computed tomograms of the bony lesion and the chest (Fig. 44-54); arteriograms, especially in renal cell carcinoma or hyponephroma; gastrointestinal radiographic series; barium enemas; intravenous pyelography; and cystography. Should the findings of one or more studies be normal, each should be considered as only a part of the workup and further tests should be obtained as indicated.

ISOTOPES

Bone scans are an invaluable diagnostic tool in the patient with a suspected malignant lesion who has had a previous

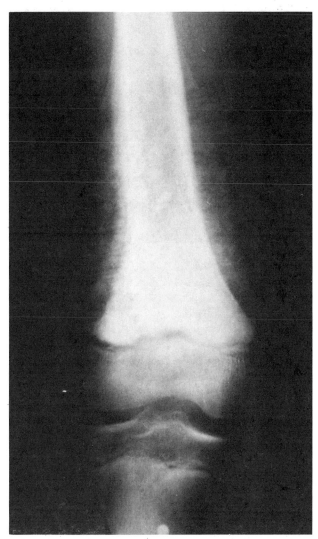

Fig. 44-53. Routine anterior-posterior film of 12-year-old with 1-month history of pain and swelling of distal right femur. Picture shows classic "sunburst"-like distal femoral metaphysis of osteogenic sarcoma and Codman's triangle toward diaphyseal region.

Fig. 44-54. Axial tomogram of primary malignant lesion of distal right femur.

tumor elsewhere and subsequently has pain at a site distant from the primary lesion. Frequently an area of isotope concentration is detected that is totally distant to the primary site and shows evidence of either bony or pulmonary metastasis (Fig. 44-55). False-negative results of bone scans may occur in patients with metastasis if the tumor has such rapid growth that the bone and the vasculature have not had sufficient time to respond.

The value of the bone scan is that it adds to overall detection of lesions undetectable by conventional radiographs, since 30% to 50% loss of bone substance is necessary for a lesion to be seen on the conventional views.

ARTERIOGRAMS

An arteriogram is useful for outlining the size of the tumor and the vessels supplying the tumor. Several characteristics of the arteriogram may point toward malignancy: rapid arterial filling with a tumor blush, increased vascular channels, increased pooling of the contrast dye, and increased size of the vessels feeding the area of the tumor (Fig. 44-56). Selective embolization of tumor vessels by means of the arteriogram catheter has been useful on occasion.

The incidence of complications of arteriography when performed with the patient under local anesthesia is small (less than 2% to 5%); allergy and thrombosis occur most often.

BIOPSY

Prior to actual biopsy the patient should have a complete evaluation including staging of the lesion. The type of biopsy selected may be one of the following: aspiration, incisional, excisional, wide excisional, and radical excisional.

For lesions of the thoracic and lumbar spine that are not readily accessible to surgical intervention without considerable systemic stress to the patient, a Craig needle biopsy may often lead to the diagnosis of a malignant tumor and further planning of the patient's treatment. The Craig needle biopsy yields a 3-mm wide core of tissue with the length dependent on the depth of the bone biopsied. A negative

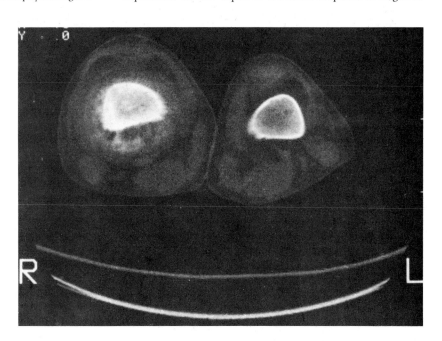

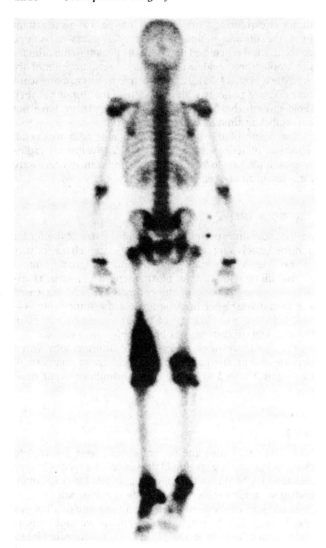

Fig. 44-55. Bone scan of increased uptake by tumor in distal right femur (same patient as in Figure 44-53).

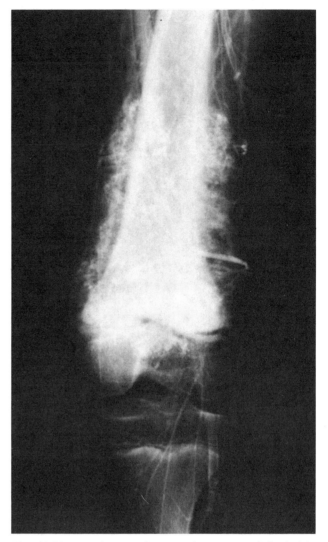

Fig. 44-56. Arteriogram of osteogenic sarcoma of distal right femur.

result of biopsy of the spine or a bone should not be taken as conclusive since the tumor may not have been penetrated. Multiple samples should always be obtained to prevent a false-negative result. I have found the Craig needle biopsy of a vertebral body to be 90% accurate in lesions of the thoracic and lumbar spine.

FROZEN SECTIONS

Frozen section can frequently be performed in benign and malignant bone and soft tissue tumors, especially in the latter. A cytologic smear of the tumor surface is often helpful in establishing a rapid diagnosis if a definitive procedure is to be performed on the basis of results of the smear or frozen section. However, when one is dealing with bone and a clear-cut diagnosis cannot be made on the basis of a cytologic smear or a frozen section, then a permanent section should be made after decalcification and staining; this requires approximately 2 days of laboratory processing. Whenever the diagnosis is in doubt, definitive surgery should be delayed until an accurate tissue diagnosis can be obtained.

SERUM ALKALINE PHOSPHATASE DETERMINATIONS

Patients with malignant bone tumors exhibit varying elevations of serum alkaline phosphatase in proportion to the amount of new bone formation or osteoid produced by the bone tumor, whether primary or metastatic. The alkaline phosphatase levels may return to normal after surgery, but that observation is not necessarily indicative of cure and does not correlate with survival. However, progressively increasing alkaline phosphatase levels in the patient with a primary metastatic bone disease indicate progression of the metastatic lesion, local recurrence, or metastatic recurrence.

REPRESENTATIVE BONE TUMORS

CHONDROBLASTOMA

The chondroblastoma is an epiphyseal lesion that is usually eccentric in its location. It occurs in the first 2 decades of life and involves the immature skeletal epiphysis before the epiphyseal plate is closed. It is most often seen in the proximal humerus, proximal tibia, and distal femur.

Clinical Manifestations. The patient often presents with a history of painful swelling with decreased range of motion in the involved joint. Roentgenograms typically show a lesion in the epiphysis that is osteolytic and contains calcific deposits. The chondroblastoma usually has a demarcated discrete margin. At biopsy the lesion is grossly vascular with a gritty appearance. Histologically, a pattern of chondroid material with occasional giant cells and osteoid tissue in calcified areas is seen.

Treatment. Treatment is curettage of the lesion and packing with autogenous cancellous bone graft, which usually gives excellent results.

OSTEOID OSTEOMA

Osteoid osteoma is diaphyseal and usually involves males in their first to third decades. There is a propensity for involvement of the bones of the lower extremity. The osteoma classically involves the cortex but may involve the medulla of the bone. It exhibits exuberant reactive bone and has a radiolucent nidus.

Clinical Manifestations. The patient presents with pain, which is often nocturnal and relieved by salicylates.

Treatment. Complete resection, if possible, usually provides a cure.

OSTEOMAS

Osteomas are small rare tumors found primarily around the skull. They occur in membranous formed bone, may be seen occasionally around the femur, and are most often called traumatic osteomas. These tumors are dense, peripheral, and termed *ivory exostoses*. The bone of an osteoma may form from abnormal growth or imperfect remodeling. Various names are given to the lesion depending on the site and the origin.

BENIGN OSTEOBLASTOMAS

The benign osteoblastoma is an uncommon avascular osteoid- and bone-forming tumor; 50% involve the posterior spinal elements. The patient is usually 20 to 50 years of age and may present with spinal cord compression and subsequent paraplegia if surgery is not performed. The lesions may have a lucent, hazy appearance and may be expansile and eccentric. They usually exhibit a reactive but not an exuberant rim. They may be seen in metaphyseal or diaphyseal regions of the long bones and may present as soft tissue masses. The lesions are usually vascular and deep red and can vary considerably in size. The tissue is strewn with abundant osteoblasts and is highly vascular, with sheets of osteoid and primitive osseous tissue. The lesion varies in density on the roentgenogram depending on the degree of ossification.

Clinical Manifestations. In general the patient presents with a dull, aching pain, occasional weakness, and paresthesia, which develops gradually.

Treatment. Treatment consists of total excision of the lesion followed by resolution of the neurologic deficits.

GIANT CELL TUMORS

Giant cell tumors, which were previously called osteoblastomas, are located in the area of the old epiphysis and occur after the physis is closed. They are eccentric and after a period of time extend into the metaphyseal regions. They occur most often in areas of remodeling bone. Giant cell tumors exhibit a thin reactive rim to no rim at all and are expansile. They most often present as a radiolucent-appearing lesion, especially in the long bones of the proximal tibia, distal femur, and distal radius. The age range at the time of presentation is usually 16 to 50 years of age.

Giant cell tumors must be differentiated from giant cells of hyperparathyroidism, unicameral bone cyst, aneurysmal bone cyst, and histiocytic granulomatosis. They are most often seen about areas of hemorrhage and spicules of old bone and walls of small cysts. In comparison, Langhans' giant cells, which are characteristic of tuberculosis, contain a smaller number of peripherally placed nuclei; foreign body giant cells are even smaller and contain fewer (usually under 15) various-sized centrally placed nuclei.

Malignant giant cell tumors of bone probably represent a sarcomatous metaplasia that occurs in previously benign giant cell tumors. These can also be described as an osteolytic form of osteogenic sarcoma, and the malignant changes originating in the benign giant cell tumor may follow previous disturbances of the tumor by irradiation or curettage.

The histologic appearance that determines malignancy is based primarily on the stromal appearance of the tumor, which may show varying degrees of typical features of mitotic activity, pleomorphism, and hyperchromatism.

Clinical Manifestations. Clinically these patients present with a history of pain, decreased function around the joint, painful range of motion, and progressive asymmetrical swelling. The characteristic finding of giant cell tumors is the very abundant giant cell. The cells usually contain centrally placed uniform nuclei with a surrounding halo of eosinophilic material.

Treatment. The operative treatment of very small lesions that are benign in appearance consists of curettage and bone grafting, but such localized treatment may be followed by a 40% to 60% rate of recurrence. Recurrences and larger primary tumors are best treated by *en bloc* resection and allografting for excision of the bone and turn-up.

UNICAMERAL BONE CYSTS

Unicameral bone cysts are most often found in the proximal humerus and proximal femur (66% cases). These lesions occur particularly in the metaphyseal area of the femur and humerus during the years of active bone growth.

Clinical Manifestations. The patients usually present with a pathologic fracture associated with a minor injury. Frequently they have had no previous symptoms and the lesion is found incidentally on the roentgenogram. These cysts are thought to originate from a remnant of synovial tissue encapsulated in the bone as it was formed embryologically.

Roentgenographically, a characteristic expanding lesion is seen in the metaphysis with a thinning of the cortex to a thin shell. The lesion is loculated into relatively large cystic areas, is expansile, and is centrally located, as opposed to the aneurysmal bone cyst, which is more eccentrically located. The prognosis depends on the proximity of the lesion to the epiphyseal plate and on the age at which the patient presents.

At surgery these cysts are seen to contain a clear, yellowish fluid with a thin, fine, fibrous layer lining the cyst. The cysts are avascular. Histologically there is a thin fibrous framework in continuity with the wall of the lesion with little cellular activity unless a pathologic fracture has occurred.

The unicameral bone cysts must be differentiated from the following four disorders:

1. A giant cell tumor appears most often in the epiphysis in an older age-group with less involvement of the metaphyseal area.
2. Osteitis fibrosa cystica, a generalized form of von Recklinghausen's disease, occurs during adolescence in the metaphysis and seems to spread more often down the shaft. The histologic appearance of biopsy of osteitis fibrosa cystica is completely different from that of the unicameral bone cyst although degeneration may be seen in both lesions.
3. Simple bone cysts must be separated from hydatid disease, which occurs in the long bones of adults and forms localized solid masses of material, replacing the marrow in cancellous and cortical components of bone and extending into the soft tissues.
4. Brodie's abscess is a low-grade osteomyelitis in which purulent material is found at biopsy that is entirely different from the biopsy specimen of a unicameral bone cyst or simple bone cyst.

Treatment. In the past, treatment has been primarily surgical, directed toward obliteration of the cavity by curettage and then bone grafting is used to restore continuity after pathologic fractures have healed.

Approximately 65% of our most recent cases have improved with one intracystic injection of methylprednisolone (Depo-Medrol). This has resulted in progressive healing of lesions, with a second injection of methylprednisolone required in only about 30% of the cases.

ANEURYSMAL BONE CYSTS

An aneurysmal bone cyst is a benign lesion that may represent an intermediate phase of other bone tumors and consists primarily of a mass of vascular spaces enclosed in a shell of periosteal new bone. The cysts are usually single and present radiographically with a "soap bubble" lobulated, expansile, eccentric appearance. Frequently they may attain sufficient size to grow outward and displace the soft tissues and may be surrounded by a faint outline of periosteal new bone. Aneurysmal bone cysts are located in the vertebral bodies, the skull, and the long bones, where they are most often evident in the metaphysis or metaphyseal-diaphyseal junction. These lesions are most commonly seen in the second and third decades of life.

At surgery the thin outer wall or shell of the aneurysmal bone cysts can be penetrated easily and a reddish-brown friable material that is interspersed with gritty particles of bone is encountered. The tumor is highly vascular and may bleed profusely as the spongy bone and marrow are replaced by small to large pools of blood enclosed in fibro-osseous septums.

Histologically, there is a thin layer of connective tissue lining the vascular spaces containing occasional nuclear giant cells with some calcium deposits. At the periphery the shell displays active periosteal new bone formation.

Clinical Manifestations. A patient may present with pain, local swelling, and limitation of motion. There are occasions in which a history of trauma may be elicited, but in cases involving the vertebral bodies the patients may present with scoliosis, long tract signs, and weakness since the lesion involves the posterior arch and may compress the cord.

Treatment. Treatment is primarily operative. Small lesions may regress spontaneously, but large lesions may be curetted and the defect filled with bone graft.

FIBROUS DISEASES OF BONE

NONOSSIFYING FIBROMA

Nonossifying fibromas are usually benign fibrous growths within a small area of bone. They are seen in about a third of the population, most often in the bones of the lower extremity. Usually they are incidental findings and only occasionally do they grow to sufficient size to produce a pathologic fracture. These fibromas are located eccentrically in the cortical regions of the metaphysis of the distal femur and proximal and distal tibias. They are often indolent and appear in the immature skeleton with a reactive rim. Frequency is approximately equal in both sexes.

Roentgenographically the lesion is sharply defined, translucent, and lobulated, with a thin border of increased density. Histologically, a thin cortex covers a soft, rubbery, gray, yellow, or reddish-brown tissue. Deposits of hemosiderin may be found within the lesion interspersed with a fibrous tissue of varying cellularity. Trabeculations are conspicuously absent, and the diagnosis is established roentgenographically.

Clinical Manifestations. Occasionally the lesions may be of sufficient size to produce a pathologic fracture as a first symptom. Bony swelling accompanied by pain on palpation may also be present.

Treatment. Treatment depends on the size; if the fibromas are of sufficient size to produce pathologic fracture, the treatment of choice would be to curette and pack the evacuated area with an autogenous cancellous graft. The operated area is protected with a cast postoperatively until sufficient bone healing occurs.

FIBROUS DYSPLASIA

Fibrous dysplasia may be monostotic or polyostotic; the latter type is known as Albright's disease. It may involve the skull or flat bones or the long bones in the metaphyseal or diaphyseal regions. It can be eccentric or central in its location within the bone. The condition begins in childhood and progresses into adulthood. Both sexes appear to be equally affected. Radiographically the affected bone is irregular, with a thin cortex bulging outward due to the underlying abnormal tissue. The lesion may have a ground-glass appearance, a thin reactive shell, and a lobulated appearance.

Involvement of the hips characteristically produces a coxa vara or "shepherd's crook" deformity. Pathologic fractures are frequent in this lesion, and the tissue observed at surgery is dense and fibrous with imbedded fibrous bone trabeculations. Bony structure is replaced by avascular fibrous tissue, which is irregular. Surgical removal of the cortex reveals a reddish-gray to gray, tough, fibrous tissue, which is dense and contains imbedded fibrous bone trabeculae. Osteoclastic activity is minimal, and the characteristic picture histologically is that of fibroblast laying down bone.

Clinical Manifestations. Clinically the fibrous dysplasia begins in early childhood or adolescence and may be asymptomatic. The initial complaint may be a limp or a pain in the leg or a shortening of one leg when compared with the other.

In the polyostotic form, which seems to involve one side of the body primarily, early puberty may occur in females, along with multiple pigmented areas of skin (café-au-lait lesions).

Treatment. Treatment classically has been curettage and packing of the bony space with an autogenous cancellous iliac crest graft followed by external support. In the presence of a pathologic fracture the patient should be allowed to wait 7 to 10 days before a bone graft is attempted, and he should be informed that there is a 20% to 30% recurrence rate.

OSTEOCHONDROMAS

Clinical Manifestations. Osteochondromas are found in bone that is preformed in cartilage. They are usually peripheral and metaphyseal and point away from the physis. The tumor is found most often in the adolescent and young adult and is characterized by a prominent mass that may or may not be associated with pain. They are frequently located at the adductor tubercle of the femur, in the proximal humerus, and in the proximal and the distal tibia. Roentgenographically they may be pedunculated or sessile with the cartilage cap poorly visualized; calcification may be present in the cap. The firm lobulated mass, which varies in size, is encapsulated and often continuous with the periosteum of the adjacent bone. On removal of the fibrous capsule a shiny, smooth cartilaginous surface is exposed. Beneath the cartilaginous cap the interior of the tumor consists of cancellous bone and fatty marrow. The osteochondroma enlarges in the same manner as the epiphyseal plate by the process of endochondral ossification and continues during the growth period of the individual. A very thick cartilaginous layer of more than 1 cm may have a poorer prognostic significance as do increasing size in the mature individual whose epiphyses have closed and the rapid, progressive onset of pain associated with tumor growth. The cancellous bone of the interior of the osteochondroma is continuous with that of the parent bone. These lesions may be single or multiple; the latter are known as multiple hereditary exostoses or multiple osteochondromatoses.

Treatment. Surgical intervention is indicated for repeated painful lesions, repeated rapid growth associated with pain (there is a malignant change in 2% to 10% of the cases), and interference with joint function. *En bloc* resection to prevent recurrence and remove the tumor at its base is the procedure of choice.

ENCHONDROMA

Enchondromas are formed from bones that arise from enchondral bone growth. They may be single or multiple, with the latter being known as Ollier's disease. They are benign tumors of childhood and young adults and occur in a central location of bone arising close to the old epiphyseal plate. Older patients present with lesions around the hands or feet. The common sites are the humerus, the femur, and the phalanges. They may be central or subperiosteal in location, are usually expansile, and may have calcific stippling. Enchondromas have a potential for undergoing malignant transformation, especially when associated with the large long bones and the pelvis, in which there is a 20% to 25% chance of malignant degeneration.

Roentgenographically, enchondromas appear as small to moderately large translucent, lobulated or nonlobulated areas that are well demarcated from surrounding bone. Erosion of the cortex of the large tubular bones suggests malignant transformation or change.

Histologically the tumor is surrounded by a fibrous capsule. The neoplastic tissue is composed of bluish-white translucent cartilage containing white areas of calcification and cysts containing a gelatinous or myxomatous substance. The tumor shows stages of cartilage formation from embryonic tissue.

Clinical Manifestations. The patients present with localized swelling and may occasionally have pathologic fractures in the hand. Frequently, when enchondromas involve the long bones no symptoms are present. Pain in the regions associated with enchondroma may be an indication of secondary sarcomatous transformation.

Treatment. The basic therapeutic approach is surgical. The enchondroma is removed and the cavity that is created is filled with autogenous cancellous bone. If malignancy is diagnosed, amputation may be advised.

CHONDROSARCOMA

Chondrosarcoma may be primary or secondary. Primary chondrosarcoma arises in bone. The lesion, which is usually centrally located, arises by malignant transformation from either a primary tumor or from an enchondroma. The long bones most often affected are the femur, tibia, and humerus; however, other bones such as the ribs and innominate bone may be sites of origin for primary chondrosarcoma.

The majority of primary chondrosarcomas occur in the age range of 30 to 60 years, with a slight predilection for males (60% of cases). Clinically, the patient is often aware of a long-term swelling, most often in the long bones, which may or may not be painful. These patients usually have a slowly enlarging mass, which in the later stages may become mildly to moderately painful. In general chondrosarcomas are very slow growing and metastasis occurs late in their development. Early metastatic changes are most often due to local erosion and extension into blood vessels. Metastasis of chondrosarcomas usually occurs to the lungs in the late stages of the disease or with highly malignant lesions.

Clinical Manifestations. Physical examination usually reveals a long bone of the femur, tibia, or humerus that is progressively enlarging and mildly tender. The skin and overlying soft tissue may not exhibit any changes until the lesion is quite large. If the chondrosarcoma is noted proximally or in proximity to a joint, there is often limitation of motion.

Roentgenologic changes in tumors that are located centrally include irregular mottling and calcific stippling, frequently with irregular destruction of the cortex. Although chondrosarcomas may be central, peripheral, or extraskeletal, the peripheral chondrosarcomas show much more calcific densities than do the benign osteochondromas. There is a calcification in chondrosarcomas that extends away from the tumor in irregular patches.

Histologically, primary chondrosarcoma shows a marked nuclear material and many cells in relation to the amount of cartilage matrix. Frequently, the cells are multinucleated with marked pleomorphism. Chondrosarcomas exhibit a peculiar behavior in that those that appear to be of a low grade quite frequently exhibit very malignant behavior while those of a high grade histologically may not be very aggressive. Thus, cartilage tumors may be very unpredictable in their clinical course.

Treatment. Owing to late metastases characteristic of chondrosarcomas, wide excision and resection of the lesion should be performed, or if resection is impossible, then amputation may be indicated. If the tumor is of sufficiently small size that resection is possible, reconstructive surgery should be considered. For a massive tumor, amputation is preferable. Cartilage tumors are notoriously radioresistant and do not respond well to chemotherapy.

SECONDARY CHONDROSARCOMAS

Malignant secondary cartilage tumors may arise from a preexisting chondroma or osteochondroma and in Ollier's disease (multiple enchondromatosis). These tumors may be periosteal or central if they arise from these preexisting lesions. They are most often seen in patients 35 to 60 years of age and are more frequently located about the pectoral and pelvic girdles. They are also seen in the distal femur and the proximal tibia.

Clinical Manifestations. The patient may complain of chronic, vague discomfort of 1 to 15 years' duration with progressively increasing swelling and pain. Frequently, early secondary chondrosarcomas can be seen arising from a preexisting lesion; but if the tumor is of long duration, the original lesion may be obscured. Pathologic fractures occur in a very small percentage of these patients (5% to 10%).

Treatment. Since the diagnosis of secondary chondrosarcoma is made only from the biopsy material rather than from the roentgenographic or gross appearance, the 5-year survival rate approaches 40% to 50%. With any cartilage tumor that is considered to have malignant potential, wide excisional biopsy is the method of choice unless the lesion is inaccessible for excision, in which case radical surgery in the form of amputation should be considered. Chemotherapy and irradiation for chondrosarcomas are generally not as effective as definitive surgery, such as wide excision or ablation.

OSTEOGENIC SARCOMA

Osteogenic sarcomas arise from cells associated with bone-forming mesenchyme. The tumor may be primarily osteolytic or osteoblastic, depending on how much tumor bone is formed. The location of this tumor is most often in the metaphysis of the femur, followed by the proximal end of the tibia and the proximal humerus. Other less common sites are the pelvis, the radius, and the ulna. The short bones of the hands and feet are seldom involved. These tumors are highly malignant and metastasize by vascular invasion. When the patient has had the symptoms for any length of time, pulmonary metastases are quite frequent; they often occur soon after definitive ablative surgery is performed or may be seen at the time of initial presentation. This very malignant tumor affects males more often than females. Previously, the 5-year survival rate was 10% to 20%; more recent studies, however, favor a 50% to 60% rate. The tumor occurs most often in the second and third decades of life, but it may occur at any age.

Histologically the diagnosis of osteogenic sarcoma is established by the presence of tumor cells laying down osteoid. Frequently the lesions may have a cartilaginous or a fibrous component, but one diagnostic characteristic is the appearance of cells that are very pleomorphic and

mitotic laying down tumor osteoid. Grossly the tumor is soft to firm, is blue-white or gray-blue and has a gritty sensation. Although the lesion is most often noted in the metaphysis, the diaphyseal side of the tumor has a Codman's triangle due to the raised periosteum with new bone formation that is triangular in shape. Pathologic fractures are uncommon because of the patient's guarding and limitation of weight-bearing, but they will occur in patients seen late in the course of their disease.

Clinical Manifestations. The patient usually complains of pain, limitation of motion of the proximal joint, rather rapid progressive enlargement of the affected parts, weight loss, and malaise. The serum alkaline phosphatase level is elevated. The characteristic sunburst appearance is not always present in osteogenic sarcoma but is diagnostic when seen. Perforation of the bony cortex and formation of bone beneath the periosteum indicate malignant tumor.

Treatment. Treatment is operative and is combined with adjuvant chemotherapy. When the diagnosis of osteogenic sarcoma has been confirmed by biopsy, radical amputation is performed through the joint above the bone that is involved with the lesion. For a lesion in the proximal tibia an amputation above the knee would be sufficient; for one in the distal femur a hip disarticulation is usually satisfactory. There are trials of *en bloc* resection followed by adjuvant chemotherapy being performed in an attempt to salvage the extremity, but the results are not conclusive. Amputation at the time of biopsy can be performed between double tourniquets, and a cytologic smear of the lesion is helpful. The first tourniquet is put up proximal to the lesion and the biopsy is performed; the tourniquet remains inflated while a second tourniquet is applied proximal to the first if possible. If a hip disarticulation is performed, the first tourniquet is not deflated at any time until the amputation is completed. These patients develop pulmonary metastases, even with chemotherapy, and thoracotomy may be advisable to remove the metastases to the lungs. Recent data indicate improved 5-year survival rates in patients with osteogenic sarcomas treated by surgery and chemotherapy.

PAROSTEAL OSTEOSARCOMA

Parosteal osteosarcoma, sometimes called juxtacortical osteogenic sarcoma, is a rarer lesion than osteogenic sarcoma and is composed of malignant ossifying tissue. These lesions grow slowly over a longer period of time than other osteogenic sarcomas. They are seen most often in the third to fourth decades of life. The posterior distal femur is the site of these tumors in over 50% of cases. The bulk of the mass of this tumor may appear separated from the bone but may also be attached to one surface. The lesion in parosteal osteosarcoma is thought to arise from the surface of the bone rather than from within as does pure osteogenic sarcoma. The 5-year survival rates are much better in parosteal osteosarcoma than in osteogenic sarcoma. The treatment of choice appears to be *en bloc* resection followed by prostheses or fibular strut grafts with chemotherapy. Severe malignancy is best treated by amputation.

EWING'S SARCOMA

Ewing's tumors, which were first described in 1921, are primarily metaphyseal or diaphyseal round cell tumors that are expansile and have an onionskin or lamination appearance of the periosteum in 30% to 40% of the cases.

They may occur in the flat bones of the pelvis and ribs and may be permeative, but they are more frequently found in the diaphyseal region of the bone than in the metaphyseal region. There is a variable endosteitis response. These lesions are seen most often in the second and third decades of life. Most often the tumor arises from medullary or intracortical areas of the bone, infiltrating and destroying the involved bone.

Clinical Manifestations. These patients often present with malaise, leukocytosis, fever, and weight loss. Pain with palpable tumor and swelling constitute the symptoms, which may occur late in the course of the disease. The most common disease to be confused with Ewing's tumor is pyogenic bone infection. Although the serum alkaline phosphatase level is often normal, the leukocyte count and sedimentation rate are often elevated in patients with Ewing's sarcoma.

Histologically, Ewing's sarcoma appears as sheets of small proliferating, round, dark, basophilic-staining cells with little stroma. Because of this appearance Ewing's sarcoma may simulate other malignant lesions of bone, metastatic neuroblastoma, and inflammatory bone changes.

Treatment. The primary therapy is irradiation followed by chemotherapy. Amputation or ablation may be considered for pathologic fractures when the disease cannot be controlled by irradiation or when complications arise secondary to irradiation. The 5-year survival rate for Ewing's sarcoma remains relatively poor (12% to 20%). If the lesion is distal in an extremity, amputation may be the treatment of choice; whereas if it is in the more proximal aspect of the extremities, irradiation and chemotherapy are used.

RETICULUM CELL SARCOMA—LYMPHOMA OF BONE

Reticulum cell sarcoma occurs most often in the fourth to fifth decades of life and arises in both the long and short bones as well as in the flat bones of the skeleton. The lesion appears to be medullary with a motheaten or permeative appearance in the bone. It may occur in the diaphyseal or metaphyseal region of the bone and often penetrates the cortex. Patients may present with pathologic fractures.

Clinical Manifestations. The most common presenting symptoms of patients with reticulum cell sarcoma are progressive pain and disability with tenderness in the involved areas. Reticulum cell sarcoma is a small round cell tumor that must be differentiated from Ewing's sarcoma and is most often called a lymphoma of bone.

Treatment. Treatment consists of operation, which may include biopsy and then stabilization of the bone to prevent pathologic fracture, irradiation, and chemotherapy. The reported 5-year survival rates with this treatment have averaged about 40%.

MULTIPLE MYELOMA

Myeloma arises from the constituents of the medullary canal and the marrow of the bone and most frequently involves the spine, the flat bones, and the skull. It is an infiltrative, diffuse lesion with little or no reactive margin. Myeloma is probably the most common primary malignant bone tumor. It usually occurs after the fourth decade, and the patient who presents with anemia, malaise, osteoporosis, and compression fractures should be examined for myeloma. Pathologic fractures are the presenting symptoms in these patients in over 50% of the cases.

Clinical Manifestations. Patients complain of pain, progressive weakness, malaise, and anemia. There may be a nephrosis accompanied by proteinuria, with the possibility of Bence-Jones protein in the urine. Serum protein electrophoresis, bone biopsy, and other laboratory metabolic studies are necessary in diagnosing this disease.

Histologically, the pathologic findings are plasma cells with a characteristic "spoke wheel" or "cogwheel" appearance.

Treatment. Treatment may consist of operation and biopsy to determine the diagnosis, followed by stabilization of the possible impending pathologic fracture. It is preferable to use intramedullary rods over plates with impending pathologic fractures. Radiotherapy combined with chemotherapy is used for treatment of the systemic disease.

FIBROSARCOMA

Fibrosarcoma of bone is a malignant spindle cell tumor that may be central or eccentric. The tumor is most often seen in middle-aged patients and in those in the later decades of life. The most frequent locations are the ends of the long bones, the femur, the tibia, and the humerus. Appearance is one of a lytic motheaten lesion, with little or no reactive rim but commonly with cortical breakthrough.

Clinical Manifestations. The patients often present with severe progressive pain or pathologic fracture with slow swelling. A biopsy of the tumor will appear grossly to be a thick fibrous tissue that can be confused with other benign fibrous lesions of bone. Malignant fibrosarcomas can occur with a fibrous appearance and few neoplastic malignant features or with very malignant neoplastic features. The characteristic histologic pattern of fibrosarcoma is the chevron of interdigitating cells in a herringbone pattern.

Treatment. Treatment for fibrosarcoma is usually radical surgery or ablation. These tumors are not sensitive to radiation, and chemotherapy is of little value.

MALIGNANT FIBROUS HISTIOCYTOMA

This is a destructive lesion of bone that may appear with the same characteristics as a fibrosarcoma. It is seen most often in the middle to later decades of life and may occur within bone or the soft tissues. These lesions have a very malignant potential with a poorer prognosis than fibrosarcoma of bone. They present with pathologic fractures in the large majority of cases.

Histologically they have a characteristic whorl pattern. The treatment of choice is ablative surgery with chemotherapy.

SYNOVIAL SARCOMA

Malignant synovioma is an uncommon tumor found most often in the lower extremities with occurrence near the knee joint or in the pararticular soft tissues in approximately 90% of the cases. Most often young adults under the age of 40 are affected.

Clinical Manifestations. Clinical history and findings include soft tissue swelling and limitation of motion of the associated joint with pain on motion. Radiographically, these tumors can appear as sharply demarcated lesions, punched-out destroyed areas, or irregular amorphous deposits or calcification within soft tissue. Histologically, the tumor is biphasic, with two predominating cell types.

Treatment. Treatment is operative with possible ablation, but more recent studies and results suggest radical excision followed by inguinal lymph node resection and chemotherapy. Irradiation may be used, but a common complication of its use is severe lymphedema with restriction of motion about the knee. Metastases may occur to the lungs. Treatment is usually multiphasic and consists of chemotherapy, surgical excision, and lymph node section.

RHABDOMYOSARCOMAS

Rhabdomyosarcomas are very malignant tumors found in striated muscle; they are divided into four types: (1) alveolar, (2) pleomorphic, (3) embryonal, and (4) botryoid.

Clinical Manifestations. The patient with rhabdomyosarcoma often presents with a vague muscle discomfort, usually in the thigh. A palpable mass is often found. Microscopically there are different presenting cells depending on which type of tumor is present.

Treatment. Treatment for a soft tissue tumor of this nature should usually include a thorough workup and staging, with resection planning depending on the type and stage of the lesion. Unfortunately, wide resection has not been particularly helpful and even amputation at the joint above and elimination of the muscle compartment involved by the tumor have not always been followed by survival. The tumor is poorly responsive to chemotherapy and irradiation. The 5-year survival rate depends on the type of cell involved.

LIPOSARCOMA

Liposarcoma is a rare tumor that most often involves the soft tissues about the pelvic and pectoral girdles. It is usually slow growing and is lobulated with a yellow-white to a yellow-gray appearance.

Histologically, there is an abundance of lipoblasts in relation to the amount of lipid material, with some varying pleomorphic giant cells and interlacing spindle cells and mitotic figures.

Clinical Manifestations. These patients most commonly present with a mass. Pain is localized and vague, and restriction of motion and deformity may depend on the size of the presenting mass and its relation to the proximal joint.

Liposarcomas of bone may show destruction, whereas liposarcomas of the soft tissues may not show any bone destruction.

Treatment. The treatment is primarily ablative resection. The response to chemotherapy or radiotherapy is poor.

BIBLIOGRAPHY

AEGETER E, KIRKPATRICK JA JR: Orthopedic Disease, 3rd ed. Philadelphia, W B Saunders, 1968

BARNES R, CATTO M: Chondrosarcoma of bone. J Bone Joint Surg [Br] 44:662, 1962

BHANSALI SK, DESAI PB: Ewing's sarcoma. J Bone Joint Surg [Am] 45:541, 1963

CAMPBELL CJ: Benign and Expanding Lesions of Bone. American Academy of Orthopaedic Surgeons Instructional Course Lectures, vol 15, p 189. Ann Arbor, MI, J W Edwards, 1958

CAMPBELL CJ, COHEN J, ENNEKING WF: New therapies for osteogenic sarcoma. J Bone Joint Surg [Am] 57:143, 1975

COLEY BL, HIGINBOTHAM HL: Giant cell tumor of bone. J Bone Joint Surg 20:870, 1938

COPELAND MM: Cartilaginous tumors of bone. American Academy of Orthopedic Surgeons Instructional Course Lectures, vol 8, p 131. Ann Arbor, MI, J W Edwards, 1951

COPELAND MM: Tumors of cartilaginous origin. Clin Orthop 7:9, 1952

COVENTRY MB, DAHLIN DC: Osteosarcoma. J Bone Joint Surg [Am] 39:741, 1951

DAHLIN DC: Bone Tumors: General Aspects on 6221 Cases. Springfield, IL, Charles C Thomas, 1978

DAHLIN DC, COVENTRY MB: Osteogenic sarcoma: A study of six hundred cases. J Bone Joint Surg 49:101, 1967

FERGUSON AB: Roentgenology of benign tumors of bone. American Academy of Orthopaedic Surgeons Instructional Course Lectures, vol 8, p 113. Ann Arbor, MI, J W Edwards, 1951

GESCHICTER CF, COPELAND MM: Parosteal osteoma of bone. Ann Surg 133:790, 1951

GREENFIELD GP: Radiology of Bone Diseases. Philadelphia, J B Lippincott, 1975

HARRIS WH, DUDLEY HR, JR, BARRY RJ: The natural history of fibrous dysplasia: An orthopaedic, pathological and roentgenographic study. J Bone Joint Surg [Am] 44:207, 1962

HENDERSON ED, DAHLIN DC: Chondrosarcoma of bone. J Bone Joint Surg [Am] 45:1450, 1963

HODGES FJ, MacINTYRE RS: Roentgenologic diagnosis and treatment of giant cell tumors of bone. American Academy of Orthopaedic Surgeons Instructional Course Lectures, vol 6, p 15. Ann Arbor, MI, J W Edwards, 1949

HUVOS AG: Bone Tumors: Diagnosis, Treatment and Prognosis. Philadelphia, W B Saunders, 1979

JAFFE HL: Osteoid osteoma of benign osteoblastic tumor composed of osteoid and atypical bone. Arch Surg 31:709, 1935

JAFFE HL: Pathology: Problem of Ewing sarcoma of bone. Bull Hosp Joint Dis 6:82, 1945

JAFFE HL: Tumors and Tumorous Conditions of the Bones and Joints. Philadelphia, Lea & Febiger, 1958

LARSSON SE, LORENTZON R, BOQUIST L: Giant cell tumor of bone. J Bone Joint Surg [Am] 57:167, 1975

LICHTENSTEIN L: Bone Tumors. St. Louis, C V Mosby, 1975

LICHTENSTEIN L: Diseases of Bone and Joint. St. Louis, C V Mosby, 1975

LICHTENSTEIN L, SAWYER WR: Benign osteoblastoma. J Bone Joint Surg [Am] 46:755, 1964

MIRRA JM: Bone Tumors: Diagnosis and Treatment. Philadelphia, J B Lippincott, 1980

MOORE TM et al: Symposium on tumors of the musculoskeletal system, Orthopaedic Clinics of North America. Philadelphia, W B Saunders, 1977

MURPHY FP, DAHLIN DC, SULLIVAN CR: Articular synovial chondromatosis. J Bone Joint Surg [Am] 44:77, 1962

PHEMISTER DB: Editorial: Local resection of malignant tumors of bone. Arch Surg 63:115, 1951

SCHAJOWICA F: Tumors and Tumorlike Lesions of Bone and Joints. New York, Springer-Verlag, 1981

SHERMAN MS: Cartilaginous tumors of bone. American Academy of Orthopaedic Surgeons Instructional Course Lectures, vol 12, p 233. Ann Arbor, MI, J W Edwards, 1955

SLOWICK FA, JR, CAMPBELL CJ, KETTLEKAMP DB: Aneurysmal bone cyst: An analysis of thirteen cases. J Bone Joint Surg [Am] 50:1142, 1968

SOULE EH: Lipomatous tumors: Classification, pathology, and diagnosis. American Academy of Orthopaedic Surgeons Instructional Course Lectures, vol 14, p 311. Ann Arbor, MI, J W Edwards, 1957

WILSON PD, LANCE EM: Surgical reconstruction of the skeleton following segmental resection for bone tumors. J Bone Joint Surg [Am] 47:1629, 1965

Urology is the surgical specialty that deals with the urinary organs in males and females and the genital system in males. A urologist is primarily a surgeon, but, because of his familiarity with the genitourinary system, he is often the specialist who is most competent to manage medical problems involving these structures. The medical counterpart of the urologic surgeon is the nephrologist, who is a subspecialist in the field of internal medicine or pediatrics.

ANATOMY

KIDNEY

The kidneys are paired structures that lie in the upper lumbar retroperitoneum (Fig. 45-1). The functional unit of the kidney is the nephron. Each kidney consists of approximately 1 million nephrons couched in a sparse fibrous stroma and surrounded by a thin fibrous capsule. The kidneys measure approximately 11 cm in long axis. Each is surrounded by fat and is enclosed within a fascial envelope (Gerota's fascia). Blood supply is from paired renal arteries, which arise from the aorta. Anomalous accessory arteries are common. Paired renal veins return blood to the inferior vena cava. These vessels enter the medially placed renal hilus, which is also occupied by the renal collecting system, calyces, and renal pelvis. Of the structures in the renal hilus, the pelvis is most posterior, the renal vein is anterior, and the renal artery is between.

URETERS

The ureters are tubular structures that are continuous with the renal pelvis and drain into the bladder at its base (see Fig. 45-1). The ureter consists of a smooth-muscle coat surrounding a lumen that is lined by transitional epithelium.

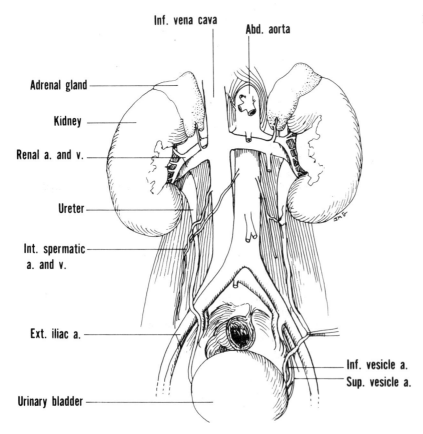

Fig. 45-1. Anatomy of the retroperitoneum.

Ureteral length varies from 24 cm to 34 cm in adults. The caliber of the lumen is 4 mm to 10 mm, with physiologic points of narrowing at the ureteropelvic junction, the level of the iliac vessels, and the ureterovesical junction.

BLADDER

The bladder is a saccular structure that occupies the anterior portion of the true pelvis (Fig. 45-2). It is composed of a meshwork of smooth muscle and is lined by transitional epithelium. The trigone of the bladder marks the site of entry of the ureters. This area is located on the posteroinferior bladder wall near the bladder neck. The ureters normally enter the bladder obliquely and pursue a course under the bladder mucosa for a distance of 1.5 cm to 2 cm. This arrangement results in a valve mechanism that prevents reflux of urine. For descriptive purposes, the bladder may be divided into seven areas: vesical neck, trigone, base or fundus, two lateral walls, anterior wall, and dome or vertex. The external surface of the fundus and dome of the bladder is covered with peritoneum.

PROSTATE

The prostate is a firm, rubbery structure composed of glandular elements and a fibromuscular stroma that contains an abundance of elastic fibers and smooth muscle (see Fig. 45-2). It is shaped as a truncated cone, with its base at the bladder neck and its apex abutting the urogenital diaphragm. Its size varies. The average measurements follow: length, 3.4 cm; width, 4.4 cm; and thickness, 2.6 cm. The prostate may be divided into various lobes, but these are not distinguishable clinically. Developmentally, it is divided into two lateral lobes, which surround the urethra and fuse anteriorly. However, the posterior wedge of prostate above the course of the ejaculatory ducts may be separately designated as the median lobe and that below the ducts as the posterior lobe. The periurethral glands contribute little to the mass of the prostate but are embryologically distinct and clinically important because of their propensity to undergo hyperplasia in older men. The prostatic urethra is 3 cm to 4 cm in length.

SEMINAL VESICLES

The seminal vesicles are paired saccular structures that lie above the prostate against the base of the bladder (see Fig. 45-2). They produce an important constituent of seminal fluid, which is discharged through the ejaculatory ducts. Normal seminal vesicles are not perceptible on rectal palpation.

TESTES

The testes are ovoid structures that, on the average, measure 4 cm to 5 cm in length, 2.5 cm from side to side, and 3 cm from front to back (see Fig. 45-2). The testes consist of seminiferous tubules and interstitial cells of Leydig surrounded by the tunica albuginea. All important connections are by way of the spermatic cord. Arterial supply is primarily from the internal spermatic arteries, which arise from the aorta. The right internal spermatic vein drains into the vena cava, and the left internal spermatic vein drains into the left renal vein. Lymphatics follow the course of the vasculature and drain into periaortic lymph nodes. Spermatozoa, which are produced in the seminiferous tubules, migrate

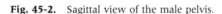

Fig. 45-2. Sagittal view of the male pelvis.

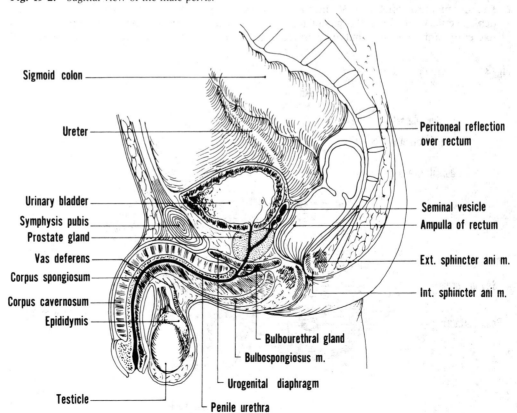

through the efferent ducts into the epididymis at its superior portion, the head. The epididymis is a soft, comma-shaped structure that invests the posterior and superior portion of the testes. It is an irregularly twisted tube that leads at its inferior portion (the tail) into the vas deferens.

PENIS

The penis consists of three cavernous bodies that are encased in a dense fascia (Buck's fascia) and covered by a loose layer of nonfatty connective tissue and skin (Fig. 45-3). The bulk of the penis is composed of the paired corpora cavernosa, which give the penis its erectile capacity. In the pendulous portion, the corpora cavernosa lie side by side and are attached in the median septum. Proximally, they diverge to become attached to the pubic arch and the urogenital diaphragm. The corpus spongiosum rests in the ventral groove of the corpora cavernosa. The distal extremity of the corpus spongiosum is expanded into the soft, conical glans penis. The expanded proximal portion is called the bulb; it abuts the inferior layer of the urogenital diaphragm. The anterior urethra traverses the corpus spongiosum and may be divided into pendulous and bulbous portions.

EMBRYOLOGY

KIDNEY

In ontogeny of humans, the development of the kidney recapitulates phylogeny in three phases. The nephrogenic cord arises by longitudinal fusion of the intermediate mesoderm and gives rise in sequence to the following:

1. The pronephros develops as seven paired segments; they can be identified by the 28th day and completely regress by the fifth week.
2. The mesonephros consists of 30 units that arise from the nephrogenic cord along the advancing wolffian duct. Excretory units develop that may produce urine, but these units regress. The prime role of the mesonephros is in the later development of the ureter and genital systems.
3. The metanephros consists of the caudal portion of the nephrogenic cord (metanephric blastema) and the ureteral bud, which is an outgrowth of the caudal portion of the mesonephric duct. As the ureteral bud grows dorsally, the cranial end swells and branches ultimately to form the calyces and collecting tubules from the fifth to the 14th week. During this process, the branching ureteral bud induces differentiation of the definitive kidney in the metanephric blastema. The unit ascends owing to unfolding of the embryo and longitudinal growth. The blood supply successively arises from higher levels on the aorta and rotation occurs so that the hilus finally achieves a medial position.

BLADDER

The bladder develops from the caudal portion of the hindgut, the cloaca. At 4 weeks, the urorectal septum grows down to the cloacal membrane, dividing the cloaca into the dorsal rectum and the urogenital sinus. The portion of the urogenital sinus cranial to the opening of the mesonephric duct will develop into the bladder and entire urethra in the female and into the bladder and posterior urethra in the male.

GENITAL SYSTEM

The genital system consists of the gonads, the internal ductal system, and the external genitalia. The testes or ovaries develop from a common indifferent gonad. The external genitalia arise from the urogenital sinus. In the male, the internal ductal system develops from the mesonephric (wolffian) ducts. In the female, the internal genital organs develop from the paramesonephric (müllerian) ducts. The direction of development of the gonad (male or female) orchestrates

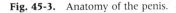

Fig. 45-3. Anatomy of the penis.

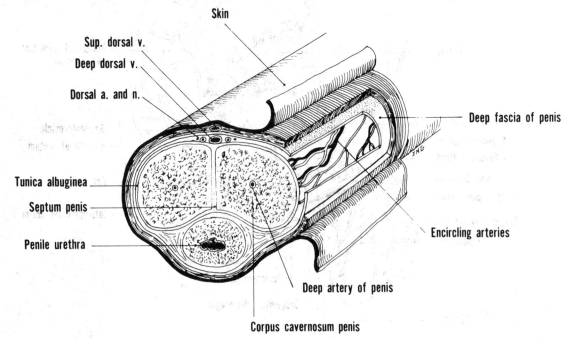

the development of the internal ductal system and the formation of the external genitalia. Up to the 17-mm stage of development, the sex of the embryo cannot be determined by examination.

PHYSIOLOGY OF THE GENITOURINARY SYSTEM

KIDNEY

The most important physiological function of the kidneys is the regulation of the composition of the blood. The kidney is also an endocrine organ that produces hormones such as renin, prostaglandins, and erythropoietin. Each kidney is an aggregate of about 1 million functional units called nephrons, which are bound together by a fibrous capsule and couched in a sparse fibrous stroma. All qualitative functions of the organ are inherent in each of these functional units. The study of renal physiology, therefore, is the study of a typical, ideal nephron. External influences on the kidney are all mediated through effects on some component of this unit (Fig. 45-4).

The formation of urine begins in the glomerulus. The glomerulus is composed of a leash of capillaries invaginated into Bowman's capsule, which is a layer of flattened epithelial cells continuous with the tubular epithelium. Functionally, the glomerulus is a semipermeable membrane that permits filtration. The glomerulus performs no work. Energy to operate this function is supplied by the myocardium in maintenance of an effective filtration pressure. The forces opposing glomerular filtration are the intracapsular pressure and the osmotic pressure of plasma proteins. Porosity of the glomerular membrane does not vary in the normal state. Glomerular filtrate is isotonic to plasma. It contains all the components of plasma, except its colloids, in concentrations equal to plasma except for the small gradient in electrically active ions as a result of Donnan's equilibrium. In the average human, 180 liters of glomerular filtrate are formed daily. This means that the tubule is presented with 180 liters of filtrate, 1100 g of NaCl, 150 g of glucose, 380 g of $NaHCO_3$, and considerable quantities of phosphate, calcium, magnesium, amino acids, and so forth, most of which have to be preserved for the body economy. The total extracellular fluid volume of the body is reworked 16 times a day.

The tubule does not work on the basis of hydrostatic pressure gradients. Energy to perform the work of the tubule is derived from metabolism in the tubular cell. The functions of the tubule can be simply stated as active reabsorption, passive reabsorption, and active excretion.

In general, the proximal tubule is responsible for reabsorption and excretion of the bulk of the glomerular filtrate. Seventy to 80% of filtered sodium ion, all of the filtered potassium ion, and about half of HCO_3 reabsorption occur in the proximal tubule. Active reabsorption of a great variety of nonelectrolytes takes place proximally. Since the proximal tubule is freely permeable to water, water passively follows these osmotically active substances, and the total volume of "urine" that leaves the proximal tubule is only 20% to 30% of the glomerular filtrate. Also, in the proximal tubule,

Fig. 45-4. The nephron.

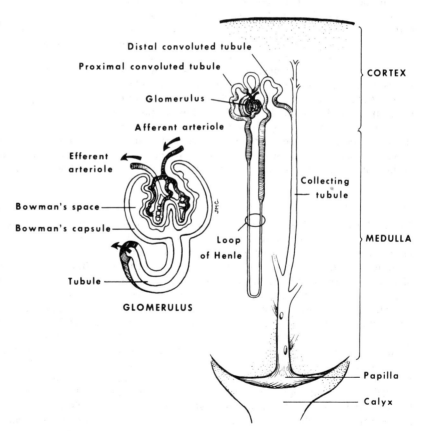

endogenous and exogenous waste products are excreted. Examples of substances reabsorbed are amino acids, phosphate, calcium, uric acid, ascorbic acid, and acetoacetic acid. Examples of excretory products are phenol-sulfonphthalein, hippuric acid, penicillin, 5-hydroxyindoleacetic acid, Diodrast, and creatinine in small amounts. The distal tubule is charged with the final responsibility of fine regulation and has to do with sodium reabsorption, H^+ and K^+ excretion, ammonia production, and the regulation of urine concentration.

It should be emphasized that the proximal tubule does not work against an osmotic gradient. Since it is freely permeable to water, the reabsorbed solution is isotonic to serum. Hence, a larger volume can be transported with a minimum of energy expenditure. The distal tubule works against osmotic gradients as well as concentration gradients, since it has limited and variable permeability to water. The fine regulation of the composition of the final urine by the loop of Henle and the distal tubule involves much less quantitative change than that which occurs in the proximal tubule but requires proportionately greater energy expenditure because of the osmotic and concentration gradients that must be opposed. The capability to excrete final urine that is more dilute or more concentrated than plasma depends upon three factors: (1) the ability to transport Na^+ against a concentration gradient, leaving "free water" in the distal tubule and achieving hypertonicity in the interstitial fluid of the medulla; (2) the anatomical arrangement of the blood vessels supplying the medulla—the vasa recta—which, by the countercurrent mechanism, permits Na^+ and urea to be trapped effectively in the interstitium of the medulla to maintain hypertonicity; and (3) the variable permeability of the distal convoluted tubule and the collecting tubule under the influence of the antidiuretic hormone. Free water may be excreted in dilute urine when antidiuretic hormone production is suppressed by water excess in plasma, leaving these tubules impermeable to water. Water is reabsorbed osmotically into the hypertonic interstitium of the medulla in dehydration to produce concentrated urine because antidiuretic hormone is increased to increase the permeability of the collecting tubule to water. The maximum concentration that can be achieved in the distal convoluted tubule is isotonicity.

URINE TRANSPORT AND MICTURITION

The production of urine is complete when the urine passes from the collecting tubule into the calyx at the renal papillae. From this point, the urine is not essentially changed during the time required for its passage to the outside. The transport of urine is the sole function of the outflow tract. Superficially considered, this might appear to be a simple function. However, the complex process that nature provides must work efficiently to avoid obstruction to which the kidney is functionally and anatomically vulnerable and to avoid the ascent of bacteria, which are omnipresent at the surface. The social nicety of continence, which the bladder normally provides, is a valuable social asset. Urine is not simply drained passively through a series of conduits but is propelled by the activity of smooth muscle through structures that are delicately controlled and balanced.

URETERAL PHYSIOLOGY

The pyelocalyceal system and ureter function as a peristaltic unit to transport urine to the bladder. They receive autonomic innervation but are capable of functioning when completely denervated. The transplanted kidney is an example. The normal stimulus of ureteral peristalsis appears to be the pressure of urine high in the renal calyces. The electrical component of the peristaltic wave is transmitted through the smooth muscle of the pelvis and ureter and is accompanied by sequential relaxation and contraction of the smooth muscle of these structures. Severe colicky pain results from the stimulation of spastic contractions against an obstruction to urine flow.

BLADDER PHYSIOLOGY

The urinary bladder is a saccular structure with a smooth-muscle coat (detrusor) and a transitional epithelial lining. The detrusor has the capacity to adapt to an increasing volume of urine without a concomitant rise in intravesical pressure until capacity is reached, at which point proprioceptive receptors activate the micturition reflex. The motor neurons to the bladder are parasympathetic and have their origin at the levels of S2, S3, and S4 in the spinal cord. The spinal cord micturition reflex is regulated by inhibitory and facilitory centers in the central nervous system, some of which are under voluntary control. Striated muscles of the pelvic floor, particularly the external urinary sphincter, play a role in urinary continence and must relax for normal urination to occur. Motor neurons for these muscles lie in the anterior horn of sacral spinal segments S2, S3, and S4. The internal urinary sphincter, or bladder neck, is not a separate anatomical or functional structure but is a part of the detrusor muscle of the bladder. The anatomical arrangement of muscular bundles around the bladder neck provides for continence at this level when the bladder is in the resting state. Sympathetic innervation provides sensory function in micturition and appears to have a motor function in the smooth-muscle contraction associated with ejaculation and in maintaining tonus in the bladder neck during the filling phase of micturition.

REPRODUCTIVE SYSTEM

A detailed discussion of reproductive physiology in the male is beyond the scope of this text. A brief review follows.

Spermatozoa are produced in the seminiferous tubules of the testes. These tubules are lined by germinal epithelium. The most primitive precursor of spermatozoa is the stem cell, or type A spermatogonium. Through an elaborate series of cell divisions and maturation, the mature spermatozoa evolve. Important contributions are made to this process by the Sertoli cells of the seminiferous tubules and by the interstitial cells of Leydig. Maturation of spermatozoa in the testes is under endocrine control and depends upon a delicate homeostatic balance between the testes, thyroid, adrenal, pituitary, and hypothalamus. The male hormone, testosterone, is produced by the interstitial cells of Leydig under the influence of the luteinizing hormone of the anterior pituitary. Testosterone is essential in the embryo for the morphological differentiation and development of the genital organs. It plays a critical role in sexual maturation at puberty. In the adult, it is essential to support the process of spermatogenesis, the production of seminal fluid, and the maintenance of sexual potency. The process of maturation of spermatozoa continues during the migration through the ductal system, which includes the epididymis, vas deferens, and ejaculatory ducts. Seminal fluid produced by the seminal vesicles and prostate serves a vital role in providing a vehicle for the transport of spermatozoa and for the nutritional sustenance that supports survival and final maturation.

Penile erection (potency) is a neurovascular phenomenon that requires hormonal support. When this mechanism is defective, it is most often due to psychological factors, but hormone deficiency, neurologic impairment, and vascular disease cause sexual impotence in a significant number of males. Orgasm is the normal culmination of the sexual act. It consists in a pleasurable psychic phenomenon that affords emotional release of sexual tension, as well as various somatic manifestations, such as ejaculation.

DIAGNOSTIC UROLOGY

A high degree of diagnostic accuracy is possible in urology because of the availability of excellent endoscopic instruments, precise radiographic studies, and laboratory tests. Proper urologic diagnostic evaluation begins with a careful medical history and physical examination.

SIGNS AND SYMPTOMS

Normal urination is a painless function that occurs three to four times daily and, occasionally, once at night. The normal person can inhibit micturition until a suitable time and place are available. On volition, a forceful urinary stream is initiable within 1 to 2 seconds; normally, the stream is continuous and uninterrupted until the bladder is emptied. Increased frequency of urination, urgency (inability to hold urine after the sensation of bladder filling is initiated), and dysuria (painful or difficult urination) are typically observed in such conditions as cystitis, vesical calculi, renal tuberculosis, prostatism, and urethral stricture. Hesitancy in starting urination, a decrease in size and force of the urinary stream, abdominal straining, and an interrupted stream should lead the physician to suspect an obstruction of the urethral channel, which may be due to cicatricial contraction at the vesical neck, enlargement of the prostate, or stricture of the urethra. Urinary incontinence is abnormal except in infancy and early childhood. Incontinence associated with urgency and frequency and occurring at intervals during the day and especially at night may be a manifestation of disease involving the central nervous system, for example, multiple sclerosis, cerebrovascular accidents, or spinal cord tumor. In women, the involuntary loss of urine when coughing, straining, or sneezing is suggestive of relaxation of the ligaments and muscles supporting the bladder neck. This condition is called stress incontinence and is usually attributed to injury sustained during childbirth. Continuous involuntary dribbling of urine may be associated with urinary retention with overflow incontinence, sometimes called paradoxical incontinence. Continuous leaking of urine also is seen in persons who have suffered injury to the sphincter mechanisms through surgery or other trauma.

Hematuria is a very important sign of genitourinary disease. It may indicate cancer of the genitourinary tract as well as a wide range of benign diseases (Fig. 45-5). Hematuria should be described as either gross or microscopic. In addition, it is important to note whether it is associated with pain, fever, or other symptoms or whether it is asymptomatic (painless). In certain conditions, blood may appear only in the initial portion of the voided urine or only in the terminal portion. In most cases, it will be distributed throughout the urinary stream. In this event, it

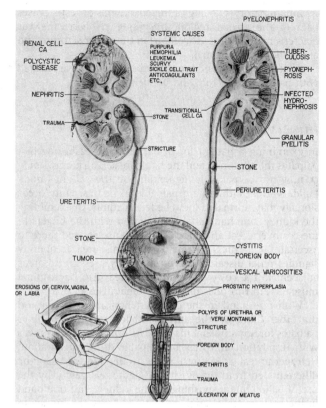

Fig. 45-5. Causes of hematuria.

is called total hematuria. Descriptions of the color of the blood, the estimated volume, and the presence or absence of clots provide important historical information. Far too many patients with cancer of the urinary tract are seen belatedly by the urologist because the importance of hematuria is not recognized by the physician who first sees the patient.

Pneumaturia, or air in the urine, is associated with enterourinary tract fistulas and very rarely with infections caused by *Bacterium aerogenes, Escherichia coli,* and certain yeasts. Fecaluria associated with pneumaturia is pathognomonic of a connection between the intestinal and the urinary systems.

Diseases of the kidney may cause characteristic pain. Equally as often, the discomfort or pain may be suggestive of disease in some other organ. Typical renal colic originates in the flank and may radiate anteriorly to the epigastrium; it is an intermittent, sharp, excruciating type of pain often associated with nausea and vomiting. Nonobstructive calculous disease of the kidney may produce a dull, boring discomfort in the epigastrium, which is frequently interpreted as evidence of a peptic ulcer or cholecystic disease. Ureteral colic can be characterized as an intermittent, sharp pain radiating along the course of the ureter into the scrotum or the labium majus. This type of pain may be produced by the passage of a calculus down the ureter.

The pain associated with disease of the bladder may be a vague and generalized suprapubic discomfort often seen in patients with urinary retention or subacute cystitis. The suprapubic pain may be more sharp in patients with interstitial cystitis, carcinoma of the bladder, or bladder stones. Irritation at the bladder neck is often associated with pain referred to the distal urethra.

Inflammatory swelling of the epididymis or testis causes pain in the scrotal region. Infections involving the vas deferens may produce discomfort in the upper scrotum and along the inguinal canal.

Acute prostatitis and prostatic abscess may be associated with pain in the rectum and perineal region.

PHYSICAL FINDINGS

In examining a patient for urinary tract disease, one first palpates the abdomen and the flank areas. The kidneys may or may not be palpable, depending on the patient's body build. Normal kidneys are palpable in infants. Only occasionally may normal kidneys be felt in adults. In examining the kidney, one hand should be placed with the fingers in the costovertebral angle area and pressure applied there to ascertain tenderness. Tenderness in this area frequently signifies renal disease. Pain produced by pressure to areas adjacent to the costovertebral angle area (*e.g.,* sacrospinal muscle, 12th rib) does not signify renal disease.

With one hand in the costovertebral angle region and the other hand on the anterior abdomen, the examiner palpates for any unusual masses. The normal kidney moves with respiration and may be palpable during inspiration. Retroperitoneal structures, such as the kidney, may be differentiated from masses in the peritoneal cavity by the use of ballottement: pushing on the kidney with one hand in the costovertebral angle region will cause the kidney to be felt by the other hand pressing against the abdomen. A mass in the peritoneal cavity (*e.g.,* liver, spleen, bowel neoplasm) usually cannot be ballotted.

Percussion and palpation are most useful procedures for ascertaining the presence of a distended bladder and other suprapubic masses.

In examining the penis, the foreskin is retracted first, and the urethral meatus, the glans, and the coronal sulcus are inspected closely for abnormalities. The shaft of the penis is then palpated for induration and nodules.

The scrotum and its contents are next in the order of examination. The spermatic cord is palpated, first high in the scrotum for the presence of varicocele, spermatocele, beaded vas deferens, or nodules. The testis and the epididymis are then felt carefully for unusual firmness, nodularity, or large masses. Scrotal masses should be transilluminated with an intense light source in a dark room. Transmission of light through the mass may be taken as evidence of a cystic lesion.

The rectal examination is used to determine the status of the prostate gland, the seminal vesicles, and the rectum. The normal prostate is a slightly tender, elastic, and firm body felt through the anterior rectal wall. Three longitudinal grooves or sulci may be palpated on the posterior aspect of the prostate, two laterally and one centrally. The seminal vesicles lie above and lateral to the prostate, beginning at the base of the prostate and running superolaterally from the prostate at an angle of about 45°. Normal seminal vesicles are soft and cystic and may or may not be detectable by palpation. A stony hard nodular prostate suggests carcinoma, tuberculosis, or calculi. A smooth hard prostate with obliteration of the sulci is indicative of infiltrating prostatic neoplasm. Early carcinoma may manifest itself as an isolated circumscribed small nodule. Marked tenderness of the prostate can be caused by acute prostatitis: An extremely tender, bulging, tense prostate suggests abscess.

A tense, exquisitely painful seminal vesicle indicates seminal vesiculitis.

While performing the rectal examination, one should test for integrity of the sacral spinal cord by attempting to elicit the bulbocavernous reflex and sensory changes in the saddle area if neurologic disease is suspected. The observations made with these examinations may be extremely helpful in determining the presence of neurologic deficits responsible for abnormalities in urination and continence.

LABORATORY TESTS

URINALYSIS

Examination of the urine is the most commonly performed laboratory examination in urology and is one of the most important. A wide range of medical and surgical diseases may be diagnosed or suspected on the basis of findings in the urine. Proper collection of the specimen by a clean technique is important, and the examination should be performed soon after collection. Microscopic examination of an unspun wet smear and examination of the centrifuged sediment are performed for detection of cellular elements such as red blood cells and white blood cells, casts, and bacteria. Tests for protein, pH, glucose, hemoglobin, and bilirubin are important. Urinary sediment may be stained with methylene blue or Gram's stain for better identification of cellular elements and bacteria. Cytologic techniques may permit the identification of malignant cells in the urine sediment.

URINE CULTURE

Conclusive diagnosis of urinary tract infection and identification of the offending organism depend on the culture of a properly collected specimen. A clean voided midstream specimen is most commonly used. However, in females, skin contamination is a frequent problem. Bacterial colony count performed on a fresh specimen may distinguish between skin contamination and true urinary tract infection. In general, counts of less than 10,000/ml suggest contamination, and counts of 100,000 or greater provide conclusive evidence of active infection. Occasionally, specimens should be obtained by catheterization or by suprapubic needle aspiration to validate the significance of a positive culture. Cultures for tuberculosis should be obtained in patients who have "sterile pyuria" and in patients who have radiographic changes in the kidneys suggesting tuberculosis.

PROSTATOVESICULAR SMEAR

Secretions may be obtained from the prostate and seminal vesicles by massage. Presence of white blood cells in excess of 5 per high-powered field on a direct smear suggests inflammatory disease in the prostate and seminal vesicles. Cultures may be obtained of these secretions to identify the offending organism. Occasionally, special cultures for *Mycoplasma* and *Chlamydia* may be indicated in cases of prostatitis of obscure etiology.

SEMEN ANALYSIS

Semen analysis is usually the first step in the laboratory investigation of male infertility. The specimen should be examined soon after its collection into a chemically clean container. Important measurements include the sperm count, volume, viscosity, and motility and morphology of spermatozoa.

BLOOD UREA NITROGEN (BUN) AND SERUM CREATININE

The BUN and creatinine are the most commonly employed measures of renal function. Creatinine clearance may be calculated by the timed measurement of creatinine excretion and simultaneous measurement of the serum creatinine. This provides a more precise quantitation of renal function.

SERUM ACID PHOSPHATASE

The serum acid phosphatase is an important screening test for prostatic cancer, and its elevation suggests spread of the cancer beyond the confines of the prostatic capsule. Other conditions may rarely cause elevation of the serum acid phosphatase.

RADIOGRAPHIC EXAMINATION

EXCRETORY UROGRAPHY

Parenteral injection (usually intravenous) of iodinated contrast media that are rapidly cleared by the kidney permits the opacification of urine for radiographic study (Fig. 45-6). This procedure has great utility in urologic diagnosis, since it provides important information about the function of each kidney and the anatomy of the kidney and the outflow tracts. It is a safe procedure to perform, although severe allergic reactions may rarely occur. The excretory urogram, or intravenous pyelogram, is an essential part of the evaluation of a wide range of urologic conditions, including hypertension, hematuria, calculi, neoplastic disease, obstructive uropathy, trauma, infections, congenital abnormalities, neurologic disease, and many others. The preliminary film or scout film of the abdomen is an essential part of this radiographic study. The performance of intravenous pyelograms should be under the direction of a physician who understands the clinical requirements in the patient being studied so that appropriate modifications may be made to enhance the quality of the study.

RETROGRADE PYELOGRAPHY

When the excretory urogram fails to provide the desired anatomical information about the kidney and its ureter because of impaired function, obstruction, or extravasation, contrast media may be injected directly into the ureter by way of a catheter introduced through a cystoscope (Fig. 45-7). Retrograde pyelograms and ureterograms are used only when the excretory urogram fails to provide adequate anatomical information.

CYSTOURETHROGRAPHY

The bladder may be more clearly demonstrated radiographically by the instillation of contrast media through a catheter. This is the best test to demonstrate bladder diverticula and vesicoureteral reflux. Cystograms are often monitored with fluoroscopy as the bladder fills and as the patient voids the contrast media to provide visualization of the bladder neck and urethra. The radiographic recording of the voiding sequence is particularly important in the investigation of outflow tract obstruction (Fig. 45-8).

RENAL ARTERIOGRAPHY

The injection of contrast media into the arterial supply to the kidney, usually by the transfemoral catheter technique, has proved to be a valuable tool in urologic investigation (Fig. 45-9). It is a necessary part of the evaluation of renal hypertension and provides the most accurate nonoperative method of distinguishing between benign and malignant renal masses. It provides the most precise evaluation of the extent of injury to the kidney in renal trauma.

LYMPHOGRAPHY

Several urologic cancers, notably carcinoma of the testes, carcinoma of the bladder, and carcinoma of the prostate,

Fig. 45-6. Excretory pyelograms made by administering radiopaque material intravenously and then obtaining roentgenograms of the kidneys, the ureters, and the bladder after the material has been excreted by the nephrons into the collecting system.

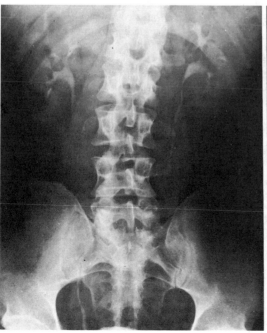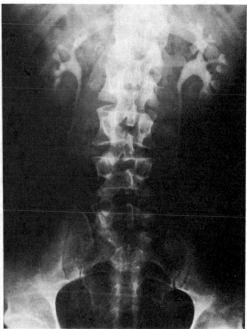

frequently metastasize by way of lymphatics. Injection of contrast media into pedal lymphatics may demonstrate the retroperitoneal lymph nodes and provide preoperative evidence of metastatic disease.

OTHER RADIOGRAPHIC TECHNIQUES

In selected cases, contrast media may be injected percutaneously into renal cysts to verify that the cyst is benign. Venacavography is important in renal tumors to rule out vena caval invasion by these growths. Retrograde instillation of contrast media into the urethra is useful in radiographic detection of strictures, carcinoma of the urethra, and diverticula. Disease in the seminal vesicles may be demonstrated by injecting contrast media into the vas deferens to fill the seminal vesicles and ejaculatory ducts.

RADIOISOTOPE RENOGRAPHY

Radioisotopes may be used to perform renograms and renal scans to assess renal function and anatomy.

ULTRASONOGRAPHY

Ultrasound scanning has the advantage of being noninvasive and entirely safe. The procedure is particularly useful in evaluating renal masses, screening patients in renal failure for ureteral obstruction, and searching for abdominal fluid collections such as blood, pus, or urine.

COMPUTED TOMOGRAPHY

Computed tomography (CT scan) has rapidly assumed an important role in uroradiology.

Fig. 45-7. Retrograde pyelogram, demonstrating calyces, infundibula, pelves, and ureters of both kidneys. Observe the ureteral catheters through which radiopaque sodium iodide has been injected.

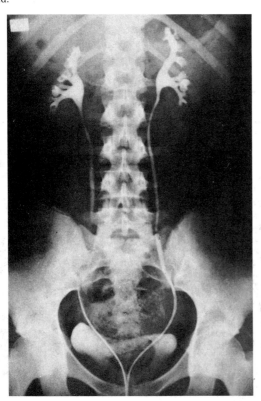

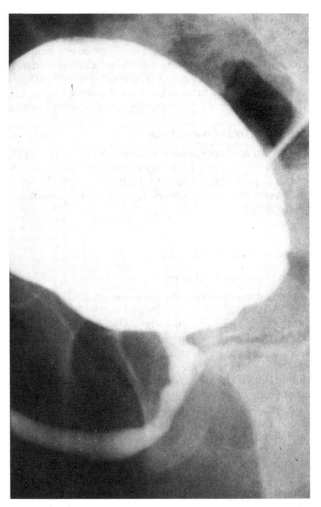

Fig. 45-8. Normal voiding cystourethrogram.

INSTRUMENTAL EXAMINATION

Evaluation of the lumen of the urethra in males and females may be accomplished by the use of calibrated instruments such as catheters and bougies. These instruments are useful in detecting acquired and congenital strictures and stenoses.

Endoscopic instruments provide the most useful tool in the hands of the urologist for evaluation of the lower urinary tract. These instruments embody an optical system that provides visualization, a method of illumination that usually is by way of fiberoptics, and operative attachments that permit diagnostic and therapeutic manipulation. Catheters can be inserted through these instruments into the ureters for radiographic diagnostic procedures and for the selective collection of specimens from individual kidneys. Various forceps are available for the crushing of stones and for obtaining biopsy specimens of lesions of the bladder and prostate. Resection of bladder tumors and resection of the prostate can be accomplished by use of the electrosurgical unit (Fig. 45-10).

Cystometry is the measurement of intravesical pressure changes that occur as the bladder is filled and as it empties. This procedure is essential in evaluation of bladder physiology, especially when neurologic impairment is suspected.

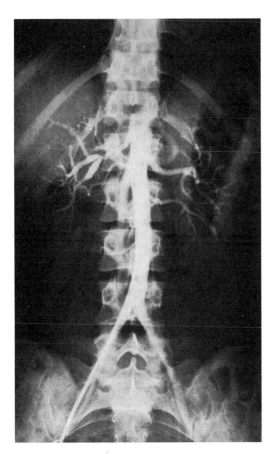

Fig. 45-9. Arteriogram depicting the renal arteries and their branches in addition to the aorta and the splenic, hepatic, mesenteric, and iliac vessels. Observe the stenosis of the right renal artery and the poststenotic dilation of its two main branches.

CONGENITAL ABNORMALITIES

Anomalous development attains its highest incidence in the urogenital tract, being found in 30% to 40% of malformed persons. Autopsy studies have shown that more than 10% of all human subjects are born with some anomaly of the urogenital tract. Well-recognized peaks occur in the incidence of genitourinary disease in the very young and the very old. The high rate of occurrence of urologic disease in the very young is almost entirely due to the frequency of congenital abnormalities.

Embryologically and anatomically, the urinary and genital tracts must be considered as a single system. The reasons for this are their common origin from the mesodermal intermediate cell mass of the embryo and the incorporation of the primitive excretory ducts of the pronephros and mesonephros into the male genital organs and their relation to the primitive cloaca. Because of this intimate embryologic development of the genital and urinary systems in each sex, it is understandable that anomalies in either system, the genital or the urinary, are often associated with anomalies in the other.

In at least 90% of cases, the cause of congenital malformations is unknown. Some defects are due to hereditary factors with predictable inheritance patterns. In these cases, genetic counseling is of great importance to apprise potential parents of the risk involved for their progeny. Irradiation exposure in the early stages of pregnancy might produce malformations, but the risk has not been quantitated and has probably been exaggerated in most discussions of the subject. Certain viral illnesses may induce abnormalities in the developing embryo. Rubella (German measles) in the first trimester of pregnancy is known to cause congenital abnormalities, and the genitourinary system may be involved. Certain drugs may have teratogenic effects. Thalidomide is a well-known example of drugs with this potential. Genital development is under hormonal control, and these hormone-sensitive embryologic structures may be altered by maternal ingestion of sex hormones.

Congenital abnormalities have a wide range of manifestation. Some of these abnormalities are of a biochemical nature. Congenital enzyme deficiencies may alter the function of the renal tubule. However, it is more common to think of genitourinary abnormalities in terms of the gross anatomical defects that are produced. The significance of these defects also has a wide range. Many anomalies are innocuous. Variations in the renal blood vessels may have no effect on health. Variations in the anatomy of the drainage system may produce no clinical sequelae. At the other end of the spectrum are anomalies that are uniformly fatal. Congenital absence of the kidneys is such an example. Other anomalies may be disabling and potentially lethal but may be amenable to effective treatment. These lesions are of most interest to clinicians, since accurate diagnosis and proper treatment produce benefits for the patient.

Fig. 45-10. Use of a cystoscope with an electrosurgical unit makes possible extirpation of tumor under direct examination.

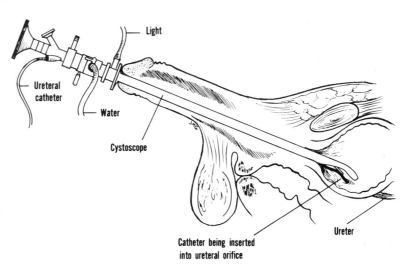

Light

Ureteral
catheter

Water

Cystoscope

Catheter being inserted
into ureteral orifice

Ureter

DELETERIOUS EFFECTS OF CONGENITAL ANOMALIES

RENAL FAILURE

Bilateral renal agenesis is a lethal anomaly. In polycystic disease, renal function is usually normal into adulthood but gradually deteriorates until renal failure occurs later in life.

OBSTRUCTIVE UROPATHY

The most common threat posed by abnormalities of the urinary system is obstruction. Because the formation of urine and micturition begin prior to birth, the ravages of obstruction may be present in the newborn. Severe obstruction may damage the kidneys prior to birth. More subtle degrees of obstruction may not be recognized until clinical manifestations occur later in life.

URINARY INCONTINENCE

The uncontrollable leakage of urine may result from a variety of congenital abnormalities. Ectopic opening of the ureters outside of the bladder, patent urachal fistulas, exstrophy of the urinary bladder, and congenital neurologic lesions may be at fault.

INFERTILITY

Impaired reproductive capacity in men may be the result of faulty gonadal development or failure of the testes to descend into the scrotum. Defects in the transport system for spermatozoa from the testes to the ejaculatory ducts may also cause infertility.

SEXUAL DYSFUNCTION

Neurologic abnormalities that impair the ability to achieve erection, endocrine abnormalities, and anomalies of the penis may cause sexual disability.

MALIGNANCY

Malignant neoplasms may be congenital in origin. Wilms' tumor of the kidney is an example. Certain congenital abnormalities may predispose to the formation of acquired cancer. Exstrophy of the urinary bladder exposes the bladder mucosa to chronic irritation, which may give rise to adenocarcinoma. Phimosis, which prevents retraction of the prepuce and impairs hygiene, may lead to the development of squamous cell carcinoma of the penis in later life. Undescended testes have a risk of malignancy (which most frequently occurs after puberty) that is 20 to 40 times as great as in the normal scrotal testes.

COSMETIC IMPAIRMENT

The appearance of the external genitalia is of sensitive psychological importance. These defects are most obvious in the male and may lead to psychiatric disease. Hypospadias is the most common example.

HYPERTENSION

Congenital stenosis of the renal arteries may cause high blood pressure.

INFECTION

Infection that results from congenital abnormality is usually secondary to obstruction. However, stasis of urine may occur as a result of congenital diverticula of the bladder and of congenital megaloureter when no obstruction is demonstrable. This stasis may predispose to infection. Vesicoureteral reflux predisposes to infection and often occurs in the absence of obstruction.

DIAGNOSTIC PROBLEMS

Some congenital abnormalities are important only because they may be mistaken for clinically significant disease. Ectopic kidneys may be mistaken for retroperitoneal tumors, and, on rare occasions, unwary surgeons have removed these structures ill-advisedly. Deviations in size and shape of the kidney may erroneously suggest the presence of an intrarenal mass.

URINARY TRACT INFECTIONS

Urinary tract infections are second in frequency of occurrence to infections of the respiratory tract. Because of this high incidence and because of the potential for serious sequelae, these infections constitute an important public health problem. In discussing this subject, a definition of terms is important to avoid confusion. Infection may predominantly involve one structure in the urinary system, and it is appropriate in these cases to speak of cystitis, urethritis, pyelonephritis, and so forth. On most occasions, however, the extent of involvement cannot be so well defined on the basis of clinical tests and the nonspecific designation *urinary tract infection* has utility.

SPECIFIC

Mycobacterium tuberculosis is an organism that causes chronic granulomatous infection that may involve various human organs. Involvement of the urinary tract is usually due to hematogenous spread from primary infection in the lung or intestinal tract. In our society, intestinal tuberculosis is rare, owing largely to universal pasteurization of milk and quality control of the dairy industry. Pulmonary tuberculosis is on the wane because of public health measures. As a result, genitourinary tuberculosis is uncommon. Approximately 10% of patients in tuberculosis sanatoriums have urinary tract involvement.

Other specific infections of the kidney include actinomycosis, candidiasis, syphilis, echinococcosis, filariasis, and schistosomiasis.

NONSPECIFIC

As commonly used, *urinary tract infection* implies disease caused by the invasion of the urinary tract by acute pyogenic organisms. These organisms are commonly found in the colon and on the skin of the perineum in the absence of disease. A list of the common offenders is given in Table 45-1. Each organism in this group has individual characteristics, such as its sensitivity to antibiotics, the severity of the changes it induces in the urinary tract, and the circumstances under which it is likely to cause infection. Virulence of these organisms may vary even within the same species. In general, we consider that these organisms are ubiquitous and that exposure is unavoidable. Factors in the host that permit these organisms to become invasive of the urinary tract receive most of our attention when we consider pathogenesis, treatment, and prevention.

Nonspecific chronic urinary tract infections are chronic not by virtue of the nature of the infective organism, as is

TABLE 45-1 RESULTS OF URINE CULTURE IN PATIENTS WITH ACUTE URINARY TRACT INFECTIONS

ORGANISM	%
E. coli	32
Klebsiella	22
Enterococci	17
Proteus	14
Pseudomonas	6
Miscellaneous	9

the case with tuberculosis, but because of the persistence or frequent occurrence of infections over a long period.

The normal urinary tract is resistant to bacterial infection. The nature of this resistance is not completely understood. The dynamics of the drainage system are surely an important factor in this resistance. The normal flow of urine from the kidneys to the bladder makes it difficult for bacteria to "swim upstream." The ureterovesical valve mechanism that normally prevents the regurgitation of urine from the bladder up to the kidney helps to prevent the ascent of organisms when bladder infection is present. The "washout phenomenon," accomplished by intermittent complete emptying of the bladder, is a critical factor in the protection against infection. Prostatic secretions and the bladder mucosa itself have some antibacterial activity, the nature of which has not been defined. An important research objective in understanding the pathogenesis of urinary tract infection in humans is a better understanding of the normal defense mechanisms.

Theoretically, bacteria can gain access to the urinary tract by several routes. Bacterial contamination may occur from instrumentation. From the colon, bacteria may spread to the urinary tract by way of the bloodstream, by lymphatic vessels, and by spread over epithelial surfaces. Most urinary tract infections come about by the ascent of bacteria from the skin of the perineum up the urinary passageway. Cultures taken from the skin around the urethral opening and from the distal part of the urethra in normal persons most often do not yield pathogenic organisms. The colonization with pathogenic organisms on skin in this area does not necessarily result in urinary tract infection, but may often be a prerequisite condition. It might truly be considered that susceptibility to urinary tract infection in some patients may be related to conditions of the skin of the perineum that permit the replacement of the normal skin bacteria by pathogenic organisms. The incidence of infection in females is ten times as great as in males, and this increase in susceptibility is probably due to the fact that the female urethra is much shorter than that of the male and the female urethral meatus is exposed to bacterial contamination more readily. Urinary tract infections are common in young females, and the incidence declines with advancing age until sexual activity begins, at which time the frequency of infection again shows an increase. Elderly men have more infections than their young counterparts because of the prevalence of prostatic disease.

DIAGNOSIS

The diagnosis of acute urinary tract infection is usually suspected on the basis of symptoms. In children, this initial step of suspecting the disease poses a particular problem, since abnormalities in the voiding pattern of infants are sometimes difficult to detect. Furthermore, infants are unable to verbalize their complaints. Urinalysis is an important test for children with fever of undetermined cause. In older children and adults, bladder symptoms usually predominate in acute urinary tract infection. These are manifest as increased frequency of urination, a feeling of urgency to urinate, and burning pain associated with the act of micturition. Occasionally, fever may accompany acute urinary tract infection, and this is particularly true when the kidney is involved in acute pyelonephritis. Backache, pain in the flank, chills and fever, and blood in the urine may all be symptoms and signs of acute urinary tract infection. The severity of symptoms usually parallels the virulence of the infection. Some patients with low-grade infections may be free of urologic complaints. Having suspected the diagnosis of acute urinary tract infection, one must prove the diagnosis by examination of the urine. Microscopic examination of a freshly collected specimen may reveal pus cells and the presence of bacteria. The urine sediment may be stained to increase the visibility of these cells. The etiology may be established by urine culture. False-positive cultures may be obtained if there is faulty collection of the specimen, which is more likely to occur in females. Efforts are made to obviate this problem in diagnosis by exercising care in the collection of the voided specimen, by obtaining catheterized specimens in selected cases, and by performing bacterial colony counts. In addition to confirming the diagnosis, urine culture helps to guide therapy by providing information about the antibiotic sensitivity of the offending organism.

Further urologic evaluation is important in selected patients to rule out underlying disease. Most males should be evaluated with their first episode of infection, since uncomplicated simple infection is relatively uncommon in males. The typical episode of acute cystitis in females may reasonably be treated without further investigation for the first episode or two, since the possibility of underlying disease is small. Patients with high fever, chills, and loin pain, suggesting kidney involvement, should be investigated after the first episode. Urologic investigation relies heavily on radiographic examinations such as excretory urography and voiding cystourethrography. Cystoscopy is required in some patients to evaluate the lower urinary tract.

TREATMENT

Management of acute urinary tract infection should be designed to treat symptoms and to eradicate the offending organism. Patients with acute cystitis often have distressing symptoms. Relief of these symptoms comes with cure of the infection, but more immediate relief may be obtained with administration of anticholinergic drugs, which reduce the unpleasant frequency and urgency that these patients experience. Mild sedatives may be helpful. The azo dyes and methylene blue seem to have a soothing effect on the bladder mucosa and are often prescribed in combination with anticholinergic drugs for symptomatic relief. Sitting in a tub of warm water temporarily reduces discomfort.

Spontaneous recovery from acute urinary tract infection is possible and even likely in uncomplicated cases. It is generally agreed, however, that acute urinary tract infection should be treated to shorten the duration of infection and reduce the risk of complications. Acute urinary tract infection responds dramatically and promptly to appropriate antibacterial medications. Ideally, an antibiotic should be selected on the basis of tests that show the sensitivity of the offending organism. Since culture and sensitivity testing requires 48 hours to perform, it is necessary in most cases to begin treatment on an empirical basis with a drug that has a high probability of success. Provision should be made to change medication if an ineffective drug has been chosen as demonstrated by lack of clinical response or by the culture of a resistant organism.

Treatment of acute uncomplicated urinary tract infection is uniformly successful. If response is not prompt, the question is immediately raised whether the antibiotic chosen is inappropriate or whether there is some underlying complicating factor that makes the disease more resistant to treatment. About half of the patients who are treated for an episode of acute urinary tract infection have another infection within 1 year. In some patients, the frequency of acute infections justifies long-term, continuous drug therapy.

OBSTRUCTIVE UROPATHY

Since the function of the urinary system is the formation and the transport of urine, it is no surprise that blockage to the drainage of urine might be disruptive of the proper functioning of this system. Obstruction plays an important role in the full spectrum of urologic disease. The term *obstructive uropathy* refers to the functional and anatomical abnormalities that result from obstruction *per se*. Many diseases that cause obstruction pose a threat to the patient's health aside from the obstruction of urinary drainage. The most notable example of a disease with this potential is cancer, which may be either primary in the urinary tract, such as adenocarcinoma of the prostate and transitional cell carcinoma of the urinary bladder, or extrinsic to the urinary tract, such as carcinoma of the cervix and carcinoma of the rectum. In these diseases, obstructive uropathy may be most important as a symptom or sign. On the other hand, other diseases are often encountered that are important only because they cause obstruction to urinary drainage. Certain congenital abnormalities, acquired strictures, and benign enlargement of the prostate belong in this category. A discussion of all of the diseases that have the potential to cause obstruction in the urinary tract is almost a discussion of the entire field of urology.

The effect of obstruction on the urinary tract is determined by the level at which the obstruction occurs, the severity of the obstruction, and the duration of the obstruction. Obstruction is important clinically for four reasons: It causes symptoms; it causes acute changes in kidney function; it causes permanent, irreversible anatomical and functional changes in the kidney and urinary drainage system; and it predisposes to infection.

The symptomatic manifestation of obstruction depends entirely on the level of the obstruction and the nature of the disease by which it is caused. Ureteral colic caused by the passage of a kidney stone is one of the most severe pains encountered in clinical medicine. Obstruction of the ureter with a surgical ligature, however, may cause only mild, vague discomfort. Symptoms due to obstruction of the bladder outlet are commonly encountered. *Prostatism* is the term that refers to the symptom complex of diminished size and force of the urinary stream, hesitancy, increased frequency of urination, terminal dribbling of urine, and the discomfort that attends these symptoms.

Diagnosis of obstruction at a level above the bladder is best made by radiographic examination. The intravenous pyelogram may give evidence of obstruction. If there is no excretion of contrast material demonstrated on the intravenous pyelogram, cystoscopy and retrograde pyelography are often required. Isotope studies are commonly employed to determine the extent of renal functional impairment.

Evaluation of obstruction of the bladder often entails radiographic studies such as the intravenous pyelogram and voiding cystourethrogram, catheterization of the bladder to check for urethral obstruction and to measure residual urine, bladder pressure studies, and cystoscopic examination. The diagnostic evaluation should assess the severity of the obstruction and the nature of the disease process that has caused the obstruction. A substantial part of urologic practice is involved in the evaluation and treatment of obstructive uropathy.

URINARY CALCULI

Calculous disease of the urinary tract is a unique phenomenon that has no counterpart in any other organ system. Stones do occur in other structures, such as the gallbladder and the salivary glands, but the process by which these stones are formed and the clinical manifestations are quite different from those found in the urinary tract. Urinary stones are organized bodies with a crystalline structure and organic matrix and are composed of various molecules that have limited solubility. All of these substances are normally excreted by the kidney, often in a state of supersaturation. In health, microscopic crystals may be seen, depending on the state of hydration and the concentration of these substances, but stone growth does not occur. The formation of an organized stone represents a disease process and, as a disease, has certain deleterious effects. The most important and the most direct ill effect is obstruction of urinary drainage, which causes impairment of renal function and hydronephrotic atrophy. Stones may cause pain. Most often this pain is due to obstruction, but inflammatory reaction to the stone may also play a part. Calculous disease is often complicated by infection. Again, the likelihood of infection is increased by obstruction and stasis of urine. This relationship of stones with infection is further complicated by the fact that infection may induce the formation of stones. The abrasive effect of stones on the lining of the urinary tract may cause hematuria.

These damaging effects of urinary stones occur because the stone is a foreign body in the urinary tract. The size and location of the stone and the complications that occur, such as obstruction, pain, and infection, dictate treatment that is often surgical. The chemical composition of stones and the nature of the disease process that leads to stone formation are most important in determining preventive treatment.

PATHOGENESIS

The chain of events that leads to the formation of a urinary stone is related to the chemical nature of the stone involved. Certain general considerations, however, are common to the formation of all calculi. Supersaturation is a prerequisite for stone formation. Therefore, factors influencing concentration are important. The amount of water excreted is important in determining concentration of excreted solutes, as is the amount of solute that the kidney is called on to excrete. This may be influenced by dietary and metabolic factors. The *p*H of the urine influences the formation of certain stones, since it influences the solubility of the constituents.

The original formation of most urinary calculi occurs on, or in, the renal papillae. It is at this site, in the terminal portion of the collecting tubule, where urine achieves its maximum concentration. Retention of the stone embryo by adherence or stasis is a necessary factor in permitting stone growth to occur.

Almost all calculi that occur in the human urinary tract are included in one of the five categories shown in Figure 45-11. Diagnostic evaluation of the pathogenesis of stone disease ideally begins with the analysis of a recovered stone if one is available for examination. The unique pathogenesis of the various types of stones and their preventive treatment are discussed separately.

TYPES

CALCIUM OXALATE STONE

Calcium oxalate is the most common type of calculus encountered in the United States. Uncomplicated calcium oxalate stones are seldom large and are most often recognized when they drop into the ureter to cause ureteral colic. Calcium oxalate has a very limited solubility that is not influenced greatly by urine *p*H. Both calcium and oxalate are normally excreted in the urine. Oxalate is a normal end product of metabolism. Most urinary oxalate is of endogenous origin and is slightly influenced by the ingestion of foods, such as spinach, that are high in oxalate content. Precipitation of calcium oxalate might occur because of an excess concentration of either calcium or oxalate. Excessive excretion of oxalate occurs in an inherited condition called primary oxaluria, but this condition is quite rare. A discussion of calcium metabolism is not permissible within the scope of this text because of its complexity, but it can be fairly said that any condition that causes excessive excretion of calcium in the urine might predispose to calcium oxalate

stones. The ingestion of calcium in the human diet varies greatly.

The first line of regulation of calcium excretion is the regulation of absorption from the gut. Under the influence of parathyroid hormone, absorption is determined largely by the metabolic needs of the body, and the excess of ingested calcium is excreted largely in the stool without causing a corresponding rise in urinary excretion. Dietary intake of calcium may play a role in calcium stone formation, but usually the role is not dominant. Abnormality in the intestinal absorption of calcium may give rise to hypercalciuria. Excess excretion of parathyroid hormone causes hypercalciuria and is probably responsible for about 5% of calcium oxalate stones. Abnormal resorption of bone may cause excessive excretion of calcium in the urine. This may occur after extensive fractures, with prolonged immobilization, and in malignant disease in which bone destruction occurs. Some cases of calcium oxalate stone remain idiopathic. Treatment to prevent recurrence of calcium oxalate stones is often empirical. The therapeutic regimen of magnesium oxide and pyridoxine is reported to reduce the frequency of stone formation. The administration of phosphates has likewise been successful. The administration of thiazide diuretics reduces renal excretion of calcium and, in selected patients, helps to control calcium stone formation. The management of the patient with frequent recurrence of calcium oxalate stones requires the attention of a urologist or internist who has a special interest in this problem. Vigorous preventive measures are not required for the patient who sporadically forms calcium oxalate stones, since after the first stone, there is only a 30% to 40% chance of another attack. The simple expedients of increasing water intake and decreasing ingestion of dairy products are sometimes sufficient to prevent further stone formation.

CALCIUM PHOSPHATE STONE

Again, both calcium and phosphate are normally found in the urine, and the combination has limited solubility. The excretion of phosphate varies considerably with diet. As in calcium oxalate stones, calcium seems to be the important variable. Because of this factor, calcium oxalate and calcium phosphate stones have an etiologic kinship, and an admixture is commonly found in a single calculus. Conditions that result in hypercalciuria predispose to calcium phosphate stone formation, and the approach to preventive treatment of uncomplicated calcium phosphate stones is much the same as for calcium oxalate stones. High *p*H (alkalinity) of the urine predisposes to calcium phosphate stone formation. Because of this fact, calcium phosphate, in its several crystalline forms, often complicates infection with organisms that elevate urine *p*H. Certain bacteria, notably *Proteus*, have the ability to split the molecule of urea to yield ammonia, which causes marked alkalinity of the urine. The most rapid and the most pernicious stone growth occurs in this circumstance, resulting in large stones that are very difficult to manage. The stone that forms on the surface of foreign bodies such as catheters in the urinary tract is predominantly calcium phosphate.

MAGNESIUM AMMONIUM PHOSPHATE STONE

Magnesium ammonium phosphate stones occur almost exclusively in urine that is infected with urea-splitting organisms because the high urine *p*H is required for their formation. The soft, puttylike calculous matter that comprises infected stones is predominantly magnesium am-

Fig. 45-11. Classification of urinary calculi is shown according to chemical composition, with relative frequency of occurrence.

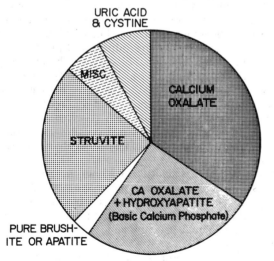

URIC ACID & CYSTINE

MISC.

CALCIUM OXALATE

STRUVITE

CA OXALATE + HYDROXYAPATITE (Basic Calcium Phosphate)

PURE BRUSH-ITE OR APATITE

BRUSHITE – Calcium Acid Phosphate
APATITE   – Basic Calcium Phosphate
STRUVITE – Magnesium Ammonium Phosphate

monium phosphate. Magnesium ammonium phosphate (struvite) and calcium phosphate (apatite) often occur as a mixture in this circumstance. Prevention requires that infection be controlled and the *p*H of the urine be lowered.

URIC ACID STONE

Uric acid is normally excreted in the urine as an end product of metabolism. Conditions such as gout, which result in increased excretion of uric acid, may cause precipitation of uric acid stones. These stones are unique in that they cast no shadow on x-ray films, since their radiodensity is the same as that of soft tissue of the body. Uric acid is more soluble in alkaline solution. Most uric acid stones may be prevented by increased intake of water and by the alkalinization of urine. Sodium citrate is often used for this purpose. Allopurinol is a drug that inhibits the enzyme xanthine oxidase, thereby preventing formation of uric acid. This drug effectively prevents formation of uric acid stones.

CYSTINE STONE

Cystine is an amino acid. The condition of cystinuria is an inherited defect in the tubular reabsorption of the amino acids cystine, lysine, arginine, and ornithine. The magnitude of loss of these amino acids is not great enough to pose any nutritional problem. The only adverse effect of cystinuria is the formation of cystine stones because of the limited solubility of cystine. The severity of the stone-forming tendency is related to the magnitude of cystine loss in the urine. Preventive treatment consists of high intake of water, alkalinization of the urine, low-methionine diet, and administration of D-penicillamine, which forms a soluble complex with cystine.

GENITOURINARY TRAUMA

The organs of the genitourinary system occupy protected positions within the trunk of the body. Because of this protection, injuries do not often occur in minor accidents. The kidney is protected by the lower rib cage, the vertebral column, and the thick muscles of the posterior abdominal wall. The ureter courses alongside the vertebral column anterior to the paraspinous muscles and the transverse processes of the vertebrae. In its lower portion, the ureter, along with the urinary bladder and part of the urethra, is protected by the bony pelvis. Injuries are more common in a highly industrialized society because of the exposure to heavy machines and the frequency of automobile accidents. When injuries to the urinary tract occur, the patient often has multiple injuries. All physicians who care for injured patients should possess a knowledge of the fundamentals of urologic traumatology.

CLASSIFICATION

It is useful to consider the nature of the trauma in classifying urologic injuries.

PENETRATING INJURIES

Gunshot wounds and stab wounds comprise the majority of penetrating injuries. Injuries sustained in military combat are most often penetrating. Penetrating injuries are frequently seen in the emergency room of most large city general hospitals but are less common in ordinary urologic practice.

NONPENETRATING INJURIES

In the United States, nonpenetrating injuries are mostly a product of automobile accidents and crushing injuries of various sorts. Blunt trauma is more common than penetrating wounds.

IATROGENIC INJURIES

Instrumentation of the urethra, bladder, and ureters may produce injury. Injury may be sustained in the course of abdominal operations or childbirth.

COMPLICATIONS

Serious loss of blood often occurs in injuries to the kidney. Bleeding is less significant in injuries to the bladder and ureter.

When there is disruption of the drainage system by trauma, leakage of urine may occur. This leakage predisposes to infection and may impair renal function. When leakage of urine occurs, a permanent opening between the urinary tract and another epithelial surface may result. One of the most commonly occurring fistulas is vesicovaginal after hysterectomy.

The patient with a perforated bladder, disruption in continuity of the urethra, or a large amount of clotted blood in the bladder may be unable to void. This requires immediate corrective measures.

Healing of injuries of the ureter or urethra may result in cicatricial obstruction (stricture).

Localized collections of blood (hematoma) or urine may become infected and form abscesses.

Injuries to pelvic nerves or vessels may result in sexual impotence in the male. Sexual disability may result from direct injuries to the penis and testicles.

Partial occlusion of the renal artery or one of its branches as a result of trauma may cause hypertension due to increased renin production.

DIAGNOSIS

The most important step in diagnosis is to suspect the injury. The nature of the trauma may provide important clues. In penetrating injuries, the path of the missile may be predictive. If there is fracture of the lower rib cage or transverse processes of the lumbar vertebrae, if there is bruising of the abdominal wall overlying the kidney, or if there is injury to the bony pelvis, one should look carefully for urologic injury. Hematuria is the most consistent sign of genitourinary injury. The presence of blood in the urine, no matter how slight, should never be overlooked in the injured patient. Urine specimens should be carefully collected to avoid the spurious introduction of red blood cells by traumatic instrumentation. The presence of hematuria always demands urologic investigation.

If the patient has difficulty voiding, the possibility of injury should be considered. A palpable mass in the lower abdomen or in the flank may suggest bladder or kidney injury with extravasation of urine or blood. Unexplained sepsis in the injured patient should prompt a search for urologic injury.

Proof of the diagnosis of genitourinary injury and its precise anatomical definition is dependent on radiographic procedures. The importance of a prompt and precise diagnosis cannot be overemphasized and can best be obtained by adequate preoperative evaluation. The genitourinary system is difficult to explore at the time of open surgery. The lack of preoperative evaluation places the urologist at a distinct disadvantage. An intravenous pyelogram is the first diagnostic study to be performed in most of these patients after the initial laboratory work and physical examination. This x-ray study provides important functional and anatomical information about the patient's urinary tract. Cystoscopy and retrograde pyelograms are reserved for those special circumstances in which the intravenous pyelogram fails to give adequate anatomical information. The retrograde urethrogram is performed by injecting contrast media into the urethral meatus and filling the urethra in a retrograde fashion. This is mandatory in all patients with suspected urethral injury. The bladder is best demonstrated by cystogram in which a catheter is introduced into the bladder to provide for filling of the bladder with contrast media. Demonstration of the blood supply to the kidney or to the pelvic viscera may be accomplished by arteriograms. Renal scan may help define the extent of the injury to the kidney.

MANAGEMENT

Recognition and proper treatment of urologic injuries are important to avoid the acute and the chronic complications that have been discussed. Errors in management are most often due to errors in diagnosis. Management of specific injuries is discussed under the heading of various organs.

NEUROLOGIC DISEASES OF THE GENITOURINARY SYSTEM

The nervous system plays an important role in the proper functioning of the genitourinary system. Neurologic connections and their functional counterparts (muscles, glands) involve complex interrelationships between somatic sensory and motor fibers, autonomic (sympathetic and parasympathetic) sensory and motor fibers, and spinal cord and central nervous system ganglia and pathways. A knowledge of the neurologic aspects of urologic disease is important in interpretation of signs and symptoms and in understanding the disease states that result from neurologic impairment. The kidneys and ureters have an abundant autonomic nerve supply, but there are no clinically significant disease states that result from deficiency of innervation of these structures. In contrast, neurologic deficits cause severe disruption in the function of the urinary bladder and in sexual function.

The bladder and its outflow tract serve two important functions: the storage and expulsion of urine and the provision of urinary continence. The essential functional components of the apparatus that normally accomplishes these functions are the smooth muscle of the bladder and urethra, the skeletal muscle of the external urinary sphincter and pelvic floor, and the intrinsic elasticity of the urethra. The muscular components are under complex neurologic control. For effective emptying, the smooth-muscle wall of the urinary bladder (detrusor) must mount a sustained, coordinated contraction that elevates intravesical pressure to a level that overcomes outlet resistance. To keep this pressure from reaching pathologic levels, there must be concomitant relaxation of the muscles that oppose urine flow. Continence of urine is possible because the normal bladder permits expansion of its capacity, within limits,

without contracting and because there is sustained tone in the muscles that oppose urine flow and in the elastic wall of the membranous urethra.

CLASSIFICATION

Classification of the types of neurogenic bladder disorders might be based on etiologic factors, except that the range of neurologic manifestations of the various diseases that might affect bladder function is very wide. Classification also might be based on the neuroanatomy of the pathologic lesions. However, clinical definition of the area of involvement is often imprecise, and the reflection of this involvement on the clinical behavior of the affected bladder is not predictable. The most useful classification, from the clinical standpoint, is one based upon the observed behavior of the neurologically impaired bladder (*e.g.*, pressure studies, roentgenograms), since this factor is a major determinant of clinical management.

UNINHIBITED NEUROGENIC BLADDER

The bladder of the young child is the best example of the uninhibited bladder. Acquired disease such as cerebral arteriosclerosis, cerebrovascular accidents, brain tumors, multiple sclerosis, and others may result in uninhibited bladder dysfunction.

REFLEX NEUROGENIC BLADDER

Reflex neurogenic bladder dysfunction is often referred to as spastic neurogenic bladder or upper motor neuron lesion. The micturition reflex center in the sacral cord is intact, and the sensory and motor limbs of the reflex are functional. More or less complete loss of central connections that coordinate the micturition reflex is sustained. This type bladder is most often seen in patients with spinal cord injury (paraplegia) but may arise from vascular accidents involving the cord, tumors of the spinal cord, herniated nucleus pulposus (ruptured disk), and congenital abnormalities.

AUTONOMOUS NEUROGENIC BLADDER

Autonomous neurogenic bladder results from disruption of the spinal cord reflex center. This may occur with injuries to the sacral cord and the cauda equina. Injury to the peripheral nerves secondary to extensive operations in the pelvis can produce similar results. Bladder tone is diminished, and uninhibited spastic contractions are absent.

SENSORY PARALYTIC BLADDER

In sensory paralytic bladder, the micturition reflex is abnormal because of deficient input of sensory impulses. The most common cause for this disorder is diabetic neuropathy.

MOTOR PARALYTIC BLADDER

When motor fibers predominantly are involved, the bladder loses its tone. Vesical sensory function remains intact, but the micturition reflex may occur at increasingly larger capacity as bladder decompensation progresses. This lesion may occur as a result of poliomyelitis, trauma, extensive pelvic operations, neoplasms, and discogenic disease.

DIAGNOSTIC EVALUATION

The diagnostic evaluation of the patient with suspected neurogenic bladder dysfunction begins with a careful history and physical examination. Often the cause for the bladder disability is readily apparent. No problem is encountered in establishing the cause in the patient whose spinal cord has been severed. On the other hand, dysfunction of the urinary bladder may be the first clinical manifestation of more subtle neurologic disease, such as multiple sclerosis or diabetic neuropathy. Physical examination should include a complete neurologic evaluation in search for other manifestations of nervous system involvement. Care must be exercised to rule out obstructing lesions that may masquerade as neurogenic dysfunction. Drug-induced alteration in bladder function may be quite difficult to distinguish from neurologic disease. Anticholinergic agents, which are often taken for gastrointestinal disease, may adversely affect the function of the bladder. Certain tranquilizing drugs, antihistamines, and adrenergic agents are frequent offenders.

Urodynamic studies are essential in evaluation of patients with suspected neurologic disease. These studies include cystometrics, in which pressures are recorded as the bladder is filled. Concomitant electromyography of muscles of the perineum helps define the reciprocal relationship of the mechanisms of continence. Voiding flow rates are measured. Radiographic evaluation with voiding cystourethrograms is an important adjuvant. Finally, cystoscopy may be useful in selected patients.

TREATMENT

Patients with neurogenic bladder dysfunction may be managed conservatively if reflex activity of the bladder permits adequate emptying. If these patients are incontinent, measures (such as the use of external catheters) must be taken to control wetness. Reflex emptying may be augmented by surgery designed to decrease bladder outlet resistance. Most often, this involves transurethral incision of the spastic external sphincter. Indwelling catheter drainage or intermittent catheterization may be required. Supravesical urinary diversion, most notably by ileal conduit, occasionally is advised. However, the frequency with which urinary diversion is performed in management of dysfunctional bladder has been greatly diminished in recent years by the demonstrated effectiveness of intermittent self-catheterization in managing the decompensated bladder.

SEXUAL DISABILITY IN MALES

Sexual function in the male may be subdivided into the sensory perception of sexual stimuli, the ability to achieve an erection (potency), the ability to have orgasm, and the production of semen. In urologic practice, impotence is one of the most common patient complaints. Impotence may be defined as the inability to achieve erection of the penis in response to erotic stimuli and to maintain turgidity through the successful performance of the sexual act. Penile erection is a neurovascular phenomenon that is strongly influenced by psychological factors and by the endocrine environment.

Impairment of function of the erectile bodies (corpora cavernosa) may result from injury, Peyronie's disease, priapism, and congenital disorders. Vascular disease or endocrine disorders may cause impotence. Impotence may result from central nervous system disease, such as head injuries, brain or spinal cord tumors, strokes, multiple sclerosis, and tabes dorsalis, or from localized spinal cord lesions, such as meningomyelocele, spinal cord tumors, and spinal cord injury. The most notable example is the sexual dysfunction of the paraplegic, in whom erections may occur but are totally divorced from erotic psychic stimuli, devoid of pleasurable sensations, and unpredictable in duration and utility for sexual purposes. Peripheral neuropathy such as that seen in diabetics may produce impotence. It is commonly known that operations on the prostate may result in impotence, owing to damage to the peripheral nerve supply. The standard operations for benign prostatic hyperplasia carry only a small risk, whereas radical prostatectomy almost invariably causes impotence. Impotence may result from pelvic surgery, such as abdominal perineal resection for cancer of the rectum, and from injuries to the pelvis from external trauma. When the membranous urethra is injured as a result of fractures of the bony pelvis, the incidence of impotence is 30%.

Evaluation of the patient with impotence should include a careful history and physical examination. In selected patients, psychological evaluation is indicated. Laboratory evaluation should include a complete blood count, automated blood chemistries (SMA 18), and serum testosterone. Penile blood pressure should be determined using the Doppler stethoscope. Monitoring of nocturnal penile tumescence is particularly helpful in distinguishing psychogenic from organic impotence, since nocturnal erections during rapid eye movement (REM) sleep are not impaired by psychological factors.

Major improvements have been made in recent years in the therapy for impotence. Sex therapy for psychogenic impotence has greatly changed since the pioneering work of Masters and Johnson, and results have improved. Specific therapy for organic impotence depends upon the discovery of a cause. Endocrine disorders may be amenable to therapy. Elimination of offending drugs, such as alcohol, certain antihypertensives, and tranquilizers, may be helpful. For patients whose impotence is refractory to specific therapy, rehabilitation may be provided by penile implants. Semirigid rods of varying design and inflatable prostheses may be surgically inserted into the corpora cavernosa to provide enough stiffness to permit intromission.

MALE CONTRACEPTION

The past decade has seen dramatic changes in attitudes about birth control measures. This has been manifest by increased demand by an informed public for professional assistance in birth control, more willingness on the part of private physicians and public agencies to provide this assistance, relaxation of restrictions in hospitals, and liberalization of laws governing birth control techniques. Vasectomy has become an increasingly popular choice for permanent contraception and is an important modality worldwide in public efforts at population control. Liability for negligence in the performance of vasectomy is the same as for any operative procedure. Informed consent of the patient is mandatory and should involve detailed explanation of the procedure and of the immediate and delayed complications that might occur. Consent of the spouse is strongly advisable. Success of the operation should not be promised. Provision should be made for follow-up to demonstrate the absence of spermatozoa in semen specimens collected monthly until two successive specimens are negative.

The search for a safe and effective contraceptive pill for men continues.

CHRONIC RENAL FAILURE

In the United States, approximately 35,000 to 50,000 patients die each year of chronic renal disease. Uremia, for many of these patients, is merely the terminal event in the course of a fatal illness such as diabetes mellitus, cancer, arteriosclerosis, heart disease, acute disseminated lupus erythematosus, and others. Approximately 10,000 to 15,000 of these patients with renal failure might survive and lead normal or near-normal lives with restoration of renal function. However, until recent years, the ultimate prognosis for most of these patients was hopeless, since the course of most medical renal diseases cannot be reversed. The development of chronic dialysis (artificial kidney) and transplantation has drastically altered the prospect for the patient who has lost the function of his own kidneys, and has opened up entirely new fields of medical practice.

HEMODIALYSIS

The concept of hemodialysis is not new. In 1877, peritoneal dialysis was studied in experimental animals. Abel and colleagues reported the first use of an artificial kidney experimentally in 1913. In 1947, Kolff established the basis for the use of the artificial kidney in clinical medicine with the use of cellophane tubing as a dialyzing membrane. In the ensuing years, improvements in the apparatus were effected and hemodialysis was widely used in the treatment of acute renal failure due to reversible kidney disease.

Chronic dialysis does not restore the patient to optimal health and productivity. Mortality rates are higher for patients on dialysis than for the general population. Most of these patients are anemic because of the loss of erythropoietin production by the kidneys, repeated loss of blood in the dialysis procedure, and other factors. Cardiovascular complications, such as high blood pressure and heart failure, are common. These patients are more susceptible to infection than is the general population.

KIDNEY TRANSPLANTATION

Successful transplantation restores the patient with renal failure to an acceptable state of health, although immunosuppressive therapy is attended by many complications. Reference should be made to recent publications for complication and survival statistics, since these figures will undoubtedly change from year to year. A major breakthrough in results of transplantation awaits the discovery of methods to control rejection without toxicity to the recipient. The surgical technique of kidney transplantation has become well standardized and perfected with experience.

DISEASES OF THE KIDNEY

CONGENITAL ANOMALIES

The kidney may become arrested in its ascent during embryologic development and occupy a position anywhere between the pelvis and the renal fossa. Occasionally, the kidney may be displaced across the midline. This is called crossed ectopia. Most ectopic kidneys are also malrotated. There may be fusion between the two kidneys, resulting in a horseshoe or pancake configuration (Fig. 45-12). There

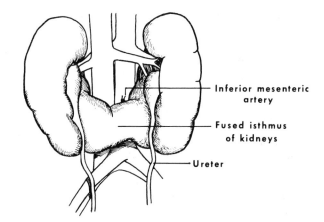

Fig. 45-12. Horseshoe kidney anomaly.

is an increased incidence of outflow tract obstruction in ectopic and malrotated kidneys. These anomalous kidneys may be mistaken for retroperitoneal neoplasms.

Renal agenesis is the congenital absence of a kidney. This is a rare anomaly. Hypoplasia refers to defective development of a kidney resulting in a small, poorly functioning structure. The distinction between hypoplasia and atrophy is often difficult.

Simple cyst is probably a congenital defect of the nephron unit. It is often single and usually unilateral. Cysts are thin-walled lesions with endothelial lining containing clear, straw-colored fluid, which is presumed to be a transudate. Simple cysts may rarely be complicated by infection, rupture, ureteral obstruction, and pain. Most often, the lesion is asymptomatic, and the most important clinical significance is that the mass must be distinguished from solid tumors, which are most often malignant. Nephrotomography and sonography may be used. Selective renal arteriography is the most reliable diagnostic test, since solid tumors most often have a demonstrable blood supply and simple cysts do not. Needle aspiration of the cyst is often performed after arteriography to confirm the diagnosis. CT scanning is helpful in some cases. In equivocal cases, surgical exploration is required.

Polycystic kidney disease is hereditary and may be divided into adult and infantile types. The infantile type is an autosomal recessive disease and leads to early renal failure. The adult type is autosomal dominant and usually does not become symptomatic until middle age. Gradual erosion of renal function can be expected. Hypertension, hematuria, and infection may complicate the cystic disease. In the advanced stage of development, polycystic kidneys consist of innumerable cysts of varying size with a great increase in the external dimensions of the kidney.

Multicystic kidney is a form of renal dysplasia in which there is atresia of the ureter and a small cluster of irregular cysts replacing the renal parenchyma. The opposite kidney is usually normal. The clinical classification of renal cysts is shown in Table 45-2.

Congenital hydronephrosis is one of the most common abdominal masses in newborns. It is often caused by congenital ureteropelvic junction obstruction (Fig. 45-13). Obstruction at this site may result from congenital stricture, adynamic ureteral segment, high implantation of the ureter on the renal pelvis, and angulation of the proximal ureter due to anomalous renal vessels. When obstruction is minimal, progressive renal damage may not occur and no treatment is required. Obstruction may be so severe that complete hydronephrotic atrophy occurs. In this event, nephrectomy may be necessary. Pyeloplasty to correct the obstruction should be performed when obstruction is causing damage to the kidney and when there appears to be significant salvageable renal function.

INFECTIONS

Pyelonephritis is an acute infection of the kidney usually caused by coliform organisms that reach the kidney by ascent through the outflow tract. It is usually attended by chills and fever and pain in the flank. Bladder symptoms may predominate. Presence of urinary tract infection is established by urinalysis and urine culture. Outflow tract obstruction, vesicoureteral reflux, urinary calculi, and anatomical lesions should be suspected in patients with pyelonephritis. Chronic pyelonephritis is a diagnosis usually applied to the chronic changes that occur in the kidney as a result of prolonged or frequently recurrent acute infections.

Renal carbuncle is a localized abscess of the renal parenchyma usually resulting from blood-borne *Staphylococcus aureus* infection. It is most often seen in diabetics.

Perinephric abscess is a suppurative infection in the perinephric fat which may result from hematogenous seeding of organisms or, more often, from infection in the kidney, especially in the presence of obstruction.

Tuberculosis of the kidney is secondary to pulmonary or gastrointestinal tuberculosis. Seeding of a glomeruli occurs during the hematogenous phase of primary tuberculosis. If the lesions progress, caseous necrosis occurs and seeding of the outflow tract and prostate may occur. Genitourinary tuberculosis should be suspected in patients with sterile pyuria. Treatment is usually medical and is similar to treatment for pulmonary tuberculosis.

Papillary necrosis is a condition in which ischemic

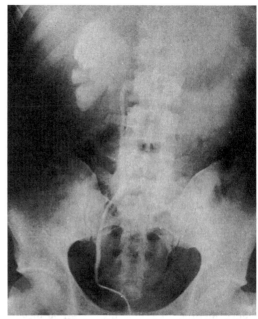

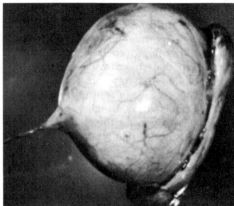

Fig. 45-13. (*Top*) Right hydronephrosis due to ureteropelvic obstruction. Ureter is normal in caliber except at the ureteropelvic junction. (*Bottom*) Actual specimen of a hydronephrotic kidney due to congenital narrowing of the ureter at the ureteropelvic junction. The pelvis is tremendously dilated with a relatively small cap of parenchyma.

necrosis of the renal papillae occurs. Analgesic abuse, diabetes, sickle-cell disease, and infection have been associated with the condition. As the papillae slough, obstruction to the drainage of the kidney may occur. Infection often complicates the condition. Rapid destruction of the kidney may be anticipated unless internal drainage is provided.

NEOPLASMS

Renal cell carcinoma is the most common of malignant tumors of the kidney in adults (Fig. 45-14). It is rare in children and is more frequent in men than in women. The tumor may invade locally and metastasize by way of the bloodstream and the lymphatics. Hematogenous metastases predominate, most commonly being found in lungs, liver, and bones. Regional lymph nodes are involved in approximately 30% of patients. Unfortunately, signs and symptoms are usually meager until the disease is advanced. Gross hematuria is the most frequent presenting complaint. Di-

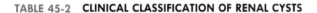

TABLE 45-2   CLINICAL CLASSIFICATION OF RENAL CYSTS

I. Renal dysplasia
   1. Congenital unilateral multicystic kidney
   2. Segmental and focal renal dysplasia
   3. Renal dysplasia associated with congenital lower tract obstruction
II. Congenital polycystic kidney disease
   1. Infantile type
   2. Adult type
III. Cystic disorders of the renal medulla
   1. Renal cystic disease with congenital hepatic fibrosis
   2. Medullary cystic disease
   3. Sponge kidney
IV. Simple cyst
V. Calyceal cyst
VI. Cysts associated with neoplasm
   1. Cystic degeneration of parenchymal tumors
   2. Malignant change occurring in wall of simple cyst
   3. Cystadenoma and multilocular cysts
VII. Cysts secondary to nonmalignant renal pathology
VIII. Peripelvic cyst
IX. Perinephric cyst
X. Miscellaneous

(Spence HM, Singleton R: Cysts and cystic disorders of the kidney: Types, diagnosis, treatment. Urol Surv 22:131, 1972)

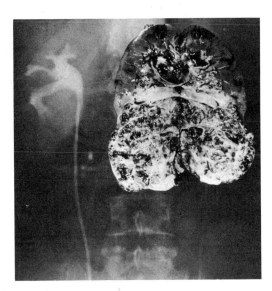

Fig. 45-14. Right retrograde pyelogram demonstrates a tumor deformity. Bivalved kidney specimen shows a hypernephroma involving the lower half of the kidney and accounting for the pyelographic abnormality.

agnosis of a mass in the kidney is best established by intravenous pyelography. Renal arteriography or CT scan may confirm the diagnosis. Metastatic survey should include chest film, bone scan, and inferior venacavogram. Radical nephrectomy is the treatment of choice and offers the only known chance for cure. The overall 5-year survival rate of patients with renal cell carcinoma is approximately 35%.

Angiomyolipoma (hamartoma) is a benign tumor of the kidney that may rarely be confused with renal cell carcinoma. It occurs frequently in patients with tuberous sclerosis.

Wilms' tumor (embryoma) is the most common of malignant tumors of the kidney in childhood. It is a highly malignant mixed tumor consisting of tissues of connective tissue origin and epithelial structures. It is usually discovered as a palpable mass by the mother or an examining physician. Treatment of the primary tumor is radical nephrectomy. Adjunctive therapy with irradiation and chemotherapy is important in improving survival.

Transitional cell carcinoma is the most common tumor of the renal pelvis and ureter. The transitional epithelium of the renal pelvis and ureter may give rise to malignant tumors that are similar to lesions that occur in the bladder. Squamous cell carcinoma may occur because of metaplastic changes. Clinical behavior of these tumors is dependent on the degree of cellular differentiation and the extent of invasion. Well-differentiated, noninvasive tumors carry a favorable prognosis. Poorly differentiated, invasive tumors are almost uniformly fatal because of early metastases. Hematuria is most commonly the presenting complaint. Diagnosis may be suspected on the basis of an intravenous pyelogram. Cytologic examination of the urine may demonstrate exfoliated malignant cells. The usual treatment is radical nephroureterectomy. Well-localized, noninvasive tumors may be amenable to local resection.

TRAUMA

Penetrating and nonpenetrating injury to the kidney may occur. Penetrating injuries occur more frequently in war-

time, and nonpenetrating injuries are more commonly encountered in civilian practice. Injury to the kidney should be suspected if the injured patient is found to have hematuria. The intravenous pyelogram is an important test in evaluation of these injuries, and findings may suggest the need for further studies, such as retrograde pyelography or renal arteriography. Minimal injuries to the kidney are classified as contusions. More severe lacerations may involve tears in the renal capsule or in the mucosa of the collecting system, or both. Major vascular injuries may occur. The most immediate problem encountered in management of renal trauma is hemorrhage. Bleeding from the injured kidney usually stops spontaneously short of exsanguination, but continued bleeding may be massive and necessitate urgent surgical intervention. Other complications include extravasation of urine, necrosis of a variable amount of renal parenchyma, and infection in devitalized tissue and hematoma. If surgery is required, the transperitoneal approach should be selected so that the abdomen may be explored for unsuspected injuries and so that renal vessels may be identified early in the operation for control of bleeding. In most cases, preservation of renal function should be possible, but nephrectomy is occasionally required when the kidney is fragmented. In this event, it is well to know the status of the opposite kidney.

STONES

Most urinary calculi originate in the kidney. Stones that remain encysted in a renal calyx usually do not require surgical removal unless complicated by obstruction of a calyx or infection. Stones that drop out of the calyx into the renal pelvis require surgical removal because of the likelihood of obstruction at the ureteropelvic junction. Staghorn calculi of the kidney are most often associated with urea-splitting infection. These stones constitute one of the most difficult surgical problems in urology because of the technical difficulty of removing all of the stone fragments without damaging the kidney. Untreated, these stones cause gradual destruction of the kidney, owing to pyelonephritis and obstruction.

DISEASES OF THE URETER

CONGENITAL ANOMALIES

Ureteral duplication (double ureter) is a common anomaly. Duplication may be complete or incomplete. The duplication anomaly is most often innocuous. However, in patients with duplicated ureters, there is an increased incidence of vesicoureteral reflux into the lower pole ureter. Likewise, there is an increased risk of ureterocele and ectopia involving the ureter which drains the upper pole of a duplicated system.

Ectopic ureteral orifice occurs as a developmental defect and may be found in an abnormal location in the bladder or urethra. In females, the opening may present on the vulva or into the vagina, cervix, or uterus. Ectopic ureters may drain into the seminal vesicles in males. Kidneys drained by ectopic ureters usually are developmentally defective and hydronephrotic. Urinary incontinence is the most common presenting complaint in females with ectopic ureters. Incontinence does not occur in males.

Ureterocele is a cystlike protrusion of mucosa of the terminal ureter into the lumen of the bladder. Internally it is lined with ureteral mucosa and externally with bladder mucosa. The orifice is usually small and obstructive. As a result, most ureteroceles are associated with ureterectasis and hydronephrosis.

Retrocaval ureter is a vascular anomaly in which abnormal development of the vena cava leaves the ureter in a retrocaval position. Drainage of the kidney is impaired, and hydronephrosis occurs. Treatment usually is division of the ureter, with reanastomosis lateral to the vena cava.

Congenital stricture of the ureter is usually associated with atresia of the smooth muscle of the ureteral wall. It occurs most often in the upper third of the ureter.

Adynamic ureteral segment is a condition in which there is defective ureteral peristalsis in a segment of the ureter. The segment is usually located at the ureteropelvic junction or at the ureterovesical junction. This defect causes a functional obstruction of urine flow. The lesion has been compared to Hirschsprung's disease of the colon but does not occur in association with that disease and does not share the absence of ganglion cells as an etiologic factor. Pyeloplasty is often required to correct obstructions encountered at the ureteropelvic junction. When the lesions occur at the ureterovesical junction, a large, dilated, tortuous ureter may be produced, which has been called primary megaureter. The condition may be managed conservatively unless deterioration in renal function is demonstrated.

Normally, backflow of urine from the bladder into the ureter is prevented by a valve mechanism at the ureterovesical junction. When this valve mechanism is incompetent, usually because the intravesical submusocal tunnel of the ureter is too short, reflux may occur. Reflux may be caused by defective development of the submucosal portion of the ureter, bladder outlet obstruction, surgical injury to the ureteral orifice, bladder infection, and neurologic disease of the bladder. Reflux is associated with an increased risk of urinary tract infection. When an infection occurs in the bladder in the presence of reflux, organisms have free access to the kidney. The significance of reflux in the absence of infection is debatable. Some children "outgrow" reflux. When reflux appears to be a permanent condition, particularly if it is associated with frequent infections or anatomical changes in the upper urinary tracts, surgical correction by reimplantation of the ureter into the bladder, creating a longer submucosal tunnel, is the accepted treatment.

NEOPLASMS

Ureteral tumors are quite rare. Transitional cell carcinoma of the ureter may occur.

TRAUMA

In contrast to injuries of the kidney, ureteral trauma is seldom caused by external violence. Approximately 90% of ureteral injuries are iatrogenic. These injuries most often occur in the course of pelvic surgery, most notably, the performance of hysterectomy. If the diagnosis of ureteral injury is suspected in the postoperative patient or in trauma victims, an intravenous pyelogram should be performed. Retrograde pyelography is often required to define the location and severity of the defect. Injury may be attended

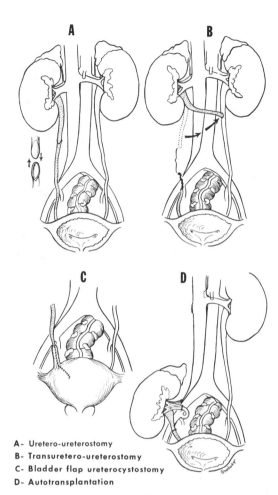

A- Uretero-ureterostomy
B- Transuretero-ureterostomy
C- Bladder flap ureterocystostomy
D- Autotransplantation

Fig. 45-15. Operative repair of ureteral injuries.

by obstruction or by extravasation of urine. Healing of ureteral injuries usually results in stricture and may be associated with continued leakage of urine through a fistula to the skin or vagina. Most ureteral injuries require surgical repair. The surgical requirements depend on the level at which the ureter is injured and whether or not there has been loss of length (Fig. 45-15).

STONES

Stones in the ureter are, with rare exceptions, displaced kidney stones and may be composed of any of the components discussed in the section on urinary calculi. Most stones small enough to gain access to the ureter through the ureteropelvic junction may be expected to pass spontaneously. However, approximately 30% of these stones require surgical removal. The diagnosis may be suspected in most patients because of the typically severe pain of ureteral colic, which usually begins in the flank and subsequently radiates to the lower abdominal quadrant or to the scrotum or vulva. Microscopic examination of urine reveals red blood cells. The intravenous pyelogram usually confirms the diagnosis (Fig. 45-16). Because of the extreme severity of the pain that some patients experience with ureteral stones, priority should be given to establishing a presumptive diagnosis on first examination so that narcotics may be safely and expeditiously administered. Conservative

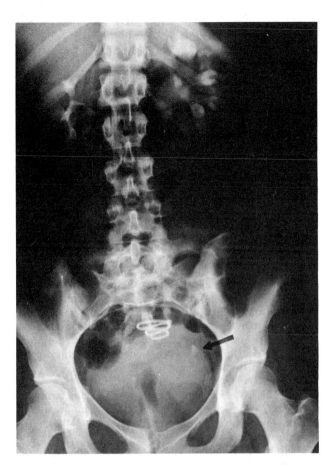

Fig. 45-16. Intravenous pyelogram showing opaque calculus in the distal ureter (*arrow*) with mild obstructive changes in the left kidney. An intrauterine contraceptive device projects over the sacrum.

treatment of these patients consists of administration of analgesics and adequate hydration. All the patient's urine should be strained for recovery of the stone if it is passed. Urinary infection is a serious complication in these patients and should be suspected in patients with fever. The end point of management must be the delivery of the stone from the ureter. If this does not occur spontaneously, surgical removal is required. The decision to abandon conservative treatment of ureteral stones is based on consideration of the following factors:

Size of the stone. In the great majority of patients, stones less than 5 mm in size should pass. Spontaneous passage becomes less likely if the stone exceeds 5 mm.

Progress of the stone. Progress of the stone is determined by radiographs during the period of observation.

Severity of obstruction. The severity is measured by intravenous pyelogram or renogram.

Infection. Acute pyelonephritis above an obstructing calculus creates a surgical and medical emergency.

Pain. Although pain is the dominant clinical feature of ureteral stones, it can most often be managed with analgesics and seldom should be taken as justification for operative intervention.

Surgery for stones. Stones may be extracted from the ureter by cystoscopic manipulation with a stone basket or by open surgery (ureterolithotomy).

DISEASES OF THE BLADDER

CONGENITAL ANOMALIES

When the allantois, which connects the urogenital sinus with the umbilicus in the embryo, is incompletely obliterated, its patency may result in a vesicocutaneous fistula at the umbilicus, a cystic mass in the lower abdominal wall, or a diverticulum of the dome of the bladder.

Bladder diverticula usually result from bladder outlet obstruction with sustained elevated intravesical pressure, but congenital diverticula without obstruction are occasionally seen.

Exstrophy is a congenital abnormality in which the bladder is open ventrally onto the abdominal wall (Fig. 45-17). There is a complete ventral defect of the anterior bladder wall and urethra. The rami of the pubic bones are widely separated, as are the rectus muscles. Surgical closure may be accomplished but seldom is successful in achieving urinary continence. Most children with exstrophy eventually require urinary diversion.

INFECTIONS

Cystitis is one of the most common ailments seen in urologic practice. It occurs much more commonly in females. The diagnosis is suggested by symptomatic manifestations such as urinary frequency, urgency, and dysuria. It may be accompanied by hematuria. Diagnosis is established by examination of urine. Uncomplicated cystitis usually reponds promptly to appropriate antibacterial therapy. Less commonly, noninfectious inflammatory lesions of the bladder may be encountered, such as interstitial cystitis, urethrotrigonitis syndrome, and irradiation cystitis.

Fig. 45-17. Exstrophy of the urinary bladder. The umbilicus is in the upper part of the lesion. The open bladder may be seen on the abdominal wall. The small, epispadiac penis is visible below the bladder.

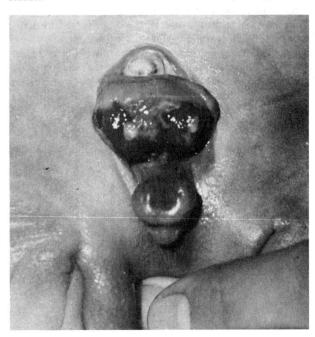

NEOPLASMS

Most bladder tumors arise from the transitional epithelium. Transitional cell carcinomas are most common. Squamous cell carcinoma comprises approximately 5% to 10% of malignant tumors of the bladder. Adenocarcinoma may arise from a urachal remnant at the dome of the bladder or from submucosal glands in the vicinity of the bladder neck. Transitional cell carcinoma of the bladder occurs more frequently in men than in women, and its frequency increases with age. Carcinoma of the bladder is quite rare in children. Hematuria is usually the first sign of bladder cancer, although symptoms of bladder irritability may predominate. The diagnosis is established by cystoscopy and biopsy of the tumor. For purposes of determining prognosis and selecting appropriate therapy, it is important to know the grade and stage of the tumor. Grade is based on the degree of cellular differentiation, with grade I being well differentiated, grade IV being anaplastic, and grades II and III being intermediate. The stage of the tumor refers to the degree of local invasion and the presence or absence of metastases (Fig. 45-18). The stage of the tumor seems to correlate best with prognosis. Treatment must be individualized. Small, superficial tumors are often amenable to transurethral resection. Larger, more invasive tumors may require radical cystectomy. Radiotherapy may be selected as definitive treatment in some patients. Preoperative irradiation followed by radical cystectomy probably provides the best chance for cure of advanced bladder cancer at present.

TRAUMA

Nonpenetrating trauma may injure the bladder by either of two mechanisms. When a blow is delivered to the lower abdomen over a full bladder, rupture may occur, owing to sudden increase in intravesical pressure. This perforation is usually through the peritoneal surface of the bladder. When there is fracture of the bony pelvis, spicules of bone may penetrate the bladder. In this event, extravasation is into the retroperitoneum. Suspecting injury to the bladder in the traumatized patient is of paramount importance, since delay in diagnosis may invite serious complications. When the diagnosis is suspected, a cystogram is performed to demonstrate the extravasation. The usual treatment is to close the bladder and to drain it with an indwelling catheter. Occasionally, bladder injuries may be successfully managed by catheter drainage of the bladder without operative closure of the perforation. The bladder may also be injured in the course of difficult childbirth or during operations in the pelvis. Vesicovaginal fistula may result from these obstetric and gynecologic injuries.

STONES

Bladder stones are most often the result of obstruction or neurologic impairment that produces stasis and infection in the urinary bladder. Patients who wear indwelling catheters for long periods are prone to form bladder calculi. Bladder stones may be crushed with an instrument inserted through the urethra and the fragments irrigated out through the instrument (litholapaxy), or they may be removed by suprapubic incision (vesicolithotomy).

DISEASES OF THE FEMALE URETHRA

Urethral diverticulum occurs in the urethrovaginal septum. This is usually an acquired disease that probably results from infection in periurethral glands. The patient may note frequency of urination, dysuria, and intermittent purulent discharge from the urethra. Diverticulum may be palpable through the anterior wall of the vagina. Purulent secretions may be expressed from the urethra by massage in this area. Diagnosis is confirmed by urethrogram and by urethroscopy. Diverticula of the female urethra are usually excised by a transvaginal approach.

Urethritis is a very common disease in females and is usually accompanied by cystitis. Most infections are due to coliform organisms. Acute urethritis may occur in the course of gonorrheal infections.

Urethral caruncle is a hyperemic, edematous protrusion of mucosa and submucosa of the posterior lip of the urethral meatus; it is most often seen in postmenopausal women. The lesion is tender, may bleed, and causes dysuria. It is a benign lesion but must be differentiated from urethral carcinoma.

Carcinoma of the urethra in females is a rare lesion. In the distal third of the urethra, adenocarcinoma and squamous cell carcinoma may occur. Transitional cell carcinoma may be found in the proximal portion of the urethra.

Urethral injury due to external violence is rare. It is more likely to be encountered in difficult obstetric cases or in vaginal surgery.

Cystourethrocele is a prolapse of the bladder and urethra into the anterior wall of the vagina as a result of relaxation of the supporting structures in the pelvic sling. This usually is a result of childbirth. The most important clinical manifestation of this condition is stress incontinence.

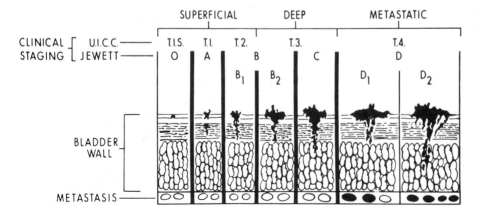

Fig. 45-18. Classification of carcinoma of the bladder.

DISEASES OF THE PENIS AND MALE URETHRA

CONGENITAL ANOMALIES

Phimosis is a condition in which tightness of the prepuce prevents its retraction over the glans penis. Paraphimosis is a condition in which the prepuce, having been retracted over the glans penis, cannot be reduced. Each of these conditions may be definitively treated with circumcision. Paraphimosis may be a surgical emergency if the blood supply to the glans penis is strangulated.

Hypospadias is a congenital anomaly involving the urethra and penis. Hypospadias is due to incomplete masculinization of the fetus. The defect is characterized anatomically by an opening of the urethra on the ventral shaft of the penis proximal to the glans penis, ventral curvature of the penis, and an incomplete prepuce, which gives a "hooded" appearance (Fig. 45-19). The defect is most important because of its psychological impact on the patient. In addition, the penile curvature may cause sexual disability. Direction of the urinary stream from the standing position may be difficult. Surgical repair is indicated and should usually be performed at about 2 years of age. Circumcision of the newborn with hypospadias should be avoided because the skin of the prepuce is useful in repair of the defect.

Penile curvature is most commonly due to hypospadias, but, occasionally, penile curvatures are seen in the absence of urethral anomalies.

Epispadias is a condition in which the urethra is defective dorsally. It is often associated with exstrophy of the bladder. Unlike hypospadias, epispadias is a defect that is not related to masculinization of the fetus. Epispadias often involves the urinary sphincter and produces urinary incontinence. Congenital strictures of the anterior urethra are rare.

Posterior urethral valves are one of the most common causes of obstructive uropathy in male infants. These valves are thin mucosal folds, most often located at the level of the verumontanum in the posterior urethra (Fig. 45-20).

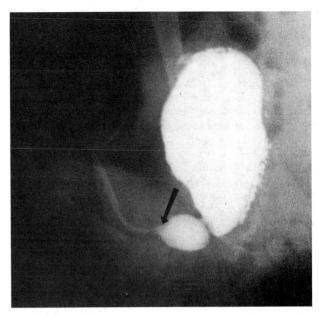

Fig. 45-20. Voiding cystourethrogram showing (*arrow*) posterior urethral valves.

The kidney, ureters, and bladder are often severely damaged in these patients because of the severity of the obstruction.

INFECTIONS

Balanitis is an inflammatory skin condition of the glans penis, usually due to nonspecific infection in patients who have redundant foreskin or phimosis. Primary venereal lesions in the male are often located on the penis. These include syphilis, chancroid, lymphopathia, and condyloma acuminatum.

Herpes progenitalis is a skin lesion of the prepuce or glans penis. It is caused by herpes simplex virus.

Urethritis in the male may be due to *Neisseria gonorrhoeae* or to nonspecific organisms. The disease is characterized by a purulent urethral discharge and dysuria. It may be associated with prostatitis or cystitis. Diagnosis of gonorrhea is established by Gram's stain of a smear of the urethral discharge. Positive findings are gram-negative intracellular diplococci. For reliable culture, the specimen must be planted promptly upon chocolate agar in an atmosphere of 10% carbon dioxide. Gonorrhea is usually treated with penicillin.

Nonspecific urethritis may be caused by a variety of bacterial organisms and often complicates the post-treatment course of patients with gonorrhea. *Mycoplasma* and *Chlamydia* organisms have also been implicated as etiologic agents.

NEOPLASMS

Squamous cell carcinoma of the penis is most often seen in older men who have not been circumcised. It has a tendency to invade the erectile tissue of the penile shaft and to metastasize to inguinal lymph nodes. Penectomy is usually required. Irradiation may be effective in selected cases.

Carcinoma of the anterior urethra in males is quite rare. When seen, it often complicates long-standing inflammatory stricture disease.

Transitional cell carcinoma of the posterior urethra is

Fig. 45-19. Anatomic features of hypospadias. (*A*) Curvature of the penis due to chordee. (*B*) Hooded foreskin. (*C*) Proximal opening of the urethra.

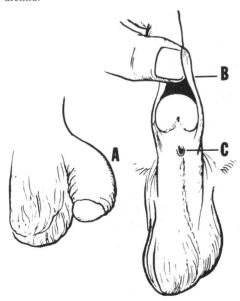

occasionally encountered, usually in the presence of carcinoma of the urinary bladder.

TRAUMA

The male urethra is most commonly injured by instrumentation, and most of these injuries are iatrogenic. Such injuries may cause bleeding and infection. Delayed development of urethral strictures is the most serious complication. Straddle injuries are those sustained in falls astride a hard object that forces the bulbous urethra against the undersurface of the pubis. Such injuries may be treated by indwelling catheter, suprapubic urinary diversion, or surgical exploration with repair. Stricture formation is a common complication.

Membranous urethral injuries are most often encountered in patients who sustain fracture of the bony pelvis. When there is displacement of the central portion of the pubis, the prostate is distracted because of its attachment to the pubis by the puboprostatic ligament. Since the membranous urethra is firmly anchored in the urogenital diaphragm, the urethra may be avulsed at this level. This is a serious injury that should be suspected in all patients with pelvic fracture who have difficulty voiding or who have bloody discharge from the urethra. Urethral instrumentation should be avoided in these patients. The diagnosis is established by retrograde urethrography (Fig. 45-21). Opinions differ as to the best treatment. Some urologic surgeons favor immediate repair of the injury. Others favor temporary suprapubic cystostomy to divert the urine, with plans for delayed repair after the patient's recovery from the injury.

Penile injuries are often due to self-mutilation in patients

Fig. 45-21. Retrograde urethrogram. The arrow indicates the point of transection of the membranous urethra. Contrast medium is extravasated into the retroperitoneal space above this point. Note the fractures of the pubic rami.

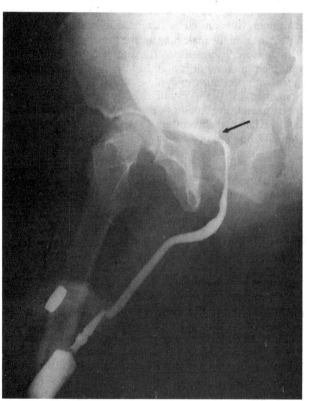

with psychiatric illness and sometimes result from lovers' quarrels. Penile replants after traumatic amputation have been tried, with limited success. Forceful angulation of the erect corpora cavernosa may result in "fracture" with laceration of the tunica albuginea. If the penile skin is avulsed in accidents, which usually involve heavy machinery, split-thickness skin grafting is the treatment of choice.

URETHRAL STRICTURES

Urethral strictures in the male may be the residuum of gonorrheal infection or may be due to trauma. These strictures cause obstruction and predispose to infection. Periurethral abscess and urinary extravasation may occur as complications. Strictures may be treated with periodic urethral dilation, internal urethrotomy, or urethroplasty.

PRIAPISM

Priapism is a sustained, painful erection of the penis that is not associated with erotic stimuli. After resolution of the priapism, most men are impotent. Surgical intervention is advisable in some patients to evacuate clotted blood from the erectile bodies and to divert venous drainage.

DISEASES OF THE PROSTATE AND SEMINAL VESICLES

INFECTIONS

Prostatitis and seminal vesiculitis often occur simultaneously and are difficult to separate on the basis of clinical examination. Prostatitis most often occurs as a complication of urethritis. Gonorrhea, nonspecific urethritis, and urethral infections secondary to catheterization may lead to prostatitis. Less frequently, the prostate may be infected by hematogenous spread. Acute prostatitis may be caused by organisms of the coliform group *N. gonorrhoeae,* staphylococci, streptococci, *Mycoplasma,* and *Chlamydia.* Acute prostatitis may be manifest by general malaise, fever, and chills. The urinary symptoms of frequency, urgency, and dysuria are usually prominent. Backache and perineal discomfort are often present. Treatment is with antibiotics.

Chronic prostatitis may be due to specific infections such as tuberculosis, but most often it is a lingering result of infection with acute pyogenic organisms. The condition causes vague backache and perineal discomfort and often is complicated by acute exacerbations of urinary tract infection. The chronicity of this infection is attributed largely to the fact that effective concentrations of antibiotics in the prostatic secretions are difficult to achieve. Prostate massage may be important adjunctive therapy in patients with chronic prostatitis.

PROSTATE STONES

Prostate stones are concretions that form in prostatic acini. These are probably not urinary stones. They are frequently seen in patients with long-standing chronic prostatitis.

BENIGN PROSTATIC HYPERPLASIA

Benign prostatic hyperplasia is one of the most common of urologic diseases, occurring to some degree in the majority of men over 50 years of age. The cause of this condition is not certain, but it is related to endocrine changes that induce hyperplasia of stromal and glandular elements in the prostate. Symptoms are almost entirely related to obstruction, although hematuria may occasionally be the presenting complaint. The diagnosis of benign prostatic hyperplasia can often be established on the basis of rectal palpation. The most important objective of the urologic evaluation of the patient with benign prostatic hyperplasia is the assessment of the severity of the obstruction. For this purpose, intravenous pyelography, measurement of residual urine, and cystoscopy are often required. The condition must be differentiated from carcinoma of the prostate. Surgery is the only effective treatment. Transurethral resection is an operation in which the gland is removed piecemeal through an endoscopic instrument called a resectoscope. Open approaches include suprapubic, retropubic, or perineal prostatectomy (Fig. 45-22). The choice of operative procedure is largely the surgeon's preference but is strongly influenced by the size of the prostate. In general, small glands are best managed by transurethral resection, and the large glands are best treated by open prostatectomy.

ADENOCARCINOMA OF THE PROSTATE

Adenocarcinoma of the prostate is the most common genitourinary malignancy. It occurs predominantly in older men. It has the capacity to grow and invade locally and to metastasize by blood and lymphatics. There is a strong predilection for metastases to bone, and these metastases have the unique characteristic of being osteoblastic. Presenting symptoms are usually related to bladder outlet obstruction or to metastatic disease. Such symptoms are quite often not manifest until the disease is locally advanced. Early diagnosis of cancer of the prostate is dependent upon routine rectal examination in asymptomatic persons. A strong presumptive diagnosis can usually be made on the basis of rectal palpation. Diagnosis is confirmed by needle biopsy of the prostate. Radical prostatectomy offers the best chance for cure of localized disease. Obstruction of the bladder outlet can be relieved by transurethral resection in those patients who are not candidates for curative treatment. Approximately 75% of prostatic cancers respond with some degree of regression to antiandrogen treatment, which may

PROSTATIC CANCER	
Clinical	Decreased stream force and size, hesitation, frequency, terminal dribbling, urinary retention
Dx	Rectal examination, needle biopsy of prostate
Rx	Radical prostatectomy Palliative: transurethral prostatic resection, orchiectomy, estrogens, radiation therapy

take the form of bilateral orchiectomy or the administration of estrogen. Radiotherapy is an alternative treatment that may be curative. The importance of careful routine palpation of the prostate in the early detection of prostatic carcinoma should be emphasized.

ADENOCARCINOMA OF THE SEMINAL VESICLE

Adenocarcinoma of the seminal vesicle is a rare lesion and is often difficult to distinguish from carcinoma of the prostate.

DISEASES OF THE TESTES AND SPERMATIC CORD

Cryptorchidism (undescended testis) is a failure of the testis to descend into the scrotum during embryologic development. The condition is more common in premature infants than in term infants. Fibrosis of the seminiferous tubules with permanent impairment of spermatogenesis occurs if the testis remains undescended through puberty. The risk of development of testis tumor in undescended testis is approximately 40 times as great as in the normal scrotal testes. Patent processus vaginalis is found in association with cryptorchidism and may result in inguinal herniation. The condition may be unilateral or bilateral. Spontaneous descent may occur following birth. Most urologists feel that cryptorchidism should be treated by surgery (orchiopexy) soon after 1 year of age.

Hydrocele is the development of fluid collection in the tunica vaginalis.

Torsion of the spermatic cord is an important cause of acute painful swelling of the scrotum in young males. In these patients, the testis is usually abnormally mobile because of anomalous development of the tunica vaginalis, which completely envelops the testis and epididymis, giving a "clapper in a bell" effect. If strangulation of blood supply to the testis occurs, the condition represents an acute surgical emergency, since testicular infarction may be expected within a few hours of onset. The opposite testis should always be explored and fixed in position by sutures when torsion is diagnosed, because the anomaly of the tunica vaginalis is often bilateral.

Varicocele is dilatation of the veins of the pampiniform plexus. It occurs more often on the left side, owing to the fact that the valves of the left internal spermatic vein are often deficient. This vein empties into the renal vein, while the right internal spermatic vein drains into the vena cava. Varicocele is usually of no significance but may be associated with infertility in some patients. Rarely, retroperitoneal tumors may cause the acute development of varicocele.

Fig. 45-22. Suprapubic prostatectomy.

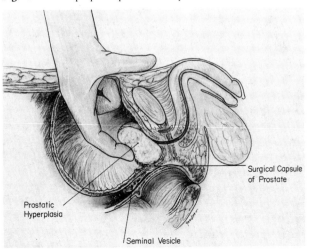

Prostatic Hyperplasia

Surgical Capsule of Prostate

Seminal Vesicle

TABLE 45-3 CLASSIFICATION OF TUMORS OF THE TESTIS*

I. Germinal Tumors (96.5% of testis tumors)
  A. Seminoma, pure
  B. Embryonal carcinoma, pure or with seminoma
  C. Teratoma, pure or with seminoma
  D. Teratoma with either embryonal carcinoma or cho-riocarcinoma or both and with or without seminoma
  E. Choriocarcinoma, pure or with either seminoma or embryonal carcinoma or both
II. Nongerminal Tumors (3.5% of testis tumors)
  A. Gonadal (strictly)
    1. Interstitial cell tumors
    2. Androblastomas
    3. Rete carcinomas
  B. Tumor similar to counterparts elsewhere in the body: fibromas, angioma, neurofibromas, adenomatoid tumors, and fibrosarcoma
      Other nongonadal tumors (rhabdomyoma, rhab-domyosarcoma, chondroma, chondrosarcoma) probably represent a one-sided development of teratomas

(*Classifications from Dixon FJ, Moore RA: Tumors of the male sex organs. In Atlas of Tumor Pathology, Section 8, Fascicles 31b and 32. Washington, DC, Armed Forces Institute of Pathology, 1952)

Epididymitis is a frequent complication of prostatitis. The usual route of infection is retrograde spread of organisms through the vas deferens. It is the most common cause of acute painful swelling of the scrotum in men. It must be distinguished from testis tumors. Treatment is with antibiotics, bed rest, and scrotal elevation.

Orchitis may occur as a complication of epididymitis. However, the most common cause of acute primary orchitis is mumps.

Testis tumor most commonly occurs in men between 25 and 35 years of age. Tumors arising from the interstitial cells of Leydig and Sertoli's cell are rarely seen. Most of the testis tumors arise from the germinal epithelium, and all of these tumors should be considered malignant except for teratomas that occur before puberty. The histologic types of germinal tumors of the testis are seminoma, embryonal carcinoma, teratoma, and choriocarcinoma (Table 45-3). The diagnosis is usually suspected because of discomfort and enlargement of the testis. Needle biopsy and transscrotal incisional biopsy should never be performed, because of the hazards of local seeding of the tumor. When the diagnosis is suspected, inguinal exploration should be carried out, with early isolation and tamponade of the spermatic cord at the internal inguinal ring. Radical orchiectomy is usually effective in control of the local tumor. However, metastases often occur early in the course of this disease. Retroperitoneal lymph nodes are the most common site of early spread, and lung metastases are common. Seminoma is quite radiosensitive, and metastatic disease may be definitively treated with radiotherapy. Nonseminomatous germ cell tumors are usually managed by a combination of retroperitoneal lymph node dissection and multiple-drug chemotherapy. Cure rates in this disease have been dramatically improved by the advent of effective chemotherapy.

Tumors of the spermatic cord are rare. Adenomatoid tumor is a benign neoplasm of the epididymis. Adenocarcinoma of the epididymis is extremely rare. Solid tumors of the spermatic cord are likewise rare and, when seen, arise from fibrous tissue, neural elements, or fat in the cord. Forty percent of these tumors are malignant.

BIBLIOGRAPHY

BORS E, COMARR AE: Neurological Urology. Baltimore, University Park Press, 1971
BRASH JC (ed): Cunningham's Textbook of Anatomy, 9th ed. New York, Oxford University Press, 1951
BROCKIS JG, FINLAYSON B (ed): Urinary Calculus. New York, Champlain Books, 1981
GLENN JF (ed): Diagnostic Urology. New York, Harper & Row, 1964
GUYTON AC: Textbook of Physiology, 4th ed. Philadelphia, W B Saunders, 1971
HARRISON JH, GITTES RF, PERLMUTTER AD et al (eds): Campbell's Urology, 4th ed. Philadelphia, W B Saunders, 1981
HEPTINSTALL RH: Pathology of the Kidney. Boston, Little, Brown & Co, 1966
JOHNSON DE: Testicular Tumors. New York, Medical Examination Publishing, 1972
JOHNSTON JH, GOODWIN WE: Reviews in Paediatric Urology. Amsterdam, Excerpta Medica, 1974
KELALIS PP, KING LR (eds): Clinical Pediatric Urology. Philadelphia, W B Saunders, 1976
MASTERS WH, JOHNSON VE: Human Sexual Response. Boston, Little, Brown & Co, 1971
ROUS SN: Understanding Urology. New York, S Karger, 1973
SMITH DR: General Urology. Los Altos, CA, Lange Medical Publications, 1981
STAMEY TA: Pathogenesis and Treatment of Urinary Tract Infections. Baltimore, Williams & Wilkins, 1980
WITTEN DM, MYERS GH, UTZ DC (eds): Emmett's Clinical Urography, 4th ed. Philadelphia, W B Saunders, 1977

Robert R. Smith

Neurosurgery

4b

From a historical perspective, neurosurgery is both an ancient and a modern surgical discipline. It was practiced several thousand years ago along the banks of the Nile River, but because the customs of the day prescribed retribution against the physician whose treatment failed, surgical disciplines failed to flourish under Egyptian rule. Trephination, or opening of the skull, was apparently a practice of many ancient peoples. Skulls with uniform openings have been found in archaeologic diggings both in Europe and in South America. Why ancient surgeons perforated the cranium of their patients is uncertain. Since in some cases fracture lines are located near the trephine openings, trauma may have been a factor.

After a relative dark age, the renaissance of neurosurgery came in the late 19th and early 20th centuries. Harvey Cushing, Victor Horsely, and Walter Dandy were pioneers in the advancement of neurosurgery, and many of the operations first performed by these surgeons were based largely on clinical examinations. Pioneers in neurology, such as Babinski and Jackson, also helped surgeons understand the relationship of the central nervous system (CNS) lesion to signs and symptoms. Finally, the development of air ventriculography as well as angiography, myelography, isotope encephalography, and more recently, computerized tomography have made the advancement of neurosurgical techniques possible.

Like wounds anywhere, cranial or spinal operations may lead to bleeding, wound hematoma, or infection. All surgical cases share the risk of postoperative deep vein thrombosis. In patients with paralyzed limbs, however, fatal pulmonary embolization occurs at 5 to 6 times the expected rate. Hypoventilation and hypotension, complications to be avoided in all patients, may potentiate brain ischemia and brain edema in patient with a central nervous system lesion. Overall, infections probably occur less frequently in neurosurgical cases than in surgical wounds elsewhere, but the effects are often more devastating. The wound abscess, while tolerated within the thoracic or abdominal cavity, finds little room for safe expansion in the intracranial space. Many factors, including the blood–brain barrier, must be taken into consideration in treating central nervous system infections. Some agents such as chloramphenicol cross the barrier in significant levels, whereas others such as the penicillins and cephalosporins are poorly transported across the barrier. There is still no convincing evidence that prophylactic antibiotics are of any significant benefit in the clean case; in fact, their use seems to increase the likelihood of development of resistant strains. The bony enclosure of the nervous system and its susceptibility to pressure must be taken into consideration, and postoperative cerebral edema must be treated with considerable respect.

Inappropriate release of antidiuretic hormone, which is associated with some head injuries and strokes, contributes to the problem of brain edema and intracranial mass by causing water retention. When intracranial pressure develops asymmetrically, the brain shifts away from the mass through an opening in the membranous or bony compartment. The cerebellar tonsils may be forced through the foramen magnum, causing compression of the respiratory and cardiac centers of the medulla oblongata. Apnea in sleep and profound cardiac changes may take place suddenly and unexpectedly. The unilateral supratentorial mass may shift the medial aspects of the temporal lobe downward and medially, causing compression of the midbrain, third cranial nerve, and the vessels that supply this area. Secondary hemorrhages in the brain stem due to temporal lobe herniation lead to coma, decerebracy, and even death.

EVALUATION OF THE NEUROSURGICAL PATIENT

Obtaining the neurologic history and performing the neurologic examination should not be done perfunctorily but with purpose. In no other field of medicine are the rewards so great to the careful practitioner. Special diagnostic tests are often indicated in addition to the routine examination, but with a proper history and neurologic examination these can be applied to their best advantage. Screening tests are expensive, some are not without complications, and false positives and false negatives occur with all. It should be ascertained whether the patient's symptoms developed spontaneously or with trauma, whether the onset was abrupt or insidious, and whether there was progression or regression of symptoms. It can never be assumed in the patient with a brain lesion that all aspects of the history are accurate, and family members should also be consulted. Possible defects in the patient's judgment and memory may make his version unreliable. Because neurologic syndromes may have genetic backgrounds, a careful family history is also an important part of the evaluation.

THE NEUROLOGIC EXAMINATION

Although heart rate and blood pressure are both maintained after irreversible brain damage, the modulation of these vital signs occurs through CNS mechanisms, and CNS irritation and compression may alter the rate and amplitude of the pulse and the blood pressure. *Cushing's hypertensive response* is mediated through posterior brain mechanisms. Pressure applied directly or indirectly to the medulla oblongata initiates the response. It is accompanied by increasing hypertension and elevated catecholamines in the blood and urine, but this reflex is not a reliable early warning sign. Hypotension may result from cardiac or neural causes or from hypervolemia. With loss of sympathetic innervation of peripheral vessels due to hypothalamic, medullary, or spinal injury, systemic vasodilatation results. When accompanied by blood loss, profound shock may be present, although generally the pressure stabilizes at 70 to 80 mmHg in patients with normal intravascular filling.

Blood gas receptors in the aortic and carotid bodies transmit information to groups of cells located in the medulla oblongata. Increased CO_2 or decreased O_2 stimulates these cells to increase respiration, whereas decreased CO_2 or increased O_2 causes the opposite response. Cortical centers also influence these cells of the respiratory center, but this pathway is unresponsive to blood gas alterations. The involuntary respiratory pathway is located in the anterior quadrants of the spinal cord and upper medulla. Irreversible damage of this pathway may leave voluntary cortical respiration intact but cause apnea in sleep.

A number of schemes have been offered to describe the conscious state (Table 46-1). The initial examiner should describe the best response and record his findings so that any subsequent examiner can also evaluate the patient's progress.

In the alert patient, the neurologic examination should begin with the patient seated on the edge of the examining

TABLE 46-1   STATE OF CONSCIOUSNESS (Classification used at University of Mississippi Medical Center)

STATE OF CONSCIOUSNESS	DEFINITION
Alert	Patient responds quickly to verbal questions and answers appropriately. He is oriented as to time, place, and person.
Lethargic	Patient opens his eyes and attempts to answer but drifts back into sleep when unstimulated.
Stuporous	Patient is arousable when pinched or stimulated. He withdraws his extremities to avoid painful stimulus. He may be combative.
Coma	No response is obtained to verbal stimulation. Painful stimulation of the extremities produces a decerebrate response with plantar flexion of the lower extremities and hyperpronation of the upper extremities.
Light Coma	Patient does not speak or open his eyes upon verbal stimulation. Deep pain produces withdrawal, however.
Deep Coma	There is no response to stimulation. All reflexes are hypoactive or absent.

table. The first cranial nerve is tested by asking the patient to identify odors. The second, third, fourth, and sixth cranial nerves may be examined together. The visual field examination is done by confrontation. Simultaneous testing is also necessary to detect minor deficits. The patient is asked to fix both eyes on the examiner while simultaneous testing is carried out. Papilledema is a sign of increased intracranial pressure but may not be present early, particularly if the pressure developed suddenly and recently. Distention of the veins of the retina and loss of venous pulsation are the earliest signs, followed by elevation of the disc margin. In later stages, veins rupture, and hemorrhages or even exudates are noted in the adjacent retina. Fifth nerve function is tested by evaluating sensory function of the face and by testing the muscles of mastication. The seventh nerve innervates the muscles of facial expression and has a sensory component that carries taste sensation from the anterior two thirds of the tongue. Peripheral lesions usually involve fibers to the upper part of the face, and the affected eyelids do not close entirely. Hearing may be examined using a quiet watch tick, by rubbing the fingers together, or by asking the patient to identify tuning fork vibrations. Examination of the ear canal should also be a part of this examination. The ninth and tenth cranial nerves are examined by noting phonation and observing retraction of the palate. The gag reflex should be tested bilaterally.

Weakness of the trapezius or sternocleidomastoid muscles is used to identify eleventh nerve lesions, and a midline protruded tongue is an indication that the twelfth nerve is functional.

The *motor system* may be evaluated generally and then more specifically according to the patient's complaints.

Proximal motor weakness is usually determined by drift of the outstretched extremity, whereas distal weakness may be evaluated more critically by comparing the patient's grip with that of the examiner. Bulk and tone, spasticity and rigidity, and the presence of fasciculations should also be a part of the motor examination. Likewise, the deep tendon reflexes should be a part of this examination, and pathologi reflexes such as Hoffmann and Babinski signs should 'sought.

Pain mechanisms, vibratory sense, appreciation of ' and cold, and joint position are all part of the se' examination. Special tests, such as sterognosis, n' writing, and two-point discrimination, should be en' to evaluate cortical function. Heel to toe walki' movement of the extremities, and the Romberg tes. to evaluate cerebellar function.

SPECIAL DIAGNOSTIC TESTS

The *lumbar puncture* allows evaluation of subarachnoid space pressure, cellular content, bacterial contamination, and the biochemical make-up of cerebrospinal fluid (CSF). Certain prerequisites must be met before lumbar puncture can be carried out safely. Careful neurologic examination must be performed and the optic fundus should be examined critically for increased intracranial pressure. Skull radiographs should be made and examined for evidence of increased intracranial pressure or unilateral mass. When other diagnostic tests such as angiography or CT scanning are planned, they should be carried out before performing lumbar puncture because they may provide evidence that mitigates against the procedure. Removal of CSF causes changes in dynamics within the intracranial or spinal cavity and may lead to sudden precipitous deterioration in neurologic function. Contraindications for puncture include infection at the puncture site, papilledema, a shifted pineal gland, or evidence of a spinal neoplasm.

Preferably the puncture should be carried out caudal to the L2–3 interspace. The conus medullaris may extend as far caudal as the lower body of L1. The L4–5 interspace provides the best access to CSF. Either a midline or a paramedian approach using a 19- or 20-gauge needle is recommended.

If blood is found on lumbar puncture, a few drops should be collected in a tube for a comparison. A vessel traumatized on entry usually seals, and the fluid clears in subsequent specimens. If all specimens are contaminated with blood, one tube should be centrifuged and the supernate examined. Xanthochromia confirms the presence of prior hemorrhage in the subarachnoid space.

Angiography is still useful in evaluating the vascular components of CNS lesions and in the evaluation of patients with vascular disease of the CNS. Techniques depend upon the experience of the angiographer, but the catheter technique is now used in most centers. Overall, complications occur in less than 1% of all studies. Pneumoencephalography and ventriculography are rarely performed today because the CT scan provides a clear view of the ventricular system.

Myelography is indicated when there is a need to visualize the contents of the spinal subarachnoid space and when the adjacent bony structure must be evaluated. After lumbar puncture, contrast material, either water-soluble or oil-based, is injected into the spinal subarachnoid space. The patient is placed in various positions as the material is manipulated under fluoroscopic control to gain visualiza-

ti

is us
pressure hy   impaired. Normally,   r, but
when absorption is impan..,   aricular
system may still be apparent at 36 in 	..ger. The electroencephalogram (EEG) is a harmless and painless method of evaluating the feeble electrical activity of the brain. Normally, electrical activity from the cerebral cortex is synchronous, and in most individuals, an alpha rhythm of 9 to 13 waves/second can be identified. Slower waves at 2 to 4/second are usually regarded as abnormal and indicate structural damage of the cerebral cortex. If the EEG and radionuclide brain scan are both normal, the likelihood of a patient having a cerebral tumor is less than 1%. However, the CT scan now rivals the accuracy of angiography and isotope scanning and is comparable in cost. *Electromyography* (EMG) and *nerve conduction studies* are useful in evaluating muscle and nerve disorders. The EMG is indicated when there is doubt about whether atrophy has occurred on the basis of nerve or muscle pathology. It also can be helpful in determining whether malfunction is due to disuse, pain, malingering, hysteria, or motor neuron disease. Specific myopathies, such as myotonic dystrophy, produce characteristic patterns.

The nerve conduction velocity is the distance an impulse travels along the nerve per unit time and is affected by lesions of the lower motor neuron generally. Conduction velocity is normal in myopathic states, but defects in both the myelin sheath and the peripheral axon prolong the conduction velocity.

PERIPHERAL AND CRANIAL NERVE LESIONS

Even minor injuries of peripheral nerves often produce bizarre pain syndromes and functional deficits far beyond the anatomic confines of the lesion. The discussion of these injuries must begin on a pessimistic note. The peripheral nerve actually consists of thousands of axons, each connected to a specific distal receptor and surrounded by a myelin sheath and bundle of fibrous tissue, the sheath of Schwann. Each nerve is further divided into fascicles by perineurium and enclosed by a thick fibrous epineurium (Fig. 46-1). It has long been recognized that the quality of any sensory phenomenon rests upon which receptors are excited, not upon the method used for excitation. For instance, pacinian corpuscles are quite sensitive to mechanical stimulation but are resistant to thermal excitation. Free nerve endings are also highly selective, responding to

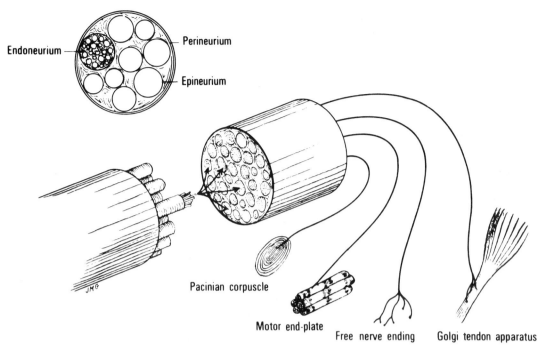

Fig. 46-1. The peripheral nerve consists of thousands of axons, each connected to a specific distal receptor. (Smith RR: Essentials of Neurosurgery. Philadelphia, J B Lippincott, 1980)

mechanical stimuli such as pinching or cutting. It is now also recognized that some nerves transmit their message in a coded form to discriminate between the various forms of excitation and to transmit information about intensity. The appreciation of the stimuli depends largely on subcortical sites in the reticular formation and thalamus. The intensity of the stimulus must be interpreted by the cerebral cortex, and localization of sensation also requires cortical input.

The various nerve functions are served by fibers of varying sizes. Large fibers 12 μ to 20 μ in diameter transmit efferent motor and afferent stretch receptors. The smallest unmyelinated fibers conduct slow pain response and transmit autonomic signals. Fast pain, on the other hand, is conducted by the larger fibers at speeds of up to 20 m/second. Some nerve injuries selectively affect fibers of a particular size. The compression neuropathies, for instance, influence small myelinated fibers, leaving only unmyelinated C fibers operating.

Because of the unique anatomy and physiology of the peripheral nerve, which contains thousands of axons of varying size and structure, various injuries may produce characteristic patterns. Nerve concussion may be compared to brain concussion in which a physiologic transmission of the impulse is blocked but anatomic continuity is preserved. Missile injuries, compression injuries, and stretch injuries produce nerve concussion often referred to as *neuropraxia.* Edema and demyelination may play some role. A second degree of injury occurs when the axon fiber itself is destroyed but the endoneural tubes are preserved. After division of the axon, progressive wallerian degeneration occurs. The nutrients are propelled from the central cell down the remaining axon, and the axon buds cross the injury site in only a few days. Meanwhile, Schwann cells and connective tissue proliferate in the distal stump while a *neuroma,* consisting of tangled axons and connective tissue, forms about the proximal stump. The mechanism that causes the regenerating axon to cross the gap and enter the appropriate

tubule is unknown but may perhaps be based on pure random order. Aberrant regeneration occurs when fibers destined to terminate on one muscle or sensory structure instead regenerate to the motor end plate of another muscle or sensory element. Motor fibers regenerating in contact with sensory receptors serve no useful function and cannot conduct afferent stimuli. Aberrant regeneration of sensory fibers may cause the patient to perceive sensory stimuli as a noxious impulse. Sensory aberration of various types occurs after peripheral nerve injuries. The burning pain that follows partial division of the peripheral sensory nerve was termed *causalgia* by Mitchell. Color change, atrophy, and autonomic dysfunction accompany this painful syndrome, which responds favorably to sympathectomy. *Sympathetic dystrophy* is similar to true causalgia but does not respond to autonomic section. The neuroma that forms after division of a nerve may also be painful on pressure. The *phantom limb syndrome* occurs following the loss of a limb, usually in civilian injuries. The pain is accompanied by a striking conceptual sensation of the amputated limb. Peculiar distortion of the missing part is described, and vermification may be experienced on the amputated limb.

The proper timing for repair of peripheral nerve injury is somewhat controversial. Primary or immediate repair of the damaged nerve is advised when the wound is not contaminated and the risk of infection is minimal. More extensive and grossly contaminated injuries necessitate delay of a month to 6 weeks. During this time, some collagenation of the distal sheath probably takes place. Peripheral nerve repair should be carried out using the operating microscope. If a neuroma is present, it must be excised. However, nerve action potentials, determined at the operating table, help in the evaluation of whether axons have penetrated the neuroma and are entering the distal stump. After injury the nerve regenerates at a rate of about 1 mm/day, or, in the case of motor axons, about 1 inch/month. The smaller axons perhaps regenerate much faster. The first signs of regeneration can be determined when the autonomic fibers return to the sweat glands of the extremity. *Tinel's sign* is also a useful clinical means of evaluating recovery of sensory axons. Percussing the distal nerve trunk indicates at what point the sensory axons have penetrated, because the patient experiences paresthesias in the normal distribution of those fibers.

ENTRAPMENT SYNDROMES AND PERIPHERAL NERVE INJURIES

The brachial plexus is made up of anterior and posterior rootlets of the fifth, sixth, seventh, and eighth cervical and the first thoracic root. The upper fibers supply the musculature of the upper arm and thorax, and the lower roots supply the musculature of the lower arm and hand. Stretch injuries involving the upper plexus (Erb's palsy) are brought about by injuries that force the shoulder downward and the head in the opposite direction. This common injury in newborns occurs upon delivery of the difficult shoulder. Stretch injuries of the lower plexus (Klumpke's paralysis) take place with an arm extended above the head, usually in some type of wringer. The roots, in either instance, may be avulsed from the spinal cord, producing a characteristic radiographic picture. The cervical rib syndrome, scalenus anticus syndrome, and thoracic outlet syndrome are terms used to describe compression of the plexus at the thoracic outlet. Cervical ribs are found in approximately 1% of the population, but 90% of this group never have symptoms. The diagnosis is usually made when vascular symptoms are noted. Raynaud's disease or loss of pulse on abduction of the arm are characteristic findings. In Adson's maneuver obliteration of the pulse and reproduction of the pain are caused by hyperabduction of the arm and rotation of the head. Neoplasms may invade the lower brachial plexus from the apex of the lung, and Horner's syndrome may be present as a distinctive feature of this pain syndrome.

The *axillary nerve* assumes a lateral position as it passes through the axilla and eventually passes posterior to the humerus to innervate the deltoid muscle. The most frequent cause of injury is dislocation of the head of the humerus and deltoid muscular atrophy, and inability to abduct the arm is the most important diagnostic feature. The musculocutaneous nerve supplies the biceps and brachialis muscles and is injured most often from missile and knife wounds of the upper extremity. A cutaneous portion supplies the radial forearm. Injuries of the *ulnar nerve* produce weakness of the flexor carpi ulnaris, flexion of the fourth and fifth fingers, and weakness of abduction and adduction of the hand. Weakness of the adductor pollicis muscle is a primary feature of Froment's sign. Injuries around the elbow joint result in hyperostosis, which entraps the ulnar nerve, causing neuroma formation. The so-called *tardy ulnar palsy* that develops secondary to elbow trauma is heralded by tingling in the fourth and fifth fingers followed by motor and permanent sensory impairment. Electromyography is useful when it demonstrates increased latency across the injured segment of the nerve. Surgical transplantation of the nerve to a more anterior position is often required and brings relief in many cases.

The *median nerve* is the primary flexor of the hand and is often injured at the antecubital fossa and in the wrist. The *carpal tunnel syndrome* occurs in those who repeatedly extend their wrist in their work. Dysesthesias of the thumb, forefinger, and middle finger on extension of the hand are characteristic clinical signs. The carpal tunnel syndrome is often the first sign of diabetes, rheumatoid arthritis, hypothyroidism, and acromegaly. It also occurs in pregnancy. Immobilization of the wrist in slight flexion in a well-padded splint will often alleviate symptoms temporarily. However, division of the transverse carpal ligament in the wrist and hand provides gratifying results in properly selected cases.

The *radial nerve* innervates the muscles that dorsiflex the wrist. The most common injury is associated with fracture of the humerus. Along with dorsiflexion weakness, this injury causes sensory loss on the dorsum of the hand. Honeymooners' palsy and Saturday night palsy are the result of compression of the radial nerve by a new spouse or a bar rail. At the wrist, the superficial branch is susceptible to injury by laceration, and a painful neuroma may result. In many of the compression neuropathies such as Saturday night palsy, recovery follows spontaneously depending on the degree of injury sustained. In simple concussion injuries, the sensory and motor function returns within a day or so. When the myelin sheath has been denuded, several weeks are often required. Injuries of the axon cylinder recover at the rate of 1 mm/day for the largest fibers.

In the lower extremity, the *ilioinguinal nerve* may be injured during herniorrhaphy as it pierces the internal oblique muscle in its course to the inguinal canal. The *lateral femoral cutaneous nerve* is often traumatized as it penetrates the inguinal fascia, giving rise to the condition known as meralgia paraesthetica. Paresthesia and pain in the lateral thigh are described, and there may be sensory loss in the anterior lateral thigh. Obesity, tight girdles, and occupational trauma are factors in development. Removing the source of irritation is much more effective than surgical transsection or neurolysis of the lateral femoral cutaneous nerve. The *obturator nerve* is occasionally injured from gun and knife wounds of the pelvis. The surgeon or gynecologist may also injure the nerve, and it is often entrapped by the obturator hernia. Pain radiating into the medial thigh is the usual complaint. The *femoral nerve* passes deep to the inguinal ligament innervating the iliacus muscle, the extensors of the knee and leg, and the flexors of the hip. Climbing stairs and other activities requiring strong extensor action are impaired early. The *sciatic nerve*, because of its relation to the femoral head, is susceptible to injury by posterior dislocation of the hip. The injection of caustic materials into the buttock also occasionally produces sciatic injury. The nerve supplies the hamstring muscle group and the primary flexors of the knee. It divides just above the popliteal space, giving rise to the *posterior tibial* and *common peroneal* nerves. The posterior tibial nerve supplies the skin of the plantar aspect of the foot and the posterior tibial muscles. The common peroneal nerve branches into deep and superficial components. The deep branch innervates dorsiflexors of the foot and toes, and its injury causes a complete foot drop. The superficial branch innervates the peroneal group of muscles that evert the foot. The common peroneal nerve is susceptible to compression and stretch injuries as it passes round the fibula.

Compression neuropathies are generally mononeuropathies, and pressure fragmentation of the myelin sheath is the most common histologic finding. When more than one nerve is involved, an underlying metabolic factor should be suspected. Weight loss with atrophy of subcutaneous fat, alcoholism, collagen disorders, malnutrition, diabetes, exposure to heavy metals, and nutritional deficiencies predispose nerves to compressive neuropathies.

HEAD AND SPINAL CORD INJURIES

HEAD INJURIES

Injuries related to the head (Tables 46-2 and 46-3) are a common cause of death and disability in most industrial countries. Progress made in diagnostic and surgical skills, anesthesia, and aseptic techniques has been more than compensated by the increasing complexity of tools and weapons. Many more patients with these injuries survive to become productive again, but larger numbers survive with mental and physical handicaps.

As in any severe injury the airway should be the first concern in the patient with a critical head or spinal wound. Hypoxia and hypercarbia increase intracranial blood volume and pressure. Blood from the nasopharynx, teeth, dentures, and gastric contents all enter the trachea when the cough reflex is impaired, and in the patient who is comatose the muscular relaxation alone may cause significant airway obstruction. A flail chest injury may accompany a head or spinal wound. In the patient with a spinal cord injury, paralysis of the intercostal muscles causes weakness of lung expansion and loss of vital capacity. Diaphragmatic respiration may also be impaired, and when the spinal injury is central to the phrenic rootlets at C3, C4, and C5, these injuries are most often fatal. Incomplete injuries may compromise tidal volume to a lesser extent. A good voluntary cough usually implies sufficient pulmonary reserve to maintain a normal Po_2, providing pneumonia, pneumothorax, or other pulmonary complications do not intervene. A rough clinical approximation of tidal volume can be obtained by having the patient take a deep breath and count. This allows continuing clinical evaluation of vital capacity. Measurement of arterial Po_2 and Pco_2, however, is a much more reliable index of pulmonary function.

Definite rules for establishment of an airway cannot be given because of the many causes for the initial trauma. The unconscious patient with a severe head injury frequently needs an endotracheal airway or a tracheostomy. Before

TABLE 46-2 HEAD INJURIES

Scalp
   Laceration
   Contusion
   Avulsion

Skull Fracture
   Open, closed
   Linear, depressed
   Basilar fractures

Cerebral
   Concussion
   Contusion
   Laceration
   Penetration wound

Mass Lesions
   Extradural hematoma
   Subdural hematoma
   Subarachnoid hemorrhage
   Intracerebral hematoma

attempting to extend the spine to perform this maneuver, a radiograph should be obtained and the neurologic examination done. Often the insertion of tongs in the patient with unstable cervical fracture will permit some extension without further compromise of the spinal canal.

An old axiom states that head injury alone does not cause shock. When profound shock is present, bleeding into the chest cavity, abdomen, or the retroperitoneal space should be suspected. Blood loss around a long bone fracture or even a scalp laceration, however, may produce shock. Loss of sympathetic tone, which occurs in spinal injuries and injuries of the hypothalamus itself, causes mild forms of shock, usually without systemic manifestations. When there is associated blood loss or dehydration, the fall in peripheral blood pressure may be enough to result in cerebral or cardiac ischemia. Replacing volume usually restores systemic pressure to near normal levels.

When blood loss results from a scalp laceration and there is profound hemorrhage, sutures that are well placed through the galea and scalp and securely tied will often arrest the hemorrhage. Before closing a scalp laceration, it is essential to inspect the wound visually or with the gloved finger. All foreign material must be removed and the cranium inspected for fractures. Intracranial hemorrhage in adults is not sufficient to affect circulating blood volume, but in infants, whose relative cranial size is much larger in proportion to body weight, intracranial blood loss may be of practical importance.

EVALUATING THE COMATOSE PATIENT

Even in poorly responsive patients a nearly complete neurologic examination can be obtained. In recording the mental state, the maximum motor response to a given stimulus should be recorded for future reference in head injury evaluation. The cranial nerve examination must not be neglected even in the uncooperative patient. Pupillary reaction usually indicates that optic pathways from the retina to the brain stem are intact. Cortical blindness may be present even when the pupil is reactive. Threatening motions directed at the various angles to the retina give some information about visual fields. Although papilledema is detected late when masses are present, large subhyaloid hemorrhages suggest intracranial bleeding. When the head is rotated rapidly from side to side, the eyes normally remain fixed vertically and do not follow head movement. This so-called ''doll's eye'' response indicates interaction between the vestibular nuclei, the sixth nerve nuclei, the third nerve nucleus, and the peripheral cranial nerves themselves. A brain stem lesion accompanied by the loss of these responses indicates an unfavorable prognosis. The fifth nerve can be tested by painfully stimulating the supraorbital ridge, and a facial grimace indicates normal seventh cranial nerve function. The remaining cranial nerves are difficult to examine in the unresponsive patient. The motor system can be evaluated grossly by painful stimulation or by vigorously massaging the sternum. Prompt withdrawal with good motor power confirms a functional pathway. Spinal reflexes persist long after cerebral cortical death, however, and unless the movement is clearly functional, it should be interpreted without optimism. Pathologic reflexes such as a Hoffman or Babinski sign indicate an injury in the corticospinal system. Only when a great deal of movement is present can coordination be evaluated.

A comment is in order here about the severely brain-traumatized patient and the concept of brain death. Many

TABLE 46-3   A SCHEMA FOR THE PATIENT WITH AN ACUTE HEAD INJURY

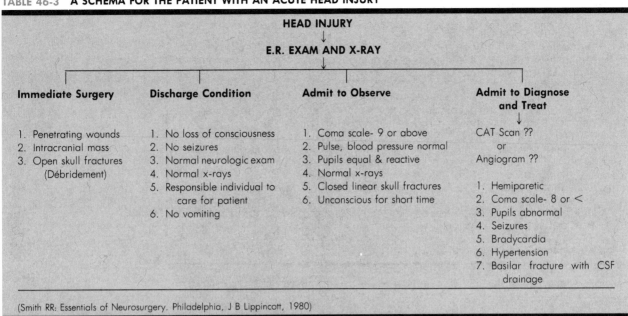

HEAD INJURY
↓
E.R. EXAM AND X-RAY
↓

Immediate Surgery	Discharge Condition	Admit to Observe	Admit to Diagnose and Treat

1. Penetrating wounds
2. Intracranial mass
3. Open skull fractures
  (Débridement)
	1. No loss of consciousness
	2. No seizures
	3. Normal neurologic exam
	4. Normal x-rays
	5. Responsible individual to
	  care for patient
	6. No vomiting
		1. Coma scale- 9 or above
		2. Pulse, blood pressure normal
		3. Pupils equal & reactive
		4. Normal x-rays
		5. Closed linear skull fractures
		6. Unconscious for short time
			CAT Scan ??
			or
			Angiogram ??
			
			1. Hemiparetic
			2. Coma scale- 8 or <
			3. Pupils abnormal
			4. Seizures
			5. Bradycardia
			6. Hypertension
			7. Basilar fracture with CSF
			  drainage

(Smith RR: Essentials of Neurosurgery. Philadelphia, J B Lippincott, 1980)

states have recently enacted laws allowing one of more physicians to declare death in the absence of cortex and brain stem function and electrocortical silence. In some states a "customary practice" is in effect, whereas in others, the medicolegal climate requires that a strict interpretation of the prevailing laws be enforced. The acquisition of good kidneys is optimally achieved by removal while circulation is intact. Good renal function should have prevailed until death. The judgment of brain death can be made in a patient with a neurologic lesion by physicians in attendance, but the members of the transplant team should not be involved in the decision process. The diagnosis is made in patients who are comatose with dilated fixed pupils, absent reflexes, no response to external stimuli, and no spontaneous respiration. Electroencephalography demonstrating isoelectric patterns and angiography substantiate the diagnosis. Once the diagnosis has been made, permission of the next of kin should be obtained, although prior commitment with a donor card is accepted now in most states.

MANAGEMENT DECISIONS

Once evaluation is complete and a working diagnosis is established, the management plan is formulated on the basis of whether immediate surgery is required or a period of observation is needed. Radiographs of the skull are essential in the care of many patients. Hematomas involving the extradural, subdural, or intracerebral compartment require immediate evacuation. Open skull fractures and penetrating wounds require débridement. Patients with signs of increased intracranial pressure, neurologic deficits, seizures, closed skull fractures, basilar fractures, and CSF leaks require admission for observation. Fortunately, many patients with head injuries do not need hospitalization or immediate surgery but, after routine evaluation, emergency room management, and tetanus prophylaxis may be discharged and observed as outpatients. The requirements for early discharge are (1) no loss of consciousness, or unconsciousness for only a few minutes, (2) normal findings on neurologic examination, (3) normal skull radiographic find-

ings, (4) no seizures, (5) no vomiting, and (6) the presence of a reliable individual to care for the patient at home. On discharge, instructions are given to the attendant about examination at intervals. The patient should be awakened every 2 hr to 3 hr, and speech, mental alertness, movement, and strength of the extremities should be evaluated. The instructions listed in Figure 46-2 should be given to the patient, and the attendant should verify responsibility in the matter.

SPINAL CORD INJURIES

Fracture and dislocations of the 24 true movable vertebrae in the spine can occur at any level. The spinal cord terminates at the caudal end of L1, and the loose nerve roots of the cauda equina fill the lumbar spinal canal, where they are somewhat less susceptible to injury. In the cervical area, however, the spinal cord almost fills the canal, and dislocations usually produce profound deficits. In addition to displaced bone fragments, the intervertebral disk may herniate to the spinal canal, causing severe cord compression. Cord compression also results from narrowing of the canal as seen in the degenerative changes of the spine associated with spondylosis. Unfortunately, many spinal injuries result in immediate and total paralysis from which there is little useful recovery. There are a number of incomplete spinal injury syndromes, however, in which recovery occurs to some extent. Ipsilateral paresis and contralateral loss of sensation mark the *Brown-Séquard's syndrome*. Vibratory and joint sensibilities are diminished on the ipsilateral side. Although true cord hemisection rarely results from trauma, modified varieties of this syndrome exist when the lateral half of the cord is damaged. The *anterior spinal cord syndrome* may be associated with a ruptured disk or dislocated vertebral body. Paralysis occurs below the level of the lesion with loss of temperature, touch, and pain sensibilites. Joint position is usually preserved. In the *central cord syndrome*, the center of the cord is affected, and because the cervical fibers are located in the deepest

During the next few weeks, you may have a problem with your head injury which was not known when you first saw a doctor.

- If you or your relations notice any of these conditions, you should come to the Outpatient Clinic: severe headache, vomiting, dizziness, difficulty in concentrating, unusual trouble in remembering things or in recognizing your family or friends, unusual weakness, unusual drowsiness or sleepiness, or should you have a convulsion.

- Do not drink alcoholic beverages. Do not take narcotic drugs or sedatives. You may take aspirin or other simple pain relieving medications. Rest for 24 hours.

- If stitches were put in your scalp, be sure you understand when you are to return to have the wound checked or have the stitches taken out.

- Show these instructions to someone who will be with you during the next few weeks so he/she can help you if necessary. During the next 24 hours, someone should wake you up every three hours while you are asleep and carry out the tests described by the doctor.

The emergency room telephone number is _____.

Fig. 46-2. Instructions used by the Department of Neurosurgery, University of Mississippi Medical Center. (This advice is very important. One of the most common serious and potentially fatal mistakes made in the emergency ward is to send home or back to jail an apparently drunk patient who has sustained major head injury.—Ed)

lamella, the hands and upper extremities suffer most. There is relative sparing of lower extremity function because the sacral fibers are most peripherally placed (Fig. 46-3).

Both complete and incomplete injuries of the spinal cord may result in a neurogenic bladder. Ordinarily, the bladder fills to a capacity of 150 to 200 ml, and the desire to void follows. When the spinal cord is transsected above the conus medullaris, the so-called upper motor neuron bladder develops. It is characterized by reduced capacity but good voiding pressure. Immediately after the spinal injury, a period of spinal shock ensues in which bladder reflex mechanisms do not develop, and catheter drainage is essential. Later, however, automatic voiding can be expected in most patients with upper motor neuron lesions.

The lower motor neuron bladder is associated with injury of the sacral spinal cord or the cauda equina and lumbosacral roots. This deficit is characterized by dribbling and overflow incontinence after the bladder has filled to capacity. Intermittent or continuous catheter drainage may be the only alternative in some of these cases.

Spinal injuries affect primarily young men and are accompanied by profound neurologic deficits. Little can be done for the spinal cord injury *per se*. Decompression, stabilization of bony elements, realignment, and care for the complications of paraplegia and quadriplegia seem to be the physician's most significant contributions toward care. Ultimately, the public must be informed and appeals made for help in preventing these tragic accidents.

LESIONS OF THE INTERVERTEBRAL DISK

Back pain, alone or associated with sciatica, has plagued humans for thousands of years. Herniation of the nucleus pulposus is recognized today as one of the most common causes of debilitating back pain and sciatica. Cervical disk rupture is much less common than lumbar disease, and thoracic ruptures are fortunately rare. Herniation of the intervertebral disk is a disease of the fourth and fifth decades. Low back pain, often of brief and minor nature, is described

by most of those who suffer from the disorder. This pain initially results from stretching of pain fibers in the posterior longitudinal ligament. Standing, bending, and lifting accentuate the discomfort, which projects deep in the midline or over the sacroiliac articulation. Later, radicular pain develops in approximately one third of those affected as the nerve root overlying the disk becomes elevated and stretched. Initially, only mechanical findings are present. In the cervical region, lateral herniation is the rule, but if midline hernias develop, the spinal cord rather than the specific nerve root may be affected. Motor or sensory function of the upper extremity or bladder or bowel function may be impaired.

Fig. 46-3. Incomplete traumatic spinal lesions. (*A*) Central cord syndrome. (*B*) Brown-Séquard syndrome. (*C*) Anterior spinal cord syndrome.

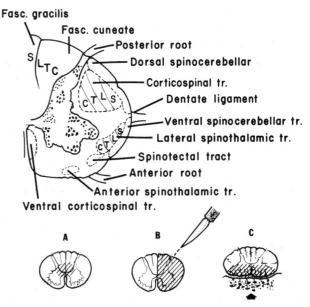

Fasc. gracilis
Fasc. cuneate
Posterior root
Dorsal spinocerebellar
Corticospinal tr.
Dentate ligament
Ventral spinocerebellar tr.
Lateral spinothalamic tr.
Spinotectal tract
Anterior root
Anterior spinothalamic tr.
Ventral corticospinal tr.

A   B   C

Diagnosis

Spasm of the erector spine muscle causes loss of lordotic curvature (*straightening*) that is normally present both in the cervical and the lumbar spine. Palpation of the spastic muscle discloses tenderness, and deep palpation presses the nerve root, reproducing the pain syndrome. The motion of the spine is limited (*stiffness*), and *scoliosis* may be present if the herniation is unilateral. Mechanical *stretch* signs are usually present. In Lasègue's test, elevation of the straightened extremity stretches the nerve root over the herniated intervertebral disk, reproducing the pain pattern. Pain is usually felt in the buttock or radiates down the distribution of the sciatic nerve. Flexion of the leg at the point of pain will usually relieve the pain caused by nerve root compression, whereas dorsiflexion of the foot aggravates it. Abduction and external rotation of the leg at this point help to differentiate primary hip joint disease from that associated with herniated intervertebral disk.

Routine spinal x-ray films may show narrowing of the interspace and osteophytic bone reaction, but it is not unusual if they are completely normal. Myelography is not particularly helpful in the patient with simple backache, nor should it be used as a screening device. The myelogram is positive in about 80% of cases of significant ruptures of the lumbar disc but is falsely positive in 10% to 15% of cases. It is also useful in diagnosis of lesions of the cervical area, but the findings are much more subtle because of the far lateral ruptures. In many cases, the diagnosis is made on the basis of a careful examination and a CT scan of the area of the spine in question. The specific neurologic findings associated with disk rupture are indicated in Figure 46-4.

Treatment

A course of bedrest should be required in virtually all patients with clinical evidence of intervertebral disk rupture. Only those with profound neurologic deficits, loss of bladder and bowel function, or foot drop should be considered for earlier operative treatment. A firm but not overly hard bed should be prescribed; the horizontal position ordinarily quickly relieves pressure from the intervertebral disk and promotes pain relief. Healing occurs slowly, however, and a great deal of patience is required on the part of both the patient and the physician. The patient is usually allowed bathroom privileges, but meals should be served in bed. Mild analgesics such as propoxyphene or aspirin may be

required for the first day or so, and muscle relaxants facilitate the adjustment to the bedrest setting. A pillow placed beneath the knees will help to alleviate severe leg pain, and a short course of steroids may also be effective in patients with acute pain. It is not clear whether traction is of any major benefit in the lumbar area, but there may be psychological benefit, and it may serve to keep the patient in bed. No more than 20 pounds should be applied by pelvic traction. Spinal manipulation has been recommended primarily by chiropractors but certainly should be avoided in the acute phase of the illness. In the chronic phase, flexion exercises and other physical therapy measures may be effective. Walking and swimming help to restore mobility to the spine, but jogging, cycling, and horseback riding should be avoided. Lifting weights greater than 25 pounds should be discouraged until the patient has been pain-free for several months. Overall, however, 80% recover when these conservative measures are applied aggressively.

Operative treatment should be reserved for those who fail to respond to a conservative program and for those who have lingering major motor disabilities. Other indications for surgery include (1) progressive paralysis, (2) extremely severe protracted attacks of sciatica, (3) repeated attacks causing lengthy incapacity, (4) economic hardships that would result from continued conservative treatment for an indefinite period. Treatment consists of a unilateral partial laminectomy, excision of the ligaments, and removal of the protruding intervertebral disk. Decompression of the nerve root should also be carried out at the same time by removal of bone coverings. If patients are properly selected, over 90% will achieve good relief from leg pain. Back pain is more difficult to treat, however. Of patients who will be compensated if they remain ill or sustain a disability, only 60% will return to productivity, even with the best of surgical technique. Bracing is also sometimes helpful in patients in whom movement seems to activate pain.

THE SURGICAL RELIEF OF PAIN

Pain serves a protective warning function, but it may in itself become a destructive force for which surgical relief may be required. Analgesics such as alcohol and opiates produce relief of pain, but there is wide variability in pain threshold among different persons, and the relief is often related to tolerance.

TRIGEMINAL NEURALGIA

Trigeminal neuralgia (tic douloureux) occurs in older people and affects one or more divisions of the trigeminal nerve, usually on one side of the face. The diagnosis is made primarily on clinical data, which include the following: (1) paroxysmal pain lasting only a few seconds, (2) trigger zones on the face, (3) pain confined to the distribution of one or more divisions of the nerve, (4) any particular pain occurring on only one side of the midline, (5) no neurologic deficit. The etiology of the disorder is unknown, but focal demyelinization in the nerve has been implicated. In some cases, a tortuous vessel, A-V malformation, or neoplasm irritates the nerve adjacent to the brain stem or in Meckel's cave. CT scan and basilar views of the skull are useful in differentiating these organic lesions from the idiopathic variety.

Initial treatment should be conservative, consisting of

Fig. 46-4. The specific nerve root findings associated with rupture of cervical and lumbar disks. (Smith RR: Essentials of Neurosurgery. Philadelphia, J B Lippincott, 1980)

DISC	NERVE ROOT	MOTOR	SENSORY	REFLEX
C5–C6	C6	Biceps		Biceps
C6–C7	C7	Triceps		Triceps
L3–L4	L-4	Quadriceps		Patella
L4–L5	L5	Ant. Tibialis Ext. Hallucis Long.		0
L5–S1	S1	Gastrocnemius Soleus		Achilles

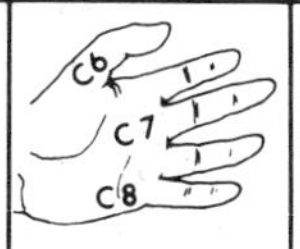

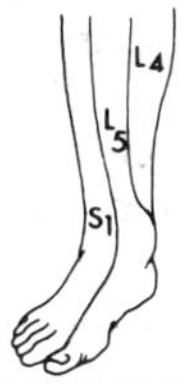

phenytoin or carbamazepine. The latter agent is extremely toxic, and bone marrow function must be monitored closely. Disorientation and ataxia are associated with the former drug. About half of the patients treated with either of these agents receive relief, but the effect may be short-lasting. Local anesthetic and alcohol injections may be given diagnostically and to relieve the pain for short intervals (6 months to 1 year). These therapies have the advantage of allowing patients to experience facial sensory loss before permanent procedures that would leave a permanent deficit are carried out.

When peripheral injections fail, the nerve can be evulsed operatively. Alternatively, percutaneous thermocoagulation of the gasserian ganglia can be carried out. In this technique, an 18-gauge needle is passed lateral to the oral cavity into the foramen ovale. Under fluoroscopy, the needle is advanced until CSF flows. An electrode is placed in the gasserian ganglia, and after stimulation to identify the divisions of the nerve, an electrolytic lesion is made. Sensory loss is generally incomplete. Microvascular decompression is aimed at relieving compression of the nerve by neoplasms and tortuous blood vessels. Probably most of those who complain of trigeminal neuralgia have such a lesion, and isolation of the nerve with a small strip of muscle affords relief.

RELIEF OF MALIGNANT PAIN

Somatic pain from the extremities and trunk is transmitted in the lateral spinothalamic tract, the division of which affords relief in the short term. Why *spinothalamic tractotomy* affords only temporary relief is unknown, but perhaps alternate pathways develop. Two methods are currently employed to perform cordotomy. In one, an open operation is performed, and in the other an electrode is placed transcutaneously in the spinothalamic tract. The percutaneous technique can be extended to many patients in poor medical condition, and it allows, to some extent, selective ablation of lumbar, thoracic, or cervical pain fibers. With either method, bladder dysfunction occurs in about 5% of patients who undergo unilateral cordotomy. Bilateral lesions in the cervical area may lead to apnea in sleep and are thus infrequently performed.

Rhizotomy refers to a division of a nerve root and *neurectomy* to the division of the nerve proper. These procedures are favored to relieve local pain of a superficial type. The pain produced by thoracic wall and abdominal wall neoplasms responds favorably to these operations. Intercostal nerve blocks using alcohol also afford relief from thoracic wall pain. Surgical procedures may be directed at the pain response center in the brain. Two areas have been found suitable targets, the frontal lobe and the cingulum. These areas seem to transmit pain responses from the thalamus and limbic system. The operation can be performed openly or stereotaxically by placing coagulating electrodes through a burr hole. Each of these operations also affects personality. *Cingulotomy* produces fewer changes, although the imaginative capacity of the individual is blunted. A *frontal lobotomy* or leucotomy, in which the fibers are divided, always impairs attentiveness and intelligence. Following lesions of this type patients rarely complain spontaneously of pain but will readily admit to it when asked. The pain is usually not as destructive, however, and often the patient is able to carry on a relatively normal life. Recently, techniques have been developed in which the pain-inhib-

iting pathways of the brain and spinal cord are stimulated electrically. Electrical stimulation of the gray matter in the periaqueductal area produces an analgesic effect peripherally. A bare-tipped electrode is introduced near the third ventricle and posterior commissure, and if temporary relief follows stimulation, the electrode is implanted subcutaneously and connected to a power source providing a continuous pulse current.

INTRACRANIAL HEMORRHAGE

Of all stroke deaths in the United States, about half are caused by intracranial bleeding, although thrombotic strokes are more often debilitating. The anatomic features of the cerebral arteries probably contribute to their tendency to rupture and bleed. The larger vessels are confined to the subarachnoid space with little connective tissue to support them. The muscularis layer, which is relatively thin, consists of a spiral network of smooth muscle cells, and defects in this layer are prominent.

SUBARACHNOID HEMORRHAGE

The term subarachnoid hemorrhage is applied to bleeding occurring principally in the subarachnoid space and blood found on lumbar puncture. It is more a clinical entity than a distinct pathologic one. Although bleeding in the subarachnoid space frequently results from trauma, the most common cause of spontaneous bleeding is an intracranial aneurysm (Fig. 46-5). Clinically, the signs may be relatively minor. Some patients experience a warning sign, the sentinel headache, which precedes the major hemorrhage by about 2 weeks. The headache is of sudden onset and is associated with nuchal rigidity and often accompanied by nausea, vomiting, and transient loss of consciousness. Depending on the source and cause of the hemorrhage, other signs may be present. Hemorrhage in and around the sylvian fissure causes contralateral paresis or sensory disturbances, and aphasia may be a feature of hemorrhage of the left hemisphere.

The CT scan outlines the cause of the subarachnoid hemorrhage with a high degree of accuracy, and the angiogram is the diagnostic procedure of choice. It should be performed soon after the initial bleeding episode and prior to ischemic complications that intervene owing to vasospasm.

The cause of cerebral aneurysms is widely debated. Hypertension must have some role in their development because those afflicted with coarctation of the aorta, polycystic renal disease, and renal artery stenosis share a propensity to develop aneurysms early in life. True saccular or berry aneurysms seem to enlarge progressively to about 6 mm, at which time they hemorrhage. Peak age for aneurysm rupture is between 55 and 65 years of age, but these aneurysms are frequently found incidentally, unruptured at postmortem examination. Those less than 5 mm in diameter usually have not ruptured by the time they are discovered. Traumatic aneurysms arise from a vessel subjected to trauma, and mycotic aneurysms develop 3 to 4 weeks after septic embolization, usually from an infected heart valve. Aneurysms may develop on any of the intracranial vessels, but the carotid artery and anterior communicating branches seem to be implicated most often. Internal carotid aneurysms consistently cause paralysis of the third cranial nerve, and pupillary dilatation is a distinctive feature of this lesion. The

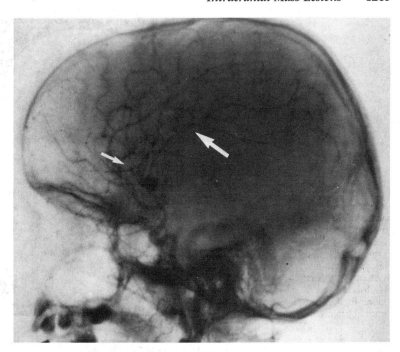

Fig. 46-5. Ruptured aneurysm of the middle cerebral artery (*small arrow*). This artery is displaced upward by adjacent hematoma (*large arrow*). The patient in this case, a 9-year-old boy, also had renal artery stenosis and hypertension.

pupil is spared in the third nerve paralysis associated with diabetes mellitus.

VASCULAR MALFORMATIONS

Vascular anomalies are probably congenital in virtually every case, although they may enlarge throughout life. They cause symptoms relative to their mass occasionally, but hemorrhage and seizures are the most common presenting complaints. In general, the peak age for hemorrhage from an arteriovenous malformation is much younger than that for aneurysms, and over half of the patients have bled by the age of 30. More than 25% can be expected to rebleed over a 20-year interval with a mortality of about 12%. Most arteriovenous malformations can be diagnosed easily with the CT scan and with rapid sequence imaging on the nuclide scan, but the angiogram is the diagnostic procedure of choice.

HYPERTENSIVE HEMORRHAGE

For many years hypertensive hemorrhages were thought to occur exclusively in the basal ganglia internal capsule, and it is known that this is their predominant site. Others, however, are known to occur in the temporal lobe and in the cerebellum; if detected early, a favorable outcome is to be expected in this location. Pathologic anatomy of the blood vessel is uncertain, but perhaps microaneurysms develop in hypertensive patients.

CAROTID CAVERNOUS FISTULAS

Carotid cavernous fistulas usually result from traumatic injury of the carotid artery within the cavernous sinus. They may arise, however, from aneurysms or small defects in the carotid artery that could rupture. A continuous murmur is audible over the eye, and increased pressures within the retinal vein follow. Glaucoma complicates most cases, and the intraocular pressure may actually exceed retinal artery pressure, leading to ischemic changes in the retinal cells.

The treatment consists of blocking the fistula as close to its origin as possible. Recently, the use of the detachable balloons best satisfies the goals of therapy, sparing carotid artery circulation but obliterating the fistulous communication.

EPIDURAL AND SUBDURAL HEMATOMAS

It is important to understand the essential difference between epidural and subdural hematoma (Fig. 46-6). Although there can be considerable overlap in both clinical signs and the pathology found, by and large the epidural hematoma (between the skull and the dura), arises within hours after injury, often from a blow to the head with rupture of the middle meningeal artery. Symptoms from a hematoma of significant size will usually appear within a few hours. In contrast, although the subdural hematoma may likewise be manifest promptly, in other instances it may be weeks or even months before swelling of the hematoma from edematous fluid produces neurologic changes, and the original injury may have been forgotten and the patient pronounced drunk if he is known to drink. This late onset poses a serious hazard of delay in diagnosis and operation, with at times disastrous results.

To sum up, intracranial hemorrhage is a serious disorder associated with high rates of death and disability. Little is to be gained by procrastination or conservatism. The surgical treatment is both specific and effective. Only by progressively pursuing the diagnosis can recurrent hemorrhage from these devastating lesions be prevented.

INTRACRANIAL MASS LESIONS

Intracranial mass lesions may be manifest principally by the symptoms and clinical findings of increased intracranial pressure. Mass lesions include *tumors, hemorrhage* (into the "tight bony box"), *abscess,* and *cysts.* In some parts of the Middle East, a common indication for craniotomy is echinococcal cyst. In addition, nonparasitic cysts may occur within the skull. Hematomas have been discussed above;

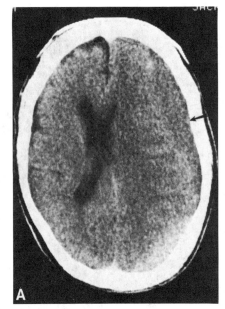
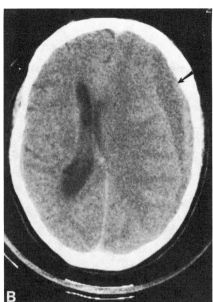

Fig. 46-6. The acute, subacute, and chronic subdural hematoma can usually be diagnosed easily by CT scan. In the acute phase, the well-formed clot is seen as increased density. As it liquefies, it becomes isodense (*A*) and has nearly the same density as a normal brain. In unilateral cases, a shift of the ventricular system away from the side of the lesion is observed. As the hematoma becomes more liquid, it is less dense than the normal brain (*B*).

INTRACRANIAL MASS LESIONS	
Etiology	Tumors and cysts Hematomas or abscesses
Dx	History and physical examination, plain roentgenograms, EEG, CT scan, arteriography, radionuclide brain scan
Rx	Reduce increased intracranial pressure; otherwise depends on lesion

brain tumor, abscess, and cyst will now be considered. The presence and probable nature of the mass lesion are suggested by clinical findings, skull roentgenograms, CT scans, arteriograms, and other investigative tools.

BRAIN TUMOR

Central nervous tumors occur in about 1% to 2% of the population, and of these, unfortunately, the gliomas comprise almost 50% (Table 46-4). In cancer in children, brain tumors are second only to leukemia in frequency. Symptoms are produced mainly by increased intracranial pressure, but local irritative and destructive effects may be a first sign. Brain tumor headaches are more common upon waking and clear during the day. They occur in over 90% of patients with brain tumors. Unlike migraine headaches, they are recognized as a new phenomenon by the patient and are often nonlocalizing. Vomiting is ordinarily a late sign of an intracranial neoplasm, but papilledema occurs in one half of all patients with tumors.

Because of their destructive effects, brain tumors may cause localizing findings depending on the major site of occurrence. Frontal lobe neoplasms cause apathy and a lack of drive and ambition. Defects in the three Ts—tact, tenacity, and tension—sum up the effect of large lesions occupying the frontal lobe. The temporal lobe is involved in about half of all infiltrating neoplasms of the nervous system. A seizure during which the patient experiences sudden unexplained tastes or smells, usually of an unpleasant nature, is described as an uncinate fit. Chewing movements, salivation, or expectoration may be a part of the seizure. These lesions may also lead to episodic aggressive behavior or even violent uncontrollable rage. The epileptic nature of the attack is rarely recognized.

The parietal lobe includes the postcentral gyrus and is concerned with discrimination of sensory function. Lesions deep in the parietal lobe produce lower quadrantic opposite visual field defects through involvement of the geniculocalcarine tract. Construction apraxia may be a prominent feature of parietal lobe neoplasms in which the patient is unable to design the face of a clock or to draw figures.

Occipital lobe lesions interfere with vision and with following movements of the eyes. About half of all patients with parietal lobe lesions have homonymous loss of vision in the opposite field.

TABLE 46-4   CNS TUMORS

TYPE	PREVALENCE	(%)
Gliomas		50
Astrocytomas (grades 1 and 2)	25	
Glioblastomas (grades 3 and 4 astrocytomas)	55	
Oligodendrogliomas	5	
Ependymomas	6	
Papillomas	1	
Colloid cysts	2	
Medulloblastomas, ganglioneuromas, neuroblastomas	6	
Meningiomas		15
Neuromas (schwannomas, neurinomas)		2
Pituitary tumors		8
Metastasis		20
Other		5

(Smith RR: Essentials of Neurosurgery. Philadelphia, J B Lippincott, 1980)

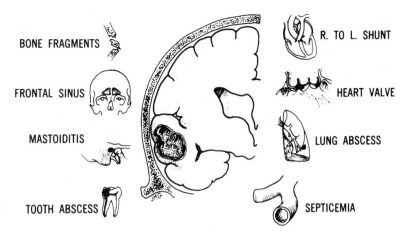

Fig. 46-7. Origins of the intracranial abscess. (Smith RR: Essentials of Neurosurgery. Philadelphia, J B Lippincott, 1980)

Tumors located in the cerebellum and posterior cranial fossa cause symptoms by obstruction of CSF outflow and by local destructive effects on the medulla and cerebellum. There may be a tremor on finger to nose testing and inability to check rapid movements. Midline neoplasms cause a wide-based gait and ataxia. Acoustic tumors, meningiomas, and cholesteatomas occur in the cerebellopontine (CP) angle and cause tinnitus as one of the first symptoms. Unilateral loss of hearing follows. The fifth nerve may also be affected.

Tumors of the pituitary gland have several distinct phases in their growth patterns. The first is associated with excessive hormonal production. In phase 2, the normal pituitary is gradually destroyed, and panhypopituitarism develops. Hypogonadism, hypothyroidism, and hypoadrenalism are first signs. In the male, loss of libido is the first symptom, but in the female, amenorrhea occurs before sex drive is impaired. In the third phase, the tumor erupts through the diaphragm of the sella into the intracranial compartment. Headaches, if present, usually abate at this time. The tumor enlarges further, however, compressing the optic chiasm, and visual impairment follows. Bitemporal visual loss is a distinctive feature of the pituitary tumor, but some neoplasms cause diffuse changes in visual acuity or may involve only one optic nerve and cause unilateral visual loss. In the fourth and final phase of growth, the tumor enlarges into the third ventricle and blocks absorption from the foramen of Monro, leading rapidly to increased intracranial pressure, hydrocephalus, and death if untreated.

Benign cranial tumors can usually be totally resected, and recurrences are unusual. Surgical therapy for cerebral gliomas has advanced little in the past half century. Only recently, radiation therapy and chemotherapy have been added to the therapeutic armamentarium. Nevertheless, few long-term survivals have been seen among those with the more highly malignant neoplasms. For the present, removal of all gross neoplasm followed by radiation or chemotherapeutic agents such as CCNU offers the best chance for survival.

BRAIN ABSCESS (AND CYSTS)

Intracranial abscess is now less common but still carries a formidable mortality when treatment is delayed. At one time 80% of brain abscesses were caused by ear infection, and most of the remainder resulted from frontal sinus involvement (Fig. 46-7). At present, brain abscess is most often seen in congenital heart disease (especially tetralogy of Fallot or subacute bacterial endocarditis), pulmonary infection, and immunosuppressed renal transplant patients.

Clinical signs are those due to increased intracranial pressure—headache, nausea and vomiting, dizziness, lethargy, and focal or generalized seizures.

Management consists of adequate decompression of the abscess, often by aspiration through an appropriately placed burr hole or craniectomy, followed by instillation of antibiotic solution into the cavity. Systemic antibiotics are continued for several weeks, and the closing of the cavity is monitored with serial CT scans.

BIBLIOGRAPHY

Basbaum AI, Fields HH: Endogenous pain control mechanisms, review and hypothesis. Ann Neurol 4:451, 1978

Cushing H: Some experimental and clinical observations concerning states of intracranial pressure. Am J Med Sci 124:375, 1902

Jennet B, Teasdale G, Brookman R: Predicting outcome in individual patients after severe head injuries. Lancet I:1031, 1976

Richardson DE, Acic H: Pain reduction by electrical brain stimulation in man. Neurosurgery 47:178, 1977

Simeone RA (ed): Operative nerve injuries and their repair. Surg Clin North Am 52:5, 1972

Smith RR: Aneurysms and Carotid Cavernous Fistula. (The Clinical Neurosciences, Section II. Neurosurgery). (In press)

Smith RR: Essentials of Neurosurgery. Philadelphia, J B Lippincott, 1980

Walker AE: A History of Neurological Surgery. Baltimore, Williams & Wilkins, 1951

Wintzen AR: The clinical course of subdural haematoma. A retrospective study of aetiological, chronological and pathological features in 212 patients and a proposed classification. Brain 103:855, 1980

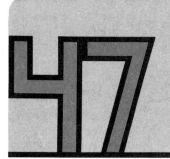

Gynecologic Surgery

The surgeon who deals with gynecologic problems must be aware of several important principles. First, a thorough knowledge of female reproductive physiology is essential. Second, emotional factors are intrinsic to gynecologic disorders and involve concepts of femininity, reproductive ability, and sexual function. Third, the majority of common gynecologic conditions are usually best managed by nonoperative means, although a knowledge of general and gynecologic surgical principles is essential, should operation be indicated. Fourth, complex gynecologic problems often require cooperative efforts with other specialists, such as internists, radiologists, or urologists.

EVALUATION OF THE GYNECOLOGIC PATIENT

When a patient presents a gynecologic complaint, it is desirable to proceed in a systematic manner toward diagnosis and management. This means determining the subjective and objective findings, developing a problem list, and outlining a plan of treatment.

SUBJECTIVE ASSESSMENT

Gynecologic complaints may be specific (*i.e.,* bleeding, discharge, pain) or they may relate to reproductive functions such as menstruation, fertility, or dyspareunia.

Every gynecologic history should contain information on the following subjects (whether obtained as part of the presenting complaint or ascertained separately):

1. Menstrual history. Specifically, the menstrual history includes the age at onset or cessation of menstruation, length of cycle, duration and amount of flow, and date of last two normal menstrual periods. Recent menstrual changes, bleeding between the periods, pain at the time of menstruation, and amount and type of vaginal discharge should also be noted.
2. Obstetrical history. The number of children; their feeding in infancy and present health; the date of the last delivery; the number and causes, if known, of abortions; and any complications of pregnancy, delivery, or abortion make up the obstetric history.
3. Psychosexual history. The psychosexual history includes past, present, and future sexual function and expectations; contraceptive practices; and attitudes toward female functions such as menstruation, birth, breast feeding, motherhood, and coitus. Many physicians are reluctant to ask questions in this sensitive area. However, the information is essential to good future management.

OBJECTIVE ASSESSMENT

Once the physician has obtained a history, he will have formed some idea of the possible nature of the problem. Knowledge of the physical findings of each condition (see below for specific disorders) will enable him to pay special attention to certain parts of the examination. However, it is important to develop and maintain a routine so that no area is missed.

GENERAL PHYSICAL EXAMINATION

The general physical examination should be brief but relevant to the patient's complaints. It serves the purpose of completeness and of instilling the confidence necessary for conducting a good pelvic examination. Particular attention should be paid to the examination of the breasts because of the importance of early detection of breast cancer.

PELVIC EXAMINATION

Equipment for an adequate gynecologic examination includes a gynecologic examining table, drapes, a stool for the examiner, a good light source, and a waste receptacle. A small movable table is useful to hold specula (Pederson, medium Graves, virginal and large), long forceps, malleable uterine sounds, uterine dressing forceps, tenacula, cotton swabs, and lubricant. A good biopsy forceps and cotton tampons to control bleeding are helpful. Equipment for obtaining cytologic studies should be readily available.

Pelvic and rectal examinations are disagreeable but not painful to the average woman. The procedure should be explained in a step-by-step fashion. Examination should be conducted quietly, gently, and without haste. The patient frequently finds it easier to relax if she is encouraged to breathe slowly and deeply, concentrating on expiration. An attendant should be readily available during the examination both from the medicolegal standpoint and to give reassurance to the patient. A glove should be worn on the internal examining hand. Inspection and palpation of the external genitalia are followed by a speculum examination of the cervix, using no lubricant. Specimens for cytologic studies should then be taken. The number of specimens varies with the cytopathologist concerned. In general, it is important to remember that cytologic studies can give information not only about possible malignant cells but also about infections and hormonal status. Ideally, specimens should be obtained from the lateral vaginal wall (for hormonal status); from the ectocervix, using a tongue blade or Ayre spatulum; and from the endocervix, using a moistened cotton swab or by aspiration with a glass or metal tube.

A vaginoabdominal examination is then performed, and the cervix, the uterine fundus, the fallopian tubes, and the ovaries are palpated. The dominant hand is best used for the abdominal part of the examination, and one or two fingers of the less dominant hand are used for the vaginal part. Finally, a rectovaginoabdominal examination is performed, usually with the middle finger in the rectum and the index finger in the vagina. The dominant hand is again used on the abdomen. By this means, the paracervical tissue, the cul-de-sac, and the rectovaginal septum may be palpated.

SPECIAL PROBLEMS IN EXAMINATION

Bleeding

Some women are reluctant to undergo examination while they are bleeding. If bleeding is part of a regular menstrual period, examination may be postponed, if feasible. If the bleeding is abnormal, or if there is likely to be no other opportunity to see the patient, examination should be carried out. Often, observation of the site of bleeding is helpful in diagnosis. Cytologic specimens (at least cervical scrapings) may usually be obtained if the bleeding is not excessive by first gently sponging out blood from the upper vagina and cervix.

Children

With girls under the age of puberty the cooperation of the mother or another female relative is helpful. Gentleness and explanation are even more necessary than in the adult. Rectal examination is almost always possible but is not sufficient if vaginal bleeding or discharge has occurred or if there is a possibility of a foreign body in the vagina. Vaginal examination can often be accomplished by the use of a urethroscope or lighted vaginoscope, although anesthesia may be necessary for full evaluation.

Periodic Examination

Regular examinations have been widely recommended as a method of detecting cancer and other diseases in their early stages. Physicians who are concerned with gynecologic disorders are frequently called on to undertake such examinations. The usual interval in the adult female of reproductive or postmenopausal age is once yearly, although more frequent examinations may be advisable for women in certain high-risk categories or for those who have specific disorders that need evaluation from time to time.

The extent of the annual examination depends on the amount of care the patient may be receiving from other physicians. Ideally, she should be seen by only one physician who serves to screen her for abnormalities and then to refer her to an appropriate specialist for any specific difficulties he may discover that are outside his field of competence.

Under these circumstances, the annual examination should consist of a brief general examination, including particularly examination of the breasts, a pelvic examination, cytologic studies of the vagina and cervix and laboratory work appropriate to the patient's age and other findings. One of the benefits of the periodic examination is the opportunity to listen to any problems (including sexual) that the patient may have and to instruct her in preventive health techniques such as self-examination of the breasts, diet, and exercise.

PROBLEM SOLVING

The further analysis of the clinical findings, including the pelvic examination and the selection of appropriate laboratory studies, depends on two types of essential knowledge. The first may be described as a branching problem-solving exercise, and the second consists of information about specific and general gynecologic diseases.

Gynecologic symptoms are relatively few in number and often indicate the likelihood of a particular disorder or suggest the direction that further examination or study should take. Below is an outline of symptoms and the lines of thought and investigation to which they lead. Only the preliminary steps of problem solving are shown in the interest of clarity. Obviously, it is possible to refine the branching extensively so as to obtain a more precise diagnosis. Symptoms are listed roughly in order from the lower end of the genital tract upward, ending in more general and nonspecific complaints:

A. Vulvar Itching
   1. If associated with discharge, it suggests a vulvovaginal infection such as candidiasis or trichomoniasis.
   2. If prolonged and associated with a lump, it suggests vulvar dystrophy or carcinoma.
   3. If unaccompanied by discharge or a lump, it suggests psychosexual or emotional problems.
B. Vulvar Lump or Mass
   1. With no pain or other symptoms, it suggests a benign or malignant tumor.
   2. With ulceration (with or without pain) it suggests infection such as syphilis, chancroid, granulomatous disease, or even carcinoma.
C. Vulvar or Perineal Pain
   If this is the primary symptom, without others, it may present a difficult diagnostic problem and leads to consideration of disease higher in the genital tract, deep-seated local problems, or difficulties related to sexual function.
D. Vaginal Discharge
   1. If thin and bloody, it suggest atrophic vaginitis or disease higher in the genital tract. In children, foreign body in the vagina must be considered.
   2. If profuse and of unpleasant odor, it suggests local

infection in the vagina or cervix such as gonorrhea, candidiasis, or trichomoniasis.
   3. If associated with fecal or urinary odor, it suggests a fistula.
   4. If associated with vulvar itching, it suggests vulvovaginal infection such as candidiasis or trichomoniasis.
   5. If it is not as profuse or unpleasant as the patient states or the associated symptoms do not fit into the categories described above, the possibility of a psychosexual or emotional problem must be considered.
E. Mass in Vagina
   Identification of the nature of a vaginal mass or protrusion is difficult for the patient.
   1. If associated with rectal symptoms, it suggests a rectocele.
   2. If associated with urinary symptoms, it suggests a cystocele or urethrocele.
   3. If associated with pain on intercourse (dyspareunia) or minimal symptoms, it suggests uterine descensus or vaginal tumor.
F. Vaginal Bleeding
   This is the most common gynecologic symptom. It is axiomatic that entirely regular menstrual cycles do not occur throughout the reproductive age for any woman and that irregularities are often of great concern to the individual woman. A common problem for the patient and the gynecologist is to determine whether the irregularities reported are within normal limits or not. Clues to the possibility of abnormal conditions being present may be as follows:
   1. Failure to menstruate at all by the end of the normal age of puberty (primary amenorrhea) suggests genetic problems or congenital anomalies.
   2. Cessation of menstruation (secondary amenorrhea) or scanty menstruation (oligomenorrhea) during the reproductive age suggests pregnancy, endocrine problems, or incipient menopause.
   3. Excessive menstruation (menorrhagia) suggests a general disorder or blood dyscrasia in younger women or myomas or hyperplasia of the endometrium in older women.
   4. Irregular bleeding (intermenstrual, prepubertal, or postmenopausal) is by far the most common problem and suggests many different conditions, examples of which include carcinoma of the cervix (especially if bleeding follows coitus), endometrial polyps, submucous myomas, carcinoma of the endometrium, abnormal ovarian function, ovarian tumors, or general endocrinologic or emotional causes.
G. Pelvic Pain
   1. If associated with fever, it may suggest pelvic inflammatory disease or an accident occurring in an ovarian cyst or tumor (torsion, infection, hemorrhage, or rupture).
   2. If associated with menstruation (dysmenorrhea), it may have originated with menstruation (primary dysmenorrhea) and may be due to congenital anomalies or be of emotional origin or it may have begun later in reproductive life (secondary dysmenorrhea) and suggest pelvic disorders such as infection or endometriosis.
   3. If associated with coitus, it may be accompanied by symptoms of other pelvic disease, suggesting a retroflexed uterus, infections, endometriosis or tumors; or it may be accompanied by no other symptoms or

obvious signs, suggesting psychosexual or emotional origins.

H. Lower Abdominal Mass

1. If not accompanied by pain, it suggests an ovarian, uterine, or extragenital mass.
2. If accompanied by pain or other symptoms, it suggests the same but includes in addition the possibility of infection or an accident occurring in a cyst or tumor.

I. Rectal or Urinary Symptoms

1. If associated with a vaginal mass (see above), they suggest the presence of a cystocele, urethrocele, or rectocele.
2. If associated with lower abdominal pain, pelvic pain or other symptoms, they suggest uterine or ovarian tumors or infections.
3. If associated with unusual vaginal discharge, they may suggest fistula.

J. General Symptoms

These features comprise nausea, vomiting, weight loss, malaise, and a variety of other symptoms. Their presence often indicates a wider diagnostic search than is encompassed by pelvic disease.

1. If associated with a pelvic mass, they suggest carcinoma of the ovary or possibly of the uterus.
2. If associated with no pelvic mass, they may suggest an extragenital, endocrinologic, or emotional problem.

PLAN OF MANAGEMENT

Once the patient's problems have been identified, as far as is possible from the history, examination, and laboratory tests, a plan of management should be developed for each current problem. This should include immediate therapy such as possible operative procedures, medication, diet, activity, patient education, and emotional and social support. Long-term plans should also be outlined.

RECORDS

The gynecologic record should accurately reflect the process of care. A problem-oriented format is appropriate and should include the collection of a data base, the development of a numbered list of problems, initial plans, and progress notes. This format can be adapted to both inpatient and outpatient care. It is particularly valuable when the patient presents with a number of complex problems.

GYNECOLOGIC DISORDERS

CONGENITAL ABNORMALITIES

The abnormalities of congenital origin found in the female genital tract are most easily understood by reference to their embryologic development. The three structures concerned are the wolffian body or mesonephros, the müllerian ducts, and the urogenital sinus. The wolffian body forms the ovary; the unfused müllerian ducts, the tubes; the fused müllerian ducts, the uterus, the cervix, and the upper vagina; and the urogenital sinus, the lower vagina and the squamous epithelium of the vagina and the cervix.

Abnormalities of the ovary are rare and consist of the failure of descent of the ovary into the true pelvis or aplasia of one or both ovaries. Supernumerary ovaries have also

been reported rarely. Aplasia, atresia, and duplication of the tubes are very uncommon.

Failure of one or both müllerian ducts to develop or fuse accounts for abnormalities of the uterus (Fig. 47-1). Failure of development leads to absence of the uterus. Incomplete development with normal fusion may give rise to hypoplasia of the uterus. Failure of fusion may take various forms, ranging from complete duplication of uterus and cervix down to minor septums or indentations of the top of the uterus. These anomalies may have varying clinical significance, particularly in regard to obstetrics.

Failure of fusion of the müllerian ducts may also lead to a vagina that is completely duplicated or has a partial septum. Complete failure of development in this area may lead to partial or complete absence of the vagina.

Abnormalities of the external genitalia include imperforate hymen, double vulva, or urethral abnormalities such as hypospadias. Enlargement of the clitoris, often leading to confusion regarding sex identity, may be related to genetic abnormalities such as intersex states or to congenital adrenal hyperplasia. Genital tract abnormalities are often associated with other congenital anomalies, especially those of the urinary tract. An interesting anomaly in the vulva is the occasional presence of breast tissue.

CLINICAL FEATURES

Failure of the genital system to develop normally may be noted at birth, when it may be difficult to determine the sex of the infant from the appearance of the external genitalia; at puberty, when menstruation does not occur or the absence of a vaginal opening is noted when coitus is attempted; and during reproductive life when repeated abortions or problems with labor and delivery occur.

When the external genitalia are ambiguous in infancy, it is important to determine, if possible, exactly which component of the female genital system is present and whether or not it is normal. Apart from enlargement of the clitoris or duplication of the labia, fusion of the labia may occur rarely, giving rise to hydrocolpos or hydrometrocolpos. Determination of genetic sex by examination of buccal smears and by more detailed chromosome analysis is often very helpful.

In adolescence, the failure of menstruation to occur at the usual age may be due to congenital abnormalities and

Fig. 47-1. Congenital anomalies of the uterus. Effects of failure of fusion of müllerian ducts.

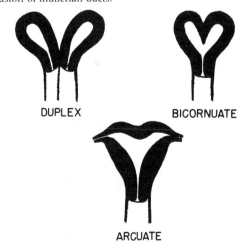

DUPLEX　　　BICORNUATE

ARCUATE

lead the patient (and her mother) to the physician. Occasionally attempts at coitus (or even self-exploration), in the absence of menarche, may be the presenting symptom. Primary amenorrhea alone may be due to a number of causes and may have associated general and endocrinologic abnormalities. If primary amenorrhea is accompanied by the absence of a vaginal opening, it may be associated either with an imperforate hymen but normal lower and upper genital tracts or with absence of the vagina and uterus with or without normal ovaries. In the former case the retention of blood in the vagina (hematocolpos), cervix (hematotrachelos), uterine cavity (hematometra), and tubes (hematosalpinx) (Fig. 47-2) may result in symptoms of increasing pain and discomfort with each menstrual period. Distention of the lower abdomen may also occur, and difficulty in urination may be noted. Sometimes the symptoms may suggest an acute abdominal condition. When the uterus and vagina are absent, no such symptoms are present.

The most important point in diagnosis is to perform a careful and detailed examination of the external and internal genitalia. If an imperforate hymen is present, a blue bulging membrane is usually seen. The distended vagina, cervix, uterus, and fallopian tubes may also be felt. They may, in addition, be demonstrated by a flat plate roentgenogram of the abdomen or with contrast material inserted into the rectum or bladder.

During reproductive life, the first symptoms of abnormality of the genital tract may be discovered when the patient presents a sterility problem, has repeated abortions, or has some difficulty with labor and delivery. In such cases, in addition to the usual methods of examination, hysterosalpingography is valuable.

TREATMENT

In infancy, once the nature of the external genitalia has been ascertained, a plan of management must be made promptly because it is most important to establish the child's sex of rearing. Reconstructive measures may then be undertaken as needed. The only immediate procedure is separation of the fused labia. This operation can be done simply and is followed with the regular use of estrogenic cream for several days to prevent recurrence. In adolescence the imperforate hymen may readily be treated by cruciate incision or total excision. Infection may follow hematocol-

Fig. 47-2. Effects of retention of menstrual flow with imperforate hymen.

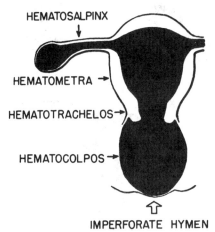

pos; and, if treatment is delayed, there may be permanent effects on the patient's reproductive capacity.

When the vagina and uterus are absent, but the ovaries are normal, with normal development of secondary sexual characteristics, the construction of a new vagina is important for establishment of the patient's ability to have coitus, even though she will not be able to bear children. The time at which the new vagina is created depends on detailed discussion with the patient and on the ensuring of her complete cooperation in maintaining patency, which is the most difficult part of the management. Good anatomical results may be expected in 60% to 70% of cases, although good function (*i.e.,* sexual satisfaction) may be higher than this.

The new vagina can be created in several ways:

Persistent pressure indentation of the perineum (Frank method). This is suitable when there is already a vaginal dimple.

Use of the labia to create a new vaginal tube (Williams procedure).

Dissection of a space between the rectum and the urethra (a modification of this technique is to free the pelvic peritoneum and bring it down to line the newly developed space) and its maintenance by an obturator (made of a sponge or lightweight material), covered by a condom with or without a skin graft. The obturator must be worn continuously at first and then intermittently (usually at night) for a number of months to ensure a good result. This requires great persistence on the part of the patient and the physician.

The most difficult problems of vaginal agenesis occur when a functioning uterus is present and some or all of the vagina is absent. Although the principles of management are the same, the results are less satisfactory.

During reproductive life, problems are most likely to arise from a septate or double uterus. An arcuate uterus does not usually require treatment. A bicornuate or even a duplex uterus may be unified by incising the medial margins of both horns, possibly removing the septum, if present, and resuturing in an anteroposterior fashion so as to enlarge the cavity.

DISEASES OF THE LOWER GENITAL TRACT

Anatomically, the lower genital tract consists of the vulva and the lower half of the vagina. Its arterial supply comes from the branches of the internal pudendal artery, and its lymphatics go primarily to the superficial inguinal nodes. Functionally, the upper vagina and the cervix up to the external os must also be considered as a part of the lower genital tract, since their squamous epithelium is derived from the urogenital sinus. However, the müllerian origin of the vaginal tube has resulted in its arterial supply coming from the internal iliac arteries and its lymphatics going primarily to the nodes surrounding these vessels. Thus, this area has to be considered somewhat as a separate entity as well as being a part of the lower genital tract.

Physiological changes occur with age in the lower genital tract, especially in the thickness of the epithelium and in the acidity of the vaginal fluid. Thus, in the newborn, owing to the maternal estrogens that have passed through the placenta, the vaginal epithelium is thick, and the pH is low. Soon afterward it reverts to the childhood type, consisting only of basal layers of cells and having a higher pH. At puberty the epithelium becomes thicker and undergoes cyclical changes. Greater cornification is noted in the proliferative phase of the cycle. The *p*H is generally in the range of 4.5 to 5.0, although it is somewhat higher just after menstruation. After menopause the epithelium reverts to the childhood type.

Changes also occur as the result of sexual activity and childbirth. With penetration of the vagina, the hymen is stretched or broken and often only skin tags (carunculae myrtiformes) remain. With delivery of the child through the lower genital tract the vagina, introitus, and perineum are greatly stretched. How well they return to their original elastic state may depend on genetic factors (largely unknown), on obstetric factors, such as the size of the infant and the difficulty of the labor, and on obstetric management.

DISORDERS RELATED TO TRAUMA

Traumatic disorders of the lower genital tract may be due to direct trauma, indirect trauma, or pelvic relaxation.

Direct Trauma

Injury to the lower genital tract is rare. It may result from forcible rupture of the hymen, perforation by instruments, damage due to the retention of foreign bodies, or vehicular or similar accidents. Recognition is usually aided by the history and confirmed by thorough examination. Treatment depends on the type of injury.

Indirect Trauma

Indirect trauma occurs more frequently and consists chiefly of fistulas. The common ones include vesicovaginal, urethrovaginal, ureterovaginal, and rectovaginal. They may be due to childbirth, operative injury, radiation, or tumor.

In *vesicovaginal fistula* there is a constant discharge of urine from the vagina with irritation and infection of the vulva and the perineal skin. When the fistula is large, it is usually obvious on pelvic examination. When it is small, insertion of methylene blue into the bladder and subsequent observation of it in the vagina may be conclusive.

Since these fistulas do not tend to heal spontaneously, treatment is usually surgical. They may be closed from the vaginal or transvesical approach or from a combined approach. The first is usually preferable. The primary object is to close separately the bladder mucosa, the fascia between bladder and vagina, and the vaginal mucosa. Where the cervix has been removed, colpocleisis of the upper vagina by denuding the anterior and posterior walls and then sewing them together, excluding the fistula, is the simplest and best procedure.

Urethrovaginal fistula is a rare condition. If it is small and continence is maintained, symptoms may consist only of misdirection of the urinary stream. Provided that some urethral wall remains, repair over a catheter is satisfactory. Large fistulas present problems similar to those of large vesicovaginal fistulas.

Ureterovaginal fistula has become more common following the more radical surgical procedures used in the treatment of pelvic malignancy. Although some close spontaneously, kidney function may be lost and operative repair is usually indicated. This is discussed in the section on urology.

In *rectovaginal fistula* discharge of feces through the vagina is the chief symptom. When the fistula is small, this may be intermittent, occurring only when the patient has diarrhea. Vaginal, vulvar, and perineal infections may follow. Although a small rectovaginal fistula may occasionally close spontaneously, surgical repair is usually the only possible treatment. It follows the same principles for repair as does a vesicovaginal fistula: it may be performed from the vaginal approach, or, if the fistula is high, a combined abdominoperineal or pull-through type of procedure may be done. It is frequently advisable to divert the fecal stream by means of a loop sigmoid or transverse colostomy before proceeding to the repair. When radiation and excessive scarring make future repair impossible, it is better to perform a permanent end sigmoid colostomy.

DISPLACEMENTS OF THE UTERUS AND PELVIC RELAXATION

Normal Position and Support of the Pelvic Organs

The uterus normally lies between the rectum and the bladder with its long axis almost in the horizontal plane so that it covers the top of the empty bladder. In this situation the cervix points almost directly backward, and the corpus bends forward slightly from the cervix. The uterus is held in this position by the fascial planes of the pelvic floor (Fig. 47-3), by the uterine ligaments, and by the pressure of the abdominal contents. The fascial planes of the pelvic floor consist of an area of fibromuscular thickening concentrated around the base of the broad ligament; this is variously called the cardinal or Mackenrodt's ligament. The ligaments of the uterus act as guy ropes to keep the organ in position. The broad ligaments hold it in the middle of the pelvis and

Fig. 47-3. Fascia and muscles of the pelvic floor (seen from below).

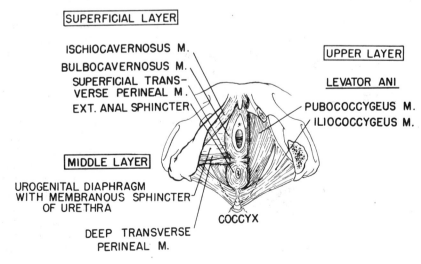

SUPERFICIAL LAYER

ISCHIOCAVERNOSUS M.
BULBOCAVERNOSUS M.
SUPERFICIAL TRANS-
VERSE PERINEAL M.
EXT. ANAL SPHINCTER

MIDDLE LAYER

UROGENITAL DIAPHRAGM
WITH MEMBRANOUS SPHINCTER
OF URETHRA

DEEP TRANSVERSE
PERINEAL M.

UPPER LAYER

LEVATOR ANI

PUBOCOCCYGEUS M.
ILIOCOCCYGEUS M.

COCCYX

keep it up. The uterosacral ligaments pull the cervix back. The round ligaments may exert some effect on holding the fundus forward, but the weight of the abdominal contents is probably of most importance in this regard.

The pelvic organs, including the bladder, the urethra, and the rectum, are also supported by the muscles and the fascia of the pelvic floor. These consist of three layers: (1) the upper pelvic diaphragm of the levator ani muscles; (2) the triangular ligament, extending forward from the deep transverse perinei muscles at the base; and (3) the superficial pelvic diaphragm, consisting of the superficial transverse perinei, the bulbocavernosus, and ischiocavernosus muscles.

Childbirth and age normally result in changes in the position of the pelvic organs. Some weakening of the ligaments may be expected to follow vaginal delivery, with consequent slight descent of the uterus and increased relaxation of the walls of the vagina. After menopause the fundus of the uterus commonly loses its forward inclination and lies in the midposition so that it extends straight upward from the cervix.

Displacements of the Uterus

Anterior and lateral displacements of the uterus occur occasionally, but they are usually the result of an enlarging tumor or abscess and are not of clinical importance in themselves.

Posterior displacements of the uterus are of more significance, although not as much as was thought 40 years ago. They may be divided into three types (Fig. 47-4); (1) retrocession, where the whole uterus is displaced toward the back of the pelvis; (2) retroversion, where the cervix is tilted forward so as to point anteriorly on vaginal examination but retains its relationship with the corpus; and (3) retroflexion, where the corpus is bent backward on the cervix. The most important displacement is retroflexion, but all three may be found together or separately and may be of varying degrees.

Retrocession and retroversion are more likely to occur in older and especially parous women. Retroflexion is more commonly of congenital origin or associated with adnexal inflammation, endometriosis, or tumors and cysts of the uterus or adnexa.

Clinical Features. Retrocession and retroversion seldom cause symptoms. Retroflexion, congenitally present in 20%

to 30% of women, may also be asymptomatic or may contribute to backache or dyspareunia (often worse just before menstruation), dysmenorrhea, or possibly abortion, because of an unfavorable location for nidation or incarceration of the enlarging uterus. Symptoms of acquired retroflexion are similar but are often overshadowed by those of the primary and associated disorder.

Diagnosis. The diagnosis is made readily on pelvic examination, unless the patient is very obese or holds herself very tense. Sometimes it may be made more difficult by the presence of a myoma on the anterior surface of the uterus or of an adnexal mass that lies behind the uterus and simulates the retroflexed corpus.

Treatment. If there are no symptoms, no treatment is needed. Congenital retroflexion, without evidence of associated disease, used to be treated by knee-chest exercises (to permit the uterus to drop forward) or manual replacement and maintenance of the uterus in the anteflexed position with a Smith or Hodge pessary. Based on the results, uterine suspension was often performed. Now these procedures are seldom indicated except when combined with others used for a specific disorder such as endometriosis. The principles of operative treatment in such circumstances include shortening the round ligaments and changing the direction of their pull by attaching them to the back of the uterus (Baldy-Webster), and shortening the round ligaments by attaching them to the abdominal wall (Gilliam).

Pelvic Relaxation

Pelvic relaxation includes the following conditions, which may occur together or separately:
1. Prolapse of the uterus (descensus uteri)
2. Prolapse of the intestine into the pouch of Douglas (enterocele)
3. Prolapse of the bladder into the anterior vaginal wall (cystocele)
4. Prolapse of the urethra into the anterior vaginal wall (urethrocele)
5. Prolapse of the rectum into the posterior vaginal wall (rectocele)
6. Weakness of the perineum (relaxed vaginal outlet)

These conditions occur most commonly, but not invariably, in parous and older women. Primarily, they are due to an exaggeration of the normal relaxation of the pelvic ligaments and support that occurs during childbirth and after the menopause. A contributing factor may be traumatic prolonged labor, although the importance of this is difficult to estimate.

Clinical Features. Prolapse of the uterus may be divided conveniently into three stages (Fig. 47-5). First-degree prolapse occurs when the cervix descends below its normal position in the vaginal canal. In second-degree prolapse, the cervix reaches the introitus. In third-degree prolapse the cervix is outside the introitus. The term *procidentia* may be used when the whole uterus protrudes. The exact degree of prolapse of the uterus may not be realized on examination unless the patient is asked to stand or strain down vigorously; straining may be reproduced by pulling the cervix down with a tenaculum. The descent of the cervix may be felt by the patient as a lump in the vagina, which is noticed on prolonged standing or straining. If the cervix becomes irritated or eroded as a result of its descent, vaginal discharge or bleeding may be noted.

Enterocele, in addition to accompanying other types of prolapse, may occur by itself following vaginal hysterectomy.

Fig. 47-4. Retrodisplacements of the uterus.

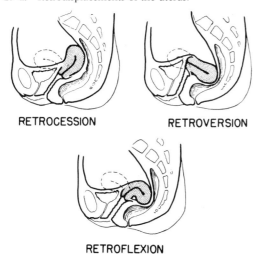

RETROCESSION   RETROVERSION

RETROFLEXION

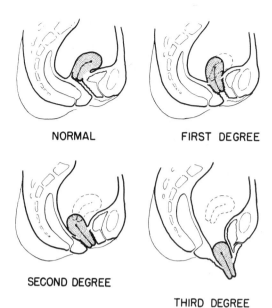

Fig. 47-5. Degrees of prolapse of the uterus.

It usually does not cause symptoms until it is felt as a protruding mass. Incarceration occurs only very rarely.

Cystocele and urethrocele are frequently associated. They may be asymptomatic, but, since they predispose to the retention of urine, infection commonly occurs. In the case of urethrocele this leads to burning and frequency of urination. On occasion a urethral diverticulum may develop. In the case of cystocele, frequency and urgency of urination, together with suprapubic pain, occur. Infection is commonly recurrent and eventually may involve the upper urinary tract. If marked cystocele is associated with prolapse of the uterus, obstruction of the lower ureter may occur with resulting hydronephrosis and decreased renal function.

Minor degrees of *rectocele* do not normally cause symptoms. If the rectocele is large, fecal material may be retained in it and the patient may have trouble expelling it unless she manually pushes the rectocele back.

Weakness of the perineum is due to damage to the smaller muscles, such as may occur during childbirth. By itself it usually causes no symptoms, except perhaps for a sensation of gaping at the introitus. Sexual symptoms (of which the patient may complain) are unlikely to be solely due to perineal relaxation. Other contributing factors should be sought. If the anal sphincter has been divided, incontinence of feces may result, especially if the stools are loose.

Involuntary discharge of urine on straining, coughing, laughing, or sneezing (stress incontinence) is a common concomitant of pelvic relaxation. Much investigation has been devoted to elucidating its cause. That it is not necessarily the result of age or parity is shown by the study of Crist and associates, who found that 31% of 695 nulliparous women reported some degree of stress incontinence.

Diagnosis. The diagnosis of pelvic relaxation is usually made readily on examination. The anterior vaginal wall may be observed by having the patient strain down while pushing the posterior wall backward. The posterior wall may be observed by having the patient strain down while pushing the anterior wall forward.

Stress incontinence presents a special problem in diagnosis. Mechanical stress incontinence, as included under the general term of pelvic relaxation, is due primarily to inadequate support of the bladder base. An important concept is that the posterior urethrovesical angle becomes much greater than the usual 90° to 100° (type 1) or the angle of inclination of the urethra to the perpendicular is greatly increased (type II).

Mechanical stress incontinence can be tested during pelvic examination by manually restoring and maintaining the normal posterior urethrovesical angle (vesical neck elevation test). Confirmation of the anatomical deformity can be obtained from a cystourethrogram. Other causes of incontinence should be excluded by urine culture, cystometrography, cystoscopy, and intravenous pyelography.

Treatment. Prophylaxis of pelvic relaxation by good obstetric practice is very important. During the second stage of labor the fascial supports of the uterus, the bladder and the rectum, and the small muscles of the perineum are greatly stretched and may even tear. Any technique that prevents these fibers rupturing or stretching beyond their capacity to return to normal is of value. In the past 2 or 3 decades it has been felt by obstetricians in this country that shortening of the second stage of labor by performing an episiotomy and extracting the infant by forceps applied at the pelvic outlet would achieve this objective. A logical approach in most normal women would seem to be by antepartum perineal muscle exercises (Fig. 47-6). If these are combined with adequate preparation of the patient for the second stage of labor, and gradual delivery is allowed, good perineal muscle tone may be restored post partum. Of course, this does not preclude the use of forceps if the second stage is abnormally prolonged or if the patient is unable to take advantage of such exercises.

In line with the prophylaxis of pelvic relaxation, the primary treatment for minor or moderate relaxation, especially in women of childbearing age, should be by nonoperative measures. This involves the patient's learning to contract the pubococcygei and the other perineal muscles effectively. She can conveniently be asked to stop the flow of urine each time she voids or, alternatively, to contract and draw in the perineal muscles 8 to 10 times in succession three times daily. The strength of the perineal muscles may be tested by using a perineometer, a type of intravaginal balloon with a gauge to indicate squeezing pressure. If the patient is simply asked to contract the muscles on the examining hand, a good indication of their strength may be obtained. Perineal exercises are particularly valuable when the patient has some stress incontinence and may be useful in improving sexual responsiveness.

When the anatomical changes are very marked, or nonoperative treatment has not produced improvement, operation is indicated. Before this is done any urinary tract infection should be investigated and treated. Vaginal infection also should be treated, and in the postmenopausal woman improvement of the condition of the vaginal mucosa may be obtained by the use of estrogens, preferably as a vaginal cream, before operation.

Fig. 47-6. Direction of muscle contraction in perineal exercises.

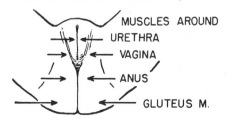

MUSCLES AROUND
URETHRA
VAGINA
ANUS
GLUTEUS M.

Repair of the prolapsed uterus is often best handled by vaginal hysterectomy, when childbearing is no longer desired or marked prolapse is present. Lesser procedures, such as amputation of the cervix and fixation of the lower part of the parametria to the cervix (Manchester-Fothergill operation), may occasionally be used in the younger patient.

In the older and debilitated patient who is a poor operative risk, prolapse occasionally may be treated satisfactorily by occlusion of the vagina (LeFort procedure: colpocleisis). This involves denudation and approximation of the anterior and the posterior vaginal walls, leaving lateral channels for drainage when the uterus is still present. Local anesthesia can be used, and the procedure may not be as traumatic as the other procedures described above.

When operation cannot be performed for any reason, relief of symptoms may be obtained by the use of a pessary. Several ring or inflatable types are available. They act by distending the vagina and suspending the cervix at a higher level than before and work best if perineal relaxation is minimal. Pessaries should be removed and replaced every 6 to 8 weeks and the vagina inspected for possible ulceration.

Repair of a cystocele and urethrocele (anterior colporrhaphy) or a rectocele (posterior colporrhaphy) consists of excising the excess vaginal mucosa over the organ concerned, plicating the fascia, and resuturing the vagina. Repair of a rectocele usually should be combined with repair of the perineum with some narrowing of the introitus. Unnecessarily tight posterior perineorrhaphies may lead to postoperative dyspareunia. Repair of the anal sphincter can be combined with a perineorrhapy by identifying the divided ends of the muscle and suturing them together.

Special problems in vaginal repair occur with enterocele or when stress incontinence is marked. As in the repair of any hernia, the sac of the enterocele must be dissected out and the peritoneum securely closed. Frequently, it is difficult to add any support to the repair from below, since the uterosacral ligaments are attenuated. In the primary repair of an enterocele an attempt should be made to close these as well as possible. However, in recurrent enterocele, obliteration of the posterior cul-de-sac from the abdominal approach may be indicated (Moschcowitz procedure).

Operation for stress incontinence is indicated if conservative measures such as exercises have not improved the symptoms. Operations are more likely to be successful if other than mechanical causes have been excluded and if the normal urethrovesical relationships are restored. If cystocele or urethrocele is present, vaginal repair (anterior colporrhaphy) with creation of a new vesicourethral junction is appropriate. If there is no relaxation, suprapubic urethrovesical suspension may be used. Recurrent mechanical stress incontinence may require special "sling" procedures, using rectus fascia or synthetic materials.

INFECTIONS

Gonorrhea

Gonorrhea is caused by the diplococcus *Neisseria gonorrhoeae,* which is identified by the fact that it is intracellular, gram-negative, and oxidase-positive on culture (Fig. 47-7). It is transmitted primarily by sexual intercourse, although occasionally infection may occur by contact with an infected towel, toilet seat, or douche nozzle.

Gonorrhea affects primarily the lower genital tract. Squamous epithelium is resistant, but the organism flourishes in the glands of the urethra (Skene's glands), the vulva

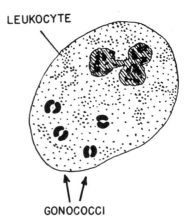

Fig. 47-7. Gonococci within a leukocyte.

(Bartholin's glands), and the cervix. Secondary invasion of the uterus and the tubes by the surface route and spread to distant parts of the body may occur, especially at the time of menstruation. These serious consequences will be considered among the diseases of the upper genital tract.

Clinical Features. The acute stage is relatively mild and may not be noticed by the patient. Within a few days after infection, dryness and irritation of the vagina are noticed. There may be some urinary frequency and burning on urination. A small amount of discharge appears. These symptoms may become more marked or may pass away. The vagina and the vulva appear reddened, and there may be more or less purulent discharge.

Spontaneous cure of the acute infection may occur, but it is likely to become subacute and chronic. In this case the organism is maintained in the cervical glands, Bartholin's glands, and Skene's glands. The clinical appearance is one of continuous purulent discharge and irritation of the vagina and the vulva from the pus, associated with urethritis. From both the acute and the chronic stages infection of the upper genital tract may result, and this remains a constant hazard while the infection is untreated.

In children the organism affects primarily the vagina and the vulva. A persistent purulent vaginal discharge occurs. There is usually no spread to the upper genital tract.

Diagnosis. The diagnosis can be made initially by Gram stain and more definitively by anaerobic culture.

Treatment. Penicillin is the best treatment for gonorrhea and has the advantage of being effective for simultaneously incubating syphilis. Gonococcal resistance to antibiotics is relative rather than absolute. The preferred regimen consists of 4.8 million units of aqueous procaine penicillin G given intramuscularly, divided into two doses. In addition, 1 g probenecid should be given orally, preferably 30 minutes before the injection. Alternatively tetracycline hydrochloride may be given in a dose of 1.5 g initially by mouth and 0.5 g four times daily for 4 days. Slightly less effective are oral ampicillin, 3.5 g, or amoxicillin, 3 g, each with 1 g probenecid by mouth. Patients who are allergic to the penicillins or probenecid should be treated with oral tetracycline as above. Patients who cannot tolerate tetracycline may be treated with spectinomycin hydrochloride, 2 g, in one intramuscular injection.

Local treatment in the acute stage should be confined to rest, local washing with soap and warm water, and careful attention to avoid infecting other persons: the latter involves avoidance of intercourse as well as sterilization and disposal of infected linen, until cure is established. The tracing and the treatment of contacts are also important.

It is frequently difficult to be sure that cure of the infection has actually occurred. Ideally, at least two negative cultures should be obtained. It is best to take at least one of these immediately after menstruation when the infection commonly becomes active again.

In chronic cases both diagnosis and treatment are more difficult. Eradication of the foci of infection in Skene's, Bartholin's, and the cervical glands may be necessary. Such treatment, especially in the cervix, is not without danger of infection of the upper genital tract.

In children antibiotics are the best method of treatment, but in resistant cases it may be advisable to attempt to convert the vaginal epithelium to the adult type by administration of estrogens.

Trichomoniasis

Trichomoniasis is caused by the flagellated protozoan, *Trichomonas vaginalis*. The organism is quite common, particularly among women with poor personal hygiene. It may exist for long periods in the vagina without causing symptoms. It has also been found in the upper genital tract, in urine, and in the bloodstream. In males it has been found in the urine, the prostatic secretion, and the semen. Thus, although the infection is primarily vaginal, it may also be generalized. How a quiescent infection is changed into an active infection is not well understood, although psychosomatic factors may be important.

Clinical Features. The patient complains of a profuse irritating vaginal discharge that frequently has a foul odor. Frequency and burning on urination are commonly noted. On examination a foamy yellow discharge is seen in the vagina. The vagina itself is reddened and may show punctate red spots. The cervix also may be involved.

Diagnosis. The motile organism may be detected by microscopic examination of a small amount of discharge mixed with saline (Fig. 47-8). The use of lubricant for examination may destroy the motility of the organism and make diagnosis more difficult. A large number of pus cells compared with epithelial cells may indicate a more severe and resistant infection.

Treatment. The preferred method of treatment is to use the oral trichomonacide metronidazole 250 mg three times daily for 7 to 10 days, or two doses of 1 g 12 hours apart. Cure rates of 90% or better may be expected with metronidazole. The patient's sex partner should also be treated in the same manner.

Fungal Infections

Infection by *Candida albicans* or other fungi is relatively common, especially in pregnancy.

Clinical Features. Itching of the vulva usually is more prominent than discharge. The vagina and the vulva may appear inflamed on examination, and patches of white cheesy material are seen clinging to the epithelium.

Diagnosis. A small amount of discharge may be mixed with 10% potassium hydroxide (to obliterate the cellular elements) and examined microscopically. The fungi are seen as fine branching and budding threads (Fig. 47-9).

Treatment. Candidiasis can be effectively treated by the intravaginal insertion of nystatin tablets, 2% miconazole cream, or chlortrimazole tablets or cream. For the occasional resistant case, repeated painting of the vagina with 1% aqueous gentian violet may be effective. Treatment of the sex partner with fungicidal cream may also be necessary.

Herpes Genitalis

Herpesvirus type II (HSV II) infections of the lower genital tract have become much more common. They are sexually transmitted with an incubation period of 2 to 12 days. Small vesicles develop on the vulva that break down into very painful ulcers. The diagnosis is made by culture of the virus or by the appearance on a smear of multinucleated giant cells with perinuclear halos. The infection subsides in 7 to 21 days, but recurrence is common. There is currently no satisfactory cure. Some symptomatic relief can be given.

Other Infections

Syphilis, chancroid, granuloma inguinale, and lymphogranuloma venereum may also affect the lower genital tract. These are identified by the demonstration of the specific organism involved or, in the case of lymphogranuloma, by the Frei test. As a rule they do not spread to involve the upper genital tract, although marked and prolonged local changes may result.

A common cause of vaginitis is *Gardnerella vaginalis*. A

Fig. 47-8. *Trichomonas vaginalis.*

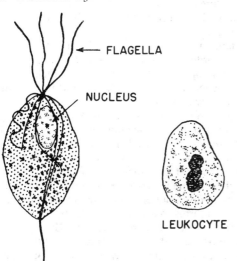

FLAGELLA

NUCLEUS

LEUKOCYTE

Fig. 47-9. *Candida.*

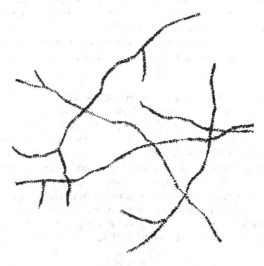

persistent vaginal discharge with an unpleasant odor is noted. The disorder is diagnosed by exclusion of *Trichomonas* and *Candida* and by identification of "clue" cells or epithelial cells coated with bacteria so that they appear stippled. Treatment with metronidazole for 7 days is effective.

Sometimes no specific cause can be found for the discharge of which the patient complains, and culture reveals only a mixed group of organisms. In this connection it is well to remember that vaginal discharge is frequently a symptom of psychosomatic disturbance and that attention to these factors, particularly in relation to the patient's sexual feelings, may be curative. Local treatment may consist of intravaginal application of bacteriostatic sulfa creams and attempts to restore the normal acidity of the vagina by acid jellies or by vinegar douches.

BENIGN CYSTS AND TUMORS

Condylomata Acuminata

These lesions appear as single or multiple projections on the perineum and vulva and may extend into the vagina and cervix. Microscopically they are seen to be papillomas. They are of viral origin and are often associated with chronic irritation or vaginal discharge of any sort. They are now found much more frequently than in the past. They may grow to a large size, especially during pregnancy. Single or small condylomata acuminata may be treated with single or repeated applications of 25% podophyllin (protecting the surrounding skin with mineral oil and washing off the podophyllin within 1 hour) or with cryosurgery. Infection present in the lower genital tract should also be treated vigorously. Larger or resistant growths may require extensive cauterization or surgical removal. Laser therapy is also effective. Condylomata may be confused with verrucous carcinoma and may often themselves have malignant potential. Careful follow-up is therefore necessary.

Urethral Caruncle

Caruncle is the term given to a small red growth that develops just at or inside the external urinary meatus. Pathologically, these lesions have the appearance of granulomas, although in some there may be evidence of papilloma formation. They are not true tumors and in general do not become malignant. Clinically, they may give no symptoms at all, or the patient may notice pain in the area, burning on urination, or bleeding. They may be 1 to 2 mm to more than 1 cm in diameter. Care should be taken to avoid confusion in diagnosis with eversion of the mucosa of the urethra, which is common, or with carcinoma of the urethra, which is very rare. Treatment, if indicated, is by excision or cauterization, and adequate anesthesia, usually general, is needed for both of these procedures.

Cysts and Abscesses of Bartholin's Glands

Obstruction of the duct of Bartholin's gland is common. This leads to retention of secretions (cyst) or pus (abscess). Abscess may be a common sequel of gonorrheal infection, although it is more likely to be due to nonspecific causes.
Clinical Features. A cyst may cause no symptoms except the sensation of a mass in the vulvar region. Abscess formation is accompanied by pain, redness, tenderness, and fever. Tender inguinal nodes are often palpable.
Diagnosis. A Bartholin's cyst lies at the posterior end of the introitus, as contrasted to other labial cysts, which lie more

anteriorly and laterally, and with abscesses resulting from perianal infections, which are felt more posteriorly.
Treatment. An abscess should be opened widely and antibiotics given. A permanent cure may be attempted even in the acute case by suturing the margins of the abscess to the adjacent skin. This type of management by marsupialization is most satisfactory for the definitive treatment of Bartholin's cysts and is simpler than excision.

Other Cysts and Tumors

A wide variety of cysts and tumors are seen in this area. The most common are vaginal inclusion cysts, cysts of wolffian duct remnants, or tumors arising from the skin of the vulva, especially fibromas and hydroadenomas. Simple surgical excision is the treatment of choice.

MALIGNANT TUMORS

Cancer of Vulva and Surrounding Structures

Cancer of the vulva comprises between 3% and 4% of all cancers of the female genital tract. Over 95% are squamous cell carcinomas, although melanomas, adenocarcinomas of Bartholin's gland, and basal cell carcinomas are found occasionally. The lesion may start anywhere on the external genitalia. Multiple origins are not uncommon. From the initial point the disease may extend backward to the rectum, anteriorly into the urethra, or upward into the vagina. Metastasis takes place to the inguinal nodes, often to the opposite side or bilaterally, and thence to the femoral and the deep pelvic nodes.
Clinical Features. The symptoms of cancer of the vulva are few in the early stages. It is primarily a disease of older women, the average age at presentation being at least 60 years. Frequently, there is a history of some chronic epithelial dystrophy. Slight itching or burning of the vulva may be noted, with bleeding only rarely being observed. Often the feeling of a hard lump in this region may be the only thing to bring the patient to a physician. Examination reveals one or more suspiciously hard nodules, parts of which may be ulcerated and may bleed easily. Inguinal nodes are frequently palpable, but this may be due to inflammation rather than to metastatic tumor, unless the nodes are very hard and fixed.
Diagnosis. The diagnosis can usually be suspected on examination but should always be confirmed by adequate biopsy before definitive treatment is started. This can often be done with the use of local anesthesia as an outpatient procedure.
Treatment. It is important to delineate the extent of the disease according to an acceptable staging classification. The system developed by the Cancer Committee of the International Federation of Gynecology and Obstetrics, although not ideal, is widely used.

Surgery provides the best treatment available at present. When the lesion is intraepithelial, wide local excision is usually preferable, especially in younger women. Occasionally when the intraepithelial lesions are widespread, vulvectomy and skin graft may be performed. The use of the laser in intraepithelial lesions is currently under evaluation. When invasion is present, the most logical approach, and one that conforms to accepted standards of cancer surgery, is that originally recommended by Way. The inguinal nodes, the tissue between the inguinal region and the vulva, and the vulva itself are removed *en bloc* in one procedure (Fig.

47-10). Extraperitoneal removal of the nodes above the inguinal ligament (up to the bifurcation of the aorta) is advisable if inguinal nodes (or Cloquet's node) show cancer on frozen section. Morley reports an overall 5-year survival rate of 67% in one large series. When regional lymph nodes were positive, the survival rate was 38%. The procedure is a formidable one, since many of the patients are old, debilitated, and affected by intercurrent disease. Even in the best hands these incisions do not heal well and later postoperative swelling of the legs is common, although usually temporary. In some poor-risk patients it may be well to stage the procedure, although this sacrifices the principle of removal of the cancer and metastatic nodes in continuity.

The significance of microinvasion is not as clear as in carcinoma of the cervix with regard to the involvement of lymph nodes. When only one area of invasion is seen less than 5 mm below the basement membrane and vascular and lymphatic spaces are not involved, vulvectomy alone or wide local excision may be appropriate, especially in elderly or poor-risk women.

In patients who are considered to be too poor risks to stand any surgical procedure or in recurrent disease, radiation may be of palliative and possibly of curative value; it is used best in the form of implantation of radium needles usually with external irradiation.

The above type of procedure is applicable to most invasive vulvar carcinomas. For more extensive lesions it may be necessary to perform an anterior, posterior, or total exenteration, in addition to vulvectomy and regional lymphadenectomy. It may be noted that it is quite practical to remove up to half of the urethra without the patient's becoming incontinent, and a large portion of the vagina also may be removed from below without difficulty.

A basal cell carcinoma of the vulva does not need extensive vulvectomy, and a wide local excision is sufficient. The same is true for a rare condition, Paget's disease of the vulva.

Cancer of the Vagina

Primary cancer of the vagina is rare, comprising from 1% to 2% of all cancers of the female genital tract. Metastatic cancer of the vagina may occur from cervix, endometrium, ovary, or other organs. Primary cancer is almost always of the squamous cell type. It tends to grow in the long axis of the vagina, and because of its proximity to the rectum on the posterior wall and to the bladder on the anterior wall it may involve either of these organs at an early stage. It also spreads laterally to the paravaginal and paracervical tissues. Metastases may pass to both iliac (from the upper half) and inguinal (from the lower half) nodes. Carcinoma of the urethra, usually of the transitional cell type, is often difficult to distinguish from primary carcinoma of the vagina. Intraepithelial neoplasia of the vagina is now being reported more frequently.

Clinical Features. Painless vaginal bleeding or discharge are usually the first symptoms, although pain and particularly dyspareunia are not uncommon. Usually it is found in the postmenopausal woman, but it may occur at an earlier age. Examination reveals a hard nodule infiltrating the vaginal wall. Ulceration and a tendency to bleed easily on manipulation are common.

Diagnosis. Diagnosis is made on the basis of clinical examination and biopsy.

Treatment. Treatment is difficult because of the close proximity of the bladder and rectum. The tumor is relatively radiosensitive and irradiation (external and internal) remains the primary method of treatment. Five-year survival rates from collected series are reported to be 74% for Stage I, 45% for Stage II, 16% for Stage III, and 9% for Stage IV (according to the staging classification of the International Federation of Gynecology and Obstetrics). Radical surgical procedures (exenteration) have been recommended by some authors, but long-term data on the results of these are insufficient for evaluation. Intraepithelial disease is managed by local excision, laser therapy, or intravaginal use of 5-fluorouracil cream.

Clear-Cell Adenocarcinoma

In recent years attention has been drawn to the relationship between the ingestion of diethylstilbestrol (DES) during pregnancy and the subsequent development of abnormalities of the genital tract in the female offspring. A very high proportion of these girls are found, during adolescence, to have ridges and furrows on the cervix and areas of columnar epithelium in the cervix or vagina. Clear-cell adenocarcinoma has been found in a few such patients. It is important that girls whose mothers took DES during pregnancy be examined, preferably after menarche, by means of a speculum, cytologic studies, and colposcopy. Specific treatment is usually not given but patients should be followed regularly, since the eventual outcome of these abnormalities is not yet known. When a frank invasive adenocarcinoma is discovered, the best treatment appears to be surgical by

Fig. 47-10. Skin incision for radical vulvectomy and bilateral inguinal node dissection.

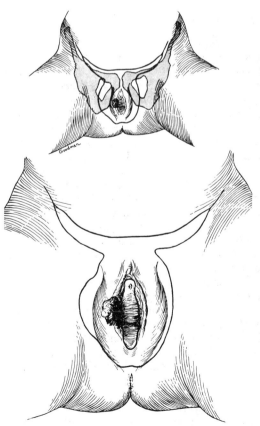

radical hysterectomy, with or without vaginectomy. In such exposed girls, abnormalities of the upper genital tract and reproductive difficulties have also been noted.

OTHER DISEASES

Atrophic Vaginitis

Often found in postmenopausal women and in premenopausal women who have lost ovarian function, atrophic vaginitis is due primarily to lack of estrogens. Clinically, it is characterized by a thin, irritating vaginal discharge, which at times may be bloody. It is an important cause of dyspareunia. On examination the vaginal mucosa is reddened and presents many petechiae. Provided that cancer of the upper and the lower genital tracts has been excluded, treatment with oral estrogens or intravaginal applications of estrogenic cream usually is helpful.

Vulvitis

The vulva is subject to a variety of acute and subacute inflammations due to irritants or allergents such as tight clothing, synthetic fabrics, perineal pads, soaps, detergents, deodorants, or various medications. The patient complains of burning, chafing, irritation, discharge, itching, and occasional bleeding. On examination the vulva appears red and inflamed with minimal discharge or bleeding. Possible irritants should be discontinued. Cotton underwear should be used, and in severe cases application of cold witch hazel or Burow's solution is helpful. White patches suggestive of dystrophy should be biopsied. Additional measures include keeping the area dry and using cortisone ointment.

Vulvar Dystrophies

Vulvar dystrophies cause a variety of symptoms and visible changes. The former include itching, burning, and occasional bleeding, often of long standing. On examination the vulva and perineal skin appear white, red, raised, or fissured. Biopsy of all suspicious areas is essential to identify the underlying condition and to exclude cancer and is best done in the office using local anesthesia and a 3- or 4-mm Keyes punch. Suture closure is not usually necessary; pressure and a styptic such as Monsel's solution is sufficient. Areas appropriate for biopsy can be delineated by staining with toluidine blue and colposcopy.

Two varieties of dystrophy are common. The first is lichen sclerosus, which is characterized by thin epithelium and acellular subepithelial tissue containing inflammatory cells. Treatment is by 3% testosterone in petrolatum. A second type is hypertrophic dystrophy in which the epithelium is thickened and shows hyperkeratosis, acanthosis, and an inflammatory infiltrate. Treatment with cortisone cream is usually effective. Occasionally, mixed dystrophies with elements of both disorders are seen, requiring alternation of therapies. Neither of these conditions are premalignant *per se*, but varying degrees of epithelial atypia are sometimes found in hypertrophic dystrophy, which requires wide local excision and careful follow-up.

Pruritus Vulvae

Itching is a common concomitant of vulvitis and vulvar dystrophy. A specific cause for the itching should be identified when possible. Abnormal glucose metabolism should be checked by a glucose tolerance test. Treatment may be difficult. Local applications to relieve itching, dietary advice, and attention to psychological factors may be important.

As a last resort, local injection of alcohol around the vulva may be used.

DISEASES OF THE CERVIX

TRAUMA

Lacerations of the cervix are an inevitable result of delivery. They occur usually at 3 or 9 o'clock and occasionally at other sites. Immediate dangers are hemorrhage or extension into the broad ligament. Later, if the laceration has extended high in the cervical canal, incompetence of the internal os of the cervix may result.

INFECTIONS

Infections of the cervix, especially acute infections, often accompany those of the lower genital tract such as trichomoniasis, candidiasis, gonorrhea, or those due to nonspecific causes. Chronic cervicitis can be diagnosed histologically in the majority of cervices, especially in parous women, by the presence of inflammatory cells. Tuberculosis or other granulomatous processes occur rarely.

Clinical Features. The symptoms of acute infection of the cervix are indistinguishable from those due to infection of the vulva and vagina (*i.e.*, discharge, itching, and irritation). On inspection, in acute cases, the cervix is red and covered with discharge. Chronic cervicitis frequently has no definite clinical features.

Diagnosis. The diagnostic measures are the same as for infections of the vulva and vagina.

Treatment. Acute cervicitis is treated similarly to acute vulvovaginitis. Treatment of chronic cervicitis *per se* is rarely indicated. When discharge is significant but not related to dysplasia of the cervix, cryosurgery may be used.

BENIGN TUMORS

Cervical Polyps

The most common benign tumors of the cervix, polyps are small pedunculated growths that arise from the endocervix or, more rarely, from the external surface of the cervix. They are often multiple and are composed of a connective tissue stroma covered by columnar epithelium, which is thrown into many folds. Inflammatory changes are common, and frequently the tip is congested. Squamous metaplasia of the epithelium is common, but malignant change occurs in less than 1%.

Clinical Features. There may be no symptoms, or the patient may notice slight vaginal bleeding or discharge. Examination of the cervix usually will show the lesion. Polyps are soft and sometimes may be missed on palpation.

Diagnosis. The important conditions to be distinguished from cervical polyps are endometrial polyps, pedunculated submucous myomas, and cancer of the cervix. Other benign tumors are occasionally seen in the cervix.

Treatment. If irregular vaginal bleeding has occurred, particularly in the postmenopausal woman, dilation and curettage should be performed to exclude intrauterine causes. The polyp itself may be twisted off and the base cauterized with silver nitrate or by cryotherapy to control bleeding. All polyps should be examined microscopically to rule out malignant changes.

Cervical Intraepithelial Neoplasia

During the past 10 years cytologic and colposcopic studies have considerably clarified the process of cervical dysplasia and neoplasia, even though the precise causes and their mechanisms are not understood. The most important concept is the behavior of the squamocolumnar junction and the transformation zone, which is described in detail by Coppleson and associates. Where the columnar epithelium meets the squamous epithelium (transformation zone) metaplasia is constantly occurring. In early life this junction may be situated well out on the visible portion of the cervix. During reproductive life its level may fluctuate, and after the menopause it may recede into the endocervical canal. The normal metaplastic process may result in the ducts of the cervical glands being covered by the new epithelium, with the subsequent development of the small or large cysts (nabothian cysts). In some women, for genetic or other reasons, atypical metaplasia occurs, and an abnormal transformation zone develops. This gives rise to the finding of abnormal cells on cytologic studies and abnormal findings on colposcopic examination. These changes potentially lead to carcinoma *in situ* and eventually after an uncertain time interval to invasive carcinoma. An appropriate name for this sequence of events is cervical intraepithelial neoplasia (CIN). CIN I is equivalent to mild dysplasia; CIN II, to moderate dysplasia; and CIN III, to severe dysplasia or carcinoma *in situ*.

An important unsolved question is the reversibility of the process. Dysplasia, carcinoma *in situ*, and invasive carcinoma appear to be a continuum, especially since all stages may be seen in sections of the same cervix (Fig. 47-11). There is no doubt that in infections such as trichomoniasis, dysplastic changes occur and later disappear. It seems likely that these changes may regress if they are only mild, but if they are moderate or severe they are, in the long run, irreversible. The time intervals in the steps of progression have not been determined. However, the average age of women discovered to have invasive carcinoma is about 10 years greater than those with carcinoma *in situ*.

Clinical Features. It is almost axiomatic that women with dysplasia of the cervix have few or no symptoms and that the severity of the symptoms bears no relation to the degree of dysplasia. Therefore, early detection of these changes in the asymptomatic women becomes very important. Improvement in methods of detection gives promise of greatly reducing or eradicating the most serious end-result of dysplasia, invasive carcinoma.

Detection. Cytologic studies form the basis of screening. Ideally, women should have these performed annually if they are over the age of 18 or are sexually active. The procedure is technically simple and can be performed by a nurse-clinician, but it should be accompanied by a screening pelvic examination. For complete study, smears should be taken from the ectocervix and from the endocervix. Smears should be fixed promptly. They are usually stained by Papanicolaou's method or a modification thereof. The original Papanicolaou classification is commonly used for reporting. In this, five classes are recognized: (I) normal; (II) slightly abnormal, possibly due to inflammatory changes; (III) suspicious; (IV) occasional malignant cells, and (V) many malignant cells. Experienced cytopathologists now frequently report the specific atypicalities represented by the cells they see (*e.g.*, inflammatory changes; mild, moderate, or severe dysplasia; carcinoma *in situ*; or invasive carcinoma). However, it is still essential to obtain a tissue diagnosis before treatment is begun. It also should be pointed out that properly taken specimens for cytologic studies will also provide information about the patient's hormonal status

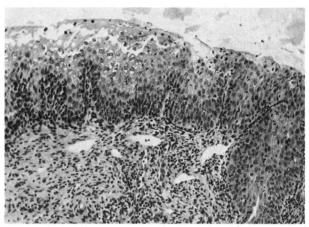

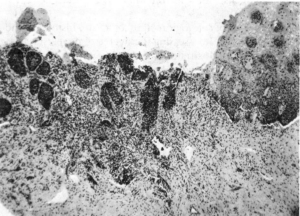

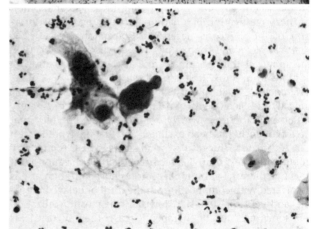

Fig. 47-11. Epithelium of the cervix, showing transition from normal stratified squamous type to intraepithelial carcinoma (*top*) and to invasive carcinoma (*center*). Cervical smear (*bottom*) shows malignant cells with large, irregular, dark-staining nuclei.

and the presence or absence of bacteria or other infectious organisms.

Diagnosis. Wider use of the colposcope has greatly facilitated the diagnosis of CIN. Previously, only random or four-quadrant biopsies could be taken. Unless there was an obvious lesion, these were necessarily blind. By means of the colposcope the surface of the cervix can be examined at a magnification of from 9 to 40 times and areas of abnormality can be selected for spot biopsy with an appropriate instrument. Colposcopic examination is best used in women who have abnormal results of cytologic screening studies and in whom there is no obvious gross lesion that can be biopsied. The degree of CIN is often evaluated colposcopically.

Careful histologic examination of biopsies is essential. Although opinion with regard to individual lesions may vary, there is fairly good agreement that in mild dysplasia the basal cell layers of the epithelium are replaced by abnormal cells. These abnormalities are characterized by lack of cellular differentiation, lack of cellular polarity, numerous and atypical mitotic figures, and pleomorphism of cells with variably enlarged hyperchromatic nuclei. In moderate dysplasia about half of the epithelium is involved; in severe dysplasia two thirds to almost all the layers are replaced by abnormal cells. Often the last cannot be distinguished from carcinoma *in situ,* which is variously diagnosed according to the malignant appearance of the cells or to the complete replacement of all layers of the epithelium with neoplastic cells, but with retention of an intact basement membrane.

Correlation of cytologic, colposcopic, and histologic findings is important in assessing the degree of neoplasia. If the findings from all studies are congruent (*e.g.,* cytologic findings of moderate dysplasia, colposcopic changes characteristic of moderate dysplasia, and histologic findings showing moderate dysplasia) treatment may begin without further investigation. If, however, microinvasion is found on any one study (even if the others do not support it), it is important to find an explanation and to exclude invasive cancer, since the treatment of the latter is much more radical. If there is any doubt about the completeness of any of the studies (*e.g.,* if the endocervix cannot be seen by colposcopy, if the area of abnormality is very large, or if biopsy results are inconclusive while the cytologic studies are persistently reported as showing invasive carcinoma), further investigation by dilation and curettage and conization of the cervix is necessary. Conization involves the removal of a cone-shaped piece of cervix and endocervix, including all the abnormal area, and the examination of sections from 8 to 12 blocks of tissue.

Treatment. CIN should usually be treated. An exception is mild dysplasia related to infection. Outpatient cryosurgery is currently the most widely used technique. Provided that invasive cancer has been excluded and that the whole lesion can be treated, the results in all degrees of CIN are very good, with a less than 5% recurrence rate. Conization is an effective therapy, although it requires hospitalization and is associated with complications in the form of delayed bleeding and cervical stenosis. However, diagnostic conization can sometimes also be therapeutic. Laser therapy for CIN is under investigation.

INVASIVE CANCER OF THE CERVIX

The causes of invasive cancer of the cervix and its precursor CIN are not fully understood. Specific genetic factors have not been clearly established, although a metabolic or other predisposition may be possible. Menstrual patterns, vaginal discharge, and the use of contraceptives have not been implicated. Of importance may be more than one sexual partner and possibly early age of first coitus. Infection with herpesvirus type II is also important since antibodies to several viral proteins are higher in patients with CIN and invasive carcinoma than in controls.

Pathologic Features

Over 90% of cervical cancers are of the squamous cell variety. The remainder are glandular (adenocarcinoma), mixed (adenosquamous or adenoacanthoma), or sarcomatous.

Cervical cancer spreads locally in the first instance to the cervix and to the paracervical tissue. Extension to the uterine cavity and to the vagina may occur early. Then the disease extends laterally as far as the pelvic wall and may involve the bladder anteriorly or the rectum posteriorly. Lymphatic spread occurs primarily to the internal iliac, obturator, external iliac, and common iliac nodes. The importance of spread to the para-aortic nodes is beginning to be appreciated. The incidence of spread to nodes in the pelvis, according to data collected from the literature by Delgardo, is 14.2% for Stage I. Node involvement is reported to be about 30% for Stage II and about 50% for Stage III. Distant metastases usually occur late and are found most commonly in the liver, the lungs, the bones, and the intestinal tract.

Clinical Features

About one third of patients with early invasive (Stage I) carcinoma of the cervix have no symptoms. In fact, many far advanced lesions frequently give the unsuspicious patient little cause for concern. When symptoms occur, they almost always consist of irregular bleeding, which is intermenstrual in the woman of childbearing age and frequently follows coitus or other trauma such as douching. Discharge sometimes occurs. With involvement of the bladder or the rectum, symptoms may be referable to these organs. If the disease extends to the pelvic wall, swelling of the leg(s), pain in the back, or pain down the leg(s) may be reported. It is to be noted that these symptoms may be due to associated inflammatory changes in the paracervical tissues and not primarily to the cancer.

Diagnosis, Grading, and Staging

The diagnosis is made by a punch biopsy from a grossly obvious lesion, by a colposcopically directed biopsy, or by a cone biopsy.

Attempts to gauge the malignant potentialities of a particular tumor, based on the degree of cell differentiation seen in biopsy or excised specimens, have not so far been very satisfactory.

Clinical staging of the disease has been of great value in prognosis and in comparing the results of treatment from different centers. The most commonly used classification is that of the International Federation of Gynecology and Obstetrics:

Stage 0	Carcinoma *in situ,* intraepithelial carcinoma
Stage I	Carcinoma strictly confined to the cervix (extension to the corpus should be disregarded)
Stage Ia	Microinvasive carcinoma (early stromal invasion)
Stage Ib	All other cases of Stage I. Occult cancer should be marked *occ.*
Stage II	Carcinoma extends beyond the cervix but has not extended onto the pelvic wall. Carcinoma involves the vagina, but not the lower third
Stage IIa	No obvious parametrial involvement
Stage IIb	Obvious parametrial involvement
Stage III	Carcinoma has extended onto the pelvic wall. On rectal examination there is no cancer-free space between the tumor and the pelvic wall. Tumor involves the lower third of the

vagina. All cases with hydronephrosis or nonfunctioning kidney are included.

Stage IIIa No extension onto the pelvic wall

Stage IIIb Extension to the pelvic wall or hydronephrosis, nonfunctioning kidney, or both

Stage IV Carcinoma has extended beyond the true pelvis or has clinically involved the mucosa of the bladder or rectum. Bullous edema as such does not permit a case to be allotted to Stage IV.

Stage IVa Spread of the growth to adjacent organs

Stage IVb Spread to distant organs

It has been found that experienced clinicians usually will agree on the staging of a particular lesion. However, such staging depends only on examination and does not take into account the malignant potentialities of the tumor or its spread to lymph nodes, both of which greatly affect the outcome.

As in all clinical staging systems further information on the extent of the disease may be acquired at operation or in the pathology laboratory. For consistency's sake the original clinical staging is retained, although it has been suggested that the time of staging could be identified by the addition of C (clinical), S (surgical), or P (pathologic).

Treatment

Treatment is best conducted in a center where adequate facilities are available, where sufficient patients are seen annually, and where there are experienced specialists in gynecologic oncology and radiotherapy who work cooperatively together. All patients with invasive cervical cancer should have adequate diagnostic workups before treatment is decided in order to exclude metastases and to serve as a baseline for posttreatment studies. This workup should include, at a minimum, for Stage I disease an intravenous pyelogram and, in addition, for Stages II, III, and IV, cystoscopy, proctoscopy, and an attempt to identify abnormal lymph nodes by abdominal computed tomographic (CT) scan or lymphangiogram.

The responsible physicians should decide the stage of the patient's disease and plan treatment according to her individual requirements. It is helpful to have specific protocols for management. Follow-up during and after therapy should also be a joint venture between the gynecologists and the radiotherapists. Since the course of treatment and aftercare is often prolonged, it is beneficial to the patient if other professionals, such as nurse-clinicians specializing in oncology, social workers, home care nurses, or chaplains are included in the support team.

Surgical treatment for invasive cancer consists of a radical hysterectomy with wide excision of the parametrial, paracervical, and paravaginal tissues and of the upper vagina, with removal of the pelvic lymph nodes from the bifurcation of the aorta to the inguinal ligament. Although this is a major surgical procedure, the operative mortality in good hands has been 1% or less. The main complications are shortening of the vagina, bladder atony, and fistula formation. In particular, ureterovaginal fistula is reported to occur following 1% to 5% of operations.

Radiotherapy involves the use of external radiation by cobalt teletherapy or other megavoltage units, together with the application of radium to the cervix by means of an applicator consisting of a tandem inserted into the uterus and ovoids or a plaque placed in the upper vagina. Various techniques are available. Radium may be applied in single or divided doses or may precede or follow external radiation. Of great recent interest has been the use of afterloading devices to enable more accurate placement of the radium sources and to reduce the radiation danger to personnel. The total dose of radiation varies with the technique used and the stage of the disease, but it is important that it be calculated carefully to avoid damage to normal tissue. The long-term complications of radiotherapy are mainly vaginal shortening and constriction, hemorrhagic cystitis, radiation proctitis leading occasionally to rectovaginal fistula, and radiation enteritis.

Various combinations of radiation therapy and operation have been described. The most commonly used—radium application followed by radical hysterectomy for relatively early disease—seems to offer little advantage over either method used separately. Studies in this area would be helpful.

Stage I. Stage Ia disease is variously defined. If it is limited to those cases in which the malignant cells penetrate less than 3 mm below the basement membrane without vascular or lymphatic permeation, simple hysterectomy is sufficient treatment, since the chance of lymph node metastases is probably considerably less than 5%. Certainly if the lesion is questionably invasive, it should be treated as carcinoma *in situ*. Judgment must be reserved on the proper definition and appropriate management of microinvasive disease.

For patients with Stage Ib disease (and possibly Stage IIa) either radical hysterectomy or radiotherapy may be used. If the patient is relatively young and in good general health, the choice of treatment may depend on which method is readily available. A good program of radiotherapy will achieve better success than inadequate surgery, and vice versa. Surgery may have some advantage for these patients, since the ovaries can be preserved, the lymph nodes, for which radiation therapy is only 50% effective, can be excised and the patient's treatment is completed at one time, rather than being continued over 6 to 12 weeks. In a randomized prospective study the authors found that the end results for both methods were similar.

Stages II, III, IV. For patients with Stage II, III, or IV lesions, surgery is contraindicated, since it is difficult to excise the tumor completely and it may involve the removal of contiguous organs. Variations in the standard techniques of radiotherapy may be needed in these stages, such as extension of the radiation ports to the para-aortic area or increased radiation dose to the pelvis because of the large bulk of the tumor.

When invasive carcinoma of the cervix is discovered in a pregnant patient, it should be managed without regard to the pregnancy unless, by preserving the pregnancy for a few more weeks, a viable infant can be obtained. Results of treatment during pregnancy do not differ greatly from those in the nonpregnant woman. If intraepithelial carcinoma is discovered during pregnancy, and invasion is excluded, radical treatment is not indicated. The pregnancy should be allowed to proceed to term and vaginal delivery to occur. Further investigation should then be carried out 6 to 18 weeks post partum.

Adenocarcinoma responds to radiation in a way similar to squamous cell carcinoma, and the same treatment considerations apply to it.

The results of treatment of cancer of the cervix vary according to different authors. In general, provided that a patient receives adequate treatment, one may expect a 5-year survival rate of 80% to 90% for Stage I, 60% for Stage II, 30% to 40% for Stage III, and 10% or less for Stage IV lesions. Intraepithelial cancer should be virtually 100% curable.

RECURRENT AND RADIORESISTANT CANCER OF THE CERVIX

Close follow-up of patients is important during and after therapy. Persistent or recurrent disease may be suspected on pelvic examination when extension of the original tumor mass with nodularity is noted. Cytologic studies should be obtained regularly; they are of limited value in the first 6 months after radiation therapy. Aspiration and cytologic study of the parametria are useful and can be performed in the office. Core needle biopsy under anesthesia may also be diagnostic.

Whether continued active growth of cancer is due to resistance or recurrence makes little difference. When an adequate course of radiation has been given, this type of treatment can offer little more, except perhaps in areas where little therapy has been given (*e.g.,* pelvic nodes). However, the development of more radical surgical procedures during the past 30 years has made it possible to offer selected patients among this previously doomed group a chance of survival. These procedures involve anterior exenteration (removal of uterus and bladder), posterior exenteration (removal of rectum and uterus), and total pelvic exenteration. All types of postoperative complications are common. Moreover, the patient is left with a considerable permanent disability owing to the artificial stomas. Therefore, such operations should not be performed unless actively growing cancer is present and the patient has received all possible treatment by other means, and finally unless there is a chance of cure. Furthermore, the patient must have the emotional stamina and the home circumstances to cope with the stomas. Under these conditions it would seem worthwhile to offer the patient what represents her only chance of survival.

Chemotherapy has little to offer the patient with recurrent cancer of the cervix. *Cis*-Platinum has been found to give a 20% to 30% response, but other agents or combinations of agents are so far of little proved value.

Terminally ill patients with recurrent cancer of the cervix are likely to have ureteral obstruction, local hemorrhage, fistulas, widespread metastases, and inanition. However, much can be done surgically, medically, and psychologically to prolong life and decrease suffering.

INFECTIONS OF THE UPPER GENITAL TRACT

Infections of the upper genital tract may affect the uterus (endometritis), tubes (salpingitis), ovaries (oophoritis), or the structures lying beside the uterus (parametritis). Frequently, all the pelvic organs, including the pelvic peritoneum, are involved to a greater or lesser degree. The general term *pelvic inflammatory disease* is used commonly for this type of infection.

Infection usually reaches the upper genital tract from the vagina or the cervix. The following conditions may help to break down the normal barrier of the internal os of the cervix and cause the ascent of infection: pregnancy and delivery, including abortion; menstruation; sexual intercourse; and instrumentation of the cervical canal. More rarely, infection may occur from the bloodstream or may be spread from neighboring intra-abdominal organs.

Four common types of infection occur:

1. Puerperal. This usually is due to an anaerobic Streptococcus or Enterobacteriacae such as *Escherichia coli* or *Klebsiella pneumoniae* and occurs following abortion or normal delivery. Spread is through the parametria, forming a pelvic cellulitis.
2. Gonococcal. This follows acute or chronic infection of the lower genital tract. Spread in this instance occurs along the surface of the uterus and along the tubes.
3. Nonspecific. This may be primary and related to the causes listed above or may follow insertion of an intrauterine device or a long-standing and unsuspected gonococcal infection. Enterobacteriaceae (including especially *E. coli*) are common single agents, but multiple organisms are often involved, with anaerobes playing an important part.
4. Tuberculous. This is due to the *Mycobacterium tuberculosis* and commonly involves the fallopian tubes first. It is usually chronic and may be associated with tuberculosis elsewhere in the body.

ACUTE PELVIC INFLAMMATORY DISEASE

The most common cause of lower abdominal pain and fever is acute pelvic inflammatory disease. Precipitating factors are important, as noted above. When the complications of pregnancy are absent, gonorrhea or its secondary invaders are the most likely causes in young women who are sexually active. The symptoms include the following:

1. Abdominal pain, which is usually in the lower abdomen and bilateral, although it may be unilateral or generalized, and in gonorrhea it may be very severe
2. Vaginal discharge
3. Malaise and fever
4. Nausea, vomiting, and abdominal distention, which occur if the infection has spread widely through the peritoneal cavity

Examination of the abdomen may show lower abdominal tenderness, rigidity and rebound tenderness, or possibly signs of peritonitis, such as distention and diminished peristalsis. Pelvic examination confirms the presence of discharge. The uterus may be enlarged and soft if the patient has been pregnant. The cervix is acutely tender on motion. If the adnexal areas can be adequately examined, acute tenderness in the region of one or both tubes will be noted. In the puerperal type an area of tender brawny induration may be felt extending out from the uterus on one or both sides.

Diagnosis. Gram stain of the endocervix and aerobic and anaerobic cultures should be obtained. If an abscess is present, it should be aspirated and cultured. Culdocentesis and culture of peritoneal fluid may occasionally be helpful, although the procedure is painful. Laparoscopy is sometimes useful. The common conditions to be considered in the differential diagnosis include the following:

1. Appendicitis. Pain is commonly localized in the right lower quadrant, the temperature is lower, and intestinal symptoms are more prominent.
2. Tubal pregnancy. Fever is absent, and symptoms and signs of pregnancy are present. The pregnancy test may be positive. Leukocytosis is usually minimal or absent. If the tubal pregnancy has ruptured, culdocentesis may be productive of nonclotting blood.

3. Accident occurring in an ovarian cyst or uterine tumor. A tender mass may be palpable.
4. Renal tract disease, such as pyelitis or stone. The symptoms and signs are usually unilateral. Pain may be referred to the groin or thigh. The urine shows leukocytes or erythrocytes.
5. Diverticulitis. Pain is usually on the left side, unless rupture has occurred. Fever may be less. Pelvic findings are minimal.

Treatment. Conservative treatment is usually in order. Rest in bed is important. Any intrauterine device should be removed. Adequate doses of antibiotics are necessary. When gram-negative intracellular diplococci are seen on the gram stain, aqueous procaine penicillin G, 4.8 million units, is given intramuscularly at two sites with 1 g probenecid by mouth. When multiple organisms are suspected from results of the gram stain or if there is acute generalized disease, intravenous penicillin with an aminoglycoside is preferred. Failure to respond in 48 to 72 hours necessitates the addition of clindamycin so that most categories of organisms can be covered. Supportive therapy in the form of intravenous fluids, gastric suction, or blood transfusion may be indicated.

Operative treatment is not primarily indicated, and any sort of instrumentation of the uterus is to be avoided. On occasion it may be impossible to differentiate pelvic inflammation from an acute intra-abdominal condition such as appendicitis. In this case it is safer to explore the patient; but if salpingitis is found, nothing should be done. Evacuation of the uterus may be advisable in postabortal infections.

CHRONIC PELVIC INFLAMMATORY DISEASE

Chronic pelvic inflammatory disease is a troublesome condition both to diagnose and to treat. It is important to avoid labeling a patient as having chronic gonorrheal pelvic inflammatory disease without sufficient proof of the cause.

Pathologic Features. The following pathologic changes commonly occur in the course of the disease:
1. Recurrent attacks of infection (acute or subacute) in tubes, ovaries, or parametria, with persistent chronic inflammation between the attacks.
2. Development of adhesions between the pelvic organs themselves or between the pelvic and other intra-abdominal organs.
3. Closure of the cornual and fimbriated ends of the tube with formation of a serous (hydrosalpinx) or purulent (pyosalpinx) collection within the tube.
4. Involvement of both tube and ovary in a tubo-ovarian abscess.
5. Rupture of a hydrosalpinx, pyosalpinx, or tubo-ovarian abscess into the peritoneal cavity.

Clinical Features. A history of one or more attacks of acute inflammation is suggestive.

The patient with uncomplicated chronic pelvic inflammatory disease or with pelvic adhesions resulting from the disease may complain of chronic vaginal discharge, pelvic pain and backache, menstrual irregularities and secondary dysmenorrhea, and generalized weakness and tiredness.

Examination may disclose slight fever. Some lower abdominal tenderness is frequently present. Pelvic examination confirms the presence of a purulent vaginal discharge and lower genital tract infection. The cervix may be tender on motion. Thickness of the adnexal areas may be noted with a sense of adherence in the pelvis. The uterus may be fixed in retroflexion.

The presence of a hydrosalpinx, a pyosalpinx, or a tubo-ovarian abscess may cause the patient to notice a tender mass in the lower abdomen, and this may be palpable on pelvic examination.

Closure of the tubes, from previous infection, may result in involuntary sterility.

Rupture of a pelvic abscess presents an acute picture of shock with low blood pressure and rapid weak pulse. The abdomen is rigid, with generalized tenderness and diminished or absent peristalsis.

Diagnosis. Uncomplicated chronic pelvic inflammatory disease and adhesions have to be distinguished from endometriosis, disease of the lower intestinal tract, and disease of the bladder.

Adnexal masses due to inflammatory disease may be confused with tubal pregnancy, tumors of the ovary or the uterus, and extragenital conditions such as diverticulitis or tumors of the colon or the retroperitoneal space.

Rupture of a pelvic abscess may give symptoms similar to those produced by rupture of any other intra-abdominal organs, such as a tubal pregnancy, appendix, or peptic ulcer.

Treatment. The treatment of uncomplicated chronic pelvic inflammatory disease is primarily conservative. This is important, since many of these patients are young, and surgery, to be effective, usually involves sacrifice of childbearing function. The following measures are of value:
1. Antibiotics. These are of most value in acute inflammation but may be given a trial in chronic disease. Penicillin or a semisynthetic analog and an aminoglycoside can be used initially.
2. Local heat by means of hot vinegar douches, heating pads to the abdomen, or short-wave or microwave diathermy.
3. Abstinence from intercourse or douching at the time of menstruation.
4. Adequate rest and emphasis on superior diet with supplemental administration of vitamins and iron.
5. Local treatment of disease of the lower genital tract. It should be remembered that procedures on the cervix are likely to cause a flare-up of upper genital tract infection. They should be performed only when the disease is quiescent.

Surgical treatment is indicated in the following instances:
1. Abscess presenting vaginally or rectally. Drainage may be performed by opening the posterior cul-de-sac between the uterosacral ligaments, breaking up loculations with the finger, and inserting a drainage tube.
2. Rupture of a pelvic abscess. Immediate laparotomy may be lifesaving. If the patient's condition permits, hysterectomy with bilateral salpingo-oophorectomy should be strongly considered. Otherwise, excision of the abscess or simple drainage is indicated.
3. Adnexal mass. Any adnexal mass over 6 cm in size requires operation and excision. It is never possible to be entirely sure on clinical examination that one is dealing with an abscess and not an ovarian tumor. If localized disease is found on one side in a young woman, local excision may be possible. However, more radical procedures are frequently necessary.
4. Severe disability due to recurrent disease or persistent inflammation which has not responded to conservative measures. Surgery should be resorted to only after careful deliberation, since such procedures in order to be curative

usually mean removal of both tubes and ovaries and the uterus.

5. Sterility due to closed tubes.

TUBERCULOSIS

Although the picture of pelvic inflammation produced by tuberculosis is frequently indistinguishable from that found with other types of infection, it does present certain particular features. For example, the infection is commonly a descending one from the tubes to the uterus and often is associated with tuberculosis elsewhere in the body. It may give no symptoms, or the patient's only complaints may be of menstrual irregularity or sterility.

The diagnosis is frequently impossible preoperatively. When the diagnosis is suspected, cultures of menstrual blood or of curettings are valuable.

Treatment is primarily by the use of antibiotics, such as isoniazid, ethambutol, and rifampicin, together with the commonly accepted measures for the treatment of the disease as a whole (*i.e.*, rest and superior diet). Surgery may be indicated if the pelvic masses cause acute symptoms or if they do not respond to antibiotics. In any case the patient should be protected by antibiotics before and after operation.

TUMORS OF THE UPPER GENITAL TRACT

BENIGN TUMORS OF THE BODY OF THE UTERUS

Myoma

Myomas are the most common tumors of the female genital tract. They are present in fully 20% of women over the age of 35. They are more common in nulliparous than in parous women, and in black than in white patients. Their etiology is unknown. Hormonal imbalance may play a part in their development, since they grow during the late years of a woman's reproductive life and decrease in size after the menopause.

Pathologic Features. Although the short term *myoma(s)* is acceptable, *leiomyoma* most accurately describes these tumors, since they are composed of interlacing bundles of smooth muscle fibers with a varying admixture of fibrous tissue. They are frequently multiple and may grow to a very large size. They may be located underneath the peritoneal covering of the uterus (subserosal), within the uterine wall (intramural), or just beneath the endometrium (submucous) (Fig. 47-12). They may be found also in the cervix, and both the subserosal and the submucous types may become pedunculated. The subserous myoma may begin to receive some of its blood supply from the omentum or other organs and may eventually become detached from the uterus (parasitic myoma). Myomas may also develop from smooth muscle tissue in the genital tract that is located outside the uterus.

Secondary changes are common and consist of the following:

1. Hyalinization: very common but of little practical importance

2. Cyst formation: common in large myomas, and due to lack of blood supply in the center

3. Calcification: a common change in myomas of long duration

4. Necrosis: may occur in the center of the tumor or on the surface as in submucous myomas

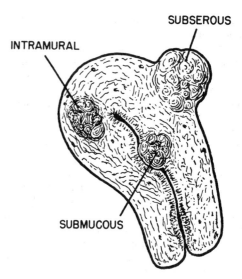

Fig. 47-12. Sites of myomas in the uterus.

5. Sarcomatous change: occurs in well under 1% of all myomas

Clinical Features. Myomas may give no symptoms until they attain a large size. When symptoms occur, they may be divided into the following groups:

1. Menstrual disturbances: menorrhagia, dysmenorrhea, and intermenstrual bleeding (the last is most common with submucous tumors)

2. Pressure symptoms: a vague sense of pressure in the lower abdomen or the back or of bladder irritability or constipation

3. General effects: Tiredness, weakness, and malaise

4. Acute accidents: Necrosis, or twisting of the pedicle of a pedunculated tumor, may cause acute lower abdominal pain, with fever and leukocytosis; minor symptoms of this sort are common in myomas associated with pregnancy.

If the tumor is large, abdominal examination will reveal a hard, nodular mass arising from the pelvis. Pelvic examination will show the uterus to be irregularly enlarged and firm. Anemia is commonly present even in the absence of menorrhagia.

Diagnosis. Myomas that project to the side of the uterus may be confused with adnexal masses. Acute accidents in myomas have to be distinguished from pelvic inflammatory disease, accidents in ovarian tumors, endometriosis, tubal pregnancy, and other intra-abdominal disorders such as acute appendicitis or diverticulitis. The possibility of pregnancy or of pregnancy associated with a myoma always must be kept in mind.

Treatment. Myomas can be cured only by surgical excision. No hormonal or medical treatment will cause them to shrink or disappear. However, they are frequently small and asymptomatic: the chance of malignant change occurring is small, and spontaneous regression in size occurs after the menopause. For these reasons continued observation with examination every 6 months in the premenopausal years and every 12 months postmenopausally is advisable in the vast majority of patients with myomas. Surgery should be performed only for the following indications:

1. Size. Any tumor larger in size than a 3-month pregnancy generally should be removed. A sudden increase in size on repeated examinations is also an indication for operation.

2. **Pressure.** Radiographic evidence of pressure on ureters or colon makes operation advisable.
3. **Symptoms.** It is important to be sure that the symptoms complained of really are due to myomas.
4. **Acute accidents.** Twisting of the pedicle of a pedunculated myoma may require operation.
5. **Sterility or repeated abortions.**

The importance of investigating any abnormal bleeding that is reported in association with myomas, so as to exclude cancer, cannot be overemphasized. This may include cytologic studies, appropriate biopsy of the cervix, endometrial biopsy, or dilation and curettage.

Myomectomy is of value where preservation of reproductive function is of importance. Even in the case of tumors that are of considerable size and are numerous, the persistent surgeon can restore the uterus to a remarkably normal appearance. Bleeding may be quite severe, although it can be controlled by temporary compression of the uterine arteries or by the intrauterine injection of vasopressin. Complications in the form of adhesions are more likely than with a hysterectomy. Myomas are estimated to recur in 15% to 45% of cases after myomectomy, and hysterectomy may eventually be necessary in some of these. However, the preservation of normal menstrual function and the possibility of retaining or increasing the patient's ability to have children are strong recommendations in favor of myomectomy.

Hysterectomy is the operation of choice for large or severely symptomatic myomas in the woman who no longer desires children or in whom the tumor is too large or too adherent to the surrounding structures to make myomectomy practical. Both corpus and cervix should be removed (total hysterectomy) (Fig. 47-13). If the patient's condition is not good enough to permit the extra dissection required to remove the cervix (a rare event), the corpus alone may be excised (supracervical hysterectomy). When the cervix is not removed, regular postoperative examinations must be performed to watch for the possible development of cancer in the stump.

The removal of ovaries at the time of hysterectomy for benign disease, such as myomas, is under debate. At age 40 the chance of a woman developing cancer in a retained ovary (a disease with a poor prognosis) is about 0.9%. Against this risk has to be placed the loss of ovarian function, the possible dangers of vascular disease, osteoporosis, and other unknown effects. On balance, conservation of ovaries, if normal, is appropriate as long as the woman is still menstruating at the time of operation. When bilateral oophorectomy is necessary, oral estrogen replacement can be given.

Endometrial Polyps

Endometrial polyps are common growths made up of endometrium, which may undergo cyclical changes, or more commonly of a proliferative or even atrophic type of epithelium. They may occur in premenopausal and postmenopausal women and may be multiple. Sometimes they project down into the cervical canal on a pedicle. They may be associated with adenocarcinoma in another area of the uterine cavity.

The importance of endometrial polyps is that they may cause slight irregular bleeding that has to be distinguished from that due to cancer. Frequently, however, they may cause no symptoms.

Treatment is by division or avulsion of the pedicle and thorough curettage to remove the base. Sometimes polyps may be missed on routine curettage unless the uterine cavity is explored with placental forceps in addition to the usual curette.

MALIGNANT TUMORS OF THE BODY OF THE UTERUS

Cancer of the corpus uteri is now the most frequent invasive cancer of the female genital tract in the United States. It is especially important in older women, since the average age of those with the disease is over 60 years. Adenocarcinoma is the type found most often, comprising about 95% of the total. Squamous metaplasia occurs in about 20% of adenocarcinomas (adenoacanthoma). Occasionally the squamous elements are malignant (adenosquamous tumor); these are considered to be more aggressive neoplasms. When adenocarcinoma of the corpus occurs in younger women (20 to 45), it is often associated with general endocrine and ovarian dysfunction.

Adenocarcinoma

A number of factors have been found to be associated with adenocarcinoma of the corpus uteri and may contribute to its development, although exact mechanisms are unknown. A comprehensive study in this area was reported by Wynder and associates. For example, general characteristics found to be associated with the disease include obesity, tallness, and endocrinologic abnormalities; factors possibly associated with the disease include heredity, low parity, breast cancer, hypertension, and elevated blood sugar levels. More specifically, possible endocrine factors include heavy menstrual bleeding, premenstrual breast swelling, late menopause, and hypothyroidism. Considerable attention has been paid to the possibility that oversecretion of estrogen or production of an abnormal estrogen may be important. Evidence for this is the relatively common occurrence of ovarian stromal hyperplasia or an estrogen-producing ovarian tumor in association with adenocarcinoma of the uterus. Also it has been repeatedly observed that the risk for developing endometrial carcinoma is increased severalfold for women who still have a uterus and take estrogens for a long time.

Fig. 47-13. Hysterectomy, showing upper vagina divided and uterus about to be removed.

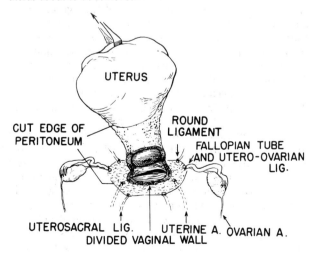

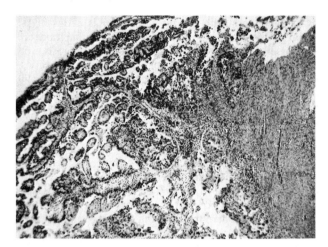

Fig. 47-14. Adenocarcinoma of the corpus uteri.

Pathologic Features. Characteristically, the microscopic picture is one of abnormal endometrial glands invading the stroma (Fig. 47-14). These glands are of irregular shape and size and commonly appear back to back, with the epithelium of one directly touching the epithelium of another. The cell nuclei are large, irregular, and hyperchromatic. Histologic grading of the tumor is a useful guide to treatment and prognosis. Well-differentiated lesions offer a better outlook than those that are poorly differentiated.

Adenocarcinoma of the body of the uterus spreads into the myometrium, down into the cervix and the vagina, and into the parametrial tissues. Local metastases to tubes and ovaries are common, but distant metastases to lungs and liver occur late in the course of the disease. Metastases to pelvic lymph nodes occur in 11% of patients with Stage I lesions, being more frequent when the lesion is poorly differentiated, the uterus is larger, or the outer half of the myometrium is involved. Spread to para-aortic lymph nodes occurs in 5.7% of patients with Stage I disease. In patients with Stage II disease, lymph node metastases occur in about 35% of cases.

Detection. Screening techniques are presently not available for cancer of the corpus uteri. Cytologic studies, even when adenomatous elements are carefully scrutinized, are positive in only 30% to 50% of cases. Periodic sampling of the endometrial cavity by curettage or aspiration biopsy does not appear feasible in the average woman because of the occasional difficulty in entering the uterine cavity due to cervical stenosis; discomfort: and, occasionally, inadequacy of the specimen obtained. However, screening by endometrial sampling of patients determined to be at high risk may prove to be worthwhile. In the long run, detection of abnormalities of estrogen secretion or metabolism may provide a useful screening technique.

Clinical Features and Diagnosis. Adenocarcinoma of the corpus uteri should be the primary consideration when irregular vaginal bleeding occurs in postmenopausal women (1 year or more after the cessation of normal menstruation). Therefore, all postmenopausal bleeding deserves adequate investigation. It is important to know if the patient is taking estrogens. Discharge, pain, local pressure symptoms, or general debility, and anemia may be noted if the disease is far advanced. On examination, softening and enlargement of the uterus may be found. Especially characteristic is the distention of the lower uterine segment.

Fractional curettage of the endocervix and the endometrium, determination of the depth of the uterus from the external os of the cervix to the fundus, and examination under anesthesia provide the most reliable diagnosis. In some instances the same information can be obtained by office endocervical curettage and endometrial aspiration biopsy, but this may be painful and may give an inadequate sample from the endometrium.

Patients with carcinoma of the corpus uteri require adequate medical evaluation since they are usually older and are likely to have associated diseases. Investigation for metastatic disease should be individualized, since the majority (75%) of patients have early (Stage I) disease. Treatment should be decided by the gynecologic oncology team, since expertise in all methods of therapy is essential to give the patient the best chance of survival.

The clinical staging classification approved by the International Federation of Gynecology and Obstetrics is widely accepted and should be used. It employs the size of the uterus and the differentiation of the tumor as originally emphasized by Gusberg and associates:

Stage I   Cancer is confined to the uterus.

Stage Ia   The length of the uterine cavity is 8 cm or less.

Stage Ib   The length of the uterine cavity is more than 8 cm.

G1:   Highly differentiated adenomatous carcinoma

G2:   Differentiated adenomatous carcinoma with partly solid areas

G3:   Predominantly solid or entirely undifferentiated carcinoma

Stage II   Cancer involves corpus and cervix.

Stage III   Cancer extends outside the uterus but not outside pelvis.

Stage IV   Cancer involves bladder or rectum or extends outside pelvis.

There are two problems with regard to clinical staging. First, it is difficult to find agreement on the grading of the tumor, since the international classification does not take into account the degree of cellular atypicality. Second, it is often uncertain whether the cervix is involved or tumor cells have "floated" from the uterine cavity onto the endocervical curettings.

Treatment. Combinations of radiation therapy and operation have been used for many years in the management of all patients with adenocarcinoma of the corpus uteri. Radical hysterectomy is impractical because of the age and poor condition of many patients. However, the advantages of a primary surgical approach to patients with clinical Stage I disease are now being recognized, since the additional information obtained permits radiation therapy (with the slight risks involved) to be omitted in some instances or to be directed to specific areas where it can do the most good. On our service patients with Stage I Grade 1 lesions receive a total abdominal hysterectomy and bilateral salpingo-oophorectomy as sufficient therapy. For Stage I Grade 2 and 3 lesions, operative sampling of pelvic and para-aortic nodes gives useful additional data. Postoperatively, if spread to the pelvic organs, to the outer half of the myometrium, or to the pelvic or para-aortic nodes has been demonstrated, postoperative radiation therapy (4500 to 5000 rads) is given to the whole pelvis, and to the para-aortic nodes, if indicated. When less than one half of the myometrium is involved, radioactive sources are applied to the vaginal vault 4 to 6 weeks after operation for a surface dose of about 7000 rads. For Stages II and III, external and internal radiation therapy, similar to that given for carcinoma of the cervix, is followed in 6 weeks by a total abdominal hysterectomy and bilateral salpingo-oophorectomy. Patients with Stage IV disease are managed by local radiation therapy to control symptoms such as bleeding or pain together with hormone therapy (progestins) or possibly combination chemotherapy.

In patients with any stage of the disease who are very poor operative risks the intrauterine insertion of radium (usually by the multiple source packing technique of Heyman), with or without external radiation, gives reasonable promise of success.

Overall survival rates at 5 years for adenocarcinoma of the endometrium are about 90% in Stage I, 50% in Stage II, 40% in Stage III, and 10% in Stage IV. Since the majority of patients reported in recent series have fallen in Stage I (75% to 80%), the prognosis for this type of cancer, with adequate treatment, is quite good.

Recurrent adenocarcinoma of the uterus presents a difficult problem in management. Although the occasional case can be treated by exenterative surgery, this is not usually practical because of the extent of the disease and the patient's poor general condition. Local recurrence in the vagina, a common site, may be treated by the application of radioactive sources, and external radiotherapy may be of some value in pelvic recurrence. The use of the synthetic progestins gives remissions in 20% to 30% of patients with extensive recurrent disease, especially those with lung metastases. The maximum duration of the response is probably about 2 years. Analysis of estrogen and progesterone receptors in the tumor tissue is useful. The use of antiestrogens and single or multiple chemotherapy is also under study.

Other Malignant Tumors of the Uterus

Sarcomas of the uterus are classified as follows:
A. Leiomyosarcomas
B. Endometrial stromal cell sarcoma
C. Mixed mesodermal sarcoma
   1. Homologous
   2. Heterologous
D. Other
   1. Blood vessel sarcoma
   2. Lymphoma
   3. Unclassified sarcoma

Sarcomas constitute about 5% of tumors of the corpus uteri. Leiomyosarcoma and mixed mesodermal sarcoma are the most frequent. Spread occurs to the pelvic and para-aortic lymph nodes and by way of the bloodstream especially to the lungs. Symptoms are similar to those for endometrial carcinoma in general, although they may arise later in the course of the disease. Treatment is primarily surgical by means of total hysterectomy. The addition of bilateral salpingo-oophorectomy probably does not improve survival rates. However, at operation the pelvic and para-aortic lymph nodes should be sampled.

Prognosis depends largely on the stage of the disease. For example, if leiomyosarcoma is discovered in the specimen and has not extended outside the uterus, the outlook is usually good (75% 5-year survival or better). If mixed mesodermal sarcoma is confined to the uterus (Stage Ia), the 5-year survival rate is about 50%. In Stages II and III the survival rate is very low (10% or less).

For Stage I disease the value of preoperative or postoperative radiation therapy is uncertain. For higher stages it

may have some palliative value. Among chemotherapeutic agents, doxorubicin (Adriamycin) is relatively effective, albeit temporarily. It is probably best used for advanced or recurrent disease.

Sarcoma botryoides, occurring in young girls and older women, is probably a mixed mesodermal sarcoma. Occasional primary squamous cell carcinoma of the uterus has been reported.

TUMORS OF THE FALLOPIAN TUBE

Tumors of any sort in the fallopian tube are rare. The most important are the malignant ones: papillary carcinoma and sarcoma. Usually they are discovered accidentally during laparotomy. Surgical removal of the uterus and both tubes and ovaries is the best treatment. Additionally, irradiation or chemotherapy may be used as for cancer of the ovary.

TUMORS OF THE OVARY

The ovary has the potentiality of developing many different kinds of cysts and tumors. The following is a classification of the more common ones:

  I. Nonneoplastic Cysts. These follicle cysts and corpus luteum cysts are extremely common and usually of small size.

  II. Neoplastic Cysts
    A. Mucinous Cysts. These cysts may grow to a very large size. They often are multilocular and contain a clear, viscid fluid. Microscopically, they are lined by a single layer of columnar epithelium, with basal nuclei. Goblet cells are common (Fig. 47-15).
    B. Serous Cysts. These cysts are slightly less common than the mucinous cysts and usually are not as large. Microscopically, they are lined by flatter epithelium, which is frequently ciliated and bears a close resemblance to the epithelium of the fallopian tube (Fig. 47-16).
    C. Dermoid Cysts (Cystic Teratomas). These tumors are derived from embryonal tissue and often show derivatives of all three germ layers, although ectodermal elements predominate. They comprise 11% of all ovarian tumors and are bilateral in 12% of cases. Grossly, dermoid cysts present a thick white capsule and characteristically contain a large amount of thick, yellow sebaceous material. Microscopically, they are lined by squamous epithe-

Fig. 47-15. Mucinous cyst of the ovary.

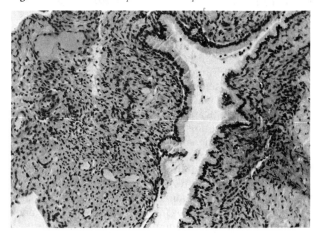

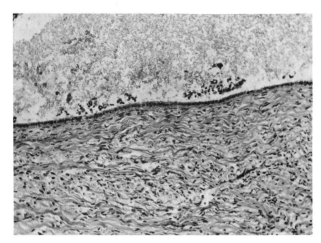

Fig. 47-16. Serous cyst of the ovary.

lium; skin appendages, such as hairs, sebaceous glands, and sweat glands, are usually present. Cartilage, ciliated epithelium lining small ducts, thyroid tissue, and other embryonic remnants may be seen. Calcification is commonly present (in about 25%), and well-developed teeth may occur. This feature, combined with the radiolucency produced in some instances by the sebaceous material in the cyst, may enable the diagnosis to be made preoperatively by roentgenography. Malignant change, usually squamous cell carcinoma, is found in less than 1% of dermoid cysts.

III. Benign Solid Tumors

   A. Fibromas. These are usually small asymptomatic tumors, although occasionally they may grow to a large size. Sometimes they are associated with ascites and hydrothorax (Meigs's syndrome). The cause of this phenomenon is obscure, but the accumulation of fluid usually disappears on removal of the fibroma. Varieties of fibroma include adenofibroma and cystadenofibroma.

   B. Brenner tumors. These tumors probably arise from the so-called Walthard cell rests that are found anywhere on the ovaries, the fallopian tubes, or the surrounding ligaments. Microscopically, Brenner tumors are composed of fibrous tissue in which are situated nests of epithelial cells of a uniform type. Cyst formation is not uncommon. Very rarely, malignant Brenner tumors have been reported.

IV. Primary Malignant Epithelial Tumors. These tumors of the ovary may be solid, cystic, or both. Mucinous, serous, endometrioid, and clear-cell (mesonephroid) forms are described. Often the same tumor contains more than one histologic type.

V. Stromal Cell Tumors. These include granulosa-theca cell tumors (feminizing), Sertoli-Leydig cell tumors (arrhenoblastomas), hilar cell or adrenal rest tumors (masculinizing), and gynandroblastomas (mixed type). Stromal cell tumors are uncommon. They should be considered malignant, but to a lesser degree than epithelial tumors.

VI. Germ Cell Tumors. These include solid immature and mature teratomas, dysgerminomas, endodermal sinus tumors, choriocarcinomas, and mixed types. They are the most common ovarian tumors in children and adolescents. Dysgerminoma is the least malignant.

VII. Metastatic Tumors. Metastases to the ovary can occur from tumors of the endometrium, the intestinal tract, the breast, and elsewhere in the body. The most noteworthy type is the so-called Krukenberg tumor, of which the primary tumor arises in the stomach or elsewhere in the intestinal tract. In this the ovarian metastases are frequently the most impressive part of the malignancy.

Complications. The following complications of ovarian cysts and tumors occur frequently and are of importance because they change the clinical picture of a simple cyst or tumor and add further diagnostic problems:

1. Size. Ovarian cysts may grow to an enormous size and then may cause marked abdominal distention with increased symptoms and interference with respiration. Large cysts may be confused with a distended bladder, pregnancy, other intra-abdominal tumors, and distention due to ascites.

2. Torsion. Many cysts and tumors are pedunculated, and the pedicle may become twisted, with subsequent interference with the blood supply and necrosis and gangrene of the tumor. The patient may notice sudden or gradual onset of pain, and on examination tenderness over a cystic mass, fever, and leukocytosis are commonly found. The clinical picture is very similar to that found in myomas with twisted pedicles, tubo-ovarian abscess, or ectopic pregnancy.

3. Hemorrhage. Common in or from cysts, occasionally it may be so severe as to cause shock similar to that found with ruptured ectopic pregnancy.

4. Rupture. This may occur spontaneously or as a result of injury or examination. Signs of peritoneal irritation occur similar to those found with any ruptured viscus, although evidence of infection and hemorrhage is usually absent.

5. Infection. Occasionally it occurs in ovarian cysts, especially dermoids, either from local ascending infection or from the bloodstream.

Clinical Features. Since there may be no symptoms, ovarian cysts or tumors may only be discovered on routine pelvic examination. If symptoms occur, they may be quite varied and due to the growth itself or its indirect effects. They include the following:

1. Palpation of a lower abdominal mass by the patient.

2. Pain. This may be dull and localized to one side or the other in the lower abdomen. It is often related to the size of the tumor, or it may be more acute and generalized if a complication has occurred.

3. Pressure on the bladder or bowel. Constipation or bladder or bowel irritability may depend on the location and size of the ovarian growth.

4. Menstrual abnormalities. A functional cyst such as a corpus luteum or follicle cyst may cause delayed menstruation or irregular vaginal bleeding. A functioning tumor, such as a granulosa cell tumor, may cause precocious bleeding in a young girl or postmenopausal bleeding in an older woman. A masculinizing tumor such as a Sertoli-Leydig cell tumor may cause amenorrhea. Associated with these menstrual changes may be extragenital effects such as breast engorgement with feminizing tumors and hirsutism and development of male habitus with masculinizing tumors.

5. General symptoms. Weight loss, malaise, and weakness may be associated with disseminated ovarian cancer.

Physical examination primarily involves determining the characteristics of the mass, which are listed below:

1. Size. Size is not diagnostic. Very large cystic tumors are not necessarily malignant.
2. Shape. A sausage-shaped mass suggests a lesion of the tubes, whereas a rounded mass suggests an ovarian lesion.
3. Tenderness. A tender mass suggests the presence of a complication or infection.
4. Consistency. A cystic tumor is more likely to be benign whereas one that is solid or part solid and part cystic is more likely to be malignant. Bilaterality is often indicative of malignancy.
5. Fixation. This suggests infection or a malignant tumor that has spread outside its capsule.
6. Associated nodularity in the cul-de-sac and ascites. This suggests the presence of malignant tumor with metastases.

Diagnosis. Roentgenograms of the abdomen may show calcification, suggesting a cystic teratoma or rarely a carcinoma. Paracentesis may permit cytologic studies of the ascitic fluid. In the case of small cysts, laparoscopy may be helpful: laparoscopic biopsy may be used when ovarian enlargement is questionable or when there is primarily an endocrinologic or sterility problem or endometriosis is suspected. Biopsy specimens should not be taken if large cysts are present or if there is suspicion of malignancy, for fear of spreading fluid or tissue containing malignant cells.

Other conditions that may be confused with ovarian cysts and tumors include myomas, especially subserous pedunculated myomas, hydrosalpinx, pyosalpinx, tubo-ovarian abscess, endometriosis, and extragenital masses, such as tumors of the colon, diverticulitis, pelvic kidney, and retroperitoneal tumors. Ultrasonography and CT scans may be helpful in identifying the site and size of a pelvic or adnexal mass. However, they are superfluous if surgical exploration is indicated due to the size of the mass or suspicion of malignancy.

Treatment. Surgery provides the only satisfactory treatment. Therefore the question is, when to operate. As a general rule, ovarian cysts or tumors that are causing symptoms or are asymptomatic and have an estimated diameter of over 6 cm should be removed. In a woman under 30 years of age, observation of an asymptomatic cyst of this size for 3 or even 6 months is justifiable, since it may disappear spontaneously. In the menopausal or postmenopausal woman the discovery of a cyst even smaller than 6 cm in diameter, especially if it has not been noted on a previous examination, may be an indication for removal. Aspiration of ovarian cysts through the abdominal wall or the vagina is not advised because of the danger of spreading malignant cells. Ovarian masses that are definitely felt to be solid should usually be removed, even if less than 6 cm in diameter, in the woman who is over 30 years of age; in the younger woman, if observation is chosen it should probably last no longer than 6 to 8 weeks.

The surgical approach to all ovarian tumors should be similar. A vertical lower abdominal incision is used, extending, if necessary, above the umbilicus. A low transverse (Pfannenstiehl) incision is recommended only in young patients in whom the possibility of cancer is very remote, since it provides inadequate exposure for exploration and management. Immediately after opening the peritoneal cavity ascitic fluid or saline washings from the cul-de-sac and lateral gutters is obtained for cytologic study. The retroperitoneal area, intestines, and upper abdomen, in-cluding the undersurface of the diaphragms are thoroughly explored. Whether the tumor is malignant or benign is established by gross examination or frozen section study of metastatic nodules or the primary lesion.

Since accurate staging is essential to future management and prognosis, any suspicious lesion should be biopsied. Specifically, the diaphragm can be biopsied under direct vision using, for example, a laparoscope and laparoscopic biopsy forceps. When the disease appears to be confined to the pelvis, biopsy of para-aortic nodes is important to exclude Stage III disease. If biopsy is not feasible, aspiration with a long 22-gauge needle and cytologic examination of the aspirate are useful.

If the cyst is clearly benign and the patient is young, the cyst alone should be removed when possible and ovarian tissue conserved even if it appears to be small in amount. When cysts are likely to be bilateral, as with dermoids, the opposite ovary should usually be bisected to exclude a small dermoid within it.

Where the diagnosis is in doubt at operation, it is probably best in a younger woman to do the minimum procedure, whereas with an older woman the tumor should be treated as if it were malignant.

Cancer of the Ovary

Once the diagnosis of cancer of the ovary has been made at the operating table, the lesion should be staged and treatment should be planned.

Staging. The staging classification of the International Federation of Gynecology and Obstetrics is generally used and is as follows:

Stage I   Growth limited to the ovaries

Stage Ia   Growth limited to *one* ovary; no ascites
   (i) No tumor on the external surface; capsule intact
   (ii) Tumor present on the external surface and/or capsule ruptured

Stage Ib   Growth limited to *both* ovaries; no ascites
   (i) No tumor on the external surface; capsule intact
   (ii) Tumor present on the external surface and/or capsule(s) ruptured

Stage Ic   Tumor either Stage Ia or Stage Ib, but with ascites present or positive findings on peritoneal washings

Stage II   Growth involving one or both ovaries with pelvic extension

Stage IIa   Extension or metastases to the uterus or tubes

Stage IIb   Extension to other pelvic tissues

Stage IIc   Tumor either Stage IIa or Stage IIb, but with ascites present or positive findings on peritoneal washings

Stage III   Growth involving one or both ovaries, with intraperitoneal metastases outside the pelvis or positive retroperitoneal nodes
   Tumor limited to the true pelvis with histologically proven malignant extension to small bowel or omentum

Stage IV   Growth involving one or both ovaries, with distant metastases. If pleural effusion is present, there must be positive cytology to allot a case to Stage IV
   Parenchymal liver metastases equal Stage IV

Special category — Unexplored cases that are thought to be ovarian carcinoma

Treatment. The primary treatment for ovarian cancer is total abdominal hysterectomy, bilateral salpingo-oophorectomy and removal of the greater omentum; the last is done because of the possibility of gross or microscopic metastases. If the whole tumor cannot be removed, it is important to excise as much as possible. If residual nodules are 1.5 cm or less in diameter, the prognosis is improved. Care should be taken to avoid perforating a potentially malignant tumor during removal, since this disseminates malignant cells in the peritoneal cavity.

Epithelial cancer of the ovary is sensitive to radiation and at least four chemotherapeutic agents: alkylating drugs, doxorubicin, *cis*-platinum, and hexamethylmelamine. Randomized studies are now in progress under the auspices of the Gynecologic Oncology Group and others so that firm data on their efficacy may be expected. In the meantime, Stage I may be appropriately managed by single drug alkylating agent chemotherapy or by the intraperitoneal instillation of chromic phosphate P_{32}. Stage II disease, which is not commonly encountered, can be managed either by one of the above methods or, if residual disease remains in the pelvis, by whole abdominal radiation therapy. Multiple chemotherapy (as well as maximum tumor reduction) has improved the short- and long-term survival in Stage III and IV disease and should be used in most such cases. Various combinations such as cyclophosphamide and doxorubicin or cyclophosphamide, doxorubicin, and *cis*-platinum have been reported to be effective, in spite of the considerable side-effects that accompany their use.

The prognosis of epithelial ovarian cancer depends on the type of tumor, its degree of histologic differentiation, the stage of the disease, and the amount of tumor left behind. For all epithelial tumors the approximate 5-year survival rates are as follows: for Stage I, 70%; for Stage II, 40%; for Stage III, 10% to 20%; and for Stage IV, 0 to 5%. In a special category are "borderline" epithelial tumors, in which the cellular criteria for malignancy are present but there is no invasion. Results in these patients are much better than in the usual invasive tumor (100% 5-year survival in Stages I and IIa). The prognosis for stromal cell tumors is somewhat better; about 75% of these patients survive for 5 years. Germ cell tumors, in general, except for dysgerminomas, have a poorer outlook.

The terminal events in ovarian cancer usually consist of partial or complete intestinal obstruction, widespread metastases, and inanition.

MENSTRUAL DISORDERS

Menstruation may be defined as the periodic discharge of bloody fluid from the uterus, occurring during the reproductive phase of a woman's life.

The mean length of the menstrual cycle, as calculated from the first day of one menstruation to the first day of the next, is about 28 days. Variations from 24 to 35 days are common. Variability is greatest up to age 25, declines to minimum between ages 35 and 39, and increases again slightly from 40 to 44.

The usual duration of the flow is from 2 to 7 days. The mean amount of blood lost is reported to be 25 to 50 ml. There is considerable variation between women but some consistency for each woman. It is often difficult both for the woman and her physican to estimate accurately the actual amount of flow.

In the healthy woman the menstrual flow varies at different periods of her life and may be affected by many factors, both physiological and psychological. The latter are of interest. Motherly women tend to menstruate more copiously or more frequently than less motherly women. Anxiety and elation can cause increased flow; depression may be accompanied by decreased flow. Sudden emotional shock, such as imprisonment, change in environment, or fear of pregnancy, can stop menstruation completely. Frequently, the menstrual cycle can be influenced by hypnosis, simple suggestion, administration of placebos, or superficial psychotherapy.

The events of the menstrual cycle are governed by a complex hormonal control involving primarily the pituitary and the ovaries. In addition, other endocrine organs such as the thyroid and the adrenal glands, as well as nutritional and other factors, are concerned with the menstrual cycle. It must be remembered that the evidence for many of the details, such as the exact mechanism of ovulation and of the onset of bleeding, is not complete. This is a rapidly changing field in which newer methods of measuring hormone levels in body fluids, such as by radioimmunoassay, are leading to important advances. Menstruation is also associated with many systemic changes. These involve almost all organs of the body and are probably related to the basic endocrinologic changes.

MENARCHE

The first menstruation occurs from 10 to 16 years of age (menarche). A regular rhythm is not usually established for several months or years. There is a high proportion of anovulatory cycles at this time, and lowered fertility exists as compared with that 3 or 4 years later.

Menarche is a time of great emotional changes and instability in the adolescent girl. Preparation for and understanding of this by parents and school authorities can make the transition to adulthood easier. Certainly, no attempt should be made to adjust the early irregular cycles with hormones, and detailed investigation should be undertaken only if excessive bleeding occurs. Provided that skeletal growth is occurring and that the child is normal, there should be no great concern about amenorrhea until the age of 16 is reached.

MENOPAUSE

The period of life around the end of cyclic menstruation is termed the *perimenopause*. Actual cessation of flow (menopause) occurs at about 50 years of age. In the latter part of a woman's reproductive life, anovulatory cycles (lack of progesterone) again become more common. Then estrogen secretion decreases and menstruation ceases. Concurrently there is a rise in pituitary gonadotropins. Following menopause the ovary produces decreasing amounts of estrogens but continues to secrete testosterone even in slightly greater amounts than before the menopause. The circulating level of androstenedione is about half the premenopausal level and this is secreted by the adrenal. Circulating estradiol levels are very much less than in the woman of reproductive age, measuring 10 to 20 pg/ml, and are probably derived from testosterone. Estrone forms a greater proportion of the total estrogens with a circulating level of about 30 pg/ml. It is mostly derived from the peripheral conversion of androstenedione, which appears to take place chiefly in adipose tissue. As a result of the hormonal changes the secondary sexual characteristics gradually atrophy.

Clinical Features. About 20% of women pass through the menopause with virtually no symptoms, 60% have mild to moderate symptoms, and 20% have considerable difficulty. Typically there is a decrease in flow, shorter menstrual periods, and a longer cycle. Rarely (1 in 10 women) menstruation stops suddenly. In some women excessive and irregular bleeding may occur.

The hot flash is the primary symptom of the perimenopause. Its exact cause is not known. Characteristically, the patient experiences a sensation of warmth, often in the shoulders, the neck, and the face, which is associated with blushing and followed by perspiration. The number and severity of the flashes vary greatly.

Varying degrees of nervousness, tension, headache, insomnia, and depression may be reported, although there is real question whether these are in fact related to the menstrual changes.

Treatment. The symptoms are interwoven with psychosomatic factors, including feelings of uselessness, boredom, or unhappiness. Therefore, an adequate social history is essential in evaluating the menopausal patient.

Assuming that no organic changes are found, the principles of treatment should include reassurance, encouragement of participation in social and other activities involving physical exercise, provision of adequate diet and supplementary vitamins, and specific therapy. Mild sedatives may be sufficient. If, however, the patient has marked disability from hot flashes or from lack of vaginal lubrication causing painful intercourse (usually after the menopause), substitution therapy with estrogens is indicated. These should be used in small doses initially (0.1 mg diethylstilbestrol or 0.3 mg conjugated estrogens) and given intermittently (*e.g.*, for 21 of 28 days or 5 days each week). Use of unopposed estrogens, especially if continued, may carry some risk of the development of endometrial hyperplasia and even adenocarcinoma. Moreover, side effects such as breast soreness can be troublesome. Added to this is the fact that the patient must continually take medication and may even become dependent on it. Therefore, consideration should be given to the use of a progestin such as medroxyprogesterone acetate for the last 7 to 10 days of estrogen administration in a 21-day cycle. The lifelong use of estrogens, as recommended by some authors, even with progestins added, has yet to be shown to be of benefit. It is probably better to use estrogen (and progesterone) replacement therapy for 6 to 12 months and then gradually taper it off and discontinue it. It can be resumed if symptoms recur. If a hysterectomy has been performed, one of the dangers of prolonged estrogen use (adenocarcinoma of the endometrium) is removed and extended administration is more practical. When the chief symptom is vaginal dryness, the use of an estrogen cream intravaginally every few days may be appropriate.

PREMENSTRUAL TENSION

Many women suffer from premenstrual tension. In few is it severe enough to cause them to seek medical aid. The cause of it is not entirely established, but probably it is due in large part to retention of excess fluid just before menstruation. This causes a sensation of being bloated, and, often, nervous irritability and insomnia. In addition, increased emotional instability and decreased aptitude for mechanical and intellectual tasks may be noted at this time.

Provided that a thorough gynecologic examination discloses no abnormalities, treatment is essentially symptomatic. It consists of attempts to remove excess water by laxatives and diuretics; dietary advice (especially vitamin B complex), and mild sedatives or tranquilizers. In severe cases temporary suppression of ovulation by oral administration of hormones or addition of progesterone in the last part of the cycle may be helpful.

DYSMENORRHEA

About 50% of all women have some pain during menstruation, usually on the first day. In perhaps 15% it is severe enough to cause them to go to bed. Clinically, it is convenient to divide the condition into primary dysmenorrhea, which has been present since the menarche, and secondary dysmenorrhea, which develops later in the reproductive life.

Although the exact cause of primary dysmenorrhea is not known, prostaglandins appear to play some part in the myometrial contractions of dysmenorrhea. Emotional factors are probably important, and cervical stenosis and retroflexion of the uterus may sometimes be responsible. Nutritional factors play a part, and the importance of hormones is shown by the fact that an anovulatory cycle is usually not accompanied by dysmenorrhea. Secondary dysmenorrhea may be due to many factors, such as myomas, pelvic inflammatory disease, and endometriosis.

A complete pelvic evaluation is important in every case. This includes postmenstrual sounding of the uterus to exclude cervical stenosis.

In primary dysmenorrhea, when no organic cause can be demonstrated, simple explanation of the physiology of menstruation, consideration of family interactions, psychological support, and symptomatic treatment can be of great value. The last consists of advice in regard to nutrition and hygiene, sedatives or tranquilizers, antispasmodics, and analgesics. Antiprostaglandins are often helpful. Suppression of ovulation for 2 to 3 months by means of estrogens or a combination of estrogen and progestin may be necessary. Frequently, patience and understanding are required to arrive at a satisfactory plan of treatment. In secondary dysmenorrhea, the treatment of any associated disease is of first importance.

MENSTRUAL IRREGULARITY

Irregular vaginal bleeding in its various forms is the most common and may be the only gynecologic complaint. It is important to determine from the history whether the patient is reporting a normal variation of her menstrual pattern or clearly unusual bleeding. It should be remembered that some women note a slight amount of vaginal bleeding at the time of ovulation: this may be due to the sudden drop of estrogens at this time and may not be abnormal.

Diagnosis. It is helpful to keep in mind the many possible causes of irregular vaginal bleeding:

  I. Specific causes
    A. Constitutional
      1. Blood dyscrasias
      2. Systemic diseases such as tuberculosis, nephritis
    B. Diseases of the vagina
      1. Trauma
      2. Foreign body
      3. Vaginitis
      4. Tumors (benign and malignant)
    C. Diseases of the cervix
      1. Infections and erosions

2. Polyps
3. Tumors (benign and malignant)
D. Diseases of the uterus
   1. Infections
   2. Polyps
   3. Adenomyosis
   4. Myoma
   5. Other tumors (benign and malignant)
E. Diseases of the fallopian tubes and ovaries
   1. Infections
   2. Ovarian cysts
   3. Ovarian tumors (benign and malignant)
F. Complications of early pregnancy
   1. Ectopic pregnancy
   2. Abortions
   3. Trophoblastic disease

II. General causes
A. Endocrine factors (congenital or acquired)
   1. Ovarian dysfunction (*e.g.,* ovarian dysgenesis, failure of ovulation)
   2. Adrenal cortical dysfunction or tumor
   3. Thyroid disorder
   4. Pituitary dysfunction or tumor
B. Emotional factors
   1. Anxiety states
   2. Emotional shock
   3. Deeper psychological causes
C. Nutritional factors

It is of fundamental importance to discover the cause of the abnormal bleeding before proceeding to treatment, and particularly before performing an exploratory operation that might lead to removal of any pelvic organs.

Histological examination of the endometrium may be helpful in diagnosing the cause of menstrual irregularity. Tissue can be obtained by endometrial aspiration or biopsy or by curettage. The first may result in insufficient material being available for complete study, but it is valuable, for example, in determining whether secretory endometrium is present. Curettage may be adequately performed with the patient under local anesthesia, but general anesthesia may be needed to permit adequate examination if the pelvic findings are indeterminate because of the patient's age, muscular resistance, or obesity.

Adequate curettage should include four steps: (1) scraping the endocervical canal with a small sharp curette (Novak); (2) determining the depth of the uterus, using a sound, from the external os to the top of the endometrial cavity; (3) dilation of the cervical canal with Hegar or similar dilators; and (4) thorough scraping of all parts of the endometrial cavity, together with the use of a polyp forceps to remove large or projecting pieces of tissue. Curettage carries a slight risk of perforating the uterus, particularly in pregnant and postmenopausal women. Suspected perforation should generally be treated conservatively, unless bleeding or signs of peritonitis follow.

Tests of thyroid function; pituitary follicle-stimulating hormone (FSH), prolactin, plasma estrogen, progesterone, or testosterone levels; or adrenocortical function may be carried out before or after curettage. Additional genetic or psychological investigations may be helpful.

Treatment. Treatment should be directed to the specific cause of the menstrual irregularity, if this can be determined. Sometimes, even if no cause can be found, the curettage itself is curative. If irregularity persists, attention should be directed to general factors such as nutritional and psychological problems. Often hormonal replacement with estrogen or progestins for several cycles, depending on the pathologic findings, will cause menstruation to revert to a more normal pattern. Radical procedures such as hysterectomy may occasionally be necessary but should be reserved for those cases in which repeated curettages and medical treatment have failed to regulate the cycle or in which excessive bleeding has occurred, leading to anemia.

AMENORRHEA

Amenorrhea presents special problems. When the patient has never menstruated, this is termed *primary amenorrhea.* Detailed investigation for genetic and congenital abnormalities is necessary, and treatment depends on the cause found. The term *secondary amenorrhea* is used when menstruation has begun and may have continued for several years but then ceases. Causes may be varied and include pituitary tumors, hypothalamic disorders, emotional disturbances, major endocrinologic abnormalities, premature gonadal (ovarian) failure, inability of the end organ (uterus) to respond to hormonal stimulation (Asherman's syndrome), or suppression of function following the use of oral contraceptives. Extensive investigation is usually necessary and treatment depends on the cause. The use of drugs such as clomiphene or gonadotropins to stimulate ovulation may be very helpful, especially when lack of ovulation leads to amenorrhea and infertility.

FERTILITY AND INFERTILITY

FERTILITY

The widespread acceptance of methods of fertility control has posed new issues for the gynecologic surgeon. These include family planning methods and their complications, termination of pregnancy, and sterilization.

Contraception

The gynecologic surgeon is commonly asked for help in controlling fertility and in the spacing of children. It is important that he be familiar with all methods so that the patient can be given advice most suited to her as an individual or referred to someone else who can assist her. The provision of adequate contraceptive advice requires a complete pelvic examination and cytologic studies, as well as thorough discussion with the patient. Regular follow-up is essential.

The family planning methods available today include rhythm, barrier techniques, oral contraceptives, and intrauterine devices (IUDs). Their failure rate is commonly measured by the Pearl index, which is the number of pregnancies/100 women years of exposure. These rates, as currently known, are given in parentheses after each method discussed in the following list. The first figure refers to the theoretical rate, that is, the failure rate that might be expected if the method were always used correctly; the second figure refers to the actual use, allowing for human error and omission.

1. Rhythm method (13/21). Whether a fixed "unsafe" time is used or unfertile days are calculated by a combination of observation of cervical mucus and basal body temperature is immaterial. No physical dangers result from the use of this method.
2. Barrier methods. These include the use of a condom

with spermicide (less than 1/5), diaphragm and spermicide (3/17), or spermicidal foam (3/22). No physical harm results from these except possible allergy to spermicidal substances.

3. Oral contraceptives (less than 0.5/4–10). Although oral contraceptives are the most effective method they carry risks of several nonsurgical complications, including hypertension, increased thrombosis, and depression.

4. Intrauterine devices (1–3/5). In addition to dysmenorrhea, excess menstrual flow, and expulsion, IUDs carry the risk of perforation and pelvic infection. Perforation is usually suspected when the tail of the IUD can no longer be felt or seen. It can usually be located by ultrasonography. If it is in the uterus, it can be removed by an endometrial curette or through the hysteroscope. If it is outside the uterus, it can be extracted through the laparoscope or by laparotomy. Pelvic infection is more common among users of IUD than in the general female population and more frequent in nulliparous than in parous women. The presence of a tender adnexal mass in association with an IUD provides the diagnosis. Treatment is by removal of the IUD, administration of appropriate antibiotics, and, occasionally, surgical intervention, in which case salpingo-oophorectomy and possibly hysterectomy may be necessary.

Termination of Pregnancy

Where abortion is legally acceptable, patients may seek it in the first or second trimester. In the first trimester (under 12 weeks from conception), pregnancy may be terminated on an outpatient basis by suction curettage (the preferred method) or by a regular curettage. It is essential that the diagnosis of pregnancy be established and appropriate examinations and laboratory tests be performed before termination is undertaken. Complications of this procedure are rare (*i.e.,* incomplete evacuation, prolonged bleeding, and infection) and the end results are usually satisfactory. In the second trimester, up to 20 weeks' gestation, termination is best performed by intra-amniotic injection of hypertonic saline or by the use of prostaglandins. Delivery of the fetus usually occurs spontaneously but may require completion by a curettage if delay in delivery of the placenta or excess bleeding occurs. Rh-negative patients should receive anti-D globulin after an abortion.

Tubal Ligation

Tubal ligation (sterilization) may be requested, in most jurisdictions, by any patient who is over the age of consent or, in some instances, by *emancipated minors,* a term whose definition varies in different states. Specific indications are no longer required nor is it necessary to obtain the permission of the husband. Tubal ligation may be performed post partum through a vertical abdominal incision or as an interim procedure by laparoscopic cautery-excision or occlusion by a plastic band, by a small 2- to 3-cm transverse suprapubic incision (minilaparotomy), or through a colpotomy. The main purpose is to excise a portion of each tube and obliterate the ends remaining by cautery or catgut ligature. Failure rates vary from 0.2% to 2%. Occasional complications occur but are least likely with laparoscopic plastic bands or with minilaparotomy. It is essential that the patient understand that reanastomosing divided tubes is difficult and even with excellent microsurgical techniques the success rate (*i.e.,* pregnancy) is no better than 50%.

INFERTILITY

Involuntary sterility occurs in about 10% of all marriages in the United States. Study of a particular problem involves a consideration of all the possible factors concerned, and the application of a plan of investigation and treatment that includes both partners. When no contraceptives are used, 70% of couples conceive in 6 months and half of the remainder will conceive within 2 years. Therefore, 1 year of unprotected coitus without a pregnancy is an appropriate time after which a young couple should seek help. It may be advisable for an older couple to seek help after 6 months of infertility.

Causes

The mechanism of fertilization in humans is still virtually unknown. Clinically, certain barriers to conception can be identified; some are obvious and some are more subtle.

Specific Genitourinary Tract Disorders. Any factor that may prevent the production or transport of the sperm or the ovum or prevent the meeting of the two for fertilization may be a cause of sterility. In the male this means defective spermatogenesis, obstruction of the vas deferens or urethra by trauma or infection, or inability to deposit the sperm in the vagina. In the female this involves deformities of the vagina that may prevent penetration, diseases of the cervix or uterus, obstruction of the tubes, or defective oogenesis.

General Factors. The general health of both partners is important. Debilitating disease in either male or female, or even mild infections, such as a cold, may be a barrier to conception. Nutritional factors also may be important. Also, it has been established that certain women may develop antibodies to sperm, although the precise significance of this remains to be determined.

Psychological Factors. Personality disturbances seem to be characteristic of both males and females in infertile couples. The relationship of the couple and their interpersonal conflicts may also be important.

Valuable data on coital physiology and relationships have been obtained by Masters and Johnson.

Investigation

The study of sterility should be accomplished within a reasonable period. The steps that should be taken have been discussed in detail by Speroff and colleagues.

The history and examination usually starts with the woman, since it is most often she who comes first to her physician for study, although it is most helpful to have her partner accompany her. The usual gynecologic history should be taken, and special emphasis should be placed on her general condition, details of her relationship with her partner, and possible psychological factors. This is followed by a general physical examination and a pelvic examination. Her partner also should undergo a general physical examination, with special attention being paid to the genitalia and to psychological factors. Additional study in both partners should include blood count, urinalysis, chest roentgenogram, serology, tests of thyroid function, and nutritional evaluation. The last should include actual calculation of average daily intake of proteins and certain key vitamins and minerals, in comparison with the standards recommended by the National Research Council.

Semen analysis is done best on a specimen produced by masturbating, after 3 days' abstinence, into an open-mouthed bottle. Analysis should include estimation of volume (normal 3 to 5 ml), motility (at least 50% progressive motility), cell count (more than 30 million/ml), and morphology (60% or more of normal forms). Since masturbation is distasteful to some men on religious or other grounds, the Huhner test, obtained at about the expected time of ovulation, may be used as a substitute for this. It does not give a true picture of the sperm count. However, if the mucus taken from inside the cervical canal within 6 hours after coitus contains 5 to 20 spermatozoa per high-power field with 50% motility and few abnormal forms when examined microscopically, the male is likely to be fertile. Additional information given by the postcoital test is that if active spermatozoa are seen there may be assumed to be no obvious hostility of the cervical mucus to the sperm.

Apart from the rather indefinite symptom of pain felt by some women at this time, ovulation can be detected only by indirect methods. These depend on the presence of a functioning corpus luteum and include absence of the "ferning" pattern when cervical mucus is spread on a slide, allowed to dry, and examined microscopically; decrease in the number of cornified cells seen in a cervical or vaginal smear; a rise in the basal body temperature (Fig. 47-17); the finding of secretory endometrium in an endometrial biopsy taken just before or preferably immediately after the onset of menstruation; and a rise in serum progesterone levels.

Tests of tubal patency may be determined by hysterosalpingography. In addition to showing the site of any obstruction of the fallopian tubes, this test may also reveal any congenital abnormalities within the uterine cavity that might be acting as a barrier to fertility.

Many authors feel that a sterility workup is incomplete without the performance of a laparoscopy. This procedure permits the ovaries to be seen and biopsied if necessary; adhesions around the tubes and tubal abnormalities can be identified; and tubal patency can be determined by injecting indigo carmine or methylene blue dye into the uterine cavity and observing its exit from the tubes.

Treatment

There is a high spontaneous cure rate in sterility. This emphasizes the fact that discussion of the problem and the progress of investigation with both partners is the first step in treatment. This should be combined with simple explanations about the mechanism of intercourse, conception and timing of intercourse, and detailed nutritional advice.

Oligospermia or azoospermia may be extremely difficult to treat, and referral to a competent urologist is advised. Even when the sperm count is very low the couple should

not be discouraged, since conception is possible and not infrequent under these circumstances.

In the woman, conditions that can be managed conservatively should be handled first. These include infections of the lower genital tract, diseases of the cervix, and minor disorders of the upper genital tract. Anovulation may be treated, with careful monitoring, by clomiphene or human chorionic gonadotropin. Major surgical procedures such as myomectomy and plastic reconstruction of the fallopian tubes should be adopted only if it seems that nothing else will help the couple. The development of microsurgical techniques for tuboplasty has improved the success rate.

If, after adequate investigation has been completed, no specific causes for a couple's sterility have been found, the patients should be informed of this. Either no further treatment is advisable—and the couple has a small chance of achieving a pregnancy under these circumstances—or the possibilities of artificial insemination may be considered. Adoption may be suggested through an appropriate adoption agency.

ENDOMETRIOSIS

Endometriosis is produced by the growth of ectopic islands of endometrial glands or stroma. It may be divided into internal and external types. In the former, which is commonly termed *adenomyosis,* the islands are found in the myometrium; in the latter they appear on ovaries, fallopian tubes, uterine ligaments, cervix, and peritoneum and even as far away from the uterine cavity as umbilicus, appendix, intestine, vagina, and vulva. Distant locations such as the lungs and the skin of the arm and the thigh have been reported.

Endometriosis occurs during the reproductive life, between the ages of 25 and 45, and rarely in the postmenopausal woman. It is more frequent among the higher socioeconomic groups and in whites than blacks.

The exact cause of endometriosis has not been determined. Three main theories have been used to explain the ectopic location of the endometrial tissue: (1) transtubal regurgitation of menstrual blood and endometrial particles, (2) lymphatic dissemination, and (3) metaplasia of embryonic coelomic epithelium. There is little concrete evidence to support the third theory. The first, which was advanced originally by Sampson in 1921, has received support from the production of experimental endometriosis in monkeys by causing the menstrual flow to be directed into the peritoneal cavity. The idea of lymphatic dissemination has received some support from the occasional finding of endometriosis in pelvic nodes removed during the course of radical pelvic surgery. Sampson's theory is the most attractive but does not explain all cases, and it may be that more than one mechanism is responsible. Hormonal and psychological factors have also been implicated, but it is uncertain how they act.

Pathologic Features. The ectopic endometrial tissue undergoes cyclical changes, as does normal endometrium. Blood-filled (chocolate) cysts may form, or the tissue may rupture into the surrounding peritoneum or other tissues, resulting in acute symptoms or in the formation of adhesions, which may be particularly dense (Fig. 47-18).

Clinical Features. Internal endometriosis usually produces secondary and increasing dysmenorrhea with menstrual irregularities. On examination the uterus may be found to

Fig. 47-17. Basal temperature chart shows postovulatory temperature rise.

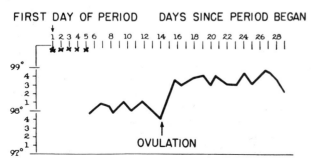

FIRST DAY OF PERIOD   DAYS SINCE PERIOD BEGAN

OVULATION

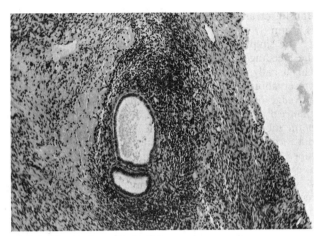

Fig. 47-18. Endometriosis of the ovary.

be symmetrically enlarged, firm, and especially tender during the premenstrual and menstrual phases of the cycle.

External endometriosis is commonly associated with internal endometriosis but may exist by itself. In addition to the symptoms of internal endometriosis the patient may complain of persistent backache, especially premenstrually but also throughout the cycle. Dyspareunia is common. Sterility may result from blockage of the tubes and from pelvic adhesions. Examination will commonly show the uterus to be retroflexed and fixed. Nodules may be palpable on the uterosacral ligaments or elsewhere in the pelvis. The ovaries may be enlarged and tender. Involvement of the intestine may rarely give rise to symptoms and signs of intestinal obstruction. Thus endometriosis should be considered in the differential diagnosis of carcinoma of the colon and the rectum and of diverticulitis.

Diagnosis. Examination in the premenstrual phase of the cycle is important, since enlargement of the endometrial nodules usually occurs premenstrually. Chronic pelvic inflammatory disease with pelvic adhesions is the most common source of confusion in diagnosis. Ovarian cysts due to endometriosis have to be distinguished from other ovarian cysts and tumors; the latter are frequently not tender. Laparoscopy is essential for diagnosis. Brownish, hemorrhagic, or purplish to black areas are seen on the vesicouterine fold, in the cul-de-sac, or on the ovaries. Laparoscopic biopsies are helpful but not essential when the typical findings are present.

Treatment. Endometriosis is practically always a disease of the childbearing age. Many patients are anxious to have children. Therefore, whenever possible, attempts should be made to preserve this function. Treatment may be divided into no treatment, endocrine and symptomatic treatment, conservative operation, and radical operation.

In some cases endometriosis may be discovered on routine examination and may be symptomless. No treatment is advisable in such instances, but repeated regular examinations are essential. Several staging systems for estimating the severity of endometriosis have been suggested and are summarized by Malinak.

When symptoms are mild, and no cysts large enough to necessitate laparotomy are found, conservative treatment should be tried. Symptomatic relief of dysmenorrhea may be offered by any one of a number of measures, such as therapy with analgesics, mild sedatives, antiprostaglandins,

and diuretics; attention to diet; and local application of heat to the abdomen. The management of patients with moderate or severe symptoms when surgical treatment is not indicated (*i.e.*, no large masses or acute problems are present) is discussed by Andrews. Hormonal therapy is useful and may consist of androgens in small doses; progestins (medroxyprogesterone acetate) for several months; pseudopregnancy using estrogen and progestin combinations for 6 to 9 months; or pseudomenopause, using danazol, for about 6 months. Varying rates of improvement and subsequent pregnancies are reported. Follow-up laparoscopy is useful. The side-effects of these hormonal agents make these regimens difficult for the patient to follow.

If conservative therapy does not help, or if the patient has an ovarian mass of significant size, laparotomy should be performed. In a young woman who is anxious to have children, only as much tissue as is necessary should be removed. This frequently consists of removing the cyst, or one tube and ovary, and cauterizing or excising any endometrial implants that may be found. Adhesions are freed, and suspension of a retrodisplaced uterus is recommended. Division of the pelvic (presacral) nerves at the brim of the pelvis, from one ureter to the other, can also be performed to relieve menstrual distress and backache. The use of a progestin before and after operation may be advisable.

Radical operation consists of bilateral salpingo-oophorectomy and total hysterectomy. It should be reserved for older women who have had a conservative surgical procedure done or have no desire for more children, or rarely for those younger women in whom it is impossible to save any pelvic organ because of extensive involvement and adhesions.

ECTOPIC PREGNANCY

Ectopic pregnancy is a potential major threat to the patient's life and may be confused with many other gynecologic disorders. The exact incidence of ectopic pregnancy is difficult to determine, since many cases may go unrecognized. Its most common site is in the fallopian tube, but it may occur on the ovary, the cervix, the uterine ligaments, or in the abdominal cavity (Fig. 47-19).

The mechanism by which the fertilized ovum implants in the tube rather than the uterus is uncertain. Conditions that cause partial blockage of the tube may predispose to tubal pregnancy. Such are pelvic inflammatory disease and adhesions or tumors arising within or outside the tubal lumen. Patients with sterility problems due to tubal factors

Fig. 47-19. Sites of tubal pregnancies.

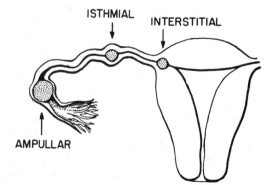

are more likely to have tubal pregnancies (1.7%). Attention has been called to the higher incidence of ectopic pregnancy in women with IUDs.

Pathologic Features. Tubal pregnancies may be located in the lateral (ampullar), middle (isthmial), or medial (interstitial) part of the tube. Very few ectopic pregnancies reach full development, although these have been reported. They may either rupture or undergo spontaneous degeneration. Rupture may occur into the peritoneal cavity or into the uterus. Occasionally, rupture and secondary implantation on another abdominal organ may occur. Rupture occurs later with the ampullar type and is usually earlier and attended with greater hemorrhage in the interstitial type.

Clinical Features. In a typical case the patient presents with the symptoms of early pregnancy (amenorrhea, breast fullness, frequency of urination, constipation, nausea). She may also notice some slight vaginal bleeding and lower abdominal pain, which is persistent and unilateral. On examination the cervix may be blue and the uterus soft and enlarged, although perhaps not to the degree expected from the length of amenorrhea. An acutely tender adnexal mass is noted.

Rupture into the uterus gives moderate to marked vaginal bleeding and intermittent lower abdominal and back pain. The picture is similar to that of abortion of an intrauterine pregnancy.

Rupture into the peritoneal cavity causes sudden lower abdominal pain, which soon becomes generalized and may spread to the shoulder. Examination may show evidence of shock with a low blood pressure and a weak and rapid pulse. The abdomen may be tender and present generalized rebound tenderness and rigidity with diminished or absent peristalsis. Pelvic examination is often difficult because of the abdominal tenderness, but an adnexal mass may be felt and a semisolid hematoma may be palpable in the cul-de-sac.

Spontaneous degeneration may cause little except regression of the previous symptoms and signs.

Diagnosis. The typical picture of either unruptured or ruptured ectopic pregnancy is relatively clear cut. Unfortunately, not all cases are typical. In an unruptured ectopic pregnancy, a pregnancy test may be of help and laparoscopy is of considerable value. Conditions to be considered in the differential diagnosis include intrauterine pregnancy with a large corpus luteum, abortion, pelvic inflammation with a hydrosalpinx or pyosalpinx or tubo-ovarian abscess, myoma, and ovarian cyst or tumor.

In a ruptured ectopic pregnancy, culdocentesis is a valuable diagnostic procedure. The posterior cul-de-sac is punctured with an 18-gauge needle attached to a syringe. Aspiration of nonclotting blood indicates intraperitoneal hemorrhage and, when associated with appropriate symptoms and signs, is strongly suggestive of ruptured ectopic pregnancy. Other intra-abdominal emergencies may be confused with ruptured ectopic pregnancy. These include ruptured ovarian cyst or pelvic abscess, ruptured appendix, or perforated peptic ulcer.

Treatment. Since the danger of rupture is ever present, there is no place for expectant treatment. Once the diagnosis of ectopic pregnancy has been established the patient should be operated on promptly. If shock is present, blood transfusion should be started as soon as possible, but it is not wise to wait until shock has been controlled completely before starting the operation because that time may never come, and control of the hemorrhage is vital. It is of the utmost importance to have suitable blood available for transfusion and preferably running by the time the operation is begun.

The simplest operative procedure necessary to control the bleeding and remove the pregnancy should be done. This usually involves removal of the tube, with, if possible, preservation of the ovary. Many authors recommend that a wedge of the uterine horn be removed to prevent the chance of a subsequent pregnancy developing in the remnant of the tube. Reconstruction of the involved tube is generally not recommended since pregnancy can occur in the other tube. However, it may be attempted when one tube has already been removed or is occluded, and the patient is very anxious to become pregnant. The area should be reperitonealized as well as possible, and excess blood removed from the peritoneal cavity.

In the rare instance of an advanced abdominal pregnancy, it may be well to wait until the infant is viable before performing laparotomy, since living children have been obtained by this procedure. If the placenta can be removed easily, this should be done. However, it may be adherent to many organs and, in this case, should be left *in situ,* since catastrophic bleeding may occur during attempts at removal. If the placenta is left in place, it may eventually be absorbed. Equally likely is the persistence of a mass, often cystic, for which a secondary operation may be required.

After removal of an ectopic pregnancy, subsequent pregnancy is quite possible, although the chances of a second ectopic pregnancy are somewhat increased.

BIBLIOGRAPHY

ANDREWS WC: Medical versus surgical treatment of endometriosis. Clin Obstet Gynecol 23:917, 1980

AURELIAN L, KESSLER II, ROSENHEIM NB, BARBOUR G: Viruses and gynecologic cancer. Cancer 48(suppl):455, 1981

BOLTEN KA: Practical colposcopy in early cervical and vaginal cancer. Clin Obstet Gynecol 10:808, 1967

CIBILS LA: Gynecologic Laparoscopy. Philadelphia, Lea & Febiger, 1975

COHEN MR: Laparoscopic diagnosis and pseudomenopause treatment of endometriosis with danazol. Clin Obstet Gynecol 23:901, 1980

COPPLESON M, PIXLEY E, REID B: Colposcopy: A Scientific and Practical Approach to the Cervix in Health and Disease, 2nd ed. Springfield, IL, Charles C Thomas, 1978

CREASMAN WT, BORONOW RC, MORROW CP DISAIA PJ, BLESSING J: Adenocarcinoma of the endometrium: Its metastatic lymph node potential. Gynecol Oncol 4:239, 1976

CRIST T, SHINGLETON HM, KOCH GG: Stress incontinence and the nulliparous patient. Obstet Gynecol 40:13, 1972

DELGARDO G: Squamous cell carcinoma of the cervix: The choice of treatment. Obstet Gynecol Surv 33:174, 1978

EVANS TN: The artificial vagina. Am J Obstet Gynecol 99:944, 1967

FRANKLIN RR, DUKES CD: Antispermatozoal antibody and unexplained infertility. Am J Obstet Gynecol 89:6, 1964

GUSBERG SB, JONES HC, TOVELL HMM: Selection of treatment for corpus cancer. Am J Obstet Gynecol 80:374, 1960

HALLBERG L, NILSSON L: Constancy of individual menstrual blood loss. Acta Obstet Gynecol Scand 43:352, 1965

HERBST AL, BERN HA: Developmental Effects of Diethylstilbestrol (DES) in Pregnancy. New York, Thieme-Stratton, 1981

KATZENSTEIN AA, MAZUR MT, MORGAN TE, KAO MS: Proliferative serous tumors of the ovary. Am J Surg Pathol 2:339, 1978

KEGEL AH: Physiologic therapy for urinary stress incontinence. JAMA 146:915, 1951

McCALL ML: Posterior culdeplasty. Obstet Gynecol 10:595, 1957

McMASTER AJ: Management of sexual dysfunction in office practice. In Ryan GM (ed): Ambulatory Care in Obstetrics and Gynecology. New York, Grune & Stratton, 1980

MALINAK LR: Infertility and endometriosis: Operative technique, clinical staging and prognosis. Clin Obstet Gynecol 23:925, 1980

MASTERS WH, JOHNSON VE: Human Sexual Response. Boston, Little, Brown & Co, 1965

MATTINGLY RF: TeLinde's Operative Gynecology, 5th ed. Philadelphia, J B Lippincott, 1977

MOIR JC: The Vesico-vaginal Fistula, 2nd ed. London, Bailliere, Tindall & Cassell, 1967

MORLEY GW: Cancer of the vulva: A review. Cancer 48(suppl):597, 1981

NEUGARTEN BL, KRAINES RJ: Menopausal symptoms in women of various ages. Psychosom Med 27:266, 1965

NEWTON M: Radical hysterectomy or radiotherapy for stage I cervical cancer: A prospective comparison with 5- and 10-year follow-up. Am J Obstet Gynecol 123:535, 1975

NEWTON N: Maternal Emotions. New York, Paul B Hoeber, 1955

NISWANDER KR: Obstetrics: Essentials of Clinical Practice. Boston, Little, Brown & Co, 1981

OSTERGAARD DR: Gynecologic Urology and Urodynamics: Theory and Practice. Baltimore, Williams & Wilkins, 1980

PETERSON WF, PREVOST EC, EDMUNDS FT et al: Benign cystic teratomas of the ovary: A clinicostatistical study of 1,007 cases with a review of the literature. Am J Obstet Gynecol 70:368, 1955

PRIDE GL, SCHULTZ AE, CHUPREVICH TA, BUCHLER DA: Primary invasive squamous cell carcinoma of the vagina. Obstet Gynecol 53:218, 1979

RUTLEDGE AL: Psychomarital evaluation and treatment of the infertile couple. Clin Obstet Gynecol 22:255, 1979

RUTLEDGE FN, SMITH JP, WHARTON JT, O'QUINN AG: Pelvic exenteration: Analysis of 296 cases. Am J Obstet Gynecol 129:881, 1977

SONEK M, NEWTON M: Colposcopy in the evaluation of patients with abnormal cytologic smears. In Taymor ML, Green TH Jr (eds): Progress in Gynecology, vol 6. New York, Grune & Stratton, 1975

SPEROFF L, GLASS RH, KASE NG: Clinical Endocrinology and Infertility, 2nd ed. Baltimore, Williams & Wilkins, 1978

WAY S, HENNIGAN M: Late results of extended vulvectomy for carcinoma of the vulva. J Obstet Gynaecol Br Commonw 73:594, 1966

WELANDER C, GRIEM ML, NEWTON M ET AL: Staging and treatment of endometrial carcinoma. J Reprod Med 8:41, 1972

WYNDER EL, ESCHER GC, MANTEL N: An epidemiological investigation of cancer of the endometrium. Cancer 19:489, 1966

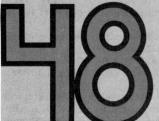

James D. Hardy

Perioperative Clinical Notes: Preoperative and Postoperative Orders, an Evening Rounds Checklist, and Common Postoperative Complications

A smoothly functioning surgical service does not come about by chance. Behind the scenes there is intelligent, intensive, and continuous activity. The purpose of this chapter is to survey some of the important details.

PREOPERATIVE ORDERS

The preoperative orders have become less and less stereotyped as the years have passed. Of course, each projected operation may require not only the routine blood and urine examination but also special chemistry tests. Special equipment, frozen sections, and roentgen studies may be needed before operation and in the operating room. Blood for transfusion should have been crossed and matched. Special skin or bowel preparation, for example, may have been necessary.

However, the only single item of preparation that *must* have been achieved is that the patient have an empty stomach so that there will be little risk of vomiting at the time of anesthesia induction, with the hazard of potentially disastrous aspiration of gastric contents into the lungs. This is usually achieved by the order "nothing by mouth after midnight." Most anesthesiologists want the patient to have had an atropinelike compound injected intramuscularly to diminish oral and tracheobronchial secretions. Otherwise, almost anything else can be taken care of in the operating room if it is found not to have been done before. Preoperative opiates and sedatives are used less and less, though we believe that a mild tranquilizer is useful in most patients.

REPRESENTATIVE POSTOPERATIVE ORDERS

VITAL SIGNS

Take and record pulse rate, respiratory rate, and blood pressure every 15 minutes for 2 hr; then every 30 minutes for 4 hr; then every hour for 12 hr. Take the rectal temperature every 2 hr. Call physician if change in patient's condition. (The importance of frequent checking of these "vital signs" in the early postoperative period lies not only in their importance *per se;* in taking these measurements so that they can be recorded on the chart for the inspection of all, the nurse will inevitably note the mental status of the patient, whether the intravenous is running dry, whether the wound is bleeding excessively, whether the catheter, nasogastric tube, or T-tube is functioning properly, whether the patient is vomiting, and so on.) These orders might be modified if the patient were being monitored in an ICU after leaving the Recovery Room, if arterial blood gas measurements were indicated, or for still other reasons.

INTRAVENOUS FLUIDS

Finish bottle of blood that is now running. (Central venous pressure measurements?)

500 ml one half normal saline in 5% dextrose

Ringers lactate as required to maintain urine volume (to be decided by physician)

INTAKE–OUTPUT RECORD

Record hourly urine volume if patient is catheterized.

CONTROL OF PAIN

Analgesic (usually morphine or meperidine in proper dosage)

AIRWAY AND VENTILATION

Turn patient frequently and urge coughing and deep breathing. Aspirate nasopharynx and trachea as required, using ''sterile'' technique.

AMBULATION?

Bed patient until fully reacted. May later stand to void if necessary. Up tonight or tomorrow (if appropriate)

VOIDING?

Call physician if patient is unable to void after 12 hr. (Attendant may stand the patient up or have him try to void while sitting on the commode or placing the penis in warm water and running water from the faucet, and so on. If catheterization is required a second time, a Foley catheter should be left in place until the patient is truly ambulatory. Women generally have less postoperative urinary tract dysfunction than men.)

INFECTION: PROPHYLAXIS OR CONTROL

Antibiotics?

EQUIPMENT

Connect various tubes to appropriate receptacles (*e.g.*, nasogastric tube to continuous suction, indwelling urethral catheter to drainage bottle, T-tube to drainage bottle or continue chest tubes to underwater closed drainage).

Again, special operations may require special orders, and some of these are noted in connection with consideration of specific operations elsewhere in this volume. The orders given above apply to the majority of patients who have just had routine major surgery, but they are only representative and must be modified to meet the given situation in a given hospital.

ORDERS REVISED

It is an important practice to reevaluate periodically all orders issued for the patient. The ones no longer needed are discarded, and antibiotics and opiates especially may be discontinued. The phrase *Orders Revised* is then written across the order sheet and the few remaining orders that are to be continued are listed below it. This bit of service housekeeping is of help to the patient, the nurses, and the physicians in charge. Each member of the team can now see at a glance what orders are in effect.

AN EVENING ROUNDS CHECKLIST

The object here is to review the objectives of evening rounds and to offer several checklists of points to be considered before and after certain representative operations.

GENERAL CONSIDERATIONS

The physician will plan to achieve the following objectives:

I. New Admissions and Those Under Study
   A. Initial evaluation
   B. Plan and begin arrangements for appropriate studies or therapy. Proceed with a target date for operation in mind. Tentatively schedule the operation if indicated.
   C. Reevaluate the current progress of preoperative studies and the therapy of patients admitted previously.

II. Preoperative Patients (for tomorrow)
   A. History and physical examination completed and recorded
   B. Essential laboratory data recorded on chart (blood work, urinalysis, chest roentgenogram, ECG, etc.)
   C. General physical status at the moment (febrile? dehydrated?)
   D. Preoperative orders written (anesthesia personnel contacted?)
   E. Blood ready for transfusion
   F. X-ray films available
   G. Patient, family (certainly of children), and, if appropriate, referring physician informed
   H. Case posted on operating schedule
   I. Special x-ray film in operating room or frozen section examinations scheduled
   J. Any other special equipment requirements in the individual case
   K. Operative permit signed and witnessed

III. Postoperative Patient (consider requirements according to which postoperative day [POD] is involved)
   A. Day of Operation: Points of Importance
      1. Examine patient briefly (check vital signs and perform auscultation of chest to determine quality of pulmonary ventilation). Is sedation adequate?
      2. Intake–output status
      3. Nurses' notes, monitoring data, blood gases
      4. Clinical chart
      5. Wound drainage excessive?
      6. Chest film? (Physician should inspect personally.)
      7. Bladder distention, intestinal distention, vomiting? (catheterize? nasogastric tube?)
      8. Repeat hemoglobin or hematocrit determination, if indicated.
      9. Consider special features of the individual case.
      10. Order sheet. Are the written orders being executed?
      11. Studies required tomorrow (plasma chemistries, blood count, chest roentgenogram?)
   B. Days Postoperative: Think particular requirements.
      1. Rewrite orders? Oral intake?
      2. Ambulate patient?

3. Remove chest tubes, urinary catheter, nasogastric tube, T-tube (after cholangiogram), drains, dressings, cast, sutures or other materials?
4. Plasma chemistry, urine, and blood count rechecks?
5. Stop antibiotics, opiates, anticoagulants, intravenous medications, precautions concerning infections, warm moist dressings, etc.?
6. Anticipate any complication.
7. Begin clearing the way for patient discharge.

All these findings in early postoperative patients should be recorded in the progress notes. These are a few of the innumerable details that must be thought of and taken care of. On the following pages are listed further reminders for several common operations that will serve individually as prototypes of procedures involving the several anatomic or physiological areas of the body. Certain of these points have been mentioned elsewhere in this book; however, it is useful to list them again here.

REPRESENTATIVE SPECIFIC OPERATIONS

THYROIDECTOMY (NECK OPERATION)

Preoperative
1. Rule out toxicity (clinical examination, T_3, TSH, T_4, radioiodine uptake).
2. Examine vocal cords by indirect laryngoscopy?
3. Chest roentgenogram for substernal extension.
4. Cross-match blood if likely to be needed.
5. Write routine preoperative orders (including sedation and atropine dosage unless written by anesthesiologist).
6. Schedule frozen section if carcinoma suspected.

Postoperative
1. *Vital Signs:* Respiratory difficulty suggests tracheal obstruction. Rapid pulse and respirations, with fever, suggest element of thyrotoxicity. Treat with IV sodium iodide, oxygen therapy, and sedation, and use digitalization and intravenous hydrocortisone, reserpine, or propranolol as indicated. Also scan nurses' notes, clinical temperature chart, and progress notes for clues and trends.
2. *The Wound:* Is drainage excessive or bloody? Is there a deep fullness of the neck? If there is any indication of respiratory difficulty, reopen wound, and if necessary reintubate or perform tracheostomy under local anesthesia. *Do not use Pentothal.* Normally, remove drains at end of 24 hr and sutures at 48 hr to 72 hr.
3. *Vocalization:* Ask patient to speak. If hoarse, examine cords with laryngeal mirror.
4. *Tingling or Tetany:* These findings suggest hypoparathyroidism. Check for positive Chvostek's sign, and draw blood for determination of serum calcium level.
5. *Intake–Output:* Are fluids in? Urine? Diet as tolerated after day of surgery.
6. *Ambulation:* Has patient been gotten out of bed?

THORACOTOMY (CHEST OPERATION)

Preoperative
1. Diagnostic workup complete? (History, physical examination, plain and special chest roentgenograms, sputum studies, bronchoscopy, mediastinoscopy, lung function tests, skin tests?)
2. Adequate blood for transfusion
3. Chest roentgenograms available for surgery
4. Preoperative orders written

Postoperative
1. *Vital Signs:* Reacted? Hypotension and tachycardia suggest hypovolemia due to inadequate replacement of losses at surgery or to continuing hemorrhage. Respiration as reflected in arterial blood gas values, chest x-ray film, and other data. Endotracheal tube and assisted ventilation as necessary, usually for 24 hr or less. (Prolonged intubation increases risk of tracheal injury and subsequent stricture.)
2. *Wound and Tube Drainage:* The thoracotomy incision rarely separates, and wound hemorrhage and serious infection are unusual. Half the skin sutures are removed on about the sixth POD and the rest on the eighth or later, as indicated after wound inspection.

   Thoracotomy tube drainage is exceedingly important following pulmonary, esophageal, mediastinal, or cardiac surgery. Is the column of fluid in the underwater drainage tube or tubes oscillating with each respiration? Is the bloody drainage excessive? Is air leakage (following lobectomy or segmental resection) excessive? If tubes are not functioning, they must be opened by stripping and perhaps instillation of sterile saline solution, or replaced. Continuing hemorrhage may require reoperation.
3. *"Cough Out":* Use "sterile" nasotracheal catheter suction where required after endotracheal tube out. Chest physiotherapy.
4. *Chest X-ray Film:* Valuable as are inspection and auscultation (the dressings may somewhat impede palpation and percussion), a chest film taken soon after operation and one again late that evening are invaluable in the early detection of hemorrhage, atelectasis, or pneumothorax. Each must be effectively treated promptly if good lung expansion is to be maintained. Either the surgeon or his house officer should personally examine these films.
5. *Intake–Output:* Check adequacy of blood and of other fluids, and urine output.
6. *Ambulation and Nutrition:* Ambulate and give diet as tolerated beginning with first POD. Continue frequent and aggressive measures to prevent atelectasis until lung is well expanded (check with serial films).

ABDOMINAL AORTIC ANEURYSM RESECTION

Preoperative
1. Site and size of aneurysm localized by history, physical examination, AP and lateral plain films of the lumbar spine, sonography, and, at times, aortogram or CT scan.
2. Assess general condition especially heart, lungs, kidneys.
3. Cross-match 3000 ml of blood.
4. Pass alimentary tube and insert Foley catheter immediately preoperatively.
5. Have fabric grafts available.
6. Schedule operative arteriograms with radiology department, if anticipated.
7. Anesthesia consult
8. Routine preoperative orders

Postoperative
1. *Vital Signs:* Reacted? Scan nurses' notes and clinical

temperature chart for clues and trends in monitoring data.

2. *Lower Extremities: Pulses* should be present in the femoral arteries and more distally if they were present below preoperatively.
3. *Intake–Output:* Blood and fluid infusion adequate but not excessive? Urine output?
4. Nasogastric suction to prevent distention
5. Ambulate on individual basis. *Diet* as tolerated when nasogastric tube removed.

BILIARY TRACT SURGERY

Preoperative

1. Establish presence of gallstones.
2. Rule out other diseases.
3. Assess general physical status.
4. Differential diagnosis—and therapy—in jaundiced patient, where indicated. Prothrombin levels and vitamin K administration. May need fresh frozen plasma.
5. Pass nasogastric tube prior to or at operation.
6. Schedule operative cholangiography if indicated.
7. Cross-match to laboratory ("hold").
8. Routine preoperative orders

Postoperative

1. *Vital Signs:* Reacted? Hypotension and rapid thready pulse must be investigated. Depressed respirations may reflect excessive sedation. Efficiency of pulmonary ventilation? Inspection, percussion, and auscultation of lungs. Also check nurses' notes and clinical temperature chart for clues and trends. Chest x-ray?
2. *Wound Drainage:* Excessive bloody drainage may require transfusion. Gross blood indicates an unligated vessel and reoperation may be in order. Copious bile may reflect severed accessory bile duct, injured common duct, or slipped ligature on cystic duct. Leakage around T-tube may be disturbing, but usually ceases when T-tube is removed. Early cholangiogram may be reassuring in regard to the last. The T-tube may be pulled after 7 days, because by then a drainage tract has been formed. Change dressing if needed. Check security of T-tube.
3. *Nausea, Vomiting, or Hiccups:* These findings often reflect gastric retention. If nasogastric tube is in place, check for patency and effectiveness of suction source. If no tube was used initially introduce one now, aspirate gastric contents, and irrigate with saline solution. The tube may then be left in place or withdrawn.
4. *Intake–Output:* Have the ordered fluids been infused? Has the patient passed urine if not catheterized?
5. *Distention and Gas Pains:* Peristalsis audible? Passing flatus? Hot water bottle to abdomen? Rectal tube to facilitate passage of gas. Enema?
6. *Ambulation:* Within 24 hr to 48 hr after operation, depending on patient.

GASTRIC OPERATIONS

Preoperative

1. Demonstrate pathology and chronicity with history, physical examination, gastroscopy, and GI series.
2. Routine laboratory work plus plasma chemistry values
3. Gastric analysis. Serum gastrin level?
4. Decompress a dilated stomach, often for 2 to 3 days.
5. Fluid and blood replacement when needed
6. Assess general physical status.

7. Cross-match with 1500 ml blood.
8. Pass nasogastric tube on morning of operation if not needed previously.
9. Routine preoperative orders

Postoperative

1. *Vital Signs:* Reacted? Hypotension and rapid thready pulse must be investigated. Suspect inadequate blood replacement at surgery or continuing concealed hemorrhage. Central venous pressure, hematocrit, and hemoglobin measurements are helpful. Blood transfusion usually suffices, and reoperation is not often required. Atelectasis, pulmonary embolus, coronary occlusion, or other possibilities must be considered. Sudden abdominal pain with fever several days following operation may be due to blowout of a suture line, with peritoneal soiling, or to pancreatitis. Chest roentgenogram?

   Examine pulmonary ventilation with *auscultation,* and have patient cough while gentle but firm manual compression of the wound is maintained. Also check nurses' notes, clinical temperature chart, and progress notes for clues and trends.
2. *The Wound:* Later, since wound drainage is not usually employed unless the procedure was quite difficult or a duodenal closure less than satisfactory, excessive serous or serosanguineous drainage through the incision often denotes partial or complete separation of the wound. This uncommon complication is especially to be considered when abdominal distention, hiccups, excessive coughing, vomiting, or wound infection is present.
3. *Nasogastric Tube Drainage:* Volume? Excessively bloody? Is tube patent? Vomiting around tube? Presence of bile establishes patency of common bile duct (and proximal stoma in Billroth II subtotal gastrectomy).
4. *Intake–Output:* Transfusion complete? Required solutions infused? Urine volume adequate?
5. *Abdominal Pain:* Pancreatitis? Gastric retention? Proximal loop syndrome? Suture line leakage? Abscess? Dumping? Gas pains? Flatus? Peristalsis?
6. *Routine.* Other considerations.

FRACTURE OR SOFT TISSUE TRAUMA WITH OR WITHOUT CAST

1. Is extremity spontaneously painful after fracture is immobilized? Remove or bivalve cast or dressings and inspect.
2. Are toes cold or numb? Suspect ischemic condition. Physical examination or arteriogram to detect arterial injury.
3. Sensation and power satisfactory under circumstances? Suspect nerve injury or compression, in addition to possible ischemia.
4. Patient febrile and "toxic"? Inspect wound for infection. Antibiotics and further débridement and drainage, if not previously adequate. Tetanus prophylaxis.
5. Do the repeat films show that satisfactory alignment of the fragments is being maintained?
6. Does the balanced traction need readjusting?
7. Routine problems of patient care: diet, urination, bowel movements, etc.

SOME COMMON POSTOPERATIVE COMPLICATIONS

Many and, indeed, most patients pass through their operative experience without developing any particular postoperative problems or complications. However, some patients must be operated on in emergency situations when preparations are necessarily somewhat incomplete; or the patient may be elderly and already have advanced cardiac, renal, pulmonary, or other disease. Therefore, on any truly active surgical service patients must be cared for who inevitably may be expected to have certain difficulties and therapeutic challenges during the postoperative period, regardless of the specific operative maneuvers performed. It is the purpose here to survey briefly some of the common postoperative problems that may be anticipated in an overall patient population. In general, the complications will be considered in the order of their usual occurrence, from the time the patient leaves the operating room until the patient has been discharged from the hospital to return home.

DISORDERS OF CONSCIOUSNESS

It is always disturbing when the patient fails to awaken from the effects of a general anesthetic agent as soon as he might ordinarily be expected to. With few exceptions, such postoperative coma may be due to any of the causes that produce this condition under other circumstances; however, with adequate preoperative screening, states such as diabetes mellitus, uremia, electrolyte imbalance, and brain injury or tumor should have been excluded or treated. Thus, in most previously healthy subjects the cause of prolonged failure to awaken from the anesthetic agent will be among the following:

1. Excessive dosage of anesthetic agent or prolonged detoxification or excretion of agent
2. Hypoxia during anesthesia–operation
3. Shock from any cause
4. Stroke
5. Fluid and electrolyte imbalance
6. Hypothermia

There are numerous other possible causes of prolonged failure to awaken from the anesthetic agent, but the most common and important are prolonged effects of the anesthetic agent or brain damage (though not necessarily severe or lasting) during the operation.

Even so, most such patients gradually awaken, perhaps even 24 hr to 48 hr later, and appear to be normal in every respect. However, when prompt awakening does not occur following operation, the situation should be viewed with serious concern, and every effort made to support the respiration and circulation as necessary until the neurologic status can be further determined. Since most patients who manifest these changes awaken gradually and without further dysfunction, a hopeful attitude should be adopted in discussion with the relatives of the patient while the precise neurologic status and prognosis are being determined.

POSTOPERATIVE BLEEDING

Hemorrhage from the wound or into the previous operative field is one of the most common of significant complications following operation, and it is also one of the most preventable. In modern surgery it is no longer permissible, in most circumstances, to close the wound without having achieved complete hemostasis. Time should be taken to ligate or coagulate bleeding points as the operation progresses and with a thorough search again at the time of closure. Even so, occasionally it is necessary to close a wound with less

than perfect hemostasis, owing to development of a diffuse oozing over a large raw surface or following incomplete resection of a tumor or still other circumstances. In this case the wound should be drained and the blood volume maintained postoperatively with appropriate monitoring. Patients who have received a large volume of blood transfused rapidly (*e.g.*, for massive blood loss in trauma) may develop a diminished capacity for blood clotting. This may be due to a low platelet count, hypothermia produced by the infusion of inadequately warmed blood, and at times many other factors. (Give fresh frozen plasma and platelets?)

Postoperative bleeding and abnormal blood coagulation are discussed in detail elsewhere. Suffice it to say here that if no obvious coagulation defect exists—and, often, even when it does—it may be useful to re-explore the wound. A specific arterial bleeder may be found. Or, in diffuse oozing, at many sites oozing may have ceased, and the relatively few persistent bleeders can now be coagulated and the wound thoroughly irrigated and then closed again, following which the bleeding may slow to a tolerable rate and finally cease. In sum, if the blood clots on standing and the platelet count is adequate, postoperative bleeding is probably due to unligated blood vessels that should be exposed and dealt with appropriately.

SHOCK IN THE RECOVERY ROOM

The two most common causes of shock immediately following operation are inadequate blood volume or inadequate respiration that impairs cardiac rhythm or strength of contraction. Other causes include myocardial infarction, pulmonary embolism, sepsis, stroke, and, rarely, adrenocortical insufficiency.

DYSPNEA, CYANOSIS, AND HYPOXIA

The obtunded patient who, owing to inadequate respiratory minute ventilation in the recovery room, becomes seriously hypoxic and acidotic may not exhibit dyspnea—and cyanosis is notoriously difficult to detect. Therefore, the most accurate, dependable, and widely used method for documenting the adequacy of respiration in the recovery room is the frequent measurement of arterial blood gas values and *p*H. The most frequent cause of inadequate respiration in the immediate postoperative period is the persistent effects of the anesthetic agent or of narcotizing drugs, leading to inadequate minute volume respiration. This is reflected in a reduced arterial P_{O_2} and an elevated arterial P_{CO_2}, leading to respiratory acidosis. The required increase in the minute volume of respiration is best achieved by the insertion of a nasotracheal tube and the use of assisted mechanical ventilation until the patient is fully recovered from the narcotizing effects of drugs of any sort. When the patient has already exhibited serious hypoxia, it is usually not safe to depend on an attendant to insist that the patient breathe adequately to avoid further danger. The patient should be reintubated immediately.

Other causes of early postoperative hypoxia include atelectasis, pneumothorax, aspiration of gastric contents during operation, excessive fluid administration, and left heart failure. The best protection against inadequate respiratory activity is to leave the endotracheal tube in place until the patient is adequately awake and then to remove the tube after the arterial blood gases have been found adequate without ventilatory assistance.

OLIGURIA

In most truly major operations a catheter is placed in the bladder at the beginning of the operation to permit monitoring of urine formation during the course of the procedure. Therefore, because it is after such large operations that postoperative renal insufficiency is most likely to occur, the patients who develop it will usually have had an indwelling catheter inserted previously, and the patency of this catheter should be checked. Of course, oliguria or even anuria may develop in a patient who has had a relatively small operation, owing to unusual factors, but this is not often the situation.

The most frequent cause of oliguria following operation is a low cardiac output for whatever reason. The commonest cause of a low cardiac output is an inadequate circulating blood volume, the hypovolemia usually being due to unreplaced blood volume losses during operation or to continuing losses (detected or undetected). The diminished blood volume may at times be due to reduced plasma volume secondary to excessive third space losses. In any event, the inadequate plasma or blood volume can be corrected by transfusion of whole blood, or infusion of plasma or electrolyte solution as required.

The low cardiac output may be due not to an inadequate circulating blood volume but to inadequate function of the heart itself, associated with inadequate blood volume or, at times, excessive blood volume. However, if low blood volume is not the problem, and if cardiac function appears to be satisfactory with or without digitalization, the problem of acute renal damage must be considered. A gradually diminishing rate of hourly urine formation most often reflects volume deficit with a diminishing cardiac output, but an increasingly severe oliguria may also represent acute renal failure. The management of acute renal failure is considered elsewhere.

POSTOPERATIVE PAIN AND ITS CONTROL

It is appreciated today that the relatively large doses of morphine and meperidine that were used in the past are less appropriate than smaller doses of opiate used more frequently. Unless the patient is still intubated and on assisted ventilation, a relatively large dose of opiate for the relief of pain may result in diminished minute volume of respiration, with resulting hypoxia and hypercarbia.

It is important to appreciate that perceived pain varies considerably from one patient to another, and certainly different patients react with different intensity to a given pain stimulus. Some patients with major operations virtually never require analgesic drugs, while others demand such medication almost continuously. Each patient must be treated as an individual, with the total merits and requirements of his case being the only factor under consideration.

If the patient has excessive abdominal pain after perhaps the first 24 hr postoperatively, the possibility of intra-abdominal pathology such as gangrenous bowel or other complication should be considered. Ordinarily, once the immediate effects of the operation have subsided over the first 24 hr postoperatively, most patients are reasonably comfortable as long as they lie quietly and make no particular muscular movement. Under these circumstances, excessive pain may represent a serious complication and should be so considered.

POSTOPERATIVE FEVER

Most patients exhibit a mild degree of body temperature elevation following the stress of anesthesia–operation, but this should not usually exceed 100°F (37.8°C). The most likely sources, in sequence of their probable appearance, are lungs, urinary tract, and the wound—"wind, water, wound." Phlebitis or antibiotic therapy may be causative.

Most commonly, significant fever in the early postoperative period is caused by pulmonary complications, chiefly atelectasis and pneumonitis. Routine pulmonary toilet and effective breathing exercises should reduce the incidence of these particular complications to as low a level as possible, though patients with chronic pulmonary emphysema and infection associated with smoking will require an excessive amount of such attention. Pulmonary management should be initiated preoperatively.

During the later postoperative days other possible causes of postoperative fever must be considered as well—urinary tract infection, wound infection, deep leg vein phlebitis and thrombosis, phlebitis due to intravenous catheters, infection with indwelling endotracheal tube, infection within a coelomic cavity and usually in the site or near the site of the operation, and still other, less common factors. Basically, in the absence of brain damage or heat stroke, a significant fever usually represents infection, and the problem consists of identifying the source of the infection and instituting appropriate management.

NAUSEA AND VOMITING

Postoperative nausea and vomiting are less common than they were before the currently used general anesthetic agents were available, but these symptoms still occur with considerable frequency. Quite aside from the discomfort to the patient, postoperative vomiting entails a number of hazards and threats to a smooth postoperative course. First, gastric contents may well be aspirated into the lungs, if an empty stomach has not been maintained with an indwelling nasogastric tube and continuous suction. Even if the tube has been in place, commonly some residual material will have collected and at times the tube is not functioning at all. Second, severe retching places undue stress on the various suture lines that were made at the time of the operation, with the serious risk of wound separation. Third, the excessive exertions of the patient during the vomiting process may so elevate the blood pressure as to set up bleeding in the operative field, not to mention the possibility of a coronary occlusion or stroke in the elderly patient.

Postoperative nausea should be controlled with the currently available agents for this purpose. The phenothiazine derivatives [*e.g.,* prochlorperazine (Compazine), chlorpromazine (Thorazine), promethazine (Phenergan)] usually are effective. If the patient is nauseated, a nasogastric tube should usually be inserted and the stomach emptied of fluid, which may be excessive in volume, even approaching the volume that might cause *acute gastric dilatation.*

With nasogastric suction and appropriate medication the nausea and vomiting are usually adequately controlled and gradually subside.

INTESTINAL DYSFUNCTION

After a major operation, most patients experience a certain degree of *adynamic ileus,* which is of course much more prominent in patients who have undergone abdominal operations, especially prolonged abdominal operations. The ileus may be even more severe and protracted if the operation was for perforation of a hollow viscus with widespread peritonitis. The degree of ileus varies widely from patient to patient, even those in whom the same operation was performed. Ileus may be quite protracted in some patients who therefore are unable to manage oral intake for excessively long periods. In our opinion, it is not beneficial to attempt to force oral intake during the first 48 hr following a really major operation. Numerous studies have documented abnormal motility and absorptive functions of the gastrointestinal tract following major injury (*e.g.*, major operations and trauma), and there is a greater danger of vomiting and pulmonary aspiration than there is of starvation during the first 2 days postoperatively. The most effective way to diminish the duration of postoperative ileus is to minimize the length of the intra-abdominal operation, to minimize the trauma to the intestine during the course of the procedure, to achieve good hemostasis, to avoid contamination of the peritoneal cavity at the time of performing various anastomoses, to maintain nasogastric suction until active bowel sounds are present and flatus has been passed postoperatively (in patients where a nasogastric tube is indicated), and then to allow oral intake on a gradual basis beginning with clear liquids.

If adynamic ileus persists for as long as 5 to 7 days, an abnormal situation clearly exists and one must consider the possible causes of what amounts in effect to intestinal obstruction. A common cause of protracted adynamic ileus postoperatively is infection within the abdomen, often peritonitis. In other cases, the infection may be localized at or near the site of operation, or may be from a subdiaphragmatic, hepatic or subhepatic, or pelvic abscess. In addition, inflammatory fibrinous adhesions may have formed and these too may contribute. By and large, however, prolonged ileus—especially if associated with fever, leukocytosis, and occasionally jaundice—suggests intra-abdominal sepsis. Incidentally, the early fibrinous adhesions may later merge into fibrous adhesions to produce mechanical small bowel obstruction (adhesions rarely produce colon obstruction).

In some elderly patients, adynamic ileus may gradually lead to *fecal impaction*. Therefore, when alimentary tract activity is judged to be abnormal, a rectal examination should be performed to exclude the possibility of impacted feces, especially since preoperative enemas have largely been abandoned on most surgical services unless the operation to be performed involves the colon itself or the pelvic organs. Moreover, barium used for alimentary tract visualization preoperatively may have become impacted in the colon. Fecal impaction may be broken up manually but often requires the instillation of repeated enemas of mineral oil, to soften the bolus of feces so that it can be manually extracted, since the patient may be incapable of expelling the material. Occasionally, opiates or even anesthesia is required, to reduce the pain that accompanies the manual maneuvers to extract the most distal portion of the fecal material so that additional saline enemas, following the oil enemas, can effect complete cleansing of the colon and rectum. The fecal impaction of course represents a form of mechanical intestinal obstruction, and mechanical intestinal obstruction should always be suspected after the first few days, as noted above. The value of appropriate physical examination and roentgenograms of the abdomen is to be emphasized.

The development of *postoperative diarrhea* may reflect a wide range of possible etiologic factors. If the operation performed was for mechanical small bowel obstruction and the small bowel contained large volumes of fluid at operation, postoperative diarrhea may reflect the fact that intestinal absorption is still abnormal and that the fluid is passing through instead of being absorbed. This is by no means uncommon following the relief of low small bowel obstruction. Postoperative diarrhea may be produced by the form or contents of nutrients offered or of drug therapy or may be secondary to the type of intestinal operation that was performed. Resection of terminal ileum may result in malabsorption of bile salts. However, if the patient is febrile and obviously toxic and the diarrhea is excessive, the possibility of *pseudomembranous enterocolitis,* which is a serious development that carries a significant mortality rate, must be considered. This type of enterocolitis may be due to a variety of causes; however, it is most often associated with the administration of broad-spectrum antibiotics. For a time it appeared to be the result of the reduction of the normal bacterial flora of the lower alimentary tract, permitting vast overgrowth of staphylococci. More recently, however, it appears to be the antibiotic *per se* or overgrowth of *Clostridium difficile* (sensitive to vancomycin) that is a common cause of this condition. Treatment consists of stopping all previous antibiotic therapy and making cultures of the stools to determine whether major bacterial overgrowth has occurred, general support of the patient, and administration of antibiotics that appear to be appropriate therapy for the organisms that are present. The condition has appeared to be more common in patients whose immunologic defenses have been reduced by immunosuppressive drugs, such as those who have undergone kidney allotransplantation. The signs and symptoms of this condition are first a watery diarrhea, which is often followed by a bloody diarrhea, with passage of a cast of the intestine. The mucosa itself may show advanced disintegration, and overwhelming toxemia may be the cause of death.

Finally, an important cause of postoperative bloody diarrhea is the presence of devitalized small bowel or large bowel. If there is any possibility that the vasculature to a segment of bowel was inadequate at the time of operation, immediate reoperation is indicated if the patient shows signs of fever, a rapid pulse, hypotension, an elevated white blood cell count or an increasingly tender abdomen.

FLUID AND ELECTROLYTE IMBALANCES

The most common postoperative problems of fluid imbalance represent (1) inadequate completion of replacement of deficits present preoperatively, as in alimentary tract obstruction, (2) excessive fluid administration during operation, and (3) inadequate renal function postoperatively. Otherwise, careful routine maintenance (Chapter 2) should prevent excessive overhydration or underhydration, using the appropriate guides for postoperative fluid administration.

POTASSIUM IMBALANCE

The importance of *hypokalemia* has been increasingly appreciated in recent years, and the incidence of serious cardiac arrhythmias due to abnormalities in serum potassium concentrations has been controlled much more effectively.

BODY WATER CONTENT

In the days immediately following the operation the patient should be weighed each morning and, if indicated, each evening. Excessive overhydration or underhydration will be apparent from such measurements. Plasma chemistry determinations should initially be requested daily following major operative procedures, and appropriate adjustments made in water and electrolyte administration.

MAGNESIUM DEFICIT

A low serum magnesium level is rare in the absence of severe and prolonged alimentary tract fluid losses. It is well to remember that tetany may be caused by either hypocalcemia or hypomagnesemia, as well as alkalosis or still other factors.

POSTOPERATIVE PSYCHOSIS

Some patients become deranged mentally and even maniacal postoperatively. Certainly, they exhibit such disorders of mental activity that they must be restrained, and members of the family become gravely concerned.

First, the arterial blood gas values should be determined to exclude hypoxemia or hypercarbia as the cause of the disorientation. Once this has been done, other causes must be considered. Delirium tremens may develop in an alcoholic patient whose addiction may not have been known to the medical staff previously. This is best treated with Librium (chlordiazepoxide hydrochloride), 50 mg by mouth every 4 hr; either paraldehyde or chlorpromazine (or both) may also be employed. Acute psychotic reaction to the stress of the operation itself may occur, and this can be controlled usually with adequate doses of chlorpromazine or some other suitable agent, preferably with the guidance of a psychiatrist. Drug withdrawal must be considered, for it may be found that the patient was taking large amounts of certain mood-altering or tranquilizing agents preoperatively. Restoration of such therapy, at least temporarily, may bring about a normal mental state.

Perhaps the most common cause of postoperative mental disturbance, certainly in the more elderly portion of the patient population, is cerebrovascular atherosclerosis—the so-called *organic brain syndrome.* These patients function adequately until they have been subjected to the overall effects of anesthesia–operation, following which they may become very disturbed and quite out of contact with their surroundings. They do not tolerate heavy doses of sedatives or tranquilizing agents, and they also tolerate poorly restraint of their arms and legs, which may actually be necessary on occasion, despite the presence of attendants or members of the family. However, the family can usually be reassured that this deranged state will gradually improve. It is usually helped by having a member of the family present in the room, and the patient generally improves still further when he has recovered sufficiently from the operation to permit him to return home to more familiar surroundings. Unfortunately, very occasionally the patient with organic brain syndrome who was in a normal state preoperatively fails to recover sufficiently following the operation and may require institutional care permanently.

Thus the possible causes of acute postoperative "psychosis" encompass a wide range of possibilities, and the patient must be protected against harm to himself while the possible cause or causes of the mental disturbance are being searched for and treated appropriately.

HICCUPS (SINGULTUS)

Hiccups can be very uncomfortable, even painful, and certainly disturbing to the patient if prolonged. Hiccups are due to diaphragmatic spasm against a closed glottis and usually affect only one side of the diaphragm. Occasional or isolated hiccups are of no significance; however, the condition can persist until the patient is exhausted. The etiology is varied, but often gastric distention or subdiaphragmatic infection will be found. At other times the hiccups appear to be due to a general metabolic alteration affecting the brain. In many instances no specific cause is ever found. The patient may hiccup only when awake and be free of hiccups while sleeping.

The first therapeutic maneuver in the early postoperative patient is to make certain that the stomach is empty, by passing a nasogastric tube if one is not present and functioning adequately. Having thus excluded gastric distention, several drugs—chlorpromazine, carbamazepine, diazepam (Valium)—may be used in dosage appropriate for the given patient. Chlorpromazine has proved to be effective in the majority of patients so treated, in our experience, but certain intractable instances require other agents as noted above.

STRESS ULCERATION

This postoperative complication is discussed elsewhere in this volume, and it is mentioned here only as one of the more serious postoperative complications. In about two thirds of the patients who develop this complication serious infection is present. Apparently, bacterial products contribute in some way to the development of many stress ulcers. Stress ulceration may consist of a single ulcer in the duodenum, but more often it consists of multiple small ulcers or erosive gastritis involving much of the stomach. Preventive measures include avoidance of infection, instillation of antacids into the stomach in patients who are at special risk, and monitoring of gastric pH every 4 hours, keeping pH at >5.5. Oral or parenteral cimetidine may be useful. Operative intervention may be required, and there is a difference of opinion in regard to the optimal operative procedure to be employed; the writer prefers to use bilateral truncal vagotomy and a 50% distal subtotal gastrectomy, which amounts to an extended antrectomy. Any residual bleeding ulcers in the portion of the stomach not resected are oversewn prior to construction of a Billroth II gastrojejunostomy.

WOUND COMPLICATIONS

A discussion of postoperative complications would not be complete without consideration of wound complications. Most wounds heal satisfactorily without untoward event. However, the wound should not be unduly painful after the first 24 to 48 hr. If there is undue swelling or if the wound is unusually painful, the possibility of a hematoma or impending infection must be considered. In abdominal and thoracotomy wounds, the drainage of excessive amounts of serous or serosanguineous fluid between the skin sutures is highly suggestive that the deeper layers of the wound have separated. When this occurs, the possibility of complete wound separation and evisceration becomes very serious. Therefore, any special complaints or changes in the appearance of the wound should be examined on the basis of the material presented in Chapter 8.

Material in this chapter was modified from Hardy JD: Total Surgical Management. New York. Grune & Stratton, 1959, and is used with permission.

BIBLIOGRAPHY

HARDY JD: Complications in Surgery and Their Management, 4th ed. Philadelphia, W B Saunders, 1981

Index

Numbers followed by an *f* indicate figures; the letter *t* indicates tabular material

A

abdomen. *See also specific abdominal organs*
  abscess in, 139–140
  acute, 445
  injuries of, 644–649
    arteriogram, 158–159, 159t
    blunt, 171–173, 173t
    categorization, 146t
    computed tomography scan, 158, 158f
    diseases of, pain pattern in, 446–452
    evaluation, 169–173
    management, 169–173, 172f, 646–649
    mortality, 645t
    penetrating, 169–171, 171t, 172f
    peritoneal lavage, 160
    physical examination, 155
  innervation of, 446
  operative techniques, 461–462
  pain in, 446–452
    causes of, 449–450, 449t
    in children, 1101–1102
    clinical evaluation of, 450–452
    in intestinal obstruction, 460–461
    parietal, 447
    referred, 447–449, 447f, 448f
    transmission of, 446–447, 446f, 447f
    visceral, 447
  palpation of, 155
  pattern of skin lines in, 115f, 1127, 1127f
  percussion of, 155
  physical examination, 155, 450–451
  postoperative infections, 139–140
  trauma of. *See* injuries of
  wound separation, 120–121
  x-ray examination, 157, 461, 461f
abdominal angina syndrome, 886–887
abdominal aorta
  aneurysm of, 918–919
    operative treatment of, 918–919, 918f, 1300–1301
  coarctation of, 1017, 1017f,
  injuries of, 950–951
abdominal wall
  anatomy, 761–763, 762f, 763f
  congenital abnormalities, 741, 1104–1106

desmoid tumor, 742
disorders in children, 1104–1106
extrainguinal hernias of, 776–783
hernia. *See* hernia
infections of, 741–742
inflammatory conditions, 741–742
injuries, 172–173
insulin lipodystrophy, 741–742
lesions of, acquired, 741–743
lipoma, 742
metastasis of tumors to, 742
pain, 743
tumors of, 742
abortion, 1293
abscess(es)
  of abdomen, 139–140
  of anal canal, 611
  of appendix, 562
  of Bartholin's gland, 1276
  of breast, 340, 340f
  of chest wall, 795
  collar-button, 1123
  drainage, 53, 129
  fistula-in-ano, 609–611, 610f
  formation, 124, 129
  intracranial, 1264–1265, 1265f
  of liver, 650–652, 651t, 652t
  of lung, 797t, 815–817, 816f
  of pancreas, 681f, 686, 702
  parapharyngeal, 295
  pelvic, 1283
  in peridiverticulitis, 577–578
  peritonsillar, 293
  . of retroperitoneum, 752–753
  retropharyngeal, 295
  of small intestine, 543
  of spleen, 718
  subdural, 1263
  subphrenic
    empyema, 797t
    pleural exudate, 796t
Accelerase, 698t
acetabulum, fractures of, 1165–1166
achalasia, of esophagus, 452, 471–472, 481–484
  primary spasm versus, 484t
  treatment, 482–484, 483t
Achilles tendon
  lengthening, 1192
  tendinitis, 1188

acid
  gastric, 497–502
  output, basal, 502
acid-base balance, 23–24
  buffer systems in, 24f
  calculation of, 31–32, 31f
  in diarrhea, 457
  in preoperative patient, 245
  in shock, 31–32
acidosis, from blood transfusions, 80
  metabolic, 31
    and cardiac arrest, 59
    compensated, 24
    diagnosis, 85f
    in diarrhea, 457
    in hypovolemic shock, 43, 47, 151
    from intravenous hyperalimentation, 103t
  respiratory, 29, 85f
acne, in Cushing's syndrome, 425
acrocyanosis, 957
acromegaly, 365–366
ACTH, 364
  adenomas producing, 366
  biochemistry, 434–435
  cortisol secretion and, 364
  in Cushing's syndrome, 417–422
  levels of, in stress, 7–8
  in neuroendocrine response to injury, 7–8, 7f
  physiological effects of, 434–435
  release, regulation of, 418–419
  secretion
    diurnal rhythm and, 418–419, 419f
    stress and, 7–8
Actinomyces infections, 144
  treatment, 133t
actinomycetacea, 822t, 823f, 825
adamantinoma, of bone, 1215–1216, 1215t
Addison's disease, 404, 424–425
adenoacanthoma, 322
adenocarcinoma
  of appendix, 563
  definition, 221
  of esophagus, 486–487
  gastric, 519
  of pancreas, 691–698
  of parathyroid, 401
  of prostate, 1251

M

N

O